THE GENETIC
BASIS
OF HUMAN
CANCER

NOTICE

Medicine is an ever-changing science. As new research and clinical experience broaden our knowledge, changes in treatment and drug therapy are required. The editors and the publisher of this work have checked with sources believed to be reliable in their efforts to provide information that is complete and generally in accord with the standards accepted at the time of publication. However, in view of the possibility of human error or changes in medical sciences, neither the editors nor the publisher nor any other party who has been involved in the preparation or publication of this work warrants that the information contained herein is in every respect accurate or complete, and they are not responsible for any errors or omissions or for the results obtained from use of such information. Readers are encouraged to confirm the information contained herein with other sources. For example and in particular, readers are advised to check the product information sheet included in the package of each drug they plan to administer to be certain that the information contained in this book is accurate and that changes have not been made in the recommended dose or in the contraindications for administration. This recommendation is of particular importance in connection with new or infrequently used drugs.

THE GENETIC BASIS OF HUMAN CANCER

Editors

Bert Vogelstein, M.D.
Professor of Oncology
The Johns Hopkins University
   School of Medicine
Investigator
Howard Hughes Medical Institute
Baltimore, Maryland

Kenneth W. Kinzler, Ph.D.
Associate Professor of Oncology
Department of Oncology
The Johns Hopkins University
   School of Medicine
Baltimore, Maryland

McGraw-Hill
Health Professions Division

New York   St. Louis   San Francisco   Auckland   Bogotá   Caracas   Lisbon   London   Madrid   Mexico City
Milan   Montreal   New Delhi   San Juan   Singapore   Sydney   Tokyo   Toronto

McGraw-Hill

A Division of The **McGraw·Hill** Companies

1234567890 QPKQPK 9987

ISBN 0-07-067596-1

This book was set in Times Roman by Monotype Composition Company, Inc. The editors were Martin J. Wonsiewicz and Peter McCurdy; the production supervisor was Rick Ruzycka; the cover designer was José Fonfrias, and Jerry Ralya prepared the index. Quebecor Printing/Kingsport was printer and binder.

This book is printed on acid-free paper.

Acknowledgments
Chapters 1, 2, 3, 10, 13, 19, 21, 22, 31, and 43 were adapted from Scriver CR, Beaudet AL, Sly WS, Valle D (eds.): *The Metabolic and Molecular Bases of Inherited Disease*, 7/e, copyright © 1995 by The McGraw-Hill Companies, Inc.

Chapters 1, 2, 3, 5–10, 12–25, 27, 29–31, and 33–42 appeared in slightly different forms in *The Metabolic and Molecular Bases of Inherited Disease CD-ROM*, copyright © 1997 by The McGraw-Hill Companies, Inc.

Library of Congress Cataloging-in-Publication Data

The genetic basis of human cancer / Bert Vogelstein, Kenneth
W. Kinzler.
       p.   cm.
  Includes bibliographical references and index.
  ISBN 0-07-067596-1
  1. Cancer—Genetic aspects.   I. Vogelstein, Bert.
II. Kinzler, Kenneth W.
  [DNLM: 1. Neoplasms—genetics. 2. Cell
Transformation, Neoplastic—genetics. 3. Gene
Expression—genetics. 4. Mutagenesis—genetics.
QZ 202 G3297 1998]
RC268.4.G445   1998
616.99′4042—dc21
DNLM/DLC
for Library of Congress 97 20508
    CIP

*We would like to thank the young investigators
(postdoctoral fellows and students) whose contributions
often go unrecognized but who are largely responsible for the revolution in
cancer research that has occurred over the last two decades.*

CONTENTS

PART 1
Basic Concepts in Cancer Genetics

PART 2
Controls on Cell Growth

PART 3
Familial Cancer Syndromes

SECTION I OVERVIEW

SECTION II DEFECTS IN CARETAKERS

SECTION III DEFECTS IN GATEKEEPERS

SECTION IV MANAGING FAMILIAL CANCER SYNDROMES

PART 4
Cancer by Site

CONTRIBUTORS*

Naji Al-dosari, B.Sc.   (40)
Duke University Medical Center, Durham, North Carolina

Stylianos E. Antonarakis, M.D.   (3)
Director, Division of Medical Genetics, University of Geneva
School of Medicine, Geneva, Switzerland; Professor, Center for
Medical Genetics, The Johns Hopkins University School of
Medicine, Baltimore, Maryland

Arleen D. Auerbach, Ph.D.   (16)
Associate Professor, Human Genetics and Hematology, The
Rockefeller University, New York, New York

Stephen B. Baylin, M.D.   (41)
Professor of Oncology and Medicine, The Johns Hopkins Medical
Institutions, Baltimore, Maryland

Arthur L. Beaudet, M.D.   (1)
Investigator, Howard Hughes Medical Institute; Professor,
Departments of Molecular and Human Genetics, Pediatrics, and
Cell Biology, Baylor College of Medicine,
Houston, Texas

Sandra H. Bigner, M.D.   (40)
Director, Section of Cytogenetics, Division of Cytopathology and
Cytogenetics, Department of Pathology, Duke University Medical
Center, Durham, North Carolina

C. Richard Boland, M.D.   (17)
Professor of Medicine and Chief, Division of Gastroenterology,
University of California San Diego, LaJolla, California

Dirk Bootsma, M.D.   (13)
Professor of Genetics, Department of Cell Biology and Genetics,
Erasmus University, Rotterdam, The Netherlands

Garrett M. Brodeur, M.D.   (7, 43)
Audrey E. Evans Endowed Chair, Professor of Pediatrics,
University of Pennsylvania; Director of Oncology Research,
The Children's Hospital of Philadelphia, Philadelphia,
Pennsylvania

G. Steven Bova, M.D.   (39)
Assistant Professor, Department of Pathology, The Johns Hopkins
University School of Medicine, Baltimore, Maryland

Manuel Buchwald, Ph.D.   (16)
Senior Scientist, The Hospital for Sick Children, Professor,
Molecular and Medical Genetics, The University of Toronto,
Toronto, Ontario, Canada

Paul Cairns, Ph.D.   (37)
Department of Otolaryngology—Head and Neck Surgery,
Division of Head and Neck Cancer Research, The Johns Hopkins
University School of Medicine, Baltimore, Maryland

Webster Cavenee, M.D.   (19)
Director, Ludwig Institute for Cancer Research, University of
California, San Diego, San Diego, California

Kathleen R. Cho, M.D.   (36)
Associate Professor, Departments of Pathology, Oncology, and
Gynecology and Obstetrics, The Johns Hopkins University School
of Medicine, Baltimore, Maryland

James E. Cleaver, Ph.D.   (13)
Professor, Department of Dermatology, University of California,
San Francisco, San Francisco, California.

Bruce E. Clurman, M.D., Ph.D.   (8)
Assistant Member, Division of Clinical Research, Fred
Hutchinson Cancer Research Center, Seattle, Washington

Ann-Marie Codori, Ph.D.   (32)
Department of Psychiatry and Behavioral Sciences and the
Oncology Center, The Johns Hopkins University School of
Medicine, Baltimore, Maryland

Francis S. Collins, M.D., Ph.D.   (22)
Director, National Center for Human Genome Research, National
Institutes of Health, Bethesda, Maryland

Fergus J. Couch, Ph.D.   (30)
Research Scientist, University of Pennsylvania, Philadelphia,
Pennsylvania

David N. Cooper, B.Sc., Ph.D.   (3)
Senior Lecturer in Molecular Genetics, Charter Molecular
Genetics Laboratory, Thrombosis Research Institute, London,
England

David R. Cox, M.D., Ph.D.   (2)
Professor, Departments of Genetics and Pediatrics, Stanford
University School of Medicine, Stanford, California

Louis Dubeau, M.D., Ph.D.   (34)
Associate Professor of Pathology, USC School of Medicine,
Kenneth Norris Jr. Comprehensive Cancer Center, Los Angeles,
California

---

*The numbers in parentheses following each contributor's name indicate the chapters
written or co-written by that contributor.

Nathan A. Ellis, Ph.D. (15)
Associate Member, Department of Human Genetics,
Memorial Sloan-Kettering Cancer Center,
New York, New York

Lynne W. Elmore, Ph.D. (42)
Laboratory of Human Carcinogenesis, National Cancer Institute,
National Institutes of Health, Bethesda, Maryland

Charis Eng, M.D., Ph.D. (28)
Assistant Professor of Medicine, Harvard Medical School,
Dana-Farber Cancer Institute, Boston, Massachusetts

Eric R. Fearon, M.D., Ph.D. (11)
Division of Molecular Medicine and Genetics, Departments of
Internal Medicine, Human Genetics, and Pathology, University of
Michigan Medical Center, Ann Arbor, Michigan

Andrew P. Feinberg, M.D., M.P.H. (4)
King Fahd Professor of Medicine, Oncology, and Molecular
Biology and Genetics, The Johns Hopkins School of Medicine,
Baltimore, Maryland

Richard A. Gatti, M.D. (14)
Professor, Department of Pathology, University of California,
Los Angeles, Los Angeles, California

James German, M.D. (15)
Member, New York Blood Center, New York, New York

Eric D. Green, M.D., Ph.D. (2)
Chief, Genome Technology Branch, National Human Genome
Research Institute, National Institutes of Health, Bethesda,
Maryland

James Gusella, Ph.D. (23)
Bullard Professor of Neurogenetics, Harvard Medical School;
Director, Neurogenetics Unit, Massachusetts General Hospital,
Boston, Massachusettes

David H. Gutmann, M.D., Ph.D. (22)
Assistant Professor, Neurology, Pediatrics, and Genetics, Director,
Neurofibromatosis Program, St. Louis Children's Hospital;
Washington University School of Medicine, Department of
Neurology, St. Louis, Missouri

Daniel Haber, M.D., Ph.D. (21)
Assistant Professor of Medicine, Massachusetts General Hospital
Cancer Center; Harvard Medical School, Boston, Massachusetts

Theodora Hadjistilianou, M.D. (19)
Assistant Professor, Institute of Ophthalmological Sciences,
University of Siena, Siena, Italy

Curtis C. Harris, M.D. (42)
Chief, Laboratory of Human Carcinogenesis, National Cancer
Institute, National Institutes of Health, Bethesda, Maryland

Lora Hedrick, M.D. (35)
Assistant Professor, Departments of Pathology, Gynecology and
Obstetrics, and Oncology, The Johns Hopkins University School
of Medicine, Baltimore, Maryland

Meenhard Herlyn, D.V.M. (27)
Chairman, Program of Cellular and Molecular Biology, the Wistar
Institute, Philadelphia, Pennsylvania

Jan H.J. Hoeijmakers, M.D. (13)
Professor of Molecular Genetics, Department of Cell Biology and
Genetics, Erasmus University, Rotterdam, The Netherlands

Michael D. Hogarty, M.D. (7)
Instructor in Pediatrics, Division of Oncology, Children's Hospital
of Philadelphia, Abramson Research Center, Philadelphia,
Pennsylvania

Ralph H. Hruban, M.D. (33)
Departments of Pathology and Oncology, The Johns Hopkins
University School of Medicine, Baltimore, Maryland

William B. Isaacs, Ph.D. (39)
Associate Professor, Department of Urology, The Johns Hopkins
University School of Medicine, Baltimore, Maryland

Hans Joenje, Ph.D. (16)
Professor, Department of Human Genetics, Free University,
Amsterdam, The Netherlands

Alexander Kamb, Ph.D. (27)
Vice President of Research, Ventana Genetics, Inc.,
Salt Lake City, Utah

Scott E. Kern, M.D. (33)
Departments of Oncology and Pathology, The Johns Hopkins
University School of Medicine,
Baltimore, Maryland

Kenneth W. Kinzler, Ph.D. (12, 31)
Associate Professor of Oncology, Department of Oncology, The
Johns Hopkins University School of Medicine, Baltimore,
Maryland

Richard D. Klausner, M.D. (24)
Office of the Director, National Cancer Institute, Bethesda,
Maryland

Kenneth H. Kraemer, M.D. (13)
Research Scientist, Laboratory of Molecular Carcinogenesis,
National Cancer Institute, National Institutes of Health, Bethesda,
Maryland

Michael Krawczak, Dip. Math., Dr. Rer. Nat. (3)
Research Scientist, Abteilung Humangenetik, Medizinische
Hochschule, Hanover, Germany

W. Marston Linehan, M.D. (24)
Urologic Oncology Section, Surgery Branch, Division of Clinical
Sciences, National Cancer Institute, Bethesda, Maryland

A. Thomas Look, M.D. (5)
Chairman, Department of Experimental Oncology, St. Jude
Children's Research Hospital, Professor of Pediatrics,
University of Tennessee College of Medicine, Memphis,
Tennessee

Mack Mabry, M.D. (41)
Assistant Professor of Oncology, Division of Radiology, The
Johns Hopkins University School of Medicine, Baltimore,
Maryland

Mia MacCollin, M.D. (23)
Assistant Professor of Neurology, Harvard Medical School;
Director, Neurofibromatosis Clinic, Massachusetts General
Hospital, Boston, Massachusetts

David Malkin, M.D. (20)
Assistant Professor, Division of Oncology, Department of
Pediatrics, The Hospital for Sick Children; Faculty of Medicine,
University of Toronto, Toronto, Ontario, Canada

Roger E. McLendon, M.D. (40)
Duke University Medical Center, Durham, North Carolina

Paul S. Meltzer, M.D., Ph.D. (6)
Head, Section of Molecular Cytogenetics, Laboratory of Cancer Genetics, National Center for Human Genome Research, National Institutes of Health, Bethesda, Maryland

Tetsuro Miki, Ph.D. (18)
Geriatric Research Education and Clinical Center, University of Washington, Seattle, Washington

Richard M. Myers, Ph.D. (2)
Professor, Department of Genetics, Stanford University School of Medicine, Stanford, California

Jun Nakura, M.D., Ph.D. (18)
Department of Geriatric Medicine, Osaka University Medical School, Osaka, Japan

Barry D. Nelkin, Ph.D. (41)
Associate Professor of Oncology, The Johns Hopkins University Medical School, Baltimore, Maryland

Irene F. Newsham, Ph.D. (19)
Section Head, Ludwig Institute for Cancer Research–San Diego Branch; Assistant Professor, Department of Medicine, University of California–San Diego School of Medicine, La Jolla, California

Morag Park, Ph.D. (10)
Molecular Oncology Group, Royal Victoria Hospital, Departments of Oncology and Medicine, McGill University, Montreal, Quebec, Canada

Ramon Parsons, M.D., Ph.D. (28)
Departments of Pathology and Medicine, Columbia University Cancer Center, New York, New York

Gloria M. Petersen, Ph.D. (32)
Department of Epidemiology, School of Hygiene and Public Health; Oncology Center, School of Medicine, Johns Hopkins University, Baltimore, Maryland

Bruce A.J. Ponder, M.D. (25)
Professor of Clinical Oncology, University of Cambridge, Cambridge, England

Steven M. Powell, M.D. (38)
Assistant Professor of Medicine, Health Sciences Center, Division of Gastroenterology and Hepatology, University of Virginia, Charlottesville, Virginia

Ahmed Rasheed, Ph.D. (40)
Duke University Medical Center, Durham, North Carolina

Jonathan L. Rees, B. Med. Sci., M.B.B.S. (29)
Professor of Dermatology, University of Newcastle upon Tyne; Honorary Consultant, Royal Victoria Infirmary and Associated Hospitals NHS Trust, Newcastle upon Tyne, England

James M. Roberts, M.D., Ph.D. (8)
Member, Division of Basic Sciences, Fred Hutchinson Cancer Research Center, Seattle, Washington

Charles M. Rudin, M.D., Ph.D. (9)
Gwen Knapp Center for Lupus and Immunology Research, Department of Medicine, Section of Hematology/Oncology, The Howard Hughes Medical Institute, University of Chicago, Chicago, Illinois

Gerard D. Schellenberg, Ph.D. (18)
Research Professor, Medicine, Associate Director for Research, Geriatric Research Education and Clinical Center, Seattle Veterans Affairs Medical Center; Departments of Medicine, Neurology and Pharmacology, University of Washington, Seattle, Washington

Charles R. Scriver, M.D.C.M (1)
Alva Professor of Human Genetics and Professor of Biology and Pediatrics, McGill University, Montreal, Quebec, Canada

David Sidransky, M.D. (37)
Department of Otolaryngology—Head and Neck Surgery, Division of Head and Neck Cancer Research, The Johns Hopkins University School of Medicine, Baltimore, Maryland

William S. Sly, M.D. (1)
Alice A. Doisy Professor of Biochemistry and Molecular Biology and Professor of Pediatrics; Chair, Edward A. Doisy Department of Biochemistry and Molecular Biology, St. Louis University School of Medicine, St. Louis, Missouri

Craig B. Thompson, M.D. (9)
Gwen Knapp Center for Lupus and Immunology Research, Department of Medicine, Section of Hematology/Oncology, The Howard Hughes Medical Institute, University of Chicago, Chicago, Illinois

Jeffrey M. Trent, Ph.D. (6)
Scientific Director, NHGRI; Chief, Laboratory of Cancer Genetics, National Human Genome Research Institute, National Institutes of Health, Bethesda, Maryland

David Valle, M.D. (1)
Investigator, Howard Hughes Medical Institute; Professor of Pediatrics, Medicine, Ophthalmology, and Molecular Biology and Genetics, The Johns Hopkins University School of Medicine, Baltimore, Maryland

Bert Vogelstein, M.D. (12, 31)
Professor of Oncology, The Johns Hopkins University School of Medicine; Investigator, Howard Hughes Medical Institute, Baltimore, Maryland

Barbara L. Weber, M.D. (30)
Associate Professor of Medicine and Genetics, Director, Breast Cancer Program, University of Pennsylvania, Philadelphia, Pennsyslvania

Charles J. Yeo, M.D. (33)
Departments of Surgery and Oncology, The Johns Hopkins University School of Medicine, Baltimore, Maryland

Chang-En Yu, Ph.D. (18)
Geriatric Research Education and Clinical Center, Seattle Veterans Affairs Medical Center; Department of Neurology, University of Washington, Seattle, Washington

PREFACE

As late as the 1970s, human cancers remained a black box. Theories were abundant: Cancer was hypothesized to result from defective immunity, viruses, dysregulated differentiation, mutations. . . . In the absence of hard evidence to confirm or refute any of these theories, it was difficult to be optimistic that cancer would soon be understood, or that there was much hope for patients afflicted with disease.

This has changed dramatically as a result of the revolution in cancer research that has occurred in the last decade. If this revolution were to be summarized in a single sentence, that sentence would be "Cancer is, in essence, a genetic disease." Although cancer is complex, and environmental and other nongenetic factors clearly play a role in many stages of the neoplastic process, the tremendous progress made in understanding tumorigenesis in large part is owing to the discovery of the genes, that when mutated, lead to cancer. This book pays tribute to this revolution by assembling what is known about the genetic basis of human cancer in a single text, with chapters written by scientists who have made seminal contributions to this knowledge.

The book began as an addition to the classic textbook, *The Metabolic and Molecular Bases of Inherited Disease*. It was soon realized that there was so much information about the genetic basis of human cancer that a separate, more focused book was warranted. It is important to note at the outset that our purpose was not to record everything that is known about cancer; excellent textbooks on the clinical aspects of cancer, on biochemical issues related to cancer, on environmental aspects related to cancer, already exist. Our purpose was to focus on the genes that cause cancer, and to attempt to answer the following questions whenever possible: What fraction of a specific cancer type is associated with a clear genetic component? What are the genes involved? What is the nature of the mutations in these genes? How do these genes work? What are the implications of knowledge about genes for diagnosis and future treatment?

In these prefatory comments, we attempt to address some very basic questions about genes and cancer that hopefully will help put the book in perspective and explain its organization.

HOW IS CANCER DIFFERENT FROM OTHER GENETIC DISEASES?

The simplest genetic diseases (e.g., Duchenne muscular dystrophy) are caused by inherited mutations in a single gene that are necessary and sufficient to determine the phenotype (Fig. 1). This phenotype generally can be predicted from knowledge of the precise mutation, and modifying genes or environmental influences often play a small role. More complex are certain diseases in which single defective genes can predispose patients to pathological condi-

tions, but the defective gene itself is not sufficient to guarantee disease. For example, patients who inherit defective low density lipoprotein-encoding genes are prone to atherosclerosis, but environmental influences, particularly dietary lipids, play a large role in determining the severity of disease. Certain cancers display an obvious hereditary influence, but, like atherosclerosis, the defective gene itself is not sufficient for the development of cancer. Cancers only become manifest following accumulation of additional, somatic mutations. These occur either as a result of the imperfection of the DNA copying apparatus ($\sim 10^{-10}$ mutations/bp/somatic cell generation) or through DNA damage caused by environmental mutagens.

DO CANCERS OCCUR ONLY IN PATIENTS WHO INHERIT A DEFECTIVE CANCER GENE?

It is estimated that only a small fraction (0.1 to 10%, depending on the cancer type) of the total cancers in the Western world occur in patients with a hereditary mutation. But one of the cardinal principles of modern cancer research is that the same genes cause both inherited and sporadic (noninherited) forms of the same tu-

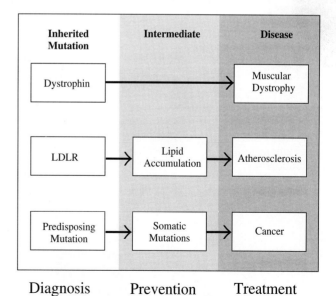

FIG. 1 Comparison of genetic diseases. Three types of genetic diseases, of increasing complexity, are illustrated. (Reprinted by permission from Kinzler and Vogelstein, *Cell*, vol. 87, p. 161, Copyright 1996, Cell Press.)

mor type (Fig. 2). This principle, first enunciated by Knudson, is well illustrated by retinoblastomas in children (Chapter 19) and colorectal tumors in adults (Chapter 31). For example, approximately 1 percent of colorectal cancer patients inherit a defective *APC* gene from one of their parents. This inherited mutation is not sufficient to initiate tumorigenesis. However, every cell of the colon from such patients is "at risk" for acquiring a second mutation, and two mutations of the right type are believed to be sufficient for initiation. The great majority of colorectal cancer patients (~99% of the total) do not inherit a mutant *APC* gene. However, these sporadic cases also require an *APC* mutation to begin the tumorigenic process. In these sporadic cases, the *APC* mutations occur somatically and occur only in isolated colorectal epithelial cells. The number of colorectal epithelial cells with *APC* mutations therefore is several orders of magnitude less in the sporadic cases than in the inherited cases, in which every cell has an *APC* mutation. Accordingly, multiple tumors often develop in patients with the hereditary mutations, instead of single, isolated tumors, and tumors develop at an earlier age in the familial patients than the sporadic patients.

What is the "second mutation" that initiates clinically apparent neoplasia in both the hereditary and sporadic types of tumors? In most known examples, the second mutation is believed to result in inactivation of the wild-type allele inherited from the unaffected parent. As described in the following, genes that, when mutated, lead to cancer predisposition, normally suppress tumorigenesis. If one allele of such a gene (e.g., *APC*) is mutated in the germ line, then the cell still has the product of the wt allele as a backup. If a somatic mutation of the wt allele occurs, however, then the resultant cell will have no functional suppressor gene product remaining, and will begin to proliferate abnormally ("clonal expansion"). One of the cells in the proliferating clone then is likely to accumulate another mutation, resulting in further loss of growth control. Through gradual clonal expansion, a tumor will evolve, with each successive mutation providing a further growth advantage, allowing its progeny to continue to replicate in microenvironments inhibitory to the growth of cells with fewer mutations.

ARE THE DNA ALTERATIONS IN CANCER DIFFERENT FROM THOSE OF OTHER GENETICALLY DETERMINED DISEASES?

Five different types of genetic alterations have been observed in tumor cells.

1. *Subtle alterations.* Small deletions, insertions, and single base pair substitutions occur in cancers just as they do in other hereditary diseases.

2. *Chromosome number changes.* Somatic losses or gains of chromosomes often are observed in cancers. Although such aneuploidy occasionally is a cause of other inherited diseases (e.g., Down syndrome), the degree of aneuploidy is much more extensive in cancers than ever observed in the phenotypically normal cells of mammals. Most cancers are aneuploid, with chromosome numbers ranging from subdiploid to supratetraploid. Molecular studies have shown that the aneuploidy observed in karyotypic studies actually underestimates the extent of gross chromosomal changes in cancer cells. Even when cancer cells appear to have two normal copies of a chromosome by karyotype, molecular analyses reveal that both chromosomes often are from the same parent. Thus, instead of one maternal and one paternal chromosome 17 per cell, the cancer cell may have no maternal chromosome 17 and two paternal chromosomes 17. This "loss of heterozygosity" (LOH) often affects more than half of the chromosomes in an individual cancer cell. LOH provides an efficient way for the cell to inactivate genes. For example, consider a cell containing two chromosomes 5, one with a mutation of a chromosome 5 tumor suppressor gene and the other with a wild-type allele of this gene. The wt copy of the gene often will prevent the cell from abnormal proliferation. If the chromosome containing this wt allele is lost, however, then the cell will be left with only the mutant copy of the suppressor gene and a selective growth advantage

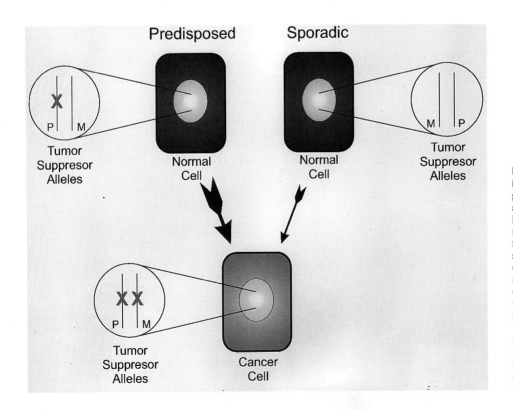

FIG. 2 Tumor suppressor gene inactivation. Tumor suppressor gene mutations are thought to initiate many forms of cancer. Both alleles of the tumor suppressor gene must be inactivated for a tumor to form. In familial cancer predisposition syndromes, a mutant allele of a suppressor gene is inherited and is present in every cell. However, tumors are not initiated until the second allele (inherited from the unaffected parent) is inactivated in a somatic cell. In nonfamilial cases, the inactivation of both alleles occurs through somatic mutations. The end result is the same: no functional suppressor gene, leading to tumor initiation.

will accrue. Such LOH events occur at much higher rates (10^{-5}/generation) than subtle mutation (~10^{-7} gene/generation), affording the cancer cell a powerful means of ridding itself of wt growth constraining genes. LOH generally occurs through the loss of an entire chromosome or through mitotic recombination. Whole chromosome losses often are associated with a duplication of the remaining chromosome, thus making this event invisible by karyotypic methods but detectable by molecular analyses using chromosomal polymorphisms as probes. Mitotic recombinations generally can be observed only through molecular analyses.

3. *Chromosome translocations.* Balanced and unbalanced translocations frequently are observed in cancers, where they occur by somatic rather than germline mutation. In common cancers of epithelial origin (e.g., breast, colon, prostate, stomach), the translocations appear to be random, with no specific breakpoints at the chromosomal or molecular levels. In contrast, leukemias and lymphomas generally contain characteristic translocations that appear to determine many of the biologic properties of the neoplasms. For example, acute promyelocytic leukemias virtually always contain a t(15;17) translocation resulting in the fusion of a retinoic acid receptor gene on chromosome 17 with another gene on chromosome 15, and chronic myelogenous leukemias always contain a t(9;22) translocation resulting in fusion of the *abl* oncogene with a gene called bcr (Chapters 5 and 6).

4. *Amplifications.* These genetic alterations are only observed in neoplastic cells in humans, and are defined by a five- to 100-fold multiplication of a small region of the chromosome (0.310 Mb). Gene amplifications generally are observed only in advanced neoplasms. The "amplicons" contain one or more genes whose expression can endow the cell with enhanced proliferative activity, and the higher expression of these genes through an increased copy number obviously is advantageous for the cancer cell.

5. *Exogenous sequences.* Certain human cancers are associated with tumor viruses, which contribute genes resulting in abnormal cell growth. Representative examples are cervical cancers (associated with human papilloma viruses; Chapter 36), Burkitt lymphomas (associated with Epstein-Barr viruses; Chapter 5), hepatocellular carcinomas (associated with hepatitis viruses; Chapter 42), and T-cell leukemias (associated with retroviruses). These exogenously introduced genes can be best considered another class of mutations that contributes to oncogenesis. Like the other mutations described earlier, no exogenous viral gene is sufficient for tumorigenesis. Such viral oncogenes simply represent one of the mutations that the cell accumulates during its progression to malignancy.

WHAT GENES ARE MUTATED IN CANCERS?

Two classes of genes are involved in cancer formation. The first, comprising oncogenes and tumor suppressor genes, directly control cellular proliferation. They can do this either by controlling the rate of cell birth (Chapter 8) or the rate of cell death (Chapter 9). Although tumorigenesis largely has been thought of as caused by increases in the rate of cell birth, it is now recognized that tumor expansion represents an imbalance between cell birth and cell death. In normal tissues, the cell birth precisely equals cell death, resulting in homeostasis. Defects in either of these processes can result in net growth, perceived as tumorigenesis.

Oncogenes are like the accelerators of an automobile; normally they result in increased cell birth or decreased cell death when expressed. A mutation in an oncogene is tantamount to having the accelerator pinned to the floor: Cell proliferation continues even when the cell's surrounding environment is giving it clear signals to stop. Mutations in oncogenes include subtle mutations that change their structure and make them constitutively active, or mutations that increase their expression to levels higher than observed in normal cells.

Continuing with this analogy, tumor suppressor genes are the "brakes" of the cell, normally functioning to inhibit cell growth. Just as do automobiles, each cell type has more than one brake, each of which can be activated under appropriate microenvironmental stimuli. It is only when several of the cell's brakes and accelerators are rendered dysfunctional through mutation that the cell entirely spins out of control, and cancer ensues.

The second class of genes (caretaker genes) does not directly control cell growth, but instead controls the rate of mutation. Cells with defective mutator genes acquire mutations in all genes, including oncogenes and tumor suppressor genes, at an elevated rate. This higher rate leads to accelerated tumorigenesis. The fact that patients (and cells) with defective mutator genes are cancer-prone provides one of the most cogent pieces of evidence that mutations in DNA lie at the heart of the neoplastic process.

IS CANCER A SINGLE DISEASE?

Tumors can be defined best as diseases in which a single cell acquires the ability to proliferate abnormally, resulting in an accumulation of progeny. "Cancers" are those tumors that have acquired the ability to invade through surrounding normal tissues. The most advanced form of this invasive process is metastasis, a state in which cancer cells escape from their original location, travel by hematogenous or lymphogenous channels, and take up residence in distant sites. The difference between a malignant tumor (cancer) and a benign tumor is the capacity of the former to invade. Both benign and malignant tumors can achieve large sizes, but the benign tumors are circumscribed and therefore generally can be removed surgically. Malignant tumors often have invaded surrounding or distant tissues prior to their detection, precluding surgical excision of the entire tumor cell mass. It is the ability of cancers to destroy other tissues through invasion that makes them lethal.

There are as many tumor types as there are cell types in the human body. Thus cancers represent not a single disease but a group of heterogeneous diseases that share certain biologic properties (in particular, clonal cell growth and invasive ability). Cancers can be classified in various ways. Most common cancers of adults are carcinomas, representing cancers derived from epithelial cells. Leukemias and lymphomas are derived from blood-forming cells and lymphoid cells, respectively. Sarcomas are derived from mesenchymal tissues. Melanomas are derived from melanocytes, and retinoblastomas, neuroblastomas, and glioblastomas are derived from stem cells of the retina, neurons, and glia, respectively.

Twenty years ago, it could not have been predicted whether all these different cancers shared common molecular pathogeneses in addition to common biologic properties. The cancer research revolution has demonstrated that they do: All result from defects in oncogenes and tumor suppressor genes. Each specific cancer arises through characteristic mutations in specific genes. Although there have been dozens of human oncogenes and tumor suppressor genes described in the literature, these genes' products appear to converge on a relatively small number of growth-controlling pathways. In some cases, the same gene is involved in multiple cancers. For example, p53 mutations commonly occur in cancers of the brain, colon, breast, stomach, bladder, and pancreas. In other cases, a defective gene appears to be associated with a single tumor type, such as the WT1 gene in childhood kidney cancers.

HOW MANY MUTATIONS ARE REQUIRED FOR CANCER FORMATION?

Epidemiologic investigations long ago revealed that the incidence of cancer increased exponentially with age (Fig. 3). Detailed modeling of age versus incidence curves are consistent with the idea that three to seven mutations are required for full development of cancers. This estimate is consistent with molecular analyses of cancers, in which it is not unusual to observe mutations of four or five different genes. Generally it is thought that benign tumors, the precursors of cancers, require fewer mutations (perhaps just two mutations to initiate a small neoplasm). As tumor cells accumulate additional mutations, the resultant clonal expansion causes tumor progression, with progressively larger and more dangerous neoplasms evolving. "Solid tumors" (i.e., those of solid organs such as the colon, bladder, brain, and breast) appear to require a greater number of mutations for their development than "liquid tumors" (i.e., leukemias). The smaller number of mutations required for leukemias may explain the shorter lag time following an initial mutagenic insult. For example, following the atomic bomb in Japan, leukemias began to appear within a few years, whereas an increased incidence of solid tumors was not evident until at least a decade later.

ORGANIZATION OF THE CANCER CHAPTERS IN THIS BOOK

It is obvious from the preceding that there are numerous interconnections between the principles underlying cancer genetics, and that any organization of chapters on cancer is arbitrary. For didactic purposes, however, the chapters were organized in four categories.

Part 1

Chapters in Part 1 focus on the basic concepts in cancer genetics.

Part 2

Chapters in this part focus on genetic and biochemical controls of cell growth.

Part 3

This part includes chapters on cancers in which heritable mutations of predisposing genes have been identified. These have been divided into those syndromes in which the responsible gene is a "caretaker" gene and those in which the responsible gene directly controls cell birth or cell death ("gatekeeper" genes).

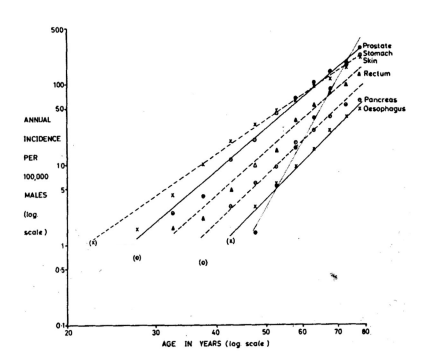

FIG. 3 Cancer incidence versus age. The log of the incidence rate and the log of age have a linear relationship, with the incidence increasing dramatically (10^3–10^7 fold) with age. (Reprinted by permission from Miller, *Cancer*, vol. 46, p 1307, copyright 1980, ACS.)

Part 4

This section includes chapters on cancers in which heritable, predisposing mutations have not been identified, or in which the responsible predisposing mutations overlap with those causing the cancers described in Part 3. The chapters in Part 4 largely emphasize somatic mutations.

Although this organization necessitates a bit of redundancy, it is hoped that the organization will satisfy those who are searching for information on specific tumor types, those who are primarily interested in specific genes, and those who are interested in acquiring a basic, general knowledge of cancer genetics.

THE GENETIC BASIS OF HUMAN CANCER

Part 1

BASIC CONCEPTS IN CANCER GENETICS

CHAPTER 1

A Human Genetics Primer

Arthur L. Beaudet ▪ Charles R. Scriver ▪ William S. Sly ▪ David Valle

DEVELOPMENT OF THE CONCEPT OF INHERITED METABOLIC DISEASE

Inborn Error Concept (Garrod)

The history of human biochemical genetics began at the turn of the twentieth century, when Sir Archibald Garrod initiated the brilliant studies of alkaptonuria that were to culminate in his Croonian Lectures in 1908[1] and in his monograph, *Inborn Errors of Metabolism*, which appeared in 1909 and in modified form in 1923.[2] With the reprinting of *Garrod's Inborn Factors in Disease* in 1989,[3] there has been increasing recognition that his work provided one of the foundation stones of modern medical thinking. A biography describing the life and contributions of Garrod was published in 1993.[4]

Garrod had observed that patients with alkaptonuria excreted large, rather constant quantities of homogentisic acid throughout their lifetimes, whereas other persons excreted none at all.[5] He observed that this condition had a familial distribution and that, while frequently one or more sibs were involved, parents and more distant relatives were normal. There was a high incidence of consanguineous marriages in the parents of his patients, as well as in the parents of similar patients studied elsewhere. On conferring with Bateson, one of the earliest of the great school of British geneticists, Garrod learned that these observations could readily be explained if the defect were inherited as a recessive condition in terms of the recently rediscovered laws of Mendel.[6,7]

From his observations of patients with alkaptonuria, albinism, cystinuria, and pentosuria, Garrod developed the concept that certain diseases of lifelong duration arise because an enzyme governing a single metabolic step is reduced in activity or missing altogether.[8] Garrod viewed the accumulation of homogentisic acid in alkaptonuria as evidence that this substance is a normal metabolite in the dissimilation of tyrosine, and he correctly attributed its accumulation to a failure of oxidation of homogentisic acid. A half-century later, Garrod's hypothesis was proved by the demonstration of a deficient activity of homogentisic acid oxidase in the liver of a patient with alkaptonuria.[9]

Similarly, the failure of pigment formation in the skin in albinism, the excretion of large amounts of cystine in the urine in cystinuria, and the appearance of pentose in the urine in essential pentosuria were viewed by Garrod as the results of blocks in normal metabolic pathways. He attributed the first instance to failure of melanin formation and the other two to excretion of metabolites accumulating proximal to a metabolic block.

One Gene-One Enzyme Concept (Beadle and Tatum)

The term *gene* was first applied to the hereditary determinant of a unit characteristic by Johannsen in 1911.[10] The relation between gene and enzyme attained clear definition in the one gene-one enzyme principle, first succinctly stated by Beadle in 1945.[11] This formulation, now a biologic precept, emerged gradually from studies of eye color in the fruit fly, *Drosophila*, by Beadle and Tatum[12,13] and Ephrussi.[14] It received extensive support from the classic studies of Beadle and Tatum on induced mutants of *Neurospora crassa*, in which the acquisition of requirements for specific metabolites in the culture medium was traced to losses of single chemical transformations, each dependent on a different enzyme.[15,16]

The one gene-one enzyme concept that developed from these experiments was well expressed by Tatum[16] as follows:

1. All biochemical processes in all organisms are under genetic control.

2. These biochemical processes are resolvable into series of individual stepwise reactions.

3. Each biochemical reaction is under the ultimate control of a different single gene.

4. Mutation of a single gene results only in an alteration in the ability of the cell to carry out a single primary chemical reaction.

The one gene-one enzyme hypothesis has since been refined[17] and extended to cover proteins that are not enzymes, as well as complex proteins composed of nonidentical polypeptide chains linked in various ways. The functional unit of DNA that controls the structure of a single polypeptide chain is frequently called a *cistron*.[18] The one gene-one enzyme principle was redefined as the one cistron-one polypeptide concept. Posttranslational cleavage to generate multiple peptides, alternative splicing, and alternative promoter sequences contribute complexities to the concept. Additional intricacies are introduced as mutations in transcription factors, gain-of-function mutations, somatic mutations, unstable mutations, and imprinting of genes are described. Some examples of the complexity and variations involved in the one gene-one enzyme concept are presented in Table 1-1.

---

*Adapted and condensed from Chapter 1: Genetics, Biochemistry, and the Molecular Basis of Variant Human Phenotypes, *The Metabolic and Molecular Bases of Inherited Disease*, © 1995, by The McGraw-Hill Companies, Inc.

Table 1-1　Complexity and Variations in the One Gene-One Enzyme Concept

Concept	Examples	Disorder
One gene-one enzyme	Phenylalanine hydroxylase	Phenylketonuria
	Hypoxanthine-guanine phosphoribosyltransferase	Lesch-Nyhan syndrome
One gene-nonenzymatic protein	Collagens	Osteogenesis imperfecta
	Spectrin/ankyrin	Spherocytosis
One gene-RNA product	Mitochondrial transfer RNA	MERRF/MELAS*
One enzyme activity requires multiple subunits from separate genes	Propionyl CoA carboxylase	Propionic acidemia
	Hexosaminidase	Tay-Sachs disease
One polypeptide chain with multiple enzymes	β subunit of hexosaminidase A and B	Sandhoff disease
	E_3 subunit of dehydrogenases	E_3 deficiency
One polypeptide chain with multiple enzyme activities	Orotate phosphoribosyl transferase and orotidine-5′-phosphate decarboxylase	Orotic aciduria
	CAD trienzyme protein	
Deficiency of one enzyme causes multiple secondary enzyme deficiencies	Cobalamin C and D	Methylmalonic acidemias
	mRNA-N-acetylglucosamine (GlcNAc): glycoprotein GlcNAc 1-phosphotransferase	I-cell disease
Posttranslational cleavage of a peptide	ACTH (adrenocorticotrophic hormone), endorphins	
Alternative promoters for transcription	Dystrophin	Duchenne dystrophy
Alternative splicing of pre-mRNA	Calcitonin	
	Muscle proteins	
DNA rearrangements prior to transcription	Immunoglobulins	Agammaglobulinemia
	T-cell receptors	Combined immunodeficiency
Posttranscriptional modification of mRNA	Apolipoproteins B-100 and B-48	Hypobetalipoproteinemia
Overlapping reading frames in DNA and RNA, suppression, frameshifting	Bacterial release factor	
	Retroviruses	

*MERRF = myoclonic epilepsy and ragged red fiber disease;
MELAS = mitochondrial myopathy, encephalomyopathy, lactic acidosis, and stroke-like episodes.

The one gene-one enzyme concept had immediate explanatory potential for the inborn errors of metabolism that Garrod had described. It appeared that inherited diseases such as alkaptonuria were produced by loss-of-function mutations in genes encoding enzymes in the same way that vitamin-dependent mutations of *Neurospora* lacked single enzymes required for vitamin synthesis. It was not until 1948 that the first enzyme defect in a human genetic disease was demonstrated by Gibson. This was the deficiency of the NADH-dependent enzyme required for the reduction of methemoglobin in recessive methemoglobinemia.[19] This was soon followed by the description in 1952 by Cori and Cori of glucose 6-phosphatase deficiency in von Gierke disease (glycogen storage disease, type I)[20] and in 1953 by Jervis of phenylalanine hydroxylase deficiency in phenylketonuria.[21]

Molecular Disease Concept (Pauling and Ingram)

Direct evidence that human mutations actually produce an alteration in the primary structure of proteins was first obtained in 1949 by Pauling and his associates.[22] Studying hemoglobin extracted from erythrocytes of patients with sickle-cell anemia, Pauling showed that sickle hemoglobin migrated differently in an electric field than did normal hemoglobin. Heterozygotes for the sickle-cell trait produced both normal and abnormal hemoglobin molecules. The subsequent studies of Ingram established that the electrophoretic abnormality arose because sickle-cell hemoglobin had a valine substituted for a glutamic acid residue at a particular point in the amino acid sequence.[23] This finding closed one era of discovery in human biochemical genetics: Inborn errors of metabolism were caused by mutant genes that produced abnormal proteins whose functional activities were altered.

The Recombinant DNA Revolution

Recombinant DNA methodology has transformed the study of human genetics. The changes trace their roots back to the description of the structure of DNA by Watson and Crick in 1953.[24] Over the ensuing two decades, the mechanisms of protein synthesis were defined, the genetic code was deciphered, and many enzymes of nucleic acid metabolism were characterized. Extensive genetic studies of *Escherichia coli, Saccharomyces cerevisiae*, bacteriophages γ and M13, bacterial plasmids, and other systems provided necessary groundwork.

By the 1970s, restriction enzymes were described,[25] and their value for preparing restriction maps was recognized.[26] The basic procedures for cloning DNA fragments in plasmid and bacteriophage vectors were described, opening the recombinant DNA era[27,28] (see Chaps. 5 and 7 in *Recombinant DNA*[29] for additional bibliography). Methods for DNA sequencing were described,[30,31] and the existence of introns and exons within genes was discovered.[32,33] Southern blotting and northern blotting became routine, and the polymerase chain reaction (PCR) brought another leap forward. The general procedures of recombinant DNA technology are well described in an introductory text entitled *Recombinant DNA*,[29] and many of the techniques are described further below.

The initial applications of recombinant DNA methodology to the study of human disease involved cloning of numerous genes in instances where the protein was characterized and/or an enzyme activity was known, as in the case of globins, phenylalanine hydroxylase, apolipoproteins, and many others. With the identification of a restriction fragment length polymorphism (RFLP) at the β-globin locus by Kan and Dozy,[34] the concept of a new and virtually inexhaustible source of genetic markers for the exploration of inherited human disease became a reality. Quickly thereafter, the feasibility of creating a linkage map of the human genome using

RFLPs was described.[35] This led to the strategy of cloning a disease gene using its map location in the genome as a mechanism for identification, a strategy initially called "reverse genetics"[36] but now more usually referred to as "positional cloning."[37] The initial successes of positional cloning took advantage of rare patients with detectable cytogenetic disorders associated with disruption or deletion of individual genes, as in the cases of Duchenne dystrophy, polyposis of the colon (Chap. 31), and neurofibromatosis (Chap. 22). Some brute force approaches in the absence of cytogenetic clues were successful, as in the cases of cystic fibrosis, myotonic dystrophy, and Huntington disease. With the progress of the human genome project, as described in Chap. 2, more and more genes and polymorphisms are being mapped to human chromosomes. This information is accessible electronically through the Genome Data Base (GDB), and it may become increasingly possible to use limited genetic mapping information for a phenotype, in combination with knowledge of genes mapping in a region, to quickly test whether a particular gene might be mutated in a human disease using what might be referred to as a positional candidate gene approach.[38]

The impact of molecular biology and recombinant DNA methodology can perhaps be measured in part by the numerous Nobel prizes[39] awarded, including those recognizing discoveries of the structure of DNA, of the genetic code, of reverse transcription by retroviruses, of restriction enzymes, of basic recombinant methods, and of DNA sequencing methods, as well as, most recently, the discovery of introns and the development of the polymerase chain reaction.

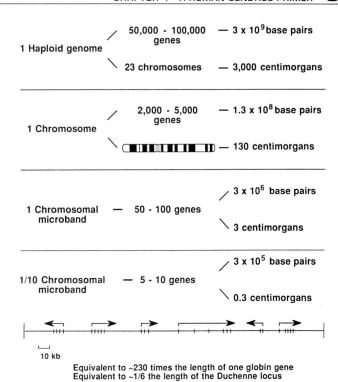

FIG. 1-1 Perspectives on the amount of DNA, number of genes, and genetic distance in the human genome. The arrows in the lowest panel indicate hypothetical transcripts, with vertical lines indicating exons within genes.

MOLECULAR BASIS OF GENE EXPRESSION

The human genome is estimated to contain about 50,000 to 100,000 genes, each of which is composed of a linear polymer of DNA (see Chap. 2 for a more detailed discussion). The genes are assembled into lengthy linear arrays, which together with certain proteins, form the rod-shaped bodies called *chromosomes*. All normal nucleated human cells other than sperm or ova contain 46 chromosomes, arrayed in 23 pairs, one member of each pair derived from each of the individual's parents. The striking discovery that genes are not continuous sequences of DNA but consist of coding sequences (exons) interrupted by intervening sequences (introns) led to a new and more complex view of gene expression.

Some approximations regarding the magnitude and organization of the human genome are presented in Fig. 1-1. The estimated 50,000 to 100,000 genes are distributed within the 3 billion base pairs of DNA that comprise a haploid genome. Linkage studies indicate that the human genome consists of approximately 3000 centimorgans in recombination distance. A *centimorgan* (1/100 of a Morgan) is a measure of genetic distance reflecting the probability of a crossover between two loci during meiosis. One centimorgan approximately equals a recombination fraction of 0.01, or a 1 percent chance of a crossover during meiosis. Thus an average chromosome would contain 2000 to 5000 genes within 130 million base pairs of DNA and would be equivalent to about 130 centimorgans of genetic material. A typical microband on a chromosome stained at the 800-band level of resolution should contain 3 to 5 million base pairs and 60 to 120 genes. This representation oversimplifies many issues. Estimates of the total number of genes are imprecise. Although the average recombination distance is estimated to be approximately one centimorgan per million base pairs of DNA, there is wide variation in this rate over shorter distances, as well as differences in recombination distance according to sex. Genes range in size from very small (1.5 kb for a globin gene) to

very large (about 2000 kb for the Duchenne muscular dystrophy locus). *Cis*-acting regulatory elements (i.e., on the contiguous DNA strand) may occur a considerable distance from the coding region, e.g., 50 kb 5′ and 20 kb 3′ to the β-globin gene,[40] thus extending the functional domains of genes and complicating the definition of boundaries.

The human genome also includes numerous nonfunctional sequences and highly reiterated sequences.[41] There are 300,000 to 500,000 copies of the *Alu* repeat sequence (the most reiterated) in the human genome. Many other reiterated sequences occur with lesser frequency. Many genes have additional nonfunctional copies (pseudogenes), and the sequence distribution of human DNA is not uniform. For example, HTF (*Hpa*II tiny fragment) islands are G-plus-C rich regions that occur near the 5′ end of constitutive genes and are thought to have some relationship to regulation of gene expression.[42] The functional significance, if any, of most of the DNA that occurs outside coding regions remains to be determined.

The Molecular Flow of Information

Much is known about how living organisms store, transmit, and use their genetic information. The picture is most detailed for prokaryotic organisms, but extensive information is also available for the more complex eukaryotic organisms. Two excellent textbooks[43,44] provide a more systematic and comprehensive treatment of cellular and molecular biology than is included here. The latest editions of the *Molecular Biology of the Gene* by Watson and colleagues[45] and *Genes V* by Lewin[46] provide a detailed view of the molecular flow of information in prokaryotic and eukaryotic organisms.

The genetic information carried on chromosomes is transmitted to daughter cells under two different sets of circumstances. One of these (mitosis) occurs each time a somatic cell (i.e., a nongerm cell) divides. Mitosis functions to transmit two identical copies of each gene to each daughter cell, thus maintaining a uniform genetic makeup in all cells of an organism. The other set of circumstances prevails when genetic information is to be transmitted from an individual to an offspring. In this case, the second process *(meiosis)* functions to produce germ cells (i.e., ova or spermatozoa) that possess only one copy of each parental chromosome, thus allowing for new combinations of chromosomes to occur when the ovum and sperm cell fuse during fertilization to restore the *diploid* state.

During the process of meiosis, the 46 chromosomes of an immature germ cell arrange themselves in 23 pairs at the center of the nucleus, each pair being composed of one chromosome derived from the mother and its homologous chromosome derived from the father. At a specified point in the meiotic process, the two partner chromosomes separate, only one of each pair going into each daughter cell, or gamete. Thus, meiosis produces gametes with a reduction in the number of chromosomes from 46 to 23, each gamete having received one chromosome from each of the 23 pairs. The assortment of the chromosomes within each pair is random, so that each germ cell receives a different combination of maternal and paternal chromosomes. During the process of fertilization, the fusion of ovum and sperm cell, each of which has 23 chromosomes, ultimately results in an individual with 46 chromosomes.

The independent assortment of chromosomes into gametes during meiosis produces an enormous diversity among the possible genotypes of the progeny. For each 23 pairs of chromosomes, 2^{23} different combinations of chromosomes can occur in gametes, and the likelihood that one set of parents will produce two offspring with the same complement of chromosomes is one in 2^{23} or one in 8.4 million (assuming no monozygotic twins). Adding even further to the enormous genetic diversity in humans is the phenomenon of *genetic recombination.*

The Structure of DNA

Most organisms store their genetic information in *deoxyribonucleic acid* (DNA). DNA is a linear polymer of four different monomeric units, collectively called *"deoxyribonucleotides"* or simply *"nucleotides,"* that are linked together in a chain by phosphodiester bonds (Fig. 1-2). A typical DNA molecule consists of two interwound polynucleotide chains, as described by Watson and Crick,[24] each containing several thousand to several million monomers (Fig. 1-3). Each nucleotide in one chain is specifically linked by hydrogen bonds to a nucleotide in the other chain. Only two nucleotide pairings are found in DNA: deoxyadenosine monophosphate with thymidine monophosphate (A-T pairs) and deoxyguanosine monophosphate with deoxycytidine monophosphate (G-C pairs). Thus, the sequence of nucleotides of one chain fixes the sequence of the other, and the two chains are therefore said to be *complementary* to each other.

The sequence of the four nucleotides along a polynucleotide chain varies among the DNAs of unrelated organisms and, indeed, is the molecular basis of their genetic diversity. Because most genetic characteristics are stably transmitted from parent to progeny, the sequence of nucleotides in DNA must be faithfully copied or replicated as the organism reproduces itself. This occurs by unwinding of the two chains and polymerization of two daughter chains along the separated parental strands. The nucleotide sequence and, hence, the genetic information are conserved during this process because each nucleotide in the daughter chains is paired specifically with its complement in the parental or template chains before polymerization occurs.

The DNA of higher organisms, separated from the great bulk of cellular components by a nuclear membrane, is wound into a tightly and regularly packed chromosomal structure consisting of

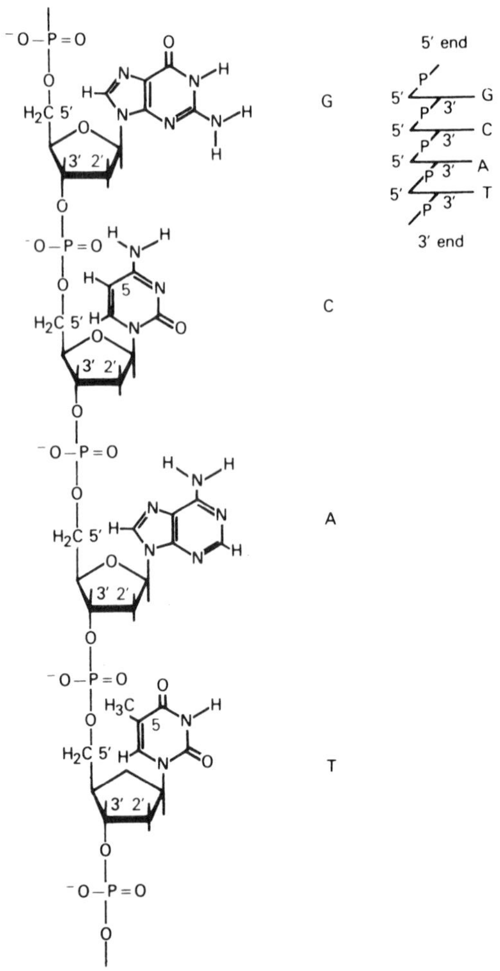

FIG. 1-2 A polynucleotide chain. One of each of the four different monomeric units of DNA is present in this tetranucleotide. The monomers of DNA are, from top to bottom, deoxyguanosine monophosphate (G), deoxycytidine monophosphate (C), deoxyadenosine monophosphate (A), and thymidine monophosphate (T). Each nucleotide consists of a phosphate group, a deoxyribose moiety, and a heterocyclic base. G and A have purine bases, and C and T have pyrimidine bases. The phosphodiester bonds that link adjacent nucleotides extend from the 3′ position of one deoxyribose moiety to the 5′ position of the next; this gives the chain a chemical polarity. An abbreviated way of writing the same sequence is shown at the top right. In RNA (see text), ribose, which contains a 2′-hydroxyl group, replaces deoxyribose, and uridine monophosphate (U) replaces T. U differs from T in the substitution of ribose for deoxyribose and in the loss of the 5-methyl group.

nucleoprotein elements called *nucleosomes.* Each of these nucleosomal elements is in turn composed of four (sometimes five) protein subunits, *histones,* that form a core structure about which are wound approximately 140 nucleotide pairs of genomic DNA. Histone structure is remarkably well conserved throughout the eukaryotic kingdom. Such conservation argues strongly that strict functional requirements, presumably related to the detailed architecture of the nucleosome, impede divergent evolution. The nucleosomes, arranged as "beads on a string," become further organized into more highly ordered structures consisting of coils of many closely packed nucleosomes that, in turn, must form the fundamental organizational units of the eukaryotic chromosome.

Nucleosomal structure may serve a variety of purposes, for example, simply compacting the enormous amount of DNA (about 6×10^9 base pairs) that makes up the human diploid genome. Aside from such a packing function, this ubiquitous structure must also be reconciled with a train of enzymes that acts on DNA to

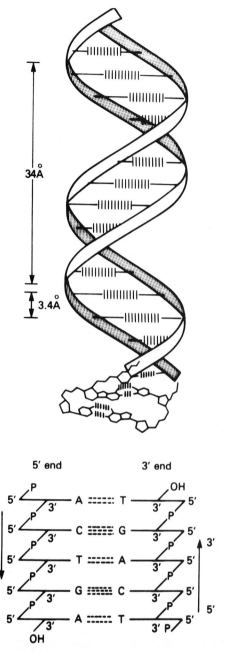

FIG. 1-3 The structure of DNA. *Top.* The two interwound hydrogen-bonded polynucleotide chains of DNA are shown. The hydrogen bonds are indicated by vertical hatches. The distance between adjacent nucleotide pairs is 3.4 Å. The distance between adjacent turns of the double helix is 34 Å, or about 10 nucleotide pairs. *Bottom.* An alterative representation in which the opposite chemical polarities of the two chains can be clearly seen.

replicate and transcribe it. Undoubtedly, these functions are subserved and modulated by other proteins that little resemble the monotonous structure of the histones and that recognize specific structural features of a DNA sequence. A fundamental question in eukaryotic molecular biology is how this nucleoprotein structure permits access to specific proteins and is made differentially available in the course of cellular growth and development.

The double-helical model of DNA immediately suggested the manner in which genes could be replicated for transmission to offspring. The actual replication process is mechanically complex but conceptually simple. The two strands of DNA separate, and each is copied by a series of enzymes that inserts a complementary base

opposite each base on the original strand of DNA. Thus, two identical double helices are generated from one.[45,46] Details of the mechanisms of DNA replication in prokaryotic and eukaryotic cells are becoming known.[47,48]

The Genetic Code

DNA makes RNA (transcription) makes protein (translation) in the accepted paradigm (Fig. 1-4). The sequence of bases in a specific gene ultimately dictates the sequence of amino acids in a specific protein. This colinearity between the DNA molecule and the protein sequence is achieved by means of the *genetic code*.[29,45,46] The four types of bases in DNA are arranged in groups of three, each triplet forming a code word or *codon* that signifies a single amino acid.

In this manner, triplet codons exist for each of the 20 amino acids that occur in proteins (Fig. 1-5); interestingly a slightly different genetic code is used in mitochondria. Inasmuch as 64 different triplets can be generated from the four bases and only 20 amino acids exist, the genetic code is said to be *degenerate*. That is, most amino acids are specified by more than one codon. Each codon, however, is completely specific. Thus the double-stranded sequence adenine-adenine-adenine (or AAA) in the transcribed (antisense) strand and thymine-thymine-thymine (or TTT) in the nontranscribed (sense) strand of DNA codes for uridine-uridine-uridine (or UUU) in mRNA, which is translated to phenylalanine in protein (Fig. 1-4).

DNA → RNA → Protein

To translate its genetic information into a protein, a segment of DNA is first transcribed into messenger ribonucleic acid (messenger RNA or mRNA). The messenger RNA contains a sequence of purine and pyrimidine bases that is complementary to the bases of the transcribed (antisense) strand of the DNA. By this mechanism each adenine of DNA becomes a uridine of RNA, each cytosine of DNA becomes a guanine of RNA, each thymine of DNA becomes an adenine of RNA, and each guanine of DNA becomes a cytosine of RNA. Thus, each DNA triplet codon is translated into a corresponding RNA triplet codon.

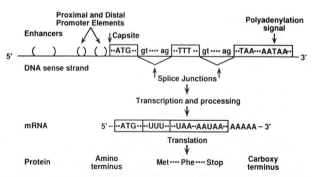

FIG. 1-4 Prototypical eukaryotic gene. In schematic form, a cellular gene is depicted in which exons or coding regions (boxes) are separated by intervening sequences (introns). Introns begin with the dinucleotide GT and end with AG. A short motif of AATAA (or modified versions) direct endonucleolytic cleavage and polyadenylation of nascent RNAs. Promoter elements, shown as empty parentheses, lie upstream from the start of the gene and are often multiple in nature. Common promoter elements include motifs such as TATA and CCAAT (TATA and CAT boxes) and GGCGGG (the Sp1 nuclear factor binding site). Additional sequences, known as enhancers, augment transcription and can lie either before, within, or downstream from the gene. After transcription, the RNA is processed to yield mature mRNA, which is translated to yield protein.

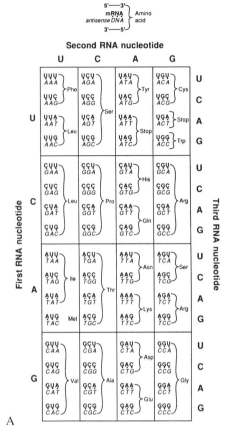

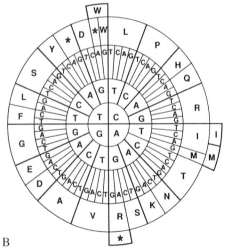

FIG. 1-5 The eukaryotic nuclear genetic code. *A.* The RNA codons appear in boldface type; the complementary DNA codons are in italics. A = adenine, C = cystosine, G = guanine, T = thymine, U = uridine (replaces thymine in RNA). In RNA, adenine is complementary to thymine of DNA; uridine is complementary to adenine of DNA; cytosine is complementary to guanine and vice versa. "Stop" = peptide chain termination. The three-letter and single-letter abbreviations for the amino acids are as follows: Ala (A) = alanine; Arg (R) = arginine; Asn (N) = asparagine; Asp (D) = aspartic acid; Cys (C) = cysteine; Gln (Q) = glutamine; Glu (E) = glutamic acid; Gly (G) = glycine; His (H) = histidine; Ile (I) = isoleucine; Leu (L) = leucine; Lys (K) = lysine; Met (M) = methionine; Phe (F) = phenylalanine; Pro (P) = proline; Ser (S) = serine; Thr (T) = threonine; Trp (W) = tryptophan; Tyr (Y) = tyrosine; Val (V) = valine. *B.* The outermost complete circle represents the amino acid in single letter code or a stop codon (*); the DNA sense strand for the triplet codon for each amino acid is given on the radial, starting with the first base of the codon in the center. Differences in the mitochondrial genetic code are shown in the outermost boxes.

The messenger RNA for each gene undergoes extensive processing in the cell nucleus, including splicing to remove intronic sequences. It then crosses the nuclear membrane and enters the cytoplasm, where it serves as a template for the synthesis of a specific protein.[45,46] To translate the messenger RNA code into a protein, the messenger RNA binds to a complex structure called a ribosome, which is composed of a different type of RNA (ribosomal RNA or rRNA) and a large number of proteins. In order to be inserted into its proper place in the protein sequence, each of the 20 amino acids is attached in the cytoplasm to an additional type of RNA (transfer RNA or tRNA). Each amino acid is attached to a specific set of transfer RNAs (Fig. 1-6).[49] Each transfer RNA contains an "anticodon loop," which includes a sequence of three bases that is complementary to a specific codon in the corresponding mRNA. For example, phenylalanine is attached specifically to a tRNA whose anticodon loop contains the sequence AAA, which is complementary to the mRNA codon UUU, which codes for phenylalanine.

Under the influence of a host of cytoplasmic factors (initiation factors, elongation factors, and termination factors), peptide bonds are formed between the various amino acids that are aligned along the mRNA (Fig. 1-7). Eventually, a terminator codon is reached and the completed polypeptide is released from the ribosome. Inasmuch as the primary sequence of bases in the coding regions of the DNA determines the corresponding primary sequence of amino acids in the protein, the gene and its protein are said to be *colinear*. This means that alterations of the sequence of bases in the gene can result in alterations of the protein at a specific point in its sequence.

Control of Gene Expression

The control of gene expression at a transcriptional level has been the focus of extensive research over the last decade or two. The basic elements of the transcriptional process are described in standard texts.[29,43-46] A detailed review of transcription factors including an extensive bibliography is available,[50] and a recent series of articles emphasizes many topical issues.[51] The proper rate and timing for transcription is subject to complex controls. *Cis*-acting regulatory DNA sequences are part of the same duplex DNA molecule as the coding sequence, and *trans*-acting factors (usually proteins) are encoded by other genes (usually unlinked). The *trans*-acting factors interact with the *cis* sequences to control the process of transcription. Many of the *cis*-acting transcriptional control elements occur short distances upstream from the initiation site for transcription, but some have been described at greater distances upstream and downstream from the initiation site for transcription, for example, at a distance of 5 to 50 kb.

The first described family of transcription factors was the helix-turn-helix protein family that includes many bacterial proteins such as the λ repressor. Another family of DNA-binding proteins contain homeodomains. These regulatory proteins were first characterized in *Drosophila*, and many mammalian homologs are now identified. The homeodomain proteins contain a type of helix-turn-helix motif. Complex clusters of homeotic genes are now well characterized in mouse and human,[52,53] and a number of these genes have been mutated in the mouse using gene targeting methodology. Another group of transcription factors contain zinc finger motifs, as originally described for the *Xenopus* transcription factor IIIA. The steroid receptors are an important family of transcriptional regulators that bear some similarity to the zinc finger proteins but represent a distinct motif. This group of proteins is of particular importance in terms of currently known examples of human mutations in transcription factors. Yet other families of transcription factors include proteins with leucine zipper motifs or helix-loop-helix motifs. Leucine zippers are characterized by hep-

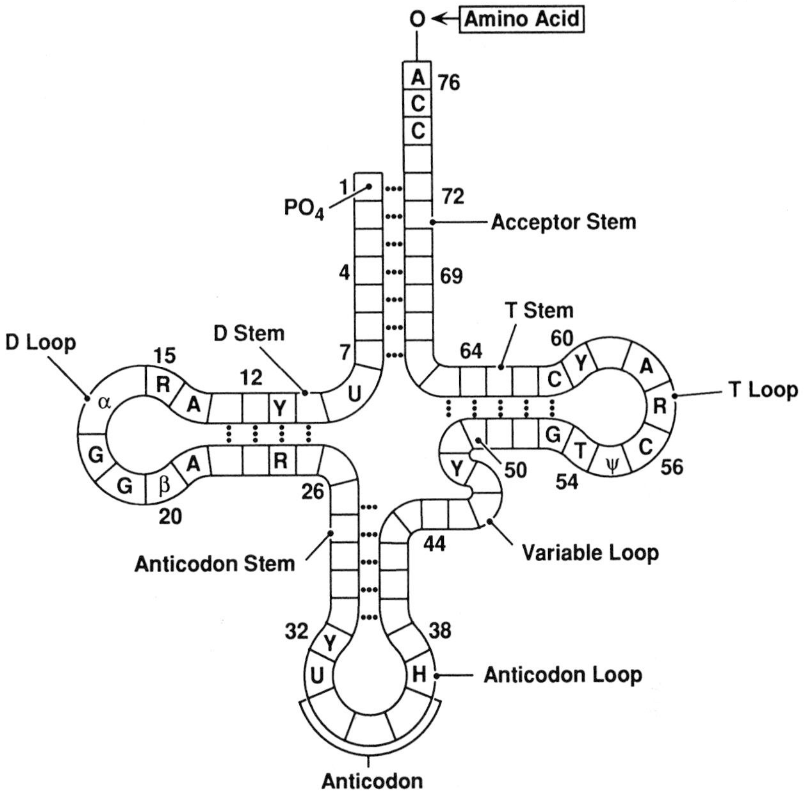

FIG. 1-6 A diagrammatic representation of a tRNA molecule. Each base in the tRNA is represented by a box. The structure is shown with interacting complementary sequences indicated by a row of dots. Each conserved loop is shown (D loop = dehydrouridylic acid loop; T loop = thymidylic acid-pseudouridylic acid-cytidylic acid loop). The anticodon position is indicated. All tRNAs end with a CCA sequence at their 3′ terminus, which serves as the amino acid acceptor portion of the molecule. The number of nucleotides in the various stems and loops is generally constant except for two parts of the D loop designated α and β (which consist of from one to three nucleotides in different tRNAs) and the variable loop (which usually has 4 or 5 nucleotides but may have as many as 21). Abbreviations are A (adenosine), G (guanosine), C (cytidine), U (uridine), R (adenosine or guanosine), Y (cytidine or uridine), T (ribothymidine), ψ (pseudouridine), H (modified adenosine or guanosine). *(From Rich and Kim.[49] Used by permission.)*

tad repeats of leucines which promote dimer formation. The leucine zipper proteins can form various heterodimers that can activate or repress transcription. The helix-loop-helix proteins also appear to form dimers that can have positive or negative regulatory effects. Considerably greater detail regarding transcription factors is available elsewhere.[75]

Regulation of gene expression also occurs at a posttranscriptional level. These processes can include regulation of export of mRNA from nucleus to cytoplasm, alternative splicing of transcripts, polyadenylation of transcripts, translation of mRNA, and stability of mRNA. A recent series of articles touches on some aspects of these processes.[54] There are numerous examples where

FIG. 1-7 The elongation reactions in protein synthesis. The figure diagrammatically represents the ribosone (60S and 40S subunits), the tRNA moieties (hairpinlike structures), and the associated mRNAs. The first elongation intermediate (upper left) shows a peptidyl tRNA, the peptide portion of which is represented by leucine and three dots, at the donor site on the ribosome interacting with a leucine codon, AUU. In the presence of GTP and elongation factor 1 (EF-1), Tyr-tRNA binds to the next available codon at the receptor site. The peptide is transferred to the oncoming Tyr-tRNA by an enzymatic activity associated with the 60S subunit of the ribosome. The next step involves release of the deacylated tRNA (leucine) and the translocation of the mRNA and the newly elongated peptidyl tRNA to the donor site, exposing the next available codon, CAU, for recognition. The later reaction requires elongation factor 2 (EF-2) and consumes GTP. The entire process is repeated until a termination codon is encountered, and the finished peptide is released in the presence of appropriate termination factors.

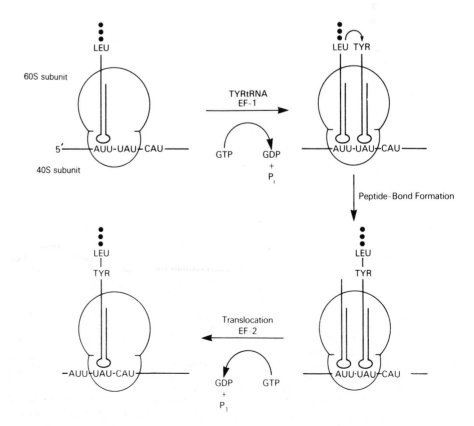

gene function is regulated through alternative splicing[18a] including control of immunoglobulin secretion, production of calcitonin versus calcitonin gene-related peptide, and modulation of the structure and function of troponin-T. Considerable regulation is also possible at a posttranslational level.[54]

MUTATION AS THE ORIGIN OF NORMAL VARIATION AND GENETIC DISEASE

A mutation traditionally has been defined as a stable, heritable change in DNA. Note that this definition does not depend on the functional significance of the change. It implies a change in primary nucleotide sequence, and other changes, such as those involving methylation, are usually referred to as epigenetic events. Mutations that occur in somatic cells may be most relevant to cancer or aging and otherwise may be of little phenotyic importance. Mutations occurring in germ cells are of greatest importance in terms of their impact on offspring. The concept that mutations are stable changes remains generally true, but the discovery of expanding triplet repeat mutations emphasizes that mutations can be unstable in either somatic or germ cells. Some mutations are genetically lethal and cannot be passed from one generation to the next, while others are less deleterious and are tolerated in the descendants under permissive conditions. From the viewpoint of evolution, mutations are essential for the generation of sufficient genetic diversity to permit species to adapt to their environment through the mechanism of natural selection. Chap. 3 is devoted to a detailed discussion of human mutation, and only a brief treatment is provided here.

Mutations are quite diverse in nature (Table 1-2). Some involve gross alterations (millions of base pairs) in the structure of a chromosome; these include duplications, deletions, and translocations of a portion of one chromosome to another. Mutations can even involve the entire genome (three billion base pairs), as in triploidy, where there is a third copy of the whole chromosome complement. On the other hand, mutations can be minute, involving a deletion, insertion, or replacement of a single base. Single-base or very small mutations are called *point mutations*. If deletions or insertions of one or two bases occur in a coding region, they give rise to *frameshift mutations* because they alter the reading frame of the genetic code such that every triplet distal to the mutation in the same gene is altered. Frameshift mutations grossly alter the protein sequence and frequently result in termination of the peptide chain shortly beyond the mutation site because a termination codon occurs in the altered reading frame. Small deletions or insertions can also affect transcription, splicing, or RNA processing, depending on their location.

When one base is replaced by another in the coding region, the point mutations may be of three types: (1) a *synonymous* or *silent mutation* (comprising about 23 percent of random base substitutions in coding regions), in which the base replacement leads not to a change in the amino acid but only to the substitution of a different codon for the same amino acid (e.g., a replacement of a single base pair in the DNA so that a codon for phenylalanine will be transcribed into RNA not as UUU but as UUC, which still codes for phenylalanine); (2) a *missense mutation* (about 73 percent of base substitutions in coding regions), in which the base replacement changes the codon to a codon for a different amino acid (e.g., the replacement of a base pair in DNA in the codon for phenylalanine such that it will be transcribed into RNA not as UUU but as UUA, which codes for leucine); and (3) a *nonsense mutation* (about 4 percent of base substitutions in coding regions), in which the base replacement changes the codon to one of the termination codons (e.g., the replacement of a base pair in the codon for tyrosine such that it is transcribed into RNA not as UAU but as the stop codon UAA).[55] Occasionally a base substitution in the coding region will alter RNA splicing either by creating a cryptic splice site or by interfering with the function of a normal splice site. For missense mutations, the single-letter amino acid code is often used to indicate substitutions, such that R560T indicates replacement of arginine (R) at position 560 by threonine

Table 1-2 Common Mechanisms of Mutation

Type	Usual Effect	Examples
Large Mutation		
Deletions	Null*	Duchenne dystrophy
		Contiguous gene
Insertions	Null	Hemophilia A/LINE repeat
Duplications	Null, gene disrupted	Duchenne dystrophy
	Dosage, gene intact	Charcot-Marie-Tooth
Inversions	Null	Hemophilia A
Expanding repeat	Null	Fragile X
	? Gain of function	Huntington
Point Mutation		
Silent (in or out of coding)	None	Cystic fibrosis
Missense or in-frame deletion	Null, hypomorphic, altered function, gain function, benign	Globin
		Cystic fibrosis
Nonsense	Null	Cystic fibrosis
Frameshift	Null	Cystic fibrosis
Splicing (ag/gt)†	Null	Globin
Splicing (outside ag/gt)†	Hypomorphic	Globin
Regulatory (TATA, other)	Hypomorphic	Globin
Regulatory (poly A site)	Hypomorphic	Globin

*"Null" indicates no functional gene product.
†"ag/gt" indicates mutations in the almost absolutely canonical first two and last two base pairs of each intron, while "outside ag/gt" indicates splicing mutations in less canonical sequences of introns or exons.

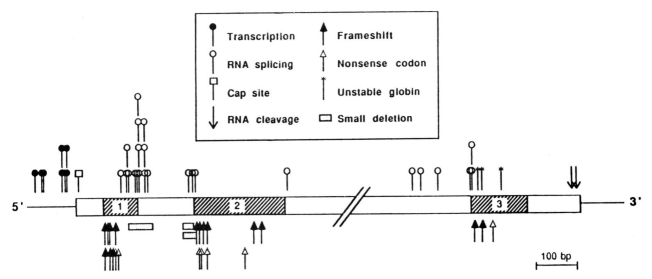

FIG. 1-8 Point mutations in β-thalassemia. The β-globin gene is shown with numbered hatched areas representing the coding regions of exons. Boxed open areas between the exons are introns, and boxed open areas at the 5′ and 3′ ends of the gene are untranslated regions that appear in the messenger RNA. The various types of mutations are depicted by different symbols. *(From Kazazian and Boehm.[57] Used by permission.)*

(T). A systematic approach to nomenclature for human mutations has been suggested.[56]

In addition to these point mutations, there are larger deletions which may affect a portion of a gene, an entire gene, or a set of contiguous genes. Such deletion mutations may interrupt or remove the coding region of a gene, causing its protein product to be absent. Alternatively, a deletion can bridge between the coding regions of two genes, producing a fusion that results in the production of a hybrid protein containing the initial sequence of one protein followed by the terminal sequence of another protein. This type of mutation is caused particularly by unequal crossing-over between tandemly repeated homologous genes, such as the globin genes (Chap. 3). The range of mutations seen at the human β-globin locus provides a good perspective on the extent of heterogeneity of mutations that can occur. Over 200 missense mutations causing amino acid substitutions with various phenotypes are known at the β-globin locus. Various δβ and βδ fusions are known. Numerous transcriptional, splicing, and RNA processing mutations cause β-thalassemia,[57] as shown in Fig. 1-8. The reciprocal products of deletions caused by unequal crossing-over are duplications, and such duplications are now well documented as the most common form of defect causing type IA Charcot-Marie-Tooth disease. Insertions in genomic DNA also occur by retrotransposition, as exemplified by the appearance of LINE repeat sequences in the factor VII gene as a cause of hemophilia. Inversions affecting the factor VIII gene appear to be a common cause of severe hemophilia A.[58]

The discovery of expanding repeat mutations, nearly all of which are triplet repeats, provides a relatively new mechanism of mutation. These mutations are known to cause fragile X mental retardation, myotonic dystrophy, spinobulbar muscular atrophy,[59] Huntington disease, spinocerebellar ataxia type 1, and other disorders. As described in greater detail in these chapters and in Chap. 3, these triplet repeat sequences can occur in the 5′ untranslated, coding, or 3′ untranslated regions. Longer repeat sequences are generally associated with a more severe and/or earlier-onset phenotype, and repeat sequences slightly longer than found in normal individuals may function as premutations in asymptomatic individuals. The premutant or mutant expanded triplet repeats are unstable and may show greater instability when transmitted from females, as in the case of fragile X and myotonic dystrophy, or when transmitted from males, as in the case of Huntington disease and spinocerebellar ataxia. For three neurodegenerative disorders (Huntington disease, spinobulbar muscular atrophy, and spinocerebellar ataxia type I), the expanded triplet repeat encodes a polyglutamine tract in the protein, but the mechanism by which this mutation causes neurodegeneration is not yet delineated. Expanding triplet repeat mutations are now well documented as at least one mechanism underlying the phenomenon of anticipation, in which the phenotype of a disease tends to worsen over successive generations in a single family.

The type and frequency of human mutations is a complex topic. Mutations causing chromosomal aneuploidy occur at increasing frequency with advancing age of the mother. Some classes of smaller mutations occur at increasing frequency with advancing age of the father, although the molecular nature of the mutations seen with advanced paternal age is just becoming known. Some loci, such as those for Duchenne muscular dystrophy and achondroplasia, are subject to very high rates of new mutation. In the instance of Duchenne dystrophy, this may be related in part to the unusually large size of the gene. The structure of the gene, its position within the genome, and the constraints on the gene product may contribute along with other factors to the frequency of new mutations causing phenotypic effects at a locus. The occurrence of 5-methylcytosine, particularly at the sites of CpG base pairs, provides sites of increased mutational frequency, owing to the occurrence of spontaneous deamination of 5-methylcytosine to yield a thymine base. This propensity leads to an increased frequency of RFLPs for at least some restriction enzymes that have CpG pairs in the recognition site[60] and accounts for certain mutational hot spots causing hemophilia A and many other human disorders (Chap. 3). The availability of recombinant DNA techniques has led to an increasingly exact definition of the nature of new mutations, of whether they arose from a maternal or paternal gamete, and of whether the mutation is of recent or ancient origin. Mutations that are widespread in the population but are descended from a single event can be recognized by the occurrence of specific haplotypes of RFLPs surrounding the mutations. A haplotype is a group of genetic markers linked together on a single chromosome, such as a group of close RFLP markers[57] or a group of HLA alleles.

When mutations occur in germ cells, the altered expression of the mutant gene is manifest only in subsequent generations and does not affect the phenotype of the individual in whom the mutation occurs. Usually such *new mutations* are sporadic events in human populations. On the other hand, when a mutation occurs in somatic cells at an early developmental stage, it may affect the individual harboring the mutation, but is not passed to subsequent generations. The individual harboring such a somatic cell mutation is said to be a *mosaic* because two populations of cells are present: normal cells and cells harboring the mutant gene. Mutations occurring in an early germ line cell can give rise to gonadal mosaicism, so that numerous mutant gametes may be descended from a single event. Gonadal mosaicism is well documented at the molecular level in osteogenesis imperfecta and in Duchenne muscular dystrophy. The molecular basis for the relatively common occurrence of gonadal mosaicism for osteogenesis imperfecta, compared to its rarity for other disorders such as achondroplasia, is unknown, but mutations arising exclusively at meiosis (e.g., unequal crossing-over) should not show gonadal mosaicism. Mutations associated with advanced paternal age are also unlikely to involve gonadal mosaicism. Somatic mutations that occur in individual cells much later do not result in mosaicism but play a major role in the development of cancers.

In the clinical context, human mutations can be thought of as falling into two general categories. One group of mutations are relatively ancient, and the same mutation is found in numerous individuals in many different populations, as in the case of sickle cell anemia, the Z allele for α1-antitrypsin deficiency, and the common mutation for cystic fibrosis. These ancient mutations tend either to be recessive, so that the mutant allele persists in the population through heterozygotes, or to be relatively benign. The presence of the same mutant allele in large numbers of individuals has implications for strategies of DNA diagnosis and screening as discussed below. It seems possible that a genetic predisposition to many common adult disorders might ultimately be shown to be associated with ancient mutations, which could be screened for in the population using molecular methods. In contrast to mutations of ancient origin, other human mutations tend to be recent or even to have occurred in the first diagnosed individual in a family. This circumstance is most common for dominant, deleterious mutations and for X-linked mutations that impair or completely prevent reproduction in males. These mutations tend to be extremely heterogeneous, with a different mutation in each family studied and with only rare recurrence of exactly identical mutations. This scenario is typical for disorders such as Duchenne muscular dystrophy, neurofibromatosis, retinoblastoma, and many other dominant disorders which affect reproductive fitness.

GENETIC DIVERSITY IN HUMANS: GARROD'S CHEMICAL INDIVIDUALITY AND THE CONCEPT OF POLYMORPHISM

Garrod recognized that the aberrant metabolism seen in a condition such as alkaptonuria might imply far more extensive chemical individuality, and he wrote[6]:

> If it be, indeed, the case that in alkaptonuria and the other conditions mentioned we are dealing with individualities of metabolism and not with the results of morbid processes the thought naturally presents itself that these are merely extreme examples of variations of chemical behavior which are probably everywhere present in minor degrees and that just as no two individuals of a species are absolutely identical in bodily structure neither are their chemical processes carried out on exactly the same lines.

Garrod further said that "diathesis is nothing else but *chemical individuality*" that he described as follows[60a]:

> . . . the factors which confer upon us our predispositions to and immunities from the various mishaps which are spoken of as diseases, are inherent in our very chemical structure; and even

in the molecular groupings which confer upon us our individualities, and which went to the making of the chromosomes from which we sprang.

It becomes increasingly apparent that individuals have both molecular and biochemical individuality. While there is often a tendency in medicine to regard patient populations as a homogeneous group of "wild-type individuals" or normal humans with "normal values" for all determinants, this is an erroneous concept. The aggregate effect of our genes determines to a large extent who dies of myocardial infarction on a high-fat diet, who develops cancer upon smoking, who only carries *Meningococcus* in the nasopharynx while another develops meningitis, who develops postoperative thromboembolism, and perhaps who is susceptible to alcoholism. These are risks that are substantially influenced by the genotype of the individual. R.J. Williams[60b] emphasized the hypothesis that "everyone is a deviate" as follows:

> The existence in every human being of a vast array of attributes which are potentially measurable (whether by present methods or not), and probably often uncorrelated mathematically, makes quite tenable the hypothesis that practically every human being is a deviate in some respects.

Garrod's concept of chemical individuality has found its explanation over the past three decades with the realization that the gene for a given protein frequently exists in different forms in different normal individuals. Subsequently it was recognized that even more extensive variation exists in the DNA sequence of genomes between individuals. The widespread nature of this genetic diversity first became apparent when it became possible to study enzymes by electrophoresis of crude cell extracts and thereby to detect structurally variant forms of enzymes without the necessity of purification. With the use of this technique, studies by Harris in humans[61] and by Lewontin and Hubby in *Drosophila*[62] demonstrated that many proteins existed in two or more forms in the population. These multiple forms are due to the existence in the population of multiple genes (called *alleles*) at the same genetic locus coding for the same protein. At each genetic locus, each individual possesses two alleles, one derived from each parent. If the two alleles are identical, the individual is said to be *homozygous*; if they differ, the individual is *heterozygous*. The various alleles have been derived from a single precursor allele by mutations that have occurred during the evolution of the species; in general, they differ from each other only in the substitution of one base for another (missense mutations). In the vast majority of cases, the proteins produced by both alleles at a given locus are equally functional, that is, the amino acid difference is "neutral" or nearly so from the standpoint of natural selection.

Based on population studies of 71 enzymes and other proteins that lend themselves to analysis by electrophoresis or other techniques, Harris found that 28 percent of genetic loci show multiple alleles in the population.[55] Moreover, the average individual is detectably heterozygous at 7 percent of his or her loci. Since most detection methods require a change in the charge of the protein, they can detect only about one-third of the actual base changes that are possible, since only one-third result in a substitution of an amino acid with a different charge. Thus, all individuals may actually be heterozygous at as many as 20 percent of their loci.

At most genetic loci (such as the locus for the β chain of hemoglobin), one standard allele accounts for the vast majority of the alleles in the population, and the alternate alleles are rare. At other genetic loci (such as the locus for the α chain of haptoglobin, a plasma protein), no single allele is sufficiently common to be designated as standard or normal. This latter situation represents an extreme example of genetic polymorphism. A polymorphic locus (or nucleotide site) is one at which the most common allele has a frequency of less than 0.99. By definition, when a polymorphism exists at a genetic locus, at least 2 percent of the population must be heterozygous at that locus.[55] Note that this definition is concerned only with the frequency of variants at a locus and not with the functional consequences of the variant.

The appreciation of polymorphism has been extended by the discovery of extraordinary variation at the DNA sequence level. Attention was focused on DNA polymorphism by the discovery of RFLPs by Kan and Dozy.[34] Extensive subsequent data suggest that approximately 1 in 100 to 1 in 200 base pairs in the human genome is polymorphic; this is consistent with heterozygosity at 1 in 250 to 1 in 500 base pairs.[63] A site is defined as polymorphic when at least 1 percent of the chromosomes have a sequence different from that of the majority. Although perhaps not an ideal usage, the term *allele* is now often extended to describe any nucleotide variation, such as DNA fragment size differences detected as RFLPs, even when not associated with an expressed gene locus. It is possible to detect single-base DNA polymorphisms that represent synonymous differences or amino acid polymorphisms in coding regions, but polymorphism at a DNA level occurs with even greater frequency outside of coding regions in parts of the genome that may have little or no effect on gene expression. The polymorphism within the genome extends beyond single-base differences to include insertions, deletions, and variations in numbers of tandemly repeated sequences. These are often referred to as variable number tandem repeats (VNTR) if the repeats are of a longer sequence or as short tandem repeats (STR) if the repeats are very short, such as di- or trinucleotide repeats.

With the recognition of the extensive amount of polymorphism in DNA (millions of nucleotide differences between two random haploid genomes), including variation in nonexpressed sequences, it becomes obvious that most DNA polymorphism is not associated with phenotypic effects. Presumably a modest fraction of genomic polymorphism is associated with effects on the phenotype that account for variations such as ethnic differences and human individuality without a significant effect on health or disease. Another portion of the polymorphism would be associated with phenotypic variation that might have relatively subtle and complex effects on susceptibility to disease. These variations would include genes affecting susceptibility to hypertension, atherosclerosis, malignancy, psychiatric illness, and infection. These genetic differences would provide the basis for polygenic and multifactorial disorders to be discussed below. Finally, a few genetic variations have such profound effects on the phenotype that they give rise to a disease condition in a relatively consistent manner (i.e., in the universal environment with minimal modifying effects from the remainder of the genome). These few genetic variations are referred to as single-gene or monogenic disorders. However, even the phenotype caused by these single gene disorders is often subject to modification by the genotype at other loci and by environmental factors. As knowledge increases, this becomes clearer, and it is exemplified by the effect of the number of α-globin loci on the phenotype when the β-globin locus is mutant in sickle cell anemia.[64,65] Other examples can be found in the disorders of apolipoproteins, where the phenotype is affected by the genotype at other loci and by environmental factors. Likewise, cancer susceptibility depends on the complex interaction of genotypic and environmental factors.

GENETIC LINKAGE AND THE HUMAN GENE MAP

The most recent update of McKusick's catalog, *Mendelian Inheritance in Man*, lists almost 6000 loci, and about 75 percent of the expressed loci are associated with a disease phenotype,[66] indicating that about 4500 single-gene-determined human diseases are known to exist. This implies that at least 4500 of the 50,000 to 100,000 human genes have undergone mutation so as to cause human disease. The chromosomal location of more than 2500 of these genes is now known.

The ability to locate genes relative to each other on the human chromosomes grew out of the pioneering studies of Morgan and his school in the first two decades of this century.[67] Using the fruit fly *Drosophila melanogaster*, Morgan demonstrated that genes are aligned in a linear manner on the chromosomes and that if two genes are close together on the same chromosomes, they do not assort independently at meiosis but are transmitted to the same gamete more than 50 percent of the time. Such genes are said to be *linked*. When two genes on a single chromosome are far apart, they are not genetically linked, even though they are physically linked by being on the same continuous chromosome. This lack of linkage is due to the phenomenon of *crossing-over*.

During the process of meiosis, when homologous chromosomes are paired, bridges frequently form between corresponding regions of the chromosome pair. These bridges, or *chiasmas*, are regions in which the two chromosomes break at identical points along their length and subsequently rejoin, the distal segments having been switched from one homologous chromosome to the other. During this process of crossing-over, no net change in the amount of genetic material occurs. However, a *recombination* of genes does occur. For example, consider a chromosome with two loci, A and B, located at opposite ends of the same chromosome. On this particular chromosome, the A locus has a rare *x* allele and the B locus has a rare *y* allele, in contrast to the common *X* and *Y* alleles at the A and B loci, respectively. Without the phenomenon of recombination, every offspring that inherited the *x* allele at the A locus would also inherit the *y* allele at the B locus. However, if recombination occurs, the A locus with the *x* allele would then be on the opposite chromosome from the B locus with the *y* allele. In that case, any offspring that inherited the *x* allele at the A locus would not inherit the *y* allele at the B locus.

Crossing-over in humans occurs with great frequency in every meiosis, and the resulting recombination of genes may occur at any point on a chromosome. The farther apart two genes are on the same chromosome, the greater is the likelihood that a crossing-over will occur in the space between them. When two genes are on the opposite ends of a long chromosome, the probability of recombination is so great that their respective alleles are transmitted to offspring almost independently of one another, just as if the two gene loci were on different chromosomes. On the other hand, gene loci that are close together on the same chromosome are said to be *linked*, so that there is a great likelihood that offspring will inherit the same combination of alleles that is present on the parental chromosome.

Assignment of a locus to a specific chromosome can be based on a variety of established methods, which have been reviewed in detail by McKusick and Ruddle.[68–70] Many genes have been mapped by linkage of traits in large families with multiple alleles at two loci (e.g., linkage of the nail-patella syndrome and the ABO blood group). Somatic cell hybrids have been used extensively to assign genes to particular chromosomes based on the concordance of the presence of the human gene product with the presence of the human chromosome (e.g., thymidine kinase segregates with chromosome 17). More recently, many genes are mapped following the isolation of cDNA or genomic DNA clones. The cloned DNA can be used with a hybrid cell panel to assess the concordance of the DNA hybridizing sequence with a particular chromosome. Alternatively, the cloned DNA can be used for synthesis of probes to be used for *in situ* hybridization with human chromosomes.[71] The opportunity for linkage studies has been greatly enhanced by the availability of numerous polymorphic DNA probes, and the genes for many common human diseases have been mapped to specific chromosomes and isolated using positional cloning strategies.

CATEGORIES OF GENETIC DISORDERS

Genetic diseases fall into one of the three categories. (1) *Chromosomal disorders* involve the lack, excess, or abnormal arrangement of one or more chromosomes, producing large amounts of excessive or deficient genetic material and affecting many genes. (2) *Mendelian or monogenic disorders* are determined primarily by a single mutant gene. Accordingly, these disorders display simple (Mendelian) inheritance patterns that can be classified into autosomal dominant, autosomal recessive, or X-linked types. (3) *Multifactorial disorders* are caused by an interaction of multiple genes and multiple exogenous or environmental factors. Although many of these multifactorial disorders, such as diabetes mellitus, gout, and cleft lip and palate, show familial clustering, the inheritance pattern is complex and the risk to relatives is much less than in the single-gene (Mendelian) disorders. Each of the above three categories of genetic disease presents different problems with respect to causation, prevention, diagnosis, genetic counseling, and treatment.

Although it is useful to consider these categories of genetic disorders, this classification necessarily represents an oversimplification. For example, small chromosomal deletions may cause the simultaneous presence of multiple Mendelian or monogenic disorders. This is exemplified by the occurrence of patients with visible deletions in the short arm of the X chromosome in association with Duchenne muscular dystrophy, chronic granulomatous disease, retinitis pigmentosa, and the McLeod phenotype.[72] These deletions may be submicroscopic and yet be large enough to cause the simultaneous presence of phenotypes such as Duchenne muscular dystrophy, ornithine transcarbamoylase deficiency, and glycerol kinase deficiency. Deletions of the retinoblastoma locus on chromosome 13 may be visible or submicroscopic and may extend to nearby loci such as esterase D (Chap. 19). Thus, these defects bridge the gap between chromosomal and monogenic disorders. The phenotype caused by chromosomal disorders obviously is due to the altered expression of single genes within the abnormal region. Chromosomal translocations may interrupt single genes, as exemplified by some females with X autosomal translocations causing Duchenne muscular dystrophy.

The phenotypes of many of the monogenic disorders discussed in this volume are modified by the genes at other loci and by environmental factors. Figure 1-9 emphasizes the effect of nongenetic factors and modifying genes on monogenic phenotypes. There are relatively few monogenic disorders where the single locus *entirely* determines the disease phenotype. Similarly, there are relatively few environmental insults where the genotype does not in some way modify the risk. For example, the genotype undoubtedly influences which infants will survive in a famine. In theory, some disorders might be polygenic, which would imply an effect of multiple genes without a major contribution by exogenous or environmental factors. In practice, most polygenic disorders are very likely to be subject to exogenous factors and therefore be of multifactorial cause. The monogenic disorders have provided an excellent starting point for attempts to understand human genetic disease. The future will increasingly involve the greater challenge of understanding the much more common multifactorial disorders.

Chromosomal Disorders

The *karyotype* of an individual (i.e., the number and structure of the chromosomes) can be ascertained from readily accessible somatic cells, such as peripheral blood lymphocytes or skin fibroblasts, by growing them in tissue culture until active proliferation occurs and then preparing single metaphase cells for examination by microscopy. By the 1970s, it became possible to identify each

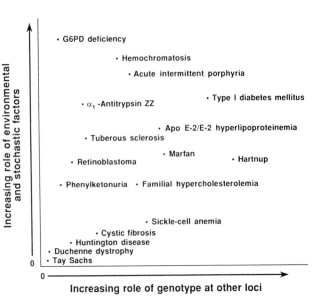

FIG. 1-9 Depiction of estimated roles of modifier genes and nongenetic factors in influencing the phenotypes for "monogenic" disorders. Extensive variation is due to allelic heterogeneity, and the intent is to indicate crude estimates of the contributions that might occur in addition to allelic variation.

individual chromosome by special staining methods using fluorescent dyes or Giemsa staining after treatment with proteolytic enzymes (trypsin). These techniques produce characteristic *banding patterns* for each chromosome (Fig. 1-10). The number of chromosomes in normal individuals is 46, of which 44 are the 22 pairs of *autosomes* and the other 2 are the *sex chromosomes*. Females have two X chromosomes (XX), and males have one X chromosome and one Y chromosome (XY). Each of the 22 pairs of autosomes and the 2 sex chromosomes can be distinguished on the basis of size, location of the centromere (which divides the chromosome into arms of equal or unequal length), and the unique banding pattern (Fig. 1-10). More details regarding cytogenetic concepts[73] and methodology[74,75] are available elsewhere, and selected chromosomal disorders are discussed in Chaps. 16 through 20.

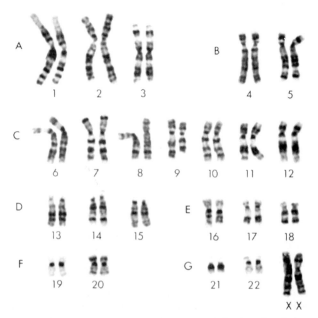

FIG. 1-10 A trypsin G-banded normal human female karyotype. (*Courtesy of David H. Ledbetter.*)

Most chromosomal disorders found in humans can be classified into one of four groups: (1) excess or loss or one or more chromosomes *(aneuploidy)*; (2) breakage and loss of a piece of a chromosome *(deletion)*; (3) breakage of two chromosomes, with transfer and fusion of parts of the broken fragments onto each other *(translocation)*; and (4) abnormal splitting of the centromere during mitosis so that one arm is lost and the other is duplicated to form one symmetric chromosome with two genetically identical arms *(isochromosome formation)*. In addition, chromosomal *mosaicism* may occur, such that a single individual may possess two cell lines, or *clones*, each differing in its chromosomal constitution. For example, many patients with the Turner syndrome have been shown to possess some cells with a 45,X constitution and other cells with a normal 46,XX. Their karyotype is symbolized 45,X/46,XX.

Chromosomal aberrations occur with extremely high frequency in various malignancies. In these instances, the constitutional karyotype is usually normal, but the tumor cells show abnormal findings. Numerous chromosomal translocations are now known to be found with some specificity for a variety of tumors.[75,77–79] In some instances, a constitutional genetic abnormality may represent a first step in a two-step process leading to malignancy. The second step in this process occurs in a single somatic cell and may often be a gross chromosomal aberration that contributes to the development of a tumor. This is best documented for retinoblastoma (Chap. 19) but also occurs in Wilms tumor (Chap 21), polyposis of the colon (Chap. 31), von Hippel-Lindau disease,[80] and other disorders. The locus involved in hereditary tumors is often also involved in sporadic tumors, as documented for colon tumors, retinoblastoma, renal cell carcinoma, and other tumors.

Monogenic Disorders

Having already acknowledged that very few phenotypes are entirely determined by a single locus, it is still very useful to discuss so-called monogenic disorders. Disorders caused by single mutant genes ordinarily show one of three simple (or Mendelian) patterns of inheritance: (1) autosomal dominant, (2) autosomal recessive, and (3) X-linked. With few exceptions, each of the approximately 4500 known Mendelian diseases is rare. As a group, these disorders constitute an important cause of morbidity and death, accounting directly for more than 5 percent of all pediatric hospital admissions.[76] The overall population frequency of monogenic disorders is about 10 per 1000 live births, with dominant conditions accounting for about 7 in 1000, recessive conditions for about 2.5 in 1000, and X-linked conditions for about 0.4 in 1000.[76]

If a particular disease shows one of the three Mendelian patterns of inheritance, its pathogenesis, no matter how complex, must be due to an abnormality at a single site in the genome and usually involves a single protein molecule. For example, in sickle cell anemia, the entire clinical syndrome, including such seemingly unrelated disturbances as anemia, pain crises, nephropathy, and predisposition to pneumococcal infections, is the physiologic consequence of having a single base change at a specific site in the gene that codes for the β-chain of hemoglobin, causing the substitution of a valine for a glutamic acid in the sixth amino acid position in the protein sequence.

In many Mendelian disorders, the protein altered by the mutation is not yet known. In such cases only the distal physiological effects of the mutation are recognizable. Nevertheless, it is safe to assume that a single primary defect exists whenever a disease is transmitted by a single-gene mechanism and that the various manifestations of the disease can all be related to the mutational event by a more or less complicated "pedigree of causes." In recent years, positional cloning techniques and other molecular methods have led to the cloning of many disease genes, in all cases confirming the monogenic interpretation.

The basic biochemical lesions in monogenic disorders involve defects in a wide variety of proteins, including enzymes, receptors, transport proteins, peptide hormones, immunoglobulins, collagens, transcription factors, and coagulation factors. There are now hundreds of human diseases whose biochemical defects have been defined. Many of the biochemical defects identified in earlier years involved enzymes, but proteins of all types are now included, owing largely to the impact of recombinant DNA methods. Most of these disorders are discussed in detail in this book and are tabulated at the end of this chapter. Although genetic defects can involve genes that do not encode a protein (e.g., defects in genes for transfer RNA), these are rare.

Significance of "Dominant" or "Recessive." Unless otherwise specified, the terms *dominant* and *recessive* refer to the clinical phenotype associated with a particular allele. The distinction between dominant and recessive medical disorders is extremely useful for clinical diagnosis, for linkage analysis, and for genetic counseling. However, there are a number of subtleties and complexities involving the use of these terms. The situation is relatively simple in cases where heterozygous individuals are indistinguishable from one or the other type of homozygote. In this case, the dominant trait (disease) or allele (mutation) is the one that prevails in the heterozygote. In true recessive disorders, the phenotype in heterozygotes is indistinguishable from normal. In true dominant disorders, heterozygous individuals have a disease phenotype indistinguishable from that of homozygous-affected individuals. Although many recessive medical disorders appear on the surface to qualify as true recessives, heterozygotes for at least some of these conditions may have subtle differences in phenotype which may be accentuated by environmental factors. These subtle phenotypic consequences may be advantageous or disadvantageous. Despite their overall clinical "normality," individuals who are heterozygous for recessive loss-of-function alleles often have demonstrable metabolic differences and always have differences at the protein level. Many of these complexities are exemplified by sickle cell anemia, which is usually considered to be a recessive disorder for clinical purposes in that heterozygotes are nearly entirely normal, healthy individuals. Despite the general lack of phenotypic effect in heterozygotes, a selective advantage for resistance to malaria is well documented in heterozygotes. Heterozygotes are also known to have subtle physiological abnormalities affecting renal concentrating ability and cardiopulmonary physiology at high altitude. These subtle phenotypic effects in heterozygotes for recessive disorders may be more common than is generally recognized and may contribute to phenotypes more often considered to be of multifactorial etiology. For example, it has been suggested that heterozygotes for ataxia telangiectasia and other DNA-repair disorders are at increased risk of malignancy.[81] Heterozygosity for homocystinuria is implicated as a risk factor in vascular disease,[82] and debate continues as to whether heterozygosity for α1-antitrypsin deficiency predisposes to pulmonary disease.[83] Heterozygosity for known recessive disorders contributes to the biochemical and medical individuality of humans.

The situation is different for dominant phenotypes. Very few conditions qualify as true dominants, although there is evidence that Huntingdon chorea is one. Homozygotes for dominant disorders are identified relatively rarely, but, when they are recognized, their disease often is much more severe than for heterozygotes, indicating that most such disorders involve semidominant (incompletely or partially dominant) traits and alleles. This is well documented for many disorders (e.g., familial hypercholesterolemia, achondroplasia, and some forms of porphyria). Some traits are referred to as codominant, and this term is perhaps most appropriate for a circumstance such as AB blood group where various alleles may be demonstrated biochemically with negligible phenotypic effect.

Additional complexities arise from the fact that the phenotypic consequences of being heterozygous may be inconsistent, resulting in uncertainty as to whether a disorder is better considered as a dominant or recessive trait. There may be circumstances where heterozygotes display symptoms in only a very small fraction of cases or where heterozygotes have extremely subtle and mild symptoms which might not typically qualify as a disease diagnosis. Homozygotes for these traits typically would have more obvious disease symptoms, and there could be uncertainty regarding whether to classify such disorders as dominant or recessive. From a clinical and counseling vantage point, most medical disorders fall clearly into the dominant or recessive category, but this classification is an arbitrary division of a continuum rather than a true biologic demarcation.

Mutant alleles may involve either a total or a partial loss of function, often referred to as null and hypomorphic alleles, respectively. Mutant alleles may retain a substantially altered function or gain a totally novel function. In general, most loss-of-function alleles are recessive, particularly those involving a protein with a catalytic function. This generalization is confirmed by the fact that most enzyme deficiencies in humans and most null mutations produced in mice by gene targeting show no obvious phenotype in heterozygotes. However, a significant fraction of null alleles can have phenotypic effects and cause human disease, typically because half of the normal level of the protein in question is insufficient for normal physiology. Tumor suppressor genes provide a notable exception to this premise; null alleles often predispose to cancer in a dominant manner due to somatic inactivation of the remaining normal allele. Whether a mutation generates a dominant or recessive disorder is determined by two factors: (1) the effect of the mutation on the function of the gene product and (2) the tolerance of the biological system for a functional perturbation of that particular gene product.

The term *dominant negative* has become popular for describing alleles that code for a mutant protein that interferes in one way or another with the function of a normal protein being produced from the other chromosome in a heterozygous situation. Dominant negative alleles are particularly likely to occur when proteins are involved in subunit structures or when proteins are involved in complex interactions with other proteins or nucleic acids. Numerous examples of complex mechanisms that can underlie dominant negative alleles are described elsewhere.[84] In general, the term *dominant negative* is appropriate when a mutant allele causes a more severe phenotype than that caused by a null allele. This results from an adverse effect of the product of the abnormal allele on the function of the product from the normal allele. Again, excellent examples are found in the case of collagen and osteogenesis imperfecta, where many missense mutations interfere with fiber assembly and cause lethal osteogenesis imperfecta in heterozygotes, while null alleles cause a much milder form of the disease. Most dominant negative mutations might be considered as altered function alleles or as a particular subset of gain-of-function alleles. In other instances, gain-of-function alleles might acquire totally new properties that have little or nothing to do with the normal function of the protein. Amyloidosis may represent a reasonably good example of such an instance, where the abnormal folding properties of the mutant protein lead to a harmful, extracellular deposition of material which appears to be unrelated to the normal function of the protein. The expanded polyglutamine tracts in the mutant alleles for Huntington disease, spinocerebellar ataxia, and spinobulbar muscular atrophy may represent clear gain-of-function alleles, but the pathogenesis is not yet understood.

Exceptions to the Rules (Unstable Mutations, Uniparental Disomy, and Imprinted Genes. Traditional thinking regarding single-gene disorders involves numerous assumptions that are generally correct. These include the tenets that mutations are stable, that an offspring inherits one allele from each parent for an autosomal locus, that both alleles at an autosomal locus are equally expressed, and that an individual who is heterozygous at a locus is equally likely to transmit either allele to offspring. Ordinary approaches to genetic counseling, linkage analysis, and interpretation of genetic data assume the above to be true. Evidence of relatively rare, but biologically fascinating, examples of exceptions to these rules now abound.

The clearest examples of unstable mutations involve the expanding triplet repeats causing fragile X syndrome, myotonic dystrophy, Huntington disease, spinobulbar muscular atrophy, and spinocerebellar ataxia type 1. Previously the significance of anticipation (defined as the worsening of a disease phenotype over generations within a family) was unclear, with most workers considering the phenomenon to be entirely an artifact involving ascertainment bias.[85] While the concept of a premutation was clear, molecular documentation for such was unavailable. Expanding triple mutations have demonstrated that premutations can exist in the population as modest expansions of triple repeats (perhaps including minor sequence variations). These premutations do not themselves cause a phenotypic effect but are prone to further expansion, which can cause disease. The phenomenon of anticipation can now be clearly demonstrated to have a molecular basis, with an increasing number of repeats correlated with earlier onset of disease and/or a more severe phenotype. It seems likely that other examples of premutation and anticipation will be defined, involving similar and different molecular underpinnings, and thinking regarding Mendelian disorders must take this into account.

The recognition that individuals can inherit two copies of part or all of a chromosome from one parent and no copy from the other parent represents a dramatic departure from Mendelian inheritance.[86] While this phenomenon of *uniparental disomy* is relatively rare, it can contribute to the occurrence of well-known clinical disorders (e.g., Prader-Willi and Angelman syndromes). The significance of uniparental disomy is in large part related to the phenomenon of imprinting whereby the maternal copy of a gene and the paternal copy of a gene may be differentially expressed. The biological and medical significance of imprinting is discussed in greater detail in Chap. 4 and elsewhere.[87,88]

There are some semantic questions and related conceptual issues regarding imprinting. This is because the phenomenon is not completely understood genetically or biochemically. The term *imprinting* implies some reversible modification of the genome causing differential expression of alleles at a locus. Imprinting may be suspected if the phenotype of the offspring is affected by the sex of the parent transmitting a particular allele. However, it may be better to consider such phenotypic observations as "parent-of-origin effects" that may be due to sex-specific mutational effects, imprinting, or other less well characterized mechanisms. Although there are differences in usage of terminology, imprinting at a molecular level might be defined as differences in phenotype or expression which occur when the identical primary nucleotide sequence is maternally or paternally derived. Consideration of the earlier onset of Huntington disease in offspring of affected males is instructive, although complete data are not available. If one assumes that the phenotype is entirely dependent on the genotype at the time of fertilization without regard to whether the mutant allele was paternally or maternally derived, there would be a parent-of-origin effect owing to a greater propensity for expansion in male gametes in Huntington disease, but molecular imprinting would not be present. This would be the case if differences related to maternal versus paternal transmission depended entirely on the expansion of triplet repeat mutations prior to fertilization. In contrast, if a specific allele length behaved differently after fertilization—perhaps involving a difference in its propensity for further somatic variation depending on whether it was maternally or paternally derived—there would be an imprinting effect. The data regarding whether triplet repeat mutations expand before or after fertilization are still being gathered,[89] and it is possible that imprinting and sex-specific mutation effects are interrelated. The situation regarding imprinting may be simpler in the case of paragangliomas, Angelman syndrome, Prader-Willi syndrome, and dwarfism caused by IGF2 deficiency in the mouse, since the mutations involved are presumed to be stable.

Another issue is the tendency to state that a gene is maternally or paternally imprinted when what is meant is that the gene is maternally or paternally repressed or silenced. It appears preferable to consider that a locus is imprinted if there is differential expression of the maternal and paternal alleles. In most of the known cases, this involves either paternal expression with maternal repression or maternal expression with paternal repression. However, many additional situations can be envisioned involving high expression and low expression, use of alternative promoters for paternal or maternal alleles, and other variations. Thus, it seems preferable to avoid the terms *maternally* or *paternally imprinted* to mean maternally or paternally repressed, although this usage is not rare. It would be more appropriate to state that the SNRPN and IGF2 loci are paternally expressed or maternally repressed (or silenced) and that the H19 and Angelman loci are paternally repressed (or silenced) or maternally expressed.

Autosomal Dominant Disorders. Dominant diseases are manifest in the heterozygous state, that is, when only one abnormal gene *(mutant allele)* is present and the corresponding allele on the homologous chromosome is normal. By definition, the gene responsible for an autosomal dominant disorder must be located on one of the 22 autosomes; hence, both males and females can be affected. Since alleles segregate independently at meiosis, there is a 1 in 2 chance that the offspring of an affected heterozygote will inherit the mutant allele.

Figure 1-11 shows typical pedigrees for autosomal dominant traits. The following features are characteristic: (1) Each affected individual has an affected parent (unless the condition arose by a new mutation in the sperm or ovum that formed the individual or unless the mutant allele is present but without phenotypic effect in the affected parent, as discussed in the section "Penetrance and Expressivity" below). (2) An affected individual will have a 50 percent probability for each offspring of affected or unaffected status. (3) Normal children of an affected individual will have only normal offspring. (4) Males and females are affected in equal proportions. (5) Either sex is equally likely to transmit the condition to male and female offspring, with male-to-male transmission occurring. (6) Vertical transmission of the condition through successive generation occurs, especially when the trait does not impair the reproductive capacity. Dominant disorders can be inherited in a sex-limited or sex-modified pattern, as exemplified by autosomal dominant breast/ovarian cancer restricted to females[90] and by familial male precocious puberty restricted to males.[91]

New Mutations. While there is a 50 percent risk that each offspring of an individual with an autosomal dominant condition will inherit the disease, it is not necessarily true that each affected person must have an affected parent. In every autosomal dominant disease, a certain proportion of affected persons owe their disorder to a new mutation rather than an inherited one. Since a rough estimate of the frequency of mutation is 5×10^{-6} mutations per gene per generation, one would expect that about 1 in 100,000 newborn persons would have a new mutation at any given genetic locus.

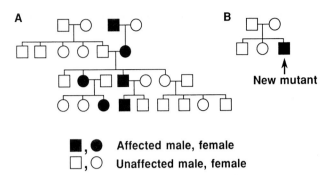

FIG. 1-11 Pedigree pattern for an autosomal dominant trait. Note the *vertical* pattern of inheritance; compare new-mutation and inherited pedigrees.

Many of these mutations either will not impair the function of the gene product or will involve a recessive function, so that the mutation will be clinically silent. Others, however, will cause a defective gene product that gives rise to a dominant trait, since a dominant trait, by definition, requires a mutation in only one of a pair of alleles. The parent in whose germ cells the mutation arose will be clinically normal. The sibs of the affected individual usually will be normal since the mutation will have affected one or only a few of the germ cells. Given the nature of germ cell proliferation, it is most probable that a mutation will occur at one of the later cell divisions since they are more numerous, but various numbers of gametes may be descended from a single mutational event. Since these mutant gametes still are likely to represent a small minority of gametes, and since humans have few offspring, the probability of a recurrence of the disorder among the siblings of a new-mutation individual is quite low. The presence of the identical mutation in siblings when neither parent has the mutation in somatic cells can occur through gonadal mosaicism. It is possible to assess the proportion of gonadal mosaicism by molecular analysis of sperm in some cases. Individuals affected with new mutations are able to transmit the disease, and their offspring are at 50 percent risk for the condition.

The proportion of patients with dominant disorders that represent new mutations is inversely proportional to the effect of the disease on biologic fitness. The term *biologic fitness* refers to the ability of an affected individual to produce children who survive to adulthood and reproduce. In the extreme case, if a dominant mutation produces absolute infertility, then all observed cases will, of necessity, represent new mutations, and it will be impossible to prove the genetic transmission of the trait. Thanatophoric dysplasia likely represents such an example, and molecular analysis could document such mutations. In moderately severe disorders, as in tuberous sclerosis, the severe mental retardation reduces biologic fitness to about 20 percent of normal, and the proportion of cases owing to new mutations is about 80 percent.[92] In dominant disorders such as familial hypercholesterolemia, in which there is negligible if any reduction in biologic fitness, almost all affected persons have a family pedigree showing classic vertical transmission. The incidence of a dominant disorder depends on the biologic fitness and on the mutation frequency for the locus, which is widely variable. Although the proportion of cases owing to new mutation is directly related to biologic fitness, genetic counseling and reproductive planning now can alter this proportion.

Many new mutations appear to occur in the germ cells of fathers who are relatively old.[73,93] Such a "paternal age effect" is seen, for example, in the Marfan syndrome, in which the average age of fathers of sporadic or "new mutation" cases (37 years) is higher than the mean age of fathers generally (30 years) and also higher than the age of fathers who transmit the Marfan disease owing to an inherited mutation (30 years).[94] The increased mutation rate associated with advanced paternal age may be caused by the large number of gene replications required for sperm production over many years. Differences in mutation rates for male and female gametes are discussed further in the section "X-Linked Disorders" below.

Before one concludes that a dominant disorder in a given patient with unaffected parents is the result of a new mutation, it is important to consider two other possibilities: (1) The gene may be carried by a parent in whom the mutant allele is not penetrant (discussed below). (2) Nonpaternity may have occurred (i.e., the father is someone other than the putative father); this is found in about 3 to 5 percent of randomly studied children in many cultures.

Penetrance and Expressivity. These terms are frequently the subject of confusion and slight variations in usage. In the autosomal dominant medical context, penetrance is the proportion of heterozygotes for a given mutation that present with *any* of the phenotypic features of the disorder induced by the mutation under a defined set of circumstances. Although penetrance at a given age can be discussed, as in the case of Huntington disease, variation in age of onset is most often considered an aspect of variable expression. In some cases, penetrance will depend on environmental exposure, as in glucose 6-phosphate dehydrogenase deficiency. In the medical context, the concept of penetrance can be usefully distinguished in a clinical and a molecular way. Penetrance is the question at issue when the apparently unaffected offspring of an affected individual wishes to know the probability that they nevertheless carry the mutant gene and could produce affected offspring. The mutant gene is not penetrant if an individual carrying it shows absolutely no phenotypic effects. The presence or absence of the mutant gene can be determined in molecular terms, and a person lacking it can be distinguished from one carrying it but showing no penetrance. In this medical and genetic counseling context, the ability to determine penetrance depends on diagnostic methods. For example, a new magnetic resonance imaging technique might demonstrate findings not previously recognizable. In the biologic context, the gene can be considered penetrant if it affects the function of the individual.

Expressivity or *variability in clinical expression* refers to the range of phenotypic effects in individuals with a mutant genotype. This variability can include the type and severity of symptoms as well as variation in the age of onset of symptoms. Variability in clinical expression is illustrated dramatically by the multiple endocrine adenoma-peptic ulcer syndrome.[95] Patients in the same family inheriting the same abnormal gene may have hyperplasia or neoplasia of one or all of a wide variety of endocrine tissues, such as the pancreas, parathyroid glands, pituitary gland, and adipose tissue. The resulting clinical manifestations are extremely diverse; different members of the same family may develop peptic ulcers, hypoglycemia, kidney stones, multiple lipomas of the skin, or bitemporal hemianopsia. This variability can make it hard to recognize that each family member suffers from the same genetic abnormality. In the case of many of the dominant disorders characterized by tumor formation, chance second mutations in tumor suppressor genes may explain some of the clinical variability (Part 3).

Variation in age of onset is seen in disorders such as Huntington chorea and adult polycystic kidney disease. These disorders often do not become manifest clinically until adult life, even though the mutant gene is present from the time of conception. Regarding variation in age of onset as one form of variation in expression is somewhat arbitrary. In one sense, it cannot be said finally that the mutant gene was never penetrant in individuals until they have had a maximal clinical evaluation and until they have completed their life and died from other causes. Lack of penetrance can be considered the absolute mildest end of the spectrum of expression, such

that no phenotypic effects whatsoever are observed. In the clinical context, variation in expression can be distinguished from penetrance as the question at issue when an affected individual wishes to know whether their offspring will have mild or severe symptoms if born affected. In molecular terms, analysis of the single gene locus usually will not answer this question (i.e., predict variation in expression within a family), but it can determine whether the mutant gene is present and not penetrant. Thus, molecular and biochemical analysis of the monogenic locus can uncover lack of penetrance, but cannot predict variability in expression within a family (unstable triplet repeat mutations are an exception).

The factors underlying lack of penetrance and variability in expression are similar and fall into three main categories: (1) the genotype at other loci or other variations at the same locus; (2) exogenous or environmental factors; and (3) stochastic factors. Genetic modifier effects are undoubtedly common, but few are delineated at a molecular level. Effects within the same locus can be seen with mutations in α-spectrin, where a polymorphism causing low expression can moderate the phenotype of hereditary elliptocytosis when in *cis* with a mutation but will worsen the phenotype when found in *trans* in a heterozygote for a pathologic mutation. In the case of cystic fibrosis, the phenotypic severity of the R117H mutation varies through a *cis* effect on the level of functional mRNA mediated by a splice junction polymorphism that influences skipping of an exon.[96] The genotype at the α-globin locus affecting the sickle cell anemia phenotype[64,65] and the genotype at various loci affecting the monogenic hyperlipidemias are examples of effects by modifier genes. The phenotypes in monogenic hyperlipidemias, the porphyrias, and hemochromatosis are affected by diet, alcohol use, smoking, and exercise; these are examples of the impact of environmental and exogenous factors. Stochastic factors are important in at least some instances, as exemplified by the severity and distribution of lesions among identical twins with disorders such as retinoblastoma, neurofibromatosis, and tuberous sclerosis. Differences in phenotypic expression owing to variable X inactivation among identical twin females heterozygous for an X-linked disorder represent another example of a stochastic effect. Although the issues of penetrance and expressivity are most easily discussed in the context of autosomal dominant disorders, these principles are also relevant to chromosomal disorders, autosomal recessive disorders, X-linked disorders, and multifactorial disorders.

Biochemical Bases of Dominant Traits. Historically, the biochemical bases for recessive disorders were frequently identified as enzyme deficiencies, while the biochemical defects for dominant disorders remained enigmatic. This has since changed as the biochemical and/or molecular defects for disorders such as familial hypercholesterolemia, amyloidosis, hereditary spherocytosis, osteogenesis imperfecta, hereditary retinoblastoma, neurofibromatosis, Marfan syndrome, and Huntington disease are being determined. A number of mechanisms can account for an abnormal phenotype in the presence of one normal gene and one mutant gene. One mechanism is simply that a half normal level of gene product is insufficient to maintain a normal phenotype, as discussed above. This is likely to be true when the gene product regulates a complex metabolic pathway, as with membrane receptors and rate-limiting enzymes in biosynthetic pathways under feedback control (e.g., familial hypercholesterolemia and dominant porphyrias). In some cases, a dosage effect owing to gene duplication can cause a dominant phenotype, as in the case of the common mutation in type IA Charcot-Marie-Tooth disease. Another mechanism involves abnormalities of structural proteins that are involved in a complex network of direct protein interactions. Dominant negative mutations are instances where the molecules of mutant gene product interfere with the functioning of the molecules of normal gene product.[84] Many of the instances involving structural proteins have a dominant negative component, and in these cases missense mutations may be more deleterious than null mutations, as in osteogenesis imperfecta. Another mechanism for dominant phenotypic effects is when heterozygous defects become homozygous at a single-cell level owing to second somatic mutations (e.g., tumor suppressor genes). These defects may be considered dominant at the pedigree level and recessive at the single-cell level. Another mechanism is the occurrence of a null or other mutation in the only active copy of an imprinted gene, as for Angelman syndrome. Conceptually, it is useful to distinguish dominant mutations that generate a product having a new biologic property that creates a harmful effect from those that merely represent a deficiency of the normal gene product. In the former group, restoration of a normal level of the gene product would not negate the effect of the mutant gene.

Disorders Involving Imprinted Genes. If an autosomal locus is imprinted such that it is expressed from one allele and repressed from the other, there is no question of a dominant or recessive effect, since the gene is functionally hemizygous. These disorders may be thought of by clinicians as more similar to dominant pedigrees, since disease may occur over multiple generations. The best-documented instances of familial disorders involving imprinted genes are hereditary paragangliomas[97] and Angelman syndrome.[98,99] For hereditary paragangliomas, the phenotype is expressed only when the mutant allele is inherited from the father. In contrast, the Angelman phenotype is expressed only when the mutant allele is inherited from the mother.

An inherited dwarfism is known in mice that is based on loss-of-function mutations in the Igf2 gene, which is paternally expressed and maternally repressed in the mouse. Imprinting can also affect the phenotype in sporadic or new mutation cases of disease, as is now well documented for Prader-Willi syndrome, Angelman syndrome, and Beckwith-Weidmann syndrome (see Chap. 4).

Autosomal Recessive Disorders. Autosomal recessive conditions are those that are clinically apparent only in the homozygous or compound heterozygous state, that is, when both alleles at a particular genetic locus are mutant alleles. By definition, the gene responsible for an autosomal recessive disorder must be located on one of the 22 autosomes; thus, both males and females can be affected.

Figure 1-12 shows two pedigrees for families with an autosomal recessive trait. Monoplex families (pedigree A) are the most common, but families with multiple affected individuals occur, and the following features are characteristic: (1) The parents are clinically normal. (2) Only sibs are affected, and vertical transmission does not occur. (3) Males and females are affected in equal proportions.

Characteristics of Autosomal Recessive Traits. The relative rarity of recessive genes in the population and the fact that two abnormal genes must be present for clinical expression combine to create special conditions for autosomal recessive inheritance: (1) The more infrequent the mutant gene in the population, the stronger the likelihood that affected individuals are the product of consanguineous matings (see below). (2) If both parents are carriers for the same autosomal recessive gene, the probability for an offspring with disease is 0.25, for a heterozygote (carrier) offspring is 0.50, and for a noncarrier normal offspring is 0.25. (3) If an affected individual mates with a heterozygote (as may occur with a common mutant gene or a consanguineous marriage), there is a 50 percent probability of disease for each child, and a pedigree simulating dominant inheritance may result. (4) If two individuals with the same recessive disease mate, all their children will be affected.

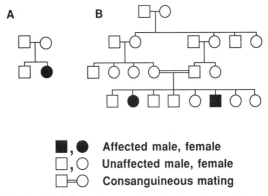

**,● Affected male, female
□,○ Unaffected male, female
□–○ Consanguineous mating

FIG. 1-12 Pedigree pattern for an autosomal recessive trait. Note the *horizontal* pattern of inheritance and consanguinity in the multiplex pedigree *(B)* in comparison to the more common monoplex pedigree *(A)*.

The clinical picture in autosomal recessive disorders tends to be more uniform than for dominant diseases, and onset often occurs early in life. As a general rule, recessive disorders are usually diagnosed in children, while dominant diseases have a trimodal age of symptomatology and are more often encountered in adults.[66]

In recessive inheritance, the probability is that only one in four children in a sibship will be affected; hence, multiple cases may not occur in a family. This is especially true in societies in which families tend to be small. Consider, for example, 16 families in which both parents are heterozygous for the same recessive disorder, such as cystic fibrosis. If each family has 2 children, the probability is that 9 of the 16 families will have no affected children, 6 will have 1 affected and 1 normal child, and only 1 of the 16 families will have 2 affected children. Because of the tendency toward small families in many contemporary societies, physicians usually see sporadic or isolated cases of a recessive disease without an affected sib to alert them to the possibility of a genetic disorder. Fortunately because of the relatively uniform clinical picture of recessive disorders and because many can be diagnosed directly by biochemical or molecular tests, the diagnosis of a genetic disease can usually be made even when no other members of a family are clinically affected. Autosomal recessive disorders can be inherited in a sex-limited manner, as exemplified by testosterone 5α-reductase deficiency, where only chromosomal males are phenotypically abnormal.

Biochemical Defects. The basic biochemical lesions underlying many autosomal recessive disorders have been identified. Mutations that give rise to recessive diseases often involve enzymatic as opposed to nonenzymatic proteins. In these conditions, recessive inheritance occurs because a mutation that destroys the catalytic activity of an enzyme generally does not impair the health of a heterozygote (i.e., an individual who has one mutant allele specifying a functionless enzyme and one normal allele on the partner chromosome specifying a normal enzyme). In this situation, each cell in the body usually produces about 50 percent of the normal number of active enzyme molecules. However, normal regulatory mechanisms function to avert any clinical consequences of this 50 percent deficiency, so that heterozygotes for enzyme defects usually are clinically normal, as discussed above. Frequently such compensation involves nothing more complicated than a simple two- to threefold increase in the substrate concentrations for the enzyme. The concentration of a substrate is usually maintained at a point below saturation for the enzyme that metabolizes it. When the enzyme level is reduced 50 percent, as in a heterozygote for a functionless gene at that locus, the residual 50 percent of enzyme molecules can be made to function twice as fast as normal, simply by allowing the substrate concentration to increase twofold. If the twofold increase in substrate does not otherwise affect metabolism adversely, the heterozygote is clinically normal. On the other hand, when an individual inherits functionless alleles at both loci specifying an enzyme, the reduction in enzyme activity is too great for a compensatory mechanism to overcome the deficiency, and a disease results.

The genetic enzyme deficiencies that produce recessive diseases tend to involve enzymes that participate in catabolic pathways. Frequently these enzymes degrade organic molecules that are ingested in the diet, such as galactose (galactosemia), phenylalanine (phenylketonuria), and phytanic acid (Refsum syndrome). A special class of such catabolic diseases is one in which the deficiency affects an acid hydrolase that occurs within lysosomes. In these *lysosomal storage disorders*,[100] the substrate, usually a complex lipid or polysaccharide, accumulates in swollen lysosomes in specific organs, giving the cells a foamy appearance. Examples of such lysosomal diseases include the mucopolysaccharidoses such as Hurler syndrome (α-iduronidase deficiency) and the sphingolipidoses such as Gaucher disease (glucocerebrosidase deficiency).

Population Genetics. In general, recessive diseases are rare because the reduced biologic fitness of homozygotes acts to remove the mutant gene from the population. A few lethal recessive disorders, such as cystic fibrosis, thalassemia, and sickle-cell anemia, are common. To explain this paradox, it has been postulated that the biologic fitness of heterozygotes is greater than that of noncarriers for these genes. In such a case, the frequency of the gene in the population depends on the balance between the increased fitness of the relatively numerous heterozygotes and the reduced fitness of the less common homozygotes. A small selective advantage of the heterozygote over the normal person results in a high gene frequency and hence a high birth frequency of homozygotes even when the disease is lethal.[101] Thus, about 1 in 20 to 25 Caucasians is heterozygous (a carrier) for the genetically lethal disease cystic fibrosis, and the disease occurs in about 1 in 2500 Caucasian births. In order to maintain such a high gene frequency, heterozygotes for cystic fibrosis may have a selective advantage over noncarriers, but the nature of such a potential advantage is unknown. A selective advantage for the mutant gene might involve the viability of heterozygotes or a reproductive advantage. There could be a slight transmission ratio distortion (meiotic drive), i.e., gametes carrying the mutant gene could have a slightly greater probability of achieving fertilization compared to gametes with the normal gene.[102] It has been argued that disorders might achieve a frequency as high as that seen with cystic fibrosis occasionally without a selective advantage, that is, by chance. There is evidence from haplotype data that individuals carrying the common ΔF508 allele are descended from a single mutational event,[103] but this does not resolve why the mutant gene is so frequent. In sickle cell anemia, another recessive disorder with a high frequency among certain populations, heterozygotes are known to have increased resistance to falciparum malaria.

Consanguinity. By definition, a recessive disease requires the inheritance of a mutant allele at the same genetic locus from each parent. When the genes are rare, the likelihood of any two parents being carriers for the same defect is small. If the parents have a common ancestor who carried a recessive gene, then the likelihood that two of the descendants would each have inherited the gene becomes relatively great. The less frequent the recessive gene, the stronger becomes the likelihood that an affected individual may have resulted from such a consanguineous mating. On the other hand, certain recessive genes are so common in the population that the likelihood of two random parents being carriers is great enough to minimize the role of consanguinity. For common traits such as

sickle cell anemia, phenylketonuria, cystic fibrosis, and Tay-Sachs disease, all of which have a high carrier frequency in certain populations, consanguinity is usually not present in the parents.

New Mutation. Although new mutations for recessive disorders occur, they rarely can be identified in a clinical setting. This is because a new mutation usually will only generate an asymptomatic heterozygote. Only generations later will the descendants of individuals with that mutation be involved in a mating where both parents are heterozygotes. In addition, the selective pressure to eliminate deleterious recessive traits from the population is less because these traits are easily passed on in heterozygous form. A large portion of recessive disease may be due to mutations that occurred many, many generations ago, as has become clear from haplotype analysis of mutations causing phenylketonuria, β-thalassemia, sickle cell anemia, Tay-Sachs disease, cystic fibrosis, and other disorders.

X-Linked Disorders. The genes responsible for X-linked disorders are located on the X chromosome; therefore, the clinical risk and severity of the disease are different for the two sexes. Since a female has two X chromosomes, she may be either heterozygous or homozygous for a mutant gene, and the trait may therefore demonstrate either recessive or dominant expression. Expression in females is often variable and heavily influenced by random X inactivation. Males, on the other hand, have only one X chromosome, so they can be expected to display the full syndrome whenever they inherit the gene, regardless of whether the gene produces a recessive or dominant trait in the female. Thus, the terms *X-linked dominant* or *X-linked recessive* refer only to the expression of the gene in women.

An important feature of all X-linked inheritance is the absence of male-to-male (i.e., father-to-son) transmission of the trait. This follows because a male must always contribute this Y chromosome to his sons; hence, he can never contribute his X chromosome. On the other hand, a male contributes his sole X chromosome to all his daughters, and so all daughters of a male with an X-linked trait must inherit the mutant gene.

GENETIC HETEROGENEITY

Genetic heterogeneity may result from the existence of a series of different mutations at a single locus (*allelic heterogeneity*) or from mutations at different genetic loci (*nonallelic or locus heterogeneity*). For example, phenotypes such as Charcot-Marie-Tooth neurogenic atrophy, congenital sensorineural deafness, and retinitis pigmentosa all have autosomal dominant, autosomal recessive, and X-linked forms. This will involve nonallelic heterogeneity in many cases, but allelic variation also can account for dominant and recessive variation at a single locus. A clinically similar bleeding disorder can be caused by mutations at either of two loci on the X chromosome, one leading to a deficiency of factor VIII (classic hemophilia, hemophilia A) and the other causing a deficiency of factor IX (Christmas disease, hemophilia B). That both allelic and nonallelic heterogeneity may underlie a clinical phenotype is exemplified by the syndrome of hereditary methemoglobinemia, which was once regarded as a homogeneous clinical entity. The disorder is the result of at least 10 different mutations occurring at three distinct gene loci: two at the locus coding for the α-chain of hemoglobin, three at the locus coding for the β-chain of hemoglobin, and at least five at the NADH dehydrogenase locus. It is increasingly obvious that most, if not all, hereditary diseases, when carefully analyzed, are genetically heterogeneous.

MULTIFACTORIAL GENETIC DISEASES

The common chronic diseases of adults (such as essential hypertension, gout, coronary heart disease, diabetes mellitus, peptic ulcer disease, and schizophrenia), as well as the common birth defects (such as cleft lip and palate, spina bifida, and congenital heart disease), have long been known to "run in families." These disorders are described as *multifactorial genetic diseases*. It is useful to emphasize the existence of etiologic heterogeneity in these disorders. For cleft lip and palate, some cases are due to single-gene defects, some to chromosome abnormalities, and most, apparently, to multiple genetic and environmental factors. Multifactorial etiology implies that multiple factors enter into the causation of most *individual cases*. Similarly, the etiology of coronary artery disease can be considered to be heterogeneous, with a small proportion due primarily to single-gene defects (e.g., familial hypercholesterolemia) while most are multifactorial (i.e., multiple factors contribute to the etiology of individual cases). Multifactorial etiology implies the interaction of multiple genes with multiple environmental factors in the etiology of individual cases to produce familial aggregation without a simple Mendelian pattern.[104,105]

In the multifactorial genetic diseases, there are *constitutional (polygenic) components*, consisting of multiple genes at independent loci whose effects interact in a cumulative fashion. An individual who inherits a particular combination of these genes has a relative risk that may combine with an *environmental component* to cross a "threshold" of biologic significance such that the individual is affected with a multifactorial disease.[104,105] In order for another individual in the same family to express the same syndrome, a similar combination of genes must be inherited. Since sibs share half their genes, the probability of a sib inheriting the same combination of genes is $(1/2)^n$, where n is the number of genes required to express the trait (assuming that none of the genes are linked).

Inasmuch as the precise number of genes responsible for polygenic traits is unknown, the risk of inheritance for a relative of an affected individual is difficult to calculate, and risk estimates are based on empirical risk figures (i.e., on a direct tally of the proportion of affected relatives in previously reported families). In contrast to the monogenic disorders, in which 25 or 50 percent of the first-degree relatives of an affected proband are at genetic risk, multifactorial genetic disorders are generally observed empirically to affect no more than 5 to 10 percent of first-degree relatives. Moreover, in contrast to Mendelian traits, the recurrence risk of multifactorial conditions varies from family to family, and its estimation is significantly influenced by two factors: (1) the number of affected persons already present in the family, and (2) the severity of the disorder in the index case. The greater number of affected relatives and the more severe their disease, the higher the risk to other relatives. For example, the risk of cleft lip in the sibs of a child with unilateral cleft lip is about 2.5 percent. But if the lesion in the index case is bilateral, the risk in the sibs rises to 6 percent.[104,105]

Multifactorial etiology is thought to be important for many diseases that occur beyond adolescence, and diseases with later age of onset may have decreased heritability on average.[106] For example, a review of nine multifactorial diseases provided evidence compatible with a decline in the impact of the genes on disease with increasing age.

The hypothesis of a polygenic component in the inheritance of multifactorial diseases has been given a sound basis over the years by the demonstration that at least 28 percent of all gene loci harbor polymorphic alleles that vary among individuals (discussed above). Such a large degree of variation in normal genes undoubtedly provides the substrate for variations in genetic predisposition with which environmental factors can interact. So far, the genetic loci most strikingly associated with predisposition to specific diseases are those that constitute the major histocompatibility locus or HLA (human leukocyte antigen) system. The HLA gene complex is located on the short arm of chromosome 6. It consists of multiple closely linked but distinct loci (A, B, DR, DQ, and DP). The products of these genes are proteins that are found on the surface of cells and are involved in cellular immune recognition. Each HLA locus in the population consists of multiple alleles, each of which produces an immunologically distinct protein. For example, an individual may inherit any 2 of more than 36 alleles at the HLA-B locus. The inheritance of certain alleles predisposes to the development of certain diseases when the individual is exposed to an environmental challenge.

Multifactorial disorders are heterogeneous in etiology in the sense that the relative contribution of the polygenic factors ("risk genes") and environmental factors will vary greatly from patient to patient. As discussed above, among common phenotypes that are largely multifactorial, a small proportion of cases may be due to monogenic or chromosomal abnormalities. For example, although coronary heart disease is usually of multifactorial etiology, about 5 percent of subjects with premature myocardial infarctions are heterozygotes for familial hypercholesterolemia, a single-gene disorder that produces atherosclerosis in the absence of an extraordinary environmental factor. However, even in a single-gene disorder such as familial hypercholesterolemia, other loci [e.g., the genes for apolipoprotein B, apolipoprotein (a), lipoprotein lipase, and apolipoprotein E] could easily influence the phenotype, and nongenetic factors (diet and smoking) certainly modify the risk. The complexity of the etiology for coronary artery disease is detailed in part in Table 1-3. Numerous interrelated biochemical and genetic factors affect the risk, as well as numerous nongenetic factors. An appreciation of this etiologic heterogeneity and careful investigation of each patient are necessary prerequisites for counseling families at risk for these disorders.

Methods for unraveling the molecular basis of multifactorial etiology are changing with the availability of detailed genetic maps in the human, mouse, and other organisms. Many newer studies focus on analysis of candidate genes using association studies, sib-pair analysis, and other complex strategies.[107–109] The advantages of focusing on molecular variations that are important in gene function as opposed to functionless variants has been emphasized.[107] The overall complexity of various approaches is daunting.[109] Despite these difficulties, significant progress is being made towards identifying major loci for a number of multifactorial diseases, such as hypertension,[110] for which genetic variation in angiotensinogen is reported to influence risk in humans.[111] There is evidence for involvement of the region encoding insulin and insulin-like growth factor 2 in addition to the known role of the HLA cluster in the etiology of insulin-dependent diabetes mellitus.[112] The use of recombinant inbred[113] and recombinant congenic[114] strains of mice and other animals also should prove valuable for deciphering the molecular basis of multifactorial phenotypes. Morton has presented an interesting perspective on the future of genetic approaches to multifactorial disorders.[109]

INTERACTION BETWEEN SINGLE GENETIC AND ENVIRONMENTAL FACTORS

In addition to polygenic states, many single-gene mutations are known to create abnormal responses to environmental factors. Some of the best examples of this interaction between genes and environmental factors are those monogenic disorders that produce clinically significant and often life-threatening idiosyncratic re-

Table 1-3 Risk Factors for Atherosclerosis and Coronary Artery Disease

LDL receptor genotype	Aging
Apolipoprotein E genotype	Male sex
Familial hypertriglyceridemia	Smoking
Familial combined hyperlipidemia	Hypertension
Lipoprotein Lp(a)	Obesity
Other apolipoprotein variants	Diet
Other gene disorders (e.g., acid lipase)	Diabetes mellitus
Increased LDL	Inactivity?
Decreased HDL	Stress?

sponses to drugs. There is significant genetic variation in the response to some widely used drugs such as isoniazid, some β-adrenergic blockers, and tricyclic antidepressants. Other disorders with important interactions between genotype and drugs include glucose 6-phosphate dehydrogenase deficiency, acute intermittent porphyria, hemochromatosis, and muscle diseases with susceptibility to malignant hyperthermia.

Misinterpretation of adverse drug reactions may result in serious harm to patients, and unusual or idiosyncratic reactions should be considered to be genetically determined until proven otherwise. Fortunately, therapy for the pharmacogenetic disorders is straightforward: avoidance of the noxious drug by the patient and relatives.

In addition to drugs, other factors in the environment may aggravate specific genetic traits. Cigarette smoke has particularly deleterious effects on persons homozygous (and possibly heterozygous) for α1-antitrypsin deficiency, who are predisposed to the development of emphysema. Patients with xeroderma pigmentosum are unusually sensitive to the ultraviolet light in sunlight (Chap. 13). Avoidance of milk at an early age prevents at least the life-threatening complications of galactosemia. Undoubtedly, diet is an important variable for many or most forms of hyperlipidemia and cardiovascular disease. Unfortunately, a modern society is also subjected to an endless array of novel environmental exposures. The current widespread use of aspartame is an example of a special risk for phenylketonuria patients.

Recombinant DNA Techniques

Recombinant DNA techniques have transformed the perspectives for studying human genetic disease and have revolutionized biologic research. Practical technical manuals[115] and an excellent introduction and overview of recombinant DNA techniques[29] are available. Many of the methods for analysis of the human genome and for positional cloning are discussed in considerably greater detail in Chap. 2.

Molecular Cloning. Cloning refers to the process by which a DNA molecule is joined to another DNA molecule (termed a *vector*) that can replicate autonomously in a specially designed host, usually a bacterium or yeast. Many variations on this general scheme have been developed, some of which are described briefly below. Many of these methods rely on the use of restriction endonucleases,[116,117] enzymes that recognize specific sequences in double-stranded DNA and generate predictable cleavages at or near those sites. In addition to their usefulness in recognizing landmarks along DNA by virtue of their sequence specificity, many restriction enzymes have the additional property of generating overhanging "sticky ends" that permit efficient joining (annealing) of unrelated but similarly digested DNA molecules. Annealed molecules may be covalently joined by enzymes known as DNA li-

gases. Using this strategy, a fragment of DNA (an insert) can be ligated into a plasmid vector, as shown in Fig. 1-13.

Numerous innovative vector cloning systems have been developed in recent years. The precise details of each are beyond the scope of this presentation. In part, the choice of the system is determined by the nature of the DNA clones desired. The sizes of DNA fragments accepted by particular vector systems vary from short molecules (a few to several thousand nucleotides), to moderate size molecules (several thousand to tens of thousands of nucleotides), to large molecules (a few million nucleotides). A large fraction of cloning is performed in either plasmid or bacteriophage vectors, which are described briefly.

Plasmids are closed circular double-stranded DNA molecules that are most useful for cloning smaller DNA fragments. Plasmid vectors employed in cloning generally contain an origin of DNA replication to permit maintenance in bacterial cells, a selectable marker (usually an antibiotic resistance gene) used to identify bacterial clones harboring the plasmid, and convenient restriction enzyme sites into which fragments are introduced. A typical scheme for cloning in a plasmid vector, such as the commonly used pBR322 and pUC19 vectors, is illustrated in Fig. 1-13. In general, DNA fragments of fewer than 10,000 nucleotides (10 kb) are conveniently manipulated in these vectors.

Given the large size of the human genome (6×10^9 nucleotides), cloning of moderately large DNA segments is experimentally advantageous, as it reduces the number of independent recombinant clones needed to encompass the entire genome. A collection of clones sufficient in number to theoretically include virtually all sequences in the starting tissue is often referred to as a "library." One of the most convenient, and most widely used, vectors for cloning mammalian genes has been bacteriophage γ (Fig. 1-14). This double-stranded DNA virus contains approximately 50,000 nucleotides (50 kb) as its genetic information and infects and propagates efficiently in *Escherichia coli* as a host. The central portion of the viral DNA genome is expendable and can be replaced by foreign DNA sequences. Joining of vector DNA, specially designed with suitable restriction enzyme sites, and donor DNA can be performed by simple procedures, after which encapsidation of the recombinant DNA molecule (donor DNA linked to vector) into the viral protein coat can be accomplished in the test tube by a method known as in vitro packaging. Following infection of a bacterial lawn, recombinant phages generate plaques when lysis of host cells occurs. Efficient procedures for screening individual plaques have been developed, such that millions of independent clones can be readily examined in a matter of days. Most often, this screening process uses radiolabeled DNA fragments as hybridization probes, generated either from previously cloned segments or from chemically synthesized DNA. Phage DNA, transferred by adsorption to fibers, is denatured *in situ* and allowed to anneal (or hybridize) to a complementary DNA strand of a probe. On average, each bacteriophage clone can accommodate roughly 15 to 20 kb of foreign DNA. Methods for the production of essentially random DNA fragments of this size permit assembly of a genomic library. Approximately 5×10^5 independent clones represents a human library equivalent. Often segments initially isolated in bacteriophage clones are subcloned into plasmid vehicles.

For a large-scale analysis of the human genome, considerably larger DNA fragments need to be cloned to complement chromosome mapping studies. Vectors known as cosmids, which have features in common with both bacteriophage and plasmid vectors, allow the cloning of DNA molecules roughly 40 kb in length, about twice the maximum length for a bacteriophage. Cloning systems using the yeast artificial chromosome (YAC) method have been developed to accept DNA fragments up to a million base pairs (a megabase or Mb), and this system is described in greater detail in Chap. 2. Numerous positional cloning successes have depended

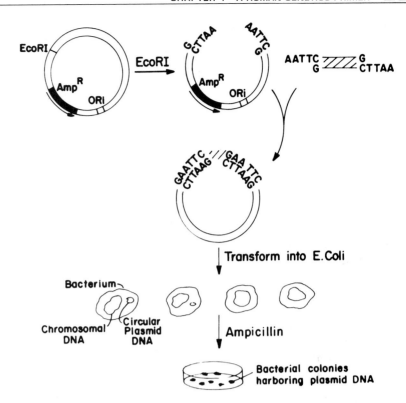

FIG. 1-13 Scheme for cloning a restriction fragment in a plasmid vector. The plasmid vector is depicted at the top left and the fragment to be subcloned at the top right. Amp[R] is an ampicillin-resistant gene, and ORi is an origin of replication for the plasmid.

heavily on the use of YAC clones. A small number of YAC libraries covering the human genome are now available in multiple laboratories around the world. The day is fast approaching when the human genome will be available in a series of overlapping YAC clones, and this goal has already been approximated for chromosomes 21 and Y,[118,119] and to some extent for the entire genome.[120]

Since only a subset of cellular DNA is eventually expressed into mRNA, cloning of mRNA, or its complementary copy known as cDNA, offers another strategy by which reagents for, and specific information about, particular genes can be obtained. The cloning of mRNA molecules rests on the use of the RNA-dependent DNA polymerase reverse transcriptase[121] to copy mRNA into cDNA.[122] Again, several procedures, one of which is depicted in Fig. 1-15, have been developed to clone cDNA synthesized in vitro.[123] The cDNA may be cloned in plasmid or bacteriophage

vectors that have been engineered to accept appropriately prepared cDNA molecules, to express the encoded products, and to provide various convenience features for investigators.

Identification of Recombinant Clones. Many different strategies and methods can be used to identify and then isolate a desired recombinant among the numerous clones represented in a genomic or cDNA library. In practice, the approach is usually dictated by the presumed abundance of the gene sequence under question (particularly if an mRNA is sought), the nature of its product, and the reagents and starting material available to the investigator.

The most common screening approach employs nucleic acid hybridization, whereby replicas of plasmid colonies or phage plaques are lysed *in situ* on nitrocellulose or nylon membranes, denatured, immobilized, and then incubated with radiolabeled DNA (or RNA) fragments specific for a desired gene sequence. If, for

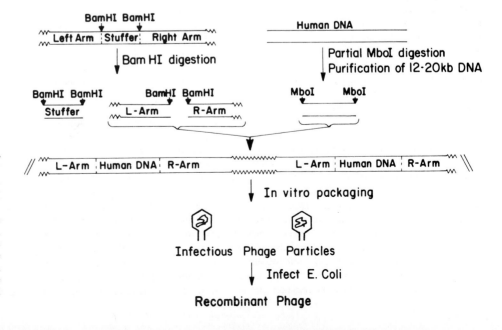

FIG. 1-14 Generation of a genomic "library" in bacteriophage. Phage DNA is depicted in the upper left. Digestion with *Bam*HI liberates a nonessential "stuffer" fragment which is discarded. Human DNA fragments of 12 to 20 kb in length resulting from partial digestion with *Mbo*I can be annealed and ligated into *Bam*HI sites of the bacteriophage arms. Since *Mbo*I cleaves at a four-base recognition sequence (GATC), partial digestion approximates random DNA fragmentation. The overhang GATC resulting from *Mbo*I digestion anneals with the same overhang of *Bam*HI digested DNA.

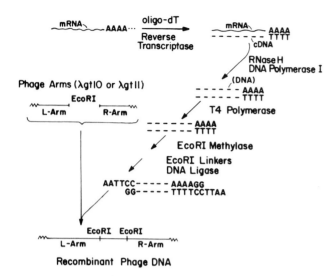

FIG. 1-15 Protocol for cDNA cloning. The method outlined schematically above (see Gubler and Hoffmann[123]) is highly efficient and maximizes generation of full-length cDNA transcripts.

example, a cDNA clone for a specific RNA transcript has bene previously isolated and a genomic clone is desired, the cDNA clone may be radiolabeled by a variety of enzymatic procedures and used to identify the desired gene in the bacteriophage library. Related cDNA or genomic sequences can often be identified by using a previously cloned DNA as a probe, but with reduced stringency of hybridization (or washing) of the filters to permit isolation of homologous members. Often a short stretch of peptide sequence has been determined for a protein of interest, but its cDNA or genomic sequence has not been isolated. Synthetic oligonucleotides[124] encoding either all possible mRNA sequences on the basis of codon degeneracies or a so-called best guess sequence can be used as a hybridization probe to screen libraries. The success of such synthetic probes rests on the much higher stability of matched than mismatched hybrid nucleic acids.[124] Alternatively, degenerate oligonucleotides can be used as primers in the polymerase chain reaction (see below) to amplify and clone homologous sequences.

Where no structural data are available for a protein, methods have been developed to identify the desired clone by expression of the protein in either bacterial or mammalian cells. In one of the most widely exploited and convenient methods, cDNAs are expressed as C-terminal fusions to E. coli β-galactosidase contained in a bacteriophage vector.[125] Upon indication of β-galactosidase synthesis, colonies are screened with antibody to the desired product. If the epitope of the antibody is available in the fusion protein made in E. coli, appropriate clones may be identified with few false positives. Generally, additional methods are required to establish that the antibody-selected clones do, in fact, encode the desired product rather than another polypeptide bearing a related or shared epitope.

The function of a desired cDNA or genomic fragment may also be used to identify a recombinant clone. For example, if a biologic assay is available for a protein, such as a hormone or growth factor, a library of cDNA may be constructed in a vector that permits expression of the cDNA inserts when DNA is introduced (or transfected) into mammalian cells. Upon assay of culture media from transfected cells and subsequent sib selection of the clones from the positive pools, a single recombinant can be identified. The success of this approach relies on the availability of a sensitive and reliable bioassay. Introduction of genomic DNA directly into mammalian cells by a process known as transfection has also been used successfully when the desired gene can be expressed in the host

cells and manifested as a cell-surface molecule detectable with an antibody or as a pheynotypic alteration (such as malignant transformation in the instance or an oncogene).[126] Several procedures have been devised to recover the mammalian cell clone harboring the foreign DNA of interest and to isolate this segment from the host cell.

Finally, positional cloning strategies have been used to isolate numerous human genes, beginning in 1986 (Table 1-4). Positional cloning strategies isolate a gene on the basis of its genetic and physical map location in the human genome. These strategies are described in detail elsewhere[37] and in Chap. 2. Strategies for cloning a gene on the basis of some knowledge of the protein or its functional properties are usually referred to as functional cloning, in comparison to positional cloning. Positional cloning strategies are laborious, and extraordinary resources were required to clone genes for which no cytogenetic clues were available, as in the case of cystic fibrosis and Huntington disease. The availability of dense linkage maps of the human genome and the promise of an overlapping YAC library of the human genome offer the hope of reducing the effort required for positional cloning, but the burden remains substantial. In reality, positional cloning is replaced to some extent by a process of positional localization followed by inspection of candidate genes in a region.[38] This positional-candidate strategy is based in part on the fact that large numbers of random cDNA clones are being isolated and partially sequenced.[127] In instances where a partial cDNA sequence identifies homologies that, in turn, provide insights into function, it may be possible to identify candidate genes for a disease that maps to a particular region. Genetic mapping of the cDNA fragments is an important part of this process, which is proceeding,[127] although at a slower pace. Syntenic mapping data from the mouse can also be used as part of this positional candidate strategy. Examples of genes cloned using positional information in conjunction with knowledge of candidate genes include familial hypertrophic cardiomyopathy, Waardenburg syndrome, Charcot-Marie-Tooth disease, and amyotrophic lateral sclerosis.[128] The identification of defects in a human mutator gene as a cause of hereditary nonpolyposis colon cancer is an excellent example of rapid and complementary observations involving de-

Table 1-4 Some Examples of Inherited Disease Genes Identified by Positional Cloning

Disease	Year	Chromosome
Chronic granulomatous disease	1986	X
Duchenne musclar dystrophy	1986	X
Retinoblastoma (Chap. 19)	1986	13
Cystic fibrosis	1989	7
Wilms tumor (Chap. 21)	1990	11
Neurofibromatosis type 1 (Chap. 22)	1990	17
Testis determining factor	1990	Y
Choroideremia	1990	X
Fragile X	1991	X
Familial polyposis coli	1991	5
Kallmann syndrome	1991	X
Aniridia	1991	11
Myotonic dystrophy	1992	19
Lowe syndrome	1992	X
Norrie syndrome	1992	X
Menkes disease	1993	X
X-linked agammaglobulinemia	1993	X
Glycerol kinase deficiency	1993	X
Adrenoleukodystrophy	1993	X
Huntington disease	1993	4
Spinocerebellar ataxia	1993	6
Tuberous sclerosis	1994	16

tection of somatic instability of short tandem repeats in tumors, mapping of a phenotype to chromosome 2, use of degenerate PCR to clone a human homolog of a bacterial mutator gene, mapping of the human cloned gene to chromosome 2, and detecting mutations in affected families (Chap. 17).

Analytic Methods. Highly sensitive and specific analytic methods have formed the basis for much of the experimental work that is fundamental to the analysis of human genes responsible for disease. Two widely used procedures are known as Southern[130] and northern blot[131,132] analysis.

The former, named after its originator, combines restriction endonuclease digestion of DNA, electrophoresis of the resulting fragments and their transfer to a solid membrane support, and hybridization of nucleic acid to identify specific DNA fragments in a mixture (Fig. 1-16). Single genes or parts of genes can be detected within total human DNA, a collection of some 10^5 to 10^6 fragments. Three sorts of information are derived from Southern blots. First, the presence or absence of a specific fragments(s) can be determined. The result often resolves whether a particular gene is present in the cellular DNA of a patient who cannot synthesize a given protein product. Second, the size(s) of detected DNA fragments provides information regarding the position of flanking restriction enzyme cleavage sites and directly reflects the physical "map" of the DNA region. Changes in restriction sites between individuals may reflect either normal variation with no phenotypic effect or a functionally significant alteration in the gene or its flanking DNA. Restriction fragment length polymorphisms (RFLP) provide useful genetic markers within families and populations and are the basis for genetic linkage analysis, which permits construction of large-scale human gene maps[133,134] (see Chap. 2). Third, the copy number of a particular DNA fragment may be estimated by comparison with normal control samples. For an autosomal gene, the deletion of a single copy results in a signal of one-half normal intensity. Additional copies of a gene, resulting either from the presence of additional chromosomes (for example, in XXY versus XY) or from amplification of gene sequences (for example, in cancers associated with amplification of oncogenes) are similarly detectable by band intensity.

Northern blot analysis, a procedure similar in principle, involves electrophoresis of RNA under denaturing conditions, its subsequent transfer to a solid support, and detection of specific transcripts by hybridization (Fig. 1-16). This method yields information on the size and abundance of RNA transcripts and is especially useful in revealing the distribution of particular mRNAs in tissue or cell samples and structural or quantitative derangements in samples from affected patients.

Numerous additional methods for analysis of large genomic regions, including pulsed-field gel electrophoresis, are discussed in Chap. 2. Methods for analysis of RNA are most relevant to mutation detection and are discussed further in that context below.

Polymerase Chain Reaction (PCR) for DNA Amplification. The polymerase chain reaction (PCR) finds extraordinarily broad applications for cloning DNA and RNA sequences and for analysis of mutations. The technique is based on knowing the nucleic acid sequence for a region that, for a diagnostic application, is to be analyzed repeatedly from different individuals. Oligonucleotide primers are prepared that are complementary to opposite strands of the DNA and are separated by up to a few hundred base pairs (Fig. 1-17). The oligonucleotide primers are incubated with the target DNA to be amplified and with a DNA polymerase that synthesizes a complementary strand in a 5′-to-3′ direction. Considerable specificity is provided by the requirement that primers must lead to convergent synthesis for amplification to be effective. The reaction is subjected to a series of temperature variations, including a denatur-

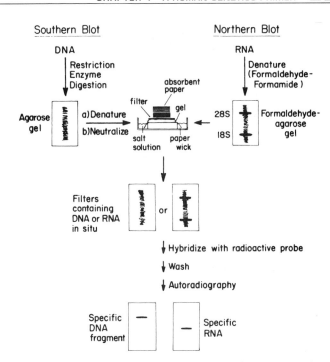

FIG. 1-16 Procedures for Southern and northern blot analysis.

ing temperature where double-stranded DNA is dissociated to single-stranded DNA, an annealing temperature where oligonucleotide primers hybridize to target DNA, and a polymerization temperature for the synthetic step. The reaction is now carried out using a thermostable polymerase such that the polymerase remains active during the temperature cycles (usually ranging from 45 to 95°C). After a number of such cycles, typically 20 to 30 or more, tens to hundreds of thousands of copies of the original target sequence have been synthesized, as depicted in Fig. 1-17. The bulk of the product is a double-stranded DNA fragment of specific length. The technique is so sensitive that it can be used to amplify and analyze DNA from a single human sperm containing one duplex target DNA molecule. PCR is easily performed with minimal sample preparation starting with crude and even degraded samples, allowing analysis from whole blood, dried blood filters, mouthwash, old tissue sections, and other sources. Molecular diagnosis with PCR can include: (1) determining the presence or the absence of an amplified product, (2) digesting the amplified product with a restriction enzyme, (3) hybridizing the PCR product with allele-specific oligonucleotides, (4) direct sequencing of the PCR product, and (5) many other methods of analysis of the PCR product. Many variations and modifications have been devised to take advantage of the PCR concept for research applications. For reverse transcription-PCR (RT-PCR), single-stranded cDNA is synthesized from mRNA using reverse transcriptase, and the cDNA is amplified using PCR. RT-PCR is often useful for analysis of expression and for characterization of mutations. PCR can be used to amplify and isolate DNA from a crude source, so that virtually any sequence available in data banks can be available to a laboratory. PCR can be used to amplify and clone related sequences using homology PCR and degenerate primers similar to the best-guess oligomers described above for hybridization. Single-stranded DNA can be synthesized by altering the ratio of the oligonucleotide primers. Other applications include preparation of recombinant DNA constructs, mutagenesis of cloned DNA, detection of rare nucleotide sequences, and detection of nucleotide sequences of infectious agents. The PCR method offers extremely rapid analysis (single day), ease of automation, relatively low cost, and extraordinary specificity.

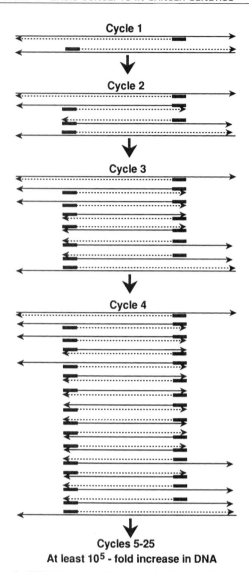

FIG. 1-17 Polymerase chain reaction for amplification of DNA. The target DNA is shown as a solid line in cycle 1. Newly synthesized DNA is indicated by dotted lines in each cycle. Primer oligonucleotides are indicated by solid rectangles. Each DNA strand is marked with an arrow indicating 5′-to-3′ orientation.

The most basic information obtainable from a cloned DNA segment is its nucleotide sequence. Two elegant methods, the dideoxy-chain termination procedure of Sanger et al.[30] and the chemical degradation procedure of Maxam and Gilbert,[31] permit rapid, highly accurate determination of DNA sequence. Methods for automating these basic techniques have been developed, and large-scale DNA sequencing projects are an important part of the human genome initiative. The methods for DNA sequencing are described in greater detail elsewhere[29] and in Chap. 2. Newer methods, such as techniques for solid-phase sequencing, are also being explored, and it is the ultimate goal of the human genome project to determine the entire nucleotide sequence for the human genome and for the genome of other organisms.

Expression cloning strategies are an important approach to the analysis of gene products. Using specially adapted vectors, it is possible to express human proteins in a variety of host-vector systems, including expression in bacteria, yeast, insect cells, and cultured mammalian cells. Each of these systems has its own advantages and disadvantages, with yeast and bacteria often being the most convenient and cheapest, but insect or mammalian cells

sometimes being required for proper functioning of proteins that undergo complex posttranslational modification. Expression cloning is extremely valuable for functional analysis, as exemplified by the expression of the cystic fibrosis transmembrane conductance regulator in cells, followed by analysis of the chloride channel properties of this protein. Functional properties can also be analyzed using the ability of human proteins to complement mutations in organisms such as yeast or *Drosophila*, as exemplified by the extensive functional analysis of the neurofibromatosis protein in yeast[135] and by the ability of a human equivalent gene to perform a regulatory function of the *deformed* locus in *Drosophila*.[136] Functional analysis of a mutant form of a protein is often the ultimate proof that a particular mutation causes disease and is not a benign variant. Using in vitro mutagenesis, a mutation identified in a patient can be introduced into an expression construct, and the functional properties (enzyme activity or other) of the expressed construct, and the functional properties (enzyme activity or other) of the expressed mutant protein can be tested. Expression cloning also offers the opportunity for producing large amounts of recombinant protein that can be crystallized and analyzed using x-ray diffraction and other methods. Although the crystallographic structure is as yet known for only a small fraction of the gene products discussed in this book, this type of information will increase rapidly in the next few years. Expression cloning also opens the opportunity for producing recombinant proteins for therapeutic use.

Analysis of Mutations. Mutation analysis is a central aspect of much of the current work in human molecular genetics, and excellent reviews of the methodology are available.[137–139] The challenge of detecting unknown mutations is significantly different from diagnostic testing for the presence of known mutations. Large mutations are more readily detected, but more discriminating methods are required to detect point mutations. The best-characterized methods for detecting unknown mutations include ribonuclease cleavage, denaturing gradient-gel electrophoresis (DGGE), carbodimide modification, chemical cleavage of mismatches, single-strand confirmation polymorphism (SSCP) analysis, heteroduplex analysis, and sequencing of DNA (Fig. 1-18). These methods involve chemical or enzymatic recognition of mismatches in nucleic acid duplexes, electrophoretic separation of single- or double-stranded DNA, or sequencing. DNA sequencing can be performed directly on PCR products or on individual clones or pools of clones. The sensitivity for detection of mutations varies from 80 to virtually 100 percent, and analysis can be performed on genomic DNA or mRNA (cDNA) depending on specific circumstances.[138] In the case of ancient mutations that are widely distributed in the population, diagnostic methods focus on the presence or absence of particular mutations. These methods include allele-specific oligonucleotide (ASO) hybridization, allele-specific amplification, ligase amplification or assay, primer extension sequencing, and restriction enzyme analysis (including artificial introduction of restriction sites) (Fig. 1-18).[137] These methods all depend on a hybridization or enzymatic reaction to distinguish nucleic acid sequences differing by as little as a single base.

Identification of disease-causing mutations is an important aspect of the positional cloning or positional candidate cloning strategy (see Chap. 2) and often provides the major evidence that a candidate gene is in fact the disease-causing locus. Typically, after a disease gene is cloned, there is a burst of activity identifying dozens if not hundreds of disease-causing mutations. Diagnosis and genetic counseling are greatly facilitated if the mutation or mutations in a family can be identified and analyzed in individual family members. Such mutation information will also allow for prognostication based on genotype-phenotype correlations in some instances.

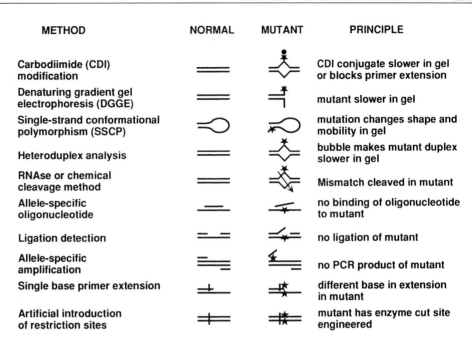

METHOD	NORMAL	MUTANT	PRINCIPLE
Carbodiimide (CDI) modification			CDI conjugate slower in gel or blocks primer extension
Denaturing gradient gel electrophoresis (DGGE)			mutant slower in gel
Single-strand conformational polymorphism (SSCP)			mutation changes shape and mobility in gel
Heteroduplex analysis			bubble makes mutant duplex slower in gel
RNAse or chemical cleavage method			Mismatch cleaved in mutant
Allele-specific oligonucleotide			no binding of oligonucleotide to mutant
Ligation detection			no ligation of mutant
Allele-specific amplification			no PCR product of mutant
Single base primer extension			different base in extension in mutant
Artificial introduction of restriction sites			mutant has enzyme cut site engineered

FIG. 1-18 Methods for detection of mutations. The asterisk represents the position of the mutation. *(Modified from Cotton.[137] Used by permission.)*

ANIMAL MODELS

Much of the remarkable progress in genetic research over the last two decades has resulted from reductive strategies focusing on specific genes or proteins. Ultimately, however, geneticists must understand how individual genes and their protein products function in the intact organism, interacting with other genes and gene products in the complex networks which achieve normal development and physiological homeostasis. In particular, medical geneticists want to understand how defects in one or a few genes disrupt normal development and/or physiological homeostasis to produce genetic disease; that is, they want to understand pathogenesis and use this knowledge to devise rational and effective treatments for their patients. These goals require integrative rather than reductive strategies and are likely to depend heavily on the use of animal models of genetic disease.

Until recently, identification of animals with genetic disorders depended on the recognition by astute observers of deviant phenotypes arising spontaneously, as the result of random mutagenesis methods, or as products of selective breeding strategies aimed at producing animals with phenotypes such as obesity or hypertension.[140,141] Although inefficient, these methods led to the identification of useful models for a host of human genetic disorders in a variety of animal species. In particular, breeders of the laboratory mouse, *Mus musculus*, identified scores of spontaneously arising mutants, many of which have been established as models of human genetic diseases.[140,150]

Fortunately, recent advances in technologies for the manipulation of mouse gametes and pluripotent embryonic stem cells have opened the way for the rational, preplanned development of specific models, greatly reducing dependence on serendipity.[142–144,151] Models of disorders caused by dominant negative and dominant gain-of-function alleles can be produced by straightforward transgenic methods (Fig. 1-19). These approaches do not require homologous integration of the introduced DNA and, depending on the characteristics of the involved biologic system, may be achieved with only a modest level of expression of the transgene. Models of disorders involving keratins (epidermolysis bullosas),[149,152] collagens (skeletal dysplasias),[148] and lipoproteins (hyperlipidemias)[147,153] have all been produced in this way.

Alternatively, specific target genes can be disrupted completely ("gene knockout") or altered in more subtle ways by homologous recombination in embryonic stem (ES) cells (Fig. 1-19).[142–145] Cloned, isogenic versions of the gene of interest are modified as desired to produce a targeting construct containing selectable markers. The targeting construct is introduced into ES cells in culture, usually by electroporation, and homologous recombinants are identified, by a combination of clonal selection and molecular methods. The heterozygous, recombinant ES cell clones are injected into mouse blastocytes to produce chimeric mice, which are bred to produce animals heterozygous or homozygous for the modified gene. The technology for this general method has advanced rapidly over the last few years, so that it is now reasonable to expect that virtually any gene can be targeted. With allowance for usual technical problems and the generation times of mice, the entire process can be accomplished in approximately 12 to 18 months. Although these methods have been established for mice, they presumably could be transferred to other species as the appropriate stem cell lines and embryo manipulation procedures are developed.

Animal models of human genetic diseases identified by any of the above methods are extraordinarily valuable for a variety of uses. First, they serve as reagents to identify genes responsible for monogenic and multifactorial disorders. Again, the mouse leads the way, particularly because of the extensive knowledge of mouse genetics. Human and murine genetic maps of phenotypes and gene loci are well developed.[154] The resolution of the human/mouse homology is increasing rapidly, so that the map location of a gene or phenotype in one species is highly predictive for the other.[154] A phenotype or gene mapped in humans can be related immediately to a phenotype or gene localized in mouse and vice versa. For example, localization of the human piebald phenotype to 4q12, a region known to contain the c-*kit* gene and to correspond to a region of mouse chromosome 5 where the dominant-white spotting (*W*) phenotype, known to be allelic with the murine c-*kit* gene, was located, immediately and correctly implicated c-*kit* mutations as the cause of piebaldism in humans.[155,156]

A second use of animal models is to assist in sorting out the genetic and environmental contributions to complex mutifactorial traits. For example, genetic linkage methods are used to identify the genes responsible for multifactorial traits such as hypertension and obesity in rat and murine models, usually developed by selective breeding.[141,157] The possible contribution of candidate genes identified in this way can then be examined in the corresponding

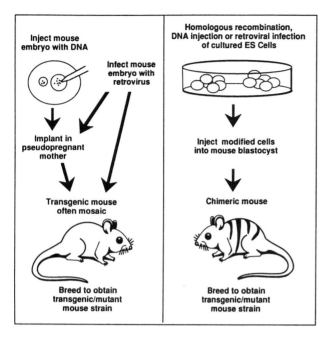

FIG. 1-19 Various strategies for producing transgenic and mutant mice. DNA can be injected into the male pronucleus of fertilized mouse eggs, followed by implantation in pseudopregnant mothers. Mouse embryos can be infected with retroviruses in vivo or in vitro. Transgenic mice may be mosaic, but the transgene can be recovered in nonmosaic form in the offspring of these mice. These strategies are depicted on the left. On the right, cultured embryonic stem (ES) cells can be modified by homologous or nonhomologous recombination or by retroviral infection. The modified cells can be selected and injected into a mouse blastocyst to produce a chimeric mouse, with subsequent recovery of the mutation in the germ line of the offspring of the chimeric mouse. *(From Beaudet AL: in Harrison's Principles of Internal Medicine 12th ed. New York, McGraw-Hill, 1994, p 349. Used by permission.)*

human disorders. The final proof that the genes identified contribute to a particular multifactorial trait can be obtained from transgenic and gene knockout experiments. Several genes thought to be involved in atherosclerosis have been tested in this way. Overexpression of the human LDL receptor or human apolipoprotein E (apo E) protected mice against massive cholesterol overloading, while overexpression of lipoprotein (a) [Lp(a)] or knockout of apolipoprotein E predisposes mice to artherosclerosis.[153,158,159] These same animals also can be used to examine the contribution of certain environmental variables such as diet, pregnancy, and pharmaceuticals to the multifactorial phenotype.

A third use of animal models is to elucidate the pathogenesis of specific disorders. As discussed above, achieving a full understanding of how a particular molecular or biochemical defect produces a particular clinical phenotype often requires an integrative approach only possible with in vivo systems. Low disease frequency, genetic heterogeneity, variation in clinical severity, and difficulty in obtaining samples of affected tissues at all stages of a disease are some of the problems that make these studies difficult to perform in human patients. Animal models provide an excellent alternative experimental system. For example, although we have considerable knowledge regarding the clinical features, biochemical abnormalities, and molecular defects in phenylketonuria, we still are unsure of the mechanism(s) by which elevation in blood phenylalanine produces the principal phenotypic feature, severe mental retardation. The recently described Pah[hph-5] mouse appears to be an excellent model for phenylketonuria; homozygous animals have less than 3 percent of normal hepatic phenylalanine hydroxylase activity, and phenylalanine supplementation of the

drinking water results in severe hyperphenylalaninemia and excretion of phenylketones in the urine.[146] It seems likely that studies of neurotransmitter metabolism and myelin formation in these animals finally may provide insight into the pathogenesis of the mental retardation in human phenylketonuria.

An observation from certain gene knockout experiments is particularly relevant to understanding pathogenesis: null mutations in some genes cause markedly different phenotypic consequences in humans and mice.[140,144] For example, mice with a complete knockout of the hypoxanthine phosphoribosyl transferase (HPRT) gene exhibit little, if any, of the mental defects and self-injurious behavior characteristic of human patients with the same genetic defect (the Lesch-Nyhan syndrome), and the dystrophin deficient *mdx* mouse does not have the obvious, progressive muscle weakness characteristic of the cognate human disorder, Duchenne muscular dystrophy. These examples of discordance in clinical phenotypes are every bit as interesting and useful as models with well-matched phenotypes. Metabolic and genetic redundancy, short absolute life span, and environmental differences are all possible explanations for this lack of concordance.[140,160] It should be obvious that elucidation of the basis for these species-dependent differences in response to a particular genetic defect will reveal important information about pathogenesis.

A final and increasingly important use of animal models is to develop treatments for genetic diseases. This includes a variety of conventional therapies such as nutritional manipulations, pharmacologic interventions, and organ transplantation. In addition, the recent explosion in activity in gene therapy research is linked closely to availability of animal models. Gene therapy successes have been reported in animal models for hypercholesterolemia,[161,162] cystic fibrosis,[163] ornithine transcarbamoylase deficiency,[164,165] and clotting factor deficiencies.[166] The scope and value of these studies is well exemplified by the comprehensive studies by Birkenmeier and colleagues[166a,167–169] and others[170] on the therapeutic approaches for treating mucopolysaccharidosis type VII in a murine model. In careful and well-controlled studies, these investigators have examined the efficacy of enzyme infusions, bone marrow transplantation, and germ-line and somatic gene therapies of various durations and in animals of various ages. Studies of this type set the stage for similar, exciting treatment trials for human genetic disease.

ACKNOWLEDGMENTS

This chapter represents the cumulative contributions of past editors, of *The Metabolic and Molecular Bases of Inherited Disease* including John B. Stanbury, James B. Wyngaarden, Donald S. Fredrickson, Joseph L. Goldstein, and Michael S. Brown. Sections are also included from Chap. 2 of the previous edition, contributed by Stuart H. Orkin. The contributions of Andrea Ballabio to the sections on molecular diagnosis, originally prepared with ALB for *Harrison's Principles of Internal Medicine* (13th edition, McGraw-Hill), are gratefully acknowledged.

REFERENCES

1. Garrod AE: Inborn errors of metabolism (Croonian Lectures). *Lancet* **2**:1, 1908.
2. Garrod AE: *Inborn Errors of Metabolism.* London, Oxford University Press, 1923.
3. Scriver CR, Childs B: *Garrod's Inborn Factors in Disease.* New York, Oxford University Press, 1989.

4. Bearn AG: *Archibald Garrod and the Individuality of Man*. New York, Clarendon Press, 1993.
5. Garrod AE: A contribution to the study of alkaptonuria. *Proc R Med Chir Soc* **2**:130, 1899.
6. Garrod AE: The incidence of alkaptonuria: A study in chemical individuality. *Lancet* **2**:1616, 1902.
7. Mendel G: *Versuche über Pflanzenhybriden*. Leipzig, Engelmann, 1901.
8. Bearn AG, Miller ED: Archibald Garrod and the development of the concept of inborn errors of metabolism. *Bull Hist Med* **53**:315, 1979.
9. LaDu BN, Zannoni VA, Laster L, Seegmiller JE: The nature of the defect in tyrosine metabolism in alcaptonuria. *J Biol Chem* **230**:251, 1958.
10. Johannsen W: The genotype conception of heredity. *Am Nat* **45**:129, 1911.
11. Beadle GW: Biochemical genetics. *Chem Rev* **37**:15, 1945.
12. Beadle GW, Tatum EL: Experimental control of developmental reactions. *Am Nat* **75**:107, 1941.
13. Beadle GW, Tatum EL: Genetic control of biochemical reactions in *Neurospora. Proc Natl Acad Sci USA* **27**:499, 1941.
14. Ephrussi B: Chemistry of "eye color hormones" of *Drosophila. Q Rev Biol* **17**:327, 1942.
15. Beadle GW: Genes and chemical reactions in *Neurospora. Science* **129**:1715, 1959.
16. Tatum EL: A case history of biological research. *Science* **129**:1715, 1959.
17. Horowitz NH, Leupold U: Some recent studies bearing on the one gene one enzyme hypothesis. *Symp Quant Biol* **16**:65, 1951.
18. Benzer S: The elementary units of heredity, in McElroy WD, Glass B (eds): *The Chemical Basis of Heredity*. Baltimore: Johns Hopkins University Press, 1957, p 70.
18a. Smith CWJ, Patton JG, Nadal-Ginard B: Alternative splicing in the control of gene expression. *Annu Rev Genet* **23**:527, 1989.
19. Gibson QH: The reduction of methaemoglobin in red blood cells and studies on the cause of idiopathic methaemoglobinaemia. *Biochem J* **42**:13, 1948.
20. Cori GT, Cori CF: Glucose-6-phosphatase of the liver in glycogen storage disease. *J Biol Chem* **199**:661, 1952.
21. Jervis GA: Phenylpyruvic oligophrenia: Deficiency of phenylalanine oxidizing system. *Proc Soc Exp Biol Med* **82**:514, 1953.
22. Pauling L, Itano HA, Singer SJ, Wells IC: Sickle cell anemia: A molecular disease. *Science* **110**:543, 1949.
23. Ingram VM: A specific chemical difference between the globins of normal human and sickle cell anaemia haemoglobin. *Nature* **178**:792, 1956.
24. Watson JD, Crick FHC: Molecular structure of nucleic acids: A structure for deoxyribose nucleic acid. *Nature* **171**:737, 1953.
25. Kelly TJ Jr, Smith HO: A restriction enzyme from *Hemophilus influenzae*. II. Base sequence of the recognition site. *J Mol Biol* **51**:393, 1970.
26. Danna K, Nathans D: Specific cleavage of simian virus 40 DNA by restriction endonuclease of *Hemophilus influenzae. Proc Natl Acad Sci USA* **68**:2913, 1971.
27. Cohen S, Chang A, Boyer H, Helling R: Construction of biologically functional bacterial plasmids *in vitro. Proc Natl Acad Sci USA* **70**:3240, 1973.
28. Jackson D, Symons R, Berg P: Biochemical method for inserting new genetic information into DNA of simian virus 40: Circular SV40 DNA molecules containing lambda phage genes and the galactose operon of *Escherichia coli. Proc Natl Acad Sci USA* **69**:2904, 1972.
29. Watson JD, Gilman M, Witkowski J, Zoller M: *Recombinant DNA* 2d ed. New York, Freeman, 1992.
30. Sanger F, Nicklen S, Coulson AR: DNA sequencing with chain-terminating inhibitors. *Proc Natl Acad Sci USA* **74**:5463, 1977.
31. Maxam AM, Gilbert W: A new method for sequencing DNA. *Proc Natl Acad Sci USA* **74**:560, 1977.
32. Berget SM, Moore C, Sharp P: Spliced segments at the 5′ termini of adenovirus-2 late mRNA. *Proc Natl Acad Sci USA* **74**:3171, 1977.
33. Chow LT, Gelinas RE, Broker TR, Roberts RJ: An amazing sequence arrangement at the 5′ ends of adenovirus 2 messenger RNA. *Cell* **12**:1, 1977.
34. Kan YW, Dozy AM: Polymorphism of DNA sequence adjacent to human β-globin structural gene: Relationship to sickle mutation. *Proc Natl Acad Sci USA* **75**:5631, 1978.

35. Botstein D, White RL, Skolnick M, Davis RW: Construction of a genetic linkage map in man using restriction fragment length polymorphisms. *Am J Hum Genet* **32**:314, 1980.
36. Orkin SH: Reverse genetics and human disease. *Cell* **47**:845, 1986.
37. Collins FS: Positional cloning: Let's not call it reverse anymore. *Nat Genet* **1**:3, 1992.
38. Ballabio A: The rise and fall of positional cloning? *Nat Genet* **3**:277, 1993.
39. U.S. Department of Health and Human Services: *Nobel Laureates*, Bethesda, MD, NIH Publication, 1992.
40. Grosveld F, van Assendelft GB, Greaves DR, Kollias G: Position independent, high level expression of the human β-globin gene in transgenic mice. *Cell* **51**:975, 1987.
41. Jelinek WR, Schmid CW: Repetitive sequences in eukaryotic DNA and their expression. *Annu Rev Biochem* **51**:813, 1982.
42. Bird AP: CpG-rich islands and the function of DNA methylation. *Nature* **321**:209, 1986.
43. Alberts B, Bray D, Lewis J, Raff M, Roberts K, Watson JD: *Molecular Biology of the Cell* 2d ed. New York, Garland, 1989.
44. Darnell J, Lodish H, Baltimore D: *Molecular Cell Biology* 2d ed. New York, Scientific American Books, 1986.
45. Watson JD, Hopkins NH, Roberts JW, Steitz JA, Weiner AM: *Molecular Biology of the Gene* Vols 1, 2, 4th ed. Menlo Park, Benjamin/Cummings, 1990.
46. Lewin B: *Genes V*. New York, Oxford University Press, 1994.
47. Kornberg A, Baker TA: *DNA Replication* 2d ed. New York, Freeman, 1992.
48. DePamphilis ML: Eukaryotic DNA replication: Anatomy of an origin. *Annu Rev Biochem* **62**:29, 1993.
49. Rich A, Kim SH: The three-dimensional structure of transfer RNA. *Sci Am* **238**(1):52, 1978.
50. Pabo CO, Sauer RT: Transcription factors: Structural families and principles of DNA recognition. *Annu Rev Biochem* **61**:1053, 1992.
51. Evans RM, Newport J: Nucleus and gene expression. *Curr Opin Cell Biol* **5**:383, 1993.
52. McGinnis W, Krumlauf R: Homeobox genes and axial patterning. *Cell* **68**:283, 1992.
53. Deschamps J, Meijlink F: Mammalian homeobox genes in normal development and neoplasia. *Crit Rev Oncog* **3**:117, 1992.
54. Hinnebusch A, Hochstrasser M: Post-transcriptional processes. *Curr Opin Cell Biol* **5**:941, 1993.
55. Harris H: *The Principles of Human Biochemical Genetics* 3d ed. Amsterdam, North-Holland, 1980.
56. Beaudet AL, Tsui L-C: A suggested nomenclature for designating mutations. *Hum Mutat* **2**245, 1993.
57. Kazazian Jr HH, Boehm CD: Molecular basis and prenatal diagnosis of β-thalassemia. *Blood* **72**:1107, 1988.
58. Lakich D, Kazazian Jr HH, Antonarakis SE, Gitschier J: Inversions disrupting the factor VIII gene are a common cause of severe haemophilia A. *Nat Genet* **5**:236, 1993.
59. La Spada AR, Wilson EM, Lubahn DB, Harding AE, Fischbeck KH: Androgen receptor gene mutations in X-linked spinal and bulbar muscular atrophy. *Nature* **352**:77, 1991.
60. Barker D, Schafer M, White R: Restriction sites containing CpG show a higher frequency of polymorphism in human DNA. *Cell* **36**:131, 1984.
60a. Garrod AE: *Inborn Factors in Disease*. London, Oxford University Press, 1931.
60b. Williams RJ: *Biochemical Individuality*. New York, Wiley, 1956.
61. Harris H: Enzyme polymorphisms in man. *Proc R Soc Lond (Biol)* **174**:1, 1966.
62. Lewontin RC, Hubby JL: A molecular approach to the study of genetic heterozygosity in natural populations. II. Amount of variation and degree of heterozygosity in natural population of *Drosophila pseudoobscura. Genetics* **54**:595, 1966.
63. Cooper DN, Smith BA, Cooke HJ, Niemann S, Schmidtke J: An estimate of unique DNA sequence heterozygosity in the human genome. *Hum Genet* **69**:201, 1985.
64. Embury SH, Dozy AJ, Miller J, Davis JR, Kleman KM, Presiler H, Vichinsky E, Lande WN, Lubin B, Kan YW, Mentzer WC: Concurrent sickle cell anemia and α-thalassemia. Effect on severity of anemia. *N Engl J Med* **306**:270, 1982.
65. Higgs DR, Aldridge BE, Lamb J, Clegg JB, Weatherall DJ, Hayes RJ, Grandison Y, Lowrie Y, Mason KP, Serjeant BE, Serjeant GR: The interaction of α-thalassemia and homozygous sickle cell disease. *N Engl J Med* **306**:1441, 1982.

66. Costa T, Scriver CR, Childs B: The effect of Mendelian disease on human health: A measurement. *Am J Med Genet* **21**:231, 1985.
67. Morgan TH: The relation of genetics to physiology and medicine, in Baltimore D (ed): *Nobel Lectures in Molecular Biology 1933–1975.* New York, Elsevier, 1977, p 3.
68. McKusick VA, Ruddle FH: The status of the gene map of the human chromosomes. *Science* **196**:390, 1977.
69. Ruddle FH: A new era in mammalian gene mapping: Somatic cell genetics and recombinant DNA methodologies. *Nature* **294**:115, 1981.
70. Ruddle FH: The William Allan memorial award address: Reverse genetics and beyond. *Am J Hum Genet* **36**:944, 1984.
71. Polymeropoulos MH, Xiao H, Glodek A, Gorski M, Adams MD, Moreno RF, Fitzgerald MG, Venter JC, Merril CR: Chromosomal assignment of 46 brain cDNAs. *Genomics* **12**:492, 1992.
72. Francke U, Ochs HD, deMartinville B, Giacalone J, Lindgren V, Disteche C, Pagon RA, Hofker MH, van Ommen G-JB, Pearson PL, Wedgwood RJ: Minor Xp21 chromosome deletion in a male associated with expression of Duchenne muscular dystrophy, chronic granulomatous disease, retinitis pigmentosa, and McLeod syndrome. *Am J Hum Genet* **37**:250, 1985.
73. Vogel F, Motulsky AG: *Human Genetics: Problems and Approaches* 2d ed. Berlin, Springer-Verlag, 1986.
74. Rooney DE, Czepulkowski BH: *Human Cytogenetics: A Practical Approach.* Vol. 1. *Constitutional Analysis* 2d ed. New York, Oxford University Press, 1992.
75. Rooney DE, Czepulkowski BH: *Human Cytogenetics: A Practical Approach.* Vol. 2. *Malignancy and Acquired Abnormalities* 2d ed. New York, Oxford University Press, 1992.
76. Galjaard H: *Genetic Metabolic Diseases: Early Diagnosis and Prenatal Analysis.* Amsterdam, Elsevier, 1980.
77. Rowley JD, Mitelman F: Principles of molecular cell biology of cancer: Chromosome abnormalities in human cancer and leukemia, in DeVita VT Jr, Hellman S, Rosenberg SA (eds): *Cancer: Principles and Practice of Oncology.* Philadelphia, Lippincott, 1993, p 67.
78. Solomon E, Borrow J, Goddard AD: Chromosome aberrations and cancer. *Science* **254**:1153, 1991.
79. Mitelman F: *Catalogue of Chromosomal Aberrations in Cancer* 4th ed. New York, Wiley-Liss, 1991.
80. Seizinger BR, Rouleau GA, Ozelieu LJ, Lane AH, Farmer GE, Lamiell JM, Haines J, Yuen JWM, Collins D, Majoor-Krakauer D, Bonner T, Mathew C, Rubenstein A, Halperin J, McConkie-Rosell A, Green JS, Trofatter JA, Ponder BA, Eierman L, Bowmer MI, Schimke R, Oostra B, Aronin N, Smith DI, Drabkin H, Waziri MH, Hobbs WJ, Martuza RL, Conneally PM, Hsia YE, Gusella JF: Von Hippel-Lindau disease maps to the region of chromosome 3 associated with renal cell carcinoma. *Nature* **332**:268, 1988.
81. Heim RA, Lench NJ, Swift M: Heterozygous manifestations in four autosomal recessive human cancer-prone syndromes: Ataxia telangiectasia, xeroderma pigmentosum, Fanconi anemia, and Bloom syndrome. *Mutat Res* **284**:25, 1992.
82. Ueland PM, Refsum H: Plasma homocysteine, a risk factor for vascular disease: Plasma levels in health, disease, and drug therapy. *J Lab Clin Med* **114**:473, 1989.
83. Feld RD: Heterozygosity of α1-antitrypsin: A health risk? *Crit Rev Clin Lab Sci* **27**:461, 1989.
84. Herskowitz I: Functional inactivation of genes by dominant negative mutations. *Nature* **329**:219, 1987.
85. Sutherland GR, Richards RI: Anticipation legitimized: Unstable DNA to the rescue. *Am J Hum Genet* **51**:7, 1992.
86. Engel E: Uniparental disomy revisited: The first twelve years. *Am J Med Genet* **46**:670, 1993.
87. Hall JG: Genomic imprinting. *Curr Opin Genet Dev* **1**:34, 1991.
88. Hall JG: Genomic imprinting: Review and relevance to human diseases. *Am J Hum Genet* **46**:857, 1990.
89. Nelson DL, Warren ST: Trinucleotide repeat instability: When and where? *Nat Genet* **4**:107, 1993.
90. Editorial: Breast cancer on the brink. *Nat Genet* **5**:101, 1993.
91. Shenker A, Laue L, Kosugi S, Merendino JJ Jr, Minegishi T, Cutler GB Jr: A constitutively activating mutation of the luteinizing hormone receptor in familial male precocious puberty. *Nature* **365**:652, 1993.
92. Bundey S, Evans K: Tuberous sclerosis-A genetic study. *J Neurol Neurosurg Psychiatr* **32**:591, 1969.
93. Jones KL, Smith DW, Harvey MAS, Hall BD, Quan L: Older paternal age and fresh gene mutation: Data on additional disorders. *J Pediatr* **86**:84, 1975.
94. Murdoch JL, Walker BA, McKusick VA: Parental age effects on the occurrence of new mutations for the Marfan syndrome. *Ann Hum Genet* **35**:331, 1972.
95. Thakker RV: The molecular genetics of the multiple endocrine neoplasia syndromes. *Clin Endocrinol* **38**:1, 1993.
96. Kiesewetter S, Macek M Jr, Davis C, Curristin SM, Chu C-S, Graham C, Shrimpton AE, Cashman SM, Tsui L-C, Mickle J, Amos J, Highsmith WE, Shuber A, Witt DR, Crystal RG, Cutting GR: A mutation in CFTR produces different phenotypes depending on chromosomal background. *Nat Genet* **5**:274, 1993.
97. Heutink P, van der Mey AG, Sandkuijl LA, van Gils AP, Bardoel A, Breedveld GJ, van Vliet M, van Ommen GJ, Cornelisse CJ, Oostra BA: A gene subject to genomic imprinting and responsible for hereditary paragangliomas maps to chromosome 11q23-qter. *Hum Mol Genet* **1**:7, 1992.
98. Wagstaff J, Knoll JHM, Glatt KA, Shugart YY, Sommer A, Lalande M: Maternal but not paternal transmission of 15q11-13-linked nondeletion Angelman syndrome leads to phenotypic expression. *Nat Genet* **1**:291, 1992.
99. Meijers-Heijboer EJ, Sandkuijl LA, Brunner HG, Smeets HJM, Hoogeboom AJM, Deelen WH, van Hemel JO, Nelen MR, Smeets DFCM, Niermeijer MF, Halley DJJ: Linkage analysis with chromosome 15q11-13 markers shows genomic imprinting in familial Angelman syndrome. *J Med Genet* **30**:853, 1993.
100. Neufeld EF: Lysosomal storage diseases. *Annu Rev Biochem* **60**:257, 1991.
101. Cavalli-Sforza LL, Bodmer WF: *The Genetics of Human Populations.* San Francisco, Freeman, 1971.
102. Charlesworth B: Driving genes and chromosomes. *Nature* **332**:394, 1988.
103. Kerem B, Rommens JM, Buchanan JA, Marklewicz D, Cox TK, Chakravarti A, Buchwald M, Tsui L-C: Identification of the cystic fibrosis gene: Genetic analysis. *Science* **245**:1073, 1989.
104. Carter CO: Genetics of common disorders. *Br Med Bull* **25**:52, 1972.
105. Carter CO: Principles of polygenic inheritance. *Birth Defects* **13**:69, 1977.
106. Childs B, Scriver CR: Age at onset and causes of disease. *Perspect Biol Med* **29**:437, 1986.
107. Sobell JL, Heston LL, Sommer SS: Delineation of genetic predisposition to multifactorial disease: A general approach on the threshold of feasibility. *Genomics* **12**:1, 1992.
108. Sribney WM, Swift M: Power of sib-pair and sib-trio linkage analysis with assortative mating and multiple disease loci. *Am J Hum Genet* **51**:773, 1992.
109. Morton NE: The future of genetic epidemiology. *Ann Med* **24**:557, 1992.
110. Bell J: Ace (or PNMT?) in the hole. *Hum Mol Genet* **1**:147, 1992.
111. Jeunemaitre X, Soubrier F, Kotelevtsev YV, Lifton RP, Williams CS, Charru A, Hunt SC, Hopkins PN, Williams RR, Lalouel J-M, Corvol P: Molecular basis of human hypertension: Role of angiotensinogen. *Cell* **71**:169, 1992.
112. Julier C, Hyer RN, Davies J, Merlin F, Soularue P, Briant L, Cathelineau G, Deschamps I, Rotter JI, Froguel P, Boitard C, Bell JI, Lathrop GM: Insulin-IGF2 region on chromosome 11p encodes a gene implicated in HLA-DR4-dependent diabetes susceptibility. *Nature* **354**:155, 1991.
113. Neumann PE: Inference in linkage analysis of multifactorial traits using recombinant inbred strains of mice. *Behav Genet* **22**:665, 1992.
114. Groot PC, Moen CJA, Dietrich W, Stoye JP, Lander ES, Demant P: The recombinant congenic strains for analysis of multigenic traits: Genetic composition. *FASEB J* **6**:2826, 1992.
115. Sambrook J, Fritsch EF, Maniatis T: *Molecular Cloning. A Laboratory Manual* 2d ed. Coldspring Harbor, NY, Cold Spring Harbor Laboratory, 1989.
116. Roberts RJ, Macelis D: Restriction enzymes and their isoschizomers. *Nucleic Acids Res* **20**:2167, 1992.
117. Roberts RJ, Macelis D: Rebase restriction enzymes and methylases. *Nucleic Acids Res* **21**:3125, 1993.
118. Chumakov I, Rigault P, Guillou S, Ougen P, Billault A, Guasconi G, Gervy P, LeGall I, Soularue P, Grinas L, Bougueleret L, Bellanne-Chantelot C, Lacroix B, Barillot E, Gesnouin P, Pook S, Vaysseix G, Frelat G, Schmitz A, Sambucy J-L, Bosch A, Estivill X, Weissenbach J, Vignal A, Riethman H, Cox D, Patterson D, Gardiner K, Hattori M, Sakaki Y, Ichikawa H, Ohki M, LePaslier D, Heilig R, Antonarakis S,

Cohen D: Continuum of overlapping clones spanning the entire human chromosome 21q. *Nature* **359**:380, 1992.

119. Foote S, Vollrath D, Hilson A, Page DC: The human Y chromosome: Overlapping DNA clones spanning the euchromatic region. *Science* **258**:60, 1992.

120. Cohen D, Chumakov I. Weissenbach J: A first-generation physical map of the human genome. *Nature* **366**:698, 1993.

121. Temin H, Baltimore D: RNA-directed DNA synthesis and RNA tumor viruses. *Adv Virus Res* **17**:129, 1972.

122. Efstratiadis A, Kafatos FC, Maxam AM, Maniatis T: Enzymatic in vitro synthesis of globin genes. *Cell* **7**:279, 1976.

123. Gubler U, Hoffmann B: A simple and very efficient method for generating cDNA libraries. *Gene* **25**:283, 1983.

124. Wallace RB, Schold M, Johnson MJ, Dembek P, Itakina K: Oligonucleotide directed mutagenesis of the human beta-globin gene: A general method for producing specific point mutations in cloned DNA. *Nucleic Acids Res* **9**:1194, 1983.

125. Young R, David RW: Efficient isolation of genes by using antibody probes. *Proc Natl Acad Sci USA* **92**:1194, 1983.

126. Weinberg RA: Oncogenes of spontaneous and chemically induced tumors. *Adv Cancer Res* **36**:149, 1982.

127. Adams MD, Kerlavage AR, Fields C, Venter JC: 3,400 new expressed sequence tags identify diversity of transcripts in human brain. *Nature Genet* **4**:256, 1993.

128. Rosen DR, Siddique T, Patterson D, Figlewicz DA, Sapp P, Hentati A, Donaldson D, Goto J, O'Regan JP, Deng H-X, Rahmani Z, Krizus A, McKenna-Yasek D, Cayabyab A, Gaston SM, Berger R, Tanzi RE, Halperin JJ, Herzfeldt B, Van den Bergh R, Hung W-Y, Bird T, Deng G, Mulder DW, Smyth C, Laing NG, Soriano E, Pericak-Vance MA, Haines J, Rouleau GA, Gusella JS, Horvitz HR, Brown RH Jr: Mutations in Cu/Zn superoxide dismutase gene are associated with familial amyotrophic lateral sclerosis. *Nature* **362**:59, 1993.

129. Fishel R, Lescoe MK, Rao MRS, Copeland NG, Jenkins NA, Garber J, Kane M, Kolodner R: The human mutator gene homolog MSH2 and its association with hereditary nonpolyposis colon cancer. *Cell* **75**:1027, 1993.

130. Southern EM: Detection of specific sequences among DNA fragments separated by gel electrophoresis. *J Mol Biol* **98**:503, 1975.

131. Thomas PS: Hybridization of denatured RNA and small DNA fragments transferred to nitrocellulose. *Proc Natl Acad Sci USA* **77**:5201, 1980.

132. Alwine JC, Kemp DJ, Stark GR: Method for detection of specific RNAs in agarose gels by transfer to diazobenzyloxymethyl-paper and hybridization with DNA probes. *Proc Natl Acad Sci USA* **74**:5350, 1977.

133. Weissenbach J, Gyapay G, Dib C, Vignal A, Morissette J, Millasseau P, Vaysseix G, Lathrop M: A second-generation linkage map of the human genome. *Nature* **359**:794, 1992.

134. NIH/CEPH Collaborative Mapping Group: A comprehensive genetic linkage map of the human genome. *Science* **258**:67, 1992.

135. Nakafuku M, Nagamine M, Ohtoshi A, Tanaka K, Toh E-A, Kaziro Y: Suppression of oncogenic Ras by mutant neurofibromatosis type 1 genes. *Proc Natl Acad Sci USA* **90**:6706, 1993.

136. Malicki J, Clanetti LC, Peschle C, McGinnis W: A human HOX4B regulatory element provides head-specific expression in *Drosophila* embryos. *Nature* **358**:345, 1992.

137. Cotton RGH: Current methods of mutation detection. *Mutat Res* **285**:125, 1993.

138. Grompe M: The rapid detection of unknown mutations in nucleic acids. *Nat Genet* **5**:111, 1993.

139. Dianzani I, Camaschella C, Ponzone A, Cotton RGH: Dilemmas and progress in mutation detection. *Trends Genet* **9**:403, 1993.

140. Darling SM, Abbott CM: Mouse models of human single gene disorders I: Non-transgenic mice. *Bioassays* **14**:359, 1992.

141. Johnson PR, Greenwood MRC, Horwitz BA, Stern JS: Animal model of obesity: Genetic aspects. *Annu Rev Nutr* **11**:325, 1991.

142. Frohman MA, Martin GR: Cut, paste, and save: New approaches to altering specific genes in mice. *Cell* **56**:145, 1989.

143. Capecchi M: Altering the genome by homologous recombination. *Science* **244**:1288, 1989.

144. Smithies O: Animal models of human genetic diseases. *Trends Genet* **9**:112, 1993.

145. Sedivy JM, Joyner AL: *Gene Targeting*. New York, Freeman, 1980.

146. McDonald JD, Bode VC, Dove WF, Shedlovsky A: Pah^hph-5: A mouse mutant deficient in phenylalanine hydroxylase. *Proc Natl Acad Sci USA* **87**:1965, 1990.

147. Lawn RM, Wade DP, Hammer RE, Cheisa G, Verstuyft JG, Rubin EM: Atherogenesis in trangenic mice expressing apolipoprotein(a). *Nature* **360**:670, 1992.

148. Jacenko O, LuValle PA, Olsen BR: Spondylometaphyseal dysplasia in mice carrying a dominant negative mutation in a matrix protein specific for cartilage-to-bone transition. *Nature* **365**:56, 1993.

149. Fuchs E, Esteves RA, Coulombe PA: Trangenic mice expressing a mutant keratin 10 gene reveal the likely genetic basis for epidermolytic hyperkeratosis. *Proc Natl Acad Sci USA* **89**:6906, 1992.

150. Lyon M, Searle AG: *Genetic Variants and Strains of the Laboratory Mouse* 2d ed. New York, Oxford University Press, 1989.

151. Hogan B, Costantini F, Lacy E: *Manipulating the Mouse Embryo: A Laboratory Manual*. Cold Spring Harbor, Cold Spring Harbor Laboratory, 1986.

152. Fuchs E, Coulombe PA: Of mice and men: Genetic skin diseases of keratin. *Cell* **69**:899, 1992.

153. Breslow JL: Transgenic mouse models of lipoprotein metabolism and atherosclerosis. *Proc Natl Acad Sci USA* **90**:8314, 1993.

154. Copeland NG, Jenkins NA, Gilbert DJ, Eppig JT, Maltais LJ, Miller JC, Dietrich WF, Weaver A, Lincoln SE, Steen RG, Stein LD, Nadeau JH, Lander ES: A genetic linkage map of the mouse: Current applications and future prospects. *Science* **262**:57, 1993.

155. Giebel LB, Spritz RA: Mutation of the KIT (mast/stem cell growth factor receptor) protooncogene in human piebaldism. *Proc Natl Acad Sci USA* **88**:8696, 1991.

156. Fleischman RA: Human piebald trait resulting from a dominant negative mutant allele of the c-kit membrane receptor gene. *J Clin Invest* **89**:1713, 1992.

157. Cicila GT, Rapp JP, Wang J-M, St. Lezin E, Ng SC, Kurtz TW: Linkage of 11β-hydroxylase mutations with altered steroid biosynthesis and blood pressure in the Dahl rat. *Nature Genet* **3**:346, 1993.

158. Brown MS, Goldstein JL: Koch's postulates for cholesterol. *Cell* **71**:187, 1992.

159. Scott J: Arterial hardening in mice. *Nature* **360**:631, 1992.

160. Erickson RP: Why isn't a mouse more like a man? *Trends Genet* **5**:1, 1989.

161. Chowdhury JR, Grossman M, Gupta S, Chowdhury NR, Baker JR Jr, Wilson JM: Long term improvement of hypercholesterolemia after ex vivo gene therapy in LDLR-deficient rabbits. *Science* **254**:1802, 1991.

162. Ishibashi S, Brown MS, Goldstein JL, Gerard RD, Hammer RE, Herz J: Hypercholesterolemia in low density lipoprotein receptor knockout mice and its reversal by adenovirus-mediated gene delivery. *J Clin Invest* **92**:883, 1993.

163. Hyde SC, Gill DR, Higgins CF, Trezise AEO, MacVinish LJ, Cuthbert AW, Ratcliff R, Evans MJ, Colleldge WH: Correction of the ion transport defect in cystic fibrosis transgenic mice by gene therapy. *Nature* **362**:250, 1993.

164. Jones SN, Grompe M, Munir MI, Veres G, Craigen WJ, Caskey CT: Ectopic correction of ornithine transcarbamylase deficiency in sparse fur mice. *J Biol Chem* **265**:14684, 1990.

165. Morsy MA, Alford EL, Bett A, Graham FL, Caskey CT: Efficient adenoviral-mediated ornithine transcarbamylase expression in deficient mouse and human heptocytes. *J Clin Invest* **92**:1580, 1993.

166. Kay MA, Rothenberg S, Landen CN, Bellinger DA, Leland F, Toman C, Finegold M, Thompson AR, Read MS, Brinkhous KM, Woo SLC: In vivo gene therapy of hemophilia B: Sustained partial correction in factor IX-deficient dogs. *Science* **262**:117, 1993.

166a. Birkenmeier EH, Ben-Zeev O, Schotz MC, Sweet HO, Davisson MT, Gordon JI: Murine mucopolysaccharidosis type VII. Characterization of a mouse with β-glucuronidase deficiency. *J Clin Invest* **83**:1258, 1989.

167. Wolfe JH, Sands MS, Barker JE. Gwynn B, Rowe LB, Vogler CA, Birkenmeier EH: Reversal of pathology in murine mucopolysaccharidosis type VII by somatic gene cell transfer. *Nature* **360**:749, 1992.

168. Birkenmeier EH, Barker JE, Vogler CA, Kyle JW, Sly WS: Increased life span and correction of metabolic defects in murine mucopolysaccharidosis type VII after syngeneic bone marrow transplantation. *Blood* **78**:3081, 1991.

169. Kyle JW, Birkenmeier EH, Gwynn B, Vogler C, Hoppe PC, Hoffman JW, Sly WS: Correction of murine mucopolysaccharidosis VII by human beta-glucuronidase transgene. *Proc Natl Acad Sci USA* **87**:3914, 1990.

170. Moullier P, Bohl D, Heard J-M, Danos O: Correction of lysosomal storage in the liver and spleen of MPS VII mice by implantation of genetically modified skin fibroblasts. *Nat Genet* **4**:154, 1993.

CHAPTER 2

The Human Genome Project and Its Impact on the Study of Human Disease

Eric D. Green ▪ David R. Cox ▪ Richard M. Myers

1. For many human diseases, the fundamental defect resides in a simple alteration in the genome—the master "blueprint" of DNA that orchestrates the basic operation of a cell and an organism. Genetic studies often provide the ability to define at a molecular level the nature of such DNA alterations (i.e., mutations). Knowledge of the normal and abnormal forms of genes is invaluable for understanding the basis of many human genetic diseases.

2. The haploid human genome consists of ~3 billion bp of DNA that are distributed among 24 distinct chromosomes (22 autosomes and two sex chromosomes). Within this vast array of nucleotides is encoded an estimated 50,000 to 100,000 genes and the necessary elements that control the regulation of their expression.

3. Analyzing a genome involves the construction of various types of maps that reflect different features of the DNA, with the major classes being cytogenetic maps, physical maps, and genetic maps. The highest-resolution physical map is the DNA sequence map, which reflects the precise order of nucleotides along the chromosome. Important technologic advances have produced a number of powerful methods that greatly facilitate the ability to analyze genomes.

4. The Human Genome Project (HGP) is a large, coordinated effort to elucidate the genetic architecture of the genomes of human and, in parallel, several model organisms. The initial phase of this endeavor involves the establishment of relatively low-resolution maps of these genomes, with the long-term goal of determining their precise nucleotide sequences and identifying the encoded genes.

5. The products of the HGP will provide a complete working knowledge of the organization of human DNA and that of several model organisms as well as an "infrastructure" (in the form of biologic, informational, and technologic tools) that will markedly advance the sophistication level of many areas of biomedical inquiry. From a clinical viewpoint, this infrastructure will facilitate the identification and characterization of genes that directly and indirectly lead to human disease, thereby improving the ability to diagnose and treat affected individuals.

GENETICS AS A PARADIGM FOR STUDYING HUMAN BIOLOGY AND DISEASE

Diseases are associated with alterations of normal biologic processes and can be caused by infectious agents, environmental influences, inherent genetic anomalies, or combinations of these factors. Human disease classically is studied by comparing affected tissues with their unaffected counterparts. Such studies may reveal biochemical and physiological differences, and this information can, in some cases, be used to formulate prospective therapies. Although this paradigm has led to the successful treatment of many diseases, it frequently fails to identify the fundamental etiology of the disease. Indeed, the differences observed in affected tissues are often owing to secondary effects rather than consequences of the primary defect. However, in cases where changes in the DNA sequence are responsible for the disorder, it is possible to identify the fundamental defect by a completely different route. Studying diseases by a genetic approach takes advantage of the fact that all human beings have an almost identical DNA "blueprint." Alterations (or mutations) at one or a few positions in the DNA sequence of this blueprint are necessary and sufficient to cause the symptoms of certain genetic diseases. The identification of such causative mutations provides an opportunity to study and understand the fundamental biologic defect of the disease.

In humans, genetic studies often start by identifying traits, usually diseases, that appear to cluster in families. Of course, not all diseases that appear multiple times in the same family are genetic in origin, and possible contributions from nongenetic factors must also be considered. In the case of familial disorders, the challenge resides in identifying what is often a single base pair change among the ~3 billion bp in the haploid genome. Causative mutations for only a few of the thousands of human genetic diseases have been identified by using hints from physiological or biochemical differences between affected and unaffected individuals. Because this approach is difficult to apply to the majority of genetic diseases, an alternative strategy, called "positional cloning," has been developed that allows the identification of disease genes without relying on knowledge or suppositions about the gene product.[1-5] In this strategy, disease genes are isolated on the basis of their location in the genome (see Background on Positional Cloning, below).

A positional cloning strategy has been used to isolate the genes for numerous genetic diseases (see http://www.ncbi.nlm.nih.

gov/dbEST/dbEST_genes), including relatively common ones such as cystic fibrosis,[6-8] Huntington disease,[9] and hereditary hemochromatosis.[10] To date, however, the strategy has been successfully applied to those diseases caused by defects in a single gene. Many common diseases (e.g., cancer, cardiovascular, autoimmune, psychiatric) have a genetic etiology, but the inheritance is complex, such that mutations in more than one gene are likely required to produce the phenotype.[11,12] Such genes are extremely difficult to identify by use of a traditional positional cloning approach. In addition to the problem of identifying multiple genes, these diseases are complicated by the frequent absence of a strict correlation between genotype and phenotype; instead an interplay exists between genetic and environmental factors. Nevertheless, there is hope that new experimental technologies can be used in conjunction with powerful statistical tools to better understand these complex diseases.[11,12] If this turns out to be the case, advances in genetics will have an even greater effect on human health.

All the steps involved in disease gene isolation are labor-intensive and require the marshaling of extensive resources and a variety of skills. A central rationale for the Human Genome Project (HGP)—an intense, international effort to map, clone, and sequence all of the DNA in the human genome—is to simplify the task of identifying disease genes.[13-16] In this chapter, we discuss how the knowledge and materials generated by the HGP and related efforts are being used to advance our understanding of genetic diseases and human biology, including cancer. Because it is important that the reader is aware of some basic concepts and the language of the geneticist, we first provide some background on DNA structure and function, the general "anatomy" of the human genome, and information about genes and other relevant sequences. The major emphasis of the chapter is to describe the experimental approaches that are being used to generate maps, to determine DNA sequences, to find genes, and to identify mutations that are responsible for disease. The strategic basis of the HGP and how this concerted endeavor is impacting the study of genetic diseases and other biological problems is discussed. We also describe the important role of studying the genomes of model organisms and how this has facilitated the development of technologies for genomic analysis and for elucidating gene function. Finally, the potential effects of the HGP on the diagnosis and treatment of genetic diseases are outlined, and the important ethical, legal, and social issues that are coming to the forefront as a consequence of the HGP are highlighted.

STRUCTURE AND ORGANIZATION OF THE HUMAN GENOME

DNA Basics

DNA is a macromolecule composed of a linear array of deoxyribonucleotides, each of which consists of three components: a nitrogenous base, a sugar (deoxyribose), and phosphate. Each base is linked to adjacent bases on the same strand by the sugar and phosphate groups. The bases in DNA are either purines [adenine (A) and guanine (G)] or pyrimidines [cytosine (C) and thymine (T)], and together these nucleotides constitute the "four-letter alphabet" of DNA that is universal among organisms. In the Watson-Crick helical structure of double-stranded DNA, first reported in 1953,[17] pairing occurs between a purine base on one strand and a pyrimidine base on the opposite strand (G pairs with C, A pairs with T), thereby making each strand complementary to the other. It is the order of these bases that encodes the genetic information contained within DNA. Physical lengths of DNA are frequently

discussed in individual base pairs (bp), thousands of base pairs (kilobase pairs, or kb), or millions of base pairs (megabase pairs, or Mb). An excellent source of background information on DNA biochemistry and recombinant *DNA* technology is *Recombinant DNA* by Watson et al.[18]

General Structure of the Human Genome

The human genome contains ~3,000 Mb of DNA[19] (Figure 2-1) divided among 22 autosomes and 2 sex chromosomes (X and Y), which range in size from ~50 to 260 Mb,[19] as well as the DNA present in mitochondria.[19] Human somatic cells are typically diploid (containing 22 pairs of autosomes and one pair of sex chromosomes), whereas germ cells (i.e., sperm and egg) are haploid (containing a single copy of each autosome and one sex chromosome). The physical length of DNA contained in each human cell is remarkably large, theoretically stretching out to a length of about 1 meter if fully "unpacked" from its associated proteins. The amount of encoded information within the genome is even

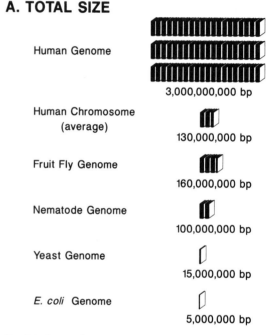

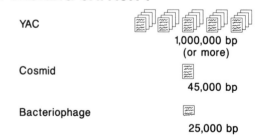

FIG. 2-1 Relative sizes of genomes, chromosomes, and cloned DNA segments. *A.* The estimated total sizes of the various DNA sources are indicated, along with schematic representations using books that contain the written DNA sequence. Each book represents ~50 million bp of DNA. *B.* The total cloning capacities of a YAC, a cosmid, and a bacteriophage clone are indicated, along with schematic representations using pages of books that contain the written DNA sequence. Each page represents ~50,000 bp of DNA, which reflects about 16-times the number of characters on a typical page of this book. *(Adapted from Green and Waterston.[13] Used by permission.)*

more daunting. In fact, a listing of the nucleotide sequence of the ~3,000 Mb in single-letter symbols (G, A, T, C) would fill ~13 sets of the *Encyclopaedia Britannica*[20] or ~750 megabytes of computer disk space.[21]

Subchromosomal Organization of Human DNA

Structural Components of Chromosomes. Human chromosomes are highly organized structures. At the molecular ends of each chromosome are telomeres, sequences thought to stabilize the chromosome, prevent fusion with other DNA, and permit DNA replication without loss of chromosomal material.[22] The DNA within a telomere consists of stretches of highly reiterated, simple repeats, with the predominant motif in human telomeres being 5′TTAGGG3′.[23] Various human telomeres have been isolated in cloned form,[24–30] allowing more precise dissection of their molecular features and corresponding function. Each chromosome also contains a single centromere, defined functionally by the site of attachment of the spindle apparatus during mitosis.[22] Human centromeres contain large blocks of repetitive DNA, called "alphoid DNA,"[31–33] which, together with other sequences, span for several megabases. Like telomeres, the cloning and characterization of human centromeric DNA will likely provide greater insight about the role of specific repetitive sequences in chromosome function.

Interspersed Repetitive DNA Sequences. In contrast to the large and extended blocks of repetitive DNA present in human telomeres and centromeres, most of the remaining regions of human chromosomes are associated with repetitive sequences that are interspersed among unique segments of DNA. The two major classes of interspersed repeated sequences in human DNA are the short interspersed nucleotide element (SINE) and the long interspersed nucleotide element (LINE). The major SINE is the *Alu* sequence, a ~300-bp segment that is estimated to be present on average every 3 to 10 kb (occurring upwards of 10^6 times in the genome). The major LINE is the L1 sequence, a segment that spans up to 6.4 kb in length. Often, only a portion of an L1 sequence is found at a particular site, with an estimated 10^4 to 10^5 L1 copies (complete or partial) present in the genome. Together, *Alu* and L1 sequences are thought to account for 10 to 20 percent of human DNA. In general, copies of the same repeat (*Alu* or L1) present at different sites in the genome are very similar in sequence (but typically not identical). However, prototypic "consensus" sequences have been established for the most common human repeats,[34] thereby allowing their identification within stretches of human DNA sequence.

Coding versus Noncoding DNA. Within the human genome are an estimated 50,000 to 100,000 genes, which can be as small as 100 bp (e.g., tRNA[Tyr] gene) to over 2.3 Mb (e.g., dystrophin gene). However, most human genes are thought to be between 1 and 200 kb in size. The coding portions of genes represent a small component of genomic DNA. In fact, some estimates predict that less than 10 percent of human DNA reflects coding sequences and their regulatory elements;[35,36] however, a more precise assessment of this figure awaits more detailed analysis. The remaining noncoding DNA in the human genome consists of repetitive and other sequences whose importance is not completely understood and likely not fully appreciated.

Gene Structure. Human genes (also called "transcription units") are complex structures containing several major compo-

nents. Exons are the segments of DNA in a gene that include the sequences that encode amino acids. Between adjacent exons of the same gene are intervening sequences known as introns, which in some cases may extend for hundreds of kilobase pairs. Following generation of the corresponding messenger RNA (mRNA) from a gene by transcription, the introns are removed from the mRNA in a series of steps known as splicing. The processed mRNA is then used to direct the sequential and precise addition of amino acids to yield a specific polypeptide chain by a process known as translation. Because different mRNAs can be produced from the same gene by alternate splicing of the primary transcript, there are likely a larger number of gene products being made than there are genes, thereby adding to the complex and combinatorial nature of the genome. Interestingly, some introns have been found to contain whole, smaller genes transcribed from the DNA strand opposite to that used for expression of the larger gene.[37,38] Also associated with genes are adjacent regulatory sequences (including promoters, enhancers, inhibitory sequences, and others) that interact with cellular proteins and other components to determine when, where, and to what level transcription (i.e., gene expression) occurs.

CpG Islands. The dinucleotide CpG (i.e., 5′CG3′) is relatively underrepresented in the human genome (in contrast to the dinucleotide GpC). Among the various enzymes that cleave DNA at precise sequences (called "restriction enzymes") is a class that cuts relatively infrequently within the human genome (called "rare cutters"), most of which contain a CpG dinucleotide within their recognition sequence. Many such rare-cutting restriction enzymes will not cleave the DNA if the nucleotides within the recognition sequence have been modified by the addition of a methyl group (i.e., if they are methylated). Interestingly, at the 5′ end of many human genes are DNA segments that contain an overabundance of unmethylated CpG dinucleotides.[39] These genomic regions are called "CpG islands" (or "HTF islands" for "*Hpa*II tiny fragments," since numerous small DNA fragments are produced from such segments by digestion with the restriction enzyme *Hpa*II). Thus, a major site for cleavage by methylation-sensitive, rare-cutting restriction enzymes are undermethylated CpG islands that essentially "mark" the 5′ ends of many (but not all) genes.[39]

Distribution of Genes, CpG Islands, and Repetitive DNA. The distribution of genes, CpG islands, and interspersed repetitive sequences is not uniform across human chromosomes. Rather, several interesting patterns that provide some insight about chromosomal organization are evident.[40,41] Chromosome preparations can be stained with various agents and examined microscopically; for example, revealing the presence of lighter- and darker-staining regions (or bands) following Giemsa staining (see Cytogenetic Maps, below). There is evidence that Giemsa-negative (light) bands tend to harbor a greater proportion of housekeeping and tissue-specific genes, contain a greater frequency of CpG islands, consist of DNA sequence with a higher GC content, and have more SINEs. In contrast, Giemsa-positive (dark) bands tend to harbor fewer genes, contain a lower frequency of CpG islands, consist of DNA sequence with a lower GC content, and have more LINEs. Another level of chromosomal organization is the grouping of DNA into blocks that span over 300 kb in length with relatively homogeneous GC compositions, referred to as "isochores." Interestingly, the composition of genes in different isochores is not uniform, with the highest gene content being associated with the GC-richest isochores.[42–44] Furthermore, there is evidence that many of the isochores containing the most genes are located near the ends of human chromosomes (in the subtelomeric regions).[44,45]

CRITICAL TECHNOLOGIES FOR GENOME MAPPING

Central to the HGP has been the development of a number of technologies that are critical for analyzing genomes. A basic understanding of these methods and approaches is necessary to comprehend the experimental bases of most current genome mapping and sequencing efforts. Virtually all of the techniques described in the following represent standard tools in the armamentarium of investigators performing genome analysis and searching for human disease genes.

Basic Recombinant DNA Techniques

The isolation and characterization of DNA involve the utilization of a fundamental set of experimental techniques that have been refined over the past two decades.[46] Most often, the source DNA (e.g., human DNA) is purified and fragmented to yield more manageable-sized pieces. The tools most often used for the latter step are restriction enzymes, each of which cleaves double-stranded DNA at a defined sequence of nucleotides. The size of the recognition sequence varies among restriction enzymes (typically, 4–8 nucleotides), with those requiring a fewer number of nucleotides cutting more often than those requiring a greater number (the latter being the rare cutters described in CpG Islands, above). Often, it is necessary to reproduce one or more of the resulting DNA fragments, thereby obtaining sufficient quantities for detailed studies. One way this can be done is by "cloning," whereby foreign DNA is inserted into a rapidly growing organism that is "tricked" into synthesizing the incorporated DNA along with its own. Another way DNA can be reproduced is by PCR.

Polymerase Chain Reaction

Few experimental techniques have made as dramatic an impact on as many biomedical areas as the polymerase chain reaction (PCR).[47–49] In the simplest view, PCR involves the in vitro enzymatic synthesis of large amounts of a specific DNA sequence. The target DNA is defined by two short (typically 18–25 bases), single-stranded oligonucleotides ("primers") that anneal to complementary sequences on opposite strands of the template DNA and initiate ("prime") synthesis back towards one another. The synthesized DNA thus consists of the two oligonucleotides and the sequence between them. Following DNA synthesis, the sample is heated (to > 90°C), causing the double-stranded DNA molecules to become single-stranded (denature). On cooling, unused oligonucleotides (which are present in excess) anneal to available target DNA molecules, and DNA synthesis is once again allowed to proceed.

The standard cycle of events (DNA synthesis, denaturation, primer annealing) is sequentially repeated 25 to 40 times, with the products of each cycle serving as templates during subsequent cycles. Such a scheme results in the exponential accumulation (or amplification) of the target DNA sequence defined by the two flanking primers, with the production of as many as a million copies of the DNA product. The size of the DNA segment that can be amplified typically is between 60 and 4000 bp, although larger DNA stretches (upwards of 10–30 kb) can be amplified under special conditions. It is important to stress that the critical aspect of PCR is the specificity of the oligonucleotide primers. The ability to amplify a particular DNA segment often depends on selecting an appropriate pair of primers that will uniquely and faithfully anneal to the target DNA sequence under the proper conditions, even when present in a complex mixture such as a whole genome.

Like other areas of molecular biology, several important advances have catalyzed the explosive growth of PCR in genome research.[50–52] These include: (1) the purification of a number of thermostable DNA polymerases (including the cloning of some of the corresponding genes), which allow the repeated cycles of DNA synthesis to occur by simple thermal cycling without the need to add fresh enzyme after each denaturation step;[53] (2) the development of more efficient and automated methods for chemically synthesizing oligonucleotide primers; and (3) the construction of more advanced instrumentation that improves the efficiency with which PCR assays can be subjected to thermal cycling. As a result, PCR now represents a routine technique utilized in virtually all genetic studies as well as an increasing number of clinical laboratories. In addition, because of its speed, high sensitivity, and suitability for automation, PCR is being used to perform a wide array of tasks inherent to the study of genomes.[50–52]

DNA Cloning Systems

Standard Bacterial Cloning Systems. Traditional DNA cloning systems are based in prokaryotic cells, typically the bacterium *Escherichia coli*. For example, plasmids are extrachromosomal DNA molecules that can be engineered to contain relatively small (typically less than 10 kb) pieces of exogenous DNA.[46] A modified form of plasmids, called "cosmids," can accommodate cloned DNA segments upwards of 40 to 45 kb in size (Figure 2-1).[46,54] Bacteriophages are viruses that infect bacteria, and certain types, such as phage lambda, can be modified to carry up to 25 kb of foreign DNA (Figure 2-1).[46] Because of their capacity for "intermediate" amounts of cloned DNA, cosmid (and to some extent bacteriophage) clones have played a major role in genome mapping for a number of years. For example, strategies for utilizing cosmids to isolate and map extended intervals of human chromosomes have been developed and implemented for several targeted genomic regions;[55–60] however, these efforts have rarely resulted in contiguous cloned coverage extending much beyond 300 to 500 kb (which represents a minor fraction of even the smallest human chromosome; see Figure 2-1). Nonetheless, cosmid and bacteriophage clones serve a critical supplementary role in the study of human DNA and the isolation of genes of interest.

Yeast Artificial Chromosomes. The yeast artificial chromosome (YAC) cloning system was developed in 1987[61] to allow the isolation and study of DNA segments that are significantly larger than those cloned in traditional bacterial-based systems.[62–65] In this case, the host is the yeast *Saccharomyces cerevisiae* (a eukaryotic cell), and the cloned DNA is contained within a linear artificial chromosome (rather than an extrachromosomal DNA molecule) (Figure 2-2). The cloned DNA contained in YACs can range in size from less than 100 kb to over 1,000 kb, which is ~10 to 20 times larger than the capacity of standard bacterial cloning systems (Figure 2-1). A number of large, comprehensive YAC libraries have been constructed from human genomic DNA,[66–71] and these clones have been used extensively for mapping various regions of the human genome.[72–95] YAC libraries have also been constructed for use in studying the genomes of other organisms, such as the mouse,[71,96–98] the nematode worm *Caenorhabditis elegans*,[99,100] the fruit fly *Drosophila melanogaster*,[101] the plant *Arabidopsis thaliana*,[102] and many others. Screening YAC libraries for

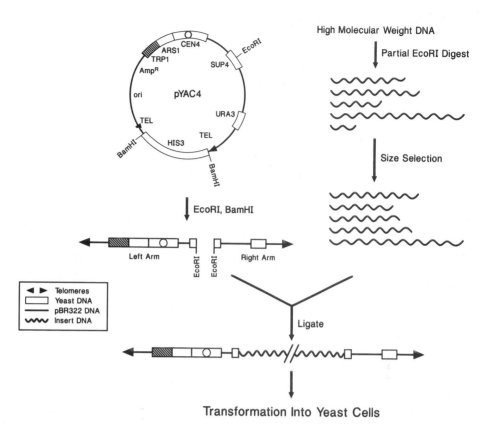

FIG. 2-2 Yeast artificial chromosome (YAC) cloning system. The YAC cloning vector (shown here is pYAC4, although others have been developed) contains all of the structural elements necessary for the propagation of a chromosome in yeast. In this case, digestion of the plasmid vector with *Eco*RI and *Bam*HI yields two vector arms (left and right), each containing appropriate telomere sequences and yeast selectable markers. The left (but not the right) vector arm also contains appropriate sequences for centromere function (CEN4) and the initiation of DNA replication (ARS1). For cloning into YACs, high-molecular-weight DNA (e.g., human DNA) is carefully prepared, partially digested with a restriction enzyme (e.g., *Eco*RI in the case of the pYAC4 vector), and size selected to yield large DNA fragments. The insert DNA and vector arms are then ligated, and the resulting material is transformed into appropriately prepared yeast cells. The system is designed such that the only yeast cells that grow are those that have incorporated a DNA molecule consisting of a left vector arm, a right vector arm, and a cloned DNA segment between them. *(Adapted from Burke et al.[61] Used by permission.)*

clones of interest was initially performed by the traditional approach of DNA–DNA hybridization with a specific probe.[67] However, a strategy for identifying YACs within complex libraries using PCR was developed[103] and now represents the most common approach for screening YAC libraries.

Several features of YAC cloning make it well-suited for use in isolating and mapping large genomic regions. First, by providing a means to obtain larger pieces of cloned DNA, YACs simplify the process of constructing maps of extended chromosomal regions and of isolating large genes in an intact form. This capability has been demonstrated for a number of regions of the human genome with particular medical relevance, including the isolation of YACs spanning the cystic fibrosis gene on chromosome 7,[72,73] the dystrophin gene on the X chromosome,[74,75] the HLA class I segment on chromosome 6,[76] the Huntington disease gene on chromosome 4, and many others.[77,78] A second important feature of YAC cloning is the ability to use the yeast host for reconstructing large human genes by the sequential "pasting" together (recombination) of smaller, overlapping YACs, as has been performed to yield single YACs containing the entire 250-kb cystic fibrosis gene,[72] the 230-kb *BCL2* protooncogene,[104] and the 2.3-Mb dystrophin gene.[105] Finally, as a eukaryote, yeast seems to provide a more hospitable environment for replicating some of the DNA of other eukaryotes and, hence, is capable of cloning certain DNA segments that were previously unclonable in bacteria.[99,100] For these various reasons, YAC cloning represents the most widely utilized system for isolating and mapping human chromosomes.

YAC cloning is not, however, without its associated problems. One disadvantage is the difficulty in purifying large amounts of YAC DNA away from the endogenous yeast DNA. Thus, it often becomes necessary to isolate smaller-insert, bacterial-based clones corresponding to the YAC insert prior to performing manipulations such as DNA sequencing, gene identification, and other routine experimental procedures. A more troubling problem associated with YACs is the frequent presence of two unrelated

segments of DNA within a single cloned insert. Such "chimeric" YACs constitute half (or more) of the clones in many libraries made from human genomic DNA.[106] Although chimeric clones do not prevent the utilization of YACs for mapping large regions of human DNA, they can hinder the efficiency and accuracy with which the maps are constructed. A major mechanism by which chimeric YACs form involves recombination between homologous regions (e.g., repetitive DNA) present in unrelated DNA segments.[106] Such yeast-based recombination events likely lead to another problem observed with YACs—the deletion of internal segments of the cloned insert. In the case of chimeric YACs, two different approaches have been successfully utilized to decrease the problem: (1) the construction of YACs from individual human chromosomes isolated from the remainder of the human genome either by recovery in a human-rodent hybrid cell line (see Somatic Hybrid Cell Lines, below), which requires subsequent screening for the human DNA-containing YACs that exist within a background of rodent DNA containing YACs,[107–112] or by separation using the technique of flow-sorting (see Generation of STSs, below)[113]; and (2) the use of recombination-defective yeast strains as hosts.[97,114] The latter approach also has proven effective at reducing the occurrence of internal deletions in YAC inserts.

Larger-Insert Bacterial Cloning Systems. The described limitations with YAC cloning are related directly to the use of yeast as the host system. Thus, there is significant interest in establishing and refining cloning systems that provide a large cloning capacity but that are based in bacteria (thereby allowing the convenient purification of large amounts of the cloned DNA). Among these are the bacteriophage P1 system, with a cloning capacity of ~75 to 100 kb[115–117] as well as the bacterial artificial chromosome (BAC)[118] and P1-derived artificial chromosome (PAC)[119] systems, both with cloning capacities upwards of 200 to 300 kb. In particular, BACs and PACs are increasingly being used for mapping and sequencing human DNA.

Pulsed-Field Gel Electrophoresis

An important adjunct technology that played a critical role in the development of YACs and other large-insert DNA cloning systems is a technique that allows the separation of large DNA molecules. Conventional approaches for gel electrophoresis (typically in agarose gels) can resolve DNA molecules that are up to ~50 kb in size; however, such techniques are incapable of separating significantly larger DNA fragments. To overcome this limitation, methods have been developed whereby the direction of the electric field applied to the DNA within an agarose gel is periodically alternated.[120–122] This technique, called "pulsed-field gel electrophoresis," can be used to separate DNA fragments up to ~10 Mb in size. Numerous refinements and modifications of the basic approaches for pulsed-field gel electrophoresis have been made, making it a routine and straightforward method.[123] As a result, pulsed-field gel electrophoresis has been utilized to study the genomes of model organisms such as yeast,[124,125] to establish long-range restriction maps of human DNA by using rare-cutting restriction enzymes,[126–130] to characterize the DNA in large-insert clones such as YACs,[61,131–133] and to detect certain types of mutations causing human genetic diseases.[134]

Fluorescence In Situ Hybridization

An important step in the characterization of a cloned DNA segment is the identification of the approximate site in the genome from which it originated (e.g., its location on a particular chromosome). The most direct route for obtaining such information involves hybridizing the DNA segment to preparations of intact chromosomes from metaphase cells using protocols that allow the structural features of the condensed chromosomes to be preserved.[135–137] If the DNA probe is labeled appropriately, microscopic examination of the chromosomes can be used to identify the position(s) of hybridization, thereby allowing assignment of the DNA to a particular subchromosomal region. Previously, radioactive labels were employed, which required lengthy exposure of the chromosomes to film and resulted in poor precision of the chromosomal assignments. Major advances in this technology have occurred in recent years, and these have included the use of fluorescent tags to label the DNA probes and fluorescence microscopy to establish the positions of hybridization,[138] a technique referred to as "fluorescence in situ hybridization (FISH)" (Figure 2-3).[138]

Continued improvements in the protocols used for performing FISH analysis have greatly enhanced the technology. In general, the basic approaches have become more efficient and reliable, making them easier to implement.[135,136,139,140] The ability to resolve closely spaced DNA segments has also improved. For example, standard FISH analysis with metaphase-chromosome preparations can be used to discriminate between regions separated by ~5 to 10 Mb.[139,140] However, with fluorescent tags of different colors and the use of interphase cells (with their highly extended chromosomes), more closely spaced DNA segments can be resolved, in some cases those only ~100 kb (or less) apart.[141–143] Since FISH analysis provides the means to establish the position of a cloned DNA segment relative to the source chromosome, this technique is playing an important role in genome mapping by spatially organizing clones being used for constructing long-range maps of human chromosomes (see Cytogenetic Maps, below).

Chromosome Microdissection

A useful approach for isolating DNA segments from cytogenetically defined regions of a genome is chromosome microdissec-

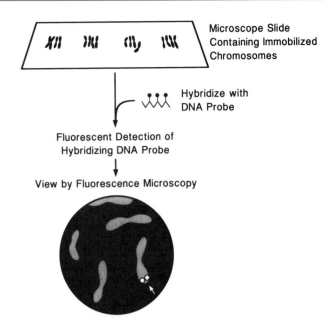

FIG. 2-3 Establishing the chromosomal position of a DNA segment by fluorescence in situ hybridization (FISH). Intact chromosomes from cells at metaphase are carefully immobilized on a microscope slide. An appropriate DNA probe (e.g., genomic clone) is labeled with a detectable moiety, such as biotin (depicted as dark circles) and hybridized to the immobilized chromosomes. The position(s) of the hybridizing DNA probe is then detected by using an appropriate fluorescence-based system (e.g., fluorescently labeled avidin, which binds to biotin). Using fluorescence microscopy, the hybridizing probe (indicated by the white arrow) typically appears as two bright yellow spots (one on each chromatid) against an orange background of the chromosome. The approximate chromosomal position of the hybridizing probe can be assessed by parallel examination of the same metaphase chromosomes following appropriate staining. *(Adapted from Hozier and Davis.[135] Used by permission.)*

tion. In this method, cytogenetically distinct subchromosomal regions are microscopically excised and isolated from the remaining genomic DNA. Although microdissection was initially applied to the large and more easily manipulated polytene chromosomes of the fruit fly *D. melanogaster,*[144] (see Studying the Genomes of Model Organisms, below), the application of PCR has markedly enhanced the power of this approach, allowing its use with human DNA.[144] For example, DNA can be microdissected from a single band of a human chromosome, appropriately processed, and amplified by PCR (Figure 2-4).[145–148] The resulting amplified DNA can then be subcloned and individual clones used as hybridization probes or DNA sequencing templates (see Generation of Sequence-Tagged Sites, below). Microdissection-based strategies can be used to isolate targeted segments of the human genome, for example, from regions that are poorly represented by existing markers.

Somatic Hybrid Cell Lines

Various somatic cell lines have been constructed that contain the entire genome of the host species (e.g., rodent) along with some amount of foreign DNA from another species (e.g., human). In particularly useful cases, the foreign DNA consists of a single, intact chromosome. For example, such monochromosomal human–rodent hybrid cell lines have been derived for virtually every human chromosome.[149] In some cases, sets of hybrid cell lines, each containing a defined portion (but not all) of a particular human chromosome, are also available. Human–rodent hybrid cell lines thus provide access to more limited parts of the human genome.

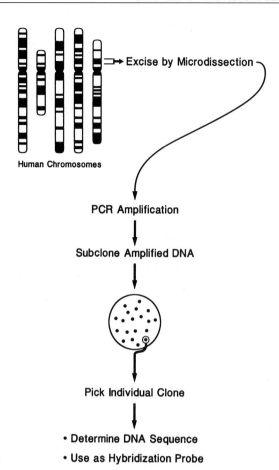

FIG. 2-4 Cytogenetically targeted isolation of DNA segments by chromosome microdissection. Human metaphase chromosomes are carefully prepared, stained, and examined microscopically. An appropriate band(s) is carefully cut (or scraped) away with a specialized micromanipulator, and the DNA carefully recovered. Either a single sample or multiple cuts of the same band from different copies of the chromosome are then used as template for PCR amplification. A number of different strategies for this amplification step have been described,[145–148] and these vary in the processing of the microdissected DNA and the choice of PCR primers. The amplified DNA is then subcloned into an appropriate vector, and individual clones are used for DNA sequencing (e.g., for subsequent STS development) or as hybridization probes.

Of course, the human DNA is not "pure," rather it is mixed within a background of the entire rodent genome (which is roughly the size of the human genome). The stability of human DNA within human–rodent hybrid cell lines varies widely, especially since there is often no selective pressure for the rodent cells to retain the human DNA. As a result, investigators must be cautious when using such cell lines, and this typically requires the routine assessment of the presence and intactness of the human chromosome (or fragment) in the cell line (e.g., by cytogenetic analysis). Human–rodent hybrid cell lines have been used extensively to generate genomic clones (e.g., cosmids, BACs, YACs) from more limited regions of the human genome. The resulting clones provide both direct access to the target DNA (see Yeast Artificial Chromosomes, above) and starting material for the development of new DNA markers (see Generation of Sequence-Tagged Sites, below).

DNA Sequencing

A number of techniques have been developed for determining the precise sequence of nucleotides within a stretch of DNA.

Some of these methods have been successfully utilized to establish extensive amounts of DNA sequence data, whereas others remain in more developmental stages.[150] The approach described by Sanger and coworkers in 1977,[151] termed "dideoxy chain-termination sequencing," is the most widely utilized sequencing method. This technique involves the in vitro synthesis of DNA molecules in the presence of artificial (dideoxy) nucleotides, which prevent chain extension when incorporated into the growing DNA strand. The resulting population of DNA molecules, which terminate at different nucleotide positions, are then analyzed by gel electrophoresis. The relative migration of the various DNA fragments can be used to deduce the overall sequence of the starting DNA template. Detection of the DNA fragments can be accomplished by incorporation of radioactive or fluorescent groups[152,153] into the DNA (Figure 2-5). Following radioactive sequencing, the gels are exposed to x-ray film to allow detection of the DNA fragments. In con-

A.

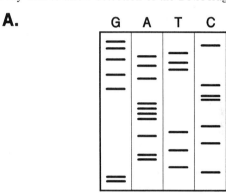

B.   GGCTAATCATCAAAACCGCAGTATGATGCG

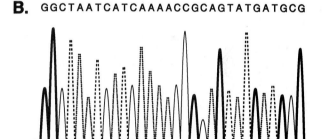

C.   GGCTAATCAT
CAAAACCGCA
GTATGATGCG

FIG. 2-5 DNA sequencing by the dideoxy chain-termination method. The dideoxy chain-termination method of DNA sequencing yields a population of DNA segments with different lengths, each terminated by a particular type of dideoxy nucleotide (i.e., G, A, T, or C) that "marks" the position of that base in the starting template.[151] The resulting products are then separated by gel electrophoresis. *A.* Detection of radioactively labeled DNA fragments by autoradiography is shown. In this case, each lane contains the DNA fragments generated with a single type of dideoxy nucleotide, with the presence of a band at a particular "rung" position of the sequencing "ladder" reflecting the base (G, A, T, or C, from left to right) at that position in the starting DNA template (the corresponding sequence is shown in panel C). *B.* Automated detection of fluorescently labeled DNA fragments is illustrated. In this case, a laser is used to detect the migration of the fluorescently labeled dideoxy-terminated DNA fragments[152] as they are electrophoresed through the gel. Each type of peak (indicated by thick, dotted, dashed, and thin lines) reflects the base (G, A, T, and C, respectively) at that position in the starting DNA template (the corresponding sequence is shown in panel C).

trast, fluorescent sequencing involves the automated, real-time detection of DNA fragments during electrophoresis by laser-based instrumentation.[152,154] At the present time, fluorescence-based dideoxy sequencing is the most commonly used approach for high-throughput generation of DNA sequence data.

GENOME MAPS: TYPES AND STRATEGIES FOR CONSTRUCTION

Genome maps are linear representations of DNA that reflect the organization of landmarks based on some coordinate system. The assembly of such maps is critical for attaining a global understanding of genome structure and function. There are three major classes of genome maps: cytogenetic maps, physical maps, and genetic maps (Figure 2-6). In each case, the coordinates that serve as the basis of the map are determined by the experimental methods used to measure the intervening distances between landmarks. Importantly, the various mapping approaches have characteristic resolution ranges (Figure 2-7) that dictate the utility of the resulting maps. The development of integrated cytogenetic, physical, and genetic maps represents a central activity of the HGP.

Cytogenetic Maps

A cytogenetic map represents the appearance of a chromosome when properly stained and examined microscopically. Particularly important is the resulting appearance of differentially staining bands that render each chromosome uniquely identifiable (Figures 2-6 and 2-7). Individual bands can be specifically discerned and are associated with well-defined names.[155] The most conventional cytogenetic maps depict the 23 chromosomes of the haploid human genome as containing a total of 350 to 500 bands at metaphase (with the amount of DNA split about equally between light and dark bands), with each band containing an average of ~5 to 10 Mb of DNA. More sophisticated, higher-resolution methods can be used to detect and represent over 1000 bands in the human genome.[135]

Cytogenetic maps have played a classic role in the diagnosis and study of human genetic diseases. A karyotype, for example, is a visual representation of an individual's chromosomes, which may reveal deletions, rearrangements, translocations, or other abnormalities. In some cases, the close association between such a cytogenetic abnormality and a particular genetic disorder has served as the starting point for the isolation of the defective gene [e.g., familial adenomatous polyposis (Chap. 31), retinoblastoma (Chap. 19), chronic granulomatous disease,[156] Duchenne muscular dystrophy,[157] fragile X syndrome[158]].

On the surface, cytogenetic maps would appear to have a limited role in genome mapping, in that they provide relatively low-resolution (e.g., ~5–10 Mb) representations of chromosomes (Figure 2-7) and they are "observational" in nature, providing neither cloned DNA for additional study nor significant assistance in obtaining it. However, cytogenetic mapping serves an important adjunct role in the construction of detailed genomic maps. By dividing the human genome into distinguishable units of ~5 to 10 Mb each, cytogenetic maps provide a framework for the construction of other types of maps. For example, cloned DNA segments can be assigned efficiently to individual chromosomal bands by FISH analysis (see FISH, above), thereby providing the ability to coalign (or integrate) other types of maps (e.g., physical and genetic) with the established cytogenetic maps.[159,160] Similarly, FISH analysis can be used to monitor the quality of the evolving physical maps. For example, while mapping a particular chromosomal region, newly obtained clones can be analyzed by FISH. Hybridization of the DNA to some other region of the genome would alert the investigator to a likely problem. In addition, the orientation of evolving maps with respect to the centromere and telomeres potentially can be established by FISH analysis using representative clones from each end of the map.[143] Thus, although the fundamental cytogenetic map of the human genome essentially is complete, efforts continue at localizing genes and other DNA segments to precise chromosomal positions by FISH analysis. The resulting information will facilitate the assembly of highly detailed maps of human chromosomes.

Physical Maps

Physical maps of DNA consist of ordered landmarks at known distances from one another (much like a travel map indicating distances between cities along a highway). The construction of phys-

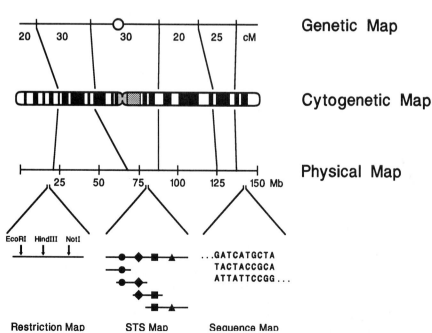

FIG. 2-6 Schematic representations of genetic, cytogenetic, and physical maps of a human chromosome. For the genetic map, the positions of several hypothetical genetic markers are indicated, along with the distances in centimorgans (cM) between them. The circle indicates the position of the centromere. For the cytogenetic map, the classic Giemsa-banding pattern of a chromosome is shown. For the physical map, the approximate physical locations of the above genetic markers are indicated, along with the relative distances between them in megabase pairs (Mb). The three types of physical maps (restriction, STS, and sequence) depicted along the bottom are discussed in the text. (*Adapted from Green and Waterston.[13] Used by permission.*)

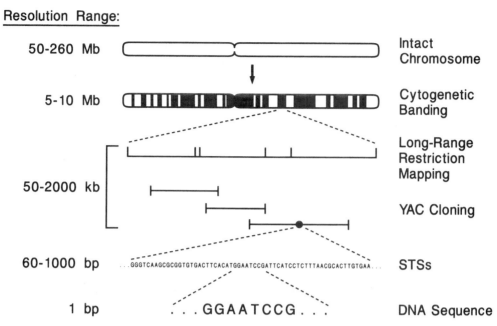

Resolution Range:

50-260 Mb	Intact Chromosome
5-10 Mb	Cytogenetic Banding
50-2000 kb	Long-Range Restriction Mapping
	YAC Cloning
60-1000 bp	STSs
1 bp	DNA Sequence

FIG. 2-7 Characteristic resolution ranges encountered in genome mapping. In the human genome, individual chromosomes range in size from ~50 to 260 Mb. When properly stained and examined microscopically, the characteristic cytogenetic banding pattern gives a unique appearance to each chromosome, with each band spanning ~5 to 10 Mb in length. Physical mapping techniques, such as long-range restriction mapping by pulsed-field gel electrophoresis (in conjunction with rare-cutting restriction enzymes) or YAC cloning, can provide analytical capabilities in the ~50 to 2000 kb size range. Individual DNA landmarks typically represent much smaller segments of DNA (e.g., ~60 to 1000 bp for an STS). The highest level of resolution is the single base pair of DNA sequence. *(Adapted from Rossiter and Caskey.[16] Used by permission.)*

ical maps is performed either on the total genomic DNA of an organism or after breaking down the genome into smaller pieces. The latter process involves the fragmentation and cloning of the DNA, whereby the DNA fragments can be purified in large amounts and more readily analyzed. However, by fragmenting the DNA, the order of the DNA segments is lost, leaving the challenge of putting the pieces back together to create a composite map. Hence, the analogy often is made to a jigsaw puzzle; however, a DNA mapping puzzle has some important differences. Instead of just one copy of every DNA fragment, many copies are present within a collection of clones. Also, the same DNA segment may be present on a number of different-sized, overlapping fragments (resulting from different "cuts" of the starting DNA).

In putting together the puzzle of a DNA region, individual pieces (or clones) are analyzed for landmarks and compared with other pieces. When a match is found, the two clones can be overlaid conceptually (or overlapped), and because the clones typically are not identical (only overlapping), a slightly larger segment is reconstructed. A set of ordered, overlapping clones is called a "contig," since the clones together reflect a contiguous segment of DNA, and information about the contig can be used to construct a contig map of the DNA. Neighboring contigs are often linked together in an effort to assemble larger contigs. Thus, a typical physical map consists of an ordered set of DNA landmarks as well as a set of overlapping clones that together contain the corresponding DNA segment.

Restriction Sites as Landmarks. Various types of landmarks can be used to construct physical maps of DNA. A simple one is the restriction site, which reflects the site of cleavage by a specific restriction enzyme(s) (Figure 2-6). Since a large number of restriction enzymes are available, each recognizing and cutting DNA at a defined sequence, detailed restriction maps can be constructed by using several different enzymes. Establishing the physical distances (in base pairs) between restriction sites within individual clones provides a "pattern" of sites (or "fingerprint")

that can be used to establish the overlap relationships among different clones. Such an approach has proven effective at constructing physical maps of the DNA from several model organisms, with their smaller and less complex genomes.[125,161–163] Although detailed restriction maps have been constructed for targeted (and relatively limited) regions of human DNA, this physical mapping approach can be particularly challenging when applied to larger genomic segments such as whole chromosomes. Similarly, long-range restriction maps of human DNA have been constructed by using rare-cutting restriction enzymes and pulsed-field gel electrophoresis;[126–128,130] however, the resulting maps typically are not very detailed. In addition, since the analysis is performed with uncloned, total genomic DNA, such a mapping approach fails to provide direct access to the DNA itself.

Sequence-Tagged Sites as Landmarks. A recently envisioned landmark—termed a "sequence-tagged site (STS)"[164]—now plays a dominant role in assembling physical maps of human DNA. STSs are defined as short stretches (e.g., ~60–1000 bp) of unique DNA sequence that can be specifically detected by a PCR assay (Figure 2-8); in essence, STSs are the physical DNA landmarks and PCR is the experimental method used to detect them. STS maps simply represent the relative order and spacing of STSs within a region of DNA (Figures 2-6 and 2-8).[72,165] STSs provide several key advantages over other, more traditional landmarks (e.g., hybridization probes) that make them well-suited for use in physical mapping. First, the use of PCR as the front-line analytical tool for detecting DNA landmarks is highly desirable, because of its high sensitivity, specificity, and efficiency. Second, all of the relevant information about an STS (e.g., the sequence of the two oligonucleotide primers, reaction components, temperature-cycling parameters) can be stored and accessed in electronic form, thereby making that STS experimentally accessible to any laboratory; that is, the DNA segment corresponding to a particular STS can be obtained simply by synthesizing the appropriate oligonucleotide primers and performing PCR under the described condi-

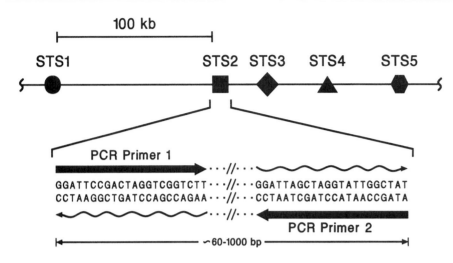

FIG. 2-8 Sequence-tagged sites (STSs) and STS maps. An STS is a unique DNA sequence in the size range of ~60 to 1000 bp that can specifically be detected by a PCR assay employing two oligonucleotide primers (indicated by thick arrows). A physical map of a human chromosome can be represented with STSs as landmarks (depicted as unique symbols), each of which is associated with a specific PCR assay. *(Adapted from Green and Olson[72] and Green and Green.[165] Used by permission.)*

tions.[166] This facilitates the merging and integration of STS maps constructed in different laboratories, since separate maps can be cross-referenced for any STS and the data conveniently merged together to produce a more refined map. Third, with an STS map, the corresponding DNA region can be isolated readily in cloned form from any genomic library by using PCR assays associated with the appropriate STSs. This ability is particularly important, since the development of newer, more powerful cloning systems can be utilized immediately with existing STSs to reassemble contigs consisting of the newer clones. Such a capability is not as easily provided with other types of landmarks (e.g., restriction sites, hybridization probes).

Generation of Sequence-Tagged Sites. To produce detailed physical maps of complex DNA sources (such as human chromosomes), tens of thousands of STSs must be developed. The generation of an STS involves determining a small amount (~100–300 bp) of DNA sequence, developing a PCR assay that will specifically amplify the corresponding DNA segment (including the design and synthesis of the two oligonucleotide primers), and demonstrating that the site is functionally "unique" within the genome.[166,167] A key step in this process is the generation of DNA sequence, which can either be obtained from a totally random piece of the source genome or from a more targeted segment (the latter being technically more involved).

The generation of DNA segments from targeted genomic regions (e.g., individual human chromosomes) typically involves the same general techniques that have been utilized for developing other types of targeted DNA markers, such as hybridization probes. Several such methods have been utilized. One approach involves the use of human–rodent hybrid cell lines containing a single human chromosome or portion thereof (see Somatic Hybrid Cell Lines, above). A number of strategies can be used to isolate the human DNA away from the rodent DNA background. For example, lambda or cosmid clones derived from such hybrid cell lines can be screened for the presence of human-specific repetitive sequences. Since most segments of human DNA present in large-insert lambda (15–25 kb) or cosmid (35–45 kb) clones should contain at least one repetitive sequence (e.g., *Alu*), clones containing human DNA can be identified by hybridization with radioactively-labeled human DNA probes.[166,167] Alternatively, segments of human DNA within the hybrid cell lines can be amplified by using a variant type of PCR, called "*Alu*-PCR" (Figure 2-9).[168,169] In this method, total DNA from the hybrid cell line is used as template in PCR assays employing oligonucleotide primers specific to consensus *Alu* sequences.[34] The PCR products generated are enriched for DNA segments residing between adjacent *Alu* re-

peats.[168,169] *Alu*-PCR thus can be used to amplify the human but not the rodent DNA, and the resulting DNA segments then can be utilized for developing STSs.[167,170,171] A second approach for generating targeted DNA segments is chromosome microdissection followed by PCR amplification of the dissected DNA (see Chromosome Microdissection, above),[145–148] which can be used to develop STSs from single or multiple chromosomal bands.[172] A third approach for isolating targeted genomic regions employs the technique of flow-sorting,[173–175] which separates individual chromosomes based on quantitation of the laser-induced fluorescence following staining. The purity of a flow-sorted DNA preparation depends on a number of factors, including the specific chromosome of interest and the cell type utilized (e.g., human cell lines vs. human–rodent hybrid cell lines). Typically, flow-sorting yields very small quantities of DNA, which then must be subcloned prior to analysis.[173–175] Although flow-sorted DNA has been used successfully for developing STSs from individual chromosomes,[87,166,167,176] the presence of irrelevant DNA segments in some cases has hindered the utility of this approach.[166,167]

Efficient strategies for developing STSs have been established and utilized in many large-scale physical mapping projects.[87,95,165–167,176] In the case of the human genome, large collections of STSs have been developed in a genome-wide fashion[95,177,178] and in a targeted fashion for a number of individual chromosomes, including 3,[179] 4,[176] 5,[180] 7,[166] 11,[87–89] 12,[91] 21,[83] 22,[85,86,181] X,[182,183] and Y.[81–82] It is also important to note that extensive collections of PCR-based genetic markers (see below) have been developed from human[177,184–189] and mouse[190–193] DNA, each of which represents an STS that can be used also for building physical maps of the corresponding DNA.

Yeast Artificial Chromosome-Based Sequence-Tagged Site-Content Mapping. The major approach that has been employed for constructing physical maps of human chromosomes utilizes STSs as the landmarks and YACs as the source of cloned DNA.[72,165] Because of their large insert size, YACs simplify the process of assembling contigs covering extended segments of a chromosome (much as jigsaw puzzles made of larger pieces are easier to assemble than those made of smaller pieces). In this strategy, YAC clones are isolated from appropriate libraries (typically by using a PCR assay corresponding to an STS[103]) and analyzed for the presence of a set of STSs (Figure 2-10). Each clone then can be represented by its STS content as well as its size, with the latter measured by pulsed-field gel electrophoresis.[131–133] Two clones are assumed to overlap if they both contain one or more common STSs. By establishing the relative overlaps among a group of YACs, contig maps can be deduced that reflect both the relation-

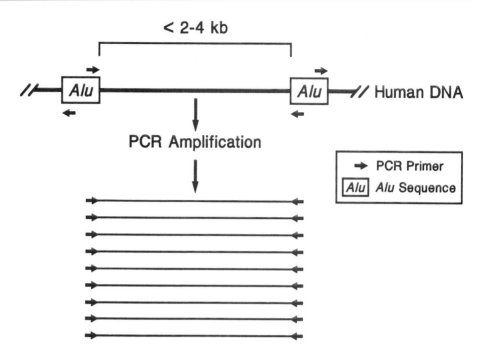

FIG. 2-9 Amplification of DNA by *Alu*-PCR. Interspersed repetitive sequences in human DNA, such as *Alu* repeats, are often closely spaced to one another (due to their high frequency in the genome). These repeated sequences represent potential annealing sites for PCR primers (depicted as horizontal arrows), in particular those that point outward from the repeats and are complementary to known consensus *Alu* sequences. When two *Alu* repeats are in close enough proximity to one another (e.g., <2 to 4 kb apart), the region between them can be amplified by *Alu*-PCR.[168,169] The resulting PCR product consists of the outer-most portions of the *Alu* sequences together with the intervening segment of human DNA. Typically, *Alu*-PCR is performed on samples of human DNA that contain numerous *Alu* repeats, resulting in the amplification of a heterogeneous array of different PCR products.

ships among the clones as well as the order and relative spacing of the STSs (Figure 2-10). This general strategy, called "STS-content mapping,"[72,165] has been used to construct large YAC contigs corresponding to a number of regions of the human genome, including segments encompassing important disease genes[72-78] (such as the cystic fibrosis and Huntington disease genes shown in Figure 2-11) and whole human chromosomes.[81-86,88-91,95] As expected, the larger DNA inserts provided by YACs have had a profound impact on the efficiency with which contigs can be assembled as well as the overall continuity in cloned coverage attained (especially when compared to bacterial cloning systems).

Radiation Hybrid Mapping. Other experimental approaches are available for establishing the relative order of landmarks (such as STSs) along a chromosome. One particularly powerful technique, called "radiation hybrid mapping," exploits the ability to recover fragments of human chromosomes in rodent cells (Figure 2-12).[194-197] In this method, human chromosomes in cultured cells are fragmented by irradiation, and the individual pieces are recovered by fusion of the irradiated cells to a rodent cell line. Each of the resulting stable cell lines typically contains numerous, disjointed fragments of the starting chromosome(s). A set of individual radiation hybrid cell lines (typically, ~100) are isolated, each of which contains a different assortment of human chromosomal fragments. The set of cell lines then is analyzed for the presence or absence of DNA markers. An efficient approach for this analysis is to use PCR for detecting a set of STSs. The relative spacing between two STSs can be deduced based on analyzing their coexistence within the collection of cell lines. Closely spaced markers tend to be present together in a larger fraction of cell lines compared to markers that are far apart on a chromosome (Figure 2-12) or that are on separate chromosomes. Statistical analysis can be used to order the markers and to estimate the relative distances between them,[194,196-201] allowing the assembly of a radiation hybrid map (Figure 2-13). One important utility of this approach is the mapping of STSs also being used for assembling YAC contigs.[95] In this case, the resulting STS-based radiation hybrid map can be used to confirm the STS order deduced by YAC-based STS-content mapping, to help order disjointed YAC contigs, and to orient YAC contigs relative to the centromere and telomeres.

Other Annotations to Physical Maps. In addition to restriction sites and STSs, other landmarks can be used to annotate a physical map of DNA. For example, cloned hybridization probes can be used to analyze clones and assemble contig maps. Similarly, as genes are identified, their physical locations within the genome can be established[202-204] (also see http://www.ncbi.nlm.nih.gov/SCIENCE96). Finally, the physical positions of landmarks used for constructing other types of maps (e.g., genetic maps) can be determined, thereby allowing precise correlation between the different representations of the same DNA region.

DNA Sequence Maps. The highest resolution physical map is the DNA sequence map, which depicts the precise order of nucleotides along a stretch of DNA (Figures 2-6 and 2-7). Increasingly, the complete (i.e., genomic) DNA sequence is being established for many large segments of human chromosomes. Eventually, the complete sequence of virtually all of the ~3,000-Mb human genome will be established; however, such an accomplishment is a long way off, with less than 5 percent determined to date. Of course, the resulting human DNA sequence will represent a composite of many different people. Interestingly, the DNA sequence among individuals typically differs only once every 1000 to 2000 nucleotides.[205] These infrequent differences, though, are responsible for much of the marked heterogeneity in phenotype that occurs within the human population.

Expressed-Sequence Tags. In contrast to complete (i.e., genomic) DNA sequence maps, sequence data generated from cDNA clones (cloned DNA copies of mRNA molecules) provide an enriched source of information about the small part of the genome that encodes protein. The refinement of methods for automated, production-scale DNA sequencing coupled with the construction of high-quality cDNA libraries (see Isolation of Disease Genes by Positional Cloning, below) has resulted in the efficient generation of large numbers of sequences from randomly selected cDNA clones [called "expressed-sequence tags" (ESTs), since they correspond to partial tags of expressed sequences]. Literally hundreds of thousands of ESTs have been generated to date,[206,207] with a large fraction of these being deposited into public databases[208,209] (e.g., dbEST, see http://www.ncbi.nlm.nih.gov/dbEST/index.html).

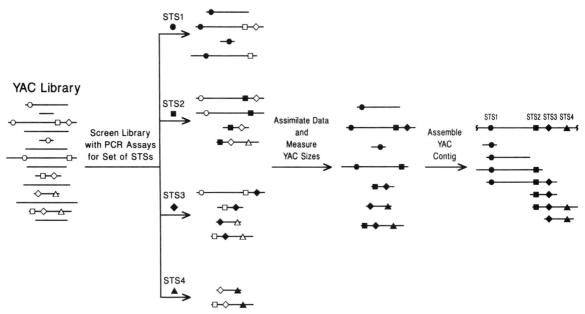

FIG. 2-10 General strategy for constructing YAC-based STS-content maps. A YAC library, consisting of clones of various sizes and unknown compositions of STSs (depicted as open symbols), is screened for a set of available STSs using a PCR-based screening method.[103] For each group of isolated clones, only the STS whose corresponding PCR assay was used to perform the library screen is known to be present in the YACs (depicted as filled-in symbols). However, the data about which YACs contain which STSs can then be assimilated and the size of each YAC measured by pulsed-field gel electrophoresis. The resulting information can be used to establish the overlap relationships among the clones and to assemble a YAC contig, from which an STS-content map can be abstracted. In the example illustrated, the relative order of the STSs as well as some information about the spacing between them can be deduced. *(Adapted from Green and Olson[72] and Green and Green.[165] Used by permission.)*

ESTs can be used as a vehicle for mapping the corresponding genes in the genome. Most often, an STS is generated from the EST sequence[95,178,210,211] and mapped by either YAC-based STS-content mapping[95] and/or radiation hybrid mapping.[95,178,197] The latter strategy was recently used for mapping over 16,000 human genes to individual chromosomal regions (see http://www.ncbi.nlm.nih.gov/SCIENCE96).[178]

The generation and mapping of large sets of ESTs provides a powerful resource for a wide array of applications, including the isolation of human disease genes by positional cloning and the study of gene function in various animal species.[212] However, ESTs are not without their limitations. For example, the data associated with an EST provides little to no information about the structure or regulation of the corresponding gene. Similarly, there is no insight about complex situations such as the production of multiple mRNAs from the same gene or the production of the same mRNA from multiple genes. Finally, ESTs are limited to those mRNA molecules that are present during the construction of a cDNA library, with rare transcripts or those not expressed in the tissue at the time of harvesting being difficult to identify. Thus, although large-scale EST generation provides an important source of biologically relevant DNA sequence, it should be regarded as a supplement (rather than a substitute) to complete genomic sequencing.

Genetic Maps

Genetic maps (also known as "linkage maps" or "meiotic maps") reflect the relative locations of genetic (as opposed to physical) markers within an interval of DNA. These maps have a more abstract meaning than do physical or cytogenetic maps, since the order and spacing between markers is related to the complex events involved in the transmission of DNA from one generation to the next.

Theory of Genetic Mapping. Most human cells contain two sets of homologous chromosomes, one inherited paternally and one inherited maternally. Thus, for a particular DNA segment (or marker), there can exist two alleles—one on each of the two homologous chromosomes. During the formation of germ cells, the diploid set of chromosomes are divided up during a process known as meiosis, which results in the generation of gametes with only one of each of the pairs of homologous chromosomes (23 chromosomes total). Markers on nonhomologous chromosomes assort randomly during meiosis. Markers on homologous chromosomes tend to be inherited together (i.e., they are "linked"). Often, a recombination event occurs between two homologous chromosomes (i.e., there is an exchange of chromosomal segments between the homologues inherited from the mother and the father), resulting in two new "hybrid" chromosomes—each containing portions of the starting homologous chromosomes (Figure 2-14). Following such a recombination event, some previously linked markers may no longer cosegregate.

Genetic mapping is simply the process of measuring the probability that two closely spaced markers on a chromosome will remain together during meiosis. This is accomplished by using a number of families to measure the frequency of recombination between markers. The greater the frequency of recombination between two markers, the larger the genetic distance separating them, and vice versa (Figure 2-14). The resulting genetic map depicts the genetic distance between different markers and, therefore, their relative order (Figures 2-6 and 2-13). The unit of measure in human genetic maps is the centimorgan (cM), with 1 cM corresponding to a probability of 1 percent that a recombination event will occur in a single meiosis (i.e., one recombination event, on average, every 100 meioses). The human genome consists of ~3,300 cM in genetic distance. The correlation between genetic distance and physical distance varies throughout the genome, since some regions are more susceptible to recombination than others. As a rough guide, 1 cM in genetic distance is thought to correspond to ~1 Mb in physical distance.

Genetic Markers. Genetic markers serve the function of discriminating between homologous chromosomes, thereby allow-

A.

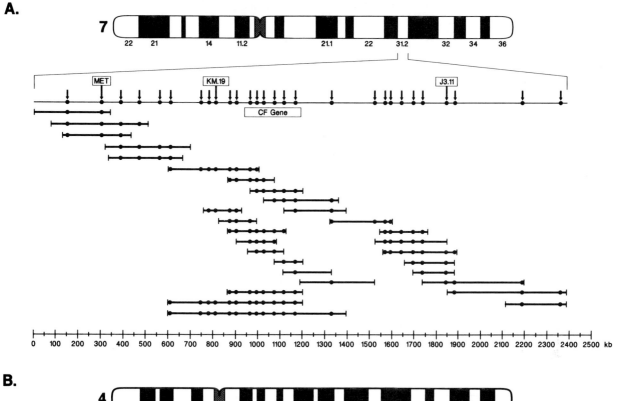

B.

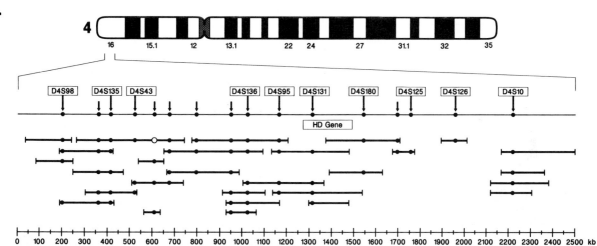

FIG. 2-11 YAC-based STS-content maps of the human cystic fibrosis and Huntington disease regions. YAC contigs spanning two of the most intensively studied regions of the human genome, the cystic fibrosis region of chromosome 7 (panel A) and the Huntington disease region of chromosome 4 (panel B), are depicted. The positions of STSs are indicated by vertical arrows, while the length of each horizontal bar represents the size of a particular YAC. In each case, the overlap relationships between YACs were established by the presence of one or more common STSs (depicted as dark circles). In panel B, the single open circle reflects the absence of that STS in that YAC, which is likely a result of an internal deletion within the cloned insert. The deduced STS-content map is depicted below the cytogenetic map of each chromosome (with the names of some key markers indicated). The approximate positions of the 250-kb cystic fibrosis (CF) gene and the 220-kb Huntington disease (HD) gene are depicted. *(Panel A was adapted from Green and Waterston,[13] Green and Green,[165] and Green and Olson;[72] panel B was adapted from Zuo et al.[77] Used by permission.)*

ing recombination events to be detected. To be useful, a genetic marker must display variance among different copies of the same chromosome (i.e., it must be polymorphic), thereby allowing it to be followed during its passage through different generations. The informativeness of a genetic marker reflects the actual likelihood that it will be different on two homologous chromosomes. Several types of markers are available for constructing genetic maps. One type of genetic marker is an inherited disease itself (e.g., premenopausal breast cancer, Huntington disease, neurofibromatosis, cystic fibrosis, sickle cell anemia). Other biologic features can also serve as genetic markers (e.g., blood cell surface antigens, serum proteins, tissue markers). However,

most markers being used for genetic mapping are DNA sequence differences that are neutral with respect to the phenotypic status of the organism.

There are several major classes of DNA sequence-based genetic markers. Restriction fragment length polymorphisms (RFLPs) reflect sequence variation that results in DNA fragments of different sizes following restriction digestion of DNA, Southern blotting,[213] and hybridization with an appropriate probe (Figure 2-15).[214-217] Since most RFLPs reflect two or very few different variants among individuals, these markers are often not particularly informative, thereby limiting their usefulness. Another class of genetic markers consists of tandemly repeated DNA

A. Radiation Hybrids: Construction and Analysis

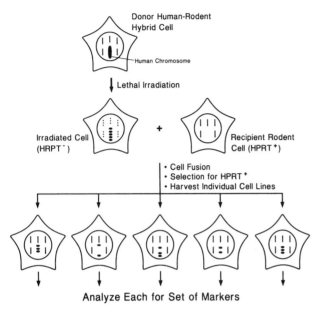

B. Radiation Hybrid Mapping Strategy

- Determine order and distance between markers
- Frequency of breakage proportional to distance between markers

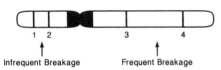

FIG. 2-12 Radiation hybrid mapping of human chromosomes. Radiation hybrid mapping involves the analysis of cell lines containing irradiated fragments of a human chromosome for the presence of a particular set of markers.[194–197] Depicted here is the construction of radiation hybrid cell lines from a human–rodent hybrid cell line containing a single human chromosome. This process involves the lethal irradiation of the donor human–rodent hybrid cell line and fusion of the irradiated cells with a recipient rodent cell line (panel A). Following appropriate selection (e.g., for the presence of the enzyme hypoxanthine phosphoribosyltransferase or HPRT), individual clonal cell lines (typically ~100) are harvested and analyzed for DNA markers present on the starting human chromosome (e.g., a set of STSs). The resulting data indicate which cell lines contain which markers, and statistical methods can be used to deduce the likely order and relative distance separating each of the markers.[194–201] The fundamental principle in the analysis of radiation hybrid mapping data (panel B) is that the frequency of radiation-induced chromosomal breaks between markers is proportional to the distance between them. Thus, in the example shown, more cell lines should be found containing both markers 1 and 2 than containing both markers 3 and 4.

sequences. Included among these markers are those containing a variable number of tandem repeats[218] (VNTRs) or "minisatellites," with each repeat containing ~11 to 60 bp (Figure 2-15). The latter polymorphisms are most often detected by agarose gel electrophoresis, Southern blotting,[213] and hybridization with an appropriate probe. Since a greater number of alleles typically are encountered (reflecting different numbers of repeated units), these markers generally are more informative than RFLPs.

RFLPs and VNTRs largely are being supplanted by a new type of genetic marker, termed the "short tandem repeat"[219–221] (STR) or "microsatellite." These sequence polymorphisms are based on differences in the lengths of DNA tracts composed of tandemly repeated di-, tri-, or tetranucleotides (typically repeated a total of 5 to 30 times) (Figure 2-15). STRs are particularly useful for genetic mapping because they tend to be more informative than other types of genetic markers. For detecting an STR, PCR primers that

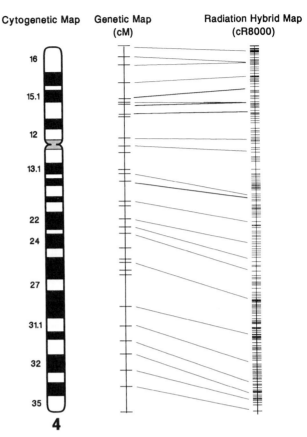

FIG. 2-13 Cytogenetic, genetic, and radiation hybrid maps of human chromosome 4. A classic cytogenetic map of human chromosome 4 is shown along with partially integrated genetic and radiation hybrid maps containing 32 and 209 markers, respectively. cR_{8000} refers to the unit of measure for the radiation hybrid map, reflecting the X-ray dose used to create the radiation hybrid cell lines (see Figure 2-12).

flank the tandem repeat are used to amplify the entire segment, and the size of the variable fragment is measured by gel electrophoresis (Figure 2-16). Thus far, the most commonly encountered STR in the human genome consists of the dinucleotide CA (or GT on the opposite strand). STRs are being met with widespread use, because of their high informativeness, frequent occurrence in the human genome (e.g., estimated every 30–60 kb for CA repeats), and efficient detection by PCR-based analyses (with its need for small amounts of DNA and potential for automation). Also, it is important to note that since each STR is associated with a unique PCR assay (i.e., an STS), it can be easily localized on the physical map, thereby allowing better correlation between genetic and physical maps.

A final class of genetic markers that currently is being investigated is the single-nucleotide polymorphism. In this case, a single base is variant at a particular site, typically being one of two different nucleotides (i.e., biallelic). Such polymorphisms can be detected by PCR amplification of the surrounding DNA followed by analysis with methods such as DNA sequencing or the more sophisticated, highly efficient technique called the "oligonucleotide ligation assay" (which can be used to detect specific single-base changes in DNA).[222–224] Although individual single-nucleotide polymorphisms suffer from their inherent limited informativeness, analyzing groups of such polymorphisms clustered close together on a chromosome has proven effective for genetic mapping studies.[222]

Construction of Genetic Maps. The process of constructing genetic maps of human DNA is a particularly complicated and te-

A. Meiotic Recombination

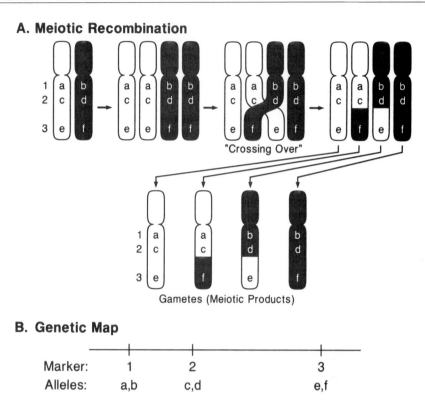

"Crossing Over"

Gametes (Meiotic Products)

FIG. 2-14 Basis of genetic mapping. (Panel A) During meiosis, each chromosome lines up with its homologous partner and is replicated. Paired chromosomes can break and rejoin with each other at one or more points (called "crossing over" or "meiotic recombination"), leading to the exchange of DNA. Thus, such a recombination event can result in the reassortment of alleles that were previously on the same chromosome. Three hypothetical markers (1, 2, and 3) on the chromosome, each with two alleles (a/b, c/d, and e/f, respectively) are indicated. A cross-over event is depicted as occurring between markers 2 and 3, yielding two recombinant chromosomes ("a, c, f" and "b, d, e") among the four meiotic products. (Panel B) The depicted genetic map is based on the measured meiotic recombination events, such as that shown in panel A. The distance between markers reflects the frequency with which they are inherited together (that is, the closer two markers are to one another, the less likely a recombination event will occur between them, and vice versa). (*Adapted from Rossiter and Caskey.[16] Used by permission.*)

B. Genetic Map

Marker:	1	2	3
Alleles:	a,b	c,d	e,f

dious process, because many of the features found with other experimental organisms (e.g., large numbers of offspring, controlled matings, relatively rapid generation times) are not available. Nonetheless, by utilizing multigeneration families with large sibships, living parents, and living grandparents, sufficient data can be generated to build useful genetic maps. A French research group [C.E.P.H. (Centre d'Etude du Polymorphisme Humain)] has been established to facilitate the distribution of cells and DNA from such families.[225] Thus, different investigators around the world can use the same families for constructing genetic maps, thereby allowing the different sets of data to be more readily integrated.

Provided with genetic markers and DNA from large families, the process of constructing genetic maps is now well established. Each DNA sample is tested by Southern blotting and hybridization (for RFLPs and VNTRs) or PCR (for STRs) (Figure 2-15), and the resulting data are carefully recorded. Sophisticated computational tools have been developed for assessing the inheritance patterns of the markers and for depicting the deduced genetic maps.[226] The first comprehensive genetic map of the human genome was reported in 1987 and included markers (predominantly RFLP-based) spaced an average of 10 cM apart.[227] Even this early-generation map provided a 95 percent chance that a given segment of the genome would be genetically linked to a mapped marker. As part of the HGP, higher-resolution (2–5 cM) genetic maps consisting of STR-type markers have been constructed for all human chromosomes.[184-189]

A highly specialized genetic mapping technique involves PCR amplification of DNA from single sperm cells.[228-232] This application has the potential to extend the power of genetic mapping in humans, since a greater number of meiotic events can be studied (given the large numbers of individual sperm cells that can be analyzed). Such an approach may allow the construction of higher resolution genetic maps for some genomic regions than could be achieved through the analysis of families.

Uses of Genetic Maps. High-resolution genetic maps greatly assist the search for genes associated with human diseases. In fami-

lies that include affected members, the disease gene itself can serve as one genetic marker whose linkage to other genetic markers can be measured. Successful identification of more and more closely linked markers allows the region of the genome containing the disease gene to be limited to an interval that eventually can be dissected by physical mapping techniques. The general process whereby an unknown gene is first localized relative to its genetic position and then cloned is called "positional cloning" (see Background on Positional Cloning, below).

In addition to facilitating the localization of disease genes, genetic maps can be used as frameworks for assembling physical maps and for studying important aspects of inheritance. Although genetic and physical maps provide different information about the corresponding DNA, they are colinear with respect to the order of markers. Thus, genetic mapping can complement physical mapping by helping to order physical landmarks based on knowledge of their genetic positions. Interestingly, there is no uniform relationship between genetic distances (recombination frequencies) and physical distances. For human DNA, the correlation of 1 cM to 1 Mb represents an estimated average, with considerable variation occurring throughout the genome. For example, the relative recombination frequencies per physical length of DNA are higher near the ends of chromosomes (telomeres) and lower near the centromeric regions. Higher-resolution genetic and physical maps eventually may allow the molecular bases for these observations to be uncovered.

STUDYING THE GENOMES OF MODEL ORGANISMS

Mapping and eventually sequencing the human genome will, in principle, reveal all the information needed for the biological development of a human being. However, the ability to interpret most of this information will be heavily dependent on parallel studies of model organisms. Experimentation in humans is rightly limited by ethical considerations, not to mention many practical

Method of Detection:

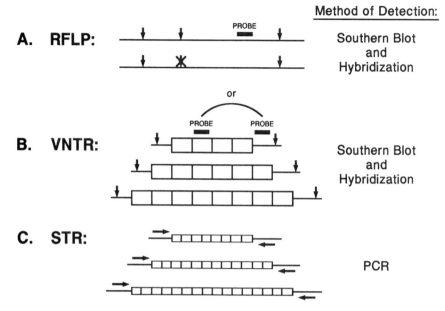

A. RFLP: — Southern Blot and Hybridization

B. VNTR: — Southern Blot and Hybridization

C. STR: — PCR

FIG. 2-15 Genetic markers and their detection. The three major types of genetic markers commonly used for genetic mapping are depicted, along with the experimental method used for their detection. *A.* RFLPs are typically associated with the variable presence of a restriction site(s) (indicated by vertical arrows) in a stretch of DNA and are detected by using an appropriate hybridization probe. *B.* VNTRs reflect variable sizes of DNA tracts harboring a repeated DNA segment, and again typically are detectable following digestion with a restriction enzyme and hybridization with an appropriate probe. *C.* In contrast to Southern blotting/hybridization detection used for RFLPs and most VNTRs, STRs consist of smaller simple-sequence (e.g., di-, tri-, or tetranucleotide) repeats, which can be detected by PCR with primers (depicted as horizontal arrows) that flank the repeated region (see Fig. 2-16). (*Adapted from Rossiter and Caskey.[16] Used by permission.*)

factors. In contrast, model organisms such as bacteria, yeasts, worms, flies, and mice can be manipulated easily, especially genetically. Importantly, the knowledge gained from mapping the genomes of these other organisms is directly relevant to understanding the human genome and many aspects of human biology, both in the normal and abnormal state[212] (see Comparative Study of the Biology of Humans and Other Organisms, below).

The model organisms have another important feature: Most have much smaller genomes than humans. This feature makes comprehensive genome analysis far more straightforward. As illustrated in Figure 2-1, the genomes of *E. coli,* yeast, nematode, and fruit flies are roughly 1/600, 1/200, 1/30, and 1/20 the size of the human genome, respectively. With smaller genomes, newly developed methods can be tested more readily. Indeed the experiences gained mapping the yeast[162, 233] and nematode[163] genomes have heavily influenced the strategies adopted for studying the human and mouse genomes. The smaller genomes of *E. coli,* yeast, nematode, and fruit flies also appear to be densely packed with genes, so that the relative amount of information derived from systematic DNA sequencing is high. Importantly, these smaller genomes actually contain many of the same genes that are found in the human genome,[212] making their study of particular interest.[212] The genomes of numerous different organisms[101,161–163,193,233–244] are being analyzed to provide insight about their structure and function; however, the organisms discussed in the following have been designated for priority study under the umbrella of the HGP.

From the earliest days of molecular biology, studies with the simple prokaryote *E. coli* have revealed many of the fundamental processes of life. A physical map of the single, circular chromosome in the form of overlapping bacteriophage clones was finished in 1987.[161] Systematic efforts have produced the DNA sequence for virtually all of the ~5 Mb in the *E. coli* genome.[234,243,245,246] With the DNA sequence of this very simple organism, it should be possible to identify many of the essential functions needed to maintain independent life.

Eukaryotic organisms, with their DNA compartmentalized into nuclei, are evolutionarily very distant from *E. coli.* The yeast *S. cerevisiae,* with a genome size of ~15 Mb, is the simplest model organism with a nucleus.[247] Comparison between it and *E. coli* should reveal the additional basic functions that distinguish eukaryotes from prokaryotes. The 16 chromosomes in *S. cerevisiae* can be separated by pulsed-field gel electrophoresis,[124] a set of overlapping bacteriophage clones has been assembled representing

most of the genome,[162] and both long-range[125] and high-resolution[233] restriction maps are complete for each chromosome. The yeast physical map has proven extremely valuable to many researchers, including those involved in the systematic sequencing of the entire yeast genome. In 1996, the sequence of the yeast genome was completed[248–252] (see http://genome-www.stanford.edu/Saccharomyces). Of note, major progress in mapping the genome of the related yeast *Schizosaccharomyces pombe*[235,236] is also being made, which is of interest because of important similarities in chromosomal structure and function between this organism and that of mammals.

Next in terms of complexity are the nematode *C. elegans* and the fruit fly *D. melanogaster,* with genomes of ~100 Mb (in six chromosomes) and ~160 Mb (in four chromosomes), respectively. As multicellular animals, these organisms share with mammals specialized cell types, such as nerve, muscle, intestine, and gonad. With the combination of molecular and mutational capabilities in the context of detailed biological information, these two organisms have become powerful systems for studying the role of many genes in development and behavior. For *C. elegans,* a detailed physical map and corresponding clone set for virtually the entire genome has been assembled with cosmids and YACs.[99,100,163] These materials represent the starting points for an ongoing, large-scale sequencing effort[253,254] (see http://www.sanger.ac.uk/~sjj/C.elegans_Home.html), which by 1998 should provide the first complete DNA sequence of a multicellular organism. For *D. melanogaster,* a well-established cytogenetic map has been available since the 1930's, in the form of the famous polytene chromosomes of the salivary gland. These structures represent a thousand or more aligned copies of each chromosome in an extended conformation, so that segments as close as 20 kb can be resolved, thereby providing a framework for organizing map information. Physical mapping and sequencing of the Drosophila genome is well underway (see http://morgan.harvard.edu/).[101,237–239]

Among the model organisms, the mouse (as a mammal) is the most closely related to humans in terms of developmental program and biologic complexity. This animal provides the closely related features of mammalian development and physiology, but in a system that is powerful in terms of its potential for genetic manipulation. The availability of fully inbred strains and a generation time of a few months make classical genetic studies feasible.[193,244,255] Furthermore, the ability to manipulate the mouse germline, including the capacity to add or delete specific genes to create transgenic mice, has provided the potential to establish the function of many genes present in mouse and humans. Also im-

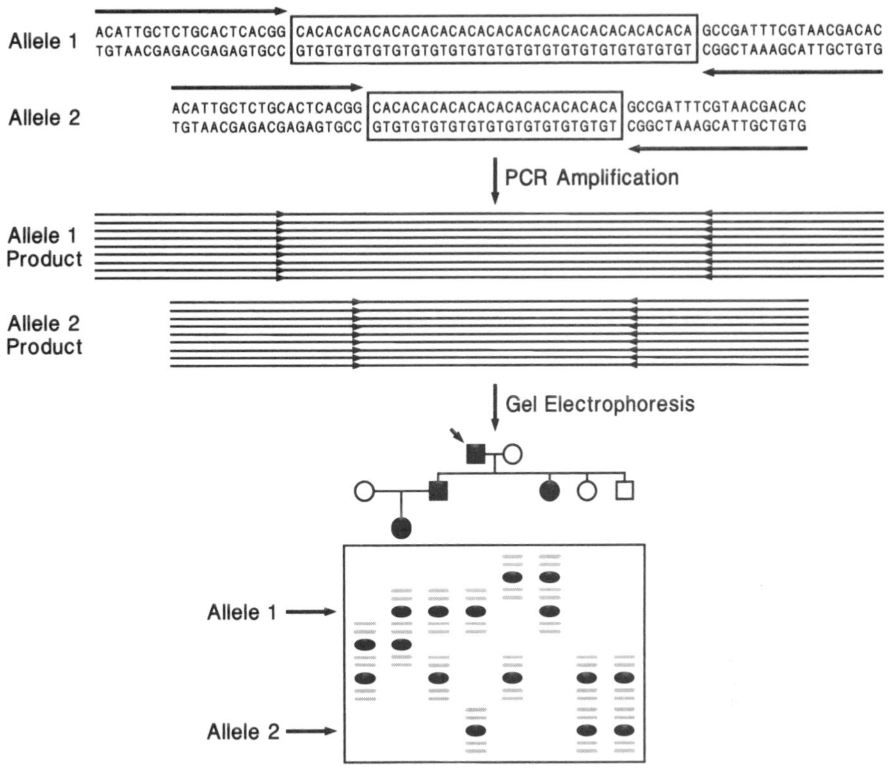

FIG. 2-16 Short tandem repeat (STR) genetic marker based on a variable number of CA repeats. Regions of the genome containing stretches of repeated CA dinucleotides are often polymorphic with respect to the number of repeat units.[219-221] One hypothetical segment is depicted, along with PCR primers (indicated by horizontal arrows) that can be used to amplify the CA-repeat unit. The two alleles (1 and 2) present in the family member indicated with an arrow are shown. PCR amplification of the STR yields products of different sizes, which can be resolved on high-resolution polyacrylamide gels. The results of analyzing a hypothetical family for this genetic marker reveal the presence of multiple alleles, which is characteristic of STRs. A common finding with PCR amplification of CA repeats is the presence of shadow (or stutter) bands (depicted as light lines) smaller and/or larger than the expected product. *(Adapted from Germino and Somlo.[5] Used by permission.)*

portant is the close evolutionary homology in the arrangement of gene segments along the chromosomes.[242,244,255-258] These features have prompted a systematic effort to construct physical and genetic maps of the mouse genome,[190-193] which is roughly the same size as the human genome. A long-term goal is to establish, in parallel, the complete DNA sequence of both the mouse and human genomes, which by important comparative analyses, will allow more precise identification of genes and their regulatory elements.[244,259,260]

THE HUMAN GENOME PROJECT

History of the Human Genome Project

The official beginning of the Human Genome Project (HGP) in the United States was heralded on October 1, 1990. However, the intellectual and administrative process responsible for the project's initiation had already been operating for a number of years before this.[261,262] Detailed historical accounts of the HGP have been compiled.[261-269] In brief, the origins of the HGP are thought by most to date back to a meeting in Alta, Utah in 1984, where the discussion focused on the analysis of DNA for the purpose of detecting mutations among atomic bomb survivors.[270] Shortly after this meeting, the concept of a comprehensive program of genome study was entertained by two groups. First, a 1985 conference in Santa Cruz, California, was convened to examine the feasibility of sequencing the genome.[271] Second, Charles DeLisi initiated discussions within the Department of Energy on the merits of genome-wide sequencing.[272] Because of their interest in health effects of radiation and other types of environmental hazards, the Department of Energy viewed establishing the sequence of the human genome as a viable means for monitoring DNA sequence changes. Furthermore, Delisi viewed the Department of Energy, with its expertise in a diversity of comple-

mentary fields (e.g., analytical chemistry, applied physics, engineering, computer science) and experience at directing large-scale projects, as representing a strong participant for such an endeavor.[272] Additional support for the HGP came independently from Renato Dulbecco, who argued in 1986 that sequencing the human genome and identifying all the encoded genes would be an efficient way to expedite cancer research.[273] Importantly, he stressed that it would be more desirable to elucidate all of this information at once, rather than obtaining it piecemeal over an extended period of time.

Two highly influential reports published in 1988 guided the development of the structure and scope of the early phases of the HGP in the United States—one by the Committee on Mapping and Sequencing the Human Genome of the National Research Council[274] and the other by a committee operating under the auspices of the U.S. Congress Office of Technology Assessment.[275] Together, these reports called for a systematic effort of genome mapping and sequencing, provided recommendations about the scope and goals of the effort, outlined the roles for both the National Institutes of Health and the Department of Energy in administering the project in the United States, and recommended funding levels for the endeavor. Of note, the general program outlined by these reports has remained fundamentally unchanged, despite advances in the technologies used for genome analysis. Amid all these discussions was a significant amount of debate within the scientific community as to the merits of the HGP,[36,276-286] although most of the negative aspects of this have since waned. The Department of Energy initiated their formal program in 1987. The Office for Human Genome Research at the National Institutes of Health was created in 1988. Later that year, this office became the National Center for Human Genome Research (NCHGR). Appropriations for both the Department of Energy and National Institutes of Health programs were initiated in 1988 (although the Department of Energy's program started the previous year using funds diverted from other sources). The first set of formal goals for the project in the United States were established in 1990,[287] at which time the project officially began.

Although the historic roots of the HGP largely are based in the United States, the project is international in structure. In addition to the National Institutes of Health and Department of Energy orchestrating the HGP in the United States, there are other analogous agencies coordinating efforts underway in other countries, particularly England, France, Canada, Japan, and Germany. As a result, there now is extensive evidence of international coordination and collaboration in many genome mapping and sequencing projects that are being performed under the auspices of the HGP.

Scientific Plan of the Human Genome Project

In the United States, the currently planned HGP has a 15-year timetable. Various goals have been set,[265–267,269,287] with the expectation that these will be transient in nature because of the anticipated advances in technologies for genome analysis.[289] Several general points about these goals should be made. First, a major emphasis of the initial phase of the HGP has been the development of high-quality genetic and physical maps for each human chromosome, along with rigorous attempts to integrate these maps with each other and with the cytogenetic map. Included in the goals are the establishment of genetic maps with highly polymorphic markers placed, on average, every 2 to 5 cM (or less) and the development of 100–kb-resolution STS maps for all human chromosomes. To accomplish the latter requires the development and mapping of more than 30,000 STSs across the human genome. Second, for DNA sequencing, the initial emphasis has been to improve the efficiency of existing methods, to develop new technologies, and to begin systematic sequencing on model organisms, with human genomic sequencing slated for the later phases of the project. Third, the goals of the HGP have included support for a range of associated activities, including those addressing important ethical, legal, and social issues (see Ethical, Legal, and Social Implications of the Human Genome Project, below), those supporting the training of individuals capable of advancing genome research, those aiming to provide public education about genetics, and those promoting the development and transfer of relevant genome technologies. For example, the involvement of investigators with expertise outside biology (e.g., engineering, chemistry, physics) is viewed as critical.[290]

Studying Model Organisms in the Human Genome Project

The inclusion of "human" in the Human Genome Project is, of course, a misnomer, since it does not accurately reflect the broadness of the overall initiative. In fact, a central component of the HGP is the parallel mapping and sequencing of model organisms. The initial phase of the HGP includes completing physical maps and initiating large-scale DNA sequencing for *E. coli, S. cerevisiae, C. elegans,* and *D. melanogaster.* This early emphasis on DNA sequencing relates to the more densely-packed genomes of these organisms, which is already providing information directly applicable to the study of human DNA sequence[212] (see Comparative Study, below).

Role of Informatics in the Human Genome Project

A critical component of the HGP is the development of capabilities for storing and analyzing the tremendous amounts of complex information being generated. The HGP includes explicit support for this discipline (commonly referred to as "informatics"). An important aspect of informatics is the development of computer databases for storing the resulting genetic and physical mapping data, along with the ability to conveniently access this information electronically (increasingly via the World Wide Web). For example, the Genome Data Base (GDB), which operates under the auspices of the Johns Hopkins University Welch Medical Library, has been established to assimilate mapping data on the human genome (DNA markers, clone information, maps) (see http://gdbwww.gdb.org).[291] DNA sequence data are being deposited into dedicated sequence databases (e.g., GenBank; see http://www.ncbi.nlm.nih.gov).[292] The aim of these databases is to provide a viable means of storing, communicating, cross-referencing, and disseminating the mapping and sequencing data. A second aspect of informatics is the development of software tools for analyzing the mapping and sequencing data. Examples include programs that help establish the validity of genetic [226] and physical maps, that compile large stretches of primary DNA sequence data,[293] and that detect the general features of genes within DNA sequence by looking for specific base compositions of coding sequences, exon–intron boundaries, and other characteristics.[294–301]

Highlights of the Human Genome Project

Despite its recent start, the HGP has already made a number of important strides toward the attainment of its goals. Several examples can be used to illustrate the general level of accomplishment. First, markedly improved genetic maps of the human[184–189] and mouse[190–193] genomes based on STR markers have been completed. Second, major progress has been made in constructing a 100-kb STS map for all human chromosomes.[81–83,86,90,91,95,159] Third, the DNA sequence of *S. cerevisiae* has been established[248–252] (e.g., see http://genome-www.stanford.edu/Saccharomyces), whereas similar efforts for *E. coli*[234,243,245,246] and *C. elegans*[253,254] are nearing completion. Most striking, however, is the realization that the human genome likely will be sequenced shortly after we enter the next century.[302,303] For the latter effort, successful increases in the scale of DNA sequencing have been accomplished by subtle improvements in instrumentation, optimizing experimental methods, and refining the maintenance of a large-scale operation. Finally, the anticipated rewards of deriving genomic maps and sequence for the study of biology[212] and human disease (see Impact of the Human Genome Project, below) are being realized.

IMPACT OF THE HUMAN GENOME PROJECT ON THE STUDY OF HUMAN DISEASE

The HGP promises to provide a number of interrelated benefits to biology and clinical medicine. These will include an improved ability to isolate, characterize, and manipulate the genes involved in normal human biology and human disease. With the parallel study of the genomes of model organisms, greater insight and experimental potential will be attained with respect to the genes that are present in a diverse array of animal species. In addition to the isolation of disease genes, the HGP will impact other aspects of clinical medicine,[13,16,304–315] including those involved in diagnosing, preventing, and treating human diseases.

Impact of the Human Genome Project on the Positional Cloning of Human Disease Genes

Background on Positional Cloning. Thousands of genes are known to cause disease when present in a mutated form (see http://www.ncbi.nlm.nih.gov/omim). Of course, the number of genes that influence human diseases in more indirect fashions is likely to be much higher. A major effort of modern molecular genetics is to identify the genetic defects that can result in pathologic states.

The identification and isolation of human disease genes has largely occurred using one of two basic strategies: functional cloning and positional cloning (Figure 2-17).[1–3] With functional cloning, the disease gene is isolated as a result of pre-existing knowledge of the fundamental physiological defect, which provides sufficient insight about the function of the defective gene or its protein product. Often, successful cloning of the gene is preceded by the purification of its protein product (with subsequent amino acid sequencing or antibody generation) or by acquiring sufficient information about its function (e.g., the cloning of genes involved in DNA repair disorders).[316] Thus, in functional cloning, mapping the gene follows its isolation (Figure 2-17). Classic examples of disease genes identified by a functional cloning strategy include β-thalassemia,[317] Lesch-Nyhan syndrome,[318–321] phenylketonuria,[322] and glucose-6-phosphate dehydrogenase (G6PD) deficiency.[323]

For most of the myriad genetic disorders (including the probable thousands not yet discovered), there is no significant prior understanding about the function of the defective gene. In most cases, direct analysis of the altered biochemical state fails to provide sufficient insight into the nature of the genetic defect to allow gene isolation. For studying these more typical diseases, the strategy of positional cloning has been refined over the past decade[1–5] and successfully utilized for identifying and isolating numerous disease genes (see http://www.ncbi.nlm.nih.gov/dbEST/dbEST_genes). With positional cloning, isolation of the gene follows the establishment of its "position" within the genome by genetic and/or physical mapping techniques. In most cases, these efforts proceed with limited knowledge of the gene's function or the nature of the pathophysiological process. Genetic mapping typically is the front-line tool used for delimiting the region of the genome to a point that allows molecular cloning of the interval, analysis for encoded genes, and identification of causative mutations. Thus, for positional cloning, mapping precedes cloning (moving in the opposite direction as functional cloning), and gene function is defined only after the gene has been isolated and characterized (Figure 2-17). Although this process was originally called "reverse genetics,"[324–327] this somewhat incorrect terminology has now been largely abandoned.[1]

Isolation of Disease Genes by Positional Cloning. The identification and isolation of disease genes by a positional cloning strategy can be conceptually divided into the series of steps depicted in Figure 2-18, each of which is discussed below.

The starting point for a positional cloning effort is the collection of pedigrees in which the defective gene is found in multiple

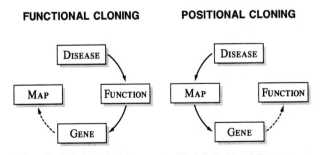

FIG. 2-17 Functional versus positional cloning of disease genes. In functional cloning, the study of gene function precedes gene identification. In positional cloning, gene mapping precedes gene identification. The last step in each case (gene mapping and defining gene function, respectively) is not critical for the isolation of the disease gene itself. (*Adapted from Collins.[1] Used by permission.*)

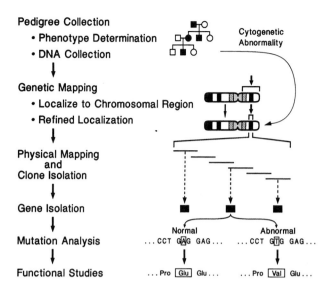

FIG. 2-18 Positional cloning of human disease genes. The major steps involved in the isolation and characterization of human disease genes by a positional cloning strategy are depicted, with additional details provided in the text. In the hypothetical example shown, a single base change (A → T) results in an amino acid change (Glu → Val) in the resulting protein, which in turn causes the disease. Remarkably, such a single base pair change in the ~3-billion-bp human genome can be lethal.

affected individuals, preferably in several generations. Of critical importance is the establishment of the correct phenotype for as many family members as possible and the isolation of DNA from these individuals. Discrepancies between an individual's phenotype and genotype can result from: (1) an incorrect diagnosis (i.e., phenotype assignment); (2) genetic heterogeneity (defects in more than one gene can lead to the phenotype); (3) incomplete penetrance (some individuals inheriting the defective gene do not express the phenotype, or at least not at the time of diagnosis); or (4) a mix-up of the DNA sample(s). Thus, significant effort must be invested during the collection of family resources to minimize errors, especially those caused by preventable mistakes.

In the next stage of positional cloning, the general region of the genome containing the defective gene is identified. In the ideal case, the disease is closely associated ("marked") with a cytogenetic abnormality(s), which immediately defines a highly delimited, candidate region harboring the gene (since such a cytogenetic alteration is likely to have interrupted the gene or regulatory element near the gene). Examples of diseases associated with cytogenetic abnormalities include genetic disorders (e.g., Duchenne muscular dystrophy,[157] neurofibromatosis,[38,328] fragile X syndrome,[158] and Lowe syndrome[329]) and a number of different forms of cancer.[330–335]

However, the great majority of genetic diseases are not associated with cytogenetic abnormalities. For these disorders, genetic mapping is performed to localize the genomic region containing the gene. At first, DNA samples from multiple family members are analyzed by using a set of genetic markers spread across the genome, searching for one that shows linkage (coinheritance) with the disease. If successful, this typically assigns the defective gene to a rough chromosomal location, usually spanning tens of millions of base pairs. More refined localization then is performed by using additional genetic markers that map nearby. The extent to which this subsequent genetic mapping allows the region to be further delimited depends on a number of factors, such as the quality of the family resources (e.g., family size, availability of DNA), as well as the number, distribution, and informativeness of the genetic markers in the region. It is important to note that a critical component of this type of genetic mapping is the use of so-phisticated computational tools for calculating the various para-meters to determine if sufficient data have been collected to allow confident establishment of linkage using the available pedi-grees.[226,336]

In the best cases, genetic mapping allows the candidate region to be limited to 1 cM; however, the corresponding physical size can vary widely because of regional and sex-specific differences in recombination rates. This provides an inherent and constant source of uncertainty. Typically, a 1-cM genetic distance corre-sponds to less than 1 to 3 Mb, and such an interval of DNA then can be analyzed by physical mapping methods and isolated by use of molecular cloning strategies. Often, the closest mapping ge-netic markers are utilized as the starting points for clone isolation. New markers (PCR- or hybridization-based) then can be derived from the ends of isolated clones and used to identify new, overlap-ping clones, and this process is repeated iteratively. The system-atic isolation of adjacent, overlapping clones by such a strategy is called "chromosome walking."[337] Additional markers also can be derived from the targeted region by other strategies (see Genera-tion of STSs, above) and used for isolating clones from the area. In ideal cases, the entire DNA interval between the flanking ge-netic markers is isolated in cloned form. The resulting clones then are used for developing additional genetic markers (to reduce fur-ther the candidate region by genetic mapping), and, importantly, for gene isolation and mutation detection.

A particularly challenging step in a positional cloning ap-proach is the identification of encoded genes within the candidate region.[203,338] A number of different strategies have been developed for detecting genes in large genomic clones (e.g., YACs, BACs, PACs, P1s, cosmids) (Table 2-1). In general, each of these meth-ods is relatively labor intensive, suffers from a number of inherent limitations, and rarely is used alone during the search for a disease gene.

One major class of techniques for identifying coding regions within cloned genomic segments employs DNA-DNA hybridiza-tion-based methods (Table 2-1). For example, small DNA frag-ments derived from larger genomic clones can be used to probe DNA from a variety of different animal species (immobilized on a membrane referred to as a "zoo blot"). Detection of cross-hy-bridizing (i.e., presumed homologous) DNA suggests the presence of sequences that may have been evolutionarily conserved and therefore likely to be essential for biologic function. The same

Table 2-1 Strategies for Identifying Genes in Large Genomic Regions

DNA–DNA Hybridization Based
  Using small DNA fragments
    Analysis of DNA from other organisms ("zoo blots")
    Analysis of RNA from individual tissues by northern blotting
    Identification of CpG islands
  Using large genomic clones (e.g., YACs, BACs, PACs, P1s, cosmids)
    Hybridization-based screening of cDNA libraries
    "Direct selection" of cDNAs using immobilized DNA
Function Based
  Exon trapping/amplification
  PolyA signal trapping
  Gene transfer and transcript identification
DNA Sequence Based
  Comparison to EST databases
  Detection of open reading frames (ORFs)
  Prediction of coding sequences
  Comparison to sequences from other species

SOURCE: Adapted from Collins FS: Positional cloning: Let's not call it reverse anymore. *Nat Genet* 1:3, 1992.

probes also can be hybridized to mRNA derived from various hu-man tissues (immobilized on a membrane referred to as a "north-ern blot"[339]) to detect the presence of expressed DNA segments. A wide survey of tissues is advisable, especially since the expression pattern of the gene generally is unknown at this stage. Finally, the probes can be used in conjunction with rare-cutting restriction en-zymes to search for the presence of CpG islands, which often (but not always) mark the 5' ends of genes.[39,340]

Alternatively, genomic clones can be used either to probe cDNA libraries directly[340,341] (made from the mRNA of particular tissues) or to capture cDNA sequences by a method known as "di-rect cDNA selection."[342–345] In the latter technique, DNA from the genomic clone is used as an "affinity matrix" to capture specifi-cally sequences present in mRNA mixtures or cDNA libraries. There are a number of important issues regarding the source of mRNA or cDNA libraries for gene isolation. First, a particular gene will be identified only if it is expressed in the tissue from which the mRNA or cDNA library was derived. Second, not all mRNA molecules are expressed at equal levels in a particular tis-sue. In fact, some genes are expressed at exceedingly low levels, and these can be particularly difficult to isolate. One route to over-come this general problem is the use of "normalized" libraries that provide a more equal representation of different cDNA clones, re-gardless of the initial concentration of the corresponding mRNA molecules.[346–350]

A second class of strategies for gene isolation exploits par-ticular aspects of gene structure or function (Table 2-1). In one approach, the presence of sequences necessary for proper re-moval of introns (called "splice junctions") is used to isolate the adjacent exon sequence by a technique called "exon ampli-fication" or "exon trapping."[351–355] Similar approaches for trap-ping the most 3'-terminal exon in a gene (using the associated polyA tract as the signal) also have been developed.[356] Alterna-tively, some genes can be isolated by transferring the cloned genomic DNA into an appropriate mammalian cell and selec-ting for the function of the gene. Of course, the latter approach requires some prior information about the likely function of the gene itself.

A final class of gene identification strategies involves the sys-tematic analysis of DNA sequence data derived from the candidate region (Table 2-1). One simple level of analysis includes the exam-ination of DNA segments that are devoid of the three-base pair sig-nals that stop protein synthesis (called "stop codons"). Such tracts are called "open reading frames" (ORFs), and each, in principle, can encode for one or more exons. Additional computational analysis of DNA sequence involves the use of more sophisticated tools for identifying sequence matches to known genes or ESTs in the public databases (see Expressed-Sequence Tags, above), for de-tecting possible exons based on surrounding splice junctions, known protein motifs, and other established features of genes, and for comparing to available DNA sequences from other organisms for the detection of evolutionarily conserved motifs.[294–300]

All genes identified within the most delimited region of DNA become candidate genes for the disease. Proof that a par-ticular gene is the correct one requires demonstration that the disease is associated with a mutation in that gene. Thus, the next stage of analysis involves the difficult task of searching for mutations within candidate genes and demonstrating that such mutations show the proper inheritance (e.g., recessive, dominant) relative to the disease. These genetic defects can range from single-base pair changes to more gross alterations (e.g., large deletions, expanded tracts of trinucleotide re-peats).[357–359] Although mutations can occur anywhere within the gene structure (including regulatory elements and introns), the majority of mutations reported to date have involved DNA sequences within coding regions.

Typically, initial screening for mutations in affected individuals involves analyzing the gene for gross rearrangements by conventional and pulsed-field gel electrophoresis. Most often, this fails to demonstrate a mutation, and the search then shifts to look for more subtle DNA alterations involving one or a few nucleotides.[360,361] A number of techniques have been developed for this purpose, including denaturing gradient gel electrophoresis (DGGE),[362–365] RNAase[366,367] or chemical[368] cleavage of mismatches, single-strand conformation polymorphism (SSCP) analysis,[369,370] and direct DNA sequencing. Ultimately, DNA sequencing must be used to establish the precise nature of any mutation. With continued improvements in the efficiency of DNA sequencing protocols, there likely will be a continued shift away from indirect screening methods and towards the use of direct sequencing for the detection of mutations in candidate genes.

An issue that must be addressed continually during the mutation detection stage of positional cloning is the discrimination between innocent sequence polymorphisms (which may simply be linked to the disease gene) and actual mutations (which cause the disease). Insight about the potential effect of a given mutation (e.g., changing an amino acid at a predicted key site in the protein) often can provide strong supportive evidence for its role in the disease. However, ultimate proof that a candidate gene is the correct one often requires evidence that the normal form of the gene corrects the abnormal phenotype and/or that the mutant form of the gene causes the abnormal phenotype.

Impact of the Human Genome Project on Positional Cloning.
Positional cloning strategies have become increasingly successful, as evidenced by the disease genes identified in recent years (see http://www.ncbi.nlm.nih.gov/dbEST/dbEST_genes). The basic infrastructure being established by the HGP in the form of high-quality maps, technologies, and reagents is dramatically simplifying the process of positional cloning, making it more efficient, cost-effective, and efficacious.

Virtually every step of a positional cloning strategy is being improved as a result of the HGP. First, improvements in genetic mapping in the form of higher-resolution genetic maps, better sets of informative STR markers, and more efficient methods for genotype analysis are allowing more precise assignments of disease gene positions, even with the limited family resources that are available for many disorders. Similarly, the generation of comprehensive physical maps and, importantly, the availability of complete clone sets for each chromosome is dramatically reducing the time it takes to isolate and characterize candidate regions. Finally, technical developments in DNA sequencing already are having a dramatic impact, with the movement toward routine sequencing of all candidate regions, the increased availability of pre-existing DNA sequence data (including hundreds of thousands of ESTs), the improved computational tools for detecting genes by sequence analysis, and the accumulation of sequence information from model organisms to aid in the identification of important human genes.

Together, these improvements are providing greater amounts of information about genes throughout the genome. When a positional cloning effort points to a genomic segment, any gene known to exist in that region becomes a candidate gene. In turn, each candidate gene can be studied in an attempt to correlate its features with the disease phenotype (e.g., expression pattern, identifiable protein domains) and to search for possible mutations. In ideal cases, the steps involving cloning the region and isolating the genes can be skipped altogether, if one of the known genes from the region is found to be the correct one. This variant of positional cloning has been termed the "positional candidate gene" approach,[2] since it combines information about map position and available data about the gene. This approach

has already been used successfully, leading to the identification of the genes causing retinitis pigmentosa,[371,372] familial hypertrophic cardiomyopathy,[373] malignant hypothermia,[374] Marfan syndrome,[376–378] early onset Alzheimer disease,[379] spinal and bulbar muscular atrophy,[380] Waardenburg syndrome,[381,382] Charcot-Marie-Tooth disease,[383–386] amyotrophic lateral sclerosis,[387] and many forms of hereditary cancer (e.g., melanoma, hereditary nonpolyposis colorectal cancer, and Li-Fraumeni syndrome [Chapters 27, 17, and 20]. This approach inevitably will become more successful as the HGP evolves, owing to the increase in density of known genes at mapped positions throughout the genome.

In general, the successful examples cited earlier and listed at http://www.ncbi.nlm.nih.gov/dbEST/dbEST_genes reflect diseases that are either relatively common (thereby providing large pedigrees and adequate DNA samples) or associated with readily visible cytogenetic alterations that assisted in the localization of the gene. Most of the remaining genetic diseases will prove to be far more complicated to study—in particular, those that are rare (and have limited family resources), are caused by defects in more than one gene (polygenic diseases),[11,12] or result from combined genetic and nongenetic components (multifactorial). Perhaps the greatest impact of the HGP will be on the ability to characterize the genetic bases for these latter types of diseases. In these cases, higher-density genetic and physical maps will prove invaluable for isolating causative genes by positional cloning. For example, with polygenic disorders, genetic analysis is inherently difficult in humans, in part because of the small pedigree sizes and lack of controlled matings. Improved maps, genetic markers, and clone sets should help to overcome such limitations, making characterization of the genetic bases of such disorders more approachable.[11,12]

Comparative Study of the Biology of Humans and Other Organisms

A major component of the HGP is mapping and sequencing the genomes of model organisms whose biologic properties have been examined for decades by geneticists, biochemists, and physiologists (see Studying Model Organisms in the Human Genome Project, above). Studying the genomes of model organisms already is playing an important role in developing the strategies, technologies, and infrastructure needed for analyzing human DNA. A strong argument can be made that the actual mapping and sequencing of the human genome will be simpler than the difficult and challenging process of determining the functions of genes and mechanisms of genetic disease pathology. However, the knowledge gained from research on model organisms will provide a framework that should facilitate efficient utilization of the reagents and information produced from human genome studies. The strong emphasis on studying model organisms within the HGP is based on the fundamental feature of biology that all organisms share the same general type of DNA blueprint, with a tremendous degree of conservation of gene structure and function existing across a diverse array of organisms. This fact, combined with the vast stores of information already available about the biology of model organisms, will insure that their study plays a critical role in understanding human gene function.[212]

There are numerous examples of how studying genes in bacteria, yeast, worms, fruit flies, mice, and other organisms provided important insights into the function of particular human genes. Generally, DNA sequence information is obtained for a human gene, and homology with an already-studied gene from a model organism provides valuable insight about possible gene function. It is perhaps most remarkable that some human genes can functionally substitute for their counterparts in organisms as distant as the yeast *S. cerevisiae*. A sampling of cases where sequence homology and/or cross-species functional studies have proven valuable includes:

1. The yeast *STE6* gene, which encodes a protein required for secreting a peptide pheromone factor involved in yeast mating,[388] is highly homologous in DNA sequence to the human *MDR1* (multidrug resistance) gene, which encodes a protein that confers resistance of tumor cells to a number of chemotherapeutic agents.[389] This strong sequence similarity motivated researchers to transfer the mouse homologue of the *MDR1* gene into a mutant yeast strain defective in the *STE6* gene, where the mammalian gene was found to correct the mutant phenotype in the yeast.[390]

2. The yeast *KEX2* gene, which encodes a protease that is involved in the secretion of a yeast mating factor, shows strong sequence homology to a human gene called c-*fur*, whose function was unknown at the time of its discovery.[391] This sequence similarity prompted researchers to test the biochemical properties of the c-*fur* gene product, which was found to be a member of a protease gene family involved in processing a number of hormones and growth factors.[391,392] Because of their key role in the biosynthesis of many important molecules, there are now intense efforts to modify the activities of these proteases with pharmacologic agents.

3. The gene defective in neurofibromatosis type 1, a common autosomal dominant disease associated with a constellation of symptoms, including characteristic neurofibromas, was cloned[38,328] and found to have strong homology with the mammalian RAS GTPase activating protein ("GAP")[393,394] and two yeast genes called *IRA1* and *IRA2*.[394,395] Gene transfer experiments showed that a segment of the mammalian neurofibromatosis type 1 gene can complement (correct) the function of defective *IRA* genes in yeast.[394]

4. The human *ERCC-3* gene encodes a presumed DNA helicase involved in repairing specific types of DNA damage, and defects in this gene are responsible for two rare genetic diseases: xeroderma pigmentosum and Cockayne syndrome.[396] A Drosophila gene called *"haywire"* appears to encode the fly equivalent of the human gene, and mutations in *haywire* result in some of the same effects as that seen in xeroderma pigmentosum.[397] Although comparisons between the two species are not completely parallel, it is likely that much can be learned about the human disease by genetic manipulation of flies. For instance, genetic studies of the fly mutant already have indicated that the product of the *haywire* gene interacts with another gene (or gene product) and produces different symptoms in flies containing different alleles. This information may help to explain the variability in symptoms seen in different xeroderma pigmentosum and Cockayne patients.

5. There are many cases in which the close evolutionary relationship between mice and humans has been exploited to understand the functioning of particular human genes. The general approach for these cross-species comparisons has been to insert foreign DNA sequences into the mouse germline to create transgenic mice. In these experiments, a human gene (either wild-type or mutant) can be transferred into mice, or the resident mouse homologue of a human gene can be altered (either changed to a mutated form or destroyed by a "knockout"). The effects of such changes in living mice are then ascertained, and inferences about the normal function of the human gene can be made. In addition, given the similarities between the species, it may be possible to develop pharmacologic agents for treating human diseases in cases where a mouse model for a pathologic state can be established. An interesting example of a mouse model for a human genetic disease is that for cystic fibrosis.[398–400]

As the HGP reaches full stride and larger amounts of DNA sequence information become available, the connections between human and model organism genes will increase at a dramatic pace. It is quite apparent now that a large fraction of the genes in yeast, nematode, and fruit fly have counterparts in humans. Thus, knowledge of the complete DNA sequence of humans and several model organisms can be regarded as the ultimate framework for making inferences about the evolution of genes and for deciphering the basic functions of DNA. In addition to cross-species comparisons, a related benefit of the HGP will be to facilitate the study of human diversity by comparative sequence analysis of individuals from distantly related populations, thereby advancing our understanding of human evolution.[401–403]

Advances in Molecular Diagnostics Resulting from the Human Genome Project

Molecular diagnostics can be broadly defined as the testing of DNA (or RNA) within a clinical context,[404–408] and this medical discipline is rapidly growing in scope and importance. The applications of molecular diagnostics span a wide range of human diseases, including tests for hereditary,[404,407,409–412] neoplastic,[413–415] and infectious diseases.[416–417] In these situations, the standard tools of molecular biology are simply being applied to answer specific clinical questions.

The HGP will accelerate the growth of molecular diagnostics in two respects. First, by facilitating the identification of disease genes (see Impact of the Human Genome Project, above), an increasing number of mutations associated with human pathology will be characterized. With this growing insight about the genetic basis of disease will come increased opportunities to make diagnostic and prognostic assessments based on examination of an individual's DNA. A natural consequence of identifying a gene by positional cloning and the obligate identification of mutations will be the ability to test for those mutations in a clinical setting. Second, many of the same methods and instruments being developed to construct physical and genetic maps of the human genome are finding immediate utility for studying DNA in a clinical setting. The resulting technologies (e.g., PCR, DNA sequencing, mutation detection) as well as their automation should, therefore, revolutionize molecular diagnostics. A prelude of this phenomenon is already evident with PCR, which has seen rapid introduction into the clinical laboratory.[414–418] Among existing PCR-based clinical assays are those that allow testing for genetic diseases (e.g., Duchenne muscular dystrophy,[419–421] cystic fibrosis[223,422]) and malignancies.[414,415] Thus, the rapid advances in understanding the genetic bases of diseases in conjunction with the explosion in technologic developments occurring with the HGP will dramatically enhance the ability to make diagnoses at a DNA level.

Prospects for Therapeutic Benefits from the Human Genome Project

The HGP promises to transform the ability to understand human genetic diseases by providing a unique interplay between genetics and clinical medicine. For all of the reasons outlined in the preceding, physicians and scientists should gain greater insight into the genetic components that contribute to disease processes and acquire better means for establishing whether a patient has inherited a genetic lesion. However, the full impact of the HGP should extend beyond these areas, and, in the long run, enhance the ability to treat patients with genetic abnormalities.

Several interrelated aspects of the HGP offer the potential for impacting patient care in a positive fashion. First, for some genetic disorders, presymptomatic knowledge of an inherited defect will provide meaningful opportunities for the use of preventive measures (e.g., lifestyle alterations, increased surveillance to aid early diagnosis, targeted intervention) that may serve to minimize the morbid effects of a mutation. As the HGP progresses, an increasing number of genes that cause such inherited diseases will be uncovered, along with the development of techniques to detect efficiently their corresponding mutations. Second, the improved capacities to define the precise molecular defects causing a disease should markedly advance the understanding of its pathophysiological bases. Such knowledge should facilitate the ability to design rational treatments for the disease, which could range from the design of better pharmacologic agents (based on insight gained about the structure of the corresponding protein), the exogenous synthesis and delivery of a missing gene product, or the introduction of the normal form of a gene into an affected patient (i.e., gene therapy).[423,424] Finally, it should be stressed that the potential for such therapeutic advances likely will be further enhanced with the development of appropriate animal models for genetic diseases. Towards that end, the parallel developments in characterizing the genomes of model organisms should improve the ability to study the relevant disease processes in animals, where pharmacologic interventions and gene therapy protocols can be more readily tested (see Comparative Mapping, above).

Ethical, Legal, and Social Implications of the Human Genome Project

One of the early anticipated benefits of the HGP—the ability to identify and isolate genes that play important roles in human disease—has already become a reality. Of course, in most cases cloning of a human disease gene is only the first step in the long process of developing a rational therapy based on knowledge of the mutant gene. Since the development of therapies will almost always lag behind the generation of new diagnostic assays, the identification of disease genes will typically provide the ability to identify individuals at risk for disorders for which there are limited therapeutic options. How such information will or should be used by patients, physicians, and society raises a number of issues that require immediate, thoughtful consideration.[425-429]

In 1990, the National Center for Human Genome Research at the National Institutes of Health in conjunction with the Department of Energy established a joint working group to study the ethical, legal, and social issues of human genome research (called the "ELSI program"). The ELSI working group, which consists of individuals representing a broad range of expertise (including medical geneticists, ethicists, theologians, lawyers, and social scientists), aims to anticipate and address the implications of mapping and sequencing the human genome and to develop policy options for assuring that the resulting information is used in a beneficial fashion. The ELSI program has targeted three high-priority areas for study: (1) the issues surrounding the introduction of new genetic testing into clinical practice; (2) the access to personal genetic information by parties outside the setting of clinical medicine; and (3) the professional and public understanding of genetic issues and concepts.

With respect to the introduction of new genetic tests into clinical practice, the ELSI program has focused on the establishment of clinical practice protocols, quality control mechanisms, basic research guidelines, and technology assessment criteria. Perhaps the most important issue regarding new genetic tests is defining the appropriate standard of care that should be used. The ELSI program is sponsoring a number of pilot research projects to study genetic testing. The results of such studies should have important consequences for population-wide genetic screening of various disorders, such as familial forms of cancer.

Regarding the use of and access to personal genetic information, major areas of focus by the ELSI program include improving the protection against employment discrimination on the basis of genetic information, developing industry-wide guidelines regulating the use of genetic information by private insurers, and establishing uniform standards for forensic DNA testing.

Finally, for educational programs on human genetics, there are plans within the HGP to train more rigorously the health care professionals who now are expected to interpret the new DNA-based diagnostic tests, to increase public genetic literacy through both the schools and the media, to encourage public discussion about genetic issues, and to target genetic education efforts at the appropriate public policy makers.

Adequate consideration of ethical, legal, and social issues concerning human genome research will be critical for the successful integration of genetic information into the mainstream of medical practice. The program laid out by the ELSI working group provides a foundation on which other groups and individuals can build in the years ahead. Further information and discussion on this topic is provided in Chapter 32.

CONCLUSION

The HGP fundamentally is an endeavor that aims to develop tools for the study of biology and medicine. These tools reflect both an information resource in the form of physical maps, genetic maps, and DNA sequence of the genomes of humans and model organisms, as well as an ever-growing number of experimental reagents and approaches. Together these tools are being used to establish a new and powerful foundation of knowledge that will revolutionize biomedical science by opening the way for research that previously was unapproachable. The more direct impact of the HGP on clinical medicine will be first, a dramatic acceleration in the ability to study a large range of genetic diseases, and second, the development of more powerful approaches for analyzing the DNA of patients. In the long run, though, the greatest impact of the HGP on the practice of medicine will be in providing future generations of scientists and clinicians an unprecedented resource that will allow them to define better the role of specific genes in the pathogenesis of inherited diseases, and, potentially, to treat humans in more sophisticated and beneficial ways.

REFERENCES

1. Collins FS: Positional cloning: Let's not call it reverse anymore. *Nature Genet* **1**:3, 1992.
2. Ballabio A: The rise and fall of positional cloning? *Nat Genet* **3**:277, 1993.
3. Collins FS: Positional cloning moves from perdition to traditional. *Nat Genet* **9**:347, 1995.
4. Tsui L-C, Estivill X: Identification of disease genes on the basis of chromosomal localization, in Davies KE, Tilghman SM (eds): *Genome Analysis (Volume 3: Genes and Phenotypes).* Cold Spring Harbor, NY, Cold Spring Harbor Laboratory Press, 1991, p 1.
5. Germino GG, Somlo S: A positional cloning approach to inherited renal disease. *Semin Nephrol* **12**:541, 1992.
6. Rommens JM, Iannuzzi MC, Kerem B, Drumm ML, Melmer G, Dean M, et al: Identification of the cystic fibrosis gene: Chromosome walking and jumping. *Science* **245**:1059, 1989.

7. Riordan JR, Rommens JM, Kerem B, Alon N, Rozmahel R, Grzel-czak Z, et al: Identification of the cystic fibrosis gene: Cloning and characterization of complementary DNA. *Science* **245**:1066, 1989.

8. Kerem B, Rommens JM, Buchanan JA, Markiewicz D, Cox TK, Chakravarti A, et al: Identification of the cystic fibrosis gene: Genetic analysis. *Science* **245**:1073, 1989.

9. The Huntington's Disease Collaborative Research Group: A novel gene containing a trinucleotide repeat that is expanded and unstable on Huntington's disease chromosomes. *Cell* **72**:971, 1993.

10. Feder JN, Gnirke A, Thomas W, Tsuchihashi Z, Ruddy DA, Basava A, et al: A novel MHC class I-like gene is mutated in patients with hereditary haemochromatosis. *Nat Genet* **13**:399, 1996.

11. Lander ES, Schork NJ: Genetic dissection of complex traits. *Science* **265**:2037, 1994.

12. Bell JI: Polygenic disease. *Curr Opin Genet Dev* **3**:466, 1993.

13. Green ED, Waterston RH: The human genome project: Prospects and implications for clinical medicine. *JAMA* **266**:1966, 1991.

14. McKusick VA: Genomic mapping and how it has progressed. *Hosp Pract* **26**:74, 1991.

15. Caskey CT, Rossiter BJF: The human genome project: Purpose and potential. *J Pharm Pharmacol* **44**:198, 1992.

16. Rossiter BJF, Caskey CT: The human genome project and clinical medicine. *Oncology* **6**:61, 1992.

17. Watson JD, Crick FHC: Molecular structure of nucleic acids: A structure for deoxyribose nucleic acid. *Nature* **171**:737, 1953.

18. Watson JD, Gilman M, Witkowski J, Zoller M: *Recombinant DNA.* New York, W.H. Freeman and Company, 1992.

19. Morton NE: Parameters of the human genome. *Proc Natl Acad Sci USA* **88**:7474, 1991.

20. McKusick VA: Mapping and sequencing the human genome. *N Engl J Med* **320**:910, 1989.

21. Olson MV: The human genome project. *Proc Natl Acad Sci USA* **90**:4338, 1993.

22. Tyler-Smith C, Willard HF: Mammalian chromosome structure. *Curr Opin Genet Develop* **3**:390, 1993.

23. Moyzis RK, Buckingham JM, Cram LS, Dani M, Deaven LL, Jones MD, et al: A highly conserved repetitive DNA sequence, (TTAGGG)ₙ, present at the telomeres of human chromosomes. *Proc Natl Acad Sci USA* **85**:6622, 1988.

24. Riethman HC, Moyzis RK, Meyne J, Burke DT, Olson MV: Cloning human telomeric DNA fragments into *Saccharomyces cerevisiae* using a yeast artificial-chromosome vector. *Proc Natl Acad Sci USA* **86**:6240, 1989.

25. Brown WRA: Molecular cloning of human telomeres in yeast. *Nature* **338**:774, 1989.

26. Dobson MJ, Brown WRA: Cloning human telomeres in yeast artificial chromosomes, in Anand R (ed): *Techniques for the Analysis of Complex Genomes.* London, Academic Press, 1992, p. 81.

27. Cross SH, Allshire RC, McKay SJ, McGill NI, Cooke HJ: Cloning of human telomeres by complementation in yeast. *Nature* **338**:771, 1989.

28. Cheng J-F, Smith CL: YAC cloning of telomeres. *Genet Anal Tech Appl* **7**:119, 1990.

29. Cheng J-F, Smith CL, Cantor CR: Isolation and characterization of a human telomere. *Nucl Acids Res* **17**:6109, 1989.

30. Bates GP, MacDonald ME, Baxendale S, Sedlacek Z, Youngman S, Romano D, et al: A yeast artificial chromosome telomere clone spanning a possible location of the huntington disease gene. *Am J Hum Genet* **46**:762, 1990.

31. Choo KH, Vissel B, Nagy A, Earle E, Kalitsis P: A survey of the genomic distribution of alpha satellite DNA on all the human chromosomes, and derivation of a new consensus sequence. *Nucl Acids Res* **19**:1179, 1991.

32. Waye JS, Willard HF: Nucleotide sequence heterogeneity of alpha satellite repetitive DNA: A survey of alphoid sequences from different human chromosomes. *Nucl Acids Res* **15**:7549, 1987.

33. Devilee P, Slagboom P, Cornelisse CJ, Pearson PL: Sequence heterogeneity within the human alphoid repetitive DNA family. *Nucl Acids Res* **14**:2059, 1986.

34. Jurka J, Walichiewicz J, Milosavljevic A: Prototypic sequences for human repetitive DNA. *J Mol Evol* **35**:286, 1992.

35. Ohno S: An argument for the genetic simplicity of man and other mammals. *J Hum Evol* **1**:651, 1972.

36. Gall JG: Human genome sequencing. *Science* **233**:1367, 1986.

37. Levinson B, Kenwrick S, Lakich D, Hammonds Jr G, Gitschier J: A transcribed gene in an intron of the human factor VIII gene. *Genomics* **7**:1, 1990.

38. Wallace MR, Marchuk DA, Andersen LB, Letcher R, Odeh HM, Saulino AM, et al: Type 1 neurofibromatosis gene: Identification of a large transcript disrupted in three NF1 patients. *Science* **249**:181, 1990.

39. Bird AP: CpG-rich islands and the function of DNA methylation. *Nature* **321**:209, 1986.

40. Bickmore WA, Sumner AT: Mammalian chromosome banding: An expression of genome organization. *Trends Genet* **5**:143, 1989.

41. Korenberg JR, Rykowski MC: Human genome organization: *Alu,* Lines, and the molecular structure of metaphase chromosome bands. *Cell* **53**:391, 1988.

42. Mouchiroud D, D'Onofrio G, Aissani B, Macaya G, Gautier C, Bernardi G: The distribution of genes in the human genome. *Gene* **100**:181, 1991.

43. Bernardi G: The vertebrate genome: Isochores and evolution. *Mol Biol Evol* **10**:186, 1993.

44. Bernardi G: The human genome: Organization and evolutionary history. *Ann Rev Genet* **29**:445, 1995.

45. Saccone S, De Sario A, Della Valle G, Bernardi G: The highest gene concentrations in the human genome are in telomeric bands of metaphase chromosomes. *Proc Natl Acad Sci USA* **89**:4913, 1992.

46. Sambrook J, Fritsch EF, Maniatis T: *Molecular Cloning: A Laboratory Manual.* Cold Spring Harbor, NY, Cold Spring Harbor Laboratory Press, 1989.

47. Mullis K, Faloona F, Scharf S, Saiki R, Horn G, Erlich H: Specific enzymatic amplification of DNA in vitro: The polymerase chain reaction. *Cold Spring Harb Symp Quant Biol* **LI**:263, 1986.

48. Mullis KB, Faloona FA: Specific synthesis of DNA *in vitro* via a polymerase-catalyzed chain reaction, in Wu R (ed): *Methods in Enzymology (Volume 155).* San Diego, Academic Press, 1987, p. 335.

49. Saiki RK, Scharf S, Faloona F, Mullis KB, Horn GT, Erlich HA, et al: Enzymatic amplification of b-globin genomic sequences and restriction site analysis for diagnosis of sickle cell anemia. *Science* **230**:1350, 1985.

50. Nelson DL: Applications of polymerase chain reaction methods in genome mapping. *Curr Opin Genet Dev* **1**:62, 1991.

51. Rose EA: Applications of the polymerase chain reaction to genome analysis. *FASEB J* **5**:46, 1991.

52. Erlich HA, Arnheim N: Genetic analysis using the polymerase chain reaction. *Ann Rev Genetics* **26**:479, 1992.

53. Saiki RK, Gelfand DH, Stoffel S, Scharf SJ, Higuchi R, Horn GT, et al: Primer-directed enzymatic amplification of DNA with a thermostable DNA polymerase. *Science* **239**:487, 1988.

54. Wahl GM, Lewis KA, Ruiz JC, Rothenberg B, Zhao J, Evans GA: Cosmid vectors for rapid genomic walking, restriction mapping, and gene transfer. *Proc Natl Acad Sci USA* **84**:2160, 1987.

55. Evans GA, Lewis KA: Physical mapping of complex genomes by cosmid multiplex analysis. *Proc Natl Acad Sci USA* **86**:5030, 1989.

56. Nizetic D, Zehetner G, Monaco AP, Gellen L, Young BD, Lehrach H: Construction, arraying, and high-density screening of large insert libraries of human chromosomes X and 21: Their potential use as reference libraries. *Proc Natl Acad Sci USA* **88**:3233, 1991.

57. Stallings RL, Torney DC, Hildebrand CE, Longmire JL, Deaven LL, Jett JH, et al: Physical mapping of human chromosomes by repetitive sequence fingerprinting. *Proc Natl Acad Sci USA* **87**:6218, 1990.

58. Tynan K, Olsen A, Trask B, de Jong P, Thompson J, Zimmerman W, et al: Assembly and analysis of cosmid contigs in the CEA-gene family region of human chromosome 19. *Nucl Acids Res* **20**:1629, 1992.

59. Baxendale S, MacDonald ME, Mott R, Francis F, Lin C, Kirby SF, et al: A cosmid contig and high resolution restriction map of the 2 megabase region containing the Huntington's disease gene. *Nat Genet* **4**:181, 1993.

60. Zuo J, Robbins C, Baharloo S, Cox DR, Myers RM: Construction of cosmid contigs and high-resolution restriction mapping of the Huntington disease region of human chromosome 4. *Hum Mol Genet* **2**:889, 1993.

61. Burke DT, Carle GF, Olson MV: Cloning of large segments of exogenous DNA into yeast by means of artificial chromosome vectors. *Science* **236**:806, 1987.

62. Hieter P, Connelly C, Shero J, McCormick MK, Antonarakis S, Pavan W, et al: Yeast artificial chromosomes: promises kept and pending, in Davies KE, Tilghman SM (eds): *Genome Analysis (Volume 1: Genetic and Physical Mapping).* Cold Spring Harbor, NY, Cold Spring Harbor Laboratory Press, 1990, p. 83.

63. Schlessinger D: Yeast artificial chromosomes: Tools for mapping and analysis of complex genomes. *Trends Genet* **6**:248, 1990.

64. Burke DT: The role of yeast artificial chromosome clones in generating genome maps. *Curr Opin Genet Dev* **1**:69, 1991.

65. Schlessinger D, Kere J: YAC-based mapping of genome structure, function, and evolution, in Davies KE, Tilghman SM (eds): *Genome Analysis (Volume 4: Strategies for Physical Mapping).* Cold Spring Harbor, NY, Cold Spring Harbor Laboratory Press, 1992, p. 131.

66. Burke DT, Olson MV: Preparation of clone libraries in yeast artificial-chromosome vectors, in Guthrie C, Fink GR (eds): *Methods in Enzymology (Volume 194: Guide to Yeast Genetics and Molecular Biology).* San Diego, Academic Press, 1991, p. 251.

67. Brownstein BH, Silverman GA, Little RD, Burke DT, Korsmeyer SJ, Schlessinger D, et al: Isolation of single-copy human genes from a library of yeast artificial chromosome clones. *Science* **244**:1348, 1989.

68. Imai T, Olson MV: Second-generation approach to the construction of yeast artificial-chromosome libraries. *Genomics* **8**:297, 1990.

69. Albertsen HM, Abderrahim H, Cann HM, Dausset J, Le Paslier D, Cohen D: Construction and characterization of a yeast artificial chromosome library containing seven haploid genome equivalents. *Proc Natl Acad Sci USA* **87**:4256, 1990.

70. Anand R, Riley JH, Butler R, Smith JC, Markham AF: A 3.5 genome equivalent multi access YAC library: Construction, characterisation, screening and storage. *Nucl Acids Res* **18**:1951, 1990.

71. Larin Z, Monaco AP, Lehrach H: Yeast artificial chromosome libraries containing large inserts from mouse and human DNA. *Proc Natl Acad Sci USA* **88**:4123, 1991.

72. Green ED, Olson MV: Chromosomal region of the cystic fibrosis gene in yeast artificial chromosomes: A model for human genome mapping. *Science* **250**:94, 1990.

73. Anand R, Ogilvie DJ, Butler R, Riley JH, Finniear RS, Powell SJ, Smith JC, Markham AF: A yeast artificial chromosome contig encompassing the cystic fibrosis locus. *Genomics* **9**:124, 1991.

74. Coffey AJ, Roberts RG, Green ED, Cole CG, Butler R, Anand R, et al: Construction of a 2.6-Mb contig in yeast artificial chromosomes spanning the human dystrophin gene using an STS-based approach. *Genomics* **12**:474, 1992.

75. Monaco AP, Walker AP, Millwood I, Larin Z, Lehrach H: A yeast artificial chromosome contig containing the complete Duchenne muscular dystrophy gene. *Genomics* **12**:465, 1992.

76. Geraghty DE, Pei J, Lipsky B, Hansen JA, Taillon-Miller P, Bronson SK, et al: Cloning and physical mapping of the *HLA* class I region spanning the *HLA-E-to-HLA-F* interval by using yeast artificial chromosomes. *Proc Natl Acad Sci USA* **89**:2669, 1992.

77. Zuo J, Robbins C, Taillon-Miller P, Cox DR, Myers RM: Cloning of the Huntington disease region in yeast artificial chromosomes. *Hum Mol Genet* **1**:149, 1992.

78. Bates GP, Valdes J, Hummerich H, Baxendale S, Le Paslier DL, Monaco AP, et al: Characterization of a yeast artificial chromosome contig spanning the Huntington's disease gene candidate region. *Nat Genet* **1**:180, 1992.

79. Schlessinger D, Little RD, Freije D, Abidi F, Zucchi I, Porta G, et al: Yeast artificial chromosome-based genome mapping: Some lessons from Xq24-Xq28. *Genomics* **11**:783, 1991.

80. Little RD, Pilia G, Johnson S, D'Urso M, Schlessinger D: Yeast artificial chromosomes spanning 8 megabases and 10-15 centimorgans of human cytogenetic band Xq26. *Proc Natl Acad Sci USA* **89**:177, 1992.

81. Vollrath D, Foote S, Hilton A, Brown LG, Beer-Romero P, Bogan JS, et al: The human Y chromosome: A 43-interval map based on naturally occurring deletions. *Science* **258**:52, 1992.

82. Foote S, Vollrath D, Hilton A, Page DC: The human Y chromosome: Overlapping DNA clones spanning the euchromatic region. *Science* **258**:60, 1992.

83. Chumakov I, Rigault P, Guillou S, Ougen P, Billault A, Guasconi G, et al: Continuum of overlapping clones spanning the entire human chromosome 21q. *Nature* **359**:380, 1992.

84. Korenberg JR, Chen X-N, Mitchell S, Fannin S, Gerwehr S, Cohen D, et al: A high-fidelity physical map of human chromosome 21q in yeast artificial chromosomes. *Gen Res* **5**:427, 1995.

85. Collins JE, Cole CG, Smink LJ, Garrett CL, Leversha MA, Soderlund CA, et al: A high-density YAC contig map of human chromosome 22. *Nature* **377**:367, 1995.

86. Bell CJ, Budarf ML, Nieuwenhuijsen BW, Barnoski BL, Buetow KH, Campbell K, et al: Integration of physical, breakpoint and genetic maps of chromosome 22. Localization of 587 yeast artificial chromosomes with 238 mapped markers. *Hum Mol Genet* **4**:59, 1995.

87. Smith MW, Clark SP, Hutchinson JS, Wei YH, Churukian AC, Daniels LB, et al: A sequence-tagged site map of human chromosome 11. *Genomics* **17**:699, 1993.

88. Quackenbush J, Davies C, Bailis JM, Khristich JV, Diggle K, Marchuck Y, et al: An STS content map of human chromosome 11: Localization of 910 YAC clones and 109 islands. *Genomics* **29**:512, 1995.

89. Qin S, Nowak NJ, Zhang J, Sait SNJ, Mayers PG, Higgins MJ, et al: A high-resolution physical map of human chromosome 11. *Proc Natl Acad Sci USA* **93**:3149, 1996.

90. Gemmill RM, Chumakov I, Scott P, Waggoner B, Rigault P, Cypser J, et al: A second-generation YAC contig map of human chromosome 3. *Nature* **377**:299, 1995.

91. Krauter K, Montgomery K, Yoon S-J, LeBlanc-Straceski J, Renault B, Marondel I, et al: A second-generation YAC contig map of human chromosome 12. *Nature* **377**:321, 1995.

92. Bellanne-Chantelot C, Lacroix B, Ougen P, Billault A, Beaufils S, Bertrand S, et al: Mapping the whole human genome by fingerprinting yeast artificial chromosomes. *Cell* **70**:1059, 1992.

93. Cohen D, Chumakov I, Weissenbach J: A first-generation physical map of the human genome. *Nature* **366**:698, 1993.

94. Chumakov I, Rigault P, Le Gall I, Bellanne-Chantelot C, Billault A, Guillou S, et al: A YAC contig map of the human genome. *Nature* **377**:175, 1995.

95. Hudson TJ, Stein LD, Gerety SS, Ma J, Castle AB, Silva J, et al: An STS-based map of the human genome. *Science* **270**:1945, 1995.

96. Rossi JM, Burke DT, Leung JCM, Koos DS, Chen H, Tilghman SM: Genomic analysis using a yeast artificial chromosome library with mouse DNA inserts. *Proc Natl Acad Sci USA* **89**:2456, 1992.

97. Chartier FL, Keer JT, Sutcliff MJ, Henriques DA, Mileham P, Brown SDM: Construction of a mouse yeast artificial chromosome library in a recombination-deficient strain of yeast. *Nat Genet* **1**:132, 1992.

98. Kusumi K, Smith JS, Segre JA, Koos DS, Lander ES: Construction of a large-insert yeast artificial chromosome library of the mouse genome. *Mammalian Genome* **4**:391, 1993.

99. Coulson A, Waterston R, Kiff J, Sulston J, Kohara Y: Genome linking with yeast artificial chromosomes. *Nature* **335**:184, 1988.

100. Coulson A, Kozono Y, Lutterbach B, Shownkeen R, Sulston J, Waterston R: YACs and the *C. elegans* genome. *BioEssays* **13**:413, 1991.

101. Hartl DL: Genome map of *Drosophila melanogaster* based on yeast artificial chromosomes, in Davies KE, Tilghman SM (eds): *Genome Analysis (Volume 4: Strategies for Physical Mapping).* Cold Spring Harbor, NY, Cold Spring Harbor Laboratory Press, 1992, p. 39.

102. Schmidt R, Dean C: Towards construction of an overlapping YAC library of the *Arabidopsis thaliana* genome. *BioEssays* **15**:63, 1993.

103. Green ED, Olson MV: Systematic screening of yeast artificial-chromosome libraries by use of the polymerase chain reaction. *Proc Natl Acad Sci USA* **87**:1213, 1990.

104. Silverman GA, Green ED, Young RL, Jockel JI, Domer PH, Korsmeyer SJ: Meiotic recombination between yeast artificial chromosomes yields a single clone containing the entire BCL2 protooncogene. *Proc Natl Acad Sci USA* **87**:9913, 1990.

105. Den Dunnen JT, Grootscholten PM, Dauwerse JG, Walker AP, Monaco AP, Butler R, et al: Reconstruction of the 2.4 Mb human DMD-gene by homologous YAC recombination. *Hum Mol Genet* **1**:19, 1992.

106. Green ED, Riethman HC, Dutchik JE, Olson MV: Detection and characterization of chimeric yeast artificial-chromosome clones. *Genomics* **11**:658, 1991.

107. Abidi FE, Wada M, Little RD, Schlessinger D: Yeast artificial chromosomes containing human Xq24-Xq28 DNA: library construction and representation of probe sequences. *Genomics* **7**:363, 1990.

108. McCormick MK, Shero JH, Cheung MC, Kan YW, Hieter PA, Antonarakis SE: Construction of human chromosome 21-specific yeast artificial chromosomes. *Proc Natl Acad Sci USA* **86**:9991, 1989.

109. Lee JT, Murgia A, Sosnoski DM, Olivos IM, Nussbaum RL: Construction and characterization of a yeast artificial chromosome library for Xpter-Xq27.3: a systematic determination of cocloning rate and X-chromosome representation. *Genomics* **12**:526, 1992.

110. Scherer SW, Tompkins BJF, Tsui L-C: A human chromosome 7-specific genomic DNA library in yeast artificial chromosomes. *Mammal Gen* **3**:179, 1992.

111. Qin S, Zhang J, Isaacs CM, Nagafuchi S, Jani Sait SN, Abel KJ, et al: A human chromosome 11 YAC library. *Genomics* **16**:580, 1993.

112. Green ED, Braden VV, Fulton RS, Lim R, Ueltzen MS, Peluso DC, et al: A human chromosome 7 yeast artificial chromosome (YAC) re-

source: construction, characterization, and screening. *Genomics* 25:170, 1995.

113. McCormick MK, Campbell E, Deaven L, Moyzis R: Low-frequency chimeric yeast artificial chromosome libraries from flow-sorted human chromosomes 16 and 21. *Proc Natl Acad Sci USA* 90:1063, 1993.

114. Vilageliu L, Tyler-Smith C: Structural instability of YAC clones and the use of recombination-deficient yeast host strains, in Anand R (ed): *Techniques for the analysis of complex genomes.* London, Academic Press, 1992, p 93.

115. Sternberg N: Bacteriophage P1 cloning system for the isolation, amplification, and recovery of DNA fragments as large as 100 kilobase pairs. *Proc Natl Acad Sci USA* 87:103, 1990.

116. Sternberg NL: Cloning high molecular weight DNA fragments by the bacteriophage P1 system. *Trends Genet* 8:11, 1992.

117. Shepherd NS, Pfrogner BC, Coulby JN, Ackerman SL, Vaidyanathan G, Sauer RH, et al: Preparation and screening of an arrayed human genomic library generated with the P1 cloning system. *Proc Natl Acad Sci USA* 91:2629, 1994.

118. Shizuya H, Birren B, Kim U-J, Mancino V, Slepak T, Tachiiri Y, et al: Cloning and stable maintenance of 300-kilobase-pair fragments of human DNA in *Escherichia coli* using an F-factor-based vector. *Proc Natl Acad Sci USA* 89:8794, 1992.

119. Ioannou PA, Amemiya CT, Garnes J, Kroisel PM, Shizuya H, Chen C, et al: A new bacteriophage P1-derived vector for the propagation of large human DNA fragments. *Nat Genet* 6:84, 1994.

120. Schwartz DC, Cantor CR: Separation of yeast chromosome-sized DNA by pulsed field gradient gel electrophoresis. *Cell* 37:67, 1984.

121. Carle GF, Frank M, Olson MV: Electrophoretic separations of large DNA molecules by periodic inversion of the electric field. *Science* 232:65, 1986.

122. Chu G, Vollrath D, Davis RW: Separation of large DNA molecules by contour-clamped homogenous electric fields. *Science* 234:1582, 1986.

123. Birren B, Lai E: *Pulsed Field Gel Electrophoresis: A Practical Guide.* San Diego, Academic Press, 1993.

124. Carle GF, Olson MV: An electrophoretic karyotype for yeast. *Proc Natl Acad Sci USA* 82:3756, 1985.

125. Link AJ, Olson MV: Physical map of the *Saccharomyces cerevisiae* genome at 110-kilobase resolution. *Genetics* 127:681, 1991.

126. Evans GA: Physical mapping of the human genome by pulsed field gel analysis. *Curr Opin Genet Dev* 1:75, 1991.

127. Smith DR: Genomic long-range restriction mapping. *Methods: A Companion to Methods in Enzymology* 1:195, 1990.

128. Poustka A: Physical mapping by PFGE. *Methods: A Companion to Methods in Enzymology* 1:204, 1990.

129. Burmeister M: Strategies for mapping large regions of mammalian genomes, in Burmeister M, Ulanovsky L (eds): *Methods in Molecular Biology (Volume 12: Pulsed-Field Gel Electrophoresis).* Totowa, NJ, Humana Press, 1992, p. 259.

130. Bickmore W: Analysis of genomic DNAs by pulsed-field gel electrophoresis, in Anand R (ed): *Techniques for the Analysis of Complex Genomes.* London, Academic Press, 1992, p. 19.

131. Chandrasekharappa SC, Marchuk DA, Collins FS: Analysis of yeast artificial chromosome clones, in Burmeister M, Ulanovsky L (eds): *Methods in Molecular Biology (Volume 12: Pulsed-Field Gel Electrophoresis).* Totowa, NJ, Humana Press, 1992, p. 235.

132. Bentley DR: The analysis of YAC clones, in Anand R (ed): *Techniques for the analysis of complex genomes.* London, Academic Press, 1992, p 113.

133. Nelson DL: Current methods for YAC clone characterization. *Genet Anal Tech Appl* 7:100, 1990.

134. Den Dunnen JT, van Ommen G-JB: Application of pulsed-field gel electrophoresis to genetic diagnosis, in Mathew C (ed): *Methods in Molecular Biology (Volume 9: Protocols in Human Molecular Genetics).* Clifton, NJ, Humana Press, 1991, p. 313.

135. Hozier JC, Davis LM: Cytogenetic approaches to genome mapping. *Anal Biochem* 200:205, 1992.

136. Trask BJ: Gene mapping by *in situ* hybridization. *Curr Opin Genet Dev* 1:82, 1991.

137. Trask BJ: Fluorescence *in situ* hybridization: Applications in cytogenetics and gene mapping. *Trends Genet* 7:149, 1991.

138. Pinkel D, Straume T, Gray JW: Cytogenetic analysis using quantitative, high-sensitivity, fluorescence hybridization. *Proc Natl Acad Sci USA* 83:2934, 1986.

139. Cherif D, Julier C, Delattre O, Derre J, Lathrop GM, Berger R: Simultaneous localization of cosmids and chromosome R-banding by fluorescence microscopy: application to regional mapping of human chromosome 11. *Proc Natl Acad Sci USA* 87:6639, 1990.

140. Lichter P, Chang Tang C-J, Call K, Hermanson G, Evans GA, Housman D, et al: High-resolution mapping of human chromosome 11 by *in situ* hybridization with cosmid clones. *Science* 247:64, 1990.

141. Lawrence JB, Villnave CA, Singer RH: Sensitive, high resolution chromatin and chromosome mapping in situ: Presence and orientation of two closely integrated copies of EBV in a lymphoma line. *Cell* 52:51, 1988.

142. Stock W, Chandrasekharappa SC, Neuman WL, Le Beau MM, Brownstein BH, Westbrook CA: Characterization of yeast artificial chromosomes containing interleukin genes on human chromosome 5. *Cytogenet Cell Genet* 61:263, 1992.

143. Trask BJ, Massa H, Kenwrick S, Gitschier J: Mapping of human chromosome Xq28 by two-color fluorescence in situ hybridization of DNA sequences to interphase cell nuclei. *Am J Hum Genet* 48:1, 1991.

144. Johnson DH: Molecular cloning of DNA from specific chromosomal regions by microdissection and sequence-independent amplification of DNA. *Genomics* 6:243, 1990.

145. Ludecke H-J, Senger G, Claussen U, Horsthemke B: Cloning defined regions of the human genome by microdissection of banded chromosomes and enzymatic amplification. *Nature* 338:348, 1989.

146. Ludecke H-J, Senger G, Claussen U, Horsthemke B: Generation of region-specific probes by microdissection and universal enzymatic DNA amplification, in Anand R (ed): *Techniques for the Analysis of Complex Genomes.* London, Academic Press, 1992, p. 215.

147. Kao F: Microdissection and microcloning of human chromosome regions in genome and genetic disease analysis. *BioEssays* 15:141, 1993.

148. Meltzer PS, Guan X, Burgess A, Trent JM: Rapid generation of region specific probes by chromosome microdissection and their application. *Nat Genet* 1:24, 1992.

149. National Institute of General Medical Sciences (U.S. Department of Health and Human Services): *1992/1993 Catalog of Cell Lines: NIGMS Human Genetic Mutant Cell Repository.* (NIH Publication 92-2011), 1992.

150. Adams MD, Fields C, Venter JC, (eds): *Automated DNA Sequencing and Analysis.* San Diego, Academic Press, 1994.

151. Sanger F, Nicklen S, Coulson AR: DNA sequencing with chain-terminating inhibitors. *Proc Natl Acad Sci USA* 74:5463, 1977.

152. Smith LM, Sanders JZ, Kaiser RJ, Hughes P, Dodd C, Connell CR, Heiner C, Kent SBH, Hood LE: Fluorescence detection in automated DNA sequence analysis. *Nature* 321:674, 1986.

153. Prober JM, Trainor GL, Dam RJ, Hobbs FW, Robertson CW, Zagursky RJ, et al: A system for rapid DNA sequencing with fluorescent chain-terminating dideoxynucleotides. *Science* 238:336, 1987.

154. Hunkapiller T, Kaiser RJ, Koop BF, Hood L: Large-scale and automated DNA sequence determination. *Science* 254:59, 1991.

155. *ISCN: an international system for human cytogenetic nomenclature. Birth Defects: Original Article Series (Volume 21, No. 1).* New York, Karger, 1985.

156. Royer-Pokora B, Kunkel LM, Monaco AP, Goff SC, Newburger PE, Baehner RL, et al: Cloning the gene for an inherited human disorder—chronic granulomatous disease—on the basis of its chromosomal location. *Nature* 322:32, 1986.

157. Monaco AP, Neve RL, Colletti-Feener C, Bertelson CJ, Kurnit DM, Kunkel LM: Isolation of candidate cDNAs for portions of the Duchenne muscular dystrophy gene. *Nature* 323:646, 1986.

158. Verkerk AJMH, Pieretti M, Sutcliffe JS, Fu Y-H, Kuhl DPA, Pizzuti A, et al: Identification of a gene (FMR-1) containing a CGG repeat coincident with a breakpoint cluster region exhibiting length variation in fragile X syndrome. *Cell* 65:905, 1991.

159. Green ED, Idol JR, Mohr-Tidwell RM, Braden VV, Peluso DC, Fulton RS, et al: Integration of physical, genetic and cytogenetic maps of human chromosome 7: Iisolation and analysis of yeast artificial chromosome clones for 117 mapped genetic markers. *Hum Mol Genet* 3:489, 1994.

160. Bray-Ward P, Menninger J, Lieman J, Desai T, Mokady N, Banks A, et al: Integration of the cytogenetic, genetic, and physical maps of the human genome by FISH mapping of CEPH YAC clones. *Genomics* 32:1, 1996.

161. Kohara Y, Akiyama K, Isono K: The physical map of the whole E. coli chromosome: application of a new strategy for rapid analysis and sorting of a large genomic library. *Cell* 50:495, 1987.

162. Olson MV, Dutchik JE, Graham MY, Brodeur GM, Helms C, Frank M, et al: Random-clone strategy for genomic restriction mapping in yeast. *Proc Natl Acad Sci USA* 83:7826, 1986.

163. Coulson A, Sulston J, Brenner S, Karn J: Toward a physical map of the genome of the nematode *Caenorhabditis elegans. Proc Natl Acad Sci USA* 83:7821, 1986.

164. Olson M, Hood L, Cantor C, Botstein D: A common language for physical mapping of the human genome. *Science* 245:1434, 1989.

165. Green ED, Green P: Sequence-tagged site (STS) content mapping of human chromosomes: Theoretical considerations and early experiences. *PCR Methods Applic* 1:77, 1991.

166. Green ED, Mohr RM, Idol JR, Jones M, Buckingham JM, Deaven LL, et al: Systematic generation of sequence-tagged sites for physical mapping of human chromosomes: Application to the mapping of human chromosome 7 using yeast artificial chromosomes. *Genomics* 11:548, 1991.

167. Green ED: Physical mapping of human chromosomes: Generation of chromosome-specific sequence-tagged sites, in Adolph KW (ed): *Methods in Molecular Genetics (Volume 1: Gene and Chromosome Analysis, Part A).*San Diego, Academic Press, 1993, p. 192.

168. Nelson DL, Ledbetter SA, Corbo L, Victoria MF, Ramirez-Solis R, Webster TD, et al: *Alu* polymerase chain reaction: a method for rapid isolation of human-specific sequences from complex DNA sources. *Proc Natl Acad Sci USA* 86:6686, 1989.

169. Nelson DL: Interspersed repetitive sequence polymerase chain reaction (IRS PCR) for generation of human DNA fragments from complex sources. *Methods: A Companion to Methods in Enzymology* 2:60, 1991.

170. Cole CG, Goodfellow PN, Bobrow M, Bentley DR: Generation of novel sequence tagged sites (STSs) from discrete chromosomal regions using Alu-PCR. *Genomics* 10:816, 1991.

171. Klein V, Piontek K, Brass N, Subke F, Zang KD, Meese E: Identification of chromosome-specific sequence-tagged sites by *Alu*-PCR. *Genet Anal Tech Appl* 10:6, 1993.

172. La Pillo B, Karpinski S, Ludecke H-J, Horsthemke B: Detailed characterization of a human 8q24.1 microdissection library and generation of "sequence-tagged sites." *Cytogenet Cell Genet* 63:185, 1993.

173. Deaven LL, Van Dilla MA, Bartholdi MF, Carrano AV, Cram LS, Fuscoe JC, et al: Construction of human chromosome-specific DNA libraries from flow-sorted chromosomes. *Cold Spring Harb Symp Quant Biol* LI:159, 1986.

174. Collins C, Kuo WL, Segraves R, Fuscoe J, Pinkel D, Gray JW: Construction and characterization of plasmid libraries enriched in sequences from single human chromosomes. *Genomics* 11:997, 1991.

175. Shimizu N, Minoshima S: Gene mapping and fine-structure analysis of the human genome using flow-sorted chromosomes, in Adolph KW (ed): *Advanced Techniques in Chromosome Research.* New York, Marcel Dekker, 1991, p. 135.

176. Goold RD, diSibio GL, Xu H, Lang DB, Dadgar J, Magrane GG, et al: The development of sequence-tagged sites for human chromosome 4. *Hum Mol Genet* 2:1271, 1993.

177. Sheffield VC, Weber JL, Buetow KH, Murray JC, Even DA, Wiles K, et al: A collection of tri- and tetranucleotide repeat markers used to generate high quality, high resolution human genome-wide linkage maps. *Hum Mol Genet* 4:1837, 1995.

178. Schuler GD, Boguski MS, Stewart EA, Stein LD, Gyapay G, Rice K, et al: A gene map of the human genome. *Science* 274:540, 1996.

179. Naylor SL, Moore S, Garcia D, Xiang X, Xin X, Mohrer M, et al: Mapping 638 STSs to regions of human chromosome 3. *Cytogenet Cell Genet* 72:90, 1996.

180. Grady DL, Robinson DL, Gersh M, Nickerson E, McPherson J, Wasmuth JJ, et al: The generation and regional localization of 303 new chromosome 5 sequence-tagged sites. *Genomics* 32:91, 1996.

181. Hudson TJ, Colbert AME, Reeve MP, Bae JS, Lee MK, Nussbaum RL, et al: Isolation and regional mapping of 110 chromosome 22 STSs. *Genomics* 24:588, 1994.

182. Ciccodicola A, Cinti C, Esposito T, Campanile C, Casamassimi A, Miano MG, et al: Sequence-tagged sites (STSs) from YAC insert-ends and X-specific flow-sorted chromosomes. *Mammal Gen* 5:511, 1994.

183. Nelson DL, Ballabio A, Cremers F, Monaco AP, Schlessinger D: Report of the sixth international workshop on human X chromosome mapping 1995. *Cytogenet Cell Genet* 71:307, 1995.

184. Weissenbach J, Gyapay G, Dib C, Vignal A, Morissette J, Millasseau P, et al: A second-generation linkage map of the human genome. *Nature* 359:794, 1992.

185. Gyapay G, Morissette J, Vignal A, Dib C, Fizames C, Millasseau P, et al: The 1993-94 Genethon human genetic linkage map. *Nat Genet* 7:246, 1994.

186. Dib C, Faure S, Fizames C, Samson D, Drouot N, Vignal A, et al: A comprehensive genetic map of the human genome based on 5,264 microsatellites. *Nature* 380:152, 1996.

187. Murray JC, Buetow KH, Weber JL, Ludwigsen S, Scherpbier-Heddema T, Manion F, et al: A comprehensive human linkage map with centimorgan density. *Science* 265:2049, 1994.

188. Buetow KH, Weber JL, Ludwigsen S, Scherpbier-Heddema T, Duyk GM, Sheffield VC, et al: Integrated human genome-wide maps constructed using the CEPH reference panel. *Nat Genet* 6:391, 1994.

189. Utah Marker Development Group: A collection of ordered tetranucleotide-repeat markers from the human genome. *Am J Hum Genet* 57:619, 1995.

190. Dietrich W, Katz H, Lincoln SE, Shin H, Friedman J, Dracopoli NC, et al: A genetic map of the mouse suitable for typing intraspecific crosses. *Genetics* 131:423, 1992.

191. Dietrich WF, Miller JC, Steen RG, Merchant M, Damron D, Nahf R, et al: A genetic map of the mouse with 4,006 simple sequence length polymorphisms. *Nat Genet* 7:220, 1994.

192. Dietrich WF, Miller J, Steen R, Merchant MA, Damron-Boles D, Husain Z, et al: A comprehensive genetic map of the mouse genome. *Nature* 380:149, 1996.

193. Dietrich WF, Copeland NG, Gilbert DJ, Miller JC, Jenkins NA, Lander ES: Mapping the mouse genome: Current status and future prospects. *Proc Natl Acad Sci USA* 92:10849, 1995.

194. Cox DR, Burmeister M, Price ER, Kim S, Myers RM: Radiation hybrid mapping: a somatic cell genetic method for constructing high-resolution maps of mammalian chromosomes. *Science* 250:245, 1990.

195. Cox DR, Myers RM: Bridging the gaps. *Curr Biol* 2:338, 1992.

196. Walter MA, Spillett DJ, Thomas P, Weissenbach J, Goodfellow PN: A method for constructing radiation hybrid maps of whole genomes. *Nat Genet* 7:22, 1994.

197. Gyapay G, Schmitt K, Fizames C, Jones H, Vega-Czarny N, Spillett D, et al: A radiation hybrid map of the human genome. *Hum Mol Genet* 5:339, 1996.

198. Boehnke M, Lange K, Cox DR: Statistical methods for multipoint radiation hybrid mapping. *Am J Hum Genet* 49:1174, 1991.

199. Lunetta KL, Boehnke M: Multipoint radiation hybrid mapping: comparison of methods, sample size requirements, and optimal study characteristics. *Genomics* 21:92, 1994.

200. Lange K, Boehnke M, Cox DR, Lunetta KL: Statistical methods for polyploid radiation hybrid mapping. *Gen Res* 5:136, 1995.

201. Lunetta KL, Boehnke M, Lange K, Cox DR: Experimental design and error detection for polyploid radiation hybrid mapping. *Gen Res* 5:151, 1995.

202. Little PFR: Gene mapping and the human genome mapping project. *Curr Opin Cell Biol* 2:478, 1990.

203. Hochgeschwender U: Toward a transcriptional map of the human genome. *Trends Genet* 8:11, 1992.

204. Southern EM: Genome mapping: cDNA approaches. *Curr Opin Genet Dev* 2:412, 1992.

205. Kwok PY, Carlson C, Yager TD, Ankener W, Nickerson DA: Comparative analysis of human DNA variations by fluorescence-based sequencing of PCR products. *Genomics* 23:138, 1994.

206. Hillier L, Lennon G, Becker M, Bonaldo M, Chiapelli B, Chissoe S, et al: Generation and analysis of 280,000 human expressed sequence tags. *Genome Res* 6:807, 1996.

207. Adams MD, Kerlavage AR, Fleischmann RD, Fuldner RA, Bult CJ, Lee NH, et al: Initial assessment of human gene diversity and expression patterns based upon 83 million nucleotides of cDNA sequence. *Nature* 377:3, 1995.

208. Boguski MS, Schuler GD: Establishing a human transcript map. *Nat Genet* 10:369, 1995.

209. Boguski MS: The turning point in genome research. *Trends Biochem Sci* 20:295, 1995.

210. Wilcox AS, Khan AS, Hopkins JA, Sikela JM: Use of 3′ untranslated sequences of human cDNAs for rapid chromosome assignment and conversion to STSs: Implications for an expression map of the genome. *Nucl Acids Res* 19:1837, 1991.

211. Berry R, Stevens TJ, Walter NAR, Wilcox AS, Rubano T, Hopkins JA, et al: Gene-based sequence tagged sites (STSs) as the basis for a human gene map. *Nat Genet* 10:415, 1995.

212. Tilghman SM: Lessons learned, promises kept: A biologist's eye view of the genome project. *Gen Res* 6:773, 1996.

213. Southern EM: Detection of specific sequences among DNA fragments separated by gel electrophoresis. *J Mol Biol* **98**:503, 1975.

214. Botstein D, White RL, Skolnick M, Davis RW: Construction of a genetic linkage map in man using restriction fragment length polymorphisms. *Am J Hum Genet* **32**:314, 1980.

215. White R, Leppert M, Bishop DT, Barker D, Berkowitz J, Brown C, et al: Construction of linkage maps with DNA markers for human chromosomes. *Nature* **313**:101, 1985.

216. Donis-Keller H, Barker DF, Knowlton RG, Schumm JW, Braman JC, Green P: Highly polymorphic RFLP probes as diagnostic tools. *Cold Spring Harb Symp Quant Biol* **LI**:317, 1986.

217. Lander ES, Botstein D: Mapping complex genetic traits in humans: New method using a complete RFLP linkage map. *Cold Spring Harb Symp Quant Biol* **LI**:49, 1986.

218. Nakamura Y, Leppert M, O'Connell P, Wolff R, Holm T, Culver M, et al: Variable number of tandem repeat (VNTR) markers for human gene mapping. *Science* **235**:1616, 1987.

219. Weber JL, May PE: Abundant class of human DNA polymorphisms which can be typed using the polymerase chain reaction. *Am J Hum Genet* **44**:388, 1989.

220. Litt M, Luty JA: A hypervariable microsatellite revealed by in vitro amplification of a dinucleotide repeat within the cardiac muscle actin gene. *Am J Hum Genet* **44**:397, 1989.

221. Weber JL: Human DNA polymorphisms based on length variations in simple-sequence tandem repeats, in Davies KE, Tilghman SM (eds): *Genome Analysis (Volume 1: Genetic and Physical Mapping)*. Cold Spring Harbor, NY, Cold Spring Harbor Laboratory Press, 1990, p. 159.

222. Nickerson DA, Whitehurst C, Boysen C, Charmley P, Kaiser R, Hood L: Identification of clusters of biallelic polymorphic sequence-tagged sites (pSTSs) that generate highly informative and automatable markers for genetic linkage mapping. *Genomics* **12**:377, 1992.

223. Nickerson DA, Kaiser R, Lappin S, Stewart J, Hood L, Landegren U: Automated DNA diagnostics using an ELISA-based oligonucleotide ligation assay. *Proc Natl Acad Sci USA* **87**:8923, 1990.

224. Landegren U, Kaiser R, Sanders J, Hood L: A ligase-mediated gene detection technique. *Science* **241**:1077, 1988.

225. Dausset J, Cann H, Cohen D, Lathrop M, Lalouel J, White R: Centre d'Etude du Polymorphisme Humain (CEPH): collaborative genetic mapping of the human genome. *Genomics* **6**:575, 1990.

226. Ott J: *Analysis of Human Genetic Linkage*. Baltimore,. Johns Hopkins University Press, 1985.

227. Donis-Keller H, Green P, Helms C, Cartinhour S, Weiffenbach B, Stephens K, et al: A genetic linkage map of the human genome. *Cell* **51**:319, 1987.

228. Li H, Gyllensten UB, Cui X, Saiki RK, Erlich HA, Arnheim N: Amplification and analysis of DNA sequences in single human sperm and diploid cells. *Nature* **335**:414, 1988.

229. Cui X, Li H, Goradia TM, Lange K, Kazazian Jr HH, Galas D, et al: Single-sperm typing: determination of genetic distance between the G-gamma-globin and parathyroid hormone loci by using the polymerase chain reaction and allele-specific oligomers. *Proc Natl Acad Sci USA* **86**:9389, 1989.

230. Arnheim N, Li H, Cui X: PCR analysis of DNA sequences in single cells: Single-sperm gene mapping and genetic disease diagnosis. *Genomics* **8**:415, 1990.

231. Li H, Cui X, Arnheim N: Analysis of DNA sequence variation in single cells. *Methods: A Companion to Methods in Enzymology* **2**:49, 1991.

232. Zhang L, Cui X, Schmitt K, Hubert R, Navidi W, Arnheim N: Whole genome amplification from a single cell: Implications for genetic analysis. *Proc Natl Acad Sci USA* **89**:5847, 1992.

233. Riles L, Dutchik JE, Baktha A, McCauley BK, Thayer EC, Leckie MP, et al: Physical maps of the six smallest chromosomes of *Saccharomyces cerevisiae* at a resolution of 2.6 kilobase pairs. *Genetics* **134**:81, 1993.

234. Koonin EV, Mushegian AR, Rudd KE: Sequencing and analysis of bacterial genomes. *Curr Biol* **6**:404, 1996.

235. Mizukami T, Chang WI, Garkavtsev I, Kaplan N, Lombardi D, Matsumoto T, et al: A 13 kb resolution cosmid map of the 14 Mb fission yeast genome by nonrandom sequence-tagged site mapping. *Cell* **73**:121, 1993.

236. Hoheisel JD, Maier E, Mott R, McCarthy L, Grigoriev AV, Schalkwyk LC, et al: High resolution cosmid and P1 maps spanning the 14 Mb genome of the fission yeast *S. pombe*. *Cell* **73**:109, 1993.

237. Merriam J, Ashburner M, Hartl DL, Kafatos FC: Toward cloning and mapping the genome of *Drosophila*. *Science* **254**:221, 1991.

238. Hartl DL, Lozovskaya ER: The *Drosophila* genome project: current status of the physical map. *Comp Biochem Physiol* **103B**:1, 1992.

239. Hartl DL, Ajioka JW, Cai H, Lohe AR, Lozovskaya ER, Smoller DA, et al: Towards a *Drosophila* genome map. *Trends Genet* **8**:70, 1994.

240. Paterson AH, WIng RA: Genome mapping in plants. *Curr Opin Biotechnol* **4**:142, 1993.

241. Schmidt R, Dean C: Physical mapping of the *Arabidopsis thaliana* genome, in Davies KE, Tilghman SM (eds): *Genome Analysis (Volume 4: Strategies for Physical Mapping)*. Cold Spring Harbor, NY, Cold Spring Harbor Laboratory Press, 1992, p. 71.

242. O'Brien SJ, Womack JE, Lyons LA, Moore KJ, Jenkins NA, Copeland NG: Anchored reference loci for comparative genome mapping in mammals. *Nat Genet* **3**:103, 1993.

243. Rudd KE: Maps, genes, sequences, and computers: An *Escherichia coli* case study. *ASM News* **59**:335, 1993.

244. Meisler MH: The role of the laboratory mouse in the human genome project. *Am J Hum Genet* **59**:764, 1996.

245. Daniels DL, Plunkett III G, Burland V, Blattner FR: Analysis of the *Escherichia coli* genome: DNA sequence of the region from 84.5 to 86.5 minutes. *Science* **257**:771, 1992.

246. Burland V, Plunkett III G, Daniels DL, Blattner FR: DNA sequence and analysis of 136 kilobases of the *Escherichia coli* genome: organizational symmetry around the origin of replication. *Genomics* **16**:551, 1993.

247. Botstein D, Fink GR: Yeast: an experimental organism for modern biology. *Science* **240**:1439, 1988.

248. Goffeau A, Barrell BG, Bussey H, Davis RW, Dujon B, Oliver SG, et al: Life with 6000 genes. *Science* **274**:546, 1996.

249. Hieter P, Bassett Jr DE, Valle D: The yeast genome—a common currency. *Nature Genet* **13**:253, 1996.

250. Johnston M: Genome sequencing: the complete code for a eukaryotic cell. *Curr Biol* **6**:500, 1996.

251. Dujon B: The yeast genome project: what did we learn? *Trends Genet* **12**:263, 1996.

252. Walsh S, Barrell B: The *Saccharomyces cerevisiae* genome on the World Wide Web. *Trends Genet* **12**:276, 1996.

253. Sulston J, Du Z, Thomas K, Wilson R, Hillier L, Waterston R, et al: The *C. elegans* genome sequencing project: a beginning. *Nature* **356**:37, 1992.

254. Wilson R, Ainscough R, Anderson K, Baynes C, Berks M, Fulton L: 2.2 Mb of contiguous nucleotide sequence from chromosome III of *C. elegans*. *Nature* **368**:32, 1994.

255. Cox RD, Lehrach H: Genome mapping: PCR based meiotic and somatic cell hybrid analysis. *BioEssays* **13**:193, 1991.

256. Nadeau JH: Maps of linkage and synteny homologies between mouse and man. *Trends Genet* **5**:82, 1989.

257. O'Brien SJ: Mammalian genome mapping: lessons and prospects. *Curr Opin Genet Develop* **1**:105, 1990.

258. DeBry RW, Seldin MF: Human/mouse homology relationships. *Genomics* **33**:337, 1996.

259. Hood L, Koop B, Goverman J, Hunkapiller T: Model genomes: the benefits of analysing homologous human and mouse sequences. *Trends Biotechnol* **10**:19, 1992.

260. Koop BF, Hood L: Striking sequence similarity over almost 100 kilobases of human and mouse T-cell receptor DNA. *Nature Genet* **7**:48, 1994.

261. Watson JD, Jordon E: The human genome program at the National Institutes of Health. *Genomics* **5**:654, 1989.

262. Watson JD: The human genome project: past, present, and future. *Science* **248**:44, 1990.

263. Cook-Deegan RM: The genesis of the human genome project, in Friedmann T (ed): *Molecular Genetic Medicine (Volume 1)*. San Diego, Academic Press, Inc. 1991, p 1.

264. Watson JD, Cook-Deegan RM: Origins of the human genome project. *FASEB J* **5**:8, 1991.

265. Jordan E: Organization and long-range plan. *Anal Chem* **63**:420A, 1991.

266. Engel LW: The human genome project: history, goals, and progress to date. *Arch Pathol Lab Med* **117**:459, 1993.

267. Jordan E: Invited editorial: the human genome project: where did it come from, where is it going? *Am J Hum Genet* **51**:1, 1992.

268. Haq MM: Medical genetics and the human genome project: a historical review. *Tex Med* **89**:68, 1993.

269. Cantor CR: Orchestrating the human genome project. *Science* **248**:49, 1990.

270. Cook-Deegan RM: The Alta Summit, December 1984. *Genomics* **5**:661, 1989.

271. Sinsheimer RL: The Santa Cruz Workshop—May 1985. *Genomics* **5**:954, 1989.
272. DeLisi C: The human genome project. *Am Sci* **76**:488, 1988.
273. Dulbecco R: A turning point in cancer research: sequencing the human genome. *Science* **231**:1055, 1986.
274. National Research Council (Committee on Mapping and Sequencing the Human Genome): *Mapping and Sequencing the Human Genome.* Washington, D.C., National Academy Press, 1988.
275. Office of Technology Assessment: Mapping *Our Genes—Genome Projects: How Big? How Fast?* Washington, D.C., 61-OTA-BA-373, 1988.
276. Watson JD: The human genome initiative: a statement of need. *Hosp Pract* **26**:69, 1991.
277. Gilbert W: Towards a paradigm shift in biology. *Nature* **349**:99, 1991.
278. Berg P: All our collective ingenuity will be needed. *FASEB J* **5**:75, 1991.
279. Yager TD, Nickerson DA, Hood LE: The human genome project: creating an infrastructure for biology and medicine. *Trends Biochem Sci* **16**:454, 1991.
280. Martin RG: We gnomes find the project an atlas but no treasure. *New Biol* **2**:385, 1990.
281. Rechsteiner MC: The human genome project: misguided science policy. *Trends Biochem Sci* **16**:455, 1991.
282. Davis BD, Colleagues: The human genome and other initiatives. *Science* **249**:342, 1990.
283. Tauber AI, Sarkar S: The human genome project: has blind reductionism gone too far? *Perspect Biol Med* **35**:221, 1992.
284. Rosenberg LE: The human genome project. *Bull N Y Acad Med* **68**:113, 1992.
285. Richardson WC: Summary, conference on the human genome project: an agenda for science & society. *Bull N Y Acad Med* **68**:162, 1992.
286. Koshland DE: Sequences and consequences of the human genome. *Science* **246**:189, 1989.
287. U.S. Department of Health and Human Services, U.S. Department of Energy: *Understanding Our Genetic Inheritance. The U.S. Human Genome Project: The First Five Years, FY 1991-1995 (DOE/ER-0452P).* Springfield. National Technical Information Service, 1990.
288. Collins F, Galas D: A new five-year plan for the U.S. human genome project. *Science* **262**:43, 1993.
289. Lander ES: The new genomics: global views of biology. *Science* **274**:536, 1996.
290. Olson MV: A tale of two cities. *Anal Chem* **63**:416A, 1991.
291. Fasman KH, Letovsky SI, Cottingham RW, Kingsbury DT: Improvements to the GDB Human Genome Data Base. *Nucl Acids Res* **24**:57, 1996.
292. Benson DA, Boguski MS, Lipman DJ, Ostell J: GenBank. *Nucl Acids Res* **24**:1, 1996.
293. Dear S, Staden R: A sequence assembly and editing program for efficient management of large projects. *Nucl Acids Res* **19**:3907, 1991.
294. *Methods in Enzymology Volume 266: Computer Methods for Macromolecular Sequence Analysis* (Doolittle RF, ed). San Diego, Academic Press, Inc. 1996.
295. *Methods in Enzymology Volume 183: Molecular Evolution: Computer Analysis of Protein and Nucleic Acid Sequences* (Wu R, ed). San Diego,. Academic Press, Inc. 1990.
296. Pearson WR, Lipman DJ: Improved tools for biological sequence comparison. *Proc Natl Acad Sci USA* **85**:2444, 1988.
297. Altschul SF, Gish W, Miller W, Myers EW, Lipman DJ: Basic local alignment search tool. *J Mol Biol* **215**:403, 1990.
298. Uberbacher EC, Mural RJ: Locating protein-coding regions in human DNA sequences by a multiple sensor-neural network approach. *Proc Natl Acad Sci USA* **88**:11261, 1991.
299. Hutchinson GB, Hayden MR: The prediction of exons through an analysis of spliceable open reading frames. *Nucl Acids Res* **20**:3453, 1992.
300. Green P, Lipman D, Hillier L, Waterston R, States D, Claverie J: Ancient conserved regions in new gene sequences and the protein databases. *Science* **259**:1711, 1993.
301. Smith RF, Wiese BA, Wojzynski MK, Davison DB, Worley KC: BCM search launcher—an integrated interface to molecular biology data base search and analysis services on the World Wide Web. *Genome Research* **6**:454, 1996.
302. Olson MV: A time to sequence. *Science* **270**:394, 1995.
303. Boguski M, Chakravarti A, Gibbs R, Green E, Myers RM: The end of the beginning: the race to begin human genome sequencing. *Genome Research* **6**:771, 1996.
304. Guyer MS, Collins FS: The human genome project and the future of medicine. *AJDC* **147**:1145, 1993.
305. Watson JD, Cook-Deegan RM: The human genome project and international health. *JAMA* **263**:3322, 1990.
306. Annas GJ: The human genome project as social policy: implications for clinical medicine. *Bull N Y Acad Med* **68**:126, 1992.
307. Charo RA: Effect of the human genome initiative on women's rights and reproductive decisions. *Fetal Diagn Ther* **8**:148, 1993.
308. Whittaker LA: The implications of the human genome project for family practice. *J Fam Pract* **35**:294, 1992.
309. Sachs BP, Korf B: The human genome project: implications for the practicing obstetrician. *Obstet Gynecol* **81**:458, 1993.
310. Sawicki MP, Samara G, Hurwitz M, Passaro E Jr: Human genome project. *Am J Surg* **165**:258, 1993.
311. Gordon J: The human genome project promises insights into aging. *Geriatrics* **44**:89, 1989.
312. Gardiner RM: The human genome: a prospect for paediatrics. *Arch Dis Child* **65**:457, 1990.
313. Cantor CR: Implications of the human genome project for clinical neurosurgery. *Clin Neurosurg* **37**:173, 1991.
314. Caskey CT: DNA-based medicine: prevention and therapy, in Kevles DJ, Hood L (eds): *The Code of Codes: Scientific and Social Issues in the Human Genome Project.* Cambridge, Harvard University Press, 1992, p. 112.
315. Hood L: Biology and medicine in the twenty-first century, in Kevles DJ, Hood L (eds): *The Code of Codes: Scientific and Social Issues in the Human Genome Project.* Cambridge, Harvard University Press, 1992, p. 136.
316. Wevrick R, Buchwald M: Mammalian DNA-repair genes. *Curr Opin Genet Develop* **3**:470, 1993.
317. Orkin SH, Nathan DG: The molecular genetics of Thalassemia, in Harris H, Hirschhorn K (eds): *Advances in Human Genetics (Volume 11).* New York, Plenum Press, 1981, p. 233.
318. Brennand J, Chinault AC, Konecki DS, Melton DW, Caskey CT: Cloned cDNA sequences of the hypoxanthine/guanine phosphoribosyltransferase gene from a mouse neuroblastoma cell line found to have amplified genomic sequences. *Proc Natl Acad Sci USA* **79**:1950, 1982.
319. Jolly DJ, Esty AC, Bernard HU, Friedmann T: Isolation of a genomic clone partially encoding human hypoxanthine phosphoribosyltransferase. *Proc Natl Acad Sci USA* **79**:5038, 1982.
320. Jolly DJ, Okayama H, Berg P, Esty AC, Filpula D, Bohlen P, Johnson GG, Shively JE, Hunkapillar T, Friedmann T: Isolation and characterization of a full-length expressible cDNA for human hypoxanthine phosphoribosyltransferase. *Proc Natl Acad Sci USA* **80**:477, 1983.
321. Melton DW, Konecki DS, Brennand J, Caskey CT: Structure, expression, and mutation of the hypoxanthine phosphoribosyltransferase gene. *Proc Natl Acad Sci USA* **81**:2147, 1984.
322. Kwok SCM, Ledley FD, DiLella AG, Robson KJH, Woo SLC: Nucleotide sequence of a full-length complementary DNA clone and amino acid sequence of human phenylalanine hydroxylase. *Biochem* **24**:556, 1985.
323. Persico MG, Viglietto G, Martini G, Toniolo D, Paonessa G, D'Urso M, et al: Isolation of human glucose-6-phosphate dehydrogenase (G6PD) cDNA clones: primary structure of the protein and unusual 5' non-coding region. *Nucl Acids Res* **14**:2511, 1986.
324. Orkin SH: Reverse genetics and human disease. *Cell* **47**:845, 1986.
325. Ruddle FH: The William Allan Memorial Award address: reverse genetics and beyond. *Am J Hum Genet* **36**:944, 1984.
326. Orkin SH: "Forward" and "reverse" genetics of inherited human disorders: the Thalassemia syndromes and chronic granulomatous disease. *Harvey Lect* **83**:57, 1989.
327. Friedmann T: Opinion: the human genome project—some implications of extensive "reverse genetic" medicine. *Am J Hum Genet* **46**:407, 1990.
328. Cawthon RM, Weiss R, Xu G, Viskochil D, Culver M, White R, et al: A major segment of the neurofibromatosis type 1 gene: cDNA sequence, genomic structure, and point mutations. *Cell* **62**:193, 1990.
329. Attree O, Olivos IM, Okabe I, Bailey LC, Nelson DL, Nussbaum RL, et al: The Lowe's oculocerebrorenal syndrome gene encodes a protein highly homologous to inositol polyphosphate-5-phosphatase. *Nature* **358**:239, 1992.
330. de Klein A, van Kessel AG, Grosveld G, Bartram CR, Hagemeijer A, Stephenson JR, et al: A cellular oncogene is translocated to the Philadelphia chromosome in chronic myelocytic leukaemia. *Nature* **300**:765, 1982.

331. Zieman-van der Poel S, McCabe NR, Gill HJ, Espinosa III R, Patel Y, Diaz MO, et al: Identification of a gene, *MLL*, that spans the breakpoint in 11q23 translocations associated with human leukemias. *Proc Natl Acad Sci USA* **88**:10735, 1991.

332. Djabali M, Selleri L, Parry P, Bower M, Young BD, Evans GA: A trithorax-like gene is interrupted by chromosome 11q23 translocations in acute leukaemias. *Nature Genet* **2**:113, 1992.

333. Barr FG, Galili N, Holick J, Biegel JA, Rovera G, Emanuel BS: Rearrangement of the PAX3 paired box gene in paediatric solid tumour alveolar rhabdomyosarcoma. *Nature Genet* **3**:113, 1993.

334. Solomon E, Borrow J, Goddard AD: Chromosome aberrations and cancer. *Science* **254**:1153, 1991.

335. Shiloh Y, Mor O, Manor A, Bar-Am I, Rotman G, Avivi L, et al: DNA sequences amplified in cancer cells: an interface between tumor biology and human genome analysis. *Mutation Res* **276**:329, 1992.

336. Ploughman LM, Boehnke M: Estimating the power of a proposed linkage study for a complex genetic trait. *Am J Hum Genet* **44**:543, 1989.

337. Stubbs L: Long-range walking techniques in positional cloning strategies. *Mammalian Genome* **3**:127, 1992.

338. Hochgeschwender U, Brennan MB: Identifying genes within the genome: new ways for finding the needle in a haystack. *BioEssays* **13**:139, 1991.

339. Thomas PS: Hybridization of denatured RNA and small DNA fragments transferred to nitrocellulose. *Proc Natl Acad Sci USA* **77**:5201, 1980.

340. Elvin P, Butler R, Hedge PJ: Transcribed sequences within YACs: HTF island cloning and cDNA library screening, in Anand R (ed): *Techniques for the Analysis of Complex Genomes.* London, Academic Press Limited, 1992, p 155.

341. Elvin P, Slynn G, Black D, Graham A, Butler R, Markham AF, et al: Isolation of cDNA clones using yeast artificial chromosome probes. *Nucl Acids Res* **18**:3913, 1990.

342. Lovett M, Kere J, Hinton LM: Direct selection: a method for the isolation of cDNAs encoded by large genomic regions. *Proc Natl Acad Sci USA* **88**:9628, 1991.

343. Parimoo S, Patanjali SR, Shukla H, Chaplin DD, Weissman SM: cDNA selection: efficient PCR approach for the selection of cDNAs encoded in large chromosomal DNA fragments. *Proc Natl Acad Sci USA* **88**:9623, 1991.

344. Tagle DA, Swaroop M, Lovett M, Collins FS: Magnetic bead capture of expressed sequences encoded within large genomic segments. *Nature* **361**:751, 1993.

345. Morgan JG, Dolganov GM, Robbins SE, Hinton LM, Lovett M: The selective isolation of novel cDNAs encoded by the regions surrounding the human interleukin 4 and 5 genes. *Nucl Acids Res* **20**:5173, 1992.

346. Travis GH, Sutcliffe JG: Phenol emulsion-enhanced DNA-driven subtractive cDNA cloning: isolation of low-abundance monkey cortex-specific mRNAs. *Proc Natl Acad Sci USA* **85**:1696, 1988.

347. Patanjali SR, Parimoo S, Weissman SM: Construction of a uniform-abundance (normalized) cDNA library. *Proc Natl Acad Sci USA* **88**:1943, 1991.

348. Ko MSH: An 'equalized cDNA library' by the reassociation of short double-stranded cDNAs. *Nucl Acids Res* **18**:5705, 1990.

349. Soares MB, Bonaldo MF, Jelene P, Su L, Lawton L, Efstratiadis A: Construction and characterization of a normalized cDNA library. *Proc Natl Acad Sci USA* **91**:9228, 1994.

350. Bonaldo MF, Lennon G, Soares MB: Normalization and subtraction: two approaches to facilitate gene discovery. *Genome Research* **6**:791, 1996.

351. Duyk GM, Kim S, Myers RM, Cox DR: Exon trapping: a genetic screen to identify candidate transcribed sequences in cloned mammalian genomic DNA. *Proc Natl Acad Sci USA* **87**:8995, 1990.

352. Auch D, Reth M: Exon trap cloning: using PCR to rapidly detect and clone exons from genomic DNA fragments. *Nucl Acids Res* **18**:6743, 1990.

353. Buckler AJ, Chang DD, Graw SL, Brook JD, Haber DA, Housman DE, et al: Exon amplification: a strategy to isolate mammalian genes based on RNA splicing. *Proc Natl Acad Sci USA* **88**:4005, 1991.

354. Hamaguchi M, Sakamoto H, Tsuruta H, Sasaki H, Muto T, Terada M, et al: Establishment of a highly sensitive and specific exon-trapping system. *Proc Natl Acad Sci USA* **89**:9779, 1992.

355. Andreadis A, Nisson PE, Kosik KS, Watkins PC: The exon trapping assay partly discriminates against alternatively spliced exons. *Nucl Acids Res* **21**:2217, 1993.

356. Krizman DB, Berget SM: Efficient selection of 3′-terminal exons from vertebrate DNA. *Nucl Acids Res* **21**:5198, 1993.

357. Caskey CT, Pizzuti A, Fu Y-H, Fenwick Jr RG, Nelson DL: Triplet repeat mutations in human disease. *Science* **256**:784, 1992.

358. Richards RI, Sutherland GR: Heritable unstable DNA sequences. *Nature Genet* **1**:7, 1992.

359. Nelson DL, Warren ST: Trinucleotide repeat instability: when and where? *Nature Genet* **4**:107, 1993.

360. Landegren U: Detection of mutations in human DNA. *Genet Anal Tech Appl* **9**:3, 1992.

361. Cotton RGH, Malcolm ADB: Mutation detection. *Nature* **353**:582, 1991.

362. Fischer SG, Lerman LS: DNA fragments differing by single base-pair substitutions are separated in denaturing gradient gels: correspondence with melting theory. *Proc Natl Acad Sci USA* **80**:1579, 1983.

363. Myers RM, Lumelsky N, Lerman LS, Maniatis T: Detection of single base substitutions in total genomic DNA. *Nature* **313**:495, 1985.

364. Myers RM, Maniatis T, Lerman LS: Detection and localization of single base changes by denaturing gradient gel electrophoresis, in Wu R (ed): *Methods in Enzymology (Volume 155).* San Diego, Academic Press, Inc. 1987, p. 501.

365. Sheffield VC, Cox DR, Lerman LS, Myers RM: Attachment of a 40-base-pair G+C-rich sequence (GC-clamp) to genomic DNA fragments by the polymerase chain reaction results in improved detection of single-base changes. *Proc Natl Acad Sci USA* **86**:232, 1989.

366. Winter E, Yamamoto F, Almoguera C, Perucho M: A method to detect and characterize point mutations in transcribed genes: amplification and overexpression of the mutant c-Ki-*ras* allele in human tumor cells. *Proc Natl Acad Sci USA* **82**:7575, 1985.

367. Myers RM, Larin Z, Maniatis T: Detection of single base substitutions by ribonuclease cleavage at mismatches in RNA:DNA duplexes. *Science* **230**:1242, 1985.

368. Cotton RGH, Rodrigues NR, Campbell RD: Reactivity of cytosine and thymine in single-base-pair mismatches with hydroxylamine and osmium tetroxide and its application to the study of mutations. *Proc Natl Acad Sci USA* **85**:4397, 1988.

369. Orita M, Suzuki Y, Sekiya T, Hayashi K: Rapid and sensitive detection of point mutations and DNA polymorphisms using the polymerase chain reaction. *Genomics* **5**:874, 1989.

370. Orita M, Iwahana H, Kanazawa H, Hayashi K, Sekiya T: Detection of polymorphisms of human DNA by gel electrophoresis as single-strand conformation polymorphisms. *Proc Natl Acad Sci USA* **86**:2766, 1989.

371. Dryja TP, McGee TL, Reichel E, Hahn LB, Cowley GS, Berson EL, et al: A point mutation of the rhodopsin gene in one form of retinitis pigmentosa. *Nature* **343**:364, 1990.

372. Farrar GJ, Kenna P, Jordan SA, Kumar-Singh R, Humphries MM, Humphries P, et al: A three-base-pair deletion in the peripherin-*RDS* gene in one form of retinitis pigmentosa. *Nature* **354**:478, 1991.

373. Geisterfer-Lowrance AAT, Kass S, Tanigawa G, Vosberg H-P, McKenna W, Seidman JG, et al: A molecular basis for familial hypertrophic cardiomyopathy: a β cardiac myosin heavy chain gene missense mutation. *Cell* **62**:999, 1990.

374. MacLennan DH, Duff C, Zorzato F, Fujii J, Phillips M, Worton RG, et al: Ryanodine receptor gene is a candidate for predisposition to malignant hyperthermia. *Nature* **343**:559, 1990.

375. Malkin D, Li FP, Strong LC, Fraumeni JFJ, Nelson CE, Friend SH, et al: Germ line p53 mutations in a familial syndrome of breast cancer, sarcomas, and other neoplasms. *Science* **250**:1233, 1990.

376. Lee B, Godfrey M, Vitale E, Hori H, Mattei M-G, Hollister DW, et al: Linkage of Marfan syndrome and a phenotypically related disorder to two different fibrillin genes. *Nature* **352**:330, 1991.

377. Maslen CL, Corson GM, Maddox BK, Glanville RW, Sakai LY: Partial sequence of a candidate gene for the Marfan syndrome. *Nature* **352**:334, 1991.

378. Dietz HC, Cutting GR, Pyeritz RE, Maslen CL, Sakai LY, Francomano CA, et al: Marfan syndrome caused by a recurrent *de novo* missense mutation in the fibrillin gene. *Nature* **352**:337, 1991.

379. Goate A, Chartier-Harlin M-C, Mullan M, Brown J, Crawford F, Hardy J, et al: Segregation of a missense mutation in the amyloid precursor protein gene with familial Alzheimer's disease. *Nature* **349**:704, 1991.

380. La Spada AR, Wilson EM, Lubahn DB, Harding AE, Fischbeck KH: Androgen receptor gene mutations in X-linked spinal and bulbar muscular atrophy. *Nature* **352**:77, 1991.

381. Tassabehji M, Read AP, Newton VE, Harris R, Balling R, Strachan T, et al: Waardenburg's syndrome patients have mutations in the human homologue of the *Pax-3* paired box gene. *Nature* **355**:635, 1992.

382. Baldwin CT, Hoth CF, Amos JA, da-Silva EO, Milunsky A: An exonic mutation in the *HuP2* paired domain gene causes Waardenburg's syndrome. *Nature* **355**:637, 1992.

383. Patel PI, Roa BB, Welcher AA, Schoener-Scott R, Trask BJ, Suter U, et al: The gene for the peripheral myelin protein PMP-22 is a candidate for Charcot-Marie-Tooth disease type 1A. *Nature Genet* **1**:159, 1992.

384. Valentijn LJ, Bolhuis PA, Zorn I, Hoogendijk JE, van den Bosch N, Baas F, et al: The peripheral myelin gene *PMP-22/GAS-3* is duplicated in Charcot-Marie-Tooth disease type 1A. *Nature Genet* **1**:166, 1992.

385. Timmerman V, Nelis E, Van Hul W, Nieuwenhuijsen BW, Chen KL, Van Broeckhoven C, et al: The peripheral myelin protein gene *PMP-22* is contained within the Charcot-Marie-Tooth disease type 1A duplication. *Nature Genet* **1**:171, 1992.

386. Matsunami N, Smith B, Ballard L, Lensch MW, Robertson M, Chance PF, et al: Peripheral myelin protein-22 gene maps in the duplication in chromosome 17p11.2 associated with Charcot-Marie-Tooth 1A. *Nature Genet* **1**:176, 1992.

387. Rosen DR, Siddique T, Patterson D, Figlewicz DA, Sapp P, Brown Jr RH, et al: Mutations in Cu/Zn superoxide dismutase gene are associated with familial amyotrophic lateral sclerosis. *Nature* **362**:59, 1993.

388. Kuchler K, Sterne RE, Thorner J: *Saccharomyces cerevisiae STE6* gene product: a novel pathway for protein export in eukaryotic cells. *EMBO J* **8**:3973, 1989.

389. McGrath JP, Varshavsky A: The yeast *STE6* gene encodes a homologue of the mammalian multidrug resistance P-glycoprotein. *Nature* **340**:400, 1989.

390. Raymond M, Gros P, Whiteway M, Thomas DY: Functional complementation of yeast *ste6* by a mammalian multidrug resistance *mdr* gene. *Science* **256**:232, 1992.

391. Fuller RS, Brake AJ, Thorner J: Intracelluar targeting and structural conservation of a prohormone-processing endoprotease. *Science* **246**:482, 1989.

392. Barr PJ: Mammalian subtilisins: the long-sought dibasic processing endoproteases. *Cell* **66**:1, 1991.

393. Bollag G, McCormick F: Differential regulation of rasGAP and neurofibromatosis gene product activities. *Nature* **351**:576, 1991.

394. Ballester R, Marchuk D, Boguski M, Saulino A, Letcher R, Collins F, et al: The *NF1* locus encodes a protein functionally related to mammalian GAP and yeast *IRA* proteins. *Cell* **63**:851, 1990.

395. Han J-W, McCormick F, Macara IG: Regulation of Ras-GAP and the neurofibromatosis-1 gene product by eicosanoids. *Science* **252**:576, 1991.

396. Weeda G, van Ham RCA, Vermeulen W, Bootsma D, van der Eb AJ, Hoeijmakers JHJ: A presumed DNA helicase encoded by *ERCC-3* is involved in the human repair disorders xeroderma pigmentosum and Cockayne's syndrome. *Cell* **62**:777, 1990.

397. Mounkes LC, Jones RS, Liang B-C, Gelbart W, Fuller MT: A Drosophila model for xeroderma pigmentosum and Cockayne's syndrome: *haywire* encodes the fly homolog of *ERCC3*, a human excision repair gene. *Cell* **71**:925, 1992.

398. Dorin JR, Dickinson P, Alton EWFW, Smith SN, Geddes DM, Porteous DJ, et al: Cystic fibrosis in the mouse by targeted insertional mutagenesis. *Nature* **359**:211, 1992.

399. Snouwaert JN, Brigman KK, Latour AM, Malouf NN, Boucher RC, Koller BH, et al: An animal model for cystic fibrosis made by gene targeting. *Science* **257**:1083, 1992.

400. Whitsett JA, Dey CR, Stripp BR, Wikenheiser KA, Clark JC, Engelhardt J, et al: Human cystic fibrosis transmembrane conductance regulator directed to respiratory epithelial cells of transgenic mice. *Nature Genet* **2**:13, 1992.

401. Cavalli-Sforza LL, Wilson AC, Cantor CR, Cook-Deegan RM, King M-C: Call for a worldwide survey of human genetic diversity: a vanishing opportunity for the human genome project. *Genomics* **11**:490, 1991.

402. Bowcock A, Cavalli-Sforza L: The study of variation in the human genome. *Genomics* **11**:491, 1991.

403. Kidd JR, Kidd KK, Weiss KM: Forum: human genome diversity initiative. *Hum Biol* **65**:1, 1993.

404. Antonarakis SE: Diagnosis of genetic disorders at the DNA level. *N Engl J Med* **320**:153, 1989.

405. Grody WW, Gatti RA, Naeim F: Diagnostic molecular pathology. *Mod Pathol* **2**:553, 1989.

406. Phillips JA III: Diagnosis at the bedside by gene analysis. *South Med J* **83**:868, 1990.

407. Rossiter BJF, Caskey CT: Molecular studies of human genetic disease. *FASEB J* **5**:21, 1991.

408. Arends MJ, Bird CC: Recombinant DNA technology and its diagnostic applications. *Histopathology* **21**:303, 1992.

409. Mathew CG: Diagnosis of genetic disorders with linked DNA markers, in Mathew C (ed): *Methods in Molecular Biology (Volume 9: Protocols in Human Molecular Genetics)*. Clifton, NJ, The Humana Press, Inc. 1991, p. 389.

410. Navidi W, Arnheim N: Using PCR in preimplantation genetic disease diagnosis. *Hum Reprod* **6**:836, 1991.

411. Lubin MB, Lin HJ, Vadheim CM, Rotter JI: Genetics of common diseases of adulthood. *Clin Perinatol* **17**:889, 1990.

412. Goldberg JD: Basic principles of recombinant DNA use for prenatal diagnosis. *Semin Perinatol* **14**:439, 1990.

413. Young BD, Cotter FE: Molecular diagnostics of cancer, in Mathew C (ed): *Methods in Molecular Biology (Volume 9: Protocols in Human Molecular Genetics)*. Clifton, NJ, The Humana Press, Inc. 1991, p. 327.

414. Lyons J: The polymerase chain reaction and cancer diagnostics. *Cancer* **69**:1527, 1992.

415. Kawasaki ES: The polymerase chain reaction: its use in the molecular characterization and diagnosis of cancers. *Cancer Invest* **10**:417, 1992.

416. Eisenstein BI: The polymerase chain reaction: a new method of using molecular genetics for medical diagnosis. *N Engl J Med* **322**:178, 1990.

417. Peter JB: The polymerase chain reaction: amplifying our options. *Rev Infect Dis* **13**:166, 1991.

418. Reiss J: The polymerase chain reaction and its potential role in clinical diagnostics and research. *J Intern Med* **230**:391, 1991.

419. Chamberlain JS, Gibbs RA, Ranier JE, Caskey CT: Detection of gene deletions using multiplex polymerase chain reactions, in Mathew C (ed): *Methods in Molecular Biology (Volume 9: Protocols in Human Molecular Genetics)*. Clifton, NJ, The Humana Press, Inc. 1991, p. 299.

420. Chamberlain JS, Gibbs RA, Ranier JE, Nguyen PN, Caskey CT: Deletion screening of the Duchenne muscular dystrophy locus via multiplex DNA amplification. *Nucl Acids Res* **16**:11141, 1988.

421. Multicenter Study Group: Diagnosis of Duchenne and Becker muscular dystrophies by polymerase chain reaction. *JAMA* **267**:2609, 1992.

422. Fujimura FK: Cystic fibrosis gene analysis: recent diagnostic applications. *Clin Biochem* **24**:353, 1991.

423. Miller AD: Human gene therapy comes of age. *Nature* **357**:455, 1992.

424. Mulligan RC: The basic science of gene therapy. *Science* **260**:926, 1993.

425. Durfy SJ: Ethics and the human genome project. *Arch Pathol Lab Med* **117**:466, 1993.

426. Byk C: The human genome project and the social contract: a law policy approach. *J Med Philos* **17**:371, 1992.

427. Vicedo M: The human genome project: towards an analysis of the empirical, ethical, and conceptual issues involved. *Biol Philos* **7**:255, 1992.

428. Murray TH: Ethical issues in human genome research. *FASEB J* **5**:55, 1991.

429. Collins FS: Medical and ethical consequences of the human genome project. *J Clin Ethics* **2**:260, 1991.

CHAPTER 3

The Nature and Mechanisms of Human Gene Mutation*

David N. Cooper • Michael Krawczak • Stylianos E. Antonarakis

1. There are various kinds of mutations in the human genome and many potential mechanisms for their production.

2. Single base-pair substitutions account for the majority of gene defects. Among them, the hypermutability of CpG dinucleotides represents an important and frequent cause of mutation in humans.

3. Point mutations may affect transcription, translation, and mRNA splicing and processing. Mutations in regulatory elements are of particular significance since they often reveal the existence of DNA domains that are bound by regulatory proteins. Mutations that affect mRNA splicing likewise contribute to our understanding of the splicing mechanism.

4. We describe mechanisms of gene deletion and the DNA sequences that may predispose to such lesions as well as mechanisms for insertions, duplications, or inversions with representative examples.

5. Retrotransposition is a rare but biologically fascinating phenomenon that can lead to abnormal phenotypes if the double-stranded DNA is inserted in functionally important regions of a gene. LINE and *Alu* repetitive elements and pseudogenes have been shown to function as retrotransposons, and their *de novo* insertion in the genome can produce disease.

6. The expansion of trinucleotide repeats represents a novel category of mutations in humans. There is a growing list of disorders due to abnormal copy number of trinucleotides (CAG and CGG) within the 5′ or 3′ untranslated regions or coding sequences of genes. However, the pathophysiological effects of the expansion of the trinucleotide repeat are unknown.

7. Understanding the spectrum of human mutations is essential for the efficient identification and interpretation of germline and somatic mutations. The nature of inherited mutations described below provides an important knowledge-base for the analysis of mutations in inherited predispositions to cancer. Likewise, many of these same principles will apply to the somatic mutations that lead to sporadic cancer. For additional consideration of mutational mechanisms that lead to cancer, see Part IIIB—Defects in Caretakers.

The study of naturally occurring gene mutations is important for a number of reasons, not the least being that the process of mutational change is fundamental to an understanding of the origins of genetic variation and the mechanisms of evolution. Knowledge of the nature, relative frequency, and DNA sequence context of different gene lesions improves our understanding of the underlying mutational mechanisms and provides valuable insights into the intricacies of DNA replication and repair. In addition, the understanding of the ground rules for assessing and predicting the relative frequencies and locations of specific types of gene lesions may contribute to improvements in the design and efficacy of mutation search strategies. Over the past 15 years, the application of novel DNA technologies has permitted very rapid progress in the analysis and diagnosis of human inherited disease by the characterization of the underlying gene lesions. Many different types of mutation (single base-pair substitutions, deletions, insertions, duplications, inversions) have been detected and characterized in a large number of different human genes. The incidence/prevalence of human genetic diseases is very variable; therefore, it is not surprising that the nature, frequency and location of pathological gene lesions in the human genome are nonrandom. This nonrandomness is largely sequence-dependent; thus, some DNA sequences are not only more mutable than others, but they also mutate in specific ways and at characteristic frequencies. In this chapter, the various types of human gene mutations and their underlying etiologic mechanisms will be discussed in the order presented in Table 3-1.

Table 3-1 Different Categories of Human Mutations Discussed in This Chapter

---

Single base-pair substitutions
    Types of nucleotide substitutions and hypermutable nucleotides
    mRNA splice junction mutations
    mRNA processing (other than splicing) and translation mutations
    Regulatory mutations
Deletions
Insertions
Duplications
Inversions
Expansion of unstable repeat sequences

SINGLE BASE-PAIR SUBSTITUTIONS

Types of nucleotide substitutions

A database containing reports of single base-pair substitutions in the coding regions of human genes causing genetic disease (up until September 1997) characterized by DNA sequencing has been maintained by the first two authors of this chapter and currently includes 7271 entries (this database is referred to as HGMD throughout this chapter). Earlier versions of this list have been published.[2] Only one example of each single base-pair substitution was recorded, owing to the difficulty in determining whether repeated mutations are identical-by-descent or truly recurrent. Regarding missense mutations, evidence for causality comes from one or more of the following sources:

1. Occurrence of the mutation in a region of known structure or function;

2. Occurrence of the lesion in an evolutionarily conserved residue;

3. Previous independent occurrence of the mutation in an unrelated patient;

4. Failure to observe such a mutation in a large sample of normal controls;

5. Novel appearance and subsequent cosegregation of the gene lesion and disease phenotype through a family pedigree;

6. Demonstration that a mutant protein produced in vitro possesses the same biochemical properties and characteristics as its in vivo counterpart;

7. Reversal of the pathological phenotype in the patient/cultured cells by replacement of the mutant gene/protein with its wild-type counterpart.

The spectrum of point mutations logged in HGMD is summarized in Table 3-2. Mutations occurring in CpG dinucleotides account for 2133 (29.3 percent) of the total. Therefore, they represent a major cause of human genetic disorders (see below). However, if

Table 3-2 All Types of Nucleotide Substitutions, Including the Methylation-Mediated Deamination of 5-Methylcytosine, in HGMD

Point Mutations Causing Human Genetic Disease Other Than CG to TG or CA

Initial Nucleotide	Nucleotide Resulting from Single Base-Pair Change				
	T	C	A	G	Total
T		**654**	271	312	1237
C	**692**		371	340	1403
A	201	163		**538**	902
G	619	453	**982**		2054
Total	1512	1270	1624	1190	5596

Point Mutations in CG Dinucleotides Consistent with Methylation-Mediated Deamination of 5-Methylcytosine

Mutation	N
CG to TG	940
CG to CA	735

A = adenine; C = cytosine; G = guanine; T = thymidine. Boldface type denotes transitions.

only CG to TG and CG to CA transitions (i.e., consistent with methylation-mediated deamination) are considered, this figure falls to 1675 (23.0 percent). Analysis of Table 3-2 yields transversion (T to A or G, A to T or C, G to C or T, T to C or A) and transition (T to C, C to T, G to A, A to G) frequencies of 37.5 percent and 62.5 percent, respectively. There is therefore a highly significant excess of transitions as compared with the expected frequency (33 percent). Most but not all of this excess can be attributed to the hypermutability of the CpG dinucleotide; when CpG mutation data are removed (36.9 percent of all transitions) from the analysis, the excess of transitions is still significant (51.2 percent vs. 33 percent expected).

DNA Polymerase Fidelity and Single Nucleotide Substitutions. DNA replication occurs as a result of an accurate yet error-prone multistep process. The final accuracy depends on the initial fidelity of the replicative step and the efficiency of subsequent error-correction mechanisms.[4] Since DNA polymerases are involved in replication, recombination, and repair processes (Table 3-3),[6] their base incorporation fidelity is probably a critical factor in determining mutation rates in the cell. In order to test the hypothesis that nonrandom base misincorporation during DNA replication is a major contributory factor in human mutations, Cooper and Krawczak[2] compared the base substitutions from Table 3-2 (i.e., the observed spectrum of mutations that cause human genetic disease) with the in vitro measured base substitution error rates (data from ref. 5 and other studies) exhibited by vertebrate DNA polymerases α, β, and δ. A significant correlation between these two sets of values was observed for polymerase β but not for polymerases α or δ. In this comparison, any consideration of the efficacy of the different proofreading and postreplicative mismatch-repair mechanisms was excluded. This is because the purified polymerase preparations used in vitro lacked the 3' to 5' exonuclease activities thought to be responsible for proofreading in vivo. The result obtained for DNA polymerase β is consistent with the postulate that a substantial proportion of the nucleotide substitutions causing human genetic disease are due to misincorporation of bases during DNA replication.

Slipped Mispairing and Single Nucleotide Substitutions. An alternative model, the slipped mispairing model for single base-pair mutagenesis,[7] seeks to explain nucleotide misincorporation through transient misalignment of the primer-template caused by looping out of a template base. During replication synthesis, the template strand slips back one base, resulting in the misincorporation of the next nucleotide on the primer strand. After realignment of both primer and template strand, the mismatch may be corrected in favor of the misincorporated base (Fig. 3-1). "Misalignment" or "dislocation" mutagenesis is thought to be mediated by runs of identical bases or by other repetitive DNA sequences in the vicinity. If misincorporation mediated by one-base-pair slippage is important, then a substantial proportion of point mutations should exhibit identity of the newly introduced base to one of the bases flanking the mutation site. In HGMD this is actually the case for 1374 (identical to 5' base) and 1266 (identical to 3' base) of the 5596 point mutations not readily explicable by methylation-mediated deamination. Nevertheless, when the expected numbers of mutations exhibiting nearest-neighbor identity are calculated assuming that all three possible base changes at a given site are equally likely, no significant excess is noted. (Expected numbers are 1369 mutations with identity to the 5' flanking nucleotide and 1319 identical to the 3' nucleotide.) Thus, one-base slippage does not appear to be an important mechanism of template-mediated mutagenesis in human genes.

Table 3-3 Eukaryotic DNA Polymerases

	α	β	γ	δ	ε
Catalytic polypeptide	165 kDa	40 kDa	140 kDa	125 kDa	255 kDa
Associated subunits	70, 58, 48 kDa	None	Unknown	48 kDa	Unknown
Cellular localization	Nuclear	Nuclear	Mitochondrial	Nuclear	Nuclear
Associated activities					
$3' \rightarrow 5'$ Exonuclease	None	None	Yes	Yes	Yes
Primase properties	Yes	None	None	None	None
Processivity	Medium	Low	High	Low	High
Fidelity	High	Low	High	High	High
Major characteristics	Principal replicative DNA polymerase, lagging strand DNA synthesis	Short-patch DNA repair	Mitochondrial DNA polymerase	Leading-strand DNA synthesis	UV-induced repair synthesis

SOURCE: Modified from Wang.[6]

CpG Dinucleotides as Hotspots for Nucleotide Substitutions (Methylation-mediated deamination of 5-methylcytosine)

CpG Distribution in the Vertebrate Genome and its Origins. In eukaryotic genomes, 5-methylcytosine (5mC) occurs predominantly in CpG dinucleotides, the majority of which appear to be methylated.[8,9] Methylation of cytosine results in a high level of mutation due to the propensity of 5mC to undergo deamination to form thymine (Fig. 3-2). Deamination of 5mC probably occurs with the same frequency as either cytosine or uracil. However, whereas uracil DNA glycosylase activity in eukaryotic cells is able to recognize and excise uracil, thymine being a "normal" DNA

base is thought to be less readily detectable and hence removable by cellular DNA repair mechanisms. One consequence of the hypermutability of 5mC is the paucity of CpG in the genomes of many eukaryotes, the heavily methylated vertebrate genomes exhibiting the most extreme "CpG suppression."[9] In vertebrate genomes, the frequency of CpG dinucleotides is between 20 and 25 percent of the frequency predicted from observed mononucleotide frequencies.[10,11] The distribution of CpG in the genome is also nonrandom: About 1 percent of the vertebrate genome consists of a fraction that is rich in CpG and that accounts for about 15 percent of all CpG dinucleotides (reviewed in ref. 12). In contrast to most of the scattered CpG dinucleotides, these "CpG islands" represent unmethylated domains and in many cases appear to coincide with transcribed regions. The evolution of the heavily methylated vertebrate genome has been accompanied by a progressive loss of CpG dinucleotides as a direct consequence of their methylation in the germ line.

The CpG Dinucleotide and Human Genetic Disease. An excess of C-to-T transitions was first reported by Vogel and Röhrborn[13] in a study of the mutations responsible for hemoglobin variants in humans. Further studies confirmed the existence of this phenomenon.[14] Many additional studies in eukaryotes (reviewed in ref. 2) have now shown that the CpG dinucleotide is specifically associated with a high frequency of C-to-T and G-to-A transitions. The G-to-A transitions arise as a result of a 5mC-to-T transition on the antisense DNA strand followed by miscorrection of G to A on the sense strand. A high frequency of polymorphism has also been detected in the human genome by restriction enzymes containing CpG in their recognition sequences.[15] CpG was found by molecular analysis to be a hotspot for mutation first in the factor VIII gene[16,17] and subsequently in a wide range of different human genes. From the relative dinucleotide mutabilities as estimated by Cooper and Krawczak[2] (see below for a description), it follows that the CG to TG or CA substitutions are approximately 11 times more likely than any other substitution in the CG dinucleotide. The observed frequency of CG-to-TG and CG-to-CA mutation varies in different human genes; for example, it is less than 10 percent in the β-globin (HBB) and HPRT genes, but it is greater than 50 percent in the ADA and HYH7 genes. In two studies concerning the coagulation factor VIII and IX genes in which almost all mutations in a given set of patients have been identified, it was found that approximately 35 percent of nucleotide substitutions were CG to TG

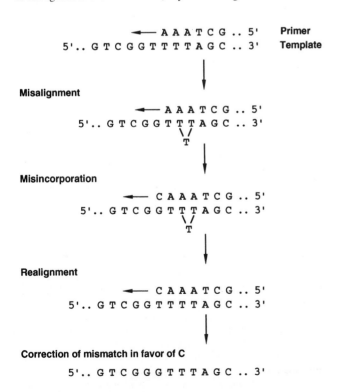

FIG. 3-1 Schematic representation of the slipped mispairing model for single nucleotide substitutions.

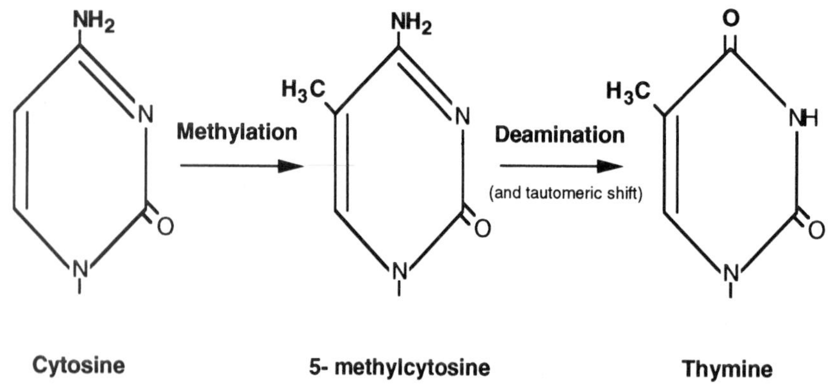

FIG. 3-2 Schematic representation of the molecules for cytosine, 5-methylcytosine, and thymine and the chemical events for the transformation of cytosine to thymine.

or CG to CA.[18–20] In the assumed absence of a detection bias (see below), this variation is due either to differences in germ-line DNA methylation and/or relative intragenic CpG frequency. The distribution of CpG mutations within a gene may also be nonrandom. For example, 9 of 122 single base-pair substitutions in exon 7 of the protein C (PROC) gene occur in a CpG; by contrast, 0 of 13 point mutations reported in exons 5 and 6 are in CpG dinucleotides,[21] although these exons contain a larger number of CpG. This observation is perhaps indicative of differences in cytosine methylation in the germ line in different exons of the same gene. CpG hypermutability in inherited disease implies that these sites are methylated in the germ line and thereby rendered prone to 5mC deamination. That 5mC deamination is directly responsible for these mutational events is evidenced by the fact that several cytosine residues known to have undergone a germ-line mutation in the LDL receptor gene (hypercholesterolemia) and the tumor protein 53 (TP53) gene (various types of tumor) are indeed methylated in the germ line.[22]

The frequency of CG to TG or CA mutations may be different in the male versus female germ line because there is a profound difference in DNA methylation in the germ cells of the two sexes; the oocyte is markedly undermethylated, whereas sperm is heavily methylated.[23,24] Thus, it may be that CG-to-TG or CG-to-CA mutations occur more commonly in male germ cells. Table 3-4 shows the germ-line origin of mutations in factor IX deficiency. In this data set, there is a sevenfold male predominance of transitions at the CpG dinucleotide[25] (the authors in Ref. 25 discuss the various biases in obtaining the data for such analysis and the need for more data collection). Pattinson et al.[27] in a small sample have noted differences between ethnic groups in the mutation frequency at specific CpG sites within the factor VIII gene. By contrast, the pattern of germ-line CpG mutation in the factor IX gene appeared to be in-

distinguishable between Asians, mostly of Korean origin, and Caucasians.[28] This finding argues for the absence of population-specific methylation patterns, and is consistent with no differences in methylation between individuals from different ethnic backgrounds.[29] In a random sample of CpG transitions in the factor IX gene causing hemophilia B, the majority (82 percent) occurred at 9 sites that correspond to functionally critical and evolutionarily conserved amino acid residues, whereas the remainder occurred at 11 poorly conserved sites.[30] This disproportionately high number of CpG mutations at conserved residues was explained in terms of selection retaining CpG dinucleotides at these locations despite the attendant high risk of deleterious mutation. The authors concluded that consideration of the ratio of CpG to non-CpG mutation might thus lead to overestimation of the intrinsic mutability of the CpG dinucleotide. However, the demonstration that similar values for the relative mutability of CpG may be derived from both clinical and evolutionary studies[2,31] argues against the validity of this postulate. Further, Koeberl et al.[20] have shown, as expected, that all factor IX missense mutations, not merely those that occur in CpG dinucleotides, tend to be located in evolutionarily conserved residues.

Are other mechanisms also responsible for CpG deamination? The suggestion that CpG deamination may result from endogenous enzymatic activity has been mooted by Steinberg and Gorman.[31a] They found that some 70 percent of their (independent) mouse lymphoma cell mutants possessed a specific CGG to TGG substitution converting Arg 334 to Trp in the gene encoding protein kinase regulatory subunit. In 5 percent of these mutants, a second mutation (CGT to TGT) was found converting Arg 332 to Cys. The co-occurrence of these two mutations at such a high frequency argues for some type of enzymatic mechanism and against two independent methylation-mediated deamination events. Such a mechanism could involve a deaminase, although no such activity has yet been purified. The relevance of the observation to human gene mutation is doubtful since (1) there are no known examples, including CpG dinucleotides, of pathological base changes in humans that occur with such a high proportional frequency and (2) although a very few isolated examples of double mutation have been reported as causes of human genetic disease, these do not involve CpG dinucleotides. Shen et al.[32] have reported that DNA methyltransferase is capable of including C-to-T transitions directly in prokaryotes and the mutation frequency was sensitive to the concentration of the methyl donor, S-adenosylmethionine. The importance of this putative deamination mechanism in eukaryotes is at present unclear.

Table 3-4 Germ-Line Origin of Mutations in the Clotting Factor IX Gene*

	Male	Female	M/F Ratio	p Value
All base substitutions	20	16	2.5	4.99×10^{-3}
All deletions	3	11	0.55	NS
Transitions				
At CpG	10	3	6.7	1.65×10^{-3}
Non-CpG	5	4	2.5	NS
Transversions	5	9	1.1	NS
Deletions				
Small (<50 bp)	1	8	0.25	NS
Large (>50 bp)	2	3	1.3	NS
Insertions	1	1		
Total	24	28		

*Modified from Ketterling et al.[25] with the addition of the Kling et al.[26] cases. The observed M/F ratio was corrected for the expected 1:2 (the expected ratio is z:1 + z, where z denotes the probability of an x-linked recessive mutation to have at least one affected male descendant. Since $z \leq 1$, the ratio of 1:2 is a conservative estimate).

Non-CpG Point Mutation Hotspots

Based upon the point mutations in HGMD not readily explicable by methylation-mediated deamination, a total of 30 codons in 16 different genes were identified as potential "hotspots" for single base-pair substitutions. These residues were characterized either by a single base being affected by at least two nonidentical substitutions or by mutations affecting two or three nucleotides within that codon. Since a variety of DNA sequence motifs are known to play an important role in the breakage and rejoining of DNA, and could therefore represent potential determinants of single base-pair mutagenesis, the DNA sequence environment of the aforementioned mutations has been analyzed. Some trinucleotide and tetranucleotide motifs are significantly overrepresented within 10 bp on either side of the mutation hotspots. These motifs are TTT, CTT, TGA, and TTG and CTTT, TCTT, TTTG. In addition, Cooper and Krawczak[2] screened a region of $\pm$10 bp around 219 non-CpG base substitution sites with known sequence environment for triplets and quadruplets that occurred at significantly increased frequencies. Only one trinucleotide was found again to occur at a frequency significantly higher than expected: CTT, the topoisomerase I cleavage site consensus sequence described by Bullock et al.[33] CTT was observed 36 times in the vicinity of a point mutation, whereas the expected frequency was 20. By contrast, two tetranucleotides were significantly overrepresented at the screened positions. TCGA was observed 17 times (7 expected; this was probably because *Taq*I restriction enzyme was used for detection of the mutations) while TGGA was observed 25 times (12 expected). The latter motif fits perfectly with the deletion hotspot consensus sequence drawn up previously for human genes,[34] which, in turn, resembles the putative arrest site for DNA polymerase α.[35] Thus, it may be that the arrest or pausing of the polymerase at the replication fork disposes the replication complex to misincorporation of nucleotides as well as deletions.

A Nearest Neighbor Analysis of Single Base-Pair Substitutions

Methylation-mediated deamination as a primary cause of point mutation is characterized by increased rated of CG to TG and CG to CA transitions. However, the relative likelihoods of point muta-

tions at other dinucleotides may also be quite variable, as is suggested by the nearest neighbor frequencies observed in HGMD (Table 3-5). (Note that each point mutation can be regarded as occurring within two distinct dinucleotides depending on whether one considers the 5′ or the 3′ neighboring base.) In Table 3-5, considerable differences are apparent with respect to nucleotides occurring adjacent to sites of point mutation. For example, G residues are clearly overrepresented as 3′ flanking nucleotides when T is mutated, and a mutated G is often flanked by another G residue on the 5′ side.

Is There a Bias in Clinical Detection and Reporting of the Mutations?

That observed relative rates of base substitution are influenced by nucleotides flanking the mutation site is explicable by the nonrandomness of both the initial mutation event and the mutation repair process. However, a further contributory factor may be differences in the phenotypic consequences of specific point mutations, and thus in the likelihood of their coming to clinical attention. In-depth studies of the phenotypic effect of large numbers of different missense mutations in a specific gene are few. One such study for missense mutations in the factor IX gene[28a] showed that mutations at "generic" residues (amino acid residues conserved in factor IX of other mammalian species and in three related serine proteases) would invariably cause disease. Mutations at factor IX-specific residues (residues conserved in the factor IX of other mammalian species but not in three related serine proteases) were some sixfold less likely to cause disease, whereas mutations at nonconserved residues were 33 times less likely to result in a hemophilia B phenotype. Bottema et al.[28a] estimated that 40 percent of all possible missense changes would cause hemophilia B, implying that 60 percent of residues serve merely as "spacers" to maintain the relative position of critical amino acid residues and probably do not fulfill any specific (known) function. Thus, detectable mutations, identified by virtue of their effect on protein structure and function

Table 3-5 Nearest Neighbor Frequencies on the 3′ and 5′ Sides of Point Mutations Causing Human Genetic Disease*

(a) Mutated Base	3′ Neighboring Base				
	T	C	A	G	Total
T	202	240	164	631	1237
C	235	354	619	1135 (195)	2343 (1403)
A	311	218	209	164	902
G	493 (374)	613 (457)	732 (547)	951 (676)	2789 (2054)
	1241 (1122)	1425 (1269)	1724 (1539)	2881 (1666)	7271 (5596)

(b) 5′ Neighboring Base	Mutated Base				
	T	C	A	G	Total
T	182	509 (314)	161	669	1521 (1326)
C	438	716 (350)	295	998 (263)	2447 (1346)
A	347	519 (355)	173	345	1384 (1220)
G	270	599 (384)	273	777	1919 (1704)
	1237	2343 (1403)	902	2789 (2054)	7271 (5596)

*Figures in brackets denote observed nearest neighbor frequencies when CG → TG (a) and CG → CA (b) transitions are excluded.

and subsequently on clinical phenotype, appear to be a subset of a rather larger number of mutations, many of which have no clinical effect, at least in the case of hemophilia B. It may not, however, be possible to extrapolate from this finding in hemophilia B (in which <5 percent normal factor IX activity must be present to generate a clinically abnormal phenotype) to other genetic disorders. It would seem reasonable to suppose that the phenotypic consequences of a given point mutation would be determined by the magnitude of the amino acid exchange as assessed by the resulting structural perturbation of the protein. Thus, specific amino acid substitutions might come to clinical attention more readily, depending on the severity of the resulting phenotype. Several methods have been reported for assessing the relative net effect of a specific amino acid exchange.[35a,36] Perhaps the best comparative measure of amino acid relatedness available is that devised by Grantham,[36] who combined the three interdependent properties of composition, polarity, and molecular volume to assign each amino acid pair a mean chemical difference. Cooper and Krawczak[2] observed that the likelihood of clinical detection increases with chemical difference. However, the phenotypic consequences of a given mutation must depend not only on the nature of the amino acid substitution, but also on the location of that substitution within the protein. In general, and with the exception of charged residues, most amino acids that make critical interactions (e.g., disulfide bonds, hydrophobic forces, hydrogen bonds, etc.) are rigid or buried within the protein structure, and their mutational substitution will be profoundly destabilizing. Therefore, any assumption that the probability of clinical detection of a specific amino acid substitution depends merely on the corresponding chemical difference is an oversimplification.

Relative Dinucleotide Mutabilities

In order to account for the nearest neighbor dependence of point mutations, Cooper and Krawczak[1,2] introduced a novel parameter—the relative dinucleotide mutability, rdm. This quantity is proportional to the rate at which a particular dinucleotide is affected by point mutation at one of its two bases. For any pair of dinucleotides, d and d′, which differ at exactly one position, rdm (d to d′) was defined as the ratio of the observed frequency of d to d′ among known point mutations and its random expectation, assum-

ing that all point mutations are equally likely. Since the latter value depends on dinucleotide frequencies within coding regions, the analysis had to be restricted to dinucleotides starting either at position 1 or 2 of a codon, respectively. This was because dinucleotide frequencies can be computed from tabulated codon usage[37] only for these positions. Although dinucleotides overlapping neighboring codons were thus systematically excluded, a bias was regarded as being unlikely to result for the rdm. Table 3-6 summarizes the results of the nearest neighbor analysis of HGMD in the form of rdm values standardized by rdm(TT to CT).

Strand Difference in Base Substitution Rates

A noteworthy feature of Table 3-6 is that it reveals some asymmetry, suggesting a strand difference for single base-pair substitutions. For example, rdm(CT to CC) and rdm(AG to GG) differ by more than threefold. Since the latter transition is complementary to the former, these two figures should coincide if point mutagenesis were acting similarly on both DNA strands. A screening of HGMD yielded 18 pairs of substitutions, complementary to each other, that exhibit the same feature. These are listed in Table 3-7 together with their expected frequencies, assuming both equal rdm values and a constant number of observations for each pair, and making allowance for the genetic code and variable likelihoods of detection. A strand difference in mutation rates has already been described by Wu and Maeda.[38] By comparison of nonfunctional sequences near the β-globin genes of six primate species, they demonstrated that purine to pyrimidine (R to Y) transversions occurred approximately 1.5 times more frequently than their pyrimidine to purine counterparts. However, complementary transitions were found to occur at equal frequencies. These findings are compatible with the mutational spectrum from HGMD: R to Y was observed 11% more frequently than Y to R, and both T-to-C and A-to-G transitions account for some 10 percent of the mutations in Table 3-2. A slightly different result was obtained for G-to-A transitions, which are 1.4 times more frequent than C-to-T transitions. Nevertheless, the rdm values in Table 3-6 reveal that strand differences in mutation rates depend on the nucleotides flanking the site of mutation. For example, whereas CT to CC is more than 3 times more likely than AG to GG, TA is 30 percent more likely to mutate to TG than to CA. A

Table 3-6 Relative Dinucleotide Mutabilities

d	Newly Introduced 5′ Base				Newly Introduced 3′ Base				rdm(d)
	T	C	A	G	T	C	A	G	
TT	—	1.00	0.28	0.39	—	0.64	0.22	0.34	0.85
CT	0.96	—	0.28	0.34	—	1.69	0.24	0.45	1.16
AT	0.41	0.20	—	1.72	—	1.27	0.38	0.33	1.16
GT	0.90	0.72	2.91	—	—	0.59	0.38	0.33	1.64
TC	—	0.77	0.32	0.18	1.08	—	0.41	0.61	0.93
CC	0.93	—	0.43	0.30	1.85	—	0.46	0.35	1.26
AC	0.20	0.32	—	0.78	1.28	—	0.46	0.44	0.94
GC	0.48	0.80	2.34	—	1.26	—	0.56	0.28	1.67
TA	—	0.93	0.30	0.34	0.16	0.21	—	1.19	1.00
CA	1.24	—	0.59	0.45	0.12	0.49	—	1.46	1.42
AA	0.14	0.20	—	0.74	0.11	0.14	—	0.92	0.48
GA	0.45	0.60	2.73	—	0.28	0.12	—	0.60	1.16
TG	—	1.65	0.35	0.49	0.58	0.60	1.82	—	1.65
CG	9.09	—	0.73	0.72	1.18	1.39	13.83	—	7.44
AG	0.09	0.22	—	0.50	0.24	0.31	1.01	—	0.52
GG	0.46	0.73	3.13	—	0.83	0.51	1.91	—	2.38

d, Original dinucleotide; rdm(d), Sum of values in each row, standardized so that rdm(TA) = 1.00.

Table 3-7 Strand Difference in Point Mutagenesis*

Substitution	Obs	Exp	Complementary Substitution	Obs	Exp	p Value
TT-AT	31	18.8	AA-AT	25	37.2	5.65×10^{-4}
TT-GT	56	36.7	AA-AC	24	43.7	$<10^{-5}$
TC-TT	89	171.7	GA-AA	353	270.3	$<10^{-5}$
CT-CC	181	103.6	AG-GG	85	162.4	$<10^{-5}$
CT-CA	29	16.2	AG-TG	25	37.9	1.34×10^{-4}
CT-CG	58	40.1	AG-CG	42	59.9	2.56×10^{-4}
CC-CT	143	213.8	GG-AG	612	541.2	$<10^{-5}$
CC-TC	176	262.7	GG-GA	319	232.3	$<10^{-5}$
CC-AC	73	106.0	GG-GT	137	104.0	$<10^{-5}$
CC-CG	33	56.1	GG-CG	129	106.0	1.41×10^{-4}
CA-CT	13	30.4	TG-AG	96	78.6	1.98×10^{-4}
CA-TA	414	472.0	TG-TA	258	200.0	$<10^{-5}$
CG-CC	72	51.1	CG-GG	58	78.9	1.74×10^{-4}
CG-CA	344	248.9	CG-TG	940	1035.1	$<10^{-5}$
GT-TT	104	70.3	AC-AA	101	134.7	$<10^{-5}$
GT-AT	281	212.0	AC-AT	97	166.0	$<10^{-5}$
GC-GT	100	156.0	GC-AC	352	296.0	$<10^{-5}$
GC-CC	103	70.5	GC-GG	34	66.5	$<10^{-5}$

*Expected frequencies were calculated assuming that rdm values of complementary substitutions are equal. The sum of observed and expected values was held fixed within a row. Only pairs with a significant chi-square test result are reported (48 comparisons, $p < 10^{-3}$ yields an overall p of 0.05).

disparity between the likelihoods of CG-to-TG and CG-to-CA transitions is also evident from inspection of Table 3-7. This observation strongly suggests that, at least within gene coding regions, the two strands are differentially methylated and/or differentially repaired. Holmes et al.[39a] have demonstrated in vitro, the existence of a strand-specific correction process in human and Drosophilia cells whose efficiency depends on the nature of the mispair. Such differential repair could also account for the observed strand differences in mutation frequency.

SINGLE BASE-PAIR SUBSTITUTIONS IN HUMAN MRNA SPLICE JUNCTIONS

Single base-pair substitutions (point mutations) affecting mRNA splicing are nonrandomly distributed, and this nonrandomness can be related to the phenotypic consequences of mutation (for review see ref. 39). Naturally occurring point mutations that affect mRNA splicing fall into three main categories: (1) Mutations within 5′ or 3′ consensus splice sites. Such lesions usually reduce the amount of correctly spliced mature mRNA and/or lead to the utilization of alternative splice sites in the vicinity. This results in the production of mRNAs that either lack a portion of the coding sequence ("exon skipping") or contain additional sequence of intronic origin ("cryptic splice site utilization"). (2) Mutations within an intron or exon that may serve to activate cryptic splice sites and lead to the production of aberrant mRNA species. (3) Mutations within a branch-point sequence.

Splice-Junction Mutations Causing Human Genetic Disease

Splicing defects are not an uncommon cause of human genetic disease. The vast majority of known gene lesions that affect splicing are point mutations within 5′ and 3′ splice sites (ss). Krawczak et al.[39] collected from the literature a total of 101 different examples of point mutation in the vicinity of exon-intron splice junctions of human genes that alter the accuracy or efficiency of mRNA splicing and were responsible for a specific disease phenotype. These lesions were reported in the literature before June 1991, at which time 558 different point mutations were known to occur within human gene coding sequences. Point mutations causing a defect in mRNA splicing therefore appear to represent some 15 percent of all point mutations causing human genetic disease. This is only slightly higher than the frequency of splice site (including cryptic splice site) mutation observed in the factor IX gene (30/278 = 10.8 percent[40]). Of the 101 different splice site mutations of ref. 39, 62 affected 5′ ss (donor splice site), 26 were located in 3′ ss (acceptor splice site) and 13 resulted in the creation of novel splice sites. Fig. 3-3 shows the consensus splice site sequences of mammalian genes. For both the wild-type and mutated splice sites, "consensus values" (CV[41]) were calculated that reflect the similarity of any one splice site to the consensus sequence. A splice site containing the least frequent bases at each position would yield a CV of 0, whereas splice sites containing only the most frequent bases would have a CV of unity. CV for the wild-type splice sites (CVN) studied were from 0.7 to 1 with a mean of about 0.83 for the 5′ and 3′ ss. While mean CVN were not much different from random expectation, sequences with either extremely small or extremely high CVN were lacking. These findings suggested that splice sites

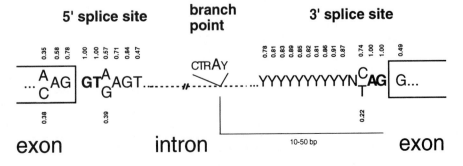

FIG. 3-3 Consensus sequences for the 5′ ss (donor site), 3′ ss (acceptor site) and the branch point. Numbers corresponding to the nucleotides represent frequencies of each given nucleotide in the collections of Padget et al.[44] and Shapiro and Senapathy.[41]

that are less than optimal in terms of their similarity to the consensus sequence are especially prone to the deleterious effects of mutation, but that splice sites with an already extremely low degree of similarity are not further functionally impaired by single base changes.

Location and Spectrum of Splice Site Mutations

A similar analysis was also conducted for the CV of mutated splice sites (CVM[39]). Observed CVM for both 5' ss and 3' ss turned out to be considerably smaller than expected under the assumption of a random distribution of point mutations within the affected splice sites, allowing for the relative dinucleotide mutabilities of Table 3-6. The CVM were from 0.48 to 0.74 for the 3' ss and from 0.5 to 0.84 for the 5' ss. Comparison of the number of mutations reported at particular splice site positions with their corresponding expectations, based on data from human gene coding regions indicated that point mutations at 5' ss are significantly overrepresented at position +1, and that the relative frequencies of observed in vivo mutations at the different positions within 5' ss reflect broadly their evolutionary conservation (Table 3-8). The sequence spectrum of mutations at 5' ss also deviates significantly from randomness. Fifty cases (81 percent) involve the substitution of the G residue at position +1, and in 64 percent of these cases, the substituting base was an A. Mutations in 3' ss were reported much less frequently than in 5' ss. However, as with 5' ss, point mutations in 3' ss were found to be distributed differently from expected, mainly due to the overrepresentation of mutations at positions -2 and -1.

It appears very likely that the observed nonrandomness of mutation within splice sites is a reflection of relative phenotypic severity (and hence detection bias) rather than any intrinsic difference in the underlying frequency of mutation. The replacement of G residues at positions +1 and +5 of 5' ss would be predicted to reduce significantly the stability of base pairing of the splice site with the complementary region of U1 snRNA. Binding to U1 snRNA is essential for the pre-mRNA to be folded correctly before cleavage and ligation can occur within the spliceosome. The same argument holds true for the six guanine replacements observed at position -1.[42] Only three examples of mutations at the +3 residue of 5' ss were noted; the corresponding residue in U1 snRNA is pseudouridine rather than a cytosine. No examples of mutation were found at the +4 adenine residue whose U1 counterpart is also pseudouridine. Thus, the spectrum of 5' ss mutations observed in vivo suggests an important role for U1 sRNA binding.

Mutations Creating Novel Splice Sites

A different category of mutation affecting mRNA splicing is provided by single base-pair substitutions outside actual splice sites

that create novel splice sites that substitute for the wild-type sites. This category may contain more mutations than currently appreciated because very few sequence data exist for introns as compared with coding regions, and investigation of the mRNA (instead of the DNA) is a prerequisite for assessing the phenotypic consequences of an observed base change located outside the coding sequence and the normal splice sites. A total of 13 mutations creating novel splice sites were collected in the survey of Krawczak et al.[39]; in all but one case, the novel splice site was situated upstream of the original wild-type site. One intriguing finding for mutations creating novel 3' acceptor splice sites should be noted: All six mutations introduced an adenine at position -2, but never a guanine at position -1. Since the A nucleotide at position -2 is also overrepresented with respect to its relative frequency of mutation, this might further reflect a particular requirement for an adenine residue at this position. CV for the activated cryptic splice sites (CVA) were calculated when possible; in 8 of 12 cases, the CVA was as high as or higher than the wild-type CVN, suggesting that the novel splice sites successfully compete with the wild-type sites for splicing factors. For mutations in the vicinity of 3' splice sites, the relative proportion of cryptic splice site-utilizing mRNA appeared to correlate positively with the CVA:CVN ratio, whereas at 5' splice sites, the distance to the wild-type site may also play an important role.

Phenotypic Consequences of Splice Site Mutation in Vivo

The phenotypic consequences of naturally occurring point mutation in the (internal) 5' ss of seven human genes were studied by Talerico and Berget,[43] who observed exon skipping in six cases as compared with only one case (β-globin gene) of cryptic splice site usage. These initial results suggested that exon skipping might be the preferred in vivo phenotype, an assertion confirmed by many subsequently reported examples. One major mRNA species was usually observed, and this invariably lacked either the exon upstream of the mutated 5' ss or downstream of the mutated 3' ss. A detection bias is nevertheless possible since a single exon-skipped transcript might be easier to detect/identify than a number of less frequent transcripts each resulting from the use of a different cryptic splice site. Several instances of the detection of small amounts of residual wild-type mRNA from the cells of patients with a 5' ss defect have also been reported. All these involve the mutation of bases outside the invariant GT dinucleotide, suggesting that normal splicing is still possible in such cases, albeit at greatly reduced efficiency. The choice between exon skipping and cryptic splice site usage may be visualized merely as a decision about whether to utilize the next available legitimate splice site or the next best, albeit illegitimate, sequence in the immediate vicinity. This choice

Table 3-8 Observed and Expected Frequencies of Point Mutations at Different Positions in 5' and 3' Splice Sites

5' Splice Sites				3' Splice Sites			
Pos	Obs	Exp	P	Pos	Obs	Exp	P
-2	0	6.4	7.37×10^{-3}	-6	0	2.6	0.090
-1	6	11.8	0.059	-5	0	3.2	0.056
+1	29	14.5	1.53×10^{-3}	-4	0	2.7	0.083
+2	8	3.9	0.029	-3	3	2.5	0.740
+3	3	5.6	0.252	-2	10	1.3	$<10^{-5}$
+4	0	4.4	0.029	-1	10	3.5	1.75×10^{-4}
+5	13	9.1	0.155	+1	0	4.0	0.029
+6	2	5.2	0.139	+2	0	3.4	0.047

Pos = position; Obs = observed frequency; Exp = expected frequency; p Values are from individual chi-square tests for particular positions.

may be made on the basis of the presence/absence of sites capable of competing with the mutated splice site for splicing factors. Krawczak et al.[39] studied the regions both upstream and downstream of their collection of mutations in an attempt to correlate sequence properties with the observed phenotypic consequences of mutation. These authors presented evidence that indicated that, at least for 5′ ss mutations, cryptic splice site usage is favored under conditions in which a number of such sites are present in the immediate vicinity and these sites exhibit sufficient homology to the splice site consensus sequence for them to be able to compete successfully with the mutated splice site. Fig. 3-4 schematically represents the consequences of splice mutations with reference to representative examples. Exon skipping as a consequence of nonsense mutations in the skipped exon[55,59] is discussed below under nonsense mutations.

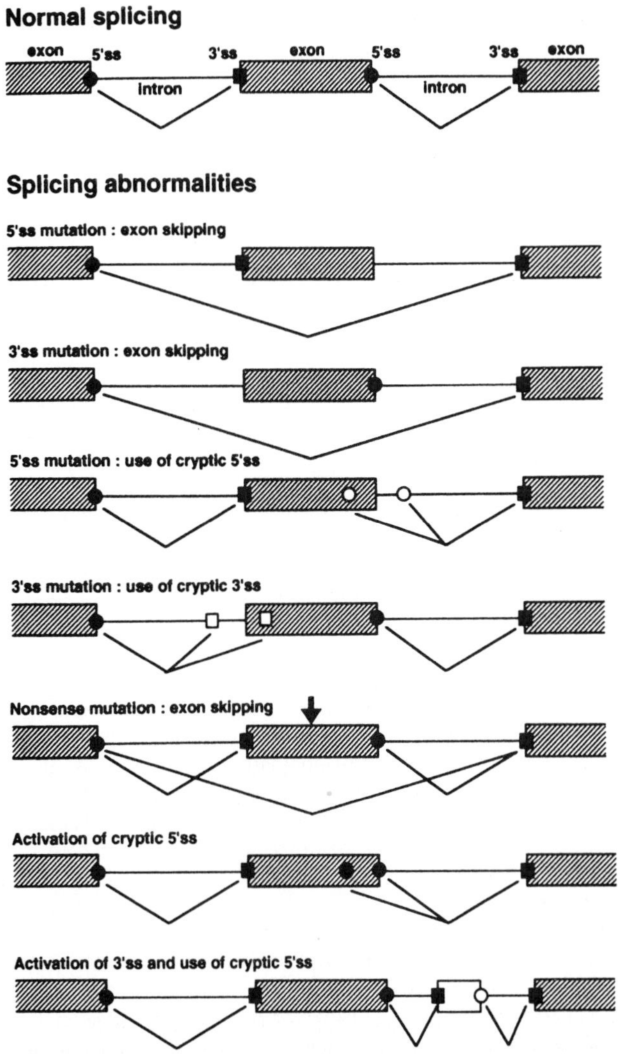

Normal splicing

Splicing abnormalities

5's mutation : exon skipping

3's mutation : exon skipping

5's mutation : use of cryptic 5'ss

3's mutation : use of cryptic 3'ss

Nonsense mutation : exon skipping

Activation of cryptic 5'ss

Activation of 3'ss and use of cryptic 5'ss

FIG. 3-4 Examples of exon skipping and utilization of cryptic splice sites as a result of mutations in splice sites. Solid square and circle denote normal or activated 3′ ss and 5′ ss, respectively. Open square and circle represent cryptic 3′ ss and 5′ ss, respectively. The arrow denotes a nonsense mutation. Examples of exon skipping due to 5′ ss mutations are reported in Weil et al.,[45] Weil et al.,[46] Grandchamp et al.,[47] Carstens et al.,[48] and Wen et al.;[49] exon skipping due to 3′ ss mutations are reported in Tromp and Prockop[50] and Dunn et al.;[51] use of cryptic 5′ ss due to 5′ ss mutations are reported in Treistman et al.,[52] and Atweh et al.;[53] use of cryptic 3′ ss due to 3′ ss mutations are reported in Carstens et al.,[48] and Su and Lin;[54] exon skipping due to nonsense mutations are reported in Dietz et al.;[55] and activation of cryptic 5′ ss and 3′ ss are reported in Orkin et al.,[56] Nakano et al.,[57] and Mitchell et al.[58]

Mutations within the Pyrimidine Tract

Three in vivo mutations have so far been detected in the 3′ ss-associated pyrimidine tracts of the steroid 21-hydroxylase B (CA21HB) and β-globin genes causing adrenal hyperplasia and β-thalassemia, respectively.[60–62] It is not clear how and why these mutations, at nucleotides -7, -8, and -13, respectively, exert a pathological influence on efficient mRNA splicing. It may be that some 3′ ss are more susceptible to the effects of pyrimidine loss than others by virtue of the relative length of the pyrimidine tract.

Mutations at the Branch Point

An intermediate stage in eukaryotic RNA splicing is the formation of a lariat structure by utilizing an A (adenosine) residue approximately 10 to 50 nucleotides from the 3′ ss. A weak consensus sequence, CTRAY, for this branch point has been observed in mammalian genes. After lariat structure formation, the first downstream AG dinucleotide is usually chosen as the acceptor splice site.[63] In a family with X-linked hydrocephalus, an A-to-C mutation 19 nucleotides upstream from a normal splice acceptor site of exon Q of the CAM-L1 gene on Xq28 was found that segregated with the disease phenotype.[64] The mutation resulted in several RNA species including those with exon Q skipping, those with insertion of 69 bp due to utilization of a cryptic splice site, and those with normal splicing. It is not yet clear whether the mutation was responsible for the X-linked hydrocephalus in this family.

Mutations in *Alu* Sequences and Creation of New 5′ ss

The creation of 3′ ss consequent to a point mutation in a member of the *Alu* family of human repetitive elements has been noted by Mitchell et al.[65] Analysis of the ornithine aminotransferase mRNA of a patient with gyrate atrophy revealed a 142 nucleotide insertion at the junction of exons 3 and 4. The patient possessed a much reduced level (5 percent) of abnormal mRNA in his fibroblasts and an even smaller amount of normal-sized mRNA. An *Alu* sequence is normally present in intron 3 of the ornithine δ-aminotransferase (OAT) gene, 150 bp downstream of exon 3. The patient was homozygous for a C-to-G transversion in the right arm of this *Alu* repeat, which served to create a new 5′ splice site. This activated an upstream cryptic 3′ ss (the polyT complement of the *Alu* polyA tail followed by an AG dinucleotide) and a new "exon," containing the majority of the right arm of the *Alu* sequence, was recognized by the splicing apparatus and incorporated into the mRNA. The "splice-mediated insertion" of an *Alu* sequence in reverse orientation may yet prove to be no unusual mechanism of insertional mutagenesis since *Alu* sequences are interspersed through many coding sequences, the sequence requirements for a functional 3′ splice site are far from stringent, and the reverse complement of a consensus *Alu* repeat contains at least two cryptic 3′ ss and several potential 5′ ss.

MRNA PROCESSING (OTHER THAN SPLICING) AND TRANSLATION MUTATIONS

Mutations affecting mRNA processing and translation may exert their pathological effects at any one of the various stages in the expression pathway between transcriptional initiation and translation. Mutations other than those affecting mRNA splicing will now be described and their phenotypic consequences assessed.

Cap Site Mutants

The transcription of an mRNA is initiated at the cap site (+1), so named because of the posttranscriptional addition of 7-methylguanine at this position to protect the transcript from exonucleolytic degradation. Wong et al.[66] have described an A-to-C transversion at the cap site in the β-globin gene of an Indian patient with β-thalassemia. Kozak[67] collated known eukaryotic mRNA sequence data and showed that the cap site is an adenine in 76 percent of cases. A cytosine residue at position +1 was noted in only 6 percent of cases. However, it is not clear whether it is transcription of the β-globin gene that is severely reduced in the above patient or whether transcriptional initiation occurs efficiently but at a different, incorrect site. In the latter case, the resulting transcript could be either incomplete or unstable.

Mutations in Initiation Codons

A number of examples of mutations in Met (ATG) translational initiation codons have been reported, with a preponderance of Met-to-Val substitutions. The consequences for mRNA transcription and translation have not been well studied. It is particularly useful to compare and contrast the two ATG mutations reported in the α_1- and α_2-globin genes, respectively. The α_1-globin gene mutation was associated with a reduction in the steady state α_1-globin mRNA level to one-fourth normal.[68] The corresponding α_2-globin mRNA level consequent to the α_2-globin gene lesion was similarly reduced to one-third normal.[69] The α_2-globin gene mutation results in a greater reduction in α-globin synthesis and a more severe α-thalassemia phenotype than its α_1-globin counterpart. This is presumably because, in normal individuals, the ratio of α_2:α_1 mRNA produced from the two genes is 2.6, reflecting the relative importance of the α_2-globin gene in α-globin synthesis. The observed reductions in steady state mRNA levels are reminiscent of the consequences of nonsense mutations (see below). Mitchell et al.[58] reported a normal amount of OAT mRNA in Lebanese gyrate atrophy patients homozygous for an initiation codon mutation.

Is the mutant mRNA translated? The answer is likely to be determined by a complex interplay of the different structural features of an mRNA that serve to modulate its translation (reviewed by Kozak[70]). Until fairly recently it was thought that an AUG codon was an absolute requirement for translational initiation in mammals. However, some exceptions are now known—for example, ACG, CUG (reviewed by Kozak[70])—indicating that some mutations might be tolerated more than others. The scanning model of translational initiation predicts that the 40S ribosomal subunit initiates at the first AUG codon to be encountered within an acceptable sequence context (GCC A/G CCAUGG is believed to be optimal[70]). Ribosomes may be capable of utilizing mutated AUG codons, albeit with reduced efficiency, or they may be able to initiate translation at the next best available site downstream.[71] The phenotypic consequences of a given ATG mutation are thus likely to depend on the nature of the mutational lesion, the tolerance of the ribosome with respect to translational initiation codon recognition, the presence of alternative downstream ATG codons with flanking translational initiation site consensus sequence, and the functional importance of the absent N-terminal end of the protein.

Creation of a New Initiation Codon

Another type of mutation that interferes with correct initiation is the creation of a cryptic ATG codon (in the context of a favorable Kozak consensus sequence), in the vicinity of the one normally used. An example of this type of lesion is provided by the G-to-A transition at position +22 (relative to the cap site) of the β-globin

gene causing β-thalassemia intermedia.[72] This cryptic initiation codon is 26 bp 5′ to the normal ATG codon and its use would lead to a frameshift and premature termination 36 bp downstream. Although the relative extent of utilization of the two ATG codons in this patient is not known, the comparatively mild clinical phenotype suggests that at least some β-globin is correctly initiated and translated.

Mutation in Termination Codons

The first reported example of a mutation in a termination codon was that in the α_2-globin gene causing Haemoglobin Constant Spring, an abnormal hemoglobin that occurs frequently in Southeast Asia.[73,74] The associated α-globin chain is 172 amino acids in length, rather than the normal 141 amino acids, as a result of a TAA to CAA transition in the termination codon. In this patient, translation extends into the 3′ noncoding region of the α_2-globin mRNA. The resulting mRNA is highly unstable, resulting in low production of hemoglobin in the red cells of heterozygous carriers.[75] Several other mutations are known to occur in the α_2-globin termination codon, and a similar phenotype to Hb_CONSTANT SPRING is observed.[76] Elongated proteins may also be generated by a second mechanism—a frameshift mutation close to the natural termination codon that results in the extension of translation until the next available downstream termination codon. A number of examples of this type of lesion are known to cause β-thalassemia.[77–81,61] All give rise to an imbalance in α- and β-globin chain synthesis and inclusion body (containing precipitated α and β chains) formation and are associated with the dominant form of the disease.

Polyadenylation/Cleavage Signal Mutations

All polyadenylated mRNA in higher eukaryotes possess the sequence AAUAAA, or a close homologue, 10 to 30 nucleotides upstream of the polyadenylation site. This motif is thought to play a role in 3′ end formation through endonucleolytic cleavage and polyadenylation of the mRNA transcript. Several single base-pair substitutions are now known in the cleavage/polyadenylation signal sequences of the α_2- and β-globin genes, and all of these cause a relatively mild form of thalassemia due to the reduction of HbA$_2$ synthesis to 3 to 5 percent of the normal level. In the β-globin gene mutants, cleavage and polyadenylation at the normal site are markedly reduced but do still occur at <10 percent of the normal level as judged by both in vivo and in vitro assays.[82,83] These mutants are characterized by a novel species of β-globin mRNA 1500 nucleotides in length and 900 nucleotides larger than the wild-type transcript. This results from the use of an alternative cleavage/polyadenylation site (AATAAAA) 900 bp 3′ to the mutated site; polyadenylation occurs within 15 nucleotides of this cryptic site. This abnormal mRNA may be highly unstable since it was extremely difficult to isolate. Several other polyadenylated mRNA species up to 2900 bp in length have been reported in an Israeli patient with a polyadenylation site mutation[84]; the β$^+$-thalassemia phenotype exhibited by this patient was consistent with the translation of these extended mRNA species. An unusual T-to-C substitution causing β-globin gene, 12 bp upstream of the AATAAA polyadenylation signal, in an Irish family.[72] It is thought that this lesion may serve to destabilize the β-globin mRNA.

Nonsense Mutations and Their Effect on mRNA Levels

Nonsense mutations obviously cause premature termination of translation and truncated polypeptides. However, these lesions may also exert their effects at the transcriptional level. Benz et al.[85] first noticed that some patients with β-thalassemia who had nonsense codons in the β-globin gene exhibited very low levels (<1 percent normal) of β-globin mRNA in erythrocytes. Subsequently, a considerable number of nonsense or frameshift mutations from a variety of different genes have been shown to be associated with dramatic reductions in the steady state level of cytoplasmic mRNA. However, this rule is not completely inviolable; a few nonsense mutations are associated with normal levels of cytoplasmic mRNA that appears to be efficiently translated to generate a truncated protein (e.g., LDLR, Lehrman et al.[86]; apo C-II, Fojo et al.[87]; β-globin, Liebhaber et al.[88]). Moreover, considerable variation in mRNA levels is apparent between different nonsense codons within the same gene: Thus, measured reticulocyte β-globin mRNA varies from <1 percent normal in a patient with β-thalassemia who had a 1-bp frameshift deletion at codon 44 (Kinniburgh et al.[89]) to 15 percent normal in a patient with a nonsense mutation in codon 17 (Chang and Kan[90]). Brody et al.[100] observed that mutations that cause premature termination in the terminal exon of the OAT gene have no effect on mRNA level, but termination in the penultimate exon or earlier is associated with markedly reduced levels of mRNA. Decreased in vitro accumulation of cytoplasmic mRNA has been reported to be associated with several nonsense mutations in the β-globin gene but not with missense mutations.[91–95] One potential explanation for the observed effect of nonsense mutations on mRNA metabolism is that mRNA that are not completely translated are not protected properly from RNase digestion on the ribosome and are therefore likely to exhibit an increased turnover rate. Consistent with this postulate, the β-globin mRNA bearing the codon 44 mutation appears to be highly unstable.[96] Moreover, Daar and Maquat[97] reported that all triosephosphate isomerase I (TPI1) gene nonsense and frameshift mutations tested in vitro exhibited a reduced mRNA stability but did not alter the rate of transcription. However, at least for the β-globin codon 39 mutation, the decreased steady state levels of both nuclear and cytoplasmic mRNA have been shown not to be due to increased mRNA instability in the cytoplasm.[91,92,94]

The mechanism by which an in-frame termination codon results in a decrease in concentration of steady state cytoplasmic mRNA is not at all understood. One or more parameters could be affected—the transcription rate, the efficiency of mRNA processing or transport to the cytoplasm, or mRNA stability. Urlaub et al.[98] showed that whereas nonsense mutations in the dihydrofolate reductase (DHFR) gene located prior to the final exon resulted in drastically reduced (ten- to twentyfold) mRNA levels, nonsense mutations in the last exon of the gene yielded normal levels of DHFR mRNA. Nuclear run-on studies and experiments with the transcriptional inhibitor actinomycin demonstrated that the low mRNA levels resulted neither from a reduced rate of transcription nor from decreased mRNA stability. Similar results were obtained for nonsense mutations artificially introduced into the TPI1 gene and expressed in vitro.[99] Urlaub et al.[98] proposed two explanatory models that imply some form of coupling between processing and/or transport of the mRNA and translation: (1) Translational translocation model. This model proposes that translation of the mRNA on the ribosome would begin as soon as the mRNA emerged from the nuclear pore and would serve to pull the pre-mRNA physically through the splicing apparatus and through the pores in the nuclear membrane. Nonsense mutations would halt the pulling process leaving the RNA molecule vulnerable to RNase digestion. However, nonsense mutations occurring in the last exon would not be recognized until the translocation of the mRNA from the nucleus was virtually complete. (2) Nuclear scanning of translation frames model. In this model, pre-mRNA are scanned within the nucleus for nonsense mutations prior to their translocation through the nuclear membrane. Detection of an in-frame termina-

tion codon would then result in a slowing down of mRNA splicing/translocation. Such a mechanism might be an intrinsic part of the mRNA splicing process since open-reading frame recognition could be important for exon definition. The translational translocation model would predict a probability gradient from 5′ to 3′ with a gradually increasing likelihood that an mRNA containing a termination codon would be successfully transported across the nuclear membrane. In support of this hypothesis are the several examples of normal levels of mRNA transcripts derived from genes bearing termination codons in their 3′-most exons (see Brody et al.[100] for the OAT gene example) and the TPI1 and DHFR examples that may imply links between pre-mRNA splicing, mRNA transport, and translation. However, counter examples, such as the β-globin gene codon 17 and 44 nonsense codons quoted above, argue against its validity in all cases since they are inconsistent with a perfect linear relationship between the relative position of the nonsense mutation and the level of mRNA produced by the mutant allele. The problem with invoking any one model alone is that it cannot adequately explain the observed inconsistencies between studies regarding the possible position effect associated with nonsense mutations in vivo and the role of changes in mRNA stability if they occur. In practical terms, the common finding of greatly reduced or absent cytoplasmic mRNA associated with nonsense mutations has important implications for mutation screening. Attempts to obtain mRNA for RT-PCR amplification and DNA sequencing[101,102] may be thwarted in patients with nonsense mutations by a cellular mechanism that links mRNA processing/transport to translation.

Nonsense Mutations and Exon Skipping

Deitz et al.[55] and Naylor et al.[59] have reported exon skipping in exons that contain nonsense mutations. In a patient with Marfan syndrome, exon B of the fibrillin gene that contained a TAT to TAG nonsense mutation was completely skipped.[55] The exon skipping was discovered by RT-PCR analysis of fibroblast mRNA. Two additional examples of this phenomenon have been reported by the same authors in the OAT transcripts of patients with gyrate atrophy: exon 6 was skipped when a Trp 178 to Stop mutation was present in this exon; similarly, exon 8 with a Trp 275 to Stop mutation was skipped. The skipping of the exons with nonsense codons in the OAT cases was partial, that is, there were RNA species which contained the nonsense mutation-containing exons. The authors proposed a mechanism of "reading" pre-mRNA exon sequences in frame either by direct coupling between translation and RNA processing or by a scanning function of ribosome-like molecules in the nucleus. Naylor et al.[59] reported similar observations associated with two different nonsense mutations in exons 19 and 22 in the factor VIII (F8) gene in patients with hemophilia A. Partial skipping has been observed with the exon 19 nonsense mutation whereas in the case of the exon 22 nonsense codon, only PCR products lacking exon 22 were observed. The mechanism that accounts for these observations is unknown.

REGULATORY MUTATIONS

Most pathological lesions underlying human genetic disease lie within gene coding regions. A different class of molecular lesion is that represented by regulatory mutations. These lesions disrupt the normal processes of gene activation and transcriptional initiation and serve either to increase or decrease the level of mRNA/gene product synthesized rather than altering its nature. The vast majority of regulatory mutations so far described are found in gene promoter regions—the 5′ flanking sequences that contain constitutive promoter elements, enhancers, repressors, the determinants of tissue-specific gene expression and other regulatory elements. Mutations in the regulatory elements may have several consequences such as alteration (reduction or increase) of the amount of mRNA transcript and alteration of the developmental expression of a gene. In the majority of regulatory mutations, the mRNA produced is qualitatively normal and therefore mutation detection methods based on RT-PCR will fail to recognize these lesions. On the other hand, the detection of mutations in potential unknown regulatory elements may predict the existence of such elements. Some representative examples of mutations in regulatory elements in the human genome will be discussed.

Mutations in DNA Motifs in the Immediate 5′ Flanking Sequences

Single base-pair substitutions that occur in the promoter region 5′ to the β-globin gene causing β-thalassemia give rise to a moderate reduction in globin synthesis. The known naturally occurring mutations are highly clustered around two regions that have been implicated in the regulation of the human β-globin gene. One is a CACCC motif located between -91 and -86 relative to the transcriptional initiation site and the other is the TATA box found at about -30. Mutations have been described in the CACCC motif at positions -92, -90, -88, -87, -86, and the TATA motif at positions -31, -30, -29, -28, of the β-globin gene.[52,103–111] Almost all these mutations are associated with a mild clinical phenotype. The CACCC box binds one or more erythroid specific nuclear factors involved in the developmental activation of β-globin gene transcription. A -101 mutation occurs in the second upstream CACCC motif between -105 and -101 of the β-globin gene.[112] Matsuda et al.[113] have reported a T-to-C transition at position -77 of the δ-globin gene in Japanese patients with δ-thalassemia. This lesion occurs at the second position of an inverted binding motif (TTATCT) for the DNA binding protein GATA1. Gel retardation and CAT expression assays demonstrated that this mutation appears to impair δ-globin gene expression by abolishing GATA1 binding to its recognition sequence.

Mutations in cis-acting regulatory elements can also increase gene expression. The best examples of such mutations have been observed in hereditary persistence of fetal hemoglobin (HPFH), which is usually a heterozygous condition in which inherited gene lesions cause a marked but variable increase in HbF (α_2, γ_2) synthesis above the normal adult level of <1 percent. The molecular analysis of HPFH has revealed both deletion and nondeletion forms. The nondeletion form of HPFH is caused by point mutations within the highly homologous promoter regions of the γ-globin genes. There are three examples of mutation at homologous positions in the ^Aγ- and ^Gγ-globin genes at positions -114, -175 and -202.[114–119] The -202 mutation occurs within a GGGGCCCC motif reminiscent of the GC box (GGGCGG) that serves as a binding site for the transcription factor Sp1. The T-to-C mutations at -175 occur within an ATGCAAAT motif (-182 to -175) known as the octamer, found in the promoters of genes encoding immunoglobulins, histones and snRNA. The -175 lesion has been shown to increase promoter activity between 3 and 20 times in erythroid cells.[120–124] This lesion appears to reduce or abolish the ability of the ubiquitous octamer binding protein (OTF-1, which is thought to be a repressor of γ-globin gene transcription) to bind at this site[124–127] and alters the binding of GATA1.[120,123–125] Using gel retardation assays, Fucharoen et al.[116] have demonstrated that the -114 mutation abolishes the binding of CP1 to the distal CCAAT motif of the ^Gγ-globin gene, although the lesion does not affect the binding of erythroid-specific factors.

Hemophilia B$_{\text{LEYDEN}}$ is a factor IX variant characterized by severe childhood hemophilia ameliorated at puberty probably under the influence of testosterone[128] and is an example of developmental specificity of regulatory mutations. The amelioration in clinical phenotype is foreshadowed by an increase in plasma factor IX activity/antigen values from <1 percent to between 30 and 60 percent normal. Several mutations have been found in positions -20, -6, +6, +8, and +13 relative to the transcriptional initiation site in such patients.[129–137] Reitsma et al.[130] noted that the region from -5 to +23 possesses significant homology with the region immediately upstream, from -31 to -6. All mutated sites occur within the region of homology. Crossley and Brownlee[138] demonstrated that the +13 mutation lies within a binding site (+1 to +18) for the CCAAT/enhancer binding protein (C/EBP) and serves to abolish binding of C/EBP to this site. Other transcription factors have been shown to bind in the -32 to +23 region.[139] Hirosawa et al.[133] demonstrated that mutations at -20 and -6 were associated with lowered expression of the factor IX gene and that restoration of expression in a concentration-dependent fashion was observed on treatment of the cultured cells with androgen. Crossley et al.[139] found that an AGCTCAGCTTGTACT motif between -36 and -22, with strong homology to the androgen-response element (ARE) consensus sequence, is functional. It would appear that, before puberty, several transcription factors (including C/EBP, LF-A1/HNF4, and a further protein that binds to the -6 site) are involved in potentiating the expression of the factor IX gene. Since mutations interfering with the binding of any of these factors lead to the abolition of factor IX gene transcription, these proteins probably act in concert. It is assumed that at puberty, when a testosterone-dependent mechanism mediated by the ARE comes into play, the binding of all three transcription factors ceases to be an absolute requirement for transcription to occur.

Mutations Outside the Immediate 5′ Flanking Sequences

In addition to known mutations in the remote promoter element known as the "locus control region" (LCR; see below), Berg et al.[140] have reported a +ATA/-T mutation at -530 that is associated with reduced β-globin synthesis. This lesion reportedly results in a ninefold increase in the binding capacity of BP1, a protein that may therefore possess the properties of a repressor.

Regulatory mutations have also been reported in the 3′ flanking sequences of genes. A G-to-A transition 69 bp 3′ to the polyadenylation site appears to be responsible for drastically reducing the expression of the δ-globin gene causing δ-thalassemia.[141] The lesion occurs within a motif homologous to the consensus recognition sequence for the erythroid-specific DNA binding protein GATA1. Gel retardation assays have shown that the G-to-A transition resulted in an increased binding affinity for GATA1.[141]

Mutation in Remote Promoter Elements

The first indication that mutations at a considerable distance 5′ to the transcriptional initiation site could affect the expression of a downstream gene came from van der Ploeg et al.[142]: A >40-kb deletion of the ^Gγ-, ^Aγ- and δ-globin genes was found in a Dutch case of γδβ-thalassemia, but this deletion had left the β-globin gene intact, together with at least a 2.5-kb 5′ flanking sequence (Fig. 3-5). The implication was that the removal of sequences far upstream of the β-globin gene had resulted in suppression of its transcriptional activity. Kioussis et al.[143] then showed that while the β-globin gene in this patient was identical in sequence to that of the wild-type, the surrounding chromatin appeared to be in an

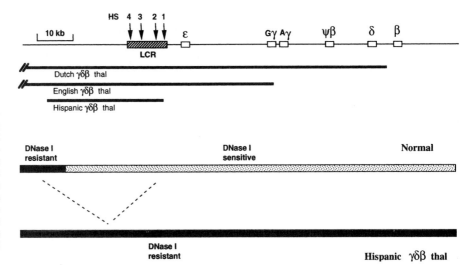

FIG. 3-5 Schematic representation of the deletions in the β-globin gene cluster that eliminate the LCR and result in silencing of the normal β-globin gene. The extent of the deletions is shown as thick black line. The LCR and its four DNase hypersensitive sequences (HRS) are depicted. The bottom part of the figure shows the conversion of the entire β-globin gene cluster to a DNase I-resistant state as a result of the Hispanic γγβ-thal deletion.

inactive conformation as judged by DNase 1 sensitivity and methylation analysis. Curtin et al.[144] reported a 90-kb deletion of the β-globin gene cluster in an English patient with γδβ-thalassemia; the ε- and part of the ^{G}γ-globin gene were deleted but ^{A}γ-, ψβ-, δ- and β-globin genes were intact. A deletion more than 25 kb upstream of the β-globin gene therefore served to abolish its expression. Driscoll et al.[145] described an important 25-kb deletion in a Hispanic patient with γδβ-thalassemia; the deletion was located between 9.5 and 39 kb upstream of the ε-globin gene and included three of the four erythroid cell-specific DNase 1 hypersensitive sites 5′ to the ε-globin gene. All the globin genes, including the ε-globin gene remained intact; the β-globin gene, some 60 kb downstream from the 3′ deletion breakpoint, was nevertheless nonfunctional. Grosveld et al.[146] showed that DNA containing the four erythroid-specific hypersensitive sites was capable of directing a high level of position-independent β-globin gene expression in vitro. The LCR 5′ to the ε-globin gene is thought to organize the β-globin gene cluster into an active chromatin domain and to enhance the transcription of individual globin genes. The Hispanic γδβ-thalassemia deletion results in an altered chromatin structure throughout more than 100 kb in the β-globin gene cluster as revealed by a change in the sensitivity to DNase 1 digestion (see Fig. 3-5). A similar LCR is also present in the α-globin gene cluster at chromosome 16pter-p13.3.[146a] Hatton et al.[147] reported a 62-kb deletion causing α-thalassemia encompassing the embryonic α-like ζ$_2$-globin gene that left the other genes and pseudogenes of the α-globin gene cluster intact. While the sequences of the α$_1$- and α$_2$-globin genes were found to be normal, they nevertheless appeared to be transcriptionally inactive. Several other examples of similar deletions 5′ to the α-globin gene cluster have now been reported.[148–151] These deletions exhibit an area of overlap between 30 and 50 kb upstream of the α-globin genes. This region contains several DNase 1 hypersensitive sites (two erythroid-specific) and is capable of directing the high-level expression of an α-globin gene both in stably transfected mouse erythroleukemia cells and when integrated into the genomes of transgenic mice.[152,153]

GENE DELETIONS

Gene deletions have so far been found to be responsible for at least 159 different inherited conditions in human,[2] and these may be broadly categorized on the basis of the length of DNA deleted. Some deletions consist of only one or a few basepairs, whereas others may span several hundred kilobases.

Gross Gene Deletions

The nonrandomness of human gene deletion is apparent at two distinct levels. First, in some X-linked recessive conditions of similar incidence, the frequency of gene deletion does not always correlate with the size and complexity of the underlying gene. For example, some 2.5 to 5 percent of patients with hemophilia A possess deletions of the factor VIII gene (26 exons spanning 186 kb genomic DNA[154,155]), whereas 84 percent of patients with steroid sulfatase (STS) deficiency possess deletions of the STS genes (10 exons spanning 146-kb genomic DNA[156]). Second, "hotspots" for deletion breakpoints have been reported within several human genes, including the Duchenne muscular dystrophy (DMD) gene,[157–160] the growth hormone-1 (GH1) gene,[161,162] the LDLR gene[163] and the α$_1$-globin gene.[164] These observations are consistent with deletional events in human genes being nonrandom. There are two main types of recombination events giving rise to gross gene deletions—homologous unequal recombination mediated either by related gene sequences or repetitive sequence elements and nonhomologous recombination involving DNA with minimal sequence homology. Homologous unequal recombination involves the cleavage and rejoining of nonsister chromatids at homologous but nonallelic DNA sequences and generates fusion genes if the recombination breakpoints are intragenic. By contrast, nonhomologous or illegitimate recombination can occur between two sites that show little or minimal sequence homology.

Homologous Unequal Recombination Between Gene Sequences

Homologous recombination describes recombination occurring at meiosis or mitosis between identical or very similar DNA sequences. Homologous unequal recombination involves the recombination at homologous but nonallelic DNA sequences. This type of homologous recombination is thought to be one cause of deletions of the α-globin genes underlying α-thalassemia. The α$_1$- and α$_2$-globin genes have evolved comparatively recently by gene duplication[165] and are thus virtually identical in sequence. These genes also possess flanking regions of homology (see regions x and z in Fig. 3-6) whose sequence similarity may have been maintained during evolution by gene conversion and unequal crossing-over. These "homology boxes" serve to potentiate homologous unequal recombination through incorrect chromosome alignment at meiosis. Recombinations between homologous x boxes, which are 4.2-kb apart (the "leftward crossover"), have been noted to produce chromosomes with a 4.2-kb deletion and only one α-globin

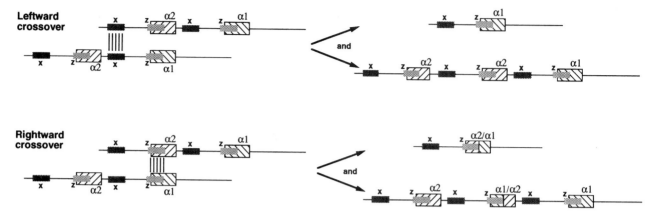

FIG. 3-6 Homologous unequal recombination between the "homology boxes" x and z in the human α-gene region. The leftward crossover is due to the misalignment of the x boxes, whereas the rightward crossover is caused by misalignment of the z boxes. The recombination events cause either deletions or duplications as shown.

gene[166] and chromosomes with three α-globin genes.[167] Recombinations between homologous z boxes that are 3.7 kb apart (the "rightward crossover") generate chromosomes with a 3.7-kb deletion as well as the reciprocal product chromosomes carrying three α-globin genes.[168] Such recombination events may be common, since their product chromosomes have been reported in many different ethnic groups.[165] In every case, the breakpoints are located within the x or z homology boxes.

Homologous Unequal Recombination Between Repetitive Sequence Elements

Recombination with *Alu* Repetitive Elements. Repetitive DNA sequences are thought to be capable of producing gene deletions by promoting unequal crossovers. The most abundant repetitive element in the human genome is the *Alu* repeat. There are up to 10^6 copies of *Alu* elements in the human genome with an average spacing of 4 kb.[169–171] They are about 300 bp in length and consist of two similar regions between 120 and 150 bp long separated by a short A-rich region. Each *Alu* element is between 70 and 98 percent homologous to the *Alu* consensus sequence. Most of the *Alu* sequences have a polyA tail at their 3′ ends and are flanked by direct repeats (4 to 20 bp). *Alu* sequences are known to contain an internal RNA polymerase III promoter.[172]

Alu repetitive sequences flanking deletion breakpoints have been noted in a considerable number of human genetic conditions. *Alu* sequence-mediated deletions are of essentially three types.

1. Recombination between an *Alu* element and a nonrepetitive DNA sequence that may not possess sequence homology with the *Alu* repeat;

2. Recombination between *Alu* sequences oriented in opposite directions;

3. Recombination between *Alu* sequences oriented in the same direction (Fig. 3-7).

The best examples of the involvement of *Alu* sequences occur in the LDLR and complement component 1 inhibitor (C1I) genes. All but one of the breakpoints associated with five LDLR gene deletions known to date occur within an *Alu* repeat sequence (of which there are a total of 21 within the LDLR gene region). A 5.5-kb deletion[173] involves the formation of a stem-loop structure mediated by inverted repeats on the same DNA strand and derived from oppositely oriented *Alu* sequences in intron 15 and exon 18. A similar mechanism has been postulated for a 5.0-kb LDLR gene deletion[174] but, in this case, while the 3′ breakpoint lies within an *Alu* repeat, the 5′ breakpoint is located in exon 13; two pairs of inverted repeats (10/11 and 7/8 matches) flank the deletion breakpoints and are thought to potentiate the formation of the stem-loop structure. Three other LDLR gene deletions[175–177] are bounded by *Alu* repeats in the same orientation. Here the deletion is proposed to occur by meiotic (or mitotic) recombination between chromosomes misaligned at the highly homologous *Alu* sequences. In the vast majority of cases in which two *Alu* sequences have been implicated in the deletion event, they occur in the same orientation. Therefore homologous unequal recombination between similarly oriented *Alu* family members, misaligned at meiosis, is probably the most common mechanism of *Alu*-mediated deletion. A clustering of deletion breakpoints within the left arm of *Alu* repeats was first noted by Lehrman et al.,[178] and has been confirmed on a much larger sample size.[2] However, the reasons for this nonrandomness are less clear. Lehrman et al.[178] pointed out that the majority of the left arm breakpoints lie within the region bounded by the RNA polymerase III promoters A and B and speculated that an

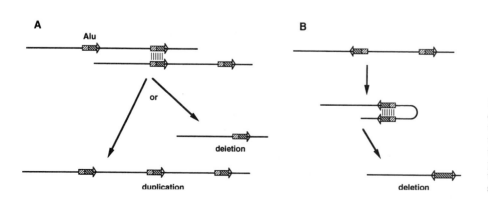

FIG. 3-7 Homologous unequal crossing-over mediated by *Alu* repetitive elements. *Alu*s in the same orientation can mediate unequal crossovers that can cause both deletions and duplications. *Alu*s in the reverse orientation can mediate crossovers via a loop structure that can cause deletions.

open conformation brought about by promoter activity could increase the propensity for recombination to occur. While breakpoints within the right arm of the *Alu* sequence are indeed much less common, Ariga et al.[179] have claimed that the breakpoints that do occur within the right arm are invariably located within the region homologous to the sequence between promoters A and B. A similar situation to that found in the LDLR gene pertains in the C1I gene, which possesses a total of 17 *Alu* repeats within a 17-kb region.[180] Deletions and partial deletions of the C1I gene appear to account for 15 to 20 percent of the lesions that cause type 1 hereditary angioneurotic edema, and a high proportion of these occur within *Alu* sequences. Clustering of breakpoints is evident; Stoppa-Lyonnet et al.[181] have shown that 5/5 deletions/duplications occurred within the first *Alu* sequence element preceding exon 4. However, the breakpoints of these rearrangements were distributed over the entire *Alu* sequence element and were not themselves further clustered.

In contrast to these examples, Henthorn et al.[182] collated data on over 30 deletions in the β-globin cluster but noted the presence of *Alu* sequences at only four breakpoints and concluded that the occurrence of deletion breakpoints in *Alu* sequences within the β-globin gene region was not significantly different from that expected by chance alone. However, it could be argued that this was due to the relative paucity of *Alu* sequences (only 8 in 60 kb) within the gene cluster. Kornreich et al.[183] reached similar conclusions by studying the association between *Alu* sequences and deletion breakpoints in the gene (GLA) encoding α-galactosidase A, a deficiency that causes Fabry disease. Although 12 *Alu* repeats are found in the 12-kb gene region (about 30 percent of the GLA gene comprises *Alu* repeat sequences), deletions were relatively infrequent (only 5 of 130 patients possessed a partial gene deletion); three breakpoints occurred within an *Alu* sequence, and only one resulted from an *Alu-Alu* recombination. Finally, no correlation has been found between the locations of deletion breakpoints and *Alu* sequences in the human HPRT gene.[184] The authors suggested that this might be because the truncated 130 to 210-bp *Alu* repeats in the HPRT gene rarely exhibited more than 30-bp sequence identity, much lower than the 200 to 300-bp sequence identity normally required to promote efficient intrachromosomal recombination in mammalian cells.[185]

Recombination Within Non-*Alu* Repeats. Most gene deletions are not mediated by *Alu* repeat sequences. Indeed, although the 66-kb human growth hormone gene cluster contains some 48 *Alu* sequences, these do not appear to be the cause of the high frequency of clustered GH1 gene deletions causing familial growth hormone deficiency.[161] Vnencak-Jones and Philips[162] studied 10 such patients and showed that in 9 the crossovers had occurred within two 99 percent homologous 594-bp regions flanking the GH1 gene. Other types of repetitive sequence element are also thought to mediate homologous unequal recombination. Approximately 90 percent of individuals with ichthyosis have a deletion at their steroid sulfatase (STS) locus.[186] Yen et al.[187] reported that 24 of 26 patients with STS deletion had breakpoints clustered within or around a number of low-copy repetitive sequences flanking the STS gene (called "S232 type repeats"), suggesting that the high frequency of deletion at this locus may be due to recombination between these repetitive sequences. In their study of some 30 deletions of the β-globin gene cluster, Henthorn et al.[182] noted breakpoints within five long interspersed repeat (LINE) elements. However, this was no higher than random expectation and thus it is unnecessary to invoke an important role for LINE elements in the causation of deletions at this locus. Sequence analysis of deletion breakpoints located within the intron 43 deletion hotspot in the dystrophin (DMD) genes of two unrelated DMD patients has revealed the presence of a transposon-like element belonging to the THE-1 family.[188] Finally, the long terminal repeats of the RTVL-H family have been found to mediate homologous unequal recombinations events.[189]

Gene Fusions Caused by Homologous Unequal Recombination. The classic example of a gene fusion is that of hemoglobin Lepore. First reported by Gerald and Diamond,[190] this hemoglobin, which is synthesized in reduced amounts, is an abnormal molecule, with the first 50 to 80 amino acid residues of δ-globin at its N-terminal and the last 60 to 90 amino acid residues of β-globin at its C-terminal. Three different examples of Hb$_{LEPORE}$ have now been described in which the fusion junction occurs at different points.[191–198] The recombination of Hb$_{LEPORE/BOSTON}$ genes have occurred within a 59-bp region of DNA (extending from codon 87 to the eleventh nucleotide in intron 2) where the δ- and β-globin gene sequences are almost identical, resulting in the deletion of ≈7 kb of intervening DNA.[194] Three haplotypes have been reported for Hb$_{LEPORE/BOSTON}$ chromosomes,[199,200] strongly supporting the view that this gene rearrangement has occurred independently on several different occasions. A similar fusion of ^{A}γ- and β-globin genes due to a 22.5-kb deletion has occurred in Hb$_{KENYA}$.[201–203] These gene fusions appear to have arisen by homologous unequal recombination during meiosis between one globin gene on one chromosome and a misaligned globin gene on the other chromosome. This mechanism would predict the existence of a second abnormal chromosome; an anti-Lepore fusion gene encoding an N-terminal β-globin fused to C-terminal δ-globin. Consistent with this interpretation, several anti-Lepore hemoglobins have been described.[204–207] Another well-characterized example of the creation of fusion genes by homologous unequal recombination is provided by visual dichromacy (red-green color blindness). The genes involved are those encoding the red and green visual pigments that are highly homologous and linked in tandem on chromosome Xq28.[208] Several other examples of fusion genes generated by unequal recombination between highly homologous, closely linked genes have also been described: between the cytochrome P$_{450}$ genes CYP11B1 and CYP11B2, causing glucocorticoid-suppressible hyperaldosteronism,[209] between the glucocerebrosidase (GBA) gene and a linked GBA pseudogene causing type 1 Gaucher disease[210] and between the α- and β-myosin heavy chain genes (MYHCA and MYHCB) causing familial hypertrophic cardiomyopathy.[211] Guioli et al.[212] have reported a different mechanism for the generation of a fusion gene in a patient with Kallmann syndrome carrying an X;Y translocation. This translocation resulted from recombination between the Kallmann gene (KALX) on chromosome Xp22.3 and its homologue (KALY) on chromosome Yq11.21. The two sequences possess ~92 percent sequence homology, and the breakpoint occurred within an identical 13-bp region. The KALX/Y fusion gene contained the entire KALX gene except the last exon, but no transcription of the novel gene was detectable.

Nonhomologous Recombination. Nonhomologous (illegitimate) recombination occurs between two sites that show minimal sequence homology. This kind of recombination can explain gross DNA rearrangements, sharing only a few nucleotides at the breakpoints, that are also common in mammalian cells. To account for this type of deletion we postulate that sequences, originally remote from one another, are brought into close proximity through their attachment to chromosome scaffolding. This would serve to explain the observed periodicities in deletions—for example, the similarity in size but not position of some α- and β-globin gene deletions.[164,213] However, Higgs et al.[165] found no association between matrix-associated regions and the deletion breakpoints in either globin gene cluster. Several types of junction have been noted in cases of nonhomologous recombination: "flush junctions" resulting from simple breakage and rejoining[213]; "insertional junctions," which contain novel nucleotides[214]; and "junctions with limited homology."[215,215a,216a] This last category of junction was first noted by Efstratiadis et al.[216] in deletions involving the β-globin gene family. These authors proposed that short (2 to 8 bp) direct repeats flanking deletions were involved in their generation. Since these short regions of homology were not long enough to support meiotic recombination between chromosomes, it was postulated that the deletions arose instead by slipped mispairing during DNA replication. Consistent with this postulate, one direct repeat was usually lost in the deletion event. Woods-Samuels et al.[217] noted two to three base-pair homologies at the breakpoints of three different deletions in the factor VIII gene and summarized the sequence features identified at 46 rearrangement junctions from large deletions that have been characterized in the human genome: 48 percent shared 2- to 6-bp homology at the breakpoint junction and in 22 percent, nucleotides were inserted at the junction. In only 17 percent was the deletion due to *Alu-Alu* recombination.

GENE CONVERSION

Gene conversion is the "modification of one of two alleles by the other."[218] The end result is very similar to that consequent to a double unequal crossing-over event. The difference between the two processes is that the modification of one allele (the target) after gene conversion is nonreciprocal, leaving the other allele (the source) unchanged. Gene conversion has been best studied in yeast.[219] In practice, it is usually not possible to distinguish the two mechanisms of interallelic recombination since in humans, it would be highly unusual to be able to examine both recombination products. Moreover, the haplotypes created by gene conversion and double unequal crossing-over are expected to be identical. The process of gene conversion may involve the whole or only a part of a gene and can occur either between alleles or between highly homologous but nonallelic sequences. Examples of the latter include the $^A\gamma$ and $^G\gamma$-globin genes[220–222] and the α_1- and α_2-globin genes.[223] The mechanism underlying gene conversion remains elusive but must presumably entail close physical interaction between the homologous DNA sequences. Gene conversion has been invoked in instances in which it is necessary to account for the association of the same disease-causing mutation with two or more different haplotypes—for example, β^E-globin alleles in Southeast Asian populations[224] and the β^S-globin mutation in African populations.[225] In the latter example, the β^S mutation was found on 16 different haplotypes, which could be subdivided into four groups that could not be derived from each other by less than two crossing-over events. Similarly, Kazazian et al.[226] and Pirastu et al.[227] invoked gene conversion to explain the spread of the nonsense mutation at codon 39 of the β-globin gene to a considerable number of different haplotypes in Mediterranean β-thalassemia patients. Zhang et al.[228] described five different β-globin gene mutations causing β-thalassemia in the Chinese population that occurred on more than one haplotype. It was considered unlikely that all cases should have occurred either by recurrent mutation on different haplotypes or through multiple recombination events. Matsuno et al.[229] reported that a frameshift mutation at codons 41 and 42 in the β-globin gene occurred in association with two different haplotypes in two ethnically distinct groups—Chinese and Southeast Asians. These authors pointed out that six of seven β-thalassemia mutations known to occur on very different haplotypes were located in a 451-bp region between codon 2 and position 16 of intron 2. Similarly, Powers and Smithies[222] have shown that gene conversion events between the $^G\gamma$ and $^A\gamma$-globin genes usually involve less than 300 bp in length. Matsuno et al.[229] also noted the existence of a chi sequence (GCTGGTGG) (known to promote recombination in both *Escherichia coli* and in mouse immunoglobulin genes[230]) at the 5′ end of exon 2 near to the site of the proposed gene conversion. Examples of gene conversion involving the steroid 21-hydroxylase (CYP21B) gene and the closely linked and

highly homologous (98 percent) pseudogene (CYP21A) have been reported by several investigators.[60,231–234] These events often bring in more than one mutation present in the source sequences. Amor et al.[232] noted the presence of six chi-like sequences (GCTGGGG) in the region of the CYP21A and CYP21B genes, which they speculated might play a role in the gene conversion events.

SHORT GENE DELETIONS

Short Gene Deletion Database

A total of 1828 independent human gene deletions of 20 bp or less have been logged in HGMD, which greatly extends earlier versions of this database.[235] This size range was selected because deletion endpoints are close enough to permit the study of putative sequence elements involved in the deletion process, deletions arising by mechanisms other than homologous recombination were thought likely to predominate in this size range, and most known short gene deletions have been discovered during DNA sequencing studies so that the sample is likely to be unbiased. For every deletion, 10 bp of DNA flanking the deletion breakpoints were noted so as to permit the analysis of the local DNA sequence environment. Excluded are deletions of the mitochondrial genome which, by virtue of its rapid replication time and own distinct DNA polymerase, may not be directly comparable to deletions occurring within the nuclear genome. The distribution of deletion lengths is given in Fig. 3-8. In 44.5 percent (814 of 1828) the deletion involved only one nucleotide and in 28.8 percent (527 of 1828) two or three nucleotides; 1565 (85.6 percent) resulted in an alteration of the reading frame. Some of the DNA sequences in SDDB share specific properties that may predispose them to deletion-type mutation. For significance assessment, observations made in SDDB were compared to results from both simulation studies using 10,000 DNA sequences generated randomly according to codon usage for human genes by Wada et al.[37] and to a random sample of 29 human cDNA sequences.

Local DNA Sequence Environment. Mononucleotide frequencies were found to differ from those derived from codon usage data[37] in that nucleotides T and A were overrepresented whereas C and G were underrepresented. Nucleotides immediately flanking the deletion breakpoints revealed a significant excess of T and deficiency of C residues. A total of 13 codons were overrepresented in frame within the DNA sequences examined: TTT, CTT, CCT,

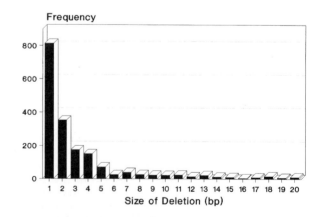

FIG. 3-8 Size distribution of short (<20bp) human gene deletions.

AGT, GGT, TTA, ATA, GTA, TCA, AAA, GAA, AGA and TAG. Several 3- and 4-bp motifs were found to be significantly overrepresented in a region of 10 bp both upstream and downstream of the deletions regardless of frame. The most dramatic examples are: TTT (721 observed vs. 496 expected), AAA (1072 observed vs. 727 expected), AGA (1124 observed vs. 879 expected), AAGA (416 observed vs. 249 expected), AAAA (346 observed vs. 204 expected), AGAA (396 observed vs. 255 expected), TTTT (208 observed vs. 117 expected), GTAA (119 observed vs. 56 expected), TTCT (237 observed vs. 150 expected), TCTT (206 observed vs. 132 expected).

Direct Repeats and the Generation of Short Deletions. A variety of different mechanisms for the generation of gene deletions involving the misalignment of short direct repeats have been proposed. Most replication-based models are essentially adaptations of the slipped mispairing hypothesis proposed by Streisinger et al.[236] The basic mechanism is as follows (Fig. 3-9): Two direct repeats, R1 and R2, occur in close proximity to one another with complementary sequences R1′ and R2′ on the other strand. As replication proceeds, the DNA duplex becomes single-stranded at the replication fork, permitting illegitimate pairing between R2 and the complementary R1′ sequence. As a result, a single-stranded loop is formed containing the R1 repeat and sequence lying between R1 and R2. DNA repair enzymes may then excise this loop and rejoin the broken ends of the DNA strand. The next round of replication would then generate one deleted and one wild-type duplex. Direct repeats (2 bp or more) could be found flanking and/or overlapping all gene deletions logged in HGMD. The most frequent length of a direct repeat was 3 bp (793 of 1828; 43.4 percent) while a sizable proportion (8691 of 1828; 47.5 percent) were between 4 and 11 bp (Fig. 3-10). The latter occurred more often than expected by chance alone. A strong positive correlation holds between the length of the flanking direct repeats and the amount of DNA deleted and the likelihood of deletion also appears to increase with the length of the repeat motif. The observations made from HGMD are thus consistent with the model of slipped mis-

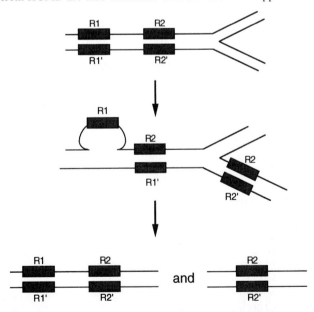

FIG. 3-9 Slipped mispairing model for the generation of deletions during DNA replication.[216] *Top panel*: double-stranded DNA containing R1 and R2 direct repeats. *Middle panel*: double-stranded DNA becoming single-stranded at replication fork and R2 repeat basepairs with complementary R1′ repeat producing a single stranded loop. *Bottom panel*: loop excised and the new double-stranded DNA molecules. One of the two products contains only one of the repeats and lacks the sequences between R1 and R2.

pairing. In accord with the postulate of Efstratiadis et al.,[216] the deletion of one whole repeat copy plus the sequence between the repeats was observed in 534 of 1019 (52.7 percent) deletions spanning two or more base pairs.

Slipped mispairing can in principle also account for the generation of minus-one-base frameshift mutations. The production of a frameshift error by these means must involve at least two separate steps: (1) a misalignment occurs within a run of identical bases followed by (2) further incorporation events that fix the misaligned bases(s). Various lines of evidence from in vitro studies now support the validity of this model and demonstrate that deletions/frameshifts can arise during DNA synthesis: (1) Vertebrate polymerases α and β produce many more frameshifts at runs of bases than at nonruns.[7,237] With pol β, hotspots occur predominantly at runs of pyrimidines (particularly TTTT) rather than purines, although this effect is less pronounced with pol α. (2) The frequency of frameshift mutations is roughly proportional to the length of the run.[7] (3) The frequency of pol β-dependent frameshift mutation at a run sequence is decreased by experimental interruption of that run.[5] Kunkel and Soni[238] have proposed an alternative mechanism to account for the generation of frameshift mutations at DNA replication: If a misincorporated nucleotide is complementary to the next base 3′, then its translocation to the next position will lead to a frameshift if the misaligned intermediate is rapidly stabilized by further base pairing. Analysis of all 814 minus-one-base frameshifts from HGMD revealed that the deleted base was identical to one of its neighbors in 500 cases. In addition, there are 238 deletions that possess a run of identical bases of 3 bp or more. Both of these observations represent a significant excess over expectation. Therefore, a considerable proportion of minus-one-base frameshift mutations causing human genetic disease may be due to slipped mispairing within runs of identical bases.

Palindromes (Inverted Repeats) and Quasipalindromes in the Vicinity of Short Gene Deletions. Ripley[239] proposed a mechanism of deletion mediated by quasipalindromic (imperfect inverted repeat) sequences. A palindrome possesses self-complementarity within the same DNA strand, which allows this strand to fold back on itself to form a hairpin or cruciform structure. The imperfect self-complementarity of quasipalindromic sequences allows them to form misaligned secondary structures. The nonpalindromic portions of these structures then provide templates for frameshifts and short deletions through the exonucleolytic removal of unpaired bases followed by repair DNA synthesis (Fig. 3-11). This model has been shown to possess predictive value at least in *E. coli*[240] A search for palindromic sequences that could potentiate the looping out of single-stranded DNA revealed that 1447 of 1828 sequences listed in HGMD contain at least one pair of inverted repeats 3 bp in length; these flank or span the deletion in 1387 cases. There are 128 examples of flanking and/or overlapping inverted repeats of at least 6 bp. A typical case is provided by a 8-bp inverted repeat associated with a lactate dehydrogenase B (LDHB) gene deletion[241]; one repeat was completely removed at the 5′ end of the deletion, whereas the other abuts immediately on the 3′ end of the deletion. However, in general, the exact location of the deleted base(s) was not predictable from the location of inverted repeats. Thus, 421 sequences possessed both direct and inverted repeats of 4 bp or longer flanking and/or overlapping the deletion; the presence of the latter may influence the nature of the deletion regardless of whether it occurs through classic mispairing or via the intrarepeat loop mechanism.

Role for Symmetric Elements? Sequence motifs that possess an axis of internal symmetry (e.g., CTGAAGTC, GGACAGG) and vary in length between 5 and 18 bp, termed "symmetric elements,"[235] were noted in 1527 of the sequences in HGMD. Sym-

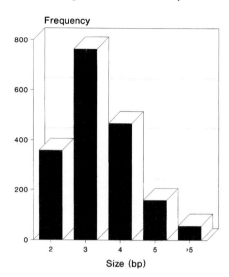

Longest Direct Repeat

Longest Inverted Repeat

FIG. 3-10 Size distribution of the longest direct (*left*) and inverted (*right*) repeats flanking and/or overlapping short human gene deletions.

metric elements spanning 5 bp or more therefore also appear to be overrepresented in the vicinity of short human gene deletions; their potential significance is unclear, however.

Deletion Hotspots in Human Genes? By examining the similarities of DNA sequences among deletions, Krawczak and Cooper[235] previously identified a consensus sequence—TG(A/G)(A/G)(T/T)(A/C)—which appears to be common to deletion "hotspots" found in different human genes. This consensus sequence is similar to the core motifs, TGGGG and TGAGC, found in the tandemly repeated immunoglobulin switch (Sμ) regions,[241a] and to putative arrest sites for polymerase α, which often contain a GAG motif. Indeed, one arrest site specifically mentioned by Weaver and DePamphilis [(T/A)GGAG[35]] fits perfectly with the deletion hotspot consensus sequence. The arrest of DNA synthesis at the replication fork may increase the probability of occurrence either of a slipped mispairing event or the formation of secondary structure intermediates potentiated by the presence of inverted repeats or symmetric elements. Monnat et al.[184] have sought a variety of sequence motifs in their study of 10 somatic deletions of the human HPRT gene causing Werner syndrome. The same collection of motifs was used for a search of the 1828 deletions and flanking sequences in HGMD. Only three of these sequence motifs appear to be overrepresented in the vicinity of short human gene deletions—polypyrimidine runs (C or T) of at least 5 bp, polypurine runs (A or G) of at least 5 bp, and the deletion hotspot consensus sequence mentioned above. Analysis of the precise localization of the deletions logged in HGMD revealed that 17 codons from seven different genes could be identified as "deletion hot spots" [antithrombin III (AT3) codon 244; cystic fibrosis trans membrane regulator

(CFTR) codons 141, 506, 1175, 1200; factor VIII codon 339; factor IX codons 7 and 182; α2-globin codon 30; β-globin codons 5, 36, 40, 42, 73, 125, and 150; protein C codon 76]. To be classified as a deletion hotspot, the DNA sequence in and around a codon had to be affected by at least two different (and therefore independent) mutations. Either a deletion hotspot consensus-like motif or a run of at least five pyrimidines was found in the vicinity of all these deletion hotspots. That polypyrimidines are significantly associated with deletions is not particularly surprising: Polymerase β-associated deletions occur predominantly in pyrimidine runs and thus, if DNA repair synthesis were a significant cause of frameshift mutation in vivo, it would be expected that the mutational spectrum of human gene deletions might show similarities to the pol β-associated mutational spectrum observed in vitro. Nevertheless, several differences between these mutational spectra are also apparent. Over 95 percent of pol β-associated frameshift deletions are 1 bp in length,[7] whereas only 44.5 percent of the deletions from HGMD are of this size. Although 988 deletions included or flanked a pyrimidine run, only 219 (44.9 percent) of these represented losses of a single base pair. This proportion compares to the deletions not associated with pyrimidine runs (595 of 1340; 44.4 percent). Finally, while 76 percent of all nonrun single-base-pair losses in vitro involved a G residue, the corresponding figure for human gene mutations is 30.3 percent (i.e., not significantly higher than random expectation).

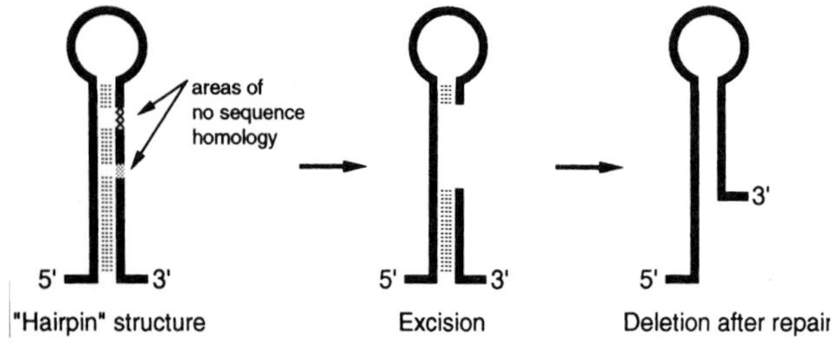

INSERTIONS

Small Insertions

That insertional mutagenesis might be nonrandom was strongly suggested by the findings of Fearon et al.,[242] who reported 10 independent examples of DNA insertion within the same 170-bp intronic region of the DCC ("deleted in colorectal carcinoma") gene. The majority of well-characterized (i.e., sequenced) gene insertions in humans appear to be of between one and a few base pairs. Examples of short insertions leading to human genetic disease have been analyzed by Cooper and Krawczak[34] to determine whether they occur nonrandomly, and whether this nonrandomness corresponds to mechanisms of mutagenesis similar to those involved in the generation of short gene deletions. These authors took a representative sample of 20 short insertion-type mutations,

FIG. 3-11 Schematic representation of the excision-repair mechanism for deletions mediated by hairpin structures due to palindrome or quasipalindrome DNA sequences.

that is, insertions of less than 10 bp. Nearly half of these (9 of 20) were insertions of a single base. All mutations interrupted the reading frame of the protein except for three examples of a three-base insertion in which the novel codons were inserted between existing codons. Three of the insertions were complex mutations, since between one and five base pairs were also deleted at the site of insertion.

Insertions Due to Slipped Mispairing. In principle, slipped mispairing at the replication fork[216,236] mediated by direct repeats can account for insertion just as for deletion-type mutations: An insertion takes place when the newly synthesized strand disconnects from the primer strand during replication synthesis and slips or folds back so that pairing between different direct repeat copies becomes possible. If synthesis is resumed so as to stabilize this mispairing, an extra copy plus nucleotide(s) from between the direct repeats is inserted behind the second repeat. Of the insertions considered by Cooper and Krawczak,[34] at least three occurred within runs of the same base while three were duplications of tandemly repeated sequences. The data were, however, too sparse to confirm any relationship with the DNA sequence environment. Nevertheless, pause sites for DNA polymerase α are known to be hotspots for nucleotide insertion.[243]

Insertions Mediated by Inverted Repeats. Analogous to the process of slipped mispairing between direct repeats, the formation of temporary secondary DNA structures may also be mediated by neighboring inverted repeats. In this situation, the newly synthesized DNA strand, instead of annealing to a direct repeat copy on the primer strand, snaps back and anneals to itself via the two inverted repeats. If DNA synthesis is then resumed, an insertion would result behind the second palindromic copy. Imperfect self-complementarity can also mediate formation of partially misaligned secondary structures.[239] The nonpalindromic portions of these structures may then provide templates for either deletions (by endonucleolytic removal of bases) or putatively insertions (by gap repair). DNA sequences flanking two insertions considered by Cooper and Krawczak[34] contain such quasipalindromes, and would correctly predict the insertion of the appropriate base (thymine) at the appropriate site [Leu 100 of the HBD gene and Cys 1146 of the type I α1-collagen (COL1A1) gene].

Insertions Mediated by Symmetric Elements. Inspection of the insertions collated by Cooper and Krawczak[34] reveals that 8 of 20 of these sequences possess symmetric elements overlapping the site of insertion. With one exception, these insertions all represent inverted duplications of sequence motifs derived from either the 5′ or the 3′ end of the symmetric element. This finding is suggestive of a common endogenous mechanism of insertional mutagenesis.

Large Insertions

To date, the largest "foreign" DNA sequence inserted into a gene is 220 kb into the DMD gene[244]; however, neither the inserted sequence nor the breakpoint junctions have been further characterized. One well-characterized insertion is that of the highly repetitive LINE elements into the factor VIII gene causing severe hemophilia A.[245] The insertion of these elements into exon 14 in the factor VIII genes of two patients involved the duplication of the target sites, a normal occurrence in such cases[246,247] and consistent with a retrotransposition mechanism. A schematic representation of retrotransposition is shown in Fig. 3-12. Patient JH27 of ref. 245 was shown to possess a 3785-bp truncated LINE element complete with 57-bp polyA tract. The insertion produced a target site duplication of 12 to 15 bp. The LINE element in patient JH-28 of ref. 245 was slightly shorter (2132 bp) but more complex; one portion of LINE element sequence (nucleotides 4020 to 5114) was preceded by another (nucleotides 5115 to 6161) in reverse (3′ to 5′) orientation; there was a polyA tail of 77 residues. Dombroski et al.[248] have shown that the LINE element found in exon 14 of patient JH27 is an exact but truncated copy of a full-length LINE element with open reading frames (ORF) found at chromosome 22q11.1-q11.2, which, since it is itself flanked by a target site duplication, may also be the product of a retrotransposition event. Another patient JH25 had an insertion of a truncated LINE element in intron 10 of factor VIII gene.[249] The element, which was 681 bp long, had a 66-bp polyA tail and target site duplication of 13 to 17 bp, and did not cause any abnormality since it was found in several members of the patient family including his normal maternal grandfather (i.e., the mutation in the factor VIII gene responsible for hemophilia A in this family was not the insertion of the LINE element). The involvement of LINE elements in insertional mutagenesis has also been reported in two other human conditions: ᴬγδβ-thalassemia due to a large deletion in which insertion of about 50 bp from a LINE element has been noted[250] and breast cancer cell lines in which such elements have been inserted in the MYC gene.[251]

The highly repetitive *Alu* sequence family has also been shown to be capable of retrotransposition both in vitro[252] and in vivo. Insertional inactivation of the NF1 gene by an *Alu* element causing neurofibromatosis type 1 was reported by Wallace et al.[253] The insertion, which occurred *de novo*, was localized to intron 5, just 44 bp upstream of exon 33. The 320 bp *Alu* repeat was inserted in reverse orientation into a 26-bp stretch of A and T residues. Sequencing of reverse transcripts of the patient's mRNA revealed skipping of exon 6. While the exact mechanism responsible for this interference with splicing is not clear, these findings are consistent with a defect in branch point recognition. Insertions of *Alu* elements into the human MLV12 oncogene associated with hematopoietic neoplasia B-cell lymphoma,[254] the cholinesterase gene causing acholinesterasemia,[255] and the factor IX gene causing severe he-

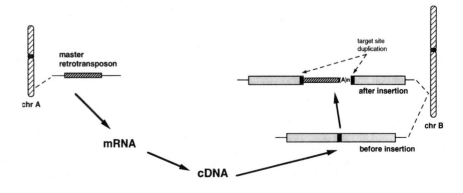

FIG. 3-12 Schematic representation of retrotransposition.

mophilia B[256] have also been reported. The *Alu* element inserted in the MLVI2 locus was 308 bp long, contained a polyA tail of 26 residues and produced an A-rich target site duplication of 8 bp. The insertion of the 342-bp-long *Alu* element into the cholinesterase gene[255] occurred in an AT-rich region of exon 2. There was a 38-bp-long polyA tail and a target site duplication of 15 bp. The inserted *Alu* element belonged to the evolutionarily recent subfamily IV. The insertion of the 322-bp-long *Alu* element in the factor IX gene[256] occurred in exon 5 and produced a Stop codon within the inserted sequence. There was a target site duplication of 15 bp and a polyA tract of 78 residues. The *de novo* inserted *Alu* sequences in the NF1 and factor IX genes both belong to the same subfamily (*Alu* HS), which is the most recent subfamily in the evolution of *Alu* sequences.

The observation that both *Alu* sequences[257] and LINE elements[245] exhibit a preference for integration at AT-rich sequences is reminiscent of the AT-rich insertional target sequences of retroviruses.[258,259] Indeed, the two LINE element target sites in the factor VIII gene[245] are 90 percent homologous to a 10-nucleotide motif (GAAGACATAC) present in one of the highly favored retroviral insertion target sequences reported by Shih et al.[259] If the generality of this observation is supported by further data, then insertions of specific DNA sequences will have been shown to be as nonrandom as the insertion of a few base pairs.

DUPLICATIONS

The duplication of either whole genes or their constituent exons have played an important role in the evolution of the mammalian genome. However, gene duplication events may also result in disease. The largest duplication reported to date for a single gene is a 400-kb internal duplication of the DMD gene involving exons 13 to 42.[261] Despite this gross alteration in the structure of the gene (and of the resulting protein: ≈600 kDa instead of 400 kDa), the patient manifested the relatively mild Becker form of muscular dystrophy. Other gene duplications and partial duplications have been reported, and these vary in size from 45 bp (COL2A1) to 20 kb (HPRT), from a part of an exon (LPL) to an entire gene (HBG2). Usually, the duplicated material exists in tandem with the original sequence, but a particular HPRT gene duplication has been reported by Yang et al.[262] that is unusual in that a segment of the gene containing exons 2 and 3 has been placed in the middle of an intron 1 fragment.

One frequent mechanism of gene duplication is homologous unequal recombination. This may take different forms depending on the nature of the DNA sequence at the breakpoints. Thus, homologous unequal recombination in the β-globin gene cluster was demonstrated to have occurred between the HBG1 and HBG2 genes whereas in the LDLR gene, it occurred between pairs of *Alu* sequences.[178] In the COL2A1 gene, alignment of two copies of the duplicated exon, in the manner that must have preceded a particular recombination-duplication event, demonstrated 78 percent nucleotide sequence homology around the recombination site.[263] In principle, unequal crossing over caused by homologous recombination between repetitive sequence elements could lead either to the deletion or the duplication of exons. That the exons found to be duplicated in the C1I[181,264] and COL2A1[263] genes of some patients are deleted in others with deficiencies of these proteins would seem to support this model of mutagenesis. However, other duplication junctions appear to possess little or no homology with each other (e.g., GLA,[183] factor VIII,[265] DMD[266,267]). In the lipoprotein lipase (LPL) gene, recombination has occurred between an *Alu* sequence and a region of exon 6 but the sequenced breakpoints exhibited no obvious homology.[268]

One of the best-characterized duplications is in the factor VIII gene in a family with hemophilia A.[169] The patient had a deletion of 39 kb of exons 23 to 25; however, his normal mother had 23 kb of intron 22 duplicated and reinserted between exons 23 and 24. Since the mother passed on a 39-kb deletion allele to two of her offspring, she must have been a germ-line mosaic for the normal, deletion, and duplication alleles. DNA polymorphism analysis suggested that the deletion and duplication events had occurred on the same chromosome. Gitschier[269] proposed a model in which the duplication had occurred first, either in a grandpaternal gamete or during the mother's early embryogenesis, and the deletion then occurred, probably mediated by the close proximity of the 23 kb direct repeats, through recombination. The deletion occurred at a pair of CATT sequences normally 39 kb apart in the factor VIII gene. Short repeated sequences are known to mediate recombination events in vertebrate genomes; both (CAGA)n and (CAGG)n repeats have been noted in the region of the recombination hotspots found within the murine MHC gene complex.[270] Several possible topoisomerase I cleavage sites were noted in the vicinity of the factor VIII gene duplication described by Casula et al.[271] Topoisomerase activity has been implicated in several cases of nonhomologous recombination.[33] Other examples of topoisomerase cleavage sites have been reported to be associated with gene duplications[183,267]; potential sites for topoisomerases I and II were found exactly coincident with the breakpoints of a duplication in the dystrophin gene.[267] The significance of these findings remains to be elucidated.

The frequency of gene duplication is difficult to assess on account of the relatively small sample size. As with gene deletions, the frequency of gene duplication is likely to vary dramatically between genes. However, several estimates of the frequency of (partial) gene duplication are available for the dystrophin gene from large studies of patients with Duchenne/Becker muscular dystrophy (DMD/BMD): 6.7 percent,[272] 5.5 percent,[266] and 1.5 percent.[273] Thus, for the DMD gene, a gene for which a disproportionately high rate of large deletions has been reported (>60 percent of total mutations), the duplication frequency is probably 5 to 10 percent of the deletion frequency. A much higher frequency of duplication (uncharacterized and evidenced only by hybridization band intensity) may be found in the CYP21B gene causing 21-hydroxylase deficiency: Haglund-Stengler et al.[274] found 11 gene deletions and 9 gene duplications in their study of 43 unrelated patients. However, at other loci, where gene deletions are much less frequent, gene duplications may well be so rare as not to be found. Why are gene duplications usually so much rarer than deletions? One possibility is that deletions are on average more likely to be deleterious and hence more likely to come to clinical attention. This is considered unlikely since with DMD/BMD, for example, it is the maintenance of the reading frame that determines the disease phenotype rather than the nature of the lesion itself.[260,261,266,275] A second possibility is that not all mechanisms involved in deletion creation would generate duplications as reciprocal products. Finally, it is possible that duplications are relatively unstable and revert or "decay" to deletions quite rapidly. The factor VIII partial gene deletion is a case in point. Another example is that of the exon 2+3 duplication in the HPRT gene; cells bearing this gene lesion reverted to wild-type in culture through the loss of the duplicated exons.[262,276] Two similar HPRT gene duplications have been reported as spontaneous mutations in the human myeloid leukemia cell line HL60[276] and these were also found to be highly unstable, exhibiting a reversion rate ≈100 times higher than the rate of gene duplication. It would seem, therefore, that once duplicated, the enlarged DNA sequence provides the substrate (a premutation) for further rounds of homologous unequal recombination.

Very large duplications also appear to arise from recombination mediated by repeated DNA sequences. Pentao et al.[277] have reported that the duplication on chromosome 17p in one patient with Charcot-Marie-Tooth disease type 1A is a tandem repeat of 1.5 Mb. A repeated element of 17 kb, termed "CMT1A-REP," flanks the 1.5-Mb CMT1A monomer unit on normal chromosome 17p and was present in an additional copy on the chromosome with the CMT1A duplication. The authors proposed that the CMT1A duplication arose from unequal crossing over due to misalignment at these CMT1A-REP repeat sequences during meiosis.

INVERSIONS

Inversions appear to be an extremely unusual form of gene mutation. Two examples involving the β-globin gene cluster will be given here: The first is a complex rearrangement of the β-globin gene cluster found in a patient with Indian $^A\gamma\delta\beta$-thalassemia.[278] Two segments—0.83 kb and 7.46 kb, respectively—were deleted, while the intervening segment was inverted and reintroduced between the $^A\gamma$ and δ gene loci. Jennings et al.[278] suggested that this mutation may have been made possible by the chromatin folding pattern of the cluster region bringing the $^A\gamma$ gene into close proximity with the δ- and β-globin genes. Interestingly, this rearrangement serves to enhance the expression of the upstream fetal $^G\gamma$ gene. A similar example of an inversion has been reported in the apo A1/C3/A4 gene cluster in a patient with premature atherosclerosis and a deficiency of both apo AI and apo CIII.[279] The inversion was 6 kb in length, with breakpoints in exon 4 of the Apo A-I gene and intron 1 of the Apo C-III gene. This inversion resulted in the reciprocal fusion of portions of the two genes and contains exons 1 to 3 of exon 4 from the Apo A-I gene plus exons 2 to 4 and intron 1 from the Apo C-III gene; the fusion gene is expressed as a stable mRNA. In the process, however, 9 bp from the Apo A-I and 21 bp from the Apo C-III gene were deleted. Since *Alu* sequences were also noted in the vicinity of the breakpoints of this inversion, Karathanasis et al.[279] speculated that they might be involved in the stabilization of a stem-loop structure prior to the inversion event. A final example of an inversion is provided by a Turkish patient with δβ⁰-thalassemia and a complex rearrangement of the β-globin gene cluster.[280] The rearrangement consists of a deletion of 11.5 kb, including the β- and δ-globin genes, a second 1.6-kb deletion downstream of the first, and a 7.6-kb inversion of the intervening sequence, including the LINE element downstream of the β-globin gene.

Perhaps the most important inversion event is that involving the factor VIII gene causing severe haemophilia A. The high frequency (~40 percent) of the inversion in these patients provides an explanation for our initial inability to detect the pathological lesion in about half of all severe haemophilia A patients[19] and the impossibility of performing PCR amplification across the exon 22/23 boundary using cDNA derived from these patients.[59] A CpG island, located within intron 22, acts as a bidirectional promoter for two transcribed genes, F8A and F8B. The F8A gene lacks introns and is transcribed in the opposite direction to the factor VIII gene. Two additional homologues of the F8A gene (the A genes), which are also transcribed, exist ~500 kb upstream of the factor VIII gene. These genes are transcribed in the opposite direction to F8A. It is now known that homologous infra-chromosomal recombination occurs between one or other of the upstream A genes and the F8A gene, generating an inversion of the intervening factor VIII gene sequence.[280a,280b] Such inversions result in the separation of exons 1–22 from exons 23–26 by some 200 to 500 kb. Most inversions (90 percent) involve the distal of the two A genes; this unique mutational mechanism is estimated to occur with a frequency of 7.2 ×

10^{-6} per gene per gamete per generation (D. S. Millar and D. N. Cooper, unpublished results).

EXPANSION OF UNSTABLE REPEAT SEQUENCES

A novel mechanism of mutation has been shown to arise through the instability and expansion of certain trinucleotide repeat sequences.[281–283] At least a half dozen disorders due to trinucleotide repeat expansion have been described. This mechanism was first reported as a cause of the fragile X syndrome, one of the most frequent causes of inherited mental retardation, which is associated with the presence of a fragile site on the X chromosome at q27.3. The gene underlying the fragile X syndrome[284–287] was found to contain (putatively upstream of the Met initiation codon and 250 bp downstream of the CpG island) an ≈90-bp CGG repeat sequence.[287] A length variation of the trinucleotide repeat in the region was noted[285,286] that appeared to correlate with the expression of the fragile X phenotype. Indeed, the (CGG)n repeat exhibited copy number variation of between 6 and 54[288] in normal healthy controls although the bulk of individuals possessed between 25 and 35 repeat copies.[289] By contrast, phenotypically normal transmitting males exhibited a repeat copy number of between 52 and >200 (the "premutation") while affected males possessed 300 and sometimes in excess of 1000 copies (the "full mutation"[289–293]). The instability of both the premutation and the full mutation is further exemplified by the existence of somatic mosaicism for different copy number alleles in some individuals.[289, 294] The studies of Rousseau et al.[290] and Fu et al.[289] have allowed several conclusions about the expansion of repeat copy number during genetic transmission: Alleles with a repeat copy number <46 exhibit no meiotic instability. The premutation represents a small increase in CGG copy number but is not associated with methylation of the gene region or with mental impairment. However, individuals bearing the premutation exhibit a high probability of having either affected children or grandchildren. Expansion of premutations to full mutations only occurs during female meiotic transmission. The probability of repeat expansion correlates with the repeat copy number in the premutation allele. The tendency was to increase repeat copy number rather than to decrease it; the ratio of probabilities was given as 64:3.[289] Since the premutation must precede the appearance of the full mutation, all mothers of affected children carried either a full mutation or a premutation; no case of direct conversion of normal copy number to full mutation has been observed.[291] The full mutation was not detected in daughters of normal transmitting males, although small increases in CGG copy number were observed in the daughters. All male patients with the fragile X syndrome possessed the full mutation, and all male individuals with the full mutation were mentally retarded. Moreover, 53 percent of females carrying the full mutation also exhibited symptoms of mental retardation. Although the transition from premutation to full mutation was always associated with the expansion of the (CGG)n repeat, examples of contraction were also observed and were reportedly associated with regression from a full mutation to a premutation.[289,291] Fu et al.[289] estimated that ≈1 of 500 females in the general population might possess a repeat copy number within the premutation range. Richards et al.[295] have presented evidence for a founder haplotype in the normal population that is associated with a much higher than average CGG repeat copy number.

A second example of a disease that exhibits expansion of unstable repeat sequences is myotonic dystrophy. This progressive disorder of muscle weakness is inherited as an autosomal dominant trait and exhibits a unique property termed "anticipation" to denote the earlier onset and increasing severity of the disease in successive generations.[296] Novel restriction fragments have been found to be associated with the myotonic dystrophy (DM) gene in a majority of patients.[297–299] The size increase correlated with increasing severity and, contrary to the situation observed in the fragile X syndrome, enlargement was seen after transmission by either sex. In pedigrees exhibiting anticipation, the fragment size increased in successive generations. The molecular basis of the instability was shown to derive from a (CTG)n repeat sequence within the 3′ untranslated region (UTR) of the DM gene 500 bp from the polyadenylation site.[296,300–303] Some 40 percent of normal controls were found to possess 5 CTG repeats, most of the remainder bearing between 10 and 14 repeats, and a few with any number up to 35 repeats. By contrast, minimally affected myotonic dystrophy patients possessed at least 50 CTG repeats, whereas the more severe cases exhibited expansion of the repeat sequence up to 5 kb. The size of the (CTG)n repeat correlated both with severity and age of onset; indeed, families in which the severity of the disease had increased in successive generations exhibited a dramatic parallel expansion in repeat copy number. Similarly, infants with severe congenital myotonic dystrophy and their mothers exhibit a greater degree of amplification of CTG repeats than in the noncongenital population. In one reported case, transmission of the affected chromosome from father to son was associated with a contraction rather than an expansion of repeat size,[304] and the son was asymptomatic. Therefore, this may provide an explanation for the incomplete penetrance manifested by myotonic dystrophy. As with the fragile X syndrome, linkage disequilibrium is apparent in heterogeneous populations between myotonic dystrophy and DNA polymorphisms in the vicinity,[298,302] implying either the existence of only one or at most a few mutations or that the chromosomal environment predispose to mutation at the DM locus. Since linkage disequilibrium has been reported between the same polymorphic alleles in both Japanese and Caucasian populations,[305] myotonic dystrophy patients from these populations may share a common ancestor. How expansion of the (CTG)n repeat within the 3′ UTR causes the myotonic dystrophy phenotype is still unclear. If it abolishes expression of the mutant allele, then myotonic dystrophy might arise through the level of the DM gene product falling below a certain threshold level. Alternatively, the repeat expansion might prevent the binding of a protein involved in the negative regulation of DM gene expression.

Other examples of trinucleotide repeat expansion disorders include Kennedy disease,[306–308] Huntington disease,[309] spinocerebellar ataxia types 1, 2, 3 and 6,[310] Friedreich's ataxia,[312] and progressive myoclonus epilepsy.[313]

The number of examples of this type of mutation will almost certainly increase and may provide explanations at the molecular level for a variety of intriguing phenomena in human genetics, such as variable expression and multifactorial inheritance.[311]

MUTATIONS IN CANCER

A common finding in a diverse array of cancers is genetic instability. Its relationship to tumorigenesis is particularly well understood in hereditary non-polyposis colon cancer (HNPCC), a syndrome characterized by predisposition to colorectal carcinoma and other cancers of the gastrointestinal and urological tracts (Chap. 31). In HNPCC, genetic instability at microsatellite sequences [RER+ ("replication error positive")] has been linked to defects in several mismatch repair (MMR) genes.[314,314a] Mutation rates in RER+ cells are two to three orders of magnitude higher than in normal RER− cells.[314] Multiple mutations are necessary for malignancy, and

MMR deficiency greatly speeds up the process of accumulating mutations at those loci which are critical for tumor progression. The target genes of the genome-wide hypermutability evident in MMR-deficient cells are now beginning to be identified. Perhaps the best example is that of the gene encoding TGFβ receptor II which is intimately involved in cellular growth regulation. Colorectal tumors are generally insensitive to the growth suppressing hormone TGFβ and in colorectal tumors manifesting MI, this insensitivity is almost invariably due to frameshift mutations within a microsatellite sequence (polyadenine tract) embedded within the TGFβ receptor II gene.[315–317] Similarly, the target sequence of mutations within the transcription factor E2F-4 gene is a $(CAG)_{13}$ trinucleotide repeat within the putative transactivation domain.[318] Thus, mutation-bearing genes which contribute to the development of colorectal neoplasia may be identified firstly through their involvement in the negative regulation of cell growth and secondly on the basis of their containing repetitive sequences which represent likely targets for mutation in RER+ cells. Some of the mutated genes are directly involved in growth regulation (e.g. APC[319], E2F-4[318], IGF2R[320]) or in promoting apoptosis (e.g., BAX[321]) and are therefore likely to play a role in tumor progression. MMR genes may themselves represent mutational targets[321a] ("the mutator that mutates the other mutator") which increases genomic instability still further. Other genes are not involved in these processes (e.g., HPRT[322]) and their mutation merely represents the consequence of a general genome-wide increase in mutability. It should be noted that the instability resulting from the deficiency of a mismatch repair enzyme is qualitatively different from the instability associated with the triplet repeat expansion disorders in which the local DNA structure appears to be critical in promoting expansion.[323]

Mutations may predispose to neoplasia directly but recent findings show that predisposition may also be indirect. A T → A transversion at nucleotide 3920 in the *APC* gene occurs in about 6% of Ashkenazi Jews and about 28% of Ashkenazim with a family history of colorectal cancer.[324] This lesion is considered unlikely to predispose to cancer directly by altering the function of the encoded protein. Rather, this transversion generates an $(A)_8$ mononucleotide tract from an existing AAATAAAA sequence motif, thereby creating a hypermutable site within the *APC* coding sequence. The induced instability of this region manifests itself in terms of a high frequency of frameshift insertions in somatic tissues which have probably arisen through DNA slippage during the replication process.

Krawczak et al.[325] demonstrated that the bulk of the spectrum of somatic single base-pair substitutions in the *TP53* gene strongly resembles that of their germline counterparts seen in other human genes. The latter set of mutations have, however, arisen in a tissue that is usually well protected against exogenous mutagens and carcinogens: the germ cells. Since spectral similarity is strongly suggestive of the involvement of similar mutational mechanisms, it would appear that many *TP53* mutations in the soma have arisen directly or indirectly as a consequence of endogenous cellular mechanisms (DNA repair and replication?) rather than through the action of exogenous mutagens. The similarity noted between the cancer-associated mutational spectrum of *TP53* and germline gene mutations was consistent with the idea that cancer is a critical mediator of negative selection against excessive germline mutation. Sommer[326] has speculated that for such a mediator function to work, there must be a correlation between germline and somatic mutation rates. If specific mutations were to occur that enhanced the rates of both germline and somatic mutation, a consequent increase in the incidence of cancer before the end of the normal reproductive period would serve to militate against their survival. It follows that *TP53* may act as a critical sensor that is built into the genome's molecular warning system and which, through carcinogenesis, kills the individual and saves the species.[326]

REFERENCES

1. Krawczak M, Cooper DN: The human gene mutation database. *Trends Genet* **13**:121, 1997.
2. Cooper DN, Krawczak M: *Human Gene Mutation*. Oxford, BIOS Scientific, 1993.
3. Cooper DN, Youssoufian H: The CpG dinucleotide and human genetic disease. *Hum Genet* **78**:151, 1988.
4. Loeb LA, Kunkel TA: Fidelity of DNA synthesis. *Annu Rev Biochem* **52**:429, 1982.
5. Kunkel TA, Alexander PS: The base substitution fidelity of eukaryotic DNA polymerases. *J Biol Chem* **261**:160, 1986.
6. Wang TSF: Eukaryotic DNA polymerases. *Annu Rev Biochem* **60**:513, 1991.
7. Kunkel TA: The mutational specificity of DNA polymerase-β during *in vitro* DNA synthesis. *J Biol Chem* **260**:5787, 1985.
8. Grippo P, Iaccarino M, Parisi E, Scarano E: Methylation of DNA in developing sea urchin embryos. *J Mol Biol* **36**:195, 1968.
9. Cooper DN: Eukaryotic DNA methylation. *Hum Genet* **64**:315, 1983.
10. Bird AP: DNA methylation and the frequency of CpG in animal DNA. *Nucleic Acids Res* **8**:1499, 1980.
11. Nussinov R: Eukaryotic dinucleotide preference rules and their implications for degenerate codon usage. *J Mol Biol* **149**:125, 1981.
12. Bird AP: CpG-rich islands and the function of DNA methylation. *Nature* **321**:209, 1986.
13. Vogel F, Röhrborn G: Mutationsvorgänge bei der Entstehung von Hämoglobinvarianten. *Humangenetik* **1**:635, 1965.
14. Vogel F, Kopun M: Higher frequencies of transitions among point mutations. *J Mol Evol* **9**:159, 1977.
15. Barker D, Schäfer M, White R: Restriction sites containing CpG show a higher frequency of polymorphism in human DNA. *Cell* **36**:131, 1984.
16. Youssoufian H, Kazazian HH, Phillips DG, Aronis S, Tsiftis G, Brown VA, Antonarakis SE: Recurrent mutations in hemophilia A give evidence for CpG mutation hotspots. *Nature* **324**:380, 1986.
17. Youssoufian H, Antonarakis SE, Bell W, Griffin AM, Kazazian HH: Nonsense and missense mutations in hemophilia A: Estimate of the relative mutation rate at CG dinucleotides. *Am J Hum Genet* **42**:718, 1988.
18. Higuchi M, Kazazian HH, Kasch L, Warran TC, McGinniss MJ, Phillips JA, Kasper C, Janco R, Antonarakis SE: Molecular characterization of severe hemophilia A suggests that about half the mutations are not within the coding regions and splice junctions of the factor VIII gene. *Proc Natl Acad Sci USA* **88**:7405, 1991.
19. Higuchi M, Antonarakis SE, Kasch L, Oldenburg J, Economou-Petersen E, Olek K, Arai M, Inaba H, Kazazian HH: Molecular characterization of mild to moderate hemophilia A: Detection of the mutation in 25 of 29 patients by denaturing gradient gel electrophoresis. *Proc Natl Acad Sci USA* **88**:8307, 1991.
20. Koeberl DD, Bottema CDK, Ketterling RP, Lillicrap DP, Sommer SS: Mutations causing hemophilia B: Direct estimate of the underlying rates of spontaneous germ-line transitions, transversions and deletions in a human gene. *Am J Hum Genet* **47**:202, 1990.
21. Reitsma PH, Poort SR, Bernardi F, Gandrille S, Long GL, Sala N, Cooper DN: Protein C deficiency: A database of mutations. *Thromb Haemost* **69**:77, 1993.
22. Rideout WM, Coetzee GA, Olumi AF, Jones PA: 5-Methylcytosine as an endogenous mutagen in the human LDL receptor and p53 genes. *Science* **249**:1288, 1990.
23. Monk M, Boubelik M, Lehnert S: Temporal and regional changes in DNA methylation in the embryonic, extraembryonic and germ lineages during mouse embryo development. *Development* **99**:371, 1987.
24. Driscoll DJ, Migeon BR: Sex differences in methylation of single copy genes in human meiotic germ cells; implications for X-inactivation, parental imprinting, and origin of CpG mutations. *Somat Cell Mol Genet* **16**:267, 1990.
25. Ketterling RP, Vielhaber E, Bottema CDK, Schaid DJ, Sexauer CL, Sommer SS: Germ-line origin of mutation in families with hemophilia B: The sex ratio varies with the type of mutation. *Am J Hum Genet* **52**:152, 1993.
26. Kling S, Ljung R, Sjorin E, Montandon J, Green P, Giannelli F, Nilsson IM: Origin of mutation in sporadic hemophilia B. *Eur J Haematol* **48**:142, 1992.
27. Pattison JK, Millar DS, Grundy CB, Wieland K, Mibashan RS, Martinowitz U, McVey J, Tan-Un K, Vidaud M, Goossens M, Sampietro M, Krawczak M, Reiss J, Zoll B, Whitmore D, Bradshaw A, Wensley R, Ajani A, Mitchell V, Rizza C, Maia R, Winter P, Mayne EE, Schwartz M, Green PJ, Kakkar VV, Tuddenham EGD, Cooper DN: The molecular genetic analysis of hemophilia A; a directed-search strategy for the detection of point mutations in the human factor VIII gene. *Blood* **76**:2242, 1990.
28. Bottema CDK, Ketterling RP, Yoon H-S, Sommer SS: The pattern of factor IX germ-line mutation in Asians is similar to that of Caucasians. *Am J Hum Genet* **47**:835, 1990.
28a. Bottema CDK, Ketterling RP, Li S, Yoon H-P, Phillips JA, Sommer SS: Missense mutations and evolutionary conservation of amino acids: Evidence that many of the amino acids in factor IX function as "spacer" elements. *Am J Hum Genet* **49**:820, 1991.
29. Behn-Krappa A, Hölker I, Sandaradura de Silva U, Doerfler W: Patterns of DNA methylation are indistinguishable in different individuals over a wide range of human DNA sequences. *Genomics* **11**:1, 1991.
30. Green PM, Montandon AJ, Bentley DR, Ljung R, Nilsson IM, Giannelli F: The incidence and distribution of CpG → TpG transitions in the coagulation factor IX gene. A fresh look at CpG mutational hotspots. *Nucleic Acids Res* **18**:3227, 1990.
31. Cooper DN, Krawczak M: Cytosine methylation and the fate of CpG dinucleotides in vertebrate genomes. *Hum Genet* **83**:181, 1989.
31a. Steinberg RA, Gorman KB: Linked spontaneous CG → TA mutations at CpG sites in the gene for protein kinase regulatory subunit. *Mol Cell Biol* **12**:767, 1992.
32. Shen J-C, Rideout WM, Jones PA: High frequency mutagenesis by a DNA methyltransferase. *Cell* **71**:1073, 1992.
33. Bullock P, Champoux JJ, Botchan M: Association of crossover points with topoisomerase I cleavage sites: A model for non-homologous recombination. *Science* **230**:954, 1985.
34. Cooper DN, Krawczak M: Mechanisms of insertional mutagenesis in human genes causing genetic disease. *Hum Genet* **87**:409, 1991.
35. Weaver DT, DePamphilis ML: Specific sequences in native DNA that arrest synthesis by DNA polymerase α. *J Biol Chem* **257**:2075, 1982.
35a. Epstein CJ: Non-randomness of amino-acid changes in the evolution of homologous proteins. *Nature* **215**:355, 1967.
36. Grantham R: Amino acid difference formula to help explain evolution. *Science* **185**:862, 1974.
37. Wada K, Wada Y, Doi H, Ishibashi F, Gojobori T, Ikemura T: Codon usage tabulated from the GenBank genetic sequence data. *Nucleic Acids Res* **19**(Suppl):1981, 1991.
38. Wu C-I, Maeda N: Inequality in mutation rates of the two strands of DNA. *Nature* **327**:169, 1987.
39. Krawczak M, Reiss J, Cooper DN: The mutational spectrum of single base-pair substitutions in mRNA splice junctions of human genes: Causes and consequences. *Hum Genet* **90**:41, 1992.
39a. Holmes J, Clark S, Modrich P: Strand-specific mismatch correction in nuclear extracts of human and *Drosophila melanogaster* cell lines. *Proc Natl Acad Sci USA* **87**:5837, 1990.
40. Giannelli F, Green PM, High KA, Sommer S, Lillicrap DP, Ludwig M, Olek K, Reitsma PH, Goossens M, Yoshioka A, Brownlee GG: Haemophilia B: Database of point mutations and short additions and deletions—third edition. *Nucleic Acids Res* **20**:2027, 1992.
41. Shapiro MB, Senapathy P: RNA splice junctions of different classes of eukaryotes: Sequence statistics and functional implications in gene expression. *Nucleic Acids Res* **15**:7155, 1987.
42. Krainer AR, Maniatis T: Multiple factors including the small nuclear riboproteins U1 and U2 are necessary for the pre-mRNA splicing *in vitro*. *Cell* **42**:725, 1985.
43. Talerico M, Berget SM: Effect of 5′ splice site mutations on splicing of the preceding intron. *Mol Cell Biol* **10**:6299, 1990.
44. Padget RA, Grabowski PJ, Konarska MM, Seiler S, Sharp PA: Splicing of messenger RNA precursors. *Annu Rev Biochem* **55**:1119, 1986.
45. Weil D, D'Alessio M, Ramirez F, Eyre DR: Structural and functional characterization of a splicing mutation in the pro-alpha 2(1) collagen gene of an Ehlers-Danlos type VII patient. *J Biol Chem* **265**:16007, 1990.
46. Weil D, Bernard M, Combates N, Wirtz MK, Hollister DW, Steinmann B, Ramirez F: Identification of a mutation that causes exon skipping during collagen pre-mRNA splicing in an Ehlers-Danlos syndrome variant. *J Biol Chem* **263**:8561, 1988.
47. Grandchamp B, Picat C, de Rooij F, Beaumont C, Wilson P, Deybach JC, Nordmann Y: A point mutation G to A in exon 12 of the PBGD gene results in exon skipping and is responsible for acute intermittent porphyria. *Nucleic Acids Res* **17**:6637, 1989.
48. Carstens RP, Fenton WA, Rosenberg LR: Identification of RNA splicing errors resulting in human ornithine transcarbamylase deficiency. *Am J Hum Genet* **48**:1105, 1991.

49. Wen JK, Osumi T, Hashimoto T, Ogata M: Molecular analysis of human acatalasemia: Identification of a splicing mutation. *J Mol Biol* **211**:383, 1990.

50. Tromp G, Prockop DJ: Single base mutation in the pro-alpha-2(I) collagen gene that causes efficient exon skipping of RNA from exon 27 to exon 29 and synthesis of a shortened but in frame pro-alpha-2(I) chain. *Proc Natl Acad Sci USA* **85**:5254, 1988.

51. Dunn JM, Phillips RA, Zhu X, Becker A, Gallie BL: Mutations in the RB1 gene and their effects on transcription. *Mol Cell Biol* **9**:4596, 1989.

52. Treistman R, Orkin SH, Maniatis T: Specific transcription and RNA splicing defects in five cloned β thalassemia genes. *Nature* **302**:591, 1983.

53. Atweh GF, Wong C, Reed R, Antonarakis SE, Zhu D, Ghosh PK, Maniatis T, Forget BG, Kazazian HH Jr: A new mutation in IVS1 of the human beta-globin gene causing beta-thalassemia due to abnormal splicing. *Blood* **70**:147, 1987.

54. Su TS, Lin LH: Analysis of a splice acceptor site mutation which produces multiple splicing abnormalities in the human argininosuccinate synthase gene. *J Biol Chem* **265**:19716, 1990.

55. Dietz HC, Valle D, Francomano CA, Kendzior RJ, Pyeritz RE, Cutting GR: The skipping of consecutive exons *in vivo* induced by nonsense mutations. *Science* **259**:680, 1993.

56. Orkin SH, Kazazian HH, Antonarakis SE, Ostrer H, Goff SC, Sexton JP: Abnormal processing due to the exon mutation of the beta-E-globin gene. *Nature* **300**:768, 1982.

57. Nakano T, Suzuki K: Genetic cause of a juvenile form of Sandhoff disease: Abnormal splicing of beta-hexosaminidase beta chain gene transcript due to a point mutation within intron 12. *J Biol Chem* **264**:5155, 1989.

58. Mitchell GA, Brody LC, Looney J, Steel G, Suchanek M, Dowling C, Kaloustian V der, Kaiser-Kupfer M, Valle D: An initiator codon mutation in ornithine-δ-aminotransferase causing gyrate atrophy of the choroid and retina. *J Clin Invest* **81**:630, 1988.

59. Naylor JA, Green PM, Rizza CR, Giannelli F: Analysis of factor VIII mRNA reveals defects in everyone of 28 hemophilia patients. *Hum Mol Genet* **2**:11, 1993.

60. Higashi Y, Tanae A, Inoue H, Hiromasa T, Fujii-Kariyama Y: Aberrant splicing and missense mutations cause steroid 21-hydroxylase deficiency in humans: Possible gene conversion products. *Proc Natl Acad Sci USA* **85**:7486, 1988.

60a. Higashi Y, Tanae A, Inoue H, Furjii-Kariyama Y: Evidence for frequent gene conversion in the steroid 21-hydroxylase P-450C21 gene: Implications for steroid 21 hydroxylase deficiency. *Am J Hum Genet* **42**:17, 1988.

61. Murru S, Loudianos G, Deiana M, Camaschella C, Sciarratta GV, Agosti S, Parodi MI, Cerruti P, Cao A, Pirastu M: Molecular characterization of β-thalassemia intermedia in patients of Italian descent and identification of three novel β-thalassemia mutations. *Blood* **77**:1342, 1991.

62. Beldjord C, Lapoumeroulie C, Pagnier J, Benabadji M, Krishnamoorthy R, Labie D, Bank A: A novel beta-thalassemia gene with a single base mutation in the conversed polypryimidine sequence at the 3-prime end of IVS2. *Nucleic Acids Res* **16**:4927, 1988.

63. Sharp P: Splicing of messenger RNA precursors. *Science* **235**:767, 1987.

64. Rosenthal A, Jouet M, Kenwrick S: Aberrant splicing of neural cell adhesion molecule L1 mRNA in a family with X-linked hydrocephalus. *Nature Genet* **2**:107, 1992.

65. Mitchell GA, Labuda D, Fontaine G, Saudubray JM, Bonnefont JP, Lyonnet S, Brody LC, Steel G, Obie C, Valle D: Splice-mediated insertion of an Alu sequence inactivates ornithine δ-aminotransferase: A role for Alu elements in human mutation. *Proc Natl Acad Sci USA* **88**:815, 1991.

66. Wong C, Dowling CE, Saiki RK, Higuchi R, Erlich HA, Kazazian HH: Characterization of β-thalassaemia mutations using direct genomic sequencing of amplified single copy DNA. *Nature* **330**:384, 1987.

67. Kozak M: Compilation and analysis of sequences upstream from the translational start site in eukaryotic mRNAs. *Nucleic Acids Res* **12**:857, 1984.

68. Moi P, Cash FE, Liebhaber SA, Cao A, Pirastu M: An initiation codon mutation (AUG to GUG) of the human α1-globin gene. *J Clin Invest* **80**:1416, 1987.

69. Pirastu M, Saglio G, Chang JC, Cao A, Kan YW: Initiation codon mutation as a cause of α thalassemia. *J Biol Chem* **259**:12315, 1984.

70. Kozak M: Structural features in eukaryotic mRNAs that modulate the initiation of translation. *J Biol Chem* **266**:19867, 1991.

71. Neote K, Brown CA, Mahuran DJ, Gravel RA: Translation initiation in the HEXB gene encoding the β-subunit of human β-hexosaminidase. *J Biol Chem* **265**:20799, 1990.

72. Cai S-P, Eng B, Francombe WH, Olivieri NF, Kendall AG, Waye JS, Chui DHK: Two novel β-thalassemia mutations in the 5′ and 3′ noncoding regions of the β-globin gene. *Blood* **79**:1342, 1992.

73. Clegg JB, Weatherall DJ, Milner PG: Haemoglobin Constant Spring—a chain termination mutant? *Nature* **234**:337, 1971.

74. Milner PF, Clegg JB, Weatherall DJ: Haemoglobin H disease due to a unique haemoglobin variant with an elongated α chain. *Lancet* **1**:729, 1971.

75. Hunt DM, Higgs DR, Winichagoon P, Clegg JB, Weatherall DJ: Haemoglobin Constant Spring has an unstable α chain messenger RNA. *Br J Haematol* **51**:405, 1982.

76. Bunn HF: Mutant hemoglobins having elongated chains. *Hemoglobin* **2**:1978, 1978.

77. Beris PH, Miesher PA, Diaz-Chico JC, Hans IS, Kutlar A, Hu H, Wilson HB, Huisman TJH: Inclusion body β-thalassaemia trait in a Swiss family is caused by an abnormal hemoglobin (Geneva) with an altered and extended β chain carboxy terminus due to a modification in codon β114. *Blood* **72**:801, 1988.

78. Ristaldi MS, Pirastu M, Murru S, Casula L, Loudianos G, Cao A, Sciarrata GV, Agosti S, Parodi MI, Leone D, Melesendi C: A spontaneous mutation produced a novel elongated β-globin chain structural variant (Hb Agnana) with a thalassemia-like phenotype. *Blood* **75**:1378, 1990.

79. Kazazian HH, Dowling CE, Hurwitz RL, Coleman M, Adams JG: Thalassemia mutations in exon 3 of the β-globin gene often cause a dominant form of thalassemia and show no predilection for malarial-endemic regions of the world. *Am J Hum Genet* **25**(*Syppl*):950, 1989.

80. Fucharoen S, Kobayashi Y, Fucharoen G, Ohba Y, Miyazono K, Fukumaki Y, Takaku F: A single nucleotide deletion in codon 123 of the β-globin gene causes an inclusion body β-thalassaemia trait: A novel elongated globin chain β Makabe. *Br J Haematol* **75**:393, 1990.

81. Thein SL, Hesketh C, Taylor P, Temperley IJ, Hutchinson RM, Old JM, Wood WG, Clegg JB, Weatherall DJ: Molecular basis for dominantly inherited inclusion body β-thalassemia. *Proc Natl Acad Sci USA* **87**:3924, 1990.

82. Orkin SH, Cheng T-C, Antonarakis SE, Kazazian HH: Thalassemia due to a mutation in the cleavage-polyadenylation signal of the human β-globin gene. *EMBO J* **4**:453, 1985.

83. Jankovic L, Efremov GD, Petkov G, Kattamis C, George E, Yank K-G, Stoming TA, Huisman THJ: Two novel polyadenylation mutations leading to β+-thalassaemia. *Br J Haematol* **75**:122, 1990.

84. Rund D, Dowling C, Najjar K, Rachmilewitz EA, Kazazian HH, Oppenheim A: Two mutations in the β-globin polyadenylation signal reveal extended transcripts and new RNA polyadenylation sites. *Proc Natl Acad Sci USA* **89**:4324, 1992.

85. Benz EJ, Forget BG, Hillman DG, Cohen-Solal M, Pritchard J, Cavallesco C, Prensky W, Housman D: Variability in the amount of β-globin mRNA in β0-thalassemia. *Cell* **14**:299, 1978.

86. Lehrman MA, Schneider WJ, Brown MS, Davis CG, Elhammer A, Russell DW, Goldstein JL: The Lebanese allele at the low density lipoprotein receptor locus. *J Biol Chem* **262**:401, 1987.

87. Fojo SS, Lohse P, Parrott C, Baggio G, Gabelli C, Thomas F, Hoffman J, Brewer HB: A nonsense mutation in the apolipoprotein C-II Padova gene in a patient with apolipoprotein C-II deficiency. *J Clin Invest* **84**:1215, 1989.

88. Liebhaber SA, Coleman MB, Adams JG, Cash FE, Steinberg MH: Molecular basis for nondeletion α-thalassaemia in American blacks; α2 116 GAG → UAG. *J Clin Invest* **80**:154, 1987.

89. Kinniburgh AJ, Maquat LE, Schedl T, Rachmilewitz E, Ross J: mRNA-deficient β0-thalassemia results from a single nucleotide deletion. *Nuclein Acids Res* **10**:5421, 1982.

90. Chang JC, Kan YW: β0 thalassemia, a nonsense mutation in man. *Proc Natl Acad Sci USA* **76**:2886, 1979.

91. Takeshita K, Forget BG, Scarpa A, Benz EJ: Intranuclear defect in β-globin mRNA accumulation due to a premature translation termination codon. *Blood* **64**:13, 1984.

92. Humphries KR, Ley TJ, Anagnou NP, Baur AW, Nienhuis AW: β0-39 thalassemia gene: A premature termination codon causes β-mRNA deficiency without affecting cytoplasmic β-mRNA stability. *Blood* **64**:23, 1984.

93. Baserga SJ, Benz EJ: Nonsense mutations in the human β-globin gene affect mRNA metabolism. *Proc Natl Acad Sci USA* **85**:2056, 1988.

94. Baserga SJ, Benz EJ: β-Globin nonsense mutation: Deficient accumulation of mRNA occurs despite normal cytoplasmic stability. *Proc Natl Acad Sci USA* **89**:2935, 1992.

95. Atweh GF, Brickner HE, Zhu X-X, Kazazian HH, Forget BG: New amber mutation in a β-thalassemic gene with nonmeasurable levels of mutant messenger RNA *in vivo. J Clin Invest* **82**:557, 1988.

96. Maquat LE, Kinniburgh AJ, Rachmilewitz EA, Ross J: Unstable β-globin mRNA in mRNA-deficient β0-thalassemia. *Cell* **27**:543, 1981.

97. Daar IO, Maquat LE: Premature translation termination mediates triosephosphate isomerase mRNA degradation. *Mol Cell Biol* **8**:802, 1988.

98. Urlaub G, Mitchell PJ, Ciudad CJ, Chasin LA: Nonsense mutations in the dihydrofolate reductase gene affect RNA processing. *Mol Cell Biol* **9**:2868, 1989.

99. Cheng J, Fogel-Petrovic M, Maquat LE: Translation to near the distal end of the penultimate exon is required for normal levels of spliced triosephosphate isomerase mRNA. *Mol Cell Biol* **10**:5215, 1990.

100. Brody LC, Mitchell GA, Obie C, Michaud J, Steel G, Fontaine G, Robert MF, Sipila I, Kaiser-Kupfer M, Valle D: Ornithine δ-aminotransferase mutations in gyrate atrophy; allelelic heterogeneity and functional consequences. *J Biol Chem* **267**:3302, 1992.

101. Ploos van Amstel HK, Diepstraten CM, Reitsma PH, Bertina RM: Analysis of platelet protein S mRNA suggests silent alleles as a frequent cause of hereditary protein S deficiency type I. *Thromb Haemost* **65**:808, 1991.

102. Peerlinck K, Eikenboom JCJ, Ploos van Amstel HK, Sangtawesin W, Arnout J, Reitsma PH, Vermylen J, Briët E: A patient with von Willebrand's disease characterized by compound heterozygosity for a substitution of Arg 854 by Gln in the putative factor VIII-binding domain of von Willebrand factor on one allele and very low levels of mRNA from the second allele. *Br J Haematol* **80**:358, 1992.

103. Orkin SH, Antonarakis SE, Kazazian HH: Base substitution at position-88 in a β-thalassemic globin gene. Further evidence for the role of distal promoter element ACACCC. *J Biol Chem* **259**:8679, 1984.

104. Orkin SH, Kazazian HH, Antonarakis SE, Goff SC, Boehm CD, Sexton JP, Waber PG, Giardina PJV: Linkage of β-thalassemia mutations and β-globin polymorphisms with DNA polymorphisms in the human β-globin gene cluster. *Nature* **296**:627, 1982.

105. Antonarakis SE, Orkin SH, Cheng TC, Scott AF, Sexton JP, Trusko SP, Charache S, Kazazian HH: β-thalassemia in American Blacks. Novel mutations in the TATA box and an acceptor splice site. *Proc Natl Acad Sci USA* **81**:1154, 1984.

106. Cai SP, Zhang JZ, Doherty M, Kan YW: A new TATA box mutation detected at prenatal diagnosis for β-thalassemia. *Am J Hum Genet* **45**:112, 1989.

107. Takihara Y, Nakamura T, Yamada H, Takagi Y, Fukumaki Y: A novel mutation in the TATA box in a Japanese patient with β+ thalassemia. *Blood* **67**:547, 1986.

108. Lin LL, Lin KS, Lin KH, Cheng TY: A novel-34 (C to A) mutant identified in amplified genomic DNA of a Chinese β thalassemia patient. *Am J Hum Genet* **50**:237, 1992.

109. Meloni A, Rosatelli MC, Faa V, Sardu R, Saba L, Murru S, Sciarratta P, Baldi M, Tannoia N: Promoter mutations producing mild β-thalassemia in the Italian population. *Br J Hematol* **80**:222, 1992.

110. Faustino P, Osorio-Almeida L, Barbot J, Espirito-Santo D, Goncalves J, Romao L, Martins MC, Marques MM, Lavinha J: Novel promoter and splice junction defects add to the genetic, clinical or geographic heterogeneity of β thalassemia in the Portuguese population. *Hum Genet* **89**:573, 1992.

111. Huisman THJ: The β and δ thalassemia repository. *Hemoglobin* **16**:237, 1992.

112. Gonzalez-Rodondo JM, Stoming TA, Kutlar A, Kutlar F, Lanclos KD, Howard EF, Fei YJ, Aksoy M, Altay C, Gurgey A, Basak AN, Efremov GD, Petkov G, Huisman THJ: A C to T substitution at nt-101 in a conserved DNA sequence of the promoter region of the β-globin gene is associated with "silent" β thalassemia. *Blood* **73**:1705, 1989.

113. Matsuda M, Sakamoto N, Fukumaki Y: δ-thalassemia caused by disruption of the site for any erythroid-specific transcription factor, GATA-1, in the δ-globin gene promoter. *Blood* **80**:1347, 1992.

114. Collins FS, Stoeckert CJ, Serjeant GR, Forget BG, Weissman SM: Gγ β+ HPFH: Cosmid cloning and identification of a specific mutation 5′ to the Gγ gene. *Proc Natl Acad Sci USA* **81**:4894, 1984.

115. Gilman JG, Mishima N, Wen XJ, Kutlar F, Huisman THJ: Upstream promoter mutation associated with a modest elevation of fetal hemoglobin expression in human adults. *Blood* **72**:78, 1988.

116. Fucharoen S, Shimizu K, Fukumaki Y: A novel C → T transition within the distal CCAAT motif of the G-gamma globin gene in the Japanese HPFH: Implication of factor binding in elevated fetal globin expression. *Nucleic Acids Res* **18**:5245, 1990.

117. Stoming TA, Stoming GS, Lanclos KD, Fei YJ, Kutlar F, Huisman THJ: A A-gamma type of nondeletional hereditary persistence of fetal hemoglobin with a T → C mutation at position −175 to the Cap site of the A-gamma globin gene. *Blood* **73**:329, 1989.

118. Oner R, Kutlar F, Gu LH, Huisman THJ: The Georgia type of non-deletion HPFH has a C to T mutation at nucleotide −114 of the Aγ-globin gene. *Blood* **77**:1124, 1991.

119. Ottolenghi S, Nicolis S, Taramelli R, Malgaretti N, Mantovani R, Comi P, Giglioni B, Longinotti M, Dore F, Oggiano L, Pistidda P, Serra A, Camaschella C, Saglio G: Sardinian Gγ HPFH: A T to C substitution in a conserved octamer sequence in the Gγ promoter. *Blood* **71**:815, 1988.

120. Martin DIK, Tsai S-F, Orkin SH: Increased gamma-globin expression in a nondeletion HPFH mediated by an erythroid-specific DNA-binding factor. *Nature* **338**:435, 1989.

121. Lloyd JA, Lee RF, Lingrel JB: Mutations in two regions upstream of the A gamma globin fene canonical promoter affect gene expression. *Nucleic Acids Res* **17**:4339, 1989.

122. Gumucio DL, Lockwood WK, Weber JL, Saulino AM, Delgrosso K, Surrey S, Schwartz E, Goodman M, Collins FS: The −175 T → C mutation increases promoter strength in erythroid cells: Correlation with evolutionary conservation of binding sites for two trans-acting factors. *Blood* **75**:756, 1990.

123. McDonagh KT, Lin HJ, Lowrey CH, Bodine DM, Nienhuis AW: The upstream region of the human gamma-globin gene promoter. Identification and functional analysis of nuclear protein binding sites. *J Biol Chem* **266**:11965, 1991.

124. Nicolis S, Ronchi A, Malgaretti N, Mantovani R, Giglioni B, Ottolenghi S: Increased erythroid-specific expression of a mutated HPFH gammaa-globin promoter requires the erythroid factor NFE-1. *Nucleic Acids Res* **17**:5509, 1989.

125. Mantovani R, Malgaretti N, Nicolis S, Ronchi A, Giglioni B, Ottolenghi S: The effects of HPFH mutations in the human gammaa-globin promoter on binding of ubiquitous and erythroid-specific nuclear factors. *Nucleic Acids Res* **16**:7783, 1988.

126. Gumucio DL, Rood KL, Gray TA, Riordan MF, Sartor CI, Collins FS: Nuclear proteins that bind the human gamma-globin gene promoter: Alterations in binding produced by point mutations associated with hereditary persistence of fetal hemoglobin. *Mol Cell Biol* **8**:5310, 1988.

127. O'Neil D, Kaysen J, Donovan-Peluso M, Castle M, Bank A: Protein-DNA interactions upstream from the human A gamma globin gene. *Nucleic Acids Res* **18**:1977, 1990.

128. Briët E, Bertina RM, van Tilburg NH, Veltkamp JJ: Haemophilia B Leyden; a sex-linked hereditary disorder that improves after puberty. *N Engl J Med* **306**:788, 1982.

129. Reitsma PH, Bertina RM, Ploos van Amstel JK, Riemans A, Briët E: The putative factor IX gene promoter in hemophilia B Leyden. *Blood* **72**:1074, 1988.

130. Reitsma PH, Mandalaki T, Kasper CK, Bertina RM, Briët E: Two novel point mutations correlate with an altered developmental expression of blood coagulation factor IX (hemophilia B Leyden phenotype). *Blood* **73**:743, 1989.

131. Crossley M, Winship P, Brownlee GG: Functional analysis of the normal and an aberrant factor IX promoter, in *Regulation of Liver Gene Expression*. Cold Spring Harbor, NY, Cold Spring Harbor Laboratory, 1989, p 51.

132. Bottema CDK, Koeberl DD, Sommer SS: Direct carrier testing in 14 families with haemophilia B. *Lancet* **2**:526, 1989.

133. Hirosawa S, Fahner JB, Salier J-P, Wu C-T, Lovrien EW, Kurachi K: Structural and functional basis of the developmental regulation of human coagulation factor IX gene: Factor IX Leyden. *Proc Natl Acad Sci USA* **87**:4421, 1990.

134. Crossley M, Winship PR, Austen DEG, Rizza CR, Brownlee GG: A less severe form of haemophilia B Leyden. *Nucleic Acids Res* **18**:4633, 1990.

135. Gispert S, Vidaud M, Vidaud D, Gazengel C, Boneu B, Goossens M: A promoter defect correlates with an abnormal coagulation factor IX gene expression in a French family (Hemophilia B Leyden). *Am J Hum Genet* **45**(*Suppl*):A189, 1989.

136. Reijnen MJ, Sladek FM, Bertina RM, Reitsma PH: Disruption of a binding site for hepatocyte nuclear factor 4 results in hemophilia B Leyden. *Proc Natl Acad Sci USA* **89**:6300, 1992.

137. Freedenberg DL, Black B: Altered developmental control of the factor IX gene: A new T to A mutation at position +6 of the FIX gene resulting in hemophilia B Leyden. *Thromb Haemost* **65**:964, 1991.

138. Crossley M, Brownlee GG: Disruption of a C/EBP binding site in the factor IX promoter is associated with haemophilia B. *Nature* **345**:444, 1990.

139. Crossley M, Ludwig M, Stowell KM, De Vos P, Olek K, Brownlee GG: Recovery from hemophilia B Leyden: An androgen-responsive element in the factor IX promoter. *Science* **257**:377, 1992.

140. Berg PE, Mittelman M, Elion J, Labie D, Schechter AN: Increased protein binding to a –350 mutation of the human β-globin gene associated with decreased β-globin synthesis. *Am J Hematol* **36**:42, 1991.

141. Moi P, Loudianos G, Lavinha J, Murru S, Cossu P, Casu R, Oggiano L, Longinotti M, Cao A, Pirastu M: δ-thalassemia due to a mutation in an erythroid-specific binding protein sequence 3′ to the δ-globin gene. *Blood* **79**:512, 1992.

142. van der Ploeg LHT, Konings A, Oort M, Roos D, Bernini L, Flavell RA: Gamma-β-thalassaemia studies showing that deletion of the γ- and δ-genes influences β-globin gene expression in man. *Nature* **283**:637, 1980.

143. Kioussis D, Vanin E, deLange T, Flavell RA, Grosveld FG: β-globin gene inactivation by DNA translocation in gamma-β-thalassaemia. *Nature* **306**:662, 1983.

144. Curtin P, Pirastu M, Kan YW, Gobert-Jones JA, Stephens AD, Lehmann H: A distant gene deletion affects β-globin gene function in an atypical γδβ-thalassemia. *J Clin Invest* **76**:1554, 1985.

145. Driscoll MC, Dobkin CS, Alter BP: γδβ-thalassemia due to a *de novo* mutation deleting the 5′ β-globin gene activation-region hypersensitive sites. *Proc Natl Acad Sci USA* **86**:7470, 1989.

146. Grosveld F, van Assendelft GB, Greaves DR, Kollias G: Position-independent high-level expression of the human β-globin gene in transgenic mice. *Cell* **51**:975, 1989.

146a. Jarman AP, Wood WG, Sharpe JA, Gourdon G, Ayyub H, Higgs DR: Characterization of the major regulatory element upstream of the human α-globin gene cluster. *Mol Cell Biol* **11**:4679, 1991.

147. Hatton CSR, Wilkie AOM, Drysdale HC, Wood WG, Vickers MA, Sharpe J, Ayyub H, Pretorius IM, Buckle VJ, Higgs DR: α-thalassemia caused by a large (62kb) deletion upstream of the human α globin gene cluster. *Blood* **76**:221, 1990.

148. Wilkie AOM, Lamb J, Harris PC, Finney RD, Higgs DR: A truncated human chromosome 16 associated with α-thalassaemia is stabilized by addition of telomeric repeat (TTAGGG). *Nature* **346**:868, 1990.

149. Romao L, Osorio-Almeida L, Higgs DR, Lavinha J, Liebhaber SA: α-thalassemia resulting from deletion of regulatory sequences far upstream of the α-globin structural genes. *Blood* **78**:1589, 1991.

150. Romao L, Cash F, Weiss I, Liebhaber S, Pirastu M, Galanello R, Loi A, Paglietti E, Ioannou P, Cao A: Human α-globin gene expression is silenced by terminal truncation of chromosome 16p beginning immediately 3′ of the zeta-globin gene. *Hum Genet* **89**:323, 1992.

151. Liebhaber SA, Griese E-U, Weiss I, Cash FE, Ayyub H, Higgs DR, Horst J: Inactivation of human α-globin gene expression by a *de novo* deletion located upstream of the α-globin gene cluster. *Proc Natl Acad Sci USA* **87**:9431, 1990.

152. Higgs DR, Wood WG, Jarman AP, Sharpe J, Lida J, Pretorius IM, Ayyub H: A major positive regulatory region located far upstream of the human α-globin gene locus. *Genes Dev* **4**:1588, 1990.

153. Vyas P, Vickers MA, Simmons DL, Ayyub H, Craddock CF, Higgs DR: Cis-acting sequences regulating expression of the human α-globin cluster lie within constitutively open chromatin. *Cell* **69**:781, 1992.

154. Antonarakis SE, Kazazian HH Jr: The molecular basis of hemophilia A in man. *Trends Genet* **4**:233, 1988.

155. Millar DS, Steinbrecher RA, Wieland K, Grundy CB, Martinowitz U, Krawczak M, Zoll B, Whitmore D, Stephenson J, Mibashan RS, Kakkar VV, Cooper DN: The molecular genetic analysis of haemophilia A: Characterization of six partial deletions in the factor VIII gene. *Hum Genet* **86**:219, 1991.

156. Ballabio A, Carrozzo R, Parenti G, Gil A, Zollo M, Persico MG, Gillard E, Affara N, Yates J, Ferguson-Smith MA, Frants RR, Eriksson AW, Andria G: Molecular heterogeneity of steroid sulfatase deficiency: A multicenter study of 57 unrelated patients at DNA and protein levels. *Genomics* **4**:36, 1989.

157. Forrest SM, Cross GS, Speer A, Gardner-Medwin D, Burn J, Davies KE: Preferential deletion of exons in Duchenne and Becker muscular dystrophies. *Nature* **329**:638, 1987.

158. Forrest SM, Cross GS, Flint T, Speer A, Robson KJH, Davies KE: Further studies of gene deletions that cause Duchenne and Becker muscular dystrophies. *Genomics* **2**:109, 1988.

159. Den Dunnen JT, Bakker E, Klein Breteler EG, Pearson PL, van Ommen GJB: Direct detection of more than 50 percent of the Duchenne muscular dystrophy mutations by field inversion gels. *Nature* **329**:640, 1987.

160. Wapenaar MC, Kievits T, Hart KA, Abbs S, Blonden LAJ, Den Dunnen JT, Grootscholten PM, Bakker E, Verellen-Dumoulin C, Bobrow M, Van Ommen GJB, Pearson PL: A deletion hot spot in the Duchenne muscular dystrophy gene. *Genomics* **2**:101, 1988.

161. Vnencak-Jones CL, Phillips JA, Chen EY, Seeburg PH: Molecular basis of human growth hormone deletions. *Proc Natl Acad Sci USA* **85**:5615, 1988.

162. Vnencak-Jones CL, Phillips JA: Hot spots for growth hormone gene deletions in homologous regions outside of Alu repeats. *Science* **250**:1745, 1990.

163. Langlois S, Kastelein JJP, Hayden MR: Characterization of six partial deletions in the low density lipoprotein (LDL) receptor gene causing familial hypercholesterolemia (FH). *Am J Hum Genet* **43**:60, 1988.

164. Nicholls RD, Fischel-Ghodsian N, Higgs DR: Recombination at the human α-globin gene cluster: Sequence features and topological constraints. *Cell* **49**:369, 1987.

165. Higgs DR, Vickers MA, Wilkie AOM, Pretorius I-M, Jarman AP, Weatherall DJ: A review of the molecular genetics of the human α-globin gene cluster. *Blood* **73**:1081, 1989.

166. Embury SH, Miller JA, Dozy AM, Kan YW, Chan V, Todd D: Two different molecular organizations account for the single α-globin gene of the α-thalassaemia-2 genotype. *J Clin Invest* **66**:1319, 1980.

167. Trent RJ, Higgs DR, Clegg JB, Weatherall DJ: A new triplicated α-globin gene arrangement in man. *Br J Haematol* **49**:149, 1981.

168. Goossens M, Dozy AM, Embury SH, Zachariades Z, Hadjiminas MG, Stamatoyannopoulos G, Kan YW: Triplicated α-globin loci in humans. *Proc Natl Acad Sci USA* **77**:518, 1980.

169. Hwu HR, Roberts JH, Davidson EH, Britten RJ: Insertion and/or deletion of many repeated DNA sequences in human and higher ape evolution. *Proc Natl Acad Sci USA* **83**:3875, 1986.

170. Moyzis RK, Torney DC, Meyne J, Buckingham JM, Wu JR, Burks C, Sirotkin KM, Goad WG: The distribution of interspersed repetitive DNA sequences in the human genome. *Genomics* **4**:273, 1989.

171. Deininder PL: SINEs: Short interspersed repetitive DNA elements in higher eukaryotes, in Berg DE, Howe MM (eds): *Mobile DNA*. Washington, DC, American Society of Microbiology, 1989, p 619–636.

172. Jelinek WR, Schmid CW: Repetitive sequences in eukaryotic DNA and their expression. *Annu Rev Biochem* **51**:813, 1982.

173. Lehrman MA, Schneider WJ, Suedhof TF, Brown MS, Goldstein JL, Russell DW: Mutation in LDL receptor: Alu-Alu recombination deletes exons encoding transmembrane and cytoplasmic domains. *Science* **227**:140, 1985.

174. Lehrman MA, Russell DW, Goldstein JL, Brown MS: Exon-Alu recombination deletes 5 kilobases from the low density lipoprotein receptor gene producing a null phenotype in familial hypercholesterolemia. *Proc Natl Acad Sci USA* **83**:3679, 1986.

175. Hobbs HH, Brown MS, Goldstein JL, Russell DW: Deletion of exon encoding cysteine-rich repeat of low-density lipoprotein receptor alters its binding specificity in a subject with familial hypercholesterolemia. *J Biol Chem* **261**:13114, 1986.

176. Horsthemke B, Beisiegel U, Dunning A, Havinga JR, Williamson R, Humphries S: Unequal crossing-over between two Alu-repetitive DNA sequences in the low-density-lipoprotein-receptor gene. *Eur J Biochem* **164**:77, 1987.

177. Lehrman MA, Russell DW, Goldstein JL, Brown MS: Alu-Alu recombination deletes splice acceptor sites and produces secreted low density lipoprotein receptor in a subject with familial hypercholesterolemia. *J Biol Chem* **262**3354, 1987.

178. Lehrman MA, Goldstein JL, Russell DW, Brown MS: Duplication of seven exons in LDL receptor gene caused by Alu-Alu recombination in a subject with familial hypercholesterolemia. *Cell* **48**:827, 1987.

179. Ariga T, Carter PE, Davis AE: Recombinations between Alu repeat sequences that result in partial deletions within the C1 inhibitor gene. *Genomics* **8**:607, 1990.

180. Carter PE, Duponchel C, Tosi M, Fothergill JE: Complete nucleotide sequence of the gene for human C1 inhibitor with an unusually high density of Alu elements. *Eur J Biochem* **197**:301, 1991.

181. Stoppa-Lyonnet D, Duponchel C, Meo T, Laurent J, Carter PE, Arala-Chaves M, Cohen JHM, Dewald G, Goetz J, Hauptmann G, Lagrue

G, Lesavre P, Lopez-Trascasa M, Misiano G, Moraine C, Sobel A, Späth PJ, Tosi M: Recombination biases in the rearranged C1-inhibitor genes of hereditary angioedema patients. *Am J Hum Genet* **49**:1055, 1991.

182. Henthorn PS, Smithies O, Mager DL: Molecular analysis of deletions in the human β-globin gene cluster: Deletion junctions and locations of breakpoints. *Genomics* **6**:226, 1990.

183. Kornreich R, Bishop DF, Desnick RJ: α-galactosidase A gene rearrangements causing Fabry disease. *J Biol Chem* **265**:9319, 1990.

184. Monnat RJ, Hackman AFM, Chiaverotti TA: Nucleotide sequence analysis of human hypoxanthine phosphoribosyltransferase *HPRT) gene deletions. *Genomics* **13**:777, 1992.

185. Bollag RJ, Waldman AS, Liskay RM: Homologous recombination in mammalian cells. *Ann Rev Genet* **23**:199, 1989.

186. Shapiro LJ, Yen P, Pomerantz D, Martin E, Rolewic L, Mohandas T: Molecular studies of deletions at the human steroid sulphatase locus. *Proc Natl Acad Sci USA* **86**:8477, 1989.

187. Yen PH, Li X-M, Tsai S-P, Johnson C, Mohandas T, Shapiro LJ: Frequent deletions of the human X chromosome distal short arm result from recombination between low copy repetitive elements. *Cell* **61**:603, 1990.

188. Pizzuti A, Pieretti M, Fenwick RG, Gibbs RA, Caskey CT: A transposon-like element in the deletion-prone region of the dystrophin gene. *Genomics* **13**:594, 1992.

189. Mager DL, Goodchild NL: Homologous recombination between the LTRs of a human retrovirus-like-element causes a 5-kb deletion in two siblings. *Am J Hum Genet* **45**:848, 1989.

190. Gerald PS, Diamond LK: A new hereditary hemoglobinopathy (the Lepore trait) and its interaction with thalassemia trait. *Blood* **13**:835, 1958.

191. Baglioni C: The fusion of two peptide chains in hemoglobin Lepore and its interpretation as a genetic deletion. *Proc Natl Acad Sci USA* **48**:1880, 1962.

192. Barnabus J, Muller CJ: Haemoglobin Lepore Hollandia. *Nature* **194**:931, 1962.

193. Ostertag W, Smith EW: Hemoglobin-Lepore-Baltimore, a third type of a δ, β crossover (δ⁵⁰, β⁸⁶). *Eur J Biochem* **10**:371, 1969.

194. Flavell RA, Kooter JW, DeBoer E, Little PFR, Williamson R: Analysis of δβ-globin gene in normal and Hb Lepore DNA: Direct determination of gene linkage and intergene distance. *Cell* **15**:25, 1978.

195. Baird M, Schreiner H, Driscoll C, Bank A: Localization of the site of recombination in the formation of the Lepore Boston globin gene. *J Clin Invest* **58**:560, 1981.

196. Mavilio F, Giampaolo A, Caré A, Sposi NM, Marinucci M: The δβ crossover region in Lepore Boston hemoglobinopathy is restricted to a 59 base pairs region around the 5′ splice junction of a large globin gene intervening sequence. *Blood* **62**:230, 1983.

197. Chebloune Y, Poncet D, Verdier G: S1-nuclease mapping of the genomic Lepore-Boston DNA demonstrates that the entire large intervening sequence of the fusion gene is of β-type. *Biochem Biophys Res Commun* **120**:116, 1984.

198. Metzenberg AB, Wurzer G, Huisman TH, Smithies O: Homology requirements for unequal crossing over in humans. *Genetics* **128**:143, 1991.

199. Lanclos KD, Patterson J, Eframov GD, Wong SC, Villegas A, Ojwang PJ, Wilson JB, Kutlar F, Huisman THJ: Characterization of chromosomes with hybrid genes for Hb Lepore-Washington, Hb Lepore-Baltimore, Hb P-Nilotic, and Hb Kenya. *Hum Genet* **77**:40, 1987.

200. Fioretti G, De Angioletti M, Masciangelo F, Lacerra G, Scarallo A, de Bonis C, Pagano L, Guarino E, De Rosa L, Salvati F, Carestia C: Origin heterogeneity of Hb Lepore-Boston gene in Italy. *Am J Hum Genet* **50**:781, 1992.

201. Huisman THJ, Wrightstone RN, Wilson JB, Schroeder WA, Kendall AG: Hemoglobin Kenya, the product of a fusion of gamma and β polypeptide chains. *Arch Biochem Biophys* **153**:850, 1972.

202. Kendall AG, Ojwang PJ, Schroeder WA, Huisman THJ: Hemoglobin Kenya, the product of a gamma-β fusion gene: Studies of the family. *Am J Hum Genet* **25**:548, 1973.

203. Ojwang PJ, Nakatsuji T, Gardiner MB, Reese AL, Gilman JG, Huisman THJ: Gene deletion as the molecular basis for the Kenya-G-γ-HPFH condition. *Hemoglobin* **7**:115, 1983.

204. Lehmann H, Charlesworth D: Observations on hemoglobin P (Congo type). *Biochem J* **119**:43, 1970.

205. Badr FM, Lorkin PA, Lehmann H: Haemoglobin P-Nilotic: Containing β δ chain. *Nature* **242**:107, 1973.

206. Honig GR, Mason RG, Tremaine LM, Vida LN: Unbalanced globin chain synthesis by Hb Lincoln Park (anti-Lepore) reticulocytes. *Am J Hematol* **5**:335, 1978.

207. Honig GR, Shamsuddin M, Mason RG, Vida LN: Hemoglobin Lincoln Park: A βδ fusion (anti-Lepore) variant with an amino acid deletion in the δ chain-derived segment. *Proc Natl Acad Sci USA* **75**:1475, 1978.

208. Nathans J, Piantanida TP, Eddy RL, Shows TB, Hogness DS: Molecular genetics of inherited variation in human color vision. *Science* **232**:203, 1986.

209. Pascoe L, Curnow KM, Slutsker L, Connell JMC, Speiser PW, New MI, White PC: Glucocorticoid-suppressible hyperaldosteronism results from hybrid genes created by unequal crossovers between CYP11B1 and CYP11B2. *Proc Natl Acad Sci USA* **89**:8327, 1992.

210. Zimran A, Sorge J, Gross E, Kubitz M, West C, Beutler E: A glucocerebrosidase fusion gene in Gaucher disease. *J Clin Invest* **85**:219, 1990.

211. Tanigawa G, Jarcho JA, Kass S, Solomon SD, Vosberg H-P, Seidman JG, Seidman CE: A molecular basis for familial hypertrophic cardiomyopathy: An α/β cardiac myosin heavy chain hybrid gene. *Cell* **62**:991, 1990.

212. Guioli S, Incerti B, Zanaria E, Bardoni B, Franco B, Taylor K, Ballabio A, Camerino G: Kallmann syndrome due to a translocation resulting in an X/Y fusion gene. *Nature Genet* **1**:337, 1992.

213. Vanin EF, Henthorn PS, Kioussis D, Grosveld F, Smithies O: Unexpected relationships between four large deletions in the human β-globin gene cluster. *Cell* **35**:701, 1983.

214. Piccoli SP, Caimi PG, Cole MD: A conserved sequence at c-myc oncogene chromosomal translocation breakpoints in plasmacytomas. *Nature* **310**:327, 1984.

215. Roth DB, Porter TN, Wilson JH: Mechanisms of non homologous recombination in mammalian cells. *Mol Cell Biol* **5**:2599, 1985.

215a. Roth DB, Wilson JH: Nonhomologous recombination in mammalian cells: Role for short sequence homologies in the joining reaction. *Mol Cell Biol* **6**:4295, 1986.

216. Efstratiadis A, Posakony JW, Maniatis T, Lawn RM, O'Connell C, Spritz RA, DeRiel JK, Forget BG, Weissman SM, Slightom JL, Blechl AE, Smithies O, Baralle FE, Shoulders CC, Proudfoot NJ: The structure and evolution of the human β-globin gene family. *Cell* **21**:653, 1980.

216a. Gilman JG: The 12.6 kilobase DNA deletion in Dutch β⁰-thalassaemia. *Br J Haematol* **67**:369, 1987.

217. Woods-Samuels P, Kazazian HH, Antonarakis SE: Nonhomologous recombination on the human genome; deletions in the human factor VIII gene. *Genomics* **10**:94, 1991.

218. Vogel F, Motulsky AG: *Human Genetics: Problems and Approaches*, 2d ed. Berlin, Springer-Verlag, 1986.

219. Nagylaki T, Petes TD: Intrachromosomal gene conversion and the maintenance of sequence homogeneity among repeated genes. *Genetics* **100**:315, 1982.

220. Shen S, Slightom JL, Smithies O: A history of the human fetal globin gene duplication. *Cell* **26**:191, 1981.

221. Stoeckert CJ, Collins FS, Weissman S: Human fetal globin DNA sequences suggest novel conversion event. *Nucleic Acids Res* **12**:4469, 1984.

222. Powers PA, Smithies O: Short gene conversion in the human fetal globin gene region: A by-product of chromosome pairing during meiosis? *Genetics* **112**:343, 1986.

223. Liebhaber SA, Goossens M, Kan YW: Homology and concerted evolution at the α 1 and α 2 loci of human α-globin. *Nature* **290**:26, 1981.

224. Antonarakis SE, Orkin SH, Kazazian HH, Goff SC, Boehm CD, Waber PG, Sexton JP, Ostrer H, Fairbanks VF, Chakravarti A: Evidence for multiple origins of the βᴱ-globin gene in Southeast Asia. *Proc Natl Acad Sci USA* **79**:6608, 1982.

225. Antonarakis SE, Boehm CD, Serjeant GR, Theisen CE, Dover GJ, Kazazian HH: Origin of the βˢ-globin gene in Blacks: The contribution of recurrent mutation or gene conversion or both. *Proc Natl Acad Sci USA* **81**:853, 1984.

226. Kazazian HH, Orkin SH, Markham AF, Chapman CR, Youssoufian H, Waber PG: Quantification of the close association between DNA haplotypes and specific β-thalassaemia mutations in Mediteraneans. *Nature* **310**:152, 1984.

227. Pirastu M, Galanello R, Doherty MA, Tuveri T, Cao A, Kan YW: The same β-globin gene mutation is present on nine different β-thalassaemia chromosomes in a Sardinian population. *Proc Natl Acad Sci USA* **84**:2882, 1987.

228. Zhang J-Z, Cai S-P, He X, Lin H-X, Lin H-J, Huang Z-G, Chehab FF, Kan YW: Molecular basis of β-thalassaemia in South China. *Hum Genet* **78**:37, 1988.

229. Matsuno Y, Yamashiro Y, Yamamoto K, Hattori Y, Yamamoto K, Ohba Y, Miyaji T: A possible example of gene conversion with a common β-thalassaemia mutation and Chi sequence present in the β-globin gene. *Hum Genet* **88**:357, 1992.

230. Smith GR: Chi hotspots of generalized recombination. *Cell* **34**:709, 1983.

231. Harada F, Kimura A, Iwanaga T, Shimozawa K, Yata J, Sasazuki T: Gene conversion-like events cause steroid 21-hydroxylase deficiency in congenital adrenal hyperplasia. *Proc Natl Acad Sci USA* **84**:8091, 1987.

232. Amor M, Parker KL, Gloverman H, New MI, White PC: Mutation in the CYP21B gene (IIe → Asn) causes steroid 21-hydroxylase deficiency. *Proc Natl Acad Sci USA* **85**:1600, 1988.

233. Morel Y, David M, Forest MG, Betuel H, Hauptman G, Andre J, Bertrand J, Miller WL: Gene conversions and rearrangements cause discordance between inheritance of forms of 21-hydroxylase deficiency and HLA types. *J Clin Endocrinol Metab* **68**:592, 1989.

234. Urabe K, Kimura A, Harada F, Iwanaga T, Sasazuki T: Gene conversion in steroid 210-hydroxylase genes. *Am J Hum Genet* **46**:1178, 1990.

235. Krawczak M, Cooper DN: Gene deletions causing human genetic disease: Mechanisms of mutagenesis and the role of the local DNA sequence environment. *Hum Genet* **86**:425, 1991.

236. Streisinger G, Okada Y, Emrich J, Newton J, Tsugita A, Terzaghi E, Inouye M: Frameshift mutations and the genetic code. *Cold Spring Harb Symp Quant Biol* **31**:77, 1966.

237. Kunkel TA: The mutational specificity of DNA polymerases α and γ during *in vitro* DNA synthesis. *J Biol Chem* **260**:12866, 1985.

238. Kunkel TA, Soni A: Mutagenesis by transient misalignment. *J Biol Chem* **263**:14784, 1988.

239. Ripley LS: Model for the participation of quasi-palindromic DNA sequences in frameshift mutation. *Proc Natl Acad Sci USA* **79**:4128, 1982.

240. DeBoer JG, Ripley LS: Demonstration of the production of frameshift and base-substitution mutations by quasi-palindromic sequences. *Proc Natl Acad Sci USA* **81**:5528, 1984.

241. Maekawa M, Sudo K, Kanno T, Li SS-L: Molecular characterization of genetic mutation in human lactate dehydrogenase A(M) deficiency. *Biochem Biophys Res Commun* **168**:677, 1990.

241a.Gritzmacher CA: Molecular aspects of heavy-chain class switching. *Crit Rev Immunol* **9**:173, 1989.

242. Fearon ER, Cho KR, Nigro JM, Kern SE, Simons JW, Ruppert JM, Hamilton SR, Preisinger AC, Thomas G, Kinzler KW, Vogelstein B: Identification of a chromosome 18q gene that is altered in colorectal cancers. *Science* **247**:49, 1990.

243. Fry M, Loeb LA: A DNA polymerase α pause site is a hotspot for nucleotide misinsertion. *Proc Natl Acad Sci USA* **89**:763, 1992.

244. Bettecken T, Müller CR: Identification of a 220 kb insertion into the Duchenne gene in a family with an atypical course of muscular dystrophy. *Genomics* **4**:592, 1989.

245. Kazazian HH, Wong C, Youssoufian H, Scott AF, Phillips DG, Antonarakis SE: Haemophilia A resulting from *de novo* insertion of L1 sequences represents a novel mechanism for mutation in man. *Nature* **332**:164, 1988.

246. Weiner AM, Deininger PL, Efstratiadis A: Nonviral retroposons: Genes, pseudogenes and transposable elements generated by the reverse flow of genetic information. *Annu Rev Biochem* **55**:631, 1986.

247. Fanning TG, Singer MF: LINE-1: A mammalian transposable element. *Biochim Biophys Acta* **910**:203, 1987.

248. Dombroski BA, Mathias SL, Nanthakumar E, Scott AF, Kazazian HH: Isolation of an active human transposable element. *Science* **254**:1805, 1991.

249. Woods-Samuels P, Wong C, Mathias SL, Scott AF, Kazazian HH, Antonarakis SE: Characterization of a non-deleterious L1 insertion in an intron of the human factor VIII gene and evidence for open reading frame in functional L1 elements. *Genomics* **4**:290, 1989.

250. Mager DL, Henthorn PS, Smithies O: A Chinese Gγ+Aγδβ°thalassaemia deletion: Comparison to other deletions in the human β-globin gene cluster and sequence analysis of the breakpoints. *Nucleic Acids Res* **13**:6559, 1985.

251. Morse J, Rothberg PG, South VJ, Spandorfer JM, Astrin SM: Insertional mutagenesis of the myc locus by a LINE-1 sequence in a human breast carcinoma. *Nature* **333**:87, 1988.

252. Lin CS, Goldthwait DA, Samols D: Identification of *Alu* transposition in human lung carcinoma cells. *Cell* **54**:153, 1988.

253. Wallace MR, Andersen LB, Saulino AM, Gregory PE, Glover TW, Collins FS: A *de novo* Alu insertion results in neurofibromatosis type 1. *Nature* **353**:864, 1991.

254. Economou-Pachnis A, Tsichlis PN: Insertion of an Alu SINE in the human homologue of the MIvi-2 locus. *Nucleic Acids Res* **13**:8379, 1985.

255. Muratani K, Hada T, Yamamoto Y, Kaneko T, Shigeto Y, Ohree T, Furuyama J, Higashino K: Inactivation of the cholinesterase gene by Alu insertion; possible mechanism for the human gene transposition. *Proc Natl Acad Sci USA* **88**:11315, 1991.

256. Vidaud D, Vidaud M, Bahnak BR, Siguret V, Sanchez SG, Laurian Y, Meyer D, Goossens M, Lavergne JM: Hemophilia B due to a *de novo* insertion of a human-specific Alu subfamily member within the coding region of the factor IX gene. *Eur J Hum Genet* **1**:30, 1993.

257. Kariya Y, Kato K, Hayashizaki Y, Himeno S, Tarui S, Matsubara K: Revision of consensus sequence of human Alu repeats—a review. *Gene* **53**:1, 1987.

258. Umlauf SW, Cox MM: The functional significance of DNA sequence structure in a site-specific genetic recombination reaction. *EMBO J* **7**:1845, 1988.

259. Shih C-C, Stoye JP, Coffin JM: Highly preferred targets for retrovirus integration. *Cell* **53**:531, 1988.

260. Hu X, Worton RG: Partial gene duplication as a cause of human disease. *Hum Mut* **1**:3, 1992.

261. Angelini C, Beggs AH, Hoffman EP, Fanin M, Kunkel LM: Enormous dystrophin in a patient with Becker muscular dystrophy. *Neurology* **40**:808, 1990.

262. Yang TP, Stout JT, Konecki DS, Patel PI, Alford RL, Caskey CT: Spontaneous reversion of novel Lesch-Nyhan mutation by HPRT gene rearrangement. *Somat Cell Mol Gen* **14**:293, 1988.

263. Tiller GE, Rimoin DL, Murray LW, Cohn DH: Tandem duplication within a type II collagen gene (COL2A1) exon in an individual with spondyloepiphyseal dysplasia. *Proc Natl Acad Sci USA* **87**:3889, 1990.

264. Stoppa-Lyonnet D, Carter PE, Meo T, Tosi M: Clusters of intragenic Alu repeats predispose the human C1 inhibitor locus to deleterious rearrangements. *Proc Natl Acad Sci USA* **87**:1551, 1990.

265. Murru S, Casula L, Pecorara M, Mori P, Cao A, Pirastu M: Illegitimate recombination produced a duplication within the FVIII gene in a patient with mild hemophilia A. *Genomics* **7**:115, 1990.

266. Hu X, Ray PN, Murphy EG, Thompson MW, Worton RG: Duplicational mutation at the Duchenne muscular dystrophy locus: Its frequency, distribution, origin and phenotype/genotype correlation. *Am J Hum Genet* **46**:682, 1990.

267. Hu X, Ray PN, Worton RG: Mechanisms of tandem duplication in the Duchenne muscular dystrophy gene include both homologous and nonhomologous intrachromosomal recombination. *EMBO J* **10**:2471, 1991.

268. Devlin RH, Deeb S, Brunzell J, Hayden MR: Partial gene duplication involving exon-Alu interchange results in lipoprotein lipase deficiency. *Am J Hum Genet* **46**:112, 1990.

269. Gitschier J: Maternal duplication associated with gene deletion in sporadic hemophilia. *Am J Hum Genet* **43**:274, 1988.

270. Steinmetz M, Uematsu Y, Lindahl KF: Hotspots of homologous recombination in mammalian genomes. *Trends Genet* **3**:7, 1987.

271. Casula L, Murru S, Pecorara M, Ristaldi MS, Restagno G, Mancuso G, Morfini M, DeBiasi R, Baudo F, Carbonara A, Mori PG, Cao A, Pirastu M: Recurrent mutations and three novel rearrangements in the factor VIII gene of hemophilia A patients of Italian descent. *Blood* **75**:662, 1990.

272. Den Dunnen JT, Grootscholten PM, Bakker E, Blonden LAJ, Ginjaar HB, Wapenaar MC, van Paassen HMB, van Broeckhoven C, Pearson PL, van Ommen GJB: Topography of the Duchenne muscular dystrophy (DMD) gene: FIGE and cDNA analysis of 194 cases reveals 115 deletions and 13 duplications. *Am J Hum Genet* **45**:835, 1989.

273. Cooke A, Lanyon WG, Wilcox DE, Dornan ES, Kataki A, Gillard EF, McWhinnie AJM, Morris A, Ferguson-Smith MA, Connor JM: Analysis of Scottish Duchenne and Becker muscular dystrophy families with dystrophin cDNA probes. *J Med Genet* **27**:292, 1990.

274. Haglund-Stengler R, Ritzen EM, Luthman H: 21-hydroxy lase deficiency: Disease-causing mutations categorized by densitometry of 21-hydroxylase-specific deoxyribonucleic acid fragments. *J Clin Endocrinol Metab* **70**:43, 1990.

275. Roberts RG, Barby TFM, Manners E, Bobrow M, Bentley DR: Direct detection of dystrophin gene rearrangements by analysis of dystrophin mRNA in peripheral blood lymphocytes. *Am J Hum Genet* **49**:298, 1991.

276. Monnat RJ, Chiaverotti TA, Hackmann AFM, Maresh GA: Molecular structure and genetic stability of human hypoxanthine phosphoribosyltransferase (HPRT) gene duplications. *Genomics* **13**:788, 1992.

277. Pentao L, Wise CA, Chinault AC, Patel PI, Lupski JR: Charcot-Marie-Tooth type 1A duplication appears to arise from recombination at repeat sequences flanking the 1.5 Mb monomer unit. *Nature Genet* **2**:292, 1992.

278. Jennings MW, Jones RW, Wood WG, Weatherall DJ: Analysis of an inversion within the human β-globin gene cluster. *Nucleic Acids Res* **13**:2897, 1985.

279. Karathanasis SK, Ferris E, Haddad IA: DNA inversion within the apolipoproteins AI/CIII/AIV-encoding gene cluster of certain patients with premature atherosclerosis. *Proc Natl Acad Sci USA* **84**:7198, 1987.

280. Kulozik AE, Bellan-Koch A, Kohne E, Kleihauer E: A deletion/inversion rearrangement of the β-globin gene cluster in a Turkish family with δβ-thalassemia intermedia. *Blood* **79**:2455, 1992.

280a.Lakich D, Kazazian HH, Antonarakis SE, Gitschier J: Inversions of the factor VIII gene as a common cause of severe hemophilia A. *Nature Genet* **5**:236, 1993.

280b.Naylor J, Brinke A, Hassock S, Green PM, Giannelli F: Characteristic mRNA abnormality found in half the patients with severe haemophilia A is due to large DNA inversions. *Hum Mol Genet* **2**:1773, 1993.

281. Caskey CT, Pizzuti A, Fu Y-H, Fenwick RG, Nelson DL: Triplet repeat mutations in human disease. *Science* **256**:784, 1992.

282. Rousseau F, Heitz D, Mandel J-L: The unstable and methylatable mutations causing the fragile X syndrome. *Hum Mut* **1**:91, 1992.

283. Mandel J-L: Questions of expansion. *Nature Genet* **4**:8, 1993.

284. Pieretti M, Zhang R, Fu Y-H, Warren ST, Oostra BA, Caskey CT, Nelson DL: Absence of expression of the FMR-1 gene in fragile X syndrome. *Cell* **66**:817, 1991.

285. Oberlé I, Rousseau F, Heitz D, Kretz C, Devys D, Hanauer A, Boué J, Bertheas MF, Mandel JL: Instability of a 550 base pair DNA segment and abnormal methylation in fragile X syndrome. *Science* **252**:1097, 1991.

286. Yu S, Pritchard M, Kremer E, Lynch M, Nancarrow J, Baker E, Holman K, Mulley JC, Warren ST, Schlessinger D, Sutherland GR, Richards RI: Fragile X genotype characterized by an unstable region of DNA. *Science* **252**:1179, 1991.

287. Verkerk AJMH, Pieretti M, Sutcliffe JS, Fu Y-H, Kuhl DPA, Pizzuti A, Reiner O, Richards S, Victoria MF, Zhang F, Eussen BE, Van Ommen GJB, Blonden LAJ, Riggins GJ, Chastain JL, Kunst CB, Galjaard H, Caskey CT, Nelson DL, Oostra BA, Warren ST: Identification of a gene (FMR-1) containing a CGG repeat coincident with a breakpoint cluster region exhibiting length variation in fragile X syndrome. *Cell* **65**:905, 1991.

288. Kremer EJ, Pritchard M, Lynch M, Yu S, Holman K, Baker E, Warren ST, Schlessinger D, Sutherland GR, Richards RI: Mapping of DNA instability at the fragile X to a trinucleotide repeat sequence p(CCG)n. *Science* **252**:1711, 1991.

289. Fu Y-H, Kuhl DPA, Pizzuti A, Pieretti M, Sutcliffe JS, Richards S, Verkerk AJMH, Holden JJA, Fenwick RG, Warren ST, Oostra BA, Nelson DL, Caskey CT: Variation of the CGG repeat at the fragile X site results in genetic instability: Resolution of Sherman paradox. *Cell* **67**:1047, 1991.

290. Rousseau F, Heitz D, Biancalana V, Blumenfeld S, Kretz C, Boué J, Tommerup N, Van der Hagen C, DeLozier-Blanchet C, Croquette M-F, Gilgenkrantz S, Jalbert P, Voelckel M-A, Oberlé I, Mandel J-L: Direct diagnosis by DNA analysis of the fragile X syndrome of mental retardation. *N Engl J Med* **325**:1673, 1991.

291. Hirst M, Knight S, Davies K, Cross G, Ocraft K, Raeburn S, Heeger S, Eunpu D, Jenkins EC, Lindenbaum R: Prenatal diagnosis of fragile X syndrome. *Lancet* **338**:956, 1991.

292. Dobkin CS, Ding X-H, Jenkins EC, Krawczak MS, Brown WT, Goonewardena P, Willner WT, Benson C, Heitz D, Rousseau F: Prenatal diagnosis of fragile X syndrome. *Lancet* **338**:957, 1991.

293. Pergolizzi RG, Erster SH, Goonewardena P, Brown WT: Detection of full fragile X mutation. *Lancet* **339**:271, 1992.

294. Yu S, Mulley J, Loesch D, Turner G, Donnelly A, Gedeon A, Hillen D, Kremer E, Lynch M, Pritchard M, Sutherland GR, Richards RI: Fragile-X syndrome: Unique genetics of the heritable unstable element. *Am J Hum Genet* **50**:968, 1992.

295. Richards RI, Holman K, Friend K, Kremer E, Hillen D, Staples A, Brown WT, Goonewardena P, Tarleton J, Schwartz C, Sutherland GR: Evidence of founder chromosomes in fragile X syndrome. *Nature Genet* **1**:257, 1992.

296. Harper PS, Harley HG, Reardon W, Shaw DJ: Anticipation in myotonic dystrophy: New light on an old problem. *Am J Hum Genet* **51**:10, 1992.

297. Harley HG, Brook JD, Rundel SA, Crow S, Reardon W, Buckler AJ, Harper PS, Housman DE, Shaw DJ: Expansion of an unstable DNA region and phenotypic variation in myotonic dystrophy. *Nature* **355**:545, 1992.

298. Harley HG, Rundle SA, Reardon W, Myring J, Crow S, Brook JD, Harper PS, Shaw DJ: Unstable DNA sequence in myotonic dystrophy. *Lancet* **339**:1125, 1992.

299. Buxton J, Shelbourne P, Davies J, Jones C, Van Tongeren T, Aslanidis C, de Jong P, Jansen G, Anvret M, Riley B, Williamson R, Johnson K: Detection of an unstable fragment of DNA specific to individuals with myotonic dystrophy. *Nature* **355**:547, 1992.

300. Brook JD, McCurrach ME, Harley HG, Buckler AJ, Church D, Aburatani H, Hunter K, Stanton VP, Thirion J-P, Hudson T, Sohn R, Zemelman B, Snell RG, Rundle SA, Crow S, Davies J, Shelbourne P, Buxton J, Harper PS, Shaw DJ, Housman DE: Molecular basis of myotonic dystrophy: Expansion of a trinucleotide (CTG) repeat at the 3′ end of a transcript encoding a protein kinase family member. *Cell* **68**:799, 1992.

301. Fu Y-H, Pizzuti A, Fenwick RG, King J, Rajnarayan S, Dunne PW, Dubel J, Nasser GA, Ashizawa T, De Jong P, Wieringa B, Korneluk R, Perryman MB, Epstein HF, Caskey CT: An unstable triplet repeat in a gene related to myotonic muscular dystrophy. *Science* **255**:1256, 1992.

302. Mahadevans M, Tsilfidis C, Sabourin L, Shutler G, Amemiya C, Jansen G, Neville C, Narang M, Barceló J, O'Hoy K, Leblond S, Earle-MacDonald J, De Jong PJ, Wieringa B, Korneluk RG: Myotonic dystrophy mutation: An unstable CTG repeat in the 3′ untranslated region of the gene. *Science* **255**:1253, 1992.

303. Tsilfidis C, Mackenzie AE, Mrttler G, Barceló J, Korneluk RG: Correlation between CTG trinucleotide repeat length and frequency of severe congenital myotonic dystrophy. *Nature Genet* **1**:192, 1992.

304. Shelbourne P, Winquist R, Kunert E, Davies J, Leisti J, Thiele H, Bachmann H, Buxton J, Williamson B, Johnson K: Unstable DNA may be responsible for the imcomplete penetrance of the myotonic dystrophy phenotype. *Hum Mol Genet* **1**:467, 1992.

305. Yamagata H, Miki T, Ogihara T, Nakagawa M, Higuchi I, Osame M, Shelbourne P, Davies J, Johnson K: Expansion of unstable DNA region in Japanese myotonic dystrophy patients. *Lancet* **339**:692, 1992.

306. La Spada AR, Wilson EM, Lubahn DB, Harding AE, Fischbeck KH: Androgen receptor gene mutations in X-linked spinal muscular atrophy. *Nature* **352**:77, 1991.

307. Yamamoto Y, Kawai H, Nakahara K, Osame M, Nakatsuji Y, Kishimoto T, Sakoda S: A novel primer extension method to detect the number of CAG repeats in the androgen receptor gene in families with X-linked spinal and bulbar muscular atrophy. *Biochem Biophys Res Commun* **182**:507, 1992.

308. Biancalana V, Serville F, Pommier J, Julien J, Hanauer A, Mandel JL: Moderate instability of the trinucleotide repeat in spino-bulbar muscular atrophy. *Hum Mol Gen* **1**:255, 1992.

309. The Huntington's Disease Collaborative Research Group: A novel gene containing a trinucleotide repeat that is expanded and unstable on Huntington's disease chromosomes. *Cell* **72**:971, 1993.

310. Orr HT, Chung MY, Banfi S, Kwiatkowski TJ, Servadio A, Beaudet AL, McCall AE, Duvick LA, Ranum LPW, Zoghbi HY: Expansion of an unstable trinucleotide CAG repeat in spinocerebellar ataxia type 1. *Nature Genet* **4**:221, 1993.

311. Sutherland GR, Haan EA, Kremer E, Lynch M, Pritchard M, Yu S, Richards RI: Hereditary unstable DNA: A new explanation for some old genetic questions? *Lancet* **338**:289, 1991.

312. Campuzano V, Montermini L, Molto MD, Pianese L, Cossée M, Cavalcanti F, Monros E, Rosius F, Duclos F, Monticelli A, Zava F, Cañizares J, Koutnikova H, Bidichandani SI, Gellera C, Brice A, Trouillas P, DeMichele G, Filla A, DeFritos R, Palau F, Patel PI, DiDonato S, Mandel J-L, Cocozza S, Koenig M, Pandolfo M: Friedreich's ataxia: autosomal recessive disease caused by an intronic GAA triplet repeat expansion. *Science* **271**:1423, 1996.

313. Mandel J-L: Breaking the rule of three. *Nature* **386**:767, 1997.

314. Kinzler KW, Vogelstein B: Lessons from hereditary colorectal cancer. *Cell* **87**:159, 1996.

314a.Papadopoulos N, Lindblom A: Molecular basis of HNPCC: mutations of MMR genes. *Hum Mutation* **10**:89, 1997.

315. Markowitz S, et al: Inactivation of the type II TGF-beta receptor in colon cancer cells with microsatellite instability. *Science* **268**:1336, 1995.

316. Lu S-L, et al: Mutations of the transforming growth factor-beta type II receptor gene and genomic instability in hereditary nonpolyposis colorectal cancer. *Biochem Biophys Res Commun* **216**:452, 1995.

317. Parsons R, et al: Microsatellite instability and mutations of the transforming growth factor beta type II receptor gene in colorectal cancer. *Cancer Res* **55**:5548, 1995.

318. Yoshitaka T, et al: Mutations of E2F-4 trinucleotide repeats in colorectal cancer with microsatellite instability. *Biochem Biophys Res Commun* **227**:553, 1996.

319. Huang J, et al: APC mutations in colorectal tumors with mismatch repair deficiency. *Proc Natl Acad Sci USA* **93**:9049, 1996.

320. Souza RF, et al: Microsatellite instability in the insulin-like growth factor II receptor gene in gastrointestinal tumors. *Nature Genet* **14**:255, 1996.

321. Rampino N, et al: Somatic frameshift mutations in the *BAX* gene in colon cancers of the microsatellite mutator phenotype. *Science* **275**:967, 1997.

321a.Perucho M: Microsatellite instability: the mutator that mutates the other mutator. *Nature Medicine* **2**:630, 1996.

322. Eshleman JR, et al: Increased mutation rate at the hprt locus accompanies microsatellite instability in colon cancer. *Oncogene* **10**:33, 1995.

323. Goellner GM, et al: Different mechanisms underlie DNA instability in Huntington disease and colorectal cancer. *Am J Hum Genet* **60**:879, 1997.

324. Laken SJ, et al: Familial colorectal cancer in Ashkenazim due to a hypermutable tract in *APC*. *Nature Genet* **17**:79, 1997.

325. Krawczak M, Smith-Sorensen B, Schmidtke J, Kakkar VV, Cooper DN, Hovig E: The somatic spectrum of cancer-associated single base-pair substitutions in the *TP53* gene is determined mainly by endogenous mechanisms of mutation and by selection. *Hum Mutation* **5**:48, 1995.

326. Sommer S: Does cancer kill the individual and save the species? *Hum Mutation* **3**:166, 1994.

CHAPTER 4

Genomic Imprinting and Cancer

Andrew P. Feinberg

1. Genomic imprinting is an epigenetic modification of a specific parental allele of a gene, or the chromosome on which it resides, in the gamete or zygote, leading to differential expression of the two alleles of the gene in somatic cells of the offspring.

2. Evidence for genomic imprinting in normal development derives from studies over many years of the whole genome, specific chromosomal regions, and individual imprinted loci. There is now an intense search for an ever increasing list of imprinted genes that are involved in many different types of cellular processes.

3. Genomic imprinting challenges two assumptions of Mendelian genetics applied to human disease: that the maternal and paternal alleles of a gene are equivalent; and that two functional copies of a gene always are associated with health. Imprinted genes probably account for many examples of developmental malformations in humans.

4. Hydatidiform moles and complete ovarian teratomas, the genome of each of which is derived from a single parental origin, show that an imbalance of maternal and paternal genome equivalents leads to neoplastic growth.

5. Several chromosomes show parental origin-specific alterations in cancer, including losses of heterozygosity in Wilms tumor and in acute myelocytic leukemia, and gene amplification in neuroblastoma.

6. Beckwith-Wiedemann syndrome, a disorder of prenatal overgrowth and cancer, sometimes involves parental origin-specific germline chromosomal rearrangements and uniparental disomy.

7. Loss of imprinting (LOI) is a recently discovered alteration in cancer that involves loss of parental origin-specific gene expression. LOI may include activation of the normally silent copy of growth-promoting genes and/or silencing of the normally transcribed copy of tumor suppressor genes. These changes can involve a switch of a maternal chromosome to a paternal epigenotype.

8. There is a rapidly increasing number of examples of genes and tumors that show LOI. Genes include IGF2, H19, and p57^{KIP2}. Tumors include Wilms tumor, hepatoblastoma, rhabdomyosarcoma, Ewing's sarcoma; uterine, cervical, esophageal, prostate, and lung cancer; choriocarcinoma, and germ cell tumors. Thus, LOI is one of the most common alterations in human cancer.

9. Normal genomic imprinting is maintained in part by parental origin-specific, tissue-independent DNA methylation of cytosine within CpG islands, regions rich in CpG dinucleotides. Tumors with LOI show abnormal methylation of these CpG islands.

10. Normal genomic imprinting should be viewed as a developmental process, rather than as a single event. Thus, a combination of both *cis*-acting and *trans*-acting signals are likely to be important in the establishment and maintenance of normal genomic imprinting, and disruption of those same factors can be expected to play a role in LOI in cancer.

11. As normal imprinting is reversible, LOI may also be reversible and amenable to novel therapeutic approaches, such as modification with 5-aza-2'-deoxycytidine, an inhibitor of DNA methylation.

INTRODUCTION

Genomic imprinting is an epigenetic modification of a specific parental allele of a gene, or the chromosome on which it resides, in the gamete or zygote, leading to differential expression of the two alleles of the gene in somatic cells of the offspring. Alterations of genomic imprinting have recently been identified in human cancers. These alterations have generated a great deal of excitement because they appear to occur commonly in both childhood and adult malignancies, lead to altered expression of growth regulatory genes, and represent potentially reversible changes. Thus they may lead to novel forms of therapy for cancer. This chapter will present the experimental foundations on which these recent discoveries have been made, a summary of our current knowledge (which is evolving rapidly), and prospects for future discovery and application.

TYPES OF EPIGENETIC INHERITANCE

Genomic imprinting is a form of epigenetic inheritance associated with a modification of the genome, heritable by cell progeny, that does not involve a change in DNA sequence. Generally, it leads to apparently non-Mendelian properties of the gene, such as modification by the other allele or a change from one generation to the next. Examples in Drosophila include transvection at the bithorax locus, or pairing-dependent gene expression caused by *trans*-sensing of alleles.[1] The mechanism of transvection is unknown, although interaction between homologous chromosomes appears to influence expression levels from both chromosomes.[2] A second example of epigenetic inheritance is paramutation in plants, a heritable alteration of one allele caused by a second allele of the same gene on the other chromosome.[3]

A third example of epigenetic inheritance is position-effect variegation (PEV) in Drosophila. This involves, for example, the spreading of condensed heterochromatin into adjacent euchromatin at sites of chromosomal rearrangement near the white locus; this leads to variably colored eyes. Two striking features of PEV are the variability of suppression caused by the heterochromatin, leading to very high apparent pseudomutation rates, and the long distances (several Mb) over which PEV can act.[4] Some of the *trans*-acting factors that mediate PEV appear to be involved in the formation or stabilization of heterochromatin.[5,6] Thus, their homologues in mammalian cells may be important in understanding genomic imprinting.

An additional example of epigenetic inheritance, similar to PEV but acting over a much shorter distance (several kb) is telomere silencing in yeast, caused by the proximity of a gene to telomere sequences. Factors that mediate telomere silencing also are known, and in some cases mammalian homologues have been identified.[7] Two underlying themes of the various forms of epigenetic inheritance are that they appear to involve changes to chromatin, and that they act over a distance larger than that of a single gene.

GENOMIC IMPRINTING IN NORMAL DEVELOPMENT

Evidence for genomic imprinting originated from the study of the whole genome, then progressed to studies of individual chromosomes and chromosomal regions, and finally led to identification of specific imprinted genes. The definition of genomic imprinting was first introduced by Helen Crouse in 1960 in her studies of the insect Sciara, which preferentially sheds paternal chromosomes during development.[8] In the first sentence of this chapter, a modification of Crouse's original definition is used to reflect the modern emphasis on transcriptional regulation. A striking example of possible whole genome imprinting is the difference between the mule and the hinny. The mule is a cross of a maternal horse and paternal donkey. It is much larger and quite dissimilar to the hinny, which is the reciprocal cross. Of course, there are other alternative explanations for this phenotypic difference, such as mitochondrial inheritance or differing in utero environments.

A whole genome clue to the existence of genomic imprinting in humans derives from the observation of spontaneously aborted triploid human embryos, which show different histopathology depending on whether the excess of chromosomes is paternal or maternal. Embryos with two maternal genome equivalents and one paternal genome equivalent lead to cystic placentas, a large fetus with malformations, and occasionally to a term pregnancy. In contrast, embryos with two paternal genome equivalents and one maternal genome equivalent show marked growth retardation and die in utero.

Formal proof for imprinting at the level of the genome was offered by Solter and colleagues, who performed pronuclear transplantation experiments in which a maternal pronucleus was replaced with a second paternal pronucleus or vice versa.[9] Androgenotes, defined as containing a normal chromosome number that is entirely of paternal origin, show mainly extra-embryonic tissue. In contrast, gynegenotes, whose chromosomes are entirely of maternal origin, show mostly embryonic tissue. Thus, it appears that the paternal genome equivalent is comparatively more responsible for placental development, and the maternal genome equivalent is comparatively more responsible for embryo development.

Evidence for imprinting of discrete portions of the genome began with studies of X inactivation. This imprinting was first shown by analyzing PGK allele expression in mice heterozygous for a polymorphism in the phosphoglycerate kinase gene, detected as an electrophoretic variant in the protein. Although the X chromosome shows random inactivation in embryonic tissues, that is not the case in extra-embryonic tissues, which show preferential inactivation of the paternal X chromosome.[10]

The beginning of our understanding of which autosomes undergo genomic imprinting came from studies over many years, by Cattanach and colleagues, of mice with germline chromosomal translocations.[11] When these mice are bred, there is a high frequency of nondysjunction, leading to both paternal and maternal uniparental disomy (UPD) beyond the translocation breakpoint, depending on which parent harbors the translocation. The phenotypes of these animals provide an estimate that 15 percent of the genome is imprinted.[11] Studies of UPD in mice also suggest that when imprinting occurs, an excess of the paternal genome coupled with maternal loss, leads to prenatal overgrowth, and an excess of the maternal genome leads to decreased growth. Other phenotypes of UPD include embryonic lethality and behavioral disorders.[11] This work provided a critical clue toward identifying imprinted loci in mouse, and by synteny mapping, in humans. It has shown that imprinting resides at the level of genes and/or chromosomal regions. However, it has several inherent limitations. The phenotype by which animals are scored is relatively insensitive. The technique used is also relatively nonspecific, in that there might be only a single imprinted gene within the entire chromosomal region that shows UPD.

The first example of a specific imprinted gene was discovered fortuitously by Swain, Leder, and colleagues, and it did not involve an endogenous gene. It was noted that a C-*myc* transgene fused to an immunoglobulin enhancer was expressed in some tissues only when inherited from the father. When inherited from the mother, the transgene was transcriptionally silent. In addition, the silent maternally inherited copy was methylated.[12] There are now several examples of transgenes that show parental origin-specific methylation, but transcriptional silencing is less common.[13]

The first example of an imprinted endogenous gene was also discovered fortuitously, when DeChiara, Efstradiatis, and colleagues disrupted the insulin-like growth factor II (IGF2) gene in knockout experiments.[14] When the disrupted allele was inherited from the father, the animals were runted, but there was no phenotype when the disrupted allele was inherited from the mother. When female mice with the disrupted allele themselves had offspring, those animals were of normal size. In situ hybridization and RNase protection experiments confirmed that there was no IGF2 expression in tissues with a disrupted paternal allele. Thus, these experiments clearly showed that IGF2 is imprinted and expressed normally only from the paternal allele.[14] However, IGF2 is biparentally expressed in two neural tissues, the choroid plexus and the leptomeninges, since animals with a disrupted paternal allele nevertheless expressed the gene in these tissues.[14] These were milestone studies because they showed that genomic imprinting affects normal endogenous genes and also that imprinting is subject to tissue-specific regulation. Recent years have provided more direct approaches to identifying novel imprinted genes.[15] These include positional cloning efforts aimed at identifying imprinted genes near other known imprinted genes; techniques for comparing gene expression in parthenogenetic embryos to that of normal embryos;[16] and restriction landmark genome scanning,[17] which exploits a principle introduced many years ago, to analyze clonality in tumors, and involves a search for DNA methylation near a polymorphic site for which the individual is heterozygous.[18] A current inventory (at this writing) of imprinted genes in mouse and humans, which are not necessarily concordant, is provided in Table 4-1. One of the most interesting features of genomic imprinting is that it affects many different cellular processes, including intercellular signaling, RNA processing, and cell cycle control.

GENOMIC IMPRINTING IN HUMAN DISEASE

Two assumptions of Mendelian genetics applied to human disease are that the maternal allele is equivalent to the paternal allele, and that two working copies of the gene are associated with normal function. Genomic imprinting challenges the first of these assumptions, as it is a form of epigenetic inheritance that causes parental origin-specific differential gene expression. As will be described later, abnormal imprinting in cancer challenges the second assumption, because loss of imprinting causing biallelic expression of some genes may be a mechanism underlying carcinogenesis.

The literature of the 1970s and 1980s is rich in presumed examples of human genetic disorders that exhibit genomic imprinting. These reports were based primarily on pedigree studies of autosomal dominant disorders that showed parental origin-specific disease penetrance. These disease loci also often show disease anticipation; namely, the phenotype becomes progressively worse from one generation to the next. Although both of these phenomena were ascribed to genomic imprinting,[19] later studies based on molecular cloning of the responsible genes revealed that genomic imprinting was often not the mechanism, after all. The classical example is fragile X syndrome, a common cause of mental retardation, which is caused by a trinucleotide repeat expansion.[20,21] This expansion undergoes preferential enlargement in the maternal germline, accounting for differential disease penetrance as

Table 4-1 Imprinted Genes in Mouse or Humans

Gene	Expression
IGF2	Paternal
IGF2R	Maternal
H19	Maternal
SNRPN	Paternal
Znf-127	Paternal
Par-5	Paternal
Ipw	Paternal
Par-1	Paternal
Insulin	Paternal
WT1	Maternal
U2afbp-rs	Paternal
Peg 1	Paternal
Peg3	Paternal
Mas	Paternal
p57^{KIP2}	Maternal
Mash2	Maternal
XIST	Paternal
Grf1	Paternal
K$_V$LQT1	Maternal

well as anticipation. However, expression is controlled by the length of the repeat and not imprinting per se.[22] Thus, parent of origin effects may or may not be owing to genomic imprinting. This is not to fault the older studies, as the definition of genomic imprinting itself has evolved somewhat to refer to modification causing parental allele-specific expression, rather than *any* parental allele-specific modification.

Two examples of true imprinted human disease loci are in close proximity on chromosome 15. Their loss causes Prader-Willi syndrome (PWS) or Angelman syndrome (AS). Both involve mental retardation, and PWS also causes obesity and AS involves gross motor disturbances. Each disorder can be caused by uniparental disomy, PWS by maternal UPD, and AS by paternal UPD.[23,24] Similarly, PWS can be caused by intrachromosomal deletions of the paternal chromosome and AS by deletions of the paternal chromosome.[25,26] PWS can be caused by mutations or deletions in the small nuclear ribonucleoprotein polypeptide N (SNRPN) gene.[27] It has recently been shown that a mutation affecting the splicing of an untranslated upstream exon of SNRPN may also lead to Angelman syndrome, as well as abnormal imprinting of other loci.[28] Thus, on chromosome 15, abnormalities of a single gene can affect imprinting of a genomic region and disrupt multiple disease-causing genes, the phenotype depending upon the parental origin of the mutated gene. Recently mutations in UBE3A, a ubiquitin protein ligase, were also found in Angelman syndrome patients.[29]

Despite the relative paucity of known human imprinted disease genes, there are probably many more yet to be identified. This seems clear because uniparental disomy for specific chromosomes is often associated with multiple congenital anomalies.[30] Chromosomes that likely show this phenomenon include 2, 6, 7, 11, 14, 15, 16, 20, and X.[30] Again, the discovery of these potential imprinted disease-causing regions has been fortuitous, as has much of our knowledge of imprinting. For example, the first such example of UPD pointing the way to an imprinted chromosome was the discovery of a cystic fibrosis patient for whom only the mother was the carrier.[31] Molecular analysis showed that the genotype of the offspring was not owing to gonadal mosaicism, but rather to maternal UPD in the offspring. The child also had short stature and possibly Russel-Silver syndrome. This observation indicated that there is at least one imprinted locus on chromosome 7, and that the patient suffered from a deficiency of one or more genes normally expressed only from the paternal allele or duplication of genes normally expressed only from the maternal allele.[31] Not all chromosomes appear to contain disease-related imprinted loci, however, as UPD of chromosomes 4, 5, 9, 10, 13, 21, and 22 has not been associated with birth defects.[30]

INDIRECT EVIDENCE FOR GENOMIC IMPRINTING IN HUMAN CANCER

As in the study of normal genomic imprinting, the idea of a role for genomic imprinting in cancer followed a similar progression of clues regarding whole genome imprinting, involvement of individual chromosomal regions, and finally imprinting at specific loci. The earliest clues suggesting that genomic imprinting is important in cancer were the whole genome examples of the hydatidiform mole and the complete ovarian teratoma. Hydatidiform mole, a malignant tumor of extra-embryonic tissue, is caused by an androgenetic embryo arising from two paternal genome equivalents and no maternal genome equivalent.[32] This can be caused by dispermy and loss of the maternal complement or by duplication of the paternal genome and loss of the maternal equivalent.

Conversely, complete ovarian teratoma, which is a very curious benign tumor that includes differentiated hair, adipose tissue, and even teeth, arises from a parthenogenetic embryo, with two maternal genome equivalents and no paternal equivalent.[33] Parthenogenesis (literally virgin birth) is a specialized type of gynogenesis, and it specifically refers to the absence of fertilization and arises within the ovary. These two tumors, although rare, offer two important general lessons for understanding the role of imprinting in cancer. One is that it takes not only 46 chromosomes to create a normal embryo, but also a balance of maternal and paternal chromosomes; a relative imbalance of paternal to maternal genetic contribution leads to neoplastic growth. The second lesson is that when there is such an imbalance, the type of neoplasm differs depending on whether there is a maternal or paternal genomic excess.

Another tumor that appears to show imprinting effects is familial paraganglioma or glomus tumor. In all cases, the transmitting parent is the father.[34] The responsible gene has recently been localized to 11q22.3-q23.[34]

Chromosomal region-specific evidence for a role for imprinting in cancer followed from an observation several years ago involving loss of heterozygosity (LOH) in Wilms tumor. It had already been known that this most common solid tumor of childhood undergoes LOH of chromosome 11, and that the specifically involved region is 11p15.[35] Schroeder et al. noted that in each of five nonfamilial cases with LOH, it was always the maternal allele that was lost.[36] In a binomial distribution, five is the minimum number required for statistical significance. Unfortunately, the word "imprinting" did not appear anywhere in this important paper, which stimulated a great deal of speculation and study in the following years.

Sapienza and colleagues confirmed and extended this observation to other so-called embryonal tumors of childhood, all of which involve the development of malignancy within what pathologists believe is fetal tissue that is abnormally residual after birth. Examples include hepatoblastoma and rhabdomyosarcoma.[37] They proposed a model in which imprinting is involved in cancer through epigenetic silencing of a tumor suppressor gene (Figure 4-1). According to this model, a tumor suppressor gene on 11p15 is imprinted and epigenetically silenced on the paternal allele, accounting for the fact that LOH is only seen on the maternal allele (Figure 4-1). After all, LOH of the paternal allele would be inconsequential since the locus is silenced normally.[37]

However, Sapienza and colleagues also pointed out a paradox in this logic. If the locus is normally imprinted and epigenetically silenced, then everyone would have only one functional copy of the gene at birth, and then the locus would behave epidemiologically as if it had undergone a germline mutation of a tumor suppressor locus following Knudson's two-hit model of carcinogenesis. According to this model, patients with germline mutations show bilateral tumors occurring at an earlier age of onset than patients with sporadically occurring tumors, which require two sequential events to take place within a given somatic cell lineage. Thus, Sapienza reasoned, epigenetic silencing of a tumor suppressor could not be present in all cells of the body, because the tumors, such as Wilms tumor, with preferential LOH of the maternal allele, are for the most part late arising unilateral tumors. On the other hand, imprinting must take place no later than the zygote stage while there is still a topological distinction between the two parental genome equivalents. Therefore, Sapienza proposed the following solution to this conundrum: In some individuals during germline development or fertilization, aberrant imprinting occurs, preferentially affecting the paternally inherited chromosome. According to this model, imprinting is subsequently erased during development, but not completely, leaving a mosaic pattern of imprinting in various tissues. Thus, the imprint would no longer be-

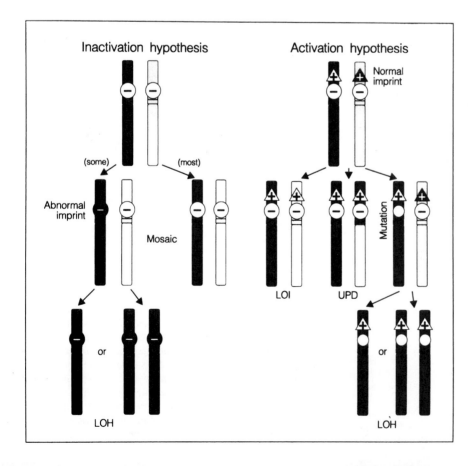

FIG. 4-1 Contrasting hypotheses of genomic imprinting in cancer. The inactivation hypothesis involves loss of expression of a tumor suppressor gene. The paternal allele is inactivated by imprinting, which displays somatic mosaicism (accounting for unilateral tumors), followed by LOH of the maternal allele (arbitrarily shown here affecting the whole chromosome). The activation hypothesis involves normal imprinting of a growth-promoting gene. Overexpression can arise from LOI of the maternal allele or UPD of the paternal allele. LOH of a distinct tumor suppressor gene would be deleterious to cell growth if it involved the transcriptionally active paternal allele of the growth promoting gene. Alternatively, both models may be correct, with LOI and LOH leading to epigenetic silencing of a tumor suppressor gene; and LOI also leading to abnormal activation of a normally silent growth-promoting gene. Dark shading, paternal chromosome; light shading, maternal chromosome; tumor suppressor gene; growth promoting gene. Reprinted from Feinberg, AP: Genomic imprinting and gene activation in cancer. *Nat Genet* 4:110–113, 1993, with permission.

have as the first hit of a two-hit Knudsonian locus (Figure 4-1).[37,38] One puzzle with this model is that it still proposes a relatively large number of cells with this epigenetic alteration, and thus the tumors might appear at an intermediate stage of frequency and age. However, parental origin-specific LOH appears to occur in quite ordinary, late occurring tumors. Furthermore, at least some tumors should not show aberrant imprinting as the first hit, but all tumors show preferential loss of the maternal allele.

There are now several examples of tumor types that show preferential LOH. Most of these involve the maternal chromosome, but not all do. For example, AML involves preferential loss of the paternal chromosome 7.[39] A summary of chromosome-specific LOH is presented in Table 4-2. However, in the study of human genetic disorders, one must be careful not to assume that parent of origin effects are owing to genomic imprinting. For example, bilateral retinoblastoma shows preferential loss of the maternal allele. However, this is owing simply to the higher mutation rate of the paternal gamete rather than imprinting, as the RB gene is not imprinted.[40]

Preferential involvement of a specific parental chromosome also applies to other types of chromosomal abnormality in cancer. For example, Haas and colleagues reported preferential involvement of the paternal chromosome 9 and the maternal chromosome 22 in the Philadelphia chromosome translocation of chronic myelogenous leukemia, based on a cytogenetic polymorphism.[41] However, subsequent studies have not shown imprinting of the rearranged BCR and ABL genes, and molecular studies have not confirmed preferential parental origin of those chromosomes.[42-44]

Other types of parental origin-specific chromosome alterations have withstood the test of time. For example, the N-*myc* gene on chromosome 2 shows preferential amplification of the paternal allele in neuroblastoma.[45] Preferential LOH of the maternal allele of chromosome 1 in neuroblastoma initially was observed by some investigators and not others.[45,46] However, this controversy was resolved when it was found that advanced tumors, showing N-*myc* amplification, also show preferential LOH of maternal chromosome 1, whereas earlier stage tumors without N-*myc* amplification do not.[47] Thus, genetic disturbances involving imprinted genes in a given type of cancer may involve multiple chromosomes concurrently. This idea of abnormal imprinting affecting multiple chromosomes is a provocative one for which there are other data. For example, Sapienza has found transmission ratio distortion, concordance of 13q loss and isochromosome 6 of the same parental origin in retinoblastoma, again consistent with a mechanism of generalized disturbance of imprinting in embryogenesis leading to increased cancer risk.[48]

Despite these intriguing observations of diverse tumors, suggesting a role for genomic imprinting in cancer, direct proof for such a role awaited the discovery of specific imprinted human genes and their altered imprinting in cancer. The guidepost toward these genes was the hereditary disorder Beckwith-Wiedemann syndrome.

Table 4-2 **Preferential Chromosomal Alterations in Cancer That Likely Involve Imprinted Genes**

Cancer	Chromosome	Alteration	Allele
Wilms tumor	11	LOH	Maternal
Rhabdomyosarcoma	11	LOH	Maternal
Osteosarcoma	13	LOH	Maternal
Acute myelocytic leukemia	7	LOH	Paternal
Neuroblastoma	1	LOH	Maternal
Neuroblastoma	2	Amplification	Paternal

BECKWITH-WIEDEMANN SYNDROME

Beckwith-Wiedemann syndrome (BWS) is a disorder of prenatal overgrowth and cancer, transmitted as an autosomal dominant trait, although most cases arise sporadically. It is reported to affect 1 in 15,000 children, although the frequency may be much higher, since close scrutiny of families of BWS patients often show subtly affected siblings or parents, and the phenotype abates with increasing age of the patient.[49,50] Its cardinal features are: macroglossia or enlargement of the tongue, macrosomia caused by prenatal overgrowth throughout gestation, abdominal wall defects (including diastasis recti, umbilical hernia), omphalocele, and craniofacial dysmorphism (including facial nevus flameus, ear pits and creases, prominent occiput, maxillary hypoplasia, widened nasal bridge, high arched palate, and occasionally mild microcephaly). In addition, BWS typically presents with neonatal hypoglycemia, caused in part by overproduction of IGF2.[49,50]

The frequency of embryonal tumors in BWS children is approximately 20 percent, a 1000-fold increase over that of the general population.[51,52] These include Wilms tumor, hepatoblastoma, rhabdomyosarcoma, and adrenocortical carcinoma.[51,52] In addition, the same organs show dysplastic changes, including adrenal cytomegaly and cysts, nephromegaly with prominent lobulation and nephrogenic rests, hepatomegaly, splenomegaly, and hyperplasia of the islets of Langerhans.[49-52]

A clue to a role for genomic imprinting is increased disease penetrance when BWS is inherited from the mother.[53] As noted earlier, parent of origin effects may or may not represent genomic imprinting. However, the tumors these children develop show preferential loss of maternal 11p15, as noted earlier, suggesting that an imprinted locus could cause BWS and also be involved in sporadically occurring tumors.[36,37] Genetic linkage analysis showed that BWS localizes to 11p15, consistent with this idea, and not to 11p13, to which the WT1 gene had been localized.[54,55]

Further support for the idea that imprinting is involved in BWS came from study of rare chromosomal translocations or inversions affecting approximately 1 percent of BWS patients. About half of these rearrangements are balanced, and by analogy to other human genetic disorders, these balanced rearrangements are likely to disrupt the coding sequence of a BWS gene. All of the balanced rearrangements have involved the maternally derived chromosome.[11,56,57] The simplest explanation is that the rearrangements are disrupting expression of a maternally expressed gene. Indeed, there are several families in which multiple individuals within the same kindred harbor the same chromosomal rearrangement, but only those inheriting the rearrangement from the mother were affected with BWS.[56,57] The other type of chromosomal rearrangement seen in BWS patients are unbalanced translocations or duplications. All of these have shown an excess of the paternally derived chromosome.[56] Thus, both paternal duplication and maternal rearrangement of chromosome 11 can lead to BWS.

More direct evidence for genomic imprinting of 11p15 in BWS came from studies of Junien and colleagues showing that some patients with BWS have paternal uniparental disomy, involving a region extending from the β-globin locus to the *ras* gene.[58] This is a very large area of at least 10 Mb and thus does not provide precise localization of an imprinted gene, but it provided an important foundation for later studies of imprinted loci on this chromosome. Curiously, all of the patients with UPD are mosaic for this abnormality.[59] Thus, it occurs postzygotically and is presumably an early embryonic lethal when present in the zygote.

Paternal UPD causes both duplication of the paternal allele and loss of the maternal allele of the involved genes. Thus, UPD by itself is consistent either with loss of function of a gene normally expressed on the maternal chromosome, or duplication of a gene normally expressed from the paternal chromosome. The balanced maternal chromosomal rearrangements in other patients could represent loss of function of a maternally expressed gene, or, alternatively, disruption of an imprinting control center, a hypothetical *cis*-acting signal that establishes the original imprinting pattern in the germline. This disruption could lead to abnormal activation of a gene or genes normally silent on the maternal chromosome, and thus functional duplication of a gene normally expressed from the paternal chromosome. Evidence for this idea derives from the fact that the balanced chromosomal rearrangements, looked at as a group, span a very large region, > 3 Mb, larger than would be expected for a single locus.[57] However, they are clustered into two distinct regions, each of which could conceivably represent a single large gene.[57] The unbalanced paternal chromosome duplications, however, are difficult to explain other than by a mechanism of increased dosage (doubling) of a gene or genes normally expressed only from the paternal chromosome. Of course, BWS may involve both duplication of paternally expressed genes and loss of maternally expressed genes. The identification of genes involved in BWS followed from the discovery of imprinted genes in human 11p15, and is described in the next section.

IMPRINTED GENES ON 11P15 AND LOSS OF IMPRINTING IN CANCER

The first human gene shown to be imprinted at the molecular level was IGF2, which was examined because of its localization to 11p15, for the reasons discussed in the preceding, and because it was known to be imprinted in the mouse. In order to test the hypothesis that IGF2 is imprinted, it was necessary to reverse transcribe (RT) the gene from RNA in a tissue that expresses it, and then PCR amplify the cDNA products. If this RT-PCR is performed on an individual heterozygous for a transcribed polymorphism (i.e., a polymorphic site is present within an exon), then one can determine whether one or both alleles are expressed. If only one allele is expressed, then one can determine if it is maternal or paternal by examining parental genomic DNA samples. In this manner, the IGF2 gene was found to be normally imprinted, with preferential expression of the paternal allele (Figure 4-2), as in the mouse.[60–63] In mouse, H19, a gene within 100 kb of IGF2 that encodes an untranslated RNA of unclear function, is oppositely imprinted, with preferential expression of the maternal allele.[64] This gene was also tested for imprinting in humans and was found to be imprinted as well, with preferential expression of the maternal allele.[60,65]

Examination of RNA from Wilms tumor (WT) led to a surprising discovery. Not one but both IGF2 alleles were expressed in 70 percent of Wilms tumors.[60,62] In addition, in 30 percent of cases, both alleles of H19 were expressed (Figure 4-2).[60] The term for this novel genetic alteration in cancer is loss of imprinting, or LOI, which simply means loss of preferential parental origin-specific gene expression, and can involve either abnormal expression of the normally silent allele, leading to biallelic expression, or silencing of the normally expressed allele, leading to epigenetic silencing of the locus.[60,66,67] Thus, in addition to the epigenetic silencing suggested earlier by Sapienza (Figure 4-1), abnormal imprinting in cancer can lead to activation of normally silent alleles of growth-promoting genes (Figure 4-1)[37,38,60,66,67]

Subsequently, a wide variety of additional tumor types have been shown to undergo LOI. At first, LOI was found in other childhood tumors, such as hepatoblastoma, rhabdomyosarcoma, and Ewing's sarcoma.[68–71] LOI of IGF2 and H19 have also now been found in many adult tumors, including uterine, cervical, esophageal, prostate, lung cancer, choriocarcinoma, and germ cell

tumors.[72–78] Thus, LOI is one of the most common alterations in human cancer. These data are summarized in Table 4-3.

Care must be used in interpreting evidence of biallelic expression of IGF2 as LOI, as IGF2 is normally expressed from both alleles of the adult or P1 promoter.[79] Nevertheless, abnormal imprinting and biallelic expression from the fetal promoters (P2–P4) has been demonstrated for most of the tumors described earlier.[69,71,72,80] Finally, LOI of IGF2 has been described in BWS, albeit in a relatively small percentage of patients.[81,82] Additional patients with large stature and Wilms tumor but not BWS per se also show LOI of IGF2.[83]

A third imprinted gene on chromosome 11p15 is p57[KIP2], encoding a cyclin-dependent kinase (CDK) inhibitor related to

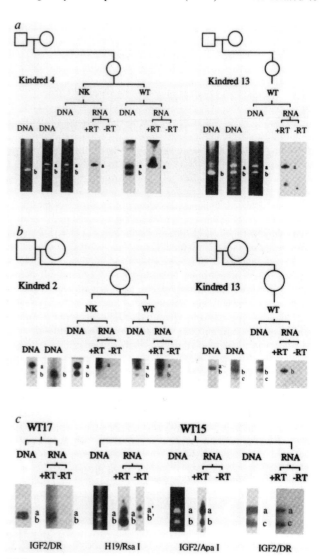

FIG. 4-2 Imprinting of H19 and IGF2 genes and loss of imprinting in cancer. A. Maternal monoallelic expression of H19 in normal kidney (NK) and Wilms tumor (WT). Both NK and WT of patient 4 and WT of patient 13 show monoallelic expression of the maternal allele. B. Paternal monoallelic expression of IGF2 in normal kidney. Kindred 2 was analyzed using an ApaI polymorphism, and kindred 13 using a dinucleotide repeat (DR) polymorphism. C. Biallelic expression of H19 and IGF2 in Wilms tumors. WT17 was analyzed using the IGF2/DR polymorphism and shows biallelic expression. WT15 was informative for all three polymorphisms. Both H19 and IGF2 show biallelic expression, as does the WT from patient 2 (see B). A single DNA-contaminated RNA sample from patient 15 was deliberately included to illustrate the larger-sized fragments (a′,b′) resulting from amplification of genomic sequences. Reprinted from Rainier S, Johnson LA, Dobry CJ, Ping AJ, Grundy PE, Feinberg AP: Relaxation of imprinted genes in human cancer. *Nature* 362:747–749, 1993, with permission.

Table 4-3   Cancers That Show Loss of Imprinting
(LOI)

Tumor Type	Gene
Wilms tumor	IGF2, H19, p57[KIP2]
Rhabdomyosarcoma	IGF2
Hepatoblastoma	IGF2
Bladder	IGF2, H19
Cervical	IGF2, H19
Prostate	IGF2
Testicular	IGF2, H19
Esophageal	H19
Breast	IGF2
Choriocarcinoma	IGF2, H19
Ovarian	IGF2
Colorectal	H19

p21[WAF1/Cip1], a target of p53.[84,85] It was mapped to 11p15, and found to be localized within 40 kb of a group of BWS balanced germline chromosomal rearrangement breakpoints, in contrast to IGF2 and H19, which are located telomeric to these breakpoints.[57,84] Nevertheless, its chromosomal location suggested that it might also be imprinted and play a role in tumors that show LOH of 11p15. Human p57[KIP2] was indeed found to be imprinted with preferential expression from the maternal allele.[86] p57[KIP2] also shows abnormal imprinting and epigenetic silencing in some tumors and BWS patients.[87] Subsequently, nonsense mutations have been described in BWS, but the frequency is quite low, only 5 percent.[88,89] Interestingly, BWS can arise from p57[KIP2] mutations transmitted from the father, although with less severity than those transmitted from the mother.[89] Thus, the phenotype must in part involve haplo-insufficiency of the gene in tissues in which it is not normally imprinted, as well as loss of function in tissues where it is imprinted.[89] This observation is the converse of that made for UBE3A, which is mutated at high frequency in Angelman syndrome but is not imprinted in most tissues,[29] yet must be imprinted in some, since it shows UPD effects.

Finally, a gene spanning a cluster of BWS balanced germline chromosomal rearrangement breakpoints has recently been identified as K_VLQT1.[131] This gene, which also causes the autosomal dominant cardiac arrhythmia long QT syndrome, spans at least 350 kb and also shows genomic imprinting, with preferential expression of the maternal allele.[131] In addition, the gene undergoes alternative splicing at the 5′ end, which involves an untranslated upstream sequence, similar to that observed upstream of the SNRPN gene.[131] Thus K_VLQT1 may be involved in imprint control similar to the function ascribed to SNRPN on chromosome 15. Interestingly, K_VLQT1 is not imprinted in the heart, explaining the lack of parent of origin effect in long QT syndrome, but marked parent of origin effect in translocation-associated BWS.[131]

How can such diverse genetic alterations lead to BWS? One possibility is that the genes involved, IGF2, p57[KIP2], and K_VLQT1 all are part of the same biochemical pathway. A second possibility is that one or more of these genes may be coordinately regulated as part of a large genomic region of multiple imprinted genes. A summary of genetic alterations in BWS is presented in Table 4-4.

THE EFFECTS OF LOI ON GENE EXPRESSION AND TUMOR CELL GROWTH

Since the time of Laennec, it has been known that cancers lose properties of their normal cellular counterparts and gain properties of other types of cells or developmental stages.[90] One of the most

intriguing aspects of LOI is that it may help to explain the abnormal gene expression patterns that are responsible for these characteristics.

Quantitative assays of gene expression in Wilms tumors with LOI reveal the following: IGF2 expression is increased approximately two-fold; H19 expression is lost; and p57[KIP2] expression is lost.[81] This is true even for tumors that show biallelic expression of H19.[87] What appears to take place in tumors with LOI is that the maternal chromosome switches to a paternal epigenotype, affecting several genes over a several hundred kilobase domain. Thus, the maternal copy of IGF2 is expressed, hence biallelic expression. Conversely, the maternal alleles of H19 and p57[KIP2] are epigenetically silenced as on the paternal chromosome, leading to little or no detectable expression of these genes overall.[81,91]

These observations suggest a unified model of LOI in some cancers, such as Wilms tumor, which explains epigenetic silencing of tumor suppressor genes as well as activation of normally silent alleles of growth-promoting genes. According to this model, LOI involves a switch in the epigenotype of a chromosomal region in the case of Wilms tumor from maternal to paternal.[81,91] Thus, IGF2 shows biallelic expression and H19 undergoes epigenetic silencing. However, this model is not meant to be universal. For example, not all tumors show a switch in expression of all three genes, IGF2, H19, and p57[KIP2]. Hepatoblastoma shows LOI of IGF2, but tumors with biallelic expression of IGF2 do not necessarily undergo epigenetic silencing of H19.[68,69]

What is the biological effect of these changes in gene expression caused by altered genomic imprinting? IGF2 is an important autocrine and paracrine growth factor.[92–99] Its mitogenic effects are mediated by signaling through the IGF1 receptor.[99] This is clearly an important pathway in cancer because blocking IGF2 at the IGF1 receptor inhibits tumor cell growth and is even the basis of an experimental therapeutic trial.[99–102] In addition, somatic mutations in the IGF2 receptor gene, which is a metabolic sink for IGF2, have been found in hepatocellular carcinoma, further supporting the idea that signaling by IGF2 is an important mitogenic growth pathway.[103]

Direct evidence for a causative role of IGF2 in tumor progression comes from studies of mice harboring an SV40 T antigen transgene under the control of a rat insulin promoter, known as *RIP-Tag* mice. These animals develop insulinomas at high frequency, and the tumors evolve through sequential stages of tumor progression.[104] When the *RIP-Tag* transgene is bred into a background of mice with homozygously knocked out IGF2 genes, they still develop tumors, but the tumors are arrested at a stage of benign neoplasia.[105] However, when the *RIP-Tag* transgene is bred into a heterozygous IGF2 knockout background, in which only the paternal allele has been disrupted, the maternal allele undergoes LOI and the tumors progress through malignancy, but the tumors are smaller.[106] Finally, when the maternal allele is knocked out, the

Table 4-4   Genetic Alterations in Beckwith-Wiedemann
Syndrome

Genetic Alteration	Allele
Balanced germline chromosomal translocations and inversions	Maternal
Unbalanced germline chromosomal translocations and duplications	Paternal
Uniparental disomy	Maternal
Loss of imprinting of IGF2	Maternal
Loss of imprinting of p57[KIP2]	Maternal
Mutation of p57[KIP2]	Maternal
Imprint-specific methylation switch (increased)	Maternal
Gene rearrangement	Maternal

tumors still show LOI, in that the neo gene is now expressed from the disrupted allele.[106] Thus, LOI is a necessary step in tumor progression in this system. This model also provides a clue to one possible effect of LOI. Tumor cells in which IGF2 has been homozygously knocked out show increased apoptosis, which is overcome by introduction into them of an IGF2 expression construct.[105] Thus, LOI may be one of the factors that allows tumors to escape the apoptosis caused by other carcinogenic mutations.

H19 is an untranslated RNA that accounts for a significant fraction (3%) of embryonic mRNA,[107] but its biological significance remains unclear. An H19 transgene was reported to be an embryonic lethal, but the lethality was caused by a small insertion in the transgene used to mark it.[108,109] An H19 expression construct caused suppression of growth in soft agar of Wilms tumor cells into which it was introduced.[110] However, H19 maps outside of the 11p15 region shown to suppress tumor growth in genetic complementation experiments.[111]

The effect of LOI on p57[KIP2] may be as important as that of IGF2 and H19. Most or all Wilms tumors undergo epigenetic silencing of p57[KIP2].[87] In some tumors, this appears to be caused by abnormal imprinting. The same effect is seen in tumors with LOH, as the normally expressed maternal allele is lost.[87] Thus, p57[KIP2] may represent an imprinted tumor gene in which epigenetic silencing is the primary carcinogenic event. Indeed, this may turn out to be the first tumor gene in which epigenetic silencing is the only carcinogenic event, if mutations in nonfamilial tumors continue not to be found.

POSSIBLE MECHANISMS OF NORMAL IMPRINTING AND LOSS OF IMPRINTING IN CANCER

DNA Methylation

Cytosine DNA methylation is a covalent modification of DNA in which a methyl group is transferred from S-adenosyl methionine to the C-5 position of cytosine by cytosine (DNA-5)-methyltransferase (referred to as DNA methyltransferase). DNA methylation occurs almost exclusively at CpG dinucleotides.[112] The pattern of DNA methylation is heritable by somatic cells and maintained after DNA replication by DNA methyltransferase, which has a 100-fold greater affinity for hemimethylated DNA (i.e., parent strand methylated, daughter strand unmethylated) than for unmethylated DNA.[112] However, developing cells in the gamete and embryo undergo dramatic shifts in DNA methylation, which involve both loss of methylation and de novo methylation.[112] It is not known what mechanism establishes the original pattern of DNA methylation.

There are two classes of cytosine DNA methylation in the genome. The first occurs throughout the body of genes that show tissue-specific expression, with methylation generally associated with gene silencing. This type of DNA methylation can occur both before and after the changes in gene expression, so they are not necessarily the cause of altered gene expression during development. Rather, they may help to "lock in" a given pattern of gene expression.[112,113]

The second class of normal cytosine methylation involves CpG islands, regions rich in CpG dinucleotides. CpG islands are almost always unmethylated in normal cells, and they are usually within the promoter or first exon of housekeeping genes.[114] However, an important exception is CpG islands on the inactive X chromosome, which are methylated. Thus, CpG island methylation, unlike non-CpG island methylation, is thought to be involved

in epigenetic silencing in general and marking of the inactive X chromosome in particular.[115]

Several recent discoveries suggest a role for DNA methylation in the control of genomic imprinting. First, some imprinted genes in mice, such as H19, show parental origin-specific, tissue-independent methylation of CpG islands. For example, the paternal CpG island in H19 is methylated and the maternal allele unmethylated, in tissues that express the gene as well as those that do not.[116,117] Thus, this methylation represents an imprinting mark on the paternal chromosome and is not secondary to changes in gene expression. Second, knockout mice deficient in DNA methyltransferase, and exhibiting widespread genome hypomethylation, do not show allele-specific methylation of the H19 CpG island and exhibit biallelic expression of H19 and loss of expression of IGF2.[118] Similar parental origin-specific methylation has also been observed for a CpG island in the first intron of the maternally inherited, expressed allele of the IGF2 receptor gene (IGF2R).[119] Methyltransferase-deficient knockout mice show loss of methylation of IGF2R and epigenetic silencing of the gene.[118]

Widespread alterations in DNA methylation in human tumors were discovered 15 years ago.[120] This remains the most commonly found alteration in human cancer, albeit an epigenetic one, and it occurs ubiquitously in both benign and malignant neoplasms.[121] The precise role of these changes has remained unclear, although both decreased and increased methylation have been found at specific sites in tumors, with an overall decrease in quantitative DNA methylation.[122-124]

Recent work using an experimental mouse model system also supports a role for DNA methylation in cancer. "Min" mice carry a mutation for the adenomatous polyposis coli (APC) gene, and thereby develop colon tumors. When bred to knockout mice deficient in DNA methyltransferase, Min mice are partially protected from the development of tumors, suggesting that cytosine DNA methylation is involved in tumorigenesis.[125] Consistent with this idea, when these mice are treated with 5-azacytidine, a specific inhibitor of DNA methylation, the incidence of tumors is markedly reduced.[125] Of course, in this model system, decreased methylation may simply protect the animals from methylcytosine to thymine transition mutations.[125] Decreased methylation may or may not also be linked to genomic imprinting, which has not yet been examined in the Min mouse system, but the studies reinforce the link between altered DNA methylation and cancer.

DNA Methylation and LOI

In humans as in mice, the paternal allele of a CpG island in the H19 gene and its promoter is normally methylated, and the maternal allele is unmethylated.[81,116,117] Thus, CpG island methylation represents an imprint-specific mark on the paternal chromosome. Because tumors with LOI of IGF2 showed reduced expression of H19, and because normal imprinting of H19 is associated with methylation of the paternal allele, the methylation pattern of H19 has been examined in tumors with LOI. In all cases showing LOI of IGF2, the H19 promoter exhibits 90 to 100 percent methylation at the sites normally unmethylated on the maternally inherited allele.[81,91] Thus, the maternal allele has acquired a paternal pattern of methylation. This is consistent with the fact that the IGF2 gene on the same (maternally derived) chromosome is expressed in these tumors, as occurs normally only on the paternally derived chromosome. In contrast, tumors without LOI of IGF2 show no change in the methylation of H19, indicating that these changes are related to abnormal imprinting and not malignancy per se.[81,91] The same alterations in methylation of the maternal allele of H19 are found in BWS patients with LOI of IGF2, indicating that LOI can precede the development of malignancy, and not arise secondarily.[81,126,127] These observations are consistent with the model presented earlier of a switch in parental epigenotype. According to this model, LOI, at least in Wilms tumor, involves a switch of the maternal chromosome to a paternal epigenotype, with activation of the maternal H19 allele, silencing of the maternal IGF2 allele, silencing of the maternal p57[KIP2] allele, and methylation of the maternal H19 allele, as on the paternal chromosome.

What is the mechanism of altered DNA methylation in cancer? One mechanism that has been proposed is increased DNA methyltransferase expression itself.[128] Based on a quantitative RT-PCR assay, a 20-fold increase in DNA methyltransferase expression was reported in human colon tumors compared to matched normal mucosa, as well as a 400-fold increase in cancer over the normal mucosa of unaffected patients.[128] However, other RT-PCR experiments showed a more modest change.[129] Furthermore, a sensitive and specific RNase protection assay (RPA) found only a 1.8 to 2.5-fold increase in MTase mRNA.[130] This small difference disappeared entirely when histone H4 was used as an internal control, as a measure of nonspecific tumor cell proliferation. Thus, the mechanism of altered methylation and genomic imprinting does not involve the known DNA methyltransferase enzyme itself.[130]

Disruption of an Imprinting Control Center

A second potential mechanism of LOI may involve disruption of an imprinting control center on chromosome 11, similar to that recently described for the PWS/AS region of chromosome 15.[28] A cluster of five BWS balanced germline chromosomal rearrangement breakpoints lies between p57[KIP2] on the centromeric side, and IGF2 and H19 on the telomeric side.[57] Thus, disruption of a gene spanning this region could cause abnormal imprinting, as well as BWS and/or cancer, at least when inherited through the germline. A gene spanning a cluster of BWS-balanced germline chromosome rearrangement breakpoints has recently been identified as K$_V$LQT1.[131] This gene spans at least 350 kb, shows genomic imprinting, and undergoes alternative splicing, similar to that observed upstream of the SNRPN gene.[130] Thus, this gene may be involved in imprint control similar to the function ascribed to SNRPN on chromosome 15.

Other Possible Factors Causing LOI

Clues to other potential mechanisms for LOI come from consideration of the factors thought to be important in establishment and maintenance of normal genomic imprinting in mouse, and of other forms of epigenetic inheritance in other species, discussed in the opening section of this chapter. One example is the loss of *trans*-acting factors, that are thought to help maintain a normal pattern of imprinting after it is established in the germline. *Trans*-acting modifiers of imprinting are likely to exist, as imprinting of transgenes is host strain-dependent.[132] The human homologues of such genes might thus act as tumor suppressor genes.

Another potential mechanism of imprinting that might be disrupted in cancer involves histone deacetylation, which is linked to X inactivation in mammals, and to telomere silencing in yeast.[133,134] Trichostatin A, a histone deacetylase inhibitor, may disrupt normal genomic imprinting.[135,136] Genes for both histone acetylase and histone deacetylase recently have been isolated.[137,138] In addition, telomere silencing in yeast also involves the action of specific genes, for example, SIR1–SIR4, at least one of which has a homologue in mammals.[7] Similarly, some examples of gene silencing in mammals may resemble position-effect variegation in Drosophila, a form of position-dependent epigenetic silencing.[139] Finally, imprinted loci on maternal and paternal

chromosomes may interact during DNA replication. Chromosomal regions harboring imprinted genes show replicate synchronously.[140] Furthermore, the two parental homologues of some imprinted genes show nonrandom proximity in late S-phase,[141] suggesting some form of chromosomal cross-talk, as has been observed for epigenetic silencing in Drosophila.[142] Although the mechanism of imprinting remains unknown, analysis of tumor cells with altered imprinting should provide an additional tool in unraveling this mystery.

In considering these diverse factors that could disrupt imprinting, it is important to view normal genomic imprinting as a developmental process, rather than as a single event (Figure 4-3). In addition to an initial mark on the chromosome, an imprinting signal likely propagates along the chromosome, similar to propagation of a signal along the inactive X chromosome. Furthermore, specific genes show tissue-specific imprinting, and the timing of silencing varies from gene to gene during early embryonic development. Thus, a combination of both *cis*-acting and *trans*-acting signals are likely to be important in the establishment and maintenance of normal genomic imprinting, and disruption of those same factors can be expected to play a role in LOI in cancer (Figure 4-3). It is also important to note that genomic imprinting normally is erased in primordial germ cells during embryonic development, and thus

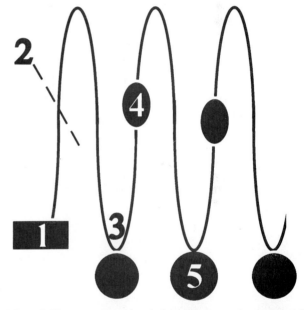

FIG. 4-3 A model of genomic imprinting as a developmental process, at which disturbances of several points might lead to loss of imprinting in cancer. An imprint organizing center (red rectangle), exerts a long-range *cis*-acting influence on IGF2 and other imprinted genes (blue ellipses), via alterations in chromatin structure (represented as DNA loops). This imprint organizing center establishes the imprinting mark as maternal or paternal. This effect is propagated outward during development similar to the organizing center on the X-chromosome. Imprinting is maintained in part by allele-specific methylation of CpG islands, as well as interactions with *trans*-acting proteins (green circles). According to this model, loss of imprinting could arise by any of several mechanisms (numbered in the figure): (1) Deletion or mutation in the imprint organizing center itself, which would lead to a failure of parental origin-specific switching in the germline; (2) separation of the imprint organizing center from the imprinted target genes, as seen in BWS germline chromosomal rearrangement cases; (3) abnormal methylation of CpG islands; (4) local mutation of regulatory sequences controlling the target imprinted genes themselves; or (5) loss of or mutations in genes for *trans*-acting factors that maintain normal imprinting. Figure modified from Feinberg AP, Kalikin LM, Johnson LA, Thompson JS: Loss of imprinting in human cancer. *Cold Spring Harbor Symp Quant Biol* 59:357–364, 1994, with permission.

the aberrant expression in tumors, of factors involved in normal imprint erasure, could also cause loss of imprinting.

IMPLICATIONS FOR CANCER TREATMENT

One of the most exciting aspects of the study of LOI in human cancer is that it is potentially reversible, given that normal imprinting involves epigenetic modifications, and imprinting is normally reversible. A recent experiment suggests that this idea shows some promise.[143] Because tumors with LOI show increased methylation of the H19 CpG island, LOI might be reversed with an inhibitor of DNA methylation, 5-aza-2′-deoxycytidine (5-aza-CdR). Two tumor cell lines exhibiting LOI were treated with 5-azaCdR for 24 hours (~1 cell division) at concentrations chosen

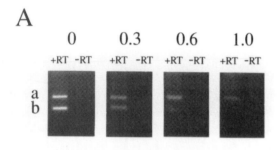

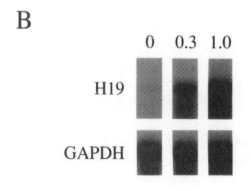

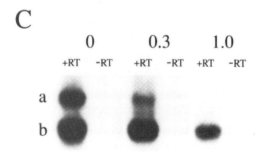

FIG. 4-4 Switch to preferential allelic expression of IGF2 by 5-aza-2′-deoxycytidine (5-azaCdR) treatment of tumor cells with LOI. RT-PCR was performed on total RNA extracted from JEG-3 choriocarcinoma cells after a single 24-hr treatment with 0, 0.3, 0.6, or 1.0 μM 5-azaCdR (indicated). Alternating lanes represent simultaneous experiments with and without reverse transcriptase. PCR products were digested with Apa I. The a and b alleles are 236 and 173 bp, respectively. Reprinted from Thompson JS, Reese KJ, DeBaun MR, Perlman EJ, Feinberg AP: Reduced expression of the cyclin-dependent kinase inhibitor p57KIP2 in Wilms tumor. *Cancer Res* in press, with permission.

to maximize methylation-related biological effects. Treatment with increasing doses of 5-azaCdR led to unequal expression of the two IGF2 alleles in both cell lines (Fig. 4-4). The cells switched from equal expression of the two alleles to predominant expression of the allele represented by the upper uncut band lacking the Apa I polymorphic site, and this effect was nonrandom and specific to one allele. Similarly, 5-azaCdR-treated tumor cells showed a marked increase in H19 expression similar to that seen in normally imprinted cells. In addition to this reactivation of overall H19 expression, H19 also switched from biallelic to monoallelic expression, again consistent with restoration of normal imprinting. Finally, methylation of the imprint-specific CpG island in H19 switched from virtually complete methylation to the expected pattern of single allele methylation.[143] In that experiment, as parental DNA was unavailable, the re-establishment of a normal imprinting pattern could have been due either to a switch of the abnormally imprinted maternal chromosome back to a normal epigenotype. It could also have been due to allele switching, in which the maternal chromosome remained paternally imprinted, but the paternal chromosome switched, to a maternal epigenotype.[143]

Nevertheless, these results are surprising and encouraging because 5-azaCdR might have been expected to show a nonspecific effect on both alleles, similar to that seen in methyltransferase-deficient knockout mice.[118] The fact that 5-azaCdR exerted a specific effect on one chromosome indicates that some imprint-specific information is still retained in tumor cells that show LOI. It further suggests that 5-azaCdR, or drugs with similar effects, may prove useful in the treatment of tumors with LOI, either alone or in conjunction with other agents, and that other strategies for intervention in the pathways regulating genomic imprinting might also eventually be exploited in the design of novel cancer treatments.

ACKNOWLEDGMENTS

This work was supported by NIH grant CA65145. The author thanks J. Barletta, L. Strichman, and G. Randhawa for helpful comments, and J. Patey for preparing the manuscript.

REFERENCES

1. Tartof KD, Henikoff S: Trans-sensing effects from Drosophila to humans. *Cell* **65**:201–203, 1991.
2. Goldsborough AS, Kornberg TB: Reduction of transcription by homologue asynapsis in Drosophila imaginal discs. *Nature* **381**:807–810, 1996.
3. Patterson GI, Thorpe CJ, Chandler VL: Paramutation, an allelic interaction, is associated with a stable and heritable reduction of transcription of the maze b regulatory gene. *Genetics* **135**:881–894, 1993.
4. Tartof KD, Bremer M: Mechanisms for the construction and developmental control of heterochromatin formation and imprinted chromosome domains. *Development* (suppl):35–45, 1990.
5. Tschiersch B, Hofmann A, Krauss V, Dorn R, Korge G, Reuter G: The protein encoded by the Drosophila position-effect variegation suppressor gene Su(var)3-9 combines domains of antagonistic regulators of homeotic gene complexes. *EMBO J* **13**:3822–3831, 1994.
6. Gerasimova TI, Gdula DA, Gerasimov DV, Simonova O, Corces VG: A drosophila protein that imparts directionality on a chromatin insulator is an enhancer of position-effect variegation. *Cell* **82**:587–597, 1995.
7. Brachmann CB, Sherman JM, Devine SE, Cameron EE, Pillus L, Boeke JD: The SIR2 gene family, conserved from bacteria to hu-

mans, functions in silencing, cell cycle progression, and chromosome stability. *Genes Dev* **9**:2888–2902, 1995.

8. Crouse H: The controlling element in sex chromosome behavior in Sciara. *Genetics* **45**:1425–1443, 1960.

9. McGrath J. Solter D: Completion of mouse embryogenesis requires both the maternal and paternal genomes. *Cell* **37**:179–183, 1984.

10. Harper MI, Fosten M, Monk, M: Preferential paternal X inactivation in extraembryonic tissues of early mouse embryos. *J Embryol Exp Morphol* **67**:127–135, 1982.

11. Cattanach BM, Beechey, CV: Autosomal and X-chromosome imprinting. *Development* (suppl):63–72, 1990.

12. Swain JL, Stewart TA, Leder, P: Parental legacy determines methylation and expression of an autosomal transgene: A molecular mechanism for parental imprinting. *Cell* **50**:719–727, 1987.

13. Sapienza C, Paquete J, Tran TH, Peterson, A: Epigenetic and genetic factors affect transgene methylation imprinting. *Development* **107**:165–168, 1989.

14. DeChiara TM, Robertson EJ, Efstratiadis, A: Parental imprinting of the mouse insulin-like growth factor-2 gene. *Cell* **64**:849–859, 1991.

15. Barlow DP, Stoger R, Herrmann BG, Saito K, Schweifer, N: The mouse insulin-like growth factor type-2 receptor is imprinted and closely linked to the Tme locus. *Nature* **349**:84–87, 1991.

16. Kuroiwa Y, Kaneko-Ishino T, Kagitani F, Kohda T, Li L.-L, Tada M, et al: Peg3 imprinted gene on proximal chromosome 7 encodes for a zinc finger protein. *Nat Genet* **12**:186–190, 1996.

17. Nagai H, Pongliktmongkol M, Kim YS, Yoshikawa H, Matsubara K: Cloning of Not I-cleaved genomic DNA fragments appearing as spots in 2D gel electrophoresis. *Biochem. Biophys. Res. Commun* **213**:258-265, 1995.

18. Vogelstein B, Fearon ER, Hamilton SR, and Feinberg AP: Use of restriction fragment length polymorphisms to determine the clonal origin of human tumors. *Science* **227**:642–645, 1985.

19. Laird CD: Proposed mechanism of inheritance and expression of the human fragile-X syndrome of mental retardation. *Genetics* **117**:587–599, 1987.

20. Oberle I, Rousseau F, Heitz D, Kretz C, Devys D, Hanauer A, Boue J, Bertheas MF, Mandel JL: Instability of a 550-base pair DNA segment and abnormal methylation in fragile X syndrome. *Science* **252**:1097–1181, 1991.

21. Fu Y, Kuhl DPA, Pizzuti A, Pieretti M, Sutcliffe JS, Richards S, et al: Variation of the CGG repeat at the fragile X site results in genetic instability: resolution of the Sherman paradox. *Cell* **67**:1047–1058, 1991.

22. Feng Y, Zhang F, Lokey LK, Chastain JL, Lakkis L, Eberhart D, et al: Translational suppression by trinucleotide repeat expansion at FMR1. *Science* **268**:731–734, 1995.

23. Nicholls RD, Knoll JHM, Butler MG, Karam S, Lalande M: Genetic imprinting suggested by maternal heterodisomy in nondeletion Prader-Willi syndrome. *Nature* **342**:281–285, 1989.

24. Knoll JHM, Nicholls RD, Magenis RE, Glatt K, Graham JM Jr, Kaplan L, et al: Angelman syndrome: three molecular classes identified with chromosome 15q11q13-specific DNA markers. *Am J Hum Genet* **47**:149–155, 1990.

25. Knoll JH, Nicholls RD, Magenis RE, Graham JM Jr, Lalande M, Latt SA: Angelman and Prader-Willi syndromes share a common chromosome 15 deletion but differ in parental origin of the deletion. *Am J Med Genet* **32**:285–290, 1989.

26. Mattei MG, Souiah N, Mattei JF: Chromosome 15 anomalies and the Prader-Willi syndrome: Cytogenetic analysis. *Hum Genet* **66**:313–334, 1984.

27. Nicholls RD: Genomic imprinting and candidate genes in the Prader-Willi and Angelman syndromes. *Curr Opin Genet Dev* **3**:445–446, 1993.

28. Dittrich B, Buiting K, Korn B, Rickard S, Buxton J, Saitoh S, et al: Imprint switching on human chromosome 15 may involve alternative transcripts of the SNRPN gene. *Nat Genet* **14**:163–170, 1996.

29. Kishino T, Lalande M, Wagstaff J: UBE3A E6-AP mutations causing Angelman syndrome. *Nat Genet* **15**:70–73, 1997.

30. Ledbetter DH, Engel E: Uniparental disomy in humans: Development of an imprinting map and its implications for prenatal diagnosis. *Hum Mol Genet* **4**:1757–1764, 1995.

31. Spence JE, Perciaccante RG, Greig GM, Willard HF, Ledbetter DH, Hejtmancik JF, et al: Uniparental disomy as a mechanism for human genetic disease. *Am J Hum Genet* **42**:217–226, 1988.

32. Kajii T, Ohama K: Androgenetic origin of hydatidiform mole. *Nature* **268**:633, 1977.

33. Linder D, McCaw B, Kaiser X, Hecht F: Parthenogenetic origin of benign ovarian teratomas. *N Engl J Med* **292**:63–66, 1975.

34. Heutink P, van Schothorst EM, van der Mey AG, Bardoel A, Breedveld G, Pertijs J, et al: Further localization of the gene for hereditary paragangliomas and evidence for linkage in unrelated families. *Eur J Hum Genet* **2**:148–158, 1994.

35. Reeve AE, Sih SA, Raizis AM, Feinberg AP: Loss of allelic heterozygosity at a second locus on chromosome 11 in sporadic Wilms' tumor cells. *Mol Cell Biol* **9**:1799–1803, 1989.

36. Schroeder W, Chao L, Dao D, Strong L, Pathak S, Riccardi V, et al: Nonrandom loss of maternal chromosome 11 alleles in Wilms tumors. *Am J Hum Genet* **40**:413–420, 1987.

37. Scrable H, Cavenee W, Ghavimi F, Lovell M, Morgan K, Sapienza C: A model for embryonal rhabdomyosarcoma tumorigenesis that involves genome imprinting. *Proc Natl Acad Sci USA* **86**:7480–7484, 1989.

38. Peterson K, Sapienza C: Imprinting the genome: Imprinted genes, imprinting genes, and a hypothesis for their interaction. *Ann Rev Genet* **27**:7–31, 1993.

39. Katz F, Webb D, Gibbons B, Reeves B, McMahon C, Chessells J, et al: Possible evidence for genomic imprinting in childhood acute myeloblastic leukaemia associated with monosomy for chromosome 7. *Br J Haematol* **80**:332–336, 1992.

40. Zhu X, Dunn JM, Phillips RA, Goddard AD, Paton KE, Becker A, et al: Preferential germline mutation of the paternal allele in retinoblastoma. *Nature* **340**:312–313, 1989.

41. Haas OA, Argyriou-Tirita A, Lion T: Parental origin of chromosomes involved in the translocation t(9;22). *Nature* **359**:414–416, 1992.

42. Riggins GJ, Zhang F, Warren ST: Lack of imprinting of BCR. *Nat Genet* **6**:226, 1994.

43. Melo JV, Yan XH, Diamond J, Goldman JM: Lack of imprinting of the ABL gene. *Nat Genet*, **8**:318–319, 1994.

44. Melo JV, Yan XH, Diamond J, Goldman JM: Balanced parental contribution to the ABL component of the BCR-ABL gene in chronic myeloid leukemia. *Leukemia* **9**:734–739, 1995.

45. Cheng JM, Hiemstra JL, Schneider SS, Naumova A, Cheung NV, Cohn SL, et al: Preferential amplification of the paternal allele of the N-myc gene in human neuroblastomas. *Nat Genet* **4**:187–190, 1993.

46. Caron H, van Sluis P, van Hoeve M, de Kraker J, Bras J, Slater R, et al: Allelic loss of chromosome 1p36 in neuroblastoma is of preferential maternal origin and correlates with N-myc amplification. *Nat Genet* **4**:191–194, 1993.

47. Caron H, Peter M, van Sluis P, Speleman F, de Kraker J, Laureys G, et al: Evidence for two tumor suppressor loci on chromosomal bands 1p35-36 involved in neuroblastoma: One probably imprinted, another associated with N-myc amplification. *Hum Mol Genet* **4**:535–539, 1995.

48. Naumova A, Hansen M, Strong L, Jones PA, Hadjistilianou D, Mastrangelo D, et al: Concordance between parental origin of chromosome 13q loss and chromosome 6p duplication in sporadic retinoblastoma. *Am J Hum Genet* **54**:274–281, 1994.

49. Engstrom W, Lindham S, Schofield P: Wiedemann-Beckwith syndrome. *Eur J Pediatr* **147**:450–457, 1988.

50. Pettenati MJ, Haines JL, Higgins RR, Wappner RS, Palmer CG, Weaver DD: Wiedemann-Beckwith syndrome: Presentation of clinical and cytogenetic data on 22 new cases and review of the literature. *Hum Genet* **74**:143–154, 1986.

51. Wiedemann HR: Tumours and hemihypertrophy associated with Wiedemann-Beckwith syndrome. *Eur J Pediatr* **141**:129, 1983.

52. Elias ER, DeBaun MR, Feinberg AP: Beckwith-Wiedemann syndrome, in Jameson JL (ed): *Textbook of Molecular Medicine.* Cambridge, Blackwell Scientific, in press.

53. Viljoen D, Ramesar R. Evidence for paternal imprinting in familial Beckwith-Wiedemann syndrome. *J Med Genet* **29**:221-225, 1992.

54. Ping AJ, Reeve AE, Law DJ, Young MR, Boehnke M, Feinberg AP: Genetic linkage of Beckwith-Wiedemann syndrome to 11p15. *Am J Hum Genet* **44**:720–723, 1989.

55. Koufos A, Grundy P, Morgan K, Aleck KA, Hadro T, Lampkin BC, et al: Familial Wiedemann-Beckwith syndrome and a second Wilms tumor locus both map to 11p15. *Am J Hum Genet* **44**:711–719, 1989.

56. Mannens M, Hoovers JMN, Redeker E, Verjaal M, Feinberg AP, Little P, et al: Parental imprinting of human chromosome region 11p15 involved in the Beckwith-Wiedemann syndrome and various human neoplasia. *Eur J Hum Genet* **2**:3–23, 1994.

57. Hoovers JMN, Kalikin LM, Johnson LA, Alders, M, Redeker, B, Law DJ, et al: Multiple genetic loci within 11p15 defined by Beckwith-Wiedemann syndrome: Rearrangement breakpoints and subchromosomal transferable fragments. *Proc Natl Acad Sci USA* **92**:12456–12460, 1995.

58. Henry I, Bonaiti-Pellie C, Chehensse V, Beldjord C, Schwartz C, Utermann G, Junien C: Uniparental paternal disomy in a genetic cancer-predisposing syndrome. *Nature* **351**:609–610, 1991.

59. Henry I, Puech A, Riesewijk A, Ahnine L, Mannens M, Beldjord C, et al: Somatic mosaicism for partial paternal isodisomy in Wiedemann-Beckwith syndrome: A post-fertilization event. *Eur J Hum Genet* **1**:19–29, 1993.

60. Rainier S, Johnson LA, Dobry CJ, Ping AJ, Grundy PE, Feinberg AP: Relaxation of imprinted genes in human cancer. *Nature* **362**:747–749, 1993.

61. Ohlsson R, Nystrom A, Pfeifer-Ohlsson S, Tohonen V, Hedborg F, Schofield P, et al: IGF2 is parentally imprinted during human embryogenesis and in the Beckwith-Wiedemann syndrome. *Nat Genet* **4**: 94–97, 1993.

62. Ogawa O, Eccles MR, Szeto J, McNoe LA, Yun K, Maw MA, et al: Relaxation of insulin-like growth factor II gene imprinting implicated in Wilms' tumour. *Nature* **362**:749–751, 1993.

63. Giannoukakis N, Deal C, Paquette J, Goodyer CG, Polychronakos C: Parental genomic imprinting of the human IGF2 gene. *Nat Genet* **4**:98–101, 1993.

64. Bartolomei M, Zemel S, Tilghman SM: Parental imprinting of the mouse H19 gene. *Nature* **351**:153–155, 1991.

65. Zhang Y, Shields T, Crenshaw T, Hao Y, Moulton T, Tycko B: Imprinting of human H19: Allele-specific CpG methylation, loss of the active allele in Wilms tumor, and potential for somatic allele switching. *Am J Hum Genet* **53**:113–124, 1993.

66. Feinberg AP: Genomic imprinting and gene activation in cancer. *Nat Genet* **4**:110–113, 1993.

67. Feinberg AP, Rainier S, DeBaun MR: Genomic imprinting, DNA methylation, and cancer. *J Natl Cancer Inst Monogr* **17**:21–26, 1995.

68. Rainier S, Dobry CJ, Feinberg AP: Loss of imprinting in hepatoblastoma. *Cancer Res* **55**:1836-1838, 1995.

69. Li X, Adam G, Cui H, Sandstedt B, Ohlsson R, Ekstrom TJ: Expression, promoter usage and parental imprinting status of insulin-like growth factor II (IGF2) in human hepatoblastoma: Uuncoupling of IGF2 and H19 imprinting. *Oncogene* **11**:221–229, 1995.

70. Zhan SL, Shapiro DN, Helman LJ: Activation of an imprinted allele of the insulin-like growth factor II gene implicated in rhabdomyosarcoma. *J Clin Invest* **94**:445–448, 1994.

71. Zhan SL, Shapiro DN, Helman LJ: Loss of imprinting of IGF2 in Ewing's sarcoma. *Oncogene* **11**:2503–2507, 1995.

72. Vu TH, Yballe C, Boonyanit S, Hoffman AR: Insulin-like growth factor II in uterine smooth-muscle tumors: Maintenance of genomic imprinting in leiomyomata and loss of imprinting in leiomyosarcomata. *J Clin Endocrinol Metab* **80**:1670–1676, 1995.

73. Doucrasy S, Barrois M, Fogel S, Ahomadegbe JC, Stehelin D, Coll J, et al: High incidence of loss of heterozygosity and abnormal imprinting of H19 and IGF2 genes in invasive cervical carcinomas: Uncoupling of H19 and IGF2 expression and biallelic hypomethylation of H19. *Oncogene* **12**:423–430, 1996.

74. Hibi K, Nakamura H, Hirai A, Fujikake Y, Kasai Y, Akiyama S, et al: Loss of H19 imprinting in esophageal cancer. *Cancer Res* **56**:480–482, 1996.

75. Jarrard DF, Bussemakers MJG, Bova GS, Isaacs WB: Regional loss of imprinting of the insulin-like growth factor II gene occurs in human prostate tissues. *Clin Cancer Res* **1**:1471-1478, 1995.

76. Kondo M, Suzuki H, Ueda R, Osada H, Takagi K, Takahashi T, et al: Frequent loss of imprinting of the H19 gene is often associated with its overexpression in human lung cancers. *Oncogene* **10**:1193–1198, 1995.

77. Hashomoto K, Azuma C, Koyama M, Ohashi K, Kamiura S, Nobunaga T, et al: Loss of imprinting in choriocarcinoma. *Nat Genet* **9**:109–110, 1995.

78. Van Gurp RJHLM, Oosterhuis JW, Kalscheuer V, Mariman ECM, Looijenga LHJ: Biallelic expression of the H19 and IGF2 genes in human testicular germ cell tumors. *J Natl Cancer Inst* **86**: 1070–1075, 1994.

79. Vu TH, Hoffman AR: Promoter-specific imprinting of the human insulin-like growth factor-II gene. *Nature* **371**:714–717, 1994.

80. Zhan S, Shapiro D, Zhan S, Zhang L, Hirschfeld S, Elassal J, et al: Concordant loss of imprinting of the human insulin-like growth factor II gene promoters in cancer. *J Biol Chem* **270**:27983–27986, 1995.

81. Steenman MJC, Rainier S, Dobry CJ, Grundy P, Horon IL, Feinberg AP: Loss of imprinting of IGF2 is linked to reduced expression and abnormal methylation of H19 in Wilms' tumor. *Nat Genet* **7**:433–439, 1994.

82. Weksberg R, Shen DR, Fei YL, Song QL, Squire J: Disruption of insulin-like growth factor 2 imprinting in Beckwith-Weidemann syndrome. *Nat Genet* **5**:143–150, 1993.

83. Ogawa O, Becroft DM, Morison IM, Eccles MR, Skeen JE, Mauger DE, et al: Constitutional relaxation of insulin-like growth factor II gene imprinting associated with Wilms' tumour and gigantism. *Nat Genet* **5**:408–412, 1993.

84. Matsuoka S, Edwards MC, Bai C, Parker S, Zhang P, Baldini A, et al: p57/KIP2, a structurally distinct member of the p21/CIP1 Cdk inhibitor family, is a candidate tumor suppressor gene. *Genes Dev* **9**:650–662, 1995.

85. Lee M-H, Reynisdottir I, Massague J: Cloning of p57/KIP2, a clini-dependent kinase inhibitor with unique domain structure and tissue distribution. *Genes Dev* **9**:639–649, 1995.

86. Matsuoka S, Thompson JS, Edwards MC, Barletta JM, Grundy P, Kalikin LM, et al: Imprinting of the gene encoding a human cyclin-dependent kinase inhibitor, p57^{KIP2}, on chromosome 11p15. *Proc Natl Acad Sci USA* **93**:3026–3030, 1996.

87. Thompson JS, Reese KJ, DeBaun MR, Perlman EJ, Feinberg AP: Reduced expression of the cyclin-dependent kinase inhibitor p57^{KIP2} in Wilms tumor. *Cancer Res* in press.

88. Hatada H, Ohashi Y, Fukushima Y, Kaneko M, Inoue Y, Komoto A, et al: An imprinted gene p57^{KIP2} is mutated in Beckwith-Wiedemann syndrome. *Nat Genet* **14**:171–173, 1996.

89. Lee MP, DeBaun M, Randhawa G, Reichard BA, Elledge SJ, Feinberg AP: Low frequency of p57^{KIP2} mutations in Beckwith-Wiedemann syndrome. *Am J Hum Genet* in press.

90. Pitot HC: *Fundamentals of Oncology.* 1981.

91. Moulton T, Crenshaw T, Hao Y, Moosikasuwan J, Lin N, Dembitzer F, et al: Epigenetic lesions at the H19 locus in Wilms' tumour patients. *Nat Genet* **7**:440–447, 1994.

92. Lahm H, Suardet L, Laurent PL, Fischer JR, Ceyhan A, Givel J-C, et al: Growth regulation and co-stimulation of human colorectal cancer cell lines by insulin-like growth factor I, II and transforming growth factor a. *Br J Cancer* **341**:346, 1991.

93. Gelato MC, Vassalotti J: Insulin-like growth factor-II: Possible local growth factor in pheochromocytoma. *J Clin Endocrinol Metab* **71**:1168–1174, 1990.

94. El-Badry OM, Minniti C, Kohn EC, Houghton PJ, Daughaday WH, Helman, LJ: Insulin-like growth factor II acts as an autocrine growth and motility factor in human rhabdomyosarcoma tumors. *Cell Growth Diff* **1**:325–331, 1990.

95. Yee D, Cullen KJ, Paik S, Perdue JF, Hampton B, Schwartz A, et al: Insulin-like growth factor II mRNA expression in human breast cancer. *Cancer Res* **48**: 6691–6696, 1988.

96. Lamonerie T, Lavialle C, Haddada H, Brison O: IGF-2 autocrine stimulation in tumorigenic clones of a human colon-carcinoma cell line. *Int J Cancer* **61**:587–592, 1995.

97. Pommier GJ, Garrouste FL, El Atiq F, Roccabianca M, Marvaldi JL, Remacle-Bonnet MM: Potential autocrine role of insulin-like growth factor II during suramin-induced differentiation of HT29-D4 human colonic adenocarcinoma cell line. *Cancer Res* **52**:3182–3188, 1992.

98. Leventhal PS, Randolph AE, Vesbit TE, Schenone A, Windebank A, Feldman EL: Insulin-like growth factor-II as a paracrine growth factor in human neuroblastoma cells. *Exp Cell Res* **221**:179–186, 1995.

99. Osborne CK, Coronado EB, Kitten LJ, Arteaga CI, Fuqua SA, Ramasharma K, et al: Insulin-like growth factor-II (IGF-II): A potential autocrine/paracrine growth factor for human breast cancer acting via the IGF-I receptor. *Mol Endocrinol* **3**:1701–1709, 1989.

100. Osborne CK, Clemmons DR, Arteaga CL: Regulation of breast cancer growth by insulin-like growth factors. *J Steroid Biochem Molec Biol* **37**:805–809, 1990.

101. Vincent TS, Hazen-Martin DJ, Garvin AJ: Inhibition of insulin-like growth factor II autocrine growth of Wilms tumor by suramin in vitro and in vivo. *Cancer Letts* **103**:49–56, 1996.

102. Miglietta L, Barreca A, Repetto L, Costantini M, Rosso R, Boccardo F: Suramin and serum insulin-like growth factor levels in metastatic cancer patients. *Anticancer Res* **13**:2473–2476, 1993.

103. De Souza AT, Hankins GR, Washington MK, Orton TC, Jirtle RL: M6P/IGF2R gene is mutated in human hepatocellular carcinomas with loss of heterozygosity. *Nat Genet* **11**:447–449, 1995.

104. Hanahan D: Heritable formation of pancreatic B-cell tumors in transgenic mice expressing recombinant insulin/simian virus 40 oncogones. *Nature* **315**:115–122, 1985.

105. Christofori G, Naik P, Hanahan D: A second signal supplied by insulin-like growth factor II in oncogene-induced tumorigenesis. *Nature* **369**:414–418, 1994.

106. Christofori G, Naik P, Hanahan D: Deregulation of both imprinted and expressed alleles of the insulin-like growth factor 2 gene during β-cell tumorigenesis. *Nat Genet* **10**:196–201, 1995.
107. Brannan CI, Dees EC, Ingram RS, Tilghman SM: The product of the H19 gene may function as an RNA. *Mol Cell Biol* **10**:28–36, 1990.
108. Brunkow ME, Tilghman SM: Ectopic expression of the H19 gene in mice causes prenatal lethality. *Genes Dev* **5**:1092–1101, 1991.
109. Pfeifer K, Leighton P, Tilghman SM: The structural H19 gene is required for its own imprinting. *Proc Natl Acad Sci USA* in press.
110. Hao Y, Crenshaw T, Moulton T, Newcomb E, Tycko B: Tumor-suppressor activity of H19 RNA. *Nature* **365**:764–767, 1993.
111. Koi M, Johnson LA, Kalikin LM, Little PFR, Nakamura Y, Feinberg AP: Tumor cell growth arrest caused by subchromosomal transferable DNA fragments from human chromosome 11. *Science* **260**:361–364, 1993.
112. Cedar H, Razin A: DNA methylation and development. *Biochim Biophys Acta* 1049:1–8, 1990.
113. Riggs AD: DNA methylation and cell memory. *Cell Biophys* **15**:1–13, 1989.
114. Bird AP: CpG-rich islands and the function of DNA methylation. *Nature* **321**:209–213, 1986.
115. Riggs AD, Pfeifer GP: X-chromosome inactivation and cell memory. *Trends Genet* **8**:169–174, 1992.
116. Ferguson-Smith AC, Sasaki H, Cattanach BM, Surani MA: Parental-origin-specific epigenetic modification of the mouse H19 gene. *Nature* **362**:751–755, 1993.
117. Bartolomei M, Webber AL, Brunkow ME, Tilghman SM: Epigenetic mechanisms underlying the imprinting of the mouse H19 gene. *Genes Dev* **7**:1663–1673, 1993.
118. Li E, Beard C, Jaenisch R: Role for DNA methylation in genomic imprinting. *Nature* **366**:362–365, 1993.
119. Stoger R, Kubicka P, Liu C-G, Kafri T, Razin A, Cedar H, et al: Maternal-specific methylation of the imprinted mouse IGF2 locus identifies the expressed locus as carrying the imprinting signal. *Cell* **73**:61–71, 1993.
120. Feinberg AP, Vogelstein B: Hypomethylation distinguishes genes of some human cancers from their normal counterparts. *Nature* **301**:89–92, 1983.
121. Goelz SE, Vogelstein B, Hamilton SR, Feinberg AP: Hypomethylation of DNA from benign and malignant human colon neoplasms. *Science* **228**:187–190, 1985.
122. Feinberg AP, Gehrke CW, Kuo KC, Ehrlich M: Reduced genomic 5-methylcytosine content in human colonic neoplasia. *Cancer Res* **48**:1159–1161, 1988.
123. Feinberg AP: Alterations in DNA methylation in colorectal polyps and cancer. *Prog Clin Biol Res* **279**:309–317, 1988.
124. Jones PA, Buckley JD: The role of DNA methylation in cancer. *Adv Cancer Res* **54**:1–23, 1990.
125. Laird PW, Jackson-Grusby L, Fazeli A, Dickinson SL, Jung WE, Li E, et al: Suppression of intestinal neoplasia by DNA hypomethylation. *Cell* **81**:197–205, 1995.
126. Reik W, Brown KW, Slatter RE, Sartori P, Elliott M, Maher ER: Allelic methylation of H19 and IGF2 in the Beckwith-Wiedemann syndrome. *Hum Mol Genet* **3**:1297–1301, 1995.
127. Reik W, Brown KW, Schneid H, Bouc YL, Bickmore W, Maher ER: Imprinting mutations in the Beckwith-Wiedemann syndrome suggested by an altered imprinting pattern in the IGF2-H19 domain. *Hum Mol Genet* **4**:2379–2385, 1995.
128. El-Deiry WS, Nelkin BD, Celano P, Yen RC, Falco JP, Hamilton SR, et al:High expression of the DNA methyltransferase gene characterizes human neoplastic cells and progression stages of colon cancer. *Proc Natl Acad Sci USA* **88**:3470–3474, 1991.
129. Schmutte C, Yang AS, Nugyen TT, Beart RB, Jones PA: Mechanisms for the involvement of DNA methylation in colon cancer. *Cancer Res* **56**:2375–2381, 1996.
130. Lee PJ, Washer LL, Law DJ, Boland CR, Horon IL, Feinberg AP: Limited upregulation of DNA methyltransferase in human colon cancer reflecting increased cell proliferation. *Proc Natl Acad Sci USA* **93**:10366-10370, 1996.
131. Lee MP, Hu R-J, Johnson LA, Feinberg AP: Human K$_V$LQT1 gene shows tissue-specific imprinting and encompasses Beckwith-Wiedemann syndrome chromosomal rearrangements. *Nat Genet* **15**:181–185, 1997.
132. Allen ND, Norris ML, Surani MA: Epigenetic control of transgene expression and imprinting by genotype-specific modifiers. *Cell* 61:353–361, 1990.
133. Wolffe AP: Inheritance of chromatin states. *Dev Genet* **15**:463–470, 1994.
134. Thompson JS, Ling X, Grunstein M: Histone H3 amino terminus is required for telomeric and silent mating. *Nature* **369**:245–247, 1994.
135. Yoshida M, Kijima M, Akita M, Beppu T: Potent and specific inhibition of mammalian histone deacetylase both in vivo and in vitro by trichostatin A. *J Biol Chem* **265**:17174–17179, 1990.
136. Efstratiadis A: Parental imprinting of autosomal mammalian genes. *Curr Opin Genet Dev* **4**:265–280, 1994.
137. Brownell JE, Zhou J, Ranalli T, Kobayashi R, Edmondson DG, Roth SY, et al: Tetrahymena histone acetyltransferase A: A homolog to yeast gcn5p linking histone acetylation to gene activation. *Cell* **84**:843–851, 1996.
138. Taunton J, Hassig CA, Schreiber SL: A mammalian histone deacetylase related to the yeast transcriptional regulator rpd3p. *Science* **272**:408–411, 1996.
139. Walters MC, Magis W, Fiering S, Eidemiller J, Scalzo D, Groudine M, et al: Transcriptional enhancers act in cis to suppress position-effect variegation. *Genes Dev* **10**:185–195, 1996.
140. Kitsberg D, Selig S, Brandeis M, Simon I, Keshet I, Driscoll DJ, et al: Allele-specific replication timing of imprinted gene regions. *Nature* **364**:459–463, 1993.
141. LaSalle JM, Lalande M: Homologous association of oppositely imprinted chromosomal domains. *Science* 272:725–728, 1996.
142. Tatof KD, Henikoff S: Trans-sensing effects from Drosophila to humans. *Cell* **65**:201–203, 1991.
143. Barletta JM, Rainier S, Strichman L, Feinberg AP: Reversal of loss of imprinting in tumor cells by 5-aza-2′-deoxycytidine. *Cancer Res* in press.
144. Feinberg AP, Kalikin LM, Johnson LA, Thompson JS: Loss of imprinting in human cancer. *Cold Spring Harbor Symp Quant Biol* **59**:357–364, 1994.

CHAPTER 5

Genes Altered by Chromosomal Translocations in Leukemias and Lymphomas

A. Thomas Look

1. **Somatically acquired chromosomal translocations activate proto-oncogenes in the hematopoietic cells of both children and adults. This mechanism of gene dysregulation contributes to well over 50 percent of all leukemias that have been characterized cytogenetically and molecularly and to a substantial proportion of lymphomas, notably the Burkitt, large cell, and follicular types.**

2. **In most instances, chromosomal translocations fuse sequences of a transcription factor or receptor tyrosine kinase gene to those of a normally unrelated gene, resulting in a chimeric protein with oncogenic properties. Repositioning of transcriptional control genes to the vicinity of highly active promoter/enhancer elements, such as those associated with immunoglobulin or T-cell receptor genes, is a second mechanism by which chromosomal translocations induce malignancy.**

3. **The vast majority of translocation-induced leukemias and lymphomas are restricted to cells of a single lineage arrested at a particular stage of development, indicating that the disrupted genes regulate vital processes limited to a subset of committed hematopoietic progenitors. Occasionally, as exemplified by leukemias arising from *MLL* gene abnormalities, more than one lineage or developmental stage is affected, suggesting the involvement of genes active in pluripotent or bipotent stem cells.**

4. **The number of fusion genes with diagnostic and prognostic relevance is increasing rapidly. The hybrid mRNAs produced by these novel structures provide specific molecular probes for identifying cases that cannot be readily diagnosed by conventional means or that require chemotherapy tailored to the risk conferred by a particular genetic lesion.**

5. **Studies in murine models, in which specific genes are mutated and homozygously inactivated in "knockout" mice or overexpressed in transgenic mice, have increasingly demonstrated the essential roles that are played in normal development and oncogenesis by genes discovered because of their proximity to the breakpoints of chromosomal translocations in the human leukemias and lymphomas.**

INTRODUCTION

The concept that cancer cells contain genetic information not found in normal cells has provided the impetus for molecular approaches to cancer research. A pivotal step in this progress was the realization that gross chromosomal changes—such as translocations, deletions, inversions, and amplifications—can perturb genes intimately involved in carcinogenesis.[1-3] Thus, a major concern over the past two decades has been the identification of consistent chromosomal abnormalities in specific types of tumor cells, the isolation of genes affected by these changes, and the elucidation of their mechanisms of action and clinical correlations. A surprising dividend of this venture, aided by technology that permits one to create homozygous null animals by inactivating individual genes (e.g., "knockout" mice), has been the discovery of proteins that not only promote cancer, but have essential functions in normal cell development as well.[4]

Specific reciprocal translocations perhaps are the best example of how cytogenetic changes pave the way for cancer induction and spread. These nonheritable abnormalities occur in a high percentage of hematologic cancers—both leukemias and lymphomas—where they disrupt signaling pathways that enhance cell survival.[4-6] Their actions can directly activate occult proto-oncogenes or, more commonly, create cell type-specific fusion proteins that contain elements of one or more transcription factors.[5,7] It is intriguing that many of the genes involved in translocation-mediated fusions have close homologues in genes controlling embryogenesis in *Drosophila* and other invertebrates, underscoring their faithful conservation in nature and their relevance to programs of early cell development.[8-10] Unfortunately, the downstream genetic programs controlled by the various transcription factors affected by chromosomal translocations largely are unknown, so that interrelationships between transcription networks and leukemogenesis remain to be assessed.

The medical benefits gained from analysis of chromosomal translocations in the leukemias and lymphomas are still modest. One of the difficulties is that fusion proteins typically are localized to the cell nucleus, making them inaccessible to most available therapies, requiring instead the introduction of therapeutic molecules into the cell. Nonetheless, the chimeric RNA and DNA of these lesions provide highly specific targets for molecular assays that can resolve interpretive ambiguities created by conventional diagnostic or cell classification methods.[11] One emerging application is the use of polymerase chain reaction-based techniques to detect chimeric RNA in residual leukemia cells.[12] Other applications include the detection of specific high-risk genetic lesions, such as the *E2A-PBX1*, *MLL-AF4*, and *BCR-ABL* fusion genes, to ensure that patients are assigned to sufficiently aggressive treatment programs.[13]

In this chapter, I summarize the molecular consequences of translocations in the human leukemias and lymphomas. Emphasis is placed on disease types with the highest frequencies of productive rearrangements and on those (often rare) types in which study of molecular aberrations has revealed novel principles of pathogenesis.

DYSREGULATION OF TRANSCRIPTIONAL CONTROL GENES

The majority of transcription factors that are altered by chromosomal translocations in the leukemias and lymphomas (Table 5-1) can be classified into four major types on the basis of recurring structural elements within their DNA- and protein-binding domains: basic region/helix-loop-helix (bHLH), basic region/leucine zipper (bZIP), zinc finger, and homeodomain.[6,7,14] Other less common but still functionally significant motifs include A-T hook, Ets-like, Runt homology, and cysteine-rich (LIM). In some cases, a transcription factor gene is rearranged to a site adjacent to a T-cell receptor (*TCR*) or immunoglobulin (*Ig*) locus, resulting in dysregulated expression of the proto-oncogenic sequences. A second, perhaps more common, mechanism involves chromosomal rearrangements that fuse transcriptional control genes into functional chimeras. Such fusions are important because they give rise to novel proteins capable of interacting with DNA and other regulatory elements, in ways that usurp normal cellular control mechanisms.[6]

The diversity of transcription factor proto-oncogenes implicated in the human leukemias and lymphoma is striking, although increasingly their essential functions can be traced to a fundamental step in cell growth, development, or survival.[7] Currently, more than 10 transcriptional control genes have been shown to play critical roles in normal hematopoiesis (Figure 5-1). Some of these factors are lineage specific, whereas others operate early in hematopoietic development, before lineage commitment. Still others are widely expressed but perform unique functions in a limited number of blood cell types, ostensibly by interacting with lineage-restricted proteins.[4] Of major pathobiological importance, many transcription factors that control blood cell differentiation are targets for productive rearrangement by translocations in the leukemias and lymphomas, reinforcing their roles as master regulators of hematopoietic cell development. In the following sections, I summarize how chromosomal translocations modify transcription factors to generate malignant cells within the hematopoietic system.

Acute Lymphoblastic Leukemias (ALL) and Non-Hodgkin Lymphomas

The frequency distributions of the various molecular abnormalities mediated by chromosomal translocations are shown diagrammatically in Figures 5-2 and 5-3, with key associations given in Tables 5-1 and 5-2.

***MYC* Activation in Burkitt Lymphoma and B-Cell Leukemia.** In Burkitt lymphoma and B-cell leukemia, arising in surface *Ig*-positive, "virgin" B lymphoblasts with moderately abundant, vacuolated cytoplasm, the principal genetic change is a juxtapositioning of the *MYC* proto-oncogene next to the *Ig* heavy-chain gene as a result of the t(8;14)(q24;q32).[15–17] *MYC* is a prototypic bHLH/leucine zipper transcription factor whose rearrangement from chromosome 8 to a site near strong *Ig* enhancer elements on chromosome 14 leads to dysregulated expression of the MYC oncoprotein. In most instances, the t(8;14) is responsible for inappropriate activation of *MYC*; however, two variants of this rearrangement can produce the same effect, except that they move *Ig*κ and *Ig*λ light-chain genes from chromosomes 2 and 22, respectively, to the *MYC* locus on chromosome 8.[18–23] The *MYC* gene often acquires point mutations in its coding or regulatory regions, probably as a result of somatic mutation that occur after translocation, which in some cases encode proteins that are unable to interact with the *Rb*-related gene, *p107*.[24–28]

A leading question since the discovery of *MYC* activation in Burkitt lymphoma/B-cell leukemia has been: How does the MYC oncoprotein transform B lymphocytes? The answer seems to lie in the effects of *MYC* dysregulation on a transcriptional network comprising at least three other factors, each also harboring bHLH/leucine zipper domains. In this cascade, MYC is able to dimerize with the MAX protein, which can bind to DNA, to itself (MAX/MAX homodimers), and to the MAD and MXI-1 family of transcription factors.[29–32] Since MYC/MAX heterodimers activate gene expression, whereas MAD/MAX heterodimers act as *trans*-repressors through an association with a protein called SIN3, and since MYC and MAD have equal affinities for MAX, increased expression of MYC in B lymphocytes is thought to disrupt the equilibrium of MAX heterodimers, leading to untimely activation of responder genes and ultimately to malignant transformation.[29,30,35–37] Experimental support for this hypothesis comes from the induction of B-cell neoplasms in transgenic mice carrying the *MYC* oncogene driven by an *Ig* gene enhancer.[38,39] An activated *MYC* gene also induces tumorigenic conversion when it is introduced in vitro into B lymphoblasts infected with human Epstein-Barr virus.[40] More recent observations implicate the ornithine decarboxylase gene, as well as the *CDC25* cell-cycle phosphatase gene, as relevant transcriptional targets of MYC/MAX heterodimers.[41,42]

***bHLH, LIM*, and *HOX11* Genes.** The role of transcription factors as the preferred targets of chromosomal translocations extends to the T-cell lymphomas and acute leukemias, in which the chromosomal breakpoints consistently appear near enhancers included in the *TCR* β locus on chromosome 7, band q34, or the α/δ locus on chromosome 14, band q11. Highly active in committed T-cell progenitors, these enhancers stimulate the expression of strategically translocated transcription factors that regulate early hematopoietic cell development or the development of other lineages, but are not normally expressed in T lymphoid cells (Table 5-1). Notable examples include the bHLH genes, *TAL1/SCL*, *TAL2/SCL2*, and *LYL1*, one of which is essential for the development of all blood cell lineages (*TAL1/SCL*).[4,43–48] The more distantly related *MYC* bHLHzip protein is dysregulated in T-cell, as well as B-cell lymphomas and leukemias.[49–51]

When rearranged near enhancers within the *TCR* β locus on chromosome 7, band q34, or the α/δ-chain locus on chromosome 14, band q11, these regulatory genes become active, and their protein products are thought to bind inappropriately to the promoter-enhancer elements of upstream target genes. The *TAL1* gene, for example, is activated by the t(1;14) or by an intragenic deletion on the 5′ side of the gene that places it under the regulation of the promoter of a gene called *SIL*; these rearrangements affect up to one-

Table 5-1 Transcriptional Control Genes Dysregulated by Chromosomal Translocations that Contribute to Human Leukemias and Lymphomas

Disease	Chromosomal Abnormality	Activated Gene	Mechanism of Activation	Predominant Structural Feature*	Invertebrate Homolog†	References
Lymphoid Leukemia/Lymphoma						
B-cell ALL/Burkitt lymphoma	t(8;14)(q24;q32)	MYC	Relocation to IgH locus	bHLHzip		[15–17]
	t(2;8)(p12;q24)	MYC	Relocation to Igκ locus	bHLHzip		[18,19,21,23]
	t(8;22)(q24;q11)	MYC	Relocation to IgL locus	bHLHzip		[20,22]
Pre-B-cell ALL	t(1;19)(q23;p13)	E2A-PBX1	Gene fusion	Homeodomain (PBX1)	exd (D), ceh-20 (C)	[118,119]
Pro-B-cell ALL	t(17;19)(q22;p13)	E2A-HLF	Gene fusion	bZIP (HLF)	giant (D), ceo-2 (C)	[158,159]
Pro B-cell ALL	t(12;21)(p13;q22)	TEL-AML1	Gene fusion	Runt homology (AML1)	runt (D)	[176–180]
T-cell ALL	t(8;14)(q24;q11)	MYC	Relocation to TCRα/δ locus	bHLHzip		[49–51]
	t(7;19)(q35;p13)	LYL1	Relocation to TCRβ locus	bHLH		[46]
	t(1;14)(p32;q11)	TAL1	Relocation to TCRα/δ locus	bHLH		[43–45]
	t(7;9)(q35;q34)	TAL2	Relocation to TCRβ locus	bHLH		[45]
	t(11;14)(p15;q11)	LMO1 (RBTN1)	Relocation to TCRα/δ locus	Cysteine-rich		[73,74]
	t(11;14)(p13;q11)	LMO2 (RBTN2)	Relocation to TCRα/δ locus	Cysteine-rich		[75,76]
	t(7;11)(q35;p13)	LMO2 (RBTN2)	Relocation to TCRβ locus	Cysteine-rich		
	t(10;14)(q24;q11)	HOX11	Relocation to TCRα/δ locus	Homeodomain		[90–93]
	t(7;10)(q35;q24)	HOX11	Relocation to TCRβ locus	Homeodomain		
Diffuse B-cell lymphoma (large cell)	t(3;14)(q27;q32)	BCL6	Relocation to IgH locus	Zinc finger (BCL6)	tramtrack (D)	[183–186]
	t(3;4)(q27;p11)	BCL6	Relocation to TTF locus	Zinc finger (BCL6)	tramtrack (D)	[184,448]
B-CLL	t(14;19)(q32;q13)	BCL3	Relocation to IgH locus	IκB homology		[449–451]
B-cell lymphoma	t(10;14)(q24;q32)	LYT10	Relocation to IgH locus	Rel homology	dorsal (D)	[452]
Lymphoplasmacytoid B-cell lymphoma	t(9;14)(p13;q32)	PAX5	Relocation to IgH locus	Paired homeobox	paired (D)	[453]

(continued)

Table 5-1 (continued)

Disease	Chromosomal Abnormality	Activated Gene	Mechanism of Activation	Predominant Structural Feature*	Invertebrate Homolog[†]	References
Myeloid Leukemia						
AML (granulocytic)	t(8;21)(q22:q22)	AML1-ETO	Gene fusion	Runt homology (AML1)	runt (D)	[197–199,454]
Myelodysplasia	t(3;21)(q26:q22)	AML1-EAP	Gene fusion	Runt homology (AML1)	runt (D)	[202]
CML (blast crisis)	t(3;21)(q26:q22)	AML1-EVI1	Gene fusion	Runt homology (AML1)	runt (D)	[201]
AML (undifferentiated)	t(3;v)(q26;v)	EVI1	Aberrant expression	Zinc finger	evi1 (D)	[254,255]
AML (myelomonocytic)	inv(16)(p13:q22)	CBFβ-MYH11	Gene fusion	Complex with AML1 (CBFβ)		[216]
AML (promyelocytic)	t(15;17)(q21:q21)	PML-RARα	Gene fusion	Zinc finger (RARα)		[218–222]
AML (promyelocytic)	t(11;17)(q23:q21)	PLZF-RARα	Gene fusion	Zinc finger (RARα)		[246]
AML (promyelocytic)	t(5;17)(q32:q12)	NPM-RARα	Gene fusion	Zinc finger (RARα)		[245]
AML	t(16;21)(p11:q22)	FUS-ERG	Gene fusion	Ets-like (ERG)		[455]
AML	t(12;22)(p13:q11)	TEL-MN1	Gene fusion	Ets-like (TEL)		[456]
Mixed-Lineage Leukemias[‡]						
Pro-B-cell ALL	t(4;11)(q21:q23)	MLL-AF4	Gene fusion	A-T hook (MLL)	trithorax (D)	[274,276,277]
AML (monocytic)	t(9;11)(p21:q23)	MLL-AF9	Gene fusion	A-T hook (MLL)	trithorax (D)	[293]
ALL/AML	t(11;19)(q23:p13.3)	MLL-ENL	Gene fusion	A-T hook (MLL)	trithorax (D)	[273,285,293]
AML	t(11;19)(q23:p13.1)	MLL-ELL	Gene fusion	A-T hook (MLL)	trithorax (D)	[285,286]
AML	t(1;11)(q21:q23)	MLL-AF1Q	Gene fusion	A-T hook (MLL)	trithorax (D)	[296]
AML	t(1;11)(1p32:q23)	MLL-AF1P	Gene fusion	A-T hook (MLL)	trithorax (D)	[457]
AML	t(6;11)(q27:q23)	MLL-AF6	Gene fusion	A-T hook (MLL)	trithorax (D)	[310]
AML	t(10;11)(p12:q23)	MLL-AF10	Gene fusion	A-T hook (MLL)	trithorax (D)	[458]
AML	t(11;17)(q23:q21)	MLL-AF17	Gene fusion	A-T hook (MLL)	trithorax (D)	[459]
AML	t(X;11)(q13:q23)	MLL-AFX1	Gene fusion	A-T hook (MLL)	trithorax (D)	[460]

Abbreviations: AML = acute myeloid leukemia; ALL = acute lymphoblastic leukemia; CML = chronic myelogenous leukemia; bHLHzip = basic region/helix-loop-helix/leucine zipper domain; bZIP = basic region/leucine zipper domain.

*Based on analysis of DNA-binding and protein interaction domain. For gene fusions, the partner contributing this structural feature is given in parentheses.

[†]Organism type is shown in parenthesis: D = Drosophila; C = C. elegans.

[‡]Only the predominant lineage is given for MLL gene rearrangements.

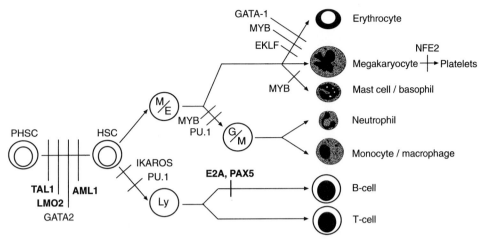

FIG. 5-1 Schematic diagram showing the relative stages at which transcription factors exert their influence on hematopoietic development. Only proteins whose activities have been demonstrated in knockout mice are shown. Factors serving as targets of chromosomal translocations in the leukemias and lymphomas are indicated in bold-face type. Note that transcription factor targets can be lineage specific (E2A) or uncommitted to a particular differentiation pathway (AML1). HSC, hematopoietic stem cell; M/E, myeloid/erythroid progenitor; Ly, lymphoid progenitor; G/M, granulocyte/macrophage progenitor. (Adapted from ref. 4 with permission.)

fourth of all cases of childhood T-cell leukemias and lymphomas.[52–58] Since the TAL1 protein can dimerize with the E2A protein through its bHLH domain to form DNA-binding complexes, and with the LMO2 protein (see the following), its ectopic expression in T-cells bearing the t(1;14) or activating deletions may aberrantly activate specific sets of target genes that are normally quiescent in T-lineage progenitors.[59–63] It is also possible that TAL1 acts by repressing E2A activity during T-cell development, because E2A/TAL1 heterodimers are inactive as transcriptional *trans*-activators.[64,65]

Interestingly, TAL1 has emerged as an essential regulator of very early stages of hematopoietic development.[66] Within the hematopoietic system, TAL1 expression is restricted to myeloid and erythroid progenitor cells, megakaryocytes, and mast cells, and as previously noted, it is not expressed by normal T lymphocytes or their progenitors.[67–70] Gene targeting experiments initially showed that mouse embryos lacking a functional *TAL1* gene were devoid of embryonic red blood cells and died at embryonic days 9–10.5 of anemia.[47,48] Additional studies of hematopoietic precursors generated by in vitro differentiation of *Tal1-l*-embryonic stem cells, and by assessing the contribution of these cells *in vivo* to the hematopoietic systems of chimeric mice, have shown that *Tal1* is required for the generation of all hematopoietic cell lineages, including T lymphocytes, suggesting that it plays an essential role in early hematopoietic development, either at the level of mesoderm induction or in maintaining the viability of multipotential hematopoietic progenitors.[66] It would not be surprising if *Tal1* were involved in a network of regulatory factors responsible for induction of the hematopoietic lineage, in view of the similar roles of related bHLH proteins as master regulators of mesodermal cell fate, such as those of the MyoD family (MyoD, Myf-5, MRF4, and myogenin), which, like the Tal1 protein, form heterocomplexes with the E12/E47 products of the *E2A* gene.[71,72]

Other types of regulatory genes can be rearranged near TCR loci, including those encoding the LMO1 and LMO2 (for cysteine-rich <u>LIM</u>-domain <u>o</u>nly) proteins (also known as RBTN1/TTG1 and RBTN2/TTG2).[73–76] Although T cells normally lack expression of either protein, LMO1 is expressed in a segmental and developmentally regulated pattern in the central nervous system, and LMO2 is coexpressed with Tal1 in several lineages, notably in erythroid and other hematopoietic progenitors.[74,77] Both LMO1 and LMO2 possess zinc finger-like structures in their LIM domains, but lack the homeobox DNA-binding domains common to other transcription factors in this family, suggesting that the LIM domain

functions in protein–protein rather than protein–DNA interactions.[78] In fact, LMO2 is coexpressed with TAL1 in several cell lineages, including erythroid progenitors, and these two proteins interact to form a transcriptional complex, both in erythroid cells and in human and murine T-cell leukemias induced by these gene products.[62,63,77,79] The functional relevance of this complex in normal development is exemplified by the fact that gene targeting experiments in mice, in which null mutations were introduced into *Lmo2*, yielded the same phenotype as those described above for *Tal1*, indicating that functional complexes are required for normal primitive erythropoiesis and likely the formation of all hematopoietic lineages.[66,77,80] Additional studies have expanded this complex to include GATA1, a zinc-finger transcription factor that is also required for erythroid cell development, and TAL1 is known to complex with E2A bHLH proteins, suggesting that multisubunit complexes minimally containing these four transcriptional regulators act in concert to regulate erythropoiesis.[81,82] Moreover, both LMO1 and LMO2 induce thymic lymphomas in transgenic mice whose thymocytes express these genes under the control of T-cell–specific or ubiquitously expressed promoters.[83–87] Although it is controversial whether *TAL1* is able to induce T-cell lymphomas in mice on its own, it has been shown to shorten the time to development of T-cell lymphomas induced by LMO2 in a double transgenic system, apparently recapitulating the cooperativity that these two proteins exhibit as a heterodimeric transcriptional regulator in human T-cell tumors.[62,63,88,89]

HOX11 is an example of a different type of developmental gene that is inappropriately placed under the control of *TCR* loci. Located on chromosome 10, band q24, this gene encodes a homeodomain transcription factor that can bind DNA and *trans*-activate specific target genes.[90–94] It is most closely related to *Hlx*, a recently described murine homeobox gene expressed in specific hematopoietic cell lineages and during mouse embryogenesis, and is distantly related to the *antennapedia* homeobox genes of *Drosophila*, which regulate segment-specific gene expression along the anterior–posterior axis of the fly embryo.[95,96] A very specific homeotic role of *Hox11* in mammalian development was demonstrated by homozygous disruption of this gene, which blocked the formation of the spleen in otherwise normal mice.[97] In the mouse, Hox11 is normally expressed in specific regions of the branchial arches and ectoderm of the pharyngeal pouches of the developing hindbrain, as well as from a single site corresponding to the splanchnic mesoderm beginning at embryonic day 11.5.[97] Because the nervous system develops normally in these mice, the

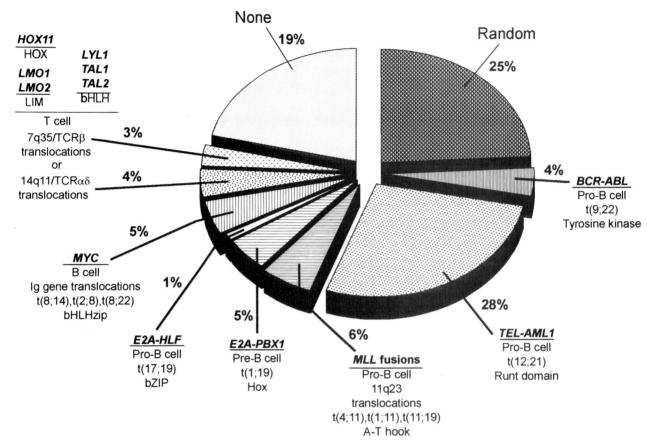

FIG. 5-2 Distribution of translocation-generated fusion genes among the commonly recognized immunologic subtypes of ALL in children and young adults. Key domains for DNA binding and protein–protein interaction of transcription factors are shown; an exception is the tyrosine kinase domain indicated for BCR-ABL. The section labeled "random" refers to sporadic rearrangements that have so far been observed only in leukemic cells from single cases. (Adapted from ref. 182 with permission.)

roles of Hox11 proteins in branchial arch and hindbrain structures appear to be compensated for by other transcription factors expressed by these cells; however, the role of Hox11 in cellular organization at the site of splenic development is absolutely essential for the genesis of this organ.[97] Further studies have shown that the splenic anlage actually develops normally in Hox11-*l*-mice, but that the developing spleen cells undergo apoptosis, suggesting that Hox11 normally acts to promote the survival of splenic precursors during organogenesis.[98] In contrast to *Lmo2* and *Tal1*, which have important roles in hematopoietic cell development, Hox11 proteins are not normally expressed in lymphoid and other types of hematopoietic cells, and hematopoietic cells are not affected by loss-of-function mutations in this gene, except in circulating erythrocytes with asplenia-related Howell-Jolly bodies.

Activation of *HOX11* by chromosomal translocations, either the t(10;14)(q24;q11) or the t(7;10)(q35;q24), in developing T cells is thought to interfere with normal regulatory cascades, thereby promoting malignant transformation. The primary oncogenic importance of aberrant expression of Hox11 in the developing thymus has been demonstrated in transgenic mice, in which this protein was redirected to the thymus, where it was associated with the development of T-cell lymphoma/leukemia at high frequencies.[99] Studies supporting a role for Hox11 in cell survival rather than lineage specification during development suggest that the protein may contribute to T-cell malignancy by abnormally blocking apoptosis of developing T cells in the thymus.[98]

***E2A* Fusion Genes.** The *E2A* gene was cloned by virtue of the fact that it encodes a protein (E12) that binds to the κE2 regulatory site of the *Ig*κ light-chain gene promoter.[100] It was subsequently shown to encode three differentially spliced products, E12, E47, and E2-5, each of which belongs to the bHLH family of transcriptional regulatory proteins.[100–104] The bHLH domain is comprised of a basic region responsible for sequence-specific DNA binding followed by a structural domain consisting of two amphipathic helices separated by a loop region of variable length (thus, helix-loop-helix), that is responsible for homo- and heterodimerization.[100,101] The bHLH family of proteins includes the *daughterless Drosophila* gene and members of the MyoD family of myogenic proteins.[71,72,105,106] DNA-binding by E2A is mediated by either homodimers or heterodimers with other bHLH proteins, with the precise binding specificity to variations of the so-called E-box sequence motif determined by the dimerization partners of each complex.[107] Recent structural analysis has supported experimental observations regarding the conformations of homo- and heterodimers formed by the E2A bHLH domains.[108] In addition, the amino-terminal sequences of E2A that are included in leukemogenic fusion proteins have been shown to contain two discrete transcriptional activation domains, called AD1 and AD2, the latter of which is also referred to as a loop-helix (LH) activation domain (see Figure 5-4).[103,109,110]

In most tissues, E2A heterodimerizes with tissue-specific bHLH family members to coordinate gene expression during development.[101,111] These binding partners include TAL/SCL family members, which heterodimerize with E2A and are themselves dysregulated in T-cell lymphomas/leukemias and aberrantly expressed as a result of translocations involving the *TCR* gene loci.[43–45,60,112] In B cells, however, E2A is able to bind E-box sequences as a homodimeric complex, apparently because of stabilization of the complex through an intermolecular disulfide bond, which is dis-

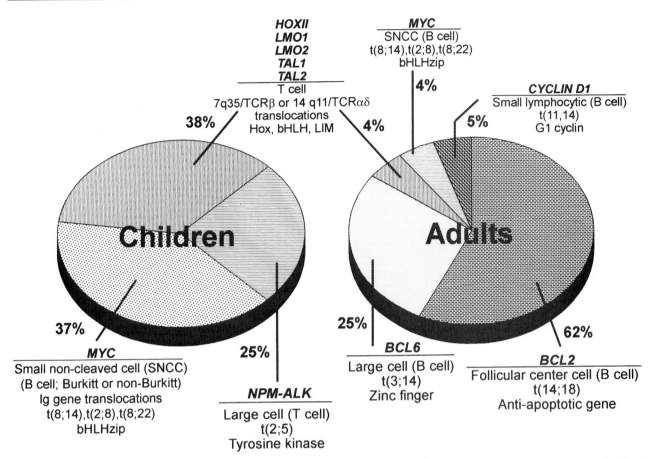

FIG. 5-3 Distribution of histologic subtypes of non-Hodgkin's lymphoma in children and adults. Chromosomal translocations and affected genes that occur in a significant fraction (but not all) of the cases within each subtype are shown. (Adapted from ref. 471 by permission.)

rupted in non-B cells.[111,113,114] The importance of E2A proteins in B-cell development is indicated by the fact that homozygous mutant mice lacking functional E2A proteins have arrested B-cell development at an early stage, but are otherwise developmentally normal.[115,116]

E2A-PBX1. The *E2A* gene participates in two fusion events with major biological and clinical implications in ALL. The first results from the t(1;19)(q23;p13) chromosomal translocation, which rearranges and joins the *E2A* gene within chromosome band 19p13.3 to the *PBX1* gene from chromosome 1, creating an *E2A-PBX1* chimera on the derivative 19 chromosome (Figure 5-3).[117–119] Because the breakpoints in the *E2A* gene consistently interrupt the ~3.5-kb intron between exons 13 and 14, the encoded E2A fusion partner invariably consists of the amino-terminal two-thirds of the molecule, which includes two transcriptional activation domains (AD1 and AD2), but not the bHLH DNA-binding–protein interaction domain.[118–120] The PBX1 segment makes up for this deficit by providing a homeodomain motif of ~60 amino acids that enables the E2A-PBX1 chimera to function as a transcription factor, driven by the potent E2A *trans*-activating domains.[121–125]

An understanding of the likely oncogenic contribution of the PBX1 fusion partner requires insight into the normal function of PBX proteins. These transcription factors are the mammalian homologues of the *Drosophila* protein, Extradenticle.[126,127] Mutations in the *exd* gene cause homeotic transformations, changes in which one body segment of the fly is transformed to resemble another segment.[128,129] Thus, the extradenticle protein may function as an obligatory cofactor in selector gene activity, by forming complexes with major homeotic fly proteins of the Antennapedia and Bithorax clusters, termed Hom, which then bind to DNA.[130–133] In view of

the close sequence homology shared by Extradenticle and PBX proteins, it is perhaps not surprising that the latter interact with specific human homologues of the Hom family, called HOX proteins, to determine the target genes recognized by PBX1.[130,132,134–139]

Given that E2A-PBX1 carries the transcriptional activation domains of E2A and the homeodomain of PBX1, how does the chimera induce malignant transformation? When Kamps and Baltimore infected bone marrow progenitors with retroviruses encoding E2A-PBX1, they reproducibly induced AML in mice repopulated with these progenitors.[140] These myeloid leukemia cells could proliferate for extended periods without maturation so long as they received granulocyte-macrophage colony-stimulating factor (GM-CSF).[141] In the absence of growth factor, the cells rapidly died. These observations are consistent with the block of differentiation characteristic of lymphoid cells carrying the t(1;19) in cases of ALL and with arrested T-cell development in lymphomas of *E2A-PBX1* transgenic mice.[142–144] Thus, a major effect of the chimera may be to arrest hematopoietic and lymphoid progenitors at particular stages of development.

Additional studies with cell transformation assays have established the specific E2A-PBX1 domains required for malignant conversion.[145] When either of the two transactivation domains of E2A are abolished, there is a loss or reduction of transforming activity. The shortest PBX1 sequence required for oncogenesis includes the homeodomain and its immediately C-terminal 25 amino acids, which also are needed for interaction with specific HOX proteins.[134] Unexpectedly, in one study, mutant proteins with deletion of the homeodomain and retention of the adjacent flanking region transformed NIH-3T3 cells and induced lymphomas in transgenic mice as efficiently as the full-length chimera.[145] Other

Table 5-2 Tyrosine Kinase and Other Genes Dysregulated by Chromosomal Translocations in Human Leukemias and Lymphomas

Disease	Chromosomal Abnormality	Activated Gene	Mechanism of Activation	Predominant Structural Feature*	Invertebrate Homolog†	References
Tyrosine Kinases						
CMML	t(5;12)(q33;p13)	TEL-PDGFRβ	Gene fusion	Tyrosine kinase		[365]
AML	t(9;12;14)(q34;p13;q22)	TEL-ABL	Gene fusion	Tyrosine kinase		[363,364]
Anaplastic large-cell lymphoma	t(2;5)(p23;q35)	NPM-ALK	Gene fusion	Tyrosine kinase		[439]
CML	t(9;22)(q34;q11)	BCR-ABL	Gene fusion	Tyrosine kinase	abl (D)	[328,334,337,338]
ALL	t(9;22)(q34;q11)	BCR-ABL	Gene fusion	Tyrosine kinase	abl (D)	[343–345]
T-cell ALL	t(1;7)(p34;q34)	LCK	Relocation to TCRβ locus	Tyrosine kinase		[461–463]
Other Genes						
Centrocytic B-cell lymphoma	t(11;14)(q13;q32)	Cyclin D1	Relocation to IgH locus	G1 cycline		[404,405,410–413]
Follicular B-cell lymphoma	t(14;18)(q32;q21)	BCL2	Relocation to IgH locus	Antiapoptotic domain	ced-9 (C)	[428–431]
AML	t(6;9)(p23;q34)	DEK-CAN	Gene fusion	Nucleoporin (CAN)		[464]
AML	t(9;9)(q34;q34)	SET-CAN	Gene fusion	Nucleoporin (CAN)		[439]
AML	t(7;11)(p15;p15)	NUP98-HOXA9	Gene fusion	Nucleoporin (NUP98)		[440,441]
AML	t(3;5)(q35;q35)	NPM-MLF1	Gene fusion	Nucleolar shuttle protein (NPM)		[446]
AML	t(10;11)(p13;q14)	CALM-AF10	Gene fusion	Clathrin assembly (CALM)	cezf (C)	[465]
T-PLL	t(x;14)(q28;q11)	C6.1B	Relocation to TCRα/δ locus	Unknown		[466]
T-cell ALL	t(7;9)(q34;q34)	TAN1	Relocation to TCRβ locus	EGF cysteine repeats	notch (D), lin-12 (C)	[467]
Pre-B ALL	t(5;14)(q31;q32)	IL-3	Relocation to IgH locus	Growth factor		[468,469]
T-cell lymphoma	t(4;16)(q26;p13)	IL2-BCM	Gene fusion	Growth factor		[470]

Abbreviations: AML = acute myeloid leukemia; ALL = acute lymphoblastic leukemia; bHLHzip = basic region/helix-loop-helix/leucine zipper domain; CML = chronic myelogenous leukemia; bZIP = basic region/leucine zipper domain.

*Based on analysis of DNA-binding and protein interaction domain. For gene fusions, the partner contributing this structural feature is given in parentheses.

†Organism type is shown in parenthesis: D = *Drosophila*; C = *C. elegans*.

‡Only the predominant lineage is given for *MLL* gene rearrangements.

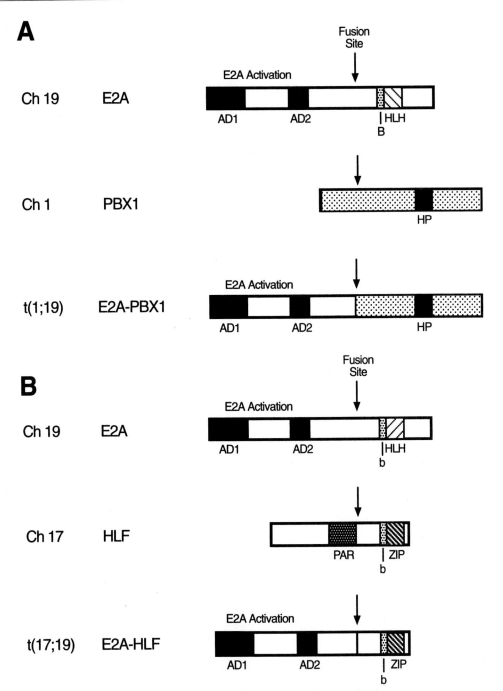

FIG. 5-4 Comparison of the structural features of two major E2A fusion proteins. The E2A portions of the chimeras are identical, retaining both the AD1 and AD2 transcriptional activation domains. The PBX1 fusion partner retains its DNA- and protein-binding domain (homeodomain) as does HLF (bZIP), providing a mechanism for recognition and activation of downstream target genes. Despite the normally wide distribution of E2A, and the lack of normal expression of the HLF and PBX1 transcription factors in hematopoietic cells, the two chimeras act specifically on B-cell precursors. HD, homeodomain; bZIP, basic leucine zipper; bHLH, basic helix-loop-helix; Ch, chromosome.

investigators have confirmed the dispensability of sequence-specific DNA binding for transformation of fibroblasts, while showing that the PBX1 homeodomain is essential for efficient arrest of myeloid cell differentiation.[146] Taken together, these observations suggest that interaction with members of the HOX family of proteins may be sufficient to target the E2A-PBX1 fusion protein to downstream target genes with critical functions in cell transformation, but not those that interfere with normal differentiation programs.[145,146]

E2A-PBX1 is one of the most common fusion genes in children with ALL, occurring in 20 to 25 percent of cases with a pre-B immunophenotype (defined by cytoplasmic but not surface expression of *Ig* genes).[142,147,148] It is also detected in adults with ALL, as well as occasional cases of pro-B-cell ALL, acute myeloid leukemia (AML), T-cell ALL, and lymphoma.[13,147–156] Patients with pre-B ALL and the t(1;19) tend to have elevated leukocytes at diagnosis and central nervous system leukemia.[13,147,148] Aside from the adverse impact of these features, the *E2A-PBX1* fusion gene was shown to be independently associated with a poor prognosis, although in recent years, intensive chemotherapy has significantly improved clinical outcome in these patients.[147,148] A prudent clinical management strategy for patients with pre-B ALL is to consider the *E2A-PBX1* fusion gene a high-risk biological feature that warrants an aggressive approach to therapy. Otherwise, these cases may be undertreated with consequent rapid development of drug-resistant disease.

E2A-HLF. A second *E2A* fusion gene is created by the t(17;19)(q21–22;13) rearrangement, which joins *E2A* to the *HLF* gene within chromosome band 17q21–22 (Figure 5-2).[157–159] The breakpoint of this translocation consistently leaves the same portion of *HLF* in the chimeric gene, but affects either intron 12 or 13 within *E2A*. The resulting hybrid protein therefore is termed type I (intron 13 breakpoint) or type II (intron 12 breakpoint), although these structural distinctions do not appear to affect the DNA-binding and transcriptional regulatory properties of E2A-HLF and will not be considered further in this section.[160,161]

The HLF (hepatic leukemia factor) component of the chimera is a novel bZIP transcription factor within the PAR subfamily of proteins (defined by a proline- and acidic amino acid-rich domain).[162–165] HLF has recently been shown to encode two proteins from alternatively spliced transcripts that are regulated by different promoters.[166] One isoform is abundant in brain, liver, and kidney, whereas the other is restricted to hepatocytes; these proteins accumulate with different circadian patterns in the liver and have distinct promoter preferences in *trans*-activation experiments. Very little is known about the normal function of the PAR proteins, including HLF, but their structural similarity with the CES-2 bZIP protein that orchestrates the death of sertoninergic nerve cells in the developing worm *C. elegans* suggests a regulatory role in cell survival, as indicated by the mechanism of E2A-HLF oncogenic activity.[167–169]

The E2A-HLF fusion product retains the entire DNA-binding/protein–protein interaction domain of HLF, as well as the two N-terminal transactivation domains of E2A.[159,160] In leukemic lymphoblasts, the chimeric protein appears to bind DNA as a homo-dimer, as one might predict given the absence of detectable levels of the known normal PAR proteins in hematopoietic precursors.[170,171] Like E2A-PBX1, the E2A-HLF oncoprotein can transform NIH-3T3 cells, dependent on the integrity of the HLF leucine zipper and the E2A transcriptional activation domains.[172] It also induces lymphoid tumors in transgenic mice.[173]

Recent experiments have provided important insight into how E2A-HLF might take control of immature lymphoid cells. When introduced into leukemic cells carrying the t(17;19), a dominant-negative form of E2A-HLF blocked the usual action of the intact chimera, and as a result the malignant cells underwent apoptosis.[167] By contrast, the dominant-negative mutant had no effect on apoptotic events in leukemic cells without the t(17;19), suggesting that E2A-HLF may increase the number of developing lymphocytes by preventing their suicide.[167] The homology between HLF and the CES-2 protein of *C. elegans*, which functions early in a genetically controlled cell death pathway, suggests that a comparable pathway operates in human B lymphoblasts and is usurped by E2A-HLF to give rise to ALL.[167,168] In this model (Figure 5-5), E2A-HLF activates a downstream target gene that is normally repressed by a CES-2-like protein, so that cell survival rather than cell death signals ensue. Thus, the leukemogenic activity of E2A-HLF may operate through an evolutionarily conserved pathway that determines the sensitivity of specific lymphoid cells to apoptotic stimuli.

The t(17;19) defines a subset (0.5–1 percent) of ALL cases with a pro-B immunophenotype.[157] In several reports, this rearrangement was linked to disseminated intravascular coagulation (DIC) and hypercalcemia at initial diagnosis.[157,159,160,174,175] Although the rarity of t(17;19)-positive ALL has hampered efforts to assess its prognostic significance, each of seven patients with molecularly identified *E2A-HLF* fusion died of leukemia, despite their enrollment on contemporary treatment protocols.[160,170,174,175] Drug resis-

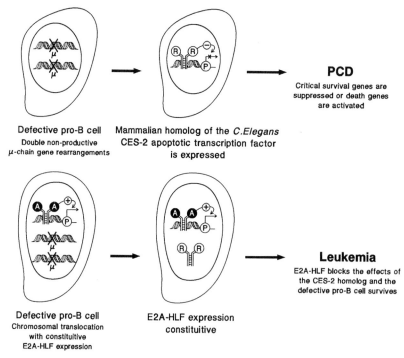

FIG. 5-5 A proposed model for the anti-apoptotic role of E2A-HLF in leukemogenesis. Leukemic cells with the t(17;19) undergo programmed cell death when E2A-HLF is inhibited through a dominant negative mechanism, suggesting that the primary effect of the hybrid oncoprotein is to prolong cell survival rather than to accelerate cell growth.[167] The close homology of the HLF bZIP domain to that of the CES-2 cell death-specification protein of the nematode *C. elegans* suggests that E2A-HLF may contribute to leukemogenesis by binding to the promoters of target genes normally regulated by a mammalian ortholog of the CES-2 protein, which causes defective pro-B cells to undergo apoptosis.[168] According to this model, E2A-HLF may activate target gene expression in contrast to the proposed repressor effects of CES-2, leading to aberrant survival through an evolutionarily conserved pathway that regulates programmed cell death during B lymphoid cell development.

tance in this type of leukemia may be augmented by the role of E2A-HLF in preventing accelerated apoptosis from therapy-induced DNA damage as well as growth factor deprivation.[167]

***TEL-AML1* Fusion Gene.** Generally considered a target of chromosomal translocations in myeloid cells, the *AML1* gene recently was found to be joined to a second transcriptional control gene, called *TEL*, as a result of the t(12;21) in cases of B-lineage ALL.[176–180] Although rarely detected by routine karyotyping (because the telomeric segments of 12p and 21q appear similar in banded metaphase preparations), the t(12;21) rearrangement is apparent by fluorescence in situ hybridization in approximately one-fourth of children with ALL, making *TEL-AML1* the most common genetic abnormality in the lymphoid leukemias.[178] The *TEL-AML1* fusion product consists of the bHLH domain of TEL linked to virtually the entire coding region of AML1, including the DNA- and protein-binding domain, which bears close amino acid identity to the Runt protein of *Drosophila*. The exact role of the TEL-AML1 oncoprotein in cell transformation remains unclear, but emerging data suggest that the primary effect relates to a compromise of AML1 transcriptional activity, which is required for normal hematopoiesis (see the section in this chapter on the involvement of the AML1–CBFβ complex in the acute myeloid leukemias).

TEL-AML1 expression is associated with a superior treatment outcome in patients with B-lineage ALL. In a recent survey of prognostic factor candidates in this disease, children with *TEL* gene rearrangements (primarily *TEL-AML1*) had a 5-year event-free survival probability of 91 percent plus or minus 5 percent (SE) compared with 64 percent plus or minus 5 percent for those with TEL in a germline configuration.[181] The prognostic strength of *TEL* rearrangement (usually as a *TEL-AML1* fusion gene) was independent of recognized good-risk features in ALL with B-lineage markers, such as the presenting leukocyte count and hyperdiploidy. Indeed, molecular detection of the *TEL-AML1* fusion gene is the first genetic assay to allow a good-risk subset of patients to be dissected from the otherwise high-risk "pseudodiploid" subset of ALL patients.[182] Thus, *TEL-AML1* was recently added to the list of genetic abnormalities requiring recognition early in the disease course (Table 5-3).

***BCL6* Activation in Diffuse Large-Cell Lymphoma.** The t(3;14)(q27;q32) and related translocations affect the long arm of chromosome 3 in diffuse large cell lymphomas of the B-cell lineage, leading to the discovery of the *BCL6* proto-oncogene, whose expression is altered in at least 30 percent of these malignancies, the vast majority of which occur in adults.[183–186] *BCL6* encodes a transcription factor containing six zinc-finger DNA-binding motifs near the carboxyl-terminus and a POZ regulatory domain near the amino-terminus. It is related to the PLZF protein that is fused to RARα as a result of the t(11;17) translocation of acute promyelocytic leukemia. (The postulated developmental roles of highly conserved zinc-finger proteins with POZ domains are discussed in the *PLZF* section of this chapter.) Like the *AML1–CBFβ* complex in the myeloid cell lineage, but unlike most genes whose expression is altered by translocation to the vicinity of the *Ig* or *TCR* genes, *BCL6* normally is expressed and developmentally regulated in cells of the same lineage in which it is linked to transformation, the B lymphocytes.[187,188] The BCL6 protein is detected in cells of the lymph node germinal center, a region in which antigen-primed B cells normally undergo transformation into either memory B cells or immunoblasts destined to become plasma cells, or die as a result of apoptosis.[189] Because BCL6 is normally downregulated before B cells exit from the germinal center, a reasonable hypothesis is that activated B lymphoblasts constitutively expressing BCL6 are unable to develop normally, and instead replicate clonally with the

considerable proliferative capacity of a large-cell lymphoma of activated B-lymphocyte origin.[190] This interpretation is supported by the fact that most *BCL6* rearrangements occur within the 5′-noncoding first exon or the first intron of the gene and result in dysregulation of expression of a structurally intact BCL6 protein.[191]

In addition to gene rearrangement mediated by chromosomal translocation, somatic point mutations of the 5′ regulatory regions of the *BCL6* gene have been identified at high frequency in both the diffuse large cell and the follicular lymphomas of B cell origin, suggesting that dysregulated expression of BCL6 may be casually linked to malignant transformation in high percentages of lymphoid tumors of these pathological subtypes.[192] Rearrangements of the *BCL6* gene have been shown to have distinct clinicopathological correlates within the adult diffuse large cell lymphomas, occurring primarily in extranodal tumors that have not spread to the bone marrow. Importantly, they independently identify a subset of patients with a favorable prognosis.[193]

Acute Myeloid Leukemias

The distribution of gene rearrangements owing to chromosomal translocations in acute myeloid leukemias (AML) of children and adolescents is shown in Figure 5-6.

Gene Rearrangements Affecting the AML1–CBFβ Complex. The AML1–CBFβ transcription factor complex (Figure 5-7) is the most frequent target of chromosomal translocations in the human leukemias, in that one of these linked proteins is expressed as an oncogenic chimera in as many as one-third of both ALL and AML cases. This regulatory complex, termed CBF because of its identity as a core binding factor (also known as PEBP2), consists of a DNA-binding subunit, AML1 (also called CBFα2 or PEBP2αB), and CBFβ (also called PEBP2β), a subunit that does not bind DNA independently but rather heterodimerizes with AML1 or one of its closely related family members.[194–196] Chromosomal translocations that modify the AML1–CBFβ complex in myeloid cells include the t(8;21), which generates *AML1–ETO*, and the t(3;21), which gives rise to *AML–EVI1*, *AML–EAP*, or *AML1–MDS1*.[197–202]

The sequence-specific DNA-binding and protein–protein interaction properties of CBF fusion proteins are provided by a large domain within AML1, showing approximately 70 percent homology with the *Drosophila* Runt and Lozenge proteins.[203] The *Drosophila* AML1 homologs participate in several developmental processes, including sex determination, segmentation and neurogenesis (Runt), and determination of photoreceptor identity during eye development (Lozenge). The sequence element recognized by AML1 is TGTGGT, an enhancer core motif that serves as a regulatory element in several viral enhancers, as well as genes whose products are involved in the regulation of hematopoiesis, such as IL-3, GM-CSF, CSF-1, myeloperoxidase, and the TCR receptors.[195,203–211] The binding affinity of AML1 is markedly increased through its heterodimerization with CBFβ, an interaction also mediated through the *runt* homology domain.[203]

The *Aml1* gene recently was inactivated in the germline of mice by homologous recombination and shown to be essential for definitive hematopoiesis of all lineages.[212,213] Homozygous null animals display normal morphogenesis and yolk sac-derived erythropoiesis, but die between embryonic days 11.5 and 12.5 because of CNS hemorrhage, postulated to be caused by a lack of platelets, possibly potentiated by abnormalities of CNS capillary endothelium.[213] Inactivation of the *Cbf*β gene in the mouse germline produced similar effects in homozygous null mice, indicating that CBFβ is required for AML1 function in vivo.[214] From these observations, it appears that the AML1-CBFβ complex is an essential

Table 5-3 Clinical Risk Assignment in the Childhood Leukemias by Genetic Classification of the Malignant Cells

Abnormality (Risk)	Method of Detection	Treatment
Hyperdiploidy, ≥53 chromosomes (good risk)	DNA flow cytometry	Antimetabolite therapy emphasizing high-dose methotrexate
TEL-AML1 fusion human gene owing to t(12;21) (good risk)	RNA-PCR to detect *TEL-AML1* fusion transcripts	Antimetabolite therapy emphasizing high-dose methotrexate
E2A-PBX1 fusion gene owing to t(1;19) (intermediate risk)	RNA-PCR to detect *E2A-PBX1* fusion transcripts	Intensified chemotherapy with alkylating agents and topoisomerase inhibitors
MLL fusion gene owing to 11q23 rearrangements and *E2A-HLF* owing to t(17;19) (high risk)	RNA-PCR to detect *MLL* and *E2A-HLF* fusion transcripts	Experimental forms of intensified chemotherapy or bone marrow transplantation
BCR-ABL fusion gene owing to t(9;22), with high leukocyte count (ultra-high risk)	RNA-PCR to detect *BCR-ABL* fusion transcripts	Bone marrow transplantation in first remission

regulator of genes required for normal hematopoietic cell development. Hence, chromosomal rearrangements that target this complex may interfere with its function in ways that produce arrested differentiation and eventually fully transformed leukemias of specific cell lineages.

The t(8;21), resulting in expression of the AML1-ETO oncoprotein, is the most frequent chromosomal abnormality in the myeloid leukemias of both children and adults; it is most often found in myeloblasts with evidence of granulocytic differentiation (M2 designation by the French-American-British classification system). The fusion protein, which retains the runt homology domain of AML1 and its ability to interact with CBFβ and the core

enhancer DNA sequence element, appears to interfere with AML1-mediated transcriptional activation.[203,215] The combinatorial versatility of the *AML1* locus is demonstrated by its fusion with sequences from either the *EVI1* gene in t(3;21)-positive chronic myeloid leukemia in blast crisis or the *EAP* (Epstein-Barr virus RNA-associated protein) gene in myelodysplastic syndrome.[201,202] Inclusion of both the Runt-homologous DNA-binding/dimerization domain of AML1 and the zinc-finger DNA-binding domains of EVI1 in the AML1-EVI1 chimeric protein affords ample opportunity for aberrant regulation of target genes. The AML1-EAP protein contains carboxyl-terminal EAP sequences fused out-of-frame to AML1 sequences, resulting in a truncated AML1 protein that

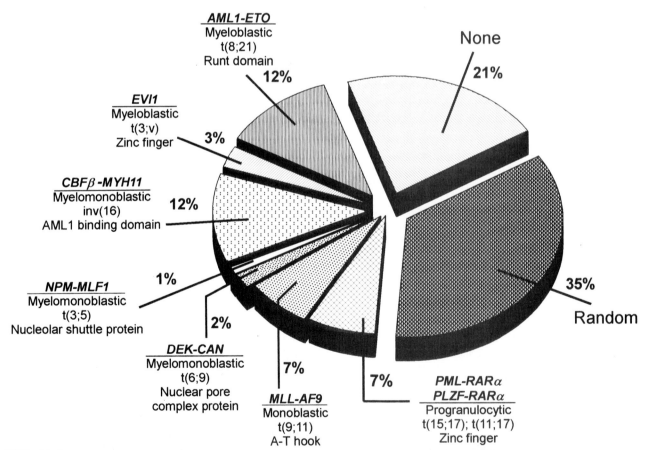

FIG. 5-6 Distribution of translocation-generated fusion genes among the various morphological subtypes of AML in children and young adults. The section labeled "random" refers to sporadic rearrangements that have so far been observed only in the leukemic cells from single cases. Key domains for DNA binding and protein–protein interaction are given for transcription factors, or the type of gene affected for nontranscription factors.

may dominantly interfere with normal AML1 function during myelopoiesis, without a contribution from a partner protein domain, as found in the other AML1 chimeras.

The CBFβ subunit is involved in another major chromosomal rearrangement in AML, the inversion 16, which affects 15 to 18 percent of AML cases, principally those with myelomonocytic differentiation and increased bone marrow eosinophils (M4-Eo designation in the French-American-British system). This rearrangement joins most of the *CBFB* gene to the carboxyl terminus of the heavy-chain gene of smooth muscle myosin (*MYHII*), resulting in formation of a CBFβ-MYHII protein.[216]

A murine model to study the effects of CBFβ-MYHII on hematopoietic cell development has been produced by inserting the human MYHII cDNA in-frame into the mouse *Cbfb* gene through homologous recombination, to "knock-in" the fused gene.[217] Mouse embryos harboring one allele of *Cbfb-MYHII* in the germline developed CNS hemorrhages at embryologic day 12.5, similar to mice lacking *Aml1* or *Cbfb*, indicating that the chimeric protein dominantly interferes with essential functions of the *Aml1–Cbfb* complex. Mice expressing Cbfb-MYHII had impairment of primitive as well as definitive hematopoiesis, however, suggesting an additional function of this fusion protein during hematopoietic cell development.[217] Since both AML1 and CBFβ normally are required for definitive hematopoiesis, the oncogenicity of their respective fusion proteins may stem from disruption of a transcriptional regulatory complex producing arrested myeloid cell differentiation; however, the basis for the phenotypic specificity of leukemias resulting from various types of AML1 and CBFβ fusion proteins is unknown (Figure 5-7). The available data imply unique activities for each chimeric protein, possibly including gain-of-function as well as loss-of-function effects, rather than global interference with the role of the heterodimeric complex.

Retinoic Acid Receptor Rearrangements

PML-RARα. Dysregulated chimeric transcription factors, which induce differentiation arrest at specific stages of development in the myeloid leukemias, offer a new class of intracellular targets for therapeutic attempts to promote differentiation of these leukemias

in vivo, so that they lose their proliferative capacity. A major example is the fusion product generated by the t(15;17)(q21;q11–22) in acute promyelocytic leukemia (APML), which links critical ligand- and DNA-binding sequences of the retinoic acid-α receptor gene (*RARα*) on chromosome 17 to sequences of the *PML* gene on chromosome 15.[218–223] In its unaltered form, the RARα protein binds to the retinoic acid ligand through a defined ligand-binding domain and to DNA through a separate zinc-finger region.[224] PML proteins, which also possess zinc-finger motifs, normally are located in novel macromolecular nuclear organelles, called PML oncogenic domains (PODs), that include at least three other proteins.[225–227] These nuclear bodies are preferential targets of proteins expressed by DNA tumor viruses, and are upregulated in activated inflammatory mononuclear cells and by interferon.[228–233] The PML-RARα fusion proteins disrupt these subnuclear structures, causing normal PML, RXR, and other nuclear proteins to disperse in an abnormal microparticulate pattern.[225–227] The fusion proteins interfere with normal myeloid cell development, possibly through adverse effects on assembly of the PODs that contain PML, and dominant inhibitory effects as a homodimeric complex with normal retinoid receptor and peroxisome-proliferator pathways, leading to arrested differentiation in the promyelocyte stage.[234–237] The oncogenic properties of PML-RARα have been demonstrated in transgenic mouse model in which expression of the fusion protein is driven by the CD11b promoter.[238] Although these mice did not develop leukemia, they did show impaired myelopoiesis. A transformation model, based on retroviral transduction of the *PML-RARα* gene into hematopoietic progenitor cells of chickens, has been developed to study mechanistic features of the fusion protein.[239]

These findings provided the mechanistic rationale for use of all-*trans* retinoic acid in patients with APML, which had already been shown to be effective in empirically initiated trials.[240–244] In response to pharmacologic doses of this compound, PML and its associated proteins are reorganized into normal-appearing nuclear PODs, with subsequent maturation of the leukemic cells into differentiated myeloid cells with limited life spans in the circulation. Resistance to all-*trans* retinoic acid generally develops within 3 to 4 months, limiting this hormone's therapeutic role to the remission induction phase of APML therapy, as an adjunct to cytotoxic chemotherapy.[243,244]

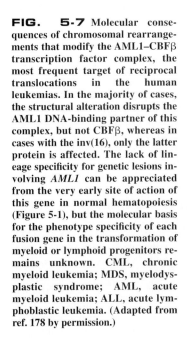

FIG. 5-7 Molecular consequences of chromosomal rearrangements that modify the AML1–CBFβ transcription factor complex, the most frequent target of reciprocal translocations in the human leukemias. In the majority of cases, the structural alteration disrupts the AML1 DNA-binding partner of this complex, but not CBFβ, whereas in cases with the inv(16), only the latter protein is affected. The lack of lineage specificity for genetic lesions involving *AML1* can be appreciated from the very early site of action of this gene in normal hematopoiesis (Figure 5-1), but the molecular basis for the phenotype specificity of each fusion gene in the transformation of myeloid or lymphoid progenitors remains unknown. CML, chronic myeloid leukemia; MDS, myelodysplastic syndrome; AML, acute myeloid leukemia; ALL, acute lymphoblastic leukemia. (Adapted from ref. 178 by permission.)

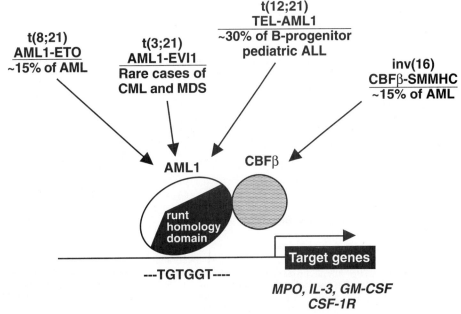

PLZF-RARα and NPM-RARα. Two variant translocations have been identified in AML that unequivocally implicate RARα in leukemias arrested at the promyelocyte stage of differentiation, as both fusion proteins involve the retinoid- and DNA-binding domains of this nuclear receptor. Very little is known about the NPM-RARα fusion protein, which was only recently identified in a single patient and links RARα in-frame to amino-terminal sequences of nucleophosmin, or NPM, a nucleolar shuttle protein that is also involved in NPM-ALK fusion proteins in large-cell lymphoma and NPM-MLF1 in AML.[245]

PLZF-RARα was first recognized several years ago, with subsequent structural and functional studies of PLZF providing intriguing insights into the potential mechanism of action.[246] PLZF is a transcription factor containing nine carboxyl-terminal zinc-finger motifs related to those of the Krüppel *Drosophila* segmentation protein, and containing an amino-terminal POZ (poxvirus and zinc-finger) protein–protein interaction domain.[247] This domain inhibits the binding of transcription factors including RARα, to DNA when linked in *cis*, suggesting that PLZF-RARα may act by sequestering RXR or other retinoid receptors within inactive multimeric complexes.[247–250] PLZF is expressed in multiple tissues during development, including elevated expression at Rhomberic boundaries in the vertebrate hindbrain.[251] It is also expressed by early hematopoietic progenitors with a punctate nuclear distribution and is downregulated during myeloid cell differentiation.[252] These findings, combined with studies showing heterodimerization of PLZF-RARα with normal PLZF through the POZ domain, suggest that normal PLZF may also play a role in normal hematopoietic cell differentiation, one that is inhibited by the fusion protein.[249]

Recently, five additional cases of APML with t(11;17)-mediated expression of PLZF-RARα fusion proteins have been reported, indicating that these patients share a proclivity with PML-RARα patients to develop life-threatening disseminated intravascular coagulation.[253] All-*trans* retinoic acid differentiation therapy is not effective in inducing remissions in patients with PLZF-RARα fusion proteins, however, indicating a clear difference that ultimately must be related to the molecular pathogenesis of these two fusion proteins, even though the proposed mechanisms through which they transform promyelocyte progenitors are quite similar.

EVI1 Gene Activation. In some cases of AML with high platelet counts, the inv(3)(q21;q26.2) or the t(3;3)(q21;q26.2) moves promoter/enhancer sequences from one site on chromosome 3 into the *EVI1* locus on the same chromosome, leading to increased gene expression.[254,255] The same effect is produced in murine myeloid leukemias by insertional mutagenesis.[256] The EVI1 protein binds to promoter/enhancer sequences containing the GATA sequence motif, and may act by interfering with regulatory signals normally mediated by the GATA family of hematopoietic transcriptional regulators.[257–260] The normal function of EVI1 is unknown, although its tissue distribution (oocytes and kidney cells) and its dominant interfering effect on normal myelopoiesis would suggest an important developmental role in regulatory pathways that interface between proliferation and differentiation.

Acute Mixed-Lineage Leukemias: MLL Fusion Genes

An extraordinarily diverse group of chromosomal translocations, deletions, and inversions affect chromosome band 11q23. In contrast to the lineage specificity of many other nonrandom rearrangements, these abnormalities occur in both lymphoid and myeloid leukemias (7–10 percent of ALL cases, 5–6 percent of AML) and

in a high percentage of the so-called mixed-lineage leukemias, defined by expression of markers of more than one hematopoietic cell lineage.[261–263] Leukemias with 11q23 translocations also account for a high percentage of acute leukemias in infants less than 1 year of age (80 percent and 45 percent of infants with ALL and AML, respectively).[264–269] Perhaps the most striking association is the presence of 11q23 translocations in as many as 85 percent of secondary leukemias in patients treated with topoisomerase II inhibitors.[270,271] Taken together, these examples of phenotypic diversity suggest that 11q23 genetic abnormalities mediate the transformation of multipotential hematopoietic stem cells, which give rise to leukemias in which the myeloid or lymphoid progenitors are blocked at various stages of development.

Molecular Biology of *MLL*. Cloning of the gene most often affected by 11q23 abnormalities fulfilled expectations based on phenotypic, cytogenetic, and clinical studies. Many of the breakpoints that occur within the 11q23 locus interrupt the *mixed-lineage leukemia* gene (*MLL*, also called *HRX, ALL-1*, and *HTRX1*), which encodes a large protein of 3968 amino acids with a predicted molecular mass of 431 kDa.[272–277] Most intriguing with regard to function are three regions of homology with the *Drosophila trithorax (trx)* gene, two associated with central zinc-finger domains and the third with a 210-amino acid carboxy-terminal region of 61 percent identity that is shared with genes of the *Polycomb* group (*Pc-G*), including *enhancer of zeste*.[273,274,278–280] *Trithorax* is a master homeotic gene regulator that positively regulates the actions of a wide spectrum of homeotic (*HOM*) genes in the *antennapedia* and *bithorax* complexes of the fly, and is required throughout embryogenesis for normal development of the head, thorax, and abdomen.[273–276,281] The amino-terminal region of the MLL protein contains three A-T hook domains, first identified in the so-called HMG (high mobility group) proteins, which are thought to help establish chromatin structure and to bind in the minor groove to DNA segments rich in A and T residues.[282] The intervening region between the A-T hooks and the zinc-finger domains includes a 47-amino acid region of homology with the noncatalytic domains of mammalian DNA methyltransferase (MT), an enzyme that acts on the hemimethylated substrate produced after DNA replication to maintain the methylation pattern of cytosine residues in the genomes of somatic cells.[283] Two additional domains have been defined based on their ability to affect transcriptional control, a *trans*-repression domain overlapping the MT-homology region and a *trans*-activation domain in the region carboxyl-terminal to the zinc-fingers.[284]

MLL Fusion Genes. Translocation breakpoints within the *MLL* gene occur exclusively in an 8.5-kb region located between exons 5 and 11, and join *MLL* sequences with genes from numerous other chromosomes to form a large fusion gene (Figure 5-8). The resulting chimeric proteins, encoded on the derivative 11 chromosome, include the amino-terminal half of MLL, with its A-T hook minor groove DNA-binding motifs, the MT homology domain, and all or part of the associated transcriptional repression domain.[273,274] Another consistent feature of MLL fusion proteins is the absence of the two zinc-finger regions and the Trithorax homology regions normally located in the carboxyl-terminal half of the protein.

In contrast to the similar regions of MLL affected by 11q23 rearrangements, an array of structurally diverse protein partners contribute amino acid segments to the MLL fusion proteins found in ALL, AML, and the mixed-lineage leukemias. Ten of the genes fused to *MLL* by 11q23 translocations have now been cloned and sequenced (Table 5-1), making it possible to examine their products for functional motifs that might provide clues to the mechanisms leading to the formation of active transforming proteins. At

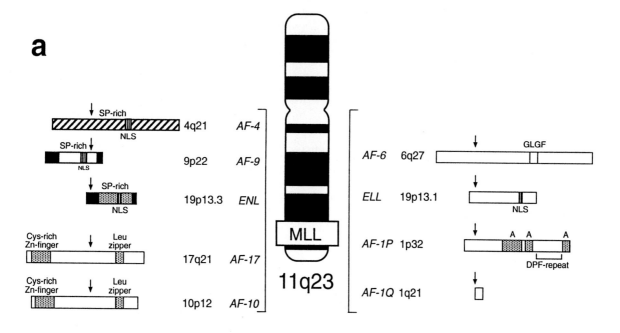

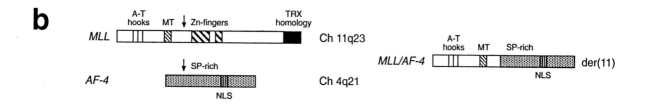

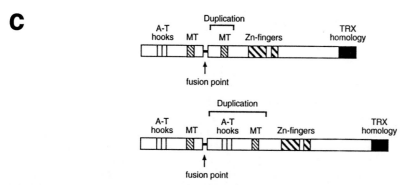

FIG. 5-8 The *MLL* gene and some of its fusion partners. The first three genes shown on the left of the ideogram (Panel A) are rich in serine and proline (SP) and contain nuclear localization signals (NLS), whereas the next two are notable for a cysteine-rich zinc-finger domain and a leucine zipper motif. The AF6 protein contains a novel glycine-leucine-phenylalanine (GLGF) domain, and AF1P is distinguished by three acidic (A) regions, together with an amino acid repeat motif (aspartic acid-proline-phenylalanine (DPF). AFIQ contributes only a minimal part of its 9-kDa total mass to its fusion with MLL, suggesting that truncation of MLL may itself contribute to leukemogenesis. Regions on the right of the breakpoints (arrows) are retained in the fusion product. Of the four major structural elements of *MLL* (Panel B), only the A-T hook and mammalian DNA methyltransferase domains are retained in the chimeric proteins. AML cases have recently been identified with "self-fusion" rearrangements (Panel C), which fuse the same amino-terminal *MLL* sequences with duplicated regions of the *MLL* gene. (Adapted from ref. 472 by permission.)

the time of its cloning, each of these fusion partners was a previously unidentified gene with unknown function. The ELL protein (also known as MEN) was originally cloned as an MLL fusion partner in translocations involving chromosome sub-band 19p13.1.[285,286] In an exciting recent development, the same protein was independently purified as an elongation factor that increases the catalytic rate of RNA polymerase II transcription.[287] This association seems unlikely to be circumstantial, in that ELL has a close functional analog called elongin (SIII), the transcription elongation factor recently shown to be regulated by the von Hippel-Lindau

(VHL) tumor suppressor.[288–291] Many questions remain to be answered before the functional significance of the MLL-ELL fusion is known; for example, is the MLL-ELL fusion protein (which contains almost all of the ELL coding sequences, fused in frame to the usual amino-terminal segment of MLL) still active as an elongation accelerator? Is ELL subject to regulation by proteins analogous to VHL? If so, does fusion with MLL block this interaction and remove ELL from positive or negative physiologic control? And, perhaps most important, which genes are controlled in their expression by ELL and how do they affect cell physiology? Although the full significance of the functional identity of this MLL fusion partner is still unknown, recognition of ELL emphasizes the potentially important roles of such proteins in chimeric constructs, particularly the potential of the chimeras to interfere with the normal roles and regulation of the fusion partner proteins, in addition to their possible inhibitory effects on the normal function of MLL itself.

Another intriguing development in research on MLL fusion genes has been the realization that the identity of the fusion partner may determine the phenotypic specificity of the chimera in hematopoietic stem cell transformation. For example, ENL, the partner gene on sub-band 19p13.3, is frequently involved in translocations affecting both ALL (especially in infants and children) and AML, whereas *ELL* is restricted to de novo and therapy-related cases of AML and is rare in children.[285,292] *ENL* is one of three related fusion partners, that include *AF-4* on chromosome band 4q21, involved in the frequent 4;11 translocations found in ALL, and *AF-9* on band 9p22, the gene affected by the 9;11 translocation important in both primary and secondary acute monocytic leukemias of children and adults. Each of these proteins appears to contribute domains with similar structural attributes to chimeric proteins, in that they contain nuclear localization signals and regions rich in serine and proline that may function as transcriptional *trans*-activation domains.[273,274,277,293–295] In support of this possibility, ENL was shown to *trans*-activate reporter gene expression in mammalian cells and yeast, through the C-terminal serine- and proline-rich region of homology between ENL and AF-9, which is included in the chimeric proteins.[295]

Some *MLL* partner genes appear to contribute functional domains to the chimeric proteins, whereas others truncate *MLL* in ways that may interfere with its normal function. *AF-10* and *AF-17*, potential examples of the first mechanism, are involved in the t(10;11)(p12;q23) and t(11;17)(q23;q21), and contain leucine zipper motifs near their carboxyl-termini and cysteine-rich zinc-finger motifs near their amino-termini. These structural elements are retained in the oncogenic fusion proteins and may provide dimerization motifs with functional significance. The alternative model is best represented by the *AF1q* gene involved in the t(1;11) (q21;q23). This 9-kDa protein lacks homology to any known protein sequence, and the minimal contribution of its sequences to the uniformly involved MLL amino-terminal region implies that loss of MLL function through haploinsufficiency or dominant negative interference may contribute to leukemogenesis.[296] This interpretation is reinforced by several cases of AML that have lacked 11q23 translocations but have contained partial internal duplications of *MLL* linking the intact gene to a duplication of its amino-terminal region.[297,298] In these rearrangements, a region beyond the A-T hook and methyltransferase domains is internally duplicated, in frame with the remainder of the coding sequences (Figure 5-4). Thus, the partially duplicated *MLL* gene product contains the N-terminal, A-T hooks, and methyltransferase domains separated from the zinc-finger motifs, indicating that dissociation of N-terminal domains of MLL from regulatory C-terminal regions is a general structural feature of oncogenic MLL fusion proteins.

Mll and Mll-Af9 in Animal Models. The murine homologue of *MLL*, *Mll*, was recently inactivated in the germline by homologous recombination, providing key insights into its function during normal development.[278] Complete loss of *Mll* was lethal during embryologic development, with the embryos lacking detectable expression of the major *Hox* genes tested, consistent with the requirement for the *Mll* fly homolog, *trithorax*, in maintenance of *Hox* gene expression in that organism. Interestingly, mice lacking function of one *Mll* allele showed a phenotype resulting from haploinsufficiency, with hematopoietic abnormalities that included anemia, thrombopenia, and reduced numbers of B cells, bidirectional homeotic transformations of the axial skeleton, and sternal abnormalities. Skeletal abnormalities appeared to be caused by shifts in the normal pattern of major *Hox* gene expression, because of inadequate *trithorax* gene dosage, so that the hematopoietic cell phenotype may have resulted from a similar mechanism, based on studies that implicate mammalian *Hox* genes in blood cell development.[299,300] Results in *Mll*-deficient mice also established a positive role for *Mll* in the regulation of *Hox* expression, consistent with its greater structural similarity to the positively acting *trithorax*, as compared to the negatively acting *Pc-G* genes. Overall, the results in *Mll*-deficient mice suggest a dual role for 11q23 translocations in human leukemogenesis, including both a gain-of-function effect mediated by the fusion oncogene, and simultaneous effects on hematopoietic cell development from haploinsufficiency owing to the loss of one normal *MLL* allele.[278]

The leukemogenicity of the *MLL-AF9* fusion gene was recently demonstrated in an animal model by generating this fusion oncogene in embryonic stem (ES) cells and using them to generate chimeric mice.[301] Although ES cells containing the *Mll-AF9* fusion gene gave rise to cells of all lineages in chimeric animals, and the cells of numerous tissues expressed the fusion gene, the only tumors to develop in the mice were acute myeloid leukemias, reinforcing the association of this fusion gene with human AML. It also appeared that the fusion gene contributed an early growth advantage to progenitors within the myeloid lineage, because circulating myeloid cells derived from the targeted ES cells were a prominent component of this cell compartment in most of the *Mll-AF9* chimeras from the time of birth. This effect was not observed in mice generated from an ES cell line modified to express a truncated and epitope-tagged *Mll* allele, implying that the disordered growth advantage imparted to myeloid cells did not arise from *Mll* haploinsufficiency but rather from expression of the Mll-Af9 fusion protein. Although leukemia induction was highly efficient in this model, the latency period ranged from 4 to 12 or more months, implying that additional mutations affecting oncogenes or tumor suppressors must occur before a fully transformed leukemic clone can emerge.[301]

Origins of Therapy-Related AML. *MLL*-associated translocations are a prominent feature of leukemias in patients treated with the epipodophyllotoxins, but the basis for this association remains uncertain.[270,271,302] An intriguing correlation has emerged from analysis of 130 breakpoints by restriction mapping and more than a dozen by genomic DNA sequencing analysis in cases of de novo or therapy-related leukemias with 11q23 translocations affecting the *MLL* gene.[303–308] That is, the centromeric portion of the 8.5-kb genomic MLL breakpoint cluster region consistently showed the largest number of breakpoints in cases of de novo leukemias, whereas the telomeric portion contained the majority of breakpoints found in therapy-related cases.[307,308] Scaffold attachment sites have been mapped in the vicinity of these breakpoint regions, as well as high affinity topoisomerase II cleavage sites, which may influence the distribution of breakpoints.[307]

With regard to the molecular mechanisms involved in the origin of 11q23 translocations in de novo and secondary AML, studies to date have focused on 1) recombination within Alu repeats, 2) involvement of V-D-J recombinase enzymes in B-lymphoid progenitors, and 3) the possible role of topoisomerase II inhibitors acting to promote breaks at consensus cleavage sites for this enzyme, which would serve as substrates for recombination events leading to *MLL* translocations in the therapy-related leukemias. The first two possibilities have gained credible support, but they do not explain the majority of cases.[298,303,304,306,309,310]

An intriguing mechanism of genetic recombination involves cleavage by topoisomerase II, as suggested by the frequent identification of *MLL* rearrangements in therapy-related cases of AML of patients treated with agents that inhibit this enzyme.[270,271,302] Antineoplastic drugs with this property include both the epipodophyllotoxin and anthracycline classes of drugs. AML linked to these agents tends to appear as an acute leukemia without a myelodysplastic phase within 6 to 24 months after diagnosis of the primary malignancy, in contrast to the longer latency periods and frequent myelodysplastic prodromes of secondary AML cases induced by alkylating agents. AML arising after treatment with a topoisomerase inhibitor typically has monoblastic or myelomonoblastic morphology, suggesting that the target cell is a myeloid progenitor cell stimulated to enter cell division by chemotherapy-induced neutropenia.[270,271,302,311–313]

Topoisomerase II catalyzes a two-step reaction involving both double-stranded DNA cleavage and strand relaxation and religation.[314] Both the epipodophyllotoxins and the anthracyclines stabilize the DNA-topoisomerase II complex after cleavage, resulting in the accumulation of double-strand DNA breaks, which are prime substrates for nonhomologous recombination.[315,316] Analysis of several 11q23 translocations has identified topoisomerase II consensus binding sites adjacent to chromosomal breakpoints.[306] Other cases of therapy-related AML lack topoisomerase II-binding sites adjacent to the breakpoints, so that additional 11q23 translocation junctions will need to be analyzed before the frequency and importance of this mechanism can be fully assessed.[303,307]

Aside from factors predisposing to nonhomologous recombination, how could topoisomerase inhibitors preferentially induce AML with characteristic MLL fusion proteins? The rapid development of these secondary leukemias suggests a collaborative mechanism in which both the drug and the fusion protein act synergistically to accelerate the multistep process leading to AML. A model incorporating the known effects of the epipodophyllotoxins on G2-phase cell cycle checkpoint control and topoisomerase II activity is shown in Figure 5-9. These compounds arrest cycling cells in G2 phase, and most committed myeloid progenitors harboring epipodophyllotoxin-induced DNA breaks are likely targeted to undergo apoptosis, based on the degree of neutropenia that accompanies a typical course of therapy with these agents (top panel, Figure 5-9). Normal myeloid progenitors arrested in G2 occasionally survive, however, with double-strand DNA breaks at the sites of topoisomerase II integration. As these lesions are repaired, some of the breaks are joined by nonhomologous recombination and result in chromosomal rearrangements. The myeloid progenitors with 11q23 translocations producing in-frame MLL fusion genes begin to proliferate because of a proliferative advantage conferred by the hybrid MLL protein and growth factors produced in response to epipodophyllotoxin-induced neutropenia. According to this model, MLL fusion proteins may exacerbate this process by relaxing cell cycle checkpoints normally activated by the presence of the integrated topoisomerase II-drug complex, leading to attenuated apoptosis and increased survival of cells with genetic damage at other loci (bottom panel, Figure 5-9). In the face of repetitive epipodophyllotoxin treatment, this could lead to the acquisition of additional genetic lesions affecting oncogenes or tumor suppressors in the expanding clone that already expresses an MLL fusion pro-

tein, with rapid progression of a multistep process culminating in overt AML.

The exceedingly high frequency of 11q23 translocations associated with infant leukemias suggests a further mechanism that could lead to *MLL* gene rearrangement and biologically active chimeric proteins. A number of pairs of infant twins have been shown to have identical *MLL* gene rearrangements.[317,318] In some cases, the leukemias had identical *Ig* gene rearrangements, consistent with transformation of a common progenitor cell that had completed V-D-J recombination. In other cases the *Ig* rearrangements differed between twin leukemias, suggesting that transformation occurred before *Ig* gene recombination and that the leukemic clones had evolved independently. Nonetheless, the identification of identical *MLL* rearrangements at the DNA sequence level in each twin indicates that the leukemic clone arose in one infant and spread through the placenta to the other sibling. The documentation of *MLL* rearrangements in utero and the high frequency of 11q23 translocations in infant leukemias (approaching 80 percent of ALL cases and 50 percent of AML) suggest that pluripotent progenitor cells with self-renewal capacity are in a proliferative state in the developing bone marrow, rendering them uniquely susceptible to transformation by chimeric MLL oncoproteins. This susceptibility may be related to patterns of gene expression or epigenetic changes in chromatin configuration that are found in subsets of progenitors that are expanding to populate the hemotopoietic system during infancy.

Myeloid progenitors similarly susceptible to the transforming effects of chimeric MLL proteins or prone to productive MLL rearrangements may be reactivated in patients undergoing therapy with epipodophyllotoxins, accounting for the rapid onset of secondary AML in children and adults treated with these agents. We have recently identified altered transcripts for the p27^{KIP1} cell cycle kinase inhibitor in leukemias expressing MLL-AF4, and have shown that MLL-AF4 induces cell cycle arrest in cell lines when its expression is driven by a conditional promoter, suggesting that hematopoietic stem cells may need to have the capacity to bypass negative cell cycle effects of this fusion protein before they become susceptible to malignant transformation.[319,320] Moreover, the short latency period between *MLL* rearrangement and overt leukemia following 11q23 translocations in infants and after epipodophyllotoxin therapy suggests that MLL fusion proteins themselves predispose susceptible hematopoeitic progenitors to undergo secondary mutations necessary for the development of a fully transformed leukemic clone.

ONCOGENIC ACTIVATION OF TYROSINE KINASES

Cellular tyrosine kinase gene products serve as growth factor receptors or intracellular signal transducers and can be aberrantly activated through a variety of mechanisms, including truncation of the ligand-binding domain of growth factor receptors, loss or replacement of carboxyl-terminal regulatory tyrosine residues, and point mutations within intact molecules.[321] In the leukemias and lymphomas, chromosomal translocations produce tyrosine kinase gene fusions that are quite specific for lymphoid progenitor cells of particular lineages and phenotypes. In two instances, the amino-terminal sequence of a functionally unrelated protein is fused to a truncated receptor tyrosine kinase. Such kinases normally occupy a proximal position in the transduction of extracellular signals required for cell proliferation, differentiation, and other biological events that determine cell fate. When activated by growth factors,

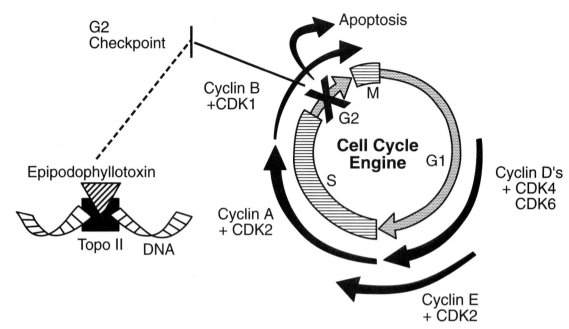

FIG. 5-9 Model accounting for the mechanisms linking epipodophyllotoxin therapy, MLL fusion proteins, cell cycle progression, and the relaxation of cell cycle checkpoints, leading to reduced levels of apoptosis in myeloid progenitor cells after genotoxic chemotherapy (hence, increased survival of cells with damaged DNA). The accelerated acquisition of additional genetic lesions in clonogenic preleukemic cells eventually culminates in overt myeloid leukemia. See text for further explanation. (Adapted from ref. 472 by permission.)

these transmembrane proteins phosphorylate themselves as well as their substrates, triggering multiple biochemical regulatory cascades. Critical steps in this process are dimerization of two adjacent receptors to initiate signal transduction and phosphorylation of high affinity-binding sites for the SH2 (Src homology) domains of GRB2 and other specific cytoplasmic signaling molecules that convert RAS proteins to their GTP-bound forms.[322]

The chimeric proteins resulting from receptor tyrosine kinase fusions invariably lack ligand-binding domains, and may lack transmembrane domains, yet they clearly function as oncogenic proteins. The mechanisms responsible for constitutive activation of a tyrosine kinase in the absence of growth factor binding appear to be related to shuttling of the chimera to a new cellular location and to constitutive activation owing to dimerization stimulated by sequences within the nonkinase fusion partner, such as a leucine zipper motif.[323,324] Thus, hybrid proteins with aberrantly activated tyrosine kinase domains represent a novel product of chromosomal rearrangements, further demonstrating the versatility of genetic mechanisms that transform hematopoietic cells.

ABL Fusion Genes in Chronic and Acute Leukemias

The Philadelphia chromosome, produced by a (9;22)(q34;q11) translocation, was first identified in patients with chronic myeloid leukemia (CML) and later shown to occur in 3 percent to 5 percent of children and 30 percent to 40 percent of adults with ALL.[325–327] This translocation results in a *BCR-ABL* chimeric tyrosine kinase oncogene, which contains sequences from the *BCR* gene upstream of the second exon of the *ABL* proto-oncogene.[328–333] Thus, t(9;22) breakpoints on the distal tip of the long arm of chromosome 9 occur in the first intron of the *ABL* proto-oncogene, which spans a distance of more than 100 kb upstream of sequences encoding the tyrosine kinase domain.[334–336] By contrast, the breakpoints on chromosome 22 are confined to a 5.8-kb region of genomic DNA known as the major breakpoint cluster region (M-bcr), which lies within *BCR*, a gene that encodes a 160-kd phosphoprotein.[337,338] The 8.5-kb fusion transcript found in CML encodes a 210-kDa hy-

brid protein that is activated as a tyrosine-specific protein kinase, as is the *v-abl* protein product.[339–342]

Although routine karyotyping does not distinguish between the t(9;22) in CML and ALL, molecular analysis of the *BCR* and *ABL* proto-oncogenes, which are rearranged in both diseases, has revealed differences that apparently mediate the phenotype specificity of these oncogenic fusion kinases.[343–345] In ALL, the rearrangement produces a shorter fusion transcript (6.5–7.0 kb) and hybrid protein (185–190 kDa) than are generated by the *BCR-ABL* fusion gene in CML (Figure 5-10).[343–345] The differences are owing to unique breakpoints on chromosome 22 in ALL cases that do not lie within the 5.8-kb region of *BCR* that contains the breakpoints in CML. Instead, they are contained within a second minor breakpoint cluster region (m-bcr) located further upstream within the *BCR* gene.[346–348] The ALL fusion protein includes amino-terminal *BCR* amino acids but lacks the internal residues that are found in the CML fusion proteins near the *BCR-ABL* junction.

The amino-terminal sequences of *ABL* are removed in oncogenic forms of the gene, and replaced by the Moloney virus *gag* gene in the case of *v-abl* and with *BCR* sequences in the *BCR-ABL* fusion gene of CML and ALL.[339–342,349–351] The products of both the *v-abl* and the *BCR-ABL* fusion genes can transform primary hematopoietic cells in vitro, providing a model system for analysis of oncogenic mechanisms.[352]

Both the P185 and P210 BCR-ABL proteins can also induce a CML-like syndrome in vivo in mice when they are expressed in hematopoietic progenitors.[353–356] Mechanistic studies of these fusion proteins have shown that RAS signaling is essential for transformation, and that multiple alternative means, including the adapters GRB2, SHC, and CRKL, are used to couple the activated ABL kinase to RAS, resulting in activation of Jun kinase.[357–359] Oncogenic signaling by BCR-ABL has also been shown to involve the cell cycle-regulated genes *MYC* and *cyclin D1*, and to constitutively activate the transcriptional signal transducer STAT5.[360–362] The emerging picture is one of multiple signaling pathways that are activated to mediate leukemic transformation by BCR-ABL; hence, selective complementation of defective mutant fusion proteins should allow the identification of genetic pathways that are in-

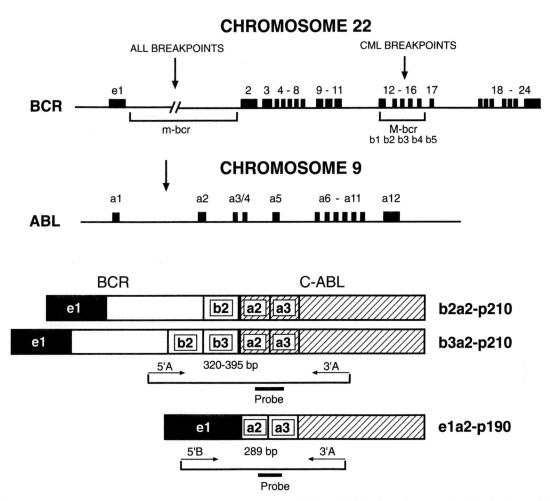

FIG. 5-10 Genomic structure of *BCR* locus on chromosome 22. Breakpoints in chronic myelogenous leukemia (CML) occur primarily in the more 3′ M-bcr region, while those in acute lymphoblastic leukemia (ALL) occur primarily in the m-bcr region. The two common BCR-ABL fusion proteins resulting from M-bcr-type breakpoints are 210 kDa (p210) in size and contain the *BCR* distal exons b1, b2, with or without b3. By contrast, breakpoints in m-bcr result in a fusion protein of 190 kDa (p190) that contains only the first BCR exon, e1. Both the p210 and p190 fusion proteins contain the same portion of ABL. (Adapted from ref. 12 by permission.)

volved in BCR-ABL-mediated hematopoietic cell transformation.[357]

A new mechanism of ABL activation in human leukemia involves a fusion between the Ets transcription factor TEL and the catalytic domain of ABL; the product of this union has been identified in two cases of acute leukemia, one myeloid and the other lymphoid.[363,364] The TEL-ABL fusion kinase resembles the TEL-PDGFβR protein previously described in association with a t(5;12) chromosomal translocation in CML.[365] As with TEL-PDGFβR, the DNA-binding domain of TEL is not incorporated into the chimeric structure. Recently, the TEL-ABL protein was shown to be a constitutively activated kinase located in the cytoskeleton, whose activity depends upon oligomerization mediated through a helix-loop-helix domain in the amino-terminus of TEL.[363]

Progress has also been made in clarifying the normal role of the ABL kinase. Studies in mice rendered *Abl* deficient by homologous recombination indicate that Abl is not required for embryogenesis; however, mice without this protein develop a wasting syndrome and die shortly after birth.[366,367] In contrast to the BCR-ABL proteins, which are cytoplasmic, normal ABL is a nuclear kinase, whose activity is tightly regulated in vivo.[368] Recent evidence suggests that the kinase is activated by DNA-damaging agents, and that it mediates growth arrest in a p53-dependent fashion.[369–373] Although the precise function of ABL is not known, the available evidence suggests that it regulates pathways that mediate cell cycle

arrest after genotoxic damage. It is fascinating that this kinase, which in many ways has functions reminiscent of a tumor suppressor, can be subverted through chromosomal translocation to function in an entirely different cytoplasmic compartment and presumably through different substrates in the malignant transformation of hematopoietic progenitors.

The exceedingly poor prognosis of ALL patients with the Philadelphia chromosome has been attributed to transformation of a primitive hematopoietic stem cell that is inaccessible to most forms of chemotherapy.[327,374–376] Long-term responses (probable cures) have been induced in a subset of children with ALL who have low white blood cell counts at diagnosis, using intensive early-phase chemotherapy, followed by repetitive treatment with pairs of non-cross-resistant drugs.[377] For most patients with BCR-ABL-positive ALL, however, the recommended strategy is allogeneic bone marrow transplantation in first remission, which is also the only known curative approach for CML.[378]

NPM-ALK In Large-Cell Lymphoma

Large-cell lymphomas constitute one-fourth of the non-Hodgkin's lymphomas that develop in children and adolescents. In a subset of these tumors, a t(2;5) chromosomal translocation links amino-terminal sequences of the ubiquitously expressed nucleophosmin

(*NPM*) gene on chromosome 5q35 to the catalytic domain of a previously unidentified tyrosine kinase gene on chromosome 2p23, now termed *ALK* (for anaplastic lymphoma kinase).[379] The NPM phosphoprotein, which shuttles between the nucleolus and the cytoplasm, consists of a putative metal binding site, two acidic amino acid clusters, and two nuclear localization signals.[380–382] NPM is highly phosphorylated during mitosis and serves as a substrate for CDC2.[383] NPM has been shown to bind to RNA, DNA, the HIV Rev protein, transcription factor YY1 and nucleolar protein p120, and is thought to play a role in ribosomal assembly, but its specific function remains undefined.[383–388]

The *ALK* gene product, a tyrosine kinase receptor of 1620 amino acids, shows greatest amino acid identity with members of the insulin receptor subfamily, leukocyte tyrosine kinase in particular (64 percent).[379] Very little is known about the normal function of ALK, with the exception of a recent study indicating that its murine homologue is exclusively expressed in cells of the central and peripheral nervous systems.[389]

The NPM-ALK chimera retains 117 amino acids from NPM and 563 from ALK. In contrast to the cell surface localization of native ALK receptors, immunofluorescence studies with Cos cells have documented both cytoplasmic and nuclear expression of the NPM-ALK chimera.[389,390] The available evidence indicates that the NPM fusion segment contributes an active promoter that drives expression of the ALK kinase domain, and a dimerization signal that stimulates its constitutive activation, leading to lymphomagenesis. The transforming potential of NPM-ALK was recently demonstrated in NIH-3T3 cells and in mice reconstituted with bone marrow cells bearing the chimeric gene.[390,391] In the latter study, half the animals developed lymphoma-like tumors that arose in the mesenteric lymph nodes and metastasized to the lungs and kidneys. In both cases, the tumors bore a T-cell immunophenotype, despite the capacity of the retroviral vector to stimulate gene expression in many types of hematopoietic cells. This selectivity agrees with the generally accepted T-cell origin of human large-cell lymphomas that harbor the t(2;5) and express NPM-ALK. Finally, experiments with NPM-ALK mutants have established a requirement for the NPM sequence in cell transformation and indicate that interaction between ALK and the GRB2 substrate may also be necessary.[390]

Discovery of the *NPM-ALK* fusion gene has definite clinical implications. About one-third of large-cell non-Hodgkin's lymphomas carry the t(2;5) chromosomal translocation, which appears to have prognostic importance.[392] It is not possible to distinguish these cases by classic histologic studies or immunophenotyping, nor do the clinical features of the patients offer diagnostic help. Thus, because of the difficulty of performing cytogenetic studies on lymphoma biopsies, assay techniques for gene abnormalities with DNA- or RNA-based polymerase chain reaction techniques or by fluorescence in situ hybridization assays with interphase cells are needed to ensure early recognition of this genetically defined tumor.[393–395]

TEL-PDGFRβ in Chronic Myelomonocytic Leukemia

An attractive hypothesis is that leukemias and lymphomas develop through an accumulation of multiple genetic changes, which eventually give rise to clonal, neoplastic growth. The transition from normal hematopoiesis to myelodysplastic syndrome (MDS) and then to overt AML affords a model in which one might establish the requirement for serial somatic mutations in the genesis of myeloid leukemia.[396] A possible paradigm for the early events in AML pathogenesis was provided by discovery of the t(5;12)(q33;p13) chromosomal translocation in chronic myelomonocytic leukemia (CMML), an MDS subtype characterized by abnormal clonal myeloid cell proliferation and progression to AML.

The t(5;12) produces a fusion transcript in which the tyrosine kinase and transmembrane domains of the platelet-derived growth factor receptor β gene (*PDGFRβ*) on chromosome 5 linked to a novel *Ets*-like gene (*TEL*) on chromosome 12. The prominent structural features of normal PDGFRβ receptors include five Ig-like extracellular loops and an interrupted intracellular tyrosine kinase domain.[397] This kinase participates in a signal transduction pathway that has a major effect on cell proliferation.[398] Mutated components of the PDGFRβ-related pathway, such as RAS, clearly have transforming potential, as does the PDGFRβ ligand, whose overexpression is associated with a myeloproliferative syndrome in mice.[399]

As emphasized in the preceding section on *AML1* gene fusion, *TEL* is a member of the *Ets* gene family and thus specifies a DNA-binding protein that recognizes the consensus motif C/A GGA A/T.[400] The distinct amino-terminal HLH domain of TEL is essential for full transactivating function, but probably does not bind DNA directly.[401] By analogy to other transcription factors, such as E2A, MYC, and MYOD, this HLH domain may be involved in protein–protein interactions.[363]

In t(5;12)-induced gene fusion, only the amino-terminal HLH domain of *TEL* is incorporated into the chimeric product, which therefore lacks a legitimate DNA-binding domain. How, then, does the TEL-PDGFRβ protein induce CMML? An obvious model is that the retained TEL HLH domain leads to dimerization (hence activation) of the PDGFRβ kinase. Another possibility, raised by retention of the PDGFRβ transmembrane domain, is that the TEL 5′ region acts as a ligand-binding domain by responding to an unknown cognate binding protein. Finally, PDGFRβ may be moved to a new location in the cell, perhaps the nucleus, through localization signals provided by TEL-binding proteins. Displacement to the nucleus could result in phosphorylation of bound transcription factors with consequent aberrant activation of critical downstream targets. Each of these models has been reviewed in detail.[402]

It therefore appears that *TEL-PDGFRβ* fusion is a pivotal early genetic change in the development of CMML. Patients who progress from this MDS subtype to AML often show numerous additional cytogenetic changes, suggesting that malignant progression results from sequential acquisition of new mutations. Identification of the t(5;12) fusion product thus represents an advance in understanding how one form of MDS predisposes to acute leukemia. Recently published evidence indicates that a variant t(5;12) translocation, the t(10;12)(q24;p13), may also generate a novel *TEL* fusion gene associated with refractory anemia, eosinophilia in the bone marrow, and increasing monocytosis.[403]

OTHER MECHANISMS OF TRANSFORMATION MEDIATED BY CHROMOSOMAL TRANSLOCATIONS

Cyclin D1 Activation in Mantle Cell Lymphoma

The t(11;14)(q13;q34) was one of the first chromosomal translocations to be dissected molecularly, based on the realization that the breakpoint on chromosome 14 occurred within the *IgH* gene and use of a probe from this gene to isolate DNA from the so-called *BCL1* region on the long arm of chromosome 11.[404,405] Although additional tumors were identified with breakpoints in this region, it initially proved difficult to identify a proto-oncogene whose expression was altered by the translocation.[406–409] This search has now ended with the identification of the gene encoding cyclin D1

(*CCND1*), located 110 kb distal to the original *BCL1* breakpoint.[410–413] Evidence that cyclin D1 is the proto-oncogene targeted by the t(11;14) includes the facts that it is the closest gene to the breakpoint cluster region on chromosome 11 and that the majority of tumors with this translocation aberrantly express this cell cycle regulatory protein.[414] Cyclin D1 is a member of a family of D-type cyclins that act in concert with their catalytic partners, the cyclin-dependent kinases (CDK4 and CDK6), to initiate the phosphorylation of the retinoblastoma protein, pRB, thus coupling growth factor-induced mitogenic signals to the biochemical machinery of the cell cycle.[415] B cells normally express two other cyclin D family members, cyclins D2 and D3, but not cyclin D1, so that cyclin D1 expression is abnormally induced in this lineage by the translocation, presumably reflecting the influence of the B-cell specific *IgH* gene enhancer from chromosome 14. The coding region of cyclin D1 is not altered by these translocations, the breakpoints of which are often 100 kb or more from the gene itself, implying that uncoupling of cyclin D1 expression from mitogenic signals that normally would regulate the levels of cyclin D2 and D3 provides a constitutive proliferative stimulus.[412,416–418] Presumably, small lymphocytes in the mantle zone of the lymph node that harbor this translocation and aberrantly express cyclin D1 are unable to exit the cell cycle on cue, and thus are unable to differentiate into Ig-secreting plasma cells.[419]

As molecular probes have become available, first for the *BCL1* locus and more recently to identify expression of the cyclin D1 mRNA and protein, it has been possible to clarify the pathologic diagnosis of B cell lymphomas harboring the t(11;14). These tumors were previously called mantle cell or diffuse small cleaved cell lymphomas, but the term mantle cell lymphoma has now been uniformly adopted by international agreement.[419–421] Comprising about 5 percent of lymphomas overall, these tumors occur primarily in elderly men, are of intermediate grade, and do not respond well to available therapies. It is now clear that virtually all mantle cell lymphomas harbor the t(11;14) and express cyclin D1, rendering newly available monoclonal antibodies that recognize this protein especially valuable as immunohistochemical reagents for more accurate diagnosis of this important subset of B-cell malignancies.[422–425]

BCL2 in Follicular Lymphoma

The *BCL2* proto-oncogene was discovered through analysis of genes that are dysregulated by the t(14;18), which is the most common chromosomal translocation among human lymphoid malignancies. The t(14;18) is found in more than 80 percent of follicular center cell lymphomas, a common and generally indolent type of B-cell lymphoma that occurs almost exclusively in adults, and in approximately 20 percent of diffuse adult B-cell lymphomas.[426,427] Molecular analysis of the breakpoints of the 14;18 translocation identified *BCL2* as the gene on chromosome 18 that is overexpressed because of its translocation into the *IgH* locus on chromosome 14.[428–431] Functional studies revealed that BCL2 defines a new class of proto-oncogene products that act to prolong cell survival, rather than through more typical effects on cell differentiation or proliferation.[432–434] It has since been learned that BCL2 is a member of a large family of highly conserved proteins that either inhibit or promote apoptosis, extending down the phylogenetic tree to the CED-9 protein, which inhibits programmed cell death in *C. elegans*.[435,436] This interesting family of proteins is discussed further in a separate chapter in this volume (see Chapter 6).

Nuclear Pore Genes in AML

Three translocations in acute myeloid leukemia have been shown to involve nuclear pore genes, the t(6;9) and a cryptic t(9;9) or inv(9) producing the *DEK-CAN* and *SET-CAN* fusion genes, and the t(7;11) producing a *NUP98-HOXA9* chimera.[437–441] The first of these to be cloned was *DEK-CAN*, which is found in children and young adults with myeloid or myelomonocytic AML (M1, M2, or M4 according to the French-American-British classification). A chimeric DEK-CAN protein is produced, comprising nearly the entire DEK protein fused to the carboxyl-terminal two-thirds of the CAN protein.[437,438] A SET-CAN fusion protein was subsequently identified in leukemic cells from a single patient, indicating a central role for CAN amino acids in the transforming capacity of these proteins, since identical portions of CAN were retained in each of the oncogenic hybrids.[439] Insight into the normal role of CAN came when a component of the nuclear pore complex, called NUP214, was independently purified and shown to be identical to CAN.[442] CAN was shown to be localized to the nuclear pore by immunofluorescence microscopy; by contrast, DEK-CAN proved to be exclusively nuclear, even though the fusion protein retains the nucleoporin-specific FXFG repeats that are thought to mediate protein–protein interactions important for nuclear transport.[443] The essential role of normal CAN in nuclear transport has been proven through studies of embryos in which the gene was inactivated by homologous recombination, and two cellular proteins have been shown to bind to CAN, of which one, a 112-kDa protein, also interacts with the nucleoporin-specific repeat of DEK-CAN and SET-CAN, suggesting that it might play a role in transformation.[444,445]

The nucleoporin connection has recently become even more intriguing with the cloning of the t(7;11) fusion gene, which encodes a hybrid protein containing the characteristic FXFG repeat region of another member of the nucleoporin complex, NUP98, fused in frame to the homeobox domain of the major HOX protein, HOXA9.[440] A current research focus is to determine whether the nucleoporin repeat regions allow these fusion proteins to interfere with protein or RNA transport across the nuclear membrane, resulting in a novel mechanistic contribution to the transformation of myeloid progenitors.[443–445] Alternatively, the presence of the HOXA9 homeodomain in the more recently identified NUP98-HOXA9 fusion protein raises the possibility that these hybrid proteins could interfere with the transcriptional regulation of genes important for myeloid cell development. According to this scenario, the nucleoporin partner may primarily contribute a protein–protein interaction and effector region to the fusion protein, with domains mediating interaction with DNA prompter/enhancer sequences coming from the other partners in these fusions. This would certainly be a plausible mechanism of transformation for the NUP98-HOXA9 fusion protein, because of the emerging evidence that the major HOX proteins contribute to hematopoietic development, as already discussed in the section on MLL fusion proteins and the role of mammalian Mll and *Drosophila* trithorax in *HOX* and *HOM-C* gene regulation.[278,299,300]

Nucleolar NPM-MLF1 Gene in AML

Another translocation specific for hematopoietic neoplasia is the t(3;5)(q25.1;q34), which occurs in a subset of myelodysplastic syndromes and acute myeloid leukemias. We recently demonstrated that the t(3;5) interrupts the *NPM* gene, encoding a nucleolar shuttle protein, which is also interrupted by the t(2;5) in large-cell lymphoma and the t(5;17) in acute promyelocytic leukemia.[245,439] In the t(3;5), the N-terminal portion of NPM is fused in-frame to sequences of a novel gene on chromosome 3 that we have named myelodysplasia/myeloid leukemia factor 1.[446] The *MLF1* gene, which is not expressed by mature blood cells, encodes a cytoplasmic protein containing no identifiable structural motifs. The NPM-MLF1 fusion protein traffics intracellularly under the direction of its NPM amino acid sequences, in that it is predominantly localized within the nucleolus of leukemic cells.[446] These features of MLF1 and NPM-MLF1 suggest that the t(3;5) may contribute to the development of acute myeloid leukemia through a previously unrecognized mechanism. Current efforts are directed toward the biochemical and biological characterization of these proteins, as well as that of *MLF2*, an *MLF1*-related gene that we have recently identified.[447]

FUTURE DIRECTIONS

What has been learned about the transforming roles of transcription factors in leukemias and lymphomas? First is the requirement for proto-oncogene activation, usually by chromosomal rearrangement (through reciprocal translocations, inversions, deletions, or tandem duplications), in which the candidate gene comes to lie in the vicinity of a *TCR* or *lg* gene or is fused with a second gene to form a chimeric protein that may retain many of the key functions of the original factor. Post-activation regulatory events remain largely unknown, although the array of factors so far identified suggests an extraordinarily diverse set of interactions. For example, heterodimerization with other proteins, as in the formation of MYC/MAX, AML1/CBFβ, TAL1/LMO2, or PBX1/HOX complexes, greatly increases the complexity of interactions between oncogenic proteins and transcriptional regulatory networks.

The key to understanding the oncogenic effects of transcription factors lies in the nature of the genes they regulate. Since the majority of these oncoproteins are ectopically expressed, one might predict that they alter the expression of tightly regulated gene programs in normal hematopoietic progenitors. Almost certainly examples will be found in which interaction of these proteins with downstream target genes either activates or represses developmental programs that are normally required only at critical times in the life cycle of the progenitor cell. In some instances, the positive or negative effects of oncogenic transcription factors are probably mediated directly through binding to enhancer sequences in target gene promoters; however, in other cases these proteins may transform cells indirectly, by binding to other transcriptional regulatory proteins and targeting them to nonfunctional or newly functional complexes.

Thus, the main challenge for the future is to identify the gene programs controlled by the various transcription factors activated by chromosomal rearrangements. Equally important will be the task of delineating subsequent interactive processes within transcriptional regulatory cascades. This is likely to be even more difficult than deciphering the molecular mechanisms regulating *Drosophila* embryogenesis, because of the greater complexity of experimental embryology and genetic analysis in vertebrate model systems. Clues to the normal roles of key gene products will continue to be provided by murine models, in which individual proto-oncogenes are targeted for inactivation by homologous recombination. The oncogenic targets of these proteins in leukemias and lymphomas may still be difficult to decipher, because chromosomal translocations often mediate aberrant expression of genes in hematopoietic cells, either as inappropriately expressed intact proteins or as chimeric proteins that contain regulatory subunits from two different proteins.

With increased knowledge of the regulatory networks affected by oncogenic transcription factors, it may be possible to develop new therapeutic strategies for human malignancies, similar to those employing all-*trans*-retinoic acid for the treatment of acute promyelocytic leukemia. Indeed, if a fusion protein is crucial to malignant growth, one could alter the disease course by interfering

with any of the multiple steps in protein synthesis and action, including oncogene transcription, RNA processing and translation, and DNA or protein–protein interactions. Fused transcription factors would appear ideal for these types of intervention, because they represent true chimeras that occur only in rare types of malignant cells. A clear advantage of this approach, which depends on a detailed understanding of the mechanisms underlying each hybrid factor's transforming properties, would be the reduced likelihood of toxicity to normal cells or the development of resistant mutants, by comparison to currently available methods of cancer therapy.

Finally, it is important to realize that aberrant activation of proto-oncogenes by chromosomal translocations are but one event in the multistep process of carcinogenesis. Future molecular research into the leukemias and lymphomas will undoubtedly uncover an array of inactivating mutations affecting tumor suppressors, which act synergistically with proto-oncogenes activated by genetic rearrangement and are required for full expression of malignant phenotypes in hematopoietic cells.

ACKNOWLEDGMENTS

I would like to thank John Gilbert for editorial review and critical comments, and Steve Morris, Anne Dejean, Cornelis Murre, T. H. Rabbitts, Nancy Speck, Paul Liu, Ethan Dmitrovsky, and Jonathan Licht for helpful comments on the manuscript. Supported in part by NIH grants CA-59571, CA-21765, CA-20180, and CA-71907, and by the American Lebanese Syrian Associated Charities (ALSAC).

REFERENCES

1. Bishop JM: The molecular genetics of cancer. *Science* **235**:305, 1987.
2. Solomon E, Borrow J, Goddard AD: Chromosome aberrations and cancer. *Science* **254**:1153, 1991.
3. Rowley JD: Molecular cytogenetics: Rosetta stone for understanding cancer—twenty-ninth G. H. A. Clowes memorial award lecture. *Cancer Res* **50**:3816, 1990.
4. Shivdasani RA, Orkin SH: The transcriptional control of hematopoiesis. *Blood* **87**:4025, 1996.
5. Rabbitts TH: Chromosomal translocations in human cancer. *Nature* **372**:143, 1994.
6. Look AT: Oncogenic role of "master" transcription factors in human leukemias and sarcomas: A developmental model, in Vande Woude G (ed): *Advances in Cancer Research.* San Diego, Academic Press, 1995, p. 25.
7. Rabbitts TH: Translocations, master genes, and differences between the origins of acute and chronic leukemias. *Cell* **67**:641, 1991.
8. Nusslein-Volhard C, Wieschaus E: Mutations affecting segment number and polarity in Drosophila. *Nature* **287**:795, 1980.
9. Nusslein-Volhard C, Frohnhofer HG, Lehmann R: Determination of anteroposterior polarity in Drosophila. *Science* **238**:1675, 1987.
10. Levine MS, Harding KW: Drosophila: The zygotic contribution, in Glover DM, Hames BD (eds): Genes and Embryos. New York, IRL, 1989, p. 39.
11. Rowley JD, Aster JC, Sklar J: The clinical applications of new DNA diagnostic technology on the management of cancer patients. *J Am Med Assoc* **270**:2331, 1993.
12. Okuda T, Fisher R, Downing JR: Molecular diagnostics in pediatric acute lymphoblastic leukemia. *Mol Diag* **1**:139: 1996.
13. Pui C-H: Childhood leukemias. *N Engl J Med* **332**:1618, 1995.
14. Papavassiliou AG: Molecular medicine transcription factors. *N Engl J Med* **332**:45, 1995.
15. Dalla-Favera R, Bregni M, Erikson J, Patterson D, Gallo RC, Croce CM: Human c-myc onc gene is located on the region of chromosome 8 that is translocated in Burkitt lymphoma cells. *Proc Natl Acad Sci USA* **79**:7824, 1982.

16. Taub R, Kirsch I, Morton C, Lenoir G, Swan D, Tronick S, Aaronson S, Leder P: Translocation of the C-*myc* gene into the immunoglobulin heavy chain locus in human Burkitt lymphoma and murine plasmacytoma cell. *Proc Natl Acad Sci USA* **79**:7837, 1982.

17. Adams JM, Gerondakis S, Webb E, et al. Cellular *myc* oncogene is altered by chromosome translocation to an immunoglobulin locus in murine plasmacytomas and is rearranged similarly in Burkitt lymphomas. *Proc Natl Acad Sci USA* **80**:1982, 1983.

18. Emanuel BS, Selden JR, Chaganti RSK, et al: The 2p breakpoint of a 2;8 translocation in Burkitt lymphoma interrupts the V kappa locus. *Proc Natl Acad Sci USA* **81**:2444, 1984.

19. Erikson J, Nishikura K, ar-Rushdi A, et al: Translocation of an immunoglobulin kappa locus to a region 3′ of an unrearranged *c-myc* oncogene enhances *c-myc* transcription. *Proc Natl Acad Sci USA* **80**:7581, 1983.

20. Hollis GF, Mitchell KF, Battey J, et al: A variant translocation places the lambda immunoglobulin genes 3′ to the *c-myc* oncogene in Burkitt's lymphoma. *Nature* **307**:752, 1984.

21. Rappold GA, Hameister H, Cremer T, et al: *C-myc* and immunoglobulin kappa light chain constant genes are on the 8q+ chromosome of three Burkitt lymphoma lines with t(2;8) translocations. *EMBO J* **3**:2951, 1984.

22. Croce CM, Thierfelder W, Erikson J, Nishikura K, Finan J, Lenoir GM, Nowell PC: Transcriptional activation of an unrearranged and untranslocated c-myc oncogene by translocation of a C lambda locus in Burkitt lymphoma. *Proc Natl Acad Sci USA* **80**:6922, 1983.

23. Taub R, Kelly K, Battey J, Latt S, Lenoir GM, Tantravahi U, Tu Z, Leder P: A novel alteration in the structure of an activated c-myc gene in a variant t(2;8) Burkitt lymphoma. *Cell* **37**:511, 1984.

24. Rabbitts TH, Hamlyn PH, Baer R: Altered nucleotide sequences of a translocated c-myc gene in Burkitt lymphoma. *Nature* **306**:760, 1983.

25. Pelicci PG, Knowles DM, 2d, Magrath I, Dalla-Favera R, Knowles DM: Chromosomal breakpoints and structural alterations of the c-myc locus differ in endemic and sporadic forms of Burkitt lymphoma. *Proc Natl Acad Sci USA* **83**:2984, 1986.

26. Taub R, Moulding C, Battey J, Murphy W, Vasicek T, Lenoir GM, Leder P: Activation and somatic mutation of the translocated c-myc gene in Burkitt lymphoma cells. *Cell* **36**:339, 1984.

27. Bhatia K, Spangler G, Gaidano G, Hamdy N, Dalla-Favera R, Magrath I: Mutations in the coding region of c-myc occur frequently in acquired immunodeficiency syndrome-associated lymphomas. *Blood* **84**:883, 1994.

28. Gu W, Bhatia K, Magrath IT, Dang CV, Dalla-Favera R: Binding and suppression of the myc transcriptional activation domain by p107. *Science* **264**:251, 1994.

29. Blackwood EM, Eisenman RN: Max: A helix-loop-helix zipper protein that forms a sequence-specific DNA-binding complex with Myc. *Science* **251**:1211, 1991.

30. Prendergast GC, Lawe D, Ziff EB: Association of Myn, the murine homolog of Max, with c-Myc stimulates methylation-sensitive DNA binding and Ras cotransformation. *Cell* **65**:395, 1991.

31. Ayer DE, Kretzner L, Eisenman RN: Mad: A heterodimeric partner for Max that antagonizes Myc transcriptional activity. *Cell* **72**:211, 1993.

32. Zervos AS, Gyuris J, Brent R: Mxi1, a protein that specifically interacts with Max to bind Myc-Mas recognition sites. *Cell* **72**:223, 1993.

33. Ayer DE, Lawrence QA, Eisenman RN: Mad-Max transcriptional repression is mediated by ternary complex formation with mammalian homologs of yeast repressor Sin3. *Cell* **80**:767, 1995.

34. Schreiber-Agus N, Chin L, Chen K, Torres R, Rao G, Guida P, Skoultchi AI, DePinho RA: An amino-terminal domain of Mxi1 mediates anti-Myc oncogenic activity and interacts with a homolog of the yeast transcriptional repressor SIN3. *Cell* **80**:777, 1995.

35. Ayer DE, Eisenman RN: A switch from Myc:Max to Mad:Max heterocomplexes accompanies monocyte/macrophage differentiation. *Gene Dev* **7**:2110, 1993.

36. Larsson LG, Pettersson M, Oberg F, Nilsson K, Luscher B: Expression of mad, mxi1, max and c-myc during induced differentiation of hematopoietic cells: Opposite regulation of mad and c-myc. *Oncogene* **9**:1247, 1994.

37. Amati B, Brooks MW, Levy N, Littlewood TD, Evan GI, Land H: Oncogenic activity of the c-Myc protein requires dimerization with Max. *Cell* **72**:233, 1993.

38. Adams JM, Harris AW, Pinkert CA, Corcoran LM, Alexander WS, Cory S, Palmiter RD, Brinster RL: The c-*myc* oncogene driven by immunoglobulin enhancers induces lymphoid malignancy in transgenic mice. *Nature* **318**:533, 1985.

39. Langdon WY, Harris AW, Cory S, Adams JM: The C-*myc* oncogene perturbs B lymphocyte development in Emu-*myc* transgenic mice. *Cell* **47**:11, 1986.

40. Lombardi L, Newcomb EW, Dalla-Favera R: Pathogenesis of Burkitt lymphoma: expression of an activated c-myc oncogene causes the tumorigenic conversion of EBV-infected human B lymphoblasts. *Cell* **49**:161, 1987.

41. Packham G, Cleveland JL: c-myc and apoptosis. *Biochim Biophys Acta* **1242**:11, 1995.

42. Galaktionov K, Chen X, Beach D: Cdc25 cell-cycle phosphatase as a target of c-myc. *Nature* **382**:511, 1996.

43. Begley CG, Aplan PD, Davey MP, Nakahara K, Tchorz K, Kurtzberg J, Hershfield MS, Haynes BF, Cohen DI, Waldmann TA, et al: Chromosomal translocation in a human leukemic stem-cell line disrupts the T-cell antigen receptor delta-chain diversity region and results in a previously unreported fusion transcript. *Proc Natl Acad Sci USA* **86**:2031, 1989.

44. Chen Q, Cheng JT, Tasi LH, Schneider N, Buchanan G, Carroll A, Crist W, Ozanne B, Siciliano MJ, Baer R: The tal gene undergoes chromosome translocation in T cell leukemia and potentially encodes a helix-loop-helix protein. *EMBO J* **9**:415, 1990.

45. Xia Y, Brown L, Yang CY, Tsan JT, Siciliano MJ, Espinosa R, III, Le Beau MM, Baer RJ: TAL2, a helix-loop-helix gene activated by the (7;9)(q34;q32) translocation in human T-cell leukemia. *Proc Natl Acad Sci USA* **88**:11416, 1991.

46. Mellentin JD, Smith SD, Cleary ML: *Lyl-l*, A novel gene altered by chromosomal translocation in T-cell leukemia, codes for a protein with a helix-loop-helix DNA binding motif. *Cell* **58**:77, 1989.

47. Shivdasani RA, Mayer EL, Orkin SH: Absence of blood formation in mice lacking the T-cell leukemia oncoprotein tal-1/SCL. *Nature* **373**:432, 1995.

48. Robb L, Lyons I, Li R, Hartley L, Kontgen F, Harvey RP, Metcalf D, Begley CG: Absence of yolk sac hematopoiesis from mice with a targeted disruption of the scl gene. *Proc Natl Acad Sci USA* **92**:7075, 1995.

49. Finger LR, Harvey RC, Moore RC, Showe LC, Croce CM: A common mechanism of chromosomal translocation in T- and B-cell neoplasia. *Science* **234**:982, 1986.

50. McKeithan TW, Shima EA, LeBeau MM, Minowada J, Rowley JD, Diaz MO: Molecular cloning of the breakpoint junction of a human chromosomal 8;14 translocation involving the T-cell receptor alpha-chain gene and sequences on the 3′ side of MYC. *Proc Natl Acad Sci USA* **83**:6636, 1986.

51. Shima EA, Le Beau MM, McKeithan TW, Minowada J, Showe LC, Mak TW, Minden MD, Rowley JD, Diaz MO: Gene encoding the alpha chain of the T-cell receptor is moved immediately downstream of c-myc in a chromosomal 8;14 translocation in a cell line from a human T-cell leukemia. *Proc Natl Acad Sci USA* **83**:3439, 1986.

52. Brown L, Cheng JT, Chen Q, Siciliano MJ, Crist W, Buchanan G, Baer R: Site-specific recombination of the tal-1 gene is a common occurrence in human T cell leukemia. *EMBO J* **9**:3343, 1990.

53. Aplan PD, Lombardi DP, Kirsch IR: Structural characterization of SIL, a gene frequently disrupted in T-cell acute lymphoblastic leukemia. *Mol Cell Biol* **11**:5462, 1991.

54. Aplan PD, Lombardi DP, Reaman GH, Sather HN, Hammond GD, Kirsch IR: Involvement of the putative hematopoietic transcription factor SCL in T-cell acute lymphoblastic leukemia. *Blood* **79**:1327, 1992.

55. Bernard O, Lecointe N, Jonveaux P, Souyri M, Mauchauffe M, Berger R, Larsen CJ, Mathieu-Mahul D: Two site-specific deletions and t(1;14) translocation restricted to human T-cell acute leukemias disrupt the 5′ part of the tal-1 gene. *Oncogene* **6**:1477, 1991.

56. Breit TM, Mol EJ, Wolvers-Tettero IL, Ludwig WD, van Wering ER, van Dongen JJ: Site-specific deletions involving the tal-1 and sil genes are restricted to cells of the T cell receptor alpha/beta lineage: T cell receptor delta gene deletion mechanism affects multiple genes. *J Exp Med* **177**:965, 1993.

57. Baer R: TAL1, TAL2, and LYL1: a family of basic helix-loop-helix proteins implicated in T cell acute leukaemia. *Sem Cancer Biol* **4**:341, 1993.

58. Bash RO, Hall S, Timmons CF, Crist WM, Amylon M, Smith RG, Baer R: Does activation of the TAL1 gene occur in a majority of patients with T-cell acute lymphoblastic leukemia? A pediatric oncology group study. *Blood* **86**:666, 1995.

59. Hsu H, Cheng J, Chen Q, Baer R: Enhancer-binding activity of the tal-1 oncoprotein in association with the E47/E12 helix-loop-helix proteins. *Mol Cell Biol* **11**:3037, 1991.

60. Hsu HL, Huang L, Tsan JT, Funk W, Wright WE, Hu JS, Kingston RE, Baer R: Preferred sequences for DNA recognition by the TAL1 helix-loop-helix proteins. *Mol Cell Biol* **14**:1256, 1994.

61. Hsu HL, Wadman I, Baer R: Formation of in vivo complexes between the TAL1 and E2A polypeptides of leukemic T cells. *Proc Natl Acad Sci USA* **91**:3181, 1994.

62. Wadman I, Li J, Bash RO, Forster A, Osada H, Rabbitts TH, Baer R: Specific in vivo association between the bHLH and LIM proteins implicated in human T cell leukemia. *EMBO J* **13**:4831, 1994.

63. Larson RC, Lavenir I, Larson TA, Baer R, Warren AJ, Wadman I, Nottage K, Rabbitts TH: Protein dimerization between Lmo2 (Rbtn2) and Tal1 alters thymocyte development and potentiates T cell tumorigenesis in transgenic mice. *EMBO J* **15**:1021, 1996.

64. Voronova AF, Lee F: The E2A and tal-1 helix-loop-helix proteins associate in vivo and are modulated by ld proteins during interleukin 6-induced myeloid differentiation. *Proc Natl Acad Sci USA* **91**:5952, 1994.

65. Hsu HL, Wadman I, Tsan JT, Baer R: Positive and negative transcriptional control by the TAL1 helix-loop-helix protein. *Proc Natl Acad Sci USA* **91**:5947, 1994.

66. Porcher C, Swat W, Rockwell K, Fujiwara Y, Alt FW, Orkin SH: The T cell leukemia oncoprotein SCL/tal-1 is essential for development of all hematopoietic lineages. *Cell* **86**:47, 1996.

67. Green AR, Salvaris E, Begley CG: Erythroid expression of the 'helix-loop-helix' gene, SCL. *Oncogene* **6**:475, 1991.

68. Kallianpur AR, Jordan JE, Brandt SJ: The SCL/TAL-1 gene is expressed in progenitors of both the hematopoietic and vascular systems during embryogenesis. *Blood* **83**:1200, 1994.

69. Mouthon MA, Bernard O, Mitjavila MT, Romeo PH, Vainchenker W, Mathieu-Mahul D: Expression of tal-1 and GATA-binding proteins during human hematopoiesis. *Blood* **81**:647, 1993.

70. Visvader J, Begley CG, Adams JM: Differential expression of the LYL, SCL and E2A helix-loop-helix genes within the hemopoietic system. *Oncogene* **6**:187, 1991.

71. Weintraub H: The MyoD family and myogenesis: redundancy, networks, and thresholds. *Cell* **75**:1241, 1993.

72. Buckingham M: Molecular biology of muscle development. *Cell* **78**:15, 1994.

73. McGuire EA, Hockett RD, Pollock KM, Bartholdi MF, O'Brien SJ, Korsmeyer SJ: The t(11;14)(p15;q11) in a T-cell acute lymphoblastic leukemia cell line activates multiple transcripts, including ttg-1, a gene encoding a potential zinc finger protein. *Mol Cell Biol* **9**:2124, 1989.

74. Greenberg JM, Boehm T, Sofroniew MV, Keynes RJ, Barton SC, Norris ML, Surani MA, Spillantini MG, Rabbitts TH: Segmental and developmental regulation of a presumptive T-cell oncogene in the central nervous system. *Nature* **344**:158, 1990.

75. Boehm T, Foroni L, Kaneko Y, Perutz MF, Rabbitts TH: The rhombotin family of cysteine-rich LIM-domain oncogenes: distinct members are involved in T-cell translocations to human chromosomes 11p15 and 11p13. *Proc Natl Acad Sci USA* **88**:4367, 1991.

76. Royer-Pokora B, Loos U, Ludwig WD: TTG-2, a new gene encoding a cysteine-rich protein with the LIM motif, is overexpressed in acute T-cell leukaemia with the t(11;14)(p13;q11). *Oncogene* **6**:1887, 1991.

77. Warren AJ, Colledge WH, Carlton MBL, Evans MJ, Smith AJH, Rabbitts TH: The oncogenic cysteine-rich LIM domain protein Rbtn2 is essential for erythroid development. *Cell* **78**:45, 1994.

78. Perez-Alvarado GC, et al: Structure of the carboxy-terminal LIM domain from the cysteine rich protein CRP. *Nat Struct Biol* **1**:388, 1994.

79. Valge-Archer VE, Osada H, Warren AJ, Forster A, Li J, Baer R, Rabbitts TH: The LIM protein RBTN2 and the basic helix-loop-helix protein TAL1 are present in a complex in erythroid cells. *Proc Natl Acad Sci USA* **91**:8617, 1994.

80. Robb L, Elwood NJ, Elefanty AG, Kontgen F, Li R, Barnett LD, Begley CG: The SCL gene product is required for the generation of all hematopoietic lineages in the adult mouse. *EMBO J* **15**:4123, 1996.

81. Osada H, Grutz G, Axelson H, Forster A, Rabbitts TH: Association of erythroid transcription factors: complexes involving the LIM protein RBTN2 and the zinc-finger protein GATA1. *Proc Natl Acad Sci USA* **92**:9585, 1995.

82. Pevny L, Simon MC, Robertson E, Klein WH, Tsai SF, D'Agati V, Orkin SH, Costantini F: Erythroid differentiation in chimaeric mice blocked by a targeted mutation in the gene for transcription factor GATA-1. *Nature* **349**:257, 1991.

83. McGuire EA, Rintoul CE, Sclar GM, Korsmeyer SJ: Thymic overexpression of Ttg-1 in transgenic mice results in T-cell acute lymphoblastic leukemia/lymphoma. *Mol Cell Biol* **12**:4186, 1992.

84. Larson RC, Fisch P, Larson TA, Lavenir I, Langford T, King G, Rabbitts TH: T cell tumours of disparate phenotype in mice transgenic for Rbtn-2. *Oncogene* **9**:3675, 1994.

85. Larson RC, Osada H, Larson TA, Lavenir I, Rabbitts TH: The oncogenic LIM protein Rbtn2 causes thymic developmental aberrations that precede malignancy in transgenic mice. *Oncogene* **11**:853, 1995.

86. Fisch P, Boehm T, Lavenir I, Larson T, Arno J, Forster A, Rabbitts TH: T-cell acute lymphoblastic lymphoma induced in transgenic mice by the RBTN1 and RBTN2 LIM-domain genes. *Oncogene* **7**:2389, 1992.

87. Neale GA, Rehg JE, Goorha RM: Ectopic expression of rhombotin-2 causes selective expansion of CD4- CD8- lymphocytes in the thymus and T-cell tumors in transgenic mice. *Blood* **86**:3060, 1995.

88. Robb L, Rasko JE, Bath ML, Strasser A, Begley CG: Scl, a gene frequently activated in human T cell leukaemia, does not induce lymphomas in transgenic mice. *Oncogene* **10**:205, 1995.

89. Kelliher MA, Seldin DC, Leder P: TAL-1 induces T cell acute lymphoblastic leukemia accelerated by casein kinase IIalpha. *EMBO J* **15**:5160, 1996.

90. Hatano M, Roberts CW, Minden M, Crist WM, Korsmeyer SJ: Deregulation of a homeobox gene, HOX11, by the t(10;14) in T cell leukemia. *Science* **253**:79, 1991.

91. Kennedy MA, Gonzalez-Sarmiento R, Kees UR, Lampert F, Dear N, Boehm T, Rabbitts TH: HOX11, a homeobox-containing T-cell oncogene on human chromosome 10q24. *Proc Natl Acad Sci USA* **88**:8900, 1991.

92. Lu M, Gong ZY, Shen WF, Ho AD: The tcl-3 proto-oncogene altered by chromosomal translocation in T-cell leukemia codes for a homeobox protein. *EMBO J* **10**:2905, 1991.

93. Dube ID, Kamel-Reid S, Yuan CC, Lu M, Wu X, Corpus G, Raimondi SC, Crist WM, Carroll AJ, Minowada J, Baker JB: A novel human homeobox gene lies at the chromosome 10 breakpoint in lymphoid neoplasias with chromosomal translocation t(10;14). *Blood* **78**:2996, 1991.

94. Dear TN, Sanchez-Garcia I, Rabbitts TH: The HOX11 gene encodes a DNA-binding nuclear transcription factor belonging to a distinct family of homeobox genes. *Proc Natl Acad Sci USA* **90**:4431, 1993.

95. Allen JD, Lints T, Jenkins NA, Copeland NG, Strasser A, Harvey RP, Adams JM: Novel murine homeobox gene on chromosome 1 expressed in specific hematopoietic lineages and during embryogenesis. *Gene Dev* **5**:509, 1991.

96. McGinnis W, Krumlauf R: Homeobox genes and axial patterning. *Cell* **68**:283, 1992.

97. Roberts CWM, Shutter JR, Korsmeyer SJ: Hox11 controls the genesis of the spleen. *Nature* **368**:747, 1994.

98. Dear TN, Colledge WH, Carlton MB, Lavenir I, Larson T, Smith AJ, Warren AJ, Evans MJ, Sofroniew MV, Rabbitts TH: The Hox11 gene is essential for cell survival during spleen development. *Development* **121**:2909, 1995.

99. Hatano M, Roberts CWM, Kawabe T, Shutter J, Korsmeyer SJ: Cell cycle progression, cell death and T cell lymphoma in HOX11 transgenic mice. [Abstract] *Blood* **80**:355a, 1992.

100. Murre C, McCaw PS, Baltimore D: A new DNA binding and dimerization motif in immunoglobulin enhancer binding, daughterless, MyoD, and myc proteins. *Cell* **56**:777, 1989.

101. Murre C, McCaw PS, Vaessin H, Caudy M, Jan LY, Cabrera CV, Buskin JN, Hauschka SD, Lassar AB, Weintraub H, Baltimore D: Interactions between heterologous helix-loop-helix proteins generate complexes that bind specifically to a common DNA sequence. *Cell* **58**:537, 1989.

102. Sun XH, Baltimore D: An inhibitory domain of E12 transcription factor prevents DNA binding in E12 homodimers but not in E12 heterodimers. *Cell* **64**:459, 1991.

103. Henthorn P, Kiledjian M, Kadesch T: Two distinct transcription factors that bind the immunoglobulin enhancer E5/E2 motif. *Science* **247**:467, 1990.

104. Henthorn P, McCarrick-Walmsley R, Kadesch T: Sequence of the cDNA encoding ITF-1, a positive-acting transcription factor. *Nuc Acids Res* **18**:677, 1990.

105. Cronmiller C, Schedl P, Cline TY: Molecular characterization of daughterless, a Drosophila sex determination gene with multiple roles in development. *Gene Dev* **2**:1666, 1988.

106. Caudy M, Vassin H, Brand M, Tuma R, Jan LY, Jan YN: Daughterless, a Drosophila gene essential for both neurogenesis and sex determination, has sequence similarities to myc and the achaete–scute complex. *Cell* **55**:1061, 1988.

107. Blackwell TK, Weintraub H: Differences and similarities in DNA-binding preferences of MyoD and E2A protein complexes revealed by binding site selection. *Science* **250**:1104, 1990.

108. Ellenberger T, Fass D, Arnaud M, Harrison SC: Crystal structure of transcription factor E47: E-box recognition by a basic region helix-loop-helix dimer. *Gene Dev* **8**:970, 1994.

109. Aronheim A, Shiran R, Rosen A, Walker MD: The E2A gene product contains two separable and functionally distinct transcription activation domains. *Proc Natl Acad Sci USA* **90**:8063, 1993.

110. Quong MW, Massari ME, Zwart R, Murre C: A new transcriptional-activation motif restricted to a class of helix-loop-helix proteins is functionally conserved in both yeast and mammalian cells. *Mol Cell Biol* **13**:792, 1993.

111. Lassar AB, Davis RL, Wright WE, Kadesch T, Murre C, Voronova A, Baltimore D, Weintraub H: Functional activity of myogenic HLH proteins requires hetero-oligomerization with E12/E47-like proteins in vivo. *Cell* **66**:305, 1991.

112. Xia Y, Hwang LH, Cobb MH, Baer RJ: Products of the TAL2, oncogene in leukemic T cells: bHLH phosphoproteins with DNA-binding activity. *Oncogene* **9**:1437, 1994.

113. Bain G, Gruenwald S, Murre C: E2A and E2-2 are subunits of B-cell-specific E2-box DNA-binding proteins. *Mol Cell Biol* **13**:3522, 1993.

114. Benezra R: An intermolecular disulfide bond stabilizes E2A homo-dimers and is required for DNA binding at physiological temperatures. *Cell* **79**:1057, 1994.

115. Bain G, Robanus-Maandag EC, Izon DJ, Amsen D, Kruisbeek AM, Weintraub BC, Krop I, Schlissel MS, Feeney AJ, van Roon M, van der Valk M, te Riele HPJ, Berns A, Murre C: E2A proteins are required for proper B-cell development and initiation of immunoglobulin gene rearrangements. *Cell* **79**:885, 1994.

116. Zhuang Y, Soriano P, Weintraub H: The helix-loop-helix gene E2A is required for B-cell formation. *Cell* **79**:875, 1994.

117. Mellentin JD, Murre C, Donlon TA, McCaw PS, Smith SD, Carroll AJ, McDonald ME, Baltimore D, Cleary ML: The gene for enhancer binding proteins E12/E47 lies at the t(1;19) breakpoint in acute leukemias. *Science* **246**:379, 1989.

118. Kamps MP, Murre C, Sun XH, Baltimore D: A new homeobox gene contributes the DNA binding domain of the t(1;19) translocation protein in pre-B ALL. *Cell* **60**:547, 1990.

119. Nourse J, Mellentin JD, Galili N, Wilkinson J, Stanbridge E, Smith SD, Cleary ML: Chromosomal translocation t(1;19) results in synthesis of a homeobox fusion mRNA that codes for a potential chimeric transcription factor. *Cell* **60**:535, 1990.

120. Mellentin JD, Nourse J, Hunger SP, Smith SD, Cleary ML: Molecular analysis of the t(1;19) breakpoint cluster region in pre-B cell acute lymphoblastic leukemias. *Genes Chrom Cancer* **2**:239, 1990.

121. Aronheim A, Shiran R, Rosen A, Walker MD: The E2A gene product contains two separable and functionally distinct transcription activation domains. *Proc Natl Acad Sci USA* **90**:8063, 1993.

122. Quong MW, Massari ME, Zwart R, Murre C: A new transcriptional-activation motif restricted to a class of helix-loop-helix proteins is functionally conserved in both yeast and mammalian cells. *Mol Cell Biol* **13**:792, 1993.

123. Van Dijk MA, Voorhoeve PM, Murre C: Pbx1 is converted into a transcriptional activator upon acquiring the N-terminal region of E2A in pre-B-cell acute lymphoblastoid leukemia. *Proc Natl Acad Sci USA* **90**:6061, 1993.

124. LeBrun DL, Cleary ML: Fusion with E2A alters the transcriptional properties of the homeodomain protein PBX1 in t(1;19) leukemias. *Oncogene* **9**:1641, 1994.

125. Lu Q, Wright DD, Kamps MP: Fusion with E2A converts the Pbx1 homeodomain protein into a constitutive transcriptional activator in human leukemias carrying the t(1;19) translocation. *Mol Cell Biol* **14**:3938, 1994.

126. Flegel WA, Singson AW, Margolis JS, Bang AG, Posakony JW, Murre C: Dpbx, a new homeobox gene closely related to the human proto-oncogene pbx1 molecular structure and developmental expression. *Mech Dev* **41**:155, 1993.

127. Rauskolb C, Peifer M, Weischaus E: Extradenticle, a regulator of homeotic gene activity, is a homolog of the homeobox-containing human proto-oncogene pbx1. *Cell* **74**:1101, 1993.

128. Weischaus E, Nusslein-Volhard C, Jurgens G: Mutations affecting the pattern of the larval cuticle in Drosophila melanogaster, III. Zygotic loci on the X chromosome and the fourth chromosome. *Arch Dev Biol* **193**:267, 1984.

129. Peifer M, Wieschaus E: Mutations in the Drosophila gene extradenticle affect the way specific homeo domain proteins regulate segmental identity. *Gene Dev* **4**:1209, 1990.

130. Chan S, Jaffe L, Capovilla M, Botas J, Mann RS: The DNA binding specificity of ultrabithorax is modulated by cooperative interactions with extradenticle, another homeoprotein. *Cell* **78**:603, 1994.

131. Rauskolb C, Wieschaus E: Coordinate regulation of downstream genes by extradenticle and the homeotic selector proteins. *EMBO J* **13**:3561, 1994.

132. Van Dijk MA, Murre C: Extradenticle raises the DNA binding specificity of homeotic selector gene products. *Cell* **78**:617, 1994.

133. Johnson FB, Parker E, Krasnow MA: Extradenticle protein is a selective cofactor for the Drosophila homeotics: role of the homeodomain and YPWM amino acid motif in the interaction. *Proc Natl Acad Sci USA* **92**:739, 1995.

134. Chang CP, Shen WF, Rozenfeld S, Lawrence HJ, Largman C, Cleary ML: Pbx proteins display hexapeptide-dependent cooperative DNA binding with a subset of Hox proteins. *Gene Dev* **9**:663, 1995.

135. Lu Q, Kamps MP: Structural determinants within Pbx1 that mediate cooperative DNA binding with pentapeptide-containing hox proteins: proposal for a model of a Pbx1-Hox-DNA complex. *Mol Cell Biol* **16**:1632, 1996.

136. Neuteboom ST, Peltenburg LT, Van Dijk MA, Murre C: The hexapeptide LFPWMR in Hoxb-8 is required for cooperative DNA binding with Pbx1 and Pbx2 proteins. *Proc Natl Acad Sci USA* **92**:9166, 1995.

137. Van Dijk MA, Peltenburg LT, Murre C: Hox gene products modulate the DNA binding activity of Pbx1 and Pbx2. *Mech Dev* **52**:99, 1995.

138. Lu Q, Knoepfler PS, Scheele J, Wright DD, Kamps MP: Both Pbx1 and E2A-Pbx1 bind the DNA motif ATCAATCAA cooperatively with the products of multiple murine Hox genes, some of which are themselves oncogenes. *Mol Cell Biol* **15**:3786, 1995.

139. Knoepfler PS, Kamps MP: The pentapeptide motif of Hox proteins is required for cooperative DNA binding with Pbx1, physically contacts Pbx1, and enhances DNA binding by Pbx1. *Mol Cell Biol* **15**:5811, 1995.

140. Kamps MP, Baltimore D: E2A-Pbx1, the t(1;19) translocation protein of human pre-B-cell acute lymphocytic leukemia, causes acute myeloid leukemia in mice. *Mol Cell Biol* **13**:351, 1993.

141. Kamps MP, Wright DD: Oncoprotein E2A-pbx1 immortalizes a myeloid progenitor in primary marrow cultures without abrogating its factor-dependence. *Oncogene* **9**:3159, 1994.

142. Privitera E, Kamps MP, Hayashi Y, Inaba T, Shapiro LH, Raimondi SC, Behm F, Hendershot L, Carroll AJ, Baltimore D, Look AT: Different molecular consequences of the 1;19 chromosomal translocation in childhood B-cell precursor acute lymphoblastic leukemia. *Blood* **79**:1781, 1992.

143. Borowitz MJ, Hunger SP, Carroll AJ, Shuster JJ, Pullen DJ, Steuber PJ, Cleary ML: Predictability of the t(1;19)(q23;p13) from surface antigen phenotype. Implications for screening cases of childhood ALL for molecular analysis. A Pediatric Oncology Group Study. *Blood* **82**:1086, 1993.

144. Dedera DA, Waller EK, LeBrun DP, Sen-Majumdar A, Stevens ME, Barsh GS, Cleary ML: Chimeric homeobox gene E2A-PBX1 induces proliferation, apoptosis, and malignant lymphomas in transgenic mice. *Cell* **74**:833, 1993.

145. Monica K, LeBrun DP, Dedera DA, Brown R, Cleary ML: Transformation properties of the E2A-PBX1 chimeric oncoprotein: Fusion with E2A is essential, but the PBX1 homeodomain is dispensable. *Mol Cell Biol* **14**:8304, 1994.

146. Kamps MP, Wright DD, Lu Q: DNA-binding by oncoprotein E2a-Pbx1 is important for blocking differentiation but dispensable for fibroblast transformation. *Oncogene* **12**:19, 1996.

147. Crist WM, Carroll AJ, Shuster JJ, Behm FG, Whitehead M, Vietti TJ, Look AT, Mahoney D, Ragab A, Pullen DJ, et al: Poor prognosis of children with pre-B acute lymphoblastic leukemia is associated with the t(1;19)(q23;p13): A Pediatric Oncology Group Study. *Blood* **76**:117, 1990.

148. Raimondi SC, Behm FG, Roberson PK, Pui C-H, Williams DL, Crist WM, Look AT, Rivera GK: Cytogenetics of pre-B-cell acute lymphoblastic leukemia with emphasis on prognostic implications of the t(1;19). *J Clin Oncol* **8**:1380, 1990.

149. Williams DL, Look AT, Melvin SL, Roberson PK, Dahl G, Flake T, Stass S: New chromosomal translocations correlate with specific immunophenotypes of childhood acute lymphoblastic leukemia. *Cell* **36**:101, 1984.

150. Michael PM, Levin MD, Garson OM: Translocation 1;19—a new cytogenetic abnormality in acute lymphocytic leukemia. *Cancer Genet Cytogenet* **12**:333, 1984.

151. Miyamoto K, Tomita N, Ishii A, Nonaka H, Kondo T, Tanaka T, Kitajima K: Chromosome abnormalities of leukemia cells in adult patients with T-cell leukemia. *J Natl Cancer Inst* **73**:353, 1984.

152. Yamada T, Craig JM, Hawkins JM, Janossy G, Secker-Walker LM: Molecular investigation of 19p13 in standard and variant translocations: The E12 probe recognizes the 19p13 breakpoint in cases with t(1;19) and acute leukemia other than pre-B immunophenotype. *Leukemia* **5**:36, 1991.

153. Secker-Walker LM, Berger R, Fenaux P, Lai JL, Nelken B, Garson M, Michael PM, Hagemeijer A, Harrison CJ, Kaneko Y, Rubin CM: Prognostic significance of the balanced t(1;19) and unbalanced der(19)t(1;19) translocations in acute lymphoblastic leukemia. *Leukemia* **6**:363, 1992.

154. Ohno H, Inoue T, Akasaka T, Okumura A, Miyanishi S, Ohashi I, Kikuchi M, Masuya M, Amano H, Imanaka T, Ohno Y: Acute lymphoblastic leukemia associated with a t(1;19)(q23;p13) in an adult. *In Med* **32**:584, 1993.

155. Vagner-Capodano AM, Mozziconacci MJ, Zattara-Cannoni H, Guitard AM, Thuret I, Michel G: t(1;19) in a M4-ANLL. *Cancer Genet Cytogenet* **73**:86, 1994.

156. Wlodarska I, Stul M, DeWolf-Peeters C, Verhoef G, Mecucci C, Cassiman JJ, Van den Berghe H: t(1;19) without detectable E2A rearrangements in two t(14;18)-positive lymphoma/leukemia cases. *Gene Chrom Cancer* **10**:171, 1994.

157. Raimondi SC, Privitera E, Williams DL, Look AT, Behm F, Rivera GK, Crist WM, Pui C: New recurring chromosomal translocations in childhood acute lymphoblastic leukemia. *Blood* **77**:2016, 1991.

158. Hunger SP, Ohyashiki K, Toyama K, Cleary ML: HLF, a novel hepatic bZIP protein, shows altered DNA-binding properties following fusion to E2A in t(17;19) acute lymphoblastic leukemia. *Gene Dev* **6**:1608, 1992.

159. Inaba T, Roberts WM, Shapiro LH, Jolly KW, Raimondi SC, Smith SD, Look AT: Fusion of the leucine zipper gene HLF to the E2A gene in human acute B-lineage leukemia. *Science* **257**:531, 1992.

160. Hunger SP, Devaraj PE, Foroni L, Secker-Walker LM, Cleary ML: Two types of genomic rearrangements create alternative E2A-HLF fusion proteins in t(17;19)-ALL. *Blood* **83**:2261, 1994.

161. Hunger SP, Brown R, Cleary ML: DNA-binding and transcriptional regulatory properties of hepatic leukemia factor (HLF) and the t(17;19) acute lymphoblastic leukemia chimera E2A-HLF. *Mol Cell Biol* **14**:5986, 1994.

162. Landschulz WH, Johnson PF, McKnight SL: The leucine zipper: A hypothetical structure common to a new class of DNA binding proteins. *Science* **240**:1559, 1988.

163. O'Shea EK, Klemm JD, Kim PS, Alber T: X-ray structure of the GCN4 leucine zipper, a two-stranded, parallel coiled coil. *Science* **254**:539, 1991.

164. Ellenberger TE, Brandl CJ, Struhl K, Harrison SC: The GCN4 basic region leucine zipper binds DNA as a dimer of uninterrupted alpha helices: Crystal structure of the protein-DNA complex. *Cell* **71**:1223, 1992.

165. Drolet DW, Scully KM, Simmons DM, Wegner M, Chu KT, Swanson LW, Rosenfeld MG: TEF, a transcription factor expressed specifically in the anterior pituitary during embryogenesis, defines a new class of leucine zipper proteins. *Gene Dev* **5**:1739, 1991.

166. Falvey E, Fleury-Olela F, Schibler U: The rat hepatic leukemia factor (HLF) gene encodes two transcriptional activators with distinct circadian rhythms, tissue distributions and target preferences. *EMBO J* **14**:4307, 1995.

167. Inaba T, Inukai T, Yoshihara T, Seyschab H, Ashmun RA, Canman CE, Laken SJ, Kastan MB, Look AT: Reversal of apoptosis by the leukaemia-associated E2A-HLF chimaeric transcription factor. *Nature* **382**:541, 1996.

168. Metzstein MM, Hengartner MO, Tsung N, Ellis RE, Horvitz HR: Transcriptional regulator of programmed cell death encoded by caenorhabditis elegans gene ces-2. *Nature* **382**:545, 1996.

169. Thompson CB: A fate worse than death. *Nature* **382**:492, 1996.

170. Inaba T, Shapiro LH, Funabiki T, Sinclair AE, Jones BG, Ashmun RA, Look AT: DNA-binding specificity and trans-activating potential of the leukemia-associated E2A-Hepatic Leukemia Factor fusion protein. *Mol Cell Biol* **14**:3403, 1994.

171. Vinson CR, Hai T, Boyd SM: Dimerization specificity of the leucine zipper-containing bZIP motif on DNA binding: prediction and rational design. *Gene Dev* **7**:1047, 1993.

172. Yoshihara T, Inaba T, Shapiro LH, Kato J, Look AT: E2A-HLF-mediated cell transformation requires both the trans-activation domain of E2A and the leucine zipper dimerization domain of HLF. *Mol Cell Biol* **15**:3247, 1995.

173. Hunger SP: Chromosomal translocations involving the E2A gene in acute lymphoblastic leukemia: Clinical features and molecular pathogenesis. *Blood* **87**:1211, 1996.

174. Devaraj PE, Foroni L, Sekhar M, Butler T, Wright F, Mehta A, Samson D, Prentice HG, Hoffbrand AV, Secker-Walker LM: E2A/HLF fusion cDNAs and the use of RT-PCR for the detection of minimal residual disease in t(17;19)(q22;p13) acute lymphoblastic leukemia. *Leukemia* **8**:1131, 1994.

175. Ohyashiki K, Fujieda H, Miyauchi J, Ohyashiki JH, Tauchi T, Saito M, Nakazawa S, Abe K, Yamamoto K, Clark SC, et al: Establishment of a novel heterotransplantable acute lymphoblastic leukemia cell line with a t(17;19) chromosomal translocation the growth of which is inhibited by interleukin-3. *Leukemia* **5**:322, 1991.

176. Golub TR, Barker GF, Bohlander SK, Hiebert SW, Ward DC, Bray-Ward P, Morgan E, Raimondi SC, Rowley JD, Gilliland DG: Fusion of the TEL gene on 12p13 to the AML1 gene on 21q22 in acute lymphoblastic leukemia. *Proc Natl Acad Sci USA* **92**:4917, 1995.

177. Romana SP, Mauchauffe M, Le Coniat M, Chumakov I, Le Paslier D, Berger R, Bernard OA: The t(12;21) of acute lymphoblastic leukemia results in a tel-AML1 gene fusion. *Blood* **85**:3662, 1995.

178. Shurtleff SA, Buijs A, Behm FG, Rubnitz JE, Raimondi SC, Hancock ML, Chan GC, Pui CH, Grosveld G, Downing JR: TEL/AML1 fusion resulting from a cryptic t(12;21) is the most common genetic lesion in pediatric ALL and defines a subgroup of patients with an excellent prognosis. *Leukemia* **9**:1985, 1995.

179. Romana SP, Poirel H, Leconiat M, Flexor MA, Mauchauffe M, Jonveaux P, Macintyre EA, Berger R, Bernard OA: High frequency of t(12;21) in childhood B-lineage acute lymphoblastic leukemia. *Blood* **86**:4263, 1995.

180. Liang D, Chou T, Chen J, Shurtleff SA, Rubnitz JE, Downing JR, Pui C, Shih L: High incidence of TEL/AML1 fusion resulting from a cryptic t(12;21) in childhood B-lineage acute lymphoblastic leukemia in Taiwan. *Leukemia* **10**:991, 1996.

181. Rubnitz JE, Downing JR, Pui C, Shurtleff SA, Raimondi SC, Evans WE, Head DR, Crist WM, Rivera GK, Hancock ML, Boyett JM, Buijs A, Grosveld G, Behm FG: TEL gene rearrangement in acute lymphoblastic leukemia: A new genetic marker with prognostic significance. *J Clin Oncol* **15**:1150, 1997.

182. Look AT: Pathobiology of the acute lymphoid leukemia cell, in Hoffman R (ed): *Hematology*, 2nd ed. New York, Churchill Livingstone, 1995, p. 1047.

183. Ye BH, Rao PH, Chaganti RS, Dalla-Favera R: Cloning of bcl-6, the locus involved in chromosome translocations affecting band 3q27 in B-cell lymphoma. *Cancer Res* **53**:2732, 1993.

184. Kerckaert JP, Deweindt C, Tilly H, Quief S, Lecocq G, Bastard C: LAZ-3, a novel zinc-finger encoding gene, is disrupted by recurring chromosome 3q27 translocations in human lymphomas. *Nat Genet* **5**:66, 1993.

185. Miki T, Kawamata N, Hirosawa S, Aoki N: Gene involved in the 3q27 translocation associated with B-cell lymphoma, BCL5, encodes a Kruppel-like zinc-finger protein. *Blood* **83**:26, 1994.

186. Ye BH, Lista F, Lo Coco F, Knowles DM, Offit K, Chaganti RS, Dalla-Favera R: Alterations of zinc-finger-encoding gene, BCL-6, in diffuse large-cell lymphoma. *Science* **262**:747, 1993.

187. Cattoretti G, Chang CC, Cechova K, Zhang J, Ye BH, Falini B, Louie DC, Offit K, Chaganti RS, Dalla-Favera R: BCL-6 protein is expressed in germinal-center B cells. *Blood* **86**:45, 1995.

188. Flenghi L, Ye BH, Fizzotti M, Bigerna B, Cattoretti G, Venturi S, Pacini R, Pileri S, Lo Coco F, Pescarmona E, et al: A specific monoclonal antibody (PG-B6) detects expression of the BCL-6 protein in germinal center B cells. *Am J Pathol* **147**:405, 1995.

189. McLennan ICM: Germinal centers. *Ann Rev Immunol* **12**:117, 1994.

190. Dalla-Fevera R, Ye BH, Cattoretti G, Lo Coco F, Chang C, Zhang J, Migliazza A, Cechova K, Niu H, Chaganti S, Chen W, Louie DC, Offit K, Chaganti RSK: BCL-6 in Diffuse Large-Cell Lymphomas, in De Vita VT, Hellman S, Rosenberg SA, (eds): *Important Advances in Oncology 1996*. Philadelphia, Lippincott-Raven, 1996, p. 139.

191. Ye BH, Chaganti S, Chang CC, Niu H, Corradini P, Chaganti RS, Dalla-Favera R: Chromosomal translocations cause deregulated BCL6 expression by promoter substitution in B cell lymphoma. *EMBO J* **14**:6209, 1995.

192. Migliazza A, Martinotti S, Chen W, Fusco C, Ye BH, Knowles DM, Offit K, Chaganti RS, Dalla-Favera R: Frequent somatic hypermutation of the 5′ noncoding region of the BCL6 gene in B-cell lymphoma. *Proc Natl Acad Sci USA* **92**:12520, 1995.

193. Offit K, Lo Coco F, Louis DC, Parsa NZ, Leung D, Portlock C, Ye BH, Lista F, Filippa DA, Rosenbaum A, Ladanyi M, Jhanwar S, Dalla-Favera R, Chaganti RSK: Rearrangement of the BCL-6 gene as a prognostic marker in diffuse large-cell lymphoma. *N Engl J Med* **331**:74, 1994.

194. Speck NA, Stacy T: A new transcription factor family associated with human leukemias. *Crit Rev Euk Gene Exp* **5**:337, 1995.

195. Wang S, Wang Q, Crute BE, Melnikova IN, Keller SR, Speck NA: Cloning and characterization of subunits of the T-cell receptor and murine leukemia virus enhancer core-binding factor. *EMBO J* **13**:3324, 1993.

196. Ogawa E, Inuzuka M, Maruyama M, Satake M, Naito-Fujimoto M, Ito Y, Shigesada K: Molecular cloning and characterization of PEBP2β, the heterodimeric partner of a novel Drosophila runt-related DNA binding protein PEBP2α. *Virology* **194**:314, 1993.

197. Miyoshi H, Shimizu K, Kozu T, Maseki N, Kaneko Y, Ohki M: t(8;21) breakpoints on chromosome 21 in acute myeloid leukemia are clustered within a limited region of a single gene, AML1. *Proc Natl Acad Sci USA* **88**:10431, 1991.

198. Gao J, Erickson P, Gardiner K, Le Beau MM, Diaz MO, Patterson D, Rowley JD, Drabkin HA: Isolation of a yeast artificial chromosome spanning the 8;21 translocation breakpoint t(8;21)(q22;q22.3) in acute myelogenous leukemia. *Proc Natl Acad Sci USA* **88**:4882, 1991.

199. Erickson P, Gao J, Chang KS, Look T, Whisenant E, Raimondi S, Lasher R, Trujillo J, Rowley J, Drabkin H: Identification of breakpoints in t(8;21) acute myelogenous leukemia and isolation of a fusion transcript. AML1/ETO, with similarity to Drosophila segmentation gene, runt. *Blood* **80**:1825, 1992.

200. Nisson PE, Watkins PC, Sacchi N: Transcriptionally active chimeric gene derived from the fusion of the AML1 gene and a novel gene on chromosome 8 in t(8;21) leukemic cells. *Cancer Genet Cytogenet* **63**:81, 1992.

201. Mitani K, Ogawa S, Tanaka T, Miyoshi H, Kurokawa M, Mano H, Yazaki Y, Ohki M, Hirai H: Generation of the AML1-EVI-1 fusion gene in the t(3;21)(q26;q22) causes blastic crisis in chronic myelocytic leukemia. *EMBO J* **13**:504, 1994.

202. Nucifora G, Begy CR, Erickson P, Drabkin HA, Rowley JD: The 3;21 translocation in myelodysplasia results in a fusion transcript between the AML1 gene and the gene for EAP, a highly conserved protein associated with the Epstein-Barr virus small RNA EBER 1. *Proc Natl Acad Sci USA* **90**:7784, 1993.

203. Meyers S, Downing JR, Hiebert SW: Identification of AML-1 and the (8;21) translocation protein (AML-1/ETO) as sequence specific DNA binding proteins: The runt homology domain is required for DNA binding and protein-protein interactions. *Mol Cell Biol* **13**:6336, 1993.

204. Nuchprayoon I, Meyers S, Scott LM, Suzow J, Hiebert S, Friedman AD: PEBP2/CBF, the murine homolog of the human myeloid AML1 and PEBP2 beta/CBF beta-proto-oncoproteins, regulates the murine myeloperoxidase and neutrophil elastase genes in immature myeloid cells. *Mol Cell Biol* **14**:5558, 1994.

205. Takahashi A, Satake M, Yamaguchi-Iwai Y, Bae SC, Lu J, Maruyama M, Zhang YW, Oka H, Arai N, Arai K, et al: Positive and negative regulation of granulocyte-macrophage colony-stimulating factor promoter activity by AML1-related transcription factor, PEBP2. *Blood* **86**:607, 1995.

206. Wotton D, Ghysdael J, Wang S, Speck NA, Owen MJ: Cooperative binding of Ets-1 and core binding factor to DNA. *Mol Cell Biol* **14**:840, 1994.

207. Hernandez-Munain C, Krangel MS: c-Myb and core-binding factor/PEBP2 display functional synergy but bind independently to adjacent sites in the T-cell receptor delta enhancer. *Mol Cell Biol* **15**:3090, 1995.

208. Manley NR, O'Connell M, Sun W, Speck NA, Hopkins N: Two factors that bind to highly conserved sequences in mammalian type C retroviral enhancers. *J Virol* **67**:1967, 1993.

209. Sun W, O'Connell M, Speck NA: Characterization of a protein that binds multiple sequences in mammalian type C retrovirus enhancers. *J Virol* **67**:1976, 1993.

210. Sun W, Graves BJ, Speck NA: Transactivation of the Moloney murine leukemia virus and T-cell receptor beta-chain enhancers of cbf and ets requires intact binding sites for both proteins. *J Virol* **69**:4941, 1995.

211. Frank R, Zhang J, Uchida H, Meyers S, Hiebert SW, Nimer SD: The AML1/ETO fusion protein blocks transactivation of the GM-CSF promoter by AML1B. *Oncogene* **11**:2667, 1995.

212. Okuda T, van Deursen J, Hiebert SW, Grosveld G, Downing JR: AML1, the target of multiple chromosomal translocations in human leukemia, is essential for normal fetal liver hematopoiesis. *Cell* **84**:321, 1996.

213. Wang Q, Stacy T, Binder M, Marin-Padilla M, Sharpe AH, Speck NA: Disruption of the Cbfa2 gene causes necrosis and hemorrhaging in the central nervous system and blocks definitive hematopoiesis. *Proc Natl Acad Sci USA* **93**:3444, 1996.

214. Wang Q, Stacy T, Miller JD, Lewis AF, Gu T, Huang X, Bushweller JH, Bories J, Alt FW, Ryan G, Liu PP, Wynshaw-Boris A, Binder M, Marin-Padilla M, Sharpe AH, Speck NA: The CBFbeta subunit is essential for CBFalpha2 (AML1) function in vivo. *Cell* **87**:697–708, 1996.

215. Meyers S, Lenny N, Hiebert SW: The t(8;21) fusion protein interferes with AML-1B-dependent transcriptional activation. *Mol Cell Biol* **15**:1974, 1995.

216. Liu P, Tarle SA, Hajra A, Claxton DF, Marlton P, Freedman M, Siciliano MJ, Collins FS: Fusion between transcription factor CBFβ/PEBP2β and a myosin heavy chain in acute myeloid leukemia. *Science* **261**:1041, 1993.

217. Castilla LH, Wijmenga C, Wang Q, Stacy T, Speck NA, Eckhaus M, Marin-Padilla M, Collins FS, Wynshaw-Boris A, Liu PP: Failure of embryonic hematopoiesis and lethal hemorrhages in mouse embryos heterozygous for a knocked-in leukemia gene CBFB-MYH11. *Cell* **87**:687–696, 1996.

218. de The H, Chomienne C, Lanotte M, Degos L, Dejean A: The t(15;17) translocation of acute promyelocytic leukaemia fuses the retinoic acid receptor alpha gene to a novel transcribed locus. *Nature* **347**:558, 1990.

219. Borrow J, Goddard AD, Sheer D, Solomon E: Molecular analysis of acute promyelocytic leukemia breakpoint cluster region on chromosome 17. *Science* **249**:1577, 1990.

220. Longo L, Pandolfi PP, Biondi A, Rambaldi A, Mencarelli A, Lo Coco F, Diverio D, Pegoraro L, Avanzi G, Tabilio A, et al: Rearrangements and aberrant expression of the retinoic acid receptor alpha gene in acute promyelocytic leukemias. *J Exp Med* **172**:1571, 1990.

221. de The H, Lavau C, Marchio A, Chomienne C, Degos L, Dejean A: The PML-RAR alpha fusion mRNA generated by the t(15;17) translocation in acute promyelocytic leukemia encodes a functionally altered RAR. *Cell* **66**:675, 1991.

222. Kakizuka A, Miller WH Jr, Umesono K, Warrell RP Jr, Frankel SR, Murty VV, Dmitrovsky E, Evans RM: Chromosomal translocation t(15;17) in human acute promyelocytic leukemia fuses RAR alpha with a novel putative transcription factor, PML. *Cell* **66**:663, 1991.

223. Kastner P, Perez A, Lutz Y, Rochette-Egly C, Gaub MP, Durand B, Lanotte M, Berger R, Chambon P: Structure, localization and transcriptional properties of two classes of retinoic acid receptor alpha fusion proteins in acute promyelocytic leukemia (APL): structural similarities with a new family of oncoproteins. *EMBO J* **11**:629, 1992.

224. Perez A, Kastner P, Sethi S, Lutz Y, Reibel C, Chambon P: PMLRAR homodimers: distinct DNA binding properties and heteromeric interactions with RXR. *EMBO J* **12**:3171, 1993.

225. Dyck JA, Maul GG, Miller WH Jr, Chen JD, Kakizuka A, Evans RM: A novel macromolecular structure is a target of the promyelocyte-retinoic acid receptor oncoprotein. *Cell* **76**:333, 1994.

226. Weis K, Rambaud S, Lavau C, Jansen J, Carvalho T, Carmo-Fonseca M, Lamond A, Dejean A: Retinoic acid regulates aberrant nuclear localization of PML-RAR alpha in acute promyelocytic leukemia cells. *Cell* **76**:345, 1994.

227. Koken MH, Puvion-Dutilleul F, Guillemin MC, Viron A, Linares-Cruz G, Stuurman N, de Jong L, Szostecki C, Calvo F, Chomienne C, Degos L, Puvion E, The HD: The t(15;17) translocation alters a nuclear body in retinoic acid-reversible fashion. *EMBO J* **13**:1073, 1994.

228. Carvalho T, Seeler JS, Ohman K, Jordan P, Pettersson U, Akusjarvi G, Carmo-Fonseca M, Dejean A: Targeting of adenovirus E1A and E4-ORF3 proteins to nuclear matrix-associated PML bodies. *J Cell Biol* **131**:45, 1995.

229. Doucas V, Ishov AM, Romo A, Juguilon H, Weitzman MD, Evans RM, Maul GG: Adenovirus replication is coupled with the dynamic properties of the PML nuclear structure. *Gene Dev* **10**:196, 1996.

230. Everett RD, Maul GG: HSV-1 IE protein Vmw110 causes redistribution of PML. *EMBO J* **13**:5062, 1994.

231. Terris B, Baldin V, Dubois S, Degott C, Flejou JF, Henin D, Dejean A: PML nuclear bodies are general targets for inflammation and cell proliferation. *Cancer Res* **55**:1590, 1995.

232. Lavau C, Marchio A, Fagioli M, Jansen J, Falini B, Lebon P, Grosveld F, Pandolfi PP, Pelicci PG, Dejean A: The acute promyelocytic leukaemia-associated PML gene is induced by interferon. *Oncogene* **11**:871, 1995.

233. Nason-Burchenal K, Gandini D, Botto M, Allopenna J, Seale JR, Cross NC, Goldman JM, Dmitrovsky E, Pandolfi PP: Interferon augments PML and PML/RARalpha expression in normal myeloid and acute promyelocytic cells and cooperates with all-trans-retinoic acid to induce maturation of a retinoid resistant promyelocytic cell line. *Blood*, in press.

234. Jansen JH, Mahfoudi A, Rambaud S, Lavau C, Wahli W, Dejean A: Multimeric complexes of the PML-retinoic acid receptor alpha fusion protein in acute promyelocytic leukemia cells and interference with retinoid and peroxisome-proliferator signaling pathways. *Proc Natl Acad Sci USA* **92**:7401, 1995.

235. Grignani F, Ferrucci PF, Testa U, Talamo G, Fagioli M, Alcalay M, Mencarelli A, Peschle C, Nicoletti I, Pelicci PG: The acute promyelocytic leukemia-specific PML-RARa fusion protein inhibits differentiation and promotes survival of myeloid precursor cells. *Cell* **74**:424, 1993.

236. Grignani F, Testa U, Fagioli M, Barberi T, Masciulli R, Mariani G, Peschle C, Pelicci PG: Promyelocytic leukemia-specific PML-retinoic acid alpha receptor fusion protein interferes with erythroid differentiation of human erythroleukemia K562 cells. *Cancer Res* **55**:440, 1995.

237. Testa U, Grignani F, Barberi T, Fagioli M, Masciulli R, Ferrucci PF, Seripa D, Camagna A, Alcalay M, Pelicci PG, et al: PML/RAR alpha+ U937 mutant and NB4 cell lines: retinoic acid restores the monocytic differentiation response to vitamin D3. *Cancer Res* **54**:4508, 1994.

238. Early E, Moore MA, Kakizuka A, Nason-Burchenal K, Martin P, Evans RM, Dmitrovsky E: Transgenic expression of PML/RARalpha impairs myelopoiesis. *Proc Natl Acad Sci USA* **93**:7900, 1996.

239. Altabef M, Garcia M, Lavaue C, Bae S, Dejean A, Samarut J: A retrovirus carrying the promyelocyte-retinoic acid receptor PML-RARalpha fusion gene transforms haematopoietic progenitors in vitro and induces acute leukaemias. *EMBO J* **15**:2707, 1996.

240. Huang ME, Ye YC, Chen SR, Chai JR, Lu JX, Zhoa L, Gu LJ, Wang ZY: Use of all-trans retinoic acid in the treatment of acute promyelocytic leukemia. *Blood* **72**:567, 1988.

241. Chen ZX, Xue YQ, Zhang R, Tao RF, Xia XM, Li C, Wang W, Zu WY, Yao XZ, Ling BJ: A clinical and experimental study on all-trans retinoic acid-treated acute promyelocytic leukemia patients. *Blood* **78**:1413, 1991.

242. Warrell RP Jr, Frankel SR, Miller WH Jr, Scheinberg DA, Itri LM, Hittelman WN, Vyas R, Andreeff M, Tafuri A, Jakubowski A, Gabrilove J, Gordon MS, Dimitrovsky E: Differentiation therapy of acute promyelocytic leukemia with tretinoin (all-trans-retinoic acid). *N Engl J Med* **324**:1385, 1991.

243. Warrell RP Jr, Maslak P, Eardley A, Heller G, Miller WH Jr, Frankel SR: Treatment of acute promyelocytic leukemia with all-trans retinoic acid: an update of the New York experience. *Leukemia* **8**:929, 1994.

244. Fenaux P, Chastang C, Chomienne C, Degos L: All transretinoic acid (ATRA) in combination with chemotherapy improves survival in newly diagnosed acute promyelocytic leukemia (APL). *Lancet* **343**:1033, 1994.

245. Redner RL, Rush EA, Faas S, Rudert WA, Corey SJ: The t(5;17) variant of acute promyelocytic leukemia expresses a nucleophosmin-retinoic acid receptor fusion. *Blood* **87**:882, 1996.

246. Chen Z, Brand N, Chen A, Chen S, Tong J, Wang Z, Waxman S, Zelent A: Fusion between a novel Krüppel-like zinc finger gene and the retinoic acid receptor-α locus due to a variant t(11;17) translocation associated with acute promyelocytic leukaemia. *EMBO J* **12**:1161, 1993.

247. Bardwell VJ, Treisman R: The POZ domain: a conserved protein-protein interaction motif. *Gene Dev* **8**:1664, 1994.

248. Chen Z, Guidez F, Rousselot P, Agadir A, Chen S, Wang Z, Degos L, Zelent A, Waxman S, Chomienne C: PLZF-RARα fusion proteins generated from the variant t(11;17)(q23;q21) translocation in acute promyelocytic leukemia inhibit ligand-dependent transactivation of wild-type retinoic acid receptors. *Proc Natl Acad Sci USA* **91**:1178, 1994.

249. Dong S, Zhu J, Reid A, Strutt P, Guidez F, Zhong HJ, Wang ZY, Licht J, Waxman S, Chomienne C, Chen Z, Zelent A, Chen SJ: Amino-terminal protein-protein interaction motif (POZ-domain) is responsible for activities of the promyelocytic leukemia zinc finger-retinoic acid receptor-alpha fusion protein. *Proc Natl Acad Sci USA* **93**:3624, 1996.

250. Licht JD, Shaknovich R, English MA, Melnick A, Li JY, Reddy JC, Dong S, Chen SJ, Zelent A, Waxman S: Reduced and altered DNA-binding and transcriptional properties of the PLZF-retinoic acid receptor-alpha chimera generated in t(11;17)-associated acute promyelocytic leukemia. *Oncogene* **12**:323, 1996.

251. Cook M, Gould A, Brand N, Davies J, Strutt P, Shaknovich R, Licht J, Waxman S, Chen Z, Gluecksohn-Waelsch S, et al: Expression of the zinc-finger gene PLZF at rhombomere boundaries in the vertebrate hindbrain. *Proc Natl Acad Sci USA* **92**:2249, 1995.

252. Reid A, Gould A, Brand N, Cook M, Strutt P, Li J, Licht J, Waxman S, Krumlauf R, Zelent A: Leukemia translocation gene, PLZF, is expressed with a speckled nuclear pattern in early hematopoietic progenitors. *Blood* **86**:4544, 1995.

253. Licht JD, Chomienne C, Goy A, Chen A, Scott AA, Head DR, Michaux JL, Wu Y, DeBlasio A, Miller WH Jr, et al: Clinical and molecular characterization of a rare syndrome of acute promyelocytic leukemia associated with translocation (11;17). *Blood* **85**:1083, 1995.

254. Morishita K, Parganas E, Bartholomew C, Sacchi N, Valentine MB, Raimondi SC, Le Beau MM, Ihle JN: The human Evi-1 gene is located on chromosome 3q24-q28 but is not rearranged in three cases of acute nonlymphocytic leukemias containing t(3;5)(q25;q34) translocations. *Onc Res* **5**:221, 1990.

255. Morishita K, Parganas E, Willman CL, Whittaker MH, Drabkin H, Oval J, Taetle R, Ihle JN: Activation of Evi-1 gene expression in human acute myelogenous leukemias by translocations spanning 300–400 kb on chromosome 3q26. *Proc Natl Acad Sci USA* **89**:3937, 1992.

256. Morishita K, Parker DS, Mucenski ML, Jenkins NA, Copeland NG, Ihle JN: Retroviral activation of a novel gene encoding a zinc finger protein in IL-3-dependent myeloid leukemia cell lines. *Cell* **54**:831, 1988.

257. Delwel R, Funabiki T, Kreider BL, Morishita K, Ihle JN: Four of the seven zinc fingers of the Evi-1 myeloid-transforming gene are required for sequence-specific binding to GA(C/T)AAGA(T/C)AA-GATAA. *Mol Cell Biol* **13**:4291, 1993.

258. Perkins AS, Fishel R, Jenkins NA, Copeland NG: Evi-1, a murine zinc finger proto-oncogene, encodes a sequence-specific DNA-binding protein. *Mol Cell Biol* **11**:2665, 1991.

259. Funabiki T, Kreider BL, Ihle JN: The carboxyl domain of zinc fingers of the Evi-1 myeloid transforming gene binds a consensus sequence of GAAGATGAG. *Oncogene* **9**:1575, 1994.

260. Kreider BL, Orkin SH, Ihle JN: Loss of erythropoietin responsiveness in erythroid progenitors due to expression of the Evi-1 myeloid-transforming gene. *Proc Natl Acad Sci USA* **90**:6454, 1993.

261. Mitelman F: *Catalog of Chromosome Aberrations in Cancer*, 5th ed. New York, Wiley-Liss, 1994.

262. Raimondi SC, Kalwinsky DK, Hayashi Y, Behm FG, Mirro J Jr, Williams DL: Cytogenetics of childhood acute nonlymphocytic leukemia. *Cancer Genet Cytogenet* **40**:13, 1989.

263. Raimondi SC: Current status of cytogenetic research in childhood acute lymphoblastic leukemia. *Blood* **70**:2237, 1993.

264. Pui C, Frankel LS, Carroll AJ, Raimondi SC, Shuster JJ, Head DR, Crist WM, Land VJ, Pullen DJ, Steuber CP, Behm FG, Borowitz MJ: Clinical characteristics and treatment outcome of childhood acute lymphoblastic leukemia with the t(4;11)(q21;q23): A collaborative study of 40 cases. *Blood* **77**:440, 1991.

265. Kaneko Y, Maseki N, Takasaki N, Sakurai M, Hayashi Y, Nakazawa S, Mori T, Sakurai M, Takeda T, Shikano T, Hiroshi Y: Clinical and hematologic characteristics in acute leukemia with 11q23 translocations. *Blood* **67**:484, 1986.

266. Heerema NA, Arthur DC, Sather H, Albo V, Feusner J, Lange BJ, Steinherz PG, Zeltzer P, Hammond D, Reaman GH: Cytogenetic features of infants less than 12 months of age at diagnosis of acute lymphoblastic leukemia: Impact of the 11q23 breakpoint on outcome: A report of the Childrens Cancer Group. *Blood* **83**:2274, 1994.

267. Pui CH, Kane JR, Crist WM: Biology and treatment of infant leukemias. *Leukemia* **9**:762, 1995.

268. Chen CS, Sorensen PH, Domer PH, Reaman GH, Korsmeyer SJ, Heerema NA, Hammond GD, Kersey JH: Molecular rearrangements on chromosome 11q23 predominate in infant acute lymphoblastic

leukemia and are associated with specific biologic variables and poor outcome. *Blood* **81**:2386, 1993.

269. Chen C, Sorensen PHB, Domer PH, Reaman GH, Korsmeyer SJ, Heerema NA, Hammond GD, Kersey JH: Molecular rearrangements on chromosome 11q23 predominate in infant acute lymphoblastic leukemia and are associated with specific biologic variables and poor outcome. *Blood* **81**:2386, 1993.

270. Pui CH, Behm FG, Raimondi SC, Dodge RK, George SL, Rivera GK, Mirro J, Kalwinsky DK, Dahl GV, Murphy SB, Crist WM, Williams DL: Secondary acute myeloid leukemia in children treated for acute lymphoid leukemia. *N Engl J Med* **321**:136, 1989.

271. DeVore R, Whitlock J, Hainsworth JD, Johnson DH: Therapy-related acute nonlymphocytic leukemia with monocytic features and re-arrangement of chromosome 11q. *Ann Intern Med* **110**:740, 1989.

272. Ziemin-van der Poel S, McCabe NR, Gill HJ, Espinosa R, Patel Y, Harden A, Rubinelli P, Smith SD, Lebeau MM, Rowley JD, Diaz MO: Identification of a gene, MLL, that spans the breakpoint in 11q23 translocations associated with human leukemias. *Proc Natl Acad Sci USA* **88**:10735, 1991.

273. Tkachuk DC, Kohler S, Cleary ML: Involvement of a homolog of Drosophila trithorax by 11q23 chromosomal translocations in acute leukemias. *Cell* **71**:691, 1992.

274. Gu Y, Nakamura T, Alder H, Prasad R, Canaani O, Cimino G, Croce CM, Cananni E: The t(4;11) chromosome translocation of human acute leukemias fuses the ALL-1 gene, related to Drosophila tritho-rax, to the AF-4 gene. *Cell* **71**:701, 1992.

275. Djabali M, Selleri L, Parry P, Bower M, Young BD, Evans G: A trithorax-like gene is interrupted by chromosome 11q23 transloca-tions in acute leukemias. *Nat Gene* **2**:113, 1992.

276. Domer PH, Fakharzadeh SS, Chen CS, Jockel J, Johansen L, Silver-man GA, Kersey JH, Korsmeyer SJ: Acute mixed-lineage leukemia t(4;11)(q21;q23) generates an MLL-AF4 fusion product. *Proc Natl Acad Sci USA* **90**:7884, 1993.

277. Morrissey J, Tkachuk DC, Milatovich A, Francke U, Link M, Cleary ML: A serine/proline-rich protein is fused to HRX in t(4;11) acute leukemias. *Blood* **81**:1124, 1993.

278. Yu BD, Hess JL, Horning SE, Brown GA, Korsmeyer SJ: Altered Hox expression and segmental identity in Mll-mutant mice. *Nature* **378**:505, 1995.

279. Simon J: Locking in stable states of gene expression: transcriptional control during Drosophila development. *Curr Opin Cell Biol* **7**:376, 1995.

280. Jones RS, Gelbart WM: The Drosophila polycomb-group gene en-hancer of zeste contains a region with sequence similarity to tritho-rax. *Mol Cell Biol* **13**:6357, 1993.

281. Mazo AM, Huang DH, Mozer BA, Dawid IB: The trithorax gene, a trans-acting regulator of the bithorax-complex in Drosophila, en-codes a protein with zinc-binding domains. *Proc Natl Acad Sci USA* **87**:2112, 1990.

282. Reeves R, Nissen MS: The A-T-DNA-binding domain of mammalian high mobility group I chromosomal proteins. *J Biol Chem* **265**:8573, 1990.

283. Ma Q, Alder H, Nelson KK, Chatterjee D, Gu Y, Nakamura T, Canaani E, Croce CM, Siracusa LD, Buchberg AM: Analysis of the murine ALL-1 gene reveals conserved domains with human ALL-1 and identified a motif shared with DNA methyltransferases. *Proc Natl Acad Sci USA* **90**:6350, 1993.

284. Zeleznik-Le NJ, Harden AM, Rowley JD: 11q23 translocations split the "AT-hook" cruciform DNA-binding region and the transcriptional repression domain from the activation domain of the mixed-lineage leukemia (MLL) gene. *Proc Natl Acad Sci USA* **91**:10610,1994.

285. Thirman MJ, Levitan DA, Kobayashi H, Simon MC, Rowley JD: Cloning of ELL, a gene that fuses to MLL in a t(11;19)(q23;p13.1) in acute myeloid leukemia. *Proc Natl Acad Sci USA* **91**:12110, 1994.

286. Mitani K, Kanda Y, Ogawa S, Tanaka T, Inazawa J, Yazaki Y, Hirai H: Cloning of several species of MLL/MEN chimeric cDNAs in myeloid leukemia with t(11;19)(q23;p13.1) translocation. *Blood* **85**:2017, 1995.

287. Shilatifard A, Lane WS, Jackson KW, Conaway RC, Conaway JW: An RNA polymerase II elongation factor encoded by the human ELL gene. *Science* **271**:1873, 1996.

288. Duan DR, Humphrey JS, Chen DY, Weng Y, Sukegawa J, Lee S, Gnarra JR, Linehan WM, Klausner RD: Characterization of the VHL tumor suppressor gene product: localization, complex formation, and the effect of natural inactivating mutations. *Proc Natl Acad Sci USA* **92**:6459, 1995.

289. Duan DR, Pause A, Burgess WH, Aso T, Chen YT, Garrett KP, Conaway RC, Conaway JW, Linehan WM, Klausner RD: Inhibition of transcription elongation by the VHL tumor suppressor protein. *Science* **269**:1402, 1995.

290. Aso T, Lane WS, Conaway JW, Conaway RC: Elongin (SIII): A mul-tisubunit regulator of elongation by RNA polymerase II. *Science* **269**:1439, 1995.

291. Kibel A, Iliopoulos O, DeCaprio JA, Kaelin WG Jr, Binding of the von Hippel-Lindau tumor suppressor protein to elongin B and C. *Science* **269**:1444, 1995.

292. Rubnitz JE, Behm FG, Curcio-Brint AM, Pinheiro RP, Carroll AJ, Raimondi SC, Shurtleff SA, Downing JR: Molecular analysis of t(11;19) breakpoints in childhood acute leukemias. *Blood* **87**:4804, 1996.

293. Nakamura T, Alder H, Gu Y, Prasad R, Canaani O, Kamada N, Gale RP, Lange B, Crist WM, Nowell PC: Genes on chromosomes 4, 9, and 19 involved in 11q23 abnormalities in acute leukemia share se-quence homology and/or common motifs. *Proc Natl Acad Sci USA* **90**:4631, 1993.

294. Chen CS, Hilden JM, Frestedt J, Domer PH, Moore R, Korsmeyer SJ, Kersey JH: The chromosome 4q21 gene (AF-4/FEL) is widely ex-pressed in normal tissues and shows breakpoint diversity in t(4;11)(q21;q23) acute leukemia. *Blood* **82**:1080, 1993.

295. Rubnitz JE, Morrissey J, Savage PA, Cleary ML: ENL, the gene fused with HRX in t(11;19) leukemias, encodes a nuclear protein with transcriptional activation potential in lymphoid and myeloid cells. *Blood* **84**:1747,1994.

296. Tse W, Zhu, W, Chen HS, Cohen A: A novel gene, AF1q, fused to MLL in t(1;11)(q21;q23), is specifically expressed in leukemic and immature hematopoietic cells. *Blood* **85**:650, 1995.

297. Schichman SA, Caligiuri MA, Gu Y, Strout MP, Canaani E, Bloom-field CD, Croce CM: ALL-1 partial duplication in acute leukemia. *Proc Natl Acad Sci USA* **91**:6236, 1994.

298. Schichman SA, Caligiuri MA, Strout MP, Carter SL, Gu Y, Canaani E, Bloomfield CD, Croce CM: ALL-1 tandem duplication in acute myeloid leukemia with a normal karyotype involves homologous re-combination between Alu elements. *Cancer Res* **54**:4277, 1994.

299. Sauvageau G, Thorsteinsdottir U, Eaves CJ, Lawrence HJ, Largman C, Lansdorp PM, Humphries RK: Overexpression of HOXB4 in hematopoietic cells causes the selective expansion of more primitive populations in vitro and in vivo. *Gene Dev* **9**:1753, 1995.

300. Lawrence HJ, Largman C: Homeobox genes in normal hema-topoiesis and leukemia. *Blood* **80**:2445, 1992.

301. Corral J, Lavenir I, Impey H, Warren AJ, Forster A, Larson TA, Bell S, McKenzie AN, King G, Rabbitts TH: An *MLL-AF9* fusion gene made by homologous recombination causes acute leukemia in chimeric mice: A method to create fusion oncogenes. *Cell* **85**:853, 1996.

302. Pui C, Ribeiro RC, Hancock ML, Rivera GK, Evans WE, Raimondi SC, Head DR, Behm FG, Mahmoud MH, Sandlund JT, Crist WM: Acute myeloid leukemia in children treated with epipodophyllotoxins for acute lymphoblastic leukemia. *N Engl J Med* **325**:1682, 1991.

303. Gu Y, Alder H, Nakamura T, Schichman SA, Prasad R, Canaani O, Saito H, Croce CM, Canaani E: Sequence analysis of the breakpoint cluster region in the ALL-1 gene involved in acute leukemia. *Cancer Res* **54**:2327, 1994.

304. Gu Y, Cimino G, Alder H, Nakamura T, Prasad R, Canaani O, Moir DT, Jones C, Nowell PC, Croce CM: The t(4;11)(q21;q23) chromo-some translocations in acute leukemias involve the VDJ recombinase. *Proc Natl Acad Sci USA* **89**:10464, 1992.

305. Felix CA, Winick NJ, Negrini M, Bowman WP, Croce CM, Lange BJ: Common region of ALL-1 gene disrupted in epipodophyllotoxin-related secondary acute myeloid leukemia. *Cancer Res* **53**:2954, 1993.

306. Negrini M, Felix CA, Martin C, Lange BJ, Nakamura T, Canaani E, Croce CM: Potential topoisomerase II DNA-binding sites at the breakpoints of a t(9;11) chromosome translocation in acute myeloid leukemia. *Cancer Res* **53**:4489, 1993.

307. Strissel Broeker PL, Super HG, Thirman MJ, Pomykala H, Yonebayashi Y, Tanabe S, Zeleznik-Le N, Rowley JD: Distribution of 11q23 breakpoints within the *MLL* breakpoint cluster region in de novo acute leukemia and in treatment-related acute myeloid leukemia: Correlation with scaffold attachment regions and topoiso-merase II consensus binding sites. *Blood* **87**:1912, 1996.

308. Domer PH, Head DR, Renganathan N, Raimondi SC, Yang E, Atlas M: Molecular analysis of 13 cases of MLL/11q23 secondary acute leukemia and identification of topoisomerase II consensus-binding

sequences near the chromosomal breakpoint of a secondary leukemia with the t(4;11). *Leukemia* **9**:1305, 1995.

309. Bernard OA, Berger R: Molecular basis of 11q23 rearrangements in hematopoietic malignant proliferations. *Gene Chrom Cancer* **13**:75, 1995.

310. Prasad R, Gu Y, Alder H, Nakamura T, Canaani O, Saito H, Huebner K, Gale RP, Nowell PC, Kuriyama K, Miyazaki Y, Croce CM, Canaani E: Cloning of the ALL-1 fusion partner, the AF-6 gene, involved in acute myeloid leukemias with the t(6;11) chromosome translocation. *Cancer Res* **53**:5624, 1993.

311. Super HJG, McCabe NR, Thirman MJ, Larson RA, Lebeau MM, Pedersen-Bjergaard J, Philip P, Diaz MO, Rowley JD: Rearrangements of the MLL gene in therapy-related acute myeloid leukemia in patients previously treated with agents targeting DNA-topoisomerase II. *Blood* **81**:3705, 1993.

312. Hunger SP, Tkachuk DC, Amylon MD, Link MP, Carroll AJ, Welborn JL, Willman CL, Cleary ML: HRX involvement in de novo and secondary leukemias with diverse chromosome 11q23 abnormalities. *Blood* **81**:3197, 1993.

313. Bower M, Parry P, Carter M, Lillington DM, Amess J, Lister TA, Evans G, Young BD: Prevalence and clinical correlations of MLL gene rearrangements in AML-M4/5. *Blood* **84**:3776, 1994.

314. Wang JC: DNA topoisomerases. *Annu Rev Biochem* **54**:665, 1985.

315. Bae YS, Kawasaki I, Ikeda H, Liu LF: Illegitimate recombination mediated by calf thymus DNA topoisomerase II in vitro. *Proc Natl Acad Sci USA* **85**:2076, 1988.

316. Sperry AO, Blasquez VC, Garrard WT: Dysfunction of chromosomal loop attachment sites: Illegitimate recombination linked to matrix association regions and topoisomerase II. *Proc Natl Acad Sci USA* **86**:5497, 1989.

317. Ford AM, Ridge SA, Cabrera ME, Mahmoud H, Steel CM, Chan LC, Greaves M: In utero rearrangements in the trithorax-related oncogene in infant leukaemias. *Nature* **363**:358, 1993.

318. Super HJG, Rothberg PG, Kobayashi H, Freeman AI, Diaz MO, Rowley JD: Clonal, nonconstitutional rearrangements of the MLL gene in infant twins with acute lymphoblastic leukemia: In utero chromosome rearrangement of 11q23. *Blood* **83**:641, 1994.

319. Fujioka K, Caslini C, Jones BG, Komuro H, Naeve CW, Look AT: Aberrant p27Kip1 transcripts identified in human leukemias expressing the MLL-AF4 fusion protein. *Blood* **88**:356A, 1996.

320. Caslini C, Murti KG, Ashmun D, Domer PH, Korsmeyer SJ, Boer JM, Grosveld GC, Look AT: Subcellular localization and cell cycle effects of the MLL-AF4 fusion oncoprotein. *Blood* **88**:557A, 1996.

321. Schlessinger J, Ullrich A: Growth factor signaling by receptor tyrosine kinases. *Neuron* **9**:383, 1992.

322. Schlessinger J: How receptor tyrosine kinases activate Ras. *Trends Biochem Sci* **18**:273, 1993.

323. Greco A, Pierotti MA, Bongarzone I, Pagliardini S, Lanzi C, Della Porta G: TRK-T1 is a novel oncogene formed by the fusion of TPR and TRK genes in human papillary thyroid carcinomas. *Oncogene* **7**:237, 1992.

324. Rodrigues GA, Park M: Dimerization mediated through a leucine zipper activates the oncogenic potential of the met receptor tyrosine kinase. *Mol Cell Biol* **13**:6711, 1993.

325. Chromosomal abnormalities and their clinical significance in acute lymphoblastic leukemia: Third International Workshop on Chromosomes in Leukemia. *Cancer Res* **43**:868, 1983.

326. Rowley JD: Biological implications of consistent chromosome rearrangements in leukemia and lymphoma. *Cancer Res* **44**:3159, 1984.

327. Ribeiro RC, Abromowitch M, Raimondi SC, et al: Clinical and biologic hallmarks of the Philadelphia chromosome in childhood acute lymphoblastic leukemia. *Blood* **70**:948, 1987.

328. Bartram CR, de Klein A, Hagemeijer A, van Agthoven T, Geurts van Kessel A, Bootsma D, Grosveld G, Ferguson-Smith MA, Davies T, Stone M, et al: Translocation of c-abl oncogene correlates with the presence of a Philadelphia chromosome in chronic myelocytic leukaemia. *Nature* **306**:277, 1983.

329. Gale RP, Canaani E: An 8-kilobase abl RNA transcript in chronic myelogenous leukemia. *Proc Natl Acad Sci USA* **81**:5648, 1984.

330. Collins SJ, Kubonishi I, Miyoshi I, Groudine MT: Altered transcription of the c-abl oncogene in K562 and other chronic myelogenous leukemia cells. *Science* **225**:72, 1984.

331. Stam K, Heisterkamp N, Grosveld G, de Klein A, Verna RS, Coleman M, Dosik H, Groffen J: Evidence of a new chimeric bcr/c-abl mRNA in patients with chronic myelocytic leukemia and the Philadelphia chromosome. *N Engl J Med* **313**:1429, 1985.

332. Canaani E, Gale RP, Steiner-Saltz D, et al: Altered transcription of an oncogene in chronic myeloid leukemia. *Lancet* **1**:593, 1984.

333. Shtivelman E, Lifshitz B, Gale RP, Canaani E: Fused transcript of abl and bcr genes in chronic myelogenous leukemia. *Nature* **315**:550, 1985.

334. Heisterkamp N, Stephenson JR, Groffen J, et al: Localization of the c-abl oncogene adjacent to a translocation breakpoint in chronic myelocytic leukaemia. *Nature* **306**:239, 1983.

335. Leibowitz D, Schaefer-Rego K, Popenoe DW, et al: Variable breakpoints on the Philadelphia chromosome in chronic myelogenous leukemia. *Blood* **66**:243, 1985.

336. Grosveld G, Verwoerd T, van Agthoven T, de Klein A, Ramachandran KL, Heisterkamp N, Stam K, Groffen J: The chronic myelocytic cell line K562 contains a breakpoint in bcr and produces a chimeric bcr/c-abl transcript. *Mol Cell Biol* **6**:607, 1986.

337. Groffen J, Stephenson JR, Heisterkamp N, et al: Philadelphia chromosomal breakpoints are clustered within a limited region, bcr, on chromosome 22. *Cell* **36**:93, 1984.

338. Heisterkamp N, Stam K, Groffen J, et al: Structural organization of the bcr gene and its role in Ph^1 translocation. *Nature* **315**:758, 1985.

339. Kloetzer W, Kurzrock R, Smith L, Talpaz M, Spiller M, Gutterman J, Arlinghaus R: The human cellular abl gene product in the chronic myelogenous leukemia cell line K562 has an associated tyrosine protein kinase activity. *Virology* **140**:230, 1985.

340. Konopka JB, Watanabe SM, Witte ON: An alteration of the human c-abl protein in K562 leukemia cells unmasks associated tyrosine kinase activity. *Cell* **37**:1935, 1984.

341. Konopka JB, Watanabe SM, Singer JW, et al: Cell lines and clinical isolates derived from Ph1-positive chronic myelogenous leukemia patients express c-abl proteins with a common structural alteration. *Proc Natl Acad Sci USA* **82**:1810, 1985.

342. Naldini L, Stacchini A, Cirillo DM, Aglietta M, Gavosto F, Comoglio PM: Phosphotyrosine antibodies identify the p210 c-abl tyrosine kinase and proteins phosphorylated on tyrosine in human chronic myelogenous leukemia cells. *Mol Cell Biol* **6**:1803, 1986.

343. Chan LC, Karhi KK, Rayter SI, et al: A novel abl protein expressed in Philadelphia chromosome-positive acute lymphoblastic leukaemia. *Nature* **325**:635, 1987.

344. Clark SS, McLaughlin J, Crist WM, et al: Unique forms of the abl tyrosine kinase distinguish Ph^1-positive CML from Ph^1-positive ALL. *Science* **235**:85, 1987.

345. Kurzrock R, Shtalrid M, Romero P, et al: A novel c-abl protein product in Philadelphia-positive acute lymphoblastic leukemia. *Nature* **325**:631, 1987.

346. Hermans A, Heisterkamp N, von Linden M, van Baal S, Meijer D, van der Plas D, Wiedemann LM, Groffen J, Bootsma D, Grosveld G: Unique fusion of bcr and c-abl genes in Philadelphia chromosome positive acute lymphoblastic leukemia. *Cell* **51**:33, 1987.

347. Walker LC, Ganesan TS, Dhut S, Gibbons B, Lister TA, Rothbard J, Young BD: Novel chimaeric protein expressed in Philadelphia positive acute lymphoblastic leukemia. *Nature* **329**:851, 1987.

348. Fainstein E, Marcelle C, Rosener A, Canaani E, Gale RP, Dreazen O, Smith SD, Croce CM: A new fused transcript in Philadelphia chromosome positive acute lymphocytic leukemia. *Nature* **330**:386, 1987.

349. Witte ON, Ponticelli A, Gifford A, et al: Phosphorylation of the Abelson murine leukemia virus transforming protein. *J Virol* **39**:870, 1981.

350. Reynolds FHJ, Oroszlan S, Stephenson JR: Abelson murine leukemia virus p120: Identification and characterization of tyrosine phosphorylation sites. *J Virol* **44**:1097, 1982.

351. Srinivasan A, Dunn CY, Yuasa Y, Devare SG, Reddy EP, Aaronson SA: Abelson murine leukemia virus: structural requirements for transforming gene function. *Proc Natl Acad Sci USA* **79**:5508, 1982.

352. Daley GQ, McLaughlin J, Witte ON, Baltimore D: The CML-specific P210 bcr/abl protein, unlike v-abl, does not transform NIH/3T3 fibroblasts. *Science* **237**:532, 1987.

353. Daley GQ, Baltimore D: Transformation of an interleukin 3-dependent hematopoietic cell line by the chronic myelogenous leukemia-specific P210bcr/abl protein. *Proc Natl Acad Sci USA* **85**:9312, 1988.

354. Elefanty AG, Hariharan IK, Cory S: bcr-abl, the hallmark of chronic myeloid leukaemia in man, induces multiple haemopoietic neoplasms in mice. *EMBO J* **9**:1069, 1990.

355. Gishizky ML, Johnson-White J, Witte ON: Efficient transplantation of BCR-ABL-induced chronic myelogenous leukemia-like syndrome in mice. *Proc Natl Acad Sci USA* **90**:3755, 1993.

356. Kelliher M, Knott A, McLaughlin J, Witte ON, Rosenberg N: Differences in oncogenic potency but not target cell specificity distinguish

the two forms of the BCR/ABL oncogene. *Mol Cell Biol* **11**:4710, 1991.

357. Goga A, McLaughlin J, Afar DE, Saffran DC, Witte ON: Alternative signals to RAS for hematopoietic transformation by the BCR-ABL oncogene. *Cell* **82**:981, 1995.

358. Senechal K, Halpern J, Sawyers CL: The CRKL adaptor protein transforms fibroblasts and functions in transformation by the BCR-ABL oncogene. *J Biol Chem*, in press.

359. Raitano AB, Halpern JR, Hambuch TM, Sawyers CL: The Bcr-Abl leukemia oncogene activates Jun kinase and requires Jun for transformation. *Proc Natl Acad Sci USA* **92**:11746, 1995.

360. Afar DE, Goga A, McLaughlin J, Witte ON, Sawyers CL: Differential complementation of Bcr-Abl point mutants with c-Myc. *Science* **264**:424, 1994.

361. Afar DE, McLaughlin J, Sherr CJ, Witte ON, Roussel MF: Signaling by ABL oncogenes through cyclin D1. *Proc Natl Acad Sci USA* **92**:9540, 1995.

362. Shuai K, Halpern J, ten Hoeve J, Rao X, Sawyers CL: Constitutive activation of STAT5 by the BCR-ABL oncogene in chronic myelogenous leukemia. *Oncogene* **13**:247, 1996.

363. Golub TR, Goga A, Barker GF, Afar DE, McLaughlin J, Bohlander SK, Rowley JD, Witte ON, Gilliland DG: Oligomerization of the ABL tyrosine kinase by the Ets protein TEL in human leukemia. *Mol Cell Biol* **16**:4107, 1996.

364. Papadopoulos P, Ridge SA, Boucher CA, Stocking C, Wiedemann LM: The novel activation of ABL by fusion to an ets-related gene, TEL. *Cancer Res* **55**:34, 1995.

365. Golub TR, Barker GF, Lovett M, Gilliland DG: Fusion of PDGF receptor beta to a novel ets-like gene, tel, in chronic myelomonocytic leukemia with t(5;12) chromosomal translocation. *Cell* **77**:307, 1994.

366. Tybulewicz VL, Crawford CE, Jackson PK, Bronson RT, Mulligan RC: Neonatal lethality and lymphopenia in mice with a homozygous disruption of the c-abl proto-oncogene. *Cell* **65**:1153, 1991.

367. Schwartzberg PL, Stall AM, Hardin JD, Bowdish KS, Humaran T, Boast S, Harbison ML, Robertson EJ, Goff SP: Mice homozygous for the ablm1 mutation show poor viability and depletion of selected B and T cell populations. *Cell* **65**:1165, 1991.

368. Van Etten RA, Jackson P, Baltimore D: The mouse type IV c-abl gene product is a nuclear protein, and activation of transforming ability is associated with cytoplasmic localization. *Cell* **58**:669, 1989.

369. Kharbanda S, Ren R, Pandey P, Shafman TD, Feller SM, Weichselbaum RR, Kufe DW: Activation of the c-ABL tyrosine kinase in the stress response to DNA-damaging agents. *Nature* **376**:785, 1995.

370. Sawyers CL, McLaughlin J, Goga A, Havlik M, Witte O: The nuclear tyrosine kinase c-Abl negatively regulates cell growth. *Cell* **77**:121, 1994.

371. Mattioni T, Jackson PK, Bchini-Hooft van Huijsduijnen O, Picard D: Cell cycle arrest by tyrosine kinase Abl involves altered early mitogenic response. *Oncogene* **10**:1325, 1995.

372. Goga A, Liu X, Hambuch TM, Senechal K, Major E, Berk AJ, Witte ON, Sawyers CL: p53 dependent growth suppression by the c-Abl nuclear tyrosine kinase. *Oncogene* **11**:791, 1995.

373. Yuan Z, Huang Y, Whang Y, Sawyers C, Weichselbaum R, Kharbanda S, Kufe D: Role for the c-ABL tyrosine kinase in the growth arrest response to DNA damage. *Nature*, **382**:272, 1996.

374. Bloomfield CD, Goldman AL, Berger AR, et al: Chromosomal abnormalities identify high-risk and low-risk patients with acute lymphoblastic leukemia. *Blood* **67**:415, 1986.

375. Jain K, Arlin Z, Mertelsmann R, et al: Philadelphia chromosome and terminal transferase-positive acute leukemia: similarity of terminal phase of chronic myelogenous leukemia and de novo acute presentation. *J Clin Oncol* **1**:669, 1983.

376. Williams DL, Harber J, Murphy SB, et al: Chromosomal translocation play a unique role in influencing prognosis in childhood acute lymphoblastic leukemia. *Blood* **68**:205, 1986.

377. Roberts WM, Rivera GK, Raimondi SC, Santana VM, Sandlund JT, Crist WM, Pui CH: Intensive chemotherapy for Philadelphia-chromosome-positive acute lymphoblastic leukaemia. *Lancet* **343**:331, 1994.

378. Thomas ED, Clift RA: Indications for marrow transplantation in chronic myelogenous leukemia. *Blood* **73**:861, 1989.

379. Morris SW, Kirstein MN, Valentine MB, Dittmer KG, Shapiro DN, Saltman DL, Look AT: Fusion of the tyrosine kinase gene ALK to the nucleolar phosphoprotein gene NPM in human t(2;5)-positive lymphomas. *Science* **263**:1281, 1994.

380. Borer RA, Lehner CF, Eppenberger HM, Nigg EA: Major nucleolar proteins shuttle between nucleus and cytoplasm. *Cell* **56**:379, 1989.

381. Szebeni A, Herrera JE, Olson MO: Interaction of nucleolar protein B23 with peptides related to nuclear localization signals. *Biochemistry* **34**:8037, 1995.

382. Chan W, Liu QR, Borjigin J, Busch H, Rennert OM, Tease LA, Chan P: Characterization of the cDNA encoding human nucleophosmin and studies of its role in normal and abnormal growth. *Biochemistry* **28**:1033, 1989.

383. Peter M, Nakagawa J, Doree M, Labbe JC, Nigg EA: Identification of major nucleolar proteins as candidate mitotic substrates of cdc2 kinase. *Cell* **60**:791, 1990.

384. Dumbar TS, Gentry GA, Olson MOJ: Interaction of nucleolar phosphoprotein B23 with nucleic acids. *Biochemistry* **28**:9495, 1989.

385. Fankhauser C, Izaurralde E, Adachi Y, Wingfield P, Laemmli UK: Specific complex of human immunodeficiency virus type 1 rev and nucleolar B23 proteins: dissociation by the Rev response element. *Mol Cell Biol* **11**:2567, 1991.

386. Feuerstein N, Mond JJ, Kinchington PR, Hickey R, Karjalainen Lindsberg ML, Hay I, Ruyechan WT: Evidence for DNA binding activity of numatrin (B23), a cell cycle-regulated nuclear matrix protein. *Biochim Biophys Acta* **1087**:127, 1990.

387. Inouye CJ, Seto E: Relief of YY1-induced transcriptional repression by protein-protein interaction with the nucleolar phosphoprotein B23. *J Biol Chem* **269**:6506, 1994.

388. Valdez BC, Perlaky L, Henning D, Saijo Y, Chan PH, Busch H: Identification of the nuclear and nucleolar localization signals of the protein p120. *J Biol Chem* **269**:23776, 1994.

389. Morris SW, Naeve C, Mathew P, James PL, Kirstein MN, Cui X, Witte DP: ALK, the chromosome 2 gene locus altered by the t(2;5) in non-Hodgkin's lymphoma, encodes a neural receptor tyrosine kinase that is highly related to leukocyte tyrosine kinase (LTK). *Oncogene* **14**:2175, 1997.

390. Fujimoto J, Shiota M, Iwahara T, Seki N, Satoh H, Mori S, Yamamoto T: Characterization of the transforming activity of p80, a hyperphosphorylated protein in a Ki-1 lymphoma cell line with chromosomal translocation t(2;5). *Proc Natl Acad Sci USA* **93**:4181, 1996.

391. Kuefer MU, Look AT, Tripp R, Behm FG, Pattengale PK, Morris SW: Retrovirus-mediated gene transfer of NPM-ALK causes lymphoid malignancy in mice. [Abstract] *Blood* **88**:450a, 1996.

392. Sandlund JT, Pui CH, Roberts M, Morris SW, Mahmoud H, Berard CW, Hutchison RE, Crist WM, Rafferty M, Raimondi SC: Clinicopathologic features and treatment outcome of children with large cell lymphoma and the t(2;5)(p23;q35). *Blood* **84**:2467, 1994.

393. Sarris AH, Luthra R, Papadimitracopoulou V, Waasdorp M, Dimopoulos MA, McBride JA, Cabanillas F, Duvic M, Deisseroth A, Morris SW, Pugh WC: Amplification of genomic DNA demonstrates the presence of the t(2;5)(p23;q35) in anaplastic large cell lymphoma, but not in other non-Hodgkin's lymphomas, Hodgkin's disease, or lymphomatoid papulosis. *Blood* **88**:1771, 1996.

394. Downing JR, Shurtleff SA, Zielenska M, Curcio-Brint AM, Behm FG, Head DR, Sandlund JT, Weisenburger DD, Kossakowska AE, Thorner P, Lorenzanz A, Ladanyi M, Morris SW: Molecular detection of the (2;5) translocation of non-Hodgkin's lymphoma by reverse transcriptase-polymerase chain reaction. *Blood* **85**:3416, 1995.

395. Mathew P, Sanger WG, Weisenburger DD, Valentine M, Valentine V, Pickering D, Higgins C, Hess M, Cui X, Srivastava DK, Morris SW: Detection of the t(2;5)(p23;q35) and NPM-ALK fusion in non-Hodgkin's lymphoma by two-color fluorescence in situ hybridization. *Blood* **89**:1678, 1996.

396. Koeffler HP: Myelodysplastic syndromes. *Hematol/Oncol Clin N Am* **6**:485, 1992.

397. Yarden Y, Escobedo JA, Kuang WJ, Yang-Feng TL, Daniel TO, Tremble PM, Chen EY, Ando ME, Harkins RN, Francke U, et al: Structure of the receptor for platelet-derived growth factor helps define a family of closely related growth factor receptors. *Nature* **323**:226, 1986.

398. Satoh T, Fantl WJ, Escobedo JA, Williams LT, Kaziro Y: Platelet-derived growth factor receptor mediates activation of ras through different signaling pathways in different cell types. *Mol Cell Biol* **13**:3706, 1993.

399. Yan XQ, Brady G, Iscove NN: Overexpression of PDGF-B in murine hematopoietic cells induces a lethal myeloproliferative syndrome in vivo. *Oncogene* **9**:163, 1994.

400. Nye JA, Petersen JM, Gunther CV, Jonsen MD, Graves BJ: Interaction of murine ets-1 with GGA-binding sites establishes the ETS domain as a new DNA-binding motif. *Gene Dev* **6**:975, 1992.

401. Rao VN, Ohno T, Prasad DD, Bhattacharya G, Reddy ES: Analysis of the DNA-binding and transcriptional activation functions of human Fli-1 protein. *Oncogene* **8**:2167, 1993.

402. Sawyers CL, Denny CT: Chronic myelomonocytic leukemia: Tel-a-kinase what Ets all about. *Cell* **77**:171, 1994.

403. Wlodarska I, Mecucci C, Marynen P, Guo C, Franckx D, La Starza R, Aventin A, Bosly A, Martelli MF, Cassiman JJ, et al: TEL gene is involved in myelodysplastic syndromes with either the typical t(5;12)(q33;p13) translocation or its variant t(10;12)(q24;p13). *Blood* **85**:2848, 1995.

404. Erikson J, Finan J, Tsujimoto Y, Nowell PC, Croce CM: The chromosome 14 breakpoint in neoplastic B cells with the t(11;14) translocation involves the immunoglobulin heavy chain locus. *Proc Natl Acad Sci USA* **81**:4144, 1984.

405. Tsujimoto Y, Yunis J, Onorato-Showe L, Erikson J, Nowell PC, Croce CM: Molecular cloning of the chromosomal breakpoint of B-cell lymphomas and leukemias with the t(11;14) chromosome translocation. *Science* **224**:1403, 1984.

406. Tsujimoto Y, Jaffe E, Cossman J, Gorham J, Nowell PC, Croce CM: Clustering of breakpoints on chromosome 11 in human B-cell neoplasms with the t(11;14) chromosome translocation. *Nature* **315**:340, 1985.

407. Louie E, Tsujimoto Y, Heubner K, Croce CM: *Am J Hum Genet (Suppl)* **41**:31, 1987.

408. Rabbitts PH, Douglas J, Fischer P, Nacheva E, Karpas A, Catovsky D, Melo JV, Baer R, Stinson MA, Rabbitts TH: Chromosome abnormalities at 11q13 in B cell tumours. *Oncogene* **3**:99, 1988.

409. Meeker TC, Grimaldi JC, O'Rourke R, Louie E, Juliusson G, Einhorn S: An additional breakpoint region in the BCL-1 locus associated with the t(11;14)(q13;q32) translocation of B-lymphocytic malignancy. *Blood* **74**:1801, 1989.

410. Lammie GA, Fantl V, Smith R, Schuuring E, Brookes S, Michalides R, Dickson C, Arnold A, Peters G: D11S287, a putative oncogene on chromosome 11q13, is amplified and expressed in squamous cell and mammary carcinomas and linked to BCL-1. *Oncogene* **6**:439, 1991.

411. Rosenberg CL, Wong E, Petty EM, Bale AE, Tsujimoto Y, Harris NL, Arnold A: PRAD1, a candidate BCL1 oncogene: mapping and expression in centrocytic lymphoma. *Proc Natl Acad Sci USA* **88**:9638, 1991.

412. Withers DA, Harvey RC, Faust JB, Melnyk O, Carey K, Meeker TC: Characterization of a candidate *bcl-1* gene. *Mol Cell Biol* **11**:4846, 1991.

413. Brookes S, Lammie GA, Schuuring E, Dickson C, Peters G: Linkage map of region of human chromosome band 11q13 amplified in breast and squamous cell tumors. *Gene Chrom Cancer* **4**:290, 1992.

414. Hall M, Peters G: Genetic alterations of cyclins, cyclin-dependent kinases, and Cdk inhibitors in human cancer, in Vande Woude GF, Klein G (eds): *Advances in Cancer Research*. San Diego, Academic Press, 1996, p. 67.

415. Sherr CJ: Mammalian G1 cyclins. *Cell* **73**:1059, 1993.

416. Rosenberg CL, Motokura T, Kronenberg HM, Arnold A: Coding sequence of the overexpressed transcript of the putative oncogene PRAD1/cyclin D1 in two primary human tumors. *Oncogene* **8**:519, 1993.

417. Rimokh R, Berger F, Bastard C, Klein B, French M, Archimbaud E, Rouault JP, Santa Lucia B, Duret L, Vuillaume M, et al: Rearrangement of CCND1 (BCL1/PRAD1) 3′ untranslated region in mantle-cell lymphomas and t(11q13)-associated leukemias. *Blood* **83**:3689, 1994.

418. Lukas J, Jadayel D, Bartkova J, Nacheva E, Dyer MJ, Strauss M, Bartek J: BCL-1/cyclin D1 oncoprotein oscillates and subverts the G1 phase control in B-cell neoplasms carrying the t(11;14) translocation. *Oncogene* **9**:2159, 1994.

419. Banks PM, Chan J, Cleary ML, Delsol G, De Wolf-Peeters C, Gatter K, Grogan TM, Harris NL, Isaacson PG, Jaffe ES, et al: Mantle cell lymphoma. A proposal for unification of morphologic, immunologic, and molecular data. *Am J Surg Pathol* **16**:637, 1992.

420. Shivdasani RA, Hess JL, Skarin AT, Pinkus GS: Intermediate lymphocytic lymphoma: clinical and pathologic features of a recently characterized subtype of non-Hodgkin's lymphoma. *J Clin Oncol* **11**:802, 1993.

421. Harris NL, Jaffe ES, Stein H, Banks PM, Chan JKC, Cleary ML, Delsol G, De Wolf-Peeters C, Falini B, Gatter KC, Grogan TM, Isaacson PG, Knowles DM, Mason DY, Muller-Hermelink H-K, Pileri SA, Piris MA, Ralfkiaer E, Warnke RA: A revised European-American classification of lymphoid neoplasms: a proposal from the International Lymphoma Study Group. *Blood* **84**:1361, 1994.

422. Banno S, Yoshikawa K, Nakamura S, Yamamoto K, Seito T, Nitta M, Takahashi T, Ueda R, Seto M: Monoclonal antibody against PRAD1/cyclin D1 stains nuclei of tumor cells with translocation or amplification at BCL-1 locus. *Jpn J Cancer Res* **85**:918, 1994.

423. de Boer CJ, van Krieken JH, Kluin-Nelemans HC, Kluin PM, Schuuring E: Cyclin D1 messenger RNA overexpression as a marker for mantle cell lymphoma. *Oncogene* **10**:1833, 1995.

424. Nakamura S, Seto M, Banno S, Suzuki S, Koshikawa T, Kitoh K, Kagami Y, Ogura M, Yatabe Y, Kojima M, et al: Immunohistochemical analysis of cyclin D1 protein in hematopoietic neoplasms with special reference to mantle cell lymphoma. *Jpn J Cancer Res* **85**:1270, 1994.

425. Yang WI, Zukerberg LR, Motokura T, Arnold A, Harris NL: Cyclin D1 (Bcl-1, PRAD1) protein expression in low-grade B-cell lymphomas and reactive hyperplasia. *Am J Pathol* **145**:86, 1994.

426. Fukuhara S, Rowley JD, Variakojis D, Golomb HM: Chromosome abnormalities in poorly differentiated lymphocytic lymphoma. *Cancer Res* **39**:3119, 1979.

427. Yunis JJ, Frizzera G, Oken MM, McKenna J, Theologides A, Arnesen M: Multiple recurrent genomic defects in follicular lymphoma. A possible model for cancer. *N Engl J Med* **316**:79, 1987.

428. Tsujimoto Y, Gorham J, Cossman J, Jaffe E, Croce CM: The t(14;18) chromosome translocations involved in B-cell neoplasms result from mistakes in VDJ joining. *Science* **229**:1390, 1985.

429. Bakhshi A, Jensen JP, Goldman P, Wright JJ, McBride OW, Epstein AL, Korsmeyer SJ: Cloning the chromosomal breakpoint of t(14;18) human lymphomas: clustering around JH on chromosome 14 and near a transcriptional unit on 18. *Cell* **41**:899, 1985.

430. Cleary ML, Sklar J: Nucleotide sequence of a t(14;18) chromosomal breakpoint in follicular lymphoma and demonstration of a breakpoint-cluster region near a transcriptionally active locus on chromosome 18. *Proc Natl Acad Sci USA* **82**:7439, 1985.

431. Cleary ML, Smith SD, Sklar J: Cloning and structural analysis of cDNAs for bcl-2 and a hybrid bcl-2/immunoglobulin transcript resulting from the t(14;18) translocation. *Cell* **47**:19, 1986.

432. Vaux DL, Cory S, Adams JM: Bcl-2 gene promotes haemopoietic cell survival and cooperates with c-myc to immortalize pre-B cells. *Nature* **335**:440, 1988.

433. Nunez G, London L, Hockenbery D, Alexander M, McKearn JP, Korsmeyer SJ: Deregulated Bcl-2 gene expression selectively prolongs survival of growth factor-deprived hemopoietic cell lines. *J Immunol* **144**:3602, 1990.

434. Korsmeyer SJ: Bcl-2 initiates a new category of oncogenes: regulators of cell death. *Blood* **80**:879, 1992.

435. Yang E, Korsmeyer SJ: Molecular Thanatopsis: A discourse on the BCL2 family and cell death. *Blood* **88**:386, 1996.

436. Hengartner MO, Horvitz HR: C. elegans cell survival gene ced-9 encodes a functional homolog of the mammalian proto-oncogene bcl-2. *Cell* **76**:665, 1994.

437. von Lindern M, Poustka A, Lerach H, Grosveld G: The (6;9) chromosome translocation, associated with a specific subtype of acute non-lymphocytic leukemia, leads to aberrant transcription of a target gene on 9q34. *Mol Cell Biol* **10**:4016, 1990.

438. von Lindern M, van Baal S, Wiegant J, Raap A, Hagemeijer A, Grosveld G: Can, a putative oncogene associated with myeloid leukemogenesis, may be activated by fusion of its 3′ half to different genes: characterization of the set gene. *Mol Cell Biol* **12**:3346, 1992.

439. von Lindern M, Breems D, van Baal S, Adriaansen H, Grosveld G: Characterization of the translocation breakpoint sequences of two DEK-CAN fusion genes present in t(6;9) acute myeloid leukemia and a SET-CAN fusion gene found in a case of acute undifferentiated leukemia. *Gene Chrom Cancer* **5**:227, 1992.

440. Borrow J, Shearman AM, Stanton VP Jr, Becher R, Collins T, Williams AJ, Dube I, Katz F, Kwong YL, Morris C, Ohyashiki K, Toyama K, Rowley J, Housman DE: The t(7;11)(p15;p15) translocation in acute myeloid leukaemia fuses the genes for nucleoporin NUP98 and class I homeoprotein HOXA9 [see comments]. *Nat Genet* **12**:159, 1996.

441. Nakamura T, Largaespada DA, Lee MP, Johnson LA, Ohyashiki K, Toyama K, Chen SJ, Willman CL, Chen IM, Feinberg AP, Jenkins NA, Copeland NG, Shaughnessy JD Jr: Fusion of the nucleoporin gene NUP98 to HOXA9 by the chromosome translocation t(7;11)(p15;p15) in human myeloid leukaemia. *Nat Genet* **12**:154, 1996.

442. Kraemer D, Wozniak RW, Blobel G, Radu A: The human CAN protein, a putative oncogene product associated with myeloid leukemogenesis, is a nuclear pore complex protein that faces the cytoplasm. *Proc Natl Acad Sci USA* **91**:1519, 1994.

443. Fornerod M, Boer J, van Baal S, Jaegle M, von Lindern M, Murti KG, Davis D, Bonten J, Buijs A, Grosveld G: Relocation of the carboxyterminal part of CAN from the nuclear envelope to the nucleus as a result of leukemia-specific chromosome rearrangements. *Oncogene* **10**:1739, 1995.

444. van Deursen J, Boer J, Kasper L, Grosveld G: G2 arrest and impaired nucleocytoplasmic transport in mouse embryos lacking the proto-oncogene CAN/Nup214. *EMBO J* **15**:5574, 1996.

445. Fornerod M, Boer J, van Baal S, Morreau H, Grosveld G: Interaction of cellular proteins with the leukemia specific fusion proteins DEK-CAN and SET-CAN and their normal counterpart, the nucleoporin CAN. *Oncogene* **13**:1801, 1996.

446. Yoneda-Kato N, Look AT, Kirstein MN, Valentine MB, Raimondi SC, Cohen KJ, Carroll AJ, Morris SW: The t(3;5)(q25.1;q34) of myelodysplastic syndrome and acute myeloid leukemia produces a novel fusion gene, NPM-MLF1. *Oncogene* **12**:265, 1996.

447. Kuefer MU, Look AT, Williams DC, Valentine V, Naeve CW, Behm FG, Mullersman JE, Yoneda-Kato N, Montgomery K, Kucherlapati R, Morris SW: cDNA cloning, tissue distribution, and chromosomal localization of myelodysplasia/myeloid leukemia factor 2 (MLF2). *Genomics* **35**:392, 1996.

448. Dallery E, Galiegue-Zouitina S, Collyn-d'Hooghe M, Quief S, Denis C, Hildebrand MP, Lantoine D, Deweindt C, Tilly H, Bastard C, et al: TTF, a gene encoding a novel small G protein, fuses to the lymphoma-associated LAZ3 gene by t(3;4) chromosomal translocation. *Oncogene* **10**:2171, 1995.

449. Ohno H, Takimoto G, McKeithan TW: The candidate proto-oncogene bcl-3 is related to genes implicated in cell lineage determination and cell cycle control. *Cell* **60**:991, 1990.

450. Wulczyn FG, Naumann M, Scheidereit C: Candidate proto-oncogene bcl-3 encodes a subunit-specific inhibitor of transcription factor NF-kappa B. *Nature* **358**:597, 1992.

451. Kerr LD, Duckett CS, Wamsley P, Zhang Q, Chiao P, Nabel G, McKeithan TW, Baeuerle PA, Verma IM: The proto-oncogene bcl-3 encodes an I kappa B protein. *Gene Dev* **6**:2352, 1992.

452. Neri A, Chang CC, Lombardi L, Salina M, Corradini P, Maiolo AT, Chaganti RS, Dalla-Favera R: B cell lymphoma-associated chromosomal translocation involves candidate oncogene lyt-10, homologous to NF-kappa B p50. *Cell* **67**:1075, 1991.

453. Iida S, Rao PH, Nallasivam P, Hibshoosh H, Butler M, Louie DC, Dyomin V, Ohno H, Chaganti RSK, Dalla-Favera R: The t(9;14)(p13;q32) chromosomal translocation associated with lymphoplasmacytoid lymphoma involves the PAX-5 gene. *Blood* **88**:4110, 1996.

454. Shimizu K, Miyoshi H, Kozu T, Nagata J, Enomoto K, Maseki N, Kaneko Y, Ohki ML: Consistent disruption of the AML1 gene occurs within a single intron in the t(8;21) chromosomal translocation. *Cancer Res* **52**:6945, 1992.

455. Ichikawa H, Shimizu K, Hayashi Y, Ohki M: An RNA-binding protein gene, TLS/FUS, is fused to ERG in human myeloid leukemia with t(16;21) chromosomal translocation. *Cancer Res* **54**:2865, 1994.

456. Buijs A, Sherr S, van Baal S, van Bezouw S, van der Plas D, Geurts van Kessel A, Riegman P, Lekanne Deprez R, Zwarthoff E, Hagemeijer A, et al: Translocation (12;22)(p13;q11) in myeloproliferative disorders results in fusion of the ETS-like TEL gene on 12p13 to the

457. Bernard OA, Mauchauffe M, Mecucci C, Van den Berghe H, Berger R: A novel gene, AF-1p, fused to HRX in t(1;11)(p32;q23), is not related to AF-4, AF-9 nor ENL. *Oncogene* **9**:1039, 1994.

458. Chaplin T, Ayton P, Bernard OA, Saha V, Della Valle V, Hillion J, Gregorini A, Lillington D, Berger R, Young BD: A novel class of zinc finger/leucine zipper genes identified from the molecular cloning of the t(10;11) translocation in acute leukemia. *Blood* **85**:1435, 1995.

459. Prasad R, Leshkowitz D, Gu Y, Alder H, Nakamura T, Saito H, Huebner K, Berger R, Croce CM, Canaani E: Leucine-zipper dimerization motif encoded by the AF17 gene fused to ALL-1 (MLL) in acute leukemia. *Proc Natl Acad SCi USA* **91**:8107, 1994.

460. Parry P, Wei Y, Evans G: Cloning and characterization of the t(X;11) breakpoint from a leukemic cell line identify a new member of the forkhead gene family. *Genes Chrom Cancer* **11**:79, 1994.

461. Tycko B, Smith SD, Sklar J: Chromosomal translocations joining LCK and TCRB loci in human T cell leukemia. *J Exp Med* **174**:867, 1991.

462. Burnett RC, David JC, Harden AM, Le Beau MM, Rowley JD, Diaz MO: The LCK gene is involved in the t(1;7)(p34;q34) in the T-cell acute lymphoblastic leukemia derived cell line, HSB-2. *Genes Chrom Cancer* **3**:461, 1991.

463. Wright DD, Sefton BM, Kamps MP: Oncogenic activation of the Lck protein accompanies translocation of the LCK gene in the human HSB2 T-cell leukemia. *Mol Cell Biol* **14**:2429, 1994.

464. von Lindern M, Fornerod M, van Baal S, Jaegle M, de Wit T, Buijs A, Grosveld G: The translocation (6;9), associated with a specific subtype of acute myeloid leukemia, results in the fusion of two genes, dek and can, and the expression of a chimeric, leukemia-specific dek-can mRNA. *Mol Cell Biol* **12**:1687, 1992.

465. Dreyling MH, Martinez-Climent JA, Zheng M, Mao J, Rowley JD, Bohlander SK: The t(10;11)(p13;q14) in the U937 cell line results in the fusion of the AF10 gene and CALM, encoding a new member of the AP-3 clathrin assembly protein family. *Proc Natl Acad Sci USA* **93**:4804, 1996.

466. Fisch P, Forster A, Sherrington PD, Dyer MJ, Rabbitts TH: The chromosomal translocation t(X;14)(q28;q11) in T-cell pro-lymphocytic leukaemia breaks within one gene and activates another. *Oncogene* **8**:3271, 1993.

467. Ellisen LW, Bird J, West DC, Soreng AL, Reynolds TC, Smith SD, Sklar J: TAN-1, the human homolog of the Drosophila notch gene, is broken by chromosomal translocations in T lymphoblastic neoplasms. *Cell* **66**:649, 1991.

468. Grimaldi JC, Meeker TC: The t(5;14) chromosomal translocation in a case of acute lymphocytic leukemia joins the interleukin-3 gene to the immunoglobulin heavy chain gene. *Blood* **73**:2081, 1989.

469. Meeker TC, Hardy D, Willman C, Hogan T, Abrams J: Activation of the interleukin-3 gene by chromosome translocation in acute lymphocytic leukemia with eosinophilia. *Blood* **76**:285, 1990.

470. Laabi Y, Gras MP, Carbonnel F, Brouet JC, Berger R, Larsen CJ, Tsapis A: A new gene, BCM, on chromosome 16 is fused to the interleukin-2 gene by a t(4;16)(q26;p13) translocation in a malignant T cell lymphoma. *EMBO J* **11**:3897, 1992.

471. Sandlund JT, Downing JR, Crist WM: Non-Hodgkin's lymphoma in childhood. *N Engl J Med* **334**:1238, 1996.

472. Downing JR, Look AT: MLL fusion genes in the 11q23 acute leukemias, in Freireich EJ, Kantarjian H (eds): *Leukemia: Advances in Research and Treatment*. Boston, Kluwer, 1995.

MN1 gene on 22q11 [published erratum appears in Oncogene 1995 Aug 17; 11(4):809]. *Oncogene* **10**:1511, 1995.

CHAPTER 6

Chromosome Rearrangements in Human Solid Tumors

Paul S. Meltzer ∎ Jeffrey M. Trent

1. Recurring sites of chromosome change represent the byproducts of molecular events which participate in the generation or progression of human cancers. Chromosome abnormalities in patients with hematopoietic cancers have proved to be of diagnostic and prognostic value, and the molecular defects for many of these abnormalities have been described (see Chap. 5). Despite the fact that solid tumors are exceedingly more common than the blood-borne cancers of humans and make a significantly greater contribution to morbidity and mortality relative to hematologic neoplasms, less is known about chromosome changes and their clinical and biologic importance in solid tumors. Nevertheless, significant information is accumulating on recurring chromosome alterations in solid tumors, including the molecular dissection of recurring breakpoints in many malignancies.

2. The pattern of chromosome alterations in human solid tumors is decidedly nonrandom. Solid tumors tend to demonstrate multiple clonal structural and numeric chromosome rearrangements, and databases are being developed to describe new karyotypic abnormalities in the context of tumor histopathology.

3. General categories of structural chromosome rearrangements in human solid tumors include chromosome translocations, deletions, and inversions, as well as changes associated with increases in the DNA sequence copy number [double minutes (dmin) and homogeneously staining regions (HSRs)].

4. Tumor-specific chromosome rearrangements have been identified in human solid tumors, and a brief discussion of chromosome alterations in many common cancers is presented.

5. Human sarcomas represent a paradigm for the molecular dissection of human solid tumors. Tumor-specific chromosome translocations have been described and characterized at the molecular level for several sarcomas, including Ewing sarcoma, alveolar rhabdomyosarcoma, synovial sarcoma, myxoid liposarcoma, and soft-tissue clear-cell sarcoma. In general, these translocations juxtapose segments of two genes which can give rise to a chimeric fusion transcript. Two closely related genes, *EWS* (on chromosome 12q13) and *FUS* (on chromosome 16p11), have been demonstrated to participate in tumor-specific translocations in several sarcomas. In each case, *EWS* or *FUS* acquires a DNA-binding domain from the translocation partner chromosome. These tumor-specific chimeric oncoproteins have transcription factor activity, and it appears that they contribute to malignant transformation by leading to dysregulated gene expression.

6. Numerous benign neoplasms, such as lipomas and leiomyomas, exhibit translocations involving members of the HMGI family of DNA-binding proteins. Multiple partner genes are involved with one of the two HMGI genes in various tumors. The disturbance of HMGI protein function appears to have a profound effect on the proliferation of mesenchymal cells in multiple lineages, yet these tumors do not become malignant.

7. The clinical value of chromosome rearrangements in the common solid tumors of adults is largely indeterminate. Recent advances and the development of new technical approaches for the analysis of complex changes in solid tumors suggest that further insights into chromosome rearrangements (and the genes dysregulated by them) may increase clinical utility.

It is now recognized that most human cancers, including solid tumors, display recurring chromosome abnormalities. However, questions remain in most cases in regard to their exact biologic significance. How do chromosomal changes relate to changes in the expression of important genes, including oncogenes? What is the significance of a recurring cytogenetic alteration when viewed against a background of other (often multiple) genetic alterations? What clinical significance, if any, do specific cytogenetic abnormalities have for solid tumors? These questions have been the focus of intense study over the past decade, and our recognition and recently our molecular understanding of chromosome abnormalities are providing significant insights into neoplasms in general and solid tumors in particular.

Significant progress has been made in tumor cytogenetics in recent years. For example, before 1981 only 1800 cases of malignancies with abnormal chromosomes were reported in all the world's literature, and less than 3 percent were from solid tumors. In contrast, by the end of 1994 there were over 22,000 published cases of neoplasms with abnormal karyotypes, and 27 percent of them were from solid tumors.[1]

With this explosion in our knowledge of human chromosome alterations in neoplasia has come the widespread acceptance of the clinical value of chromosome analysis in studies of human hematologic cancers. Specifically, chromosome analysis of malignant cells from patients with hematopoietic cancers provides diagnostic and equally importantly prognostic information independent of other laboratory and clinical features of disease.[2–4] Despite the fact that solid tumors represent almost 95 percent of the cancers of humankind, far less is known about chromosome changes and especially their clinical importance in solid tumors. This chapter focuses on features of solid tumor cytogenetics which can be related to our understanding of the biologic and clinical utility of this information.

Two recent and excellent books[2,3] survey the field of cancer cytogenetics and provide in-depth descriptions of chromosome changes by histopathologic subtype. Further, there is a useful (though didactic) description of all published cytogenetic changes in the reported literature which may be of interest to those who seek a listing of all chromosome changes.[2] Finally, a comprehensive technical manual of methods for the analysis of solid tumors has appeared.[5] No attempt will be made in this brief chapter to duplicate the wealth of detail these books contain, and the interested reader is referred to those sources for in-depth information on techniques as well as detailed karyotypic information on any tumor type.

GENERAL ASPECTS OF CHROMOSOME CHANGE IN SOLID TUMORS

The diversity of structural chromosome alterations across the spectrum of human cancers is enormous and is increasing rapidly. The central dogma underlying the study of chromosomes in cancer is that karyotypic changes are nonrandom and thus are nonuniformly distributed throughout the human genome. Specific chromosome bands are preferentially involved in rearrangements in different neoplasms, and increasingly, the underlying molecular defects are being understood. Examination of the nonrandom nature of chromosome alterations has led to the identification of over 200 recurring chromosome changes in more than 70 neoplastic disorders (including many benign proliferations).[1] Taken together, every human chromosome with the exception of the Y can now be characterized by some form of neoplasia-associated alteration.

Methodology and Clonality

Technical obstacles have been in large part responsible for the relative paucity of cytogenetic information from solid tumor samples, including difficulties in sample disaggregation, cell viability resulting from necrosis of biopsy samples, contamination of samples with normal cells, and the complexity of most tumors (especially carcinomas), which frequently display a heterogeneous pattern of chromosome change. In most solid tumors, the times of clinical manifestation and removal of the tumor mass are thought to occur at a point considerably distant from cellular transformation, resulting in the generation of significant chromosomal rearrangement and imbalances. From a technical point of view, this means that in some solid tumors no two karyotypes from the same specimen may be identical and that as few as 1 or as many as 100 chromosome rearrangements may be described within a single karyotype. To make matters even more confusing, there is also evidence that at least some tumors may arise from multiple stem cells or diverge soon after the appearance of an initiating transformation event and

then undergo clonal expansion of cell populations with unrelated karyotypes (i.e., be "polyclonal" in origin).[6–8] However, even with these complex karyotypes and heterogeneous tumor cell populations it has been possible to describe certain chromosomal abnormalities which are germinal to the development of a given tumor type. Primary chromosome aberrations frequently are found as the sole karyotypic abnormality in a neoplastic cell and reflect their presumed causal role in cellular transformation. Secondary chromosome aberrations are thought to be important in tumor progression, do not appear alone, but nevertheless display nonrandom features with distribution patterns that frequently are tumor type-dependent. It is believed that the features of genetic instability, divergence, and heterogeneity observed in most solid tumors represent significant genetic obstacles to effective patient treatment through Darwinian selection of genetically rearranged cells with a proliferative (or therapy-resistant) advantage. Despite the difficulty in analyzing solid tumors cytogenetically, there is much evidence that most cancers are monoclonal (and thus all the cells in a tumor share genetic characteristics of the original transformed cells), and therefore cancer is heritable at the cellular level.[9] This discovery, which was initially based largely on cytogenetic evidence, has been a major factor in reaching the conclusion that changes in the DNA sequences of individual cells are responsible for malignant changes in those cells.

Terminology

As was described above, the results of tumor chromosome studies are complex and challenging to summarize. The range of chromosome counts may be quite wide, for example, from hypodiploid (e.g., fewer than 46 chromosomes per cell) to hypertetraploid (more than 96 chromosomes), and it is not uncommon to find more than one modal number. It is also generally true that even in karyotyping cells with the same number of chromosomes, no two karyotypes from the same specimen are completely identical in all the numeric as well as structural abnormalities observed. Consequently, the field ordinarily describes the clonal changes which are evident and make up a composite karyotypic interpretation of the specimen. A numeric abnormality is said to be clonal if a missing chromosome is observed in at least three karyotypes and an extra chromosome is found in at least two, while a clonal structural abnormality is one that is found in two or more cells. Karyotypic anomalies which are found in a majority of cells from a tumor are said to represent the stemline population, while the abnormalities which are found in a small proportion of karyotypes are said to represent a sideline population. Multiple sidelines may (and usually do) exist in the same tumor sample. Many of the problems associated with describing complex karyotypes and multiple sidelines have been addressed by international convention according to the International System of Cytogenetic Nomenclature (ISCN),[10] and all descriptions of cancer (and constitutional) karyotypes are written in accordance with the ISCN recommendations. Table 6-1 gives representative examples of abbreviations used in chromosome nomenclature for solid tumors.

RECURRING CHROMOSOME ALTERATIONS IN HUMAN SOLID TUMORS

General Findings

Although it has been difficult to obtain information on chromosome alterations in solid tumors, many recurring cytogenetic alter-

Table 6-1 Chromosome Nomenclature

A–G	Chromosome groups
1–22	Autmosome numbers
X, Y	Sex chromosomes
/	Mosaicism; e.g., 46/47 designates a mosaic with 46-chromosome and 47-chromosome cell lines
p	Short arm of chromosome (petite)
q	Long arm of chromosome
del	Deletion
der	Derivative of chromosome
dup	Duplication
I	Isochromosome
ins	Insertion
inv	Inversion
r	Ring chromosome
t	Translocation
ter	Terminal (also may be written as pter or qter)
+ or −	When placed before the chromosome number, these symbols indicate the addition (+) or loss (−) of a whole chromosome; e.g., +21 indicates an extra chromosome 21, as in Down syndrome. When placed after the chromosome number, these symbols indicate the gain or loss of a chromosome part; e.g., 5p− indicates the loss of part of the short arm of chromosome 5, as in cri du chat syndrome.

SOURCE: Used with permission from Ref. 178.

ations have been described, and a summary of nonrandom chromosomal abnormalities is presented in Table 6-2. Representative examples of chromosome rearrangements in human solid tumors are documented in banded cells from two different cancers (Figs. 6-1 and 6-2). Examples of the utility of fluorescence in situ hybridization (FISH) as a powerful approach to identify all human chromosomes (Fig. 6-3) and for analysis of complex rearrangements (Fig. 6-4) are provided. After a brief discussion of generic classes of chromosome rearrangements, short summaries of recurring chromosome alterations of selected cancers are provided. A detailed description of human sarcomas is presented to highlight the significant and unique (to solid tumors) molecular characterization of these cancers.

Generally, abnormalities of chromosome 1 are nearly universal, and the high frequency of alterations in the majority of solid tumors has led to the suggestion that these changes represent a common event in the progression, but not genesis, of various cancers. In general, the reports of clinical relevance have been limited to studies of neuroblastoma, where deletion of 1p correlates with specific oncogene (NMYC) amplification[11,12] (see Chap. 7). In addition to structural alterations of chromosome 1, gain of chromosome 7 is one of the most common abnormalities in epithelial tumors and has been identified as a primary karyotype abnormality in a number of tumors.[1,13–18]

Cytologic Evidence of Gene Amplification

Another common category of chromosome alteration in solid tumors characterizes a clinically important mechanism for activation of oncogene overexpression: DNA sequence amplification (see Chap. 7). This increase in DNA sequence copy number change often results in cytologically recognizable chromosome alterations referred to as either homogeneously staining regions (HSRs) if integrated within chromosomes or double minutes (dmin) if extrachromosomal in nature (Fig. 6-5). Figures 6-6 and 6-7 illustrate the use of FISH technologies with chromosome microdissection to identify changes in DNA copy number recognizable within a tu-

Table 6-2 Recurring Karyotypic Abnormalities in Human Solid Tumors*

Tumor Type	Karyotype Abnormalities and Other Findings
	Malignant
Bladder (transitional cell carcinoma)	**+7; del(10)(q22–q24); del(21)(q22);** del and t of 1q21; i(5p); −9; i(11p); i(11q); del and t of 11p11–q11; del, t, and dup of 13q14
Brain, rhabdoid tumor	**−22**
Breast (adenocarcinoma)	**−17; i(1q); der(16)t(1;16)(q10;p10);** del(1)(q11–q12); del(3)(p12–p13p 14–p21); del(6)(q21–22); +7; +18; +20; del and t of 1p11–p13; t of 1q21–q23; 3q11–q13, 7q32–q36, and 11q13–q14; dup of 11q13–q14; dmins; hsrs(8p1)
Colon (carcinoma)	**+7; +20; i(1q);** inv and t of 1p11–q11; i(7q); +7; t of 7p11–q11; +8; +12; del of 12q; i(17q); t of 17p11–q11; del of 17p; −18; dmins
Ewing's sarcoma	**t(11;22)(q24;q12);** t(1;16)(q11;q11.1); +8;
Extraskeletal myxoid chondrosarcoma	**−Y;** t(9;22)(q22–31;q11–12)
Fibrosarcoma	**−Y**
Giant-cell tumors	**+8;** telomeric fusions of 11p15, 13p, 15p, 18p, 19p, 21p; fus(14p;21p); fus(15p;21p)
Glioma*	**+7; −10; −22; −X; +X; −Y;** del(22)(q11–q13); del or t of 9p; (hsr) 12q13–q14
Kidney (renal cell carcinoma)	**del(3)(p14–p21); del(3)(p11–p14);** t(3;5)(p13;q22); −3; +7; −8; +10; −Y; t(3;8)(p14;q24), t(3;11) (p13–p14;p15); i(5p); del(6)(q21–q23)
Kidney (papillary)	**+7; +17;** t(X;1)(p11;q21)
Larynx (squamous cell carcinoma)	**−Y**
Liposarcoma	**t of 12q13–q14**
Liposarcoma (myxoid)	**t(12;16)(q13;p11)**
Lung (adenocarcinoma)	**del(3)(p14p23); +7**
Lung (small-cell carcinoma)	**del(3)(p14p23); +7;** del of 5q, 6, 9p, 13q, 17p
Lung (squamous-cell carcinoma)	**+7**
Fibrous histiocytoma	**−Y**
Melanoma, cutaneous	t(1;6)(q11–q21;q11–q13); t(1;19)(q11;q13); t of 1q11–q12 that yield 1q gain; del and t of 1p11–q12; i(6p); t of 6p11–q11 that yields 6p gain; other t of 6q11–q13; t of 7q11; +7; del and t 9p
Melanoma, uveal	−3; partial del of 3; +8; i(8q)
Meningioma	**−22; +22; −Y; del(22)(q11–q13)**
Mesothelioma	del, t, dup, or inv of 3p21–p23
Nasopharynx (squamous-cell carcinoma)	**−Y**
Neuroblastoma	**del(1)(p32–p36);** t which yield del of 1p32–p36; der(1)t(1;17)(p36;?); dmins
Ovarian carcinoma	**+12, +7, +8; −X;** del(6q15–q23), del(3)(p21–p10); +3; +5; loss of 1p; gain of 1q; t(1;17)(p36;?); dmins; hsrs; hsrs of 19q13.1–q13.2
Prostate	**del(10)(q24), +7, −Y**

(continued)

Table 6-2 (continued)

Tumor Type	Karyotype Abnormalities and Other Findings
Retinoblastoma	**i(6p); del(13)(q14.1q14.1)**
Rhabdomyosarcoma	**t(2;13)(q37;q14); t(1;13)(p36;q14)**
Salivary gland (adenocarcinoma)	**del(6)(q22–q25); +8; −Y**
Squamous-cell, oral	**+7**
Synovial sarcoma	**t(X;18)(p11;q11)**
Testicular carcinoma (seminoma, teratoma)	i(12p); other structural abnormalities which yield 12p gain
Thyroid (adenocarcinoma)	**inv(10)(q11q21)**
Uterus (adenocarcinoma)	**+10;** i(1q); del or t of 1q21; del(6) (q21)
Wilms' tumor	**del(11)(p13p13); del(11)(p15p15)** i(1q); t(1;16)(q10;q10)
	Benign
Barrett esophagus	**−Y**
Colon (adenoma)	**+7;** +8; +12; del of 12q
Giant-cell tumor	**+8**
Lipoma	**t(1;12)(p33–p34;q13–q15); t(2;12)(p22–p23;q13–q15); t(3;12)(q27–q28;q13–15); t(5;12)(q33;q13–q15); t(11;12)(q13;q13–q15); del(12)(q13q15); t(12;21)(q13–q15;q21); del(13)(q12–q22)**
Neuorepithelioma	**t(11;22)(q24;q12)**
Neurinoma	**22;−Y**
Ovary (adenoma)	**+12**
Ovary (fibroma)	**+12**
Ovary (thecoma)	**+12**
Mixed salivary gland tumor (pleomorphic adenomas)	**t(1;8)(p22;q12); (3;8)(p21;q12); t(6;8)(p21–p22;q12); t(8;13)(p23;q13–q14); del(8)(q12q21–q22); t(8;9)(q12;p22); t(9;12)(p21–p24;q13–q15); inv(12)(p13q13)**
Uterus (leiomyoma)	**r(1)(p11–p36q11–q14); t(2;12)**(q35–q37;q14);del(7) (q21–q22q31–q32); **t(12;14)(q14–q15;q23–q24; +12;** other translocations of 12q13–q15; structural abnormalities with 1p36 breakpoints

NOTE: **Primary karyotype changes are in boldface type,** secondary changes are in normal type. Generic structural alterations are given by ISCN abbreviations (e.g., del for deletions, t for translocations, inv for inversions, dup for duplications (see Table 6-1).
*Includes glioma, anaplastic glioma, glioblastoma, astrocytoma, oligodendroglioma, and ependymoma.
SOURCE: Derived from Thompson.[5]

mor as well as provide specific examples of HSRs and dmin in human breast and ovarian cancers.

Transitional Cell Carcinoma of the Bladder

Among the first cytogenetic studies to demonstrate the clinical importance of cytogenetic results in a human solid tumor were reports characterizing the propensity for recurrence of bladder tumors with cytogenetic abnormalities.[19,20] Long-term follow-up demonstrated that patients with abnormal karyotypes had a greater rate of tumor recurrence than did patients with normal karyotypes (measured as the presence of detectable gross structural rearrange-

ments). More recent studies have corroborated these data, and in general, patients with diploid tumors appear to have more favorable outcomes than do patients with a mix of diploid and hyperdiploid or hyperdiploid tumors.[21]

The chromosomes most frequently altered in tumor type[2,3,22–28] include +7, del(10)(q22-24), and del(21)(q22). Other consistent chromosome alterations are listed in Table 6-2. Another recurring change characterizing bladder cancers is the loss of one copy of chromosome 9 (termed monosomy 9). These results have been confirmed by loss of heterozygosity (LOH) studies and appear to suggest that an initiating genetic defect in bladder tumors is associated with deletion of 9p.[27,28]

Brain Tumors

In this brief section no attempt is made to stratify chromosome alterations into the numerous histologic subtypes of brain (and particularly glial) tumors. In general, across all subtypes of brain cancer several examples of recurring chromosome alteration have been observed, including trisomy 7, monosomy 10, monosomy 22 or del(22)(q11-q13), and loss of one or both sex chromosomes.[2,3,29–32] Cytologic evidence of gene amplification (especially dmin) is found in up to 50 percent of brain tumors,[29,30,32] and initial observation of these changes dates back over three decades.[29] Finally, cytogenetic analysis has defined a minimal region of deletion in glial tumors, 10q25, as a likely site of a tumor-suppressor gene important in the development of this malignancy.[31]

Breast Carcinoma

Numerous studies defining the chromosome changes in breast carcinoma have been published recently, and the interested reader is referred to them for detailed information.[1–3,32–41] Briefly, among the most frequent changes in breast carcinomas are the loss of chromosome 17 in primary tumors[38] and the amplification in metastatic tumors of the band region on 17 (q13), which encodes the HER-2/neu oncogene.[42,43] More commonly, structural alterations of chromosomes 1, 3, 7, and 11 are the most frequently seen alterations.[1–3,32–41] As is true for brain cancers, another important feature of breast carcinomas is the common occurrence of gene amplification, most frequently detectable as HSRs in metastatic tumors. As was mentioned above, amplification of the HER-2/neu oncogene[42,43] is most characteristic, followed by the recent recognition of amplification of a gene or genes on the long arm of chromosome 20.[33,35,36,44,45]

Karyotypic changes in breast cancer not surprisingly increase in frequency in metastatic tumors in contrast to the changes recognized in primary tumors.[33,34,46,47] The most common numeric changes in primary tumors include loss of 17, loss of 19, and gain of chromosome 7, while the chromosomes most frequently structurally altered are chromosomes 1 and 6. Both primary and metastatic lesions often demonstrate overrepresentation of 6p and 1q, frequently with loss of 1p and 6q.[33,34,48] Although common in both primary and metastatic disease, chromosome 1 alterations are even more common in metastatic disease. These data have led to the suggestion that a permissive phenotype for generalized genomic instability may be associated with the transition to metastatic disease.[34]

Colon Cancer

Colon cancer is the paradigm in solid tumors, demonstrating associated chromosomal (and now defined genetic) changes associated with disease predisposition, initiation, and progression[1–3,49] (see

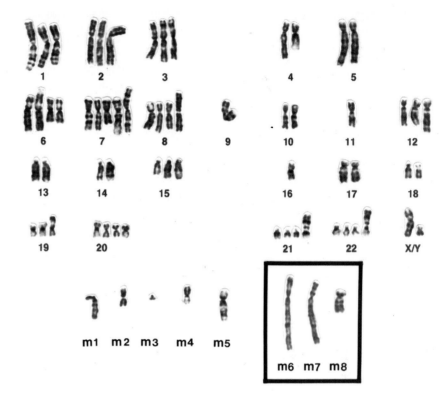

FIG. 6-1 A representative G-banded karyotype from a human malignant melanoma demonstrating numerous structural and numeric alterations. The bottom of the figure illustrates marker (m) chromosomes, which represent chromosomes rearranged beyond recognition of their normal component chromosome(s). (*Used with permission from Ref. 98.*)

Chap. 31). Cytogenetic studies were particularly useful initially in defining chromosomes that are altered with disease progression; therefore, it is not surprising that among the chromosomes most frequently altered are chromosome 5 (loss) as well as structural rearrangements most frequently involving chromosomes 1 and 6 (usually 1p21-q11 and 6q13-q16). Overall, overrepresentation of 1q, 6p, 8q, and chromosomes 7 and 13 is observed, while underrepresentation of chromosomes 17, 18, and 15 and 5 is most common.[1–3,50–55] In contrast, breast cancers studies comparing primary

to metastatic samples show a similar overall frequency and distribution of chromosome alterations.

Renal Cell Carcinoma

Nonpapillary renal cell carcinoma (RCC) is the most common form of adult kidney cancer, and cytogenetic analysis has revealed several recurring sites of chromosome change, including structural alterations of chromosome 3 (particularly 3p11-p14)

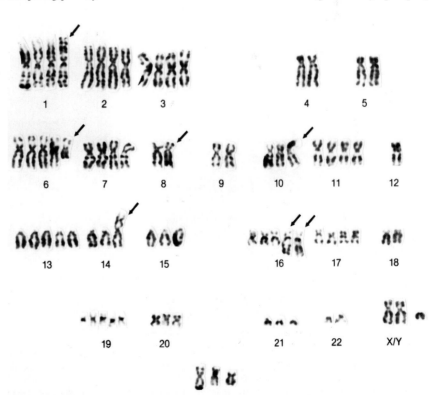

FIG. 6-2 Representative G-banded karyotype from a malignant metastatic colon adenocarcinoma demonstrating numerous structural (arrows) and numeric alterations as well as unidentifiable marker chromosomes (*Umars*).

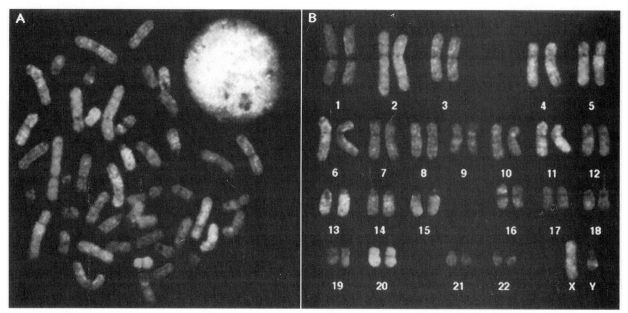

FIG. 6-3 Illustration of fluorescence in situ hybridization (FISH) of a normal human metaphase spread *(A)* and the karyotype of the same cell *(B)*. In this case, the spectral karyotyping of human chromosomes is performed after the simultaneous hybridization of 24 combi- natorially labeled chromosome painting probes *(Schröck et al: Science 273:494, 1996)*. The resulting spectral analysis assigns a unique color to each of the 24 human chromosomes. *(Picture provided by T. Ried and E. Schröck, NCHGR, NIH.)*

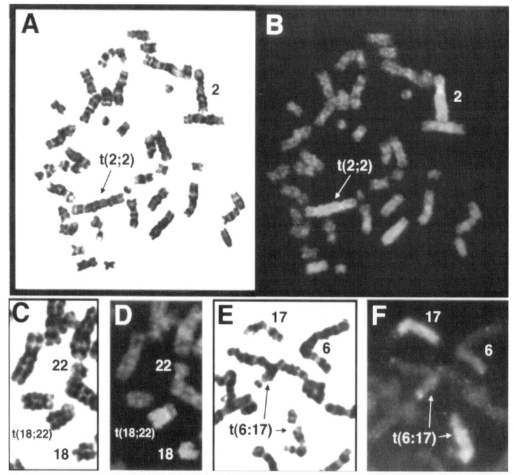

FIG. 6-4 Illustration of the application of fluorescence in situ hy- bridization (FISH) to detect complex chromosome rearrangements in malignancy. In this case, a cancer with three different translocations [t(2;2), t(18;22), and t(6;17)] was studied using probes specific for the long and short arms or each involved chromosome. *A.* G-banded metaphase. *B.* The identical metaphase in *A* hybridized with fluores- cent probes for the long arm and short arm of chromosome 2. A nor- mal copy of chromosome 2 and a rearranged chromosome 2 (arrow) were observed. *C, D.* Detection of reciprocal translocations between chromosomes 18 and 22 *(C/D)* and 6 and 17 *(E/F)*. In both cases, a par- tial G-banded metaphase is shown on the left; FISH, using probes spe- cific for each involved chromosome arm, is shown on the right.[99] *(Used with persmission from Nowell.[9])*

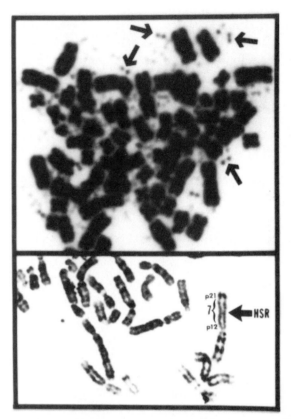

FIG. 6-5 Cytologic evidence of DNA sequence (gene) amplification. *Top.* **Example of tumor cell metaphase stained with Giemsa stain and displaying multiple copies of double minutes (dmin) (arrows). *Bottom.* Example of a tumor cell metaphase G-banded and displaying a homogeneously staining region (HSR) involving the short arm of chromosome 7 (arrow) (see text).**

and the numeric changes +7, −8, +10, and −Y.[1-3,56-60] The deletion of 3p as a simple deletion or by translocation has strongly suggested the presence of a predisposing gene to 3p25-36. The autosomal dominant disorder von Hippel-Lindau syndrome is associated with RCC alone or in combination with other phenotypic abnormalities, and this gene has been identified and characterized (see Chap. 24).

Lung Cancer

An overwhelming number of cytogenetic studies of lung cancer have characterized small-cell lung carcinoma (SCLC).[1-3,61-64] The most typical finding is del(3)(p14p23), and LOH and other biologic studies have suggested that a gene or genes important in SCLC etiology maps to 3p21-p22. SCLC, like many other solid tumors, is characterized by gain of chromosome 7, which has been reported as a sole or primary change in lung carcinomas, as well as a change that is frequently observed in adjacent normal lung tissue.[15,65] Other secondary changes include loss of 5q, 6, 9p, 13q, 17p, and 9p.[1-3] As is true of breast and brain tumors, cytologic evidence of gene amplification (principally in the form of dmin) has been observed frequently in SCLC and has been shown most frequently to involve amplification of the *myc* and *ras* oncogene families particularly L-*myc*).

In non-small-cell lung carcinomas, deletions of 3p and 5q are also the most common finding, although the frequency of 3p loss is significantly lower.[63,65,66] In general, these tumors have complex karyotypes which show loss of 3p, 5q, 8p, Y, 5p, and 10p and gain of 1q, 3q, and 7q.[1-3,65,66]

Malignant Melanoma

Several recent studies of the chromosomes in malignant melanoma have been reported. Briefly, the chromosomes most often involved in both structural and numeric abnormalities are 1, 6, 7, 9, 10, and 11.[1-3,67-72] Figure 6-8 provides an example of the distribution of breakpoints involved in structural alterations from 158 cases of melanoma.[67] Translocations or deletions of the long arm of chromosome 6 (6p11-q12) are very common in this disorder,[73,74] and recently it was recognized that apparently simple deletions in this disorder in fact represented cryptic translocations where the telomere of another chromosome was captured to stabilize the breakage event.[74a] Importantly, LOH and biologic evidence also indicate that a gene or genes on chromosome 6 is implicated in the control of tumorigenicity in this disorder.[75-77]

Abnormalities of chromosome 1 are exceedingly common, most often involving the pericentromeric region 1p12-q12.[1-3,68] The net effect of these abnormalities is usually loss of 1p segments coupled with overrepresentation of 1q, a finding common in many solid tumors. Finally, several studies have suggested a familial predisposition for a subset of malignant melanomas, with suggested linkage to 1p[78] and, more important, the identification of a hereditary melanoma gene on 9p[79-81] (see Chap. 21).

Studies from our laboratory have demonstrated that a recurring translocation t(1;6)(q11-21;q11-13) has been observed in a number of melanoma cases[73]; Fig. 6-9 shows an example of this translocation. The figure also provides an illustration of the dissection of the translocation breakpoint (a starting point for positional cloning studies). Translocation of chromosome 1 segments to chromosomes 19 and 11 has also been reported to occur in a nonrandom fashion.[82,83] Evidence of gene amplification (HSRs) has been identified in melanomas, but the frequency is very low.[98]

Neuroblastoma

Deletion of part of the long arm of chromosome 1 (resulting in net loss of 1p32-p36) is the principal change recognized in this pediatric neoplasm.[1-3,11,12] Loss of this chromosomal segment is often followed by amplification of the oncogene N-*myc*, which is accompanied by recognition of HSRs or dmin in some clinical samples (see Chap. 24 for additional information).

Ovarian Carcinoma

Descriptive cytogenetics in ovarian carcinoma has been difficult because of the complexity of the clonal changes characteristic of this tumor. More so than with any other carcinoma, highly fragmented chromosomes, quadriradials, telomeric fusions, and complexly rearranged chromosomes are found.[2,3] Nevertheless, recurring sites of chromosome change have been described, including deletions in the region 6q15-q21 and the translocation of chromosome 6 with chromosome 14, t(6;14)(q21;q24).[85,86] Although deletion or translocation of chromosome 6 has not been described as the sole primary change, the loss of 6q remains the most common abnormality described in this tumor to date. The most frequently altered chromosomes in ovarian cancer are loss of genetic material for several regions, including 3p, 6q, 11p, 17q, and 17p13.[1-3,87-89] Cytologic evidence of gene amplification in the form of HSRs and dmins and molecular evidence for specific amplification (e.g., the K-*ras* oncogene) have been seen in several studies.[90-93]

Testicular Germ-Cell Tumors

Histopathologic classification of testicular germ-cell tumors is based on the contribution of embryonic (embryonal carcinoma, im-

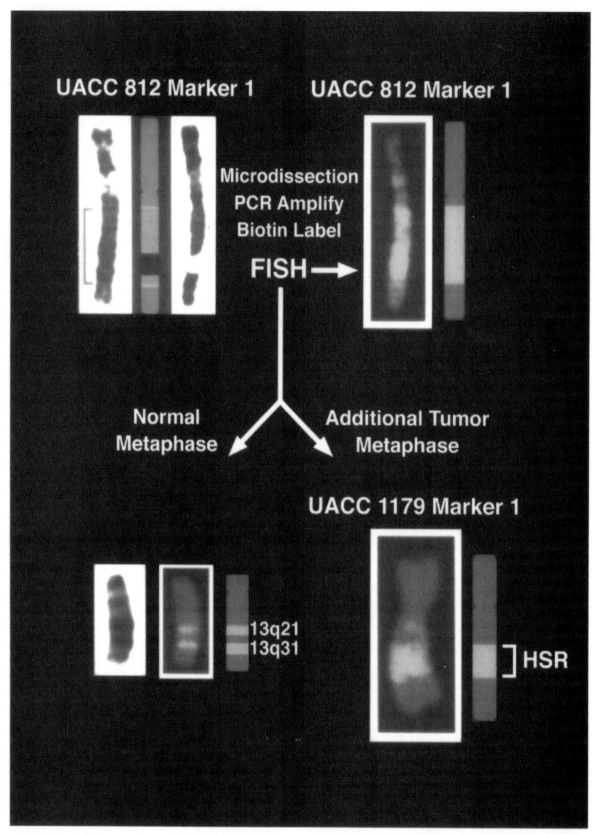

FIG. 6-6 Diagrammatic representation of the detection and characterization of HSRs from human breast cancers by chromosome microdissection (see Ref. 100). *Upper left.* G-banded HSR-bearing marker 1 (left) from case UACC812 (right). Microdissection through the HSR of marker 1. *Upper right.* After PCR amplification and biotin labeling of the dissected DNA, the PCR product is purified and hybridized by FISH back to marker 1 to confirm that the dissection product hybridized to the HSR (bracket). *Lower left.* The same microdissection probe for the HSR was used to identify the location in the normal cells of the amplified sequences. Results indicated specific hybridization to the two regions of one chromosome (13q21 and 13q31): left, G-banded chromosome 13; right, the identical chromosome after hybridization with the HSR probe. *Lower right.* The same microdissection FISH HSR probe used to hybridize to additional breast tumor cases to determine the commonality of 13q amplification. A representative example of an HSR encoding 13q amplified sequences is presented from case UACC1179 marker 1. (*Used with permission from Ref. 100.*)

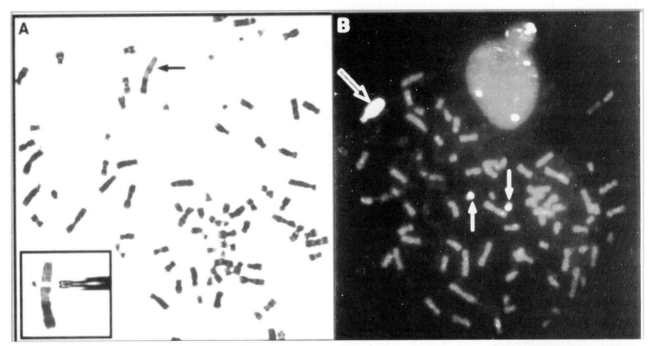

FIG. 6-7 Dissection of a fragment of a homogeneously staining region (HSR) from a human ovarian carcinoma. *A.* G-banded tumor metaphase (insert shows the dissection through the HSR to isolate DNA from the amplified region for use as a FISH probe). *B.* The same case as in *A* after FISH illustrating the HSR (thick arrow) and the normal single-copy region amplified in this tumor (19q13). (*Used with permission from Ref. 92.*)

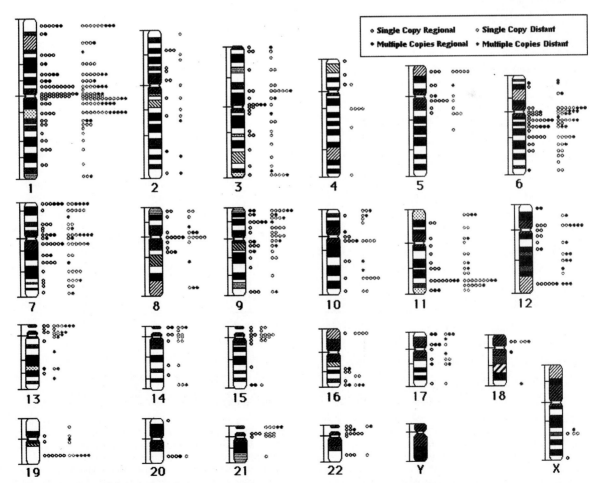

FIG. 6-8 Chromosomal breakpoints identified in clonal structural abnormalities from 158 cases of metastatic melanoma. Dark circles are from cases with tumor limited to the region of surgical dissection; light circles represent cases from patients with disseminated disease at the time of tumor biopsy. (*Used with permission from Ref. 67.*)

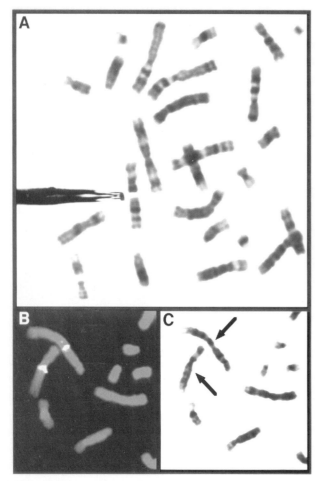

FIG. 6-9 Cytogenetic characterization of a chromosome translocation from a metastatic melanoma. *A.* G-banded tumor metaphase demonstrating a translocation between chromosomes 1 and 6 [t(1;6) (q21;q14)]. Dissection of the chromosomal breakpoint is performed with a glass needle targeted to the translocation breakpoint. *B.* FISH analysis of the dissected material hybridized to a normal human metaphase cell showing chromosome regions involved in the translocation between chromosomes 1 and 6. *C.* The cell in *B*, G-banded to confirm the specific chromosomal regions. (*Used with permission from Ref. 101.*)

mosome change.[1–3,94–96] Structural alterations involving the short arm of chromosome 12 have also been reported, but the net change is usually an increase relative to the diploid copy number of 12p and a decrease in the relative copy number of 12q. This information has been suggested to play a clinically useful role in determining patient outcome,[97] but the true clinical utility is indeterminate.

CHROMOSOME ALTERATIONS AND MOLECULAR IDENTIFICATION OF HUMAN SARCOMAS

Although the possibility that cytogenetic anomalies can serve as signposts identifying genes which play critical roles in oncogenesis has long been realized for numerous leukemias, only recently have translocations in solid tumors yielded to molecular analysis. The common epithelial malignancies of adults lack recurrent tumor-specific chromosome translocations which have been characterized at the molecular level. However, several tumor-specific translocations of sarcomas have been analyzed in this fashion (Table 6-3). In addition, specific genes are now recognized to be the targets of chromosome change in benign tumors. Certain themes have emerged from the study of these rearrangements which are well illustrated by the genetic abnormalities present in Ewing sarcoma and alterations of related genes in other cancers.

Chromosome Translocations in Ewing's Sarcoma

Specific chromosome translocations have been characterized in detail in several sarcomas, including alveolar rhabdomyosarcoma and synovial sarcoma, but Ewing's sarcoma presents the most intriguing example for detailed discussion because of the many ramifications arising from the molecular analysis of this cancer.[102–104] Ewing's sarcoma is a rare, highly malignant tumor of children and young adults which can occur in diverse anatomic sites but most frequently arises in bone. The cell of origin is uncertain, and Ewing's sarcoma can be difficult to distinguish morphologically from other so-called small round blue cell tumors, which include virtually all the solid tumors of childhood in their undifferentiated forms.[105] This difficulty helped fuel interest in the observation that a reciprocal translocation t(11;22)(q24;q12) is present in most cases of Ewing's sarcoma.[106,107] The existence of a recurrent translocation suggested that this rearrangement probably involves genes which are directly related to the pathogenesis of Ewing's sarcoma. In fact, molecular characterization of t(11;22) has provided strong support for this proposal. Positional cloning techniques revealed

mature and mature teratomas) or extraembryonic tissues (yolk sac tumors and choriocarcinomas) or combinations of both. In published cytogenetic studies of germ-cell tumors, isochromosomes for 12p [i(12p)] are the most common and earliest recognizable chro-

Table 6-3 Chromosome Translocations in Sarcomas

Tumor	Translocation	Genes
Ewing's sarcoma	t(11;22)(q24;q12)	EWS/FL1
	t(21;22)(q22;q12)	EWS/ERG
	t(7;22)(q22;q12)	EWS/ETV1
	t(17;22)(q21;q12)	EWS/ETV4
Malignant melanoma (clear cell sarcoma) of the soft parts	t(12;22)(q13;q12)	EWS/ATF-1
Desmoplastic small round cell tumor	t(11;22)(p13;q12)	EWS/WT-1
Myxoid chondrosarcoma	t(9;22)(q22–31;q11–12)	EWS/CHN
Myxoid liposarcoma	t(12;16)(q13;p11)	FUS/CHOP
	t(12;22)(q13;q12)	EWS/CHOP
Alveolar rhabdomyosarcoma	t(2;13)(q35;q14)	PAX3/FKHR
Synovial sarcoma	t(X;18)(p11;q11)	SYT/SSX

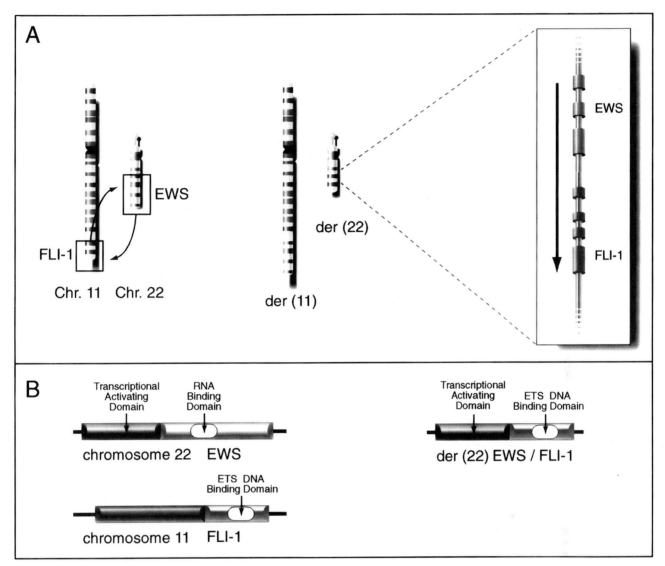

FIG. 6-10 *A.* Translocation of sequences from chromosome 11 to chromosome 22 creates a fusion protein derived from the *EWS* and *FLI-1* genes in Ewing's sarcoma. On the far right, the arrow indicates the direction of transcription and exons are represented by enlarged areas. *B.* The fusion protein contains transcriptional activating sequences from the N-terminal portion of *EWS* joined to the ETS DNA binding-domain of *FLI-1*.

that t(11;22) results in the juxtaposition of sequences from the *FLI1* gene on chromosome 11 and the *EWS* gene on chromosome 22.[129] Although both der(22) and der(11) might produce fusion transcripts, loss of der(11) in some tumors and expression analysis strongly implicate der(22) as site of the critical rearrangement. The chromosome breakpoints on chromosomes 11 and 22 occur within introns of these genes, leading to the generation of a chimeric gene in which the 5′ portion of *EWS* is fused in frame to 3′ sequences from *FLI1* (Fig. 6-10).[109]

Characterization of these genes revealed that *FLI-1* has 97 percent identity with a murine gene (*Fli-1*) first described as a target of oncogenic retroviral integration on mouse chromosome 9 in a region which is syntenic to human chromosome 11.[108] Sequence analysis demonstrates that *FLI-1* is a member of the ETS family of transcription factors, which contain a characteristic DNA-binding motif, the ETS domain.[111] The *ETS-1* proto-oncogene itself was originally defined by the presence of ETS-related sequences in the E26 avian leukosis virus.[112] The oncogenic potential of the ETS family is further suggested by the observation that *ETS-1*, which maps to 11q23, enters into amplifications in some acute leukemias.[113] The 656-amino acid protein encoded by *EWS* was

novel but contained a putative RNA-binding domain. Analysis of the genomic structure of EWS demonstrated that the gene is composed of 17 exons distributed over approximately 40 kb.[114] The first seven exons encode a repetitive polypeptide with the consensus sequence SYGQQS followed by a hinge region encoded by exons 8 through 10, while the candidate RNA-binding domain is encoded in exons 11 through 13.

The breakpoints in t(11;22) vary from case to case but always lead to replacement of the RNA-binding domain of *EWS* by the DNA-binding domain of *FLI-1* (Fig. 6-11).[115] The resultant fusion protein would be predicted to have the properties of a transcription factor with a transcriptional activation domain contributed by *EWS* and a DNA-binding domain contributed by *FLI-1*. A considerable body of experimental evidence has accumulated to support this interpretation.[116–122] The *EWS/FLI1* −1 fusion protein is localized in the nucleus and retains the DNA-binding specificity of *FLI-1*. Reporter gene assays also demonstrate that it is a potent transcriptional activator, and unlike *FLI-1*, it is able to transform NIH 3T3 cells. The *EWS* sequences clearly confer transcriptional activating function. In addition, they are likely to provide important protein interaction and regulatory functions, since the transforming prop-

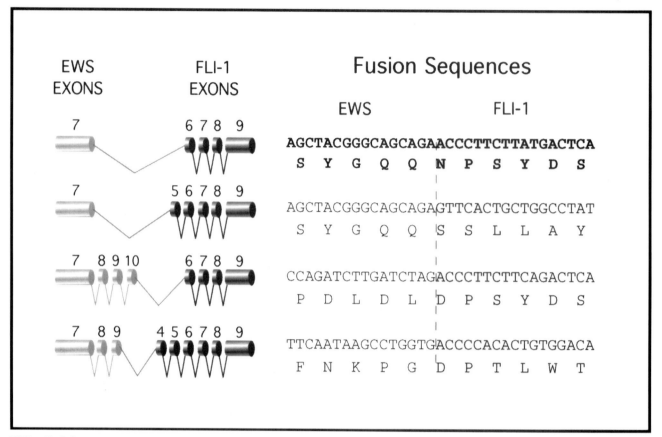

FIG. 6-11 Representative fusion transcripts identified by Zucman et al.,[142] illustrating their variability. The most common type joins exon 7 of *EWS* to exon 6 of *FLI-1*. All the variants replace the RNA-binding domain of *EWS* with the ETS DNA-binding domain of *FLI-1*.

erties of *EWS* cannot be replaced by other strong transcriptional activation domains.[123]

Important observations have emerged as additional cases of Ewing's sarcoma have been characterized. Although the *EWS* gene is consistently involved in every instance, variant translocation partners for *EWS* have been identified in a subset of cases. The most common alternative to *FLI-1* is *ERG*, a gene which maps on chromosome 21q22. *ERG* is also a member of the ETS family of transcription factors and in a fashion is quite comparable to the *EWS/FLI-1* translocation; the *EWS–ERG* fusion transfers the *ERG* DNA-binding domain to the *EWS* transcriptional activating domain.[109,124] A third variant translocation involves *EWS* with the *ETV1* gene on chromosome 7p22.[125] *ETV1* is yet another member of the ETS family, further emphasizing the importance of the ETS DNA-binding domain to the fusion proteins contributed by each of these three transcription factors. Finally, a fourth variant translocation, t(17;22)(q21;q12), has been described which joins the transactivation domain of *EWS* with a fourth member of the ETS family, the adenovirus E1A enhancer-binding protein (ETV4).[126] Of interest, ETV4 is known to activate the transcription of matrix metalloproteinase genes, potentially linking the EWS/ETV4 fusion protein with the invasive properties of the tumor.

Diagnostic Implications

Ewing's sarcoma can be difficult to distinguish from other cancers which are morphologically similar. This has led to an examination of the diagnostic importance of t(11;22). This is well illustrated by consideration of another diagnostic entity described variously as primitive neuroepithelioma (PN) and peripheral primitive neuroec-

todermal tumor of childhood (PNET). These tumors are clinically similar to Ewing's sarcoma but most frequently occur in extraosseus sites during adolescence. However, unlike Ewing's sarcoma, PN consistently expresses ultrastructural features of neural differentiation and is therefore felt to be of neural origin. Although PN can be distinguished from Ewing's sarcoma on this basis, it is now recognized that t(11;22) also is found in PN.[127,128] The presence of the same underlying molecular genetic alteration suggests that these disorders must be very closely related if not identical. Some pathologists now consider these cancers as part of an incompletely defined Ewing's sarcoma group of peripheral neuroectodermal tumors, all of which are linked by the presence of t(11;22).[129] In fact, since it is possible to determine the presence of the *EWS/FLI-1* fusion gene by either RT-PCR or interphase FISH, it is likely that testing for the presence of this molecular aberration will become part of the routine characterization of these tumors.[130–136] However, the presence of *EWS/FLI-1* transcripts in a few tumors with myogenic or biphenotypic features suggests that molecular characterization will supplement rather than replace traditional tumor markers.[137] Nonetheless, because of its pathogenic role, the presence of the t(11;22) may ultimately prove more important than markers of cell differentiation, especially if therapies are developed which are directed at the pathways triggered by the *EWS/FLI-1* transcription factor.[138] The question also arises whether the variant *EWS* translocations within Ewing's sarcoma have different clinical behavior.[115,139] Preliminary data have suggested a possible advantage for patients with *EWS–FLI-1* fusions occurring after exon 7 of *EWS* relative to the other variants, but additional data will be required to confirm this suggestion. Importantly, as illustrated by the following examples, rearrangements involving the *EWS* gene are not confined to Ewing's sarcoma.

EWS Rearrangements in Other Sarcomas

A rare tumor of young adults called malignant melanoma of the soft parts or clear-cell sarcoma of the soft parts is characterized by a tumor-specific translocation t(12;22)(q13:q12).[140,141] This tumor, which exhibits some neuroectodermal features, most frequently occurs in the tendons and aponeuroses. Molecular characterization of t(12;22) has revealed that this rearrangement also involves the *EWS* gene, which in this instance gives rise to a chimeric protein carrying sequences from the *ATF-1* gene on chromosome 12q13.[142,143] Again, in parallel with t(11;22), *ATF-1*, a transcription factor in the bZIP family, contributes its DNA-binding domain to the fusion protein.[144,145]

EWS contributes to yet another tumor-specific translocation: the t(11;22)(p13:q12) observed in desmoplastic small round-cell tumors.[110,177] This is a tumor which occurs primarily in the abdomen of adolescent males or in association with other serosal surfaces.[145,146] In this disorder *EWS* forms a chimeric protein with *WT-1*.[147–150] Remarkably, *WT-1* is the Wilms tumor gene, which was identified as the target of constitutional deletion in the Wilms tumor–aniridia syndrome.[151] *WT-1*, like the other *EWS* partners, is a transcription factor, and the *EWS–WT-1* fusion once again pairs the *EWS* transcriptional activation domain with the zinc finger DNA-binding domain of *WT-1*.

A recent report implicated *EWS* rearrangements in myxoid chondrosarcoma, which exhibits a specific chromosomal translocation, t(9;22)(q22-31;q11-12). This rearrangement links *EWS* with almost the entire coding sequence of CHN, a member of the steroid hormone receptor superfamily.[152,153] The involvement of *EWS* with multiple partners in so many different sarcomas is remarkable and is even more impressive when one considers *FUS* a homologue of *EWS*, which also is involved in tumor-specific rearrangements.

An *EWS* Homologue Also Participates in Sarcoma Translocations

Myxoid liposarcoma (MLPS) is characterized by t(12;16)(q13; p11).[154] This rearrangement gives rise to a chimeric transcription factor derived from the *CHOP* gene on chromosome 12 and a gene which has been called either *FUS* (for fusion) or *TLS* (for translocated in liposarcoma) on chromosome 16.[155–157] Remarkably, the *FUS/TLS* gene closely resembles the *EWS* gene and contains the same functional domains. *CHOP* is a transcription factor of the C/EBPb family and normally is induced in response to starvation or stress stimuli.[158] Heterodimers formed between *CHOP* and C/EBPb have reduced DNA-binding activity, and *CHOP* therefore appears to be a negative regulator.[159–162] However, in the *FUS–CHOP* chimera the bZIP domain does confer DNA-binding activity. Remarkably, cases of MLPS have been described which contain *EWS–CHOP* fusions, further emphasizing the functional similarities of *EWS* and *FUS/TLS* as well as the specificity of *CHOP* for MLPS.[163]

Several conclusions seem inevitable on consideration of the range of tumors which exhibit rearrangements of either *EWS* or *FUS/TLS*. These molecular abnormalities appear to be essential to the pathogenesis of the tumors in which they occur. Because all the fusion proteins described above are transcription factors, perturbation of the normal pattern of gene expression must be critical to the malignant transformation of normal precursor cells. Since the occurrence of these translocations is most likely a random event, the emergence of a translocation-bearing tumor clone presumably reflects both the lineage specificity and the oncogenic potency of that specific chimeric transcription factor. The precise reasons for the predominant rearrangement of ETS family genes in Ewing's sarcoma or of *CHOP* in myxoid liposarcoma remain to be elucidated but presumably relate to the underlying program of gene expression required for the differentiation of the various mesenchymal cell lineages. Elucidation of the detailed downstream biochemical effects of the oncogenic chimeric transcription factors is an important focus of continuing research. In addition, it should be emphasized that sarcomas bearing chimeric transcription factors are likely to contain additional genetic alterations, such as a p53 mutation, which are important in the evolution of the clinically evident malignant tumor.[164,165] However, based on their high incidence in tumors of a given type, it is likely that the translocations which characterize these tumors occur early in their evolution and create a fundamental disturbance of cell function essential to the tumorigenic process.

Rearrangements of the *HMGI-C* Gene in Benign Tumors

Tumor-specific translocations are not limited to malignant tumors. Benign tumors, notably lipomas and leiomyomas, may be karyotypically abnormal. Among the most frequent abnormalities observed in these tumors have been rearrangements of chromosome 12q14-q15.[166–168] Diverse partner chromosomes have been observed linked to 12q14-q15 in various tumors. In addition to lipomas and leiomyomas, rearrangements of the 12q14-q15 region have been observed in pulmonary chondroid hamartomas, pleomorphic adenomas of the salivary gland, endometrial polyps, and a variety of benign tumors of mesenchymal origin.[169–171] The frequent appearance of the 12q breakpoint was highly suggestive that a pathogenically important gene resides at that location, a suspicion borne out when the *HMGI-C* gene was mapped to the site of these breakpoints in both leiomyomas and lipomas.[172,173] *HMGI-C* is the human homologue of the murine pygmy gene and is a member of the HMGI family of small nuclear proteins, including *HMGI-C* and *HMGI(Y)*, which are characterized by the presence of a DNA-binding domain called the AT hook because of its affinity for binding to the minor groove of AT-rich DNA and inducing DNA bending.[174] The HMGI-C protein consists of only 109 amino acids encoded by five exons, with the three AT hook domains encoded by the first three exons. The third intron is large (140 kb) and is the site of the translocations which fuse sequences from almost every chromosome to the AT hook domains of *HMGI-C*.[173] HMGI proteins have not been shown to have intrinsic transcription factor activity but appear to function as accessory factors that promote the binding of other proteins to DNA.[175] In addition, *HMGI-C* is induced in NIH3T3 cells as a delayed early response gene, suggesting a possible connection between *HMGI-C* and cell cycle progression. The precise biochemical effects of the fusion proteins have not been established, and the multiple partner genes have not been fully characterized. In one case [a lipoma with t(3;12)], the partner gene contains two tandem LIM motifs, sequences which are known to function as protein interaction domains.[172,173] The second gene in the HMGI family, *HMG-I(Y)*, maps to chromosome 6p21, and variant translocations in benign tumors may involve this gene instead of HMGI-C.[176]

The *HMGI* family translocations present both parallels and sharp contrasts to those involving the *EWS* gene family. Both categories of translocation involve chimeric DNA-binding proteins which most likely exert their oncogenic effects by perturbing normal gene expression. In both cases, a critical domain is provided by either member of a two-gene family. In the case of *HMGI* this is a DNA-binding domain, while in the case of *EWS* it is the transcriptional activating domain. The benign behavior of tumors with *HMGI* translocations contrasts with the highly malignant properties of tumors with *EWS* translocations. Benign lipomas and leiomyomas do not appear to evolve into malignant tumors. It is not at all clear how the *HMGI-C* translocations confer proliferative capacity without a tendency to accumulate further genetic alterations which would promote malignant progression. Comparison of the biochemical consequences of these two categories of translocation is likely to prove important in defining the molecular features which distinguish malignant tumors from their benign counterparts.

CONCLUSION

This review has attempted to provide an update on current progress in identifying recurring sites of chromosome change in human solid tumors. Despite methodologic difficulties, a recurring and decidedly nonrandom pattern of chromosome alterations has clearly emerged. It appears likely that as additional cases of solid tumors are cytogenetically examined, the stratification of some specific histopathologic subtypes will be possible, and this may facilitate diagnostic (and possibly prognostic) analysis.

At present the clinical utility of chromosome analysis in solid tumors is largely indeterminate. However, the pinpointing of regions of the genome which are characteristically altered in solid tumors has been and will continue to be of significant benefit in targeting future molecular (and probably mechanistic) investigations. Continued study of the basic genetics of solid tumors appears to be a particularly fruitful avenue as it assuredly will add to our understanding of the causation, progression, and control of these disorders.

ACKNOWLEDGMENT

The authors would like to dedicate this chapter to Floyd Thompson, a colleague and friend who died suddenly after a brief illness last year (Fig. 6-12). Floyd was a research specialist and the director of the cytogenetic oncology laboratory of the Arizona Comprehensive Cancer Center in Tucson. Floyd was instrumental in the cytogenetic analysis of tumors from our laboratory over the past decade, much of which is featured in this chapter. Further, his work on the technical aspects of human solid tumor karyology[5] served as a keynote reference for the body of this chapter. Floyd will be remembered not just for his scientific accomplishments but also for his quick and sharp sense of humor, his willingness to laugh in spite of adversity, and his courageous outlook on life. The scientific world has lost a gifted scientist, and many researchers, including ourselves, have lost a wonderful friend.

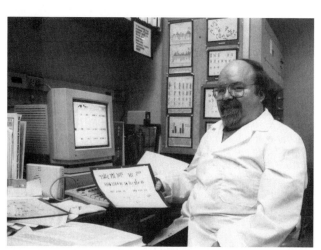

FIG. 6-12 Floyd Thompson, 1951–1996.

REFERENCES

1. Mitelman F: *Catalog of Chromosome Aberrations in Cancer*, 5th ed. New York, Wiley-Liss, 1995.
2. Sandberg AA: *The Chromosomes in Human Cancer and Leukemia*, 2d ed. New York, Elsevier, 1990.
3. Heim S, Mitelman F: *Cancer Cytogenetics: Chromosomal and Molecular Genetic Aberrations of Tumor Cells*, 2d ed. New York, Wiley-Liss, 1995.
4. De Klein A, Guerts van Kessel A, Grosveld G, et al: A cellular oncogene is translocated to the Philadelphia chromosome in chronic myelocytic leukaemia. *Nature* **300**:765, 1982.
5. Thompson FH: Cytogenetic methodological approaches and findings in human solid tumors, in Barch MJ (ed): *The ACT Cytogenetics Laboratory Manual*, 2d ed. New York, Raven Press, 1996, pp 451–488.
6. Yang JM, Thompson FH, Knox SM, Dalton WS, Salmon SE, Trent JM: Polyclonal origin of a primary breast carcinoma demonstrated by serial cytogenetic studies of a patient with a history of osteosarcoma (abstract). *Cancer Genet Cytogenet* **66**:153, 1993.
7. Pandis N, Heim S, Bardi G, Idvall I, Mandahl N, Mitelman F: Chromosome analysis of 20 breast carcinomas: Cytogenetic multiclonality and karyotypic-pathologic correlations. *Genes Chromosom Cancer* **6**:51, 1993.
8. Heim S, Caron M, Jin Y, Mandahl N, Mitelman F: Genetic convergence during serial in vitro passage of a polyclonal squamous cell carcinoma. *Cytogenet Cell Genet* **52**:133, 1989.
9. Nowell PC: Tumors as clonal proliferation. *Virchows Arch B Cell Pathol* **29**:145, 1978.
10. Mitelman F (ed): *An International System for Human Cytogenetic Nomenclature*. Basel: Karger, 1995.
11. Christiansen H, Schestag J, Christiansen NM, Grzeschik K-H, Lampert F: Clinical impact of chromosome 1 aberrations in neuroblastoma: A metaphase and interphase cytogenetic study. *Genes Chromosom Cancer* **5**:141, 1992.
12. Caron H, van Sluis P, Van Hoeve M, et al: Allelic loss of chromosome 1p36 in neuroblastoma is of preferential maternal origin and correlates with N-myc amplification. *Nat Genet* **4**:187, 1993.
13. Trent JM, Meyskens FL, Salmon SE, et al: Relation of cytogenetic abnormalities and clinical outcome in metastatic melanoma. *N Engl J Med* **322**:1508, 1990.
14. Korc M, Meltzer P, Trent J: Enhanced expression of epidermal growth factor receptor correlates with alterations of chromosome 7 in human pancreatic cancer. *Proc Natl Acad Sci USA* **83**:5141, 1986.
15. Lee JS, Pathak S, Hopwood V, et al: Involvement of chromosome 7 in primary lung tumor and nonmalignant normal tissue. *Cancer Res* **47**:6349, 1987.
16. Aly MS, Dal Cin P, Van de Voorde W, et al: Chromosome abnormalities in benign prostatic hyperplasia. *Genes Chromosom Cancer* **9**:227, 1994.
17. Arps S, Rodewald A, Schmalenberger B, Carl P, Bressel M, Kastendieck H: Cytogenetic survey of 32 cancers of the prostate. *Cancer Genet Cytogenet* **66**:93, 1993.
18. Herrmann ME, Lalley PA: Significance of trisomy 7 in thyroid tumors. *Cancer Genet Cytogenet* **62**:144, 1992.
19. Falor WH: Chromosomes in noninvasive papillary carcinoma of the bladder. *JAMA* **216**:791, 1971.
20. Falor WH, Ward RM: Prognosis in early carcinoma of the bladder based on chromosomal analysis. *J Urol* **199**:44, 1978.
21. Schapers RFM, Smeets AWGB, Pauwels RPE, Van Den Brandt PA, Bosman FT: Cytogenetic analysis in transitional cell carcinoma of the bladder. *Br J Urol* **72**:887, 1993.
22. Wang M-R, Perissel B, Taillandier J, et al: Nonrandom changes of chromosome 10 in bladder cancer—detection by FISH to interphase nuclei. *Cancer Genet Cytogenet* **73**:8, 1994.

23. Atkin NB, Baker MC: Cytogenetic study of ten carcinomas of the bladder: Involvement of chromosome 1 and 11. *Cancer Genet Cytogenet* **15**:253, 1985.

24. Gibas Z, Prout GR, Connolly JG, Pontes JE, Sandberg AA: Nonrandom chromosomal changes in transitional cell carcinoma of the bladder. *Cancer Res* **44**:1257, 1984.

25. Gibas Z, Prout GR, Pontes JE, Connolly JG, Sandberg AA: A possible specific chromosome change in transitional cell carcinoma of the bladder. *Cancer Genet Gytogenet* **19**:229, 1986.

26. Poddighe PJ, Ramaekers FCS, Smeets AWGB, Vooijs GP, Hopman AHN: Structural chromosome 1 aberrations in transitional cell carcinoma of the bladder: Interphase cytogenetics combining a centromeric, telomeric, and library DNA probe. *Cancer Res* **52**:4929, 1992.

27. Cairns P, Shaw ME, Knowles MA: Initiation of bladder cancer may involve deletion of a tumour-suppressor gene on chromosome 9. *Oncogene* **8**:1083, 1993.

28. Miyao N, Tsai YC, Lerner SP, et al: Role of chromosome 9 in human bladder cancer. *Cancer Res* **53**:4066, 1993.

29. Lubs HA, Salmon JH: The chromosomal complement of human solid tumors: II. Karyotypes of glial tumors. *J Neurosurg* **22**:160, 1965.

30. Magnani I, Guerneri S, Pollo B, et al: Increasing complexity of the karyotype in 50 human gliomas. *Cancer Genet Cytogenet* **75**:77, 1994.

31. Rasheed BKA, McLendon RE, Friedman HS, et al: Chromosome 10 deletion mapping in human gliomas: A common deletion region in 10q25. *Oncogene* **10**:2243, 1995.

32. Reifenberger G, Reifenberger J, Ichimura K, Meltzer PS, Collins PV: Amplification of multiple genes from chromosomal region 12q13–14 in human malignant gliomas: Preliminary mapping of the amplicons shows preferential involvement of CDK4, SAS, and MDM2. *Cancer Res* **54**:4299, 1994.

33. Thompson F, Emerson J, Dalton WS, et al: Clonal chromosome abnormalities in human breast carcinomas: I. 28 cases with primary disease. *Genes Chromosom Cancer* **7**:185, 1993.

34. Trent J, Yang J-M, Emerson J, et al: Clonal chromosome abnormalities in human breast carcinomas: II. 34 cases with metastatic disease. *Genes Chromosom Cancer* **7**:194, 1993.

35. Tanner MM, Tirkkonen M, Kallioniemi A, et al: Increased copy number at 20q13 in breast cancer: Defining the critical region and exclusion of candidate genes. *Cancer Res* **54**:4257, 1994.

36. Adelaide J, Penault-Llorca F, Dib A, Yarden Y, Jacquemier J, Birnbaum D: The heregulin gene can be included in the 8p12 amplification unit in human breast cancer. *Genes Chromosom Cancer* **11**:66, 1994.

37. Almeida A, Muleris M, Dutrillaux B, Malfoy B: The insulin-like growth factor I receptor gene is the target for the 15q26 amplicon in breast cancer. *Genes Chromosom Cancer* **11**:63, 1994.

38. Nagai MA, Yamamoto L, Salaorni S, et al: Detailed deletion mapping of chromosome segment 17q12–21 in sporadic breast tumours. *Genes Chromosom Cancer* **11**:58, 1994.

39. Bieche I, Champeme M-H, Lidereau R: Loss and gain of distinct regions of chromosome 1q in primary breast cancer. *Clin Cancer Res* **1**:123, 1995.

40. Pandis N, Jin Y, Gorunova L, et al: Chromosome analysis of 97 primary breast carcinomas: Identification of eight karyotypic subgroups. *Genes Chromosom Cancer* **12**:173, 1995.

41. Hoggard N, Brintnell B, Howell A, Weissenbach J, Varley J: Allelic imbalance on chromosome 1 in human breast cancer: II. Microsatellite repeat analysis. *Genes Chromosom Cancer* **12**:24, 1995.

42. Slamon DJ, Clark GM, Wong SG, Levin WJ, Ullrich A, McGuire WL: Human breast cancer: Correlation of relapse and survival with amplification of the HER-2/neu oncogene. *Science* **235**:177, 1987.

43. Slamon DJ, Godolphin W, Jones LA, et al: Studies of the HER-2/neu proto-oncogene in human breast and ovarian cancer. *Science* **244**:707, 1989.

44. Tanner MM, Tirkkonen M, Kallioniemi A, Isola J, Kuukasjorvi T, Collins C, Kowbel D, Guan X-Y, Trent J, Gray JW, Meltzer P, Kallioniemi O-P: Independent amplification and frequent co-amplification of three nonsyntenic regions on the long arm of chromosome 20 in human breast cancer. *Cancer Res* **56**:3441, 1996.

45. Guan X-Y, Xu J, Anzick SL, Zhang H, Trent JM, Meltzer PS: Hybrid selection of transcribed sequences from microdissected DNA: Isolation of genes within an amplified region at 20q11–q13.2 in breast cancer. *Cancer Res* **56**:3446, 1996.

46. Trent J: Cytogenetic and molecular biologic alterations in human breast cancer: A review. *Breast Cancer Res Treat* **5**:221, 1985.

47. Trent JM, Yang J-M, Thompson FH, Leibovitz A, Villar H, Dalton WS: Chromosome alterations in human breast cancer, in Sluyser M (ed): *Oncogenes and Hormones in Breast Cancer.* Ellis Horwood, 1987, p 142.

48. Devilee P, van Vliet M, van Sloun P, et al: Allelotype of human breast carcinoma: A second major site for loss of heterozygosity is on chromosome 6. *Oncogene* **6**:1705, 1991.

49. Vogelstein B, Fearon ER, Hamilton SR, et al: Genetic alterations during colorectal-tumor development. *N Engl J Med* **319**:525, 1988.

50. Muleris M, Zafrani B, Validire P, Girodet J, Salmon R-J, Dutrillaux B: Cytogenetic study of 30 colorectal adenomas. *Cancer Genet Cytogenet* **74**:104, 1994.

51. Muleris M, Salmon RJ, Zafrani B, Girodet J, Dutrillaux B: Consistent deficiencies of chromosome 18 and of the short arm of chromosome 17 in eleven cases of human large bowel cancer: A possible recessive determinism. *Ann Genet* **28**:206, 1985.

52. Muleris M, Salmon R-J, Dutrillaux B: Chromosome study demonstrating the clonal evolution and metastatic origin of a metachronous colorectal carcinoma. *Int J Cancer* **38**:167, 1986.

53. Thompson FH, Liu Y, Alberts D, Taetle R, Trent JM: Cytogenetic findings in 51 colorectal carcinomas: Correlations with sample site (abstract). *Am J Hum Genet* **53**:1993.

54. Muleris M, Salmon R-J, Dutrillaux A-M, et al: Characteristic chromosomal imbalances in 18 near-diploid colorectal tumors. *Cancer Genet Cytogenet* **29**:298, 1987.

55. Bomme L, Bardi G, Pandis N, Fenger C, Kronborg O, Heim S: Clonal karyotypic abnormalities in colorectal adenomas: Clues to the early genetic events in the adenoma-carcinoma sequence. *Genes Chromosom Cancer* **10**:190, 1994.

56. Berger CS, Sandberg AA, Todd IAD, et al: Chromosome in kidney, ureter, and bladder cancer. *Cancer Genet Cytogenet* **23**:1, 1986.

57. Kovacs G, Szucs S, De Reise W, Baumbartel H: Specific chromosome aberration in human renal cell carcinoma. *Int J Cancer* **40**:171, 1987.

58. Pathak S, Strong LC, Ferrell RE, Trindade A: Familial renal carcinoma with a 3;11 chromosome translocation limited to tumor cells. *Science* **217**:939, 1982.

59. Yoshida MA, Ohyashiki K, Ochi H, et al: Rearrangement of chromosome 3 in renal cell carcinoma. *Cancer Genet Cytogenet* **19**:351, 1986.

60. Henn W, Zwergel T, Wullich B, Thonnes M, Zang KD, Seitz G: Bilateral multicentric papillary renal tumors with heteroclonal origin based on tissue-specific karyotype instability. *Cancer* **72**:1315, 1993.

61. Rey JA, Bello MJ, de Campos JM, Kusak ME, Moreno S, Benitz J: Deletion 3p in two lung adenocarcinomas metastatic to the brain. *Cancer Genet Cytogenet* **25**:355, 1987.

62. Levin NA, Brzoska P, Gupta N, Gray JW, Christman MF: Identification of frequent novel genetic alterations in small cell lung carcinoma. *Cancer Res* **54**:5086, 1994.

63. Hosoe S, Ueno K, Shigedo Y, et al: A frequent deletion of chromosome 5q21 in advanced small cell and non-small cell carcinoma of the lung. *Cancer Res* **54**:1787, 1994.

64. Johansson M, Karauzum SB, Dietrich C, et al: Karyotypic abnormalities in adenocarcinomas of the lung. *Int J Oncol* **5**:17, 1994.

65. Siegfried JM, Hunt JD, Zhou J-Y, Keller SM, Testa JR: Cytogenetic abnormalities in non-small cell lung carcinoma: Similarity of findings in conventional and feeder cell layer cultures. *Genes Chromosom Cancer* **6**:30, 1993.

66. Siegfried JM, Ellison DJ, Resau JH, Miura I, Testa JR: Correlation of modal chromosome number of cultured non-small cell lung carcinomas with DNA index of solid tumor tissue. *Cancer Res* **51**:3267, 1991.

67. Thompson FH, Emerson J, Olson S, et al: Cytogenetics in 158 patients with regional or disseminated melanoma: Subset analysis of near diploid and simple karyotypes. *Cancer Genet Cytogenet* (in press).

68. Morse HG, Moore GE, Ortiz LM, Gonzalez R, Robinson WA: Malignant melanoma: From subcutaneous nodule to brain metastasis. *Cancer Genet Cytogenet* **72**:16, 1994.

69. Morse HG, Moore GE: Cytogenetic homogeneity in eight independent sites in a case of malignant melanoma. *Cancer Genet Cytogenet* **69**:108, 1993.

70. Parmiter AH, Nowell PC: Cytogenetics of melanocytic tumors. *J Invest Dermatol* **100**:254S, 1993.

71. Grammatico P, Caticala C, Potenza C, et al: Cytogenetic findings in 20 melanomas. *Melanoma Res* **3**:169, 1993.

72. Ozisik YY, Meloni AM, Altungoz O, et al: Cytogenetic findings in 21 malignant melanomas. *Cancer Genet Cytogenet* **77**:69, 1994.

73. Trent JM, Thompson FH, Meyskens FL: Identification of a recurring translocation site involving chromosome 6 in human malignant melanoma. *Cancer Res* **49**:420, 1989.

74. Guan X-Y, Cao J, Meltzer PS, Trent J: Rapid generation of region-specific genomic clones by chromosome microdissection: Isolation of DNA from a region frequently deleted in malignant melanoma. *Genomics* **14**:680, 1992.

74a.Meltzer PS, Guan X-Y, Trent JM: Telomere capture stabilizes chromosome breakage. *Nat Genet* **4**:252, 1993.

75. Millikin D, Meese E, Vogelstein B, Trent J: Loss of heterozygosity for loci on the long arm of chromosome 6 in human malignant melanoma. *Cancer Res* **51**:5449, 1991.

76. Trent JM, Stanbridge EJ, McBride HL, et al: Tumorigenicity in human melanoma cell lines controlled by introduction of human chromosome 6. *Science* **247**:568, 1990.

77. Su YA, Ray ME, Lin T, Seidel NE, Bodine DM, Meltzer PS, Trent JM: Reversion of monochromosome-mediated suppression of tumorigenicity in malignant melanoma by retroviral transduction. *Cancer Res* **56**:3186, 1996.

78. Goldstein AM, Dracopoli NC, Ho EC, et al: Further evidence for a locus for cutaneous malignant melanoma-dysplastic nevus (CMM/DN) on chromosome 1p, and evidence for genetic heterogeneity. *Am J Hum Genet* **52**:537, 1993.

79. Cannon-Albright LA, Goldgar DE, Meyer LJ, et al: Assignment of a locus for familial melanoma, MLM, to chromosome 9p13–p22. *Science* **258**:1148, 1992.

80. Kamb A, Gruis NA, Weaver-Feldhaus J, et al: A cell cycle regulator potentially involved in genesis of many tumor types. *Science* **264**:436, 1994.

81. Goldstein AM, Dracopoli NC, Engelstein M, Fraser MC, Clark WH Jr, Tucker MA: Linkage of cutaneous malignant melanoma/dysplastic nevi to chromosome 9p, and evidence for genetic heterogeneity. *Am J Hum Genet* **54**:489, 1994.

82. Morse HG, Gonzalez R, Moore GE, Robinson WA: Preferential chromosome 11q and/or 17q aberrations in short-term cultures of metastatic melanoma in resections from human brain. *Cancer Genet Cytogenet* **64**:118, 1992.

83. Parmiter AH, Balaban G, Herlyn M, Clark WH, Nowell PC: A t(1;p19) chromosome translocation in three cases of human malignant melanoma. *Cancer Res* **46**:1526, 1986.

84. Zhang J, Trent JM, Meltzer PS: Rapid isolation and characterization of amplified DNA by chromosome microdissection: Identification of IGF1R amplification in malignant melanoma. *Oncogene* **8**:2827, 1993.

85. Wake N, Hreshchyshyn MM, Piver SM, Matsui S, Sandberg AA: Specific cytogenetic changes in ovarian cancer involving chromosomes 6 and 14. *Cancer Res* **40**:4512, 1980.

86. Trent JM: *Prevalence and Clinical Significance of Cytogenetic Abnormalities in Human Ovarian Cancer.* Boston, Nijhoff, 1985.

87. Lee JH, Kavanagh JJ, Wildrick DM, Wharton JT, Blick M: Frequent loss of heterozygosity on chromosome 6q, 11, and 17 in human ovarian carcinomas. *Cancer Res* **50**:2724, 1990.

88. Bello MJ, Rey JA: Chromosome aberrations in metastatic ovarian cancer: Relationship with abnormalities in primary tumors. *Int J Cancer* **45**:50, 1990.

89. Thompson FH, Emerson J, Alberts D, et al: Clonal chromosome abnormalities in 54 cases of ovarian carcinoma. *Cancer Genet Cytogenet* **73**:33, 1994.

90. Guan X-Y, Alberts D, Burgess AC, Thompson FH, Trent JM: Chromosomal analysis of 90 cases of ovarian carcinomas (abstract). *Cancer Genet Cytogenet* **41**:291, 1989.

91. Filmus J, Trent JM, Pullano R, Buick RN: A cell line from a human ovarian carcinoma with amplification of the K-ras gene. *Cancer Res* **46**:5179, 1986.

92. Guan X-Y, Cargile CB, Anzick SL, et al: Chromosome microdissection identifies cryptic sites of DNA sequence amplification in human ovarian carcinoma. *Cancer Res* **55**:3380, 1995.

93. Sasano H, Garrett CT, Wilkinson DS, Silverberg S, Comerford J, Hyde J: Protooncogene amplification in human ovarian neoplasms. *Hum Pathol* **21**:382, 1990.

94. Gibas Z, Prout GR, Pontes JE, Sandberg AA: Chromosome changes in germ cell tumors of the testis. *Cancer Genet Cytogenet* **19**:245, 1986.

95. Oosterhuis JW, de Jong B, Cornelisse CJ, et al: Karyotyping and DNA flow cytometry of mature residual teratoma after intensive chemotherapy of disseminated nonseminomatous germ cell tumor of the testis: A report of two cases. *Cancer Genet Cytogenet* **22**:149, 1986.

96. Speicher MR, Jauch A, Walt H, et al: Correlation of microscopic phenotype with genotype in a formalin-fixed, paraffin-embedded testicular germ cell tumor with universal DNA amplification, comparative genomic hybridization, and interphase cytogenetics. *Am J Pathol* **146**:1332, 1995.

97. Bosl GJ, Dmitrovsky E, Reuter VE, et al: Isochromosome of chromosome 12: Clinically useful marker for male germ cell tumors. *JNCI* **81**:1874, 1989.

98. Bani MR, Rak J, Adachi D, Wiltshire R, Trent JM, Kerbel RS, Ben-David Y: Multiple features of advanced melanoma recapitulated in tumorigenic variants of early stage (radial growth phase) human melanoma cell lines: Evidence for a dominant phenotype. *J Cancer Res* **56**:3075, 1996.

99. Guan X-Y, Zhang H, Bittner ML, Jiang Y, Meltzer PS, Trent JM: Rapid generation of human chromosome arm painting probes (CAPs) by chromosome microdissection. *Nat Genet* **12**:10, 1996.

100. Guan X-Y, Meltzer PS, Dalton WS, Trent JM: Identification of cryptic sites of DNA sequence amplification in human breast cancer by chromosome microdissection. *Nat Genet* **8**:155, 1994.

101. Zhang J, Cui P, Glatfelter AA, Cummings LM, Meltzer PS, Trent JM: Microdissection based cloning of a translocation breakpoint in a human malignant melanoma. *Cancer Res* **55**:4640, 1995.

102. Clark J, Rocques PJ, Crew AJ, Gill S, Shipley J, Chan AM, Gusterson BA, Cooper CS: Identification of novel genes, SYT and SSX, involved in the t(X;18)(p11.2;q11.2) translocation found in human synovial sarcoma. *Nat Genet* **7**:502, 1994.

103. Shapiro DN, Sublett JE, Li B, Downing JR, Naeve CW: Fusion of PAX3 to a member of the forkhead family of transcription factors in human alveolar rhabdomyosarcoma. *Cancer Res* **53**:5108, 1993.

104. Barr FG, Galili N, Holick J, Biegel JA, Rovera G, Emanuel BS: Rearrangement of the PAX3 paired box gene in the paediatric solid tumour alveolar rhabdomyosarcoma. *Nat Genet* **3**:113, 1993.

105. Miser JS, Triche TJ, Pritchard DJ, Kinsella T: Ewing's sarcoma and the nonrhabdomyosarcoma soft tissue sarcomas of childhood, in Pizzo PA, Poplack DG (eds): *Principles and Practice of Pediatric Oncology.* Philadelphia, Lippincott, 1989, pp. 659–688.

106. Turc-Carel C, Philip I, Berger MP, Philip T, Lenoir GM: Chromosome study of Ewing's sarcoma (ES) cell lines: Consistency of a reciprocal translocation t(11;22)(q24;q12). *Cancer Genet Cytogenet* **12**:1, 1984.

107. Turc-Carel C, Aurias A, Mugneret F, Lizard S, Sidaner I, Volk C, Thiery JP, Olschwang S, Philip I, Berger MP, et al: Chromosomes in Ewing's sarcoma: I. An evaluation of 85 cases of remarkable consistency of t(11;22)(q24;q12). *Cancer Genet Cytogenet* **32**:229, 1988.

108. Ben-David Y, Giddens EB, Letwin K, Bernstein A: Erythroleukemia induction by Friend murine leukemia virus: Insertional activation of a new member of the ets gene family, Fli-1, closely linked to c-ets-1. *Genes Dev* **5**:908, 1991.

109. Zucman J, Melot T, Desmaze C, Ghysdael J, Plougastel B, Peter M, Zucker JM, Triche TJ, Sheer D, Turc CC, et al: Combinatorial generation of variable fusion proteins in the Ewing family of tumours. *EMBO J* **12**:4481, 1993.

110. Biegel JA, Conard K, Brooks JJ: Translocation (11;22)(p13;q12): primary change in intra-abdominal desmoplastic small round cell tumor. *Genes Chromosom Cancer* **7**:119, 1993.

111. Seth A, Ascione R, Fisher RJ, Mavrothalassitis GJ, Bhat NK, Papas TS: The ets gene family. *Cell Growth Differ* **3**:327, 1992.

112. Watson DK, McWilliams-Smith MJ, Nunn MF, Duesberg PH, O'Brien SJ, Papas TS: The ets sequence from the transforming gene of avian erythroblastosis virus, E26, has unique domains on human chromosomes 11 and 21: Both loci are transcriptionally active. *Proc Natl Acad Sci USA* **82**:7294, 1985.

113. Goyns MH, Hann IM, Stewart JG, Birnie GD: The c-ets-1 proto-oncogene is rearranged in some cases of acute lymphoblastic leukaemia. *Br J Cancer* **56**:611, 1987.

114. Plougastel B, Zucman J, Peter M, Thomas G, Delattre O: Genomic structure of the EWS gene and its relationship to EWSR1, a site of tumor-associated chromosome translocation. *Genomics* **18**:609, 1993.

115. Zoubek A, Pfleiderer C, Salzer-Kuntschik M, Amann G, Windhager R, Fink FM, Koscielniak E, Delattre O, Strehl S, Ambros PF, et al: Variability of EWS chimaeric transcripts in Ewing tumours: A comparison of clinical and molecular data. *Br J Cancer* **70**:908, 1994.

116. Ohno T, Rao VN, Reddy ES: EWS/Fli-1 chimeric protein is a transcriptional activator. *Cancer Res* **53**:5859, 1993.

117. Rao VN, Ohno T, Prasad DD, Bhattacharya G, Reddy ES: Analysis of the DNA-binding and transcriptional activation functions of human Fli-1 protein. *Oncogene* **8**:2167, 1993.

118. Mao X, Miesfeldt S, Yang H, Leiden JM, Thompson CB: The FLI-1 and chimeric EWS-FLI-1 oncoproteins display similar DNA binding specificities. *J Biol Chem* **269**:18216, 1994.

119. Lessnick SL, Braun BS, Denny CT, May WA: Multiple domains mediate transformation by the Ewing's sarcoma EWS-FLI-1 fusion gene. *Oncogene* **10**:423, 1995.

120. Bailly RA, Bosselut R, Zucman J, Cormier F, Delattre O, Roussel M, Thomas G, Ghysdael J: DNA-binding and transcriptional activation properties of the EWS-FLI-1 fusion protein resulting from the t(11;22) translocation in Ewing sarcoma. *Mol Cell Biol* **14**:3230, 1994.

121. Magnaghi-Jaulin L, Masutani H, Robin P, Lipinski M, Harel-Bellan A: SRE elements are binding sites for the fusion protein EWS-FLI-1. *Nucleic Acids Res* **24**:1052, 1996.

122. Braun BS, Frieden R, Lessnick SL, May WA, Denny CT: Identification of target genes for the Ewing's sarcoma EWS/FLI fusion protein by representational difference analysis. *Mol Cell Biol* **15**:4623, 1995.

123. Zinszner H, Albalat R, Ron D: A novel effector domain from the RNA-binding protein TLS or EWS is required for oncogenic transformation by CHOP. *Genes Dev* **8**:2513, 1994.

124. Sorensen PH, Lessnick SL, Lopez-Terrada D, Liu XF, Triche TJ, Denny CT: A second Ewing's sarcoma translocation, t(21;22), fuses the EWS gene to another ETS-family transcription factor, ERG. *Nat Genet* **6**:146, 1994.

125. Jeon IS, Davis JN, Braun BS, Sublett JE, Roussel MF, Denny CT, Shapiro DN: A variant Ewing's sarcoma translocation (7;22) fuses the EWS gene to the ETS gene ETV1. *Oncogene* **10**:1229, 1995.

126. Urano F, Umezawa A, Hong W, Kikuchi H, Hata J: A novel chimera gene between EWS and E1A-F, encoding the adenovirus E1A enhancer-binding protein, in extraosseous Ewing's sarcoma. *Biochem Biophys Res Commun* **219**:608, 1996.

127. Stephenson CF, Bridge JA, Sandberg AA: Cytogenetic and pathologic aspects of Ewing's sarcoma and neuroectodermal tumors. *Hum Pathol* **23**:1270, 1992.

128. Giovannini M, Biegel JA, Serra M, Wang JY, Wei YH, Nycum L, Emanuel BS, Evans GA: EWS-erg and EWS-Fli1 fusion transcripts in Ewing's sarcoma and primitive neuroectodermal tumors with variant translocations. *J Clin Invest* **94**:489, 1994.

129. Delattre O, Zucman J, Melot T, Garau XS, Zucker JM, Lenoir GM, Ambros PF, Sheer D, Turc-Carel C, Triche TJ, et al: The Ewing family of tumors—a subgroup of small-round-cell tumors defined by specific chimeric transcripts [see comments]. *N Engl J Med* **331**:294, 1994.

130. Desmaze C, Zucman J, Delattre O, Melot T, Thomas G, Aurias A: Interphase molecular cytogenetics of Ewing's sarcoma and peripheral neuroepithelioma t(11;22) with flanking and overlapping cosmid probes. *Cancer Genet Cytogenet* **74**:13, 1994.

131. Selleri L, Giovannini M, Romo A, Zucman J, Delattre O, Thomas G, Evans GA: Cloning of the entire FLI1 gene, disrupted by the Ewing's sarcoma translocation breakpoint on 11q24, in a yeast artificial chromosome. *Cytogenet Cell Genet* **67**:129, 1994.

132. Sorensen PH, Liu XF, Delattre O, Rowland JM, Biggs CA, Thomas G, Triche TJ: Reverse transcriptase PCR amplification of EWS/FLI-1 fusion transcripts as a diagnostic test for peripheral primitive neuroectodermal tumors of childhood. *Diagn Mol Pathol* **2**:147, 1993.

133. Ladanyi M, Lewis R, Garin-Chesa P, Rettig WJ, Huvos AG, Healey JH, Jhanwar SC: EWS rearrangement in Ewing's sarcoma and peripheral neuroectodermal tumor: Molecular detection and correlation with cytogenetic analysis and MIC2 expression. *Diagn Mol Pathol* **2**:141, 1993.

134. Ida K, Kobayashi S, Taki T, Hanada R, Bessho F, Yamamori S, Sugimoto T, Ohki M, Hayashi Y: EWS-FLI-1 and EWS-ERG chimeric mRNAs in Ewing's sarcoma and primitive neuroectodermal tumor. *Int J Cancer* **63**:500, 1995.

135. Scotlandi K, Serra M, Manara MC, Benini S, Sarti M, Maurici D, Lollini PL, Picci P, Bertoni F, Baldini N: Immunostaining of the p30/32MIC2 antigen and molecular detection of EWS rearrangements for the diagnosis of Ewing's sarcoma and peripheral neuroectodermal tumor. *Hum Pathol* **27**:408, 1996.

136. Downing JR, Head DR, Parham DM, Douglass EC, Hulshof MG, Link MP, Motroni TA, Grier HE, Curcio BA, Shapiro DN: Detection of the (11;22)(q24;q12) translocation of Ewing's sarcoma and peripheral neuroectodermal tumor by reverse transcription polymerase chain reaction. *Am J Pathol* **143**:1294, 1993.

137. Sorensen PH, Shimada H, Liu XF, Lim JF, Thomas G, Triche TJ: Biphenotypic sarcomas with myogenic and neural differentiation express the Ewing's sarcoma EWS/FLI1 fusion gene. *Cancer Res* **55**:1385, 1995.

138. Ouchida M, Ohno T, Fujimura Y, Rao VN, Reddy ES: Loss of tumorigenicity of Ewing's sarcoma cells expressing antisense RNA to EWS-fusion transcripts. *Oncogene* **11**:1049, 1995.

139. Zoubek A, Dockhorn-Dworniczak B, Delattre O, Christiansen H, Niggli F, Gatterer-Menz I, Smith TL, Jurgens H, Gadner H, Kovar H: Does expression of different EWS chimeric transcripts define clinically distinct risk groups of Ewing tumor patients? *J Clin Oncol* **14**:1245, 1996.

140. Stenman G, Kindblom LG, Angervall L: Reciprocal translocation t(12;22)(q13;q13) in clear-cell sarcoma of tendons and aponeuroses. *Genes Chromosom Cancer* **4**:122, 1992.

141. Mrozek K, Karakousis CP, Perez MC, Bloomfield CD: Translocation t(12;22)(q13;q12.2-12.3) in a clear cell sarcoma of tendons and aponeuroses. *Genes Chromosom Cancer* **6**:249, 1993.

142. Zucman J, Delattre O, Desmaze C, Epstein AL, Stenman G, Speleman F, Fletchers CD, Aurias A, Thomas G: EWS and ATF-1 gene fusion induced by t(12;22) translocation in malignant melanoma of soft parts. *Nat Genet* **4**:341, 1993.

143. Fujimura Y, Ohno T, Siddique H, Lee L, Rao VN, Reddy ES: The EWS-ATF-1 gene involved in malignant melanoma of soft parts with t(12;22) chromosome translocation, encodes a constitutive transcriptional activator. *Oncogene* **12**:159, 1996.

144. Vallejo M, Ron D, Miller CP, Habener JF: C/ATF, a member of the activating transcription factor family of DNA-binding proteins, dimerizes with CAAT/enhancer-binding proteins and directs their binding to cAMP response elements. *Proc Natl Acad Sci USA* **90**:4679, 1993.

145. Brown AD, Lopez-Terrada D, Denny C, Lee KA: Promoters containing ATF-binding sites are de-regulated in cells that express the EWS/ATF1 oncogene. *Oncogene* **10**:1749, 1995.

146. Rodriguez E, Sreekantaiah C, Gerald W, Reuter VE, Motzer RJ, Chaganti RS: A recurring translocation, t(11;22)(p13;q11.2), characterizes intra-abdominal desmoplastic small round-cell tumors. *Cancer Genet Cytogenet* **69**:17, 1993.

147. Ladanyi M, Gerald W: Fusion of the EWS and WT1 genes in the desmoplastic small round cell tumor. *Cancer Res* **54**:2837, 1994.

148. Brodie SG, Stocker SJ, Wardlaw JC, Duncan MH, McConnell TS, Feddersen RM, Williams TM: EWS and WT-1 gene fusion in desmoplastic small round cell tumor of the abdomen. *Hum Pathol* **26**:1370, 1995.

149. Gerald WL, Rosai J, Ladanyi M: Characterization of the genomic breakpoint and chimeric transcripts in the EWS-WT1 gene fusion of desmoplastic small round cell tumor. *Proc Natl Acad Sci USA* **92**:1028, 1995.

150. de Alava E, Ladanyi M, Rosai J, Gerald WL: Detection of chimeric transcripts in desmoplastic small round cell tumor and related developmental tumors by reverse transcriptase polymerase chain reaction: A specific diagnostic assay. *Am J Pathol* **147**:1584, 1995.

151. Call KM, Glaser T, Ito CY, Buckler AJ, Pelletier J, Haber DA, Rose EA, Kral A, Yeger H, Lewis WH, Jones C, Housman DE: Isolation and characterization of a zinc finger polypeptide gene at the human chromosome 11 Wilms' tumor locus. *Cell* **60**:509, 1990.

152. Clark J, Benjamin H, Gill S, Sidhar S, Goodwin G, Crew J, Gusterson BA, Shipley J, Cooper CS: Fusion of the EWS gene to CHN, a member of the steroid/thyroid receptor gene superfamily, in a human myxoid chondrosarcoma. *Oncogene* **12**:229, 1996.

153. Gill S, McManus AP, Crew AJ, Benjamin H, Sheer D, Gusterson BA, Pinkerton CR, Patel K, Cooper CS, Shipley JM: Fusion of the EWS gene to a DNA segment from 9q22-31 in a human myxoid chondrosarcoma. *Genes Chromosom Cancer* **12**:307, 1995.

154. Limon J, Turc-Carel C, Dal Cin P, Rao U, Sandberg AA: Recurrent chromosome translocations in liposarcoma. *Cancer Genet Cytogenet* **22**:93, 1986.

155. Aman P, Ron D, Mandahl N, Fioretos T, Heim S, Arheden K, Willen H, Rydholm A, Mitelman F: Rearrangement of the transcription factor gene CHOP in myxoid liposarcomas with t(12;16)(q13;p11). *Genes Chromosom Cancer* **5**:278, 1992.

156. Crozat A, Aman P, Mandahl N, Ron D: Fusion of CHOP to a novel RNA-binding protein in human myxoid liposarcoma. *Nature* **363**:640, 1993.

157. Rabbitts TH, Forster A, Larson R, Nathan P: Fusion of the dominant negative transcription regulator CHOP with a novel gene FUS by

translocation t(12;16) in malignant liposarcoma. *Nat Genet* **4**:175,1993.

158. Ron D, Habener JF: CHOP, a novel developmentally regulated nuclear protein that dimerizes with transcription factors C/EBP and LAP and functions as a dominant-negative inhibitor of gene transcription. *Genes Dev* **6**:439, 1992.

159. Batchvarova N, Wang XZ, Ron D: Inhibition of adipogenesis by the stress-induced protein CHOP (Gadd 153). *EMBO J* **14**:4654, 1995.

160. Ubeda M, Wang XZ, Zinszner H, Wu I, Habener JF, Ron D: Stress-induced binding of the transcriptional factor CHOP to a novel DNA control element. *Mol Cell Biol* **16**:1479, 1996.

161. Wang XZ, Ron D: Stress-induced phosphorylation and activation of the transcription factor CHOP (GADD 153) by p38 MAP kinase. *Science* **272**:1347, 1996.

162. Barone MV, Crozat A, Tabaee A, Philipson L, Ron D: CHOP (GADD 153) and its oncogenic variant TLS-CHOP, have opposing effects on the induction of G1/S arrest. *Genes Dev* **8**:453, 1994.

163. Panagopoulos I, Hoglund M, Mertens F, Mandahl N, Mitelman F, Aman P: Fusioin of the EWs and CHOP genes in myxoid liposarcoma. *Oncogene* **12**:489, 1996.

164. Komuro H, Hayashi Y, Kawamura M, Hayashi K, Kaneko Y, Kamoshita S, Hanada R, Yamamoto K, Hongo T, Yamada M, et al: Mutations of the p53 gene are involved in Ewing's sarcomas but not in neuroblastomas. *Cancer Res* **53**:5284, 1993.

165. Hamelin R, Zucman J, Melot T, Delattre O, Thomas G: p53 mutations in human tumors with chimeric EWS/FLI-1 genes. *Int J Cancer* **57**:336, 1994.

166. Sreekantaiah R, Leong SP, Karakousis CP, McGee DL, Rappaport WD, Villar HV, Neal D, Fleming S, Wankel A, Herrington PN, et al: Cytogenetic profile of 109 lipomas. *Cancer Res* **51**:422, 1991.

167. Mrozek K, Karakousis CP, Bloomfield CD: Chromosome 12 breakpoints are cytogenetically different in benign and malignant lipogenic tumors: Localization of breakpoints in lipoma to 12q15 and in myxoid liposarcoma to 12q13.3. *Cancer Res* **53**:1670, 1993.

168. Heim S, Mandahl N, Kristoffersson U, Mitelman F, Rooser B, Rydholm A, Willen H: Reciprocal translocation t(3;12)(q27;q13) in lipoma. *Cancer Genet Cytogenet* **23**:301, 1986.

169. Sreekantaiah C, Sandberg AA: Clustering of aberrations to specific chromosome regions in benign neoplasms. *Int J Cancer* **48**:194, 1991.

170. Kazmierczak B, Rosigkeit J, Wanschura S, Meyer-Bolte K, van de Ven WJ, Kayser K, Krieghoff B, Kastendiek H, Bartitzke S, Bullerdiek J: HMGI-C rearrangements as the molecular basis for the majority of pulmonary chondroid hamartomas: A survey of 30 tumors. *Oncogene* **12**:515, 1996.

171. Wanschura S, Kazmierczak B, Pohnke Y, Meyer-Bolte K, Bartnitzke S, van de Ven WJ, Bullerdiek J: Transcriptional activation of HMGI-C in three pulmonary hamartomas each with a der(14)t(12;14) as the sole cytogenetic abnormality. *Cancer Lett* **102**:17, 1996.

172. Ashar HR, Fejzo MS, Tkachenko A, Zhou X, Fletcher JA, Weremowicz S, Morton CC, Chada K: Disruption of the architectural factor HMGI-C: DNA-binding AT hook motifs fused in lipomas to distinct transcriptional regulatory domains. *Cell* **82**:57, 1995.

173. Schoenmakers EF, Wanschura S, Mols R, Bullerdiek J, van den Berghe H, van de Ven WJ: Recurrent rearrangements in the high mobility group protein gene, HMGI-C, in benign mesenchymal tumours. *Nat Genet* **10**:436, 1995.

174. Zhou X, Benson KF, Ashar HR, Chada K: Mutation responsible for the mouse pygmy phenotype in the developmentally regulated factor HMGI-C [see comments]. *Nature* **376**:771, 1995.

175. Chau KY, Patel UA, Lee KL, Lam HY, Crane-Robinson C: The gene for the human architectural transcription factor HMGI-C consists of five exons each coding for a distinct element. *Nucleic Acids Res* **23**:4262, 1995.

176. Friedmann M, Holth LT, Zoghbi HY, Reeves R: Organization, inducible-expression and chromosome localization of the human HMGI-I(Y) nonhistone protein gene. *Nucleic Acids Res* **21**:4259, 1993.

177. Parkash V, Gerald WL, Parma A, Miettinen M, Rosai J: Desmoplastic small round cell tumor of the pleura. *Am J Surg Pathol* **19**:659, 1995.

CHAPTER 7

Gene Amplification in Human Cancers: Biological and Clinical Significance

Garrett M. Brodeur ▪ Michael D. Hogarty

INTRODUCTION

Cytogenetically visible rearrangements in human cancer cells fall into three general categories: (1) deletions, with net loss of genetic material; (2) translocations, with transposition of genetic material but no net loss or gain; and (3) gene amplification, with net gain of a specific chromosomal region. Deletions are thought to represent loss of a suppressor gene, whereas translocations and gene amplification generally represent activation of a proto-oncogene. Translocations could result in inactivation of a suppressor gene, but this appears to be a rare event. Gene amplification also can involve drug resistance genes or other genes that confer a selective advantage when overexpressed. For the purposes of this chapter, gene amplification will be used to refer to an increase in copy number (more than six copies per diploid genome) of a specific, subchromosomal region (generally, 1–2 mb or less). It is not used to refer to numerical gain (generally, three to four copies per diploid genome) of whole chromosomes, chromosome arms, or very large chromosomal regions.

Gene amplification usually is apparent cytogenetically, either as extrachromosomal double-minute chomatin bodies (dmins), or as chromosomally integrated, homogeneously staining regions (HSRs). If the copy number is low (e.g., five to ten copies per cell), if the size of the amplified unit (amplicon) is small, or if the karyotype is extremely complex, gene amplification may not be evident by conventional cytogenetics. However, several different molecular approaches have been developed to allow reliable detection of gene amplification in interphase nuclei from small amounts of tumor DNA (see the following). In general, the latter techniques presuppose that the gene (or genes) that might be amplified are known.

Gene amplification almost always results in the overexpression of one or more genes contained on the amplicon. Usually there is a single gene that appears to be the target of the gene amplification, but some amplified units may contain two or more genes that could theoretically confer a selective advantage. Furthermore, in some cancers, two or more discrete regions may be amplified. However, in the majority of cases, only a single genetic region is amplified in a given tumor.

Theoretically, the amplification and consequent overexpression of a number of genes could confer a selective advantage on a cancer cell. In practice, the majority of examples that have been studied involve oncogenes or drug resistance genes. For the purposes of this chapter, we will concentrate on genes that are amplified in a substantial percentage (at least 10%) of primary tumors that have been extensively studied (at least 50 cases examined). We will discuss *MYCN* amplification in neuroblastomas in detail to illustrate certain points, because it is the most consistent and extensively studied example of oncogene amplification in a human tumor. For the sake of completeness, we will discuss amplification of drug resistance genes in human cancers, but they do not fulfill the criteria for inclusion discussed above.

AMPLIFICATION OF DRUG RESISTANCE GENES

Culturing mammalian cells under conditions of incrementally increasing concentrations of a cytotoxic drug can lead to amplification of the gene encoding the protein that is the target of that drug.[1] This has suggested the possibility that human cancer cells may become resistant to chemotherapy by amplifying certain genes,[2] like the dihydrofolate reductase (*DHFR*) gene in methotrexate resistance, or the multidrug-resistance genes (*MDR*1, *MRP*) in tumors simultaneously resistant to multiple unrelated chemotherapeutic agents.[3] Indeed, there are several reports of human tumor cells that amplified the *DHFR* gene and became resistant to methotrexate.[7,10] However, this has occurred in only a few cases, and only after prolonged clinical treatment, so the frequency with which it occurs does not meet our criteria for inclusion in this chapter. Furthermore, no reports of *MDR* or *MRP* amplification have been reported in human tumors in vivo.[11] Thus, gene amplification appears to be a fairly rare mechanism for the development of drug resistance in humans.

AMPLIFICATION OF ONCOGENES

There are an increasing number of reports of human tumors and cell lines with amplification of proto-oncogenes. A catalog of every reported tumor or cell line that was demonstrated to amplify an oncogene or related genes is beyond the scope of this chapter. Rather, we will focus on examples of gene amplification in primary tumors that occur with substantial prevalence. Inclusion of cell line studies would bias the data, because established cell lines in many systems show a higher prevalence of gene amplification than their primary tumor counterparts. For instance, amplification of *MYCN* and *ERBB1* (*EGFR*) are found in approximately 80% of cell lines established from neuroblastomas and squamous cell carcinomas, respectively, whereas they are amplified in approximately 25 and 10% of primary tumor specimens, respectively.[12–14]

Many different malignancies have been demonstrated to amplify a variety of oncogenes. These include neuroblastoma, breast, and ovarian carcinoma, small cell lung carcinoma (SCLC), and head and neck squamous cell carcinoma (*HNSCC*). In these malignancies the prevalence of gene amplification ranges from 20 to 50% (see Table 7-1), often with amplification correlating with aggressive behavior or advanced stage. In additional malignancies, such as sarcomas, hepatocellular carcinomas, malignant gliomas, and cervical and gastrointestinal cancers, data are accumulating that implicate gene amplification in their pathogenesis or progression as well (Table 7-1).

Genes amplified in human cancers are thought to confer a growth advantage to a clone, analogous to amplification in vitro of drug resistance genes under certain selective external pressures. Genes frequently amplified in cancer tissues include members of the *MYC* (*MYC, MYCN, MYCL*) and *RAS* (*HRAS, KRAS, NRAS*) families of proto-oncogenes, growth factor receptors (*ERBB1* and -2, FGFR1 and -2), and genes that are involved in cell-cycle regulation (*CCND1, CCNE, MDM2, CDK4*), in addition to other miscellaneous genes (*AKT2, MYB*) (Table 7-2).

Activation of oncogenes is a frequent mechanism of tumorigenesis, and may be accomplished by point mutation, translocation, or amplification. In many malignancies studied to date, amplification of an oncogene is strongly associated with advanced stages of disease and with a poor outcome. In neuroblastoma, for example, *MYCN* amplification is associated with rapid disease progression independent of patient age and stage.[15,17] In other malignancies, however, the presence of amplification does not always maintain significance as an independent variable for outcome when stage and histology are considered. In breast cancer, many studies have correlated the presence of *ERBB2* amplification with clinical variables such as high stage and grade, lymph node involvement, large tumor size, and steroid hormone receptor absence.[18,19] In multivariate analysis controlling for the preceding clinical data, the presence of *ERBB2* amplification does not always predict a poor outcome. It remains to be answered, therefore, whether oncogene amplification is a consequence of aggressive, deregulated cell proliferation and resulting genomic instability, or is an early cellular event that is causative of the more aggressive clinical phenotype.

In certain situations, the amplicon harbors multiple candidate genes and it may be difficult to determine a putative oncogene target among these. The most widely studied of these amplicons includes the region of 11q13 containing *CCND1* (Cyclin D1), *FGF4*, *FGF3/int*, *EMS1* as well as other candidate genes. Investigators have used molecular techniques to implicate *CCND1* based on amplification prevalence and expression patterns in the amplified tumors.[20,21] Other examples include the 12q14 amplicon in the region of *MDM2, GLI, SAS, CDK4*; and 8p12 with *FGFR1, PLAT*, and others.[22,23] Likewise, it is possible to exploit the presence of amplified domains to discover new oncogenes. Amplified DNA fragments can be cloned and mapped within the genome. From the amplified domain new genes may be sought to explain the biological significance of the amplification, as well as to elucidate their function in normal cells.[20,24]

The prevalence of gene amplification in different tumors, as well as the biological and clinical significance of amplifying particular genes, is discussed in the following, with particular emphasis on the role of *MYCN* amplification in neuroblastoma. Tumors that are presented in detail elsewhere in this volume are discussed only briefly.

MYCN Amplification in Neuroblastomas

Neuroblastomas are tumors of the peripheral nervous system that are found almost exclusively in children. The peak age at diagnosis

Table 7-1 Recurrent Oncogene Amplification in Human Cancers

Tumor Type	Gene Amplified	Frequency, Percent	References
Neuroblastoma	*MYCN*	20–25	(25,26)
Small Cell Lung Cancer	*MYC*	15–20	(57,58)
Glioblastoma	*ERBB*1(EGFR)	33–50	(118,119)
Breast Cancer	*MYC*	20	(18,19,120)
	*ERBB*2(EGFR2)	~20	(18,19)
	*FGF*R1	12	(23,51)
	*FGF*R2	12	(51)
	*CCND*1(Cyclin D1)	15–20	(19,21)
Esophageal Cancer	*MYC*	38	(121)
	*CCND*1(Cyclin D1)	25	(12)
Gastric Cancer	*KRAS*	10	(62)
	CCNE(Cyclin E)	15	(21,61)
Hepatocellular Cancer	*CCND*1(Cyclin D1)	13	(122,123)
Sarcoma	*MDM*2	10–30	(16,17)
	*CDK*4	11	(15)
Cervical Cancer	*MYC*	25–50	(125,125)
Ovarian Cancer	*MYC*	20–30	(126,127)
	*ERBB*2(*EG*R2)	15–30	(53,54)
	AKT2	12	(55)
Head and Neck Cancer	MYC	7–10	(14,15)
	*ERBB*1(EGFR)	10	(14)
	*CCND*1(Cyclin D1)	~50	(14,65)
Colorectal Cancer	*MYB*	15–20	(64)
	HRAS	29	(63)
	KRAS	22	(63)

Table 7-2 Oncogenes Amplified in Human Cancers

Gene Amplified	Locus	Tumors
AKT2	19q13	Ovarian cancer
CCND1(Cyclin D1)	11q13	HNSCC, esophageal, breast, HCC
CCNE(Cyclin E)	19q12	Gastric cancer
CDK4	12q14	Sarcoma
ERBB1(EGFR)	7p12	Glioblastoma, HNSCC
ERBB2(EGFR2)	17q11	Breast, ovarian cancer
FGFR1	8p12	Breast cancer
FGFR2	10q25	Breast cancer
HRAS	11p15	Colorectal cancer
KRAS	12p13	Colorectal, gastric cancer
MDM2	12q14	Sarcoma
MYB	6q23	Colorectal cancer
MYC	8q22	Ovarian, breast, SCLC, HNSCC, esophageal, cervical cancer
MYCN	2p24	Neuroblastoma

is 22 months, and it is rare after 10 years of age. Neuroblastomas often are localized and have a less aggressive behavior in infants, but they are frequently metastatic and have a poor prognosis in older children. The reason for this apparent discrepancy was unclear until recently. Cytogenetic and molecular analysis of these tumors has identified characteristic differences that allow these tumors to be subclassified into three groups that are distinct in terms of biological features and clinical behavior (see Chapter 22). The feature that characterizes the most aggressive subset of neuroblastomas is amplification of the *MYCN* oncogene.

Cytogenetic examination of neuroblastomas reveals that a substantial number either have extrachromosomal dmins, chromosomally integrated HSRs, or both in subpopulations of cells. These two abnormalities are cytogenetic manifestations of gene amplification. Dmins are the predominant form of amplified DNA in primary tumors, but dmins and HSRs are found with about equal frequency in neuroblastoma cell lines.[25,26] Indeed, dmins and/or HSRs occur in about 90% of neuroblastoma cell lines but only 25% of primary tumors. Evidence suggests that this represents selection *in vitro* for cell lines derived from tumors that have preexisting dmins or HSRs, and there is no evidence to date that these abnormalities develop with time in culture, at least in neuroblastomas. It is unclear why HSRs are a more common form of amplified DNA in established cell lines than they are in primary tumors.

Although cytogenetic analysis of human neuroblastomas frequently has revealed dmins or HSRs in primary tumors and cell lines, the nature of the amplified sequences was not known initially. Evidence for amplification of genes associated with drug resistance was sought, but none was found.[25,26] However, a study was undertaken to determine if a proto-oncogene was amplified in a panel of neuroblastoma cell lines. An oncogene related to the viral oncogene v*MYC*, but distinct from *MYC*, was amplified in the majority of neuroblastoma cell lines tested.[27] The amplified *MYCN* sequence was mapped to the HSRs on different chromosomes in neuroblastoma cell lines, but the normal single-copy locus was mapped to the distal short arm of chromosome 2.[28] Thus, the *MYCN* locus was amplified in neuroblastomas, regardless of whether they had dmins or an HSR, and regardless of the chromosomal location of the HSR.

In collaboration with others, we began a study of primary tumors from untreated patients to determine if *MYCN* amplification occurred. In the initial analysis of 63 primary tumors, amplification ranging from 3 to 300 per haploid genome was found in 24 tumors (38%).[29] All cases with *MYCN* amplification in this initial study came from patients with advanced stages of disease. The progression-free survival of these patients was analyzed according

to the stage of disease and *MYCN* copy number.[30] *MYCN* amplification clearly was associated with rapid tumor progression and a poor outcome, independent of the stage of the tumor.

These studies have been extended to over 3000 patients with neuroblastoma enrolled in protocols of the Children's Cancer Group (CCG) and the Pediatric Oncology Group (POG) (Table 7-3).[26,31] Examples of *MYCN* amplification seen in some of the primary tumors are shown by fluorescence *in situ* hybridization (FISH) (Figs. 7-1B, 7-1C), compared to a normal control (Fig. 7-1A). It is now clear that, among patients with less advanced stages of disease traditionally associated with a good prognosis, a minority (5–10%) have tumors with *MYCN* amplification.[26,31] Our data indicate that virtually all of these patients are destined to have rapid tumor progression and a poor outcome, similar to their counterparts with advanced stages of disease. Over 30% of patients with more advanced tumor stages had *MYCN* amplification, and they also had an expectedly poor outcome. Our findings that *MYCN* amplification is associated with a poor outcome regardless of the clinical stage of tumor is supported by independent studies from Japan and Europe.[32-34]

We analyzed the *MYCN* copy number in multiple simultaneous or consecutive samples of neuroblastoma tissue from 60 patients to determine whether or not the presence or absence of *MYCN* was consistent in different tumor samples from a given patient, or if single-copy tumors ever developed amplification at the time of recurrence.[35] Indeed, we found a consistent pattern of *MYCN* copy number (either amplified or unamplified) in different tumor samples taken from an individual patient, either simultaneously or consecutively.[35] These results suggest that *MYCN* amplification is an intrinsic biological property of a subset of neuroblastomas. Tumors that develop *MYCN* amplification generally do so by the time of diagnosis, and so cases of neuroblastoma with a single copy (per haploid genome) of *MYCN* at the time of diagnosis almost never have developed amplification subsequently.

About 25–30% of the children with neuroblastoma have *MYCN* amplification in their tumors, and virtually all of these children have rapidly progressive and fatal disease. However, in patients with single-copy tumors, there is not yet a biological marker or explanation why half of these patients do not survive. A general correlation has been demonstrated between *MYCN* copy number and expression, but a high level of *MYCN* expression in single-copy tumors does not appear to identify a subset with a particularly poor outcome.[34,36-38] It is still possible that activation of *MYCN* by mechanisms other than amplification or overexpression may play an important role. In addition, it is likely that either activation of other oncogenes, deletion of specific suppressor genes, or other genetic lesions may contribute to the poor clinical outcome in these patients.

We had sought evidence for amplification of other oncogenes, including *MYC, MYCL, NRAS, HRAS, KRAS, EGFR1, EGFR2, SIS, SRC, MYB, FOS,* and *ETS* in neuroblastomas, but none was found.[26] However, there are at least six examples of neuroblastoma cell lines or primary tumors that amplify regions that are remote from the *MYCN* locus at 2p24. These include amplification of

Table 7-3 Correlation of *MYCN* Copy Number with Stage and Survival in 3000 Neuroblastomas

Stage at Diagnosis	MYCN Amplification		Three Year Survival, Percent
Benign Ganglioneuromas	0/64	(0%)	100
Low Stages (1,2)	31/772	(4%)	90
Stage 4-S	15/190	(8%)	80
Advanced Stages (3,4)	612/1,974	(31%)	30
TOTAL	658/3000	(22%)	50

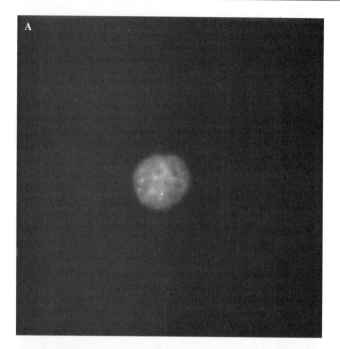

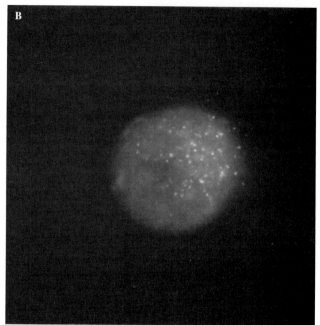

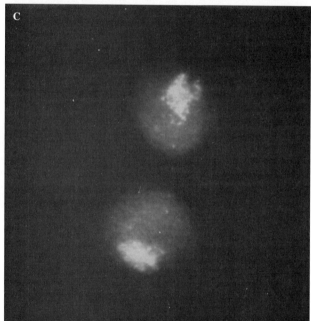

FIG. 7-1 *MYCN* amplification demonstrated by FISH analysis. *A.* **Normal interphase nucleus showing 2 dots, corresponding to the two normal homologs of *MYCN*. *B.* Interphase nucleus from a neuroblastoma cell with amplification of *MYCN* in the form of dmins. Signals are heterogeneously scattered throughout the nucleus. *C.* Interphase nucleus from a neuroblastoma cell with amplification of *MYCN* in the form of an HSR. Note the confluence of signals in a discrete area, in contrast to the randomly distributed signals in the upper right panel.** (*Courtesy of J. Biegel, Children's Hospital of Philadelphia.*)

DNA from 2p22 and 2p13 in the IMR cell line, as well as coamplification of both *MYCN* (from 2p24–32) and *MDM2* (from 12q14) in the NGP, TR, and LS cell lines.[22,39–41] Finally, there is one report of coamplification of *MYCN* and *MYC*L in a neuroblastoma cell line,[42] and this has been seen in at least one primary tumor as well (unpublished observations). These findings indicate that more than one locus can be amplified, but no neuroblastoma has been shown to amplify another gene that did not also amplify *MYCN*.

The presence of *MYCN* amplification in human neuroblastomas has been shown to correlate strongly with advanced clinical stage and poor prognosis.[26,29,30,33,34,36–38] Our recent studies showed a very strong correlation between *MYCN* amplification and 1p LOH ($p <$ .001), indicating that LOH was common in patients with amplification.[25,26,43] Both *MYCN* amplification and deletion of 1p (as detected by cytogenetic or molecular analysis) appear strongly correlated with a poor clinical outcome and with each other, but it is not yet clear if they are independent prognostic variables.[44–50] Never-

theless, they appear to characterize a genetically distinct subset of very aggressive neuroblastomas.

ONCOGENE AMPLIFICATION IN OTHER CANCERS

Breast Cancer

Breast cancer is the single most common cancer occurring in women, and represents a genetically heterogeneous disease with frequent amplification of oncogenes and allelic deletions.[18] *MYC, ERBB2,* and *CCND1* (Cyclin D1) are the most frequently amplified genes in breast cancer, each occurring in approximately 20% of cases. Genes of the fibroblast growth factor receptor family (*FGFR*1 and *FGFR*2) are also amplified in another 12% of cases, respectively, although it is not clear that their expression is increased above baseline (Table 7-2).[23,51] Many studies have attempted to correlate the presence of a particular amplified gene with outcome or other clinical prognostic factors with contradictory results, although there is support for the notion that amplification is a late event in the multi-step pathogenesis of breast cancer.[18,52]

Ovarian Cancer

In ovarian cancer, amplification of ERBB2 and MYC are each found to occur in 15–30% of samples.[53,54] ERBB2 or MYC amplification tends to occur in advanced stages of disease and is seen infrequently in early invasive or borderline ovarian epithelial tumors, again implying that these are late genetic events.[53] AKT2 is a protein serine/threonine kinase gene discovered by homology to VAKT, a viral oncogene that can cause lymphomas in mice. This oncogene is amplified independently of MYC or ERBB2 in approximately 12% of ovarian cancers and also correlates with invasiveness.[55] Although amplification of NRAS and KRAS are seen infrequently in ovarian cancers, there is some evidence that these events occur earlier based on their prevalence in low stage disease, but this remains speculative.[56]

Lung Cancer

Lung cancer is one of the most common and fatal malignancies, and its incidence is increasing in both men and women. Small cell lung carcinoma (SCLC) makes up approximately 25% of cases and has a distinct clinical course with a propensity for early metastasis. The MYC proto-oncogenes are the only genes amplified in a significant number of SCLCs (15–20% of cases), although cell lines derived from SCLC specimens more frequently have gene amplification.[14,57,58] The majority of these cases involves MYC, with amplification of MYCN and MYCL also occurring.[57–59] However, coamplification of multiple MYC family genes has not been described to date in SCLC specimens. It is possible that the propensity of SCLC cell lines to amplify MYC in vitro illustrates this cancer's underlying genetic instability and virulent phenotype. The clinical association of MYC amplification with shortened survival was seen in one study, but this has not been confirmed.[60]

Gastrointestinal Cancers

A diverse group of genetic alterations occur in gastrointestinal cancers, involving mutation or deletion of tumor suppressor genes and DNA repair genes, in addition to amplification of oncogenes. Amplification of MYC and CCND1 occurs frequently in esophageal squamous cell carcinoma, the latter gene being almost uniformly amplified in metastatic disease and correlating with clinical and pathological staging.[61] In contrast, a plethora of genetic alterations occur in gastric cancer, many presumed to induce cell proliferation via induction of growth factor production or increased growth factor receptor expression, but amplification does not occur commonly. These genetic alterations differ in poorly-differentiated and well-differentiated gastric cancers, and overall 10–15% of cases will demonstrate KRAS or CCNE amplification.[21,61,62] In colorectal cancers, cytogenetic evidence for gene amplification has long existed in the form of dmins but with no clear candidate genes. In some series, MYB, HRAS, or KRAS amplification has been found, but in the majority of colorectal cancers, none of the known oncogenes have been amplified in a significant proportion of cases.[63,64]

HNSCC, Other

In head and neck squamous cell carcinomas, amplification of the 11q13 locus with CCND1 occurs frequently, whereas MYC and ERBB1 amplification are also seen.[14,65] These findings are particularly germane in that current clinical prognostic factors are poor for HNSCC and molecular data may in the future become of significant predictive importance. In still other malignancies, gene amplification has been shown to be a prominent feature. In glioblastoma, hepatocellular carcinoma, cervical cancer, and certain sarcomas the role of oncogene amplification is being elucidated as advanced molecular analyses of these malignancies becomes more prevalent (Table 7-2).

MECHANISMS OF GENE AMPLIFICATION

The precise mechanism by which gene amplification occurs in human cancers is not known with certainty. Some information can be obtained by studying amplification of drug resistance genes in cells grown in vitro under selective pressure. However, these systems generally involve the rapid selection for resistance to an antimetabolite or other toxic compound, so it is not clear that these model systems will provide relevant information. It is more likely that the selective pressures that lead to amplification of a gene that provides a survival or growth advantage in vivo are not as profound, so the mechanisms leading to gene amplification may be quite different.

Unfortunately, only the end point of gene amplification can be studied, so it is difficult to draw firm conclusions about early events in the amplification process. Some information can be obtained by structural analysis of the amplified unit, as well as analysis of the genomic configuration of the locus that was amplified. In the majority of cases, the initial form of amplified DNA seen in human cancers is the extrachromosomal dmin. These structures lack centromeres or kinetocores, and they apparently segregate randomly in the two daughter cells after cell division. In order to remain stable, it is likely that dmin are closed circular molecules. Experimental data supporting this hypothesis have come from the study of amplified units involving the MYCN gene in human neuroblastomas, as well as other systems.

Several models have been proposed to explain the genomic amplification of specific chromosomal regions. These include the overreplication (onion skin) model, the chromosomal breakage/deletion plus episome formation model, and the duplication and crossing over model. These models were based on the analysis of genomic rearrangements that followed the rapid, stepwise selection of resistance to a particular drug. However, none of these models are consistent with what is known about the structure of DNA in tumors with spontaneous amplification of regions containing oncogenes, such as the MYCN oncogene in human neuroblastomas.

Amler and colleagues used pulsed-field gel electrophoresis (PFGE) to study the restriction pattern of MYCN amplicons using infrequently cutting enzymes and probes around the MYCN gene.[66,67] These studies led to the conclusion that the amplicons were arranged in tandem, head-to-tail arrays in the HSRs, and that most of the amplicons had a consistent restriction pattern (there was relatively little rearrangement). These conclusions were verified by Schneider and colleagues who cloned a representative amplified domain into yeast artificial chromosomes (YACs) from a cell line with 300 copies of MYCN per cell as dmins.[68] They showed that the amplicons were arranged in a head-to-tail, presumably circular arrangement, with general preservation of the germ line genomic structure. Finally, Corvi and coworkers showed the germ line copy of

MYCN was apparently intact on both homologs of chromosome 2 (i.e., it was not deleted).[69]

Based on the overreplication model, the resolution of this complex structure would result in considerable rearrangement of the amplified sequences relative to the germ line configuration. Also, a gradient of amplification should be seen, with the highest level of amplification near the gene that is the presumed target of amplification, with decreasing amplification further away from the amplification epicenter. However, the PFGE data by Amler and YAC cloning data by Schneider are inconsistent with this model, even though some variation from the germ line pattern was detected by both approaches.[66,68]

The duplication plus crossing over model would suggest that relatively intact copies of the amplicon would occur *in situ* on a given chromosome, leading to an HSR at the site of the normal gene. However, the most common form of amplified DNA is the extrachromosomal dmins, and the chromosomal locations of HSRs representing amplification of *MYCN* in neuroblastomas occur almost everywhere but at the normal chromosomal location of *MYCN* at 2p24.[70] Thus, this model does not seem applicable to what happens when *MYCN* becomes amplified in human neuroblastomas, and perhaps amplification of oncogenes in general.

Finally, the chromosomal breakage/deletion plus episome formation model would suggest that one germ line copy of the amplified region is deleted, but this was not detected in the five cell lines studied by Corvi or the cell line studied by Kanda and Shiloh.[39,69,71,72] One study by Hunt and Tereba did suggest that one germ line copy of *MYCN* was deleted from a homolog in one cell line by segregating the homologs into separate somatic cell hybrids, but this is inconsistent with data from at least six other cell lines studied by FISH.[73] It is possible that the apparent deletion may have occurred during the formation of the somatic cell hybrids, or that there may be different mechanisms by which *MYCN* amplification can occur.

In summary, none of the above models derived from the study of amplification of drug resistance genes appears to apply to the *de novo* amplification of oncogenes in human tumors in vivo. It seems likely that a variation of the breakage/deletion plus episome formation model is applicable. However, given the apparent retention of the normal parental copies of the amplified region, it is likely that some form of duplication of the amplified region occurs, followed by excision and circularization to form a dmin.[73a] Further study will be required to elucidate this mechanism, which may be difficult if a model system for *de novo* oncogene amplification cannot be found.

STRUCTURAL ANALYSIS OF AMPLICONS

General Comments about the Size/Structure of Amplified Domains

Estimates of the size of the amplified domain around the *MYCN* proto-oncogene in neuroblastomas have ranged from 300–3000 kb, based on physical, chemical and electrophoretic measurements of the amplified DNA.[70] However, all these approaches to map the size of the amplified domain have been indirect. An attempt was made to clone and map the amplified domain around *MYCN* in a representative neuroblastoma cell line NGP using cosmid and lambda vectors.[74,75] However, only 140 kb of contiguous DNA around the *MYCN* locus could be mapped, and a number of additional amplified clones were identified that were not contained in the 140 kb contiguous region. The entire 140-kb contiguous locus was amplified in a panel of 12 primary neuroblastomas with

MYCN amplification, whereas the noncontiguous fragments were amplified in subsets of them.[75] These data indicate that, although each tumor had a relatively unique pattern of amplified DNA fragments, there was core region that was consistently amplified in different tumors.

Amler and Schwab have analyzed the amplified domain of a series of neuroblastoma cell lines with *MYCN* amplification, most in the form of chromosomally integrated HSRs.[66] They analyzed the amplification domain by pulsed-field gel electrophoresis and hybridization with DNA probes that represent the 5′ and 3′ ends of the *MYCN* gene. They confirmed the heterogeneity of size of the amplified domain seen in different neuroblastomas demonstrated by earlier studies.[39,72,74,75] They also concluded that most amplified regions of DNA consisted of multiple tandem arrays of DNA segments that were several hundred kilobases in size, and that *MYCN* was at or near the center of the amplified units. Rearrangements were more commonly found in the cell lines with higher *MYCN* copy number (greater than 50–100 copies/haploid genome).

We have analyzed the amplified domain in human neuroblastomas in order to determine the size and structural organization of this region in different tumors and cell lines, as well as the core region that is consistently amplified. Because of the large size of the domain, we have used the yeast artificial chromosome (YAC) cloning vector system.[76] To date, 20 YACs have been identified which contain segments of the amplified domain from a representative neuroblastoma cell line, and the YACs can be arranged in a contiguous linear map of approximately 1.2 Mb.[68,77] In general, the YAC clones are consistent with a linear map of the region, but a few rearrangements have been identified thus far. Our data also indicate that the core of the domain amplified in different tumors is no more than 130 kb, and the amplicons of one tumor have deleted about half of this core.[78] Although it remains a formal possibility that there may be other genes near *MYCN* whose expression is important in mediating the aggressive phenotype associated with *MYCN* amplification, our data suggest that *MYCN* is the target of amplification in neuroblastomas.

Combined with the findings of Corvi and others that both homologs of *MYCN* are retained, these data are inconsistent with the deletion model of gene amplification.[79–81] Nevertheless, it is likely that a large region containing the selectable marker and an origin of replication is duplicated, excised, and circularized, forming an extrachromosomal episome (Fig. 7-2). This episome segregates randomly during cell division, but cells with more copies of the marker gene have a selective advantage and accumulate to a certain stable average number. Although there would inevitably be heterogeneity in the number of episomes per cell, the average number in a population should be relatively stable. Larger episomes or episome multimers would be visible with the light microscope and called dmins. As a rare event, the episomes would integrate into a chromosome at an apparently random site forming an HSR. Because of the secondary recombinational events, the structure of the amplified domains from HSRs would likely be more rearranged and heterogeneous.[68,77]

BIOLOGICAL SIGNIFICANCE OF GENE AMPLIFICATION

Presumably, the mechanism by which gene amplification confers a selective advantage on the cancer cells is that there is overexpression of the gene or genes contained on the amplicon. In general, this overexpression is proportional to the increase in copy number, but this is not an absolute correlation. The overexpression of the gene or genes then must confer some advantage to the cell in terms

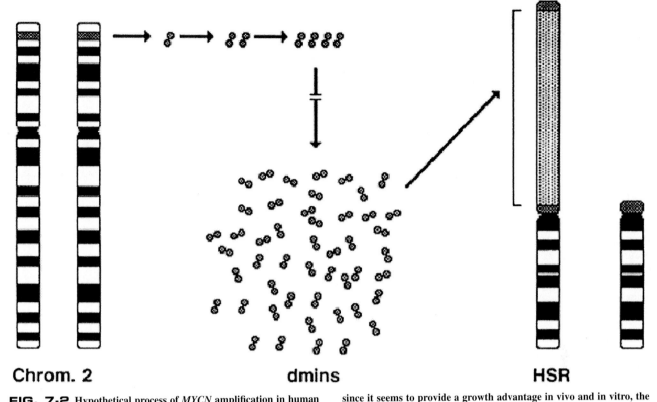

Chrom. 2   **dmins**   **HSR**

FIG. 7-2 Hypothetical process of *MYCN* amplification in human neuroblastomas. The location of the normal *MYCN* gene is shown by the shaded band, chromosome 2p24 on the left. The current data suggest that a large region of DNA containing the *MYCN* gene is duplicated on one homolog of chromosome 2 and forms an extrachromosomal element or episome, which probably is circular. It must contain an origin of replication but lacks a centromere or kinetocore, so it does not segregate evenly between daughter cells during mitosis. However, since it seems to provide a growth advantage in vivo and in vitro, the episomes accumulate in a subset of cells but remain unstable and therefore heterogeneously distributed among the cells in the population. If these episomes are large enough to be seen in the light microscope they are called dmins. As a rare event, particularly in cells in vitro with pre-existing *MYCN* amplification, the dmins linearly integrate into a chromosome at a seemingly random site.

of growth or survival. We will review briefly what is known about the likely consequences of overexpressing the most frequently amplified genes in human cancers: the *MYC* family, the *RAS* family, the *ERBB* and *FGF*R families, and the cell-cycle control genes, including the cyclins and *MDM*2.

MYC Family Amplification

The structure of the *Myc* proteins consists of a transactivating domain at the N-terminal third of the protein, followed by a basic region, helix-loop-helix region, and leucine zipper domain (B-HLH-Zip). These proteins are thought to activate transcription by binding to a hexanucleotide motif CACGTG known as an E-box. However, they do not bind well as monomers or as homodimers, but rather as heterodimers with another B-HLH-Zip protein known as *MAX*.[82] This protein lacks a transcriptional activation domain, and it can form homodimers that are thought to be transcriptionally repressive.[83–87] Thus, in a state of *MAX* excess, *MAX* homodimers predominate, and transcription is repressed. Conversely, when N-*MYC* (or C-*MYC*) are expressed at higher levels, heterodimers form, resulting in transcriptional activation. The consequence of this is progression through the cell cycle, and proliferation of the cell population. Inactivation of *MYCN* occurs when leucines in the Zip region are mutated, indicating the importance of this region in *MYCN* function.[88]

MYC oncoproteins have a short half-life (20–30 minutes), so once transcription and translation cease, the levels of *MYC* fall rapidly, and *MAX-MAX* transcriptional repression predominates. However, in tumors which amplify *MYC*, *MYCN* or *MYC*L, the level of amplification is usually one to two orders of magnitude (or more), with corresponding overexpression of the oncoprotein.[34,36–38,58] This leads to very high steady-state levels of MYC, even when it is not being actively transcribed. This in turn presumably favors a state of proliferation, with less likelihood that the cell will enter G_0 and become quiescent. This is presumably the selective advantage conferred by overexpressing this family of genes.

RAS Family Amplification

RAS genes encode a family of proteins known as G proteins, which participate in the signaling cascade initiated by the activation of tyrosine kinase receptors or other mechanisms.[89–91] *RAS* activation (by certain base pair mutations) or overexpression (usually by amplification) leads to enhanced signal transduction through the *RAF*1 serine-threonine kinase, the early response kinases (*ERK*1 and *ERK*2), and subsequent induction of transcription of immediate-early genes (e.g., *FOS*, *JUN*, *EGR*1, etc.) in the nucleus.[89–91]

The amplification and overexpression of *RAS* genes leads to constitutive signal transduction, mimicking the effects of continual activation of a growth factor receptor, like *EGFR* or *PDGFR*.[89–94] This in turn leads to continuous cell proliferation. However, the cellular background is very important, because in certain cellular milieus (such as neural cells), the predominant receptor tyrosine kinase may be signaling differentiation and not proliferation.[95–97] Activation or overexpression of *RAS* in this context would lead to differentiation of the cell, which would not promote the proliferation of tumor cells.[89–91,93] This may explain why *RAS* activation (usually by mutation) is rare in neural tumors, whereas it is one of the most common types of oncogene activation in many other tumor types.[92–94]

Amplification of the ERBB and FGFR Family

Amplification and overexpression of genes for growth factors and/or their receptors, such as those of the *EGF/EGFR* (*ERBB*) and *FGF/FGFR* families, occur in a number of human cancers.[23,51,53] The *ERBB* and *FGF* receptors are transmembrane protein tyrosine kinases involved in cell proliferation. After specific ligand binding, signal transduction occurs through phosphorylation of the SH2 domains of cytoplasmic proteins associated with the receptor. This leads to *RAS* activation, serine/threonine phosphorylations, and changes in phosphotidyl inositol metabolism with the end result being modulation of specific genes necessary for proliferation.[98,99]

Gastric cancers express a number of growth factors and receptors including *EGF, TGF-α, ERBB2*, and *FGFR2*.[61,100] *EGF* is synthesized as a transmembrane precursor with secreted protein being released by proteolytic cleavage. It has been shown to enhance growth of cells from most epithelial tumors, and in gastric cancer *EGF* amplification is associated with poor outcome.[100,101] In addition, human gastric cancers that possess both *EGF* and *EGFR* or *ERBB*2 simultaneously had a greater degree of local invasion and lymph node metastasis, further suggesting autocrine stimulation. Additionally, high levels of expression of growth factor receptor alone may result in autophosphorylation and signaling even in the absence of ligand.

Constitutive activation of these growth factor-receptor signaling pathways is a common motif in oncogenesis.[98,99] Amplification and overexpression of either ligand or receptor may cause growth stimulation in an autocrine or paracrine fashion in the appropriate cellular setting and contribute to biologic malignancy.

Amplification of the Genes Encoding Regulators of the Cell Cycle

Cells of most higher organisms maintain a stringent checkpoint control over progression from G1 into S phase and subsequent cell division. Early in G1, cells are dependent on mitogenic stimuli, but beyond a certain point a switch to intrinsic cell-cycle machinery occurs with a reduced requirement for growth factors, apparently ensuring an ordered completion of the cell division cycle. This switch-point is mediated by the D-type cyclins, though many proteins play important roles as both positive and negative regulators. These include (but are not limited to) other cyclins, cyclin-dependent kinases (CDKs), and their inhibitors (CDKIs). Activation of G1 cyclins (*CCND1* and *CCNE*) occurs via growth factor signals which induce *CCND1* phosphorylation. Activated cyclins D and E, in association with their predominant cyclin-dependent kinases CDK4 and CDK2, then sequentially phosphorylate the RB protein. This causes the release of E2F from pRB, which activates transcription of genes involved in cell proliferation.[102,103] Overexpression of *CCND1, CCNE*, or *CDK4* presumably results in a growth advantage for cells by tipping the balance in favor of G1 transition rather than quiescence. Likewise, overexpression of *MDM2* could have similar effects. *MDM2* protein binds p53, a potent cell-cycle inhibitor. By blocking p53 transcriptional activation of CDKIs such as p21, cells are more likely to enter S phase.[102,103] This loss of checkpoint control fails to allow time for repair of DNA damage caused by a multitude of insults, such as ionizing radiation, drugs, and cellular toxins. Experimentally, cells with either homozygous loss or inactivation of p53 or *CCND1* overexpression have been shown to more readily undergo gene amplification in response to selective pressures.[104–106] This enhancement of genetic instability illustrates the potential importance of cell cycle-control protein perturbations in the development of the malignant phenotype.

METHODS OF DETECTING GENE AMPLIFICATION

A variety of techniques may be used to detect gene amplification.[107] Each has certain advantages and disadvantages in terms of the amount of tumor tissue or DNA needed, the ease of performing the technique, the sensitivity of the technique to detect low levels of amplification, or the size of the amplified unit. These techniques include: conventional cytogenetics; Southern analysis; fluorescence in situ hybridization (FISH); semiquantitative PCR; and comparative genomic hybridization (CGH).

Cytogenetic Analysis

Cytogenetic analysis is a labor-intensive technique that is dependent on dividing cells in the tumor tissue or adaptation to growth in short-term culture. As a result, it is unsuccessful in the majority of solid tumors and a substantial minority of leukemias. The detection of HSRs or dmins provides evidence for gene amplification in the culture, although small HSRs or dmins may escape detection. Also, it is impossible to know with certainty which gene or chromosomal region is amplified. This is a useful technique when investigating a new tumor type but is not the most efficient or sensitive approach once it is known which gene or genes are likely to be amplified.

Southern Analysis

Southern analysis is perhaps the gold standard by which other techniques are compared. This technique relies on the preparation of DNA from tumor tissue that is relatively free of contaminating normal tissue. The DNA is digested with a restriction enzyme, electrophoresed on an agarose gel, blotted to a membrane, and hybridized with a radioactive probe corresponding to the gene or genetic region thought to be amplified.[29,35] This technique is rather labor intensive, and it requires at least 5–10 μg of DNA. Frequently an internal control gene is also hybridized so the intensity of the band of interest can be normalized for quantitative densitometry. However, this technique can miss a small percentage of amplified cells in an unamplified population. Slot-blot is a variation on this technique that requires no digestion, only 1 μg of DNA, and it is easily subjected to densitometric analysis, but low levels of amplification can be missed.

Fluorescence In Situ Hybridization (FISH)

The FISH technique is probably the most efficient and popular technique at the current time.[108,109] It requires only a small amount of tumor tissue, usually a touch prep or cytospin of several thousand cells on a slide. It can even be done on paraffin embedded tissue.[109] Hybridization to interphase nuclei takes place overnight under a coverslip, and the results can be interpreted within 48 hours. This technique can also distinguish a small percentage of amplified tumor cells in a population of normal or nonamplified tumor cells, if a counterstain to visualize the cells is implemented. It may be necessary to utilize a control probe for the centromere or opposite chromosomal arm of the region usually amplified in order to distinguish between low-level amplification and polysomy for the particular chromosome. However, this approach does require an expensive fluorescence microscope and sophisticated imaging equipment, and the probes are expensive to purchase commercially, so it is not the ideal approach for all laboratories.

An interesting variation of this technique has been developed whereby amplicons are microdissected and used as FISH hybridization probes to determine the chromosomal origin.[110] This micro-dissection approach allows the chromosomal origin of dmins or HSRs to be determined in a single hybridization without knowing a priori the genetic region that is amplified. Indeed, this approach can also identify amplification of previously unsuspected chromosomal regions. However, in addition to the technical demands of FISH, this approach also requires both successful metaphase preparation, with identification of dmins or HSRs, and the ability to perform microdissection and preparation of a microclone library. Therefore, this method will not be useful for most laboratories.

Semiquantitative PCR

The PCR technique had obvious advantages that might be applied to the detection of genomic amplification in small amounts of tumor DNA.[111–114] As long as the number of cycles of amplification is carefully controlled, and an internal control gene is used for normalization, it is possible to semiquantitatively amplify a given gene or DNA sequence and distinguish the normal copy number from multiple copies. Although some claim to detect as low as two-fold amplification, generally five- to ten-fold amplification is the limit of detection of this semiquantitative technique on primary tumor samples.[111–114]

Comparative Genomic Hybridization (CGH)

This is the newest of the approaches that has been applied to the detection of genomic amplification.[115–117] This approach has the advantage of conventional cytogenetics, in that the whole genome is surveyed, not just one or a few specific genomic regions that are known or suspected to be amplified in a given tumor type. Also, because the chromosomal location of the amplified region is known, the likely gene amplification frequently is apparent. Tumor metaphases are not needed, and only a small amount of DNA is required. However, this approach requires a sophisticated fluorescence microscope and image capturing capability, as well as software to analyze the data obtained. Furthermore, very small amplicons or low levels of amplification may be missed.

SUMMARY AND CONCLUSIONS

Gene amplification in human cells is a phenomenon that appears to be restricted to tumor cells. In the majority of cases in which the amplified genomic region has been identified, the driving force of the amplification appears to be an oncogene, usually of the *ERBB*, *MYC*, or *RAS* families. A variety of other genes have been shown to be amplified in small numbers of cases, or in tumor cell lines, but the above families are found the most consistently. Furthermore, examples of amplification of genes conferring drug resistance have been found in certain cancers at relapse, but this does not appear to be a common mechanism by which cancer cells become drug resistant in vivo.

The mechanism by which amplification of oncogenes in human cancer cells occurs is unknown, but it probably involves the duplication of a large chromosomal region, followed by deletion and circularization to form an extrachromosomal dmin. Then there is accumulation of these dmin by uneven segregation into the daughter cells during mitosis, until maximal advantage is achieved. This is presumably a consequence of the overexpression of a gene or genes on the amplicon that confer the selective advantage. The region amplified may be quite large, from 100 kb to several Mb. However, the region that is consistently amplified may contain little more than the single gene suspected of providing a growth or survival advantage.

The identification of oncogene amplification in certain human cancers provides some insight into the pathogenesis of these diseases. Indeed, in some tumor systems, oncogene amplification had been associated with a greater likelihood of invasion, metastasis and a poor outcome. Thus, the identification of oncogene amplification in human cancers may have some prognostic value. Ultimately, it may be possible to develop novel therapeutic approaches that target the amplified oncogene or the overexpressed oncoprotein. This approach may be particularly attractive if the amplified gene is mutated or chimeric, allowing the development of selective biological reagents, including antibodies, drugs, antisense, or targeted gene therapy approaches.

ACKNOWLEDGMENTS

This work was supported in part by National Institutes of Health grant RO1-CA39771.

REFERENCES

1. Schimke RT: Gene amplification in cultured cells. *J Biol Chem* **263**:5989, 1988.
2. Sobrero A, Bertino JR: Clinical aspects of drug resistance. *Cancer Surv* **5**:93, 1986.
3. Pastan I, Gottesman M: Multiple resistance in human cancer. *N Engl J Med* **316**:1388, 1987.
4. Chin JE, Soffir R, Noonan KE, Choi K, Roninson IB: Structure and expression of the human MDR (P-glycoprotein) gene family. *Mol Cell Biol* **9**:3808, 1989.
5. Ling V: P-glycoprotein and resistance to anticancer drugs. *Cancer* **69**:2603, 1992.
6. Grant CE, Valdimarsson G, Hipfner DR, Almquist KC, Cole SPC, Deeley RG: Overexpression of multidrug resistance protein (MRP) increases resistance to natural product drugs. *Cancer Res* **54**:357, 1994.
7. Curt GA, Carney DN, Cowan K, Jolivet J, Bailey BD, Drake JC, Kao CS, Minna JD, Chabner BA: Unstable methotrexate resistance in human small-cell lung carcinoma associated with double minute chromosomes. *New Engl J Med* **308**:199, 1983.
8. Horns RCJ, Dower WJ, Schimke RT: Gene amplification in a leukemic patient treated with methotrexate. *Clin Oncol* **2**:2, 1984.
9. Trent JM, Buick RN, Olson S, Horns RCJ, Schimke RT: Cytologic evidence for gene amplification in methotrexate cells obtained from a patient with ovarian adenocarcinoma. *J Clin Oncol* **2**:8, 1984.
10. Carman MD, H. SJ, Rivest RS, Srimatkandada S, Portlock CS, Duffy T, Bertino JR: Resistance to methotrexate due to gene amplification in a patient with acute leukemia. *J Clin Oncol* **2**:16, 1984.
11. Merkel DE, Fuqua SAW, Tandon AK, Hill Sm, Buzdar AU, McGuire WL: Electrophoretic analysis of 248 clinical breast cancer specimens for P-glycoprotein overexpression or gene amplification. *J Clin Oncol* **7**:1129, 1989.
12. Jiang W, Kahn SM, Tomita N, Zhang YL, Lu SH, Weinstein IB: Amplification and expression of the human cyclin D gene in esophageal cancer. *Cancer Res* **52**:2980, 1992.

13. Akama Y, Yasui W, Yokozaki H, Kuniyasu H, Kitahara K, Ishikawa T, Tahara E: Frequent amplification of the cyclin E gene in human gastric carcinomas. *Jpn J Cancer Res* **86**:617, 1995.

14. Leonard JH, Kearsley JH, Chenevix G, Hayward NK: Analysis of gene amplification in head and neck squamous carcinomas. *Int J Cancer* **48**:511, 1991.

15. Maelandsmo GM, Berner JM, Florenes VA, Forus A, Hovig E, Fodstad O, Myklebost O: Homozygous deletion frequency and expression levels of the CDKN2 gene in human sarcomas: relationship to amplification and mRNA levels of CDK4 and *CCND1*. *Br J Cancer* **72**:393, 1995.

16. Florenes VA, Maelandsmo GM, Forus A, Andreassen A, Myklebost O, Fodstad O: MDM2 gene amplification and transcript levels in human sarcomas: relationship to TP53 gene status [see comments]. *J Natl Cancer Inst* **86**:1297, 1994.

17. Leach FS, Tokino T, Meltzer P, Burrell M, Oliner JD, Smith S, Hill DE, Sidransky D, Kinzler KW, Vogelstein B: p53 mutation and MDM2 amplification in human soft tissue sarcomas. *Cancer Res* **53**:2231, 1993.

18. Garcia I, Dietrich PY, Aapro M, Vauthier G, Vadas L, Engel E: Genetic alterations of c *MYC*, *cERBB*, and *cRAS* protooncogenes and clinical associations in human breast carcinomas. *Cancer Res* **49**:6675, 1989.

19. Berns EM, Klijn JG, van Staveren IL, Portengen H, Noord*EGR* aaf E, Foekens JA: Prevalence of amplification of the oncogenes cMYC, HER2/neu, and INT in one thousand human breast tumours: correlation with steroid receptors. *Eur J Cancer* **28**:697, 1992.

20. Schuuring E: The involvement of the chromosome 11q13 region in human malignancies: cyclin D1 and EMS1 are two new candidate oncogenes: a review. *Gene* **159**:83, 1995.

21. Karlseder J, Zeillinger R, Schneeberger C, Czerwenka K, Speiser P, Kubista E, Birnbaum D, Gaudray P, Theillet C: Patterns of DNA amplification at band q13 of chromosome 11 in human breast cancer. *Genes Chromosom Cancer* **9**:42, 1994.

22. Van Roy N, Forus A, Myklebost O, Cheng NC, Versteeg R, Speleman F: Identification of two distinct chromosome 12 amplification units in neuroblastoma cell line NGP. *Cancer Genet Cytogenet* **82**:151, 1995.

23. Theillet C, Adelaide J, Louason GFB, Jacquemier J, Adnane J, Longy M, Katsaros D, Sismondi P, Gaudray P, et al.: *FGF*RI and PLAT genes and DNA amplification at 8p12 in breast and ovarian cancers. *Genes Chromsom Cancer* **7**:219, 1993.

24. Shiloh Y, Mor O, Manor A, Bar I, Rotman G, Eubanks J, Gutman M, Ranzani GN, Houldsworth J, Evans G, et al.: DNA sequences amplified in cancer cells: an interface between tumor biology and human genome analysis. *Mutat Res* **276**:329, 1992.

25. Brodeur GM, Green AA, Hayes FA, Williams KJ, Williams DL, Tsiatis AA: Cytogenetic features of human neuroblastomas and cell lines. *Cancer Res* **41**:4678, 1981.

26. Brodeur GM, Fong CT: Molecular biology and genetics of human neuroblastoma. *Cancer Genet Cytogenet* **41**:153, 1989.

27. Schwab M, Alitalo K, Klempnauer KH, Varmus HE, Bishop JM, Gilbert F, Brodeur G, Goldstein Trent JM: Amplified DNA with limited homology to *MYC* cellular oncogene is shared by human neuroblastoma cell lines and a neuroblastoma tumour. *Nature* **305**:245, 1983.

28. Schwab M, Varmus HE, Bishop JM, Grzeschik KH, Naylor SL, Sakaguchi AY, Brodeur G, Trent J: Chromosome localization in normal human cells and neuroblastomas of a gene related to c *MYC*. *Nature* **308**:288, 1984.

29. Brodeur GM, Seeger RC, Schwab M, Varmus HE, Bishop JM: Amplification of N *MYC* in untreated human neuroblastomas correlates with advanced disease stage. *Science* **224**:1121, 1984.

30. Seeger RC, Brodeur GM, Sather H, Dalton A, Siegel SE, Wong KY, Hammond D: Association of multiple copies of NMYC oncogene with rapid progression of neuroblastomas. *N Engl J Med* **313**:1111, 1985.

31. Brodeur GM: Neuroblastoma: Clinical applications of molecular parameters. *Brain Pathol* **1**:47, 1990.

32. Tsuda T, Obara M, Hirano H, Gotoh S, Kubomura S, Higashi K, Kuroiwa A, Nakagawara A, Nagahara N, Shimizu K: Analysis of N *MYC* amplification in relation to disease stage and histologic types in human neuroblastomas. *Cancer* **60**:820, 1987.

33. Nakagawara A, Ikeda K, Tsuda T, Higashi K, Okabe T: Amplification of N *MYC* oncogene in stage II and IVS neuroblastomas may be a prognostic indicator. *J Pediatr Surg* **22**:415, 1987.

34. Bartram CR, Berthold F: Amplification and expression of the N*MYC* gene in neuroblastoma. *Eur J Pediatr* **146**:162, 1987.

35. Brodeur GM, Hayes FA, Green AA, Casper JT, Wasson J, Wallach S, Seeger RC: Consistent N *MYC* copy number in simultaneous or consecutive neuroblastoma samples from sixty individual patients. *Cancer Res* **47**:4248, 1987.

36. Seeger RC, Wada R, Brodeur GM, Moss TJ, Bjork RL, Sousa L, Slamon DJ: Expression of N *MYC* by neuroblastomas with one or multiple copies of the oncogene. *Progr Clin Biol Res* **271**:41, 1988.

37. Nisen PD, Waber PG, Rich MA, Pierce S, Garvin JRJ, Gilbert F, Lanzkowsky P: N*MYC* oncogene RNA expression in neuroblastoma. *J Natl Cancer Inst* **80**:1633, 1988.

38. Slave I, Ellenbogen R, Jung W, Vawter GF, Kretschmar C, Grier H, Korf BR: *MYC* gene amplification and expression in primary human neuroblastoma. *Cancer Res* **50**;1459, 1990.

39. Shiloh Y, Shipley J, Brodeur GM, Bruns G, Korf B, Donlon T, Schreck RR, Seeger R, Sakai K, Latt SA: Differential amplification, assembly and relocation of multiple DNA sequences in human neuroblastomas and neuroblastoma cell lines. *Proc Natl Acad Sci USA* **82**:3761, 1985.

40. Corvi R, Savelyeva L, Breit S, Wenzel A, Handgretinger R, Barak J, Oren M, Amler L, Schwab M: Non-syntenic amplification of MDM2 and *MYCN* in human neuroblastoma. *Oncogene* **10**:1081, 1995.

41. Corvi R, Savelyeva L, Amler L, Handgetinger R, Schwab M: Cytogenetic evolution of *MYCN* and MDM2 amplification in the neuroblastoma LS tumor and its cell line. *Eur J Cancer* **31A**:520, 1995.

42. Jinbo T, Iwamura Y, Kaneko M, Sawaguchi S: Coamplification of the LMYC and N *MYC* oncogenes in a neuroblastoma cell line. *Jpn J Cancer Res* **80**:299, 1989.

43. Fong CT, Dracopoli NC, White PS, Merrill PT, Griffith RC, Housman DE, Brodeur GM: Loss of heterozygosity for chromosome 1p in human neuroblastomas: Correlation with NMYC amplification. *Proc Natl Acad Sci USA* **86**:3753, 1989.

44. Kaneko Y, Kanda N, Maseki N, Sakurai M, Tsuchida Y, Takeda T, Okabe I, Sakurai M: Different karyotypic patterns in early and advanced stage neuroblastomas. *Cancer Res* **47**:311, 1987.

45. Christiansen H, Lampert F: Tumour karyotype discriminates between good and bad prognostic outcome in neuroblastoma. *Br J Cancer* **57**:121, 1988.

46. Hayashi Y, Kanda N, Inaba T, Hanada R, Nagahara N, Muchi H, Yamamoto K: Cytogenetic findings and prognosis in neuroblastoma with emphasis on marker chromosome 1. *Cancer* **63**:126, 1989.

47. Maris JM, White PS, Beltinger CP, Sulman EP, Castleberry RP, Shuster JJ, Look AT, Brodeur GM: Significance of chromosome 1p loss of heterozygosity in neuroblastomas. *Cancer Res* **55**:4664, 1995.

48. Martinsson T, Shoberg P, Hedborg F, Kogner P: Deletion of chromosome 1p loci and microsatellite instability in neuroblastomas analyzed with short repeat-tandem polymorphisms. *Cancer Res* **55**:5681, 1995.

49. Gehring M, Berthold F, Edler L, Schwab M, Amler LC: The 1p deletion is not a reliable marker for the prognosis of patients with neuroblastoma. *Cancer Res* **55**:5366, 1995.

50. Caron H, van Sluis P, de Kraker J, Bokkerink J, Egeler M, Laureys G, Slater R, Westerveld A, Voute PA, Versteeg R: Allelic loss of chromosome 1p as a predictor of unfavorable outcome in patients with neuroblastoma. *New Engl M Med* **334**:225, 1996.

51. Adnane J, Gaudray P, Dionne CA, Crumley G, Jaye M, Schlessinger J, Jeanteur P, Birnbaum D, Theillet C: BEK and FLG, two receptors to members of the *FGF* family, are amplified in subsets of human breast cancers. *Oncogene* **6**:659, 1991.

52. Brison O: Gene amplification and tumor progression. *Biochim Biophys Acta* **1155**:25, 1993.

53. Fajac A, Benard J, Lhomme C, Rey A, Duvillard P, Rochard F, Bernaudin JF, Riou G: c *ERBB*2 gene amplification and protein expression in ovarian epithelial tumors: evaluation of their respective prognostic significance by multivariate analysis. *Int J Cancer* **64**:146, 1995.

54. Zhang GL, Zu KL, Yu SY: Amplification of C-MYC gene in ovarian cancer. *Chung Hua Fu Chan Ko Tsa Chih* **29**:401, 1994.

55. Bellacosa A, de Feo D, Godwin AK, Bell DW, Cheng JQ, Altomare DA, Wan M, Dubeau L, Scambia G, Masciullo V, et al.: Molecular alterations of the AKT2 oncogene in ovarian and breast carcinomas. *Int J Cancer* **64**:280, 1995.

56. Bian M, Fan Q, Huang S: Amplification of proto CMYC, H RAS, KRAS, CERBB2 in ovarian carcinoma [abstract]. *Chung Hua Fu Chan Ko Tsa Chih* **30**:406, 1995.

57. Chiba W, Sawai S, Hanawa T, Ishida H, Matsui T, Kosaba S, Watanabe S, Hatakenaka R, Matsubara Y, Funatsu T, et al.: Correlation between DNA content and amplification of oncogenes (c *MYC*, LMYC,

cERBB) and correlation with prognosis in 143 cases of resected lung cancer. *Gan To Kagaku Ryoho* **20**:824, 1993.

58. Brennan J, O'Connor T, Makuch RW, Simmons AM, Russell E, Linnoila RI, Phelps RM, Gazdar AF, Ihde DC, Johnson BE: *MYC* family DNA amplification in 107 tumors and tumor cell lines from patients with small cell lung cancer treated with different combination chemotherapy regimens. *Cancer Res* **51**:1708, 1991.
59. Wong AJ, Ruppert JM, Eggleston J, Hamilton SR, Baylin SB, Vogelstein B: Gene amplification of cMYC and N MYC in small cell carcinoma of the lung. *Science* **233**:461, 1986.
60. Johnson BE, Ihde DC, Makuch RW, Gazdar AF, Carney DN, Oie H, Russell E, Nau MM, Minna JD: *MYC* family oncogene amplification in tumor cell lines established from small cell lung cancer patients and its relationship to clinical status and course. *J Clin Invest* **79**:1629, 1987.
61. Tahara E: Genetic alterations in human gastrointestinal cancers, the application to molecular diagnosis. *Cancer* **75**:1410, 1994.
62. Ranzani GN, Pellegata NS, Previdere C, Saragoni A, Vio A, Maltoni M, Amadori D: Heterogeneous protooncogene amplification correlates with tumor progression and presence of metastases in gastric cancer patients. *Cancer Res* **50**:7811, 1990.
63. Salhab N, Jones DJ, Bos JL, Kinsella A, Schofield PF: Detection of *RAS* gene alterations and *RAS* proteins in colorectal cancer. *Dis Colon Rectum* **32**:659, 1989.
64. Greco C, Gandolfo GM, Mattei F, Gradilone A, Alvino S, Pastore LI, Casale V, Casole P, Grassi A, Cianciulli AM; Detection of *CMYB* genetic alterations and mutant p53 serum protein in patients with benign and malignant colon lesions. *Anticancer Res* **14**:1433, 1994.
65. Merritt WD, Weissler MC, Turk BF, Gilmer TM: Oncogene amplification in squamous cell carcinoma of the head and neck. *Arch Otolaryngol Head Neck Surg* **116**:1394, 1990.
66. Amler LC, Schwab M: Amplified NMYC in human neuroblastoma cells is often arranged as clustered tandem repeats of differently recombined DNA. *Mol Cell Biol* **9**:4903, 1989.
67. Amler LC, Schwab M: Multiple amplicons of discrete sizes encompassing NMYC in neuroblastoma cells evolve through differential recombination from a large precursor DNA. *Oncogene* **7**:807, 1992.
68. Schneider SS, Hiemstra JL, Zehnbauer BA, Taillon P, Le Paslier D, Vogelstein B, Brodeur GM: Isolation and structural analysis of a 1.2-megabase NMYC amplicon from a human neuroblastoma. *Mol Cell Biol* **12**:5563, 1992.
69. Corvi R, Amler LC, Savelyeva L, Gehring M, Schwab M: *MYCN* is retained in single copy at chromosome 2 band p23 during amplification in human neuroblastoma cells. *Proc Natl Acad Sci USA* **91**:5523, 1994.
70. Brodeur GM, Seeger RC: Gene amplification in human neuroblastomas: Basic mechanisms and clinical implications. *Cancer Genet Cytogenet* **19**:101, 1986.
71. Kanda N, Schreck R, Alt F, Bruns G, Baltimore D, Latt S: Isolation of amplified DNA sequences from IMR-32 human neuroblastoma cells: Facilitation by fluorescence flow sorting of metaphase chromosomes. *Proc Natl Acad Sci USA* **80**:4069, 1983.
72. Shiloh Y, Korf B, Kohl NE, Sakai K, Brodeur GM, Harris P, Kanda N, Seeger RC, Alt F, Latt SA: Amplification and rearrangement of DNA sequences from the chromosomal region 2p24 in human neuroblastomas. *Cancer Res* **46**:5297, 1986.
73. Hunt JD, Valentine M, Tereba A: Excision of N MYC from chromosome 2 in human neuroblastoma cells containing amplified N MYC sequences. *Mol Cell Biol* **10**:823, 1990.
74. Kinzler KW, Zehnbauer BA, Brodeur GM, Seeger RC, Trent JM, Meltzer PS, Vogelstein B: Amplification units containing human NMYC and cMYC genes. *Proc Natl Acad Sci USA* **83**:1031, 1986.
75. Zehnbauer BA, Small D, Brodeur Gm, Seeger R, Vogelstein B: Characterization of NMYC amplification units in human neuroblastoma cells. *Mol Cell Biol* **8**:522, 1988.
76. Schneider SS, Zehnbauer BA, Vogelstein B, Brodeur GM: Yeast artificial chromosome (YAC) vector cloning of the *MYCN* amplified domain in human neuroblastomas. *Progr Clin Biol Res* **366**:71, 1991.
77. Reiter JL, Kuroda H, White PS, Schneider SS, Taillon P, Brodeur GM: Physical mapping of the normal and amplified *MYCN* locus. *Genomics* (submitted), 1997.
78. Reiter JL, Brodeur GM: High-resolution mapping of a 130 core region of the *MYCN* amplicon in neuroblastomas. *Genomics* **32**:97, 1996.
79. Carroll S, DeRose M, Gaudray P, Moore C, VanDevanter DN, Von Hoff D, Wahl G: Double minute chromosomes can be produced from precursors derived from a chromosomal deletion. *Mol Cell Biol* **8**:1525, 1988.
80. Stark GR, Debatisse M, Giulotto E, Wahl GM: Recent progress in understanding mechanisms of mammalian DNA amplification. *Cell* **57**:901, 1989.
81. Wahl GM: The importance of circular DNA in mammalian gene amplification. *Cancer Res* **49**:1333, 1989.
82. Blackwood EM, Eisenman RN: Max: a helix-loop-helix zipper protein that forms a sequence-specific DNA-binding complex with *MYC*. *Science* **251**:1211, 1991.
83. Makela TP, Koskinen P, Vastrik I, Alitalo K: Alternative forms of Max as enhancers or suppressors of *MYC-RAS* cotransformation. *Science* **256**:373, 1992.
84. Reddy CD, Dasgupta P, Saikumar P, Dudek H, Rauscher FJ, III, Reddy EP: Mutational analysis of Max: role of basic, helix-loop-helix leucine zipper domains in DNA binding, dimerization and regulation of *MYC* transcriptional activation. *Oncogene* **7**:2085, 1992.
85. Kretzner L, Blackwood EM, Eisenman RN: *MYC* and Max proteins possess distinct transcriptional activities. *Nature* **359**:426, 1992.
86. Amati B, Dalton S, Brooks MW, Littlewood TD, Evan GI, Land H: Transcriptional activation by the human cMYC oncoprotein in yeast requires interaction with Max. *Nature* **359**:423, 1992.
87. Amati B, Brooks MW, Levy N, Littlewood TD, Evan GI, Land H: Oncogenic activity of the cMYC protein requires dimerization with Max. *Cell* **72**:233, 1993.
88. Nakajima H, Ikeda M, Tsuchida N, Nishimura S, Taya Y: Inactivation of the N MYC gene product by single amino acid substitution of leucine residues located in leucine-zipper region. *Oncogene* **4**:999, 1989.
89. Bar D: *RAS* proteins: Biological effects and biochemical targets (review). *Anticancer Res* **9**:1427, 1989.
90. Hall A: The cellular functions of small GTP proteins. *Science* **249**:635, 1990.
91. Medema RH, Boss JL: The role of p21 *RAS* in receptor tyrosine kinase signaling. *Crit Rev Oncol* **4**:615, 1993.
92. Marshall CJ: The *RAS* oncogenes. *J Cell Sci* (Suppl) **10**:157, 1988.
93. Bos JL: *RAS* oncogenes in human cancer: A review. *Cancer Res* **49**:4682, 1989.
94. Field JK, Spandidos DA: The role of *RAS* and *MYC* oncogenes in human solid tumours and their relevance in diagnosis and prognosis (review). *Anticancer Res* **10**:1, 1990.
95. Bar D, Feramisco JR: Microinjection of the *RAS* oncogene protein into PC12 cells induces morphological differentiation. *Cell* **42**:841, 1985.
96. Noda M, Ko M, Ogura A, Liu D, Amano T, Takano T, Ikawa Y: Sarcoma viruses carrying *RAS* oncogenes induce differentiation properties in a neuronal cell line. *Nature* **318**:73, 1985.
97. Hagag N, Halegoua SMV: Inhibition of growth factor differentiation of PC12 cells by microinjection of antibody to *RAS* p21. *Nature* **319**:680, 1986.
98. Bishop JM: Molecular themes in oncogenesis. *Cell* **64**:235, 1991.
99. Ullrich A, Schlessinger J: Signal transduction by receptors with tyrosine kinase activity. *Cell* **61**:203, 1990.
100. Tokunaga A, Masahiko O, Okuda T, Teramoto T, Fujita I, Mizutani T, Keyama T, Yoshiyuki T, Nishi K, Matsukura N: Clinical significance of epidermal growth factor (*EGF*), *EFG* receptor, and c *ERBB* in human gastric cancer. *Cancer* [supplement] **75**:1418, 1995.
101. Hamburger AW, White CP, Brown RW: Effect of epidermal growth factor on proliferation of human tumor cells in soft agar. *J Natl Cancer Inst* **67**:825, 1981.
102. Hartwell L: Defects in a cell cycle checkpoint may be responsible for the genomic instability of cancer cells. *Cell* **71**:543, 1992.
103. Sherr CJ: Mammalian G1 cyclins. *Cell* **73**:1059, 1993.
104. Asano K, Sakamoto H, Sasaki H, Ochiya T, Yoshida T, Ohishi Y, Machida T, Kakizoe T, Sugimura T, Terada M: Tumorigenicity and gene amplification potentials of cyclin D1 NIH3T3 cells. *Biochem Biophys Res Commun* **217**:1169, 1995.
105. Livingstone LR, White A, Sprouse J, Livanos E, Jacks T, Tisty TD: Altered cell cycle arrest and gene amplification potential accompany loss of wild p53. *Cell* **70**:923, 1992.
106. Zhou P, Jiang W, Weghorst CM, Weinstein IB: Overexpression of Cyclin D1 enhances gene amplification. *Cancer Res* **56**:36, 1996.
107. Wasson JC, Brodeur GM: Molecular analysis of gene amplification in tumors, in Dracopoli NC, Haines JL, Korf BR, Moir DT, Morton CC, Seidman CE, Seidman JG, Smith DR (eds): *Current Protocols in Human Genetics*. New York: Greene Publishing Associates, Inc., and John Wiley & Sons, Inc., 1994, p. 10.5.1.
108. Shapiro DN, Valentine MB, Rowe ST, Sinclair AE, Sublett JE, Roberts WM, Look AT: Detection of NMYC gene amplification by

fluorescence in situ hybridization. Diagnostic utility for neuroblastoma. *Am J Pathol* **142**:1339, 1993.

109. Misra DN, Dickman PS, Yunis EJ: Fluorescence in situ hybridization (FISH) detection of *MYCN* oncogene amplification in neuroblastoma using paraffin tissues. *Diag Mol Pathol* **4**:128, 1995.

110. Guan X, Meltzer PS, Dalton WS, Trent JM: Identification of cryptic sites of DNA sequence amplification in human breast cancer by chromosome microdissection. *Nat Genet* **8**:155, 1994.

111. Crabbe DC, Peters J, Seeger RC: Rapid detection of *MYCN* gene amplification in neuroblastomas using the polymerase chain reaction. *Diag Mol Pathol* **1**:229, 1992.

112. Gilbert J, Norris MD, Haber M, Kavallaris M, Marshall GM, Stewart BW: Determination of N*MYC* gene amplification in neuroblastoma by differential polymerase chain reaction. *Mol Cell Probes* **7**:227, 1993.

113. Huddart SN, Mann JR, McGukin AG, Corbett R: *MYCN* amplification by differential PCR. *Pediat Hematol Oncol* **10**:31, 1993.

114. Boerner S, Squire J, Thorner P, McKenna G, Zielenska M: Assessment of *MYCN* amplification in neuroblastoma biopsies by differential polymerase chain reaction. *Pediatr Pathol* **14**:823, 1994.

115. Kallioniemi A, Kallioniemi O, Sudar D, Rutovitz D, Gray JW, Waldman F, Pinkel D: Comparative genomic hybridization for molecular cytogenetic analysis of solid tumors. *Science* **258**:818, 1992.

116. Kallioniemi A, Kallioniemi O, Piper J, Tanner M, Stokke T, Chen L, Smith HS, Pinkel D. Gray JW, Waldman FM: Detection and mapping of amplified DNA sequences in breast cancer by comparative genomic hybridization. *Proc Natl Acad Sci USA* **91**:2156, 1994.

117. Ried T, Peterson I, Holtgreve H, Speicher MR, Schrock E, du Manoir S, Cremer T: Mapping of multiple DNA gains and losses in primary small cell lung carcinomas by comparative genomic hybridization. *Cancer Res* **54**:1801, 1994.

118. Bigner SH, Wong AJ, Mark J, Muhlbaier LH, Kinzler KW, Vogelstein B, Bigner DD: Relationship between gene amplification and chromosomal deviations in malignant human gliomas. *Cancer Genet Cytogenet* **29**:165, 1987.

119. Torp SH, Helseth E, Ryan L, Stolan S, Dalen A, Unsgaard G: Amplification of the epidermal growth factor receptor gene in human gliomas. *Anticancer Res* **11**:2095, 1991.

120. Bieche I, Champeme MH, Lidereau R: A tumor suppressor gene on chromosome 1p32 controls the amplification of *MYC* family genes in breast cancer. *Cancer Res* **54**:4274, 1994.

121. He J, Zhang RG, Zhu D: Clinical significance of c *MYC* gene in esophageal squamous cell carcinoma. *Chung Hua I Hsueh Tsa Chih* **75**:94, 1995.

122. Nishida N, Fukuda Y, Komeda T, Kita R, Sando T, Furukawa M, Amenomori M, Shibagaki I, Nakao K, Ikenaga M: Amplification and overexpression of the cyclin D1 gene in aggressive human hepatocellular carcinoma. *Cancer Res* **54**:3107, 1994.

123. Zhang YJ, Jiang W, Chen CJ, Lee CS, Kahn SM, Santella RM, Weinstein IB: Amplification and overexpression of cyclin D1 in human hepatocellular carcinoma. *Biochem Biophys Res Commun* **196**:1010, 1993.

124. Monk BJ, Chapman JA, Johnson GA, Brightman BK, Wilczynski SP, Schell MJ, Fan H: Correlation of c *MYC* and HER/neu amplification and expression with hisotpathologic variables in uterine corpus cancer. *Am J Obstet Gynecol* **171**:1193, 1994.

125. Ocadiz R, Sauceda R, Cruz M, Graef AM, Gariglio P: High correlation between molecular alterations of the c*MYC* oncogene and carcinoma of the uterine cervix. *Cancer Res* **47**:4173, 1987.

126. Baker VV, Borst MP, Dixon D, Hatch KD, Shingleton HM, Miller D: c *MYC* amplification in ovarian cancer. *Gynecol Oncol* **38**:340, 1990.

127. Bast RCJ, Boyer CM, Jacobs I, Xu FJ, Wu S, Wiener J, Kohler M. Berchuck A: Cell growth regulation in epithelial ovarian cancer. *Cancer* **71**:1597, 1993.

Part 2

CONTROLS ON CELL GROWTH

CHAPTER 8

Cell Cycle Control: An Overview

Bruce E. Clurman ▪ **James M. Roberts**

The process of cellular reproduction is known as the *cell cycle*.[1-3] Most often the cell cycle produces two progeny, or daughter cells, that closely resemble their parent and are capable of repeating the process. For this to be accomplished, three things are necessary: replication of the genome, a doubling of cell mass (this refers generally to all cellular components other than chromosomes), and a precise segregation of chromosomes plus a more or less equal distribution of other cell components to the daughter cells. The execution of these events divides the cell cycle into four phases: (1) Chromosomes are replicated during S (synthetic) phase, (2) cell constituents are segregated to daughter cells during M (mitotic) phase, and two G (gap) phases intervene between S and M, (3) G1 precedes S phase, and (4) G2 precedes mitosis (Fig. 8-1). Thus, chromosome replication and segregation are confined to discrete parts of the cell cycle, whereas the third essential component of cell reproduction—growth— occurs continuously in G1, S, G2, and M. It is during G1 and G2 that cells typically respond to the proliferative and antiproliferative signals (e.g., growth factors and cytokines) that determine whether the cell cycle ought to proceed. In this way the cell cycle has the option of stopping within G1 and G2 without interrupting the critical and precarious events of chromosome replication and chromosome segregation.

Faithful reproduction of the cell requires that these events be coordinated with one another. Thus, ordinarily mitosis does not occur until all chromosomes have been replicated and the cell has doubled in size. However, there are specialized cell cycles where these processes are uncoupled from one another (Fig. 8-2). Repeated S phases with no intervening M phases, known as endocycles, result in the increased chromosome ploidy seen in megakaryocytes. Conversely, the basic cell cycle logic of meiosis is the execution of two sequential M phases without an S phase. A third important variation is seen in the cleavage cycles that occur after fertilization of amphibian eggs. Amphibian eggs are huge cells which after fertilization undergo extremely rapid cell cycles consisting of alternating S and M phases with no cell growth. After approximately 12 cleavage cycles the embryo consists of 4000 cells, each containing a full complement of genetic material and each reduced to the size of a typical somatic cell.[4,5]

These simple examples show that each of the component processes of the cell cycle—growth, chromosome replication, and mitosis—can occur independently of the others. Since cell reproduction could not occur if these processes were executed in random order, there must be mechanisms for establishing and enforcing the normal sequence of events. This chapter will describe the molecules that control progression through the cell cycle and illustrate how their activities are linked together to orchestrate the orderly process of cell reproduction. Based on these ideas, we will suggest that cancer may be a disease of the cell cycle, a hypothesis that is elaborated in subsequent chapters.

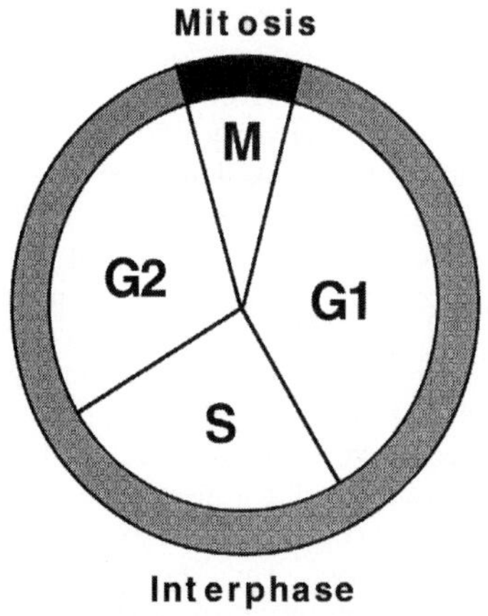

ORIGINS OF MODERN CELL CYCLE BIOLOGY

The current revolution in our understanding of cell cycle control has its origins in yeast genetics and amphibian reproductive cell physiology. It was through these seemingly independent lines of investigation that we grasped the fundamental logic of the program that controls cell reproduction, identified the genes and molecules responsible for this program, and learned how these molecules are integrated into pathways that have been evolutionarily conserved from yeast to humans.

The yeasts *Saccharomyces cerevisiae* and *Schizosacchromyces pombe* have been favorites of cell cycle research since the pioneering studies of Hartwell and Nurse.[6,7] The power of yeast as a model experimental system lies in its facile genetics. It is possible to readily isolate mutations that impair the execution of specific biological processes, such as the events of the cell cycle. Identification of the mutated gene provides information about the pro-

Mitosis

Interphase

FIG. 8-1 The four phases of the cell cycle. Interphase is composed of the S (synthesis) phase, during which DNA replication occurs, and two G (gap) phases, during which cells respond to various proliferative and antiproliferative stimuli and cell growth occurs. Chromosomes and cellular contents are then distributed to two daughter cells during M (mitosis) phase, and the resulting progeny reenter the cell cycle in G1.

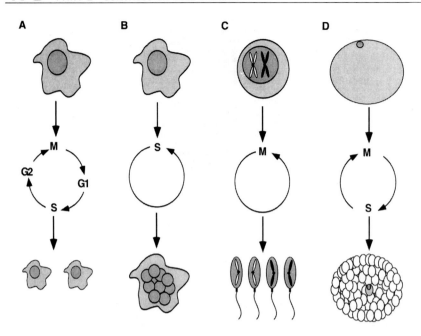

FIG. 8-2 Specialized cell cycles. *A* A normal cell cycle is depicted in which a cell gives rise to two identical daughter cells. *B.* During megakaryopoiesis, promegakaryocytes undergo repeated rounds of DNA replication in the absence of mitosis (endoreduplication), resulting in polyploid megakaryocytes with a DNA content greater than that of their progenitors. *C.* In meiosis, two successive cell divisions after DNA replication result in four haploid daughter cells. *D.* Amphibian eggs undergo 12 rapid cell cycles consisting of alternating S and M phases. No cell growth occurs during these cycles, and the large egg cell is subdivided into approximately 4000 cells, each containing a normal complement of chromosomes.

teins required for the execution of that biologic pathway. Of special utility are conditional mutations, because they effect the activity of the encoded protein product only under specific restrictive conditions, for example, elevated temperatures. Cells harboring conditional mutations can be collected and propagated by growth under permissive conditions, and the consequences of the mutation then can be determined by shifting growth to restrictive conditions.

S. cerevisiae is known as budding yeast because it reproduces by forming a bud that grows to become the daughter cell. The regular pattern of bud development provides convenient morphologic landmarks that can be used to assemble a temporal map of the cell cycle.[8] Thus, an unbudded cell is in G1, a small bud first emerges coincident with the initiation of S phase, and a cell with a large bud is in G2/M. Hartwell isolated a large group of genes required for progression through the cell cycle by identifying conditional mutations that caused a cell population to arrest with a uniform morphology (e.g., all unbudded cells). Since the morphology of a yeast cell defines its position in the cell cycle, each mutant presumably had a position-specific defect in the operation of a cell cycle event. He called these cdc (cell division cycle) mutations.[9] Thus, some cdc mutants were defective in G1-specific events (and arrested as unbudded cells), others in S phase (small budded cells), and yet others in events that take place in G2/M (large budded cells). Further analysis of nuclear morphology and the state of the mitotic spindle provided additional information about the specific processes affected by each mutation. In this way Hartwell successfully identified the vast majority of genes responsible for regulating the eukaryotic cell cycle.[10]

The characterization of cdc mutations revealed a major principle of cell cycle regulation: The orderly execution of cell cycle events results from a series of dependent relationships in which the completion of one event is required for the beginning of the next.[9] For instance, a cell with a mutation in a gene required for DNA replication stops its cell cycle in S phase and does not try to begin mitosis inappropriately (even though it should be capable of doing so). Initially, these dependencies were thought to reflect underlying biochemical pathways in which the product of one event was an essential substrate for the next. Hence, only after an upstream event occurred correctly would the substrates for the next event become available. This would be one way to ensure that cell cycle events were not executed in random order. The idea that the cell cycle is organized by dependent relationships is still considered one of the

most important in cell cycle biology; however, the explanation for dependencies has changed, as will be discussed below.

A particularly important set of dependent pathways, called cell cycle START, is initiated together at the transition from G1 into S phase.[11] Uniquely at START the yeast cell senses the external and internal signals that control its proliferation, including mating pheromone, nutrients, and cell size (Fig. 8-3).[12–14] The yeast cell responds by initiating (or failing to initiate) the three parallel pathways required for reproduction of the cell: bud emergence, DNA replication, and duplication of the spindle pole body (the spindle pole body is the yeast equivalent of the centrosome of the mitotic spindle). The coordinated regulation of these three parallel reproductive pathways indicates that completion of START represents the commitment of the cell to complete the entire program of events required for cell reproduction. Thus, genes required for START must play pivotal roles in the control of cell proliferation, and the CDC28 gene has gained particular prominence among the handful of START-specific genes.[6,15,16] Analogous to START, the R point (restriction point) in mammalian cells defines a transition within G1, after which completion of the remainder of the cell cycle becomes independent of extracellular mitogens.

In contrast to the budding yeast cell cycle, during which cell growth and cell division are linked in G1 at START, in *S. pombe* (known also as fission yeast) these processes usually are coordinated at the transition between G2 and mitosis.[17] Nurse identified cdc mutants in *S. pombe* that were unable to undergo the G2/M transition, and one, called cdc2, received special attention.[18–20] First, cdc2 is required twice during the fission yeast cell cycle, once at the G2/M transition and again at the G1/S transition (where a backup size control exists). Second, certain dominantly acting mutations of cdc2 caused cells to shorten the length of G2, enter mitosis too quickly, and consequently become smaller than normal (known as wee phenotypes). This suggests that cdc2 activity is rate-limiting for the onset of mitosis. The budding yeast cdc28 gene and the *S. pombe* cdc2 gene are homologues of one another.[17,19] Although cdc28 first was identified through its role at G1/S and cdc2 was identified by its role at G2/M, it is now known that these proteins are required at the G1/S and G2/M transitions in both types of yeast.[17,21,22] On the basis of these experiments, cdc2/cdc28 emerged as a key regulator of the cell cycle.

Complementing these genetic analyses of the yeast cell cycle were studies on the meiotic maturation of amphibian eggs. These physiologic studies led to the discovery of a natural regulator of

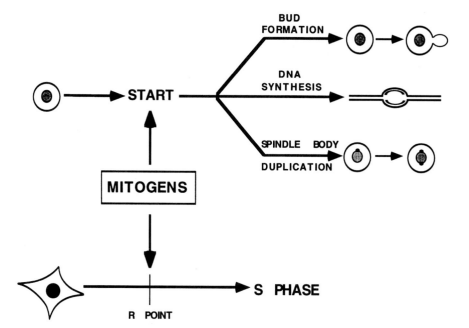

FIG. 8-3 START and the R (restriction) point define G1 transitions, after which cell cycle progression becomes mitogen-independent. At START, budding yeast initiate three independent processes required for cell duplication: bud emergence, DNA synthesis, and spindle body duplication. A variety of mitogenic and antimitogenic signals determine if cells traverse START, after which cell cycle progression no longer depends on those stimuli. At the analogous R point in mammalian cells, S-phase entry is no longer mitogen-dependent. The biochemical bases of START and the R point are discussed in the text.

cell cycle progression, an activity named maturation promoting factor (MPF).[23–25] Amphibians produce mature eggs in response to the hormone progesterone, which induces immature oocytes to emerge from a prolonged arrest in G2 and resume the meiotic cell cycle. The progesterone-stimulated oocyte completes the reductive meiotic divisions and eventually pauses again in metaphase of meiosis II, but now as a mature egg awaiting fertilization. In other words, oocyte maturation requires cell cycle progression from G2 of meiosis I to metaphase of meiosis II and is under the control of MPF. Indeed, injection of MPF isolated from a mature egg into the cytoplasm of an immature oocyte is sufficient to initiate meiotic maturation independently of a hormonal trigger (Fig. 8-4). Furthermore, MPF activity is not restricted to meiosis. MPF activity oscillates during each mitotic cycle, being high in M phase and

low in interphase.[24,26,27] This indicates that MPF is a fundamental component of cell cycle regulation in all cell cycles, mitotic as well as meiotic.

Remarkably, MPF activity continues to oscillate even in enucleated cells.[28] Because MPF activity can oscillate independently of nuclear events, it has been proposed that the MPF cycle may be an autonomous mitotic clock and that the state of the clock (the time of day) determines which cell cycle event will occur.[26,28,29] Thus, high MPF activity would permit entry into mitosis, and low MPF activity would permit cells to enter S phase. This model supplanted the earlier idea that the obligate order of cell cycle events might simply be established by substrate—product relationships. However, the notion of a mitotic clock then would require the existence of additional feedback controls to keep the clock entrained to actual progress through the cell cycle; the clock must stop if essential cell cycle events do not occur. These feedback controls do in fact exist and are known as checkpoints.[30]

Perhaps the most far-reaching advance in the cell cycle field in the last 15 years has been the demonstration that cell cycle controls are evolutionarily conserved.[31,32] This first became evident when it was discovered that the CDC2 and CDC28 genes in fission and budding yeast encode homologous proteins now known as the CDC2 protein kinase.[20] Furthermore, gene transfer experiments show that the human CDC2 gene can complement mutations in the yeast CDC2 gene.[33] This was reinforced 6 years later when MPF was purified (initially from Xenopus and later from other vertebrates), and its catalytic subunit was shown to be a homologue of CDC2.[34–38] These observations set the stage for our current paradigm of eukaryotic cell cycle control, which in its simplest form depicts the cell cycle as a CDC2 cycle (Fig. 8-5).[39] Thus, in organisms ranging from yeast to humans the catalytic activity of CDC2 and related kinases is required for each of the major transitions within the cell cycle—from G1 into S and from G2 into M.[40–46]

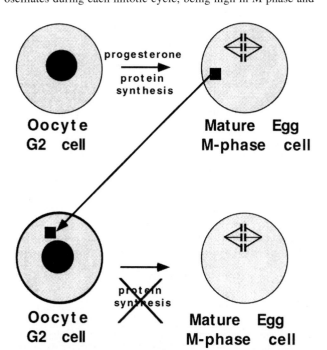

FIG. 8-4 MPF stimulates mitosis in G2 oocytes. As described in the text, injection of cytoplasm extract from an M-phase amphibian egg is sufficient to induce maturation of the recipient egg in the absence of progesterone or protein synthesis.

CYCLIN-DEPENDENT KINASE REGULATION

In budding and fission yeast, the highly regulated action of a single kinase subunit (cdc28 and cdc2, respectively) drives the cell cycle forward.[47] In higher eukaryotes, cell cycle control is more complex, and several proteins homologous to cdc2 [termed the cyclin-

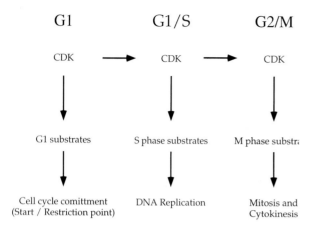

FIG. 8-5 The CDC2 cycle. The enzymatic activity of cdc2 and related kinases (CDKs) drives each of the key cell cycle transitions.

dependent kinases (cdks)] have been identified.[48] Cdks are protein kinases that vary in size between 30 and 40 kD and share greater than 40 percent sequence identity. In addition to amino acid homology, cdks share many functional and regulatory features with yeast cdc2/28.[49,50] Almost all cdks require association with protein subunits called cyclins to become active kinases. Cdks also contain conserved amino acid residues that modulate kinase activity when phosphorylated or dephosphorylated. Additionally, cdk activity is inhibited by specific regulatory molecules that bind and inhibit cdk subunits. Each of these regulatory mechanisms will be discussed in detail below. Remarkably, although differences among organisms exist, this multitiered regulatory system has been conserved from yeast to humans.

Each phase of the cell cycle is characterized by a unique pattern of cdk activity (Fig. 8-6).[51–53] In mammalian cells, eight cdks have been identified, and most are active (and required) only in specific phases of the cell cycle. Progression through G1 depends on the activities of cdk2, cdk3, and cdk4, and cdk6. The recently described cdk8 protein also may function primarily in G1 and may be involved in transcriptional regulation. Cdk2 and cdc2 are active in S phase, and cdc2 kinase activity also governs mitotic entry and exit. In distinction to its kindred, cdk5 does not appear to be intimately involved in cell cycle progression but instead may play a role in the developing nervous system, where it associates with the noncyclin activator p35.[54,55]

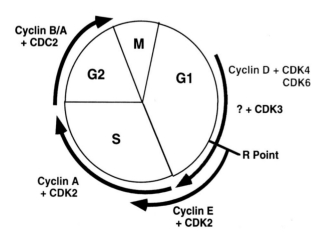

FIG. 8-6 Patterns of cyclin–cdk activity during the mammalian cell cycle. The expression patterns of the key mammalian cyclins is superimposed on the cell cycle, along with their respective cdk partners. The approximate position of the R point is shown. (*Adapted from Sherr.*)

Cyclins: Activating Subunits of CDK Enzymes

Monomeric cdk subunits essentially are devoid of enzymatic activity, and kinase activation requires the association of cdks with cyclins.[49] An active cdk thus is a hetrodimeric enzyme consisting of regulatory (cyclin) and enzymatic (cdk) subunits. The cyclins are a group of related proteins that contain a conserved region of homology (the cyclin box) and usually are expressed in a cell cycle-specific fashion. Cyclin expression is rate-limiting for cdk activation, and control of cyclin expression is a fundamental mechanism underlying cdk periodicity. In general, cyclin levels are determined by both transcriptional control and regulated proteolysis by the ubiquitin–proteasome system.

The recently solved crystal structure of cyclin A bound to cdk2 reveals that cyclins activate cdks in at least two ways. Cyclin binding induces conformational changes in the cdk that reorient the configuration of the ATP phosphate groups to facilitate phosphotransfer to protein substrates and move the T loop of the cdk out of a position that would otherwise block entry of protein substrates into the active site (Fig. 8-7).[56,57]

The specificity of cdk action at different times in the cell cycle is in large part determined by its particular cyclin subunit. This functional diversity of cyclins first was established in the yeast *S. cerevisiae*, where specific cyclins have been identified that are required for G1, S phase, and mitosis. Budding yeast express three functionally redundant G1 cyclins (cln1, cln2, and cln3) that are required for passage through START.[58–62] Although differences between the cln genes have been described, mutant yeast cells with mutated cln alleles can enter S phase as long as one of these three genes remains functional. Transcription of cln1 and cln2 is controlled by the Swi4/Swi6 transcription factor, and cln activity positively reinforces further cln expression.[63–68] Thus, CLN1 and CLN2 mRNAs rise during G1, reaching peak levels around START.

Once START has been traversed, cln activity no longer is required for subsequent cell cycle progression. Instead, other cyclins associate with and activate cdc28 during other phases of the cell cycle. Complexes containing cdc28 and the cyclins clb5 and clb6 are required for S phase, and the four B-type cyclins clb1–4 are required for mitosis.[69–71]

START marks a point of transition in the yeast cell cycle where G1 cyclin expression ends and mitotic cyclin expression begins. This transition comes about because these two classes of cyclin modulate each other's expression. Cln/cdc28 kinase activity directly increases the expression of the clb genes, and conversely clb-cdc28 kinase activity represses CLN expression.[72] Not only do G1 cyclins promote the expression of the genes for mitotic cyclins (as described below), they also increase the stability and functional activity of clb proteins. Furthermore, the cln proteins themselves are degraded rapidly after START. This is discussed in the section on cell cycle-regulated proteolysis. Together, these controls ensure ordered progression through the cell cycle by establishing alternating periods of the cycle where either G1 or mitotic cyclins are expressed and functionally active.

Mammalian cyclins C, D1, and E first were identified in a screen for mammalian genes that could complement yeast cyclin mutations.[73–75] At the same time cyclin D1 was identified as a mitogen-responsive gene in a macrophage cell line and as a gene located at a chromosome inversion breakpoint in a parathyroid tumor (and in this guise originally was named PRAD1).[76,77] A dozen mammalian cyclin genes have been identified that are both structurally and functionally homologous to yeast cyclins.[51,52] Like the yeast cyclins, many of these molecules exhibit cell cycle-dependent periodicity in their expression and activity (Fig. 8-6).

The primary mammalian G1 cyclins are the D-type cyclins and cyclin E. These cyclins associate with the cdk 4/6 and cdk2 subunits, respectively. There are three D-type cyclins (D1, D2, and

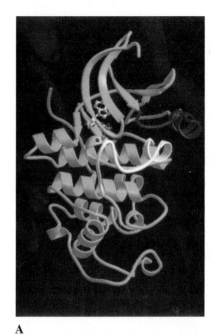

A

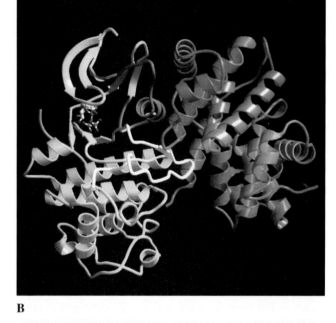

B

C

D

FIG. 8-7 Crystal structure of cdk2, cyclin A-cdk2, and cyclin A-cdk2-p27 complexes. *Top left*. The structure of monomeric cdk2. The T loop is grey, and the PSTAIRE motif is black. An ATP molecule is indicated within the active site. *Top right*. The structure of cdk2 bound to an amino terminal truncated version of cyclin A. Cyclin binding reorients the PSTAIRE helix and moves the T loop, resulting in the repositioning of ATP-phosphate groups within the complex and allowing substrate accessibility to the active site. *Bottom left*. The structure of

CAK-phosphorylated cyclin A bound to CDK2. The ball indicates the position of Thr160 within the T loop. *Bottom right*. The structure of a temary complex of the amino terminus of p27 bound to cyclin A–cdk2. Separate domains of P27 interact with both cyclin A and cdk2. The structure of this complex reveals that p27 inhibits cdk activity by distorting the structure of the active site and interacting with residues within the catalytic cleft and preventing ATP binding. *(Illustrations courtesy of N. Pavletich and reprinted with permission.)*

D3), and these are expressed in a cell type-specific fashion.[51,52,78] The G1 role of the D-type cyclins is revealed by their pattern of expression and functional properties. Cyclin D expression begins in early G1, when quiescent cells are stimulated to reenter the cell cycle, and cyclin D expression remains at high levels as long as mitogens are present. In other words, the expression of these labile proteins ($t_{1/2} < 20$ min) is not periodic intrinsically but instead depends on the presence of cell type-specific mitogens. Inhibition of cyclin D1 function blocks the cell cycle in G1, demonstrating the necessity of cyclin D for the cell cycle.[79,80] Also, enforced overexpression

of cyclin D1 shortens the G1 phase of the cell cycle and partially diminishes the mitogen requirement for cell proliferation, demonstrating that cyclin D1 levels are limiting for G1 progression.[80,81]

Cyclin E activity also is required in G1, although probably somewhat after cyclin D activity.[81–83] Cyclin E protein expression peaks at the G1-S boundary and then decays as S phase progresses.[82,84,85] Determinants of cyclin E periodicity include both transcriptional control by E2F and regulated proteolysis (see below). Overexpression of cyclin E results in G1 contraction and decreased mitogen requirements, and cyclin E kinase activity is required for S-phase entry.[81–83,86] Activation of cyclin D- and cyclin E-associated kinases biochemically may constitute the restriction point, the mammalian equivalent of START control in yeast.

Later cell cycle transitions are governed by the cyclin A and cyclin B proteins. Cyclin A associates with both the cdk2 and cdc2 subunits, and cyclin A kinase activity is required at the start of S phase and at the G2-M transition.[87–89] Cyclin B associates with cdc2, and like the yeast Clb proteins, cyclin B–cdc2 kinase activity regulates both mitotic entry and exit.[90]

The cyclin H protein associates with cdk7, and this heterodimer constitutes the cdk-activating kinase (CAK).[91] CAK also is a component of the human transcription factor TFIIH and is capable of phosphorylating the carboxy terminal domain (CTD) of RNA polymerase II. Cyclin C is classed as a G1 cyclin, although its role is not defined.[73] Cyclin C recently has been shown to associate with cdk8, and cyclin C–cdk8 complexes also have RNA polymerase II CTD kinase activity, although they do not copurify with TFIIH.[92] Phosphorylation of the CTD by cyclin—cdk complexes may couple cell cycle events to the cellular transcriptional machinery.

Comparatively little is known about the remaining cyclins identified to date, including cyclins F, G, and I. Cyclin F is the largest cyclin, with a molecular weight of 87 kD, and is most closely related to cyclins A and B. Cyclin F mRNA peaks in G2, and cyclin F protein accumulates in interphase and is destroyed during mitosis.[93] Cyclin G mRNA does not fluctuate in a cell cycle-dependent fashion but is induced by both the p53 protein and growth stimulation of quiescent cells.[94] The cyclin I protein is expressed most highly in postmitotic tissues, including muscle and neurons, and may play a unique regulatory role.[95]

Cyclin-Dependent Kinase Regulation by Phosphorylation and Dephosphorylation

In addition to cyclin binding, phosphorylation and dephosphorylation of conserved cdk residues provide another important level of control over kinase activity.[49] cdks can be activated or inactivated by phosphorylation (Fig. 8-8). The site of activating phosphoryla-

tion is a conserved threonine residue in the so-called T loop (e.g., threonine 161 in cdc2 and threonine 160 in cdk2).[56] The binding of cyclin to the cdk and phosphorylation of this residue together move the T loop away from the catalytic cleft of the enzyme, providing access to protein substrates.[96] Thr160 is phosphorylated by CAK (cyclin H–cdk7), and this phosphorylation is required for cdk activation.[97–100] CAK activity, however, is neither cell cycle-regulated nor limiting, and the major determinant of Thr160 phosphorylation probably is cyclin binding.[91]

cdks also can be phosphorylated on a specific amino terminal tyrosine residue (e.g., tyrosine 15 in cdc2 and cdk2). Tyrosine phosphorylated cdk2 is inactive catalytically even if it is phosphorylated on the activating threonine within the T loop.[98,100–103] The kinases that phosphorylate tyr15 are evolutionarily conserved and are known as the wee1 and mik1 kinases.[104–107] Conversely, dephosphorylation of tyrosine by the cdc25 phosphatase activates the cdk.[108–112] Regulation of wee1 and cdc25 is complex, but the bottom line is that the relative activities of these enzymes set a threshold for CDK activation and determine mitotic entry.[113,114] Three mammalian cdc25 homologues have been identified (cdc25a, cdc25b, and cdc25c), and each may play a unique cell cycle role.[115,116] cdc25a is active in G1 and may be induced by raf-dependent pathways.[117]

Cyclin-Dependent Kinase Inhibitors: Inhibitory Subunits of Cyclin-Dependent Kinase Enzymes

All organisms express proteins that directly bind to and inhibit cdk activity.[118,119] These cdk inhibitors (CKIs) provide another important strategy by which cdk activity is regulated in response to diverse stimuli. In budding yeast, two kinds of inhibitors have been described. One type is inducible and links the cell cycle to extracellular signals; the other type is an intrinsic component of the mitotic cycle. The best example of the first type of cdk inhibitor is the FAR1 protein. Mating pheromones induce FAR1, a protein that binds to and inhibits cln–cdc28 kinase and thereby causes the yeast cell cycle to arrest at START. Another important cdk inhibitor in budding yeast is Sic1, but it is a constitutive element in the mitotic clock and is not known to be induced by extrinsic proliferative signals.[120,121] At the conclusion of each mitosis Sic1 protein levels rise, inhibiting the clb–cdc28 kinases and facilitating the transition from anaphase to the next G1. Sic1 protein remains at high levels during G1 until activation of the cln–cdc28 kinases at START induces its degradation. This is one mechanism that links activation of the S phase clb–cdc28 kinases to passage through START.

Mammalian cells express two classes of CKIs that are distinguished by their cdk targets: The Cip/Kip family of CKIs are universal cdk inhibitors, whereas the INK4 proteins are specific cdk4/6 inhibitors (Fig. 8-9).[118] The Cip/Kip family consists of three members: p21, p27, and p57. Overexpression of these molecules causes a G1 arrest in cultured cells, and they are able to inhibit most cyclin—cdk complexes in vitro. These molecules bind to assembled cyclin—cdk complexes much more avidly than to monomeric cdk or cyclin subunits. First, p21 was identified as a component of cyclin–CDK complexes in proliferating cells and as a protein induced as cells in vitro became senescent.[123,124] Shortly thereafter, it was cloned by a number of independent approaches.[125–128] The p21 protein contains two functional domains, an amino terminal cdk interaction region that is sufficient for cdk inhibition and a carboxy terminal region that binds PCNA, a processivity factor associated with DNA polymerase delta.[129–131]

Two biologic roles have been suggested for p21.[118,122] The first is in contributing to the cell cycle arrest that occurs in cells with damaged DNA.[127] This is discussed in greater detail below. Additionally, p21 has been suggested to facilitate withdrawal from the cell cycle in cells undergoing terminal differentiation.[132,133]

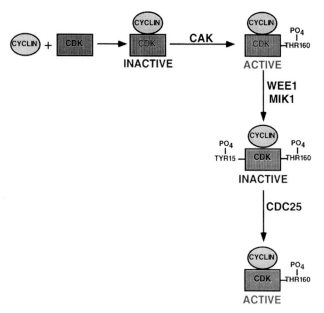

FIG. 8-8 cdk regulation by cyclin binding and cdk phosphorylation. As described in the text, activation of cdks requires cyclin binding and cdk phosphorylation at thr160 by the cdk-activating kinase (CAK). Subsequent phosphorylation of tyr15 by the wee1 and mik1 kinases and dephosphorylation by cdc25 phosphatases further regulate kinase activity.

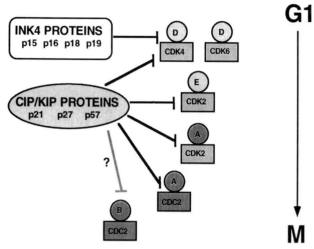

FIG. 8-9 Mammalian cdk inhibitors are classed by their cyclin—cdk targets. The Cip/Kip proteins (p21, p27, p57) are universal cdk inhibitors that inactivate all cyclin—cdk complexes (with the possible exception of cyclin B—cdc2). In contrast, the INK4 proteins (p15, p16, p18, p19) specifically bind and inhibit only cdk4/6 and cyclin D—cdk4/6 complexes.

The cdk inhibitor p27Kip1 is structurally related to p21Cip1.[134,135] p21 and p27 share significant amino terminal homology within the cdk inhibitory domain, but p27 does not contain the PCNA interaction region. Although p27 is not a p53 response gene, p27 levels respond to a variety of extracellular mitogenic and antimitogenic signals.[118] In general, p27 levels are high in nondividing cells and low in proliferating cells. The regulation of p27 is complex, with transcriptional, translational, and posttranslational mechanisms all implicated in different biologic contexts.[136]

The mechanism of cdk inhibition by p27 has been clarified by the crystal structure of p27 bound to cyclin A—cdk2 (Figure 8-7).[96] In the ternary p27—cyclin A—cdk2 complex, separate domains in p27 interact with the cyclin and the cdk. Although p27 does not significantly alter the structure of the cyclin, it may bind to a site on the cyclin that the cyclin ordinarily would use for interactions with protein substrates. In this way p27 might inhibit the phosphorylation of physiologically important substrates without inhibiting the catalytic activity of the cdk enzyme. In addition, p27 does have dramatic effects on cdk structure: p 27 disrupts the structure of the N terminal lobe of the cdk, widening and distorting the ATP binding site. In fact, p27 itself inserts into the catalytic cleft and directly interacts with the amino acids that would bind ATP. This would completely prevent binding of ATP by the cdk and therefore completely inhibit catalytic activity.

Less is known about p57, the most recently isolated family member, which was cloned by virtue of its homology with p27.[137,138] Both the amino and carboxy terminal domains of p57 are related to p27. Compared with p27, however, p57 expression is relatively restricted to terminally differentiated tissues.

The INK4 family of CKIs includes four structural proteins (p15, p16, p18, and p19), each of which contains four ankyrin repeats.[118] The first member of this family to be identified, p16, was found to be associated with cdk4 in transformed cells and subsequently was identified as a candidate tumor suppresser in familial melanoma.[138–140] INK4 proteins bind to monomeric cdk4/6 subunits, preventing their association with D-type cyclins, and INK4 proteins also can inhibit the activity of cyclin D—cdk4/6 complexes. The other INK4 proteins are expressed ubiquitously in mouse tissues and cultured cells, and the expression of p19 oscillates with the cell cycle.[141,142] Although p15 has been shown to be involved in the antiproliferative response to TGF-B, the physiologic roles of the INK4 protein remain unknown. The frequent

deletions of p15 and p16 in primary tumors and the high spontaneous tumor rate in p16-deficient mice indicate that these proteins play a critical role in maintaining normal growth control.[143]

CYCLIN-DEPENDENT KINASE SUBSTRATES

cdks promote progression through the cell cycle by phosphorylating a group of protein substrates.[53] However, compared with the enormous amount of data concerning cdk regulation, relatively little is known about cdk substrates. The most thoroughly characterized cdk substrates are cell cycle regulatory proteins themselves. For example, in budding yeast, phosphorylation of p40sic1 by the cln—cdc28 kinase leads to its ubiquitin-mediated proteolysis and progression from G1 to S phase.[120,121] In fact, a yeast strain lacking all cln genes is viable if p40sic1 also is mutated, suggesting that phosphorylation of this CKI is a key function of the cln proteins in promoting cell cycle progression.[144]

A critical regulator of cell cycle progression in higher eukaryotes, including humans, is the Rb protein. The importance of Rb in cell cycle control became evident as a result of three separate seminal observations.[145] First, the oncogenic proteins encoded by a variety of DNA tumor viruses (e.g., SV40, adenovirus, and papillomavirus) all bind to the Rb protein.[146–148] Second, the Rb gene is mutated in the germ line in patients with hereditary retinoblastoma and frequently is mutated in tumor cells in patients who develop spontaneous tumors.[149–151] Third, the Rb protein undergoes cell cycle-dependent phosphorylation during G1, and this modifies its interaction with an essential transcription factor known as E2F.[152–156] E2F transcription factors are heterodimeric proteins composed of one E2F subunit and one DP subunit that regulate the transcription of many genes required in S phase.[157–159] There are five known E2F subunits, designated E2F1—5, and three known DP subunits, designated DP1—3. When complexed with Rb, E2F is inactive or may even be a transcriptional repressor, and the cell cycle arrests in the absence of these needed gene products. E2F sequestration is regulated by the phosphorylation state of Rb; unphosphorylated Rb avidly binds E2F, whereas hyperphosphorylated Rb does not. As cells progress through G1, Rb is progressively phosphorylated at multiple sites, ultimately releasing E2F. It has since been shown that viral oncoproteins specifically bind to the unphosphorylated form of Rb and in doing so automatically release E2F from its Rb-bound inactive state.

The kinases that phosphorylate Rb are the cdks. The pRb protein contains eight consensus cdk–phosphorylation sites, and cyclin D—, E—, and A—cdk complexes have Rb kinase activity in vitro and in vivo.[160–163] Cyclin D—cdk4 complexes bind stably to Rb, and this complex disassembles once Rb is phosphorylated.[164] Cyclin D—cdk4/6 and cyclin E—cdk2 complexes probably cooperate to phosphorylate and inactivate Rb during G1. The observation that cyclin D function is dispensable in cells with mutant Rb alleles suggests that pRb phosphorylation is the critical means by which D-type cyclins promote G1 progression.[165–167] Phosphorylation of Rb by cyclin E—cdk2 also may be required prior to S-phase entry, but cyclin E is essential for cell cycle progression in Rb-mutant cells, demonstrating that other substrates of cyclin E—cdk2 also must exist.[82]

Rb is one member of a family of structurally related pocket proteins which includes p107, p130, and Rb itself.[167] All the pocket proteins bind to members of the E2F family of transcription factors, and phosphorylation of these proteins by cyclin—cdk complexes liberates E2F and thereby removes some constraints on cell proliferation.[168,169] However, neither p107 nor p130 is a tumor suppressor, and their function during the cell cycle is poorly understood.

E2F activity is essential for the G1—S transition, but it also must be inactivated for the ensuing S phase to progress normally.[170,171] E2F/DP heterodimers form stable complexes with cyclin A—cdk2, and phosphorylation of a specific DP residue by cyclin A—cdk2 suppresses E2F DNA binding. Thus, G1 cyclins activate E2F via Rb phosphorylation, and cyclin A—cdk 2 then directly inactivates E2F through DP phosphorylation. In this way sequentially acting cyclin—cdk complexes first initiate and then extinguish E2F activity, causing a pulse of E2F-dependent gene transcription at the G1—S-phase transition.

The elucidation of cdk substrates clearly remains incomplete.[172] For instance, it is thought that proteins directly involved in the initiation of DNA replication will be phosphorylated and activated by cdks at the start of S phase, although not a single such protein has been identified.[173] Almost as short is the list of cdk substrates during mitosis. The first identified mitotic cdk substrates were the nuclear lamins.[174,175] The nuclear lamina is a structure composed of intermediate filament proteins that depolymerizes at the onset of mitosis. The polymerization of lamins is regulated by phosphorylation, and lamins have been shown to be substrates for cyclin B–cdc2. Phosphorylation of lamins promotes their disassembly, and it has been proposed cyclin B—cdc2 lamin kinase activity is responsible for the breakdown of the nuclear lamina at mitosis. cdc2 kinase activity also is required for assembly of the mitotic spindle.[176] The human Eg5 protein is a kinesin-related motor protein that is needed to build a bipolar spindle. The localization of Eg5 to the spindle apparatus is dependent on phosphorylation at thr927, and this residue is phosphorylated by cyclin B—cdc2. Inhibition of Eg5 function results in a mitotic block, and one mechanism by which cyclin B—cdc2 promotes mitosis is likely to involve Eg5 phosphorylation.

PROTEOLYSIS IN CELL CYCLE REGULATION

A basic feature of the cell cycle is that its transitions are irreversible. Anaphase cells, for instance, cannot regress to metaphase,

nor can S-phase cells reverse course and go back to G1. This is accomplished by a cycle of protein destruction that complements the periodic activation of cyclin—cdk complexes. In general, protein destruction eliminates proteins that have been used in the preceding phase of the cell cycle as well as proteins that would inhibit progression into the next cell cycle phase.[177] The net effect is to cause the cell cycle to move irreversibly forward.

The paradigm for periodic protein degradation during the cell cycle is the destruction of cyclin B during mitosis (Fig. 8-10).[35,178] The abundance of cyclin B protein oscillates during each cell division cycle, being highest as cells enter mitosis and disappearing after chromosome disjunction has occurred at the transition from metaphase to anaphase.[179] This is caused by changes in the rate of its degradation. Many short-lived proteins, including cyclin B, are degraded in the proteosome, a 26S complex that contains multiple proteolytic enzymes and that specifically recognizes and degrades ubiquitinated proteins.[180] Conjugation of a protein to ubiquitin is the signal for its delivery to the proteosome, and this is accomplished in a multistep reaction in which ubiquitin ultimately is transferred through a thiol-ester linkage to lysine side chains of the target protein.[181,182] Ubiquitin, a 76-amino acid protein, first is attached through its carboxy terminus to a ubiquitin-activating enzyme called E1 in an ATP-dependent reaction. The E1-bound ubiquitin then is transferred to one of a family of carrier proteins called E2s, or ubiquitin-conjugating enzymes, that can then transfer ubiquitin to target proteins. Most eukaryotes are thought to have a single E1 gene but multiple E2 genes (at least 12 in budding yeast). Each of the E2 enzymes recognizes and transfers ubiquitin to only particular proteins, thereby imposing some degree of selectivity on the process of ubiquitin-dependent proteolysis. Further selectivity arises from the fact that conjugation of some proteins to ubiquitin requires collaboration between an E2 enzyme and an E3 enzyme called *ubiquitin ligases*.

The E2 and E3 enzymes choose proteins for ubiquitination by recognizing specific amino acids motifs.[183] A few types of motifs have been identified, each presumably recognized by certain E2 or E2/E3 combinations. The particular ubiquitination motif within cyclin B is called the cyclin destruction box.[184] A mutant version of cyclin B lacking the destruction box (called cyclin B db) is not con-

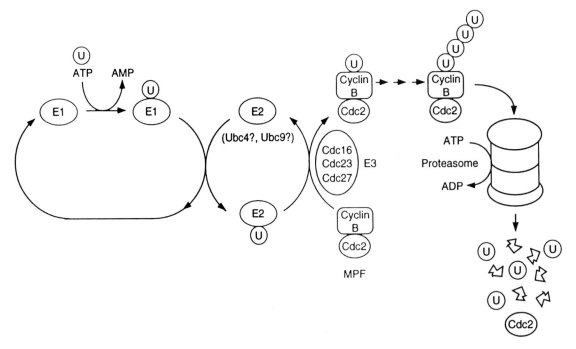

FIG. 8-10 The biochemistry of cyclin destruction. See text for details. (*Reprinted from Murray[190] with permission.*)

jugated to ubiquitin during mitosis and is not degraded.[185] Consequently, cyclin B db–cdc2 (and its MPF activity) remains active, and the cell cycle becomes blocked in mitosis.[186–188] This important experiment demonstrates that destruction of cyclin B is required for inactivation of cdc2 and MPF activity in anaphase cells and that inactivation of cdc2 is required for mitosis to be completed. Therefore, just as synthesis of cyclin B is required for a cell to enter mitosis, destruction of cyclin B is required for a cell to exit mitosis and begin a new cell cycle.[189] Cyclin A also has a destruction box and is degraded in mitosis at about the same time as cyclin B.[190]

The ubiquitination of cyclin B is controlled by an E3-like activity called the anaphase promoting complex (APC).[191] As its name implies, the APC is required not only in anaphase for the destruction of cyclin B but also earlier in mitosis at metaphase to promote the transition into anaphase.[192] It is thought that at the transition from metaphase to anaphase APC is required for the targeted ubiquitination and proteolysis of a protein necessary for cohesion between sister chromatids on the metaphase plate. APC has been characterized both genetically and biochemically and has been shown to be a 20S particle that includes at least three proteins, cdc16, cdc23, and cdc27 (which were originally discovered by Hartwell in the cdc screen described earlier).[191,193–195]

The activity of APC is regulated during the cell cycle.[177] The ability of the APC to ubiquitinate B-type cyclins is turned on during mitosis and turned off again in G1, leading directly to the periodic accumulation and destruction of these cyclins.[195–197] In this way, the duration of APC activity defines the interval in the cell cycle where the levels of B-type cyclins are kept low, and this is a key element in establishing the G1 phase of the cell cycle. Conversely, inactivation of APC is required for reaccumulation of S-phase cyclins, such as Clb5 and 6, in yeast and probably cyclin A in mammalian cells and therefore is a prerequisite for entry into S phase. Thus, cyclin—cdks and APC are complementary activities that work in parallel to control major transitions within the cell cycle. The mechanisms regulating APC are incompletely understood, but it seems that APC activity is directly coupled to cyclin/cdk activity. First, during mitosis it is thought that cyclin B/cdc2 initiates the pathway leading to its own destruction by phosphorylating and activating the APC.[177,196] Second, once activated in mitosis, APC remains active until late in G1, when it is inactivated by G1 cyclin—cdk activity.[196] In yeast this occurs coincidentally with START, and in mammalian cells it may be one of the events that lead to cell cycle commitment at the restriction point.

Protein destruction also controls the abundance of the cyclins and CKIs that regulate entry into S phase. Cyclin E in mammalian cells and the G1 cyclins in yeast (the cln proteins) are both degraded by ubiquitin-dependent proteolysis.[198–202] In both cases phosphorylation of the cyclin triggers its ubiquitination, and this is a common theme in regulated protein turnover.[203–205] Often, phosphorylation of a protein is the end result of a signal transduction pathway and can be used to allow recognition of proteins by E2 and E3 ubiquitin-conjugating enzymes. In the case of cyclin E and the cln proteins, the cyclins are directly phosphorylated by their associated cdks. Thus, cyclin E/cdk2 activity inherently is self-limited, because cdk2 activity initiates the pathway leading to cyclin E destruction. In essence, this is similar to the control of A- and B-type cyclin turnover by APC, because in each instance cyclin degradation is initiated by cdk activity.

cdk inhibitor levels are also regulated during G1 by proteolysis. In mammalian cells the cdk inhibitor p27Kip1 is eliminated from cells after mitogenic stimulation by the ubiquitin-proteosome pathway, and in budding yeast the cdk inhibitor p40Sic1 is regulated in a similar manner.[121,144,206] In fact, the cln proteins and p40Sic1 in budding yeast may both be ubiquitinated by an E2+E3 complex composed of the cdc34 and cdc53 proteins.[197,202,205] Human homologues of cdc34 and cdc53 have been identified, indicating that this

pathway for cell cycle-regulated proteolysis during G1 has been evolutionarily conserved.[207,208]

MOLECULAR BASES OF CELL CYCLE PHYSIOLOGY

Mitogenic and antimitogenic signals control cell proliferation by starting and stopping the cell cycle, but cells respond differently to these signals at different times in the cell cycle.[209] Immediately after mitosis cells enter a portion of G1 where the continued presence of mitogenic signals (or the absence of antimitogenic signals) is required for continued progression through the remainder of G1 and into S phase. However, at a fixed point in G1 the cell cycle becomes refractory to these signals, and cell division is completed even if mitogens are absent or antimitogens are present.[210] The restriction point is defined as the end of the mitogen-responsive portion of G1 (or the moment of transition to mitogen independence), and it reflects the execution of the fundamental proliferative decision made by the cell.[211,212] It has been shown that tumor cells characteristically lose restriction point control over cell cycle progression (they become constitutively mitogen-independent), highlighting the importance of this pathway in the normal regulation of cell proliferation.[213] The restriction point physiologically is analogous to START in the yeast cell cycle and shares many of its molecular components. Thus, the requirement for cdc28 at START is paralleled by a requirement for cdks in restriction point control.[214]

Mitogenic and antimitogenic signals control the cell cycle in G1 because they control the activity of the cyclins and cdks that are required for progression through G1. Growth factors and cell–substratum interactions are among the best studied mitogenic signals, and DNA damage and TGF-beta are among the best studied antimitogenic signals. All these proliferative signals alter the activity of essential G1 cyclin—cdk complexes and thereby bring about either continued cell cycle progression or cell cycle arrest.

Mitogenic growth factors have pleiotropic effects on cell cycle proteins that stimulate progression through G1 and entry into S phase.[213,215,216] They increase expression of G1 cyclins, decrease expression of cdk inhibitors, and promote assembly of G1 cyclin—cdk complexes. Growth factors increase expression of all three cyclins needed for entry into S phase—cyclin D (1, 2, and 3), cyclin E, and cyclin A—at least in part by increasing transcription of their respective genes. Cyclin D1 transcription has been shown to be under the control of at least two growth factor-modulated signal transduction pathways: the c-*myc* and *ras* pathways.[217–219] The biochemical pathways linking c-*myc* and cyclin D1 transcription are not well defined, but the effects of *ras* on cyclin D1 transcription appear to be mediated by the MAP kinase pathway.[219] Cyclin D1 transcription begins early in G1 and is followed by an increase in cyclin E gene expression. Cyclin E is one of a large group of genes that includes DNA polymerase alpha, thymidine kinase, PCNA, dihydrofolate reductase, and many others required for cell proliferation whose transcription is under control of E2F.[152–159] The induction of cyclin E gene transcription by E2F establishes a positive feedback loop for increasing cyclin E expression (Fig. 8-11).[220] In this pathway, cyclin E–cdk2 phosphorylates Rb, releasing E2F from its Rb-bound inactive state. The free E2F will promote cyclin E gene expression, resulting in increased amounts of cyclin E–cdk2 activity, increasing Rb phosphorylation, and so on. This suggests an interesting and important physiologic linkage between cyclin D and cyclin E during the mitogenic response to growth factors. Cyclin D expression is elevated directly by mitogenic growth factors, and this initiates the pathway of Rb phosphorylation and E2F-dependent gene expression. Once initiated, however, Rb

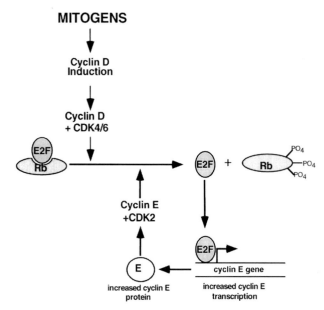

FIG. 8-11 A positive feedback loop reinforces cyclin E transcription. As described in the text, phosphorylation of Rb by cyclin D- and cyclin E-associated kinases liberates E2F, which then stimulates cyclin E transcription. Increased cyclin E–cdk2 kinase activity then results in more Rb phosphorylation and greater E2F activity. Establishment of this feedback loop renders Rb phosphorylation mitogen-independent and may be an important component of the R-point.

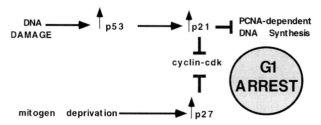

FIG. 8-12 Induction of Cip/Kip proteins by antiproliferative stimuli imposes a G1 arrest. The p21 and p27 proteins respond to different physiologic signals. In the example depicted, DNA damage results in p53 induction and increased p21 transcription, which leads to elevated levels of p21 protein and a G1 arrest via cdk inhibition. In addition, p21 inhibits DNA synthesis through the processivity factor PCNA. Similarly, mitogen deprivation induces p27 expression and cell cycle arrest via cdk inhibition.

phosphorylation can be maintained independently of cyclin D (and hence independently of mitogenic growth factors) via the autonomous feedback loop linking Rb to cyclin E. Thus, growth factors are required, through cyclin loop linking Rb to cyclin E. Thus, growth factors are required, through cyclin D, to start the program of E2F-dependent gene expression but become dispensable once cyclin E–cdk2 becomes activated and substitutes for cyclin D–cdk4 in phosphorylating Rb. Inherent in this scheme is a transition from a mitogen-dependent to a mitogen-independent route for maintaining Rb phosphorylation, and therefore it may be one molecular pathway underlying commitment to cell cycle progression at the restriction point. Cyclin A transcription also increases in growth factor-stimulated cells just before entry into S phase, but the pathways controlling cyclin A transcription are not well understood.[51]

The cdk inhibitor p27Kip1 is another key element in the cell cycle response to mitogenic growth factors. p27 is required for cells to stop dividing on schedule when growth factors are withdrawn.[221] p27 is expressed at very low levels in proliferating cells, but its expression greatly increases in cells starved for essential mitogenic growth factors.[222–224] Under these conditions p27 binds to and inactivates cyclin–cdk complexes and causes the cell cycle to stop (Fig. 8-12). If cells do not make p27, their exit from the cell cycle is delayed and they continued to proliferate in the absence of growth factors.[222] Indeed, mice engineered to contain a homozygous deletion of the p27 gene grow twice as fast as do control mice and have increased numbers of cells in all lineages.[225] Conversely, high levels of p27 are sufficient to prevent cell proliferation, and therefore mitogenic stimulation of nondividing cells requires the elimination of p27.[232] Both control of p27 mRNA translation rate and control of p27 proteolysis by the ubiquitin-proteosome pathway have been implicated in modulating p27 protein levels in response to mitogenic growth factors.[136,206]

A third mechanism by which growth factors promote cell cycle progression is through the assembly of cyclin–cdk complexes. Cyclin D–cdk4 complexes cannot assemble from their individual subunits in growth factor-starved nondividing cells.[226] An assembly

factor is induced by growth factors, although its molecular identity has not been established.

The proliferative response of a cell to environmental signals depends equally on its interactions with soluble extracellular growth factors and on more local interactions with neighboring cells and with the extracellular matrix. Appropriate interactions between specific cell surface receptors (most often the integrin family of proteins) and the extracellular matrix are absolutely required for cell proliferation, a phenomenon known as anchorage dependence. In fact, loss of anchorage dependence is the single property of transformed cells that most closely correlates with their ability to form tumors in animals. The effect of cell anchorage on cell cycle progression, like the effect of growth factors, occurs during G1. Cell anchorage is required for transcription and translation of cyclin D1, for activation of the cyclin E—cdk2 kinase, and for transcription of cyclin A.[227,228] Anchorage regulates cyclin E—cdk2 activity by controlling the levels of the p21 and p27 cdk inhibitors. Therefore, cell anchorage controls the expression and/or activity of all three cyclin—cdk complexes required for the transition from G1 to S. Cell anchorage and growth factors jointly regulate the cell cycle by modulating the activity of the cyclins and cdks required for G1 and entry into S phase.

The antiproliferative action of agents such as TGF-β, cyclic AMP,[235] and DNA damage also can be understood in terms of their effects on cell cycle proteins.[125–128,229–234,236–238] The TGF-β family of cytokines regulates diverse cellular responses, including cell proliferation, cell differentiation, and cell death.[239] The antimitogenic action of TGF-β has become a paradigm for the inhibition of cell proliferation by extracellular agents. The active form of TGF-β is a disulfide-linked protein dimer that, like other members of this cytokine family, signals by bridging together type I and type II receptor serine–threonine kinases on the cell surface. The signal from the heterodimeric type I and type II receptor complex is transduced to the nucleus by a member of the Smad family of nuclear phosphoproteins. The Smad proteins are thought to be transcription factors that promote the expression of genes required for the biologic effects of TGF-β or related cytokines. Mutations in DPC4, a member of the Smad protein family located on chromosome 18q21, have been detected in half of all pancreatic cancers, and this may reflect a role for this protein in transmitting an antimitogenic TGF-β-like signal in pancreatic cells.[240] Ultimately, the TGF-β signal has a plethora of effects on cell cycle proteins that together impose a tight blockade on progression through G1. TGF-β blocks the activation of cyclin D–cdk4 complexes by inducing expression of the cdk inhibitor p15 and by inhibiting translation of cdk4 mRNA.[232,241,242] TGF-β also blocks activation of cyclin E–cdk2, in some cases by directly inducing p21 and p27 and in other instances indirectly by promoting the redistribution of p27 from cyclin D—cdk4 complexes to cyclin E—cdk2.[232,233] The biochemical pathways that link activation of the Smad proteins to these diverse effects on cell cycle proteins have not been determined.

Normal cells will not replicate a damaged chromosome. Instead, cells pause in G1 to repair the DNA lesion, thereby avoiding duplication of a damaged DNA template and preventing the propagation of generic misinformation to daughter cells. This DNA damage response is controlled by the p53 tumor suppressor protein.[243,244] The p53 protein is stabilized in cells containing damaged chromosomal DNA, although it is not understood how DNA damage is detected by the cell or how this results in decreased turnover of the p53 protein.[245] p53 is a transcriptional transactivator, and upregulation of p53 leads to increased expression of p53-responsive genes.[246–248] Among these genes is one encoding the cdk inhibitor p21Cip, and p21 protein levels rise in cells with damaged DNA (Fig. 8-12).[127,238] Consequently, as p53 levels rise, G2 cyclin–cdk complexes contain elevated amounts of p21 and are inactivated. Additionally, p21 binds to and inactivates the DNA polymerase cofactor PCNA, and this contributes to the G1—S-phase arrest.[129,130] However, p21 does not inhibit the repair functions of PCNA, and this allows DNA repair to continue while DNA replication is blocked.[249] Mice containing an engineered homozygous deletion of the p21 gene are viable, but cells taken from these mice have a defective cell cycle response to DNA damage.[236,237]

CELL CYCLE CHECKPOINTS

Cells usually are produced only when a new cell is needed.[250] Normal cells are periodically recruited into (or released from) the proliferating state by extracellular signals, and as was discussed, this is mediated by activation (or inactivation) of cell cycle proteins. Tumor cells, in contrast, proliferate when normal cells would not. Current data show that many and possibly all cancer cells contain mutations in cell cycle regulatory proteins, perhaps partly explaining their unregulated proliferation.[251–256] In particular, one or another element in the Rb regulatory pathway, including p16, cyclin D, cdk4, E2F, or Rb itself, may be mutated in almost 100 percent of human tumors (Fig. 8-13).[251–261] Altered expression of other cell cycle regulatory proteins also is commonly observed (i.e., cyclin E and p27), but this often occurs by mechanisms other than gene mutation.[262–265]

Although mutations in cell cycle proteins may directly stimulate proliferation, other considerations suggest that these changes are not sufficient to explain the origin of tumorigenic cells. Epidemiologic, molecular, and genetic evidence suggests that multiple mutations are required to transform a normal cell into a tumor cell.[266–268] However, simple calculations show that at normal mutation rates it would be very unlikely for a cell with more than two or three mutations to arise within the lifetime of a typical person. This has suggested that increased genetic mutation rates must be a prerequisite for the evolution of malignant cells and has given rise to the idea that the defining characteristic of a tumor cell may be genetic instability.[269–272] The frequent occurrence in tumor cells of aneuploidy, DNA translocations, DNA deletions, DNA amplifications, and other genetic abnormalities may be a direct manifestation of their genetic instability.

The critical question therefore is, What controls the genetic stability of a cell? Of course, the accuracy of the enzymes that replicate and segregate chromosomes is largely responsible for the faithful propagation of genetic information. However, despite their great fidelity, these enzymes have an intrinsic, spontaneous error rate. What's more, the frequency of errors can be further elevated by exogenous agents such as chemical mutagens. Therefore, to reduce the accumulation of genetic mistakes, normal cells also continually monitor the success of DNA replication and mitosis and bring the cell cycle to a halt if these events do not occur correctly.

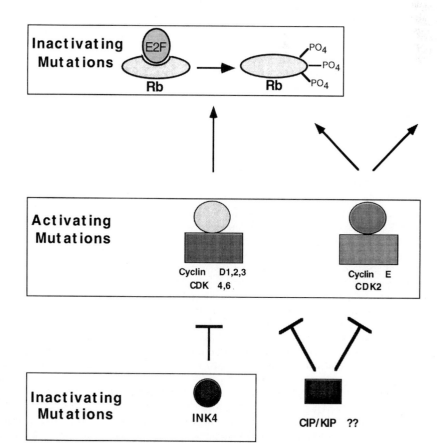

FIG. 8-13 The cyclin D–Rb pathway frequently is mutated in human tumors. Mutations that have been detected in human cancers include both inactivating (recessive) mutations in Rb and the INK4 proteins and activating (dominant) mutations in the cyclin genes. All result in the deregulation of this pathway.

Once active proliferation is suspended, the cell shifts from duplicating genetic information to repairing it and resumes proliferation only after the mistakes have been corrected. Checkpoints are the pathways that make progression through the cell cycle dependent on the accurate execution of specific cell cycle events.[30,269] More specifically, they are the biochemical links between the cyclin–cdk cycle and the macromolecular events of the cell division cycle, such as DNA replication and mitosis.

Checkpoints first were identified experimentally by Weinert and Hartwell in a landmark work describing the cell cycle response to DNA damage.[273] DNA damage causes the yeast cell cycle to pause in G2, allowing time for repair enzymes to correct the lesions and thereby preventing the cell from attempting to segregate broken chromosomes during mitosis. It was shown that this pause in G2 is controlled by the RAD9 gene, but not because the RAD9 gene is involved directly in the repair process itself. Instead, it was shown that RAD9 is part of a surveillance mechanism and that activation of the RAD9 pathway by DNA damage prevents cyclin–cdk activity from driving a cell into mitosis. The mechanism by which RAD9 blocks cyclin—cdk activity is not completely understood, but in some cells it is thought to involve tyrosine phosphorylation and catalytic inactivation of cdc2.[274-278] Thus, cells containing a mutated rad9 gene are unable to restrain cell cycle progression after DNA damage. Consequently, these mutant cells propagate damaged DNA and have greatly elevated mutation rates. Subsequent to the discovery of RAD9, a large number of other genes have been identified in yeast that together define an intricate network of pathways that make cell cycle progression dependent on the faithful duplication of chromosomes during S phase.[279,280] A different but equally robust set of pathways checks for the proper attachment of chromosomes to the mitotic spindle and delays mitosis if this has not occurred correctly.[281,282] This checkpoint is triggered by the absence of spindle-induced tension on kinetochores.[283] Once it is triggered, this checkpoint initiates a MAP kinase-dependent pathway that delays the programmed destruction of mitotic cyclins and prevents the initiation of anaphase.[284] It is likely that this pathway modulates activation of APC, the mitotic proteolytic machinery. Mutations in these checkpoint genes (the MAD and BUB genes) elevate rates of chromosome nondysjunction. Other, less well-defined checkpoint pathways are thought to monitor cell growth, cytokinesis, and centrosome duplication and prevent cell cycle progression if those events are executed incorrectly.

Normal cells use cell cycle checkpoints as fail-safe mechanisms to avoid the accumulation of genomic errors during cell division. Inactivation of checkpoint pathways is thought to underlie the genetic instability seen in tumor cells. Thus, many tumor suppressor genes may be part of checkpoint pathways, and inactivation of these genes could contribute to the clonal evolution of cancer cells by allowing the accumulation of genomic errors that would normally have resulted in cycle arrest (and repair) or cell death. Perhaps the best example is the p53 gene, the most commonly mutated gene in human tumors.[245,246,252,255,285] As was discussed, p53 governs the G1 checkpoint in human cells that prevents cells from entering S phase and replicating a damaged chromosome. Also, the gene mutated in the cancer-prone syndrome ataxia-telangiectasia is thought to be required for coordinating cell cycle progression with the repair of DNA damage during S and G2.[286,287] Human homologues of various yeast checkpoint genes are being characterized, and their relevance to genetic instability in tumor cells will soon be determined.

In conclusion, the process of tumorigenesis may begin with changes in cell cycle regulation. Mutations in cell cycle proteins contribute to tumorigenesis in two ways. First, they promote cell proliferation directly by allowing the cell to override or bypass controls that ordinarily restrict proliferation. Second, they cause the cell to ignore internal alarms that signal the presence of errors in the duplication and segregation of genetic information. This results in genetic instability and sets the stage for the evolution of malignant cells. For these reasons cancer can be thought of as a disease of the cell cycle.

REFERENCES

1. Prescott DM: *Reproduction of Eukaryotic Cells*. New York, Academic Press, 1976.
2. Murray A, Hunt T: *The Cell Cycle: An Introduction*, 1st ed. New York: Freeman, 1993.
3. Mitchison JM: *The Biology of the Cell Cycle*. London, Cambridge University Press, 1971.
4. Edgar B: Diversification of cell cycle controls in developing embryos. *Curr Opinion Cell Biol* 7:815, 1995.
5. Alberts, B, Bray D, Lewis J, Raff M, Roberts K. Watson J: *Molecular Biology of the Cell*. New York, Garland, 1989.
6. Hartwell L: Twenty-five years of cell cycle genetics. *Genetics* **129**: 975, 1991.
7. Nurse P: Universal control mechanism regulating onset of M-phase. *Nature* 344:503, 1990.
8. Hartwell L, Culotti J, Pringle J, Reid B: Genetic control of the cell division cycle in yeast. *Science* 183:46,1974.
9. Hartwell L, Mortimer K, Culotti J, Culotti M: Genetic control of the cell division cycle in yeast: V. Genetic analysis of cdc mutants. *Genetics* **74**:267, 1973.
10. Pringle JR, Hartwell LH: The Saccharomyces cerevisiae cell cycle, in Strathern JN, Jones EW, Broach JR (eds): *The Molecular Biology of the Yeast Saccharomyces*. New York, Cold Spring Harbor Laboratory Press, 1981, p 97.
11. Cross F: Starting the cell cycle: What's the point? *Curr Opinion Cell Biol* 7:790, 1995.
12. Reid B, Hartwell L: Regulation of mating in the cell cycle of Saccharomyces cerevisiae. *J Cell Biol* **75**:355, 1977.
13. Hartwell LH, Unger MW: Unequal division in Saccharomyces cerevisiae and its implications for the control of cell division. *J Cell Biol* **75**:422, 1977.
14. Johnston G, Pringle J, Hartwell L: Coordination of growth with cell division in the yeast S. cerevisiae. *Exp Cell Res* **105**:79, 1977.
15. Nasymth K: Control of the yeast cell cycle by the Cdc28 protein kinase. *Curr Opinion Cell Biol* 5:166, 1993.
16. Lorincz AT, Reed SI: Primary structure homology between the product of the yeast cell cycle control gene CDC28 and vertebrate oncogenes. *Nature* **307**:183, 1984.
17. Nurse P: Genetic control of cell size at cell division in yeast. *Nature* **256**:457, 1975.
18. Hindley J, Phear GA: Sequence of the cell division gene cdc2 from Schizosaccharomyces pombe: Pattern of splicing and homology to protein kinases. *Gene* 31:129, 1984.
19. Nurse P, Bisset Y: Gene required in G1 for commitment to cell cycle and in G2 for control of mitosis in fission yeast. *Nature* 292:558, 1981.
20. Beach D, Durkacz B, Nurse P: Functionally homologous cell cycle control genes in fission yeast and budding yeast. *Nature* 300:706, 1982.
21. Reed SI, Wittenberg C: Mitotic role for the CDC28 protein kinase of S. cerevisae. *Proc Natl Acad Sci USA* 87:5697, 1990.
22. Piggot JR, Rai R, Carter BLA: A bifunctional gene product involved in two phases of the yeast cell cycle. *Nature* **298**:391, 1982.
23. Masui H, Market CL: Cytoplasmic control of nuclear behaviour during meiotic maturation of frog oocytes. *J Exp Zool* 117:129, 1971.
24. Wasserman WJ, Smith LD: The cyclic behaviour of a cytoplasmic factor controlling nuclear membrane breakdown. *J Cell Biol* 78:R15, 1978.
25. Reynhout JK, Smith LD: Studies on the appearance and nature of a maturation-inducing factor in the ctyoplasm of amphibian oocytes exposed to progesterone. *Dev Biol* 38:394, 1974.
26. Newport J, Kirschner M: Regulation of the cell cycle during early Xenopus development. *Cell* 37:731, 1984.
27. Nelkin B, Nichols C, Vogelstein B: Protein factor(s) from mitotic CHO cells induce meiotic maturation in Xenopus laevis oocytes. *FEBS Lett* **109**:233, 1980.

28. Hara K, Tydeman P, Kirschner M: A cytoplasmic clock with the same period as the division cycle in Xenopus eggs. *Proc Natl Acad Sci USA* **77**:462, 1980.

29. Murray A, Kirschner MW: Dominoes and clocks: The union of two views of the cell cycle. *Science* **246**:614, 1989.

30. Hartwell L, Weinert T: Checkpoints: Controls that ensure the order of cell cycle events. *Science* **246**:629, 1989.

31. Cross F, Roberts J, Weintraub H: Simple and complex cell cycles. *Annu Rev Cell Biol* **5**:341, 1989.

32. Nurse P: Universal control mechanism regulating onset of M-phase. *Nature* **344**:503, 1990.

33. Lee MG, Nurse P: Complementation used to clone a human homologue of the fission yeast cell cycle control gene cdc2. *Nature* **327**:31, 1987.

34. Gautier J, Norbury C, Lohka M, Nurse P, Maller JL: Purified maturation-promoting factor contains the product of a Xenopus homolog of the fission yeast cell cycle control gene cdc2+. *Cell* **54**:433, 1988.

35. Hunt T: Maturation promoting factor, cyclin and the control of M-phase. *Curr Opinion Cell Biol* **1**:268, 1989.

36. Labbe JC, Picard A, Peaucellier G, Cavadore JC, Nurse P, Doree M: Purification of MPF from starfish: Identification as the H1 histone kinase p34cdc2 and a possible mechanism for its periodic activation. *Cell* **57**:253, 1989.

37. Labbe JC, Lee MG, Nurse P, Picard A, Doree M: Activation at M-phase of a protein kinase encoded by a starfish homologue of the cell cycle gene Cdc2. *Nature* **335**:251, 1988.

38. Dunphy WG, Brizuela L, Beach D, Newport J: The Xenopus cdc2 protein is a component of MPF, a cytoplasmic regulator of mitosis. *Cell* **54**:423, 1988.

39. Murray A: The cell cycle as a cdc2 cycle. *Nature* **342**:14, 1989.

40. Riabowol K, Draetta G, Brizuela L, Vandre D, Beach D: The cdc2 kinase is a nuclear protein that is essential for mitosis in mammalian cells. *Cell* **57**:393, 1989.

41. D Urso G, Marraccino RL, Marshak DR, Roberts JM: Cell cycle control of DNA replication by a homologue from human cells of the p34-cdc2 protein kinase. *Science* **250**:786, 1990.

42. Th'ng JPH, Wright PS, Hamaguchi J, Lee MG, Norbury CJ, Nurse P, Bradbury EM: The FT210 cell line is a mouse G2 phase mutant with a temperature-sensitive CDC2 gene product. *Cell* **63**:313, 1990.

43. Tsai LE, Lees E, Faha B, Harlow E, Riabowol K: The cdk2 kinase is required for the G1 to S transition in mammalian cells. *Oncogene* **8**:1593, 1993.

44. Fang F, Newport J: Evidence that the G1-S and G2-M transitions are controlled by different cdc2 proteins in higher eukaryotes. *Cell* **66**:731, 1991.

45. Furakawa Y, Piwnica-Worms H, Ernst TJ, Kanakura Y, Griffin JD: Cdc2 gene expression at the to S transition in human T lymphocytes. *Science* **250**:805, 1990.

46. Lamb N, Fernandex A, Watrin A, Labbe J, Cavadore J: Microinjection of the p34cdc2 kinase induces marked changes in cell shape, cytoskeletal organization and chromatin structure in mammalian fibroblasts. *Cell* **60**:151, 1990.

47. Nasymth K: Control of the yeast cell cycle by the Cdc28 protein kinase. *Curr Opinion Cell Biol* **5**:166, 1993.

48. Myerson M, Enders GH, Wu C, Su L, Gorka C, Nelson C, Harlow E, Tsai L: The human cdc2 kinase family. *EMBO J* **11**:2909, 1992.

49. Morgan D: Principle of CDK regulation. *Nature* **374**:131, 1995.

50. Lees E: Cyclin dependent kinase regulation. *Curr Opinion Cell Biol* **7**:773, 1995.

51. Sherr C: Mammalian G1 cyclins. *Cell* **73**:10591, 1993.

52. Sherr C: G1 phase progression: Cycling on cue. *Cell* **79**:551, 1994.

53. Van den Heuval S, Harlow E: Distinct roles for cyclin-dependent kinases in cell cycle control. *Science* **262**:2050, 1994.

54. Tsai L, Delalle I, Caviness V, Chae T, Harlow E: p35, a neural specific regulatory subunit of the cdk5 kinase. *Nature* **371**:419.

55. Nikoklic M, Dudek H, Kwon Y, Ramos Y, Tsai LH: The cdk5/p35 kinase is essential for neurite outgrowth during neuronal differentiation. *Gene Dev* **8**:816, 1996.

56. DeBondt, Rosenblatt J, Jarncarik J, Jones H, Morgan D, Kim S: Crystal structure of the cyclin-dependent kinase 2. *Nature* **363**:595, 1993.

57. Jeffrey PD, Russo AA, Polyak K, Gibbs E, Hurwitz J, Massague J, Paveltich NP: Crystal structure of a cyclin A-cdk2 complex at 2.3A: Mechanism of cdk activation by cyclins. *Nature* **376**:313, 1995.

58. Cross F: DAF1, a mutant gene affecting size control, pheromone arrest, and cell cycle kinetics of Saccharomyces cerevisiae. *Mol Cell Biol* **8**:4675, 1988.

59. Cross F: Cell cycle arrest caused by CLN gene deficiency in Saccaromyces cerevisiae resembles START-1 arrest and is independent of the mating-pheromone signalling pathway. *Mol Cell Biol* **10**:6482, 1990.

60. Richardson H, Wittenberg C, Cross F, Reed S: An essential G1 function for cyclin-like proteins in yeast. *Cell* **59**:1127, 1989.

61. Hadwiger J, Wittenberg C, Richardson H, Lopes M, Reed S: A family of cyclin homologs that control the G1 phase in yeast. *Proc Natl Acad Sci USA* **86**:6255, 1989.

62. Wittenberg C, Sugimoto K, Reed SI: G1-specific cyclins of S. cerevisiae: cell cycle periodicity, regulation by mating pheromone, and association with the p34-CDC28 protein kinase. *Cell* **62**:225, 1990.

63. Koch C, Nasmyth K: Cell cycle regulated transcription in yeast. *Curr Opinion Cell Biol* **6**:451, 1994.

64. Koch C, Moll T, Neuberg M, Ahorn H, Nasmyth K: A role for the transcription factors Mbp1 and Swi4 in progression from G1 to S phase. *Science* **261**:1551, 1993.

65. Dirick L, Moll T, Auer H, Nasmyth K: A central role for SWI6 in modulating cell cycle Start-specific transcription in yeast. *Nature* **357**:508, 1992.

66. Dirick L, Nasmyth K: Positive feedback in the activation of G1 cyclins in yeast. *Nature* **351**:754, 1991.

67. Cross FR, Tinkelenberg H: A potential positive feedback loop controlling CLN1 and CLN2 gene expression at the start of the yeast cell cycle. *Cell* **65**:875, 1992.

68. Dirick L, Bohm, T., Nasmyth K: Roles and regulation of cln-cdc28 kinases at the start of the cell cycle of Saccaromyces cerevisiae. *EMBO J* **14**:4803, 1995.

69. Schwob E, Nasmyth K, CLB5 and CLB6, a new pair of B cyclins involved in S phase and mitotic spindle formation in S. Cerevisiae. *Gene Dev* **7**:1160, 1993.

70. Epstein C, Cross F: CLB5: A novel B cyclin from budding yeast with a role in S phase. *Gene Dev* **6**:1695, 1992.

71. Fitch I, Dahmann C, Surana U, Amon A, Nasmyth K, Goetch L, Byers B, Futcher B: Characterization of four B-type cyclin genes of the budding yeast Saccharomyces cerevisiae. *Mol Biol Cell* **3**:805, 1992.

72. Amon A, Tyers M, Futcher B, Nasmyth K: Mechanisms that help the yeast cell cycle clock tick: G2 cyclins transcriptionally activate their own synthesis and repress G1 cyclins. *Cell* **74**:993, 1993.

73. Lew DJ, Dulic V, Reed SI: Isolation of three novel human cyclins by rescue of G1 cyclin (cln) function in yeast. *Cell* **66**:1197, 1991.

74. Koff A, Cross F, Fisher A, Schumacher J, Leguelle K, Philippe M, Roberts JM: Human cyclin E, a new cyclin that interacts with two members of the CDC2 gene family. *Cell* **65**:1217, 1991.

75. Xiong Y, Connolly T, Futcher B, Beach D: Human D-type cyclin. *Cell* **65**:691, 1991.

76. Matsushime, H, Roussel M, Ashmun R, Sherr CJ: Colony-stimulating Factor 1 regulates novel cyclins during the G1 phase of the cell cycle. *Cell* **65**:701–713, 1991.

77. Motokura T, Bloom T, Kim HG, Juppner H, Ruderman JV, Kronenberg HM, Arnold A: A BCL1-linked candidate oncogene which is rearranged in parathyroid tumors encodes a novel cyclin. *Nature* **350**:512, 1991.

78. Sherr C, Kato J, Quell D, Matsuoka M, Roussel M: D-type cyclins and their cyclin-dependent kinases: G1 phase integrators of the mitogenic response. *Cold Slpring Harbor Symp Quant Biol* **49**:11, 1994.

79. Baldin V, Lukas J, Marcotte MJ, Pagano M, Draetta G: Cyclin D1 is a nuclear protein required for cell cycle progression in G1. *Gene Dev* **7**:812, 1993.

80. Quelle DE, Ashmun RA, Shurtleff SA, Kato J, Bar-Sagi D, Roussel MF, Sherr CJ: Overexpression of mouse D-type cyclins accelerates G1 phase in rodent fibroblasts. *Genes Dev* **7**:1559, 1993.

81. Resnitzky D, Gossen M, Bujard H, Reed SI: Acceleration of the G1/S phase transition by expression of cyclin D1 and E with an inducible system. *Mol Cell Biol* **14**:1669, 1994.

82. Ohtsubo M, Theodoras AM, Schumacher J, Roberts JM, Pagano M: Human cyclin E: A nuclear protein essential for the G1 to S phase transition. *Mol Cell Biol* **15**:2612, 1995.

83. Knoblich J, Sauer K, Jones L, Richardson H, Saint R, Lehner C: Cyclin E controls S phase progression and its down-regulation during Drosophila embryogenesis is required for the arrest of cell proliferation. *Cell* **77**:107, 1994.

84. Koff A, Giordano A, Desai D, Yamashita K, Harper JW, Elledge S, Nishimoto T, Morgan DO, Franza R, Roberts JM: Formation and activation of a cyclin E/CDK2 complex during the G1 phase of the human cell cycle. *Science* **257**:1689, 1992.

85. Dulic V, Lees E, Reed SI: Association of human cyclin E with a periodic G1-S phase protein kinase. *Science* **257**:1958, 1992.

86. Ohtsubo M, Roberts JM: Cyclin-dependent regulation of G1 in mammalian fibroblasts. *Science* **259**:1908, 1993.

87. Pagano M, Pepperkok P, Verde F, Ansorge W, Draetta G: Cyclin A is required at two points in the human cell cycle. *EMBO J* **11**:961, 1992.

88. Giordano A, White P, Harlow E, Franza BR Jr, Beach D, Draetta G: A 60 kd cdc2-associated polypeptide complexes with the E1A proteins in adenovirus-infected cells. *Cell* **58**:981, 1989.

89. Girard F, Strausfeld U, Fernandez A, Lamb N: Cyclin A is required for the onset of DNA replication in mammalian fibroblasts. *Cell* **67**:1169, 1991.

90. Pines J, Hunter T: Isolation of a human cyclin cDNA: Evidence for cyclin mRNA and protein regulation in the cell cycle and for interaction with p34-cdc2. *Cell* **58**:833, 1989.

91. Niff E: Cyclin-dependent kinase 7: At the crossroads of transcription, DNA repair and cell cycle control. *Curr Opinion Cell Biol* **8**:312, 1996.

92. Tassan JP, Jaquenoud M, Leopold P, Schultz SJ, Nigg EA: Identification of human cyclin-dependent kinase 8, a putative protein kinase partner for cyclin C. *Proc Natl Acad Sci USA* **92**:8871, 1995.

93. Bai C, Richman R, Elledge SJ: Human cyclin F. *EMBO J* **13**:6087, 1994.

94. Okamoto K, Beach D: Cyclin G is a transcriptional target of the p53 tumor suppressor. *EMBO J* **13**:4816, 1994.

95. Nakamura T, Sanolawa R, Saski Y, Ayusawa D, Oishi M, Mori N: Cyclin I: A new cyclin encoded by a gene isolated from human brain. *Expt Cell Res* **221**:534, 1995.

96. Russo A, Jeffrey P, Pavelitch N: Crystal structure of the p27Kip1 cyclin-dependent kinase inhibitor bound to the cyclin A-CdK2 complex. *Nature* **382**:325, 1996.

97. Solomon MJ: The function(s) of CAK, the p34cdc2 activating kinase. *Trends Biochem Sci* **19**:496, 1994.

98. Soloman M, Glotzer M, Lee T, Phillippe M, Kirschner M: Cyclin activation of p34-cdc2. *Cell* **63**:1013, 1990.

99. Solomon MJ, Lee T, Kirschner M: Role of phosphorylation in p34CDC2 activation: Identification of an activating kinase. *Mol Biol Cell* **3**:13, 1991.

100. Solomon MJ, Harper JW, Shuttleworth J: CAK, the p34CDC2 activating kinase, contains a protein identical or closely related to p40MO15. *EMBO J* **12**:3133, 1993.

101. Gould KL, Nurse P: Tyrosine phosphorylation of the fission yeast Cdc2+ protein kinase regulates entry into mitosis. *Nature* **342**:39, 1989.

102. Moreneo S, Hayles J, Nurse P: Regulation of p34-cdc2 protein kinase during mitosis. *Cell* **58**:361, 1989.

103. Simanis V, Nurse P: The cell cycle control gene cdc2+ of fission yeast encodes a protein kinase potentially regulated by phosphorylation. *Cell* **45**:261, 1986.

104. Heald R, McLoughlin M, McKeon F: Human Wee1 maintains mitotic timing by protecting the nucleus from cytoplasmically activated Cdc2 kinase. *Cell* **74**:463–474, 1993.

105. Igarashi M, Nagata A, Jinno S, Suto K, Okayama H: Wee1+-like gene in human cells. *Nature* **353**:80, 1991.

106. Lundgren D, Walworth N, Booher R, Dembski M, Kirschner M, Beach D: mik1 and wee1 cooperate in the inhibitory tyrosine phosphorylation of cdc2. *Cell* **64**:1111, 1991.

107. Russell P, Nurse P: Negative regulation of mitosis by wee1+, a gene encoding a protein kinase homolog. *Cell* **49**:559, 1987.

108. Russell P, Nurse P: cdc25+ functions as an inducer in the mitotic control of fission yeast. *Cell* **45**:145, 1986.

109. Sadhu K, Reed S, Richardson H, Russell P: Human homolog of fission yeast cdc25 mitotic inducer is predominantly expressed in G1. *Proc Natl Acad Sci USA* **87**:5139, 1990.

110. Kumagai A, Dunphy W: The Cdc25 protein controls tyrosine dephosphorylation of the Cdc2 protein in a cell free system. *Cell* **64**:903, 1991.

111. Sebastian B, Kakizuka A, Hunter T: Cdc25 activation of cyclin-dependent kinase by dephosphorylation of threonine-14 and tyrosine 15. *Proc Natl Acad Sci USA* **90**:3521, 1993.

112. Strausfield V, Labbe JC, Fesquat O, Cavadore JC, Picard A, Sadhu, Russell P, Durec M: Dephosphorylation and activation of a p34cdc2/cyclin B complex in vitro by human cdc25 protein. *Nature* **35**:242, 1991.

113. Atherton-Fessler S, Hannig G, Piwnica-Worms H: Reversible tyrosine phosphorylation and cell cycle control. *Semin Cell Biol* **4**:433, 1993.

114. Dunphy W: The decision to enter mitosis. *Trends Cell Biol* **4**:202, 1994.

115. Jinno S, Suto K, Nagata A, Igarashi M, Kanaoka Y, Nojima H, Okayama H: Cdc25A is a novel phosphatase functioning early in the cell cycle. *EMBO J* **13**:1549, 1994.

116. Hoffmann I, Draetta G, Karsenti E: Activation of the phosphatase activity of human cdc25A by a cdk2-cyclin E dependent phosphorylation at the G1/S transition. *EMBO J* **13**:4302, 1994.

117. Galaktionov K, Jessus C, Beach D: Raf1 interaction with Cdc25 phosphatase ties mitogenic signal transduction to cell cycle activation. *Gene Dev* **9**:1046–1058, 1995.

118. Sherr C, Roberts J: Inhibitors of mammalian G1 cyclin-dependent kinases. *Gene Dev* **9**:1149, 1995.

119. Peter M, Kerskowitz I: Joining the complex: Cyclin dependent kinase inhibitory proteins and cell cycle. *Cell* **79**:181, 1994.

120. Mendenhall M: An inhibitor of p34CDC28 protein kinase activity from Saccharomyces cerevisiae. *Science* **259**:216, 1993.

121. Schwob E, Bohm T, Mendenhall M, Nasmyth K: The B-type cyclins kinase inhibitor p40sic1 controls the G1 to S phase transition in S. cerevisiae. *Cell* **79**:233, 1994.

122. Elledge S, Harper W: Cdk inhibitors: On the threshold of checkpoints and development. *Curr Opinion Cell Biol* **6**:847, 1994.

123. Xiong Y, Zhang H, Beach D: Subunit rearrangement of the cyclin-dependent kinases is associated with cellular transformation. *Gene Dev* **7**:1572, 1993.

124. Noda A, Ning Y, Venable S, Pereira-Smith O, Smith J: Cloning of senescent cell-derived inhibitors of DNA synthesis using an expression screen. *Exp Cell Res* **211**:90, 1994.

125. Harper JW, Adami GR, Wei N, Keyomarsi K, Elledge SJ: The p21 Cdk-interacting protein Cip1 Is a potent inhibitor of G1 cyclin-dependent kinases. *Cell* **75**:805, 1993.

126. Xiong Y, Hannong G, Zhang H, Casso D, Kobayashi R, Beach D: p21 is a universal inhibitor of cyclin kinases. *Nature* **366**:701, 1993.

127. El-Deiry WS, Tokino T, Velculescu VE, Levy DB, Parsons R, Trent JM, Lin D, Mercer WE, Kinzler KW, Vogelstein B: WAF1, a potential mediator of p53 tumor suppression. *Cell* **75**:817, 1993.

128. Gu Y, Turek C, Morgan D: Inhibition of CDK2 activity in vivo by an associated 20K regulatory subunit. *Nature* **366**:707, 1993.

129. Waga S, Hannon G, Beach D, Stillman B: The p21 inhibitor of cyclin-dependent kinases controls DNA replication by interaction with PCNA. *Nature* **369**:574, 1994.

130. Flores-Rozas H, Kelman Z, Dean F, Pan Z, Harper JW, Elledge S, O Donnell M, Hurwitz J: CDK-interacting protein 1 directly binds with proliferating cell nuclear antigen and inhibits DNA relication catalyzed by the DNA polymerase and holoenzyme. *Proc Natl Acad Sci USA* **91**:8655, 1994.

131. Luo Y, Hurwitz J, Massague J: Cell-cycle inhibition by independent CDK and CPNA binding domains in p21Cip1. *Nature* **375**:159, 1995.

132. Halevy O, Novitch B, Spicer D, Skapek S, Rhee J, Hannon G, Beach D, Lasser A: Correlation of terminal cell cycle arrest of skeletal muscle with induction of p21 by MyoD. *Science* **267**:1018, 1995.

133. Parker S, Eichele G, Zhang P, Rawls A, Sands A, Bradley A, Olson E, Harper JW, Elledge S: p53-independent expression of p21Cip1 in muscle and other terminally differentiating cells. *Science* **267**:1024, 1995.

134. Polyak K, Lee MH, Erdjument-Bromage H, Koff A, Roberts JM, Tempst P, Massague J: Cloning of p27kip1, a cyclin-dependent kinase inhibitor and a potential mediator of extracellular antimitogenic signals. *Cell* **78**:67, 1994.

135. Toyoshima H, Hunter T: p27, a novel inhibitor of G1-cyclin-cdk protein kinase activity, is related to p21. *Cell* **78**:67, 1994.

136. Hengst L, Reed SI: Translational control of p27Kip1 accumulation during the cell cycle. *Science* **271**:1861, 1996.

137. Lee M, Reynisdottir I, Massague J: Cloning of p57Kip2, a cyclin-dependent kinase inhibitor with unique domain structure and tissue distribution. *Gene Dev* **9**:639, 1995.

138. Matsuoka S, Edwards M, Bai C, Parker S, Zhang P, Baldini A, Harper JW, Elledge S: p57Kip2, a structurally distinct member of the p21Cip1 cdk inhibitor family, is a candidate tumor suppressor gene. *Gene Dev* **9**:650, 1995.

138a. Serrano M, Hannon GJ, Beach D: A new regulatory motif in cell-cycle control causing specific inhibition of cyclin D-Cdk4. *Nature* **366**:704, 1993.

139. Sheaff R, Roberts J: Lessons in p16 from phylum Falconium. *Curr Biol* **5**:28, 1995.

140. Kamb A: Role of a cell cycle regulator in hereditary and sporadic cancer. *Cold Spring Harbor Symp Quant Biol* **49**:39, 1994.

141. Quelle DE, Ashmun RA, Hannon GJ, Rehberger PA, Trono D, Richter KH, Walker C, Beach D, Sherr CJ, Serrano M: Cloning and

characterization of murine p16INK4a and p15INK4b genes. *Oncogene* **11**:635, 1995.

142. Hirai H, Roussel MF, Kato JY, Ashmun RA, Sherr CJ: Novel INK4 proteins, p19 and p18, are specific inhibitors of the cyclin D-dependent kinases CDK4 and CDK6. *Mol Cell Biol* **15**:2672, 1995.

143. Serrano M, Lee H, Chin L, Cordon-Cardo C, Beach D, DePinho RA: Role of the INK4a locus in tumor suppression and cell mortality. *Cell* **85**:27, 1996.

144. Schneider B, Yang Y, Futcher B: Linkage of replication to start by the CDK inhibitor sic1. *Science* **272**:560, 1996.

145. Weinberg RA: The retinoblastoma protein and cell cycle control. *Cell* **81**:323, 1995.

146. Dyson N, Howley PM, Munger K, Harlow E: The human papilloma virus-16E7 oncoprotein is able to bind to the retinoblastoma gene product. *Science* **243**:934, 1989.

147. Whyte P, Williamson NM, Harlow E: Cellular targets for transformation by the adenovirus E1A proteins. *Cell* **56**:67, 1989.

148. Whyte P, Buchkovich KJ, Horowitz JM, Friend SH, Raybuck M, Weinberg RA, Harlow E: Association between an oncogene and an anti-oncogene: The adenovirus E1A proteins bind to the retinoblastoma gene product. *Nature* **334**:124, 1988.

149. Friend SH, Horowitz JM, Gerber MR, Wang XF, Bogenmann E, Li FP, Weinberg RA: Deletions of a DNA sequence in retinoblastomas and mesenchymal tumors: Organization of the sequence and its encoded protein. *Proc Natl Acad Sci USA* **84**:9059, 1987.

150. Friend SH, Bernards R, Rogelj S, Weinberg RA, Rapaport JM, Albert DM, Dryja TP: A human DNA segment with properties of the gene that predisposes to retinoblastoma and osteosarcoma. *Nature* **323**:643, 1986.

151. Horowitz JM, Park S, Bogenmann E, Cheng J, Yandell DW, Kaye FJ, Minna JD, Dryja TP, Weinberg RA: Frequent inactivation of the retinoblastoma anti-oncogene is restricted to a subset of human tumor cells. *Proc Natl Acad Sci USA* **87**:2775, 1990.

152. Buchkovich K, Duffy LA, Harlow E: The retinoblastoma protein is phosphorylated during specific phases of the cell cycle. *Cell* **58**:1097, 1989.

153. Mittnacht S, Lees JA, Desai D, Harlow E, Morgan DO, Weinberg RA: Distinct sub-populations of the retinoblastoma protein show a distinct pattern of phosphorylation. *EMBO J* **13**:118, 1994.

154. Nevins J: E2F: A link between the Rb tumor suppressor protein and viral oncoproteins. *Science* **258**:424, 1992.

155. Sherr CJ: The ins and outs of Rb: Coupling gene expression to the cell cycle clock. *Trends Cell Biol* **4**:15, 1994.

156. Lees JA, Saito M, Vidal M, Valentine M, Look T, Harlow E, Dyson N, Helin K: The retinoblastoma protein binds to a family of E2F transcription factors. *Mol Cell Biol* **13**:7813, 1993.

157. Kaelin WG Jr, Krek W, Sellers WR, DeCaprio JA, Ajchenbaum F, Fuchs CS, Chittenden T, Li Y, Farnham PJ, Blanar MA, Livingston DM, Flemington EK: Expression cloning of a cDNA encoding a retinoblastoma-binding protein with E2F-like properties. *Cell* **70**:351, 1972.

158. Helin K, Lees JA, Vidal M, Dyson N, Harlow E, Fattaey A: A cDNA encoding a pRB-binding protein with properties of the transcription factor E2F. *Cell* **70**:337, 1992.

159. Wu CL, Zukerberg LR, Ngwu C, Harlow E, Lees JA: In vivo association of E2F and DP family proteins. *Mol Cell Biol* **15**:2536, 1995.

160. Lees JA, Buchkovich KJ, Marshak DR, Anderson CW, Harlow E: The retinoblastoma protein is phosphorylated on multiple sites by human cdc2. *EMBO J* **10**:4279, 1991.

161. Dowdy S, Hinds P, Lovic K, Reed S, Arnold A, Weinberg RA: Physical interaction of the retinoblastoma protein with human D cyclins. *Cell* **73**:499, 1993.

162. Ewen M, Sluss K, Sherr CJ, Livingston M, Matsushime H, Kato JY, Livingston DM: Functional interactions of the retinoblastoma protein with mammalian D-type cyclins. *Cell* **73**:487, 1993.

163. Hinds P, Mittnacht S, Dulic V, Arnold A, Reed S, Weinberg R: Regulation of retinoblastoma protein functions by ectopic expression of human cyclins. *Cell* **70**:993, 1992.

164. Kato JY, Matsushime H, Hiebert S, Ewen M, Sherr C: Direct binding of cyclin D to the retinoblastoma gene product and pRb phosphorylation by the cyclin D-dependent kinase, cdk4. *Gene Dev* **7**:331, 1993.

165. Bates S, Parry D, Bonetta L, Vousden K, Dickson C, Peters G: Absence of cyclin D/Cdk complexes in cells lacking functional retinoblastoma protein. *Oncogene* **9**:1633–1640, 1994.

166. Lukas J, Parry D, Aagaard L, Mann DJ, Bartkova J, Strauss M, Peters G, Bartek J: Retinoblastoma-protein-dependent cell-cycle inhibition by the tumour suppressor p16. *Nature* **375**:503, 1995.

167. Lukas J, Bartkova J, Rohde M, Strauss M, Bartek J: Cyclin D1 is dispensable for G1 control in retinoblastoma gene-deficient cells independently of cdk5 activity. *Mol Cell Biol* **15**:2600, 1995.

168. Zhu L, Enders GH, Wu CL, Starz MA, Moberg KH, Lees JA, Dyson N, Harlow E: Growth suppression by members of the retinoblastoma protein family. *Cold SLpring Harbor Symp Quant Biol* **59**:75, 1994.

169. Bandara L, Adamczewski J, Hunt T, LaThanghe N: Cyclin A and the retinoblastoma gene product complex with a common transcription factor. *Nature* **352**:249, 1991.

170. Shirodkar S, Ewen M, DeCaprio J, Morgan J, Livingston D, Chittenden T: The transcription factor E2F interacts with the retinoblastoma product and a p107-cyclin A complex in a cell cycle regulated manner. *Cell* **68**:157, 1992.

170. Dynlacht B, Flores O, Lees J, Harlow E: Differential regulation of E2F transactivation by cyclin/cdk2 complexes. *Gene Dev* **8**:1772, 1994.

171. Krek W, Ewen M, Shirodkar S, Arany Z, Kaelin W. Livingston D: Negative regulation of the growth-promoting transcription factor E2F-1 by a stably bound cyclin A-dependent protein kinase. *Cell* **78**:161, 1994.

172. Nigg EA: Targets of cyclin-dependent protein kinases. *Curr Opinion Cell Biol* **5**:187, 1993.

173. Heichman K, Roberts JM: Rules to replicate by. *Cell* **79**:1, 1994.

174. Nigg EA: Assembly-disassembly of the nuclear lamina. *Curr Opinion Cell Biol* **4**:105, 1992.

175. Heald R, McKeon F: Mutations of phosphorylation sites in lamin A that prevent nuclear lamina disassembly in mitosis. *Cell* **61**:579, 1990.

176. Blangy A, Lane HA, d'Henrit P, Harper M, Kress M, Nigg EA: Phosphorylation by p34cdc2 retulates spindle association of human Eg5, a kinesin-related motor essential for bipolar spindle formation in vivo. *Cell* **83**:1159, 1995.

177. Deshaies R: The self-destructive personality of a cell cycle in transition. *Curr Opinion Cell Biol* **7**:781, 1995.

178. Maller J: Mitotic control. *Curr Opinion Cell Biol* **3**:269, 1991.

179. Evans T, Rosenthal lE, Youngblom J, Distel D, Hunt T: Cyclin: A protein specified by maternal mRNA in sea urchin eggs that is destroyed at each cleavage division. *Cell* **33**:389, 1983.

180. Ciechanover A: The ubiquitin-proteasome proteolytic pathway. *Cell* **79**:13, 1994.

181. Hochstrasser M: Ubiquitin, proteasomes, and the regulation of intracellular protein degradation. *Curr Opinion Cell Biol* **7**:215, 1995.

182. Jentsch S, Schlenker S: Selective protein degradation: A journey's end within the proteasome. *Cell* **82**:881, 1995.

183. Rogers S, Wells R, Rechsteiner M: Amino acid sequences common to rapidly degraded proteins: The PEST hypothesis. *Science* **234**:364, 1986.

184. Glotzer M, Murray A, Kirschner M: Cyclin is degraded by the ubiquitin pathway. *Nature* **349**:132, 1991.

185. Murray AW, Solomon MJ, Kirschner MW: The role of cyclin synthesis and degradation in the control of maturation promoting factor activity. *Nature* **339**:280, 1989.

186. Ghiara JB, Richardson HE, Sugimoto K, Henze M, Lew DJ, Wittenberg C, Reed SI: A cyclin B homolog in S. cerevisiae: Chronic activation of the CDC28 protein kinase by cyclin prevents exit from mitosis. *Cell* **65**:163, 1991.

187. Surana U, Robitsch H, Price C, Schuster T, Fitch I, Futcher AB, Nasmyth K: The role of CDC28 and cyclins during mitosis in the budding yeast S. cerevisiae. *Cell* **79**:563, 1994.

188. King RW, Jackson P, Kirschner MW: Mitosis in transition. *Cell* **79**:563, 1994.

189. Juca FC, Shibuya EK, Dohrmann EE, Ruderman JV: Both cyclin A 60 and B 97 are stable and arrest cells in M phase but only cyclin B 97 turns on cyclin destruction. *EMBO J* **10**:4311, 1991.

190. Murray AW: Cyclin ubiquitination: The destructive end of mitosis. *Cell* **81**:149, 1995.

191. King R, Peters J, Tugendreich S, Rolfe M, Hieter P, Kirschner M: A 20S complex containing cdc27 and cdc16 catalyzes the mitosis-specific conjugation of ubiquitin to cyclin B. *Cell* **81**:279, 1995.

192. Holloway SL, Glotzer M, King RW, Murray AW: Anaphase is initiated by proteolysis rather than by the inactivation of maturation-promoting factor. *Cell* **73**:1393, 1993.

193. Sudakin V, Ganoth D, Dahan A, Heller H, Hershko J, Luca F, Ruderman J, Hershko A: The cyclosome, a large complex containing cyclin-selective ubiquitin ligase activity, targets cyclins for destruction at the end of mitosis. *Mol Cell Biol* **6**:185, 1995.

194. Irniger S, Piatti S, Michaelis C, Nasmyth K: Genes involved in sister chromatid separation are needed for B-type cyclin proteolysis in budding yeast. *Cell* **81**:269, 1995.

195. Seufert W, Futcher B, Jentsch S: Role of a ubiquitin-conjugating enzyme in degradation of S-phase and M-phase cyclins. *Nature* **373**:78, 1995.

196. Felix M, Labbe J, Doree M, Hunt T, Karsenti E: Triggering of cyclin degradation in interphase extracts of amphibian eggs by cdc2 kinase. *Nature* **346**:379, 1990.

197. Amon A, Irniger S, Nasmyth K: Closing the cell cycle circle in yeast: G1 cyclin proteolysis initiated at mitosis persists until the activation of G1 cyclins in the next cell cycle. *Cell* **77**:1037, 1994.

198. Clurman BE, Sheaff RJ, Thress K, Groudine M, Roberts JM: Turnover of cyclin E by the ubiquitin-proteasome pathway is regulated by CDK2 binding and cyclin phosphorylation. *Genes Dev* **1**:1464, 1996.

199. Won K, Reed S: Activation of cyclin E/CDK2 is coupled to site-specific autophosphorylation and ubiquitin-dependent degradation of cyclin E. *EMBO J* **15**:4182, 1996.

200. Lanker S, Valdivieso M, Wittenberg C: Rapid degradation of the G1 cyclin cln2 induced by CDK-dependent phosphorylation. *Science* **271**:1597, 1996.

201. Tyers M, Tokiwa G, Nash R, Futcher B: The cln2-cdc28 kinase complexes of S. cervesiae is regulated by proteolyis and phosphorylation. *EMBO J* **11**:1773, 1992.

202. Yaglom J, Linskens M, Sadis S, Rubin D, Futcher B, Finley D: p34Cdc28-mediated control of cln3 degradation. *Mol Cell Biol* **15**:731, 1995.

203. Chen Z, Hagler J, Palombella V, Melandri F, Scherer D, Ballard D, Maniatis T: Signal-induced site-specific phosphorylation targets IkBa to the ubiquitin-proteasome pathway. *Gene Dev* **9**:1586, 1995.

204. Treier M, Staszewski L, Bohmann D: Ubiquitin-dependent c-Jun degradation in vivo is mediated by the g domain. *Cell* **78**:787, 1994.

205. Willems AR, Lanker S, Patton EF, Craig KL, Nason TF, Kobayashi R, Wittenberg C, Tyers M: Cdc53 targets phosphorylated G1 cyclins for degradation by the ubiquitin proteolytic pathway. *Cell* **86**:453, 1996.

206. Pagano M, Tam SW, Theodoras A, Beer-Romero P, Del Sal G, Chau V, Yew R, Draetta G, Rolfe M: Role of the ubiquitin proteosome pathway in regulating abundance of the cyclin-dependent kinase inhibitor p27. *Science* **269**:682, 1995.

207. Plon S, Leppig KA, Do HN, Groudine M: Cloning of the human homolog of the CDC34 cell cycle gene by complementation in yeast. *Proc Natl Acad Sci USA* **90**:10484, 1993.

208. Kipreos E, Lander L, Wing J, He WW, Hedgecock E: cul-1 is required for cell cycle exit in C. elegans and identifies a novel gene family. *Cell* **85**:829, 1996.

209. Baserga R: *The Biology of Cell Reproduction.* Cambridge, MA, Harvard University Press, 1985.

210. Zetterberg A, Larson O: Kinetic analysis of regulatory events in G1 leading to proliferation of quiescence of Swiss 3T3 cells. *Proc Natl Acad Sci USA* **82**:5365, 1985.

211. Pardee AB: A restriction point for control of normal animal cell proliferation. *Proc Natl Acad Sci USA* **71**:1286, 1974.

212. Zetterberg A: Control of mammalian cell proliferation. *Curr Opinion Cell Biol* **2**:296, 1990.

213. Pardee AB: G1 events and regulation of cell proliferation. *Science* **246**:603, 1989.

214. Zetterberg A, Larsson O, Wiman K: What is the restriction point? *Curr Opinion Cell Biol* **7**:835, 1995.

215. Chao M: Growth factor signalling: Where is the specificity? *Cell* proteins. **68**:995, 1992.

216. Cantley L, Auger K, Carpenter C, Duckworth B, Graziani A, Kapeller R, Soltoff S: Oncogenes and signal transduction. *Cell* **64**:281, 1991.

217. Winston JT, Pledger WJ: Growth factor regulation of cyclin D1 mRNA expression through protein synthesis-dependent and -independent mechanisms. *Mol Biol Cell* **4**:1133, 1993.

218. Roussel MF, Theodoras AM, Pagano M, Sherr CJ: Rescue of defective mitogenic signaling by D-type cyclins. *Proc Natl Acad Sci USA* **92**:6837, 1995.

219. Albanese C, Johnson J, Watanabe G, Eklund N, Vu D, Arnold A, Pestell R: Transforming p21 ras mutants and c-Ets-2 activate the cyclin D1 promoter through distinguishable regions. *J Biol Chem* **270**:23589, 1995.

220. Hatakeyama M, Herrera R, Makela T, Dowdy S, Jacks T, Weinberg R: The cancer cell and the cell cycle clock. *Cold Spring Harbor Symp Quant Biol* **59**:1, 1994.

221. Roberts JM, Koff A, Polyak K, Firpo E, Collins S, Ohtsubo M, Massague J: Cyclins, cdks, and cyclin kinase inhibitors. *Cold Spring Harbor Symp Quant Biol* **59**:31, 1994.

222. Coats S, Flannagan WM, Nourse J, Roberts J: Requirement of p27Kip1 for restriction point control of the fibroblast cell cycle. *Science* **272**:877, 1996.

223. Nourse J, Firpo E, Flanagan M, Meyerson M, Polyak K, Lee MH, Massague J, Crabtree G, Roberts J: IL-2 mediated elimination of the p27kip1 cyclin-Cdk kinase inhibitor prevented by rapamycin. *Nature* **372**:570, 1994.

224. Firpo EJ, Koff A, Solomon M, Roberts J: Inactivation of a Cdk2 inhibitor during interleukin 2-induced proliferation of human T lymphocytes. *Mol Cell Biol* **14**:4889, 1994.

225. Fero ML, Rivkin M, Tasch M, Porter P, Carow CE, Firpo E, Polyak K, Tsai L, Broudy V, Perlmutter RM, Kaushansky K, Roberts JM: A syndrome of multi-organ hyperplasia with features of gigantism, tumorigenesis and female sterility in p27kip1-deficient mice. *Cell* **85**:733, 1996.

226. Matsushime H, Quelle D, Shurtleff S, Shibuya M, Sherr C, Kato JY: D-type cyclin-dependent kinase activity in mammalian cells. *Mol Cell Biol* **14**:2066, 1994.

227. Guadagno T, Ohtsubo M, Roberts J, Assoian R: A link between cyclin A expression and adhesion-dependent cell cycle progression. *Science* **262**:1572, 1993.

228. Zhu X, Ohtsubo M, Bohmer RM, Roberts JM, Assoian R: Adhesion-dependent cell cycle progression linked to the expression of cyclin D1 activation of cyclin E-cdk2 and phosphorylation of the retinoblastoma protein. *J Cell Biol* **133**:391, 1996.

229. Draetta G, Loef E: Transforming growth factor 1 inhibition of p34cdc2 phosphorylation and histone H1 kinase activity is associated with G1/S-phase growth arrest. *Mol Cell Biol* **11**:1185, 1991.

230. Koff A, Ohtsuki M, Polyack K, Roberts J, Massague J: Negative regulation of G1 in mammalian cells: Inhibition of cyclin E-dependent kinase by TGF-beta. *Science* **260**:536, 1993.

231. Laiho M, DeCaprio J, Ludlow J, Livingston D, Massague J: Growth inhibition by TGF-B linked to suppression of retinoblastoma protein phosphorylation. *Cell* **62**:175, 1990.

232. Reynisdottir I, Polyak K, Iavarone A, Massague J: Kip/Cip and Ink4Cdk inhibitors cooperate to induce cell cycle arrest in response to TGF-beta. *Gene Dev* **9**:1831, 1995.

233. Slingerland J, Hengst L, Pan C. Alexander D, Stampfer M, Reed S: A novel inhibitor of cyclin-cdk activity detected in transforming growth factor B-arrested epithelial cells. *Mol Cell Biol* **14**:3683, 1994.

234. Polyak K, Kato J, Solomon M, Sherr C, Massaque J, Roberts J, Koff A: p27kip1, a cyclin-cdk inhibitor, links transforming growth factor beta and contact inhibition to cell cycle arrest. *Gene Dev* **8**:9, 1994.

235. Kato JM, Matsuoka M, Polyak K, Massague J, Sherr CJ: Cyclic AMP-induced G1 phase arrest mediated by an inhibitor (p27Kip1) of cyclin-dependent kinase-4 activation. *Cell* **79**:487, 1994.

236. Brugarolas J, Chandrasekaran C, Gordon J, Beach D, Jacks T, Hannon G: Radiation-induced cell cycle arrest compromised by p21 deficiency. *Nature* **377**:552, 1995.

237. Deng C, Zhang P, Harper JW, Elledge S, Leder P: Mice lacking p21Cip1/Waf1 undergo normal development but are defective in G1 checkpoint control. *Cell* **82**:675, 1995.

238. Dulic V, Kaufman W, Wilson S, Tlsty T, Lees E, Harper JW, Elledge S, Reed S: p53-dependent inhibition of cyclin-dependent kinase activities in human fibroblasts during radiation-induced G1 arrest. *Cell* **76**:1013, 1994.

239. Massague J: TGF beta signalling: Receptors, transducers, and mad proteins. *Cell* **85**:947, 1996.

240. Hahn S, Schutte M, Hoque A, Moskaluk C, da Costa L, Rozenblum E, Weinstein C, Fischer A, Hruban R, Kern S: *Science* **271**:350, 1996.

241. Hannon G, Beach D: p15Ink4b is a potential effector of cell cycle arrest by TGFBeta. *Nature* **371**:257, 1994.

242. Ewen M, Sluss H, Whitehouse L, Livingston D: Cdk4 modulation by TGF-α leads to cell cycle arrest. *Cell* **74**:1009, 1993.

243. Kuerbitz S, Plunkett B, Walsh W, Kastan M: Wild-type p53 is a cell cycle checkpoint determinant following irradiation. *Proc Natl Acad Sci USA* **82**:7491, 1992.

244. Kastan M, Onyekwere O, Sidransky D, Vogelstein B, Craig R: Participating of p53 protin in the cellular response to DNA damage. *Cancer Res* **51**:6304, 1991.

245. Lane D: p53, guardian of the genome. *Nature* **358**:15, 1992.

246. Vogelstein B, Kinzler K: p53 function and dysfunction. *Cell* **70**:523, 1992.

247. Fields S, Jang S: Presence of a potent transcription activating sequence in the p53 protein. *Science* **249**:1046, 1990.

248. Kern S, Kinzler K, Bruskin A, Jarosz D, Friedman P, Prives C, Vogelstein B: Identification of p53 as a sequence specific DNA binding protein. *Science* **252**:1708, 1992.

249. Li R, Waga S, Hannon G, Beach D, Stillman B: Differential effects by the p21 cdk inhibitor on PCNA dependent DNA replication and DNA repair. *Nature* **371**:534, 1994.

250. Raff M: Size control: The regulation of cell numbers in animal development. *Cell* **86**:173, 1996.

251. Clurman BE, Roberts JM: Cell cycle and cancer. *J Natl Cancer Inst* **87**:1499, 1995.

252. Harlow E: An introduction to the puzzle. *Cold Spring Harbor Symp Quant Biol* **59**:709, 1994.

253. Hunter TJ, Pines J: Cyclins and cancer *Cell* **66**:1071, 1991.

254. Morgan D: Cell cycle control in neoplastic cells. *Cur Opinion Gen Dev* **2**:33, 1992.

255. Hall M, Peters G: Genetic alterations of cyclins, cyclin-dependent kinases, and CDK inhibitors in human cancer. *Adv Cancer Res* **68**:67, 1996.

256. Sherr C: Cancer cell cycles, *Science* **274**:1672, 1996.

257. Jiang WY, Zhang Y, Kahn SM, Hollstein M, Santella M, Lu S, Harris CC, Montesano R, Weinstein IB: Altered expression of the cyclin D1 and retinoblastoma genes in human esophageal cancer. *Proc Natl Acad Sci USA* **90**:9026, 1993.

258. Lee E, To H, Shew J, Bookstein R, Scully P, Lee WH: Inactivation of the retinoblastoma susceptibility gene in human breast cancers. *Science* **241**:218, 1988.

259. Mori T, Miura K, Aoki T, Nishihira T, Mori S, Nakamura Y: Frequent somatic mutation of the MTS1/CDK4I (multiple tumor suppressor/cyclin-dependent kinase 4 inhibitor) gene in esophageal squamous cell carcinoma. *Cancer Res* **54**:3396, 1994.

260. Kamb A, Gruis NA, Weaver-Feldhaus J, Liu Q, Harshman K, Tavtigian SV, Stockert E, Day RS III, Johnson BE, Skolnick MH: A cell cycle regulator potentially involved in genesis of many tumor types. *Science* **264**:436, 1994.

261. Sheaff R, Roberts J: Lessons in p16 from phylum Falconium. *Curr Biol* **5**:28, 1995.

262. Kawamata N, Morosetti R, Miller S, Park D, Spirin K, Nakamaki T, Takeuchi S, Hatta Y, Simpson J, Wilcyznski S, et al: Molecular analysis of the cyclin dependent kinase inhibitor gene p27/Kip1 in human malignancies. *Cancer Res* **55**:2266, 1995.

263. Keyomarsi K, O Leary N, Molnar G, Lees E, Fingert H, Pardee A: Cyclin E, a potential prognostic marker for breast cancer. *Cancer Res* **54**:380, 1994.

264. Pietenpol J, Bohlander S, Sato Y, Papadoupolos B, Liu C, Friedman B, Trask B, Roberts J, Kinzler K, Rowley J, Vogelstein B: Assignment of the human p27Kip1 gene to 12p13 and its analysis in leukemias. *Cancer Res* **55**:1206, 1995.

265. Ponce-Castenada M, Lee M, Latres E, Polyak K, Lacombe L, Montgomery K, Mathew S, Krauter K, Sheinfeld J, Massague J, et al: p27Kip1: Chromosomal mapping to 12p12-12p13.1 and absence of mutations in human tumors. *Cancer Res* **55**:1211, 1995.

266. Fearon E, Vogelstein B: A genetic model for colorectal tumorigenesis. *Cell* **61**:759, 1990.

18. Loeb L: Mutator phenotype may be required for multistage tumorigenesis. *Cancer Res* **54**:4590, 1990.

267. Knudson AG: Genetics of human cancer. *Annu Rev Genet* **20**:231, 1986.

268. Renan MJ: How many mutations are required for tumorigenesis? Implications from human cancer data. *Mol Carcinog* **7**:139, 1993.

269. Hartwell L, Weinert T, Kadyk L, Garvik B: Cell cycle checkpoint, genomic integrity, and cancer. *Cold Spring Harbor Symp Quant Biol* **59**:259, 1994.

270. Tlsty T, White A, Livanos E, Sage M, Roelofs H, Briot A, Poulose B: Genomic integrity and the genetics of cancer. *Cold Spring Harbor Symp Quant Biol* **59**:265, 1994.

271. Schmike R, Sherwood S, Hill A, Johnston R: Overreplication and recombination of DNA in higher eukaryotes: Potential consequences and biological implications. *Proc Natl Acad Sci USA* **83**:2157, 1986.

272. Nowell PC: The clonal evolution of tumor cell populations. *Science* **194**:23, 1976.

273. Weinert T, Hartwell L: The RAD9 gene controls the cell cycle response to DNA damage in Saccharomyces cerevisiae. *Science* **241**:317, 1989.

274. Dasso M, Newport J: Completion of DNA replication is monitored by a feedback system that controls the initiation of mitosis in vitro: Studies in Xenopus. *Cell* **61**:811–823, 1990.

275. Enoch T, Nurse P: Mutation of fission yeast cell cycle control genes abolishes dependence of mitosis on DNA replication. *Cell* **60**:665, 1990.

276. Rowley R, Hudson J, Young P: The wee1 protein kinase is required for radiation-induced mitotic delay. *Nature* **356**:353, 1992.

277. Smythe C, Newport J: Coupling of mitosis to the completion of S phase in Xenopus occurs via modulation of the tyrosine kinase that phosphorylates p34 CDC2. *Cell* **68**:787, 1992.

278. Walworth N, Davey S, Beach D: Fission yeast chk1 protein kinase links the rad checkpoint pathway to cdc2. *Nature* **363**:368, 1993.

279. Murray AW: The genetics of cell cycle checkpoints. *Curr Opin Genet Dev* **5**:5, 1995.

280. Sanchez Y, Elledge S: Stopped for repairs. *Bioessays* **17**:545, 1995.

281. Li R, Murray A: Feedback control of mitosis in budding yeast. *Cell* **66**:519, 1991.

282. Hoyt A, Totis L, Roberts BT: S cerevisiae genes required for cell cycle arrest in response to loss of microtubule function. *Cell* **66**:507, 1991.

283. Murray AW: Tense spindles can relax. *Nature* **373**:560, 1995.

284. Minshull J, Sun H, Tonks N, Murray AW: A MAP kinase-dependent spindle assembly checkpoint in Xenopus egg extracts. *Cell* **79**:475, 1994.

285. Lin J, Wu X, Chen J, Chang A, Levine AJ: Functions of the p53 protein in growth regulation and tumor suppression. *Cold Spring Harbor Symp Quant Biol* **59**:215, 1994.

286. Barlow C, Hirotsune S, Paylor R, Liyanage M, Eckhaus M, Collins F, Shiloh Y, Crawley J, Ried T, Tagle D, Wynshaw-Boris A: Atm-deficient mice: A paradigm of ataxia telangiectasia. *Cell* **85**:159, 1996.

287. Meyn MS: Ataxia-telangiectasia and cellular responses to DNA damage. *Cancer Res* **55**:5991, 1995.

CHAPTER 9

Apoptosis and Cancer

Charles M. Rudin ▪ Craig B. Thompson

1. *Apoptosis* is a descriptive term for the phenotype of cells undergoing programmed cell death. Apoptosis is a critical component of development and homeostasis in multicellular eukaryotic organisms. Apoptotic cell death can be distinguished from necrotic cell death by several criteria, including the characteristic morphology and the absence of a resulting inflammatory reaction.

2. The Bcl-2 family of proteins plays a central role in apoptotic control and is conserved evolutionarily. The realization that Bcl-2 functions to prevent apoptosis defined a new category of oncogene: the antiapoptotic gene. Apoptotic regulation is dependent on the relative balance of opposing Bcl-2 family members. Those family members may function by regulating homeostasis between key intracellular organelles and the cytoplasm.

3. The ICE-related proteases are evolutionarily conserved regulators of apoptosis. Control of ICE-related protease activity is dependent on proteolytic processing of cytoplasmic proenzymes. Some proteases have autocatalytic potential. The critical downstream targets of ICE family proteolysis have not been defined.

4. Many cell surface receptors, including the tumor necrosis factor receptor (TNFR) family, have been shown to modify the apoptotic sensitivity of cells. Different members of the TNFR family can promote or inhibit apoptosis. An apoptotic signaling pathway from one of these receptors, Fas, has been traced by direct protein–protein interaction from receptor engagement to ICE-related protease activation.

5. Cellular and viral oncogenes that stimulate proliferation are strong inducers of apoptosis. This induction of apoptosis probably is dependent on cell cycle checkpoints (tumor suppressor gene products) that detect abnormally replicating cells and trigger apoptosis. Inhibition of apoptosis therefore is frequently an essential step in the process of oncogenesis.

6. Anticancer therapies induce apoptosis in sensitive cells. Inhibition of apoptosis is a major mechanism of chemotherapeutic resistance. Chemotherapy may accelerate the mutagenesis rate and promote aneuploidy of tumors in which apoptosis has been suppressed. New therapies directed at modifying apoptotic signaling pathways may be helpful in circumventing these problems.

INTRODUCTION

The term *programmed cell death* refers to the induction of cell death by a regulated pathway inherent to the cell. It can be contrasted with necrotic cell death, which is traumatic and depends on factors entirely external to the cell. *Apoptosis* (from the Greek for falling leaves) is a descriptive term that originally was used to describe the characteristic phenotype of cells that die in the absence of evident trauma. The apoptotic phenotype has been found to be so ubiquitous among cells undergoing programmed cell death that the terms are now used interchangeably. Wyllie and colleagues in the early 1970s were among the first to observe and record a phenotype of dying cells that appeared to be conserved among widely disparate cell types and was distinct in many respects from necrotic cell death.[1,2] These initial descriptive studies spawned an enormous field of inquiry with direct implications for many problematic areas of medicine, including neurodevelopmental and neurodegenerative disease, infection, autoimmunity, and cancer.[3–7]

The study of apoptosis has had an important impact on the understanding of organismal growth and differentiation. The characteristic features of the process are conserved widely among multicellular eukaryotes.[8,9] The capacity to initiate an apoptotic pathway appears to be a shared feature of all the cells of the body, including rapidly cycling populations such as leukocytes and long-lived cells such as neurons. Apoptosis plays a crucial role in development, permitting the necessary elimination of surplus cells in the formation of many complex organs, including the brain.[10]

Several morphologic features of apoptotic cells distinguish them from cells that die in response to trauma or hypoxia.[2] Necrotic cell death is characterized by cell swelling and gross disruption of organelles and the cell membrane. Apoptotic cell death is characterized by cell contraction, blebbing of the cytoplasmic membrane, dense condensation of the nucleus, and a pathognomonic autodigestion of the genome into fragments that correspond in size to multiples of the amount of DNA found in individual nucleosomes. If electrophoresed through a polyacrylamide gel, DNA from an apoptotic cell therefore can be displayed as a ladder, with rungs corresponding to cleavage between one, two, or multiple nucleosome elements (Fig. 9-1).

Traumatic cell death leads to leakage of intracellular contents and the generation of a potent inflammatory response that is dependent on multiple cytokines and pyrogens. This response may be critical to confining infection as well as to wound healing and scar formation. In contrast, apoptotic cell death does not lead to cytokine release or the generation of an inflammatory response. Apoptotic cell remnants are recognized and engulfed by adjacent cells (frequently by cells that are not part of the phagocytic

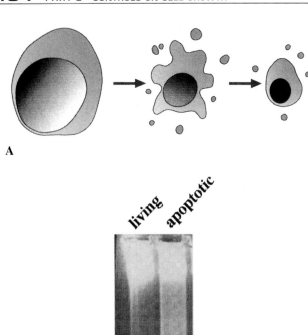

A

living apoptotic

B

FIG. 9-1 Characteristic cellular changes of apoptosis. *A.* Typical morphologic changes of apoptosis are shown, including blebbing of the cytoplasmic membrane, cell contraction, and marked condensation of the nucleus. Importantly, cytoplasmic contents are not spilled into the extracellular space. *B.* Polyacrylamide gel electrophoresis of genomic DNA from apoptotic cells. A pathognomonic laddering of DNA fragments in approximately 200-base pair increments is seen, corresponding to the amount of DNA contained within individual nucleosomes. The cells are murine lymph node cells after 0 h (living) and 48 h (apoptotic) in culture. (*Image courtesy of Patricia Noel.*)

macophage/monocyte system) without initiating an inflammatory cascade.[11–13] The ability to delete cells in an immunologically silent manner is of central importance in permitting the natural turnover and remodeling of tissues without risking autoimmune disease.

Homeostasis in any cell population requires a balance between the processes of cell proliferation and cell death (Fig. 9-2). Accumulation of abnormal numbers of a clonally related population (neoplasm) can result from either uncontrolled proliferation or inhibition of cell death. The regulatory mechanisms that control cell proliferation clearly are extensive and have been the primary focus of research on carcinogenesis for many years. Recently, it has become apparent that the mechanisms of programmed cell death are also tightly regulated, highly responsive to extracellular signals, and similarly integral to the inhibition of carcinogenesis. This

chapter outlines the known mechanisms that regulate cell death and some of the implications of dysregulated cell death on carcinogenesis and chemotherapeutic resistance.

BCL-2 AND THE ORIGINS OF THE STUDY OF APOPTOSIS AND CANCER

The *bcl-2* gene (for B-cell lymphoma/leukemia-2) initially was identified as the gene on chromosome 18q21 at the breakpoint of the t(14;18) chromosomal translocation found in the majority of B-cell follicular lymphomas (Fig. 9-3).[14–17] This genomic rearrangement juxtaposes the *bcl-2* gene with the immunoglobulin heavy chain gene enhancer, leading to marked up-regulation and constitutive expression of the *bcl-2* gene in lymphoid cells. The coding sequence of Bcl-2 is not altered by this translocation.

The role of Bcl-2 in oncogenesis remained obscure for several years after its discovery. Unlike all previously identified oncogenes, overexpression of the *bcl-2* gene did not increase the proliferative potential of cells in any of the commonly used assays for oncogenic transformation, which depend on a modulation of the growth rate of the transfected cell. The failure to induce rampant growth correlates with the phenotype of most follicular lymphomas, which have an indolent, slowly progressive natural history, have low proliferative indices, and retain many of the phenotypic characteristics of nontransformed lymphocytes.[18]

The first association between Bcl-2 and inhibition of cell death was made in 1988.[19] Stable *bcl-2* transformants of a cell line dependent on the growth factor interleukin-3 (IL-3) were found to survive for prolonged periods after withdrawal of IL-3, much longer than the parental cell line lacking the upregulated *bcl-2* gene. In addition, Bcl-2 was shown to cooperate with a more traditional oncoprotein, c-myc, to immortalize pre-B cells (see below). Bcl-2 subsequently has been found to be a potent inhibitor of apoptosis in a wide variety of experimental systems.[20]

The discovery of the function of Bcl-2 challenged the prevailing view of carcinogenesis and defined a new category of oncogene.[21] Research on oncogenesis had focused largely on the mechanisms regulating cell proliferation: Cancer was thought to arise from the products of abnormally expressed genes driving cell replication (oncogenes) or failing to inhibit cell replication (tumor suppressor genes). Bcl-2, which is overexpressed by the most common chromosomal rearrangement in lymphoid malignancy, was found to have no direct effect on replication but caused a failure to die. This realization implied for the first time that alteration of either side of the homeostatic balance can contribute not only to cell accumulation but also to carcinogenesis. Subsequent work by many groups has confirmed the carcinogenic potential of antiapoptotic gene dysregulation and has led to a broader view of the types of genetic alterations that contribute to cancer.

To place the effects of apoptotic dysregulation in cancer cells in context, the next sections summarize the current understanding of the mechanisms that regulate apoptosis in normal cells.

THE CENTRAL APOPTOTIC PATHWAY

C. elegans and the Evolutionary Conservation of Apoptotic Regulators

The striking morphologic similarity between disparate cell types undergoing apoptosis suggests that the underlying molecular

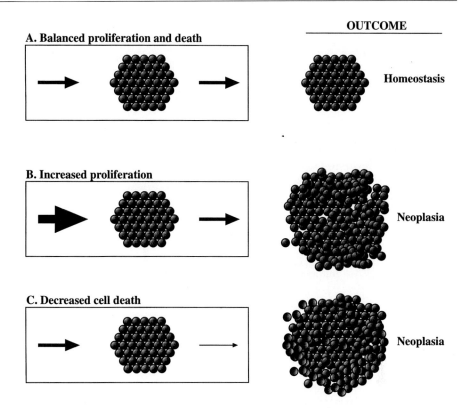

OUTCOME

A. Balanced proliferation and death

Homeostasis

B. Increased proliferation

Neoplasia

C. Decreased cell death

Neoplasia

FIG. 9-2 Dysregulation of either side of the homeostatic balance can lead to neoplasia. *A.* A population of cells in homeostatic balance replicates and dies at equal rates. Mutations that result in either an increase in the proliferative rate (*B*) or a decrease in the death rate (*C*) can lead to the accumulation of clonally related cells.

processes may be similar.[22] Many of the features of this central apoptotic control system have been defined, and the outline of this pathway provides insight into potential mechanisms for viral and cellular oncogenic transformation (Fig. 9-4).

The critical factors involved in the control of apoptosis have been defined best in the nematode *Caenorhabditis elegans*. Every cell division and cell death event in the normal pathway of *C. elegans* development is known, and this developmental pathway follows a determined, predictable program.[23] All of the 131 programmed cell death events in the developing worm are dependent on the normal function of three proteins: Ced-3, Ced-4, and Ced-9. Loss of Ced-3 or Ced-4 function or a gain-of-function mutation of the Ced-9 protein will lead to complete abrogation of cell death in *C. elegans* development.[24,25] Loss of Ced-9 function leads to in-

creased apoptotic cell death.[25] Ced-9 appears to function by suppressing inappropriate activity of Ced-3 and Ced-4.[26]

Strong evolutionary pressures would be expected to preserve the mechanisms involved in a process as fundamental to the organism as the control of cell death. Many of the proteins central to apoptotic control indeed have been highly conserved, from the roundworm to the human. Ced-9 is highly homologous to mammalian Bcl-2.[27,28] Bcl-2 expression in *C. elegans* mimics a Ced-9 gain-of-function and partially can revert a Ced-9 loss-of-function mutant. Ced-3 was found by database searching to be related to the mammalian interleukin-1b converting enzyme, ICE.[29] As discussed below, ICE-related proteins have been found to play a central role in apoptotic regulation. No mammalian homologue of Ced-4 has been identified.

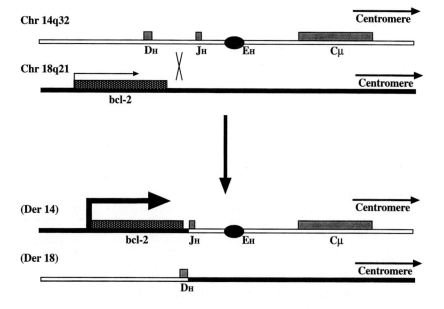

Chr 14q32

D_H   J_H   E_H   Centromere   Cμ

Chr 18q21

Centromere

bcl-2

(Der 14)

bcl-2   J_H   E_H   Centromere   Cμ

(Der 18)

Centromere

D_H

FIG. 9-3 The t(14;18) translocation characteristic of follicular lymphomas. Exons of the immunoglobulin heavy chain gene are represented by light boxes, the *bcl-2* gene by a dark box, and the heavy chain enhancer by a black oval. The translocation involves sites in the immunoglobulin heavy chain locus that normally are involved in the rearrangements necessary to generate a functional heavy chain gene and probably occurs in the pre-B-cell stage. The breakpoint in the *bcl-2* gene frequently is in the 3′ untranslated region and thus does not affect the coding sequence.

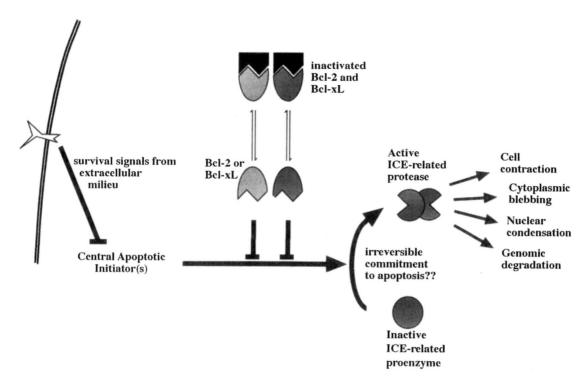

FIG. 9-4 A hypothetical model of the central apoptotic pathway. Initiation of apoptosis is held in check by survival signals received by cell surface receptors. Removal of the cell from its in vivo context or blockade of these survival signals allows induction of the apoptotic pathway, resulting in ICE-related protease activation and the characteristic morphologic changes of apoptosis. Activation of this pathway is inhibited by Bcl-2 and Bcl-x$_L$. This inhibition in turn can be overcome by interaction with proapoptotic Bcl-2 related molecules. The relative positions of the Bcl-2 family members and ICE proteases in this schema are hypothetical. Bcl-2 family members have been shown to act downstream of at least some ICE proteases. Other important apoptotic initiators include cell surface receptor-mediated cell death, DNA damage, cell cycle dysregulation, and metabolic alterations. (*Used with permission from Annual Reviews of Medicine, vol. 48, copyright 1997 Annual Reviews Inc.*)

The Bcl-2 Family

Bcl-2 overexpression is capable of inhibiting cell death in response to many disparate apoptotic signals, suggesting that it acts as the convergence of many apoptotic pathways. Bcl-2 has been found to be one of a family of related proteins, several members of which appear to play important positive and negative roles in the control of apoptosis (Table 9-1). Bcl-x was the second gene in this family to be identified.[30] The *bcl-x* gene encodes at least two protein products, differentiated by alternative mRNA splicing, that have opposite effects on apoptotic induction. The full-length Bcl-x$_L$ is homologous to Bcl-2 and has a similar ability to inhibit cell death by multiple pathways. The truncated Bcl-x$_S$ protein is able to inhibit the action of either Bcl-2 or Bcl-x$_L$ and enhances the apoptotic sensitivity of the cell. Other proapoptotic family members include Bax, Bak, and Bad, which have been shown to heterodimerize with Bcl-2 and/or Bcl-x$_L$.[31–36] Like Bcl-2, Bcl-x$_L$ has been found to be overexpressed in several tumor types.

The mechanism of action of the Bcl-2 family members has not been determined, although several important insights have been established. The structure of Bcl-x$_L$ has been determined by x-ray crystallography and NMR spectroscopy.[37] The molecular structure of Bcl-x$_L$ surprisingly is similar to that of members of the colicin family of bacterial proteins. Colicins are proteins secreted by bacteria that form pores in the surface membranes of other bacterial strains, causing cell death.[38] The relevance of this unexpected structural link between families of proteins involved in mammalian and bacterial cell death is unclear.

Bcl-2 appears to be localized to the mitochondrial outer membrane.[39–41] Recent studies have associated commitment to apoptotic cell death with loss of mitochondrial membrane potential and have shown that the membrane potential gradient can be maintained by Bcl-2 overexpression.[42–45] Many of the characteristic nuclear changes of apoptosis can be induced by the addition of dATP and cytochrome c to cytoplasmic extracts in vitro.[46] As cytochrome c normally is tightly sequestered within mitochondria, Bcl-2 family members may function by directly controlling mitochondrial membrane permeability. This model is made more attractive by the observation that mitochondria probably are derived from ancient prokaryotes, suggesting that the similarity between Bcl-2 and colicins may be meaningful.

The ICE Protease Family

Another group of proteins that has been implicated strongly in the central apoptotic pathway is the ICE-related protein family.[47,48] The ICE-related proteins, including Ced-3, are cysteine proteases that cleave at aspartate residues in a defined amino acid context. The family has at least nine mammalian members, which can be subgrouped on the basis of relatedness and target specificity (Table 9-2). Overexpression of most ICE-related proteases has been shown to trigger apoptosis in cell lines. A central role for this family of proteases in the process of apoptosis in mammalian

Table 9-1 Mammalian Bcl-2-Related Proteins

Antiapoptotic	Proapoptotic	Unclassified
Bcl-2	Bax	Mcl1
Bcl-x$_L$	Bak	Al
	Bad	
	Bcl-x$_S$	

cells has been suggested by studies using specific inhibitors of ICE-related proteases, which prevent apoptosis in response to many of the known triggers of programmed cell death.[49,50] These inhibitors include viral products such as p35 and crmA (see below) as well as synthetic oligopeptides that occupy and block the protease activity site.

Regulation of ICE-related protease activity may occur on several levels. All the ICE-related proteins are synthesized as larger inactive proenzymes that must undergo proteolytic processing to the active enzymatic form.[51] The cleavage sites in several of these proenzymes are consistent with processing by ICE-related proteases. High local concentrations of some ICE family members may be sufficient to permit autocatalysis and activation.[52] The processing sites of other family members (e.g., CPP32) are target sites for different ICE-related proteases, suggesting a sequential cascade of protease activation. Initial activation of an ICE-related protease may generate a rapidly and irreversibly amplified signal by initiating autocatalysis as well as triggering activation of downstream proteases. An additional layer of regulation may derive from alternate mRNA splicing. At least four of the ICE-related protease genes encode truncated forms as well as full-length proteases.[53–56] These truncated proteins may down-regulate protease activity by directly inhibiting the active proteases or by binding and stabilizing the proenzyme forms.

Despite strong evidence for the central position of this protein family in apoptosis, defining the roles and relative importance of the various ICE-related proteases has been difficult. There are many related (and possibly functionally similar) family members and few known downstream targets. Homozygous inactivation of the ICE gene in mice generated only select defects in apoptotic induction, suggesting functional redundancy among ICE-related proteases.[57,58] One of the known targets for the subset of ICE-related proteases most similar to Ced-3 is poly-ADP ribose polymerase (PARP), an enzyme involved in genomic repair and integrity.[59] The ICE-related proteases CPP32, FLICE, and ICE-LAP6 can all cleave PARP.[56,60,61] PARP processing has been used as a marker for the nuclear changes associated with apoptosis, but PARP cleavage recently was shown to be neither necessary nor sufficient for apoptosis.[62,63]

CELL SURFACE SIGNALS AFFECTING APOPTOSIS

Survival of most cells in the body is highly dependent on their environment.[9] Cells removed from their in vivo context frequently undergo rapid apoptosis. This suggests that in their natural context many cells continuously receive extracellular signals that decrease their apoptotic sensitivity. These survival signals may be generated by direct cell–cell contact or by locally diffused soluble factors. Externally derived factors that may increase or decrease apoptotic sensitivity include growth factors, cytokines, interleukins, glucocorticoids, androgens and estrogens, and neurotransmitters. The

cell membrane receptors that affect apoptotic sensitivity and the resultant intracellular signaling pathways initiated by engagement of these receptors are being studied intensively.

The largest family of cell surface receptors that affect apoptotic sensitivity are related to the tumor necrosis factor (TNF) receptors.[64] The family includes the two receptors for TNF (TNFR1 and TNFR2) and at least 10 other related receptors. All TNFR family members have related cysteine-rich extracellular domains, each of which interacts with one of a family of TNF-related signaling proteins. The intracellular domains of these receptors differ widely, suggesting that different signaling pathways may be initiated by engagement of each receptor. Different family members are capable of producing opposing signals, and in fact engagement of a single receptor may have different effects in different contexts. In many experimental systems, engagement of some family members (e.g., Fas, TNFR1) promotes apoptosis, whereas engagement of others (e.g., CD30, CD40, TNFR2) promotes survival.

Proapoptotic Signaling

The proapoptotic receptors Fas and TNFR1 share a related sequence in their C-terminal cytoplasmic tails known as the death domain (Fig. 9-5). Three cytoplasmic proteins have been isolated on the basis of their ability to associate with these receptors.[65–67] These proteins—RIP, TRADD, and FADD—all contain death domains responsible for association with the receptor tails. RIP and FADD associate most strongly with Fas, and TRADD binds to TNFR1. Overexpression of any of these proteins can initiate apoptosis.

FADD contains a unique N-terminal effector domain that is required for apoptotic induction.[65] In contrast, apoptotic signaling by RIP and TRADD is dependent only on the death domains, suggesting that these proteins may function primarily by recruitment of FADD or a similar effector protein to an activated receptor. TRADD serves as a link between TNFR1 engagement and multiple downstream signaling pathways.[68] The TNFR1–TRADD complex engages TRAF2 (see below), leading to NFκB activation, and also recruits FADD through association of death domains. Mutation of the FADD effector domain blocks TNFR1-mediated apoptosis; although the association between FADD and TNFR1 may be predominantly indirect (i.e., through TRADD), FADD is integral to apoptotic signaling from TNFR1.

Recently, FADD was shown to recruit an ICE family protease named FLICE (or Mach) to the activated Fas receptor.[69,70] FLICE binds FADD through an N-terminal domain homologous to the effector domain of FADD. Mutation of the ICE-related domain of FLICE blocks apoptosis in response to engagement of either Fas or TNFR1, suggesting that FLICE may be a component of both receptor complexes.[69] Activated FLICE may initiate a cascade of cysteine protease activation, leading to apoptosis. ICE activation has been implicated in this cascade; ICE-deficient mice have a selective defect in Fas-mediated apoptosis.[57,58]

Antiapoptotic Signaling

Other members of the TNFR family of cell surface receptors mediate signals that increase the apoptotic threshold of a cell. These receptors, including TNFR2, CD30, and CD40, interact with a family of related intracellular proteins known as TNF receptor-associated factors (TRAFs). TRAF1, TRAF2, and TRAF3 (CRAF1, CD40bp, CAP-1, LAP-1) have been studied the most extensively.[71–75] Two additional related proteins—CART1 and TRAF5—have been identified, but the binding properties of these factors, have not been defined.[76,77]

Table 9-2 Mammalian ICE Family Proteases

Ced-3 Subfamily	ICE Subfamily	NEDD-2 Subfamily
CPP32 (Yama/Apopain)	ICE	ICH-1
ICE-LAP3		
(Mch3/CMH-1)	ICE rel II (ICH2/TX)	NEDD-2 (mouse)
Mch2	ICE rel III	
FLICE (Mach)		
ICE-LAP6		

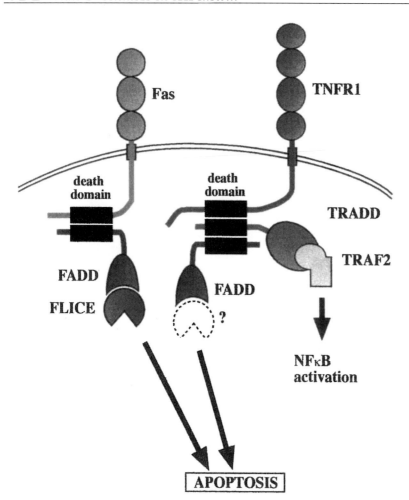

FIG. 9-5 Signaling complexes associated with the proapoptotic TNFR family members. Receptor engagement by extracellular ligand promotes receptor multimerization and initiates formation of the depicted complexes, recruiting FADD by direct interaction or through the intermediary TRADD. An ICE-related protease has not been directly associated with the TNFR1 receptor complex, but mutations of the protease domain of FLICE block TNFR1-mediated apoptosis. This suggests that FLICE plays a role in both apoptotic signaling pathways. (*Adapted from and used with permission from Annual Reviews of Medicine, vol. 48, copyright 1997 Annual Reviews, Inc.*)

TRAF proteins may form homo- or heterodimers and associate with multiple sites in the TNFR family cytoplasmic tails. TRAF1 has been shown to bind directly only to CD30 but forms indirect associations with other receptors through heterodimerization with TRAF2.[71,78] TRAF2 binds directly to TNFR2, CD30, and CD40. TRAF3 also binds directly to multiple receptors.[72–75,78] TRAF2 has been shown in some experimental systems to induce NFκB activation, whereas TRAF3 may suppress NFκB activity either directly or by inhibition of TRAF2 function.[79]

The association between TRAF binding and antiapoptotic signaling by these receptors is primarily correlative. The intracellular domains of the TNFR family of proteins are remarkably dissimilar, suggesting that proteins other than the TRAFs are involved in the signaling complexes. The effects of ligand binding to these receptors probably are dependent on many variables, including the relative numbers of (potentially competing) receptors, the particular set of intracellular second messengers available to associate with these receptors, and the downstream targets present in a given cell.

VIRAL MIMICRY AND APOPTOTIC INHIBITION

Apoptosis is an important defense against many types of viral infection. Cell suicide in response to viral infection may both inhibit successful viral replication in lytic infections and defend against viral transformation. Viruses have adapted methods to suppress apoptosis in the host that provide insight into the critical components of apoptotic regulation. Several viral proteins that regulate TNF-related signal transduction of ICE protease activity or mimic Bcl-2 activity have been identified. The fact that viruses have evolved these ways of preventing host cell death underscores the central importance of these molecules in regulating cell survival.

Recently, a family of four mammalian proteins related to the baculovirus inhibitor of apoptosis (IAP) was identified.[80–85] Baculoviruses are small DNA viruses that infect insect cells. Baculoviral IAP inhibits apoptosis in mammalian as well as insect cells, again demonstrating the evolutionary conservation of apoptotic pathways. Two IAP-related mammalian proteins, cIAP-1 and cIAP-2, were identified as proteins associating with the TNFR2/TRAF2/TRAF1 complex. A third IAP-related protein, ILP, has been shown to be a potent inhibitor of apoptosis when it is overexpressed in mammalian cells, whereas mutations in the fourth, NAIP, have been implicated in the pathogenesis of the neurodegenerative disorder spinal muscular atrophy. The binding properties of the various IAP-related proteins are distinct, and their relative roles in signaling pathways inhibiting apoptosis have not been determined. They may constitute an important link between TNFR family member ligand binding and antiapoptotic effect.

Baculovirus encodes another potent inhibitor of apoptosis, p35, that functions as a specific inhibitor of ICE-related proteases.[80] The cowpox crmA protein, although unrelated, has a similar function.[86] Mammalian proteins related to these potent and specific inhibitors have not been identified.

A number of viruses encode Bcl-2 homologues, including Epstein-Barr virus (EBV), African swine fever virus, and adenovirus.[87–89] The adenovirus homologue, E1B 19kDa, has low sequence similarity to Bcl-2 but was used as a probe to identify three novel proteins that also interact with Bcl-2.[87] These proteins may play important roles in the regulation and/or function of Bcl-2, and the low sequence conservation may help define functional domains of Bcl-2.

EBV has been linked causally to infectious mononucleosis, Burkitt lymphoma, nasopharyngeal carcinoma, AIDS-related lymphomas, and posttransplant lymphoproliferative disorder.[90] One of the necessary components of EBV transformation is the latent membrane protein LMP1. LMP1 is a transmembrane protein that is recognized and bound by the TRAF proteins and may function in part by mimicking an occupied TNFR-related antiapoptotic receptor.[72] LMP-1 inhibits apoptosis of infected lymphocytes and up-regulates endogenous Bcl-2.[91] The intracellular domain of LMP1 is complex and may activate multiple signaling pathways. BHRF1, the EBV-encoded Bcl-2 homologue, is not expressed in viral latency and therefore is unlikely to play a role in viral transformation. This protein may be critical in preventing host cell apoptosis in the lytic cycle of the virus.

ONCOGENES AND APOPTOTIC INDUCTION

A cell may acquire mutations in any of a variety of known oncogenes that in theory would confer a growth advantage to that cell. To prevent the development of neoplasia, the body must have potent mechanisms by which to inactivate such cells. Immune surveillance may play a role in detecting such transformants, but recent evidence suggests that apoptosis plays a much more critical role: The outgrowth of such potential tumor cells may be prevented by the induction of a suicide response within a premalignant cell. The isolated up-regulation of many oncogenes has been demonstrated to result in host cell apoptosis.

Cellular Oncogenes

The proto-oncogene that has been most clearly associated with apoptotic induction is c-*myc*. The c-*myc* gene encodes a transcription factor that is up-regulated in many transformed cells and induces rapid cell proliferation.[92] However, isolated c-*myc* overexpression results in apoptosis.[19,93–95] Concomitant overexpression of the *bcl-2* gene prevents apoptosis, resulting in an immortalized, transformed phenotype.[19,95] Overexpression of both c-*myc* and *bcl-2* in lymphocytes of transgenic mice results in synergistic tumorigenesis, generating lymphoid tumors much more rapidly than either transgene alone. c-myc-induced apoptosis in fibroblasts can be prevented by cytokines such as insulin-like growth factor-1 and by high-serum growth conditions.[96]

Two models of c-myc function have been proposed to explain these findings (Fig. 9-6).[96] The conflict model proposes that c-myc generates a purely growth-promoting signal. Under favorable conditions, this leads to cell proliferation, but under adverse conditions, a conflict between proliferative and inhibitory signals is generated, resulting in the triggering of apoptosis. The dual signal model proposes that c-myc concurrently generates both proliferative and apoptotic signals. Proliferation then requires the suppression of apoptosis either by cytokine signaling or by expression of antiapoptotic genes such as *bcl-2*.

The t(1;19) chromosomal translocation associated with childhood pre-B-cell leukemia generates a chimeric E2A-PBX1 transcription factor. Transgenic mice with this fusion gene under lymphocyte-specific expression demonstrate increased numbers of

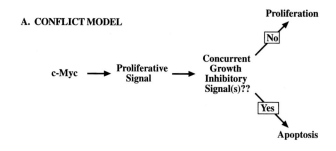

A. CONFLICT MODEL

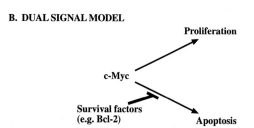

B. DUAL SIGNAL MODEL

FIG. 9-6 Two models of the signaling pathways of c-myc. *A.* The conflict model proposes that c-myc generates a purely proliferative signal. Under unfavorable growth conditions, the cell produces inhibitory factors to prevent proliferation. This conflict of opposing signals affecting cell cycle progression results in an apoptotic response. Under favorable growth conditions, no conflict arises, and the cell proliferates. *B.* The dual signal model proposes that c-myc, generates two signals, one proliferative and the other apoptotic. Proliferation in response to c-myc expression is dependent on suppression of the apoptotic response by survival signals. These signals may be generated by growth factors or antiapoptotic gene up-regulation.

cycling lymphocyte precursors but also widespread apoptosis in the same populations, resulting in greatly diminished numbers of lymphocytes.[97] All animals died of malignant leukemia/lymphoma within 5 months, presumably because of the outgrowth of cells that acquire secondary mutation(s) that prevent apoptosis.

Viral Oncogenes

Several viral oncogenes also provide insight into the association of oncogene expression with apoptosis. Human papillomavirus has been implicated as a causative agent in cervical carcinoma and other anogenital cancers. Oncogenic papillomaviruses encode a protein, E7, that inactivates the retinoblastoma gene product and is a potent stimulant of cell cycle progression.[98] E7 expression alone causes rapid induction of the cellular p53 gene (which is involved in cell cycle regulation and apoptotic induction; see below), resulting in apoptotic cell death. These viruses encode a second protein, E6, which binds to and inactivates p53, preventing cell death and thus permitting oncogenic transformation. E7 also induces apoptosis by a p53-independent pathway that is poorly understood; E6 has been shown to be similarly effective in circumventing this p53-independent apoptosis in p53-negative cells.[99]

Adenovirus E1A is another oncogenic protein that induces rapid cell proliferation in transfected cells. Like papillomavirus E7 protein, the adenovirus E1A protein alone is not transforming, because it strongly triggers apoptosis.[100] Viral oncogenes is dependent on the concurrent expression of the E1B gene, which encodes two factors that may both help circumvent apoptosis. E1B 19kDa encodes a Bcl-2 homologue, and E1B 55kDa binds to and inactivates p53.[87,101]

Tumor Suppressor Genes

Tumor suppressor gene function has been found to be much more strongly linked to apoptosis than had been imagined initially. Tumor suppressors, such as p53 and the retinoblastoma gene product pRb, participate in cell cycle regulation and can inhibit proliferation by causing stage-specific cell cycle pauses or arrests known as checkpoints.[102] Cell cycle checkpoints are thought to function to permit the repair of DNA damage and to ensure integrity of the genome before cell cycle progression. It is recognized increasingly that in addition to inhibiting the cell cycle progression of abnormal cells, checkpoints are involved in triggering apoptosis to delete potentially abnormal cells from the body.

p53 is the most commonly mutated gene in human malignancy, and germ line heterozygous mutation (the Li-Fraumeni syndrome) is associated with high rates of tumorigenesis in many tissues.[103] The p53 protein is a sequence-specific transcription factor that normally is present at very low levels but is up-regulated rapidly by DNA damage or viral infection. p53 induction in response to DNA damage causes a G1-specific cell cycle arrest.[104]

The association between p53 and apoptosis has been demonstrated in vivo and in vitro. Transfection of wild-type p53 into p53-negative tumors results in apoptosis in both solid and hematologic malignancies.[105,106] Loss of p53 in the evolution of experimentally induced tumors of the choroid plexus correlates directly with loss of apoptosis in vivo.[107] Thymocytes from mice with homozygous p53 inactivation demonstrate greatly increased resistance to apoptosis in response to gamma radiation and chemotherapeutic agents.[108,109]

How p53 activation triggers apoptosis is unknown. p53 has been shown to directly up-regulate the transcription of bax, a proapoptotic member of the *bcl-2* gene family.[110] However, Bax-deficient mice carry out p53-dependent apoptosis normally, implying that Bax regulation cannot be the primary mechanism of p53-dependent apoptotic signaling.[111] The mechanism of apoptosis induction by p53 may be indirect; strong inhibition of cell cycle progression in a cell primed for proliferation may generate a dichotomy of signals, resulting in activation of a default suicide pathway as proposed in the conflict model for c-myc (Fig. 9-6).

The retinoblastoma gene product pRb also functions as a cell cycle regulator and is inactivated in many human tumors.[112] The pRb protein interacts with at least three members of the E2F family of transcription factors, inhibiting E2F activity and preventing entry into S phase of the cell cycle. Phosphorylation of pRb by cyclin-dependent kinases releases the E2F factors, permitting E2F-mediated transcriptional regulation and S-phase entry.

Mutations of one Rb allele in mice and humans increases the likelihood of tumorigenesis in many tissues. Homozygous knock-out of the Rb gene in mice is embryonic lethal, causing massive apoptosis in the brain.[113,114] Analogously to c-*myc*, dysregulation of the controls on cell cycle progression generates not only rapid proliferation but also concurrent apoptotic induction.

The Link between Proliferative Signals and Apoptosis

In the examples of cellular and viral oncogenes discussed earlier, a surprisingly tight association was found between oncogenic proliferative signals and the triggering of apoptosis. Studies of c-myc variants have been unsuccessful in separating the proliferative and apoptotic signals generated by this protein.[93,115] The same regions of c-myc that are essential for proliferation are essential for apoptosis. Incremental increases in c-myc expression cause parallel increases in both proliferative and apoptotic signals. Both signals are equally dependent on c-myc binding to its partner, Max. This

unanticipated feature of oncogene activation suggests a fundamental mechanism for avoiding malignant transformation. Gene expression that generates potent proliferative signals may coordinately increase the apoptotic susceptibility of the cell, resulting in cell death unless strong antiapoptotic signals are present. A major function of cell cycle regulatory pathways may be to inextricably link proliferative induction to increased apoptotic sensitivity.

APOPTOSIS AND THE MULTIHIT MODEL OF ONCOGENESIS

The multihit model of oncogenesis holds that multiple genetic mutations must occur within a single cell to produce fully malignant transformation. The fact that many potentially oncogenic mutations trigger apoptosis suggests that mutations that inhibit apoptotic control are necessary for tumor cells to grow to sufficient mass to cause problems for the host. In order for the c-*myc* gene to be transforming, a prior event must have occurred to prevent apoptotic induction. Rb inactivation alone may promote p53-dependent cell death rather than tumorigenesis unless apoptosis in inhibited. Activation of oncogenes and inactivation of tumor suppressor genes may be insufficient to promote significant expansion of tumor cells without the tumor cell also acquiring defects in its ability to undergo apoptosis. Mutations in genes that affect apoptosis also may be central to the ability of tumor cells to metastasize. Metastatic cells must survive in the absence of many of the survival signals their normal counterparts receive from the extracellular milieu (Fig. 9-4).

Mutation of apoptotic control genes without secondary mutations in growth regulatory genes similarly is insufficient for tumorigenesis. The characteristic t(14;18) translocation of the *bcl-2* gene has been detected at a low frequency in normal lymphoid hyperplasia in response to infection.[116] The rearrangement has been reported to be detectable by PCR in the peripheral blood of up to 55 percent of the population, and the frequency of the rearrangement increases with age.[117] Cells carrying the translocation may represent a long-lived premalignant population that has the potential to progress to lymphoma with the accumulation of additional mutations.

Inactivation of p53 is unique in eliminating an important negative regulatory control on proliferation while making the cell more resistant to apoptosis in response to aberrant replication. The double-edged effect of p53 inactivation may explain why this mutation is seen so frequently in a wide array of human malignancies and also may explain why p53 inactivation is such a frequent target of early gene expression by oncogenic viruses.

APOPTOSIS AND CANCER THERAPY

Chemotherapeutic Resistance

One of the most important problems that arise in cancer patients undergoing treatment is the development of tumors with multidrug resistance. This can arise *de novo* but is especially prevalent in previously treated patients. The multidrug resistance phenotype can be explained in a minority of cases by up-regulation of the *mdr-1* gene, which encodes a cell membrane pump that can expel a defined collection of antineoplastic agents.[118] A more general mechanism of multidrug resistance has been elucidated that involves apoptosis control.

Traditionally, tumoricidal radiation and chemotherapy were thought to function by causing irreparable metabolic or physical damage to cancer cells, resulting in cell necrosis. However, studies of cells killed by radiation and any of a wide variety of antineoplastic agents have demonstrated that these modalities induce typical apoptotic changes in the cells.[119] Cells exposed to chemotherapy are not passively killed by the drug. Instead, most cells die because intracellular surveillance mechanisms recognize the alteration of cell processes caused by chemotherapy and induce apoptosis. These observations suggest that a major mechanism for chemotherapeutic resistance in tumors may result from the inhibition of apoptosis.

Studies of tumor cell lines in vitro as well as tumors arising in vivo have demonstrated the importance of this idea. Overexpression of Bcl-2 and Bcl-x$_L$ simultaneously can increase tumor resistance to multiple chemotherapeutic agents and radiation.[120–125] The agents tested represent essentially all major categories of antineoplastic drugs, including antimetabolites, anthracyclines, DNA crosslinking agents, topoisomerase inhibitors, and mitotic spindle inhibitors. Cells overexpressing Bcl-x$_L$ that are exposed to chemotherapeutic agents arrest at the characteristic cell cycle stages where individual drugs are known to have their effects.[125] Subsequent removal of the chemotherapeutic agents from the media permitted cell cycle progression and proliferation, confirming the viability of the treated cells. High levels of endogenous Bcl-x$_L$ expression have been reported in tumor cells after exposure of those cells to chemotherapy. Bcl-x$_L$ and Bcl-2 expression in neuroblastoma decreases apoptotic sensitivity to chemotherapy.[122,126] High-level Bcl-2 expression has been correlated with chemotherapeutic resistance in acute myeloid leukemia.[127,128]

Inactivation of p53 similarly has been associated with increased chemotherapeutic resistance, perhaps by the loss of p53-dependent apoptosis.[129] However, p53-independent mechanisms also can detect DNA damage, cause cell cycle arrest, and initiate apoptosis. Chemotherapeutic mutagens or radiation causes cell cycle arrest and apoptosis in tumors of p53-negative mice.[130] Expression of antiapoptotic control genes therefore may be a more potent mechanism of chemotherapeutic resistance than is p53 inactivation.

Antiapoptotic Gene Expression and Mutation Rate

Overexpression of antiapoptotic genes in cancer cells abrogates a major mechanism that prevents the expansion of cells that demonstrate abnormal cell cycle progression. Cells that suffer abnormal mitosis, chromosome loss, or major genomic mutation normally are prevented from attempting replication by cell cycle checkpoints that trigger apoptotic cell death. Up-regulation of antiapoptotic gene expression permits the survival and propagation of such mutant cells and thus would be expected to greatly augment the rate of accumulation of genetic errors. Since inhibition of apoptosis appears to be a common step in oncogenesis, this mechanism could explain the high degree of chromosomal instability characteristic of cancer cells.

Cancer treatments may further accelerate mutagenesis. DNA-damaging chemotherapeutic agents and radiation are inherently mutagenic. Cells exposed to high levels of these mutagens are killed unless apoptotic pathways are blocked. Antiapoptotic gene expression therefore may promote tumor evolution by allowing the propagation of chemotherapy-induced mutations.

Chemotherapeutic agents that interfere with cell cycle progression also may promote chromosomal aberrations. An example of this type of derangement is seen in cells exposed to vincristine or nicodazole, agents which inhibit mitotic spindle formation.[131] These agents induce cell cycle arrest and apoptosis in tumor cells. Cells overexpressing Bcl-xL arrest but do not die in response to

these agents and on drug removal begin to proliferate without completing mitosis, thus becoming polyploid.

Rational Cancer Treatment Design

As described here, apoptotic regulation has been found to be a critical determinant of tumorigenesis and the therapeutic responsiveness of tumors. One of the challenges that is only beginning to be addressed is the translation of this new perspective on cancer biology into meaningful changes in clinical practice. As the associations between patient outcome and the activity of various antiapoptotic genes become clearer, screening of tumors for the expression of apoptotic regulatory genes may help define prognostic categories and influence treatment decisions.

More fundamentally, the study of apoptotic mechanisms affected by malignancy offers an opportunity for the consideration of entirely new approaches to the treatment of cancer. The unexpected finding that most successful anticancer treatments, including radiotherapy, chemotherapy, and hormonal modulation, function by apoptotic induction has generated increasing interest in therapies specifically targeted to apoptotic pathways. Such treatment may have much less nonspecific toxicity than do traditional antineoplastic agents. A pilot study of anti-Bcl-2 antibodies in the treatment of B-cell lymphoma is under way.[132] Disruption of LMP-1 signaling pathways could play an important role in the treatment of EBV-associated malignancies and lymphoproliferative disorders. Modification of apoptotic pathways by influencing the activity of cell surface receptors has not been explored. Therapy designed to stimulate apoptosis in target cells may play an increasingly central role in the treatment of cancer.

CONCLUSIONS

A great deal of information about the regulation of apoptosis at the molecular level has been acquired in the years since its initial phenotypic description. In mammalian cells, although many levels of apoptotic regulation have been defined, much of the control appears to be concentrated in a central pathway consisting of highly evolutionarily conserved regulatory proteins. Determination of the apoptotic threshold of a cell is dependent on interactions between positive and negative signaling elements in this central apoptotic pathway. A variety of external conditions, including the presence of growth factors, cytokines, and the membrane proteins of neighboring cells, influence the balance of the central apoptotic regulators through multiple cell surface receptors and intracellular signaling pathways.

The control of apoptosis is integral to many aspects of cancer biology. Apoptosis serves as an essential mechanism to prevent the proliferation of cells with potentially transforming mutations. As a corollary, inhibition of apoptosis may lead to the accumulation of cells with a higher mutation rate, thus accelerating malignant transformation. Cell cycle checkpoint controls play a critical role in detecting aberrant cells and initiating apoptosis. Viral and cellular oncoproteins, by driving cell cycle progression, often are strong inducers of apoptosis.

Most antineoplastic therapies function by triggering apoptosis in sensitive cells. Resistance to treatment can result from specific inhibition of apoptotic signaling. Chemotherapy or radiation may increase the mutation rate and hasten tumor evolution in cancer cells that are resistant to apoptosis. The study of apoptosis has not had a dramatic effect on clinical practice in oncology. However, the conceptual changes that have derived from apoptosis research have potentially wide clinical ramifications. We can look forward to many more trials of cancer therapy based on the modification of the controlling pathways of apoptotic regulation.

ACKNOWLEDGMENT

We thank Therese Conway for excellent secretarial support in preparing the manuscript.

REFERENCES

1. Kerr JFR, Wyllie AH, Currie AR: Apoptosis: A basic biological phenomenon with wide-ranging implications in tissue kinetics. *Br J Cancer* **26**:239, 1972.
2. Wyllie AH, Kerr JFR, Currie AR: Cell death: The significance of apoptosis. *Int Rev Cytol* **68**:251, 1980.
3. Thompson CB: Apoptosis in the pathogenesis and treatment of disease. *Science* **267**:1456, 1995.
4. Gougeon M-L, Montagnier L: Apoptosis in AIDS. *Science* **260**:1269, 1993.
5. Mountz JD, Wu J, Cheng J, Zhou T: Autoimmune disease: A problem of defective apoptosis. *Arthritis Rheum* **37**: 1415, 1994.
6. Margolis RL, Chuang D-M, Post RM: Programmed cell death: implications for neuropsychiatric disorders. *Biol Psychiatry* **35**:946, 1994.
7. Harrington EA, Fanidi A, Evan GI: Oncogenes and cell death. *Curr Opin Genet Dev* **4**:120, 1994.
8. Ellis RE, Yan J, Horvitz HR: Mechanism and function of cell death. *Ann Rev Cell Biol* **7**:663, 1991.
9. Raff, MC: Social controls on cell survival and cell death. *Nature* **356**:397, 1992.
10. Oppenheim RW: Cell death during development of the nervous system. *Annu Rev Neurosci* **14**:453, 1991.
11. Fadok VA, Voelker DR, Campbell PA, Cohen JJ, Bratton DL, Henson PM: Exposure of phosphatidylserine on the surface of apoptotic lymphocytes triggers specific recognition and removal by macrophages. *J Immunol* **148**:2207, 1992.
12. Fadok VA, Savill JS, Haslett C, Bratton DL, Doherty DE, Campbell PA, Henson PM: Different populations of macrophages use either the vitronectin receptor or the phosphatidylserine receptor to recognize and remove apoptotic cells. *J Immunol* **149**:4029, 1992.
13. Hall SE, Savill JS, Henson PM, Haslett C: Apoptic neutrophils are phagocytosed by fibroblasts with participation of the fibroblast vitronectin receptor and involvement of a mannose/fructose-specific lactin. *J Immunol* **153**:3218, 1994.
14. Tsujimoto Y, Finger LR, Yunis J, Nowell PC, Croce CM: Cloning of the chromosome breakpoint of neoplastic B cells with the t(14;18) chromosome translocation. *Science* **226**:1097, 1984.
15. Tsujimoto Y, Gorman J, Cossman J, Jaffe E, Croce CM: The t(14;18) chromosome translocations involved in B-cell neoplasms result from mistakes in VDJ joining. *Science* **229**:1390, 1985.
16. Bakhshi A, Jensen JP, Goldman P, Wright JJ, McBride OW, Epstein AL, Korsmeyer SJ: Cloning the chromosomal breakpoint of t(14;18) human lymphomas: Clustering around JH on chromosome 14 and near a transcriptional unit on 18. *Cell* **41**:889, 1985.
17. Cleary ML, Sklar J: Nucleotide Sequence of a t(14;18) chromosomal breakpoint in follicular lymphoma and demonstration of a breakpoint cluster region near a transcriptionally active locus on chromosome 18, *Proc Natl Acad Sci USA* **82**:7439, 1985.
18. Longo DL, DeVita VT, Jaffe ES, Mauch P, Urba WJ: Lymphocytic lymphomas, in DeVita VT, Hellman S, Rosenberg SA (eds): *Cancer: Principles and Practice of Oncology*, 4th ed. Philadelphia, Lippincott, 1993.
19. Vaux DL, Cory S, Adams JM: Bcl-2 gene promotes haemopoietic cell survival and co-operates with *c-Myc* to immortalize pre-B cells. *Nature* **335**:440, 1988.
20. Yang E, Korsmeyer SJ: Molecular thanatopsis: A discourse on the BCL2 family and cell death. *Blood* **88**:386, 1996.
21. Korsmeyer SJ: Bcl-2 initiates a new category of oncogenes: Regulators of cell death. *Blood* **80**:879, 1992.
22. Arends MJ, Wyllie AH: Apoptosis: Mechanisms and roles in pathology. *Int Rev Exp Pathol* **32**:223, 1991.
23. Horvitz HR, Shaham S, Hengartner MO: The genetics of programmed cell death in the nematode Caenorhabditis elegans. *Cold Spring Harbor Symp Quant Biol* **59**:377, 1994.
24. Ellis RE, Horvitz HR: Genetic control of programmed cell death in the nematode *C. elegans*. *Cell* **44**:817, 1986.
25. Hengartner MO, Ellis RE, Horvitz HR: Cernorhabditis elegans gene ced-9 protects cells from programmed cell death. *Nature* **356**:494, 1992.
26. Shaham S, Horvitz HR: Developing Caenorhabditis elegans neurons may contain both cell-death protective and killer activities. *Gene Dev* **10**:578, 1996.
27. Hengartner MO, Horvitz HR: *C. elegans* cell survival gene ced-9 encodes a functional homolog of the mammalian proto-oncogene bcl-2. *Cell* **76**:665, 1994.
28. Vaux DL, Weissman IL, Kim SK: Prevention of programmed cell death in Caenorhabditis elegans by human bcl-2. *Science* **258**:1955, 1992.
29. Yan J, Shahm S, Ledoux S, Ellis HM, Horvitz HR: The *C. elegans* cell death gene ced-3 encodes a protein similar to mammalian interleukin-1b-converting enzyme. *Cell* **75**:641, 1993.
30. Boise LH, Gonzalez-Garcia M, Postema CE, Ding L, Lindsten T, Turka LA, Mao X, Nunes G, Thompson CB: bcl-x, a bcl-2-related gene that functions as a dominant regulator of apoptotic cell death. *Cell* **74**:597, 1993.
31. Oltvai ZN, Milliman CL, Korsmeyer SJ: bcl-2 heterodimerizes in vivo with a conserved homolog, Bax, that accelerates programmed cell death. *Cell* **74**:609, 1993.
32. Sedlak TW, Oltvai ZN, Yang E, Wang K, Boise LH, Thompson CB, Korsmeyer SJ: Multiple Bcl-2 family members demonstrate selective dimerizations with Bax. *Pro Natl Acad Sci USA* **92**:7834, 1995.
33. Farrow SN, White JHM, Martinou I, Raven T, Pun K-T, Grinham CJ, Martinou J-C, Brown R: Cloning of a bcl-2 homologue by interaction with adenovirus E1B 19K. *Nature* **374**:731, 1995.
34. Chittenden T, Harrington EA, O'Connor R, Flemington C, Lutz RJ, Evan GI, Guild BC: Induction of apoptosis by the Bcl-2 homologue Bak. *Nature* **374**:733, 1995.
35. Kiefer MC, Brauer MJ, Powers VC, Wu JJ, Umansky SR, Tomei LD, Barr PJ: Modulation of apoptosis by the widely distributed Bcl-2 homologue Bak. *Nature* **374**:736, 1995.
36. Yang E, Zha J, Jockel J, Boise LH, Thompson CB, Korsmeyer SJ: Bad, a heterodimeric partner for Bcl-xL and Bcl-2, displaces Bax and promotes cell death. *Cell* **80**:285, 1995.
37. Muchmore SW, Sattler M, Liang H, Meadows RP, Harlan JE, Yoon HS, Nettesheim D, Chang B, Thompson CB, Wong S, Ng S-C, Fesik SW: X-ray and NMR structure of human Bcl-xL, an inhibitor of programmed cell death. *Nature* **381**:335, 1996.
38. Cramer WA, Heymann JB, Schendel SL, Deriy BN, Cohen FS, Elkins PA, Stauffacher CB: Structure-function of the channel-forming colicins. *Annu Rev Biophys Biomol Struct* **24**:611, 1995.
39. Monoghan P, Robertson D, Amos T, Dyer M, Mason D, Greaves M: Ultrastructural localizations of Bcl-2 protein. *J Histochem Cytochem* **40**:1819, 1992.
40. Krajewski S, Tanaka S, Takayama S, Schibler MJ, Fenton W, Reed JC: Investigation of the subcellular distribution of the bcl-2 oncoprotein: Residence in the nuclear envelope, endoplasmic reticulum, and outer mitochondrial membranes. *Cancer Res* **53**:4701, 1993.
41. Nguyn M, Miller DG, Yong VW, Korsmeyer SJ, Shore GC: Targeting of Bcl-2 to the mitochondrial outer membrane by a COOH-terminal signal anchor sequence. *J. Biol Chem* **268**:25265, 1993.
42. Zamzami N, Susin SA, Marchetti P, Hirsh T, Gomez-Monterrey I, Castedo M, Kroemer G: Mitochondrial control of nuclear apoptosis, *Exp Med* **183**:1533, 1996.
43. Castedo M, Hirsch T, Susin SA, Zamzami N, Marchetti P, Macho A, Kroemer G: Sequential acquisition of mitochondrian and plasma membrane alterations during early lymphocyte apoptosis. *J Immunol* **157**:512, 1996.
44. Zamzami N, Marchetti P, Castedo M, Zanin C, Vayssiäre J-L, Petit PX, Kroemer G: Reduction in mitochondrial potential constitutes an early irreversible step of programmed lymphocyte death in vivol. *J Exp Med* **181**:1661, 1995.
45. Zamzami N, Marchetti P, Castedo M, Decaudin D, Macho A, Hirsch T, Susin SA, Petit PX, Mignotte B, Kroemer G: Sequential reduction of mitochondrial transmembrane potential and generation of reactive oxygen species in early programmed cell death. *J Exp Med* **182**:367, 1996.

46. Liu X, Kim CN, Yang J, Jemmerson R, Wang X: Induction of apoptotic program in cell-free extracts: Requirement for dATP and cytochrome c. *Cell* **86**:147, 1996.

47. Chinnaiyan AM, Dixit VM: The cell-death machine. *Curr Biol* **6**:555, 1996.

48. Henkart PA: ICE family proteases: Mediators of all apoptotic cell death? *Immunity* **4**:195, 1996.

49. Miura M, Zhu H, Rotello R, Hartwieg EA, Yuan J: Induction of apoptosis in fibroblasts by IL-1b-converting enzyme, a mammalian homology of the C. elegans cell death gene ced-3. *Cell* **75**:653, 1993.

50. Rabizadeh S, LaCount DJ, Friesen, PD, Bredesen DE: Expression of the baculovirus p35 gene inhibits mammalian neuronal cell death. *J Neurochem* **61**:2318, 1993.

51. Duan H, Chinnaiyan AM, Hudson PL, Wing JP, He WW, Dixit VM: ICE-LAP3, a novel mammalian homologue of the Caenorhabditis elegans cell death protein Ced-3 is activated during Fas- and tumor necrosis factor-induced apoptosis. *J Biol Chem* **369**:621, 1996.

52. Walker NP, Talanian RV, Brady KD, Dang LC, Bump NJ, Ferenz CR, Franklin S, Ghayur T, Hackett MC, Hammill LD, Herzog L, Hugunin M, Houy W, Mankovich JA, McGuiness L, Orlewicz E, Paskind M, Pratt CA, Reis P, Summani A, Terranova M, Welch JP, Xiong L, Moller A, Tracey DE, Kamen R, Wong WW: Crystal structure of the cysteine protease interleukin-1 beta-converting enzyme: A (p20/p10)2 homodimer. *Cell* **78**:343, 1995.

53. Alnemri ES, Fernandes-Alnemri T, Litwack G: Cloning and expression of four novel isoforms of human interleukin-1 beta converting enzyme with different apoptotic activities. *J Biol Chem* **270**:4312, 1995.

54. Wang L, Miura M, Bergeron L, Zhu H, Yuan J: Ich-1, an Ice/ced-3-related gene, encodes both positive and negative regulators of programmed cell death. *Cell* **78**:739, 1994.

55. Fernandes-Alnemri T, Litwack G, Alnemri ES: Mch2, a new member of the apoptotic CED-3/ICE cysteine protease gene family. *Cancer Res* **55**:2737, 1995.

56. Duan H, Orth K, Chinnaiyan AM, Poirier GG, Froelich CJ He W-W, Dixit VM: ICE-LAP6, a novel member of the ICE/Ced-3 gene family, is activated by the cytotoxic T cell protease granzyme B. *J Biol Chem* **271**:16720, 1996.

57. Li P, Allen H, Banerjee S, Frank S, Herzog L, Johnson C, McDowell J, Paskind M, Rodman L, Salfeld J, Towne E, Tracey D, Warwell S, Wei F-Y, Wong W, Kamen R, Seshadri T: Mice deficient in IL-1b-converting enzyme are defective in production of mature IL-1b and resistant to endotoxic shock. *Cell* **80**: 401, 1995.

58. Kiuda K, Lippke JA, Ku G, Hardin MW, Livingston DJ, Su MS, Flavell RA: Altered cytokine export and apoptosis in mice deficient in interleukin-1b converting enzyme. *Science* **267**:2000, 1995.

59. Lazebnik YA, Kaufmann SH, Disnoyers S, Poirer GG, Earnshaw WC: Cleavage of poly(ADP-ribose) polymerase by a proteinase with properties like ICE. *Nature* **371**:346, 1994.

60. Nicholson DW, Ali A, Thornberry NA, Vaillancourt JP, Ding CK, Gallant M, Gareau Y, Griffin PR, Labelle M, Lazebnik YA, Munday NA, Raju SM, Smulson ME, Yamin T-T, Yu VL, Miller DK: Identification and inhibition of the ICE/CED-3 protease necessary for mammalian apoptosis. *Nature* **376**:37, 1995.

61. Tewari M, Quan LT, O'Rourke K, Desnoyers S, Zeng Z, Beidler DR, Poirier GG, Salvesen GS, Dixit VM: Yama/CPP32 beta, a mammalian homolog of CED-3, is a CrmA-inhibitable protease that cleaves the death substrate poly(ADP-ribose) polymerase. *Cell* **81**:801, 1995.

62. Wang Z-Q, Auer B, Stingle L, Berghammer H, Haidacher D, Schweiger M, Wagner EF: Mice lacking ADPRT and poly(ADP-ribosyl)ation develop normally but are susceptible to skin disease. *Gene Dev* **9**:509, 1995.

63. Boise LH, Thompson CB: Bcl-xL can inhibit apoptosis in cells that have undergone Fas-induced protease activation. *Proc Natl Acad Sci USA* **94**:3759, 1997.

64. Bazzoni F, Beutler B: The tumor necrosis factor ligand and receptor families. *N Engl J Med* **334**:1717, 1996.

65. Chinnaiyan AM, O'Rourke K, Tewari M, Dixit VM: FADD, a novel death domain-containing protein, interacts with the death domain of Fas and initiates apoptosis. *Cell* **81**:505, 1995.

66. Stanger BZ, Leder P, Lee T, Kim E, Seed B: RIP: A novel protein containing a death domain that interacts with FAS/Apo-1 (CD95) in yeast and causes cell death. *Cell* **81**:513, 1995.

67. Hsu H, Xiong J, Goeddel DV: The TNF receptor 1-associated protein TRADD signals cell death and NF-kB activation. *Cell* **81**:495, 1995.

68. Hsu H, Shu H-B, Pan M-G, Goeddel DV: TRADD-TRAF2 and TRADD-FADD interactions define two distinct TNF receptor 1 signal transduction pathways. *Cell* **84**:299, 1996.

69. Boldin MP, Goncharov TM, Goltsev YV, Wallach D: Involvement of MACH, a novel MORT1/FADD-interacting protease, in Fas/APO-1- and TNF receptor-induced cell death. *Cell* **85**:803, 1996.

70. Muzio M, Chinnaiyan AM, Kischkel FC, O'Rourke K, Shevchenko A, Ni J, Scaffidi C, Bretz JD, Zhang M, Gentz R, Mann M, Krammer PH, Peter ME, Dixit VM: FLICE, a novel FADD-homologous ICE/CED-3-like protease, is recruited to the CD95 (Fas/Apo-1) death-inducing signaling complex. *Cell* **85**:817, 1996.

71. Rothe M, Wong SC, Henzel WJ, Goeddel DV: A novel family of putative signal transducers associated with cytoplasmic domain of the 75 kDa tumor necrosis factor receptor family. *Cell* **78**:681, 1994.

72. Mosialos G, Birkenbach M, Yalamanchili R, VanArsdale T, Ware C, Kieff E: The Epstein-Barr virus transforming protein LMP1 engages signaling proteins for the tumor necrosis factor receptor family. *Cell* **80**:389, 1995.

73. Chang G, Cleary AM, Ye Z, Hong DI, Lederman S, Baltimore D: Involvement of CRAF1, a relative of TRAF, in CD40 signaling. *Science* **267**:1494, 1995.

74. Hu HM, O'Rourke K, Boguski MS, Dixit VM: A novel RING finger protein interacts with the cytoplasmic domain of CF40. *J Biol Chem* **269**:30069, 1994.

75. Sato T, Irie S, Reed JC: A novel member of the TRAF family of putative signal transducing proteins binds to the cytoplasmic domain of CD 40. *FEBS Lett* **358**:113, 1995.

76. Regnier CH, Tomasetto C, Moog-Lutz C, Chenard M-P, Wendling C, Basset P, Rio MC: Presence of a new conserved domain in CART1, a novel member of the tumor necrosis factor receptor-associated protein family, which is expressed in breast carcinoma. *J Biol Chem* **270**:25715, 1995.

77. Nakano H, Oshima H, Chung W, Williams-Abbott L, Ware CF, Yagita H, Okumura K: TRAF5, an activator of NF-kB and putative signal transducer for the lymphotoxin-b receptor. *J Biol Chem* **271**:14661, 1996.

78. Gedrich RW, Gilfillan MC, Duckett CS, VanDongen JL, Thompson CB: CD30 contains two binding sites with different specificities for members of the tumor necrosis factor receptor-associated factor family of signal transducing proteins. *J Biol Chem* **271**:12852, 1996.

79. Rothe M, Sarma V, Dixit VM, Goeddel DV: TRAF2-mediated activation of NFkB by TNF receptor 2 and CD40. *Science* **269**:1424, 1995.

80. Clem RJ, Miller LK: Control of programmed cell death by the baculovirus genes p34 and iap. *Mol Cell Biol* **14**:5212, 1994.

81. Roy N, Mahadevan MS, McLean M, Shutler G, Yaraghi Z, Farahani R, Baird S, Besner-Johnston A, Lefebvre C, Kang X, Salih M, Aubry H, Tamai K, Guan X, Ioannou P, Crawford TO, de Jong PJ, Surh L, Ikeda J-E, Korneluk RG, MacKenzie A: The gene for neuronal apoptosis inhibitory protein is partially deleted in individuals with spinal muscular atrophy. *Cell* **80**:167, 1995.

82. Rothe M, Pan M-G, Henzel WJ, Ayres TM, Goeddel DV: The TNFR2-TRAF signaling complex contains two novel proteins related to baculoviral inhibitor of apoptosis proteins. *Cell* **83**:1243, 1995.

83. Duckett CS, Nava VE, Gedrich RW, Clem RJ, VanDongen JL, Gilfillan MC, Shiels H, Hardwick JM, Thompson CB: A conserved family of cellular genes related to the baculovirus iap gene and encoding apoptosis inhibitors. *EMBO J* **15**:2685, 1996.

84. Liston P, Roy N, Tamai K, Lefebvre C, Baird S, Cherton-Horvat G, Farahani R, McLean M, Ikeda JE, MacKenzie A, Korneluk RG: Suppression of apoptosis in mammalian cells by NAIP and a related family of IAP genes. *Nature* **379**:349, 1996.

85. Uren AG, Pakusch M, Hawkins CH, Puls KL, Vaux DL: Cloning and expression of apoptosis inhibitory protein homologs that function to inhibit apoptosis and/or bind tumor necrosis factor receptor-associated factors. *Proc Natl Acad Sci USA* **93**:4974, 1996.

86. Ray CA, Black RA, Kronheim SR, Greenstreet TA, Sleath PR, Salvesen GS, Pickup DJ: Viral inhibition of inflammation: Cowpox virus encodes an inhibitor of the interleukin-1b-converting enzyme. *Cell* **69**:597, 1992.

87. Boyd JM, Malstron S, Subramanian T, Venkatesh LK, Schaeper U, Elangovan B, Sa-Eipper C, Chinnadurai G: Adenovirus E1B 19kDa and Bcl-2 proteins interact with a common set of cellular proteins. *Cell* **79**:341, 1994.

88. Henderson S, Huen D, Rowe M, Dawson C, Johnson G, Rickson A: Epstein-Barr virus-coded BHRF1 protein, a viral homologue of Bcl-2, protects human B cells from programmed cell death. *Proc Natl Acad Sci USA* **90**:8479, 1993.

89. Nielan JG, Lu Z, Afonzo L, Kutish GF, Sussman MD, Rock DL: An African swine fever virus gene with similarity to the proto-oncogene bcl-2 and the Epstein-Barr virus gene BHRF1, *J Virol* **67**:4391, 1993.

90. Liebowitz D, Kieff E: Epstein-Barr virus, in Roizman B, Whitley RJ, Lopez C (eds): *The Human Herpesviruses.* New York: Raven Press, 1993, p107.

91. Henderson S, Rowe M, Gregory C, Croom-Carter D, Wang F, Long-necker R, Kieff E, Rickinson A: Induction of Bcl-2 expression by Epstein-Barr virus latent membrane protein 1 protects infected B cells from programmed cell death. *Cell* **65**:1107, 1991.

92. Evan G, Littlewood T: The role of *c-Myc* in cell growth. *Curr Opin Genet Deb* **3**:44, 1993.

93. Evan G, Wyllie A, Gilbert C, Littlewood T, Brooks M, Waters C, Penn L, Hancock D: Induction of apoptosis in fibroblasts by *c-Myc* protein. *Cell* **63**:119, 1992.

94. Langdon WY, Harris AW, Cory S: Growth of E mu-myc transgenic B-lymphoid cells in vitro and their evolution toward autonomy. *Oncogene Res* **3**:271, 1988.

95. Bissonnette RP, Echeverri F, Mahboubi A, Green DR: Apoptotic cell death induced by *c-Myc* is inhibited by bcl-2. *Nature* **359**:552, 1992.

96. Harrington EA, Bennett MR, Fanidi A, Evan GI: *c-Myc*-induced apoptosis in fibroblasts is inhibited by specific cytokines. *EMBO J* **13**:3286, 1994.

97. Dedera D, Waller E, LeBrun D, Sen-Majumdar A, Stevens M, Barsh G, Cleary M: Chimeric homeobox gene E2A-PBX1 induces prolifer-ation, apoptosis and malignant lymphomas in transgenic mice. *Cell* **74**:833, 1993.

98. Tommasino M, Crawford L: Human papillomavirus E6 and E7: Pro-teins which deregulate the cell cycle. *Bioessays* **17**:509, 1995.

99. Pan H, Griep AE: Temporally distinct patterns of p53-dependent and p53-independent apoptosis during mouse lens development. *Gene Dev* **9**:2157, 1995.

100. Rao L, Debbas M, Sabbatini P, Hockenberry D, Korsmeyer S, White E: The adenovirus E1A proteins induce apoptosis, which is inhibited by the E1B 19-kDa and Bcl-2 proteins. *Proc Natl Acad Sci USA* **89**:7742, 1992.

101. Yew PR, Berk AJ: Inhibition of p53 transactivation required for trans-formation by adenovirus early 1B protein. *Nature* **357**:82, 1992.

102. Murray AW: The genetics of cell cycle checkpoints. *Curr Opin Genet Dev* **5**:5, 1995.

103. Vogelstein B: Cancer: A deadly inheritance. *Nature* **348**:681, 1990.

104. Kuerbitz SJ, Plunkett BS, Walsh WV, Kastan MB: Wild-type p53 is a cell cycle checkpoint determinant following irradiation. *Proc Natl Acad Sci USA* **89**:7491, 1992.

105. Shaw P, Bovey R, Tardy S, Sahli R, Sordat B, Costa J: Induction of apoptosis by wild-type p53 in a human colon tumor-derived cell line. *Proc Natl Acad Sci USA* **89**:4495, 1992.

106. Yonish-Rouach E, Resnitzky D, Lotem J, Sachs L, Kimchi A, Oren M: Wild-type p53 induces apoptosis of myeloid leukaemic cells that is inhibited by interleukin-6. *Nature* **352**:345, 1991.

107. Symonds H, Krall L, Remington L, Saenz-Robles M, Lowe S, Jacks T, Van Dyke T: p53-dependent apoptosis suppresses tumor growth and progression in vivo. *Cell* **78**:703, 1994.

108. Lowe SW, Schmitt EM, Smith SW, Osborne BA, Jacks T: p53 is re-quired for radiation-induced apoptosis in mouse thymocytes. *Nature* **362**:847, 1993.

109. Clarke AR, Purdie CA, Harrison DJ, Morris RG, Bird CC, Hooper ML, Wyllie AH: Thymocyte apoptosis induced by p53-dependent and independent pathways. *Nature* **362**:849, 1993.

110. Miyashita T, Krajewski S, Krajewska M, Wang HG, Lin HK, Lieber-mann DA, Hoffman B, Reed JC: Tumor suppressor p53 is regulator of bcl-2 and bax gene expression in vitro and in vivo. *Oncogene* **9**:1799, 1994.

111. Knudson CM, Tung KSK, Tourtellote WG, Brown GAJ, Korsmeyer SJ: Bax-deficient mice with lymphoid hyperplasia and male germ cell death. *Science* **270**:96, 1995.

112. Riley DJ, Lee EY-HP, Lee W-H: The retinoblastoma protein: More than a tumor suppressor. *Annu Rev Cell Biol* **10**:1, 1994.

113. Lee EY-HP, Chang C-Y, Hu N, Wang Y-CJ, Lai C-C, Herrup K, Lee W-H, Bradley A: Mice deficient for Rb are noviable and show defects in neurogenesis and haematopoiesis. *Nature* **359**:288, 1992.

114. Jacks T, Fazeli A, Schmitt EM, Bronson RT, Goodell MA, Wein-berg RA: Effects of an Rb mutation in the mouse. *Nature* **359**:295, 1992.

115. Amati B, Littlewood T, Evan G, Land H: The *c-Myc* protein induces cell cycle progression and apoptosis through dimerisation with Max. *EMBO J* **12**:5083, 1994.

116. Limpens J, de Jong D, van Krieken JH, Price CG, Young BD, van Ommen GJ, Kluin PM: Bcl-2/JH rearrangements in benign lymphoid tissues with follicular hyperplasia. *Oncogene* **6**:2271, 1991.

117. Liu Y, Hernandez AM, Shibata D, Cortopossi GA: BCL2 transloca-tion frequency rises with age in humans. *Proc Natl Acad Sci USA* **91**:8910, 1994.

118. Gottesman MM, Pastan I: Biochemistry of multidrug resistance me-diated by the multidrug transporter. *Annu Rev Biochem* **62**:385, 1993.

119. Lowe SW, Ruley HE, Jacks T, Housman DE: p53-dependent apoptosis modulates the cytotoxicity of anticancer agents. *Cell* **74**:957, 1993.

120. Miyashita T, Reed JC: bcl-2 gene transfer increases relative resis-tance of S49:1 and WEHI7.2 lymphoid cells to cell death and DNA fragmentation induced by glucocorticoids and multiple chemothera-peutic drugs. *Cancer Res* **52**:5407, 1992.

121. Walton MI, Whysong D, O'Connor PM, Hockenberry D, Korsmeyer SJ, Kohn KW: Constitutive expression of human bcl-2 modulates ni-trogen mustard and camptothecin induced apoptosis. *Cancer Res* **53**:1853, 1993.

122. Dole M, Nunez G, Merchant AK, Maybaum J, Rode CK, Bloch CA, Castle VP: Bcl-2 inhibits chemotherapy-induced apoptosis in neuro-blastoma. *Cancer Res* **54**:3253, 1994.

123. Fisher TC, Milner AE, Gregory CD, Jackman AL, Aherne GW, Hart-ley JA, Dive C, Hickman JA: bcl-2 modulation of apoptosis induced by anticancer drugs: Resistance to thymidylate stress is independent of classical resistance pathways. *Cancer Res* **53**:3321, 1993.

124. Miyashita T, Reed JC: Bcl-2 oncoprotein blocks chemotherapy-induced apoptosis in a human leukemia cell line. *Blood* **81**:151, 1993.

125. Minn AJ, Rudin CM, Boise LH, Thompson CB: Expression of Bcl-xL can confer a multidrug resistance phenotype. *Blood* **86**:1903, 1995.

126. Dole MG, Jasty R, Cooper MJ, Thompson CB, Nunez G, Castle VP: Bcl-xL is expressed in neuroblastoma cells and modulates chemotherapy-induced apoptosis. *Cancer Res* **55**:2576, 1995.

127. Lotem J, Sachs L: Regulation by bcl-2, *c-Myc*, and p53 of suscepti-bility to induction of apoptosis by heat shock and cancer chemother-apy compounds in differentiation-competent and- defective myeloid leukemic cells. *Cell Growth D* **4**:41, 1993.

128. Campos L, Rouault J-P, Sabido O, Oriol P, Roubi N, Vasselon C, Archimbaud E, Magaud J-P, Guyotat D: High expression of bcl-2 protein in acute myeloid leukemia cells is associated with poor re-sponse to chemotherapy. *Blood* **81**:3091, 1993.

129. Lowe SW, Bodis S, McClatchey A, Remington L, Ruley HE, Fisher DE, Housman DE, Jacks T: p53 status and the efficacy of cancer ther-apy in vivo. *Science* **266**:807, 1994.

130. Strasser A, Harris AW, Jacks T, Cory S: DNA damage can induce apoptosis in proliferating lymphoid cells via p53-independent mecha-nisms inhibitable by Bcl-2. *Cell* **79**:329, 1994.

131. Minn, AJ, Boise LH, Thompson CB: Expression of Bcl-xL and loss of p53 can cooperate to overcome a cell cycle checkpoint induced by mitotic spindle damage. *Gene Dev* **10**:2621, 1996.

132. Webb A, Cunningham D, Cotter F, Hill M, Clark P, di Stefano F, Viner C, Prendeville J, Rahal S, Dziewanowska Z: Phase 1 bcl-2 anti-sense trial: Preliminary results (abstract). *Ann Oncol* **7**(3):32, 1996.

CHAPTER 10

Oncogenes

Morag Park

1. Oncogenes, which originally were identified as the transforming genes in viruses, are altered forms of normal cellular genes called proto-oncogenes. In human cancers, proto-oncogenes frequently are located adjacent to chromosomal breakpoints and are targets for mutation. The products of proto-oncogenes are highly conserved in evolution and regulate the cascade of events that maintains the ordered progression through the cell cycle, cell division, and differentiation. In a cancer cell this ordered progression is partially lost when one or more of the components of this pathway are altered.

2. The control of normal cell growth and differentiation is mediated by the interaction of growth factors and cytokines with their membrane-bound receptors. This event triggers a cascade of intracellular biochemical signals that eventually results in the activation and repression of various genes. Proto-oncogene products have been shown to function at critical steps in these pathways and include proteins such as extracellular cytokines and growth factors, transmembrane growth factor receptors, cytoplasmic proteins that transmit the signal to the nucleus, and nuclear proteins that include transcription factors and proteins involved in the control of DNA replication.

3. Accumulating evidence suggests that the activation of several oncogenes and the inactivation of several growth-suppressor genes are necessary for the acquisition of a complete neoplastic phenotype. It has been possible in experimental studies to subdivide oncogenes into several groups. One class of genes rescues cells from senescence and programmed cell death, acting as immortalizing genes. A second class of genes reduces growth factor requirements and induces changes in cell shape that result in a continuous proliferative response that is no longer regulated.

4. The use of transgenic mice provides a powerful experimental approach to the investigation of the role of oncogenes in cancer. Oncogene expression can be directed to specific tissues where a role for the oncogene in tumor formation in that tissue can be evaluated. Although transgenic mouse strains that carry a single oncogene generally show an increased incidence of neoplasia, oncogene expression usually precedes tumor formation by many months and the tumors that result frequently are clonal, implying that other events are necessary. Examination of the secondary events in tumors from oncogene-bearing transgenic mice has confirmed the conclusions derived from in vitro studies and has identified new oncogenes. When two strains of oncogene-bearing mice are crossed, the consequence of multiple oncogenes on tumor incidence can be studied in a host capable of mounting a physiologic response.

In the past 15 years the study of oncogenes has advanced our understanding of the molecular mechanisms leading to cancer. The application of techniques from many cancer research disciplines has led to the discovery of both dominantly acting transforming genes and tumor suppressor genes. The dominant transforming genes, collectively called oncogenes, are altered forms of normal cellular genes called proto-oncogenes. Proto-oncogenes are highly conserved in evolution, and their products are important regulators of normal cell growth and differentiation in species ranging from primitive eukaryotes to humans. They are localized throughout the cell and regulate the cascade of events that maintains the ordered progression through the cell cycle, cell division, and the differentiated state of the cell. In a cancer cell, this ordered progression is partially lost when one or more of the components of this pathway becomes altered as an oncogene. Mutations that alter the structure, levels, or sites of expression of the gene products in this pathway have been shown to activate their oncogenic potential.

Just as the growth-promoting proto-oncogenes are thought to regulate the proliferation of normal cells, the actions of tumor suppressor genes function normally to constrain cell growth. Genetic lesions that inactivate tumor suppressor genes therefore free the cell from the growth constraints imposed by these genes. The end result of oncogene activation or suppressor gene inactivation is deregulated cell growth. Increasing evidence suggests that the acquisition of multiple sequential alterations involving both oncogenes and tumor suppressor genes generally is required for the progression from the normal phenotype to a fully malignant phenotype. This chapter focuses on the identification, mechanisms of activation, and function of the oncogene/proto-oncogene class of growth regulators. Tumor suppressor genes are discussed in Chap. 8.

PROTO-ONCOGENES

More than 20 different viral oncogenes have been identified, each of which has a counterpart in normal cells. A list of oncogene/proto-oncogene products and their functions is provided in Table 10-1. The majority of oncogenes listed in the table have been compared at the level of their nucleotide or predicted amino acid sequences with the host proto-oncogene from which they were derived as well as with proto-oncogene homologues in other species.

Table 10-1 Oncogenes

Oncogene	Lesion	Neoplasm	Proto-Oncogene	Ref.
Growth Factors				
v-sis		Glioma/fibrosarcoma	B chain PDGF	254
int 2	Proviral insertion	Mammary carcinoma	Member of FGF family	255
KS3	DNA transfection	Kaposi's sarcoma	Member of FGF family	46
HST	DNA transfection	Stomach carcinoma	Member of FGF family	45
int-I	Proviral insertion	Mammary carcinoma	Possible growth factor	256
Receptors Lacking Protein Kinase Activity				
mas	DNA transfection	Mammary carcinoma	Angiotensin receptor	21
Tyrosine Kinases: Integral Membrane Proteins, Growth Factor Receptors				
EGFR	Amplification	Squamous cell carcinoma	Protein kinase (tyr) EFGR	257
v-fms		Sarcoma	Protein kinase (tyr) CSF-1R	258
v-kit		Sarcoma	Protein kinase (tyr) Stem cell factor R	111
v-ros		Sarcoma	Protein kinase (tyr)	40
MET	Rearrangement	MNNG-treated human osteo carcinoma cell line	Protein kinase (tyr) HGF/SFR	39
TRK	Rearrangement	Colon carcinoma	Protein kinase (tyr) NGFR	41
NEU	Point mutation	Neuroblastoma	Protein kinase (tyr)	39
	Amplification	Carcinoma of breast		
RET	Rearrangement	Carcinoma of thyroid Men 2A, Men 2B	Protein kinase (tyr) GDNFR	125
Tyrosine Kinases: Non-receptor				
SRC		Colon carcinoma	Protein kinase (tyr)	40
v-yes		Sarcoma	Protein kinase (tyr)	40
v-fgr		Sarcoma	Protein kinase (tyr)	259
v-fps		Sarcoma	Protein kinase (tyr)	40
v-fes		Sarcoma	Protein kinase (tyr)	258
BCR/ABL	Chromosome translocation	CML	Protein kinase (tyr)	258
Membrane Associated G Proteins				
H-RAS	Point mutation	Colon, lung, pancreas carcinoma	GTPase	26
K-RAS	Point mutation	AML, thyroid carcinoma, melanoma	GTPase	27
N-RAS	Point mutation	Carcinoma, melanoma	GTPase	31
gsp	Point mutation	Carcinoma of thyroid	Gsα	74
gip	Point mutation	Ovary, adrenal carcinoma	Giα	75
GEF Family of Proteins				
Dbl	Rearrangement	Diffuse B-cell lymphoma	GEF for Rho and Cdc42Hs	166
Ost		Osteosarcomas	GEF for RhoA and Cdc42Hs	260
Tiam-1	Metastatic and oncogenic	T-lymphoma	GEF for Rac and Cdc42Hs	165
Vav	Rearrangement	Hematopoietic cells	GEF for Ras?	261
Lbc	Oncogenic	Myeloid leukemias	GEF for Rho	262
Serine/Threonine Kinases: Cytoplasmic				
v-mos		Sarcoma	Protein kinase (ser/thr)	263
v-raf		Sarcoma	Protein kinase (ser/thr)	264
pim-1	Proviral insertion	T-cell lymphoma	Protein kinase (ser/thr)	265
Cytoplasmic Regulators				
v-crk			SH-2/SH-3 adaptor	142
Nuclear Protein Family				
v-myc		Carcinoma myelocytomatosis	Transcription factor	40
N-MYC	Gene amplification	Neuroblastoma: Lung carcinoma	Transcription factor	65
L-MYC	Gene amplification	Carcinoma of lung	Transcription factor	266
v-myb		Myeloblastosis	Transcription factor	267
v-fos		Osteosarcoma	Transcription factor API	268
v-jun		Sarcoma	Transcription factor API	269
v-ski		Carcinoma	Transcription factor	270
v-rel		Lymphatic leukemia	Mutant NFKB	271
v-ets		Myeloblastosis	Transcription factor	272
v-erbA		Erythroblastosis	Mutant thioredoxine receptor	257

Conserved or related protein domains, which are crucial for biochemical function and cellular localization of the oncogene or proto-oncogene protein product, have been used to classify these domains into distinct groups (Table 10-1).

The expression of proto-oncogenes in normal cells is tightly regulated, and these cells do not give rise to malignancy. The potential for proto-oncogene products to participate in tumorigenesis relates to their role in the complex signaling networks that control the growth and differentiation of normal cells.[1,2] The function of these genes is discussed later, but sites of their activity are represented conceptually in Fig. 10-1. In a normal cell, interaction of growth factors and cytokines with specific membrane receptors triggers a cascade of intracellular biochemical signals that result in the expression and repression of various genes. The relaxation of requirements of transformed cells for growth factors can be mediated by an alteration through overexpression or mutation of the gene products involved at any level of these signal transduction pathways.

DISCOVERY OF ONCOGENES

Viral Oncogenes

The majority of oncogenes were isolated as altered forms of proto-oncogenes acquired (transduced) by RNA tumor viruses (v-*onc*). An examination of human tumors by a variety of methods revealed that many of the v-*onc* genes also are altered in human tumors. The concept that there are genes capable of causing cancer (oncogenes) is based largely on studies carried out with transplantable tumors in chickens, mice, and rats.[3] The causative agent for such tumors was found to be an RNA virus. Based on the highly efficient manner in which the viruses were able to cause tumors, it was proposed that the virus carried genetic information responsible for transforming a normal cell into a tumor cell.[4]

However, there is little evidence that such viruses are causative agents for the majority of human cancers.

Retroviruses are RNA-containing animal viruses that replicate through a DNA intermediate.[5] They have been isolated from many avian and mammalian sources and can be divided into two classes on the basis of the latent period between infection and the appearance of a tumor (Fig. 10-2). Acute transforming retroviruses rapidly produce tumors in newborn animals and carry genetic information capable of inducing tumors directly (oncogene).[6] The slowly transforming retroviruses do not carry oncogenes and induce tumors by integrating themselves adjacent to a cellular gene and altering its transcriptional regulation.[7]

Activation of Oncogenes via Retroviral Transduction

The acquisition of cellular genes by acute transforming retroviruses occurs as a consequence of their mode of replication. Retroviruses first copy their RNA genome into a complementary DNA intermediate that integrates into the host's cellular genome. During transcription and production of viral genomic and messenger RNA, mature replication-proficient virus may be packaged and released from the cell, or alternatively, viral sequences are lost and replaced with a cellular proto-oncogene that is then packaged as an mRNA copy of that gene lacking introns into the virus (Fig. 10-2A).[8,9] Once transduced into a virus, the proto-oncogene sequence can rapidly undergo numerous mutational events that occur during viral replication. Since the isolation of acute transforming viruses involves screening for tumor induction and the ability of virus isolates to transform cells in culture, this results in selection for virus isolates containing proto-oncogene products (v-*onc*) that have undergone genetic alterations, such as point mutations and deletions, that directly affect protein function (Table 10-1). These genetic alterations, in conjunction with a high level of expression driven by retroviral transcriptional enhancers unleash the transforming potential of the transduced proto-oncogene.[10]

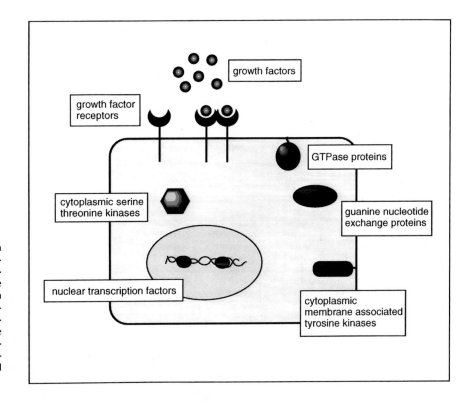

FIG. 10-1 Schematic representation of the cellular compartments where oncogene or proto-oncogene products are localized. These compartments include growth factors, transmembrane growth factor receptors, nonintegral membrane-associated proteins of the *src* tyrosine kinase gene family, the *ras* GTPase gene family, guanine nucleotide exchange proteins plus serine threonine kinase oncoproteins localized in the cytoplasm, and nuclear transcription factors.

Activation of Oncogenes by Proviral Insertion

Retroviruses that produce disease in animals after long latent periods do not contain transduced host oncogenes. The long latency period for disease caused by these retroviruses is in part a result of the low probability that the retrovirus will integrate into or adjacent to host cellular proto-oncogenes (Fig. 10-2B,C). Integration enhances proto-oncogene expression in a manner similar to that of the acute transforming retroviruses and has been shown to induce the unregulated expression of cellular homologues of known oncogenes, resulting in or contributing to neoplastic transformation.[7,11]

This activation mechanism first was demonstrated with avian leukosis virus-induced bursal lymphomas. In these tumors, transcription of the c-*myc* gene was elevated 50- to 100-fold as a result of a provirus insertion upstream from the c-*myc* proto-oncogene locus.[7] This is shown schematically in models *B* and *C* (Fig. 10-2). Several modes of oncogene activation by provirus insertion have been documented, showing that integration of proviruses can also occur downstream of c-*myc* or upstream in the opposite orienta-

tion.[11] Retroviruses that lack v-*onc* sequences can induce many different types of tumors, ranging from lymphoproliferative diseases to mammary carcinomas. The presence of a provirus integrated in the same region of the cellular genome in independently derived tumors of the same histologic type has allowed investigators to identify new cellular genes that can be activated in specific tumor lineages. With the use of this strategy, many novel oncogenes have been discovered (Table 10-1).

DETECTION OF ONCOGENES IN HUMAN TUMORS

Evidence for a genetic role of oncogenes in cancer comes from multiple sources. Many of the cancer-prone syndromes, such as Fanconi syndrome, Bloom syndrome, and ataxia-telangiectasia, show greatly increased chromosome instability.[12] Studies of colon

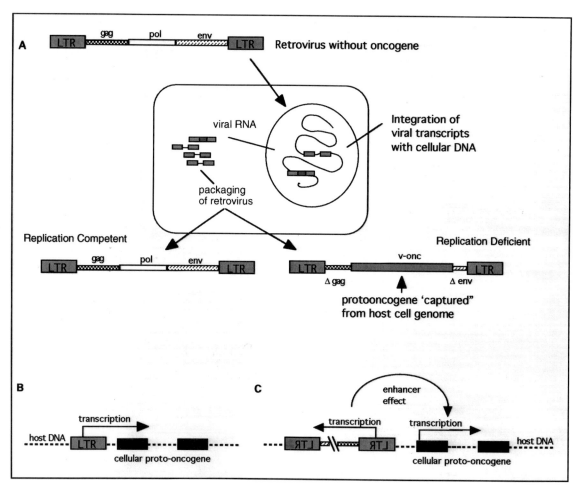

FIG. 10-2 Schematic representation of the mechanisms of activation of a host gene by insertion of a provirus and the general structure of leukemia and leukosis and acute transforming retroviral genomes. *A.* Genome of a nondefective leukemia or leukosis retrovirus, infection of a host cell, and integration into the host genome. The *gag* region encodes the internal structural proteins of the virion, the *pol* region encodes the virion RNA-dependent DNA polymerase (reverse transcriptase), and the *env* region encodes the proteins found on the surface of the virion envelope. LTR is the long terminal repeat that appears at each end of the integrated linear DNA forms. Within the LTR region are DNA sequences which define the initiation site for RNA transcription and at the 3' end encode a poly A addition site where the viral RNA polyadenylation occurs and transcription enhancer sequences that result in the production of high levels of transcripts. The LTR elements provide all the functions needed for eukaryotic transcription to take place and for

the provirus to express genomic viral RNA. *B* and *C* depict two different configurations of inserted proviral DNA. Replication-competent and -defective viruses are produced. The genome of a replication-defective acute transforming retrovirus containing v-*onc* sequences is shown. Although substantial portions of *gag, pol,* and/or *env* may be deleted in acute transforming retroviruses, they still retain the terminal noncoding LTR regions. *B.* Insertion of a proviral LTR upstream of the first coding exon as observed with c-*myc*. This insertion results in a transcript that no longer contains sequences that regulate c-*myc* expression levels. The protein coding domains (exons) of the normal host gene are shown in solid black rectangles. *C.* Integration of an intact provirus upstream (or downstream) from, for example, the *int 1* and *int 2* genes. This form of integration may not alter the gene product but generally results in increased transcription of that gene promoted by the transcriptional enhancing activity of the retroviral LTR.

cancer have shown that many cancers have accumulated multiple chromosome deletions and mutations.[13] The recent identification of the bacterial mutS and mutL DNA mismatch repair genes as genetic lesions that predispose to colon cancer further supports the role of mutation in the generation of cancer.[14,15] Several strategies were developed to identify oncogenes in human tumors. They were identified initially by using DNA transfection techniques. However, the discovery that oncogenes frequently are activated by chromosomal translocations has stimulated the isolation of genes that map to the breakpoints of nonrandom chromosomal rearrangement present in human tumors as a method to identify new candidate oncogenes.

Detection of Oncogenes by DNA Transfection

The DNA transfection assay was developed to study and identify the transforming genes of RNA or DNA tumor viruses.[16,17] The cells used as recipients in most transfection experiments are NIH3T3 cells; these cells are mouse fibroblasts in origin and are maintained as contact-inhibited, nontumorigenic cell lines. Transformation of these cells by gene transfer is monitored by changes in cell morphology in culture and loss of contact inhibition, where cells overgrow the monolayer and form focal areas of dense layers termed foci, or by a modification of this technique in which the cells that have acquired transforming genes produce tumors in nude mice (Fig. 10-3).[18–21]

To assay for transforming genes, genomic DNA prepared from human tumors or tumor cell lines is transferred to recipient NIH3T3 cells. Transfer of DNA-containing activated oncogenes occasionally gives rise to foci of morphologically altered cells that have tumorigenic properties. Foci or tumors thus obtained contain NIH3T3 cells that are transformed as a result of incorporating human DNA containing an activated oncogene. Human repetitive DNA sequences located in the vicinity of the oncogene can be distinguished from mouse sequences[22] and can be used to molecularly clone and isolate the DNA segment responsible for transformation of the NIH3T3 cells (Fig. 10-3).[23–25] Many of the human transforming genes identified in this manner are related to the *ras* family of oncogenes (Table 10-1). For instance, the transforming genes of a human bladder and lung carcinoma were shown to be homologous to the *ras* genes previously identified in the acute transforming retroviruses of the Harvey[26] and Kirsten[27] sarcoma viruses and were designated c-H-*ras*[28–30] and c-K-*ras*, respectively.[28–30] In addition, a third *ras* gene family member initially was identified in a human neuroblastoma tumor cell line and human promyelocytic leukemia cell line and was designated N-*ras* (Table 10-1).[31–35] Approximately 50 percent of colorectal cancers and 95 percent of pancreatic cancers contain mutations of a *ras* gene. A significant subset of acute nonlymphocytic leukemias, thyroid cancers, and adenocarcinomas of the lung also contain such mutations. In most other tumor types (e.g., cancers of the breast, prostate, stomach, bladder, liver, and brain), however, *ras* mutations do not occur often if at all. As *ras* genes are ubiquitously expressed and presumably have similar functions in all cells, the basis for this tissue specificity is perplexing.[36–38]

Gene transfer studies also have led to the identification of a growing number of transforming genes that are not members of the *ras* gene family and have not been identified in a retrovirus. These include the *neu, met, trk, mas, erbB-2/HER-2, ret, hst,* and KS3 oncogenes (Table 10-1).[21,39–46]

Chemical Carcinogens

Chemical carcinogens are known to be mutagenic and induce tumors in rodent models. Whereas the majority of mutations are non-

deleterious to the host, a small number trigger neoplastic development. Genes activated in chemically induced tumors were identified by the DNA transfection assay and were shown frequently to involve genes of the *ras* family. A single dose of nitrosomethylurea (NMU) or dimethylbenz(a)anthracene (DMBA), a direct-acting carcinogen, induces mammary tumors in rats, where the c-H-*ras* locus is activated in 85 and 25 percent of the cases, respectively.[47–49] Similarly, one allele of the c-H-*ras* gene is activated in 90 percent of benign papillomas induced by topical application of DMBA followed by treatment with the tumor promoters reviewed.[38,50]

The mutations identified in the activated *ras* genes are carcinogen-specific. For example, each of the *ras* oncogenes activated in NMU- but not DMBA-treated rats became activated by a single

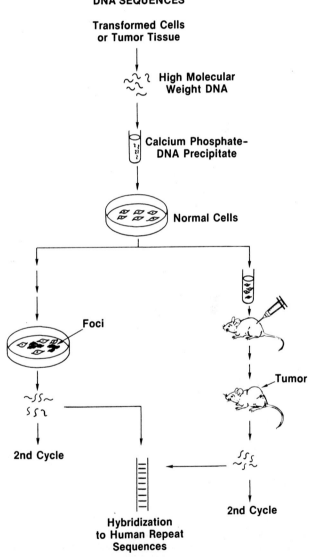

DETECTION OF TRANSFORMING HUMAN DNA SEQUENCES

FIG. 10-3 NIH3T3 DNA transfection and/or transformation assay. High-molecular-weight DNA prepared from transformed cell or tumor DNA is precipitated with calcium phosphate and added to nontransformed mouse NH3T3 cells. These cells are then assayed for tumor production in nude mice or assayed for the appearance of foci. DNA is prepared from either primary foci or tumors and is subjected to a second cycle of transfection to facilitate the loss of additional sequences that are transferred with the transforming gene. After several cycles of transfection, the majority of the foreign DNA in the focus or tumor corresponds to the transforming gene and can be isolated by recombinant DNA technology.

point mutation that caused the replacement of the guanine for an alanine base in codon 12 of the *ras* gene. These mutations result from the properties of NMU, which causes O6 methylation of the guanosine, and if this is not repaired, it will result in the replacement by an alanine during DNA replication (reviewed in Ref. 38). In contrast, DMBA forms large adducts with adenine residues, and *ras* genes activated by DMBA treatment in the mouse skin model have A-T transitions in the second base of codon 61. However, this mutation was not detected when DMBA was replaced by an alkylating carcinogen, MMNG, where G-A transitions in codon 12 were observed.[50] *Ras* genes in human tumors have been shown to be activated by similar single point mutations predominantly involving codons 12, 13, 59, and 61.

Identification of Oncogenes at Chromosomal Breakpoints

The chromosomal location of cellular proto-oncogenes determined by in situ hybridization led to the identification of several proto-oncogenes at or near chromosomal translocation break points.[51,52] In general, structural rearrangements that juxtapose two different chromosomal regions are thought to contain dominant transforming genes, whereas deletions or monosomies are thought to be the site of recessive tumor suppressor genes.

Recurrent tumor-specific chromosome translocations were first identified in cytogenetic analyses of leukemias and myelodysplasias and are considered to be involved in tumor development.[53,54] The tumor-specific chromosome abnormalities of leukemias and lymphomas usually are somatically acquired alterations. In some tumor types, such as chronic myelogenous leukemia, the same translocations consistently appear, supporting the hypothesis that these events are a prerequisite for tumor induction. Where it has been possible to characterize and molecularly isolate the genes adjacent to translocation breakpoints, candidate genes implicated in tumor initiation and progression have been identified (Table 10-2).

In many cases, breaks occur within a gene on each of the participating chromosomes, resulting in the formation of a chimeric gene that encodes a fusion protein. An example of this is chronic myelogenous leukemia (CML), which is a pluripotent stem cell disease characterized by the presence of a consistent translocation. The Philadelphia (Ph) chromosome translocation between chromosomes 9 and 22, t(9;22) (q34;qll) is present in the leukemic cells of at least 95 percent of all CML patients.[51,55] The proto-oncogene c-*abl*, which is the normal cellular homologue of the oncogene v-*abl* of Abelson murine leukemic virus (A-MuLV) (Table 10-1), is translocated from chromosome 9, band q34, into the *bcr* gene on chromosome 22 at band q11.[56] This gives rise to a chimeric gene expressing a fusion protein containing the amino terminus derived from the *bcr* protein and the carboxy terminus derived from the *abl* protein (Fig. 10-4). The resulting chimeric protein has increased catalytic activity compared with the normal protein and will transform cells in culture.[57] These alterations are discussed in more detail in Chap. 6.

Although many translocations give rise to a new protein, some, such as those involving the c-*myc* and immunoglobulin genes on the chromosome translocations 2:14, 8:14, and 22:14 observed in lymphomas, result in altered regulation of the *myc* gene.[58] Normally, the expression of this gene is tightly regulated, but in cells where the translocation has occurred, the gene is expressed constitutively.

As a consequence of technical improvements, cytogenetic abnormalities have now been identified in solid tumors (Table 10-2).[59] Such rearrangements are found in a high proportion of tumors, suggesting that they could provide much-needed markers for use in diagnosis of sarcoma types. In addition to chromosomal rearrangements, frequent chromosomal abnormalities documented in solid tumors involve the amplification or deletion of specific chromosomal regions.

Proto-Oncogene Amplification

Cellular proto-oncogenes have been found in multiple copies in various tumors and transformed cell lines. The amplified proto-oncogene copies can occur in homogeneously staining chromosomal regions or double-minute chromosomes.[60,61] Oncogene amplification also has been observed through the use of hybridization techniques in tumor cells in the absence of microscopic chromosomal changes. The mechanism of gene amplification is not fully understood; illegitimate DNA replication occurring more than once during a single cell cycle could account for the increase of multiple segments (amplification units) of DNA from 200 to 2000 kb in size.[62]

All amplified proto-oncogenes express high levels of the corresponding RNA and protein and appear to be unrearranged. The amplification unit containing the proto-oncogene DNA can be at a site distant from its normal locus as a heterogeneously staining region. The c-*myc* gene was the first proto-oncogene to be amplified. In the promyelocytic leukemia cell line HL60 as well as in the primary tumor, 8 to 30 copies of c-*myc* per cell were detected.[63,64] Other proto-oncogenes, including c-*myb*, c-*erb*B (EGFR), HER-2 (also called c-*erb*B2; corresponds to *neu* in the rat), and c-*myc* family members, have also been shown to be amplified in certain tumors or tumor cell lines (Table 10-3). The presence of multiple copies of proto-oncogenes in tumor cells has been associated with a poor prognosis. N-*myc*, which was first identified as an amplified gene in a human neuroblastoma, is present in multiple copies in 40 percent of neuroblastomas, and its amplification correlates with more advanced stages of the disease.[65,66] Amplification of members of the *myc* gene family (c-*myc*, N-*myc*, L*myc*) in small-cell lung carcinomas also may be associated with the more malignant stages of the tumor.[67] The amplified proto-oncogene frequently is tumor-specific; for example, N-*myc* or c-*myc* appears to be associated with the progression of neuroblastomas and small-cell lung carcinoma cells, the EGFR (c-*erb*B) gene has been found to be amplified in glioblastomas and several squamous carcinomas, and the related HER-2 gene is often found amplified in adenocarcinomas and in advanced, hormone-independent mammary tumors with a poor prognosis.[68-72] This suggests that increased expression of these proto-oncogenes plays a role in the development and progression of these tumors.

FUNCTIONS AND MECHANISMS OF ACTIVATION OF PROTO-ONCOGENE PRODUCTS

Conservation of Proto-Oncogenes

Homologues of proto-oncogenes have been found in all multicellular animals studied thus far, and their widespread distribution in nature indicates that their protein products play essential biologic roles. The more highly conserved domains of the protein probably are those which have a crucial structural and/or functional role, and characterization of their normal biochemical properties will provide insight into the contribution an activated oncogene makes to cell transformation. Understanding the mechanism of activation of each oncogene requires characterization of the proto-oncogene,

Table 10-2 Molecularly Characterized Neoplastic Rearrangements

Affected Gene	Translocation	Disease	Protein Type	Ref.
Gene Fusions				
c-ABL (9q34)	t(9;22) (q34;q11)	Chronic myelogenous leukemia and acute leukemia	Tyrosine kinase activated by BCR	56
BCR (22q11)				
PBX-1 (1q23)	t(1;19)(q23;p13.3)	Acute pre-B-cell leukemia	Homeodomain	273
E2A (19p13.3)			HLH	
PML (15q21)	t(15;17) (q21;q11–22)	Acute myeloid leukemia	Zn finger	274,275
RAR (17q21)				
CAN (6p23)	t(6;9) (p23;q34)	Acute myeloid leukemia	No homology	276
DEK (9q34)				
REL	ins(2;12) (p13;p11.2–14)	Non-Hodgkin's lymphoma	NF-kBfamily	277
NRG			no homology	
Oncogenes Juxtaposed with IG Loci				
c-MYC	t(8;14) (q24;q32)	Burkitt's lymphoma, BL-ALL	HLH domain	278
	t(2;8) (p12;q24)			
	t(8;22) (q24;q11)			
BCL1 (PRADI?)	t(11;14) (q13;q32)	B-cell chronic lymphocyte leukemia	PRADI-G1 cyclin	279,280
BCL-2	t(14;18) (q32;21)	Follicular lymphoma	Inner mitochondrial membrane	219,281
BCL-3	t(14;19) (q32;q13.1)	Chronic B-cell leukemia	CDC10 motif	282,283
IL-3	t(5;14) (q31;q32)	Acute pre-B-cell leukemia	growth factor	282,283
Oncogenes Juxtaposed with TCR Loci				
c-MYC	t(8;14) (q24;q11)	Acute T-cell leukemia	HLH domain	284
LYL-1	t(7;19) (q35;p13)	Acute T-cell leukemia	HLH domain	285
TAL-1/SCL/ TCL-5	t(1;14) (p32;q11)	Acute T-cell leukemia	HLH domain	286
TAL-2	t(7;9) (q35;q34)	Acute T-cell leukemia	HLH domain	287
Rhombotin 1/ Ttg-1	t(11;14) (p15;q11)	Acute T-cell leukemia	LIM domain	288
Rhombotin 2/ Ttg-2	t(11;14) (p13;q11)	Acute T-cell leukemia	LIM domain	289
	t(7;11) (q35;p13)			
HOX-11	t(10;14) (q24;q11)	Acute T-cell leukemia	Homeodomain	290,291
	t(7;10) (q35;q24)			
TAN-1	t(7;9) (q34;q34.3)	Acute T-cell leukemia	Notch homolog	280,292
Gene Fusions in Sarcomas				
FLI1, EWS	t(11;22) (q24;q12)	Ewing's sarcoma	Ets transcription factor family	59
ERG, EWS	t(21;22) (q22;q12)	Ewing's sarcoma	Ets transcription factor family	
ATV1, EWS	t(7;21) (p22;q12)	Ewing's sarcoma	Ets transcription factor family	
ATF1, EWS	t(12;22) (q13;q12)	Soft tissue clear cell sarcoma	Transcription factor	
CHN, EWS	t(9;22) (q22–31;q12)	Myxoid chondrosarcoma	Steroid receptor family	
WT1, EWS	t(11;22) (p13;q12)	Desmoplastic small round cell tumor	Wilms' tumor gene	
SSX1, SSX2, SYT	t(X;18) (p11.2;q11.2)	Synovial sarcoma	HLH domain	
PAX3, FKHR	t(2;13) (q37;q14)	Alveolar	Homeobox homologue	
PAX7, FKHR	t(1;13) (q36;q14)	Rhabdomyosarcoma	Homeobox homologue	
CHOP, TLS	t(12;16) (q13;p11)	Myxoid liposarcoma	Transcription factor	
var, HMGI-C	t(var;12) (var;q13–15)	Lipomas	HMG DNA binding protein	
HMGI-C?	t(12;14) (q13–15)	Leiomomas	HMG DNA binding protein	
Oncogenes Juxtaposed with Other Loci				
PTH deregulates	inv(11)(p15;q13)	Parathyroid adenoma	PRADI-GI cyclin	279,293
PRADI				
BTGI deregulates	t(8;12)(q24;q22)	B-cell chronic lymphocytic leukemia	MYC-HLH domain	294
MYC				

IG = immunoglobulin; TCR = T-cell receptor; HLH = helix loop helix structural domain; zn = zinc; HMG = high mobility group.

a comparison of the changes that have occurred, and systematic testing of changes that influence the transforming potential.

There essentially are only three biochemical mechanisms by which proto-oncogenes act. One mechanism involves phosphorylation of proteins on serine, threonine, or tyrosine residues.[73] Proteins of this class transfer phosphate groups from ATP to the side chain of tyrosine or serine or threonine residues. Phosphorylation serves two basic purposes in signal transduction. First, in many instances it changes the conformation and activates the enzymatic kinase activity of the protein. Second, phosphorylation of tyrosine residues generates docking sites that recruit target proteins, which the activated kinase may phosphorylate. Thus, phosphorylation

acts to potentiate signal transmission through the generation of complexes of signal-transducing molecules at the specific sites in the cell where they are required to act. For example, activation of the catalytic activity of a receptor tyrosine kinase by its ligand leads to the formation of a complex of signaling proteins at the plasma membrane where the receptor is localized.

The second mechanism by which genes act to transmit signals involves GTPases.[74,75] The prototype for this class of proteins is the *ras* gene family. In a similar manner to the kinase gene family, *ras* proteins function as molecular switches that are turned of and on via a regulated GDP/GTP cycle. *Ras* proteins have been implicated as key intermediates that relay the signal from upstream tyrosine

Normal Configuration of
Chromosomes 9 and 22

Rearranged Chromosome 9(9q+) & 22(Ph)

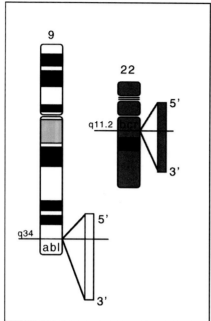
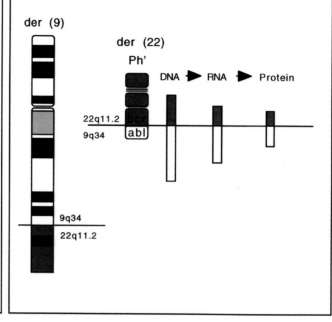

FIG. 10-4 Schematic representation of the chromosomes involved in the generation of the Philadelphia chromosome observed in >95 percent of patients with CML. A schematic presentation of the normal chromosomes 9 and 22 and one of the chromosome translocations 9q+ and 22q− are shown. The c-*ABL* proto-oncogene on the distal tip of chromosome 9q34 is translocated into the *BCR* locus on chromosome 22q11.2. This generates a chimeric gene that expresses a chimeric *BCR-ABL* message and fusion protein.

kinases to downstream serine threonine kinase pathways. Some of the conventional heterotrimeric G proteins can also transform cells when altered.[74] The third mechanism involves proteins that are localized in the nucleus. A large variety of proteins that control progress through the cell cycle and gene expression are encoded by proto-oncogenes, some of which also may be involved in DNA replication.[77,78] Thus, the relaxation of the requirements of transformed cells for growth factors could be mediated by an activated oncogene at multiple levels of the signal transduction pathway.

Growth Factors

Growth factors stimulate cells in a resting, or G0, stage to enter the cell cycle. This mitogenic response occurs in two phases; a quiescent cell is stimulated to proceed into the G1 phase of the cell cycle by competence factors and then becomes committed to DNA synthesis by progression factors (Fig. 10-5).[79] Successful transition through the G1 phase requires sustained growth factor stimulation over a period of several hours. This is followed by a critical phase where the presence of a progression factor such as insulin growth factor I is required in addition to the growth factor for successful

progression through the cell cycle (Fig. 10-5). This dual signal requirement may prevent accidental triggering of quiescent cells into the cell cycle by transient exposure to mitogenic growth factors. In some cell types, the absence of growth factor stimulation causes the rapid onset of programmed cell death, or apoptosis.[80] Certain growth factors also can promote differentiation of a progenitor cell while stimulating cell proliferation, whereas others block differentiation and promote proliferation. Therefore, innapropriate expression of a growth factor may result in constant stimulation of cell growth in addition to a block of cell differentiation.

There is much evidence to support a role for growth factors and their receptors in the development of human malignancies. The first direct correlation of an oncogene with a growth factor was revealed after a computer-assisted comparison that showed that the amino acid sequence of the v-*sis* oncogene product was highly related to the B chain of platelet-derived growth factor (PDGF) (Table 10-1).[81–83] PDGF is released from platelets during clotting and is recognized as an important serum mitogen required for mesenchymal cell growth in culture.[84] Connective tissue tumors, such as sarcomas and glioblastomas, have been shown to express the c-*sis* proto-oncogene, whereas their normal tissue counterparts do not.[85] Thus, in an autocrine fashion, the sarcoma and glial tumor

Table 10-3 Examples of Cellular Proto-Oncogenes Amplified in Human Tumors

Tumor	Oncogene	Amplification	Ref.
Small-cell lung cancer	c-*myc*	Up to 80X	67
	N-*myc*	Up to 50X	66
	L-*myc*	Up to 20X	266
Neuroblastomas	N-*myc*	Up to 250X	295
Glioblastomas	c-*erb*B1 (EGFR)	Up to 50X	296
Mammary carcinoma	c-*erb*B2 (HER2)	Up to 30X	71,72
	c-*myc*	Up to 50X	297
	cyclin D1	Up to 30X	201

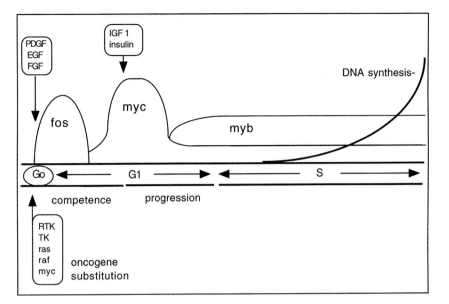

FIG. 10-5 A schematic representation of the requirements for the coordinated actions of two complementing growth factors to induce DNA synthesis. A transient increase in the expression of both c-*fos* and c-*myc* occurs after PDGF, FGF, or EGF stimulation or treatment of cells with phorbol ester (TPA or a calcium ionophore). Cells rendered competent require insulin or insulin growth factor 1 to progress through the cell cycle. Several oncogenes specifically substitute for the competence factor requirement when tested on murine fibroblasts.

cells appear to synthesize the mitogen to which they are normally responsive (Fig. 10-6). By contrast, no genetic alterations of the PDGF gene have been observed that would explain this synthesis. Until the mechanism underlying the expression of PDGF is clarified, it will be difficult to know whether this expression is a cause or an effect of neoplastic growth.

Int-2, whose expression is activated by MMTV proviral insertion in mouse mammary carcinomas, the KS3 oncogene identified in a Kaposi sarcoma, and *hst*, a transforming gene identified in a human stomach cancer by DNA transfection, are members of the basic or acidic fibroblast growth factor (FGF) family of related peptide mitogens (Table 10-1).[45,86–89] Basic FGFs are expressed by human melanoma cell lines but not by normal melanocytes that are dependent on bFGF to proliferate.[90,91] Similarly, transforming growth factor α (TGFα) is frequently produced by carcinomas that express high levels of the epidermal growth factor receptor (EGFR) and appears to function as an autocrine in this system through stimulation of EGFR.[92] Because many ligands and their receptors have not been characterized, the contribution of au-

tocrine growth stimulatory loops to human malignancies may be greater than is appreciated currently.

Growth Factor Receptors

Oncogenes derived from growth factor receptors confer on cells the ability to bypass the growth factor requirement, rendering cells growth factor-independent. By far the largest number of receptor-derived oncoproteins are derived from growth factor receptors that have tyrosine kinase activity.

Tyrosine Protein Kinases. More than 40 different protein tyrosine kinases have been identified (Table 10-1).[73] These kinases are subdivided into two main categories: those spanning the plasma membrane, such as the EPGR, and those located in the cytoplasm, many of which are associated with the plasma membrane, such as c-*src* (Fig. 10-7). All the protein-tyrosine kinases have sequence homology over a region of approximately 300 amino acids that has been defined as the catalytic kinase domain (Fig. 10-7).[93] This domain is responsible for catalyzing the transfer of the phosphate group of ATP to tyrosine residues during trans- and autophosphorylation. This kinase domain also is homologous to the *raf*, *mil*, and *mos* members, which have phosphorylation specificity for serine and threonine (Table 10-1).[94] Phosphorylation on tyrosine is a rare event in normal cells and accounts for only 0.05 percent of all protein phosphorylation, but tyrosine kinases regulate key events in signal transduction pathways that control cell shape and growth.[95]

Growth Factor Receptor Tyrosine Kinases. Many growth factors mediate their effects by means of receptors with tyrosine kinase activity. These receptors have an extracellular ligand-binding domain, a single transmembrane domain, and an intracellular catalytic domain, responsible for transducing the mitogenic signal (Fig. 10-7).[96] Binding of growth factors to cell surface receptors results in receptor dimerization and activation of their intrinsic tyrosine kinase, leading to intermolecular phosphorylation of each receptor on specific tyrosine residues.[97] This results in the recruitment of signaling molecules containing *src* homology 2 (SH2) domains, which recognize, in a sequence-specific manner, short peptide segments containing phosphotyrosine within activated receptors (Fig. 10-8).[98–101] These molecules include proteins with enzymatic activity such as phospholipase Cγ (PLCγ), phosphatidyl inositol 3-kinase (PI3K), and, the GTPase activating protein for p21 *Ras* (p120 GAP), and proteins that lack enzyme activ-

Autocrine Model

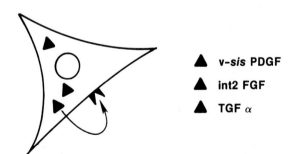

▲ v-*sis* PDGF

▲ int2 FGF

▲ TGF α

FIG. 10-6 Diagrammatic representation of an autocrine model of growth stimulation. The figure shows a cell with a nucleus that bears growth factor receptors on its surface. The cell produces and exports one of these factors (closed triangles) to the extracellular fluid. The normal growth factors and their corresponding oncogene are platelet-derived growth factor (PDGF) (v-*sis*), fibroblast growth factor (FGF) (int-2), transforming growth factor α (TGFα), and interleukin-2 and -3 (IL-2 and IL-3). Only cells that express a receptor specific for a particular growth factor will respond. For clarity, closed triangles are used to represent all the factors. In reality each growth factor has a characteristic structure and a specific receptor.

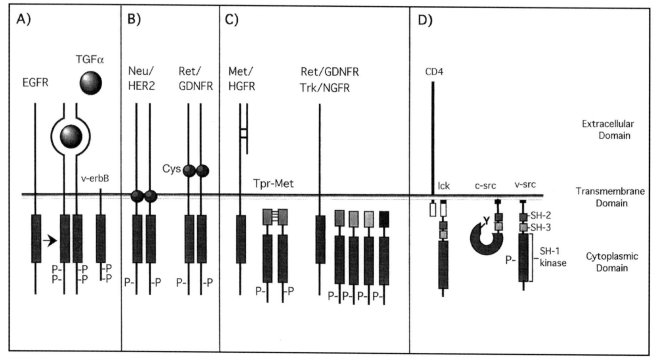

FIG. 10-7 Schematic comparison of structural features of cell surface growth factor receptor tyrosine kinases and membrane-associated tyrosine kinase oncogene products. The cytoplasmic tyrosine kinase domain is represented as cross-hatched boxes. SH-1, SH-2, and SH-3 domains are indicated as solid black boxes, and the position of carboxy terminal tyrosine residues is shown (Y). The deletion that activates v-*erb*B and the gene rearrangements that activate the *met*, *ret*, and *trk* oncogene products are illustrated. The v-*src* oncogene is generated after deletion of a negative regulatory carboxy terminal tyrosine residue in addition to point mutations within critical domains of the molecule. Single point mutations in the transmembrane domain of the HER2/Neu and the extracellular domain of the Ret/GDNFR receptor are shown as solid circles. The complex formed between CD4 and the *src* family kinase *lck* is shown. The protein domains through which *lck* and CD4 interact are represented as open boxes in these molecules. EGF = epidermal growth factor; HGF/SF = hepatocyte growth factor–scatter factor; NGF = nerve growth factor; GDNF = glial cell-derived nerve growth factor; TGFβ = transforming growth factor β.

ity and function as adaptor proteins, such as Grb2. Collectively they act to transmit signals that mediate the pleiotrophic responses to growth factors.[102,103] PLCγ hydrolyzes phosphoinositols and thereby generates diacylglycerol and inositol-3-phosphate. PI3K phosphorylates phosphoinositides and generates putative second messangers for cytoskeletal rearrangements and cellular trafficking. By contrast, Grb2 lacks enzymatic activity and contains only SH2 and SH3 domains. SH3 domains also function as protein:protein interaction motifs and recognize proline-rich domains in other proteins.[104] Grb2 serves as an adapter that binds to phosphotyrosines in activated receptors via its SH2 domain and recruits the *ras* nucleotide exchange factors Son of sevenless (mSos-1 and mSos-2) to the receptor via its SH3 domain. Sos catalyzes exchange of GDP bound to *ras* for GTP and is considered the most important step in *ras* activation.[105,106] These proteins, through a series of protein–protein interactions, in part mediated through SH2 domains and SH3 domains, form signaling complexes downstream of receptor tyrosine kinases.[104] Many of these signaling complexes regulate the activity of serine/threonine kinases, which in turn regulate through phosphorylation the activity of transcription factors. A generalized scheme for receptor signaling is presented in Fig. 10-8.

A number of oncogenes encode mutant forms of receptor tyrosine kinases. These include receptors for known factors, such as the epidermal growth factor receptor (v-*erb*B), colony stimulating factor-1 receptor (v-*fms*), hepatocyte growth/scatter factor receptor (*met*), nerve growth factor receptor (*trk*), stem cell factor receptor (*kit*), neuroregulin receptor (HER2/*Neu*), GDNF receptor (*ret*), and receptor-like proteins with unknown ligands (*ros*) (Fig. 10-7).[107–114] In the receptor-related oncogenes thus far examined, the structural changes that activate the transforming potential appear to deregulate the receptor kinase activity, and these oncoproteins transform by delivering a continuous ligand-independent signal.[115] Receptors

isolated as retrovirally transduced oncogenes, such as v-*erb*B (EGFR), v-*fms* (CSF-1R), and v-*kit* (SCFR) (Table 10-1), frequently sustain deletions of the extracellular ligand-binding domain in combination with other structural alterations, such as carboxy terminal deletions and mutations that remove negative regulatory domains and render the receptor catalytically active in the absence of ligand (Fig. 10-7).[115]

Mutations that promote ligand-independent dimerization represent a general mechanism for oncogenic activation of receptor tyrosine kinases. A single point mutation in the transmembrane domain of the *Neu/HER*2 oncogene product is sufficient for ligand-independent activation. This mutation promotes receptor dimerization and kinase activation in the absence of ligand (Fig. 10-7).[116,117] Similarly, the loss of a single cysteine residue in the extracellular domain of the *Ret* receptor in multiple endocrine neoplasia type 2A syndrome results in a constitutively activated receptor. This mutation frees a cysteine residue that is normally involved in intrareceptor disulfide bond formation and enhances receptor dimerization by the formation of intermolecular disulfide bonds promoting constitutive activation of the receptor catalytic activity (Fig. 10-7).[118,119] A similar mechanism has been demonstrated for the activation of the *Neu/HER*2 receptor in experimentally induced mammary neoplasias.[120] Alternatively, activation of the *Ret* receptor in multiple endocrine neoplasia type 2B occurs through a single point mutation in the kinase domain that increases the basal kinase activity and alters the substrate specifity of the receptor, thus altering the signal transduction pathways activated by the receptor.[119,121]

A growing class of receptor tyrosine kinase oncogenes in human tumors, including *trk*, *met*, *ret*, and PDGFR, are rendered constitutively active after genomic rearrangements that juxtapose novel sequences derived from unrelated loci with the kinase do-

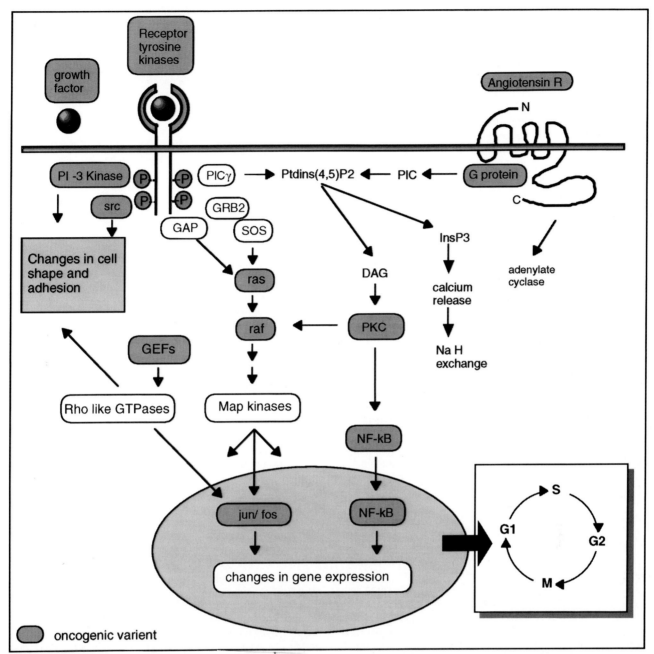

FIG. 10-8 Substrates and mitogenic signaling for receptor tyrosine kinases (RTKs) and receptors of the serpentine class (seven transmembrane domain motif). Activation of receptor tyrosine kinases by the binding of growth factors stimulates cross-phosphorylation of their kinase domains. It is believed that SH2 domain-containing proteins bind to phosphorylated tyrosine residues on activated receptors and substrates to directly interact with and become phophorylated by RTKs; GAP (GTPase activating protein), PLCγ (phospholipase C γ), PI-3 kinase (phosphatidyl inositol 3′ kinase), and *src* (tyrosine kinase) are represented. After stimulation of the serpentine class of receptors they couple with heterotrimeric G proteins and initiate their signaling pathway through activation of phospholipase C or adenylate cyclase. Secondary responses for both receptor types involve the breakdown of phosphatidyl inositol 4,5 *bis*-phosphate into diacylglycerol (DAG) and inositol triphosphate (InsP3), which stimulate protein kinase C and calcium release, respectively. Components of the signal transduction pathway that have been identified as oncogenes are shown.

main of the receptor (Fig 10-7).[41,122–124] The majority of receptor oncogenes activated by gene rearrangement are fused with a protein domain capable of protein:protein interaction and thus mediate dimerization and constitutive activation of the kinase in the absence of ligand.[115] Receptor fusion oncogenes involving *RET* and *TRK* are generated at high frequency in papillary thyroid carcinomas.[125–127] In these tumors both *RET* (10q11.2) and *TRK* (1q21) are rearranged with loci from the same chromosome, such as H4-*ret* (D10S170, Ptc) 10q21 and tropomyosin or tpr/trk (1q21–31).[122,128,129] Thus, small intrachromosomal deletions or inversions that are not readily detected cytogenetically may be a common event in the oncogenic activation of these receptor kinases in human tumors.

In addition to structural rearrangements, growth factor receptors are frequently amplified and overexpressed in human tumors. EGFR is overexpressed in squamous cell carcinomas and gliomas, *HER2/neu* in adenocarcinomas of the breast, stomach, and ovary, *met* (HGFR) in human stomach and some colon carcinomas, and *bek*, a member of the FGFR family, in human stomach carcinomas (Table 10-3).[68–72,130–132]

Growth factor receptors not derived from tyrosine kinases also have been activated as oncoproteins. Two oncogenes—*mas*, which encodes the angiotensin receptor, and the seratonin receptor—are members of a family of receptors for neurotransmitters.[133] This family includes receptors for bombesin, bradykinin, noradrenalin, and vasopressin and encodes proteins with seven transmembrane domains and a short extracellular and cytoplasmic domain. Ligand binding results in activation of heterodimeric guanine nucleotide-binding proteins (G proteins), which couple such receptors with various effectors, including adenylyl cyclase, phospholipase C, and potassium channels (Fig. 10-8).[83] Oncogenic activation of these receptors results in the generation of a continuous growth stimulatory signal. In addition, autocrine activation of these receptors also has been documented in human tumors. Bombesin-like peptides are produced by neuroectodermally derived cells of small-cell carcinoma of the lung. Growth of these tumor cells can be inhibited in some instances by antibodies against bombesin, demonstrating the dependence of these cells for secretion of the autocrine to maintain cell growth.[134] It should be reemphasized, however, that the genetic mechanisms underlying these apparent activations have not been defined, and, so conclusions about their causal role in neoplasia should be guarded. Many genes are expressed differentially in transformed cells, and only a portion of such genes actually play a direct role in the neoplastic process.

Nonreceptor Protein Tyrosine Kinases. The protein products of v-*src*, v-*fes*, v-*fps*, v-*fgr*, v-*yes*, and *lck* are associated with the plasma membrane but are not transmembrane proteins (Fig. 10-7; Table 10-1). Many of these proteins have a myristilated N-terminal glycine residue that promotes association with the plasma membrane. The cytoplasmic tyrosine protein kinase domain is in the carboxy terminus of the protein, and all the tyrosine kinase oncogene proteins are homologous in this region. The *src* subfamily has additional regions of homology not found in the receptor family. These regions include two additional domains named *src* homology 2 and 3 (SH2 and SH3) (with SH1 defined as the kinase domain) (Fig. 10-7).[135] As discussed earlier, the *src* homology 2 domain is highly conserved in proteins involved in signal transduction and recognizes phosphotyrosine residues, whereas SH3 recognizes proline-rich motifs present in signaling proteins and cytoskeletal proteins.

Association of *src* family kinases with the plasma membrane is essential for their transforming activity. Mutation of the myristilation signal in these proteins abolishes membrane association and transforming activity, indicating that their signal must be initiated at the plasma membrane, perhaps through interaction with other membrane-bound proteins.[94,136] One of the *src* family of tyrosine kinases, *lck*, binds tightly to the cytoplasmic carboxy terminal domain of the CD4 and CD8 T-cell surface molecules (Fig. 10-7).[137,138] In this structure the *lck* protein is thought to serve as the catalytic subunit for these proteins in T cells and is activated on ligand binding to either the CD4 or CD8 cell surface molecules. Indeed, all *src* family tyrosine kinases may have similar functions.

Oncogenic activation of *src*-like kinases as retrovirally transduced oncoproteins occurs through the aquisition of point mutations and/or deletion of negative regulatory protein domains located at the carboxy terminus. These alterations generate oncoproteins that phosphorylate cellular proteins on tyrosine residues in an unregulated fashion and thus deliver a continuous rather than a regulated signal. *src* or other *src*-like kinases are essential components of mitogenic signaling pathways downstream from receptor tyrosine kinases.[139] Moreover, *src* kinase activity is activated by receptor tyrosine kinases, suggesting that *src* or *src*-like kinases are activated in tumors where receptor tyrosine kinases are deregulated.[139] Indeed, activation of c-*src* has been observed in mammary tumors in transgenic mice induced by an oncogenic *Neu/HER*2 receptor.[140]

The *abl* tyrosine kinase constitutes a separate family of nonreceptor tyrosine kinases that are localized to both the nucleus and the cytoplasm. The *Bcr-abl* product has been implicated in the pathogenesis of more than 95 percent of cases of CML. In a manner similar to receptor fusion oncoproteins, *Bcr* mediates oligomerization of *Bcr-abl*, promoting constitutive activation of the *Abl* kinase and association with downstream signaling molecules.[141] Moreover, the *Bcr-abl* oncoproteins are excluded from the nucleus that may also prevent interactions with substrates that act to regulate cell growth negatively.[141]

Cytoplasmic Adaptor Proteins. The discovery that some oncogenes encode adaptor proteins that contain only SH2 and SH3 domains but lack any catalytic activity has allowed a more complete understanding of the role of these proteins in signal transduction. For example, the v-*crk* oncogene product (Table 10-1) contains only SH2 and SH3 domains but causes an increase in tyrosine phosphorylated proteins in the cell.[142,143] *Crk* and other SH2/SH3 domain-containing adapter proteins bind to phosphorylated tyrosine residues on activated receptor tyrosine kinases or other kinases via their SH2 domains and bind to other proteins via their SH3 domains. In this manner they bring together heteromeric protein complexes that allow the subsequent phosphorylation of proteins in this complex by the kinase.[144,145] This phosphorylation event, in addition to dephosphorylation events, acts as a mechanism to relay the signal from the cell surface to the nucleus.

Proteins with GTPase Activity

The role of proteins with GTPase activity in tumorigenesis was first identified through the discovery of the *ras* oncogenes that encode a previously unknown form of GTPase.[38] Three *ras* gene family members designated c-H-*ras*, c-K-*ras*, and N-*ras* involved in malignant transformation have been identified by their presence in rapidly transforming retroviruses and by DNA transfection (Table 10-1). This reflects the critical function of *ras* in mitogenic signal transduction in many cell types, and *ras* is therefore among the most intensively studied oncogenes.

In normal cells members of the *ras* family have been highly conserved throughout evolution and encode cytoplasmic proteins of 21,000 daltons (p21*ras*).[146] *ras* proteins are posttranslationally targeted to the plasma membrane through a highly conserved sequence at their amino and carboxy termini (Fig. 10-9).[147] Membrane association is essential for the function of *ras* proteins. Certain domains in *ras* proteins are homologous to the subunit of trimeric G proteins in regions involved in guanine nucleotide binding, and *ras* proteins have been shown to bind guanine nucleotides (GTP and GDP).[148] The model proposed for the p21 *ras* proto-oncogene product is that it exists in equilibrium between two conformations: active, with GTP bound, and inactive, with GDP bound (Fig. 10-9).

In the past 10 years components of signal transduction pathways have been elucidated and have placed *ras* as a crucial regulator of cell shape, motility, and growth downstream from growth factor receptors (Fig. 10-8). Activation of *ras* is coupled to ligand stimulation of growth factor receptors and is mediated by a guanine nucleotide exchange factor (GEF) (Sos). In the case of receptor tyrosine kinases, activation of *ras* is mediated by binding of the Grb2 adapter molecule via its SH2 domain to a specific phosphorylated tyrosine residue on the receptor. Grb2 pulls along the Sos protein, thus localizing it to the plasma membrane, where its substrate *ras* is localized. *Sos* then stimulates the exchange of GDP for GTP on *ras*, converting *ras* from an inactive to an active form able to interact with an effector/substrate molecule(s) (Fig. 10-9).[17,34,149–151] Conversely, the inactivation of *ras* is mediated in part by the intrinsic GTPase activity of *ras*. Usually this activity is low; however, the GTPase activity is stimulated by a GTPase-activating protein GAP, which converts the active GTP-bound form of

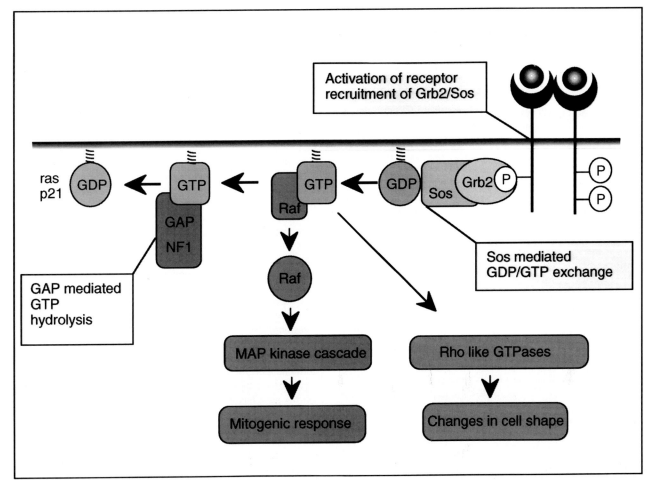

FIG. 10-9 Model for regulation of the *ras* p21 product and for GAP as a downstream effector and regulator of *ras* activity. *Ras* is localized to the inner aspect of the plasma membrane. The alternating relaxed (GDP-bound) and activated (GTP-bound) states of the p21 *ras* protein are shown in normal cells. Conversion of GDP- to GTP-bound forms is the rate-limiting step. Binding of the Grb2 adapter protein to a specific tyrosine phosphorylated residue on an activated (growth factor-stimulated) receptor tyrosine kinase translocates the Sos guanine nucleotide exchange factor to the plasma membrane, where it stimulates the exchange of GDP for GTP on *ras*. Activation of *ras* alters its conformation and allows it to interact with and recruit the *raf* serine threo- nine kinase to the membrane, where it becomes activated by an un- known (not *ras*) mechanism. Activation of *raf* activates the downstream MAP kinase signaling pathway involved in the mitogenic response. In addition, activation of *ras* stimulates changes in cell shape and motility mediated through the *Rho* family of GTPase proteins, which are part of the *ras* superfamily of small GTPase proteins. Inactivation of *ras* is in part controlled by the *ras* GTPase activating proteins (GAP and NF1). Oncogenic p21 *ras* proteins with mutations at amino acid positions 12, 13, 59, and 61 remain in their active GTP-bound states and constitu- tively activate downstream signaling pathways.

ras into the inactive GDP-bound form.[152–154] GAP also contains an SH2 domain and is recruited by activated receptor tyrosine kinases to the plasma membrane.

The activation and inactivation of *ras* proteins are carefully orchestrated. The conversion of *ras* to the GTP-bound state allows it to interact with other proteins that function as downstream effectors for *ras*. One effector for *ras* is the serine threonine kinase *raf*. Activation of *ras* recruits *raf* kinase to the membrane, where it is activated. In turn *raf* activates a linear signaling pathway involving a series of MAP kinases that culminates in the expression and activation of transcrition factors *fos* and *jun* (Fig. 10-8). These in turn form the AP1 transcription factor that induces transcrition of the c-*myc* transcription factor, which in turn regulates genes whose products control cell cycle progression, culminating in one round of DNA replication and cell division.

The *raf* protein kinase was independently isolated as a retrovirally transduced oncoprotein (Table 10-1). Inhibition of the *raf* signaling pathway by specific inhibitors or through the use of dominant negatively interfering mutants blocks transformation of fibroblasts in culture by an oncogenic *ras* protein.[155] In addition to *raf*, transformation of cells by an oncogenic *ras* also requires the

activity of members of the *Rho* family of GTPases, *Rho* and *Rac*.[156,157] Members of the *Rho* family of GTPases are involved in rearrangements in the actin cytoskeleton and are thought to regulate the morphologic changes in cell shape associated with transformation of cells by *ras* (Fig. 10-9).[158,159]

ras oncogenes have been identified in a variety of tumors. As was discussed previously, the oncogenic forms of *ras* differ from their normal counterparts by mutations that result in amino acid substitutions at positions 12, 13, 59, and 61 in the phosphate-binding domain of the protein.[38] These oncogenic *ras* proteins are locked in their active GTP-bound state through an increased exchange of GDP for GTP or through an inability to interact with or be dephosphorylated by GAPs.[90,160] They therefore have a reduced requirement for GDP/GTP exchange factors and no longer require activation by the *Sos* exchange factor.

Multiple GAP proteins that function to switch the *ras* signal off have been identified. The p120 GAP and neurofibromin (NF1) were the first to be discovered. The p120 GAP appears to control the response to *ras* to growth factor stimulation, whereas NF1 appears to control basal *ras* activity.[161,162] In humans, loss of the GAP protein NF1 results in the disease neurofibromatosis type 1. Aspects of the disease can be explained in terms of elevated *ras*-GTP and are thought to result from the loss of neurofibromin GAP activity.[163]

GTPase Exchange Factors

Support for *Rho*-like GTPases in cell transformation and tumorigenesis also has been provided by the discovery that multiple independently isolated oncogenes act as exchange factors for *Rho*-type GTP-binding proteins. *Dbl, Vav, Ect*-2, *Ost, Tim, Lbc, Lfc*, and *Dbs* were discovered by gene transfer methods by virtue of their ability to transform fibroblasts in culure (Table 10-1).[164] Tiam-1, which appears to directly influence the invasive capacity of T lymphoma cells, was identified adjacent to a proviral insertion site in retrovirally induced invasive T lymphoma variants.[165] The *dbl* oncogene was the first member of this family to be identified.[166] Amino acid sequence analysis revealed that *dbl* shares homology with a yeast cell division cycle protein *Cdc* 24, which is an exchange protein for a yeast *Rho*-like small GTP-binding protein.[167] The homology was restricted to the domain of cdc24 responsible for the GEF activity, and this result led to the discovery that *dbl* is an exchange factor for a mammalian *Rho*-like protein (cdc42).[167] All the oncogenic exchange proteins for small GTP-binding proteins that have been identified contain a similar domain that is now referred to as a *dbl* homology domain. The *Dbl* domain is essential for the transforming activity of this class of oncogenes, suggesting that their exchange activity for *Rho*-like GTP-binding proteins is essential for transformation. A full characterization of the mechanism of oncogenic activation of this family of oncoproteins has not been achieved; however, the deletion of amino terminal sequences of *dbl* or *vav* will result in oncogenic activation.[167,168] These deletions may remove a negative regulatory domain that normally acts to regulate the GEF activities of these proteins. The current thinking is that *dbl* and related proteins activate *Rho*-like GTP-binding proteins that play important roles in mediating various cytoskeletal reorganizations in cells. Unlike the signaling cascade in which the *Ras* GEF *Sos* participates, which binds to the adapter protein Grb2 and translocates *Sos* to cell surface receptor tyrosine kinases to activate *Ras* in response to growth factors, the signaling complexes coupling *dbl*-like GEFs to upstream components remain elusive.

Cytoplasmic Serine-Threonine Protein Kinases

The serine-threonine kinases studied so far are soluble cytoplasmic proteins. This class includes the *mos, cot, pim*-1, and *raf* oncogenes in addition to protein kinase C (Table 10-1). Oncogenic forms of the v-*raf* serine kinase have lost amino terminal regulatory sequences that lead to constitutive activation of the kinase activity and mitogenic MAP kinase pathway (Figs. 10-8 and 10-9). Phosphorylation of the c-*raf* protein kinase is normally tightly regulated. *raf* kinase activity is rapidly elevated when resting cells are stimulated by mitogens (Figs. 10-8 and 10-9) or by another member of the serine threonine kinase family, protein kinase C (PKC).[169] Several tumor promotors act via stimulation of the PKC family and mediate activation of the *raf* signaling pathway.[170] Although a mutant form of PKCα has been detected as an oncogene and although overexpression of PKC can affect the growth of cells in culture, mutant PKC enzymes are rare in human cancers.[171]

The *mos* oncogene is a serine kinase and functions as a cytostatic factor (CSF) in Xenopus eggs; it is required for meiotic maturation of Xenopus oocytes.[172,173] The expression of c-*mos* normally is restricted to germ cells, where its exact mechanism of action is unknown. Ectopic expression of *mos* in fibroblasts after retroviral transduction appears to lead to chromosome fragmentation, possibly as a consequence of forcing cells to prematurely enter mitosis.[174] Disruption of cell cycle timing in this manner may contribute to the aneuploid nature of many tumor cells.

Nuclear Protein Family

The products of oncogenes and proto-oncogenes localized to the nucleus are directly implicated in the control of the gene expression involved in cellular proliferation and differentiation. Many of these products have been shown to act as transcription factors and appear to be constitutively activated forms of their normal cellular counterparts.[175] For example, a complex between c-*jun* and c-*fos* corresponds to the mammalian transcription factor AP-l, which interacts after phorbol ester treatment or serum stimulation of cells with specific promoter elements to stimulate gene transcription.[176-179] The oncogenic *jun* and *fos* transcription factors carry mutations that lead to the loss of negative regulatory elements, and these factors are now constitutively active.[179] In addition to loss of negative regulatory domains, some oncogenic transcription factors, such as v-*erb*A and v-*rel*, lose positive effector domains, resulting in dominant negative proteins that appear to prevent the expression of genes required for cell differentiation.[180] The nuclear oncogene v-*erb*A was identified as a nuclear receptor for thyroid hormones triodothyronine (T_3) and thyroxine (T_4).[181-183] Thyroid hormone receptor T_3 binding is known to positively or negatively regulate the expression of a wide variety of genes.[184] Although the v-*erb*A gene has no detectable oncogenic potential of its own, it completely blocks spontaneous differentiation of erythroblasts.[185] Similarly, v-*rel* is related to the NF-kB DNA binding subunit (Table 10-1) and may transform B cells by binding to NF-kB recognition sites in DNA and blocking transcription of various genes that may be required for the differentiation of B cells.

Since at least some nuclear oncogenes have been implicated in *trans*-activating and/or *trans*-repressing gene expression, it is possible that alteration of these genes either directly (activated c-*myc*, v-*jun*, v-*erb*A) or indirectly (e.g., induction of their expression by an activated growth factor receptor) may lead to an imbalance in the delicate network of gene expression that regulates cell differentiation and growth control. Consistent with the hypothesis that nuclear oncogenes play central roles in events involved in cellular proliferation, the proto-oncogene forms of these genes normally are expressed in a variety of cell types during proliferation and have RNA and protein products with short half-lives. Because of the lability of the RNA and protein products, changes in transcription could lead to relatively rapid fluctuations in the steady-state levels of RNA and protein.[186] For example, c-*fos* and c-*myc* are expressed in replicating cells, but their expression is negligible in quiescent cells or during terminal differentiation.[187-189] When quiescent murine fibroblasts are stimulated with serum or growth factors to enter the G1 phase of growth, a transient increase in the levels of c-*myc*, c-*fos*, c-*jun*, and c-*myb* is observed (Fig. 10-5).[186,190,191] It is now accepted that these proto-oncogenes are required for cells to transit from a resting state (GO) to a state in which proliferation can proceed (G1) (c-*fos*, c-*jun*, c-*myc*) and to traverse specific points in the cell cycle.

The retroviruses that have transduced *myc, myb*, and *fos* express these genes in infected cells at levels higher than those in their cellular counterparts and in a nonregulated manner. Similarly, the amplification of the c-*myc* locus in human tumors or the rearranged c-*myc* locus in Burkitt lymphomas is no longer subjected to control, and these genes are expressed constitutively. Thus, the unregulated and/or ectopic expression of these genes in a differentiated cell substitutes for the growth factor requirement for quiescent cells to enter G1 and provides a constant proliferative signal in the absence of growth factors.

COOPERATION BETWEEN ONCOGENES

Accumulating evidence suggests that the products of proto-oncogenes and growth suppressor genes function in both common and parallel signaling pathways.[1] The activation of cooperating oncogenes and the inactivation of growth suppressor genes appear necessary for a complete neoplastic phenotype. Several events are required to influence aspects of the transformed phenotype, such as cell shape, invasiveness, and anchorage-independent growth, in addition to blocking cell differentiation and driving a cell constantly through uncontrolled cell division.

Oncogenes and the Cell Cycle

The signals from the oncogenes described above converge on a control apparatus: the cell cycle clock that controls cell proliferation. The genomic changes and mutations observed in tumor cells are now considered to result from defects in checkpoints that control the cell cycle in response to DNA damage, defects in DNA replication, or chromosome attachment to the spindle.[192]

Many regulated decision points are required for a cell to progress through the cell cycle, and it is now clear that many of these are targets for oncogene action. Based on studies in yeasts and the conserved nature of the cell cycle components, the eukaryotic cell cycle is believed to be regulated at two major decision points: a point in G1 when a cell becomes committed to DNA synthesis and the G2 mitosis (M) boundary (Fig. 10-10).[193]

Many cells in vivo are in a quiescent state (G0) with unduplicated DNA. Growth inhibitory signals are provided by soluble factors such as TGFβ, cell-to-cell contacts, and adhesion to extracellular matrix components, whereas growth stimulatory signals are provided by growth factors.[194,195] The balance between growth inhibitory signals and growth stimulatory signals forces cells to make a decision to enter G1 and initiate cell division.[196] At a checkpoint in late G1 (the restriction point) a cell decides whether the signals received are suitable for growth and progresses through G1 into S phase.[196]

The transition through the restriction point in late G1 represents a critical point where a cell decides between continued proliferation and escape from the cell cycle. It has become clear that the deregulation of this transition is critical to malignant growth. Cancer cells escape growth inhibition in several ways. One mechanism involves the activation of growth promoting genes, growth factors, receptors, *ras* genes, or nuclear oncoproteins that allow the cell to progress through G1; a second mechanism involves the loss of receptors for growth inhibitory genes such as TGFβ[197] (Fig. 10-10). Once at the restriction point at the end of G1, the entry into S phase is governed through the activation of cyclin-dependent kinases (cdks). The G1 cyclins (D and E type) regulate the G1/S boundary, whereas mitotic cyclins (A and B type) regulate the G2/M transition (Fig. 10-10). Alterations in cyclins can cause transformation. Cyclin D1 was identified as the oncogene product of PRAD1, a gene rearranged in human parathyroid carcinomas and expressed at high levels, and as the product of the *Bcl*1 oncogene, a proviral integration site.[198–200] Cyclin D1 is amplified and its mRNA is overexpressed in many tumor types.[201] Moreover, mice carrying a cyclin D1 transgene under the control of a mammary-specific promoter develop mammary hyperplasia and adenocarcinoma, whereas overexpression of cyclin D1 and c-*myc* in lymphoid cells of transgenic mice gives rise to lymphomas.[202–204]

The control of the G1-S checkpoint is regulated by the phosphorylation of the tumor suppressor gene product Rb by cyclin D- and E-dependent kinases.[205] Phosphorylated Rb is unable to form complexes with E2F-type transcription factors, which then are free to induce transcription of S-phase specific genes.[206] Regulation of this checkpoint is lost by several mechanisms. One involves the overexpression of cyclin D. Others involve the loss of function of the tumor suppressor gene *Rb* so that it no longer interacts with E2F and loss of function of an inhibitor of cyclin D (p16 INK).[207–209] Thus, the functional inactivation of *Rb* obtained through the deregulated expression of cyclin D1, inactivation of an inhibitor of cyclin D1 (p16 INK), or mutation in the *Rb* gene results in the loss of a cell cycle checkpoint and is thought to be an obligatory step for tumorigenesis.

The product of c-*mos*, a serine threonine kinase, also is implicated in cell cycle control. It activates serine kinases of the MAP kinase family and is implicated in the reorganization of microtubules that lead to formation of the spindle pole during meiosis in oocytes.[210] The aberrant expression of *mos* in somatic cells leads to

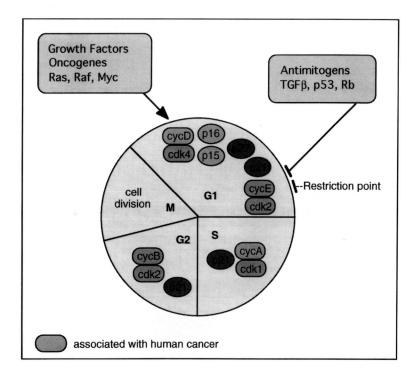

FIG. 10-10 Combinatorial interactions of cyclins and cdks during the cell cycle. Progression from G0 through G1 requires the continued presence of growth factors. This requirement is overcome by oncogenes such as *myc, ras, raf,* and tyrosine kinases. Progression through G1 can be blocked by antimitogens, TGFβ, or the p53 or Rb tumor suppressor genes. Cyclins D and E in complexes with cdks are required for progression through G1 and entry into S phase. Cyclins A and B form complexes with *cdk*2 later in the cell cycle and are involved in the progression from G2 to M. Cyclins found altered in human cancers are shown.

cells with 4N DNA content, possibly through interference with the assembly and positioning of the mitotic spindle.[174] Such an event could provide a mechanism for genetic instability that leads to the polyploid DNA content frequently observed in tumor cells.

Oncogenes and Cell Death

Whether in a normal tissue or in a tumor, the balance between cell death and proliferation governs the accumulation of cells. There is now evidence that induced suicide (apoptosis) is a major mechanism for the elimination of cells with DNA damage or an aberrant cell cycle, that is, cells that are precursors for neoplastic changes. In contrast to necrosis, which represents a pathologic response to severe cellular injury, apoptosis is a cell's normal response to physiologic signals or a lack thereof.[211] Apoptosis is an active process. Internucleosomal cleavage of DNA is a feature of apoptosis, and the resulting DNA ladder is used as an assay for apoptosis. Apoptotic cells also can be detected in tumors either cytologically or by using molecular assays on tissue sections. Thus, cell death probably accounts for the slow growth rate of some tumors.

Recently, some dominant oncogenes were shown to exhibit a surprising biologic property: the ability to induce apoptosis. The c-myc proto-oncogene, whose expression is altered or deregulated in a large percentage of tumors, can promote apoptosis as well as proliferation.[212,213] Many cytokines are both survival and proliferation signals, suggesting that their receptors transduce signals that stimulate proliferation and entry into the cell cycle as well as inhibiting apoptosis. Thus, a mechanism coupling cell proliferation with apoptosis would provide a safety net for any proliferating cell when stimulated by a mitogen, or a mutation (amplified myc) would spontaneously induce cell death when it exhausted the available cytokines (Fig. 10-11).

Many of the signals that monitor the state of the cell in response to these distinct physiologic signals converge on the p53 protein, which then signals the cell cycle clock to shut down until the problem, such as DNA damage, is corrected, or alternatively will initiate cell death through apoptosis. The p53 tumor suppressor gene encodes a transcription factor that regulates the expression of proteins that negatively regulate the cdks required for cell

cycle progression.[214–216] Thus, if induction of apoptosis were an automatic response to oncogene activation, an increase in cell number would be dependent on active suppression of apoptosis.[214] This can be achieved through loss or mutation of p53, a common event in human cancers, where cells that sustain DNA damage or oncogene activation no longer trigger apoptosis.[214] Alternatively, the deregulated expression of the Bcl-2 oncogene mediates antiapoptotic effects and specifically blocks the ability of c-myc to induce apoptosis.[217,218]

The Bcl-2 oncogene was found at the junction of the chromosome 14;18 translocation in follicular lymphoma (Table 10-1) and encodes a membrane-associated protein that is found in the endoplasmic reticulum and nuclear and outer mitochondrial membranes.[219,220] Although Bcl-2 activation alone is not sufficient for follicular lymphoma formation, Bcl-2 translocations appear to lead to cell immortalization and suggest an initiating role for Bcl-2 in the etiology of tumors through prolonged cell survival. Bcl-2 is a member of a growing family of proteins that have been conserved throughout evolution and inhibit p53-mediated apoptosis induced by growth factor deprivation, deregulated myc, or genotoxic agents.[221,222] Since Bcl-2 can inhibit apoptosis induced by a wide variety of agents the step regulated by Bcl-2 was thought to lie within a common final pathway. Indeed, Bcl-2 proteins inhibit the action of ICE-like proteases that trigger apoptosis (Fig. 10-11).[223]

Experimental Evidence for Cooperating Oncogenes

It has been possible to further subdivide the oncogenes into two groups on the basis of their phenotypes in DNA transfection assays performed in embryo fibroblast cells that have a finite life in culture. It was first demonstrated that the transforming genes of certain DNA tumor viruses [adenovirus (Ad) and polyoma virus (Py)] display different biologic activities in embryo fibroblasts. One class of genes (Ad ElA and Py large T-antigen gene) rescues embryo fibroblasts from senescence, allowing cells to be continuously maintained in culture (immortalization), whereas the second class (Ad E 1 B and Py middle T-antigen genes) morphologically alters the rescued cells and renders them tumorigenic (transformation).[224–226] It was subsequently discovered that many of the onco-

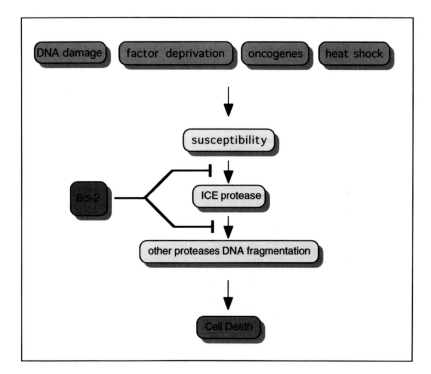

FIG. 10-11 Model for regulation of apoptosis by *Bcl-2*. Apoptosis is triggered by many agents, including DNA damage, factor deprivation, oncogene activation (e.g., *myc*), and stress such as heat shock. The ability of *Bcl-2* to inhibit cell death caused by many different agents argues for the involvement of *Bcl-2* in a final common pathway. This involves an ICE-like cysteine protease. *Bcl-2* may suppress apoptosis by preventing cleavage and activation of the cysteine protease proenzyme, interfering with proteoplytic activity, or sequestering a target protein.

genes could be assigned to either the immortalization group or the transformation group. Furthermore, members of the immortalization group, whether a gene from DNA tumor viruses (*Ad, Py*) or a v-*onc* or c-*onc* gene, act synergistically with members of the transformation group to transform embryo fibroblasts; for example, foci of transformed cells appear when embryo fibroblasts are transfected with both v-H-*ras* and v-*myc* oncogenes.[130,226,227] The v-*myc* oncogene rescues cells from senescence and therefore belongs to the immortalization-complementation group, which includes the *myc* gene family, nuclear transcription factors *fos* and *jun*, and DNA tumor virus genes *Py* large T, *Ad ElA*.[226–230] In this assay, the v-*ras* gene morphologically transforms immortalized embryo fibroblasts and belongs to the transformation-complementation group. This group contains members of the *ras* gene family and the *src* gene family, plus DNA tumor virus genes *Py* middle T-antigen gene and the *Ad ElB* gene.[36]

NIH3T3 cells have properties similar to those of embryo fibroblast cells immortalized with a member(s) of the first complementation group, and therefore these cells are particularly useful in DNA transfection assays for identifying genes of the second complementation group (e.g., *ras*). In general, the protein products of the members of the first group are found in the nucleus and generally do not alter cell morphology or anchorage requirements but appear to immortalize cells. Conversely, products of the second group are found in the cytoplasm and in most cases are associated with the cytoplasmic side of the plasma membrane. These oncoproteins can reduce growth factor requirements, induce changes in cell shape, and lead to anchorage-independent cell growth but do not immortalize cells.

TRANSGENIC MOUSE MODELS FOR CANCER

Compelling evidence for oncogene cooperation also have come from studies of transgenic mice.[231–233] Specific genes (transgenes) are introduced into the germ line of mice by microinjection of recombinant DNA into the male pronucleus of fertilized eggs.[234] Progeny from implanted transgenic embryos are scored for the presence of the transgene by analysis of DNA extracted from the tail of the newborn animal. In this system the action of activated oncogenes can be assessed in a host capable of mounting a physiologic response to tumor formation.

Transgenic mouse strains carrying a single oncogene under the transcriptional control of ubiquitous promoter elements or tissue-specific promoter elements from heterologous genes generally show a strongly enhanced level of neoplasia or hyperplasia, but frequently this occurs only in specific tissues, not in all tissues expressing the oncogene. In many cases, oncogene expression precedes tumor formation by many months. Long latencies and variable penetrance may be observed; frequently, the tumors that do arise are both rare and clonal, inferring that other events are necessary. Retroviruses carrying a single oncogene give rise to tumors; however, this occurs largely through virus spread that recruits surrounding cells into forming a polyclonal tumor. Although chronic myelogenous leukemia may be initiated solely by *bcr-abl* expression, its chronic phase may actually represent a preneoplastic syndrome. In general, there is little evidence to support the concept that in vivo expression of a single oncogene can induce polyclonal tumors.[235,236]

Tumor-prone transgenic mice provide insight into oncogene collaboration. Known or putative oncogenes can be tested for their ability to accelerate tumorigenesis. When two strains of oncogene-bearing mice are crossed, the tumor incidence often is greatly ac-

celerated and increased. Moreover, an effective way to screen for many genes that can collaborate with the transgene is provided by insertional mutagenesis with a retrovirus that lacks an oncogene (Fig. 10-2). These viruses promote tumorigenesis by chance integration next to a cellular gene, altering its transcription. Consequently, sites of integration common to several tumors are used to identify genes that have contributed to the neoplastic process.

Studies with retroviruses and transgenic mice have identified eight genes that can cooperate with *myc* to transform lymphoid cells. In mice bearing a *myc* gene coupled to an immunoglobulin heavy chain enhancer (Eu), constructed to mimic the translocations that occur in Burkitt's lymphoma, B lymphoid tumors invariably develop.[232] However, tumor onset takes place in a random fashion, and tumors are monoclonal in nature.[232,237] Despite its proliferative signal, the deregulated expression of *myc* was not sufficient for full neoplastic transformation, and both the pre-B and B cells died rapidly if deprived of growth factors in culture. Thus, additional oncogenic mutations that can collaborate with the transgene are required. Doubly transgenic progeny from Eu-*myc* and Eu-N-*ras* mice rapidly developed B-cell tumors.[238] Thus, *myc* and *ras* are effective partners in leukomagenesis as well as other tumor types. In addition to *ras*, *myc* synergizes with the *raf* and pim-1 serine threonine kinases in addition to the *abl* tyrosine kinase, the antiapoptotic gene *Bcl*-2, and the transcription factor *bmi*-1, as well as mutations in the tumor suppressor gene p53. Mutations in different genes are thought to provide complementary functions. For example, *myc* seems to prevent cells from becoming quiescent by overcoming the G1-S checkpoint, whereas *Bcl*-2 blocks apoptosis induced by the expression of *myc* and others; for example, *ras, raf*, or *pim*1 may decrease growth factor requirements.

The synergistic action of expression of v-H-*ras* and c-*myc* constructs also induces breast cancer when the transgenes are expressed in breast epithelia using the mouse mammary tumor virus (MMTV) promoter/enhancer.[239] However, in all cases tumors arise as clonal outgrowths, and nonmalignant cells expressing both oncogenes predominate. Moreover, *RAS* mutations are rare in human breast cancers. Instead, at least three proto-oncogenes have been implicated in human breast carcinogenesis. They include *myc*, the HER2/*Neu* receptor tyrosine kinase, and cyclin D1, each of which has been found amplified and overexpressed in human mammary tumors.[240,241] Similar transgenic models for breast cancer have been made involving *myc*, HER2/*neu*, and cyclin D1 under the MMTV or whey acid protein promoter/enhancer.[242,243] Female transgenic mice from each of these systems develop mammary tumors, although it is apparent that events in addition to the transgene usually are required for tumor development. Similarly, in pancreatic neoplasia induced by expression of the large T antigen of the DNA tumor virus SV40 in pancreatic islet cells, the hyperproliferation of islet cells requires the expression of insulin-like growth factor II, which is thought to be essential to block the apoptosis that accompanies the aberrant proliferation stimulated by SV40 large T antigen.[244,245]

TARGETING SIGNAL TRANSDUCTION PATHWAYS AS A METHOD FOR THERAPY

The high correlation of the clinical pattern of CML with the Ph chromosome and expression of the chimeric *bcr-abl* protein argue for a role of the *bcr-abl* gene in the development of CML. Other cellular oncogenes have been implicated in the development of human neoplasia. The HER-2 gene is amplified in mammary carcinomas with a poor prognosis, and the EGFR (c-*erbB*) and c-*myb* genes have been found to be amplified and overexpressed in certain tumors. The expression of the growth factor c-*sis* (B-chain PDGF) is increased in some human sarcoma and glioblastoma cell lines and tumors and may function as an autocrine for these tumors.

A major goal of new antitumor therapies involves interrupting the constitutive signals that drive tumor cell growth. The goal is to introduce agents that specifically turn off the signaling pathway(s) in a given tumor type. Inhibition of signaling pathways can be achieved by a variety of reagents, including small peptide-based mimics, antibodies, DNA encoding dominant negative proteins, antisense RNA, and target-specific RNA ribozymes (Table 10-4).[246,247] Most of the efforts to generate novel drugs aimed at signal transduction pathways involve attempts to design small molecules that act as specific inhibitors of enzymatic activity or protein–protein interactions interrupting the ability of docking proteins to interact with their receptors. Intensive efforts therefore have been invested in generating inhibitors of protein tyrosine kinase activity, and highly selective blockers have been synthesized.[246] Specific blockers for EGFR have been shown to block the growth of solid tumors overexpressing EGFR,[248,249] although none of these studies reported complete eradication of the tumor. However, antibodies against the HER/2*neu* receptor and EGF receptor are already in clinical trials as a treatment for breast cancer and cancers that overexpress the EGF receptor.[250,251] Complete tumor eradication was achieved in a Jak-2 kinase driven pre-B-cell acute lymphoblastic leukemia model using an inhibitor of the JAK-2 kinase.[252] More important, no toxic side effects were observed. Specificity in these systems, however, is dependent on either the restricted expression of the oncogene primarily to tumor tissue, such as Jak-2, or an apparent decrease in the redundancy of growth factor-driven signaling pathways observed in human tumors.

Other targets are designed to inhibit proteins, such as *ras* and cyclin-dependent kinases, that are involved in many mitogenic pathways. Specific inhibitors of *cdks* induce cell cycle arrest in the G1-S phase boundary of the cell cycle. Moreover, the frequency with which *ras* genes are activated in human tumors and their role as an important signal transducer for signals from protein tyrosine kinases make them an ideal target for inhibitors. One effective strategy is based on the requirement of the *ras* protein to first attach to the inner surface of the plasma membrane by linking to an isoprenyl group (farnesyl). A number of small molecules have been developed to inhibit this process in vivo,[253] and some of these molecules inhibit the growth of *ras* transformed cells in vitro; however, the central nature of *ras* action in normal cellular signaling pathways requires that inhibitors target only mutant *ras* or *ras* in tumor cells. Other strategies have been designed to interfere

with the interaction of *ras* with the exchange proteins required for its activation. Other techniques involve gene therapy designed to introduce into tumor cells genes encoding dominant negative inhibitors of *ras* that produce a mutant protein that incorporates into and blocks the signaling pathway. Although these strategies have been used successfully in tumor cells in vitro, this approach awaits further development as a suitable anticancer therapy. As every tumor usually is driven by multiple signaling pathways, a combination of strategies may be essential for complete suppression of tumor growth. Considering that oncogenes were discovered only 20 years ago, the pace of recent developments involving the molecular nature of their action has opened the gate to the ability to design specific inhibitors for each of these products.

SUMMARY

It is now accepted that cancer is a multistep process and that activation of oncogenes is involved in at least some steps in this pathway. Although the link between oncogene activation and the initiation or progression of human cancer is complex, it has been possible to identify several oncogenes in human cancers. The same rearrangements and mutations involving genes already identified by retroviral transduction have been found repeatedly in human and animal tumors. Clearly, the link between oncogene activation and the development of human cancer is complex, but the discovery of oncogenes has provided a new method, particularly in hematologic malignancies and now in sarcomas, for tumor diagnosis. Having sufficient information about the structure and function of the proteins encoded by dominant oncogenes will allow the design of specific inhibitors for each oncogene product and ultimately should lead to the development of new treatments for neoplastic disease.

ACKNOWLEDGMENTS

The author is a senior scholar of the National Cancer Institute of Canada. Work in the author's laboratory has been supported by grants from the Medical Research Council of Canada, the National Cancer Institute of Canada, and the Canadian Breast Cancer Research Initiative with funds from the Canadian Cancer Institute.

Table 10-4 Selective and Universal Targets of Signal Transduction Inhibitors

Universal Targets	Inhibitor	Selective Targets	Inhibitor
c-*src*	?	EGFR	RG 13022[6]: AG1478
Ras farnesylation	L-744,832 PD153035: Antibody 225	*Grb2* SH2 domain *Sos* SH3 domain	? ?
raf-1	?	HER-2/*neu*	AF789, Antibody to HER-2
MAPK pathway	PD 098059	PDGFR	AG 1295/6; CGP 53716
Protein kinase C transcription factors: *myc, fos*	Bryostatin ?	JAK-2 p210[Bcr-Abl]	AG490 AG1112

REFERENCES

1. Cantley LC, Auger KR, Carpenter C, Duckworth B, Graziani A, Kapeller R, Soltoff S: Oncogenes and signal transduction. *Cell* **64**:281, 1991.
2. Aaronson SA: Growth factors and cancer. *Science* **254**:1146, 1991.
3. Rous P: A sarcoma of the fowl transmissible by an agent separable from the tumor cells. *Nature* **13**:397, 1911.
4. Temin HM: On the origin of genes for neoplasia. G. H. A. Clowes Memorial Lecture. *Cancer Res* **34**:2835, 1974.
5. Gross L: *Oncogenic Viruses*. New York, Pergamon, 1970.
6. Weiss R: Experimental biology and assay of RNA tumor viruses. *RNA Tumor Viruses*, 2d ed. New York, Cold Spring Harbor Laboratory, 1984, p. 209.
7. Hayward WS, Neel BG, Astrin SM: Activation of a cellular onc gene by promoter insertion in ALV-induced lymphoid leukosis. *Nature* **290**:475, 1981.
8. Stehlin D, Varmus HE, Bishop JM, Vogt PK: DNA related to the transforming gene(s) of avian sarcoma viruses is present in normal avian DNA. *Nature* (London) **260**:170, 1976.
9. Bishop JM: Enemies within: The genesis of retrovirus oncogenes. *Cell* **23**:5, 1982.
10. Blair DG, Oskarsson MK, Wood TG, McClements WL, Fishinger PJ, Van de Woude G: A molecular model for oncogenesis. *Science* **212**:941, 1981.
11. Payne GS, Bishop JM, Varmus HE: Multiple arrangements of vital DNA and an activated host oncogene in bursal lymphomas. *Nature* **295**:209, 1982.
12. Hanawalt PC, Sarasin A: Cancer-prone hereditary diseases with DNA processing abnormalities. *Trends Genet* **2**:124, 1986.
13. Vogelstein B, Fearon ER, Scott EK, Hamilton SR, Preisinger AC, Nakamura Y, White R: Allelotype of colorectal carcinomas. *Science* **244**:207, 1989.
14. Leach FSC, Nicolaides NC, Papadopoulos N, Liu B, Jen Jet AL: Mutations of a mutS homolog in hereditary non-polyposis colorectal cancer. *Cell* **66**:519, 1991.
15. Fishel R, Lescoe MK, Rao MR, Copeland NG, Jenkins NA, Garber J, Kane M, Kolodner R: The human mutator gene homolog MSH2 and its association with hereditary nonpolyposis colon cancer [published erratum appears in *Cell* 1994 Apr 8; **77**(1):167]. *Cell* **75**:1027, 1993.
16. Hill M, Hillova J: Virus recovery in chicken cells tested with Rous sarcoma cell DNA. *Nature* **237**:35, 1972.
17. Graham FL, Van Der Eb AJ: A new technique for the assay of infectivity of human adenovirus 5 DNA. *J Virol* **52**:456, 1973.
18. Weinberg RA: Use of transfection to analyze genetic information and malignant transformation. *Biochim Biophys Acta* **651**:25, 1981.
19. Cooper GM, Okenquist S, Silverman L: Transforming activity of DNA of chemically transformed and normal cells. *Nature* **284**:418, 1980.
20. Blair DG, Cooper CS, Oskarsson MK, Eader LA, Vande Woude G: New method for detecting cellular transforming genes. *Science* **218**:1122, 1982.
21. Fasano O, Birnbaum D, Edlund L, Fogh J, Wigler M: New human transforming genes detected by a tumorigenicity assay. *Mol Cell Biol* **4**:1695, 1984.
22. Schmid CW, Jelinek WR: The alu family of dispersed repetitive sequences. *Science* **216**:161, 1982.
23. Shih C, Weinberg RA: Isolation of a transforming sequence from a human bladder carcinoma cell line. *Cell* **29**:161, 1982.
24. Pulciani S, Santos E, Lauver AV, Long LK, Aaronson SA, Barbacid M: Oncogenes in solid human tumors. *Nature* **300**:539, 1982.
25. Goldfarb MP, Shimizu K, Perucho M, Wigler M: Isolation and preliminary characterization of a human transforming gene from T24 bladder carcinoma cells. *Nature* **296**:404, 1982.
26. Harvey TT: An unidentified virus which causes the rapid production of tumors in mice. *Nature* **204**:1104, 1964.
27. Kirsten WH, Meyer LA: Morphological responses to a murine erythroblastosis virus. *J Natl Cancer Inst* **39**:311, 1967.
28. Der CJ, Krontiris TG, Cooper GM: Transforming genes of human bladder and lung carcinoma cell lines are homologous to the *ras* genes of Harvey and Kirsten sarcoma viruses. *Proc Natl Acad Sci USA* **79**:3637, 1982.
29. Parada LP, Tabin CJ, Shih C, Weinberg RA: Human EJ bladder carcinoma oncogene is a homologue of Harvey sarcoma virus *ras* gene. *Nature* **297**:474, 1982.
30. Santos E, Tronick SR, Aaronson SA, Pulciana S, Barbacid M: T24 human bladder carcinoma oncogene is an activated form of the normal human homologue of BALB- and Harvey-MSV transforming genes. *Nature* **298**:343, 1982.
31. Perucho M, Goldfarb MP, Shimizu K, Lama C, Pogh J, Wigler M: Human-tumor-derived cell lines contain common and different transforming genes. *Cell* **27**:467, 1981.
32. Murray MJ, Shilo B-Z, Shih C, Cowing D, Hsu HW, Weinberg RA: Three different human tumor cell lines contain different oncogenes. *Cell* **25**:355, 1981.
33. Hall A, Marshall CJ, Spurr NK, Weiss RA: Identification of the transforming gene in two human sarcoma cell lines as a new member of the *ras* gene family located on chromosome 1. *Nature* **303**:396, 1983.
34. Murray MJ, Cunningham JM, Parada LF, Dautry F, Lebowitz P, Weinberg RA: The HL-60 transforming sequence: A *ras* oncogene coexisting with altered myc genes in hematopoietic tumors. *Cell* **33**:749, 1983.
35. Shimizu K, Birnbaum D, Ruley MA, Fasano O, Suard Y, Edlund L, Taparowsky E, Goldfarb M, Wigler M: Structure of the Ki-ras gene of the human lung carcinoma cell line Calu-1. *Nature* **304**:497, 1983.
36. Marshall C: Human oncogenes, in *RNA Tumor Viruses*, 2d ed. New York, Cold Spring Harbor Laboratory, 1984, pp. 487–565.
37. Varmus HE: The molecular genetics of cellular oncogenes. *Annu Rev Genet* **18**:553, 1984.
38. Barbacid M: *ras* genes. *Annu Rev Biochem* **56**:779, 1987.
39. Bargamann CI, Hung M-C, Weinberg RA: Multiple independent activations of the neu oncogene by a point mutation altering the transmembrane domain of pl85. *Cell* **45**:649, 1986.
40. Cooper CS, Park M, Blair DG, Tainsky MA, Huebner K, Croce CM, Vande Woude G: Molecular cloning of a new transforming gene from a chemically transformed human cell line. *Nature* (London) **311**:29, 1984.
41. Martin-Zanca D, Hughes SH, Barbacid M: A human oncogene formed by the fusion of truncated tropomyosin and protein tyrosine kinase sequences. *Nature* (London) **319**:743, 1986.
42. Yamamoto T, Ikawa S, Akiyama T, Semba K, Nomura N, Miyajima N, Saito T, Toyoshima K: Similarity of protein encoded by the human c-erb-B-2 gene to epidermal growth factor receptor. *Nature* **319**:230, 1986.
43. Coussens L, Yang-Feng TL, Liao Y, Chen E, Gray A, McGrath JP, Seeburg PH, Libermann TA, Schlessinger J, Prancke U, Levinson AD, Ullrich A: Tyrosine kinase receptor with extensive homology to EGF receptor shares chromosomal location with neu oncogene. *Science* **230**:1132, 1985.
44. Takahashi M, Cooper GA: ret transforming gene encodes a fusion protein homologous to tyrosine kinases. *Mol Cell Biol* **7**:1378, 1987.
45. Yoshida T, Muyagawa K, Odagiri H, Sakamoto H, Little PPR, Terada M, Sugimura T: Genomic sequence of hst, a transforming gene encoding a protein homologous to fibroblast growth factors and the int-2-encoded protein. *Proc Natl Acad Sci USA* **84**:7305, 1987.
46. Bovi PD, Curatola AM, Kern FG, Greco A, Ittman M, Basilico C: An oncogene isolated by transfection of Kaposi's sarcoma DNA encodes a growth factor that is a member of the FGF family. *Cell* **50**:729, 1987.
47. Lane DP, Benchimol S: p53: Oncogene or anti-oncogene? *Gene Dev* **4**:1, 1990.
48. Megidish T, Mazurek N: A mutant protein kinase C that can transform fibroblasts. *Nature* **342**:807, 1989.
49. Zarbl H, Sukumar S, Arthur AV, Martin-Zanca D, Barbacid M: Direct mutagenesis of Ha-ras-1 oncogenes by N-nitroso-N-methylurea during initiation of mammary carcinogenesis in rats. *Nature* **315**:382, 1985.
50. Brown K, Buchmann A, Balmain A: Carcinogen-induced mutations in the mouse c-Ha-ras gene provide evidence of multiple pathways for tumor progression. *Proc Natl Acad Sci USA* **87**:538, 1990.
51. Rowley JD: Human oncogene locations and chromosome aberrations. *Nature* **301**:290, 1983.
52. Yunis J, Soreng AL, Bowe AE: Fragile sites are targets of diverse mutagens and carcinogens. *Oncogene* **1**:59, 1987.
53. Mitelman F: *Catalogue of Chromosome Aberrations in Cancer*, 2d ed. New York, Liss, 1985.
54. Rowley JD, Testa JR: Chromosome abnormalities in malignant hematologic diseases. *Adv Cancer Res* **36**:103, 1982.
55. Nowell PC, Hungerford DA: A minute chromosome in human chronic granulocytic leukemia. *Science* **32**:1497, 1960.
56. Heisterkamp N, Groffen L, Stephenson JR, Spurr NK, Goodfellow PN, Solomon E, Carritt B, Bodmer WF: Chromosomal localization of human cellular homologues of two viral oncogenes. *Nature* **299**:747, 1982.

57. De Klein A, Van Kessel AG, Grosveld G, Bartram CR, Hagemeijer A, Bootsma D, Spurr NK, Heisterkamp N, Groffen J, Stephenson JR: Cellular oncogene is translocated to the Philadelphia chromosome in chronic myelocytic leukaemia. *Nature* **300**:765, 1982.

58. Wang JYJ: Abl tyrosine kinase in signal transduction and cell-cycle regulation. *Curr Opinion Gen Dev* **3**:35, 1993.

59. Cooper CS: Translocations in solid tumors. *Curr Opinion Gen Dev* **6**:71, 1996.

60. Alitalo K, Schwab M, Lin CC, Varmus HE, Bishop JM: Homogeneously staining chromosomal regions contain amplified copies of an abundantly expressed cellular oncogene (c-myc) in malignant neuroendocrine cells from a human colon carcinoma. *Proc Natl Acad Sci USA* **80**:1707, 1983.

61. Schwab M, Aalitalo K, Klempnauer K-H, Varmus HE, Bishop JM, Gilbert F, Brodeur GM, Goldstein M, Trent J: Amplified DNA with limited homology to myc cellular oncogene is shared by human neuroblastoma cell lines and a neuroblastoma tumor. *Nature* **305**:245, 1983.

62. Shilo Y, Shipley J, Brodeur GM, Bruns G, Korf B, Donlon T, Schreck RR, Seeger R, Sakai K, Latt SA: Differential amplification, assembly, and relocation of multiple DNA sequences in human neuroblastomas and neuroblastoma cell lines. *Proc Natl Acad Sci USA* **82**:3761, 1985.

63. Collins S, Groudine M: Amplification of endogenous myc-related DNA sequences in a human myeloid leukaemia cell line. *Nature* **298**:679, 1982.

64. Dalla-Favera R, Wong-Staal F, Gallo RC: onc gene amplification in promyelocytic leukaemia cell line HL-60 and primary leukaemic cells of the same patient. *Nature* **299**:61, 1982.

65. Schwab M, Varmus HE, Bishop JM, Grzeschik KH, Naylor SL, Sakaguchi AY, Brodeur GM, Trent J: Chromosome localization in normal cells and neuroblastomas of a gene related to c-*myc*. *Nature* **308**:288, 1984.

66. Brodeur GM, Seeger RC, Schwab M, Varmus HE, Bishop JM: Amplification of N-myc in untreated human neuroblastomas correlates with advanced disease stage. *Science* **224**:1121, 1984.

67. Little CD, Nau MM, Carney DN, Gazdar AF, Minna JD: Amplification and expression of the c-*myc* oncogene in human lung cancer cell lines. *Nature* **306**:194, 1983.

68. Libermann TA, Nusbaum HR, Razon N, Kris R, Lax I, Soreq H, Whittle N, Waterfield MD, Ullrich A, Schlessinger J: Amplification, enhanced expression and possible rearrangement of EGF receptor gene in primary human brain tumors of glial origin. *Nature* **313**:144, 1985.

69. Yamamoto T, Kamat N, Kawano H, Shimizu S, Kuroki T, Toyoshima K, Rikimaru K, Nmura N, Ishizaki R, Pastan I, Gamou S, Shimizu N: High incidence of amplification of the epidermal growth factor receptor gene in human squamous carcinoma cell lines. *Cancer Res* **46**:414, 1986.

70. Yokota J, Terada M, Toyoshima K, Sugimura T, Yamato T, Battifora H, Cline MJ: Amplification of the c-*erb*B-2 oncogene in human adenocarcinomas in vivo. *Lancet* **1**:765, 1986.

71. Zhou D, Battifora H, Yokota J, Yamamoto T, Cline MJ: Association of multiple copies of the C-*erb*B-2 oncogene with spread of breast cancer. *Cancer Res* **47**:6123, 1987.

72. King CR, Kraus MH, Aaronson SA: Amplification of a novel v-*erb*B-related gene in a human mammary carcinoma. *Science* **229**:974, 1985.

73. Hunter T, Cooper JA: Protein-tyrosine kinases. *Annu Rev Biochem* **54**:897, 1985.

74. Bourne HR: G proteins and cAMP: Discovery of a new oncogene in pituitary tumors? *Nature* **330**:517, 1987.

75. Bourne HR, Sanders DA, McCormick F: The GTPase superfamily: I. A conserved switch for diverse cell functions. *Nature* **348**:125, 1990.

76. McCormick F: *ras* GTPase activating protein: Signal transmitter and signal terminator. *Cell* **56**:5, 1989.

77. Ariga H, Imamura Y, Iguchiariga SMM: DNA replication origin and transcriptional enhancer of the c-myc gene share the c-myc protein binding sequences. *EMBO J* **8**:4273, 1989.

78. Wasylyk C, Schneikert J, Wasylyk B: Oncogene v-*jun* modulates DNA replication. *Oncogene* **5**:1055, 1990.

79. Pledger WJ, Stiles CD, Aantoniades HN, Scher CD: Induction of DNA synthesis in BALBg3T3 by serum components: Re-evaluation of the commitment process. *Proc Natl Acad Sci USA* **74**:4481, 1977.

80. Westaway D, Papkoff J, Moscovici C, Varmus HE: Identification of a provirally activated c-Ha-*ras* oncogene in an avian nephroblastoma via a novel procedure: cDNA cloning of a chimaeric viral-host transcript. *EMBO J* **5**:301, 1986.

81. Doolittle RF, Hunkapiller MW, Hood LE, Devare SG, Robbins KC, Aaronson SA, Aantoniades HN: Simian sarcoma virus onc gene, v-sis, is derived from the gene (or genes) encoding a platelet-derived growth factor. *Science* **221**:275, 1983.

82. Chiu I-M, Reddy EP, Givol D, Robbins KC, Tronick SR, Aaronson SA: Nucleotide sequence analysis identifies the human c-sis proto-oncogene as a structural gene for platelet-derived growth factor. *Cell* **37**:123, 1984.

83. Waterfield MD, Scrace GT, Whittle N, Stroobant P, Johnsson A, Wasteson A, Westermark B, Heldin CH, Huang JS, Deuel TF: Platelet-derived growth factor is structurally related to the putative transforming protein p28 sis of simian sarcoma virus. *Nature* **304**:35, 1983.

84. Ross R, Glomset J, Kariya B, Harker L: A platelet-dependent serum factor that stimulates the proliferation of arterial smooth muscle cells in vitro. *Proc Natl Acad Sci USA* **71**:1207, 1974.

85. Eva A, Robbins KC, Aandersen PR, Srinivasan A, Tronick SR, Reddy EP, Ellmore NW, et al: Cellular genes analogous to retroviral oncogenes are transcribed in human tumor cells. *Nature* **295**:299, 1982.

86. Dickson C, Smith R, Brookes S, Peters SG: Tumorigenesis by mouse mammary tumor virus: Proviral activation of a cellular gene in the common integration region int-2. *Cell* **37**:529, 1984.

87. Dickson C, Peters G: Potential oncogene product related to growth factors. *Nature* **326**:833, 1987.

88. Taira M, Yoshida T, Miyagawa K, Sakamoto H, Terada M, Sugimura T: cDNA sequence of human transforming gene hst and identification of the coding sequence required for transforming activity. *Proc Natl Acad Sci USA* **84**:2980, 1987.

89. Esch F, Baird A, Ling N, Ueno N, Hill F, Denoroy L, Klepper R, Gospodarowicz D, Bzhlen P, Guillemin R: Primary structure of bovine pituitary basic fibroblast growth factor (FGF) and comparison with the amino-terminal sequence of bovine brain acidic FGF. *Proc Natl Acad Sci USA* **82**:6507, 1985.

90. Levinson AD: Normal and activated *ras* oncogenes and their encoded products. *Trends Genet* **2**:81, 1986.

91. Halaban R, Langdon R, Birchall N, Cuomo C, Baird A, Scott G, Moellmann G, McGuire J: Basic fibroblast growth factor from human keratinocytes is a natural mitogen for melanocytes. *J Cell Biol* **107**:1611, 1988.

92. Dernyck R, Goeddel DV, Ullrich A, Gutterman JU, Williams RD, Bringman TS, Berger WH: Synthesis of messenger RNAs for transforming growth factors a and b and the epidermal growth factor receptor by human tumors. *Cancer Res* **47**:707, 1987.

93. Hunter T, Cooper JA: Epidermal growth factor induces rapid tyrosine phosphorylation of proteins in A431 human tumor cells. *Cell* **24**:741, 1981.

94. Moelling K, Pfaff E, Beug H, Beimling P, Bunte T, Schaller HE, Graf T: DNA-binding activity is associated with purified myb proteins from AMV and E26 viruses and is temperature-sensitive for E26 ts mutants. *Cell* **40**:983, 1985.

95. Cooper JA, Bowen-Pope DF, Raines E, Ross R, Hunter T: Similar effects of platelet-derived growth factor and epidermal growth factor on the phosphorylation of tyrosine in cellular proteins. *Cell* **31**:263, 1982.

96. Ullrich A, Schlessinger J: Signal transduction by receptors with tyrosine kinase activity. *Cell* **61**:203, 1990.

97. Schlessinger J, Ullrich A: Growth factor signaling by receptor tyrosine kinases. *Neuron* **9**:383, 1992.

98. Pawson T, Schlessinger J: SH2 and SH3 domains. *Curr Biol* **3**:434, 1993.

99. Escobedo JA, Kaplan DR, Kavanaugh WM, Turck CW, Williams LT: A phosphatidylinositol-3 kinase binds to platelet-derived growth factor receptors through a specific receptor sequence containing phosphotyrosine. *Mol Cell Biol* **11**:1125, 1991.

100. Songyang Z, Shoelson SE, Chaudhuri M, Gish G, Pawson T, Haser WG, King F, Roberts T, Ratnofsky S, Lechlelder RJ, Neel BG, Birge RB, Fajardo JE, Chou MM, Hanafusa H, Schaffhausen B, Cantley LC: SH2 domains recognize specific phosphopeptide sequences. *Cell* **72**:767, 1993.

101. Songyang Z, Shoelson SE, McGlade J, Olivier P, Pawson T, Bustelo XR, Barbacid M, Sabe H, Hanafusa H, Yi T, Ren R, Baltimore D, Ratnofsky S, Feldman RA, Cantley YLC: Specific motifs recognized by the SH2 domains of Csk, 3BP2, fps/fes, GRB-2, HCP, SHC, Syk, and Vav. *Mol Cell Biol* **14**:2777, 1994.

102. Pawson T: Tyrosine kinases and their interactions with signalling proteins. *Curr Opinion Gen Dev* **2**:4, 1992.

103. Fantl WJ, Escobedo JA, Martin GA, Turck CW, Del Rosario M, Mc-Cormick F, Williams LT: Distinct phosphotyrosines on a growth factor receptor bind to specific molecules that mediate different signaling pathways. *Cell* **69**:413, 1992.

104. Pawson T: Protein modules and signalling networks. *Nature* **373**:573, 1995.

105. Rozakis-Adcock M, Fernley R, Wade J, Pawson T, Bowtell D: The SH2 and SH3 domains of mammalian Grb2 couple the EGF receptor to the *Ras* activator mSos1. *Nature* (London) **363**:83, 1993.

106. Gale NW, Kaplan S, Lowenstein EJ, Schlessinger J, Bar-Sagi D: Grb2 mediates the EGF-dependent activation of guanine nucleotide exchange on *Ras. Nature* **363**:88, 1993.

107. Sherr CJ, Rettenmeier CW, Sacca R, Roussel MF, Look AT, Stanley ER: The c-fms proto-oncogene product is related to the receptor for the mononuclear phagocyte growth factor, CSF-I. *Cell* **41**:665, 1985.

108. Mehment H, Morris C, Rozengurt E: Multiple synergistic signal transduction pathways regulate c-fos expression in Swiss 3T3 cells: The role of cyclic AMP. *Cell Growth Differ* **1**:293, 1990.

109. Park M, Dean M, Kaul K, Braun MJ, Gonda MA, Vande Woude G: Sequence of met proto-oncogene cDNA has features characteristic of the tyrosine kinase family of growth factor receptors. *Proc Natl Acad Sci USA* **84**:6379, 1987.

110. Bottaro DP, Rubin JS, Faletto DL, Chan AM-L, Kmieck TE, Vande Woude GF, Aaronson SA: Identification of the hepatocyte growth factor receptor as the c-met proto-oncogene product. *Science* **251**:802, 1991.

111. Besmer P, Murphy JE, George PC, Qiu F, Bergold PJ, Lederman L, Snyder HW, Brodeur D, Zuckerman EE, Hardy WD: A new acute transforming feline retrovirus and relationship of its oncogene v-kit with the protein kinase gene family. *Nature* **320**:415, 1986.

112. Durbec P, Marcosgutierrez CV, Kilkenny C, Grigourou M, Wartiowaara K, Suvanto P, Smith D, Ponder B, Costantini F, Saarma M, Sariola H, Pazchnis V: GDNF signalling through the Ret receptor tyrosine kinase. *Nature* **381**:789, 1996.

113. Takahashi M, Buma Y, Iwamoto T, Inaguma Y, Ikedi H, Hiai H: Cloning and expressing of the ret proto-oncogene encoding a tyrosine kinase with two potential transmembrane domains. *Oncogene* **3**:571, 1988.

114. Bister K, Duesberg PH: *Genetic Structure and Transforming Genes of Avian Retroviruses.* New York, Raven, 1982, pp. 3–42.

115. Rodrigues GA, Park M: Oncogenic activation of tyrosine kinases. *Curr Opinion Gen Dev* **4**:15, 1994.

116. Weiner DB, Liu J, Cohen JA, Williams WV, Greene MI: A point mutation in the *neu* oncogene mimics ligand induction of receptor aggregation. *Nature* **339**:230, 1989.

117. Martin-Zanca D, Barbacid M, Parada LF: Expression of the trk proto-oncogene is restricted to the sensory cranial and spinal ganglia of neural crest origin in mouse development. *Gene Dev* **4**:683, 1990.

118. Asai N, Iwashi T, Matsuyama M, Takahashi M: Mechanism of activation of the ret proto-oncogene by multiple endocrine neoplasia 2A mutations. *Mol Cell Biol* **15**:1613, 1995.

119. Santoro M, Carlomango F, Romano A, Bottaro DP, Dathan NA, Grieco M, Fusco A, Vecchio G, Matoskova B, Kraus MH, Di Fiore PP: Activation of RET as a dominant transforming gene by germline mutations of MEN 2A and MEN 2B. *Science* **267**:381, 1995.

120. Siegel PM, Dankort DL, Hardy WR, Muller WJ: Novel activating mutations in the neu proto-oncogene involved in induction of mammary tumors. *Mol Cell Biol* **14**:7068, 1994.

121. Carlson KM, Dou S, Chi D, Scavarda N, Toshima K, Jackson CE, Wells SA, Goodfellow PJ, Donis-Keller H: Single missense mutation in the tyrosine kinase catalytic domain of the RET proto-oncogene is associated with multiple endocrine neoplasia type 2B. *Proc Natl Acad Sci USA* **91**:1579, 1994.

122. Park M, Dean M, Cooper CS, Schmidt M, O'Brien SJ, Blair DG, Vande Woude G: Mechanism of met oncogene activation. *Cell* **45**:895, 1986.

123. Takahashi M, Ritz J, Cooper GM: Activation of a novel human transforming gene, ret, by DNA rearrangement. *Cell* **42**:581, 1985.

124. Rodrigues G, Park M: Dimerization mediated by a leucine zipper oncogenically activates the met receptor tyrosine kinase. *Mol Cell Biol* **13**:6711, 1993.

125. Feramisco JR, Clark R, Wong G, Arnheim N, Milley R, McCormick F: Transient reversion of ras oncogene-induced cell transformation by antibodies specific for amino acid 12 of ras protein. *Nature* **314**:639, 1985.

126. Greco A, Pierotti MA, Bongarzone I, Pagliardini S, Lanzi C, Della Porta G: Trk-t1 is a novel oncogene formed by the fusion of tpr and trk genes in a human papillary thyroid carcinoma. *Oncogene* **7**:237, 1992.

127. Lanzi C, Borrello MG, Bongarzone I, Migliazza A, Fusco A, Grieco M, Santoro M, Gambetta RA, Zunino F, Porta GD, Pierotti MA: Identification of the product of two oncogenic rearranged forms of the RET proto-oncogene in papillary thyroid carcinomas. *Oncogene* **7**:2189, 1992.

128. Sozzi G, Bongarzone I, Miozzo M, Cariani CT, Mondellini P, Calderone C, Pilotti S, Pierotti MA, Della Porta G: Cytogenic and molecular genetic characterization of papillary thyroid carcinomas. *Gene Chrom Cancer* **5**:1, 1992.

129. Pierotti MA, Santoro M, Jenkins RB, Sozzi G, Bongarzone I, Grieco M, Monzini N, Miozzo M, Herrmann MA, Fusco A, Hay ID, Della Porta G, Vecchio G: Characterization of an inversion on the long arm of chromosome 10 juxtaposing D10S170 and RET and creating the oncogenic sequence RET/PTC. *Proc Natl Acad Sci USA* **89**:1616, 1992.

130. Liu C, Park M, Tsao S: Over-expression of met proto-oncogene but not epidermal growth factor receptor or c-*erb*2 in primary human colorectal carcinomas. *Oncogene* **7**:181, 1992.

131. Giordano S, Ponzetto C, Di Renzo MF, Cooper CS, Comoglio PM: Tyrosine kinase receptor indistinguishable from the c-met protein. *Nature* **339**:155, 1989.

132. Hattori Y, Odagiri H, Nakatani H, Miyagawa K, Naito K, Sakamoto H, Katoh O, Yoshida T, Sugimara T, Terada M: K-sam, an amplified gene in stomach cancer, is a member of the heparin-binding growth factor receptor genes. *Proc Natl Acad Sci USA* **87**:5983, 1990.

133. Curran T, Morgan JI: Superinduction of the c-fos by nerve growth factor in the presence of peripherally active benzodiazeprines. *Science* **229**:1265, 1985.

134. Cuittitta F, Carney DN, Mulshine J, Moody TW, Fedorko J, Fischler A, Minna JD: Bombesin-like peptides can function as autocrine growth factors in human small cell lung cancer. *Nature* **316**:823, 1985.

135. Pawson T: Non-catalytic domains of cytoplasmic protein-tyrosine kinases: Regulatory elements in signal transduction. *Oncogene* **3**:491, 1988.

136. Maxwell SA, Arlinghaus RB: Serine kinase activity associated with Moloney murine sarcoma virus-124-encoded p37mos. *Virology* **143**:321, 1985.

137. Veillette A, Bookman MA, Horak EM, Bolen JB: The CD4 and CD6 T cell surface antigens are associated with the internal membrane tyrosin-protein kinase p56lck. *Cell* **55**:301, 1988.

138. Rudd CE, Trevillyan JM, Dasgupta JD, Wong LL, Schlossman SF: The CD4 receptor is complexed in detergent lysates to a protein-tyrosine kinase (p58) from human lymphocytes. *Proc Natl Acad Sci USA* **85**:5190, 1988.

139. Twamley-Stein GM, Pepperkok R, Aansorge W, Courtneidge SA: The Src family tyrosine kinases are required for platelet-derived growth factor-mediated signal transduction in NIH 3T3 cells. *Proc Natl Acad Sci USA* **90**:7696, 1993.

140. Muthuswamy SK, Siegel PM, Dankort DL, Webster MA, Muller WJ: Mammary tumors expressing the neu proto-oncogene possess elevated c-Src tyrosine kinase activity. *Mol Cell Biol* **14**:735, 1994.

141. McWhirter JR, Wang JY: Activation of tyrosine kinase and microfilament-binding functions of c-abl by bcr sequences in bcr/abl fusion proteins. *Mol Cell Biol* **11**:1553, 1991.

142. Mayer BJ, Hamaguchi M, Hanafusa H: A novel viral oncogene with structural similarity to phospholipase C. *Nature* **332**:272, 1988.

143. Matsuda M, Mayer BJ, Fukui Y, Hanafusa H: Binding of transforming protein, P47gag-crk, to a broad range of phosphotyrosine-containing proteins. *Science* **248**:1537, 1989.

144. Mayer BJ, Hanafusa H: Association of the v-crk oncogene product with phosphotyrosine-containing proteins and protein kinase activity. *Proc Natl Acad Sci USA* **87**:2638, 1990.

145. Ellis C, Moran M, McCormack F, Pawson T: Phosphorylation of GAP and GAP-associated proteins by transforming and mitogenic tyrosine kinases. *Nature* **343**:377, 1990.

146. Shih TY, Weeks MO, Young HA, Scolnick EM: Identification of a sarcoma virus-coded phosphoprotein in nonproducer cells transformed by Kirsten or Harvey murine sarcoma virus. *Virology* **96**:64, 1979.

147. Willingham MC, Pastan I, Shih TY, Scolnick EM: Localization of the src gene product of the Harvey strain of MSV to plasma membrane of transformed cells by electron microscopic immunocytochemistry. *Cell* **19**:1005, 1980

148. Hurley JB, Simon MI, Teplow DB, Robishaw JD, Gilman AG: Homologies between signal transducing G proteins and *ras* gene products. *Science* **226**:860, 1984.

149. McCormick F, Clark BFC, La Cour TFM, Kjeldaard M, Norskov-Lauritsen L, Nyborg J: A model for the tertiary structure of p21, the product of the *ras* oncogene. *Science* **228**:96, 1985.

150. Clanton DJ, Hattori S, Shih TY: Mutations of the *ras* gene product p21 that abolish guanine nucleotide binding. *Proc Natl Acad Sci USA* **83**:5076, 1986.

151. Willumsen BM, Christensen A, Hubbert NL, Papageorge AG, Lowy DR: The p21 *ras* C-terminus is required for transformation and membrane association. *Nature* **310**:583, 1984.

152. Trahey M, McCormick F: A cytoplasmic protein stimulates normal N-*ras* p21 GTPase, but does not affect oncogenic mutants. *Science* **238**:542, 1987.

153. Downward J, Riehl R, Wu L, Weinberg RA: Identification of a nucleotide exchange-promoting activity for p21*ras*. *Proc Natl Acad Sci USA* **87**:5998, 1990.

154. Zhang K, Declue JE, Vass WC, Papageorge AG, McCormick F, Lowy DR: Suppression of c-*ras* transformation by GTPase-activating protein. *Nature* **346**:754, 1990.

155. Dudley DT, Pang L, Decker SJ, Bridges AJ, Saltiel AR: A synthetic inhibitor of the mitogen-activated protein kinase cascade. *Proc Natl Acad Sci USA* **92**:7686, 1995.

156. Qiu RG, Chen J, Kim D, McCormick F, Symons M: An essential role for Rac in *Ras* transformation. *Nature* **374**:457, 1995.

157. Khosravi-Far RSP, Clark GJ, Kinch MS, Der CJ: Activation of Rac1, Rhoa and mitogen activated protein kinases is required for *Ras* transformation. *Mol Cell Biol* **15**:6443, 1995.

158. Ridley AJ, Paterson HF, Johnston CL, Diekmann D, Hall A: The small GTP-binding protein rac regulates growth factor-induced membrane ruffling. *Cell* **70**:401, 1992.

159. Ridley AJ, Hall A: The small GTP-binding protein *rho* regulates the assembly of focal adhesions and actin stress fibers in response to growth factors. *Cell* **70**:389, 1992.

160. Seeburg PH, Colby WW, Capon DJ, Goeddel DV, Levinson AD: Biological properties of human c-Ha-*ras*1 genes mutated at codon 12. *Nature* **312**:71, 1984.

161. Boguski MS, McCormick F: Proteins regulating *Ras* and its relatives. *Nature* (London) **366**:643, 1993.

162. Henkemeyer M, Rossi DJ, Holmyard DP, Puri MC, Mbamalu G, Harpal K, Shih TS, Jacks T, Pawson T: Vascular system defects and neuronal apoptosis in mice lacking *Ras* GTPase-activating protein. *Nature* (London) **377**:695, 1995.

163. Xu G, O'Connell P, Viskochil D, Cawthorn R, Robertson M, Culver M, Dunn D, Stevens J, Gesteland R, White R, Weiss R: The neurofibromatosis type 1 gene encodes a protein related to GAP. *Cell* **62**:599, 1990.

164. Cerione RA, Zheng Y: The Dbl family of oncogenes. *Curr Opinion Cell Biol* **8**:216, 1996.

165. Habets GGM, Scholtes EHM, Zuydgeest D, Van Der Kammen RA, Stam JC, Berns A, Clooard JG: Identification of an invasion-inducing gene, Tiam-1, that encodes a protein with homology to GDP-GTP exchangers for rho-like proteins. *Cell* **77**:537, 1994.

166. Eva A, Aaronson SA: Isolation of a new human oncogene from a diffuse B-cell lymphoma. *Nature* **316**:273, 1985.

167. Ron D, Zannini M, Lewis M, Wickner RB, Hunt LT, Graziani G, Tronick SR, Aaronson SA, Eva A: A region of proto-dbl essential for its transforming activity shows sequence similarity to a yeast cell-cycle gene, CDC24, and the human breakpoint cluster gene, bcr. *New Biol* **3**:372, 1991.

168. Katzav S: VAV: Captain Hook for signal transduction? *Crit Rev Oncogen* **6**:87, 1995.

169. Morrison DK, Kaplan DR, Rapp U, Roberts TM: Signal transduction from membrane to cytoplasm: Growth factors and membrane-bound oncogene products increase Raf-1 phosphorylation and associated protein kinase activity. *Proc Natl Acad Sci USA* **85**:8855, 1988.

170. Kikkawa U, Kishimoto A, Nishizuka Y: The protein kinase C family: Heterogeneity and its implications. *Annu Rev Biochem* **53**:31, 1989.

171. Housey GM, Johnson MD, Hsiao WLW, O'Brian CA, Murphy JP, Kirschmeier P: Overproduction of protein kinase C causes disordered growth in rat fibroblasts. *Cell* **52**:343, 1988.

172. Sagata N, Watanabe N, Vande Woude GF, Ikawa Y: The c-*mos* proto-oncogene product is a cytostatic factor responsible for meiotic arrest in vertebrate eggs. *Nature* **342**:512, 1989.

173. Sagata N, Daar I, Ooaskarsson M, Showalter SD, Vande Woude GF: The product of the MOS proto-oncogene as a candidate initiator for oocyte maturation. *Nature* **245**:643, 1989.

174. Fukasawa K, Vande Woude GF: Mos overexpression in Swiss 3T3 cells induces meiotic-like alterations of the mitotic spindle. *Proc Natl Acad Sci USA* **92**:3430, 1995.

175. Lewin B: Oncogenic conversion by regulatory changes in transcription factors. *Cell* **64**:303, 1991.

176. Struhl K: The DNA-binding domains of the jun oncoprotein and the yeast GCN4 transcriptional activator protein are functionally homologous. *Cell* **50**:841, 1987.

177. Distel RJ, Ro H-S, Rosen BS, Groves DL, Spiegelman BM: Nucleoprotein complexes that regulate gene expression in adipocyte differentiation: Direct participation of c-*fos*. *Cell* **49**:835, 1987.

178. Bohmann D, Bos TJ, Admon A, Nishimura T, Vogt PK, Tjian R: Human proto-oncogene c-jun encodes a DNA binding protein with structural and functional properties of transcription factor AP-I. *Science* **238**:1386, 1987.

179. Rauscher FJ II, Cohen DR, Curran T, Bos TJ, Vogt PK, Bohmann D, Tjian R, Franza BR Jr: Fos-associated protein p39 is the product of the jun proto-oncogene. *Science* **240**:1010, 1988.

180. Kiernan M, Blank V, Logest F, Vnadekerckhove J, Lottspeich F, Lebail O, Urban MB, Kourilsky P, Baeuerle PA, Israel A: The DNA binding subunit of NF-kB is identical to factor KBF1 and homologous to the rel oncogene product. *Cell* **62**:1007, 1990.

181. Sap J, Munoz A, Damm K, Glysdael J, Leutz A, Beug H, Vennstrom B: The v-erbA protein is a high affinity receptor for thyroid hormone. *Nature* **324**:635, 1986.

182. Weinberger C, Hollenberg SM, Rosenfeld MG, Evans RM: Domain structure of the human glucocorticoid receptor and its relationship to the v-erbA oncogene product. *Nature* **318**:670, 1985.

183. Weinberger C, Thompson C, Ong E, Gruold, Evans R: The C-v-*erb*A gene encodes a thyroid hormone receptor. Nature **324**:641, 1986.

184. Oppenheimer H, Samuels HH: *Molecular Basis of Thyroid Hormone Action.* New York, Academic, 1983.

185. Frykberg L, Palmieri S, Beng H, Craf T, Hayman MJ, Vennstron B: Transforming capacities of avian erythroblastosis virus mutants deleted in the v-erbA or erbB oncogenes. *Cell* **32**:227, 1983.

186. Greenberg ME, Ziff EB: Stimulation of mouse 3T3 cells induces transcription of the c-fos oncogene. *Nature* **311**:433, 1984.

187. Eisenman RN, Hann SR: Biosynthesis of *myc*-encoded proteins and regulation of *myc* gene expression, in Cooper G (ed): *Viral and Cellular Oncogenes*. Boston, Martinus Nijhoff, 1988.

188. Torelli G, Selleri L, Donelli A, Ferraro S, Emilia G, Venturelli D, Moretti L, Torelli U: Activation of c-myb expression by phytohemagglutinin stimulation in normal human T lymphocytes. *Mol Cell Biol* **5**:2874, 1985.

189. Prochownik EV, Kukowska J: Deregulated expression of c-myc by murine erythroleukemia cells prevents differentiation. *Nature* **32**:848, 1986.

190. Kruijer W, Cooper JA, Hunter T, Verma IM: Platelet-derived growth factor induces rapid but transient expression of the c-fos gene and protein. *Nature* **312**:711, 1984.

191. Muller R, Bravo R, Burckhardt J, Curran T: Induction of c-*fos* gene and protein by growth factors precedes activation of c-*myc*. *Nature* **312**:716, 1984.

192. Hartwell LH, Weinert TA: Checkpoints: Controls that ensure the order of cell cycle events. *Science* **246**:629, 1989.

193. Murray AW: Creative blocks: Cell cycle checkpoints and feedback controls. *Nature* **359**:599, 1992.

194. Wieser RJ, Oesch F: Contact inhibition of growth of human diploid fibroblasts by immobilized plasma membrane glycoproteins. *J Cell Biol* **103**:361, 1986.

195. Yamasaki H: Role of cell-cell communication in tumor suppression. *Immunol Ser* **51**:245, 1990.

196. Pardee AB: G1 events and regulation of cell proliferation. *Science* **246**:961, 1989.

197. Kimchi A, Wang X-F, Weinberg RA, Cheifetz S, Massaguo J: Absence of transforming growth factor-β receptors and growth inhibitory responses in retinoblastoma cells. *Science* **240**:196, 1987.

198. Motokura T, Bloom T, Kim HG, Jueppner H, Ruderman J, Kronenberg H, Arnold A: A novel cyclin encoded by a bcl-1-linked candidate oncogene. *Nature* **17610**:12336, 1991.

199. Motokura T, Bloom T, Kim HG, Juppner H, Ruderman JV, Kronenberg HM, Arnold A: A novel cyclin encoded by a bcl1-linked candidate oncogene. *Nature* **350**:512, 1991.

200. Withers D, Harvey R, Faust J, Melnyk O, Carey K, Meeker T: Characterization of a candidate *bcl*-1 gene. *Mol Cell Biol* **11**:4846, 1991.

201. Motokura T, Arnold A: Cyclin D and oncogenesis. *Curr Opin Genet Dev* **3**:5, 1993.

202. Wang TC, Cardiff RD, Zukerberg L, Lees E, Arnold A, Schmidt EV: Mammary hyperplasia and carcinoma in MMTV-cyclin D1 transgenic mice. *Nature* **369**:669, 1994.

203. Bodrug S, Warner B, Bath M, Lindeman G, Harris A, Adams J: Cyclin D1 transgene impedes lymphocyte maturation and collaborates in lymphomagenesis with the myc gene. *EMBO J* **13**:2124, 1994.

204. Lovec H, Grzeschiczek A, Kowalski M, Moroy T: Cyclin D1/Bcl-1 cooperates with myc genes in the generation of B-cell lymphoma in transgenic mice. *EMBO J* **13**:3487, 1994.

205. Ewen ME: The cell cycle and the retinoblastoma protein family. *Cancer Metastasis Rev* **13**:45, 1994.

206. Nevins JR: E2F: A link between the Rb tumor suppressor protein and viral oncoproteins. *Science* **258**:424, 1992.

207. Hussussian CJ, Struewing JP, Goldstein AM, Higgins PA, Ally DS, Sheahan MD, Clark WHJR, Tucker MA, Dracopol NC: Germline p16 mutations in familial melanoma. *Nature Genet* **8**:15, 1994.

208. Kamb A, Shattuck-Eidens D, Beles R, Liu Q, Gruis NA, Drig W, Hussey C, Tran T, Miki Y, Weaver-Feldhaus Jet AL: Analysis of the p16 gene (CDKN2) as a candidate for the chromosome 9p melanoma susceptibility locus. *Nature Genet* **8**:22, 1994.

209. Caldas C, Hanh SA, Da Costa LT, Redstone MS, Schutze M, Seymour AB, Weinstein CL, Hruban RH, Yeo CJ, Kern SE: Frequent somatic mutations and homozygous deletions of the p16 (MTS1) gene in pancreatic adenocarcinoma. *Nature Genet* **8**:27, 1994.

210. Zhou R, Oskarsson M, Paules RS, Schulz N, Cleveland D, Vande Woude GF: Ability of the c-mos product to associate with and phosphorylate tubulin. *Nature* **671**, 1991.

211. Kerr JFR, Harmon BV: Apoptosis: An historical perspective. *Curr Commun Cell Mol Biol* **3**:5, 1996.

212. Askew DS, Ashmun RA, Simmons BC, Cleveland JL: Constitutive c-*myc* expression in an IL-3-dependent myeloid cell line suppresses cell cycle arrest and accelerates apoptosis. *Oncogene* **6**:1915, 1991.

213. Evan GI, Wyllie AH, Gilbert CS, Littlewood TD, Land H, Brooks M, Waters CM, Penn LZ, Hancock DC: Induction of apoptosis in fibroblasts by c-myc protein. *Cell* **69**:119, 1992.

214. Lane DP: p53, guardian of the genome. *Nature* **358**:15, 1992.

215. Donehower LA, Bradley A: The tumor suppressor p53. *Biochim Biophys Acta* **1155**:181, 1993.

216. Hunter T: Breaking the cycle. *Cell* **75**:839, 1993.

217. Bissonnette R, Echeverri F, Mahboubi A, Green D: Apoptotic cell death induced by c-*myc* is inhibited by bcl-2. *Nature* **359**:552, 1992.

218. Fanidi A, Harrington E, Evan G: Co-operative interaction between c-*myc* and bcl-2 can block drug-induced apoptosis. *Nature* **359**:554, 1992.

219. Hockenberry D, Nunez G, Milliman C, Schreiber RD, Korsmeyer S:Bcl-2, an inner mitochondrial membrane protein blocks programmed cell death. *Nature* **348**:334, 1990.

220. Krajewski S, Tanaka S, Takayama S, Schibler M, Fenton W, Reed JC: Investigation of the subcellular-distribution of the Bcl-2 oncoprotein: Residence in the nuclear-envelope, endoplasmic-reticulum, and outer mitochondrial-membranes. *Cancer Res* **53**:4701, 1993.

221. Vaux DL, Weissman IL, Kim SK: Prevention of programmed cell-death in Caenorhabditis elegans by human *bcl*-2. *Science* **258**:1955, 1992.

222. Henderson S, Huen D, Rowe M, Dawson C, Johnson G, Rickinson A: Epstein-Barr virus-coded BHRF1 protein, a viral homolog of Bcl-2, protects human B-cells from programmed cell-death. *Proc Natl Acad Sci USA* **90**:8479, 1993.

223. Miura M, Zhu H, Rotello R, Hartwieg EA, Yuan J: Induction of apoptosis in fibroblasts by IL-1b-converting enzyme, a mammalian homolog of the C. elegans cell death gene ced-3. *Cell* **75**:653, 1993.

224. Shiro K, Shimojo H, Swaada Y, Vemizo Y, Fujimaga K: Incomplete transformation of rat cells by a small fragment of adenovirus 12 DNA. *Virology* **95**:127, 1979.

225. Houweling A, Van Den Elsen PJ, Van Der Eb AJ: Partial transformation of primary rat cells by the left-most 4-5 D fragment of adenovirus 5 DNA. *Virology* **105**:537, 1980.

226. Van Den Elsen P, De Pater S, Houweling A, Van Der Veer J, Van Der Eb AJ: The relationship between region Ela and Elb of human adenoviruses in cell transformation. *Gene* **18**:175, 1982.

227. Li W, Stanley ER: Role of dimerization and modification of the CSF-1 receptor in its activation and internalization during the CSF-1 response. *EMBO J* **10**:277, 1991.

228. Parada LF, Land H, Weinberg RA, Wolfe D, Rotter V: Cooperation between gene encoding P53 tumor antigen and *ras* in cellular transformation. *Nature* **312**:648, 1984.

229. Eliyahu D, Raz A, Gruss P, Givol D, Oven M: Participation of pS3 cellular tumor antigen in transformation of normal embryonic cells. *Nature* **312**:647, 1984.

230. Yancopolous GD, Nisen PD, Tesfaye A, Kohl NE, Goldfarb MP, Att FW: N-myc can cooperate with *ras* to transform normal cells in culture. *Proc Natl Acad Sci USA* **82**:5455, 1983.

231. Hanahan D: Transgenic mice as probes into complex systems. *Science* **246**:1265, 1989.

232. Adams JM, Cory S: Transgenic models of tumor development. *Science* **254**:1161, 1991.

233. Frost P, Hart I, Kerbel RS: Cancer and metastasis reviews: Transgenic mice. *Cancer Metastasis Rev* **14**:77, 1995.

234. Brinster RL, Chen HV, Trumbauer ME, Yagle MK, Palmiter RD: Factors effecting the efficiency of introducing foreign DNA into mice by microinjecting eggs. *Proc Natl Acad Sci USA* **82**:4438, 1985.

235. Weinberg RA: Oncogenes, anti-oncogenes, and the molecular bases of multistep carcinogenesis. *Cancer Res* **49**:3713, 1989.

236. Quintanilla M, Brown K, Ramsden M, Balmain A: Carcinogen-specific mutation and amplification of Ha-*ras* during mouse skin carcinogenesis. *Nature* **322**:78, 1986.

237. Adams JM, Harris AW, Pinker CA, Corcoran LM, Alexander WS, Cory S, Palmiter RD, Brinster RL: The c-myc oncogene driven by immunoglobulin enhancers induces lymphoid malignancy in transgenic mice. *Nature* **318**:533, 1985.

238. Alexander WS, Bernard O, Cory S, Adams JM: Lymphomagenesis in Em-myc transgenic mice can involve *ras* mutations. *Oncogene* **4**:575, 1989.

239. Sinn E, Muller W, Pattengale PK, Tepler I, Wallace R, Leder P: Coexpression of MMTV/v-Ha-*ras* and MMTV/c-myc genes in transgenic mice: Synergistic action of oncogenes in vivo. *Cell* **49**:465, 1987.

240. Lammie GA, Fantl V, Smith R, Schuuring E, Brookes R, Michalides C, Dickson C, Arnold A, Peters G: D11S287, a putative oncogene on chromosome 11q13, is amplified and expressed in squamous cell and mammary carcinomas and linked to BCL-1. *Oncogene* **6**:439, 1991.

241. Machotka SV, Garrett CT, Schwartz AM, Callahan R: Amplification of the proto-oncogenesint-2, c-erbB-2, and c-*myc* in human breast cancer. *Clin Chim Acta* **184**:207, 1989.

242. Cardiff RD, Muller WJ: Transgenic models of mammary tumorigenesis. *Cancer Surv* **16**:97, 1993.

243. Wang TC, Cardiff RD, Zukerberg L, Lees E, Arnold A, Schmidt FV: Mammary hyperplasia and carcinoma in MMTV-cyclin D1 transgenic mice. *Nature* **369**:669, 1994.

244. Christofori G, Naik P, Hanahan D: Insulin-like growth factor II is focally up-regulated and functionally involved as a cofactor in oncogene-induced tumorigenesis. *Nature* **368**:414, 1994.

245. Naik P, Christofore G, Hanahan D: Insulin-like growth factor II is focally up-regulated and functionally involved as a second signal for oncogene-induced tumorigenesis, in *The Molecular Genetics of Cancer* (Cold Spring Harbor Symposia on Quantitative Biology). New York, Cold Spring Harbor, 1994, pp 459–471.

246. Levitzki A, Gazit A: Tyrosine kinases inhibition: An approach to drug development. *Science* **267**:1782, 1995.

247. Gibbs JB, Oliff A: Pharmaceutical research in molecular oncology. *Cell* **79**:193, 1994.

248. Fry DW, Kraker AJ, McMichael A, Ambroso LA, Nelson JM, Leopold WR, Connors RW, Bridges AJ: A specific inhibitor of the epidermal growth factor receptor tyrosine kinase. *Science* **9**:1093, 1994.

249. Buchdunger E, Trinks U, Mett H, Regenass U, Muller M, Meyer T, McGlynn E, Pinna LA, Traxler P, Lydon NB: 4,5-dianilinophthalimide: A protein-tyrosine kinase inhibitor with selectivity for the epidermal growth factor receptor signal transduction pathway and potent in vivo antitumor activity. *Proc Natl Acad Sci USA* **91**:2334, 1994.

250. Shepard HM, Lewis GD, Sarup JC, Fenderly BM, Maneval D, Mordenti J, Figari I, Kotts CE, Palladino MAJR, Ullrich A, et al: Monoclonal antibody therapy of human cancer: Taking the HER2 proto-oncogene to the clinic. *J Clin Immunol* **11**:117, 1991.

251. Baselga J, Mendelsohn J: Receptor blockade with monoclonal antibodies as anti-cancer therapy. *Pharmacol Ther* **64**:127, 1994.

252. Meydan N, Grunberger T, Dadi H, Shahar M, Aarpaia E, Lapidot Z, Leader S, Freedman M, Cohen A, Gazit A, et al: Inhibition of recurrent human pre-B acute lymphoblastic leukemia by Jak-2 tyrosine kinase inhibitor. *Nature* **379**:645, 1996.

253. Kohl NE, Omer CA, Conner MW, Anthony NJ, Davide JP, Desolms SJ, Giuliani EA, Gomez RP, Graham SL, Hamilton K, et al: Inhibition of farnesyltransferase induces regression of mammary and salivary carcinoma in *ras* transgenic mice. *Nature Med* **1**:792, 1995.

254. Robbins KC, Devare SG, Reddy EP, Aaronson SA: In vivo identification of the transforming gene product of simian sarcoma virus. *Science* **218**:1131, 1982.

255. Peters G, Brookes S, Smith R, Dickson C: Tumorigenesis by mouse mammary tumor virus: Evidence for a common region for provirus integration in mammary tumors. *Cell* **33**:369, 1983.

256. Nusse R, Varmus HE: Many tumors induced by the mouse mammary tumor virus contain a provirus integrated in the same region of the host genome. *Cell* **31**:99, 1982.

257. Hayman MJ, Ramsay GM, Savin K: Identification and characterization of the avian erythroblastosis virus erbB gene product as a membrane glycoprotein. *Cell* **32**:579, 1983.

258. Stephenson JR, Todaro GJ: Viral-encoded transforming proteins and transforming growth factors, in Klein G (ed): *Advances in Viral Oncology*, vol 1. New York, Raven, 1982, pp 107–126.

259. Naharro G, Robbins KC, Reddy EP: Gene product of v-fgr onc: Hybrid protein containing a portion of actin and tyrosine-specific protein kinase. *Science* **223**:63, 1984.

260. Horii Y, Beeler JF, Sakagrichi K, Tachabini M, Miki T: A novel oncogene, ost, encodes a guanine nucleotide exchange factor that potentially links rho and rac signalling pathways. *EMBO J* **13**:4776, 1994.

261. Margolis B, Hu P, Katzavi S, Li W, Oliver JM, Ullrich A, Weiss A, Schlessinger J: Tyrosine phosphorylation of vav proto-oncogene product containing SH2 domain and transcription factor motifs. *Nature* **356**:71, 1992.

262. Zheng Y, Olson MF, Hall A, Cerione RA, Toksoz D: Direct involvement of the small GTP-binding protein *Rho* in *Ibc* oncogene function. *J Biol Chem* **270**:9031, 1995.

263. Ppapkoff J, Verma IM, Hunter T: Detection of a transforming gene product in cells transformed by Moloney murine sarcoma virus. *Cell* **29**:417, 1982.

264. Rapp UR, Goldsborough MD, Mark GE: Structure and biological activity of v-raf, a unique oncogene transduced by a retrovirus. *Proc Natl Acad Sci USA* **80**:4218, 1983.

265. Voronova AF, Sefton BM: Expression of a new tyrosine protein kinase is stimulated by retrovirus promoter insertion. *Nature* **319**:682, 1986.

266. Nau MM, Brooks BJ, Battey J, Sausville E, Gazdar AF, Kirsch IR, McBride OW, Bertness V, Hollis GF, Minna JD: L-myc, a new *myc*-related gene amplified and expressed in human small lung cancer. *Nature* **318**:69, 1984.

267. Klempnauer K-H, Gonda TJ, Bishop JM: Nucleotide sequence of the retroviral leukemia gene v-*myb* and its cellular progenitor c-*myb*: The architecture of a transduced oncogene. *Cell* **31**:453, 1982.

268. Curran T, Teich NM: Candidate product of the FBJ murine osteosarcoma virus oncogene: Characterization of 55,000-dalton phosphoprotein. *J Virol* **42**:114, 1982.

269. Westin EH, Gallo RC, Arya SK, Eva A, Souza LM, Baluda MA, Aaronson SA, Wong-Staal F: Differential expression of the amv gene in human hematopoietic cells. *Proc Natl Acad Sci USA* **79**:2194, 1982.

270. Stavnezer E, Gerhard DS, Binari RC: Generation of transforming viruses in cultures of chicken fibroblasts infected with an avian leukosis virus. *J Virol* **39**:920, 1981.

271. Stephens RM, Rice NR, Hiebsch RR: Nucleotide sequence of v-rel: The oncogene of reticuloendotheliosis virus. *Proc Natl Acad Sci USA* **80**:6229, 1983.

272. Nunn MF, Seeburg PH, Moscovici C: Tripartite structure of the avian erythroblastosis virus E26 transforming gene. *Nature* **306**:391, 1983.

273. Kamps MP, Murre C, Sun X, Baltimore D: A new homeobox gene contributes the DNA binding domain of the t(1;19) translocation protein in pre-B ALL. *Cell* **60**:547, 1990.

274. Borrow J, Goddard AD, Sheer D, Solomon E: Molecular analysis of acute promyelocytic leukemia breakpoint cluster region on chromosome 17. *Science* **249**:1577, 1990.

275. Kakizuka A, Miller WH Jr, Umesono K, Warrell RP Jr, Frankel SR, Murty VVVS, Dmitrovsky E, Evans RM: Chromosomal translocation t(15;17) in human acute promyelocytic leukemia fuses RARa with a novel putative transcription factor, PML. *Cell* **66**:663, 1991.

276. Von Lindern M, Ppoustka A, Lerach H, Grosveld G: The (6;9) chromosome translocation, associated with a specific subtype of acute nonlymphocytic leukemia, leads to aberrant transcription of a target gene on 9q34. *Mol Cell Biol* **10**:4016, 1990.

277. Lu D, Thompson JD, Gorski GK, Rice NR, Mayer MG, Yunis JY: Alterations at the rel locus in human lymphoma. *Oncogene* **6**:1235, 1991.

278. Leder P, Battey J, Lenoir G, Moulding C, Murphy W, Potter H, Stewart TA, Taub R: Translocations among antibody genes in human cancer. *Science* **222**:765, 1983.

279. Arnold A, Kim HG, Gaz R, Eddy RL, Fukushima Y, Byers MG, Shows TB, Kronenberg HM: Molecular cloning and chromosomal mapping of DNA rearranged with the parathyroid hormone gene in a parathyroid adenoma. *J Clin Invest* **83**:2034, 1989.

280. Ellisen LW, Bird J, West DC, Soreng AL, Reynolds TC, Smith SD, Sklar J: TAN-1, the human homolog of the drosophila notch gene, is broken by chromosomal translocations in T lymphoblastic neoplasms. *Cell* **66**:649, 1991.

281. Tsujimoto Y, Gorham J, Cossman J, Jaffe E, Croce CM: The t(14;18) chromosome translocations involved in B-cell neoplasms result from mistakes in VDJ joining. *Science* **229**:1390, 1985.

282. Haupt Y, Alaexander WS, Barri G, Klinken SP, Adams JM: Novel zinc finger gene implicated as myc collaborator by retrovirally accelerated lymphomagenesis in em-myc transgenic mice. *Cell* **65**:753, 1991.

283. Grimaldi JC, Meeker TC: The t(5;14) chromosomal translocation in a case of acute lymphocytic leukemia joins the interleukin-3 gene to the immunoglobulin heavy chain gene. *Blood* **73**:2081, 1989.

284. Shima EA, Le Beau MM, McKeithan TW, Minowaida J, Showe LC, Mak TW, Minden MD, Rowley JD, Diaz MO: Gene encoding the a chain of the T-cell receptor is moved immediately downstream of c-myc in a chromosomal 8;14 translocation in a cell line from a human T-cell leukemia. *Proc Natl Acad Sci USA* **83**:3439, 1986.

285. Mellentin JD, Smith SD, Cleary ML: lyl-1, a novel gene altered by chromosomal translocation in T cell leukemia, codes for a protein with a helix-loop-helix DNA binding motif. *Cell* **58**:77, 1989.

286. Aplan PD, Lombardi DP, Ginsberg AM, Cossman J, Bertness VL, Kirsch IR: Disruption of the human SCL locus by illegitimate V-(D)-J recombinase activity. *Science* **250**:1426, 1990.

287. Adelaide J, Mattei M-G, Marics I, Raybaud F, Planche J, De Lapeyrisre O, Birnbaum D: Chromosomal localization of the hst oncogene and its co-amplification with the int 2 oncogene melanoma. *Oncogene* **2**:413, 1988.

288. Boehm T, Baer R, Lavenir I, Forster A, Waters JJ, Nacheva E, Rabbitts TH: The mechanism of chromosomal translocation t(11;14) involving the T-cell receptor Cd locus on human chromosome 14q11 and a transcribed region of chromosome 11p15. *EMBO J* **7**:385, 1988.

289. Boehm T, Foroni L, Kaneko Y, Perutz MF, Rabbits TH: The rhombotin family of cysteine-rich LIM-domain oncogenes: Distinct members are involved in T-cell translocations to human chromosomes 11p15 and 11p13. *Proc Natl Acad Sci USA* **88**:4367, 1991.

290. Kagan J, Finger LR, Letofsky J, Finan J, Nowell PC, Croce CM: Clustering of breakpoints on chromosome 10 in acute T-cell leukemias with the t(10;14) chromosome translocation. *Proc Natl Acad Sci USA* **86**:4161, 1989.

291. Hatano M, Roberts CWM, Minden M, Crist WM, Korsmeyer SJ: Deregulation of a homeobox gene, HOX11, by the t(10;14) in T cell leukemia. *Science* **253**:79, 1991.

292. Reynolds TC, Smith SD, Sklar J: Analysis of DNA surrounding the breakpoints of chromosomal translocations involving the b T cell receptor gene in human lymphoblastic neoplasms. *Cell* **50**:107, 1987.

293. Lammie GA, Fantl V, Smith R, Schuuring E, Brookes S, Michalides R, Dickson C, Arnold A, Peters G: D11S287, a putative oncogene on chromosome 11q13, is amplified and expressed in squamous cell and mammary carcinomas and linked to BCL-1. *Oncogene* **6**:439, 1991.

294. Rimokh R, Rouault JP, Nahbi K, Gadoux M, Lafage M, Archimbaud E, Charrin C, Gentilhomme O, Germain D, Samarut J: A chromosome 12 coding region is juxtaposed to the MYC proto-oncogene locus in a t(8;12) (924;922) translocation in a case of B-cell chronic lymphocytic leukemia. *Genes Chrom Cancer* **3**:24, 1991.

295. Schwab M: Amplification of N-myc as a prognostic marker for patients with neuroblastoma (review). *Semin Cancer Biol* **4**:13, 1993.

296. Schimke RT: Gene amplification in cultured animal cells. *Cell* **37**:705, 1984.

297. Shiu RP, Watson PH, Dubik D: c-*myc* oncogene expression in estrogen-dependent and -independent breast cancer (review). *Clin Chem* **39**:353, 1993.

CHAPTER 11

Tumor Suppressor Genes

Eric R. Fearon

1. Cancers arise as the result of an accumulation of inherited and somatic mutations in proto-oncogenes, tumor suppressor genes, and DNA repair genes. Tumor suppressor genes are distinguished from the other two classes because they encode proteins that function in growth regulatory or differentiation pathways, and loss of their function contributes directly to the altered phenotype of cancer cells.

2. In contrast to the relatively straightforward approaches to the identification of oncogenic alleles in cancer, identification of tumor suppressor genes has proven quite difficult. Somatic cell genetic studies provided early compelling evidence that tumorigenicity was a recessive trait in many cancers. Based on such findings, the existence of tumor suppressor genes was inferred. Somatic cell genetic approaches also provided a means to define specific chromosomal regions containing tumor suppressor genes.

3. Knudson's epidemiological studies of retinoblastoma led to an intriguing proposal that has been termed the "two-hit hypothesis." In brief, Knudson proposed that two inactivating mutations were necessary for retinoblastoma development. The first mutation at the retinoblastoma susceptibility locus could be either a germline or somatic mutation, whereas the second mutation was always somatic. The hypothesis not only illustrated the mechanisms through which inherited and somatic mutations might collaborate in tumorigenesis, but also it linked the notion of recessive genetic determinants for cancer susceptibility to the findings from the somatic cell genetic studies.

4. More than a dozen tumor suppressor genes have been localized and identified through several experimental approaches that are often employed in concert. These approaches include cytogenetic studies of constitutional chromosomal alterations in cancer patients, linkage analyses to localize genes that predispose to cancer, and loss of heterozygosity (LOH) or allelic loss studies undertaken on matched pairs of normal and cancer tissue.

5. The authenticity of a tumor suppressor gene is most clearly established by the identification of inactivating germline mutations that segregate with cancer predisposition, coupled with the identification of somatic mutations inactivating the wild-type allele in cancers arising in those with a germline mutation. Supportive, but less compelling, evidence of a tumor suppressor role for other genes may be presented, such as the identification of somatic, inactivating mutations in a gene in one or more types of cancer or its decreased or absent expression in cancers. In large part because of the difficulties in assigning causal significance to any gene solely based on somatic alterations in its sequence and/or expression in cancers, all genes not targeted by inactivating germline mutations might be considered most appropriately as candidate tumor suppressor genes until additional data are available.

6. Although powerful insights into the cellular functions of some tumor suppressor proteins, such as *p105-RB, p53,* and *p16,* have been obtained, the functions of others remain poorly understood. It has become clear, nevertheless, that tumor suppressor proteins function in a diverse array of growth regulatory pathways. Further studies of tumor suppressor function will bridge gaps in our understanding of cancer pathogenesis and the means by which we can improve the management and treatment of cancer patients and their families.

A commonly held view is that cancers arise as the result of an accumulation of mutations in cellular genes and subsequent clonal selection of variant progeny with increasingly aggressive growth properties. A relatively small subset of the mutations are present in the germline of individuals and predispose to cancer. The vast majority of the mutations that contribute to the development and behavior of cancer are somatic and are present only in the neoplastic cells of the patient. Three classes of genes—proto-oncogenes, tumor suppressor genes, and DNA repair genes—are targeted by mutations in cancer cells. The focus of this chapter will be on tumor suppressor genes. However, brief mention will be made here of the general properties of oncogenes and DNA repair genes in an effort to compare and contrast them to tumor suppressor genes.

The relationship between proto-oncogenes and oncogenes and their functions in growth control and apoptosis were reviewed in Chapters 5, 6, and 7. More than 100 different proto-oncogenes have been identified through a variety of experimental strategies.[1,2] In general, these genes have critical roles in growth regulation, and their protein products are distributed throughout virtually all subcellular compartments. Oncogenic variant alleles present in cancers are generated by point mutation, chromosomal rearrangement, or gene amplification of the proto-oncogene sequences.

The role of DNA repair genes in cancer will be extensively discussed in subsequent chapters in the text. Like tumor suppressor genes, these genes are targeted by loss-of-function mutations. However, the DNA repair genes differ from the tumor suppressor genes in critical ways. Specifically, although protein products of many tumor suppressor genes are likely to be directly involved in growth inhibition or differentiation, many DNA repair proteins are

229

likely to have a more passive role in regulating cell growth. Their inactivation in tumor cells results in an increased rate of mutations in other cellular genes, presumably including proto-oncogenes and tumor suppressor genes. Because the accumulation of mutations in these genes appears to be rate-determining in tumorigenesis, the process of tumor progression is greatly accelerated.

As will be reviewed in the subsequent chapters that describe the gene defects in specific forms of cancer, substantial progress has been made in the identification of inherited and somatic mutations in tumor suppressor genes in cancer. Thus, these findings will not be summarized in any detail here. Rather, the primary aims of this chapter will be to review the somatic cell genetic, family, and loss of heterozygosity studies that established the existence of tumor suppressor genes; and to provide an overview of the identification and function of tumor suppressor genes.

SOMATIC CELL GENETIC STUDIES

As reviewed in Chapter 7, the identification of oncogenic alleles in human tumors has been greatly facilitated by several of their features, including the prior identification of retroviral (v-*onc*) genes and the molecular cloning and characterization of novel oncogene sequences at translocation breakpoints.[1,2] In addition, the ability of some oncogenes to generate tumorigenic properties when transferred to non-tumorigenic recipient cells not only supported the critical role of oncogene mutations in cell transformation, but also provided a clear-cut functional strategy for the identification of some oncogenic alleles.[3–6]

In contrast, the direct identification of tumor suppressor genes has proven far more difficult. For example, functional strategies for their identification have a number of theoretical and practical problems. Although the successful transfer of a functional copy of tumor suppressor gene to a tumor cell might be expected to revert aspects of its phenotype, the identification of such reverted cells in the midst of a background of fully transformed cells has proven to be a particularly arduous experimental task. Hence, the strategies for identification of tumor suppressor genes and the mutations in these genes in human cancers have been somewhat more circuitous. Nevertheless, because somatic cell genetic studies provided early, compelling evidence that tumor suppressor genes must exist, the studies will be reviewed here.

Harris and his colleagues were the first to demonstrate that the growth of murine tumor cells in syngeneic animals could be suppressed when the malignant cells were fused to non-malignant cells[7,8] However, tumorigenic revertants often arose when the hybrid cells were cultured for extended periods, and chromosome losses were found in the revertants. Harris and coworkers proposed that malignancy was a recessive trait that could be suppressed in somatic cell hybrids, and this proposal subsequently was supported by additional studies of rodent somatic cell hybrids.[8,9] Interspecies hybrids between rodent tumor cells and normal human cells also supported the proposal that tumorigenicity was a recessive trait, although the karyotypic instability of the rodent–human hybrids complicated the analysis of the human chromosomes mediating suppression. This problem was overcome by fusion of various human tumor cell lines to normal, diploid human fibroblasts.[10] Hybrids retaining both sets of parental chromosomes were suppressed for tumorigenic growth in athymic mice. Furthermore, it was demonstrated that the loss of specific human chromosomes, and not simply chromosome loss in general, correlated with reversion. Tumorigenicity could be suppressed even if activated oncogenes, such as mutant ras genes, were expressed in the hybrids.[11]

Because the loss of specific chromosomes was associated with tumorigenic reversion, it was suggested that a single chromosome and perhaps even a single gene might be sufficient to suppress the tumorigenic growth of human cancer cells in nude mice. To directly test this hypothesis, using the technique of microcell-mediated chromosome transfer, single chromosomes were transferred from normal cells to cancer cells. As predicted, the transfer of specific human chromosomes suppressed the tumorigenic growth properties of various cancer cell lines.[12–17]

Although the tumorigenic phenotype often can be suppressed following single chromosome transfer or cell fusion, other traits of the parental cancer cells, such as immortality and anchorage-independent growth, may be retained in the hybrids. Consistent with the notion that most malignant tumors arise from multiple genetic alterations, suppression of tumorigenicity thus might represent correction of only one of the alterations. Nevertheless, because the transferred genes suppressed at least some of the phenotypic properties seen in cancer cells, all genes that suppressed neoplastic growth properties in in vitro assays or in vivo tumor models often have been referred to collectively as tumor suppressor genes. As will be discussed in the following, this, in fact, may be an overly broad definition of tumor suppressor genes.

KNUDSON'S TWO-HIT HYPOTHESIS

Essentially concurrent with the somatic cell studies, Knudson undertook epidemiologic studies of retinoblastoma.[18] Although most cases of retinoblastoma were sporadic, in some families, autosomal dominant inheritance was seen. Knudson found that familial cases were much more likely than sporadic cases to develop bilateral or multifocal disease. In addition, Knudson found that the familial and bilateral/multi-focal cases, in general, had an earlier age of onset. Knudson developed a model based largely on these observations.[18] In this model, he proposed that two "hits," or mutagenic events, were necessary for retinoblastoma development in all cases. In those with the inherited form of retinoblastoma, Knudson proposed the first hit was present in the germline and thus in all cells of the body. However, inactivation of one allele of the susceptibility gene was insufficient for tumor formation, and a second somatic mutation was needed. Given the high likelihood of a somatic mutation occurring in at least one retinal cell during eye development, the dominant inheritance pattern of retinoblastoma in some families could be explained. In the nonhereditary form of retinoblastoma, both mutations were somatic and hypothesized to arise within the same cell. Although each of the two hits could have been in different genes, subsequent loss of heterozygosity studies led to the conclusion that both hits were at the same genetic locus, inactivating both alleles of the retinoblastoma (*RB1*) susceptibility gene. The significance of Knudson's hypothesis was two-fold. First, it served to illustrate the mechanisms through which inherited and somatic genetic changes might collaborate in tumorigenesis. Second, it linked the notion of recessive genetic determinants for human cancer to the somatic cell genetic studies.

IDENTIFICATION OF TUMOR SUPPRESSOR GENES

Among the strategies that have been applied successfully to tumor suppressor gene localization and identification are cytogenetic studies to identify constitutional chromosomal alterations in patients with cancer; DNA linkage approaches to localize genes involved in inherited predisposition to cancer; and loss of heterozygosity (LOH) or allelic loss studies. All of these approaches ultimately require positional cloning strategies to identify and isolate tumor suppressor genes from the chromosomal region. Because of the critical importance of these strategies to tumor suppressor gene discovery, they will be described here. Studies of the *RB1* gene have proven illustrative, and some of the seminal observations relevant to the initial characterization of the *RB1* gene will be highlighted.

Cytogenetic Studies Provide Clues to Tumor Suppressor Gene Locations

Among the successful approaches to the initial localization of chromosomal regions that may contain tumor suppressor genes have been cytogenetic studies carried out on peripheral blood lymphocytes from cancer patients. The rationale for such an approach is that chromosomal deletions, as well as some translocations, might be predicted to inactivate one of the two copies of a tumor suppressor gene in the affected region. Unfortunately, only a very small subset of cancer patients have gross constitutional chromosomal deletions or rearrangements. Nevertheless, when noted, the chromosomal defects have proven extremely valuable for implicating regions likely to contain tumor suppressor genes.

In more than 5 percent of patients with retinoblastoma, cytogenetic studies of peripheral blood lymphocytes or skin fibroblasts have revealed interstitial deletions involving band q14 of chromosome 13.[19] Similarly, those patients with the constellation of findings termed WAGR (for Wilms' tumor, aniridia, genitourinary abnormalities, and mental retardation) often have been found to have interstitial deletions of chromosome 11p13 detectable with conventional karyotypic analyses.[20] Cytogenetic studies of a mentally retarded man with hundreds of adenomatous intestinal polyps and no prior family history of polyposis revealed that the patient had an interstitial deletion involving chromosome 5q, suggesting that mutant alleles of a gene that predisposed to adenomatous polyps might map to chromosome 5q.[21] Furthermore, in some cancer patients, balanced translocations have been noted, such as those involving chromosome 17q in a very small subset of patients with neurofibromatosis type 1 (*NF-1*), suggesting the presence of the *NF-1* gene on this chromosome.[22,23]

Linkage Analysis

Although recurrent constitutional alterations of specific chromosomal regions in patients with a particular type of cancer provide compelling evidence that cancer predisposition genes may reside there, additional data are required to establish that the predisposition gene functions as a tumor suppressor. Moreover, the identification of a single cancer patient with a constitutional deletion of a particular chromosomal region, such as the patient with the chromosome 5q deletion and polyposis, does not provide proof that a Mendelian cancer predisposition gene maps to the region. In such cases, linkage analysis must be used to document that genetic markers from the implicated chromosomal region co-segregate with the inheritance of the disease phenotype in a number of large, multi-generational kindreds with a specific inherited cancer syndrome.

Localization of cancer predisposition genes for which a candidate chromosomal region has not yet been highlighted by cytogenetic studies can be accomplished using genome-wide linkage scans. Although linkage analysis can pinpoint the region containing the cancer predisposition gene to a domain much smaller than

a chromosomal band, identification of the predisposition gene ultimately requires positional cloning approaches and detailed mutational analyses. In several cancer syndromes, including familial polyposis, von Hippel-Lindau syndrome, and neurofibromatosis type 2, further localization and the eventual identification of each tumor suppressor gene was aided greatly by the fact that a subset of patients had interstitial chromosomal deletions that, although not detectable in conventional cytogenetic analyses, were readily detectable by techniques such as pulse field gel electrophoresis.[24–30]

Loss of Heterozygosity Studies

As reviewed in the preceding, cytogenetic studies of a subset of patients with retinoblastoma identified deletions involving chromosome band 13q14. Interestingly, in the patients with 13q14 deletions, it was noted that levels of esterase D, an enzyme of unknown physiological function, were approximately 50 percent of those seen in normal individuals.[31] This finding and further studies of families with inherited retinoblastoma established that the esterase D and *RB1* loci were genetically linked.[32] Subsequently, a child with inherited retinoblastoma was found to have esterase D levels approximately one-half of normal, although no chromosome 13 defects were seen in cytogenetic studies of his blood cells and skin fibroblasts.[33] Tumor cells from the patient had no esterase D activity, despite harboring a single copy of chromosome 13 that appeared intact by cytogenetic analysis. To explain the findings, it was proposed that the chromosome 13 retained in the tumor cells had a submicroscopic deletion of both the esterase D and *RB1* genes[33] Moreover, it was suggested that cells with a defect in only one *RB1* allele had a normal phenotype. The effect of the predisposing mutation, however, could be unmasked by a second event, such as the loss in the tumor cells of the chromosome 13 carrying the intact *RB1* gene. This proposal was entirely consistent with Knudson's two-hit hypothesis.

To establish the generality of these observations, others undertook studies of a panel of retinoblastomas using chromosome 13 DNA probes. On comparison of the marker patterns seen in paired normal and tumor samples, LOH or allelic loss of chromosome 13 was seen in over 60 percent of the tumors studied.[34] Loss of heterozygosity (LOH) of the 13q region containing the *RB1* locus resulted from various mechanisms (Figure 11-1). In addition, through the study of inherited cases, it was shown that the *RB1* allele retained in the tumor cells was derived from the affected parent and the wild-type *RB1* allele had been lost.[35] These data established that the unmasking of a predisposing mutation at the *RB1* locus, whether the initial mutation had been inherited or had arisen somatically, occurred by the same chromosomal mechanisms.

Genetic analysis of somatically mutated alleles of tumor suppressor genes therefore can supplement and reinforce the information derived from analysis of germline mutations. For example, the chromosome 5q region implicated in predisposition to intestinal polyposis was found to be targeted by LOH in a large fraction of adenomatous polyps and colorectal cancers.[36,37] Indeed, convincing evidence that a predisposition gene functions as a suppressor gene is provided by data demonstrating that the chromosome harboring the wild-type allele of the gene is the target of LOH and the mutant allele is specifically retained in tumors. In the vast majority of cases, LOH affects many or all of the markers on the particular chromosomal arm carrying a predisposition and/or tumor suppressor gene. For this reason, precise localization of a tumor suppressor gene rarely is achieved by LOH analysis alone.

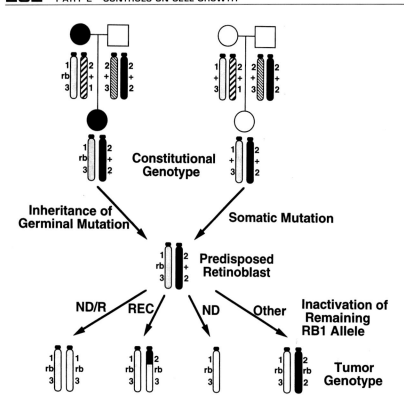

FIG. 11-1 Chromosomal mechanisms result in loss of heterozygosity for alleles at the retinoblastoma predisposition (*RB1*) locus at chromosome band 13q14. In the inherited setting (top left), the affected daughter inherits a mutant *RB1* allele (rb) from her affected mother and a normal *RB1* allele (+) from her father (constitutional genotype rb/+). DNA polymorphisms can be used to distinguish the two copies of chromosome 13 in her normal cells. (Polymorphic alleles are designated by a number.) Retinoblastoma arises after inactivation of the remaining wild-type *RB1* allele through the following mechanisms: chromosome non-disjunction and reduplication of the remaining copy of chromosome 13 (ND/R); mitotic recombination (REC); non-disjunction (ND); and other more localization mutations that inactivate the remaining *RB1* allele (OTHER). In the non-inherited (sporadic) form of the disease, a somatic mutation arises in a developing retinal cell and inactivates one of the *RB1* alleles, and the remaining *RB1* allele is inactivated by one of the mechanisms shown. Modified with permission of Elsevier Press from Cavenee W, Koufos A, Hansen M: *Mutat Res* 168:3, 1986. Please note that the figure corresponds to Figure 2-3 of Fearon ER: Oncogenes and tumor suppressor genes, in Abeloff MD, Armitage JO, Lichter AS, Niederhuber JE (eds), *Clinical Oncology*, New York, Churchill Livingstone, 1995. The figure was modified from its original form (Cavenee et al: *Mutat Res* 168:3, 1986).

CANDIDATE TUMOR SUPPRESSOR GENES

All of the tumor suppressor genes discussed in the preceding are noteworthy in that mutated alleles of the genes are present in individuals with specific inherited predispositions to cancer. These findings provide incontrovertible evidence of the importance of the genes in tumorigenesis. As reviewed, other findings, such as the demonstration of LOH of one allele of a tumor suppressor gene and somatic mutation of the remaining allele in sporadic tumors, have supported a more widespread role for these genes in cancer (Table 11-1).

It seems reasonable to suspect that germline mutations in some tumor suppressor genes may give rise to enigmatic cancer syndromes or may fail entirely to predispose to cancer. Nonetheless, these genes may be frequent targets for somatic mutations and important in human cancer. One strategy to identify tumor suppressor genes with such properties has been to identify chromosomal regions for which allelic losses can be frequently observed in sporadic cancers of various types (Table 11-1). For example, chromosome 18q very frequently is affected by LOH in colorectal and other cancer types, although no tumor predisposition genes have been localized to 18q.[38] A number of tumor suppressor genes from other chromosomal regions frequently targeted by LOH, but for which no cancer predisposition syndrome has been mapped, also have been hypothesized to exist. Among these are a gene(s) on 10q in prostate cancers and gliomas; on 8p in colorectal, breast, prostate, and other cancers; and on 1p in neuroblastomas and colorectal and other cancers. Studies of candidate tumor suppressor genes from two chromosomes frequently affected by LOH in cancer will be reviewed herein, because the studies suggest that those who would hope to identify tumor suppressor genes solely from LOH and somatic mutational analysis should proceed with some caution.

As noted, no Mendelian cancer syndrome has been mapped to chromosome 18q, although the genetic basis for cancer predisposition in many families remains to be discovered. Allelic losses of

18q are frequent in a number of cancers, including colorectal and pancreatic tumors.[37–39] Unfortunately, it is difficult to utilize LOH analysis to definitively localize the region(s) on 18q containing the tumor suppressor gene(s), because the entirety of 18q often is affected by LOH. However, homozygous deletions in cancers have proved of some utility in identifying three candidate suppressor genes on 18q. These genes are *DCC* (deleted in colorectal cancer), *DPC4* (deleted in pancreatic cancer locus 4), and *JV18-1* or *MADR2,* which encodes a *DPC4*-related protein.[40–43]

DCC is an enormous gene spanning greater than 1350 kilobases.[44] Somatic mutations in *DCC* have been detected in only a small subset of cancers, although there are both theoretical and practical difficulties associated with screening for inactivating mutations in a gene the size of *DCC*.[38,40,44] In the majority of colorectal cancers and cancer cell lines, *DCC* expression is markedly reduced or absent, consistent with the hypothesis that loss of *DCC* function may contribute to the cancer cell phenotype.[38,40,45] Somatic *DPC4* mutations have been detected in about 40 to 50 percent of pancreatic cancers.[41] *DPC4* mutations are infrequent in the other tumor types, including colorectal cancer, and their significance in these other tumor types is less clear-cut.[45–47] Similarly, mutations in the *JV18-1* gene appear to be infrequent in most colorectal cancers.[42,43] The presence of at least three different 18q genes affected by somatic, inactivating mutations in at least some cancers illustrates the difficulties that may be encountered in definitive identification of the gene(s) targeted by a common LOH event. Furthermore, the data reinforce the point that, in the absence of other supporting data, a limited cohort of somatic alterations provides rather weak evidence implicating any gene in cancer development.

In the search for the adenomatous polyposis coli (*APC*) gene at chromosome 5q21, a candidate tumor suppressor gene, termed *MCC* (for mutated in colorectal cancer) was identified prior to the cloning of *APC* gene.[48] *MCC* was found to be somatically mutated in about 10 percent of colorectal cancers, and the mutations included missense mutations affecting conserved amino

Table 11-1 Selected Tumor Suppressor Gene and Presumptive Tumor Suppressor Gene Alterations

Tumor Type/Tumor Syndrome	Chromosomal Region	Evidence*
Retinoblastoma	13q14	LA, LOH, RB1 mutation
Osteosarcoma	13q14	LA, LOH, RB1 mutation
	17p13	LA, LOH, p53 mutation
Wilms' tumor	11p13	LA, LOH, WT1 mutation
	11p15	LA, LOH
	16q	LOH
	Other(s)	LA
Rhabdomyosarcoma	17p13	LA, LOH, p53 mutation
	11p15	LOH
Hepatoblastoma	5q	APC mutation
	11p15	LOH
Colorectal	1p	LOH
	5q21	LA, LOH, APC mutation
	8p	LOH
	17p13	LOH, p53 mutation
	18q21	LOH, DCC, DPC4 mutations
	Others	LOH
Breast	17p13	LA, LOH, p53 mutation
	17q21	LA, LOH, BRCA1 mutation
	16q	LOH, E-cadherin mutation
	11p15	LOH
	11q	LOH
	13q12	LA, BRCA2 mutation
	13q14	LOH, RB1 mutation
	Others	LOH
Lung (small cell)	3p	LOH
	13q14	LOH, RB1 mutation
	17p	LOH, p53 mutation
	Others	LOH
Lung (non–small-cell)	3p	LOH
	17p13	LOH, p53 mutation
	Others	LOH
	9p21	LOH, p16/CDKN2 mutation
Bladder (transitional cell)	9p21	LOH, p16/CDKN2 mutation
	9q	LOH
	11p15	LOH
	17p13	LOH, p53 mutation
	Others	LOH
Kidney (renal cell)	3p25	LA, LOH, VHL mutation
	17p13	LOH, p53 mutation
	Others	LOH
Glioblastoma	9p21	LOH, p16/CDKN2 mutation
	10q	LOH
	17p13	LOH, p53 mutation
	Others	LOH
Melanoma	9p21	LA, LOH, p16/CDKN2 mutation
	17q	NF1 mutation
	Others	LOH
Ovarian	16q	LOH, E-cadherin mutation
	17q	LOH, BRCA1 mutation
	Others	LOH
Gastric	5q	LOH
	16q	LOH, E-cadherin mutation
	17p	LOH, p53 mutation
	18q	LOH
Pancreatic	9p21	LA, LOH, p16/CDKN2 mutation
	13q14	LOH, BRCA2 mutation
	17p13	LOH, p53 mutation
	18q21	LOH, DPC4 mutation
Neurofibromatosis type 1	17q	LA, LOH, NF1 mutation
Neurofibromatosis type 2	.22q	LA, LOH, NF2 mutation
Meningioma	22q	LOH, NF2 mutation

*LA, Linkage analysis and/or germline mutation; LOH, loss of heterozygosity.

acids, splicing mutations, and one gross rearrangement of the gene. Because the *APC* gene, and not *MCC*, was mutated in the germline of those with familial polyposis, further studies on *MCC* have lagged. The *MCC* gene may have a role in the development of a subset of colorectal cancers; however, more definitive insights into the role of the *MCC* gene in human cancer await the results of further studies. The *MCC* story provides another cautionary note for those who might hope to identify tumor suppressor genes solely by LOH and somatic mutational analysis.

Finally, there are a few other admonitions regarding the premature designation of a gene as a tumor suppressor. An increasing number of genes that have decreased or absent expression in cancers are being discovered. In response, these genes are sometimes termed tumor suppressors. Similarly, other genes that antagonize the tumorigenic or in vitro growth properties of cancer cell lines may be termed tumor suppressors. Undoubtedly, some of these genes may prove critical in growth regulation and perhaps even targets for loss-of-function mutations in human cancer. However, it should be kept in mind that the altered expression of many genes in cancers may not result from specific inactivation by mutational mechanisms, but may simply reflect the altered growth properties of cancer cells. Finally, as is the case for the gene encoding the retinoblastoma cousin *p107* and the *p21/WAF1/CIP1* gene, some genes may have particularly potent growth suppressive properties in cancer cells, but may be rarely, if ever, mutated

in human cancer. In the end, it is the sum total of the mutational and functional data that establishes whether a gene has a causal role in tumorigenesis and is appropriately designated as a tumor suppressor gene.

TUMOR SUPPRESSOR FUNCTION

About a dozen tumor suppressor genes with critical roles in cancer predisposition have been identified and cloned, and other candidate tumor suppressor genes have been suggested (Table 11-2). Although the cellular functions of a number of the tumor suppressor proteins, such as *p105-RB, p53,* and *p16*, are becoming increasingby well understood, others remain largely undefined. It is clear, however, that the tumor suppressor proteins will exhibit a variety of functions and act at many sites within the cell (Table 11-2). Some tumor suppressor proteins have been shown to directly or indirectly antagonize the function of proto-oncogenes in growth regulation.

Many of the tumor suppressor gene products appear to be expressed at roughly equivalent levels in virtually all adult tissues. Thus, the basis for the restricted tumor spectrum seen in those harboring a germline mutation in a tumor suppressor allele is rather puzzling. For example, patients with an *RB1* germline mutation are

Table 11-2 Tumor Suppressor Genes and Candidate Tumor Suppressor Genes

Cancer Syndrome	Gene	Principal Tumors	Protein Product Localization	Mode of Action
Retinoblastoma	*RB1*	Retinoblastoma, Osteosarcoma	Nucleus	Transcriptonal regulator/factor
Li-Fraumeni	*p53*	Sarcomas, breast and brain tumors	Nucleus	Transcripton factor
Familial adenomatous polyposis	*APC*	Adenomatous polyps, colon cancer	Cytoplasm	?Regulates β-catenin function
Wilms' tumor	*WT-1*	Nephroblastoma	Nucleus	Transcription factor
Neurofibromatosis type 1	*NF-1*	Neurofibromas, sarcomas, gliomas	Cytoplasm	p21ras-GTPase activator
Neurofibromatosis type 2	*NF-2*	Schwannomas, meningiomas	Cytoplasm (juxta-membrane)	Cytoskeleton membrane link
von-Hippel Lindau	*VHL*	Renal cell (clear cell) pheochromocytomas, hemangiomas	Nucleus	Regulates transcriptional elongation
Familial melanoma and pancreatic cancer	*p16*	Melanoma, pancreatic cancer, ?other	Nucleus	Cyclin-dependent kinase inhibitor
Familial breast cancer	*BRCA1*	Breast and ovarian cancer	?Nucleus	Unknown
	BRCA2	Breast and ?other	Unknown	Unknown
Tuberous sclerosis	*TSC2*	Renal and brain tumors	?Golgi	p21rap-GTPase activator

Presumed/Candidate Tumor Suppressor Genes not yet Associated with a Cancer Syndrome

	DPC4	Pancreatic, and some others, including colon	Cytoplasm	TGF-β signaling
	E-cadherin	Gastric, breast, endometrial, ovarian, others	Trans-membrane	Cell-cell, adhesion
	α-catenin	Prostate, lung, ?others	Cytoplasm (juxta-membrane)	Cytoskeletal linker protein
	DCC	Colorectal, brain, neuroblastoma, ?others	Trans-membrane	?Netrin receptor
	TGF-βII R	Colorectal, ?others	Transmembrane	Receptor for TGF-β signaling

at elevated risk for the development of only a rather limited number of tumor types, including retinoblastoma in childhood, and osteosarcomas, soft tissue sarcomas, and melanoma later in life. *RB1* germline mutations fail to predispose to more common cancers, despite the fact that somatic *RB1* mutations have been observed in a sizeable fraction of breast, small cell lung, bladder, and prostate cancers.[49] Similarly, somatic mutations in the *p53* and *p16* genes are very prevalent in many different types of cancer.[50–52] Yet, those with *p53* germline mutations are predisposed to a relatively limited number of cancers, including breast cancer, sarcomas, brain tumors, and lymphomas.[49,53] Similarly, those with germline *p16* mutations are predisposed to a very narrow spectrum of tumors, including melanoma and pancreatic cancer.

Although a detailed molecular explanation for these rather mysterious observations has not yet been provided, several new findings have provided clues. In some cell types, loss of *p105-RB* function has been shown to lead to increased cell death, rather than transformation.[54,55] Hence, inactivation of both *RB1* alleles may provide a growth advantage in only a limited number of cell types, unless other oncogene or tumor suppressor gene mutations already have arisen in the cells. Similarly, given that those with germline *p53* mutations do not appear to be predisposed to most common cancers, loss of *p53* function does not appear to be critical to the early developmental stages of many common epithelial cancers, including lung and colon cancer.[50] Rather, mutations that inactivate *p53* function may only provide selective growth at later stages of tumorigenesis, such as when neoplastic cells confront growth arrest or apoptosis signals stemming from environmental stresses to which the cells are exposed.[56]

SUMMARY

As reviewed above, there is now a compelling body of evidence to support the importance of tumor suppressor genes in cancer. Evidence for the existence of tumor suppressor genes emerged gradually from somatic cell genetic and epidemiological studies, as well as studies of chromosome losses in tumor cells using cytogenetic and molecular genetic techniques. In the last decade, more than a dozen well-documented and candidate tumor suppressor agenes have been identified. The genes are inactivated in the germline in some patients, and, in such cases, their inactivation strongly predisposes to cancer. More often, tumor suppressor genes are inactivated by somatic mutations arising during tumor development. As will be reinforced in the subsequent chapters of this text, although we have learned much about the tumor suppressor genes, much work remains. A more complete description of tumorigenesis undoubtedly will emerge with the identification of additional tumor suppressor genes, the detailed characterization of their normal cellular functions, and the elucidation of germline and somatic mutations that inactivate these genes in human tumors. These findings not only will provide new insights into cancer pathogenesis, but also ultimately should prove of critical importance in improving the management and treatment of patients and families with cancer.

REFERENCES

1. Bishop JM: Molecular themes in oncogenesis. *Cell* **64**:235, 1991.
2. Rabbitts TH: Chromosomal translocations in human cancer. *Nature* **372**:143, 1994.
3. Shih C, Shilo B-Z, Goldfarb MP, et al: Passage of phenotypes of chemically transformed cells via transfection of DNA and chromatin. *Proc Natl Acad Sci USA* **76**:5714, 1979.
4. Parada LF, Tabin CJ, Shih C, et al: Human EJ bladder carcinoma oncogene is homologue of Harvey sarcoma virus ras gene. *Nature* **297**:474, 1982.
5. Der CJ, Krontiris TG, Cooper GM: Transforming genes of human bladder and lung carcinoma cell lines are homologues to the *ras* genes of Harvey and Kirsten sarcoma viruses. *Proc Natl Acad Sci USA* **79**:3637, 1982.
6. Santos E, Tronick SR, Aaronson SA, et al: T24 human bladder carcinoma oncogene is an activated from of the normal human homologue of *BALB-* and Harvey *MSV* transforming genes. *Nature* **298**:343, 1982.
7. Harris H, Klein G: Malignancy of somatic cell hybrids. *Nature* **224**:1314, 1969.
8. Harris H: The analysis of malignancy by cell fusion: The position in 1988. *Cancer Res* **48**:3302, 1988.
9. Klinger HP: Suppression of tumorigenicity. *Cytogenet Cell Genet* **32**:68, 1982.
10. Stanbridge EJ, Der CJ, Doerson CJ, et al: Human cell hybrids: analysis of transformation and tumorigenicity. *Science* **215**:252, 1982.
11. Geiser A, Der CJ, Marshall CJ, Stanbridge EJ: Suppression of tumorigenicity with continued expression of the c-Ha-*ras* oncogene in EJ bladder carcinoma X human fibroblast hybrid cells. *Proc Natl Acad Sci USA* **83**:5029, 1986.
12. Saxon PJ, Srivastan ES, Stanbridge EJ: Introduction of human chromosome 11 via microcell transfer controls tumorigenic expression of HeLa cells. *EMBO J* **5**:3461, 1986.
13. Weissman BE, Saxon PJ, Pasquale SR, et al: Introduction of a normal human chromosome 11 into a Wilms' tumor cell line controls its tumorigenic expression. *Science* **236**:175, 1987.
14. Shimizu M, Yokota J, Mori N, et al: Introduction of normal chromosome 3p modulates the tumorigenicity of a human renal cell carcinoma cell line YCR. *Oncogene* **5**:185, 1990.
15. Trent JM, Stanbridge EJ, McBride HL, et al: Tumorigenicity in human melanoma lines controlled by introduction of human chromosome 6. *Science* **247**:568, 1990.
16. Oshimura M, Hugoh H, Koi M, et al: Transfer of human chromosome 11 suppresses tumorigenicity of some but not all tumor cell lines. *J Cell Biochem* **42**:135, 1990.
17. Tanaka K, Oshimura M, Kikuchi R, et al: Suppression of tumorigenicity in human colon carcinoma cells by introduction of normal chromosome 5 or 18. *Nature* **349**:340, 1991.
18. Knudson AG, Jr: Mutation and cancer: Statistical study of retinoblastoma. *Proc Natl Acad Sci USA* **68**:820, 1971.
19. Francke U: Retinoblastoma and chromosome 13. *Cytogenet Cell Genet* **16**:131, 1976.
20. Riccardi VM, Hittner HM, Francke U, et al: The aniridia-Wilms' tumor association: The clinical role of chromosome band 11p13. *Cancer Genet Cytogenet* **2**:131, 1980.
21. Herrera L, Kakati S, Gibas L, et al: Brief clinical report: Gardner syndrome in a man with an interstitial deletion of 5q. *Am J Med Genet* **25**:473, 1986.
22. Fountain JW, Wallace MR, Bruce MJ, et al: Physical mapping of a translocation breakpoint in neurofibromatosis. *Science* **244**:1085, 1989.
23. O'Connell P, Leach R, Cawthon R, et al: Two von Recklinghausen neurofibromatosis translocations map within a 600 kb region of 17q11.2. *Science* **244**:1087, 1989.
24. Groden J, Thlivers A., Samowitz W, et al: Identification and characterization of the familial adenomatous polyposis coli gene. *Cell* **66**:589, 1991.
25. Joslyn G, Carlson M, Thlivers A, et al: Identification of deletion mutations and three new genes at the familial polyposis locus. *Cell* **66**:601, 1991.
26. Kinzler KW, Nilbert MC, Su L-K, et al: Identification of FAP locus genes from chromosome 5q21. *Science* **253**:661, 1991.
27. Nishisho I, Nakamura Y, Miyoshi Y, et al: Mutations of chromosome 5q21 genes in FAP and colorectal cancer patients. *Science* **253**:665, 1991.
28. Latif F, Tory K, Gnarra J, et al: Identification of the von Hippel-Lindau disease tumor suppressor gene. *Science* **260**:1317, 1993.
29. Trofatter J, MacCollin M, Rutter J, et al: A novel moesin-, ezrin-, radixin-like gene is a candidate for the neurofibromatosis 2 tumor suppressor. *Cell* **72**:791, 1993.

30. Rouleau GA, Merel P, Luchtman M, et al: Alteration in a new gene encoding a putative membrane-organizing protein causes neurofibromatosis type 2. *Nature* **363**: 515, 1993.

31. Sparkes RS, Sparkes MC, Wilson MG, et al: Regional assignment of genes for human esterase D and retinoblastoma to chromosome band 13p14. *Science* **208**:1042, 1980.

32. Sparkes RS, Mruphree AL, Lingua RW, et al: Gene for hereditary retinoblastoma assigned to human chromosome 13 by linkage to esterase D. *Science* **219**:971, 1983.

33. Benedict WF, Murphree AL, Banerjee A, et al: Patient with chromosome 13 deletion: Evidence that the retinoblastoma gene is a recessive cancer gene. *Science* **219**:973, 1983.

34. Cavenee WK, Dryja TP, Phillips RA, et al: Expression of recessive alleles by chromosomal mechanisms in retinoblastoma. *Nature* **305**:779, 1983.

35. Cavenee WK, Hansen MF, Nordenskjold M, et al: Genetic origin of mutations predisposing to retinoblastoma. *Science* **228**:501, 1985.

36. Solomon E, Voss R, Hall V, et al: Chromosome 5 allele loss in human colorectal carcinomas. *Nature* **328**:616, 1987.

37. Vogelstein B, Fearon ER, Hamilton SR, et al: Genetic alterations during colorectal-tumor development. *N Engl J Med* **319**:525, 1988.

38. Cho KR, Fearon ER: *DCC*: Linking tumor suppressor genes and altered cell surface interactions in cancer? *Curr Opin Genet Dev* **5**:72–78, 1995.

39. Hahn SA, Seymour AB, Shamsul Hoque ATM, et al: Allelotype of pancreatic adenocarcinoma using xenograft enrichment. *Cancer Res* **55**:4670, 1995.

40. Fearon ER, Cho KR, Nigro JM, et al: Identification of a chromosome 18q gene that is altered in colorectal tumors. *Science* **247**:49, 1990.

41. Hahn, S.A., Schutte, M., Shamsul Hoque ATM, et al: *DPC4*, a candidate tumor suppressor gene at human chromosome 18q21.1. *Science* **271**:350, 1996.

42. Riggins GJ, Thiagalingam, Rozenblum E, et al: Mad-related genes in the human. *Nat Genet* **13**:347, 1996.

43. Eppert K, Scherer SW, Ozcelik H, et al: MADR2 maps to 18q21 and encodes a *TGF-β* regulated MAD-related protein that is functionally mutated in colorectal carcinoma. *Cell* **86**:543, 1996.

44. Cho RK, Oliner JD, Simons JW, et al: The *DCC* gene: Structural analysis and mutatioins in colorectal carcinomas. *Genomics* **19**:525, 1994.

45. Thiagalingam, S., Lengauer, C., Leach, F.S., et al: Evaluation of chromosome 18q loss in colorectal cancers. *Nat Genet* **13**:343, 1996.

46. Schutte M, Hruban RH, Hedrick L, et al: *DPC4* gene in various tumor types. *Cancer Res* **56**:2527, 1996.

47. Kim SK, Fan Y, Papadimitrakopoulou Y, et al: *DPC4*, a candidate tumor suppressor gene, is altered infrequently in head and neck squamous cell carcinoma. *Cancer Res* **56**:2519, 1996.

48. Kinzler KW, Nilbert M, Vogelstein B, et al: Identification of a gene located at chromosome 5q21 that is mutated in colorectal cancers. *Science* **251**:1366, 1991.

49. Knudson AG: Antioncogenes and human cancer. *Proc Natl Acad Sci USA* **90**:10914, 1993.

50. Greenblatt MS, Bennett WP, Hollstein M, Harris CC: Mutations in the *p53* tumor suppressor gene: Clues to cancer etiology and molecular pathogenesis. *Cancer Res* **54**:4855, 1994.

51. Cairns P, Polascik TJ, Eby Y, et al: Frequency of homozygous deletion at *p16/CDKN2* in primary human tumors. *Nat Genet* **11**:210, 1995.

52. Okamoto A, Hussain SP, Hagiwara K, et al: Mutations in the *p16INK4/MTS1/CDKN2*, *p15INK4B/MTS2*, and *p18* genes in primary and metastatic lung cancer. *Cancer Res* **55**:1448, 1995.

53. Malkin D, Li FP, Strong LC, et al: Germline *p53* mutations in a familial syndrome of breast cancer, sarcomas, and other neoplasms. *Science* **250**:1233, 1990.

54. Howes KA, Ransom N, Papermaster DS, et al: Apoptosis or retinoblastoma: Alternative fates of photoreceptors expressing the HPV-16 E7 gene in the presence or absence of *p53*. *Genes & Dev* **8**:1300, 1994.

55. Williams BO, Morgenbesser SD, DePinho RA, Jacks T: Tumorigenic and developmental effects of combined germ-line mutations in Rb and *p53*. *Cold Spring Harbor Symp Quant Biol* **59**:449, 1994.

56. Graeber TG, Osmanian C, Jacks T, et al: Hypoxia-mediated selection of cells with diminished apoptotic potential in solid tumors. *Nature* **379**:88, 1996.

Part 3

FAMILIAL CANCER SYNDROMES

Section I

OVERVIEW

CHAPTER 12

Familial Cancer Syndromes: The Role of Caretakers and Gatekeepers

Kenneth W. Kinzler ▪ Bert Vogelstein

The past decade has witnessed the elucidation of the specific genetic bases of nearly twenty inherited predispositions. This information is not only yielding immediate practical benefits in the form of genetic testing but is also providing important insights into mechanisms regulating cancer susceptibility. The inheritance of a predisposition to a sporadic event such as tumor formation has always presented an interesting problem. Its complexity was compounded by studies of the age dependence of cancer incidence, suggesting multiple genetic changes were required for cancer formation. This problem prompted Knudson to postulate that individuals with an autosomally dominant cancer susceptibility inherited one genetic alteration that was rate limiting for tumor formation but that subsequent steps were required. Over the years Knudson's hypothesis was refined to include a second hit at the same locus to inactivate the remaining normal allele. The past decade has seen numerous molecular confirmations of Knudson's hypothesis (e.g., *RB*, Chap. 19; *APC*, Chap. 31) and concrete demonstration of the multiple genetic events required for tumorigenesis (e.g., colon cancer, Chap. 31). The characterization of

the genes underlying the inherited predispositions has also provided important insights into the nature of tumor suppressor genes.

It appears that most tumor suppressor genes can be broadly divided into two groups, named "gatekeepers" and "caretakers." Gatekeepers are genes that directly regulate the growth of tumors by inhibiting their growth or by promoting their death. The functions of these genes are rate limiting for tumor growth, and as a result both the maternal and paternal copies of these genes must be inactivated for a tumor to develop (Fig. 12-1). In accord with Knudson's hypothesis, predisposed individuals inherit one damaged copy of such a gene and as a result require only one additional mutation for tumor initiation. The identity of gatekeepers varies with each tissue, such that inactivation of a given gene leads to specific forms of cancer predisposition. For example, inherited mutations of *APC* lead to colon tumors (Chap. 31), whereas inherited mutations of *VHL* predispose to kidney cancers (Chap. 24). However, because these gatekeeping genes are rate-limiting for tumor initiation, they tend to be frequently mutated in

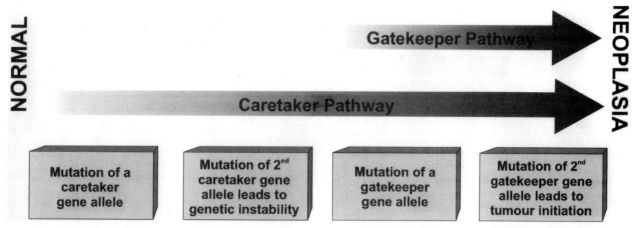

FIG. 12-1 Pathways to neoplasia. Inherited mutation of either a gatekeeper or a caretaker can predispose an individual to neoplasia. However, additional genetic changes are required to convert a predisposed cell to a neoplastic cell. In the case of the caretaker pathway, three additional mutations are generally required, though the genetic instability that follows inactivation of the second caretaker allele accelerates the accumulation of the later mutations. In the case of the gate-

keeper pathway, only one additional mutation (inactivation of the second gatekeeper allele) is required to initiate neoplasia. (Though the concepts depicted in this figure apply to all inherited cancer susceptibilities, variations do occur. For example, inherited mutations of both alleles of a proofreader gene occur in recessively inherited diseases such as xeroderma pigmentosum, and a single dominant negative mutation can substitute for two inactivation mutations of a gatekeeper gene.)

sporadic cancers through somatic mutation as well as in the germ line of predisposed individuals.

In contrast, inactivation of caretakers does not directly promote growth of tumors. Rather, inactivation of caretakers leads to a genetic instability that only indirectly promotes growth by causing an increased mutation rate. Because numerous mutations are required for the full development of a cancer, inactivation of caretakers, with the consequent increase in genetic instability, can greatly accelerate the development of cancers. Caretaker mutations in the germline occur in two different forms. In dominantly inherited diseases (e.g., HNPCC, Chap. 17), only one mutant allele of the caretaker is inherited; as with gatekeepers, the remaining allele of the caretaker gene must be mutated for phenotypic defect (i.e., increased mutation rate) to be realized (Fig. 12-1). In other cases, both alleles of the gene must be inherited in mutant form to cause susceptibility (e.g., *XP*, Chap. 13). The targets of the accelerated mutagenesis that occurs in cells with defective care-

takers are the gatekeeping tumor suppressor genes, other tumor suppressor genes (whose inactivation can lead to tumor progression), and oncogenes (genes whose activation leads to cancer). Somatic mutations of caretaker genes are only rarely found as initiating events in tumors arising in the general population presumably because such mutations would still need to be followed by several other mutations in order for a tumor to initiate (Fig. 12-1).

For the purposes of this book, we have divided cancer susceptibility syndromes into two forms, gatekeepers and caretakers, based on the predominant mechanism underlying the susceptibility. In some cases, the mechanism underlying the susceptibility is not completely characterized and the assignments were made based on the current body of evidence. For example, the BRCA1 and BRCA2 (Chap. 30) genes have been hypothesized to function as caretakers in some studies and as gatekeepers in others; further research will be required to discriminate the true role of these genes in tumor suppression.

DEFECTS IN CARETAKERS

nism are known or in the process of being clarified. Disease-causing mutations have been identified in most of the corresponding genes.

6. Several of the protein (complexes) involved in NER participate in other DNA transactions as well. All NER genes associated with TTD: XPB, XPD and TTDA are simultaneously implicated in basal transcription. The XPF complex probably has a dual involvement in a mitotic recombination pathway and later steps in NER are shaped with replication. The notion of function sharing has important implications for the clinical consequences of inherited mutations in these NER proteins. It is likely that the symptoms, which are not easy to explain on the basis of an NER defect *per se* (e.g. the brittle hair and nerve dysmyelination), are caused by subtle insufficiencies in basal transcription.

7. The first mouse models for NER deficiencies have been generated. They provide excellent tools for understanding the complex relationships between DNA repair defects and clinical consequences.

8. Prenatal diagnosis for XP, CS and TTD is possible if an unequivocal NER defect or the responsible mutations in the family have been demonstrated.

The development and maintenance of life have critically depended on the evolvement of mechanisms that ensure genetic integrity and stability. DNA, the vital carrier of genetic information, is continually subject to undesired chemical alterations. Numerous environmental or endogenous compounds and various types of radiation, such as X-rays and ultra-violet light, induce a wide variety of lesions in the bases, sugars, or phosphates that make up the DNA. Obviously, such lesions (adducts, crosslinks, breaks, etc.) interfere with the proper functioning of the genome. An intricate network of single and multi-step DNA repair systems constitutes the main protecting barrier against the deleterious consequences of DNA injury. This is illustrated by the phenotype of inherited defects in one of these repair pathways. Invariably such disorders are associated with a characteristic hypersensitivity to a specific class of genotoxic agents. In addition, the DNA lesions that persist lead to cell malfunctioning and to enhanced mutagenesis, because of the higher chance that mistakes are made upon replication of a damaged template. Somatic mutagenesis is the initiator and driving force for the multistep process of carcinogenesis. Rare inborn disorders with hallmarks characteristic for repair defects or inadequate response to DNA damage comprise the class of chromosomal instability syndromes. Well known examples are: Fanconi anemia, ataxia telangiectasia and Bloom syndrome, all of which display different manifestations of cancer proneness and increased sensitivity to specific mutagens. The prototype repair disorder is, however, xeroderma pigmentosum (XP), in which a defect in the nucleotide excision repair (NER) pathway underlies the pronounced predisposition to skin cancer and the characteristic photosensitivity of most patients. It clearly highlights the importance of the NER process. In the past decade, impressive progress has been made in unravelling the molecular intricacies of NER; for instance, all seven NER genes involved in XP (named XPA through XPG) have been cloned and their defect analyzed in patients; in addition, the NER process has been reconstituted in vitro which has enabled a stepwise dissection of the contribution of the various gene functions.

Genetic analysis of NER mutants and biochemical studies have provided evidence for the involvement of more than 20 gene products in the repair process. As discussed below these proteins have been conserved to a remarkable degree throughout the over 1.2×10^6 years of eukaryotic evolution, underlining the fundamental importance of this process. This makes it likely that the

mode of action of NER in lower eukaryotes, such as the baker's yeast *Saccharomyces cerevisiae (S. cerevisiae)*, is probably to a large extent similar to that in man. On the other hand, clear differences have become apparent with the process in the prokaryotic model organism *E. coli.*

Furthermore, intimate links between NER and other cellular processes have been disclosed, some of which were quite unexpected. Tight coordination of repair and cell cycle regulation exists: upon encountering abnormally high levels of damage a transient arrest in cell cycle progression is introduced before DNA replication or prior to cell division. This gives the repair machinery the opportunity to remove the lesions before they give rise to permanent, potentially catastrophic, changes in the genetic material. In addition, connections with recombination, replication, chromatin dynamics and the basic transcription apparatus have been unveiled.

The generation of the first NER-compromised mouse models has already been welcomed. This will be of great importance for clinical studies, for understanding the biological relevance of the NER system and for cancer research in general.

In this chapter the present knowledge of consequences of NER deficiency will be discussed. Besides XP, other disorders like Cockayne syndrome (CS) and the remarkable hair disorder trichothiodystrophy (TTD) will be covered, as both are associated with repair deficiency as well. It will become clear that the relation between the molecular defect and the clinical symptoms appears straightforward in some cases. In other instances there is a beginning of understanding, and a great deal of mystery remains.

For a comprehensive review of DNA damage and the intricate network of DNA repair systems in general, the interested reader is referred to Friedberg, Walker and Side.[1]

CLINICAL ASPECTS OF XP, CS, AND TTD

Xeroderma Pigmentosum

XP is a rare autosomal recessive disease. Affected patients (homozygotes) have sun sensitivity resulting in progressive degenerative changes of sun-exposed portions of the skin and eyes, often leading to neoplasia. Some XP patients have, in addition, progressive neurologic degeneration.[2] Obligate heterozygotes (parents) are generally asymptomatic.

History. Xeroderma, or parchment skin, was the term given by Moritz Kaposi to the condition he observed in a patient in 1863 and reported in the dermatology textbook he wrote with Ferdinand von Hebra in 1874.[3] In 1882 the term *pigmentosum* was added to emphasize the striking pigmentary abnormalities. Eye involvement, including cloudiness of the cornea, was recognized by Kaposi. In 1883, Neisser reported two brothers with cutaneous xeroderma pigmentosum and neurologic degeneration beginning in the second decade.[4] De Sanctis and Cacchione in 1932 described three sibs with cutaneous XP associated with microcephaly, progressive mental deterioration, dwarfism, and immature sexual development–the DeSanctis-Cacchione syndrome.[5]

Epidemiology. Xeroderma pigmentosum has been found in all races worldwide. The frequency is about 1 in 1 million in the United States and Europe[6] but is considerably higher in Japan (1 in 100,000)[7] and North Africa. In a literature survey of more than 800 patients[2] there were nearly equal numbers of male (54 percent) and female (46 percent) patients. Consanguinity of the patients parents was reported in 31 percent. Nearly 20 percent of the patients, including a high proportion of Japanese patients, had neurologic abnormalities.

Symptoms. The median age of onset of symptoms was between 1 and 2 years. In 5 percent of patients, onset of symptoms was delayed until after 14 years[2] (see Fig. 13-1). Initial symptoms included abnormal reaction to sun exposure in 19 percent (including severe sunburn with blistering and persistent erythema on minimal sun exposure) (Table 13-1). However, many patients sunburned normally. Freckling occurred by 2 years of age in most of the patients. The cutaneous abnormalities were usually strikingly limited to sun-exposed areas of the body (Fig. 13-2). At an early stage, the skin appears similar to that seen in farmers and sailors after many years of sun exposure: areas of increased pigment alternating with areas of decreased pigment, which display atrophy and telangiectasia. A few patients who exhibit a wide spectrum of characteristic cutaneous and ocular findings have been unambiguously diagnosed as having XP, even though the erythematous response to sun exposure was normal.[6] This may be a distinctive feature of the form of XP known as variant or pigmented xerodermoid.[6]

Premalignant actinic keratoses and malignant and benign neoplasms developed.[2] The neoplasms were predominantly basal-cell or squamous-cell carcinomas (at least 45 percent of patients, many with multiple primary neoplasms) but also included melanomas (5 percent of patients), sarcomas, keratocanthomas, and angiomas. About 90 percent of the basal-cell and squamous-cell carcinomas occured on the face, head, and neck—the sites of greatest UV exposure. The median age of onset of first skin neoplasm was 8 years, nearly 50 years younger than that in the general population of the United States (see Fig. 13-1). This represents one of the largest reductions in age of onset of neoplasia documented for any recessive human genetic disease. The frequency of basal-cell carcinomas, squamous-cell carcinomas, or melanoma of the skin was 2000 times greater than in the general poulation for patients under 20 years of age.[8] There was an approximate 30-year reduction in survival, with a 70 percent probability of surviving to age 40 years.[2] Many patients died of neoplasia.

Ocular abnormalities include photophobia, which may vary among patients from severe to absent; conjuctivitis of the interpapebral (sun-exposed) area; ectropion (turning out of the lids) due to atrophy of the skin of the eyelids; exposure keratitis; and benign and malignant neoplasms of the lids, conjunctiva, and limbus (Table 13-1). The distribution of ocular damage and neoplasms corresponds closely with the sites of UV exposure. The ocular neoplasms involved the anterior portion of the eye (lids, cornea, conjunctiva) almost exclusively. This portion of the eye shields the posterior eye (uveal tract, retina) from UV radiation: visible light is the only radiation that reaches the photosensitive cells of the retina. The frequency of ocular neoplasms was increased more than a thousandfold in patients under 20 years of age.[6] There was also a greater than 10,000 times increase in squamous-cell carcinoma of the tip of the tongue, another sun-exposed portion of the body.

The 18 percent of XP patients with neurologic abnormalities had a sex ratio, reported age, frequency of ocular abnormalities, and frequency of cutaneous neoplasms similar to those of patients with only skin and eye involvement.[6] The neurologic symptoms varied in age of onset and severity, but were characterized by progressive deterioration[9,10] (Table 13-1). Diminished deep tendon reflexes and sensorineural deafness were frequent early abnormalities. In some patients, progressive mental retardation became evident only in the second decade of life. Patients with the DeSanctis-Cacchione syndrome had neurologic and somatic abnormalities beginning in the first years of life.[5] They had microcephaly, intellectual deterioration with loss of the ability to talk, and increasing spasticity with loss of ability to walk, leading to quadriparesis, in addition to dwarfism and immature sexual development. Among the few autopsies reported, the major finding was

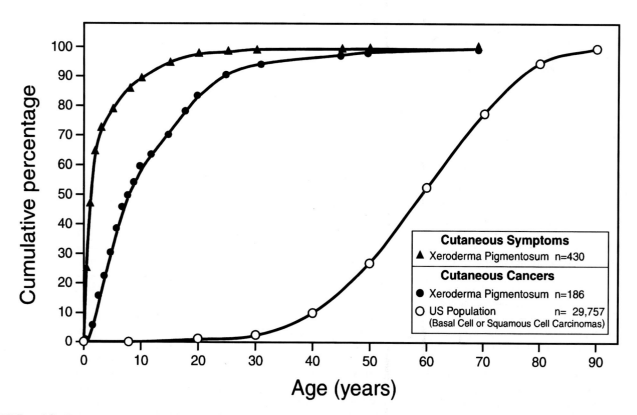

FIG. 13-1 Age at onset of XP symptoms. Age at onset of cutaneous symptoms (generally sun sensitivity or pigmentation) was reported for 430 patients. Age at first skin cancer was reported for 186 patients and is compared with age distribution for 29,757 patients with basal-cell carcinoma or squamous-cell carcinoma in the United States general population. (*From Kraemer et al.,[2] used by permission.*)

Table 13-1 Most Common Clinical Features of
Xeroderma Pigmentosum

Skin abnormalities (usually limited to sun exposed sites)
Erythema and bullae (acute sensitivity in infancy)
Freckles
Xerosis (dryness) and scaling
Areas of hyperpigmentation alternating with hypopigmentation
Telangiectasia
Atrophy
Benign lesions: actinic keratoses, keratoacanthomas, angiomas, fibromas
Malignant lesions: basal cell carcinoma, squamous cell carcinoma, melanoma
Ophthalmologic abnormalities (limited to anterior UV exposed portion of the eye)
Atrophy of lids
Conjunctivitis with photophobia, lacrimation, edema
Corneal abnormalities: keratitis, opacification, impaired vision
Neoplasms of conjunctiva, cornea and lids
Neurologic manifestations (about 20 percent of patients)
Microcephaly
Low intelligence
Progressive mental deterioration
Progressive sensorineural deafness
Abnormal motor activity
Hyporeflexia or areflexia
Primary neuronal degeneration

SOURCE: Adapted from Cleaver and Kraemer[6]

a primary neuronal degeneration with loss (or absence) of neurons, particularly in the cerebral cortex and cerebellum, without evidence of a storage process or inflammatory changes.[6] The severity of neurologic disease has been reported to correlate with the degree of sensitivity of cultured skin fibroblasts to UV inhibition of colony forming ability.[11]

XP patients have a tenfold to twentyfold increase in the frequency of internal neoplasms under the age of 20 years.[8] There are reports of patients with primary brain tumors (including two sarcomas), two with leukemia, two with lung tumors (including one patient who died at age 34 after smoking a pack of cigarettes a day for 16 years), and patients with gastric carcinomas.[6] Chemical carcinogens are suspected to play a role in these neoplasms, since cultured cells from XP patients are hypersensitive to certain DNA-binding chemical carcinogens that produce damaged DNA which is normally acted on by the NER system. These include benz[a]pyrene derivatives (found in cigarette smoke), and tryptophan pyrolysis products (found in charred food).[6]

COCKAYNE SYNDROME

CS is a rare, pleiotropic, autosomal recessive disorder with an extensive variation in symptoms and severity of the disease. Patients have cutaneous, neurologic and somatic abnormalities (see Table 13-2). Sun sensitivity of the skin is apparent in about three-fourths of affected individuals. In contrast to XP, CS patients do not have skin cancer predisposition.

The first report on this condition by Cockayne appeared in 1936[6]: dwarfism with retinal atrophy and deafness. An extensive review, comprising 140 cases, was published by Nance and Berry in 1992.[12] These authors distinguish three clinically different classes of the disease:

(1) a classical form (or CSI), which includes the majority of the patients; (2) a severe form (or CSII), characterized by early onset and severe progression of manifestations; and (3) a mild form, typified by late onset and slow progression of symptoms. Classical CS patients (CSI) (Fig. 13-3) show (1) growth failure (short stature), (2) neurodevelopmental and later neurological dysfunction, (3) cutaneous photosensitivity (with or without thin or dry skin or hair), (4) progressive ocular abnormalities (such as progressive pigmentary retinopathy and/or cataracts), (5) hearing loss, (6) dental caries, and (7) a characteristic physical appearance (cachectic dwarfism, wizened facial appearance: bird-like facies). The last four criteria are more often registered in the older children. For diagnosis of CS in the infant the presence of the first two criteria and a few of the other five criteria, together with biochemical and cellular evidence (UV sensitivity and DNA repair characteristics of CS in fibroblasts; see below) are required. Pathological calcifications have been observed in the basal ganglia and at other locations in the central nervous system. Primary dysmyelination is an important feature seen in the nervous system of CS patients, in contrast to primary neuronal degeneration in XP. The symptoms described above are much more severe and the onset much earlier in the CSII form of the disease. The characteristic facial and somatic appearance is present within the first two years of life. The prognosis is much worse than that of the classical CS patients. Death usually occurs by age 6 or 7. For details on the different forms of Cockayne Syndrome and further reference to other publications, the reader is referred to the review of Nance and Berry.[12]

Trichothiodystrophy

Trichothiodystrophy (TTD) (sulphur-deficient brittle hair) is a rare, autosomal recessive disorder. It represents a specific hair dysplasia associated with a variable range of abnormalities in organs derived from ectoderm and neuro-endoderm (Fig. 13-4). About half of the patients show photosensitivity of the skin that is due to a defect in NER.

The term *trichothiodystrophy* was introduced by Price in 1979.[14] The clinical hallmark of TTD is brittle hair, which is due to a reduced content of a class of matrix hair proteins which provide the hairshaft with its natural strength. With polarizing light microscopy, a typical tiger tail pattern of the hair is visible. On scanning electron microscopy, the hair is flattened and irregular with longitudinal ridging, and often somewhat twisted along the axis. Frequently fractures are apparent and the viscoelastic parameters of hair are different from controls.[15] The aminoacid composition of the hair proteins is dramatically changed with a strong reduction in cysteine and to a lesser extent proline, threonine and serine residues and a concomittant relative increase in aspartic acid, methionine, phenylalanine, alanine, leucine and lysine.[16] This is due to the strong reduction or complete absence of the class of ultra-high sulphur-rich matrix proteins, up to 30 percent of which are composed of cysteine residues that are involved in disulfide cross-links. In addition nails are dystrophic. Cutaneous signs include photosensitivity, ichthyosis, keratosis, erythema and collodion baby. In many cases, the brittle hair is associated with a heterogeneous complex of neuro-ectodermal abnormalities. Neurologic and developmental impairments within TTD are reminiscent of those found in CS. In a few cases, calcification of the basal ganglia and dysmyelination[17–19] have been reported, as has been observed in CS (Table 13-3). Clinical manifestations and their severity vary extensively between TTD individuals. The broad spectrum of symptoms partly explains the confusing nomencla-

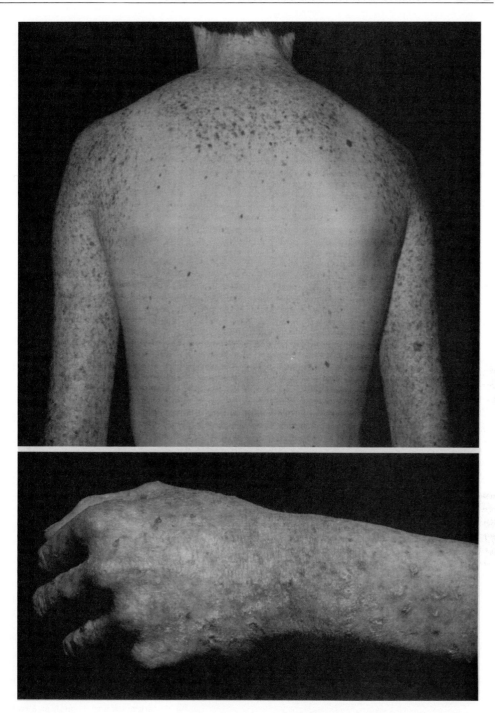

FIG. 13-2 Typical skin abnormalities in an adolescent xeroderma pigmentosum patient (complementation group XP-C). *Top*: Pigmentation abnormalities; freckling and dryness and atrophy visible at the sun-exposed areas of the skin. *Bottom*: Hand of same patient showing actinic keratosis and (pre)malignant lesions. *(Courtesy of Department of Dermatology, Erasmus University, Rotterdam.)*

ture in the literature for (probably) the same disease.[20,21] PIBIDS is an acronym for a specific combination of symptoms: *p*hotosensitivity, *i*chthyosis, *b*rittle hair and nails, *i*mpaired intelligence, *de*creased fertility and *s*hort stature. TTD also encompasses IBIDS, BIDS and *S*IBIDS (osteo*s*clerosis and IBIDS). Several other names have been used to describe cases in which a number of the above features are present in combination with brittle hair: Pollitt, Tay, Amish brittle hair, Sabinas and Marinesco-Sjögren syndromes and ONMR (onychotrichodysplasia, neutropenia, mental retardation). These patients, whether they have TTD or not, do not show photosensitivity and probably do not have a DNA repair defect. A practical classification scheme, based on a checklist of clinical abnormalities associated with TTD, is proposed by Tolmie et al.[19] and may be helpful in diagnosis of TTD patients.

A TTD patient has been described who lost the hair during an episode of pneumonia.[22] Within a period of a few months, the scalp hair returned. This peculiar phenomenon of hair loss after fever may be indicative of a thermosensitive mutaion in the gene responsible for the disorder in these patients (see below).

Xeroderma Pigmentosum–Cockayne Syndrome Complex

Ten patients have been identified with clinical features of both XP and CS.[23–25] These patients had the cutaneous pigmentary and, in most cases, neoplastic features of XP with the dwarfism, mental retardation, increased reflexes, and retinal degeneration typical of CS.

Table 13-2 Most Common Clinical Features of
Cockayne Syndrome

Growth failure
    Decreased height and weight
    Decreased head circumference (microcephaly)
Neurologic manifestations
    Delayed psychomotor development
    Increased muscle tone
    Tremor
    Limb ataxia/incoordination
    Gait abnormality
    Hearing loss
    Calcification of basal ganglia of brain
Ophthalmologic abnormalities
    Cataracts
    Optic athrophy/hypoplasia
    Pigmentary retinopathy
Dental abnormalities
    Caries
Skin abnormalities
    Photosensitivity
    Thin, dry hair

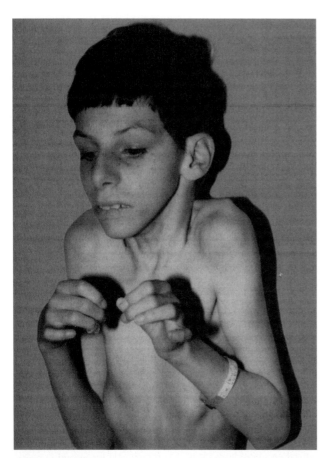

FIG. 13-3 Patient with Cockayne syndrome (CS). Growth failure, characteristic wizened facial appearance (birdlike facies), and skeletal deformation are visible. *(Photograph kindly provided by D. Atherton, Hospital for Sick Children, London. From A. Lehmann,[13] used by permission.)*

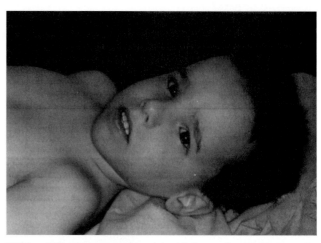

FIG. 13-4 Patient with trichothiodystrophy (TTD). Note the brittle hair as one of the crucial features of TTD. *(Photograph kindly provided by A. Sarasin, CNRS, Villejuif, France, and C. Blanchet-Bardon, Hôpital Saint-Louis, Paris. From A. Lehmann,[13] used by permis-*

BIOCHEMICAL AND CELLULAR ASPECTS OF XP, CS, AND TTD

Production of Cellular Damage by Sunlight

Sunlight is the major environmental agent that is involved in many of the clinical symptoms of XP; it does so by damaging cutaneous cells. Understanding the biochemical defects in XP requires knowledge of the way the damaging wavelengths in sunlight are absorbed by macromolecules and the nature of the damage that is produced.

The wavelengths of sunlight reaching the surface of the earth extend into the near-UV region, the shortest detectable being about 290 nm. Shorter-wavelength UV (present in solar radiation in space) is blocked from reaching the ground by ozone and other components of the atmosphere. This lower limit slightly overlaps the upper region of the absorption spectra of nucleic acids and proteins. Energy in this region of overlap is absorbed by macromolecules in the skin, producing harmful effects that include erythema, burns and actinic carcinogenesis.[26–28] Comparisons between direct sunlight and short-wavelength UV light (254 nm) indicate that sunlight in the midwestern United States is equivalent in germicidal activity to about 0.1 to 0.2 J per square meter of surface per minute (J/m²-min) of 254-nm UV light.[6] Since normal human cells in culture have a D_{37}* of only about 3 to 5 J/m² of radiation at 254 nm, the direct exposure of human proliferating cells to sunlight can result in significant amounts of cell killing.

Radiation at the UV end of the suns spectrum produces its biologic effects through absorption of quanta in molecules that have unsaturated chemical bonds, such as aromatic amino acids in proteins and purine and pyrimidine components of DNA and RNA. The action spectra for production of DNA damage (pyrimidine photoproducts), cell killing, production of aberrant chromosomes, and induction of unscheduled DNA repair synthesis (i.e., DNA synthesis not associated with the normal cell cycle; see below) are all similar, exhibiting maximum efficiency in wavelengths from 260 to 280 nm. Although there is negligible energy in this region of the sun's spectrum, there is sufficient overlap of the shortest end of the sun's spectrum with the longer-wavelength side of the absorption spectrum of DNA for significant photochemical reac-

*The D_{37} is the dose required to reduce survival to 0.37 from the initial value of 1.0, and in target theory corresponds to the dose required to produce an average of one lethal hit on the sensitive target of an irradiated organism when the survival curve is exponential.

Table 13-3 Main Clinical Symptoms of NER Syndromes

Clinical Symptoms	XP	XP/CS	CS	TTD
Photosensitivity	++	++	+*	+*
Abnormal pigmentation	++	+	−	−
Skin cancer	++	+	−	−
Progressive mental degeneration	−/+**	+	+	+
Neuronal loss	−/+**	−	−	−
Neurodysmyelination	−	++	+	+
Wizened facies	−	+	+	+
Growth defect	+/−**	+	+	+
Hypogonadism	−/+	+	+	+
Brittle hair and nails	−	−	−	+
Ichthyosis	−	−	−	+

*Also TTD and CS patients occur without photosensitivity and NER defect.
**These neurologic and growth defects are characteristic features of XP patients with the DeSanctis Cacchione Syndrome.

tion to occur. Shorter-wavelength UV is absorbed by the outer, nondividing layers of skin cells. An action spectrum of production of DNA damage in human skin shows a peak at about 302 nm.[6]

Two kinds of pyrimidine photoproducts are formed in DNA by absorption of UV light. The most frequent is the cyclobutane pyrimidine dimer (Fig. 13-5). This is formed between adjacent pyrimidines in the same strand of DNA by the formation of two bonds between the 5 positions and between the 6 positions on the pyrimidine rings. An alternative dipyrimidine photoproduct is the [6-4]pyrimidine-pyrimidone product mainly consisting of 5'TC or 5'CC (Fig. 13-5), which is formed at lower rates than the cyclobutane dimer but is also important biologically. Various estimates suggest that the [6-4] photoproduct is formed at 10 to 50 percent of the frequency of cyclobutane dimers by low doses of 254-nm light. Numerous biologic effects, such as cell killing, production of chromosome aberrations, mutagenesis, and carcinogenesis, can be attributed to these photoproducts in DNA. Other photoproducts have biologic effects in some circumstances. These include the unstable cytosine hydrate, purine photoproducts, and, at relatively high doses, locally denatured regions, DNA-protein crosslinks, and single-strand breaks.

Repair of Sunlight-Induced DNA Damage

At least three different biochemical repair systems operate in sunlight-exposed cells to safeguard DNA from permanent damage. These are excision repair, postreplication repair (which is more like a damage tolerance mechanism), and photoreactivation. These systems have been found in bacteria, yeast, amphibians, fish, rodents, marsupials, and mammals. They are especially important in the skin, where they mend damage to DNA caused by UV. Some of the repair systems can also mend damage to DNA caused by chemical carcinogens. These systems presumably protect internal tissues against the carcinogenic and mutagenic consequences of exposure to chemicals that damage DNA.

Excision repair is extremely versatile and can mend a large variety of UV light, X-ray, and chemically induced forms of damage to DNA.[6,29] Excision repair may be subdivided into nucleotide excision repair and base excision repair. The nucleotide excision repair system, which will be discussed in the next paragraph, excises damaged single strands of DNA and replaces them with a new sequence of bases, using as a template for base pairing the intact strand of DNA opposite the original damaged site.

Base excision repair removes damaged bases, leaving the sugar-phosphate backbone of the DNA intact and creating an AP

(apurinic or apyrimidinic) site. This site is subsequently converted into a strand break and repaired by short patch repair of usually one or a few nucleotides.

Postreplication repair is not a damage repair pathway per se but a damage tolerance mechanism that solves the problem the replication machinery faces when it encounters a damage in the template. This poorly defined process has been studied best in *S. cerevisiae*, where two subpathways have been distinguished.[30] The first is reinitiation of DNA replication at a more downstream location, leaving a gap opposite the lesion. After replication of the complementary strand, the newly copied information is used to fill in the gap in the other strand by recombination. This pathway is in principal error-free. The second subpathway induces translesion DNA replication. However, this process is error-prone and may be the main determinant of all damage-induced mutations. Very little is known about this pathway in mammals, and it is not sure whether it follows the same principal steps in higher species.

The third repair system, photoreactivation, simply reverts the damaged DNA to the normal chemical state without removing or exchanging any material from DNA. The photoreactivation system was thought to be specific for one form of damage induced by UV light—the cyclobutane pyrimidine dimer. Photoreactivation cleaves these dimers. Evidence is presented for a light-dependent system in *Drosophila* for repair of [6-4] photoproducts as well.[31] Photoreactivation has been demonstrated in bacteria, yeast, fish, amphibians and marsupials, but the existence and importance of this system in human tissue is still controversial.[6] A human gene has been cloned which shows significant homology with the *Drosophila* [6-4] photoproduct-lyase.[31,32]

The Nucleotide Excision Repair System

Nucleotide excision repair (NER) is one of the major and most versatile repair mechanisms that operates in the cell. This universal system eliminates a remarkably diverse array of structurally unrelated lesions, that range from UV-induced photoproducts (cyclobutane pyrimidine dimers and [6-4] photoproducts) to bulky and small chemical adducts as well as interstrand crosslinks. Thus, it is not surprising that the NER process entails multiple steps and involves the concerted action of a number of proteins. The details of this repair mechanism are best understood in the case of the UvrABC system in the bacterium *E. coli*.[33-36] Briefly, at least six distinct steps can be discerned: (1) lesion recognition and (2) lesion marcation, which involves conformational changes in DNA, are carried out by the $UvrA_2B$ complex. (3) A complex of UvrB and UvrC incises the damaged strand on both sides of the lesion at some distance, leaving the nondamaged strand intact. (4) The damage-containing oligomer is removed by the helicase action of UvrD, followed by (5) gap-filling DNA synthesis by DNA polymerase I. The process is completed by (6) the sealing of the new DNA to the preexisting strand by DNA ligase. In principle this mode of repair is error-free as it utilizes the nucleotide sequence information of the intact complementary DNA strand.

Although in outline and in concept quite simple, it is becoming increasingly apparent that the scheme of the NER repair mechanism as outlined above for *E. coli* represents a dramatic oversimplification particularly when extrapolated to eukaryotes. This notion is based on a number of observations.

First, a minimum of two in-part overlapping NER subpathways have been discovered; these are schematically represented in Fig. 13-6. One subpathway, here referred to as *transcription-coupled repair*, deals with the complication that the vital process of transcription is blocked by lesions in the template. To cope with this urgent problem transcription-coupled repair takes complete elimination of injury in the transcribed strand of active structural

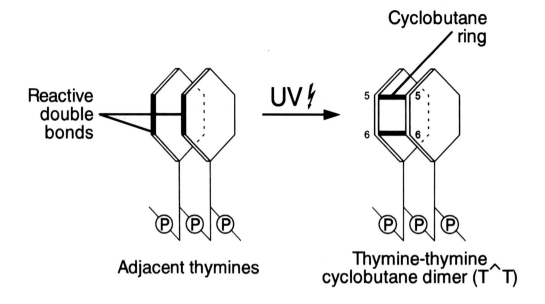

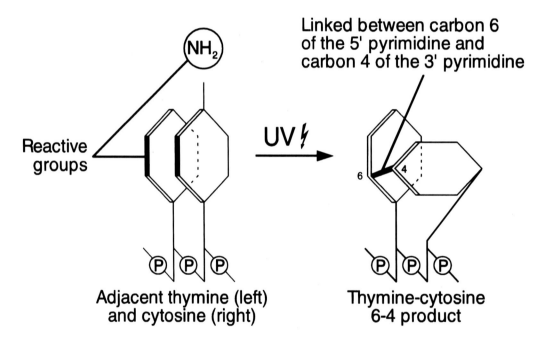

FIG. 13-5 Main UV-induced DNA lesions. *Top:* The cyclobutane pyrimidine dimer between adjacent thymines on the same strand of DNA. *Bottom:* [6-4] photoproduct between adjacent thymine and cyto- sine on same strand of DNA. These structures result in considerable distortion of the phosphodiester backbone of DNA.

genes.[37,38] This holds particularly for lesions for which repair otherwise would be too slow or inefficient. In this specialized NER subpathway, initial damage detection is thought to be carried out by RNA polymerase II, when it is blocked in front of a lesion. As part of the repair mechanism the stalled RNA polymerase complex has to be displaced to give the repair machinery access to the injury. Another branch of the NER system (here designated *global genome repair*) accomplishes the removal of lesions in the remainder of the genome, including the nontranscribed strand of active genes. Damage recognition in this repair system is performed by a specific NER protein (complex) and is for many—but not all—lesions more slow and less efficient when compared with transcription-coupled repair. The efficiency of damage recognition

by the global genome repair system varies strongly from lesion to lesion and may also vary with the chromatin conformation, the location in the genome and the state of differentiation of the cell. This is not so surprising when one realizes the tremendous task that is faced by this system in continually surveilling the 2 m of DNA double helix in every mammalian nucleus for trace amounts of a diversity of lesions.

NER is visualized under the microscope by the Unscheduled DNA Synthesis (UDS) test. Cultured fibroblasts are exposed to UV and briefly (2-3 hours) incubated in ³H-thymidine-containing medium. Cells in G_1 or G_2 phase of the cell cycle become radioactively labelled by the gap-filling DNA-synthesis step of the NER process. Following autoradiography the repair capacity of these

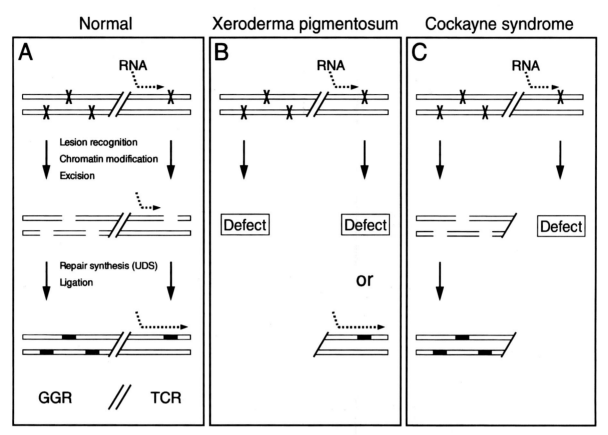

FIG. 13-6 NER pathways and defects in XP and CS. This simplified scheme shows in the left panel (normal cells) the transcription-coupled repair (TCR) pathway at the right that mends lesions in the transcribed strand of active genes; and the Global Genome Repair (GGR) pathway (left) that deals with lesions in the remaining part of the genome. In XP (middle panel) the genetic defect in most cases affects both mechanisms, in XP complementation group C only GGR is impaired. In CS (right panel) the defect is opposite of XP-C, only TCR is

cells can be quantified at the single-cell level. UDS has proven to be a powerful tool to measure NER in repair-proficient and -deficient cells (see Figs. 13-7 and 13-11).

NER Activity in XP, CS and TTD Cells

Defective DNA excision repair in UV-irradiated skin fibroblasts from some XP patients was for the first time reported by Cleaver in 1968[39] and in skin in vivo by Epstein et al.[40] The NER defect in TTD cells was first reported by Stefanini et al.[41] The defect in most XP and TTD cells is reflected by decreased levels of UDS (Fig. 13-7). Measurement of UV-induced UDS is in fact required for a definitive diagnosis of NER deficient XP and TTD. Different levels of UDS in unrelated XP patients suggested heterogeneity at the molecular level in this syndrome.[42] A number of XP patients have shown a normal response in the UDS test. They have been designated as XP variants[43] and were found to have a defect in postreplication repair.[44]

Similarly various degrees of NER deficiency have been demonstrated among TTD patients, including normal DNA repair in approximately half of the patients.[49]

UDS in CS cells is not significantly different from normal cells. However, by measuring NER in transcribed and nontranscribed gene sequences separately, a technique developed by the group of Hanawalt,[45] Venema et al.[46] have demonstrated deficient repair of the transcribed strand of active genes in CS cells (see Fig. 13-6). The less efficient global genome repair is still functional. Since transcription-coupled repair (TCR) makes a relatively small contribution to the total repair synthesis, CS fibroblasts show near-normal levels of UDS. The TCR defect prevents

the rapid recovery of RNA synthesis after UV exposure. This delayed recovery of RNA synthesis and also of S-phase DNA synthesis in CS cells following UV exposure is used as a diagnostic criterion of CS[47,48,25] in combination with clinical symptoms.

Colony-Forming Ability of XP, CS and TTD Cells

The number of cells in culture that can grow into colonies after UV irradiation can be used as an in vitro measurement of sensitivity. Heterogeneity in the response of fibroblasts of unrelated XP patients is evident (Fig. 13-8, left panel). In all cases, NER-deficient XP fibroblasts are more sensitive than normal cells, and those from patients who exhibit neurological abnormalities are generally the most sensitive.[10]

XP cells are also more sensitive to carcinogenic chemicals creating bulky DNA adducts (including benz(a)pyrene), but are normal in response to DNA methylating agents and, with a few exceptions, to X-rays.[6]

Fibroblasts of XP-variants do not exhibit a significant increase of UV-sensitivity under standard test conditions. However, a dramatic increase of sensitivity becomes apparent if XP-variant cells are incubated in the presence of caffeine after UV-exposure (Fig. 13-8, middle panel). This effect of caffeine on UV-sensitivity may be used as a diagnostic test which is specific for the XP-variant type and much simpler than the demonstration of a defective post replication repair.

The delayed recovery of RNA synthesis as a result of the TCR defect in CS cells probably causes the increased sensitivity in CS cells (Fig. 13-8, right panel). An increasing number of CS patients have been diagnosed, who do not show photosensitivity.[12] Fibro-

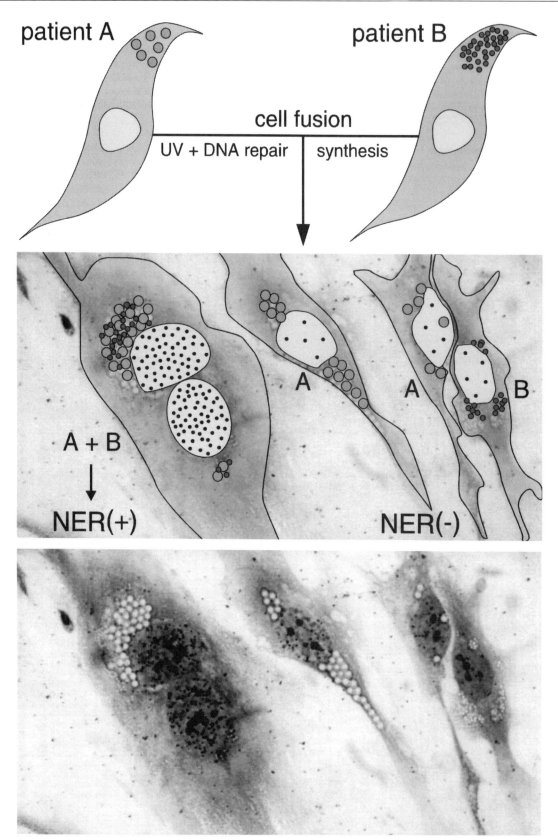

FIG. 13-7 Genetic heterogeneity in xeroderma pigmentosum studied by cell fusion and UV-induced unscheduled DNA synthesis (UDS). *Top:* A schematic representation of the micrograph presented at the bottom. Cultured fibroblasts from two unrelated patients (A and B) were fused, exposed to UV-light, pulse labeled with ³H-thymidine, fixed and autoradiographed to visualize DNA repair synthesis (UDS). Cells of patient A are marked with engulfed large latex beads and those of patient B with small beads. This marking enables the identification of the fused cells containing nuclei of both patients (heterokaryons). If the patients are mutated in different DNA repair genes (gene A and gene B) the heterokaryon will be able to perform normal levels of DNA repair synthesis (UDS is visualized by wild-type levels of autoradiographic grains in the emulsion above the nuclei). In this case patient A and B belong to two different complementation groups. *(From the Department of Cell Biology and Genetics, Erasmus University, Rotterdam, W. Vermeulen and D. Bootsma.)*

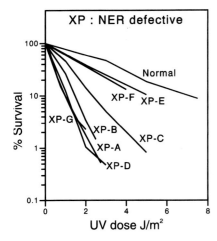

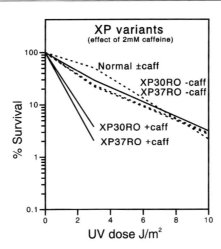

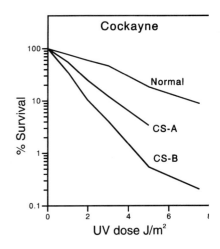

FIG. 13-8 UV sensitivity of xeroderma pigmentosum (XP) and Cockayne syndrome (CS) cells. *(Left panel)* XP cells of different complementation groups. *(Center)* XP variant cells in the presence and absence of caffeine. Caffeine sensitizes XP variant cells to UV. *(Right panel)* CS cells. *(From the Department of Cell Biology and Genetics: Raams, Jaspers, and Hoeijmakers.)*

blasts of these patients do not display increased sensitivity in the colony-formation test. Similar patterns of UV sensitivity are observed with fibroblast cultures of photosensitive and non-photosensitive TTD patients.[49] These non-photosensitive CS and TTD fibroblasts also behave like normal cells in UDS and in DNA- and RNA-synthesis recovery tests. These results suggest that these patients do not have a DNA repair defect and that their clinical symptoms have another cause. (For an explanation, see Implications for Diagnosis, below.)

CS cells are also sensitive to UV-mimetic carcinogens such as 4NQO and *N*-acetoxy-*N*-2-acetyl-2-aminofluorene but not to monofunctional alkylating agents.[50]

Mutational Events in XP, CS and TTD Cells

Cultured cells from most XP and CS patients have a normal karyotype. Distinctive spontaneous karyotypic changes characteristic for some diseases with a high cancer incidence, such as ataxia telangiectasia, Fanconi anemia, and Bloom syndrome[21] are not seen in XP patients.

XP cells show a normal frequency of spontaneous sister chromatid exchanges (SCE) but a greater than normal frequency after exposure to UV light and most chemical carcinogens.[6] Similarly, XP cells show more chromosome aberrations than normal cells after exposure to UV light and chemical carcinogens.[6]

The frequency with which cells resistant to 6-thioguanine, ouabain, diphtheria toxin, or other toxic chemicals are produced by irradiation with UV light or artificial sunlight, or by exposure to chemical carcinogens, is greater in all XP cells, including XP variants, than in normal cells.[6] This implies that the genetic defects in XP cells confer increased mutability. In the XP variant, the repair system has lost fidelity and so produces a high frequency of mutations. Evidence has been presented for increased transformation to anchorage independence (growth in suspension instead of attached to the bottom of a culture disk) after UV irradiation of XP variant cells compared to normal cells.[51]

Shuttle vector plasmids that are capable of autonomous replication in both mammalian cells and *E. coli* have been used for measuring the frequency and spectrum of mutations following exposure of transfected cells to DNA damage.[6] There were significantly fewer plasmids with tandem or multiple base substitution mutations or with single or tandem transversion mutations after transfection of UV-damaged plasmids in XP cells than in normal cells. With all cell lines, the predominant base

substitution mutation was the G:C to A:T transition, i.e., the C mutated to a T. Thus, with these human cells, the major UV photoproduct, the TT cyclobutane dimer, is not the major premutagenic lesion. This finding is consistent with the A rule: a tendency of polymerases to insert adenines opposite noninstructional lesions. Thus, insertion of A opposite TT dimers results in the correct pairing, while insertion of A opposite a C, involved in cyclobutane dimers and [6-4] photoproducts (see Fig. 13-5), results in G:C to A:T transitions.

UV-damaged viruses and plasmids have also been used as substrates to measure the capacity of NER-deficient cells to repair DNA damage by monitoring the extent of their biological recovery, e.g., by their ability to propagate in bacterial hosts.[6] The extent of this host-cell reactivation by various cell types often parallels the ability to survive UV damage. Host cell reactivation assays employing UV-damaged plasmids treated in vitro with photolyase (which selectively removes cyclobutane dimers) have been used to study repair of different types of photoproducts. While XPA cells show poor repair of all types of photoproducts, CS cells have faulty repair of cyclobutane dimers but normal repair of non-dimer photoproducts.[52,53]

GENETIC ASPECTS OF XP, CS, AND TTD

Complementation Analysis of NER Deficiency Syndromes

The clinical heterogeneity in XP and the marked differences in cellular expression of the excision repair defect in terms of unscheduled DNA synthesis in different patients[42] prompted us to devise a cell fusion assay to investigate genetic heterogeneity in XP.[54] Heterokaryons formed between fibroblasts of different XP patients exposed to ultraviolet light either showed normal or nearly normal levels of UDS (i.e., patients complement each others defects and, therefore, belong to different complementation groups; Fig. 13-7) or they exhibit the impaired levels of UDS seen in the unfused XP cells (i.e., patients are in the same complementation group). Each complementation group may represent a gene that, if mutated and in homozygous condition, causes XP.

A total of seven complementation groups has been identified in excision repair-deficient XP.[6] This number may be a low estimate of the number of genes that are expected to cause deficient DNA repair in humans. In comparison, at least 15 distinct genes involved in nucleotide excision repair (the *RAD3* epistasis group) have been identified in *S. cerevisiae,* and even this number is likely to be an underestimate.

By using the RNA-synthesis recovery test in cell fusion studies the patients with Cockayne syndrome (in its classical form, without XP features and/or without global genome repair deficiency) could be assigned to two complementation groups: CS-A and CS-B.[47,55]

The rare patients having the XP-CS complex were found to be members of complementation groups XP-B, D and G.[24] Intriguingly, there is also overlap between XP and TTD, although the clinical features are very different. Most TTD patients fall into the XP-D group.[49] Recently, one TTD family was found to belong to XP-B[56] and a third kindred constitutes a distinct NER-deficient complementation group, TTD-A,[41] not (yet) associated with XP.

Thus, both genetic heterogeneity within and genetic overlap between all NER disorders is found. A specific subset of XP groups (notably XP-D and XP-B) is associated with extreme variability ranging from XP to CS to TTD. Therefore, these disorders may in fact be considered different manifestations of one heterogeneous clinical continuum.

Characteristics of Complementation Groups

Some of the properties of the XP and TTD complementation groups are summarized in Table 13-4.

XP group A. Group A usually corresponds to the most severe clinical form of XP, in which there are both skin symptoms and central nervous system (CNS) disorders. Many patients exhibit manifestations from birth or early in life and correspond to the clinical category of the DeSantis-Cacchione syndrome with progressive neurologic degeneration.[6]

Excision repair is generally very low (<2 percent of normal) in cells of most XP-A patients and they are about 10 times more sensitive than normal to killing by UV irradiation or other carcinogens (see Fig. 13-8). The genetic defect in this group interferes with both transcription-coupled repair (TCR) and global genome repair (GGR).

There are exceptions to these general characteristics of group A cells. Cells from a British patient without CNS disorders,

XP8LO, exhibited about 30 percent of normal cellular excision repair and higher survival after UV than other group A cells.[6] A 35-year-old Egyptian male (XP13CA) had the typical low level of unscheduled synthesis, but was neurologically normal, had normal stature, and was fertile. Two other group A patients, XP12BE and XP1LO, also show milder neurologic abnormalities, whereas their cells are less UV sensitive than the majority in group A.[6] In one Italian family, group A sibs exhibited different clinical symptoms; only one had CNS signs.[6] In cell cultures, it appeared that the sib without CNS disorder had, on average, higher repair due to a subpopulation of cells with normal repair mixed with typical group A cells. Therefore, although group A patients usually have the associated neurologic abnormalities of the DeSantis-Cacchione syndrome, several are known who are neurologically normal or have less severe neurologic abnormalities.

XP group B. For many years XP group B consisted only of 1 patient (XP11BE; see Fig. 13-9).[23] This patient died of acute hypertension at age 33. She had small stature, deafness, mental retardation, immature sexual development, premature senility, absence of subcutaneous fat, and optic nerve and retinal pigment degeneration characteristic of Cockayne syndrome. She exhibited acute sun sensitivity, ocular changes, and multiple cutaneous malignancy at age 18, all typical of XP.

Two sibs (XP1BA and XP2BA) with mild features of XP and CS were recently assigned to XP-B.[58] Developmental abnormalities are nearly absent in these individuals and neurological symptoms became evident only after the second decade of life.[59]

A remarkable clinical variation is observed between these two XP-B families. The two sibs do not display any cutaneous malignancies despite a, for XP, relatively advanced age of more than 40 years, whereas patient XP11BE had skin tumors at 18 years. Nevertheless, the level of UDS representing the repair defect is similar in both families (5 to 10 percent of NER-proficient cells) and effects both TCR and GGR.

The assignment to XP-B of two sibs (TTD4VI and TTD6VI), with relatively mild clinical features of TTD and moderately impaired NER characteristics (about 40 percent UDS),[56] extends the clinical heterogeneity within this complementation group.

XP group C. Group C is one of the largest groups and is often referred to as the classic form of XP. The patients usually show only

Table 13-4 Properties of XP, CS, and TTD Complementation Groups

| Complementation group | UV Sensitivity | Residual UDS* | NER Activity | | Relative Frequency¶ | Skin Cancer | Neurologic Abnormalities | Clinical Phenotype |
			TCR**	GGR†				
XP-A	+++	<5%	−	−	High	+	++	XP
XP-B	++	3–40%	−	−	3 families	+/−	++/+	XP/CS or TTD
XP-C	+	15–30%	+	−	High	+	−	XP
XP-D	++	15–50%	−	−	Intermediate	+/−	++/−	XP, XP/CS or TTD
XP-E	±	≥50%	?	?	Rare	+/−	−	XP
XP-F	+	15–30%	−	−	Rare	+/−	−/±	XP
XP-G	++	<5–25%	−	−	Rare	+/−	++/+	XP or XP/CS
TTD-A	+	10%	−	−	1 family	−	+	TTD
CS-A	+	Normal	−	−	Intermediate	−	++	CS
CS-B	+	Normal	−	+	High	−	++	CS
XP-V§	+/±	Normal	+	+	High	+/−	−	XP

*Unscheduled DNA synthesis, expressed as percentage of repair synthesis in normal cells.
**Transcription coupled repair.
†Global genome repair.
¶The overall frequency of XP is between 10^{-5} to 10^{-6}, less than 500 cases have been classified.
§XP-variant, defect in post replication repair, proficient NER.

skin and eye disorders. These vary considerably in severity, depending on the climate. Patients of over 80 years of age have been diagnosed. Tumors of the tip of the tongue have been observed in several patients. A case of XP-C is presented in Fig. 13-2. The level of UDS varies between 15 and 30 percent of normal and XP-C cells are less sensitive to killing by UV light and chemical carcinogens than cells from group A and D (Fig. 13-8). One characteristic of repair unique to this group is that it is clustered rather than random[60] due to a selective loss in the capacity to perform GGR in the presence of normal levels of TCR.[61] Apparently, this defect is opposite of the deficiency in the classical form of CS[46] (see Fig. 13-6).

One exceptional patient (XP1MI) exhibited symptoms of XP, systemic lupus erythematosus, microcephaly and a marginal degree of mental retardation.[62] Cells from this patient had DNA repair levels typical for XP-C but were the most UV-sensitive in group C.[11] Two reported instances of CNS tumors in XP patients—XP106LO and Hawaiian patient XP15BE—are in this group.[6]

XP group D. This is a very interesting group because of the extensive clinical heterogeneity. Many XP-D patients have skin and neurological abnormalities like those in group A, although the onset of the CNS disorders may be delayed until the second decade. In addition to these classical XP patients, most of the photosensitive TTD patients have been assigned to this complementation group.[49,63] So far, no reports on the occurrence of skin cancer within this group of XP-D TTD patients have appeared. Furthermore, two patients with the combined XP-CS complex were found

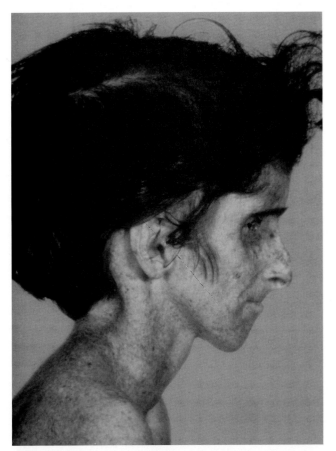

FIG. 13-9 XP patient (XP11BE). This patient, 28 years old, from complementation group B, exhibits skin, ocular, and neurologic characteristics that have been ascribed to both XP and CS. *(From Kraemer,[57] used by permission.)*

to belong to XP group D.[6] Thus XP-D is a complex group involving diverse clinical syndromes.[64] Excision repair varies from 15 percent (in XP and XP/CS cases) to above 50 percent in some TTD patients. Some evidence suggests that the amount of UDS in the XP and XP/CS cases is higher than expected from the low amount of dimer excision observed in these cells and their sensitivity to cell killing (comparable with XP-A cells, see Fig. 13-8). This is perhaps due to better repair of [6-4] photoproducts in these cells.[6]

XP group E. Patients in the rare group E exhibit mild skin symptoms and are neurologically normal.[23] The level of excision repair is high (more than 50 percent of normal), and the level relative to normal cells increases with increasing UV dose. The cells are only slightly more sensitive than normal to UV damage (Fig. 13-8). Patients have been reported from Europe and Japan. One XP-E patient (XP2RO) died from metastatic tumor of endothelial origin.

XP group F. Most representatives of group F have been described in Japan.[65] The patients had acute sun sensitivity in infancy but relatively mild symptoms with late onset of skin cancer despite a substantially reduced level of repair. Excision repair was 15 to 30 percent of normal, but increased to 60 percent with incubation. The cells appear to be more defective in repair of damage that occurs at rapid rates and at early times after irradiation such as [6-4] photoproducts.[6] They show an intermediate sensitivity to killing by UV light and a high degree of excision of pyrimidine dimers when measured at late times after irradiation. There was a marked enhancement of UV survival when cells were held in a density-inhibited condition after irradiation.[66]

XP group G. Until 1966 this rare group comprised 8 patients originating from Europe and Japan.[24] The clinical symptoms vary from mild cutaneous and no neurologic abnormalities to severe dermatological and neurologic impairment. So far only one XP-G patient (XP31KO) developed a skin tumor, which appeared at a relatively late age. The UDS level varies between <5% to 25% (in XP31KO) and cell killing by UV light resembles that of group A and D patients. One patient (XP3BR) is unusual in having a slightly increased sensitivity to killing by X-rays.[67] Four patients (XPCS1LV, XPCS2LV, XP20BE and XPCS1RO) display symptoms characteristic of CS.[12,24] Although the CS symptoms are more prominent than the XP features (small pigmented spots on trunk, limbs and face), the repair defect of these patients is typical of XP: UDS is severely reduced (<5% of normal).

XP variant. Patients in the variant group have mild to severe skin symptoms and usually have normal CNS functions. The variant form is found worldwide and is a frequently occurring and distinct group, even though it cannot often be clinically identified without cell culture studies. Originally defined as a clinically recognized XP without a defect in excision repair,[23,43] it was also described earlier under the clinical designation *pigmented xerodermoid*.[68] With careful clinical investigation, some patients in this group may be recognized by relatively mild symptoms and the absence of an enhanced erythematous response, but this is insufficient for unambiguous diagnosis, and other XP variant patients may have severel clinical symptoms.[23]

The high level of mutagenesis with near-normal levels of cell survival after UV irradiation could be interpreted as an indication, that the inherited disorder has made XP variant cells error-prone.[6] The outstanding feature of this form of XP is that after UV irradiation, replication forks appear to stop or to be interrupted during semi-conservative replication at every site of DNA damage.[44] This is interpreted as a defect in postreplication repair.

Whether the variant group is homogeneous or has multiple subgroups is not known, but the clinical heterogeneity is suggestive. The pigmented xerodermoid family of Jung et al.,[68] although biochemically identical to other XP variants, is unusual because no clinical symptoms were evident until after the age of 40, and patients lived into their eighties. These mild symptoms contrast with other variant families from comparable environments in whom the disease is quite severe.[6] One attempt at studying complementation between cells from different XP variant patients indicated a single XP variant group.[69]

TTD group A. The cells of one TTD patient (TTD1BR) complemented cells from all seven XP complementation groups and apparently represents a third TTD complementation group (TTD-A) in addition to XP-B and XP-D.[41] This patient, first described in 1982[70] and now in his twenties, has typical symptoms of TTD and has been sensitive to sunlight since early childhood. His clinical features are quite distinct from those associated with XP showing no significant freckling or other pigmentary changes and no skin tumors.[41]

CS complementation groups. Complementation analysis has disclosed two groups in the classical form of CS: CS-A and CS-B. CS is clinically heterogeneous. The clinical differentiation among CS individuals based on the age of onset and severity of the disease (CSI and CSII)[12] does not correlate with these two complementation groups. Clinical variation is further complicated by other syndromes, which resemble many of the traits observed in CS: CAMFAK (*c*ataracts, *m*icrocephaly, *f*ailure to thrive, *k*yphoscoliosis) and COFS (*c*erebro-*o*culo-*f*acial *s*yndrome). Assays of DNA repair have been normal in these syndromes.[12] Recently, two siblings were described without clear CS signs, but with CS-like biochemical DNA repair properties (increased UV sensitivity, normal UDS but a reduced post-UV RNA synthesis recovery).[71] Genetic analysis revealed that these two siblings can be assigned to a new complementation group (designated UV[s] syndrome, since they complement all known XP and CS groups).[72] Two other patients with a CS-type DNA repair defect, assigned to CS complementation group B, exhibit only XP symptoms.[73] At the other side of the spectrum, there are individuals with clear CS hallmarks (dwarfism, mental retardation, deafness and peculiar facies) but without a reduced post-UV RNA

synthesis recovery and photosensitivity.[74] These observations strengthen the notion that the syndromes XP and CS (and TTD) are closely related biochemically and may be part of a broader clinical disease spectrum.

Genetic Classification of Other Eukaryotic NER Mutants

The clinical and genetic heterogeneity in NER syndromes raised the question of whether the complementation groups represent single gene defects, inherited in a simple Mendelian fashion, or whether more than one genetic locus is involved in each patient.[75] Cloning of the responsible genes would give the answer.

An important first step on the way to cloning repair genes was the isolation of repair-deficient rodent mutant cell lines. Many of these cell lines are of Chinese hamster origin (CHO and V79 cell lines). So far, complementation analysis of these mutants has revealed at least 11 distinct complementation groups.[76,77] The main features are summarized in Table 13-5. The first five groups consist of cell lines which are extremely sensitive to UV and bulky adducts and, in that respect, resemble the XP groups A, B, D, and G. Repair in the few representatives of the remaining groups (except group 11) appears to be only partially disturbed, as in CS-A, CS-B and in XP groups C, E and F. A unique characteristic of groups 1 and 4 is their extreme sensitivity to cross-linking agents such as MMC. This suggests that the NER genes affected in these mutants act in additional systems other than NER or respond to cross-link damage in DNA. Cell fusion studies performed by Thompson[78] showed that human genes could complement the rodent repair defects in these mutant cell lines.

Another relevant class of eukaryotic NER mutants is presented by the *RAD3* epistasis group of bakers yeast *S. cerevisiae*. At least 15 complementation groups have been identified in this category of UV-sensitive yeast mutants (for review see ref. 36). The versatility of yeast genetics has permitted the cloning of almost all of the corresponding genes. The strong parallels with the mammalian system that have emerged in recent years make this organism a relevant paradigm for human NER. As shown below, there is considerable overlap between the yeast and Chinese hamster mutants and the human NER syndromes. This overlap is represented by

Table 13-5 Properties of Rodent NER Complementation Groups

Group	Representative mutant	Parental strain*	Sensitivity** UV	Sensitivity** MMC	Incision deficiency	Correcting human gene	XP or CS equivalent
1	UV20, 43-3B	CHO	++	+++	yes	*ERCC1*	not identified
2	UV5, VH-1	CHO/V79	++	+	yes	*ERCC2*	XP-D
3	UV24, 27-1	CHO	++	+	yes	*ERCC3*	XP-B
4	UV41	CHO	++	+++	yes	*ERCC4*	XP-F
5	UV135, Q31	CHO, mouse lymphoma	+(+)	±	yes	*ERCC5*	XP-G
6	UV61, US46	CHO, mouse lymphoma	+	+	partial	*ERCC6*	CS-B
7	VB11	V79	+	±	partial	?	?
8	US31	mouse lymphoma	+	+	?	*ERCC8*	CS-A
9	CHO4PV	CHO	+	+	partial	−	?
10	CHO7PV	CHO	+	+	partial	−	?
11	UVS1	CHO	+/++	+	yes	*ERCC11*†	XP-F

*CHO = Chinese hamster ovary.
**+: 2-5×; ++: 5-10×; +++: >10× wild type sensitivity; MMC = mitomycin C.
†*ERCC11* and *ERCC4* are probably identical.

the sequence homology of DNA repair genes and proteins in yeast, *Drosophila* and mammals including humans and is based on strong evolutionary conservation of DNA repair mechanisms. It is based on strong evolutionary conservation of DNA repair mechanisms and emphasizes the important function of DNA repair in maintaining life.

Cloning of Human NER Genes

Different strategies have been followed to clone human NER genes. A time-consuming but successful procedure has been transfection of genomic DNA from repair-proficient human cells or from a chromosome-specific cosmid library to repair-deficient rodent mutants followed by UV selection of repair-competent, UV-resistant transformants. The correcting gene can subsequently be isolated via standard recombinant DNA techniques. This strategy has resulted in the cloning of the human *excision repair cross complementing (ERCC)* genes that correct the rodent complementation groups 1 to 6: *ERCC1*,[79] *ERCC2*,[80] *ERCC3*,[81] *ERCC4*,[82] *ERCC5*[83] and *ERCC6*.[84]

Their possible role in NER syndromes in humans can be investigated by DNA transfection of the cloned genes into cells of the different complementation groups of XP, CS or TTD. Alternatively, the cDNA or the gene product can be microinjected into the nucleus or cytoplasm of cultured fibroblasts of NER-deficient patients. Introduction of the *ERCC2*, *ERCC3*, *ERCC5*, and *ERCC6* genes into human NER-deficient cells alleviated the specific defects in cells from XP-D,[85,86] XP-B,[87] XP-G,[88] and CS-B[89] respectively. An example is presented in Fig. 13-10.

The cloning of the *XPG* and *CSB* genes nicely demonstrates the unexpected contribution of findings in related and sometimes unrelated fields of research. The serendipitous cloning of the *XPG* gene was based on the screening of a *Xenopus laevis* cDNA expression library with antiserum from a human patient with the autoimmune disease lupus erythematosis by Clarkson and coworkers (Geneva).[88] The isolated full length frog and corresponding human cDNA turned out to be homologous to the yeast NER gene, *RAD2*. The human cDNA was able to correct the defect in cells of an XP-G patient. Independently, the *ERCC5* gene was cloned and also found to be homologous to *RAD2*.[90] Extracts of ERCC5 and XP-G cells appeared both deficient in the same protein.[91] A possible role of the *ERCC6* gene (cloned by Christine Troelstra in our laboratory[89]) in CS was suggested by an observation of Fryns c.s. (Leuven) that a CS patient had a constitutional deletion of a region of chromosome 10 to which we had mapped *ERCC6*.[92,89]

Genomic DNA transfection directly to cultured cells of patients with NER syndromes has, with one notable exception,[93] been unsuccessful. The difficulty of isolating repair-competent transformants after transfection of repair-defective human cells is due to the low amount of DNA that stably integrates in the genome of these cells. Compared to rodent cells, approximately 30 to more than one hundredfold less DNA is integrated. This raises the number of cells required to be transfected to generate one genomic transformant containing a specific gene to extremely high levels (depending on gene length, to more than 10^9 cells[94]). Therefore, the one example of successful isolation of a NER gene, the gene defective in XP group A (*XPA*), by Tanaka and coworkers[93] via very large-scale genomic DNA transfection to XP-A cells, was a formidable effort. They used an interspecies system (mouse DNA into human cells) to be able to identify and isolate the correcting (mouse) gene. This enabled the cloning of the human counterpart by cross-hybridization.

An alternative transfection approach has been the use of episomally replicating plasmid vectors carrying the Epstein-Barr virus replication origin and the gene for the Epstein-Barr virus nuclear antigen, EBNA1. With these vectors containing human cDNAs the *XPC* gene was cloned by Legerski et al.[95] and the *CSA* gene by the group of Friedberg.[96] Fusion of CS-A cells with the only rodent mutant representing complementation group 8 and transfection of the cloned *CSA* gene in these rodent mutant cells revealed the identity of *CSA* and *ERCC8* (see ref. 97 and Table 13-5).

Sequence homology based on evolutionary conservation has been used for the cloning of several other (human) DNA repair genes in different manners. One method utilizes nucleotide sequence homology to cross species barriers. Attempts to use cloned yeast NER genes for the isolation of homologous human sequences by low-stringency cross-hybridization with human DNA libraries has resulted in the cloning of two human genes homologous to *S. cerevisiae RAD6*: *HHR6A* and *HHR6B*.[98] *RAD6* encodes a protein involved in ubiquitin conjugation and is implicated in postreplication repair and damage-induced mutagenesis. The yeast protein and its two human counterparts may exert their functions by modulating chromatin structure via histone ubiquitination.[99] Alternatively, sequence conservation may permit the design of degenerate oligonucleotide primers based on conserved domains. These primers can be utilized for the cloning of homologous sequences by PCR amplification. In this manner we have recently succeeded in cloning a human cDNA with clear homology to the yeast *RAD1* gene.[100] Subsequent transfection and microinjection experiments revealed that this human *RAD1* homolog corrected the DNA repair defects in rodent group 4 and 11 mutants (revealing for the first time intragenic complementation between two rodent complementation groups) and XP-F fibroblasts.[100] Independently, the *ERCC4* gene was cloned by Thompson and collaborators (Livermore) by cosmid DNA transfection.[82]

These types of cloning strategies based on sequence conservation are enhanced by computerized database homology searching using powerful sequence-similarity search algorithms. The wealth of sequence information that is now available and will be even more so in the future, as a result of the Human Genome Project and related efforts, opens the possibility of identification of mammalian homologs of known relevant genes of lower species. This can be done by critical database screening based on conserved domains. In the last few months a large number of mammalian DNA repair genes have been identified. Most of them were not yet published when this chapter was written. Examples from our laboratory at Rotterdam are two human genes homologous to the *S. cerevisiae* NER gene *RAD23*: *HHR23A* and *B* (see also ref. 101); a human gene with homology to the photoreactivating enzyme (present in several organisms),[102] and identical to the gene independently identified by Todo c.s.[32]; and two human equivalents of the *Schizosaccharomyces pombe* DNA double-strand break-repair gene, *rad21*.[103] The same procedures also work in the other direction: from human DNA sequences to the isolation of homologs in lower eukaryotes. An example is the cloning of the *S. cerevisiae* counterpart of *CSB (ERCC6)*: *RAD26*.[104]

Another obvious procedure for cloning genes starts with the purification of the gene product, followed by designing nucleotide primers on the basis of a partial amino acid sequence obtained by microsequencing of the protein, and cloning of the gene by PCR. A gene that may be involved in XP complementation group E was cloned in this manner. The purification and characterization of this DNA damage binding protein (DDB) were reported by Hwang et al. (see ref. 105 and references therein) and the group of S. Linn.[106,107] Similarly, Hanaoka and collaborators purified the XPC protein (in a complex with another polypeptide, that turned out to be HHR23B), and subsequently cloned the cDNAs.[101]

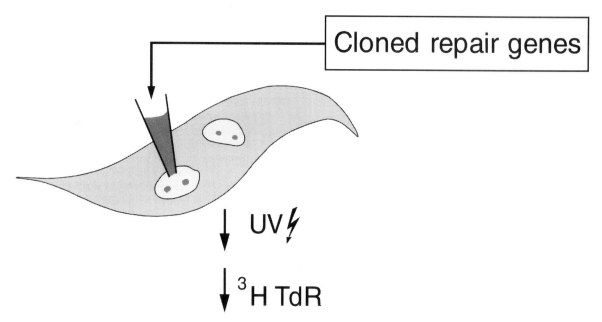

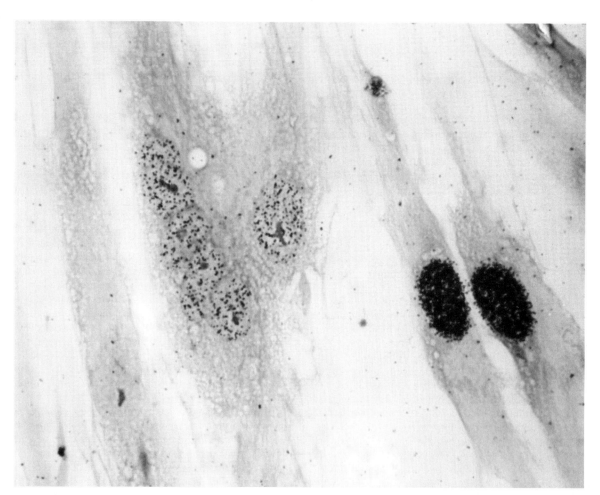

FIG. 13-10 Correction of NER defect in XP-B (XP11BE, see Fig. 13-9) multinuclear cells after microinjection of *ERCC3* in one of the nuclei. *Top:* Scheme of microinjection procedure. *Bottom:* DNA repair synthesis (UDS) is corrected to normal levels in the multinucleated cell after introduction of *ERCC3* cDNA. The low UDS level of the mononuclear fibroblast (left) reflects the NER defect of XP11BE cells. The two heavily labeled fibroblasts at the right were in S phase. *(From the Department of Cell Biology and Genetics, Erasmus University Rotterdam, W. Vermeulen.)*

MAMMALIAN NER GENES: THEIR FUNCTION IN THE NER PATHWAY AND ROLE IN NER SYNDROMES

Candidates for the NER genes involved in all seven XP complementation groups have been molecularly cloned although the responsible gene for XP-E is still uncertain. In addition, the two genes implicated in the classical form of CS have been isolated and two of the three TTD (photosensitive form) genes have been identified. Futhermore, several human NER genes have been cloned for which no human NER complementation groups are known yet but for which either a rodent mutant or a yeast NER equivalent exists.

Using in vitro NER assay systems based on cell-free extracts (developed by the groups of Wood and Sancar[108,109]) several proteins known to be involved in DNA replication have also been demonstrated to participate in the incision and/or DNA synthesis step of the NER pathway. Very recently, the core of the mammalian NER reaction was successfully reconstituted in vitro with (partly) purified components.[110,111] These in vitro systems provide valuable tools for studying the function of isolated repair proteins.

Computer-assisted comparison of the predicted amino acid sequence of the encoded proteins with known gene products present in large databases has highlighted a striking functional resemblance with NER proteins of the yeast RAD3 epistasis group. The extent of similarity suggests a golden rule: for each yeast NER protein there is a counterpart in humans and vice versa. The conclusion must be that the entire NER mechanism is strongly conserved in all eukaryotes. The primary amino acid sequence also disclosed homology with functional protein domains, such as well-characterized DNA-binding and helix-unwinding sequence motifs. This type of information provided valuable clues to the biochemical activity of the encoded polypeptides. Finally, overproduction, purification, and enzymological characterization have led to the elucidation of functional properties of several of the NER proteins and the identification of intricate complexes. Table 9-6 lists all mammalian NER genes cloned to date and summarizes their main properties.

In the following paragraphs the function of the genes involved in the NER syndromes will be discussed within the context of a model for the NER pathway that is based on currently available evidence, taking into account our still considerable ignorance. A schematic representation of the model for the multistep NER mechanism is depicted in Fig. 13-11.

Four subsequent phases are distinguished:

Damage recognition: how do cells identify lesions in the DNA? Which proteins are involved and what is their specificity?

Demarcation of the lesion: chromatin and DNA have to be made accessible to enzymes that will remove the damage.

Dual incision: nicks have to be made at both sides of the lesion in the damaged strand only.

Postincision events: the damage-containing oligomer should be removed and the gap filled in by repair DNA synthesis, followed by ligation.

Damage Recognition (XPA, XPE?) (Fig. 13-11, Table 13-6)

The first step in NER is expected to be the binding of a damage-recognition factor to the lesion, which enables the association of further repair components. Both XPA and XPE (or DDB) are candidate recognition factors, since both proteins have a high affinity for UV-damaged DNA and are involved in NER.

The XPA gene specifies a 273 amino acid protein with the sequence hallmarks of a DNA-binding Zn^{2+}-finger domain.[112] The gene product has been purified and biochemical evidence confirmed that it is a zinc metalloprotein with affinity for double-stranded (ds) and single-stranded (ss) DNA.[113–115] A marked preference has been found for a number of lesions, including [6-4] photoproducts and Cs-Pt adducts, but poor binding to cyclobutane pyrimidine dimers.[113,116] This parallels strikingly the preference of the NER pathway itself and is reminiscent of the lesion-binding spectrum of the E. coli $UvrA_2B$ complex. However, it may also reflect the limitations of in vitro studies, since in these assays the configuration of DNA is different from DNA packed into nuclear chromatin. Using the in vitro cell-free NER assay the XPA product has been functionally assigned to a step in the pre-incision stage of the reaction.[108] These data are consistent with the idea that XPA is implicated in damage recognition. Studies of mutations in XPA demonstrated that an intact Zn-finger is indispensable for proper function of the protein.[115,117,118] The S. cerevisiae homolog of XPA is RAD14.[119] RAD14 also binds preferentially to [6-4] photoproducts and chelates zinc.[120]

The other potential damage-recognition factor, DDB, was first identified in human cell lysates, by specific retention with UV-damaged oligonucleotides.[121] This DDB activity is possibly implicated in XP-E, since it is absent in extracts derived from some, but not all, XP-E patients.[122,123] Microinjection of purified DDB transiently corrects the partial NER defect in XP-E cells which lack the DDB activity.[107] The DDB activity copurified with a heterodimeric complex consisting of 124- and 41-kDa proteins.[106,124] Mutations have been described to occur in the small subunit in DDB-deficient XP-E patients.[191] Recently, structural homologs of the large subunit were found in a database search including a DDB-like polypeptide in human (van der Spek and Hoeijmakers, unpublished) and C. elegans.[125] These gene products probably represent a novel class of DNA-binding proteins. It is tempting to speculate that the relatively mild DNA repair defect in XP-E cells is due to the fact that this second human XPE-like gene might be functionally redundant to the original human XPE gene. The XP-E correcting factor has a strong preference for binding to DNA containing [6-4] photoproducts but exhibits modest discrimination of cyclobutane pyrimidine dimers and no measurable affinity for psoralen-thymine monoadducts.[126] These lesion-binding characteristics are not consistent with it being the universal damage recognition factor, but an auxiliary role is not ruled out. The striking abundance of the protein in normal cells (in the order of 10^5 copies per cell[106]), suggests that it has an additional function. A general characteristic of NER factors is that they seem to be present only in trace amounts. One possibility is that the XP-E correcting protein assists XPA in detection of some lesions, but direct interaction between these polypeptides has not been demonstrated.

Alternatively, evidence has been presented that XPA can transiently associate with the ERCC1/XPF incision complex by interaction with ERCC1,[127,128] while also binding domains for RPA [129,130] and TFIIH[131] have been reported (see below). Thus, XPA may constitute the docking protein nucleating the assembly of the NER machinery and determining its orientation toward the lesion (see below).

Detection of the primary lesion in the transcription-coupled NER subpathway is probably performed by RNA polymerase II. The transcription machinery probably subjects the DNA to a more rigorous test for intactness than achieved via the standard NER damage-recognition complex. This may explain why lesions that

Table 13-6 Main Properties of Cloned Human NER Genes

Gene*	Chromosome Location	Size Protein (aa)†	Yeast Homolog	Protein Properties‡
XPA	9q34	273	*RAD14*	Zn^{2+} finger, binds different types of damaged DNA, transient interaction with ERCC1, RPA, and TFIIH complex (?)
XPB(ERCC3)	2q21	782	*RAD25*	3′→5′ DNA helicase, subunit of TFIIH, essential for transcription initiation
XPC	3p25.1§	940	*RAD4*	Complexed with HHR23B, strong ssDNA binding, involved in global genome repair only
XPD(ERCC2)	19q13.2§	760	*RAD3*	5′→3′ DNA helicase, subunit of TFIIH, essential for transcription initiation
XPE	11	1140	Identified¶	Binds UV-damaged DNA, mutations identified in 48 kD subunit
XPF(ERCC4)	16p13.3	~905	*RAD1*	Also identical to ERCC11, complex with ERCC1 makes 5′ incision, Y structure-specific endonuclease, dual function in recombination
XPG(ERCC5)	13q32 → 33	1186	*RAD2*	Y structure-specific endonuclease, makes 3′ incision
CSA(ERCC8)	5	396	*RAD28*	5 WD repeats, involved in transcription-coupled repair only
CSB(ERCC6)	10q11→ 21	1493	*RAD26*	DNA-dependent ATP-ase (helicase?), involved in transcription-coupled repair only
ERCC1	19q13.2§	297	*RAD10*	Partial homology to UvrC and many nucleases, complex with XPF makes 5′ incision, Y-structure-specific endonuclease, dual function in recombination
HHR23A	19p13.2	363	*RAD23*	Ubiquitin-like N terminus, 2 ubiquitin-associated domains
HHR23B	3p25.1§	409	*RAD23*	As HHR23A, fraction of HHR23B complexed with XPC, complex binds ssDNA and is involved in global genome repair only
p62^TFIIH	11p14 → 15.1	548	*TFB1*	Subunit of TFIIH, essential for transcription initiation
p52^TFIIH	6p21.3	513	*TFB2*	Subunit of TFIIH, essential for transcription initiation
p44^TFIIH	5q1.3	395	*SSL1*	DNA-binding Zn^{2+} finger, subunit of TFIIH, essential for transcription initiation
p34^TFIIH	12	303	*TFB4*	Zn^{2+} finger, subunit of TFIIH, essential for transcription initiation

*Not included in this table are the genes for proteins involved in the DNA-synthesis step of the NER reaction, such as PCNA, RPA, RF-C, and DNA ligase.

†aa = amino acids.

‡Question marks indicate properties inferred but not proven.

§The *XPC* and *HHR23B* genes are located on a common 650-kb MluI fragment; *ERCC1* and *XPD(ERCC2)* are less than 250 kb apart.

¶A yeast gene encoding a product with clear overall homology to the XPE protein has been identified in the yeast genome database. In addition, a second human gene with significant similarity to XPE has been discovered (*van der Spek, Hoeijmakers, unpublished results*).

are poorly removed from the genome overall are efficiently eliminated by the transcription-coupled repair mode.

Demarcation of the Lesion (XPB, XPD) (Fig. 13-11, Table 13-6)

By analogy with the *E. coli* system, it is plausible that after damage detection the DNA and chromatin have to be made accessible for recognition by the incision protein complex(es). This may involve the induction of a strongly kinked, locally unwound—but uniform for all lesions—DNA structure as observed with the UvrA₂B complex, which overrides the aberrant lesion-specific conformation. By analogy with the recently described mechanism of action of *E. coli* photoreactivating enzyme, this may involve flipping out of the photoproduct from the DNA axis.[132] At present no proteins have been demonstrated to be associated with this presumed NER reaction intermediate. The RPA complex, composed of three subunits of 70, 34, and 11kDa, previously found to participate in initiation and elongation of DNA replication, may act at this stage. From studies involving the cell-free in vitro NER assay it appears that this trio of single-stranded DNA-binding proteins plays a role prior to or at the incision step.[108,133] As indicated in Fig. 13-11, this complex fits nicely in a model involving a melted intermediate. An additional participant in this stage of the reaction could be the TFIIH transcription/repair complex, which possesses bidirectional helicase activity (discussed in the next section).

The Role of the TFIIH Transcription-Repair Complex (Fig. 13-11, Table 13-6.) Many parallels exist between XPD and XPB

(and their yeast counterparts RAD3 and RAD25, also known as SSL2).[87] Based on identification of helicase motifs in the primary amino acid sequence Weeda et al. proposed that both proteins form a complex with bidirectional helix-unwinding activity.[87] As apparent below, this early idea has been corroborated in recent studies. The notion that null alleles of one or both genes in yeast,[134,135] *Drosophila*,[136] and mouse[192] are inviable indicates that these repair proteins must be involved in an additional process essential for viability. The nature of the latter was elucidated by a surprising discovery made by Egly and coworkers,[137] who were studying transcription initiation, an intricate process, involving the concerted action of numerous products (for a review see ref. 138). A multisubunit component required in a late stage of RNA polymerase II basal transcription initiation is TFIIH, previously also designated BTF2. It is a complex of at least nine polypeptides[139,140] (Table 13-7). The two largest subunits of this basal transcription factor were found to be the repair proteins XPB[137] and XPD.[141,142] Moreover, purified TFIIH corrects the XP-B, XP-D, and TTD-A repair defects in vivo as well as in vitro[56,143] indicating the presence of at least three repair proteins in this transcription factor and a striking relationship with NER complementation groups involving TTD.

With the cell-free NER assay it was also shown that TFIIH stimulates NER activity.[143] Since in this assay neither transcription nor translation can occur, this stimulation suggests a direct involvement of TFIIH in the NER reaction. Correcting activities of XP-B, XP-D, and TTD-A exactly co-elute with transcription and helicase activities of TFIIH.[56,143] NER-competent cell lysates and purified TFIIH fractions can be deprived of repair activity after immunoprecipitation with antibodies directed against some components of

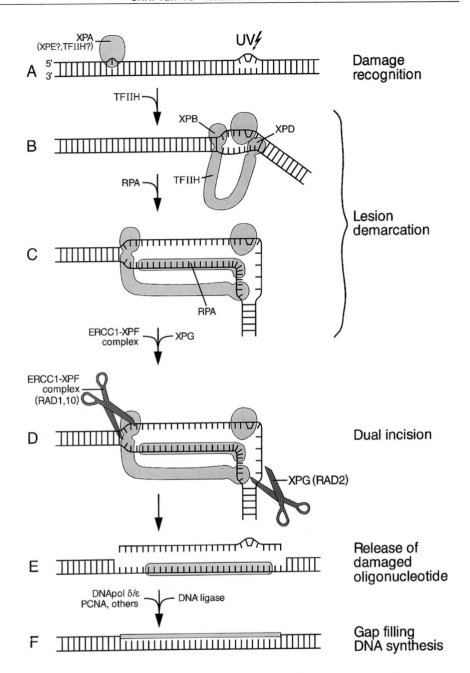

FIG. 13-11 Model for the human NER mechanism. Only the steps in the core of NER are represented, including the XP proteins active in the core. Proteins located specifically in the TCR (CSA and CSB) or GGR (XPC) subpathways are not depicted in this scheme.

TFIIH (anti-XPB, -p62, -p44, -p43; see Table 13-7).[56,144] Furthermore, mutations in the yeast SSL1 and TFB1, yeast homologs of the human TFIIH subunits p44 and p62, give rise to a UV-sensitive phenotype consistent with a function in repair.[145]

These data suggest that the entire transcription initiation factor TFIIH is involved in NER. The dual functionality of the entire TFIIH complex is also evident from recent studies with yeast TFIIH.[146-149]

Purified TFIIH displays the following activities and properties: a DNA-dependent ATPase, a protein kinase phosphorylating the carboxyterminus of the large subunit of RNA polymerase II, and a bidirectional DNA unwinding activity (see ref. 141 and references therein). The latter is due to the XPB ($3' \to 5'$) and the XPD ($5' \to 3'$) helicases. In addition, the TFIIH complex is endowed with two proteins (p44 and p34) containing one or more Zn^{2+}-finger domains that likely mediate DNA and/or protein-protein interactions[144] (Table 13-7). Studies using in vitro transcription initiation assays have not fully established the role of TFIIH in transcription

initiation. However, several plausible models can be advanced. The bidirectional helicase activity may be required for inducing a specific DNA conformation by locally opening the template[138] for load-

Table 13-7 Main Properties of Human and Yeast TFIIH Components

Human Gene	Yeast Gene	Features/Function
XPB(ERCC3)	RAD25/SSL2	$3' \to 5'$ helicase
XPD(ERCC2)	RAD3	$5' \to 3'$ helicase
p62	TFB1	Unknown
p52	TFB2	Unknown
p44	SSL1	2 Zn^{2+}-fingers
Mo 15/CDK7	Kin28	CDK-like kinase
p34	Scp34	SSL1-like Zn^{2+}-finger
CyclinH	cc11	Homology to cyclins
MAT1	TFB3	ring Zn^{2+}-finger

ing RNA polymerase onto the transcribed strand. Alternatively, or in addition, the complex may promote promoter clearance.[150]

What can be the role of the TFIIH complex in NER? Since TFIIH repair mutants show defects in both transcription-coupled as well as global genome repair (Table 13-4), the complex probably functions in the core of the NER reaction. Furthermore, it is reasonable to suppose that TFIIH catalyses a similar step in the context of NER and transcription initiation. Thus, one of the options is that it induces a melted DNA conformation required for loading a NER incision complex onto the template and/or for altering the DNA conformation around the lesion in a manner similar to UvrA$_2$B. Alternatively, or in addition, this complex may be involved in clearance of the damaged region, possibly including release of the damage-containing oligonucleotide and turnover of repair proteins (Fig. 13-11).

Dual Incision (ERCC1/XPF Complex, XPG) (Fig. 13-11, Table 13-5)

Huang and coworkers elegantly demonstrated that the mammalian NER machinery makes a dual incision in the damaged strand, involving the fifth phosphodiester bond 3′ and the 21-23 bond 5′ of the lesion.[151] Two strong candidates for this step have appeared on the scene recently. The first nominee is a protein complex consisting of the ERCC1 and XPF, ERCC4, and ERCC11 correcting activities[152,153] (see also Table 13-6). The yeast counterpart of this complex, comprising the Rad1 and Rad10 proteins, has been demonstrated to possess a ssDNA endonuclease activity, that specifically cleaves the 3′-protruding single strand at the transition from a double-strand to single-strand region,[154–156] leading to the suggestion that this heterodimer makes the 5′ incision. The yeast complex is also implicated in intrachromosomal mitotic recombination.[156–158] Both processes encompass DNA incision as an obligatory step in their reaction mechanism.

In collaboration with Wood c.s. (South Mimms, London), we have very recently shown that *ERCC4* and *XPF* (and probably *ERCC11*) are identical. Causative mutations and strongly reduced but still detectable ERCC4/ERCC11/XPF protein levels were identified in XP-F patients.[100] An ERCC1-XPF complex was purified from mammalian cells which exhibits a structure-specific endonuclease activity with similar properties as the homologous yeast RAD1-RAD10 dimer.[100] This suggests that *XPF* and *ERCC1* are involved in incision at the 5′ site of the lesion (Fig. 13-11).

Recently, it was shown that the XPG protein is one of the mammalian endonucleases involved in NER.[159] The *XPG* gene is identical to the previously cloned human *ERCC5* gene (see above) and homologous to the yeast RAD2 (Table 13-6). XPG cleaves near junctions of unpaired and duplex DNA, cutting the single strand with the 5′ end (i.e., with polarity opposite to ERCC1/XPF). Structures required for both incision enzymes can be easily envisaged as a reaction intermediate in the course of NER after lesion demarcation and local helix unwinding (Fig. 13-11). The biochemical helicase activity of the TFIIH complex might well be involved in this step.

Although the candidate endonucleases in NER genes seem to be identified, the order of cleavage action (if any) is not definitely established. It is even likely that a complete assembly of both incision factors is required for the dual incision, which may act simultaneously. Other factors are also required for an efficient excision of damaged DNA. One of them is the human single-stranded binding protein complex RPA (see above). Another possible function for RPA is that it serves as a binding factor between the different NER factors. Interactions of RPA components with XPA and XPG have been observed.[129,130]

Postincision Events (Fig. 13-11)

The final stages of the NER reaction should entail release of the damage-containing oligomer, turnover of the bound NER proteins, gap-filling DNA synthesis (used most frequently for assaying NER (UDS)), and sealing of the remaining nick by ligation. At present it is unknown which proteins carry out the first of these steps. Again, the TFIIH complex is a potential candidate since it harbors two helicases that could peel off the damage-containing 27-29-mer. Alternatively, it is possible that the DNA replication machinery carries out this reaction.

The use of the cell-free NER assay has permitted the identification of the proliferating cell nuclear antigen (PCNA) as being required for the gap-filling DNA synthesis step.[108,160] PCNA is known to stimulate DNA polymerase delta and/or epsilon in regular DNA replication. The implication of PCNA in this part of the NER reaction mechanism suggests that the repair synthesis itself is mediated by any or both of these polymerases. The final sealing of the new DNA to the preexisting strand is thought to be carried out by DNA ligase I.

It is interesting to note that mutations in the ligase I gene can give rise to a UV-sensitive phenotype.[161] So far, only one patient with a ligase I defect has been discovered, but it may well turn out that this individual (designated 46BR) belongs in a new category of NER-deficient patients.

So far, we have dealt with steps in the core of the NER reaction. As mentioned earlier two subpathways have been distinguished in NER: global genome repair (GGR) and transcription-coupled repair (TCR). Gene functions specific for these subpathways are discussed in the following paragraphs. Finally as discussed below, instead of a stepwise assembly of individual factors described above evidence has been presented in the analogous yeast system for the existence of a preassembled "repairosome."[149] Furthermore, the above tentative model does not incorporate yet the chromatin dynamics that must play a part in vivo.

Steps Specific for the GGR Pathway (XPC) (Table 13-6)

Analysis of mutants has lead to the identification of at least three genes selectively implicated in the repair of the nontranscribed bulk of the genome: *RAD7* and *RAD16* in yeast[162] and *XPC* in humans.[163]

The XPC amino acid sequence displays significant homology to the yeast RAD4 protein.[95,101] However, *rad4* null mutants, in contrast to XP-C mutants, are defective in both NER subpathways.[162] This may reflect a principal difference between mammals and yeast. The recently purified XPC protein (125 kDa) appeared to be complexed with HHR23B (43 kDa), one of the two human homologs of yeast RAD23. Intriguingly, the *XPC* and *HHR23B* genes are also located very close to each other in the genome (at chromosome 3p25, probably within 650 kb).[164] The XPC-HHR23B heterodimer has a very high affinity for ssDNA, but no associated enzymatic activities have been detected.[101] A notable feature of the HHR23 proteins is the presence of a ubiquitin-like domain in the N-terminus.[101] In some other ubiquitin-fusion proteins this moiety is thought to function as a chaperone, facilitating complex formation. Hence this domain may perform a similar role in assembling the XPC-HHR23B complex. To date, no known human NER syndromes have been associated with the *HHR23B* gene, and a simple explanation might be that the highly homologous HHR23A protein diminished the effect of loss of HHR23B function.

In keeping with the golden rule derived from the striking correspondence between yeast and mammalian NER, it would be expected that human homologues of RAD7 and RAD16 exist and that they participate in the global repair process. The RAD7 sequence does not reveal any clue to its function.[165] The *RAD16* gene, however, encodes a protein containing a special type of DNA-binding ZN^{2+} finger and an extended region with strong homology to a specific subfamily of presumed DNA helicases.[166] Interestingly, CSB, also a protein specific for transcription-coupled repair, is also equipped with such domains.[89] A characteristic of other members of this helicase subfamily is that they reside in multiprotein complexes. Genetic evidence in yeast suggests that the complex interacts with chromatin. (See ref. 167 and references therein.)

In this light, what is the role of these genes? One possibility, suggested elsewhere, is that they are involved in uncoupling essential NER components from the transcription machinery to make them available for global genome repair.[101] The TFIIH transcription repair complex is the most logical partner in this option. The strong ssDNA binding of the XPC complex could release TFIIH from the transcription-initiation machinery and makes it available for NER. On the other hand, the RAD16 protein(-complex?) may be implicated in altering chromatin structure required for global genome repair. Obviously, these speculations need to be experimentally investigated.

Steps Specific for Transcription-Coupled Repair (CSA,CSB) (Table 13-6)

Two genes involved in TCR that are defective in Cockayne syndrome are *CSA* and *CSB*. The protein sequence of CSA contains the consensus of five WD-repeats.[96] This type of motif is present in many proteins, believed to possess a regulatory, rather than a catalytic function.[168] Many of these WD-repeat proteins reside in multiprotein complexes. CSA is thought to associate with p44 (a component of TFIIH, see Table 13-7) and with CSB.[96]

CSB is a member of the closely related subfamily of putative DNA/RNA helicases, described above, to which RAD16 also belongs. A yeast homolog of this protein was unknown, but the sequence conservation seen for all other eukaryotic NER factors permitted bridging the large evolutionary gap between human and yeast. Like CSB, a yeast disruption mutant, designated *rad26*, displayed a selective defect in transcription-coupled repair.[104] Interestingly, inactivation of this NER subpathway in yeast does not induce a significant UV sensitivity, suggesting that this process is not very important for UV survival in yeast. It is feasible that CSB and the other repair members of this helicase subfamily possess a local DNA melting activity and in doing so accomplish displacement of bound proteins (e.g., nucleosomes or a stalled RNA polymerase complex) from the DNA to give repair proteins access to the lesion. The possibility exists that the CSB protein functions as a general mediator linking transcription to the total of repair pathways.

Higher Order NER Complexes

Although most of the important players in mammalian NER are identified, it is not known yet how these factors assemble on a lesion and how they interact with each other. Recently, several reports appeared in the literature dealing with proposed interactions between NER factors. However, many of these studies are either based on associations in a rather artificial environment (immobilized fusion proteins) or associations after overexpression in yeast (two-hybrid system). In both systems, transient or low-affinity interactions can be selected, which might not reflect the in vivo situation.

A central role for the XPA protein is likely in view of the very severe NER-deficient phenotype of XP-A cells. Biochemical studies with XPA suggest that this factor serves as an nucleation point in the repair reaction. Interaction of XPA (in addition to that with damaged DNA) has been described with ERCC1,[127,128,169] RPA (RPA2),[129,130] and TFIIH.[131] Binding of both ERCC1 and RPA to XPA has a synergistic effect on the DNA damage-specific binding affinity of XPA.[130,169] RPA2 is claimed to interact with XPG,[130] whereas XPG (Rad2) and XPC (Rad4) might be associated with TFIIH.[142,170] Several of these assumed interactions are dependent on isolation conditions[111] and variable or different results have been obtained by other laboratories.[56,110] Using specific isolation conditions, a NER supercomplex, designated repairosome, was purified from yeast cells.[148] The majority of the different yeast NER factors are reported to reside in this repairosome. However, this isolated complex still lacks some essential factors as it is not active in a reconstituted NER reaction. Also the amount of each of the NER factors residing in this complex is not known.

MOUSE MODELS FOR GENETIC DEFECTS IN NUCLEOTIDE EXCISION REPAIR

Introduction

Gene targeting by homologous recombination in totipotent embryonal stem (ES) cells permits the generation of mouse mutants in any cloned NER gene. This sophisticated methodology enables the development of experimental animal models for all types of NER deficiencies and associated syndromes. Genes can be fully inactivated (knockout mutants), but it is also possible to reconstruct specific partially inactivating mutations encountered in patients in the mouse genome. The use of this new genetic tool will have a major impact on clinical and fundamental research of the human NER syndromes and cancer in general. First, it will help in understanding the complex ramifications and biological relevance of NER pathways particularly with respect to understanding the mechanisms of carcinogenesis, neurodegeneration, photoimmunology and aging. Secondly, animal models for human NER syndromes will be instrumental for clinical research on these conditions, including diagnosis, prevention, and therapy. Furthermore, it may lead to the discovery of new disorders for NER genes for which no corresponding condition has been identified yet. In addition, it will help in disentangling the intricate genotype-phenotype relationships of CS and TTD. Crossing animals with different genetic lesions will permit the study of synergistic effects with other mechanisms implicated in genetic (in)stability, such as cell cycle control, complementary repair pathways, and apoptosis. Finally, since the NER system targets a very wide spectrum of DNA lesions, mice deficient in this pathway will be a valuable and sensitive model for assessing the genotoxic effect of known and unknown compounds. This paragraph presents the current status in this field, keeping in mind that new developments are occurring very rapidly.

The ERCC1 Mouse

The first NER-deficient mouse mutant was generated in the *ERCC1* gene, one of the NER genes for which no parallel human syndrome is yet known.[171] Thus, it was not *a priori* evident whether full inactivation of this function would be compatible with life, particularly since both the yeast and rodent mutants provide evidence for a dual involvement of this gene in an additional mitotic recombination repair pathway with unpredictable biological impact, as noted previously. A functional knockout mutation appeared barely viable; indeed, most ERCC1$^{-/-}$ embryos die in utero and the few mutants born are severely runted and usually die before weaning, that is within 4 weeks[193] Recent evidence indicates that the genetic makeup influences the life span and embryonal death to a considerable extent: maximal life span is extended to several months in a C57B1/6 strain and mutant embryonal death is postponed to the moment of birth in an FVB background.[193] This indicates that these two types of early death may have different causes. One of the causes of postnatal death is liver malfunctioning, probably due to increased nuclear aneuploidy. Elevated levels of aneuploid nuclei are also apparent in kidney, and there is ferritin deposition in spleen. Increased levels of p53 are reported in liver, brain, and kidney.[172] Subcutaneous fat is absent. As far as investigated, the neurologic status of the mice seems normal. Several of the above clinical features point to premature aging possibly as the result of accumulation of unremoved endogenous DNA lesions. At the cellular level replicative senescence is seen as well as increased spontaneous transformation.[193] As expected, mouse embryonal fibroblasts (MEFs) derived from the mutant mice display a total NER defect and are hypersensitive to UV and chemical genotoxins that are substrates of the NER pathway. In addition, there is cellular sensitivity to crosslinking agents presumably as the consequence of an additional defect in one of the recombination repair pathways. In order to create a milder phenotype, a mouse mutant was designed in which only the very C-terminal 7 amino acids were deleted (ERCC1^{*292}, Fig 13-12). However, apart from a extended life span to more than 6 months, most of the other features were very similar to those of the full knockout mice, indicating that the very last part of the protein is still important for its biological functions. The signs of premature senescence observed in the ERCC1$^{-/-}$ suggest that accumulation of unrepaired DNA damage contributes to early aging. The ERCC1^{*292} mice were utilized in a carcinogenesis experiment. Cutaneous application of dimethylbenz[*a*]anthracene (DMBA) at a dose easily tolerated by XPA knockout mice caused death within 3 days, revealing an extreme sensitivity to genotoxins.[193] Apart from the UV sensitivity, the clinical picture is very different from any of the human NER syndromes. The lack of similarity between the mouse and the human NER mutants may, in part, reflect species differences, but the picture may also be compounded by the dual functionality of the ERCC1 protein. In this connection, a comparison of the severe clinical phenotype of ERCC1 mutant mice with that of XPA knockout mice, described below (also harboring a complete NER defect) may be very instructive.

The XPA Mouse

A closer but still partial correspondence to the parallel human disease was noted with a mouse model for XP-A generated independently in two laboratories. Consistent with the human pathology, XPA knockout mice display cutaneous and ocular photosensitivity and a greatly increased susceptibility to UV- and DMBA-induced skin cancer.[173,174] However, in contrast to XP-A patients knockout mutant mice appear physiologically normal, are fertile, and at the age of 18 months fail to develop the neuropathology, characteristic of the human condition. One factor

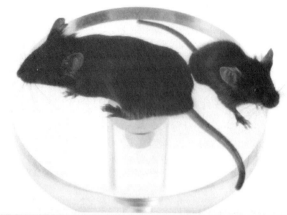

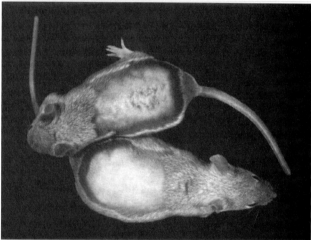

FIG. 13-12 Mouse models of NER syndromes. NER-deficient mice were obtained by targeting mouse embryonic stem cells by a DNA construct containing a mutated NER gene, followed by blastocyst injection and breeding germ line chimeras. *Top: ERCC1* mutant mouse showing growth defects (compare the small mutant mouse with its normal litter mate). This mouse is extremely sensitive to ultraviolet light and UV-mimicking agents. *Bottom:* Homozygous CSB mutant mouse representing a mouse model for Cockayne syndrome. The UV-induced erythema on the skin reflects the severe UV sensitivity of this CSB$^{-/-}$ mouse. *(From the Department of Cell Biology and Genetics, Erasmus University, Rotterdam; G. Weeda, ERCC1 mouse and B. van der Horst, CSB mouse.)*

that should be taken into account in this regard is the difference in life span. The accelerated neurodegeneration observed in XP-A human patients is manifested over the course of several years, whereas such a time period cannot be reached in the mouse model. As in the case with ERCC1 in one genetic background, approximately half of the $-/-$ embryos died in the midfetal stage (with signs of anemia),[174] whereas in another background this phenomenon was absent.[173] XPA$^{-/-}$ MEF exhibited all parameters of a total NER deficiency. This indicates that the NER phenotype is as predicted and also as observed in ERCC1$^{-/-}$ mice. The fact that, with respect to the NER defect, XPA and ERCC1 knockout mice are indistinguishable permits a valid comparison between these two phenotypes. Considering the additional function of ERCC1 in a mitotic recombination repair pathway, it is logical to conclude that the extra symptoms registered in the ERCC1$^{-/-}$ mice, such as liver and kidney aneuploidy, growth retardation, and premature aging, are a consequence of a compromise of this second function.

The XPC Mouse

A phenotype very similar to XPA mice is observed in mice carrying an inactivating mutation in the XPC gene. As in the case of XP-C patients, a normal development and clear UV hypersensitivity, and increased frequency of skin cancer were found.[175]

The CSB Mouse

Recently, we have mimicked a mutation of a known CS-B patient in the mouse genome.[194] Analysis of repair parameters in embryonic fibroblasts from the CSB mutant versus wild-type and heterozygous mice showed a specific loss of transcription-coupled repair. In agreement with the human syndrome CSB-deficient mice are photosensitive (Fig. 13-12). The other CS-like clinical features observed were mild, such as slightly retarded growth and neurologic (behavioral and motor coordination) abnormalities. Remarkably, when a GGR defect was introduced in CSB-deficient mice a strong augmentation of the CS phenotype was observed. Such XPC/CSB double mutant mice exhibit a very severe growth retardation (75 percent) are unable to walk, and die around day 18. These observations suggest that a CS defect becomes exaggerated in the absence of GGR, pointing to accumulation of endogenous damage as a contributing factor to the CS symptoms.[195]

In striking contrast to human CS, CSB-deficient mice appear clearly prone to skin cancer, when exposed to UV light or to the chemical carcinogen DMBA. Thus, in the mouse, intact GGR is not sufficient to protect from tumorigenesis. This finding could imply that CS patients may have a hitherto unnoticed cancer predisposition. Alternatively, the species difference in tumorigenesis could be due to the fact that, in man compared to rodents, the GGR pathway is more potent in eliminating cyclobutane pyrimidine dimers, the major UV-induced lesion.[194]

Mouse Mutants in the TFIIH Subunits XPB and XPD.

Like some of the other NER genes, the TFIIH complex has a dual functionality complicating the clinical outcome of a mutation in the genes involved. In the case of TFIIH, the second function entails initiation of basal transcription of all structural genes transcribed by RNA polymerase II. This is one of the most fundamental processes in the cell. Complete inactivation of such a function is most probably lethal, explaining the rarity of mutants in TFIIH genes. Recently, we have made knockout mutations in the mouse for both XPB and XPD. Although heterozygous mice were readily obtained, $-/-$ mutants were selectively absent from the offspring. Preliminary evidence suggests that death occurs at the two-cell stage when embryonal transcription has to start up.[192] This demonstrates that inactivation of these genes is lethal and that this is due to their role in transcription. Obviously, more subtle mutations have to be made mimicking the phenotype-determining allele in the corresponding human patients. This requires a more delicate and laborious strategy of gene targeting, but recently viable TTD mouse mutants were

born and their analysis will reveal the extent to which they reflect the human syndrome.

IMPLICATIONS FOR DIAGNOSIS AND TREATMENT

Clinical Heterogeneity and Pleiotropy Associated with Mutations in TFIIH

It is clear that the spectrum of diseases linked with mutations in the TFIIH subunits XPB, XPD, and TTDA is remarkably heterogeneous and pleiotropic. It includes seemingly unrelated symptoms as photosensitivity, predisposition to skin cancer, brittle hair and nails, neurodysmyelination, impaired sexual development, ichthyosis, and dental caries. The rare XP group B consists of only 4 patients: 3 had the XP/CS complex and one has TTD. The more common group D is associated with classical XP, combinations of XP and CS, and TTD[56,58,176] (Table 13-4). The clinical variability in TTD is also apparent from the fact that at least seven disorders are thought to be identical or closely related to TTD. These include the following syndromes: Pollitt (MIM 275550), Tay (242170), Sabinas (211390), Netherton (256500), ONMR (258360), Hair-Brain (234050) and the Marinesco-Sjögren (248800) syndromes.[20,21] The occurrence of TTD in three distinct NER-deficient complementation groups argues against a chance association between genetic loci separately involved in NER and in brittle hair. Consistent with the idea that these processes are intimately connected is the recent identification of point mutations in the *XPD* and *XPB* genes in TTD patients (Fig. 13-13).[177,196] The positions of the relatively large number of mapped *XPD* mutations and the three *XPB* mutations indicate that mutations resulting in XP, combined XP and CS (XP/CS), or TTD do not overlap (Fig. 13-13). Therefore, these mutations may interfere with the functions of these genes in a specific manner, resulting in the three different phenotypes.

The Clinical Features Derived from the NER Defect

In striking contrast to the pleiotropy and clinical heterogeneity selectively associated with XP-B and XP-D, the symptoms seen in the most common XP groups, A (totally deficient in NER) and C (defective in the global genome repair subpathway) are much more uniform. They involve photosensitivity, pigmentation abnormalities, predisposition to skin cancer, and, in the case of XP-A, accelerated neurodegeneration (which is not associated with neurodysmyelination), but no CS and TTD symptoms. The gene products affected in these groups are not vital and therefore do not appear to be essential for basal transcription. This indicates that these forms of XP present the manifestations of a pure NER defect. The fact that XP-C is associated with a strong cancer predisposition suggests that the global genome subpathway is of major importance for preventing mutagenesis and carcinogenesis. This may provide a plausible explanation why, in CS, no significant cancer proneness is observed; CS patients still possess a potent GGR system. The transcription-coupled repair subpathway may be important for cell survival but less relevant for preventing mutagenesis, since it accomplishes—and only for some lesions—more rapid repair in only one of the strands of an active gene.

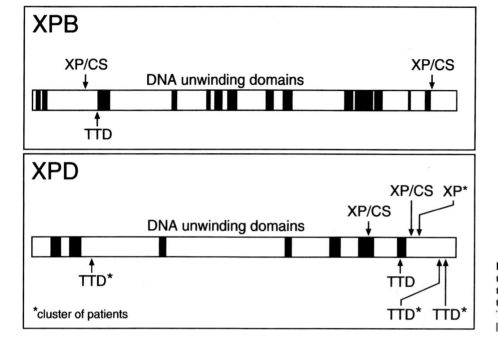

FIG. 13-13 Position of mutations in the *XPB* and *XPD* genes in patients with XP, XP/CS and TTD. Clusters of different mutations causing TTD or XP were found at specific sites [ref. 177, unpublished results].

Evidence for the Involvement of Transcriptional Defects in CS and TTD

Mutations in subunits of the multi-functional and intricate TFIIH are envisaged to have multiple effects. The selective association of TFIIH with the peculiar forms of XP and the dual role of this complex in repair and transcription make it tempting to link the unexpected TTD and CS features with the additional transcription-related function of the NER genes involved. Indeed, it would be highly unlikely that all mutations in subunits of this bifunctional complex would only affect the repair function and leave the inherent transcriptional role entirely intact. This interpretation is supported by the phenotype of a *Drosophila ERCC3* mutant, *haywire*. This mutant displays UV sensitivity, central nervous system abnormalities, and impaired sexual development, as found in XP-B.[136] Spermatogenesis in *Drosophila* is very sensitive to the level of β2-tubulin.[178] Mutations in the *Drosophila ERCC3* gene seem to affect β-tubulin expression, causing the male sterility.[136] It is therefore likely that expression of this gene in *Drosophila* (and by inference possibly in humans) is particularly sensitive to the level of transcription and thereby to subtle mutations in TFIIH. This could easily explain the immature sexual development found in TTD and CS. Expression of the myelin basic protein is known to be critically dependent on transcription. It has been demonstrated that reduced transcription of this gene in mice causes neurological abnormalities.[179] Thus, the characteristic neurodysmyelination of CS and TTD[18,180] may also relate to suboptimal transcription of this or other genes involved in myelin sheath formation. Similarly, reduced transcription of genes encoding the class of ultrahigh-sulphur proteins of the hairshaft may account for the observed reduced cysteine content in the brittle hair of TTD patients.[20] A comparable explanation is proposed for the poor enamelation of teeth in CS and TTD. Thus, mutations in TFIIH which subtly disturb its transcription function may affect a specific subset of genes whose functioning critically depends on the level or fine-tuning of transcription. It is logical to suppose that strong secondary structure in a promoter requires full unwinding capacity, i.e., a maximally active complex, to permit efficient transcription. Recent studies indicate that the requirement for basal transcription factors may vary from promoter to promoter depending on the sequence around the initiation site, the topological state

of the DNA, and the local chromatin structure.[181] These mechanisms can readily explain the pronounced clinical heterogeneity even within families. Obviously, total inactivation of the transcription is lethal; this is consistent with the observation that deletion mutants of TFIIH subunits in yeast, *Drosophila*, and mice are inviable.[56,192] The narrow window of viable mutations also explains the rarity of these TFIIH-associated diseases.

As noted previously,[182] there are many parallels between CS and TTD, suggesting that they are manifestations of a broad clinical continuum. This is consistent with the finding that mutations in different subunits of the same (TFIIH) complex give rise to a similar set of CS and TTD features. Thus, defects in *CSA* and *CSB* as well as *XPG* may also affect basal transcription, as they give rise to a comparable phenotype (see also below).

Transcription and Repair/Transcription Syndromes

A tentative model proposed for the etiology of the defects in the conglomerate of CS, TTD and related disorders is shown in Table 13-8.

In this model, mutations in TFIIH subunits inactivating only the NER function result in a XP phenotype as observed in the classical patients of XP group D. If, in addition, the transcription function is subtly affected, the combination of XP and CS features is found. Theoretically, mutations causing a (still viable) transcription problem without NER impairment may be expected as well. Indeed, recently CS (-like) patients without an associated NER defect were identified.[74] This model fits with the observation of specific sites of mutations in XPB and XPD resulting in a XP, XP/CS, or TTD phenotype (Fig. 13-13).

When CS features are due to mutations that cripple the transcription function of TFIIH, how can the differences between CS and TTD, i.e., the additional presence of brittle hair and nails in TTD be rationalized? In view of the intrinsic properties of complexes such as TFIIH it is likely that some mutations also will affect the stability of the complex. In fact, a significant proportion of TFIIH mutations in yeast yield a temperature-sensitive phenotype,[145] pointing to complex instability. It is feasible, that such type of mutations also occur among TFIIH patients. As mentioned above, an exceptional TTD individual exhibited a reversible sud-

Table 13-8 Model for the Relation between TFIIH Defects and Clinical Features

TFIIH-Related Disorder	NER	TFIIH Function*		Documented Gene Mutation
		Transcription	Stability	
XP	−	+	+	*XPD*
XP/CS	−	+/−	+	*XPD, XPB, XPG*[†]
CS (photosensitive)	+/−[‡]	+/−	+	*CSA, CSB*[†]
CS (nonphotosensitive)[§]	+	+/−	+	?
TTD (photosensitive)		+/−	+/−	*XPD, XPB, TTDA*
TTD (nonphotosensitive)[§]	+	+/−	+/−	?

*+ = normal repair or transcription function or stability of TFIIH; +/− = partially affected function/stability; − = severely impaired function.

[†]TFIIH transcription may be indirectly affected by mutations in XPG, CSA, and CSB. In addition, XPG afffects total NER; CSA and CSB affect only transcription-coupled repair.

[‡]Only the NER subpathway of transcription-coupled repair is disturbed.

[§]CS patients without a NER defect were identified (see ref. 74, as well as Jaspers, Kleijer, and Hoeijmakers, unpublished observations). There may be many disorders related to nonphotosensitive variants of TTD and CS such as Netherton syndrome, brain-hair syndrome, Pollitt syndrome, etc.

den, dramatic worsening of the brittleness of the hair formed during an episode of fever.[22] This fits with a human, temperature-sensitive TFIIH mutation. Furthermore, it suggests that transcription of the genes for cysteine-rich matrix proteins of hair and nails is affected by TFIIH instability. In other cells the steady state levels of TFIIH may be sufficient, because *de novo* synthesis is high enough to cope with the reduced $t_{1/2}$ of the complex. However, the cysteine-rich matrix proteins, are one of the last gene products produced in very large quantities in keratinocytes before they die. Thus, the hallmark of TTD may be due to a TFIIH stability problem becoming overt in terminally differentiated cells that are exhausted for TFIIH before completion of their differentiation program.

Many TTD patients are not noticeably photosensitive and have normal NER.[74] According to the scheme in Table 9-8, these patients may have a TFIIH transcription and stability problem without concomittant impairment of the NER function of the complex. These findings extend the implications to non-repair-defective disorders. Therefore, and in view of the models pronounced heterogeneity, it is possible that the Sjögren-Larsson (MIM 270200), RUD (308200), ICE (146720), OTD (257960), IFAP (308205), CAM(F)AK (212540), Rothmund-Thomson (268400), KID (242150) and COF syndromes[21,56] also fall within this category. Interestingly, some of these diseases show occurrence of skin cancer.

When the CS features in TTD are due to a basal transcription problem, this should also apply to the other complementation groups with CS patients, i.e., CS-A, CS-B, and XP-G. Although the CSA, CSB, and probably the XPG proteins are not vital and therefore not essential for transcription, they may influence TFIIH functioning indirectly (Table 13-8). For instance, CSA and CSB could have an auxiliary function for TFIIH in transcription and in transcription-coupled (but not global genome) repair. Some XP-G (XP/CS) patients are more severely affected, than XP-A patients,[24] although the latter are, in general, more defective in NER, suggesting that XPG has an additional, nonrepair function. Consistent with these considerations interactions between the CS proteins and TFIIH components have been claimed.[96,142]

In conclusion, these findings provide evidence for the presence of a wide class of disorders that can collectively be called transcription syndromes.[182] A prediction from this model is that these patients carry mutations in transcription factors that do not affect the NER process. This explanation introduces a novel concept into human genetics. It can be envisioned that similar phenomena are associated with subtle defects in translation, implying the potential existence of translation syndromes.

Patient Care

Treatment. Treatment of XP, CS, and TTD patients is purely symptomatic. The discovery of the molecular defects in these disorders has not (yet) resulted in specific modalities for treatment.

Treatment of XP patients is a multifaceted process involving early diagnosis, genetic counseling, patient and family education, and regular monitoring of the skin.[183] The diagnosis is suspected in cases with marked sun sensitivity, photophobia, and/or early onset of freckling. Laboratory tests of UV sensitivity of fibroblasts and of excision repair confirm the diagnosis. Genetic counseling is directed toward acquainting the patients and their parents with the inherited aspects of the disease and its rarity, the increased risk for parents (with the 25 percent probability that the disease will appear among subsequent offspring), and the improbability of the patients having affected children.[21,2,184]

Patients should be shielded from sunlight by protective measures, including wearing two layers of clothing, using long hairstyles, wearing broad-brimmed hats and UV-absorbing sunglasses with side shields, and use of chemical sunscreens with sun protection factor (SPF) numbers of 15 or higher. Patients should avoid direct exposure to sunlight, especially during the peak UV hours (about 10 AM to 3 PM in the continental United States), and indirect UV reflected from snow or water. Window glass and many plastic shields for fluorescent lamps will absorb UV radiation indoors. Known chemical carcinogens such as tobacco smoke should be avoided. Patients and their families should be taught to examine their skin and to recognize and bring to medical attention any lesions suspected to be malignant. Color photographs are often useful for follow-up.

Malignant skin neoplasms are treated as in patients who do not have XP by excision; electrodesiccation; and curettage, cryosurgery, or chemosurgery. XP patients have received x-ray therapy for malignant skin tumors and have had a normal response.[183] Dermabrasion or dermatome shaving has been used in patients with multiple tumors, permitting the epidermis to be repopulated by cells from the hair follicles, which are relatively shielded from sunlight.[183] Total removal of the skin of the face with grafting of skin from sun-shielded areas has been used in extreme cases. Oral retinoids have been shown to prevent new skin cancers in XP patients, but have many severe side effects.[185]

Nance and Berry[12] mention several measures that can be taken in management of CS patients including monitoring of treatable complications of this condition such as hypertension, hearing loss, and dental carries. As in XP, photosensitive CS patients should avoid excessive sun exposure and use sunscreens when outdoors. If the condition is compatible with life into the teens and twenties (in the case of CSI) the neurologic and neurosensory capacities should be periodically assessed. This assessment of intellectual, social, visual, and auditory skills can help in providing appropriate home and school services for the patient. Nance and Berry[12] also recommend physical therapy directed toward preventing contractures and maintaining ambulation in the older patient.

Although little is known about the treatment of TTD patients, the overlap of clinical symptoms in TTD and CS (neurologic and growth defects) indicates comparable management of patients suffering from these diseases.

Prenatal Diagnosis. As the NER-deficiency syndromes have autosomal recessive inheritance, parents of an affected child face a high risk of recurrence (25 percent) in subsequent pregnancies. Prenatal diagnosis is possible if the deficiency has been demonstrated unequivocally in cultured skin fibroblasts of the index patient.

Early reports of prenatal diagnosis of XP concern the analysis of unscheduled DNA synthesis (UDS) in cultured amniocytes.[186,187] This approach allows a relatively rapid diagnosis within 1 or 2 weeks after amniocentesis in the sixteenth week, as only a few cells are needed for the autoradiographic assessment of UDS. A much earlier diagnosis is however possible by chronic villus sampling (CVS) in the tenth to twelfth week of pregnancy. Autoradiographic analysis of the early outgrowths of cells from the villi then allows a first-trimester diagnosis. Successful prenatal diagnoses using chorionic villus cells have been reported for XP and TTD.[188,189,22] The TCR defect in CS can be demonstrated indirectly by measuring the recovery of RNA or DNA synthesis after UV-exposure of cultured cells. The reliability of this test for the (postnatal) diagnosis of CS using cultured skin fibroblasts has been shown extensively. Cases of prenatal diagnosis using amniocytes[48] and chorionic villus cells[188] have been reported. Because of the earlier stage of sampling, the use of chronic villus cells may be prefered but the present experience for CS is very small. Therefore, if initial results on the chorionic villus cells suggest a normal fetus, it may be considered to confirm the diagnosis by amniocentesis. Mutation analysis using DNA from uncultured chorion villi would, in principle, allow reliable and early diagnosis. This requires knowledge of the gene involved and of the mutations in the family. In general it may not be practical to search for these mutations in these rare diseases unless common mutations are known, as reported for Japanese XP-A patients.[190]

ACKNOWLEDGEMENTS

We are indebted to all members of the DNA repair group of the Medical Genetics Centre South-West Netherlands (MGC) for valuable and stimulating discussions and for providing new information for this text. We thank Dr. W.J. Kleijer, Dr. M.F. Niermeijer, and Dr. P.C. Hanawalt for a thoughtful review of the manuscript, and Rita Boucke (secretary), Mirko Kuit (photography), Wim Vermeulen, and Koos Jaspers for their help in preparing this chapter. The research of the MGC group is supported by the Dutch Cancer Society, the Netherlands Organization for Scientific Research (NWO) through the Foundation of Medical Sciences, and the Commission of the European Community.

REFERENCES

1. Friedberg EC, Walker GC, Siede W: *DNA repair and mutagenesis,* Washington, D.C., ASM Press, 1995.
2. Kraemer KH, Lee MM, Scotto J: Xeroderma pigmentosum: Cutaneous, ocular and neurologic abnormalities in 830 published cases. *Arch Dermatol* **123**:241, 1987.
3. von Hebra F, Kaposi M: *On diseases of the skin, including the exanthemata.* Tay W, trans. London, New Sydenham Society, 1874, vol 3, p 252.
4. Neisser A: Ueber das Xeroderma pigmentosum (Kaposi) lioderma essentialis cum melanosi et telangiectasia. *Viertel Dermatol Syphil* 47, 1883.
5. DeSanctis C, Cacchione A: Lidiozia xerodermica. *Riv Sper Freniatr* **56**:269, 1932.
6. See reference(s) cited in: Cleaver JE, Kraemer KH: Xeroderma pigmentosum and Cockayne syndrome, Scriver CR, Beaudet AL, Sly WS, Valle D (eds): *The metabolic and molecular bases of inherited disease. Seventh edition,* New York, The McGraw-Hill Companies, Inc., 1995, p 4393.
7. Takebe H, Nishigori C, Satoh Y: Genetics and skin cancer of xeroderma pigmentosum in Japan. *Jpn J Cancer Res (Gann)* **78**:1135, 1987.
8. Kraemer KH, Lee MM, Andrews AD, Lambert WC: The role of sunlight and DNA repair in melanoma and non-melanoma skin cancer: The xeroderma pigmentosum paradigm. *Arch Dermatol* **130**:1018, 1994.
9. Mimaki T, Itoh N, Abe J, Tagawa T, Sato K, Yabuuchi H, Takebe H: Neurological manifestations of xeroderma pigmentosum. *Ann Neurol* **20**:70, 1986.
10. Robbins JH, Brumback RA, Mendiones M, Barrett SF, Carl JR, Cho S, Denckla MB, Ganges MB, Gerber LH, Guthrie RA, Meer J, Moshell AN, Polinsky RJ, Ravin PD, Sonies BC, Tarone RE: Neurological disease in xeroderma pigmentosum. Documentation of a late onset type of the juvenile onset form. *Brain* **114**:1335, 1991.
11. Andrews AD, Barrett SF, Robbins JH: Xeroderma pigmentosum neurological abnormalities correlate with colony-forming ability after ultraviolet radiation. *Proc Natl Acad Sci USA* **75**:1984, 1978.
12. Nance MA, Berry SA: Cockayne syndrome: Review of 140 cases. *Am J of Med Genet* **42**:68, 1992.
13. Lehmann AR: Nucleotide excision repair and the link with transcription. *Trends Biochem Sci* **20**:402, 1995.
14. Price VH, Odom RB, War WH, Jones FT: Trichothiodystrophy: Sulfur-deficient brittle hair as a marker for a neuroectodermal symptom complex. *Arch Dermatol* **116**:1378, 1980.
15. Tsambaos D, Nikiforidis G, Balas C, Marinoni S: Trichothiodystrophic hair reveals an abnormal pattern of viscoelastic parameters. *Skin Pharmacol* **7**:257, 1994.
16. Van Neste DJJ, Gillespie JM, Marshall RC, Taieb A, De Brouwer B: Morphological and biochemical characteristics of trichothiodystrophy-variant hair are maintained after grafting of scalp specimens on to nuce mice. *Brit J of Dermatol* **128**:384, 1993.
17. Chen E, Cleaver JE, Weber CA, Packman S, Barkovich AJ, Koch TK, Williams ML, Golabi M, Price VH: Trichothiodystrophy: clinical spectrum, central nervous system imaging, and biochemical characterization of two siblings. *J Inves Dermatol* **103**:154, 1994.
18. Peserico A, Battistella PA, Bertoli P: MRI of a very hereditary ectodermal dysplasia: PIBI(D)S. *Neuroradiology* **34**:316, 1992.
19. Tolmie JL, de Berker D, Dawber R, Galloway C, Gergory DW, Lehmann AR, McClure J, Pollitt JR, Stephenson JPB: Syndromes associated with trichothiodystrophy. *Clin Dysmorphol* **1**:1, 1994.
20. Itin PH, Pittelkow MR: Trichothiodystrophy: review of sulfur-deficient brittle hair syndromes and association with the ectodermal dysplasias. *J Am Acad Dermatol* **22**:705, 1990.
21. McKusick VA: Mendelian inheritance in man. *11th ed.* Baltimore, The Johns Hopkins University Press, 1994.
22. Kleijer WJ, Beemer FA, Boom BW: Intermittent hair loss in a child with PIBI(D)S syndrome and trichothiodystrophy with defective

DNA repair—xeroderma pigmentosum Group D. *Am J Med Gen* **52**:227, 1994.

23. Robbins JH, Kraemer KH, Lutzner MA, Festoff BW, Coon HG: Xeroderma pigmentosum. An inherited disease with sun sensitivity, multiple cutaneous neoplasms and abnormal DNA repair. *Ann Intern Med* **80**:221, 1974.

24. Hamel BCJ, Raams A, Schuitema-Dijkstra AR, Simons P, Van Der Burgt I, Jaspers NGJ, Kleijer WJ: Xeroderma pigmentosum—Cockayne syndrome complex: a further case. *J Med Genet* **33**:607, 1996.

25. Moriwaki SI, Stefanini M, Lehmann AR, Hoeijmakers JHJ, Robbins JH, Rapin I, Botta E, Tanganelli B, Vermeulen W, Broughton BC, Kraemer KH: DNA repair and ultraviolet mutagenesis in cells from a new patient with xeroderma pigmentosum group G and Cockayne syndrome resemble xeroderma pigmentosum cells. *J Invest Dermatol* **107**:647, 1996.

26. Setlow RB: The wavelengths in sunlight effective in producing skin cancer: A theoretical analysis. *Proc Natl Acad Sci USA* **71**:3363, 1974.

27. Epstein JH: Ultraviolet carcinogenesis. *Photophysiology* **5**:235, 1970.

28. Blum HF: Carcinogenesis by ultraviolet light. Princeton, NJ, Princeton University Press, 1959.

29. Cleaver JE: Repair processes for photochemical damage in mammalian cells, Lett JT, Adler H, Zelle M (eds): *Advances in Radiation Biology*, New York, Academic Press, 1974, p 1.

30. Lawrence C: The Rad6 DNA repair pathway in *Saccharomyces cerevisiae*: What does it do and how does it do it? *Bioessays* **16**:253, 1994.

31. Todo T, Takemori H, Ryo H, Ihara M, Matsunaga T, Nikaido O, Sato K, Nomura T: A new photoreactivating enzyme that specifically repairs ultraviolet light-induced [6-4] photoproducts. *Nature* **361**:371, 1993.

32. Todo T, Ryo H, Yamamoto K, Toh H, Inui T, Ayaki H, Nomura T, Ikenaga M: Similarity among Drosophila [6-4] photolyase, a human photolyase homolog, and the DNA photolyase-blue-light photoreceptor family. *Science* **272**:109, 1996.

33. Sancar A, Sancar GB: DNA repair enzymes. *Ann Rev Biochem* **57**:29, 1988.

34. van Houten B: Nucleotide excision repair in *Escherichia coli*. *Microbiol Rev* **54**:18, 1990.

35. Grossman L, Thiagalingam S: Nucleotide excision repair, a tracking mechanism in search of damage. *J Biol Chem* **268**:16871, 1993.

36. Hoeijmakers JHJ: Nucleotide excision repair I: from *E. coli* to yeast. *Trends Genet* **9**:173, 1993.

37. Bohr VA: Gene specific DNA repair. *Carcinogenesis* **12**:1983, 1991.

38. Hanawalt P, Mellon I: Stranded in an active gene. *Curr Biol* **3**:67, 1993.

39. Cleaver JE: Defective repair replication of DNA in xeroderma pigmentosum. *Nature* **218**:652, 1968.

40. Epstein JH, Fukuyama K, Reed WB, Epstein WL: Defect in DNA synthesis in skin of patients with xeroderma pigmentosum demonstrated in vivo. *Science* **168**:1477, 1970.

41. Stefanini M, Vermeulen W, Weeda G, Giliani S, Nardo T, Mezzina M, Sarasin A, Harper JL, Arlett CF, Hoeijmakers JHJ, Lehmann AR: A new nucleotide-excision-repair gene associated with the disorder trichothiodystrophy. *Am J Hum Genet* **53**:817, 1993.

42. Bootsma D, Mulder MP, Pot F, Cohen JA: Different inherited levels of DNA repair replication in xeroderma pigmentosum cell strains after exposure to ultraviolet irradiation. *Mutat Res* **9**:507, 1970.

43. Cleaver JE: Xeroderma pigmentosum: Variants with normal DNA repair and normal sensitivity to ultraviolet light. *J Invest Dermatol* **58**:124, 1972.

44. Lehmann AR, Kirk-Bell S, Arlett CF, Paterson MC, Lohman PHM, de Weerd-Kastelein EA, Bootsma D: Xeroderma pigmentosum cells with normal levels of excision repair have a defect in DNA synthesis after UV-irradiation. *Proc Natl Acad Sci USA* **72**:219, 1975.

45. Bohr VA, Smith CA, Okumoto DS, Hanawalt PC: DNA repair in an active gene: removal of pyrimidine dimers from the *DHFR* gene of CHO cells is much more efficient than in the genome overall. *Cell* **40**:359, 1985.

46. Venema J, Mullenders LHF, Natarajan AT, Van Zeeland AA, Mayne LV: The genetic defect in Cockayne syndrome is associated with a defect in repair of UV-induced DNA damage in transcriptionally active DNA. *Proc Natl Acad Sci USA* **87**:4707, 1990.

47. Tanaka K, Kawai K, Kumahara Y, Ikenaga M, Okada Y: Genetic complementation groups in Cockayne syndrome. *Somat Cell Genet* **7**:445, 1981.

48. Lehmann AR, Francis AJ, Gianelli F: Prenatal diagnosis of Cockaynes syndrome. *Lancet I*:486, 1985.

49. Stefanini M, Lagomarsini P, Giliani S, Nardo T, Botta E, Peserico A, Kleijer WJ, Lehmann AR, Sarasin A: Genetic heterogeneity of the excision repair defect associated with trichothiodystrophy. *Carcinogenesis* **14**:1101, 1993.

50. Wade MH, Chu EHY: Effects of DNA damaging agents on cultured fibroblasts derived from patients with Cockaynes syndrome. *Mutat Res* **59**:49, 1979.

51. McCormick JJ, Kately-Kohler S, Watanabe M, Maher VM: Abnormal sensitivity of human fibroblasts from xeroderma pigmentosum variants to transformation to anchorage independence by ultraviolet radiation. *Cancer Res* **46**:489, 1986.

52. Barrett SF, Robbins JH, Tarone RE, Kraemer KH: Defective repair of cyclobutane pyrimidine dimers with normal repair of other DNA photoproducts in a transcriptionally active gene transfected into Cockayne syndrome cells. *Mutat Res* **255**:281, 1991.

53. Parris CN, Kraemer KH: Ultraviolet induced mutations in Cockayne syndrome cells are primarily caused by cyclobutane dimer photoproducts while repair of other photoproducts is normal. *Proc Natl Acad Sci USA* **90**:7260, 1993.

54. De Weerd-Kastelein EA, Keijzer W, Bootsma D: Genetic heterogeneity of xeroderma pigmentosum demonstrated by somatic cell hybridization. *Nature New Biology* **238**:80, 1972.

55. Lehmann AR: Three complementation groups in Cockayne syndrome. *Mutat Res* **106**:347, 1982.

56. Vermeulen W, van Vuuren AJ, Chipoulet M, Schaeffer L, Appeldoorn E, Weeda G, Jaspers NGJ, Priestley A, Arlett CF, Lehmann AR, Stefanini M, Mezzina M, Sarasin A, Bootsma D, Egly J-M, Hoeijmakers JHJ: Three unusual repair deficiencies associated with transcription factor BTF2(TFIIH). Evidence for the existence of a transcription syndrome. *Cold Spring Harbor Symp Quant Biol* **59**:317, 1994.

57. Kraemer KH: Xeroderma pigmentosum, Demis DJ, McGuire J (eds): *Clinical Dermatology 4*, Philadelphia, Harper & Row, 1980, p 1.

58. Vermeulen W, Scott RJ, Potger S, Muller HJ, Cole J, Arlett CF, Kleijer WJ, Bootsma D, Hoeijmakers JHJ, Weeda G: Clinical heterogeneity within xeroderma pigmentosum associated with mutations in the DNA repair and transcription gene ERCC3. *Am J Hum Genet* **54**:191, 1994.

59. Scott RJ, Itin P, Kleijer WJ, Kolb K, Arlett C, Muller H: Xeroderma pigmentosum-Cockayne syndrome complex in two new patients: absence of skin tumors despite severe deficiency of DNA excision repair. *J Am Acad Dermatol* **29**:883, 1993.

60. Manebridge JN, Hanawalt PC: Domain-limited repair of DNA in ultraviolet fibroblasts from xeroderma pigmentosum complementation group C, in Friedberg EC, Bridges BA (eds): *Cellular Responses to DNA Damage*. New York, Alan R. Liss, Inc., 1983, p 195.

61. Venema J, Van Hoffen A, Natarajan AT, Van Zeeland AA, Mullenders LHF: The residual repair capacity of xeroderma pigmentosum complementation group C fibroblasts is highly specific for transcriptionally active DNA. *Nucleic Acids Res* **18**:443, 1990.

62. Hananian J, Cleaver JE: Xeroderma pigmentosum exhibiting neurological disorders and systemic lupus erythematosus. *Clin Genet* **17**:39, 1980.

63. Lehmann AR, Arlett CF, Broughton BC, Harcourt SA, Steingrimsdottir H, Stefanini M, Malcolm A, Taylor R, Natarajan AT, Green S: Trichothiodystrophy, a human DNA repair disorder with heterogeneity in the cellular response to ultraviolet light. *Cancer Res* **48**:6090, 1988.

64. Wood RD: Seven genes for three diseases. *Nature* **350**:190, 1991.

65. Arase S, Kozuka T, Tanaka K, Ikenaga M, Takebe H: A sixth complementation group in xeroderma pigmentosum. *Mutat Res* **59**:143, 1979.

66. Nishigori C, Fujiwara H, Uyeno K, Kawaguchi T, Takebe H: Xeroderma pigmentosum patients belonging to complementation group F and efficient liquid recovery of ultraviolet damage. *Photodermatol Photoimmunol Photomed* **8**:146, 1991.

67. Arlett CF, Harcourt SA, Lehmann AR, Stevens S, Ferguson-Smith MA, Mosley WN: Studies on a new case of xeroderma pigmentosum (XP3BR) from complementation group G with a cellular sensitivity to ionizing radiation. *Carcinogenesis* **1**:745, 1980.

68. Jung EG: New form of molecular defect in xeroderma pigmentosum. *Nature* **228**:361, 1970.

69. Jaspers NGJ, Jansen-v.d., Kuilen G, Bootsma D: Complementation analysis of xeroderma pigmentosum variants. *Exp Cell Res* **136**:81, 1981.

70. Jorizzo JL, Atherton DJ, Crounse RG, Wells RS: Ichthyosis, brittle hair, impaired intelligence, decreased fertility and short stature (IBIDS syndrome). *Br J Dermatol* **106**:705, 1982.

71. Itoh T, Ono T, Yamaizumi M: A new UV-sensitive syndrome not belonging to any complementation groups of xeroderma pigmentosum or Cockayne syndrome: Siblings showing biochemical characteristics of Cockayne syndrome without typical clinical manifestations. *Mutat Res* **314**:233, 1994.

72. Itoh T, Fujiwara Y, Ono T, Yamaizumi M: UVs syndrome, a new general category of photosensitive disorder with defective DNA repair, is distinct from xeroderma pigmentosum variant and rodent complementation group 1. *Am J Hum Genet* **56**:1267, 1995.

73. Itoh T, Cleaver JE, Yamaizumi M: Cockayne syndrome complementation group B associated with xeroderma pigmentosum phenotype. *Hum Genet* **97**:176, 1996.

74. Lehmann AR, Thompson AF, Harcourt SA, Stefanini M, Norris PG: Cockaynes syndrome: Correlation of clinical features with cellular sensitivity of RNA synthesis to UV irradiation. *J Med Genet* **30**:679, 1993.

75. Lambert WC, Lambert MW: Co-recessive inheritance: a model for DNA repair, genetic disease and carcinogenesis. *Mutat Res* **145**:227, 1985.

76. Thompson LH, Busch DB, Brookman K, Mooney CL: Genetic diversity of UV-sensitive DNA repair mutants of Chinese hamster ovary cells. *Proc Natl Acad Sci USA* **78**:3734, 1981.

77. Collins AR: Mutant rodent cell lines sensitive to ultraviolet light, ionizing radiation and cross-linking agentsA comprehensive survey of genetic and biochemical characteristics. *Mutat Res* **293**:99, 1993.

78. Thompson LH: Somatic cell genetics approach to dissecting mammalian DNA repair. *Environ Mol Mutagen* **14**:264, 1989.

79. Westerveld A, Hoeijmakers JHJ, van Duin M, de Wit J, Odijk H, Pastink A, Wood RD, Bootsma D: Molecular cloning of a human DNA repair gene. *Nature* **310**:425, 1984.

80. Weber CA, Salazar EP, Stewart SA, Thompson LH: Molecular cloning and biological characterization of a human gene, *ERCC2*, that corrects the nucleotide excision repair defect in CHO UV5 cells. *Mol Cell Biol* **8**:1137, 1988.

81. Weeda G, Van Ham RCA, Masurel R, Westerveld A, Odijk H, De Wit J, Bootsma D, Van Der Eb AJ, Hoeijmakers JHJ: Molecular cloning and biological characterization of the human excision repair gene *ERCC*. *Mol Cell Biol* **10**:2570, 1990.

82. Thompson LH, Brookman KW, Weber CA, Salazar EP, Reardon JT, Sancar A, Deng Z, Siciliano MJ: Molecular cloning of the human nucleotide-excision-repair gene *ERCC4*. *Proc Natl Acad Sci USA* **91**:6855, 1994.

83. Mudgett JS, MacInnes MA: Isolation of the functional human excision repair gene *ERCC 5* by intercosmid recombination. *Genomics* **8**:623, 1990.

84. Troelstra C, Odijk H, De Wit J, Westerveld A, Thompson LH, Bootsma D, Hoeijmakers JHJ: Molecular cloning of the human DNA excision repair gene *ERCC-6*. *Mol Cell Biol* **10**:5806, 1990.

85. Weber CA, Thompson LH, Salazar EP: Characterization of ERCC2 and its correction of xeroderma pigmentosum group D, in Proceedings of the American Association for Cancer Research Special Conference on Cellular Responses to Environmental DNA Damage, Banff, Canada, December 1, 1991.

86. Flejter WL, McDaniel LD, Johns D, Friedberg EC, Schultz RA: Correction of xeroderma pigmentosum complementation group D mutant cell phenotypes by chromosome and gene transfer: involvement of the human *ERCC2* DNA repair gene. *Proc Natl Acad Sci USA* **89**:261, 1992.

87. Weeda G, Van Ham RCA, Vermeulen W, Bootsma D, Van der Eb AJ, Hoeijmakers JHJ: A presumed DNA helicase encoded by *ERCC-3* is involved in the human repair disorders xeroderma pigmentosum and Cockaynes syndrome. *Cell* **62**:777, 1990.

88. Scherly D, Nouspikel T, Corlet J, Ucla C, Bairoch A, Clarkson SG: Complementation of the DNA repair defect in xeroderma pigmentosum group G cells by a human cDNA related to yeast RAD2. *Nature* **363**:182, 1993.

89. Troelstra C, van Gool A, de Wit J, Vermeulen W, Bootsma D, Hoeijmakers JHJ: *ERCC6*, a member of a subfamily of putative helicases, is involved in Cockaynes syndrome and preferential repair of active genes. *Cell* **71**:939, 1992.

90. MacInnes MA, Dickson JA, Hernandez RR, Learmont D, Lin GY, Mudgett JS, Park MS, Schauer S, Reynolds RJ, Strniste GF, Yu JY: Human *ERCC5* cDNA-cosmid complementation for excision repair

91. and bipartite amini acid domains conserved with RAD proteins of *S. cerevisiae* and *S. pombe*. *Mol Cell Biol* **13**:6393, 1993.

91. O'Donovan A, Wood RD: Identical defects in DNA repair in xeroderma pigmentosum group G and rodent ERCC group 5. *Nature* **363**:185, 1993.

92. Fryns JP, Bulcke J, Verdu P, Carton H, Kleczkowska A, van den Berghe H: Apparent late-onset Cockayne syndrome and interstitial deletion of the long arm of chromosome 10 (del(10)(q11.23q21.2)). *Am J Med Genet* **40**:343, 1991.

93. Tanaka K, Satokata I, Ogita Z, Uchida T, Okada Y: Molecular cloning of a mouse DNA repair gene that complements the defect of group A xeroderma pigmentosum. *Proc Natl Acad Sci USA* **86**:5512, 1989.

94. Hoeijmakers JHJ, Odijk H, Westerveld A: Differences between rodent and human cell lines in the amount of integrated DNA after transfection. *Exp Cell Res* **169**:111, 1987.

95. Legerski R, Peterson C: Expression cloning of a human DNA repair gene involved in xeroderma pigmentosum group C. *Nature* **359**:70, 1992.

96. Henning KA, Li L, Iyer N, McDaniel L, Reagan MS, Legerski R, Schultz RA, Stefanini M, Lehmann AR, Mayne LV, Friedberg EC: The Cockayne syndrome group A gene encodes a WD repeat protein that interacts with CSB protein and a subunit of RNA polymerase II TFIIH. *Cell* **82**:555, 1995.

97. Itoh T, Shiomi T, Shiomi N, Harada Y, Wakasugi M, Matsunaga T, Nikaido O, Friedberg EC, Yamaizumi M: Rodent complementation group 8 (ERCC8) corresponds to Cockayne syndrome complementation group A. *Mutat Res* **362**:167, 1996.

98. Koken MH, Reynolds P, Jaspers-Dekker I, Prakash L, Prakash S, Bootsma D, Hoeijmakers JH: Structural and functional conservation of two human homologs of the yeast DNA repair gene RAD6. *Proc Natl Acad Sci USA* **88**:8865, 1991.

99. Jentsch S: The ubiquitin-conjugation system. *Ann Rev Genet* **26**:179, 1992.

100. Sijbers AM, de Laat WL, Ariza RR, Biggerstaff M, Wei YF, Moggs JG, Carter KC, Shell BK, Evans E, de Jong MC, Rademakers S, de Rooij J, Jaspers NGJ, Hoeijmakers JHJ, Wood RD: Xeroderma pigmentosum group F caused by a defect in a structure-specific DNA repair endonuclease. *Cell* **86**:811, 1996.

101. Masutani C, Sugasawa K, Yanagisawa J, Sonoyama T, Ui M, Enomoto T, Takio K, Tanaka K, van der Spek PJ, Bootsma D, Hoeijmakers JHJ, Hanaoka F: Purification and cloning of a nucleotide excision repair complex involving the xeroderma pigmentosum group C protein and a human homolog of yeast RAD23. *EMBO J* **13**:1831, 1994.

102. Spek van der PJ, Kobayashi J, Bootsma D, Takao M, Eker APM, Yasui A: Cloning, tissue expression, and mapping of a human photolyase homolog with similarity to plant blue-light receptors. *Genomics* **37**:177, 1996.

103. McKay MJ, Troelstra C, van der Spek PJ, Kanaar R, Smit B, Hagemeijer A, Bootsma D, Hoeijmakers JHJ: Sequence conservation of Schizosaccharomyces pombe double strand break DNA repair gene rad 21. *Genomics* **36**:305, 1996.

104. van Gool AJ, Verhage R, Swagemakers SMA, van de Putte P, Brouwer J, Troelstra C, Bootsma D, Hoeijmakers JHJ: *RAD26*, the functional *S. cerevisiae* homolog of the Cockayne syndrome B gene *ERCC6*. *EMBO J* **13**:5361, 1994.

105. Hwang BJ, Liao JC, Chu G: Isolation of a cDNA encoding a UV-damaged DNA binding factor defective in xeroderma pigmentosum group E cells. *Mutat Res* **362**:105, 1996.

106. Keeney S, Chang GJ, Linn S: Characterization of human DNA damage binding protein implicated in xeroderma pigmentosum E. *J Biol Chem* **268**:21293, 1993.

107. Keeney S, Eker APM, Brody T, Vermeulen W, Bootsma D, Hoeijmakers JHJ, Linn S: Correction of the DNA repair defect in xeroderma pigmentosum group E by injection of a DNA damage-binding protein. *Proc Natl Acad Sci USA* **91**:4053, 1994.

108. Shivji MKK, Kenny MK, Wood RD: Proliferating cell nuclear antigen is required for DNA excision repair. *Cell* **69**:367, 1992.

109. Sibghat-Ullah, Husain I, Carlton W, Sancar A: Human nucleotide excision repair in vitro: repair of pyrimidine dimers, psoralen and cisplatin adducts by HeLa cell-free extract. *Nucleic Acids Res* **17**:4471, 1989.

110. Aboussekhra A, Biggerstaff M, Shivji MKK, Vilpo JA, Moncollin V, Podust VN, Protic M, Hubscher U, Egly J, Wood RD: Mammalian DNA nucleotide excision repair reconstituted with purified components. *Cell* **80**:859, 1995.

111. Mu D, Park C-H, Matsunaga T, Hsu DS, Reardon JT, Sancar A: Reconstitution of human DNA repair excision nuclease in a highly defined system. *J Biol Chem* **270**:2415, 1995.

112. Tanaka K, Miura N, Satokata I, Miyamoto I, Yoshida MC, Satoh Y, Kondo S, Yasui A, Okayama H, Okada Y: Analysis of a human DNA excision repair gene involved in group A xeroderma pigmentosum and containing a zinc-finger domain. *Nature* **348**:73, 1990.

113. Robins P, Jones CJ, Biggerstaff M, Lindahl T, Wood RD: Complementation of DNA repair in xeroderma pigmentosum group A cell extracts by a protein with affinity for damaged DNA. *EMBO J* **10**:3913, 1991.

114. Eker APM, Vermeulen W, Miura N, Tanaka K, Jaspers NGJ, Hoeijmakers JHJ, Bootsma D: Xeroderma pigmentosum group A correcting protein from calf thymus. *Mutat Res* **274**:211, 1992.

115. Miyamoto I, Miura N, Niwa H, Miyazaki J, Tanaka K: Mutational analysis of the structure and function of the xeroderma pigmentosum group A complementing protein. *J Biol Chem* **267**:12182, 1992.

116. Jones CJ, Wood RD: Preferential binding of the xeroderma pigmentosum group A complementing protein to damaged DNA. *Biochemistry* **32**:12096, 1993.

117. Asahina H, Kuraoka I, Shirakawa M, Morita EH, Miura N, Miyamoto I, Ohtsuka E, Okada Y, Tanaka K: The XPA protein is a zinc metalloprotein with an ability to recognize various kinds of DNA damage. *Mutat Res* **315**:29, 1994.

118. Miura N, Miyamoto I, Asahina H, Satokata I, Tanaka K, Okada Y: Identification and characterization of XPAC protein, the gene product of the human *XPAC* (xeroderma pigmentosum group A complementing) gene. *J Biol Chem* **266**:19786, 1991.

119. Bankmann M, Prakash L, Prakash S: Yeast *RAD14* and human xeroderma pigmentosum group A DNA repair genes encode homologous proteins. *Nature* **355**:555, 1992.

120. Guzder SN, Sung P, Prakash L, Prakash S: Yeast DNA-repair gene *RAD14* encodes a zinc metalloprotein with affinity for ultraviolet-damaged DNA. *Proc Natl Acad Sci USA* **90**:5433, 1993.

121. Chu G, Chang E: Xeroderma pigmentosum group E cells lack a nuclear factor that binds to damaged DNA. *Science* **242**:564, 1988.

122. Kataoka H, Fujiwara Y: UV damage-specific DNA protein in xeroderma pigmentosum complementation group E. *Biochem Biophys Res Commun* **175**:1139, 1991.

123. Keeney S, Wein H, Linn S: Biochemical heterogeneity in xeroderma pigmentosum complementation group E. *Mutat Res* **273**:49, 1992.

124. Hwang BJ, Chu G: Purification and characterization of a human protein that binds to damaged DNA. *Biochemistry* **32**:1657, 1993.

125. Takao M, Abramic M, Moos M, Otrin VR, Wootton JC, Mclenigan M, Levine AS, Protic M: A 127 kDa component of a UV-damaged DNA-binding complex which is defective in some xeroderma pigmentosum group E patients is homologous to a slime mold protein. *Nucleic Acids Res* **21**:4111, 1993.

126. Reardon JT, Nichols AF, Keeney S, Smith CA, Taylor JS, Linn S, Sancar A: Comparative analysis of binding of human damaged DNA-binding protein (XPE) and *Escherichia coli* damage recognition protein (UvrA) to the major ultraviolet photoproducts T[CS]TT[Ts] TT[6-4]T and T[Dewar]T. *J Biol Chem* **268**:21301, 1993.

127. Li L, Elledge SJ, Peterson CA, Bales ES, Legerski RJ: Specific association between the human DNA repair proteins XPA and ERCC1. *Proc Natl Acad Sci USA* **91**:5012, 1994.

128. Park C-H, Sancar A: Formation of a ternary complex by human XPA, ERCC1 and ERCC4(XPF) excision repair proteins. *Proc Natl Acad Sci USA* **91**:5017, 1994.

129. Matsuda T, Saijo M, Kuraoka I, Kobayashi T, Nahatssu Y, Nagai A, Enjoji T, Masutani C, Sugasawa K, Hanaoka F, Yasui A, Tanaka K: DNA repair protein XPA binds to replication protein A (RPA). *J Biol Chem* **270**:4152, 1995.

130. He Z, Henricksen LA, Wold MS, Ingles CJ: RPA involvement in the damage and incision step of nucleotide excision repair. *Nature* **374**:566, 1995.

131. Park C-H, Mu D, Reardon JT, Sancar A: The general transcription-repair factor TFIIH is recruited to the excision repair complex by the XPA protein independent of the TFIIE transcription factor. *J Biol Chem* **270**:4896, 1995.

132. Park H-W, Kim S-T, Sancar A, Deisenhofer J: Crystal structure of DNA photolyase from *Escherichia coli*. *Science*. **268**:1866, 1995.

133. Coverley D, Kenny MK, Lane DP, Wood RD: A role for the human single-stranded DNA binding protein HSSB/RPA in an early stage of nucleotide excision repair. *Nucleic Acids Res* **20**:3873, 1992.

134. Naumovski L, Friedberg EC: A DNA repair gene required for the incision of damaged DNA is essential for viability in *Saccharomyces cerevisiae*. *Proc Natl Acad Sci USA* **80**:4818, 1983.

135. Park E, Guzder S, Koken MHM, Jaspers-Dekker I, Weeda G, Hoeijmakers JHJ, Prakash S, Prakash L: *RAD25*, a yeast homolog of human xeroderma pigmentosum group B DNA repair gene is essential for viability. *Proc Natl Acad Sci USA* **89**:11416, 1992.

136. Mounkes LC, Jones RS, Liang B-C, Gelbart W, Fuller MT: A Drosophila model for xeroderma pigmentosum and Cockaynes syndrome: *haywire* encodes the fly homolog of ERCC3, a human excision repair gene. *Cell* **71**:925, 1992.

137. Schaeffer L, Roy R, Humbert S, Moncollin V, Vermeulen W, Hoeijmakers JHJ, Chambon P, Egly J: DNA repair helicase: a component of BTF2 (TFIIH) basic transcription factor. *Science* **260**:58, 1993.

138. Conaway RC, Conaway JW: General initiation factors for RNA polymerase II. *Ann Rev Biochem* **62**:161, 1993.

139. Feaver WJ, Svejstrup JQ, Henry NL, Kornberg RD: Relationship of CDK-activating kinase and RNA polymerase II CTD kinase TFIIH/TFIIK. *Cell* **79**:1103, 1994.

140. Roy R, Adamczewski JP, Seroz T, Vermeulen W, Tassan J-P, Schaeffer L, Nigg EA, Hoeijmakers JHJ, Egly J: The MO15 cell cycle kinase is associated with the TFIIH transcription repair factor. *Cell* **79**:1093, 1994.

141. Schaeffer L, Moncollin V, Roy R, Staub A, Mezzina M, Sarasin A, Weeda G, Hoeijmakers JHJ, Egly JM: The ERCC2/DNA repair protein is associated with the class II BTF2/TFIIH transcription factor. *EMBO J* **13**:2388, 1994.

142. Drapkin R, Reardon JT, Ansari A, Huang JC, Zawel L, Ahn K, Sancar A, Reinberg D: Dual role of TFIIH in DNA excision repair and in transcription by RNA polymerase II. *Nature* **368**:769, 1994.

143. van Vuuren AJ, Vermeulen W, Ma L, Weeda G, Appeldoorn E, Jaspers NGJ, van der Eb AJ, Bootsma D, Hoeijmakers JHJ, Humbert S, Schaeffer L, Egly J-M: Correction of xeroderma pigmentosum repair defect by basal transcription factor BTF2(TFIIH). *EMBO J* **13**:1645, 1994.

144. Humbert S, van Vuuren AJ, Lutz Y, Hoeijmakers JHJ, Egly J-M, Moncollin V: Characterization of p44/SSL1 and p34 subunits of the BTF2/TFIIH transcription/repair factor. *EMBO J* **13**:2393, 1994.

145. Wang Z, Buratowski S, Svejstrup JQ, Feaver WJ, Wu X, Kornberg RD, Donahue TD, Friedberg EC: The yeast *TFB1* and *SSL1* genes, which encode subunits of transcription factor IIH, are required for nucleotide excision repair and RNA polymerase II transcription. *Mol Cell Biol* **15**:2288, 1995.

146. Feaver WJ, Svejstrup JQ, Bardwell L, Bardwell AJ, Buratowski S, Gulyas KD, Donahue TF, Friedberg EC, Kornberg RD: Dual roles of a multiprotein complex from *S. cerevisiae* in transcription and DNA repair. *Cell* **75**:1379, 1993.

147. Guzder SN, Sung P, Bailly V, Prakash L, Prakash S: RAD25 is a DNA helicase required for DNA repair and RNA plymerase II transcription. *Nature* **369**:578, 1994.

148. Svejstrup JQ, Want Z, Feaver WJ, Wu X, Bushnell DA, Donahue TF, Friedberg EC, Kornberg RD: Different forms of TFIIH for transcription and DNA repair: holo-TFIIH and a nucleotide excision repairosome. *Cell* **80**:21, 1995.

149. Wang Z, Svejstrup JQ, Feaver WJ, Wu X, Kornberg RD, Friedberg EC: Transcription factor b (TFIIH) is required during nucelotide excision repair in yeast. *Nature* **368**:74, 1994.

150. Goodrich, JA, Tjian R: Transcription factors IIE and IIH and ATP hydrolysis direct promoter clearance by RNA polymerase II. *Cell* **77**:145, 1994.

151. Huang JC, Svoboda DL, Reardon JT, Sancar A: Human nucleotide excision nuclease removes thymine dimers from DNA by incising the 22nd phosphodiester bond 5' and the 6th phosphodiester bond 3' to the photodimer. *Proc Natl Acad Sci USA* **89**:3664, 1992.

152. van Vuuren AJ, Appeldoorn E, Odijk H, Yasui A, Jaspers NGJ, Bootsma D, Hoeijmakers JHJ: Evidence for a repair enzyme complex involving ERCC1 and complementing activities of ERCC4, ERCC11 and xeroderma pigmentosum group F. *EMBO J* **12**:3693, 1993.

153. Biggerstaff M, Szymkowski DE, Wood RD: Co-correction of ERCC1, ERCC4 and xeroderma pigmentosum group F DNA repair defects *in vitro*. *EMBO J* **12**:3685, 1993.

154. Bardwell AJ, Bardwell L, Tomkinson AE, Friedberg EC: Specific cleavage of model recombination and repair intermediates by the yeast Rad1-Rad10 DNA endonuclease. *Science* **265**:2082, 1994.

155. Davies AA, Friedberg EC, Tomkinson AE, Wood RD, West SC: Role of the Rad1 and Rad10 proteins in nucleotide excision repair and recombination. *J Biol Chem* **270**:24638, 1995.

156. Fishman-Lobell J, Haber JE: Removal of nonhomologous DNA ends in double-strand break recombination: The role of the yeast ultraviolet repair gene *RAD1*. *Science* **258**:480, 1992.

157. Saffran WA, Greenberg RB, Thaler MS, Jones MM: Single strand and double strand DNA damage-induced reciprocal recombination in yeast. Dependence on nucleotide excision repair and *RAD1* recombination. *Nucleic Acids Res* **22**:2823, 1994.

158. Schiestl RH, Prakash S: *RAD10*, an excision repair gene of *Saccharomyces cerevisiae* is involved in the *RAD1* pathway of mitotic recombination. *Mol Cell Biol* **10**:2485, 1990.

159. ODonovan A, Davies AA, Moggs JG, West SC, Wood RD: XPG endonuclease makes the 3' incision in human DNA nucleotide excision repair. *Nature* **371**:432, 1994.

160. Nichols AF, Sancar A: Purification of PCNA as a nucleotide excision repair protein. *Nucleic Acids Res* **20**:2441, 1992.

161. Barnes DE, Tomkinson AE, Lehmann AR, Webster ADB, Lindahl T: Mutations in the *DNA ligase 1* gene of an individual with immunodeficiencies and cellular hypersensitivity to DNA-damaging agents. *Cell* **69**:495, 1992.

162. Verhage R, Zeeman A, de Groot N, Gleig F, Bang D, van der Putte P, Brouwer J: The *RAD7* and *RAD16* genes are essential for repair of non-transcribed DNA in *Saccharomyces cerevisiae*. *Mol Cell Biol* **14**:6135, 1994.

163. Venema J, van Hoffen A, Karcagi V, Natarajan AT, van Zeeland AA, Mullenders LHF: Xeroderma pigmentosum complementation group C cells remove pyrimidine dimers selectively from the transcribed strand of active genes. *Mol Cell Biol* **11**:4128, 1991.

164. Spek van der PJ, Smit EME, Beverloo HB, Sugasawa K, Masutani C. Hanaoka F, Hoeijmakers JHJ, Hagemeijer A: Chromosomal localization of three repair genes: the xeroderma pigmentosum group C gene and two human homologs of yeast RAD23. *Genomics* **23**:651, 1994.

165. Perozzi G, Prakash S: *RAD7* of *Saccharomyces cerevisiae*: Transcripts, nucleotide sequence analysis and functional relationship between the RAD7 and RAD23 gene products. *Mol Cell Biol* **6**:1497, 1986.

166. Bang DD, Verhage R, Goosen N, Brouwer J, Putte Pvd: Molecular cloning of *RAD16*, a gene involved in differential repair in *Saccharomyces cerevisiae*. *Nucleic Acids Res* **20**:3925, 1992.

167. Wolffe AP: Switched-on chromatin. *Curr Biol* **4**:525, 1994.

168. Neer EJ, Schmidt CJ, Nambudripad R, Smith TF: The ancient regulatory-protein family of WD-repeat proteins. *Nature* **371**:297, 1994.

169. Nagai A, Saijo M, Kuraoka I, Matsuda T, Kodo N, Nakatsu Y, Mimaki T, Mino M, Biggerstaff M, Wood RD, Sijbers A, Hoeijmakers JHJ, Tanaka K: Enhancement of damage-specific DNA binding of XPA by interaction with the ERCC1 DNA repair protein. *Biochem Biophys Res Commun* **211**:960, 1995.

170. Bardwell AJ, Bardwell L, Iyer N, Svejstrup JQ, Feaver WJ, Kornberg RD, Friedberg EC: Yeast nucleotide excision repair proteins rad2 and rad4 interact with RNA polymerase II basal transcription factor b (TFIIH). *Mol Cell Biol* **14**:3569, 1994.

171. van Duin M, Vredeveldt G, Mayne LV, Odijk H, Vermeulen W, Klein B, Weeda G, Hoeijmakers JHJ, Bootsma D, Westerveld A: The cloned human DNA excision repair gene *ERCC-1* fails to correct xeroderma pigmentosum complementation groups A through I. *Mutat Res* **217**:83, 1989.

172. McWhir J, Seldridge J, Harrison DJ, Squires S, Melton DW: Mice with DNA repair gene (ERCC-1) deficiency have elevated levels of p53, liver nuclear abnormalities and die before weaning. *Nat Genet* **5**:217, 1993.

173. Nakane H, Takeuchi S, Yuba S, Saijo M, Nakatsu Y, Ishikawa T, Hirota S, Kitamura Y, Kato Y, Tsunoda Y, Miyauchi H, Horio T, Tokunaga T, Matsunaga T, Nikaido O, Nishimune Y, Okada Y, Tanaka K: High incidence of ultraviolet-B or chemical-carcinogen-induced skin tumours in mice lacking the xeroderma pigmentosum group A gene. *Nature* **377**:165, 1995.

174. de Vries A, van Oostrom CTM, Hofhuis FMA, Dortant PM, Berg RJW, de Gruijl FR, Wester PW, van Kreijl CF, Capel PJA, van Steeg

H, Verbeek SJ: Increased susceptibility to ultraviolet-B and carcinogens of mice lacking the DNA excision repair gene *XPA*. *Nature* **377**:169, 1995.

175. Sands AT, Abuin A, Sanchez A, Conti CJ, Bradley A: High susceptibility to ultraviolet-induced carcinogenesis in mice lacking *XPC*. *Nature* **377**:162, 1995.

176. Johnson RT, Squires S: The XPD complementation group. Insights into xeroderma pigmentosum, Cockaynes syndrome and trichothiodystrophy. *Mutat Res* **273**:97, 1992.

177. Broughton BC, Steingrimsdottir H, Weber CA, Lehmann AR: Mutations in xeroderma pigmentosum group D DNA repair/transcription gene in patients with trichothiodystrophy. *Nature Genet* **7**:189, 1994.

178. Kemphues KJ, Kaufman TC, Raff RA, Raff EC: The testis-specific beta-tubulin subunit in *Drosophila* melanogaster has multiple functions in spermatogenesis. *Cell* **31**:655, 1982.

179. Readhead C, Popko B, Takahashi N, Shine HD, Saavedra RA, Sidman RL, Hood L: Expression of a myelin basic protein gene in transgenic shiverer mice: correction of the dysmyelinating phenotype. *Cell* **48**:703, 1987.

180. Sasaki K, Tachi N, Shinoda M, Satoh N. Minami R, Ohnishi A: Demyelinating peripheral neuropathy in Cockayne syndrome: a histopathologic and morphometric study. *Brain Dev* **14**:114, 1992.

181. Parvin JD, Sharp PA: DNA topology and a minimum set of basal factors for transcription by RNA polymerase II. *Cell* **73**:533, 1993.

182. Bootsma D, Hoeijmakers JHJ: DNA repair: Engagement with transcription. *Nature* **363**:114, 1993.

183. Kraemer KH, Slor H: Xeroderma pigmentosum. *Clin Dermatol* **3**:33, 1985.

184. Lynch HT, Anderson DE, Smith JL, Howell JB, Krush AJ: Xeroderma pigmentosum, malignant melanoma and congenital ichthyosis. *Arch Dermatol* **96**:625, 1967.

185. Kraemer KH, Digiovanna JJ, Moshell AN, Tarone RE, Peck GL: Prevention of skin cancer with oral 13-cisretinoic acid in xeroderma pigmentosum. *N Engl J Med* **318**:1633, 1988.

186. Ramsay CA, Coltart TM, Bl,unt S, Pawsey CA, Gianelli F: Prenatal diagnosis of xeroderma pigmentosum. Report of the first successful case. *The Lancet,* November 9:1109, 1974.

187. Halley DFF, Keijzer W, Jaspers NGJ, Niermeijer MF, Kleijer WJ, Boué A, Bootsma D: Prenatal diagnosis of xeroderma pigmentosum (group C) using assays of unscheduled DNA synthesis and postreplication repair. *Clin Genet* **16**:137, 1979.

188. Cleaver JE, Volpe JPG, Charles WC, Thomas GH: Prenatal diagnosis of xeroderma pigmentosum and Cockayne Syndrome. *Prenatal Diagnosis* **14**:921, 1994.

189. Sarasin A, Blanchet-Bardon C, Renault G, Lehmann A, Arlett C, Dumez Y: Prenatal diagnosis in a subset of trichothiodystrophy patients defective in DNA repair. *Br J Dermatol* **127**:485, 1992.

190. Matsumoto N, Saito N, Harada N, Tanaka K, Niikawa N: DNA-based prenatal carrier detection for group A xeroderma pigmentosum in a chorionic villus sample. *Prenatal Diagnosis* **15**:1675, 1995.

191. Nichols AF, Ong P, Linn S: Mutations specific to the xeroderma pigmentosum group E Ddb(-) phenotype. *J Biol Chem* **271**:24317, 1996.

192. De Boer J, Donker I, de Wit J, Hoeijmakers JHJ, Weeda G: Disruption of the mouse XPD DNA repair/basal transcription gene results in preimplantation lethality. *Cancer Research* **1997**, in the press.

193. Weeda G, Donker I, de Wit J, Morreau H. Janssens R, Vissers CJ, Nigg A, van Steeg H, Bootsma D, Hoeijmakers JHJ: Disruption of mouse *ERCC1* results in a novel repair syndrome with growth failure, nuclear abnormalities and senescence. *Curr Biol* **7**:427, 1997.

194. van der Horst GTJ, van Steeg H, Berg RJW, van Gool AJ, de Wit J, Weeda G, Morreau H, Beems RB, van Kreijl CF, de Gruijl FR, Bootsma D, Hoeijmakers JHJ: Defective transcription-coupled repair in Cockayne syndrome B mice is associated with skin cancer predisposition. *Cell* **89**:425, 1997.

195. van Gool AJ, van der Horst GTJ, Citterio E, Hoeijmakers JHJ: Cockayne syndrome: defective repair of transcription? *EMBO J* **16**:4155, 1997.

196. Weeda G, Eveno E, Donker I, Vermeulen W, Chevallier-Lagente O, Taïeb A, Stary A, Hoeijmakers JHJ, Mezzina M, Sarasin A: A mutation in the *XPB/ERCC3* DNA repair transcription gene, associated with trichothiodystrophy. *Am J Hum Genet* **60**:320, 1997.

CHAPTER 14

Ataxia-Telangiectasia

Richard A. Gatti

1. The diagnosis of ataxia-telangiectasia (A-T) is based primarily on clinical examination and should include progressive cerebellar ataxia with onset between 1 and 3 years of age. Ocular apraxia is a reliable diagnostic sign after 2 years of age. Telangiectasias often are manifested several years after the onset of ataxia; the degree of telangiectasia is quite variable from family to family. Serum alpha-fetoprotein is elevated in 95 percent of patients. Magnetic resonance imaging shows a dystrophic cerebellum. Karyotyping, if successful, reveals characteristic translocations involving chromosomes 14q11-12, 14q32, 7q35, and 7p14. Immunodeficiency and cancer, usually lymphoid, are observed in many A-T patients.

2. Because A-T patients are radiosensitive, conventional doses of radiation therapy are contraindicated. In young children with lymphoid malignancies, an underlying diagnosis of A-T should be considered before one calculates doses of radiation or radiomimetic drugs.

3. The incidence of A-T is estimated at 1 per 40,000 live births in the United States. The carrier frequency is estimated at 1 percent. Carriers are indistinguishable from normal individuals. Despite this, female carriers are thought to have a five-fold increased risk of breast cancer. Carriers may account for 5 percent of all cancer patients in the United States. Carriers are intermediate in their in vitro responses to ionizing radiation-induced DNA damage. Whether they are clinically more radiosensitive than normals is not known. Conventional wisdom suggests that exposure of A-T carriers to ionizing radiation should be minimized. However, mammograms are recommended as for noncarriers.

4. The ATM (A-T, mutated) gene and gene product(s) are very large: 3056 amino acids, 350 kDa, an ~13-kb transcript (and smaller alternatively spliced products), and 66 exons that cover ~150 kb of genomic DNA. ATM is expressed in all organs tested. The function of the gene is unknown, although sequence homology analyses suggest that it belongs to a large-molecular-weight family of protein kinases. Delayed or reduced expression of p53 in radiation-damaged A-T cells suggests that ATM interacts with proteins upstream of p53 in intracellular signaling pathways. The ATM gene product also plays a role in gametogenesis, as part of the synaptonemal complex.

5. Seventy percent of ATM mutations would result in a shortened (truncated) protein. These mutations are found over the entire gene and are best detected at present by mRNA-based techniques that first translate the mRNA to cDNA by RT-PCR before screening for mutations. The favored RT-PCR-based methods thus far have been PTT, REF, SSCP, and direct sequencing. Rapid assays that are DNA-based are being developed for the more common mutations or mutations that are common to particular ethnic populations, such as Amish, central-southern Italian, Midlands English, Costa Rican, Norwegian, and Polish. Thus far, attempts to demonstrate an increased frequency of ATM mutations in breast cancer patients have not been convincing.

6. Several related syndromes overlap with A-T. Nijmegen breakage syndrome (NBS) shares t(7;14) translocations, radiosensitivity, immunodeficiency, and cancer susceptibility with A-T, but these patients do not have ataxia, telangiectasia, or elevated AFP. NBS patients are microcephalic and mentally retarded, whereas A-T patients usually are not. Berlin breakage syndrome is very similar to NBS but sometimes includes syndactyly or anal stenosis. AT$_{Fresno}$ combines the A-T and NBS syndromes. AT$_{Fresno}$ patients have ATM mutations. NBS and BBS families link not to 11q23.1, the site of the ATM gene, but to 8q21.

7. A-T is a very pleiotropic syndrome and is not yet understandable in terms of a single common denominator. All cells show nucleomegaly on histologic examination. Purkinje cells degenerate and migrate abnormally in the cerebellum. The thymus remains embryonic. The cause of radiation hypersensitivity also must be explained by this common denominator. The ATM gene product senses double-stranded DNA breaks, and when it is defective, the DNA damage is not repaired before the next replication cycle begins. A-T cells have G1, S, and G2/M checkpoint defects. To date, all DNA repair mechanisms that have been studied in A-T cells have been normal. The ATM protein interacts with IκB-α, RPA, Chk1, c-*abl*, p53, ATR, MLH1, and Rad51.

8. Therapy for A-T patients remains restricted to supportive care, such as good pulmonary hygiene, speech therapy, aggressive physiotherapy to prevent contractures, and a few medications that can be tried in individual patients to partially alleviate drooling, tremors, and myoclonic spasms. Free-radical scavengers such as alpha-tocopheral usually are recommended despite a lack of evidence of their efficacy.

Now that the ataxia-telangiectasia (A-T) gene has been isolated, it seems more pertinent than ever to carefully review the changes that occur in the various physiologic systems which are affected in ataxia-telangiectasia, trying to relate each facet of the syndrome to the functions of the gene. With the gene in hand, many new and old hypotheses are now testable. While it is clear that the gene functions both in the cytoplasm and in the nucleus, and that elucidating these functions is the present frontier of A-T research, the next frontier will involve translating how mistakes in single cells can misdirect entire cell populations and result in cerebellar degeneration, thymic dystrophy, and tumor formation.

THE ATAXIA-TELANGIECTASIA SYNDROME

The A-T syndrome varies little from family to family in its late stages.[1–6] Its primary features include (1) progressive gait and truncal ataxia with onset from 1 to 3 years of age, (2) progressively slurred speech, (3) oculomotor apraxia, i.e., an inability to follow an object across the visual fields, (4) oculocutaneous telangiectasia, usually by 6 years of age, (5) elevated serum alpha-fetoprotein, (6) frequent infections, with accompanying serum and cellular immunodeficiencies, (7) susceptibility to cancer, usually leukemia or lymphoma, (8) hypersensitivity to ionizing radiation, contraindicating the use of conventional doses of radiation therapy for cancer, and (9) reciprocal translocations that involve chromosomes 7 and 14 almost exclusively. Other features include premature aging and endocrine abnormalities. Figure 14-1 highlights some of the major features of this complex syndrome.

Neurology and Neuropathology

The most obvious and troubling characteristic of the A-T syndrome is the progressive cerebellar ataxia. Shortly after learning to walk, A-T children begin to stagger. By 10 years of age they are confined to a wheelchair for the remainder of their lives. The ataxia begins as purely truncal but within several years involves peripheral coordination as well. Deep tendon reflexes are decreased or absent in older patients; plantar reflexes are upgoing or absent. Slurred speech and oculomotor apraxia are noted early. Both horizontal and vertical saccadic eye movements are affected. Writing is affected by 7 or 8 years of age. Choreoathetosis is found in almost all these patients. Myclonic jerking and intention tremors

are present in about 25 percent. Drooling is a frequent complaint; this can sometimes be helped with medication (see "Therapy," below). All teenage A-T patients need help dressing, eating, washing, and using the toilet. The neurologic status of some patients appears to improve from 2 to 4 years, then begins to progress again; this is probably due to the rapid neurologic learning curve of young individuals. Muscle power is normal at first but wanes with disuse, especially in the legs. Arm strength generally remains. Contractures in fingers and toes are common in older patients but may be preventable through rigorous exercise (see "Therapy," below).

The typical patient with A-T is of normal intelligence, although slow responses make it difficult to support this by timed IQ testing. Many American and British patients have finished high school with good grades; some have finished college or university. A few seem to be minimally retarded.

The most obvious lesion in the central nervous system at postmortem examination is the paucity of Purkinje cells (PCs) in the cerebellum. About 10 years ago we wished to determine whether these cells are absent from birth or degenerate afterward. Knowing that basket cells form only around preexisting PCs, we sought to visualize basket cells by Bielschowsky silver staining. We showed that normal or nearly normal numbers of basket cells were present (Fig. 14-2). We therefore concluded that PC numbers must also have been normal at birth and degenerated after birth.[7–8]

We also found evidence suggesting that PC migration and arborization are not completely normal.[8] A significant number of ectopic PCs can be found in cerebellar sections from A-T patients from both undermigration and overmigration (Fig. 14-2). PCs make their last cell division at about 13 weeks of gestation and then begin to migrate toward the pial surface. Following the tracts of climbing fibers, they arrive at the single-cell PC layer during the fifth to seventh month of gestation. Thus, this lesion of ectopic PCs would most likely be expressed by the last trimester of pregnancy. This is the earliest known manifestation of the A-T defect.

It remains possible that PCs are not the primary A-T lesion and that the observed PC defects are due to other factors, such as an absence or abnormalities of supporting cells such as basket cells, mossy fibers, parallel fibers, climbing fibers, and glial cells. Anteriograde or retrograde degeneration of PCs would then occur, with the underlying lesion being either afferent or efferent to the PCs. Recently, Becker-Catania, in our laboratory, was able to demonstrate the presence of ATM message in PCs as well as in cells of the internal and external granular layers and in neurons of the dentate nucleus. We see ATM mRNA in both healthy and affected tis-

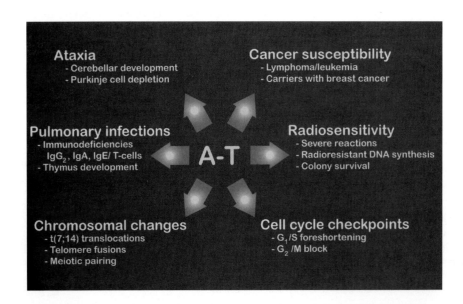

FIG. 14-1 The A-T syndrome.

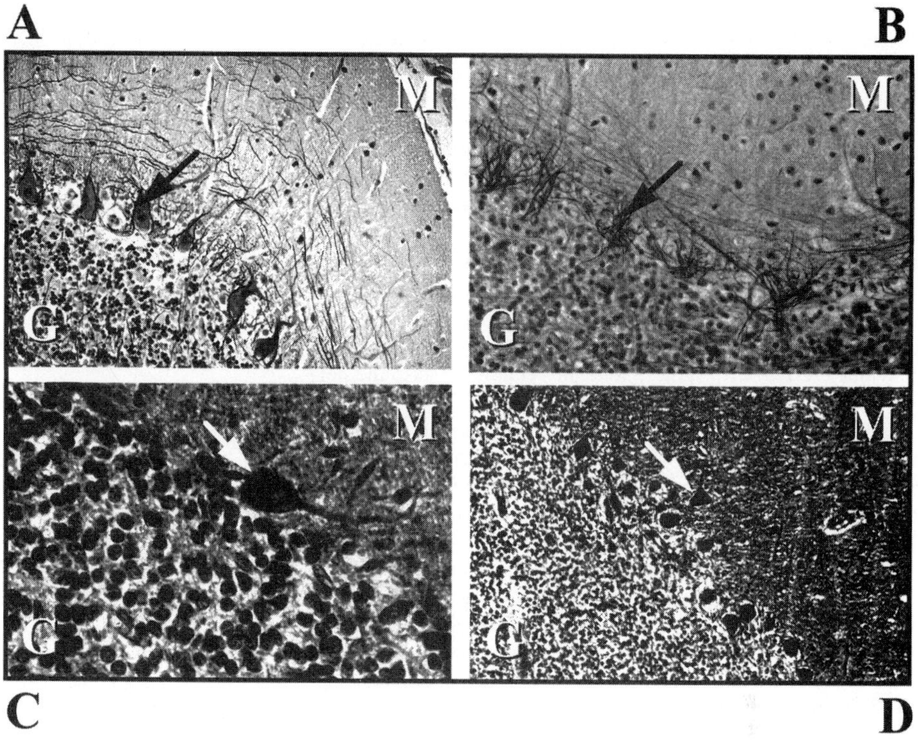

A

B

FIG. 14-2 Neuropathology. Photomicrographs of the cerebellum. M-molecular layer; G-granular cell layer. *A.* Bielschovsky stain of normal cerebellum (10×) showing basket cell fibers surrounding Purkinje cells (arrow). *B.* Bielschovsky stain of cerebellum from an A-T patient (10×) showing empty basket cells (arrow) in the Purkinje cell layer. *C.* In situ hybridization with ATM cDNA on normal infant cerebellum (40×) showing a Purkinje cell (arrow) with a positive peroxidase stain for ATM mRNA. *D.* In situ hybridization with ATM cDNA on cerebellum from an A-T patient (20×) showing ectopic (undermigrated) Purkinje cells (arrows) with a positive peroxidase stain for ATM mRNA. (Courtesy of S. Becker-Catania)

C

D

sues (Fig. 14-2). However, since most mutated ATM protein is unstable in A-T cells, the primary site of action for the ATM protein in the cerebellum remains undetermined.

Changes also have been noted in the dentate and olivary nuclei. The medulla shows neuroaxonal dystrophy.[9] Degenerative changes are seen in the substantia nigra. Diffuse demyelination in the posterior columns of the spinal cord was noted in some of the original autopsies[1] and is a progressive change. For further details of postmortem changes in A-T patients, the two lengthy reviews authored by Sedgwick and Boder should be consulted.[2,5]

Throughout the tissues of the bodies of A-T patients, nucleomegaly is a universal finding.[2,5] This is best seen in organs where nuclear morphology is usually very regular, such as the hepatic cords and renal tubules. Here it is obvious that the size of the nucleus is extremely variable in A-T tissues compared to normal. Some nuclei are very large, hyperchromatic (dark-staining), and irregular in shape. Nucleomegaly also is seen in association with normal ageing and in viral lesions. However, numerous studies have failed to demonstrate virus or viral particles in A-T cells, including an attempt by Gadjusek to inoculate primates with brain tissue extracts from two A-T patients.[5] It is entirely possible that the nucleomegaly seen in A-T tissues results from defective cell cycle checkpoints that lead to mitotic division without cell replication in random cells. Naeim et al.[10] demonstrated polyploidy (4n and 8n) in lymphoblastoid cell lines (LCLs) from A-T patients by flow cytometric cell cycle analysis.

Telangiectasia

Figure 14-3 shows a typical pattern of telangiectasia in a 12-year-old patient. Telangiectasia is discussed early in this chapter not because it is believed to be important in the pathogenesis of the disease but because its appearance aids in diagnosis. Telangiectasias can be seen not only on the conjunctiva but on the ears, over the bridge of the nose, in the anticubital fossae, and behind the knees in some patients. Occasional patients have them all over their bodies. Telangiectasias usually do not appear until about 4 to 6 years of age, and although they are a hallmark of the disorder, they sometimes do not

become obvious for several years after the onset of ataxia. Elderly individuals without A-T occasionally have similar telangiectasias in many of the same places. Boder felt that telangiectasias appear in response to ultraviolet light exposure; however, that would not explain finding them behind the knee in some patients. About 5 percent of A-T patients never develop prominent telangiectasias.

Telangiectasias are composed of dilated capillaries. The pattern of these capillaries does not resemble a response to angiogenic factors but a response of endothelial cells to a dilatory stimulus. However, Van Meir et al. have shown that at least one pathway for inhibition of angiogenesis is through p53,[11] and p53 expression is reduced in A-T cells (see "Cell Cycle Aberrations," below). Little research has been done on this. With rare exceptions,[1,12–15] telangiectasias are not found internally at surgery or at postmortem examination, nor do ATM knockout mice manifest telangiectasias.[16] However, these mice die at 2 to 4 months of age, and this may be too early to see telangiectasias. Amromin et al.[15] noted widely distributed gliovascular nodules in the cerebral white matter and to a lesser extent in the brain stem and spinal cord postmortem in a 32-year-old patient. These nodules consisted of dilated capillary loops, many with fibrin thrombi, with perivascular hemorrhages and hemosiderosis, surrounded by demyelinated white matter, reactive gliosis, and numerous atypical astrocytes. These nodules were not seen in the cerebellum and have not been observed in other postmortem examinations of younger patients.

Radiosensitivity in Vivo and in Vitro

Over the past 30 years, radiation therapists have observed that when A-T patients with cancer are treated with conventional doses of ion-

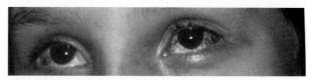

FIG. 14-3 Characteristic telangiectasias over the conjunctiva of a 12-year-old A-T patient.

izing radiation, they develop life-threatening sequelae characteristic of much higher doses.[17–21] This radiosensitivity can also be demonstrated in vitro using fibroblasts from A-T homozygotes, which are sensitive not only to ionizing radiation but to a variety of radiomimetic and free-radical-producing agents.[22,23]

Early radiosensitivity assays for A-T measure colony formation efficiency; cells are irradiated and then cultured, and the number of colonies that grow are scored after a measured time period. Fibroblasts from A-T heterozygotes form colonies with an efficiency that is intermediate between A-T homozygosity and normal[22]; the same observation can be made using neocarzinostatin.[24] In general, however, colony-forming efficiency is not a reliable way to detect individual heterozygotes.[23–26] Many other methods have been used to identify A-T heterozygotes; none are reliable because the normal and heterozygous data sets overlap.[10,27–31]

Now that A-T heterozygotes (carriers) can be identified more easily by genetic testing, in families with prior affected patients physicians are confronted with the dilemma of having to advise carriers about the risks of radiation exposure. Unfortunately, there are as yet no clinical studies on which to base such advice. For example, data are lacking on whether the in vitro radiosensitivity of heterozygotes has any clinical correlate, i.e., unusual reactions to standard radiologic procedures. One can only make the general recommendation that exposure to all types of ionizing radiation be minimized in persons suspected of being A-T carriers, remembering that two-thirds of the sibs of A-T patients are likely to be carriers as well as the parents. Whether routine dental x-rays should be recommended in A-T patients is also an unresolved issue.

ATM knockout mice that are heterozygous (ATM+/−) do not show an abnormal response to total-body irradiation.[16] Some caveats: (1) these studies are preliminary, (2) they have not been repeated or confirmed, (3) only one specific site in the ATM gene was disrupted in these experiments, and (4) knockout mouse models seldom mimic a human disease in all facets of the syndrome. Swift's epidemiologic data suggest that exposure of heterozygotes to myelograms and other diagnostic x-rays may increase their cancer risk.[32] There is also cause for concern about mammograms in female A-T carriers, who appear to be at an increased risk of breast cancer (see below). The recommendation at this writing is that mammograms be continued on the same age-dependent schedule used for noncarriers but that the most up-to-date mammography machines be employed to minimize exposure to only a few rads. The added risk of cancer to such women is only slightly increased (from 1.5 in 100 from annual mammography screening doses in noncarriers to perhaps 2 in 100 in A-T carriers), and this should be compared to a 1 in 9 natural lifetime risk and the 30 percent reduction in mortality from annual mammography screening in women over age 40.[33–35]

Epidemiologic and radiosensitivity studies of A-T family members further suggest that many cancer patients in general may be receiving the wrong doses of radiotherapy: too much for A-T heterozygotes and too little for noncarriers.[33,34,36] Considering that 5 percent of cancer patients under 46 years of age may be A-T carriers and intermediate in their radiosensitivity,[37] this issue could involve many thousands of patients annually (see "Cancer Susceptibility," below). Some x-ray dosage regimens are first tested empirically on cadres of cancer patients, and if those cadres contain up to 5 percent A-T carriers, one can easily imagine how radiation sequelae might be more apt to appear in the A-T carriers, thereby lowering the "safe" doses defined for everyone else. Once A-T carrier testing can be implemented on a wide scale, these issues may be resolved.

Although radiation damage to DNA has been used for many years as a laboratory tool for characterizing the phenotype of A-T cells, it should be remembered that A-T cells usually are not exposed to irradiation in vivo. Thus, the radiosensitivity of A-T cells is a laboratory artifact. Despite this, the complex A-T syndrome develops quite uniformly in most affected patients. From this, one might conclude that the substrate for the ATM protein is ubiquitous in the human body and that whatever DNA damage occurs must result from a naturally recurring insult to all cells. Oxidative stress and the normal production of DNA-damaging free-radical products of metabolism are certainly good candidates for the naturally recurring insult.[38] Although many attempts have been made to demonstrate defective DNA repair in A-T cells, this has not been demonstrated convincingly.[39] Recent observations suggest that it is the inability to *sense* this damage that is defective in A-T cells, not the actual mechanisms of repair.[38,40]

Cancer Susceptibility

During their shortened lifetimes, 38 percent of A-T homozygotes develop a malignancy.[41] This represents a 61- and a 184-fold increase in European-American and African-American patients, respectively, Roughly 85 percent of these malignancies are either leukemia or lymphoma. In younger patients, an acute lymphocytic leukemia is most often of T-cell origin,[42,43] although the pre-B common to ALL of childhood (HLADR+, CD10+, CD5+, and CD19+) has also been seen in A-T patients. When leukemia develops in older A-T homozygotes, it is usually an aggressive T-cell leukemia with a morphology similar to that of chronic lymphoblastic leukemia, hence the old name T-CLL[42–45]; T-cell prolymphocytic leukemia (T-PLL) is the equivalent modern nomenclature.[46] The leukemic cells often contain a translocation and/or inversion involving the T-cell receptor alpha chain gene complex at 14q11-12[47–49] (see "Chromosomal Instability," below). Myeloid leukemia has not been reported in A-T patients. Lymphomas in A-T homozygotes, in contrast to leukemias, are usually B-cell types, although T-cell lymphomas also have been observed. As A-T patients are living longer, more nonlymphoid cancers are being observed. Several of our older patients have developed breast cancer and melanoma. Cancers of the stomach and ovary have been reported.[5,42] When fibroids or leiomyomas are found in A-T females, a special effort should be made by the pathologist to quantitate high power fields for mitotic figures, since leiomyosarcomas of precocious onset have been reported.[50] For specific lists of other tumor types and frequencies, see refs. 41, 42, and 44.

A-T heterozygotes are also believed to be cancer-prone, perhaps accounting for as many as 5 percent of all cancer patients under 46 years of age in the United States.[37] They are not clinically distinguishable from normal individuals. An increased incidence of breast cancer in female A-T heterozygotes has been reported in the United States, England, and Norway.[32,51–53] In the U.S. study, the risk of breast cancer was found to be fivefold higher among the mothers of A-T homozygotes than in a comparable female population.[32,52] Based on this observation, Swift et al. estimated that between 8 and 18 percent of all breast cancer patients may be A-T heterozygotes.[37] This would imply that ATM is the most common cancer susceptibility gene in the general population. While the issue is far from settled, several recent genetic studies of breast cancer patients have failed to produce convincing evidence in support of Swift's predictions. Croce and coworkers[54] looked for ATM mutations in tumor tissue from 38 sporadic breast cancers. They first screened this material by single-stranded conformational polymorphism (SSCP) gels and then sequenced any regions suspected of harboring mutations. They found no significant mutations. We similarly screened cDNAs from nine breast cancer patients who had been radiation technologists, using a combination of protein truncation testing (PTT) and conformation sensitive gel electrophoresis (CSGE). We found no significant mutations (unpublished). Spurr and coworkers[56] looked for a link to BRCA1 and BRCA2 in 63 early-onset breast cancer families; 55 percent linked to BRCA1, and 45 percent linked to BRCA2. This implied that none linked to 11q22-23, as Wooster et al. and Cortessis et al. had reported earlier.[57,58] When asked whether their data rule out a role for ATM in breast cancer susceptibility, these workers felt that late-onset or sporadic breast cancers may still be related to ATM mutations. This interpretation would be compatible with the epidemiologic data from A-T families showing that the breast cancer seen among A-T mothers (who are obligate heterozygotes) peaks in the age group of 45 to 54,[52] not really an early-onset pattern.

FitzGerald et al.,[55] using PTT, detected ATM mutations in 2/401 women with sporadic early-onset breast cancer. They found mutations in 2/202 control samples. Recently, Athma et al.[59] have once again noted an increased incidence of breast cancer in A-T heterozygotes who were identified by haplotyping members of extended A-T families. Several independent studies of ATM knockout mice have confirmed the extreme cancer susceptibility of the homozygotes; virtually all homozygous mice died with massive, widely metastasized malignant thymic lymphomas.[16,169] Heterozygous animals have not yet shown tumors. A report by Carter et al. found significant loss of heterozygosity in sporadic breast cancers across chromosome 11q22-23.[60] Although this region includes the ATM gene, it measures ~35 cM and probably includes more than 1000 other genes as well. Thus, the contribution of ATM mutations to familial breast cancer is likely to be low, with ATM perhaps playing a more important role in a sporadic, low-penetrance form of breast cancer.

The most frequently reported cancers in American heterozygotes have been in breast, trachea/bronchus/lung, stomach, prostate, melanoma, and gallbladder.[32] In Italy and Costa Rica, gastric cancer has been especially noteworthy. Among 64 A-T parents and grandparents in Costa Rica, half the 12 cancers reported were gastric cancer.[61] (Costa Rica ranks among the top three countries in the world for stomach cancer in the general population, making it difficult to interpret these observations.) In Italian families, 7 of 20 cancers in grandparents were gastric cancer.[62] Stomach cancer has been reported in homozygotes as well,[42,44] including two families in which both affected sibs developed stomach cancer. Despite this, Morrell et al.[41] did not note any increase in stomach cancers in A-T homozygotes. Perhaps the most exciting new observation is that most individuals who develop T-PLL are probably constitutional A-T heterozygotes, the second ATM allele being somatically disabled in the leukemia cells by a second "hit".[84,129] This result would categorize ATM as a tumor suppressor gene, in addition to its growing list of other roles.

Cell Cycle Aberrations

Important checkpoints monitor the progress of the cell cycle and prevent mutagenic damage to DNA from being fixed into future cell generations. The G1 checkpoint prevents replication of a damaged DNA template; the G2 checkpoint prevents segregation of damaged chromosomes.[64] Kastan et al.[65,66] showed that A-T cells have a delayed radiation-induced increase in p53, compared to normal cells. p53, dubbed the "guardian of the genome," acts to suppress normal cell cycle progression at G1 until DNA repairs have been completed. (For reviews pertinent to A-T, see Refs. 38, 40, and 67.) It accomplishes this by binding DNA at sequence-specific sites, thereby transcriptionally activating a signal-transduction cascade. In so doing, p53 functions as a tumor suppressor. Cells from p53 knockout mice, lacking both normal alleles of p53 (p53-/-), fail to observe the G1 checkpoint; they do not experience G1 arrest after irradiation nor do they show neurologic abnormalities, immune defects, or problems with sterility.[40,67,68] The phosphorylation of replication factor A (RPA) is similarly delayed in

A-T cells after irradiation. Both p53 and RPA may be directly phosphorylated by ATM.[69] Lavin and coworkers confirmed the p53 expression delay and have demonstrated that c-*abl* binds to an SH$_3$ domain on the ATM molecule.[70] The fact that the newly cloned A-T gene has a kinase domain[71-73] and protein kinase activity[137] supports the significance of these studies. The strong association of multiple types of cancer with p53 deficiency,[67,74-77] further suggests that involvement of this pathway in apoptosis and in the pathogenesis of A-T may help explain the increased frequency of cancer.

Interestingly, p53$-/-$ mutants are not radiosensitive.[78] Thus, yet another mechanism must account for this facet of the A-T syndrome. Much work still needs to be done before the role of ATM proteins in intracellular signaling can be understood. For example, despite much evidence of the inefficiency of G1/S, S, and G2/M checkpoints in A-T cells, holding A-T cells in G0 for up to 7 days does not improve their postirradiation survival,[40] suggesting that even these checkpoint defects may not be the crucial common denominator underlying A-T pathogenesis. Recent evidence presented by Jung and associates[79,80] implicates the NF-κB and IκB-α proteins in ATM function; the ATM protein appears to phosphorylate IκB-α, thereby activating the transcription factor NF-κB.[81] These findings also support observations of increased radiation-induced apoptosis in cell lines derived from A-T patients.[40,76,77]

When DNA synthesis of irradiated fibroblasts is measured, A-T homozygotes show a characteristic dose response curve (Fig. 14-4) that is diagnostic of the disease.[82] This phenomenon is called radioresistant DNA synthesis (RDS) because unlike normal cells that temporarily halt the synthesis of new DNA after irradiation damage, A-T cells simply continue into S phase of the cell cycle. Later experiments that attempted to complement RDS and other radiomimetic features of A-T cells by transfection found, however, that these phenomena often were dissociated.[6,83] Thus, RDS most likely reflects a cell cycle checkpoint failure at S phase that is indepen-

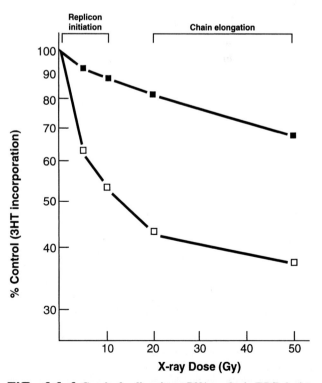

FIG. 14-4 Graph of radioresistant DNA synthesis (RDS) depicting theoretical targets of radiation at increasing doses of radiation. The major defect in A-T (black squares) is seen at very low radiation doses, affecting replicon initiation, while chain elongation appears normal in A-T, as depicted by the normal slope of that portion of the curve.

dent of other radiosensitivity phenotypes of A-T cells. Using RDS, heterozygous cells cannot be distinguished from normals.

The shape of the RDS curve (Fig. 14-4) for A-T cells has been insightfully interpreted by Painter[84] as having two components, one reflecting replicon initiation and the other reflecting chain elongation. The second component is determined by the slope of the curve above 2 kilorads (krad), and this slope does not differ in normal and A-T fibroblasts. The early component, however, is essentially missing from the A-T curves, suggesting that replicon initiation is quite abnormal. Painter further suggested that while in unirradiated normal cells initiation occurs synchronously at the origins of a cluster of replicons and that in irradiated normal cells damage to one replicon inhibits the entire cluster, in irradiated A-T cells damage to one replicon inhibits only that replicon; i.e., the damage is not sensed or translated to the rest of the cluster, and chain elongation near the growing forks is not curbed. Thus, radiation to A-T cells blocks initiation of individual replicons rather than blocking the initiation of clusters of replicons.[39,85,86] Hand and Gautschi[87] provided evidence that one single-strand break may inactivate the initiation of as many as a hundred replicons. Although Painter's interpretation of the RDS curve was put forth over 10 years ago, it remains a very attractive hypothesis for explaining one facet of the pathogenesis of A-T. Recent evidence suggests that ATM may act as part of a very large protein complex.

Immunodeficiency

At postmortem examination, virtually every A-T homozygote has a small embryonic-like thymus.[12] In the late 1960s and again in the early 1980s, many attempts were made to characterize the immunodeficiencies of A-T patients.[88] No single consistent abnormality could be identified in all A-T patients; affected sibs often differ in the degree and profile of their immunodeficiencies. In a review of British patients, Woods and Taylor[89] noted normal immunologic function in 27 of 70 patients. Only 10 percent had severe immunodeficiencies.

When the genomic arrangement of the IGH V, D, J, and H gene subfamilies was first described, we noted that the immunoglobulin (Ig) classes that were most frequently decreased in A-T patients were those with the greatest genomic distances between the variable genes and the respective heavy chain genes;[90] roughly 60 to 80 percent of A-T homozygotes manifest an IgA, IgE, and/or IgG2 deficiency.[12,88,89–95,121,122] whereas serum levels of IgM, IgG1, and IgG3 are usually normal. This suggests that B cells from these patients have a maturational problem with Ig class switching, perhaps based on a recombinase-based deficiency. On a similar note, an increased proportion of T gamma/delta cells noted in one early study suggested a maturational delay in T cells; however, this was before normal T gamma/delta cell ranges had been clearly defined and has not been generally confirmed. IgM levels are occasionally extremely high (see below); this could be based on a similar defective maturational mechanism that arrests some B cells at the IgM-producing stage. However, when V(D)J recombination was examined in A-T cells, both signal and coding joint formation were normal.[96–98] Approximately half of A-T patients with immunodeficiencies have T-cell deficiencies. CD4+/CD45RA+ (naive) T cells are decreased in some patients.[99] Responses to antigens are poor, especially allogeneic antigens.[12,88,100–105] T-cell cytotoxicity to influenza-infected target cells is reduced.[106] T lymphocytes show abnormally fast capping of FITC-labeled concanavalin A.[88] Markedly elevated cyclic AMP levels have been observed in T cells from A-T patients.[88] Neutrophil chemotaxis was reported to be decreased in some studies and normal in others. Similarly, NK cell activity and NK cell levels have been described as normal, decreased, or increased in various studies.[88,107,108] Some of these discrepancies no doubt reflect the transient immune status of patients with active infections. Although 91 percent of Costa Rican A-T patients had diminished PHA responses, 65 percent of this patient cohort has the same mutation; thus, this sample would be skewed against some features and would favor others and probably has little bearing on patients around the world with other mutations. Further analyses of this cohort are under way. Knockout ATM mice have many of these same immune defects; despite this, T and B cell precursors are present in normal numbers.[169]

Hyper-IgM with Ataxia-Telangiectasia

Elevated serum IgM levels are fairly common in A-T patients, arising perhaps as compensation for low IgA, IgE, and IgG2 levels. However, occasional A-T patients with elevated AFPs, bulbar telangiectasia, and typical progressive cerebellar ataxia have an extended syndrome that may include splenomegaly, lymphoadenopathy, neutropenia, thrombocytopenia, and congestive heart failure from high blood viscosity.[109,110] Postirradiation colony survival studies[111] in six of these families suggest a level of radiosensitivity that is intermediate between normals and that seen in other A-T patients (see "Differential Diagnosis," below). In three families, ATM mutations have already been identified (unpublished). However, in one of these families, the two affected children are discordant for hyper-IgM. In another family, the cerebellar pathology was not typical of A-T[109] in that it failed to show depletion of PCs. [It was labeled as a "variant" family for the consortium linkage studies. Despite this, we recently identified a homozygous point mutation that deletes 64 nucleotides (nt) from the cDNA.] Thus, while hyper-IgM and A-T have been observed together in a number of families, the underlying pathology and genetics remain obscure.

Alpha-Fetoprotein

Serum alpha-fetoprotein (AFP) levels are elevated in most A-T patients.[112,113] AFP is thought to have a suppressor effect on the developing immune system and on immune function.[114] Although serum AFP levels can be very useful in confirming a suspected diagnosis of A-T, approximately 5 to 10 percent of typical A-T patients have normal AFP levels. This is independent of race, sex, or complementation group and is usually concordant in affected sibs. AFP levels do not increase with patient age.[89] Serum AFP levels still elevated from infancy sometimes can be misleading in children under 2 years, in whom normal ranges have not been carefully defined by most clinical laboratories. Thus, it is best to avoid using AFP as a diagnostic criterion until after 2 years of age. Other causes of elevated AFP, such as liver disease, familial hyper-AFP, and the presence of a teratoma, are not likely to confound a diagnosis of A-T. Ishiguro et al.[115] showed that the lectin-binding profile of elevated AFPs from A-T patients was probably of hepatic origin, and although no evidence of liver disease is present at postmortem examination, other liver proteins are often increased as well, such as serum glutamic-pyruvic transaminase (SGPT), serum glutamic-oxalacetic transaminase (SGOT), alkaline phosphatase, and carcinoembryonic antigen.[90,112]

With the routine monitoring of AFP in amniotic fluid now in vogue, the question is occasionally asked whether amniotic AFP levels are elevated when the fetus has A-T. AFP levels are very high in all fetuses, peaking at about 13 weeks of gestation.[112] In two cases that had been diagnosed by prenatal testing and in which a decision had been made by the parents not to terminate the pregnancies, amniotic AFP levels were within normal ranges. A cord blood AFP was elevated in one of these patients and remained so over the next 3 years. (In the other patient, cord blood was not tested.) Thus, although the serum AFP level of a fetus is high, there appears to be no extravasation or secretion into the amniotic fluid of A-T-affected fetuses, as occurs in open neural tube defects and Down syndrome.

Chromosomal Instability

A-T homozygotes show nonrandom chromosomal aberrations in lymphocytes, such as translocations and inversions, which preferentially involve chromosomal breakpoints at 14q11, 14q32, 7q35, 7p14, 2p11, and 22q11.[43,117] These aberrations appeared to correlate generally with the regions of the T-cell receptor (TCR-alpha, -beta, and -gamma) and B-cell receptor (IGH, IGK, and IGL) gene complexes. Since these six sites contain the only gene complexes in the genome that are known to require site-specific gene rearrangement/recombination before expressing a mature protein, it was logical to examine V(D)J recombination mechanisms in A-T cells. As was noted above, signal and coding joint formation are both normal.[96–98] When we examined the chromosomes of fibroblasts from eight A-T homozygotes, all with typical 7:14 translocations in their lymphocytes, the fibroblast aberrations were totally random.[117,118] Hecht and Hecht studied almost 50,000 amniotic fluid cell metaphases; of 37 translocations in that non-AT sample, none involved chromosomes 7 and 14.[119] This is intriguing when one considers that fibroblasts and amniotic cells express the radiosensitivity defect. Heterozygotes show t(7;14) translocations in lymphocytes, but only in 1 to 2 percent of metaphases.[119]

In some patients, cell clones with the above breakpoints expand,[45,120] sometimes accounting for 100 percent of the lymphocytes that are karyotyped. Despite this, lymphocyte counts remain within the normal range for years thereafter. Some of these clones have been followed for 10 to 20 years by us and others.[48,118] These clones tend to evolve, with subclones adding new rearrangements, such as inv(14;14)(q11;q32), i(8q), and 6q-, in addition to many other smaller clones. Eventually, such patients develop T-PLL, previously referred to as T-CLL (T-cell chronic lymphblastic leukemia).[45,46] Affected sibs usually are not concordant for developing such clones, thus implicating somatic influences superimposed upon an A-T genotype.

These clonal expansions have allowed the breakpoint sites to be analyzed by molecular techniques. Three types of patients have been studied: (1) A-T patients with nonleukemic clones, (2) A-T patients with leukemic clones, and (3) non-A-T patients with similar cytogenetic translocations and T-PLL. Thanks to many years of perseverance by Taylor and coworkers[124] in trying to pinpoint the breakpoints of these translocations or inversions, a fascinating story is now emerging that is quite similar to that of *myc* in Burkitt lymphoma. The A-T expanded clones always have one of the TCR sites, usually TCR-alpha, juxtaposed to another family of genes located proximal to, but not actually within, the B-cell receptor gene complexes. The most common and best-studied translocations are those involving 14q11 (TCR-alpha) and a breakpoint cluster region ~10 Mb proximal to the IGH locus at 14q32. Within ~400 kb, at least eight such breakpoints have been identified in A-T patients with and without leukemia and in several non-A-T patients with T-PLL. This region centers on the TCL-1 (T-cell leukemia-1) gene,[123] the 1.3-kb transcript of which is preferentially expressed in immature (and leukemic) B and T cells. Circulating mature lymphocytes do not express this gene. Leukemia cells without the t(14;14) or inv(14;14) do not express TCL-1.

An occasional A-T patient has a large t(X;14)(q28;q11) clone, including at least two who have developed T-CLL/T-PLL and one without leukemia when last studied.[45] The breakpoints at Xq28

cluster to within a few kilobases in a region of ~70 kb proximal to the factor VIII gene. This region contains the genes c6.1A and c6.1B. (The latter gene is believed to be the crucial one in these translocations, since two of the breakpoints fall within the first exon of c6.1B, also known as MTCP1, "mature T-cell proliferation-1."[124–126]) Most interesting, c6.1B has homology with TCL-1 (40 percent identity, 60 percent similarity) and is a mitochrondrial protein.[127] TCL-1 and MTCP-1 also share three-dimensional structure. TCL-1 prevents apoptosis and is p53-independent. Since TCR/TCL-1 translocations do not by themselves cause leukemia, another factor must interact with the protein product or products resulting from the translocations. This factor is most likely the ATM gene product, based on the recent finding that most non-AT patients with T-PLL are constitutive A-T heterozygotes, with the leukemia cells actually carrying two defective ATM genes.[84]

Constitutional cytogenetic defects involving translocations or deletions at 11q22-23 have not been observed in A-T homozygotes, even though karyotypes of >500 patients have been examined worldwide. Many cytogenetic reports on children with suspected A-T return labeled "insufficient metaphases for analysis." This problem occurs because the lymphocyte response to mitogens, such as phytohemagglutinin (PHA), is often weak or delayed in A-T patients, and when cell cultures are harvested routinely at 48 h, few cells are dividing. Harvest results can be improved by using a double dose of mitogen and harvesting at 72 h or at several time points.

Telomeric fusions are observed frequently in A-T patients, a provocative finding considering the strong homology between ATM and the yeast Tel-1 mutant gene.[71] Tumor cells and senescent cells of normal persons can also show such fusions. Further understanding of this observation was limited until 1988, when the DNA structure of the telomere and the mechanisms of its maintainance were elucidated.[132,133] When the role of telomerase in telomere stability was introduced,[133,134] it was logical to examine telomerase levels in A-T cells. Pandita et al.[130] showed that although the telomeres of A-T cell lines are shorter than normal cells, telomerase activity was normal.

Metcalfe et al.[135] demonstrated significant telomere shortening in A-T peripheral blood lymphocytes (PBLs). PBLs from 20 A-T patients showed an average loss of 95 ± 23 bp (base pairs) per year of age, compared to a loss of 35 ± 9 bp per year in normals. The preleukemic T-cell clones described above showed an even greater loss of 158 ± 9 bp per year and are especially prone to show telomeric fusions.

Accelerated telomeric shortening is probably a characteristic of all rapidly dividing A-T cells. It is of further interest that telomeric shortening is associated with senescence of CD28−/CD8+ T cells in AIDS patients and centenarians[136]; in both situations this may account for waning T-cell immunity. A similar mechanism might explain the abnormal development and function of the immune system in A-T patients. Thus, the precocious onset of cancers such as basal cell carcinoma,[2] leiomyosarcoma,[50] and T-PLL[124] may reflect (1) the basic propensity of their cells to accelerate telomere shortening and (2) waning immunity. This would also provide a p53-independent, radiation-independent pathway to cancer susceptibility in A-T patients.

When the ATM gene was isolated and sequenced, it was noted to have strong homology to the yeast *tel1* gene, primarily through sharing a region of PI-3 kinase homology and secondarily through sharing weak homology with rad3.[137–141] (Ref. 141 contains a comprehensive analysis of homologies between kinase, rad3, RH3 and FRB domains.) Rad3 is a fission yeast gene containing helicase motifs and required for G2 arrest after DNA damage.[142,143] Of the large family of genes sharing PI-3 kinase homology with ATM, only *tel1*, *mec1* (another yeast gene), and *mei41* (of Drosophila) also share some rad3 homology. (The rad3 homology of *tel1* is admittedly weak.) A growing body of evidence suggests that *tel1*, *mec1*, and ATM perform overlapping functions. Of the three, only *mec1* is an essential gene. In yeast, *mec1* (mitosis entry checkpoint) is required for regulation of the S/M and G2/M checkpoints,[144] the rate of ongoing S phase in response to damage,[145] and meiotic recombination.[145,146] Cells with mutations in *mec1* (also called ESR1 or SAD3) proceed directly to mitosis when DNA replication is inhibited with hydroxurea and are unable to delay the onset of mitosis (G2/M) on induction of DNA damage.[147] RAD53 is also regulated by MEC1 and Tel1.[147] Although *tel1* mutants are not radiosensitive and *mec1* mutants are, *tel1/mec1* double mutants somehow synergize to increase the sensitivity to DNA damage from ionizing radiation and radiomimetic drugs.[141] The human homologue of *mec1*, called FRP1 (FRAP-related protein) or ATR (AT-related Rad3-related), has recently been cloned and maps to chromosome 3q22-q24.[141,148] It plays a reciprocal role to ATM on synapsing chromosomes during meiotic recombination,[139] interacting with Rad51 and BRCA1.

Complementation Groups

Fusion of fibroblasts from unrelated patients will often correct or "complement" their radiosensitivity.[149–151] Five complementation groups have been defined (Groups A, C, D, E, and V1).[151] The first four groups are phenotypically identical and can be distinguished from one another only by complementation studies. It was unclear whether these complementation groups represented several distinct A-T genes, perhaps forming part of a common enzymatic pathway or coding for parts of a common multimeric molecule, or alternatively, whether the complementation groups represented intragenic mutations of a single gene. It was also possible that complementation was a nongenetic phenomenon. In 1988, we localized the gene for A-T Group A (ATA) to chromosome 11q22-23.[152] In 1991, in a collaboration with Shiloh's lab, A-T Group C (ATC) was localized to the same region.[153] Between 1990 and 1994, 26 genes were shown to complement A-T fibroblasts; none localized to chromosome 11q23.1.[6,40,154,155] No convincing evidence for genetic heterogeneity was ever found in the linkage analysis studies despite such expectations. In 1995, Savitsky et al. identified part of a single gene (ATM) in which mutations were found for all four major complementation groups.[72] Most interesting is the fact that one homozygous mutation is present in both a Group C patient and a Group E patient, suggesting either that complementation groups in A-T are somewhat artifactual or that assigning patients to complementation groups is somewhat error-prone. To date, no laboratory has confirmed whether the cells from these two patients complement each other. Most likely this reflects the fact that complementation group assignment by fusion of A-T fibroblasts is extremely tedious and that no laboratory worldwide has performed such studies since around 1990.

Complementation of A-T cells by gene transfections was a commonly used approach to cloning the gene. Many genes complement various facets of the radiophenotype. These complementing genes obviously interact in some way with the ATM gene, the protein, or the signal transduction pathway. Some must bypass the ATM block in A-T cells and might provide exciting therapeutic opportunities for replacement therapy in A-T patients.[156] Despite the lack of success of the cloning experiments, complementation may provide a useful way of identifying functional domains in the ATM molecule.

Genetics

A-T is transmitted as autosomal recessive.[1–6] The incidence of A-T has been estimated at 1 in 40,000 to 100,000 live births, while the gene frequency is believed to be as high as 1 to 3 percent of the general population.[4] All races are affected. Despite the fact that the A-T gene affects so many different and apparently unrelated systems, the disease is inherited in each family as a single autosomal recessive gene defect. It is unclear why, in an autosomal recessive disorder, so many of the parents of British, Italian, and American patients are unrelated. This is borne out by the recent finding that most A-T patients worldwide are compound heterozygotes, i.e., have two different mutations.[72,157] The large size of the gene certainly provides a large target for new mutations. Recent studies also suggest that gametogenesis is abnormal in ATM knockout mice[16] and that mitotic and meiotic recombination is increased in A-T patients.[76,158] Furthermore, as was discussed above, the ATM gene shares homology with *mec1* in yeast and *mei41* in *Drosophila*,[40,141] and both are meiotic recombination defective mutants.[40,159] Whether this would affect heterozygous parents in A-T families sufficiently to influence the incidence of affected fetuses remains to be clarified. Recombination fractions in A-T families (i.e., in the parents) were normal across a 40 cM range of chromosome 11q22-23.[161]

Claims that "A-T is not always a recessive disorder"[45,160] are misleading and belie the consortium experience of having localized the ATM gene to within less than 0.5 cM by using a model that assumed autosomal recessive inheritance in 176 families from eight countries.[161,162] Families that do not link to 11q22-23 will have mutations in other genes, and other names will have to be given to those "AT-like" disorders (see "Ataxia-Telangiectasia Variants," below).

The rate of spontaneous mutations is unknown. However, of the 176 consortium families, all but 5 linked to chromosome 11q23.1.[161,162] (A sixth family with two affected children now links.) Since linkage rules out spontaneous mutations, only these five could harbor spontaneous mutations. Using the ratio of 5:176 and a gene frequency estimate of 0.01, mutation rate estimates approximate 1.5×10^{-4} percent. This is rather high even for a large gene. Of course, if the ATM gene product really affects gametogenesis,[16,139,169] it may not be appropriate to apply standard genetic algorithms, based on Hardy-Weinberg equilibrium, to the existing epidemiologic data.[163,164] It may also be that some young patients succumb to malignancies before a diagnosis of A-T can be recognized, further skewing the data.

Endocrine Defects

Very little research has been done on endocrine defects in A-T patients. This may change considering that ATM knockout mice have problems with both spermatogenesis and ovulation.[16,39,169] Gonadal streaks, absent or hypoplastic ovaries, dysgerminomas, and undeveloped fallopian tubes have been observed at postmortem examination in both mice[16] and human patients.[2] Laboratory tests of pituitary function reveal no consistent abnormality.

In stark contrast to the earlier statement that "female hypogonadism with sexual infantilism is found consistently [in A-T patients],"[2,5] most female patients followed by the author have normal menstrual cycles, and although menstruction sometimes starts late, cycles come at regular intervals. There is no other evidence as to whether these patients ovulate normally. Anecdotally, some long-lived female patients may have entered menarche prematurely. Most male patients followed by the author have developed normal secondary sex characteristics. Some patients can have erections and even ejaculate. Studies of sperm haplotyping on semen from several A-T patients have documented that some actually produce sperm. None have fathered a child.

Some patients develop an insulin-resistant diabetes, usually in the late teens. This is characterized by hyperglycemia without glycosuria or ketosis.[165,166] Other forms of diabetes, such as juvenile diabetes mellitus and late-onset diabetes, have been observed by the author quite frequently among nonaffected members of A-T families. A genetic imprinting model has been considered; however, this would not explain the pattern of diabetes in these families.

Premature Ageing

Many of the chromosomal instability syndromes, such as A-T, Fanconi anemia, xeroderma pigmentosum, and Bloom syndrome, show progeroid features.[167] Young A-T patients often have strands of gray hairs and develop keratoses, and precocious basal cell carcinoma has been reported.[2,42] Some of these findings may reflect either premature menarche or the accelerated shortening of telomeres described above[135] (see "Chromosomal Instability"). However, thymic dystrophy and lymphoid depletion are also characteristic of ageing and may be secondary to recombination defects during T-cell maturation rather than to telomeric shortening. Autoantibody formation is also found in both ageing populations and A-T patients[9,168,170] (see the discussion in Ref. 170).

Postmortem examinations of older patients also show progeric changes, such as neurofibrillary tangles in large neurons of the cerebral cortex, hippocampus, basal ganglia, and spinal cord, similar to those seen in Alzheimer disease.[15] Lipofuscin granules have been found in many neurons, satellite cells of the dorsal ganglia, and Schwann cells. Further, Marinesco bodies seen in the pigmented neurons of the substantia nigra in A-T patients are considered signs of precocious ageing.[171]

Other Findings

Among Costa Rican families with classical A-T, about 40 percent of patients have clubbing of the fingertips, a finding usually associated with poorly oxygenated blood. These A-T children do not have cardiac defects. Most, but not all, live in San José, which is 3700 feet above sea level, not high enough to aggravate most cardiac problems. The mutations in these families are known and the clubbing does not associate with a particular mutation (see "Patient Mutations," below). It is possible that as part of their A-T syndrome these patients also have a pulmonary abnormality that compromises the oxygenation of their blood, such as microscopic arteriovenous fistulas or an anomolous bronchial tree.[197] However, this is purely speculative; at this writing, we have no explanation for the clubbing in Costa Rican A-T patients.[61]

Many of the Costa Rican patients also have hypertrichosis.[61] This has been noted in other A-T patients as well.[5] Considering the diverse endocrinologic abnormalities that have been described in A-T patients (and in ATM knockout mice), hypertrichosis could reflect a mild hormonal imbalance in some patients.

Swift et al.[32] also observed a fourfold increase of ischemic heart disease among female A-T carriers. Thus, while heterozygotes are at a 3.2-fold increased mortality risk, only 44 percent and 35 percent of the deaths (men and women, respectively) were attributable to cancer; 34 percent and 35 percent of the deaths (men and women, respectively) were attributable to heart disease.

Related Syndromes

The related Nijmegen breakage syndrome (NBS)[172] and the Berlin breakage syndrome (BBS),[173] respectively assigned to complementation groups V1 and V2, do not show ataxia and do not link to chromosome 11q23.[162,174,175] They found their way into the A-T literature because they also manifest the 7;14 translocations and radioresistant DNA synthesis. NBS further includes cancer susceptibility and immunodeficiency. Telangiectasia is absent, and the

serum AFP level is normal. NBS patients have birdlike facies, microcephaly, and mental retardation (A-T patients typically are not mentally retarded). BBS very closely resembles NBS and may not represent a different syndrome or a different gene. Both link to chromosome 8q11.[253] However, NBS cells complement the RDS of BBS, implicating a second gene. Only a handful of BBS patients have been described in the literature. They have most of the signs and symptoms of NBS, with the possible addition of syndactyly, anal atresia, hypospadias, and a prominent nose. Most of the reported NBS and BBS families have been of eastern European origin.[176–178] Efforts are under way to clone the gene(s) for both syndromes.

AT_{Fresno} (ATF) combines the classical A-T syndrome with NBS, including an elevated AFP (Fig. 14-5).[179] Whenever microcephaly and mental retardation are seen in an otherwise classical A-T patient, an ATF diagnosis should be suspected. However, since ATF families link to chromosome 11q23.1 and ATM mutations have been found in three ATF families, it is unclear what the clinical importance of this diagnostic distinction will be. The same ATM mutations found in two ATF families have also been observed in classic A-T patients. If a second modifier gene were involved, it would have to link to the 11q22-23 region as well.

Ataxia-Telangiectasia Variants

There is an abundant literature describing patients who do not meet all the diagnostic criteria for A-T discussed above.[180–182] Many of these reports describe very young patients, transient ataxias, probable A-T patients without telangiectasias,[162,183,184] patients with normal AFP levels, or those with nearly normal immunologic parameters. Recent screening for ATM mutations in such "variant" families in the international consortium (families that were categorically excluded from the linkage analyses) suggests that most of these *are* A-T. In several families with classically affected patients, prominent telangiectasias have been noted in members who do not have ataxia and do not carry the two affected ATM haplotypes.[162] Some of these persons are bona fide A-T heterozygotes. Conversely, we have one family in which both affected alleles appeared in a teenager with full-blown telangieactasia but without ataxia. (This family was one of six nonlinking families in the consortium linkage analyses.) Other families have been described with intermediate radiosensitivity, a parameter that is difficult to quantitate; nonetheless, in some hands this must be considered a reliable finding that will probably relate in some way to the sites of ATM mutations in those families (see "Correlating Phenotypes with Genotypes," below). No doubt there is also a sizable population of radiosensitive individuals whose symptoms partially overlap the A-T syndrome. It will be interesting to learn whether these patients have ATM mutations or mutations in other genes that interact with

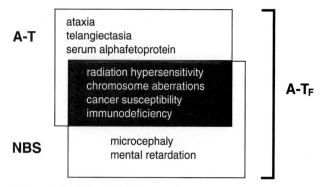

FIG. 14-5 Overlapping A-T and NBS syndromes combine to form the AT_{Fresno} syndrome.

the ATM protein. In some families with later-onset ataxia, telangiectasias often do not become very prominent. However, we recently found ATM mutations in several of these families, thus confirming them as bona fide A-T patients.

Differential Diagnosis

The most difficult challenge in making a diagnosis of A-T involves very young patients. The most common misdiagnosis is cerebral palsy, especially when there is a spastic component to the child's movements. With time, however, a diagnosis of A-T will become clear when the ataxia is notably progressive and cerebellar, eye movements demonstrate poor tracking, and speech becomes slurred. The absence of telangiectasia at this stage should not weigh against a diagnosis of A-T. Family history may be helpful if (1) a prior child exists with similar signs and symptoms and (2) the parents are related. Both factors should certainly raise suspicion about a hereditary disorder, and A-T is the most common hereditary early-onset progressive ataxia. The presence or absence of cancer in the family generally is not helpful, for it can be interpreted in many ways. Laboratory studies should include (1) serum AFP, (2) a cytogenetic search for t(7;14) translocations, and (3) an immunologic evaluation, and (4) in vitro radiosensitivity (see below). Recent evidence suggests that ATM protein levels in extracts of A-T cells may be very low or absent in many classical patients; these can be measured semi-quantitatively on Western blots.

Even if some of the above tests are not informative, a diagnosis of A-T may still be valid for the following reasons: (1) The AFP remains normal throughout life in ~5 percent of patients. As was discussed above, the serum AFP is occasionally above "normal" levels in normal children under 2 years of age and thus is not a reliable test until after that age. (2) A cytogenetic search for t(7;14) translocations or clones is often unsuccessful in A-T patients because a poor mitogenic response makes it difficult to find enough metaphases for analysis (see "Chromosomal Instability," above). Even if sufficient metaphases are found, these translocations are sometimes missed. Radiation-induced and bleomycin-induced breakage studies may be helpful but seldom contribute to making the diagnosis because of overlap between normal and A-T ranges.[89] (3) The immunologic evaluation can be normal in some A-T patients. Whether it becomes progressively more abnormal in older A-T patients is debatable; in the author's experience, this has not been apparent (see "Immunodeficiency," above). The response to allogeneic cells, the mixed lymphocyte response, is quite abnormal in some patients; however, this is a very laborious and costly test that is hard to quantitate without extensive controls and is therefore difficult to justify for strictly clinical purposes.

An MRI (magnetic resonance imaging) of the cerebellum usually will reveal marked dystrophy, even in young children (Fig. 14-6). Newer techniques for imaging the cerebellum are also being evaluated, such as functional MRI and PET scanning (positron emission tomography);[231,232] however, both depend heavily on patient cooperation and may not be applicable to very young children. Also, PET scanning uses radioactive tracers, and although the exposure doses are very small, they could theoretically contribute to cancer risk. When risk-benefit ratios are considered for procedures using ionizing radiation, difficult judgments must be made. For example, an x-ray examination to visualize the thymic shadow as part of a diagnostic workup is usually superfluous and can often be circumvented because chest x-rays are clinically indicated.

The most dangerous diagnostic situation for a young A-T patient occurs when cancer is the presenting symptom. Fortunately, this does not occur very often. Anecdotally, one child had a cerebellar astrocytoma removed at 27 months, but his unsteady gait actually worsened postoperatively. His clinicians were quite con-

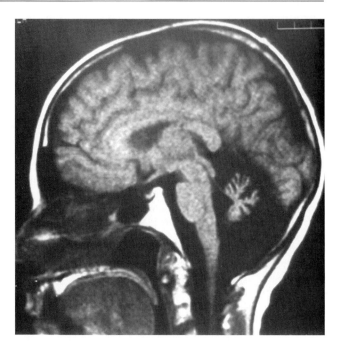

FIG. 14-6 Magnetic resonance imaging of a 6-year-old A-T patient showing markedly reduced size of the cerebellar shadow.

cerned and confused by the persistent ataxia until several years later, when the patient's younger sister began to stagger as well and a diagnosis of A-T was made on both children. Because the astrocytoma was totally resectable, no consideration was given to further therapy with chemotherapeutic agents or radiation. The patient died more than 20 years later without any sequelae of the cancer or surgery. Other children have not been so fortunate,[17–19] presenting with a malignancy and receiving conventional doses of irradiation because it was not realized that they were suffering from A-T, only to suffer iatrogenic deaths. The late Dr. Boder claimed that she could make a diagnosis of A-T in any child under 2. While this is a challenging claim, it is certainly true that most young A-T patients do have at least some suspicious neurologic findings at a very early age. Upon questioning, mothers sometimes volunteer that they noted head tilting or swaying in these infants (Fig. 14-7). Thus, it would seem prudent for pediatric oncologists and radiation oncologists to rule out the diagnosis of A-T before treating any young child with lymphoma or leukemia either by obtaining a complete history and performing a careful neurologic examination with this in mind or by obtaining a neurologic consultation as part of the workup.

While the presence of hypersensitivity to ionizing radiation has been a laboratory hallmark of the disease, clinical testing for this has not been readily available, primarily because most radiosensitivity assays use fibroblasts and establishing fibroblasts in A-T patients is painful, costly, and technically challenging. With this in mind, our laboratory established the CSA, a clonogenic assay that evaluates the colony survival fraction of LCLs from patients after the cells have received 1 Gy of ionizing irradiation.[111] From a single 10-ml heparinized blood sample that can be shipped without refrigeration, cells are transformed with Epstein-Barr virus. Once a stable cell line has been established, the cells are plated in two-cell concentrations onto 96-well tissue culture trays that are irradiated (or not irradiated) and returned to an incubator for 10 days, at which point the number of wells containing colonies larger than 32 cells is scored and compared to the colony survival fractions of normal cells. Unlike other CSAs, the CSA conditions in our laboratory were selected so that heterozygotes would score as normals, allowing more reliable detection of A-T homozygotes (Fig. 14-8).

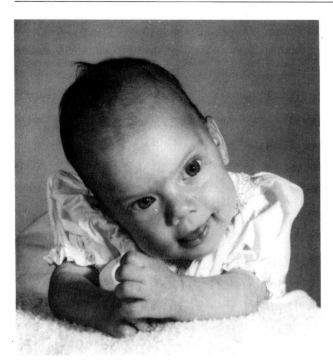

FIG. 14-7 Head-tilting in a 6-month-old infant with A-T. Staggering was not noted until she began to walk.

Recently, two referred patients with normal CSA results on repeated testing were subsequently tested for Friedreich ataxia and found to have the typical (GAA)n expansions on chromosome 9q13. Although the differential diagnosis between Friedreich ataxia (FRDA) and A-T is usually not difficult—FRDA is a later-onset ataxia (usually around puberty), and most FRDA patients have hypertrophic cardiomyopathy (by ECG testing), whereas A-T patients generally do not have cardiac problems—this experience served to underscore the value of using radiosensitivity to confirm a suspected early diagnosis of A-T. FRDA patients have normal CSA results.[111,185] Patients from all complementation groups, including NBS and BBS, have the same very reduced CSA levels that A-T patients have.

Abnormal facies other than the slowly developing smile or mask-like expression of many A-T patients should raise suspicion about other diagnoses. Severe mental retardation and inability to speak at an appropriate age are also uncharacteristic of A-T. Mental retardation is seen more commonly in lower-socioeconomic-level families and countries, perhaps because they lack the resources needed to keep A-T patients in the mainstream of family and community life. The absence of oculomotor apraxia in a 5-year-old would also be considered strong evidence against the diagnosis of A-T.

Ataxia is common to a variety of other hereditary disorders[186] (1) as a major feature with progressive ataxia–beta-lipoprotein abnormalities, hexaminidase deficiency (GM2), and cholestanolosis, (2) as a major feature with intermittent ataxia–urea cycle defects, maple syrup urine disease, isovaleric acidosis, 2-hydroxyglutaric aciduria, Hartnup disease, pyruvate dysmetabolism, and mitochondrial disease, and (3) as a minor feature of Niemann-Pick syndrome, metachromatic leukodystrophy, multiple sulfatase deficiency, late-onset globoid cell leukodystrophy, adrenoleukodystrophy, sialidosis type 1, and ceroid lipofuscinosis. The latter can be diagnosed only by biopsy of the conjunctiva or brain. Most of the other disorders listed above will show abnormalities in urinary amino acids, lysosomal hydrolases, or very long chain fatty acids. Refsum disease is characterized by retinitis pigmentosa, deafness, polyneuropathy, and ataxia.[187] (For further information, see Ref. 5.)

Determining whether a new patient's ataxia has been inherited in a dominant or a recessive manner can aid in distinguishing A-T

from olivopontocerebellar atrophy, spinocerebellar ataxia, or Joseph-Machado disease. The familial pattern for age at onset of the ataxia is also helpful, since few familial ataxias present in early childhood, as does A-T. While an occasional case of early-onset FRDA might be mistaken for A-T on this basis, neurologic examination will reveal spinal cord ataxia with a positive Romberg sign; and in the laboratory homozygosity for a (GAA)n expansion in the first intron of the FRDA gene is easily diagnosed.[188]

Aicardi et al.[189] described a group of 14 patients with a late-onset progressive ataxia, chroeoathetosis, and oculomotor apraxia without frequent infections or telangiectasia. The AFP was normal, and a search for t(7;14) translocations was negative. We agree with the authors' suggestion that these children suffered from "an unusual type of spinocerebellar degeneration," probably not A-T. However, it would be interesting to test whether any of those patients were radiosensitive, for example, by CSA.

Prenatal Diagnosis

With the fine mapping of the ATM gene, a set of highly informative genetic markers was developed that now allows accurate haplotyping within families, with basically 100 percent reliability of the fetus either being affected or not being affected. The finding of only a single A-T gene for all complementation groups also simplifies this diagnostic approach. This is in contrast to earlier attempts to perform prenatal diagnoses by trying to quantitate spontaneous chromosome breakage.[89,109–193] (see the discussion in Ref. 150), assessing radiation-induced chromosomal damage of amniocytes or fetal fibroblasts, or performing RDS, all of which were misleading at one time or another (personal communications). One hopes that these approaches have by now been abandoned.

Prenatal diagnosis by haplotyping relies on a prior affected child to identify the two affected chromosome 11q23.1 segments (i.e., haplotypes) carrying the ATM gene.[192] Figure 14-9 demonstrates the concept of haplotyping and shows how it was possible to determine that the first cousin of an affected patient was not affected. In the unusual example shown, a definitive diagnosis was possible only because (1) a prior affected child existed in the family and (2) both sets of parents were first cousins. Having DNA from a prior affected child in the family is a prerequisite for prenatal diagnosis by haplotyping, while consanguinity is not. The markers we use today are all within 1 percent recombination of the ATM gene: D11S1817,[194] D11S1819,[194] NS22 (unpublished), D11S2179,[195] and D11S1818.[194] Two of these markers are within the ATM gene itself, thereby circumventing the need for reporting the risk of recombination separating the testing markers from the actual ATM gene. Most of this testing can be performed before conception and resumed once the mother is pregnant, so that once a DNA sample is available from the fetus—either from growing amniocytes or from a chorionic villous biopsy—the entire haplotyping can be completed within a week. Because abortion guidelines vary with the country or state of residence of the mother, we ask not for the due date or the date of last menses but for the referring laboratory's deadline for reporting the results of prenatal diagnosis to the family. We also insist that the results be conveyed to the family by a genetic counselor.

Determining whether two mutations exist within the ATM gene of a child suspected of having A-T would certainly be the most definitive way of establishing the diagnosis. Unfortunately, at this writing such an approach is not feasible with rare exceptions. In families of certain ethnic backgrounds (see "Patient Mutations," below), we can perform rapid DNA assays for mutations that cover 50 to 70 percent of the mutations in that population. However, unless the patient is homozygous for that mutation—which is very

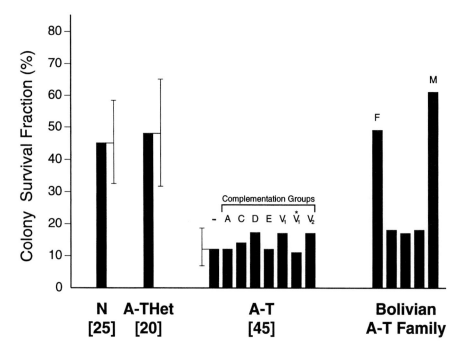

FIG. 14-8 Colony survival assay (CSA) measures radiosensitivity of LCLs to 1 Gy on patients with A-T, A-T heterozygotes, normals, and a Bolivian family with three affected children. Also included are results from patients with NBS (V1), BBS (V2), and ATF (V1*).

unlikely unless the parents are consanguineous—a second mutation must still be sought. This requires a great deal of effort either by mRNA/cDNA/RT-PCR-based screening assays or by a systematic genomic search of the 66 exons of the ATM gene. Even this approach is not 100 percent effective in finding all mutations at the present time, since some lie deep within introns and others require analysis of both genomic DNA and mRNA (see "Patient Mutations," below). Eventually, we hope to determine the mutations in most A-T families worldwide. This effort should expedite performing prenatal diagnosis by mutation analysis.

Therapy

At the present writing, no effective therapy exists for halting the progression of the ataxia.[2,5,196] Two other areas are of great concern to the health of A-T patients: (1) pulmonary infections and (2) malignancy. Pulmonary infections usually are due to the normal spectrum of microbes and are treatable by conventional approaches. Opportunistic infections do not occur in A-T patients as they do in patients with other immunodeficiency disorders. Malignancies must be treated with great care to avoid conventional doses of radiation therapy or radiomimetic agents. If possible, neurotoxic agents should be avoided.

Not all A-T patients manifest frequent pulmonary or sinus infections. Those with chronic bronchiectasis are best treated in the same way as patients with cystic fibrosis: routine chest percussion, postural drainage, and generally aggressive pulmonary hygiene. Periodic pulmonary function studies may assist in monitoring infection-prone patients. In older patients, pulmonary infections are the major cause of failing health and death. Increasing bulbar dysfunction may predispose to aspiration pneumonia. In addition to appropriate antibiotics, intravenous gamma globulin every 3 to 4 weeks may reduce the frequency of infections in infection-prone patients. There is some indication that the lungs of A-T patients may not be anatomically normal. Pump et al.[197] made a latexlike impression of one lung [using a substance called Vultex moulage (General Latex and Chemicals Ltd, Verdun, Quebec)] from a single A-T patient; they found bronchiectatic changes in many parts of the lung, with saccular dilatations throughout the bronchi.

Perhaps the most effective impact on care that the physician can make is to strongly encourage the parents of young A-T patients to institute an aggressive and engaging physical exercise program aimed at enhancing lung function, preventing contractures, and avoiding positional kyphoscoliosis. Almost all patients who have been denied such care develop severe contractures of the feet and hands. These begin in the late teens in patients who are not encouraged to routinely abandon the wheelchair for one-half hour each day, if only to do situps or repeatedly hoist themselves onto a sofa.

Physical therapists are often uneasy taking care of such patients; however, they have little reason to be since no harm can be done by regular exercise.[198] Wheelchair-bound patients should be encouraged to shift position periodically, alternating the elbow they lean on. Swimming and horseback riding are two activities that are popular among A-T patients; both minimize their handicaps.

Speech therapy is also effective, not in arresting the progression of the dysarthria but in minimizing the frustration felt by the patients when they cannot be understood by peers. Parents should encourage A-T teenagers to converse with friends on the telephone, for this forces them to enunciate.

Some of the neurologic symptoms, such as ataxia, drooling, and tremors, can be partially relieved by various agents.[196] Buspirone, a serotonergic 5-hydroxytryptophan agonist, is active in some types of cerebellar ataxia.[253] Amantidine improves balance and coordination and minimizes drooling in some patients. Methyl scopalamine and propantholine hydrochloride sometimes are effective in reducing drooling. Postural tremors may be reduced by propranolol and other beta blockers, while cerebellar tremors and myoclonus may respond to low doses of clonazepam or valproic acid. However, these agents sometimes increase the ataxia and drowsiness. Drooling also can be alleviated by ligating the salivary ducts. This may also reduce the risk of aspiration pneumonia. Clinical trials are also under way to test the efficacy of inositol and N-acetylcysteine on general symptoms. (For a review of other AT-related medications, see Ref. 196.)

When radiation therapy is planned for treating a malignancy in an A-T patient, doses should be reduced by approximately 30 percent. Some chemotherapeutic agents, especially alkylating agents,

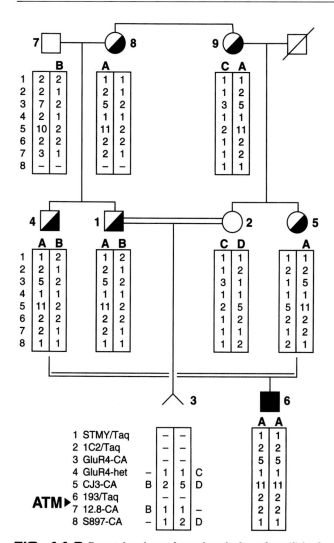

	1 STMY/Taq		–	–	
	2 1C2/Taq		–	–	
	3 GluR4-CA		–	–	
	4 GluR4-het	–	1	1	C
	5 CJ3-CA	B	2	5	D
ATM▶	6 193/Taq		–	–	
	7 12.8-CA	B	1	1	–
	8 S897-CA	–	1	2	D

FIG. 14-9 Prenatal testing to determine whether a fetus (3) is affected. By history, two brothers had married two sisters who were their first cousins. One couple (4 and 5) had an affected child (6), prompting the second couple (1 and 2) to seek prenatal testing. However, testing before conception would have identified the mother (2) as a noncarrier, thereby circumventing any further testing on the fetus. Haplotype [A] carries the affected ATM gene. The genetic markers that are currently being used for prenatal testing are given in the text.

probably should be used in reduced doses. There has been a suggestion that topoisomerase inhibitors should be avoided. Unfortunately, there is only anectodal literature on the important and recurring issue of oncologic treatment of A-T patients. Further, the intricacies of planning such a regimen depend on the type of malignancy being treated and other details that are beyond the scope of this chapter.

Occasionally the possibility of bone marrow transplantation arises, usually because a young A-T patient has developed leukemia and has an HLA-compatible sib to serve as a potential donor. Despite several such attempts over the past 20 years, the author is not aware of a single transplant with convincing documentation of long-term engraftment. This could be for several reasons, the most compelling of which would be the difficulty of establishing a safe but effective regimen for delivering the marrow-ablating irradiation or chemotherapy for the reasons touched on above. In general, hyperfractionation of radiation doses would seem prudent under such circumstances if this need were to arise. There is of course little reason to expect that bone marrow transplantation would correct the cerebellar degeneration. Stem cell transplanta-

tion might reduce the need for complete ablation but probably would also reduce the chances of engraftment.

Many A-T patients have been immunized inadvertently for smallpox, polio, and varicella, with no apparent sequelae. Nevertheless, these natural varicella infections are often quite severe. Thus, contrary to the general warning that patients with immunodeficiencies not be given live vaccines, varicella immunization would seem advisable in patients with only mild immunodeficiency.

Prognosis

Most A-T patients in the United States live well beyond 20 years. Many are now in their thirties. This is a major change from just a few years ago, when it was unusual for these patients to live beyond the teenage years. This is unfortunately still true in many other countries. The reasons for this are unclear. They could be related to better nutrition, better diagnostics, better treatment of pulmonary infections and malignancies, and more aggressive physical therapy. There is hope among A-T investigators that the young children being diagnosed today will benefit from some currently undiscovered effective therapy before their neurologic status becomes irreversible and too debilitating. We have perhaps 10 years to help such children!

MOLECULAR GENETICS

Early attempts to utilize some of the known immunlogic abnormalities in A-T patients as genetic markers for linkage analysis proved fruitless,[88] since the parameters measured often varied even in affected sibs. Linkage studies were next attempted with genetic markers such as HLA, ABO, MN, Rh, and Gm (IGH subtypes).[199,200] Although not very informative, these markers represented a starting point for preparing an exclusion map of each chromosome by which a gene is methodically excluded from each chromosome until it is localized. At about the same time (1982), White's laboratory in Salt Lake City was developing an impressive array of biallelic genetic markers—RFLPs—that would eventually cover the entire genome.[201–203] A collaboration was arranged to apply these markers to linkage analysis of the available families. This was a major intellectual departure for A-T research at that time. Botstein offered to analyze the available families for statistical power and was less than enthusiastic that linkage could be established with so few families available, especially when the complementation groups of most families were unknown and the genes for those complementation groups might be located on different chromosomes.[199] Jaspers agreed to characterize more families for complementation assignments.[150,151,204]

Meanwhile, our laboratory decided to utilize a large Amish pedigree that included four extant branches of the family with affected members for the preliminary genomic screening; this family was later assigned by Jaspers and coworkers to complementation group A.[152] Peripheral blood and skin biopsies were obtained on 61 members of this pedigree to establish lymphoblastoid cell lines and fibroblast cultures, respectively. (We had hoped to use the fibroblasts for heterozygote identification of nonaffected members to increase the genetic information on the segregation of the affected gene.[26] In retrospect, this ambitious subproject added little power to the linkage analyses.[152]) Over the next 5 years, DNAs were isolated and screened with a total of 171 RFLP markers, using numerous Southern blots containing DNA digested mainly with EcoRI, BamHI, MspI, and TaqI. In 1988, a linkage was found to a THY1/MspI polymorphism developed in our laboratory.[205]

Confirmation with another nearby marker (S11S144) from White's laboratory followed, and the Group A gene was localized to chromosome 11q22-23.[152] [The initial RFLP markers were all biallelic. No maps, yeast artificial chromosomes (YACs), bacterial artificial chromosomes (BACs), or P1 artificial chromosomes (PACs) were available in 1988. In retrospect, this "identity by descent" approach could have been streamlined significantly if microsatellite markers had been available. However, the sublocalization and isolation of the gene still would have required many additional families, mapping, markers, and cloning experiments.]

To our initial surprise, when lod scores from all A-T families were added together, regardless of complementation group assignments, the cumulative lod scores *increased*.[152,206,207] This suggested that either (1) the complementation group genes were all clustered in the 11q22-23 region, (2) most of the families were of similar complementation groups (Groups A and C were thought to include over 80 percent of the typed families), (3) the complementation groups represented intragenic mutations, or (4) complementation typing with A-T fibroblasts did not reflect Mendelian inheritance. In all our subsequent linkage analyses over the next 7 years, we never found any convincing evidence for genetic heterogeneity.[18,206–208] The cloning of a single gene for all complementation groups confirmed these early interpretations.

Localizing the A-T Gene

Subsequent to our 1988 report localizing the A-T gene or genes to 11q22-23,[152] many reports followed which confirmed and extended that observation.[153,161,162,181,206–221] When the need for positional cloning to a resolution of 0.5 cM was realized, an international consortium was organized and new biostatistical approaches were sought. Two new computer programs were developed by Lange and Sobel, based on Metropolis-coupled Markov chain Monte Carlo (MCMC) statistical methods.[222,223] The first program added almost eight logs to existing lod scores but could only handle biallelic markers; a second program was eventually developed that could handle the new multiallelic short tandem repeat (STR) markers.[223] We avoided including in the consortium database families with any variations that were considered significant so as to minimize genetic heterogeneity in the linkage studies. These were labeled "V" for possible "variant" and analyzed separately each time linkage analyses were performed. In retrospect, we are finding ATM mutations in most of those families as well.

In the final linkage studies of 176 families that had been entered into the nine-country consortium, two subsets of analyses were performed. In the first subset, incorporating all 176 bona fide families and over 40 genetic markers, the location score curve reached its peak at D11S535 with a maximum lod score of 56. In the second subset, seven nonlinking families were excluded to improve the localization of the gene. As expected, the location score curve of the second subset was shifted upward (from 56 to 73 lod units), retaining the same general shape as the curve of the first subset and peaking within the same interval (Fig. 14-10A). The 2-lod support region containing the A-T locus for the second subset was a ~500-kb interval beginning ~150 kb proximal to S384 and ending just short of S1294 (Fig. 14-10B). If we counted the number of families with recombinants in the candidate region, the same ~500-kb region of common overlap could eventually be appreciated (Fig. 14-11).

In an almost independent effort to localize the A-T gene without segregation analysis (in the event that meiotic recombination was increased in A-T—a chromosomal breakage syndrome, after all—and the linkage results might mislead the positional cloning experiments), we utilized a subset of 27 Costa Rican families to track ancestral haplotypes,[223] a form of linkage disequilibrium analysis and "identity by descent" analysis. We found that

roughly two-thirds of these purportedly "unrelated" families shared the same haplotype (haplotype [A] in Fig. 14-12). Inferred (ancestral) recombination events involving this common haplotype in earlier generations suggested that the gene was distal to D11S384/B7. Nine other haplotypes were identified within the Costa Rican population. When considered together with all other evidence (i.e., from two of the other labs), the Costa Rican study further sublocalized the "major A-T locus" to ~200 kb, between the markers D11S384 and D11S535, within which the ATM gene was found.

From 1993 to 1995, detailed YAC, BAC, and cosmid maps were made of the candidate region by several of the consortium laboratories, and, using these genomic segments, many transcripts from many cDNA libraries were isolated. Five recovery methods were used, including exon trapping,[224] the only method that did not depend on whether the A-T gene was being expressed in any particular library. The genomic map from our laboratory is shown in Fig. 14-13; it included 3 BACs, 12 cosmids, and 21 sequence-tagged sites (STSs) by the time the gene had been cloned (compare with the maps in Refs. 6 and 72).

Each of the recovered transcripts had to be sequenced so that PCR primers could be designed and used to amplify and screen for mutations, using cDNAs from 100 A-T patients as templates for PCR. Several labs found a large transcript in 1993 that was ubiquitously expressed, thus qualifying it as a good candidate A-T gene. Our laboratory called this gene CAND3 (candidate 3). Despite a very thorough search of CAND3 for mutations in about 100 A-T patients, using SSCP, heteroduplex analysis (HA), density gradient gel electrophoresis (DGGE), and direct cDNA sequencing, no mutations were found. In 1995, the ATM gene was isolated by the Israeli members of the consortium,[72,73] headed by Yosef Shiloh, from within the distal portion of the ~500-kb region defined by the linkage analyses (Fig. 14-10B).

CAND3 maps 544 bp proximal to ATM and is oriented in the opposite transcriptional direction (Fig. 14-13). Several laboratories are exploring the relationship between these two large housekeeping genes at 11q23.1.[225–227] Some of the promoter elements and regulatory sequences within the small intervening segment appear to be functional in either orientation and probably act as bidirectional promoters for ATM and CAND3. CAND3/E14/NPAT has some interesting homologies, suggesting that it is a nucleoporin protein containing cyclin-dependent kinase (cdk) phosphorylation targets and possible PI-3 kinase activity.[227] It ubiquitously expresses two transcripts of ~6 and ~5 kb, with a protein of 1427 amino acids. It is phylogenetically conserved in yeast, chicken, and mammals. Imai et al.[226] also failed to find mutations in this gene in eight Japanese A-T patients. Its relationship to the A-T phenotype remains to be discovered. (The GDB accession numbers for CAND3/E14/NPAT are Z66089, D83243, and D83244.)

Before the cloning of the gene, it was possible to establish that only a single gene was responsible for all the Costa Rican patients by pairing each of the Costa Rican haplotypes with a different one (Fig. 14-12). We further reasoned that the patients carrying haplotype [A] were carrying the same mutation. We have recently confirmed this and have developed a rapid screening test for this mutation which takes less than a day to screen hundreds of DNAs (Fig. 14-14). This provides an opportunity to compare the clinical symptoms of multiple patients with the same mutation; indeed, some of the patients are homozygous for this mutation.

The ATM Gene

The full ATM gene transcript is 13 kb (9054 nt of ORF), with 66 exons, the largest being exon 12 with 372 nucleotides (nt) (GDB accession numbers U26455, X91196, U40887-40918, and U33841 as well as the reports of Savitsky et al.,[72,140] Rasio et al.,[228] Uziel et

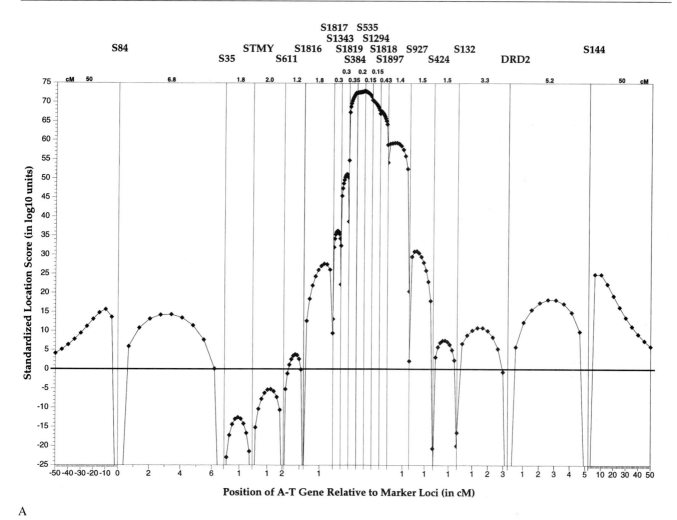

A

FIG. 14-10 Lod score curves estimated by Metropolis-coupled Markov chain Monte Carlo linkage analysis across a 30-c*M* region of chromosome 11q22-23, using 169 A-T families. *A.* Shows a peak at a lod score of 73. *B.* Demonstrates the position of the later-cloned ATM gene on a detail of the lod score peak shown in *A.* Proximal-to-distal is from left-to-right.

al.,[229] Byrd et al.,[225] Vorechovsky et al.,[54] Pecker et al.[230] and Platzer et al.[251]). It is a member of a large family of high-molecular-weight protein kinases.[72,139–141,233] Northern blots reveal expression in all tissues, with several transcripts of 10.5 (fibroblasts), 6.2, and 4.9 kb. Recent studies by Rotman and coworkers (Tel Aviv) indicate that a considerable amount of alternative splicing occurs at the 5′ end. The 3′ portion of the gene has strong homology to yeast and mammalian phosphatidylinositol 3-kinases as well as to DNA-PK. Thus, ATM appears to play a major role as an intracellular signal transducer that gives warning to the cell, via cell cycle checkpoints, of DNA damage that must be repaired before the next cell division. However, as was discussed above, another role for the ATM protein remains to be elucidated, one that is p53-independent and probably involves replicon initiation and meiotic pairing during gametogenesis. A leucine zipper domain around exon 27 suggests that the ATM protein may form homo- or heterodimers and bind DNA. An SH$_3$ domain (aa 1373–1382) binds c-*abl* in response to DNA damage.[70] A website has been created for tracking published ATM mutations: http://www.vmmc.org/vmrc/atm.htm.

Patient Mutations

Over 250 mutations in the ATM gene have already been identified. The mutations have been defined primarily in the laboratories of Shiloh,[72,234] Concannon,[235,237] Taylor,[225] and Gatti.[157,252] These labo-

ratories have used a variety of screening approaches: Shiloh and Taylor have used restriction endonuclease fingerprinting (REF), Concannon has used SSCP followed by single-strand sequencing, and we have used PTT and CSGE. Each screening approach affects the types of mutations found. Almost all the early work used mRNA as template (via reverse transcription of mRNA to cDNA). About 70 percent of ATM mutations result in truncated proteins, most of which affect splice sites.[252] Platzer et al.[251] used dye terminator methodology to sequence directly 27.3 kb of DNA on each of 72 patients; the team detected only 50 percent of mutations. A comparative discussion of mutation detection strategies for ATM is beyond the scope of this chapter. (For further details, see References 236 and 237.)

Because the 3′ half of the ATM gene was sequenced first, the distribution of mutations shown in Fig. 14-15 is slightly biased against finding equal numbers of mutations in the 5′ half. Most A-T patients are compound heterozygotes. One potential hotspot (approximately 15 percent of mutations) was identified, in exon 54.[235] Exon 54 is just proximal to the PI3-kinase homology domain. In screening cDNAs, two types of mutations were observed here: 2544del159 and 2546del9, both resulting in in-frame deletions (Fig. 14-15*B*). (The first number indicates the first codon that is affected in the cDNA mutation.) Because of the marginal effect that the 2546del9 mutation would have on the predicted protein, it can be argued that this could be a polymorphism. Wright et al.[235] addressed this issue by screening 75 parents of CEPH families for this mutation; no ex-

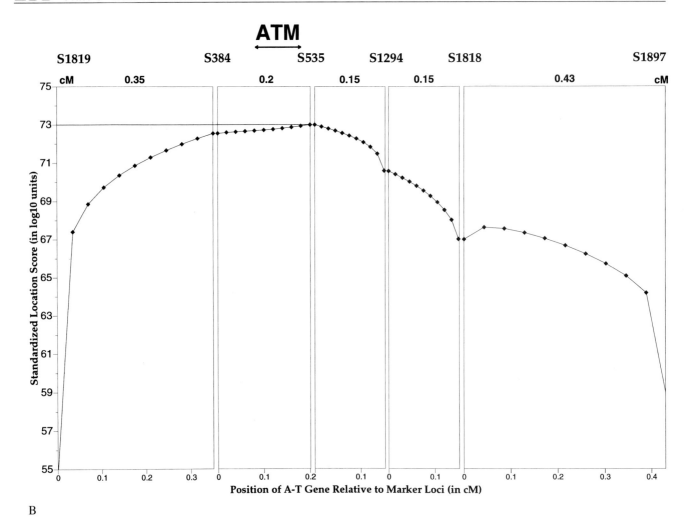

B

FIG. 14-10 *(cont.)*

amples of 2546del9 were found. Recent data from our laboratory indicate that not all the 2544del159 cDNA mutations have the same nt7638A→C mutation at the splice acceptor site. Thus, the exon 54 hotspot contains at least three different mutations. Furthermore, recent studies indicate that five of six patients with the 2546del9 mutation share haplotypes; i.e., this is an Irish–English founder effect.

Our laboratory has recently defined the three most common mutations for Costa Rican patients: haplotypes [A], [B], and [C]. These mutations account for >80 percent of affected families.[221,252] A peculiar ATC→TGAT mutation accounts for 10 of 16 affected chromosomes in Norwegian patients.[252] We have also developed simple assays for detecting the Amish nt1563delAG (codon 521) mutation in the original pedigree used to map the gene to chromosome 11q23[152,257] and for the 7518del4 (codon 2506) mutation found in seven families from central-southern Italy.[72,140] The above mutations are represented only once in Fig. 14-15, by boxes, because they are founder-effect defects, i.e., are common to multiple patients from presumably related families. We also have observed five recurring defects in Polish families; three of these appear in families that share a haplotype as defined by the microsatellite markers D11S1817, D11S1819, D11S2179, and D11S1818 (see map in Fig. 14-11).[157,252] We have also identified a second very polymorphic microsatellite marker within the ATM gene that should further improve the accuracy and turnaround time of prenatal diagnostic studies, NS22 (unpublished).

As was mentioned above, many mutations described so far have been defined in mRNA and involve deletions of one, two, or three exons (Fig. 14-16). However, when the corresponding genomic mutations have been defined, single base mutations have been found that destroy existing splice sites and sometimes create new ones. In one family, a genomic G→A mutation at 2250 nt does not change the amino acid (AAG and AAA are both lysine codons), whereas the cDNA-based PTT indicates that this "silent" mutation results in a more deleterious 126-nt deletion (Fig. 14-17). Since the last nucleotide in an exon is a "G" ~79 percent of the time,[238] the G→A change most likely disturbs the splice donor site for exon 16 so that the splice acceptor site at exon 17 skips upstream to the next acceptable splice donor site, that of exon 15. This deletes the 126 nt of exon 16, thereby truncating the protein by 42 amino acids.

Much work lies ahead in characterizing the genomic defect underlying each of these observations. Such observations may improve our understanding of evolutionary mechanisms for circumventing the deleterious effects of certain mutations. It also should be noted that many of the cDNA "deletions" shown in Fig. 14-15A will eventually be replaced by genomic "point mutations" that may not be at the same site as the cDNA mutations. Further, as demonstrated above, the true effect of some genomic mutations will be missed unless PTT studies are also performed (Fig. 14-17). While this may not be as important for identifying mutations, appreciating the true biologic significance of each mutation will allow better

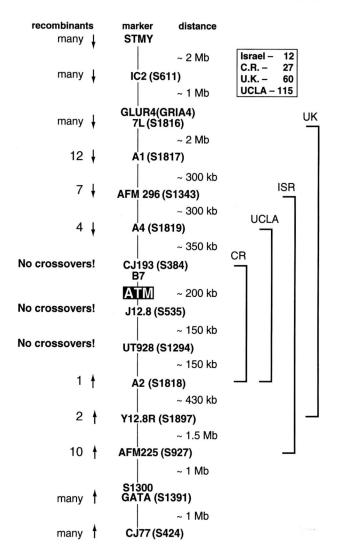

recombinants	marker	distance
many ↓	STMY	
		~ 2 Mb
many ↓	IC2 (S611)	
		~ 1 Mb
many ↓	GLUR4(GRIA4) 7L (S1816)	
		~ 2 Mb
12 ↓	A1 (S1817)	
		~ 300 kb
7 ↓	AFM 296 (S1343)	
		~ 300 kb
4 ↓	A4 (S1819)	
		~ 350 kb
No crossovers!	CJ193 (S384) B7	
	ATM	~ 200 kb
No crossovers!	J12.8 (S535)	
		~ 150 kb
No crossovers!	UT928 (S1294)	
		~ 150 kb
1 ↑	A2 (S1818)	
		~ 430 kb
2 ↑	Y12.8R (S1897)	
		~ 1.5 Mb
10 ↑	AFM225 (S927)	
		~ 1 Mb
many ↑	S1300 GATA (S1391)	
		~ 1 Mb
many ↑	CJ77 (S424)	

Box at right:
Israel – 12
C.R. – 27
U.K. – 60
UCLA – 115

FIG. 14-11 Combined linkage and physical map of 11 c*M* surrounding the most likely region for the later-cloned ATM gene (indicated). The map was based on the combined linkage analysis of 249 families (59 CEPH and 190 A-T) and pulsed field gel analyses.[220] Also depicted are the most likely regions for the ATM gene based on the number of families from the respective consortium members (see box and brackets at right) as well as the number of recombinants in the consortium families (left). These studies localized the ATM gene to within 0.5 c*M*.

correlations of phenotypes with genotypes. Furthermore, if large populations of breast and gastric cancer patients are to be screened using only archival DNA from tumors, some significant mutations may be misinterpreted as insignificant and not be included in the final analysis of any possible correlations.

Correlating Phenotypes with Genotypes

Correlating phenotypes with genotypes requires that the mutations of a large number of patients first be defined. Since most nonconsanguineous A-T patients have two distinct mutations, such studies further require that both mutations be defined before the symptoms can be compared. Another major caveat for this aspect of A-T research is that although most patients have two stable forms of mutated ATM mRNA in LCLs and PBLs, these cells do not appear to

contain stable protein. This fact makes it somewhat difficult to conceptualize how specific mutations affect phenotypes.

Recently, 10 families from the British Midlands were described with "late-onset ataxia" and intermediate radiosensitivity.[219,239] They share a common chromosome 11q23.1 haplotype that was identified during the positional cloning studies and before the shared phenotype was appreciated. The report describes a very interesting 137-bp insertion into the mRNA (a new exon!) coupled with a point mutation that enhances the efficiency of an abnormal ("cryptic") splice site. Each patient has a different second mutation, and this has not been defined in all cases. This subset of families could provide interesting insights about phenotype-genotype relationships; however, the "late-onset ataxia" data are not convincingly homogeneous, given in Table 1 of that report as years 8, 3, 3, 3, 5, 2, 2.5, 2.5, 1.8, 12, and 1.5. Considering that the average age at onset is characteristically between 1 and 3 years, only 4 of the 12 patients would qualify as late-onset. Furthermore, we have a family with three affected siblings who have the same mutation for one allele; their ages at onset were 8 months, 18 months, and 3 years. The suggestion in this report that a small subset of patients may exist with two "mild" ATM mutations that do not lead to clinically obvious A-T deserves further study.

In collaboration with Sanal and coworkers (unpublished), we have studied a family in which all four sibs are affected with A-T. Because the parents are first cousins, the children are homozygous for their mutation at 6199del9, which deletes three amino acids at codons 2067-2069, well before the region of strongest homology with PI3-K (Fig. 14-16). Table 14-1 describes the partial phenotypes of these four sibs and gives a preview of phenotype-genotype analyses. Note that this mutation is not associated with infections or immunodeficiencies in this family. The same mutation has not been seen in any other family so far.

Postlogue

Each of the first six A-T workshops has painstakingly brought us a little closer to understanding this complex disorder. Summaries were published for most of the workshops,[240–244] and books were published based on the first.[245] second,[246] fifth,[247] and sixth[248] workshops. These make interesting background reading. The recorded comments and discussions that followed the presentations at the 1984 workshop (ATW2) are still very pertinent to much of today's research.[246]

In 1981 (ATW1), a better phenotype was described. In 1984 (ATW2), the neurodegenerative nature of A-T was clarified by the presence of basket cell "footprints,"[7,8] and plans for positional cloning were developed. By 1987 (ATW3), as part of that approach, many key families around the world had been assigned to complementation groups, primarily through the work of Jaspers and coworkers.[150,151] In 1989 (ATW4), formal presentations and confirmations were made regarding the localization of an A-T gene to chromosome 11q22-23.[152] A higher-resolution map of distal chromosome 11 was already under way,[209,248] taking advantage of the burgeoning new genome projects around the world, such as the CEPH linkage mapping consortium in Paris.[203] However, at that time most investigators felt that the A-T gene would be cloned not by the slower positional cloning approach but by more direct transfection and complementation experiments. Indeed, a candidate A-T gene (ATDC) isolated by this method was much discussed at ATW5 (1992).[249,250] However, it was already becoming clear that ATDC was not the true gene, and complementational cloning was potentially misleading. The ATW6 (1994) workshop confirmed both of these conclusions, for by then 26 cDNA clones had been

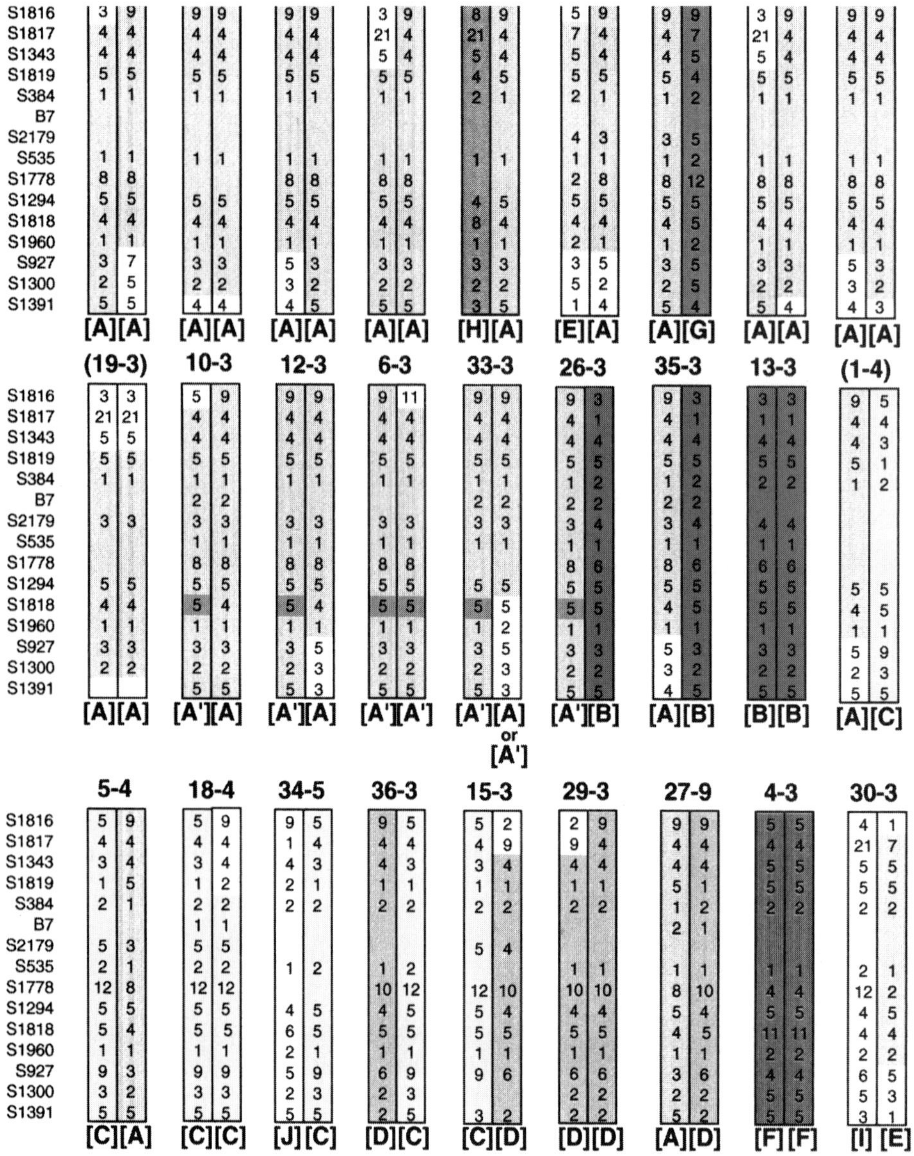

Top block

Marker	19-3 [A][A]	10-3 [A][A]	12-3 [A][A]	6-3 [A][A]	33-3 [H][A]	26-3 [E][A]	35-3 [A][G]	13-3 [A][A]	1-4 [A][A]
S1816	3 9	9 9	9 9	3 9	8 9	5 9	9 9	3 9	9 9
S1817	4 4	4 4	4 4	21 4	21 4	7 4	4 7	21 4	4 4
S1343	4 4	4 4	4 4	5 4	5 4	5 4	4 5	5 4	4 4
S1819	5 5	5 5	5 5	5 5	4 5	5 5	5 4	5 5	4 5
S384	1 1	1 1	1 1	1 1	2 1	2 1	1 2	1 1	1 1
B7									
S2179						4 3	3 5		
S535	1 1	1 1	1 1	1 1	1 1	1 1	1 2	1 1	1 1
S1778	8 8		8 8	8 8		2 8	8 12	8 8	8 8
S1294	5 5	5 5	5 5	5 5	4 5	5 5	5 5	5 5	5 5
S1818	4 4	4 4	4 4	4 4	8 4	4 4	4 5	4 4	4 4
S1960	1 1	1 1	1 1	1 1	1 1	2 1	1 2	1 1	1 1
S927	3 7	3 3	3 3	5 3	3 3	3 5	3 5	3 3	5 3
S1300	2 5	2 2	3 2	2 2	2 2	5 2	2 5	2 2	3 2
S1391	5 5	4 4	4 5	5 5	3 5	1 4	5 4	5 4	4 3

Haplotypes: [A][A] [A][A] [A][A] [A][A] [H][A] [E][A] [A][G] [A][A] [A][A]
Patients: (19-3) 10-3 12-3 6-3 33-3 26-3 35-3 13-3 (1-4)

Middle block

Marker	5-4	18-4	34-5	36-3	15-3	29-3	27-9	4-3	30-3
S1816	3 3	5 9	9 9	9 11	9 9	9 3	9 3	3 3	9 5
S1817	21 21	4 4	4 4	4 4	4 4	4 1	4 1	1 1	4 4
S1343	5 5	4 4	4 4	4 4	4 4	4 4	4 4	4 4	4 3
S1819	5 5	5 5	5 5	5 5	5 5	5 5	5 5	5 5	5 1
S384	1 1	1 1	1 1	1 1	1 1	1 2	1 2	2 2	1 2
B7		2 2				2 2	2 2		
S2179	3 3	3 3	3 3	3 3	3 3	3 4	3 4	4 4	
S535		1 1	1 1	1 1	1 1	1 1	1 1	1 1	
S1778	8 8	8 8	8 8	8 8		8 6	8 6	6 6	
S1294	5 5	5 5	5 5	5 5	5 5	5 5	5 5	5 5	5 5
S1818	4 4	5 4	5 4	5 5	5 5	5 5	5 5	5 5	4 5
S1960	1 1	1 1	1 1	1 1	1 2	1 1	1 1	1 1	1 1
S927	3 3	3 3	3 3	3 3	3 5	3 3	3 3	3 3	5 9
S1300	2 2	2 2	2 3	2 2	2 3	2 2	2 2	2 2	2 3
S1391		5 5	5 3	5 5	5 3	5 5	5 5	5 5	5 5

Haplotypes: [A][A] [A'][A] [A'][A] [A'][A'] [A'][A] or [A'] [A'][B] [A][B] [A][B] [B][B] [A][C]
Patients: 5-4 18-4 34-5 36-3 15-3 29-3 27-9 4-3 30-3

Bottom block

Marker	(col 1)	(col 2)	(col 3)	(col 4)	(col 5)	(col 6)	(col 7)	(col 8)	(col 9)
S1816	5 9	5 9	9 5	9 5	5 2	2 9	9 9	5 5	4 1
S1817	4 4	4 4	1 4	4 4	4 9	9 4	9 9	4 4	21 7
S1343	3 4	3 4	4 3	4 3	3 4	4 4	4 4	5 5	5 5
S1819	1 5	1 2	2 1	2 1	1 1	1 1	5 1	5 5	5 5
S384	2 1	2 2	2 2	2 2	2 2	2 2	1 2	2 2	2 2
B7		1 1					2 1		
S2179	5 3	5 5			5 4				
S535	2 1	2 2	1 2	1 2	1 1	1 1	1 1	1 1	2 1
S1778	12 8	12 12		10 12	12 10	10 10	8 10	4 4	12 2
S1294	5 5	5 5	4 5	4 5	5 4	4 4	5 4	5 5	4 5
S1818	5 4	5 5	6 5	5 5	5 5	5 5	4 5	11 11	4 4
S1960	1 1	1 1	2 1	1 1	1 1	1 1	1 1	2 2	2 2
S927	9 3	9 9	5 9	6 9	6 9	6 6	3 6	4 4	6 5
S1300	3 2	3 3	2 3	2 3	2 3	2 2	2 2	5 5	5 3
S1391	5 5	5 5	5 5	2 5	2 5	2 2	5 2	5 5	3 1

Haplotypes: [C][A] [C][C] [J][C] [D][C] [C][D] [D][D] [A][D] [F][F] [I][E]

FIG. 14-12 Haplotyping of 27 Costa Rican A-T patients defined by genotyping with 15 markers across 7 cM flanking the most likely region for the later-cloned ATM gene. The most prominent haplotype, haplotype [A], was found in 19 patients (70 percent), 12 of whom were homozygous for this haplotype. Subsequent studies have confirmed that these patients all carry an identical mutation, as demonstrated by the assay shown in Fig. 14-14. As haplotype [A] was inherited by different descendants of the original carrier, the genomic region that remained associated with the true region of the gene was reduced by random recombination. Thus, "ancestral haplotyping" provided further localization of the gene. Furthermore, by pairing the 10 haplotypes observed in these families, it was possible to predict that a single gene was causing the syndrome (with the exception of haplotype [F], which was never observed paired with another haplotype).

found to complement RDS, radiomimetic sensitivity, or both, but none localized to 11q22-23.[6,63,154,244] In 1995 the gene was cloned purely by positional cloning.[72]

A scientific logjam has been broken! Many new investigators have entered the field of A-T research to make antibodies, construct full-length cDNAs, and develop functional assays. However, once again, from what was to have been the pinnacle, many new peaks have been sighted.

ACKNOWLEDGMENTS

The author wishes to dedicate this chapter to Drs. Elena Boder and Robert Sedgwick, both of whom died shortly after the gene was cloned in June 1995. Almost 40 years had elapsed since their seminal observations and descriptions of the A-T syndrome. I thank them for having provided me with almost 30 years of enlightenment on A-T, their encouragement to persevere in the linkage studies, and their insights and efforts in identifying new families for our research.

The positional cloning project was initiated with funding from three major grants between 1984 and 1986 from the Ataxia-Telangiectasia Medical Research Foundation: to Richard Gatti (Los Angeles), to Yosef Shiloh (Tel Aviv), and to N. J. G Jaspers (Rotterdam). These grants allowed the first A-T families to be identified, assigned to complementation groups, and genotyped so that the linkage studies could go forward. The ATMRF provided Drs. Shiloh and Gatti with uninterrupted funding for these studies until and after the gene was cloned.

I thank Ken Lange and his four generations of graduate students in biomathematics for devising new analytic approaches in response to each obstacle we encountered, ensuring constant progress in the sublocalization of the gene. For additional support we thank the Department of Energy (ER60548) (1987 to present), the American Cancer Society (CD-328), the National Cancer Institute (CA16042), the North Atlantic Treaty Organization (ARW920385), the Ataxia-Telangiectasia Medical Trust-UK, the Ataxia-Telangiectasia Children's Project, the Joseph Drown Foundation, the Andrew Norman Foundation, the Eric Lightner Memorial Fund, and the Harry Ringel Foundation. Special thanks go to Dr. Benjamin Landing for the many years he has spent reviewing histology slides with us. Last and most impor-

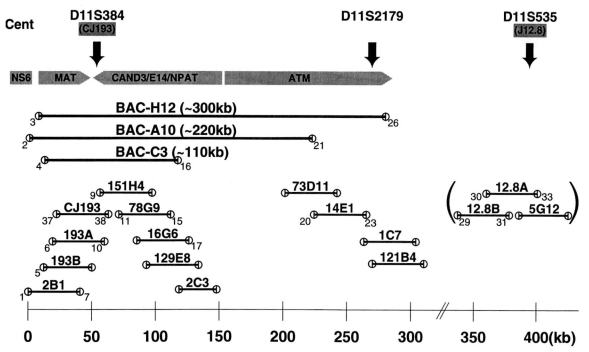

FIG. 14-13 Physical map of the genomic region localized by linkage analyses, showing cosmids, BACs, and sequence-tagged sites (numbers at ends of each cosmid or BAC) as well as the position of the later-cloned ATM gene and its relationship to other genes cloned from this region. Note the opposite transcriptional orientation of the ATM gene and the CAND3/E14/NPAT gene, with 554 bp separating the two genes (a bidirectional promoter region).

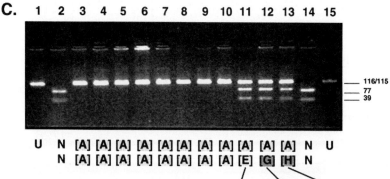

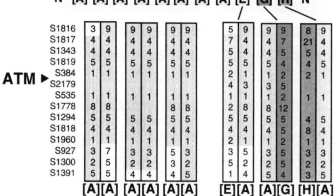

FIG. 14-14 A rapid assay for the Costa Rican haplotype [A] mutation: a deletion of a "C" at position 5908 that destroys a Sau3A1 recognition site. Thus, in haplotype [A] homozygotes, a 115-bp PCR fragment is seen on agarose gels. This fragment is also seen in heterozygotes who carry other ATM mutations.

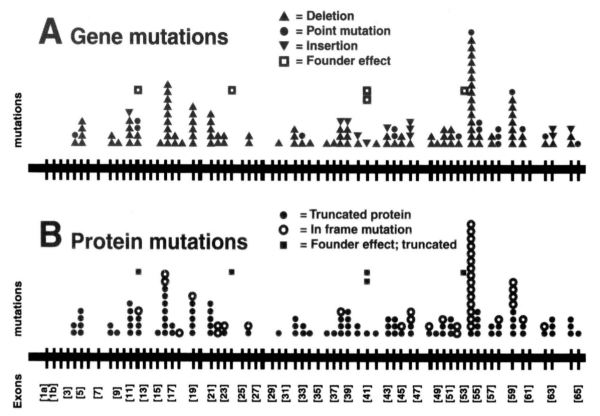

FIG. 14-15 Spectrum of ~120 ATM mutations based on studies of cDNA from cells of patients from many countries. *A.* Mutations seen in related (or probably related, because they share haplotypes) families are indicated only once (boxes) to avoid biasing the distribution. The exact position of many of these mutations will be revised once the genomic mutation sites have been defined. *B.* The majority of mutations result in truncated ATM proteins. [For an updated version of this figure, see website:

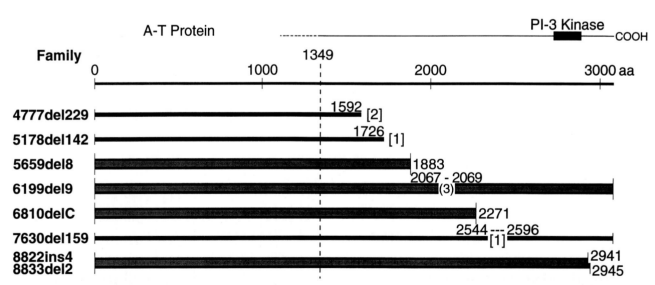

FIG. 14-16 Schematic showing some characteristic cDNA types of ATM mutations and their relationship to the most conserved portion of the PI-3 kinase domain. Bracketed numbers represent deleted exons; numbers in parentheses represent deleted codons. While most deletions result in truncation of the protein, a few do not create frameshifts, and presumably the protein continues to be translated downstream from the deletion, thereby including the presumably important PI-3 kinase domain. Thick bars represent patients with homozygous mutations. Such patients can now be analyzed for phenotype-genotype correlations (see Table 14-1).

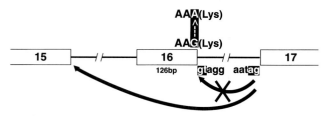

FIG. 14-17 Genomic mutation 2250G>A at the end of exon 16 should not result in a change of the lysine at codon 709. The G>A transition would be considered a "silent mutation." However, protein truncation testing (PTT) demonstrates that this mutation results in a 126-nt deletion in the cDNA. This perturbs the donor splice site of exon 16 and causes the acceptor site to skip upstream to the donor site of exon 15, thereby deleting exon 16. Since the deletion does not result in a frameshift, downstream translation of the protein is probably not affected. Thus, what might appear from genomic analysis to be an insignificant mutation is in fact a deleterious one, as evidenced by the characteristic A-T phenotype of two unrelated homozygous patients with this mutation.

Table 14-1 Phenotypes of Four Consanguineous Affected Siblings with Mutation 6199del9 [deletes codons 2067–2069 (haplotypes in parentheses)]

	Sib 1 (AC)	Sib 2 (AC)	Sib 3 (AC)	Sib 4 (AC)
Ataxia onset (year)	1	2.5	2	0.5
Walked unaided until (year)	7	7	9	7
Telangiectasia onset (year)	4	4	2.5	4
Dysarthria onset (year)	2	2.5	2.5	3
Gray hairs	0	0	0	0
Frequent infections	0	0	0	0
Serum immunoglobulins	N	N	N	N
Alpha-fetoprotein (ng/ml)	54	30	16	—

tant, the A-T patients and their families and the referring immunologists and neurologists must be acknowledged for their continuing cooperation in innumerable blood drawings, skin biopsies, and mailings.

REFERENCES

1. Boder E, Sedgwick RP: Ataxia-telangiectasia: A familial syndrome of progressive cerebellar ataxia, oculocutaneous telangiectasia and frequent pulmonary infection. *Pediatrics* **21**:526, 1958.
2. Sedgwick RP, Boder E: Ataxia-telangiectasia, in Vinken PJ, Bruyn GW (eds): *Handbook of Clinical Neurology*, vol. 14. Amsterdam, North-Holland, 1972, pp 267–339.
3. Boder E: Ataxia-telangiectasia: An overview, in Gatti RA, Swift M (eds): *Ataxia-Telangiectasia: Genetics, Neuropathology, and Immunology of a Degenerative Disease of Childhood*. New York, Liss, 1985, pp 1–63.
4. Gatti RA, Boder E, Vinters HV, Sparkes RS, Norman A, Lange K: Ataxia-telangiectasia: An interdisciplinary approach to pathogenesis. *Medicine* **70**:99, 1991.
5. Sedgwick RP, Boder E: Ataxia-telangiectasia, in de Jong JMBV (ed): *Handbook of Clinical Neurology*, vol. 16, *Hereditary Neuropathies and Spinocerebellar Atrophies*. Amsterdam, Elsevier, 1991, pp 347–423.
6. Shiloh Y: Ataxia-telangiectasia: Closer to unraveling the mystery. *Eur J Hum Genet* **3**:116, 1995.
7. Gatti RA, Vinters HV: Cerebellar pathology in ataxia-telangiectasia, in Gatti RA, Swift M (eds): *Ataxia-Telangiectasia: Genetics, Neuropathology, and Immunology of a Degenerative Disease of Childhood*. New York, Liss, 1985, pp 225–232.

8. Vinters HV, Gatti RA, Rakic P: Sequence of cellular events in cerebellar ontogeny relevant to expression of neuronal abnormalities in ataxia-telangiectasia, in Gatti RA, Swift M (eds): *Ataxia-Telangiectasia: Genetics, Neuropathology, and Immunology of a Degenerative Disease of Childhood*. New York, Liss, 1985, pp 233–255.
9. Aguilar MJ, Kamoshita S, Landing BH, Boder E, Sedgwick RP: Pathological observations in ataxia-telangiectasia: A report on 5 cases. *J Neuropathol Exp Neurol* **27**:659, 1968.
10. Naeim A, Repinski C, Huo Y, Hong J-H, Chessa L, Naeim F, Gatti RA: Ataxia-telangiectasia: Flow cytometric cell cycle analysis of lymphoblastoid cell lines in G2/M before and after gamma-irradiation. *Mod Pathol* **7**:587, 1994.
11. Van Meir EG, Polverini PJ, Chazin VR, Su Huang H-J, de Tribolet N, Cavenee WK: Release of an inhibitor of angiogenesis upon induction of wild type p53 expression in glioblastoma cells. *Nat Genet* **8**:171, 1994.
12. Peterson RD, Kelly WD, Good RA: Ataxia-telangiectasia: Its association with a defective thymus, immunological-deficiency disease, and malignancy. *Lancet* **1**:1189, 1964.
13. Centerwall WR, Miller MM: Ataxia-telangiectasia and sinopulmonary infections: A syndrome of slowly progressive deterioration in childhood. *Am J Dis Child* **95**:385, 1958.
13a. Sourander P, Bonnevier JO, Olsson Y: A case of ataxia-telangiectasia with lesions in the spinal cord. *Acta Neurol Scand* **42**:354, 1966.
14. Thieffry S, Arthuis M, Farkas-Barceton E, Vinh LeT: L'ataxia-telangiectasie: Une observation anatomo-clinique familiale. *Ann Pediatr* **13**:749, 1966.
15. Amromin GD, Boder E, Teplitz R: Ataxia-telangiectasia with a 32 year survival: A clinicopathological report. *J Neuropathol Exp Neurol* **38**:621, 1979.
16. Barlow C, Hirotsune S, Paylor R, Liyanage M, Eckhaus M, Collins F, Shiloh Y, Crawley JN, Tied T, Tagle D, Wynshaw-Boris A: Atm-deficient mice: A paradigm of ataxia-telangiectasia. *Cell* **86**:159, 1996.
17. Gotoff SP, Aminmokri E, Liebner EJ: Ataxia-telangiectasia. Neoplasia, untoward response to x-irradiation, and tuberous sclerosis. *Am J Dis Child* **114**:617, 1967.
18. Morgan JL, Holcomb TM, Morrissey RW: Radiation reaction in ataxia-telangiectasia. *Am J Dis Child* **116**:557, 1968.
19. Cunliffe PN, Mann JR, Cameron AH, Roberts KD, Ward HWC: Radiosensitivity in ataxia-telangiectasia. *Br J Radiol* **48**:374, 1975.
20. Abadir R, Hakami N: Ataxia-telangiectasia with cancer. An indication for reduced radiotherapy and chemotherapy does. *Br J Radiol* **56**:343, 1983.
21. Hart RM, Kimler BR, Evans RG, Park CH: Radiotherapeutic management of medulloblastoma in a pediatric patient with ataxia-telangiectasia. *Int J Radiat Oncol Biol Phys* **13**:1237, 1987.
22. Taylor AMR, Harnden DG, Arlett CF, Harcourt SA, Lehmann AR, Stevens S, Bridges BA: Ataxia-telangiectasia: A human mutation with abnormal radiation sensitivity. *Nature* **258**:427, 1975.
23. Shiloh Y, Tabor E, Becker Y: In vitro phenotype of ataxia-telangiectasia fibroblast strains: Clues to the nature of the "AT DNA lesion" and the molecular defect in AT, in Gatti RA, Swift M (eds): *Ataxia-telangiectasia: Genetics, Neuropathology, and Immunology of a Degenerative Disease of Childhood*. New York, Liss, 1985, pp 111–121.
24. Shiloh Y, Tabor E, Becker Y: The response of ataxia-telangiectasia homozygous and heterozygous skin fibroblasts to neocarzinostatin. *Carcinogenesis* **3**:815, 1982.
25. Paterson MC, Mac Farlane SJ, Gentner NE, Smith BP: Cellular hypersensitivity to chronic gamma-radiation in cultured fibroblasts from ataxia-telangiectasia heterozygotes, in Gatti RA, Swift M (eds): *Ataxia-Telangiectasia: Genetics, Neuropathology, and Immunology of a Degenerative Disease of Childhood*. New York, Liss, 1985, pp 73–87.
26. Weeks DE, Paterson MC, Lange K, Andrais B, Davis RC, Yoder F, Gatti RA: Assessment of chronic gamma radiosensitivity as an in vitro assay for heterozygote identification of ataxia-telangiectasia. *Radiation Res* **128**:90–99, 1991.
27. Parshad R, Sanford KK, Jones GM, Tarone RE: G2 chromosomal radiosensitivity of ataxia-telangiectasia heterozygotes. *Cancer Genet Cytogenet* **14**:163, 1985.
28. Parshad R, Sanford KK, Jones GM: Chromosomal radiosensitivity during the G2 cell cycle period of skin fibroblasts from individuals with familial cancer. *Proc Natl Acad Sci USA* **82**:5400, 1985.
29. Shiloh Y, Parshad R, Frydman M, Sanford KK, Portnoi S, Ziv Y, Jones GM: G2 chromosomal radiosensitivity in families with ataxia-telangiectasia. *Hum Genet* **84**:15, 1989.

30. Rosin MP, Ochs HD, Gatti RA, Boder E: Heterogeneity of chromosomal breakage levels in epithelial tissue of ataxia-telangiectasia homozygotes and heterozygotes. *Hum Genet* **83**:133, 1989.

31. Scott D, Jones LA, Elyan SAG, Spreadborough A, Cown R, Ribiero G: Identification of A-T heterozygotes, in Gatti RA, Painter RB (eds): *Ataxia-Telangiectasia*. Heidelberg, Springer-Verlag, 1993, pp 101–116.

32. Swift A, Morrell D, Massey RB, Chase CL: Incidence of cancer in 161 families affected by ataxia-telangiectasia. *N Engl J Med* **325**:1831–1836, 1991.

33. Norman A, Kagan AR, Chan SL: The importance of genetics for the optimization of radiation therapy. *Am J Clin Oncol* **11**:84, 1988.

34. Norman A, Withers R: Recommendation about radiation exposure for A-T heterozygotes, in Gatti RA, Painter RB (eds): *Ataxia-Telangiectasia*. Heidelberg, Springer-Verlag, 1993, pp 137–142.

35. Law J: Patient dose and risk in mammography. **64**:360, 1991.

36. Peterson RDA, Funkhouser JD, Tuck-Miller CM, Gatti RA: Cancer susceptibility in ataxia-telangiectasia, in *Leukemia*. Macmillan, 1992, pp 8–13.

37. Swift M, Sholman L, Perry M, Chase C: Malignant neoplasms in the families of patients with ataxia-telangiectasia. *Cancer Res* **36**:209, 1976.

38. Rotman G, Shloh Y: The ATM gene and protein: Possible roles in genome surveillance, checkpoint controls and cellular defense against oxidative stree. *Cancer Surv* (in press).

39. Painter R: Altered DNA synthesis in irradiated and unirradiated ataxia-telangiectasia cells, in Gatti RA, Swift M (eds): *Ataxia-Telangiectasia: Genetics, Neuropathology, and Immunology of a Degenerative Disease of Childhood*. New York, Liss, 1985, pp 89–100.

40. Meyn MS: Ataxia-telangiectasia and cellular responses to DNA damage. *Cancer Res* **55**:5991, 1995.

41. Morrell D, Cromartie E, Swift M: Mortallity and cancer incidence in 263 patients with ataxia-telangiectasia. *J Natl Cancer Inst* **77**:89, 1986.

42. Spector BD, Filipovich AH, Perry GS, Kersey JH: Epidemiology of cancer in ataxia-telangiectasia, in Bridges BA, Harnden DG (eds): *Ataxia-Telangiectasia: Cellular and Molecular Link between Cancer, Neuropathology and Immune Deficiency*. New York/London, Wiley, 1982, pp 103–107.

43. Hecht F, Koler RD, Rigas DA, Dahnke G, Case M, Tisdale V, Miller RW: Leukkaemia and lymphocytes in ataxia-telangiectasia. *Lancet* **2**:1193, 1966.

44. Gatti RA, Good RA: Occurrence of malignancy in immunodeficiency diseases. *Cancer* **28**:89, 1971.

45. Taylor AMR, Metcalfe JA, Thick J, Mak Y-F: Leukemia and lymphoma in ataxia-telangiectasia. *Blood* **87**:423, 1996.

46. Foon KA, Gale RP: Is there a T-cell form of chronic lymphocytic leukaemia? *Leukemia* **6**:867, 1992.

47. Hollis RJ, Kennaugh AA, Butterworth SV, Taylor AMR: Growth of chromosomally abnormal T cell clones in ataxia-telangiectasia patients is associated with translocation at 14q11—a model for other T cell neoplasia. *Hum Genet* **76**:389, 1987.

48. Russo G, Isobe M, Gatti RA, Finan J, Batuman O, Huebner K, Nowell PC, Croce CM: Molecular analysis of a t(14;14) translocation in leukemic T-cells of an ataxia-telangiectasia patient. *Proc Natl Acad Sci USA* **86**:602, 1989.

49. Davey MP, Bertness V, Nakahara K, Johnson JP, McBride OW, Waldmann TA, Kirsch IR: Juxtaposition of the T-cell receptor alpha-chain locus (14q11) and a region (14q32) of potential importance in leukemogenesis by a 14;14 translocation in a patients with T-cell chronic lymphocytic leukemia and ataxia-telangiectasia. *Proc Natl Acad Sci USA* **85**:9287, 1988.

50. Gatti RA, Nieberg R, Boder E: Uterine tumors in ataxia-telangiectasia. *Gynecol Oncol* **32**:257, 1989.

51. Pippard EC, Hall AJ, Baker DJP, Bridges BA: Cancer in homozygotes and heterozygotes of ataxia-telangiectasia and xeroderma pigmentosum in Britain. *Cancer Res* **48**:2929, 1988.

52. Swift M, Reitnauer PJ, Morrell D, Chase CL: Breast and other cancers in families with ataxia-telangiectasia. *N Engl J Med* **316**:1289, 1987.

53. Borresen A-L, Andersen TI, Tretli S, Heiberg A, Moller P: Breast cancer and other cancers in Norwegian families with ataxia-telangiectasia. *Genes Chrom Cancer* **2**:339, 1990.

54. Vorechovsky I, Rasio D, Luo L, Monaco C, Hammarstrom L, Webster DB, Zaloudik J, Barbanti-Brodano G, James M, Russo G, Croce CM, Negrini M: The ATM gene and susceptibility to breast cancer:

55. FitzGerald MG, Bean JM, Hegde SR, Unsal H, MacDonald DJ, Harkin DP, Finkelstein DM, Isselbacher KJ, Haber DA: Heterozygous ATM mutations do not contribute to early onset of breast cancer. *Nature Genet* **15**:307, 1997.

56. Spurr NK, Kelsell CP, Mavrakis E, Bryant SP, Crockford G, Bishop DT: Genetic heterogeneity in UK breast and ovarian cancer families. *Am J Hum Genet* **S57**:A5, 1995.

57. Cortessis V, Ingles S, Millikan R, Diep A, Gatti RA, Richardson L, Thompson WD, Paganini-Hill A, Sparkes RS, Haile RW: Linkage analysis of DRD2, a marker linked to the ataxia-telangiectasia gene, in 64 families with premenopausal bilateral breast cancer. *Cancer Res* **53**:5083, 1993.

58. Wooster R, Easton DF, Ford D, Mangion J, Ponder BAJ, Peto J, Stratton M: The A-T gene does not make a major contribution to familial breast cancer, in Gatti RA, Painter RB (eds): *Ataxia-Telangiectasia*. Heidelberg, Springer-Verlag, 1993, pp 127–136.

59. Athma P, Rappaport R, Swift M: Molecular genotyping shows that ataxia-telangiectasia heterozygotes are predisposed to breast cancer. *Cancer Genet Cytogenet* **92**:130, 1996.

60. Carter SL, Negrini M, Baffa R, Illum DR, Rosenberg AL, Schwartz GF, Croce CM: Loss of heterozygosity at 111q22-23 in breast cancer. *Cancer Res* **54**:6270, 1994.

61. Porras O, Arguendas O, Arata M, Barrantes M, Gonzalez L, Saenz E: Epidemiology of ataxia-telangiectasia in Costa Rica, in Gatti RA, Painter RB (eds): *Ataxia-Telangiectasia*. Heidelberg, Springer-Verlag, 1993, pp 199–208.

62. Chessa L, Fiorilli M: Epidemiology of ataxia-telangiectasia in Italy, in Gatti RA, Painter RB (eds): *Ataxia-Telangiectasia*. Heidelberg, Springer-Verlag, 1993, pp 191–198.

63. Lohrer HD: Regulation of the cell cycle following DNA damage in normal and ataxia-telangiectasia cells. *Experentia* **52**:316, 1996.

64. Hartwell LH, Weinert TA: Checkpoints: Controls that ensure the order of cell cycle events. *Science* **246**:629, 1989.

65. Kastan MB, Zhan Q, El-Deiry WS, Carrier F, Jacks Y, Walsh WV, Plunkett BS, Vogelstein B, Fornace AJ: A mammalian cell cycle checkpoint pathway utilizing p53 and GADD45 is defective in ataxia-telangiectasia. *Cell* **71**:587, 1992.

66. Kastan MB: Ataxia-telangiectasia: defective in a p53-dependent signal transduction pathway, in Gatti RA, Painter RB (eds): *Ataxia-Telangiectasia*. Heidelberg, Springer-Verlag, 1993, pp 163–173.

67. Donehower LA, Harvey M, Stagle BL, McArthur MJ, Montgomery CA, Butel JS, Bradley A: Mice deficient for p53 are developmentally normal but susceptible to spontaneous tumors. *Nature* **356**:215, 1992.

68. Purdie CA, Harrison DJ, Peter A, Dobbie L, White S, Howie SE, Salter DM, Bird CC, Wyllie AH, Hooper ML: Tumour incidence, spectrum and ploidy in mice with a large deletion in the p53 gene. *Oncogene* **9**:603, 1994.

69. Liu VF, Weaver DT: The ionizing radiation-induced replication protein A phosphorylation response differs between ataxia-telangiectasia and normal human cells. *Mol Cell Biol* **13**:7222, 1993.

70. Shafman T, Khanna KK, Kedar P, Spring K, Kozlov S, Yen T, Hobson K, Gatei M, Zhang N, Watters D, Egerton M, Shiloh Y, Kharbanda S, Kufe D, Lavin MF: Interaction between ATM protein and c-Abl in response to DNA damage. *Nature* **387**:520, 1997.

71. Lavin MF, Khanna KK, Beamish H, Spring K, Watters D, Shiloh Y: Relationship of the ataxia-telangiectasia protein ATM to phosphoinositide 3-kinase. *Trends Biol Sci* **20**:382, 1995.

72. Savisky K, Bar-Shira A, Gilad S, Rotman G, Ziv Y, Vanagaite L, Tagle DA, Smith S, Uziel T, Sfez S, Ashkenazi M, Pecker I, Frydman M, Harnik R, Patanjali SR, Simmons A, Clines GA, Sartiel A, Gatti RA, Chessa L, Sanal O, Lavin MF, Jaspers NGJ, Taylor MR, Arlett CF, Miki T, Weissman SM, Lovett M, Collins FS, Shiloh Y: A single ataxia-telangiectasia gene with a product similar to PI-3 kinase. *Science* **268**:1749, 1995.

73. Nowak R: Discovery of AT gene sparks biomedical research bonanza. *Science* **268**:1700, 1995.

74. Hartwell LH, Kastan MB: Cell cycle control and cancer. *Science* **266**:1821, 1994.

75. Vogelstein B: A deadly inheritance. *Nature* **348**:681, 1990.

76. Meyn MS, Strasfeld L, Allen C: Testing the role of p53 in the expression of genetic instability and apoptosis in ataxia-telangiectasia. *Int J Radiat Biol* **66**:S141–S149, 1994.

77. Lowe SW, Ruley HE, Jacks T, Housman DE: P53-dependent apoptosis modulates the cytotoxicity of anticancer agents. *Cell* **74**:957, 1993.

78. Lee JM, Bernstein A: P53 mutations increase resistance to ionizing radiation. *Proc Natl Acad Sci USA* **90**:5742, 1993.

79. Jung M, Zhang Y, Dritschilo A: Correction of radiation sensitivity in ataxia-telangiectasia cells by a truncated IkB-a. *Science* **268**:1619, 1995.

80. Jung M, Kondratyev A, Lee SA, Dimtchev A, Dritschilo A: ATM gene product phosphorylates IκB-α. *Canc Res* **57**:24, 1997.

81. Thanos D, Maniatis T: NF-kB: A lesson in family values. *Cell* **80**:529, 1995.

82. Painter RB, Young BR: Radiosensitivity in ataxia-telangiectasia: A new explanation. *Proc Natl Acad Sci USA* **77**:7315, 1980.

83. Thacker J: Cellular radiosensitivity in ataxia-telangiectasia. *Int J Radiat Biol* **66**:S87–S96, 1994.

84. Vorechovsky I, Luo L, Dyer MJS, Catovsky D, Amlot PL, Yaxley JC, Foroni L, Hammarstrom L, Webster DB, Yuille MAR: Clustering of missense mutations in the ataxia-telangiectasia gene in a sporadic T-cell leukaemia. *Nature Genet* **17**:96, 1997.

85. Painter RB: Inhibition of mammalian cell DNA synthesis by ionizing radiation. *Int J Radiat Biol* **49**:771, 1986.

86. Painter RB: Radiobiology of ataxia-telangiectasia, in Gatti RA, Painter RB (eds): *Ataxia-Telangiectasia*. Heidelberg, Springer-Verlag, 1993, pp 257–268.

87. Hand R, Gautschi JR: Replication of mammalian DNA in vitro: Evidence for initiation from fiber autoradiography. *J Cell Biol* **82**:485, 1979.

88. Gatti RA, Bick MB, Tam CF, Medici MA, Oxelius V-A, Holland M, Goldstein AL, Boder E: Ataxia-telangiectasia: A multiparameter analysis of eight families. *Clin Immunol Immunopathol* **23**:501, 1982.

89. Woods CG, Taylor AMR: Ataxia-telangiectasia in the British Isles: The clinical and laboratory features of 70 affected individuals. *Q J Med New Series* **298**:169, 1992.

90. Gatti RA: Ataxia-telangiectasia: A neuroendocrine-immune disease? Alternative models of pathogenesis, in Fabris N, Garaci E, Hadden J, Mitchison, NA (eds): *Immunoregulation*. New York, Plenum, 1983, pp 385–398.

91. Thieffry S, Arthuis M, Aicardi J, Lyon G: L'ataxie-telangiectasie. *Rev Neurol* **105**:390, 1961.

92. Oxelius V-A, Berkel AI, Hanson LA: IgG2 deficiency in ataxia-telangiectasia. *N Engl J Med* **306**:515, 1982.

93. Rivat-Peran L. Buriot D, Salier J-P, Rivat C, Dumitresco S-M, Griscelli C: Immunoglobulins in ataxia-telangiectasia: Evidence for IgG4 and IgA2 subclass deficiencies. *Clin Immunol Immunopathol* **20**:99, 1981.

94. Ammann AJ, Cain WA, Ishizaka K, Hong R, Good RA: Immunoglobulin E deficiency in ataxia-telangiectasia. *N Engl J Med* **281**:469, 1969.

95. Polmar SH, Waldmann TA, Balestra ST, Jost M, Terry WD: Immunoglobulin E in immunologic deficiency disease. *J Clin Invest* **51**:326, 1972.

96. Hsieh C-L, Lieber MR: Lymphoid V(D)J recombination: Accessibility and reaction fidelity in normal and ataxia-telangiectasia cells, in Gatti RA, Painter RB (eds): *Ataxia-Telangiectasia*. Heidelberg, Springer-Verlag, 1993, pp 143–154.

97. Hsieh CL, Arlett CF, Lieber MR: V(D)J recombination in ataxia-telangiectasia, Bloom's syndrome and a DNA ligase I-associated immunodeficiency disorder. *J Biol Chem* **268**:20105, 1993.

98. Kirsch IR; V(D)J recombination and ataxia-telangiectasia: A review. *Int J Radiat Biol* **66**:S97–S108, 1994.

99. Paganelli R, Scala E, Scarselli E, Ortolani C, Cossarizza A, Carmini D, Aiuti F, Fiorilli M: Selective deficiency of CD4+/CD45RA+ lymphocytes in patients with ataxia-telangiectasia. *J Clin Immunol* **12**:84, 1992.

100. Eisen AH: Delayed hypersensitivity in ataxia-telangiectasia. *N Engl J Med* **272**:801, 1965.

101. Oppenheim JJ, Barlow M, Waldmann TA, Block JB: Impaired in vitro lymphocyte transformation in patients with ataxia-telangiectasia. *Br Med J* **2**:330, 1966.

102. Leiken SI, Bazelon M, Park KH: In vitro lymphocyte transformation in ataxia-telangiectasia. *J Pediatr* **68**:477, 1966.

103. Epstein WL, Fudenberg HH, Reed WB, Boder E, Sedggwick RP: Immunologic studies in ataxia-telangiectasia. *Int Arch Allergy* **30**:15, 1966.

104. Hosking G: Ataxia telangiectasia. *Dev Med Child Neurol* **24**:77, 1982.

105. Waldmann TA, Misiti J, Nelson DL, Kraemer KH: Ataxia-telangiectasia: A multisystem hereditary disease with immunodeficiency, impaired organ maturation, X-ray hypersensitivity, and a high incidence of neoplasia. *Ann Intern Med* **99**:367, 1983.

106. Nelson DL, Biddison WE, Shaw S: Defective in vitro production of influenza virus-specific cytotoxic T lymphocytes in ataxia-telangiectasia. *J Immunol* **130**:2629, 1983.

107. Weaver M, Gatti RA; Lymphocyte subpopulations in ataxia-telangiectasia, in Gatti RA, Swift M (eds): *Ataxia-Telangiectasia: Genetics, Neuropatholgy, and Immunology of a Degenerative Disease of Childhood*. New York, Liss, 1985, pp 309–314.

108. Peter HH: The origin of human NK cells: An ontogenic model derived from studies in patients with immunodeficiencies. *Blut* **46**:239, 1983.

109. Sanal O, Ersoy F, Tezcan I, Gogus S: Ataxia-telangiectasia presenting as hyper IgM syndrome, in Chapel HM, Levinsky JR, Webster ADB (eds): *Progress in Immune Deficiency*, vol III. Royal Society of Medicine **173**:303, 1991.

110. Thiele EA, Bonilla F, Rosen F, Riviello JI: Ataxia telangiectasia associated with the hyper-IgM syndrome. International Neurology Conference, San Francisco, Sept. 9–11, 1994.

111. Huo YK, Wang Z, Hong J-H, Chessa L, McBride WH, Perlman SL, Gatti RA: Radiosensitivity of ataxia-telangiectasia X-linked agammaglobulinemia and related syndromes. *Cancer Res* **54**:2544, 1994.

112. McFarlin DE, Strober W, Waldmann TA: Ataxia-telangiectasia. *Medicine* **51**:281, 1972.

113. Waldmann TA, McIntire KR: Serum alpha-fetoprotein levels in patients with ataxia-telangiectasia. *Lancet* **2**:112, 1972.

114. Yamashita T, Nakane A, Watanabe T, Miyoshi I, Kasai M: Evidence that alpha-fetoprotein suppresses the immunological function in transgenic mice. *Biochem Biophy Res Commun* **201**:1154, 1994.

115. Ishiguro T, Taketa K, Gatti RA: Tissue of origin of elevated alphafetoprotein in ataxia-telangiectasia. *Dis Markers* **4**:293, 1986.

116. Gatti RA, Aurias A, Griscelli C, Sparkes RS: Translocations involving chromosomes 2p and 22q in ataxia-telangiectasia. *Dis Markers* **3**:169, 1985.

117. Kojis TL, Gatti RA, Sparkes RS: The cytogenetics of ataxia-telangiectasia. *Cancer Genet Cytogenet* **56**:143, 1992.

118. Kojis TL, Schreck RR, Gatti RA, Sparkes RS: Tissue specificity of chromosomal rearrangements in ataxia-telangiectasia. *Hum Genet* **83**:337, 1989.

119. Hecht F, Hecht BK: Ataxia-telangiectasia breakpoints in chromosome rearrangements reflect genes important to T and B lymphocytes, in Gatti RA, Swift M (eds): *Ataxia-Telangiectasia: Genetics, Neuropathology, and Immunology of a Degenerative Disease of Childhood*. New York, Liss, 1985, pp 189–195.

120. Hecht F, McCaw BK, Koler RD: Ataxia-telangiectasia—clonal growth of translocation lymphocytes. *N Engl J Med* **289**:286, 1972.

121. Berkel AI: Studies of IgG subclasses in ataxia-telangiectasia patients. *Monogr Allergy* **29**:100, 1986.

122. Roifman CM, Gelfand EW: Heterogeneity of the immunological deficiency in ataxia-telangiectasia: Absence of a clinical-pathological correlation, in Gatti RA, Swift M (eds): *Ataxia-Telangiectasia: Genetics, Neuropathology, and Immunology of a Degenerative Disease of Childhood*. New York, Liss, 1985, pp 273–285.

123. Virgilio L, Narducci MG, Isobe M, Billips LG, Cooper MD, Croce CM, Russo G: Identification of the TCL1 gene involved in T cell malignancies. *Proc Natl Acad Sci USA* **91**:12530, 1994.

124. Taylor AMR, Lowe PA, Stacey M, Thick J, Campbell L, Beatty D, Biggs P, Formstone CJ: Development of T cell leukaemia in an ataxia-telangiectasia patient following clonal selection in t(X;14) containing lymphocytes. *Leukemia* **6**:961, 1992.

125. Kenwrick S, Llevinson B, Taylor S, Shapiro A, Gitschier J: Isolation and sequence of two genes associated with a CpG island 5′ of the factor VIII gene. *Hum Mol Genet* **1**:179, 1992.

126. Soulier J, Madni A, Cacheux V, Rosenwajg M, Sigaux F, Stern M-H: The MTCP-1/c6-1B gene encodes for a cytoplasmic 8kd protein overexpressed in T cell leukaemia bearing a t(X;14) translocation. *Oncogene* **9**:3565, 1994.

127. Madani A, Soulier J, Schmid M, Plichtova R, Lerme F, Gateau-Roesch O, Garnier J-P, Pla M, Sigaux F, Stern M-H: The 8 kd protein of the putative oncogene MTCP-1 is a mitoochondrial protein. *Oncogene* **10**:2259, 1995.

128. Fu T, Virgilio L. Narducci MG, Facciano A, Russo G, Croce CM: Characterisation and localisation of the TCL-1 oncogene product. *Cancer Res* **54**:6297, 1994.

129. Knudsen AG: Hereditary cancer, oncogenes, and antioncogenes. *Cancer Res* **45**:1437, 1985.

130. Pandita TK, Pathak S, Geard C: Chromosome and associations, telomeres and telomerase activity in ataxia-telangiectasia cells. *Cytogenet Cell Genet* **71**:86, 1995.

131. Moyzis RK, Buckingham JM, Cram LS, Dani M, Deaven LL, Jones MD, Meyne J, Ratliff RL, Wu J-R: A highly conserved repetitive DNA sequence (TTAGGG)n, present in the telomeres of human chromosomes. *Proc Natl Acad Sci USA* **85**:6622, 1988.

132. Kipling D, Cooke HJ: Beginning or end? Telomere structure, genetics and biology. *Hum Mol Genet* **1**:3, 1992.

133. De Lange T, Shiue L, Myers RM, Cox DR, Naylor SL, Killery AM, Varmus HE: Structure and varability of human chromosome ends. *Molec Cell Biol* **10**:518, 1990.

134. Kim NW, Piatyszek MA, Prowse KR, Harley CB, West MD, Ho PLC, Coviello GM, Wright WE, Weinrich SL, Shay JW: Specific association of human telomerase activity with immortal cells and cancer. *Science* **266**:2011, 1994.

135. Metcalfe JA, Parkhill J, Campbell L. Stacey M, Biggs P, Byrd PJ, Taylor AMR: Accelerated telomere shortening in ataxia-telangiectasia. *Nat Genet* **13**:350, 1996.

136. Effros RB, Allsopp R, Chiu C-P, Hausner MA, Hirji K, Wang L, Harley CB, Villeponteau B, West MD, Giorgi JV: Shortened telomeres in the expanded CD28-CD8+ cell subset in HIV disease implicate replicative senescence in MIV pathogenesis. *AIDS* **10**:F17, 1996.

137. Enoch T, Norbury C: Cellular responses to DNA damage: Cell cycle checkpoints, apoptosis and the roles of p53 and ATM. *Trends Biol Sci* **20**:426, 1995.

138. Lehmann AR, Carr AM: The ataxia-telangiectasia gene: A link between checkpoint controls, neurodegeneration and cancer. *Trends Genet* **11**:375, 1995.

139. Keegan KS, Holtzmann DA, Plug AW, Christenson ER, Brainerd EE, Flaggs G, Bentley NJ, Taylor EM, Meyn MS, Moss SB, Carr AM, Ashley T, Hoekstra MF: The Atr and Atm protein kinases associate with different sites along meiotically pairing chromosomes. *Genes Development* **10**:2423, 1996.

140. Savitsky K, Sfez S, Tagle DA, Ziv Y, Sartiel A, Collins FS, Shiloh Y, Rotman G: The complete sequence of the coding region of the ATM gene reveals similarity to cell cycle regulators in different species. *Hum Mol Genet* **4**:2025, 1995.

141. Cimprich KA, Shin TB, Keith CT, Schreiber SL: cDNA cloning and gene mapping of a candidate human cell cycle checkpoint protein. *Proc Natl Acad Sci USA* **93**:2850, 1996.

142. Al-Khodairy F, Carr AM: DNA repair mutants defining G2 checkpoint pathways in Schizosaccharomyces pombe. *EMBO J* **11**:1343, 1992.

143. Seaton BL, Yucel J, Sunnerhagen P, Subramani P: Isolation and characterization of S: Pombe rad3 gene involved in the DNA damage and DNA synthesis checkpoints. *Gene* **119**:83, 1992.

144. Weinert TA, Kiser GL, Hartwell LH: Mitotic checkpoint genes in budding yeast and the dependence of mitosis on DNA replication and repair. *Gene Dev* **8**:652, 1994.

145. Paulovich AG, Hartwell LH: A checkpoint regulates the rate of progression through S phase in *S. cervisiae* in response to DNA damage. *Cell* **82**:841, 1995.

146. Kato R, Ogawa H: An essential gene, ESR1, is required for mitotic cell growth, DNA repair and meiotic recombination in Saccaromyces cerebisiae. *Nucl Acids Res* **22**:3104, 1994.

147. Sanchez Y, Desany BA, Jones WJ, Liu Q, Wang B, Elledge SJ: Regulation of RAD53 by the ATM-like kinases MEC1 and TEL1 in yeast cell cycle checkpoint pathways. *Science* **271**:357, 1996.

148. Morrow DW, Tagle DA, Shiloh Y, Collins FS, Hieter P: TEL1, an S. cerevisiae homolog of the human gene mutated in ataxia-telangiectasia, is functionally related to the yeast checkpoint gene MEC1. *Cell* **82**:831, 1995.

149. Jaspers NGJ, Bootsma D: Genetic heterogeneity in ataxia-telangiectasia studies by cell fusion. *Proc Natl Acad Sci USA* **79**:2641, 1982.

150. Jaspers NGJ, Painter RB, Paterson MC, Kidson C, Inoue T: Complementation analysis of ataxia-telangiectasia, in Gatti RA, Swift M (eds): *Ataxia-Telangiectasia: Genetics, Neuropathology, and Immunology of a Degenerative Disease of Childhood*. New York, Liss, 1985, pp 147–162.

151. Jaspers NGJ, Gatti RA, Baan C, Linssen PCML, Bootsma D: Genetic complementation analysis of ataxia-telangiectasia and Nijmegan breakage syndrome: A survey of 50 patients. *Cytogenet Cell Genet* **49**:259, 1988.

152. Gatti RA, Berkel I, Boder E, Braedt G, Charmley P, Concannon P, Ersoy F, Foroud T, Jaspers NGJ, Lange K, Lathrop GM, Leppert M, Nakamura Y, O'Connell P, Paterson M, Salser W, Sanal O, Silver J, Sparkes RS, Susi E, Weeks DE, Wei S, White R, Yoder F: Localization of an ataxia-telangiectasia gene to chromosome 11q22-23. *Nature* **336**:577, 1988.

153. Ziv Y, Rotman G, Frydman M, Dagan J, Cohen T, Foroud T, Gatti RA, Shiloh Y: The ATC (ataxia-telangiectasia Group C) locus localizes to chromosome 11q22-q23. *Genomics* **9**:373, 1991.

154. Meyn MS, Lu-Kuo JM, Herzing LBK: Expression cloning of multiple human cDNAs that complement the phenotypic defects of ataxia-telangiectasia Group D fibroblasts. *Am J Hum Genet* **53**:1206, 1993.

155. Gatti RA, Nakamura Y, Nussmeier M, Susi E, Shan W, Grody WW: Informativeness of VNTR genetic markers for detecting chimerism after bone marrow transplantation. *Dis Markers* **7**:105, 1989.

156. Fritz E, Elsea SH, Patel PI, Myen MS: Overexpression of a human protein corrects multiple aspects of the ataxia-telangiectasia phenotype. *Proc Natl Acad Sci USA* (in press).

157. Telatar M, Wang Z, Udar N, Liang T, Bernatowska-Matuszkiewicz E, Lavin M, Shiloh Y, Concannon P, Good RA, Gatti RA: Ataxia-telangiectasia: Mutations in ATM cDNA detected by protein-truncation screening. *Am J Hum Genet* **59**:40, 1996.

158. Meyn MS: High spontaneous intrachromosomal recombination rates in ataxia-telangiectasia. *Science* **260**:1327, 1993.

159. Muriel WJ, Lamb JR, Lehmann AR: UV mutation spectra in cell lines from patients with Cockayne's syndrome and ataxia-telangiectasia, using the shuttle vector pZ189. *Mutat Res* **254**:119, 1991.

160. Woods CG, Bunday SE, Taylor AMR: Unusual features in the inheritance of ataxia-telangiectasia. *Hum Genet* **84**:555, 1990.

161. Lange E, Corresen A-L, Chen X, Chessa L, Chiplunkar S, Concannon P, Dandekar S, Gerken S, Lange K, Liang T, McConville C, Polakow J, Porras O, Rotman G, Sanal O, Sheikhavandi S, Shiloh Y, Sobel E, Taylor M, Telatar M, Teraoka S, Tolun A, Udar N, Uhrhammer N, Vanagaite L, Wang Z, Wapelhorst B, Yang H-M, Yang L, Ziv Y, Gatti RA: Localization of an ataxia-telangiectasia gene to a ~500 kb interval on chromosome 11q23.1: Linkage analysis of 176 families in an international consortium. *Am J Hum Genet* **57**:112, 1995.

162. Gatti RA, Lange E, Rotman G, Chen S, Uhrhammer N, Liang T, Chiplunkar S, Yang L, Udar N, Dandekar S, Sheikhavandi S, Wang Z, Yang U-M, Polakow J, Elashoff M, Telatar M, Sanal O, Chessa L, McConville C, Taylor M, Shiloh Y. Porras O, Borresen A-L, Wegner R-D, Curry C, Gerken S, Lange K. Concannon P: Genetic haplotyping of ataxia-telangiectasia families localizes the major gene to an ~850 kb region on chromosome 11q23.1. *Int J Radiat Biol* **66**:S57, 1994.

163. Swift M, Morrell D, Cromartie E, Chamberlin AR, Skolnick MH, Bishop DT: The indicence and gene frequency of ataxia-telangiectasia in the United States. *Am J Hum Genet* **39**:573, 1986.

164. Swift M: Genetics and epidemiology of ataxia-telangiectasia, in Gatti RA, Swift M (eds): *Ataxia-Telangiectasia: Genetics, Neuropathology, and Immunology of a Degenerative Disease of Childhood*. New York, Liss, 1985, pp 133–144.

165. Barlow MH, McFarlin ED, Schalch DS: An unsual type of diabetes mellitus with marked hyperinsulinism in patients with ataxia telangiectasia. *Clin Res* **13**:530, 1965.

166. Schalch DS, McFarlin DE, Barlow MH: An unusual form of diabetes mellitus in ataxia telangiectasia. *N Engl J Med* **282**:1396, 1970.

167. Gatti RA, Walford RL: Immune function and features of aging in chromosomal instability syndromes, in Segre D, Smith L (eds): *Immunologic Aspects of Aging*. New York, Marcel Dekker, 1981, pp 449–465.

168. Terplan KL, Krauss RF: Histopathologic brain changes in association with ataxia-telangiectasia. *Neurology* **19**:446, 1969.

169. Xu Y, Ashley T, Brainerd EE, Bronson RT, Meyn MS, Baltimore D: Targeted disruption of ATM leads to growth retardation, chromosomal fragmentation during meiosis, immune defect, and thymic lymphoma. *Genes Development* **10**:2411, 1996.

170. Herndon RM: Selective vulnerability in the nervous system, in Gatti RA, Swift M (eds): *Ataxia-Telangiectasia: Genetics, Neuropathology, and Immunology of a Degenerative Disease of Childhood*. New York, Liss, 1985, pp 257–267.

171. Kamoshita S, Aguilar MJ, Landing BH: Precocious aging in ataxia-telangiectasia: Pathological evidence in the central nervous system, in *Proceedings of the First International Congress of Child Neurology*. Toronto, 1975.

172. Weemaes CMR, Hustinx TWJ, Scheres JMJC, Van Munster PJJ, Bakkeren JAJM, Taalman RDFM: A new chromosomal instability disorder: The Nijmegen breakage syndrome. *Acta Paediatr Scand* **70**:557, 1981.

173. Wegner RD, Metzger M, Hanefeld NG, Jaspers J, Baan C, Magdorf K, Kunze J, Sperling K: A new chromosomal instability disorder confirmed by complementation studies. *Clin Genet* **33**:20, 1988.

174. Stumm M, Seemanova E, Gatti RA, Sperling K, Reis A, Wegner R-D: The ataxia-telangiectasia variant genes 1 and 2 show no linkage to the AT candidate region on chromosome 11q22-23. *Am J Hum Genet* **57**:960, 1995.

175. Saar K, Chrzanowska KH, Stumm M, Jung M, Nurnberg G, Wienker TF, Seemanova E, Wegner R-D, Reis A, Sperling K. The gene for ataxia-telangiectasia-variant (Nijmegen Breakage Syndrome) maps to a 1 cM interval on chromosome 8q21. *Am J Hum Genet* **60**:605, 1997.

176. Taalman RDFM, Hustinx TWJ, Weemaes CMR, Seemanova E, Schmidt A, Passarge E, Scheres JMJC: Further delineation of the Nijmegen Breakage Syndrome. *Am J Med Genet* **32**:425, 1989.

177. Burgt I, Chrzanowska K, Smeets D, Weemaes C: Nijmegen breakage syndrome. *J Med Genet* **33**:153, 1996.

178. Chrzanowska KH, Kleijer WJ, Krajewska-Walasek M, Bialecka M, Gutkowska A, Goryluk-Kozakiewicz B, Michalkiewicz J: Eleven Polish patients with microcephaly, immunodeficiency and chromosomal instability: The Nijmegen breakage syndrome. *Am J Med Genet* **57**:462, 1995.

179. Curry CJR, O'Lague P, Tsai J, Hutchinson HT, Jaspers NGJ, Wara D, Gatti RA: AT$_{Fresno}$: A phenotype linking ataxia-telangiectasia with the Nijmegen breakage syndrome. *Am J Hum Genet* **45**:270, 1989.

180. Gatti RA: Ataxia-telangiectasia: genetic studies, in Griscelli C, Gupta S (eds): *New Concepts in Immunodeficiency*. Chichester, UK, Wiley, 1993, pp 203–229.

181. Lange E, Gatti RA, Sobel E, Concannon P, Lange K: How many A-T genes? in Gatti RA, Painter RB (eds): *Ataxia-Telangiectasia*. Heidelberg, Springer-Verlag, 1993, pp 37–54.

182. Taylor AMR, McConville CM, Woods GW, Byrd PJ, Hernandez D: Clinical and cellular heterogeneity in ataxia-telangiectasia, in Gatti RA, Painter RB (eds): *Ataxia-Telangiectasia*. Heidelberg, Springer-Verlag, 1993, pp 209–233.

183. Maserati E, Ottoline A, Veggiatti P, Lanzi G, Pasquali F: Ataxia without telangiectasia in two sisters with rearrangements of chromosomes 7 and 14. *Clin Genet* **34**:283, 1988.

184. Byrne E, Hallpike JF, Manson JI, Sutherland GR, Thong YH: Progressive multisystem degeneration with IgE deficiency and chromosomal instability. *J Neurol Sci* **66**:307, 1984.

185. Wang Z, Guo B, Meyn S, McCurdy DK, Plaeger S, Conley ME, Driscoll DA, Perlman SL, Saxon A, Gatti RA: Increased radiosensitivity of lymphoblastoid cell lines from patients with immunodeficiency syndromes. *Cancer Res* (submitted).

186. Harding A: *The Inherited Ataxias and Related Disorders*. London, Churchill Livingstone, 1984.

187. Bird, TD: Hereditary motor sensory neuropathies: Charcot-Marie-Tooth syndrome. *Neurol Clin North AM* **7**:9, 1989.

188. Campuzano V, Montermini L, Molto MD, Pianese L, Cossee M, Cavalcanti F, Monros E, Rodius F, Duclos F, Monticelli A, Zara F, Canizares J, Koutnikova H, Bidichandani SI, Gellera C, Brice A, Trouillas P, De Michele G, Filla A, De Frutos R, Palau F, Patel PI, Di Donato S, Mandel J-L, Cocozza S, Koenig M, Pandolfo M: Friedreich's ataxia: Autosomal recessive disease cased by an intronic GAA triplet repeat expansion. *Science* **271**:1423, 1996.

189. Aicardi J, Barbosas C, Andermann E, Andermann F, Morcos R, Ghanem Q, Fukuyama Y, Awaya Y, Moe P: Ataxia-ocular motor apraxia: A syndrome mimicking ataxia-telangiectasia. *Ann Neurol* **24**:497, 1988.

190. Jaspers NGJ, van der Kraan M, Linssen PCML, Macek M, Seemanova E, Kleijer WJ: First-trimester prenatal diagnosis of the Nijmegen breakage syndrome and ataxia-telangiectasia using an assay of radioresistant DNA synthesis. *Prenat Diagn* **10**:667, 1990.

191. Gianelli F, Avery JA, Pembrey ME, Blunt S: Prenatal exclusion of ataxia-telangiectasia, in Bridges BA, Harnden DG (eds): *Ataxia-Telangiectasia: Cellular and Molecular Link between Cancer, Neuropathology and Immune Deficiency*. New York/London, Wiley, 1982, pp 393–407.

192. Gatti RA, Peterson KL, Novak J, Chen X, Yang-Chen L, Liang T, Lange E, Lange K: Prenatal genotyping of ataxia-telangiectasia. *Lancet* **342**:376, 1993.

193. Kleijer WJ, van der Kraan M, Los FJ, Jaspers MGJ: Prenatal diagnosis of ataxia-telangiectasia and Nijmegen breakage syndrome by the assay of radioresistant DNA synthesis. *Int J Radiat Biol* **66**:S167, 1994.

194. Rotman G, Savitski K, Vanagaite L, Bar-Shira A, Ziv Y, Gilad S, Vchenik V, Smith S, Shiloh Y: Physical and genetic mapping at the ATA/ATC locus on chromosome 11q22-23. *Int J Radiat Biol* **66**:S63, 1994.

195. Vanagaite L, James MR, Rotman G, Savitsky K, Var-Shira A, Gilad S, Ziv Y, Uchenik V, Sartiel A, Collins FS, Sheffield VC, Richard CW III, Weissenbach J, Shiloh Y: *Hum Genet* **95**:451, 1995.

196. Perlman, SL: Treatment of ataxia-telangiectasia, in Gatti RA, Painter RB (eds): *Ataxia-Telangiectasia*. Heidelberg, Springer-Verlag, 1993, pp 269–278.

197. Pump KK, Dunn HG, Meuwissen H: A study of the bronchial and vascular structures of a lung from a case of ataxia-telangiectasia. *Dis Chest* **47**:473, 1965.

198. Hall S: *Ataxia-Telangiectasia: A Guide to Physiotherapy*. Harpenden, Herts, UK, A-T Society, 1995.

199. Gatti RA, Boehnke M, Crist M, Sparkes RS: Genetic linkage studies in ataxia-telangiectasia, in Gatti RA, Swift M (eds): *Ataxia-Telangiectasia: Genetics, Neuropathology, and Immunology of a Degenerative Disease of Childhood*. New York, Liss, 1985, pp 163–172.

200. Hodge SE, Berkel AI, Gatti RA, Boder E, Spence MA: Ataxia-telangiectasia and xeroderma pigmentosum: No evidence of linkage to HLA. *Tissue Antigens* **15**:313, 1980.

201. Botstein D, White RI, Skolnick M, Davis RW: Construction of a genetic linkage map in man using restriction fragment length polymorphisms. *Am J Hum Gen* **32**:314, 1980.

202. Donis-Keller H, Green P, Helms C, Cartinhour S, Weiffenbach B, Stephens K, Keith TP, Bowden DW, Smith DR, Lander ES, Botstein D, Akots G, Rediker KS, Gravius T, Brown VA, Rising MB, Parker C, Powers JA, Watt DE, Kauffman ER, Bricker A, Phipps P, Muller-Kahle H, Fulton TR, Ng S, Schumm JW, Braman JC, Knowlton RG, Barker DF, Crooks S, Lincoln SE, Daly MJ, Abrahamson J: A genetic linkage map of the human genome. *Cell* **51**:319, 1987.

203. Dausset J, Cann H, Cohen D, Lathrop M, Lalouel J-M, White R: Centre d'Etude du Polymorphisme Humain (CEPH): Collaborative genetic mapping of the human genome. *Genomics* **6**:575, 1990.

204. Murnane JP, Painter RB: Complementation of the defects in DNA synthesis in irradiated and unirradiated ataxia-telangiectasia cells. *Proc Natl Acad Sci USA* **79**:1960, 1982.

205. Gatti RA, Shaked R, Wei S, Koyama M, Salser W, Silver J: DNA polymorphism in the human THY-1 gene. *Human Immunol* **22**:145, 1988.

206. Sanal O, Wei S, Foroud T, Malhotra U, Concannon P, Charmley P, Salser W, Lange K, Gatti RA: Further mapping of an ataxia-telangiectasia locus to the chromosome 11q23 region. *Am J Hum Genet* **47**:860, 1990.

207. Foroud T, Wei S, Ziv Y, Sobel E, Lange E, Chao A, Goradia T, Huo Y, Tolun A, Chessa L, Charmley P, Sanal O, Salman N, Julier C, Lathrop GM, Concannon P, McConville C, Taylor M, Shiloh Y, Lange K, Gatti RA: Localization of an ataxia-telangiectasia locus to a 3-cM interval on chromosome 11q23: Linkage analyses of 111 families by an international consortium. *Am J Hum Genet* **49**:1263, 1991.

208. Sanal O, Lange E, Telatar M, Sobel E, Salazar-Novak J, Ersoy F, Concannon P, Tolun A, Gatti RA: Ataxia-telangiectasia-linkage analysis of chromosome 11q22-23 markers in Turkish families. *FASEB J* **6**:2848, 1992.

209. Charmley P, Foroud T, Wei S, Concannon P, Weeks DE, Lange D, Gatti RA: A primary linkage map of the human chromosome 11q22-23 region. *Genomics* **6**:316, 1990.

210. Charmley P, Nguyen J, Wei S, Gatti RA: Genetic linkage analysis and homology of syntenic relationships of genes located on human chromosome 11q. *Genomics* **10**:608, 1991.

211. Concannon P, Malhotra U, Charmley P, Reynolds J, Lange K, Gatti RA: Ataxia-telangiectasia gene (ATA) on chromosome 11 is distinct from the ETS-1 gene. *Genomics* **46**:789, 1990.

212. Wei S, Rocchi M, Archidiacono N, Sacchi N, Romeo G, Gatti RA: Physical mapping of the human chromosome 11q23 region containing the ataxia-telangiectasia locus. *Cancer Genet Cytogenet* **46**:1, 1990.

213. McConville CM, Byrd PJ, Ambrose HJ, Taylor AMR: Genetic and physical mapping of the ataxia-telangiectasia locus on chromosome 11q22-23, in Taylor AMR, Scott D, Arlett CF, Cole J (eds): *Ataxia-Telangiectasia: The Effect of a Pleiotropic Gene*. Taylor & Francis, 1994, pp S45–S57.

214. McConville CM, Formstone CJ, Hernandez D, Thick J, Taylor AMR: Fine mapping of the chromosome 11q22-23 region using PFGE, linkage and haplotype analysis: Localization of the gene for ataxia-telangiectasia to a 5 cM region flanked by NCAM/DRD2 and STMY/CJ52.75, ph2.22. *Nucleic Acids Res* **18**:4334, 1990.

215. McConville C, Woods CG, Farrall M, Metcalfe JA, Taylor AMR: Analysis of 7 polymorphic markers at chromsome 11q22-23 in 35

ataxia-telangiectasia families: Further evidence of linkage. *Hum Genet* **85**:215, 1990.

216. McConville CM, Byrd PJ, Ambrose H, Stankovic T, Ziv Y, Bar-Shira A, Vanagaite L, Rotman G, Shiloh Y, Gillett GT, Riley JH, Taylor AMR: Paired STSs amplified from radiation hybrids, and from associated YACs, identify highly polymorphic loci flanking the ataxia-telangiectasia locus on chromosome 11q22-23. *Hum Mol Genet* **2**:969, 1993.

217. Cornelis F, James M, Cherif D, Tokino T, Davies J, Girault D, Bernard C, Litt M, Berger R, Nakamura Y, Lathrop M, Julier C: Precise localization of a gene responsible for ataxia-telangiectasia on chromosome 11q, in Gatti RA, Painter RB (eds): *Ataxia-Telangiectasia*. Heidelberg, Springer-Verlag, 1993, pp 23–36.

218. Oskato R, Bar-Shira A, Vanagaite L, Ziv Y, Ehrlich S, Rotman G, McConville CM, Chakravarti A, Shiloh Y: Ataxia-telangiectasia: Allelic association with 11q22-23 markers in Moroccan-Jewish patients. *Am J Hum Genet* **53**:A1055, 1993.

219. Taylor AMR, McConville CM, Rotman G, Shiloh Y, Byrd PJ: A haplotype common to intermediate radiosensitivity variants of ataxia-telangiectasia in the UK. *Int J Radiat Biol* **66**:S35, 1994.

220. Uhrhammer N, Concannon P, Huo Y, Nakamura Y, Gatti RA: A pulsed-field gel electrophoresis map in the ataxia-telangiectasia region of chromosome 11q22.3. *Genomics* **20**:278, 1994.

221. Uhrhammer N, Lange E, Porras O, Naeim A, Chen X, Sheikhavandi S, Chiplunkar S, Yang L, Dandekar S, Liang T, Patel N, Udar N, Concannon P, Gerken S, Shiloh Y, Lange K, Gatti RA: Sublocalization of an ataxia-telangiectasia gene distal to D11S384 by ancestral haplotyping in Costa Rican families. *Am J Hum Genet* **57**:103, 1995.

222. Lange K, Sobel E: A random walk method for computing genetic location scores. *Am J Hum Genet* **49**: 1320, 1991.

223. Sobel E, Lange K: Metropolis sampling in pedigree analysis. *State Methods Med Res* **2**:263, 1993.

224. Buckler AJ, Chang DD, Graw SL, Brook JD, Haber DA, Sharp PA, Housman DE: Exon amplification: A strategy to isolate mammalian genes based on RNA splicing. *PNAS* **88**:4005, 1991.

225. Byrd PJ, McConville CM, Cooper P, Parkhill J, Stankovic T, McGuire GM, Thick JA, Taylor AMR: Mutations revealed by sequencing the 5′ half of the gene for ataxia-telangiectasia. *Hum Mol Genet* **5**:145, 1996.

226. Imai T, et al.: Identification and characterization of a new gene physically linked to the ATM gene. *Genome Res* **6**:439, 1996.

227. Chen X, Yang L, Udar N, Liang T, Uhrhammer N, Xu S, Bay JO, Wang Z, Dandakar U, Chiplunkar S, Klisak I, Telatar M, Yang H, Concannon P, Gatti RA: CAND3: A ubiquitously-expressed gene immediately adjacent and in opposite transcriptional orientation to the ATM gene at 11q23.1. *Mamm Genome* **8**:129–133, 1997.

228. Rasio D, Negrini M, Croce CM: Genomic organization of the ATM locus involved in ataxia-telangiectasia. *Cancer Res* **55**:6053, 1995.

229. Uziel T, Savitsky K, Platzer M, Ziv Y, Helbitz T, Nehls M, Boehm T, Rosenthal A, Shiloh Y, Rotman G: Genomic organization of the ATM gene. *Genomics* **33**:317, 1996.

230. Pecker I, Avrahan KB, Gilbert DJ, Savitsky K, Rotman G, Harnik R, Fukao T, Schrock E, Hirotsune S, Tagle DA, Collins FS, Wynshow-Boris A, Ried T, Copeland NG, Jenkins NA, Shiloh Y, Ziv Y: Identification and chromosomal localization of atm, the mouse homolog of the ataxia-telangiectasia gene. *Genomics* 1996.

231. Gao J-H, Parsons LM, Bowers JM, Xiong J, Li J, Fox PT: Cerebellum implicated in sensory acquisition and discrimination rather than motor control. *Science* **272**:545, 1996.

232. Barinaga M: The cerebellum: Movement coordinator or much more? (editoral overview). *Science* **272**:482, 1996.

233. Keith CT, Schreiber SL: PIK-related kinases: DNA repair, recombination, and cell cycle checkpoints. *Science* **270**:50, 1995.

234. Gilad S, Khosravi R, Shkedy D, Uziel T, Ziv Y, Savitsky K, Rotman G, Smith S, Chessa L, Jorgensen TJ, Harnik R, Frydman M, Sanal O, Portnoi S, Goldwicz Z, Jaspers MGJ, Gatti RA, Lenoir G, Lavin M, Tatsumi K, Wegner RD, Shiloh Y, Bar-Shira A: Predominance of null mutation in ataxia-telangiectasia. *Hum Mol Genet* **5**:433, 1996.

235. Wright J, Teraoka S, Onengut S, Tolun A, Gatti RA, Ochs HD, Concannon P: A high frequency of distinct ATM mutations in ataxia-telangiectasia. *Am J Hum Genet* **59**:839, 1996.

236. Forrest S, Cotton R, Landegren U, Southern E: How to find all those mutations. *Nat Genet* **10**:375, 1995.

237. Concannon P, Gatti RA: Diversity of ATM gene mutations detected in patients with ataxia-telangiectasia. *Hum Mutation* **10**:100, 1997.

238. Hawkins JD: *Gene Structure and Expression*, 2d ed. Cambridge, UK, Cambridge University Press, 1991, p 127.

239. McConville CM, Stankovic T, Byrd PJ, McGuire GM, Yao Q-Y, Lennox GG, Taylor AMR: Mutations associated with variant phenotypes in ataxia-telangiectasia. *Am J Hum Genet* **59**:320, 1996.

240. Gatti RA: Ataxia-telangiectasia: Immune dysfunction is one of many defects. *Immunol Today* **5**:121, 1984.

241. Lehmann A, Jaspers NJG, Gatti RA: Ataxia-telangiectasia: Meeting report. *Cancer Res* **47**:4750, 1987.

242. Lehmann AR, Jaspers NGJ, Gatti RA: Meeting report: Fourth International Workshop on Ataxia-Telangiectasia. *Cancer Res* **49**:6162, 1989.

243. Taylor AMR, Jaspers NGJ, Gatti RA: Meeting report: Fifth International Workshop on Ataxia-Telangiectasia. *Cancer Res* **53**:438, 1993.

244. Gatti RA, McConville CM, Taylor AMR. Meeting report. Sixth International Workshop on Ataxia-Telangiectasia. *Cancer Res* **54**:6007, 1994.

245. Bridges BA, Harnden DG (eds): *Ataxia-Telangiectasia: A Cellular and Molecular Link between Cancer, Neuropathology, and Immune Deficiency*. Chichester, UK, Wiley, 1982, pp 1–402.

246. Gatti RA, Swift M (eds): *Ataxia-Telangiectasia: Genetics, Neuropathology, and Immunology of a Degenerative Disease of Childhood*. New York, Liss, 1985.

247. Gatti RA, Painter RB (eds): *Ataxia-Telangiectasia*, vol 77, NATO ASI Series. Heidelberg, Springer-Verlag, 1993.

248. Julier C, Nakamura Y, Lathrop M, O'Connell P, Leppert M, Litt M, Mohandas T, Lalouel, J-M, White R: Detailed map of the long arm of chromosome 11. *Genomics* **7**:335, 1990.

249. Kapp LN, Painter RB, Yu L-C, van Loon N, Richard CW, James MR, Cox DR, Murnane JP: Cloning of a candidate gene for ataxia-telangiectasia group D. *Am J Hum Genet* **51**:45, 1992.

250. Kapp LN, Murnane JP: Cloning and characterization of a candidate gene for A-T complementation Group D, in Gatti RA, Painter RB (eds): *Ataxia-Telangiectasia*. Heidelberg, Springer-Verlag, 1993, pp 7–22.

251. Platzer M, Rotman G, Bauer D, Uziel T, Savitsky K, Bar-Shira A, Gilad S, Shiloh Y, Rosenthal A. Ataxia-telangiectasia locus: Sequence analysis of 184 kb of human genomic DNA containing the entire ATM gene. *Genome Res* **7**:592, 1997.

252. Telatar M, Teraoka S, Wang Z, Chun HH, Liang T, Castellvi-Bel S, Udar N, Borresen-Dale A-L, Chessa L, Bernatowska-Matuszkiewicz E, Porras O, Watanabe M, Junker A, Concannon P, Gatti RA: Ataxia-telangiectasia: Identification and detection of founder mutations in the ATM gene in ethnic populations. *Am J Hum Genet* (in press).

253. Trouillas P, Xie J, Adeleine P: Buspirone, a serotonergic 5-HT1A agonist, is active in cerebellar ataxia. A new fact in favor of the serotonergic theory of ataxia. *Prog Brain Res* **114**:589, 1997.

CHAPTER 15

Bloom Syndrome*

James German ▪ Nathan A. Ellis

1. Clinically, Bloom syndrome (BS) features (a) proportional dwarfism, usually accompanied by (b) a sun-sensitive erythematous skin lesion limited to the face and dorsa of the hands and forearms, (c) a characteristic facies and head configuration, and (d) immunodeficiency often associated with otitis media and pneumonia. (e) Affected males produce no spermatozoa, and females, although sometimes fertile, have an abnormally early cessation of menstrual cycles. (f) Well-circumscribed areas of dermal hypo- and hyperpigmentation are present in abnormal numbers. (g) The three major complications are chronic lung disease, diabetes mellitus, and—by far the most important and most frequent—cancer.

2. BS is a genetically determined trait transmitted in straightforward autosomal recessive fashion, and mutation at a single locus, *BLM*, causes the disorder. Many different mutations at *BLM* are segregating in various human populations, and the same phenotype (BS) can be produced by either homozygosity or compound heterozygosity of any of the mutations that have been defined at the molecular level. The mutations are predominantly null alleles; however, missense mutations have been detected as well. BS is rare in all populations, but in the Ashkenazi Jewish population one particular mutated allele, a six bp deletion and seven bp insertion resulting in premature translation termination, has, through founder effect, reached a relatively high carrier frequency of approximately 1%. Consequently, one or both parents of 31% of all persons with BS are Ashkenazi Jews.

3. The genome is abnormally unstable in the somatic cells of persons with BS, spontaneous hypermutability being the consequence. Mutations arise and accumulate in numbers manyfold greater than normal, including microscopically visible chromatid gaps, breaks, and rearrangements and mutations in specific loci. Although a complete characterization at the molecular level of the array of mutations that accumulate in BS somatic cells remains to be carried out, BS cells are known to show in particular an increased tendency for exchange to take place between chromatids, usually at what appear to be homologous sites. One consequence of this recombination is segregation of alleles at

polymorphic loci distal to the point of crossing-over, so that reduction to homozygosity of constitutionally heterozygous loci becomes a major form of mutation. One specific form of recombination that can be demonstrated in persons with BS who are compound heterozygotes is intragenic recombination: crossing-over between the two different mutated sites within *BLM* itself can result in the formation of a functionally normal gene and in the correction of the cellular phenotype of the somatic cells that comprise the progeny of a cell in which this recombinational event had occurred.

4. Many of the clinical characteristics of BS may be viewed as the direct or indirect consequences of the hypermutability of the BS cell. The hypermutability is postulated to be the cause of the small size by way of the induction of excessive cell death. Another major consequence is the proneness to neoplasia; BS more than any other known human state predisposes to the early development of cancer of the types and sites that affect the general population. BS thus is the prototype of a class of disease that may be called the somatic mutational disorders.

5. Diagnosis of BS is based on clinical observation, and the phenotype is striking. Laboratory confirmation ordinarily is by cytogenetic demonstration of the characteristically increased tendency of chromatid exchange to take place or by demonstration of the presence of mutation in *BLM*. BS is the only condition known that features a greatly increased rate of sister-chromatid exchange (SCE); blood lymphocytes in short-term culture are suitable for demonstrating this.

6. With respect to management of BS, measures to increase the size have not been found. Protection from the sun, especially during infancy and childhood, is valuable in reducing the severity of the facial skin lesion. Greater than normal surveillance for carcinoma is indicated in persons who reach adulthood. Because many are the sites and types of neoplasm that may arise, devising a surveillance program in BS is a particularly challenging matter, for both the affected person and for the physician.

7. The mapping of *BLM* to chromosome band 15q26.1 and its subsequent molecular isolation identified a nuclear protein which contains seven amino acid motifs characteristic of DNA and RNA helicases. The absence of the

---

*Portions of this chapter were adapted from two of our recent papers: (I) German, J.: Bloom's syndrome, In: Genodermatoses with Malignant Potential" (eds. Cohen, P. R. & Kurzrock, R.), Dermatologic Clinics (W. B. Saunders Co., Philadelphia) 13:7-18, 1995; (ii) Ellis, N. A. and German, J.: Molecular genetics of Bloom's syndrome. Hum. Molec. Genet. 5:1457-1463,1996.

BLM protein from the cell (the situation in BS) results in an excessive amount of mutation. The function of BLM, at present in the early stages of biochemical and molecular characterization, promises to provide fundamental understanding of how stability of the genome is maintained as the zygote expands via the cell-division cycle into the greater than 10^{17} cells that will constitute the normal size adult body.

Homozygosity or compound mutant heterozygosity at *BLM*, a gene distal on chromosome No. 15, results in a striking phenotype known as Bloom syndrome (BS).[1-5] A constant clinical feature of BS and one that makes a lasting impression on the observer is a well-proportioned small size. The additional constant feature, one not apparent from physical observation of the patient, however, is instability of the genome; BS somatic cells accumulate more mutations than any other cell type known, apparently at any and every part of the genome. The genomic instability, which is of a characteristic type and to some extent recognizable through the microscope as chromosome breakage,[6,7] is responsible for the most important complication of BS, namely cancer. The genomic instability also probably is responsible for there being fewer than normal cells in the tissues and organs of the affected person, hence the abnormally small size.

BS's rarity is responsible for its obscurity as an entity in clinical medicine; in contrast, the remarkable genomic instability and consequent hypermutability of the BS cell and the dramatic cancer proneness of the affected individual have awarded it prominence among students of mutation, DNA synthesis, DNA repair, and recombination, and among human biologists interested in the developmental consequences of mutation in somatic cells, including the consequences of crossing-over, which is greatly increased in BS. Here we shall describe the clinical entity and its genetics (autosomal recessive transmission); summarize what is known of the hypermutability of BS cells including the microscopically visible chromosome breakage, the feature that first called attention to BS as an important clinical entity and experimental model; and present its molecular genetics and mention the earliest information acquired about the protein encoded by *BLM*.

Diagnosing Bloom syndrome is always a momentous occasion for the following reason. The physician who identifies a person with BS simultaneously identifies a person who, along with the other few persons alive with this very rare disorder, is far more likely than anyone else to develop one or many of the cancers of the standard sites and types that affect humans, and at an unusually early age. Cancer emerges excessively in BS because throughout intrauterine and postnatal life an excessive number of mutations of various types arise and accumulate in the cells. However, some, possibly most, of the clinical features of BS other than cancer proneness also are attributable to this genomic instability. Consequently, BS is the prototype of a class of human disease that can be referred to as the *somatic mutational disorders*.[4,8]

Thus, despite the fact that BS is exceedingly rare it takes on inordinate significance in academic medicine and in human biology generally for two reasons. First, it displays dramatically the clinical consequences of an excessive somatic mutation rate. Any abnormality present in a person with BS, even though it may not be a recognized or constant feature of the syndrome, is brought under suspicion of being etiologically on a mutational basis, either directly or indirectly. Second, the BS cell and *BLM*, the BS gene, constitute valuable experimental materials in cell biology. It has been clear for a long time that the protein encoded by *BLM* is of pivotal importance in the maintenance of the genomic stability of somatic cells; now its exact role there can be defined because the gene recently was isolated.

THE CLINICAL ENTITY

Unpublished data in the dossiers of the 168 persons who comprise the Bloom's Syndrome Registry are the source of most of the information presented here.[9] The Registry is comprised of the vast majority of persons ever diagnosed BS up to 1991 (when it arbitrarily was closed to new accessions), and as far as can be determined is an unbiased representation of this very rare entity (Table 15-1). The mean age of those alive in the Registry is 21.6 years (range 4–44 years), and the mean age at death has been 23.6 years (range <1–49 years). Additional clinical information about BS including photographs of affected persons is to be found in references 1–5.

Table 15-1 Composition of the Population in the Bloom's Syndrome Registry, 1996

	No.		Age* (Years) Mean	Range
Persons affected with BS				
Alive	108	(64%)	21.6	4–46
Dead	60	(35%)	23.6	<1–49
Total affected persons	168			
Families				
With 1 affected with BS	116	(83%)		
With 2 affected with BS	22	(16%)		
With 4 affected with BS	2	(1%)		
Total Families	140			
Dwelling places of persons				
North America	83			
Europe	41			
Asia Minor	16			
Japan	12			
Meso- & South America	11			
Australia	3			
North Africa	2			
Ethnic origins of families				
European, non-Jewish	66			
Mixed†	34			
German	11			
Italian	9			
Dutch/Flemish	6			
British	5			
Other	4			
Jewish	42			
Ashkenazi‡	41			
Non-Ashkenazi	1			
Japanese	10			
South American Mixed	6			
African American	4			
Turkish	4			
Arab Mohammedan	2			
Mexican Mestizo	2			
Gypsy	1			
Consanguinity§				
Non-Jewish	31/105 families			
Ashkenazi Jewish**	2/35 families			
Non-Ashkenazi Jewish	1/1 families			

Note: 114 of the 168 registered persons have been examined personally by at least one registrar, i.e., by David Bloom, James German, and, or Eberhard Passarge.
*Age at present if living; age at death if dead.
†Most non-Jewish United Statesans, Canadians, and Australians are classified "Mixed."
‡One or both parents.
§Of the parents of affected individuals.
**Both parents.

The predominating and constant clinical features of BS are two (1 and 2 in the following). Only the first is obvious from physical observation:

1. An overall *small body size* with fairly normal proportioning except for a slightly disproportionately small brain/head accompanied by dolichocephaly. Subcutaneous fatty tissue is consequently sparse. The several fetuses whose size has been monitored by sonography have been much smaller than expected for their ages. The mean birth weight for males is 1906 g (range 930–3400) and for females 1810 g (range 920–2667). The mean adult height for men is 147.5 cm (range 130–162), and for women 138.6 cm (range 122–151) (Fig. 15-1).

2. An enormous *predisposition to cancer,* probably of all cell types and at all sites (covered more fully in the following).

Eleven additional features that may or may not be present in persons with BS and that vary in severity are the following. Ordinarily the presence of several of these serves to distinguish BS from other disorders that feature a striking degree of growth deficiency:

3. A *characteristic facies* (Fig. 15-2). The face is somewhat keel-shaped because of the small narrow cranium, malar hypoplasia, nasal prominence, and small mandible. The ears may appear protuberant and unusually prominent.

4. Hypersensitivity to sunlight of the areas of the skin ordinarily exposed to the sun during infancy, that is, the face and the dorsa of the hands and forearms.

5. Patchy areas of *hyper- and hypopigmentation of the skin.*

6. A *characteristic voice,* high-pitched and of a somewhat coarse, squeaky timbre.

7. A variable degree of *vomiting and diarrhea* during infancy, often rapidly leading to life-threatening dehydration. Their basis is completely obscure. Also, a large proportion of affected infants and young children show a profound lack of interest in eating. The gastrointestinal problems along with the repeated respiratory tract and ear infections make infancy a trying period for many parents of children with BS.

8. *Diabetes mellitus,* as yet neither well-characterized clinically nor studied experimentally (Table 15-2). Diabetes has been diagnosed in 20 of the 168 (11.9%) persons in the Registry, at a mean age of 24.9 years (range 11–40 years). In many ways the diabetes of BS resembles standard late-onset, non-insulin dependent diabetes; however, six of the diabetics in the Registry have required insulin therapy, and ketoacidosis has occurred in several.

9. In men, abnormally small testes accompanied by a total *failure of spermatogenesis,* and in women, an abnormally *early cessation of menstruation* accompanied by *reduced fertility.* Nevertheless, three women with BS have given birth to four normal, healthy babies.

10. *Immunodeficiency* of a generalized type, ranging from mild and essentially asymptomatic to severe, manifested by recurrent respiratory tract infections complicated by otitis media

ADULT HEIGHTS

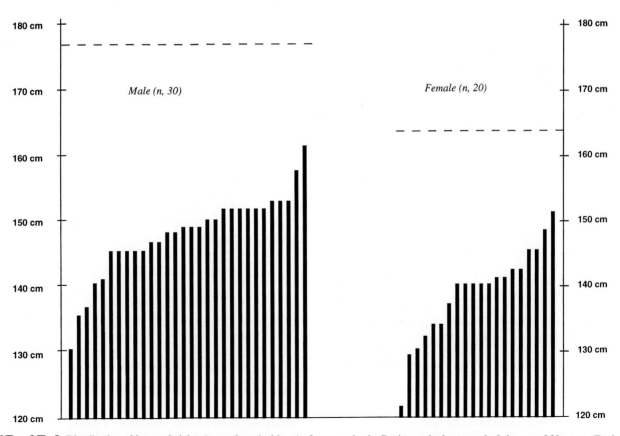

FIG. 15-1 **Distribution of known heights (tops of vertical bars) of persons in the Registry who have reached the age of 20 years. (Dashed lines show the means for normal adults.)**

and pneumonia.[10] In 20.1% of cases, at least one life-threatening bacterial infection of the respiratory tract is recorded that doubtless would have led to early death in the preantibiotic era. Inadequately treated lung infections may lead to bronchiectasis and crippling chronic lung disease that in five instances has been fatal, becoming the second commonest cause of death after cancer (Table 15-2). Serious ear infections have occurred in 29.2% of persons with Bloom syndrome and may decrease auditory acuity. The severe and recurring vomiting and diarrhea of infancy, mentioned in 70 above, conceivably is caused by bacterial infection, but this has never been studied. Although also not known to be on an infectious basis, a mild, sometimes recurring, idiopathic hepatitis has been reported in several affected individuals, and evidence of liver toxicity is a common complication when cancer chemotherapy is administered.

11. A slightly excessive incidence of *minor anatomical anomalies*, including mildly anomalous digits, pilonidal dimples, wedges of altered color of the irises, localized areas of white hair, and obstructing anomalies of the urethra. The only major anomaly has been one instance of a congenital cardiac anomaly.

12. *Restricted intellectual ability.* Intelligence in BS seems in general to be average to low-average. When limitation does exist, it varies widely in degree from minimal to severe. It is impossible to predict early in life whether a person with BS will have some degree of mental deficiency or be quite normal. Al-
though several affected individuals have been frankly moderately deficient mentally, several others have completed college, a few of them obtaining higher degrees. However, even when testing indicates normal intelligence, there tends to be a poorly defined and unexplained learning disability and short attention span in BS. Characteristically this is associated with an inability to develop a normally wide array of interests. From earliest childhood, the person with BS typically exhibits a charming, pleasant personality, but he fails to mature from a childlike judgment and gullibility, and (perhaps fortunately, in view of the grim specter of early neoplasia) he maintains an inordinate upbeat optimism. Several affected persons have displayed a strikingly poor memory. Although only conjectural at this point, the possible role played by inadequate nutrition early in life, the result of the infant's/child's lack of interest in eating (mentioned earlier) deserves investigation, because, if etiologically significant in the restriction on intellectual maturation, treatment in the form of nonvolitional feeding possibly would be preventive.

13. Any one of an array of seemingly *unrelated clinical entities or features*. Each of these has occurred in only one or a few individuals, and they are not to be considered part of the syndrome itself. They include the following: hyperlipidemia, congenital thrombocytopenia, chronic idiopathic thrombocytopenic purpura, acanthosis nigricans, mild anemia and in some cases a poorly defined dyserythropoiesis, asthma, psoriatic arthritis, and Legg-Perthes disease.

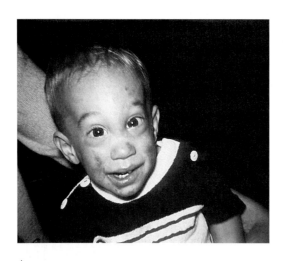

A

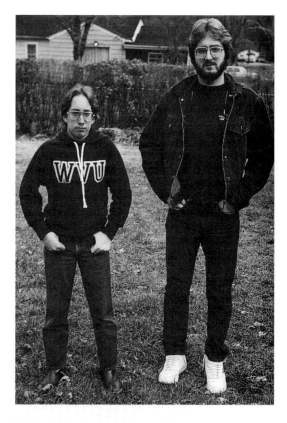

B

FIG. 15-2 51 (KeMc) in the Bloom's Syndrome Registry manifests the major clinical features of BS. His birth weight was 2160 g and his birth length 44.5 cm. He exhibited striking dolichocephaly and hypoplastic malar areas. Within the first year of life, a moderate to severe photosensitive erythematous skin lesion appeared that was limited to the face and hands. He also had a recurring fissure of the lower lip. (*A*) 51(KeMc) at about 18 months showing the facial erythematous skin lesion. (*B*). On left, 51(KeMc) at age 17, exhibiting small body size (height 147 cm, weight 4100 g) and the photosensitive facial skin lesion, and on right his unaffected brother at age 19. The unaffected brother is just under 6 feet tall. 51(KeMc), who is healthy at age 27, was successfully treated for acute undifferentiated leukemia at age 12.

Table 15-2 The Serious Medical Complications in the 168 Persons in the Bloom's Syndrome Registry, April, 1996

	Number of Persons Affected	Death from the Complication	Age at Diagnosis Mean	Range
Chronic lung disease	7	5		
Diabetes mellitus	20	0	24.9	11–40
Cancer*				
Persons with 1 or >1 primaries	71	50	24.7	2–48
Persons with 2 or >2 primaries	19			
Persons with 3 or >3 primaries	5			
Persons with 4 or >4 primaries	3			
Persons with 5 primaries	2			

*A total of 100 cancers diagnosed, in 71 of the 168 persons in the Registry.

The Skin in BS

In BS, two unrelated skin lesions coexist.

A Sun-Sensitive Facial Lesion. The clinically more important skin lesion of BS is a sun-sensitive erythema that is limited almost exclusively to the face, usually unassociated with dyspigmentation. The cheeks and nose are the areas most often affected, explaining the early erroneous confusion of BS and lupus. The dorsa of the hands and forearms may be mildly affected. In exceptionally severe cases, the erythema does extend to the ears, sides, and back of the neck, the suprasternal area, and very rarely and in mild degree onto the shoulders or upper chest. However, effectively ruling out the diagnosis BS is any prominent erythematous, telangiectatic lesion that affects trunk, the lower extremities, arms, and, or, buttocks, even though the face might be affected also.

The clinical onset of the facial skin lesion most often is as persistent erythema that follows the infant's first significant exposure to sunlight, which most often has been during the first or second summer of life. In one exceptional case, the lesion did not appear until age 12. This sun-sensitive skin lesion varies in severity and may be completely absent. The severity of the erythema when present ranges from a faint blush during the summertime to a disfiguring, flaming red lesion of irregular distribution over the bridge of the nose, cheeks, and other facial areas. Crying may accentuate what appears on first examination to be a minimal or absent lesion. The lower eyelids often are hyperemic, and atrophy of the lower lids with loss of eyelashes is common. In many cases, blistering and encrustation and a recurring fissure of the lower lip during summertime becomes a particularly aggravating aspect of the lesion.

The severity and extent of the skin lesion usually is disclosed by early childhood. Often parents intuitively protect a child from the sun when they realize that hypersensitivity is present, which may explain the failure of progression in severity at later ages in many patients. Similarly, in sibships with multiple affected children, the rigorous protection from the sun of later-born affecteds is frequently associated with a mild or absent skin lesion. Ordinarily, if there is to be a skin lesion, it makes its appearance during the first two years of life. (It is not congenital, as originally described—"congenital telangiectatic erythema resembling lupus erythematosus in dwarfs."[11]) Although some form of sun sensitivity quite clearly exists early in life in BS, the few objective tests of nonfacial skin that have been carried out by dermatologists have failed either to characterize the defect or even detect its existence.

Furthermore, several adults with BS report that they enjoy sunbathing and tanning, and that they are unaware of any sun-hypersensitivity of other than facial skin. However, the lesion in the area that was symptomatic early in life persists, as does the continued accentuation of it by sun exposure.

Usually, careful examination of the affected area reveals an accompanying telangiectasia varying in degree from minimal to prominent. It usually is absent during infancy. Even when the erythema is minimal to absent, careful examination often reveals a faint degree of telangiectasia at the margin of the upper lip or about the irregular patches of atrophic skin and dyspigmentation. In 6 of the 168 registered cases, prominent telangiectasia of the bulbar conjunctiva—as prominent as in the entity ataxia-telangiectasia—has been present, unrelated to the severity of the skin lesion.

Histologic study of the characteristic sun-sensitive skin lesion in BS has been made in a few cases but has contributed little to an understanding of the pathogenesis; biopsy is not indicated for diagnostic purposes. In fact, the pathogenesis of the sun-sensitive skin lesion of BS is obscure. In males, the lesion is more severe than in females, and relatively greater underdiagnosis of BS itself in females probably contributes to their slight underrepresentation in the Bloom's Syndrome Registry—93 males versus 75 females.

A Non-Sun-Sensitive Lesion Not Limited to the Face. A second skin abnormality exists in BS, clinically and presumably pathogenetically completely different from the sun-sensitive lesion. It consists of prominent well-circumscribed areas of hyperpigmentation—the cafe-au-lait spots of normal people but present in BS in excessive numbers and often quite extensive. In addition, circumscribed areas of hypopigmentation usually are present. These lesions may appear anywhere on the body but are most commonly found on the trunk. The hyperpigmented lesions vary in diameter from a few millimeters to many centimeters, and in an occasional person are linear and extend extensively over the back of the thorax. Most often, the several hyperpigmented lesions tend to have similar degrees of brownness, but an occasional spot in a given patient may be considerably darker than the others. Sometimes the brownish spots, large ones and small, are found in a localized cluster. Well-demarcated hypopigmented areas also are highly characteristic of BS but usually are less conspicuous than the hyperpigmented lesions. Exceptionally, a hypopigmented area can, like a hyperpigmented one, be extensive, covering an area many centimeters in diameter. In affected individuals of sub-Saharan African ancestry, the hyper-and hypopigmented areas are more prominent than in lighter-complexioned persons, some appearing quite black and others strikingly white. It usually is in early childhood that the pigmentary changes are first noted, rather than in infancy.

Neoplasia[4,12]

At any time in the life of a person with BS a neoplasm is much more likely to appear than in other people of the same age. The four most impressive aspects of the neoplasia proneness of BS are the great frequency with which both benign (not discussed further here) and malignant neoplasms arise, the wide variety of anatomic sites and cellular types, the exceptionally early age at which neoplasms become clinically apparent, and the frequency with which multiple neoplasms arise in one person, which partly is the consequence of careful surveillance for cancers of affected persons by themselves, their families, and their physicians that in turn makes possible early treatment and cures.[4]

The cancers that have arisen in the 168 persons in the Registry are summarized[4,12] in Table 15-3, along with the age ranges at which they were diagnosed. The distribution of sites and types of cancer in BS resembles that in the general population; but in BS they have arisen at a greatly increased frequency and in the case of the carcinomata and acute myelogenous leukemias decades earlier than expected. The mean age at diagnosis of cancer has been 24.7 years (range 2–48 years). It has been responsible for the death of 50 of the 61 persons in the Registry who have died.

Then, the study of BS at the cellular, chromosomal, and DNA levels should facilitate the analysis of the changes responsible for the initiation and progression of the generality of human cancer. The two hypotheses in such work are that among the changes that take place spontaneously in BS cells are the very ones that are responsible, as in other people, not just for neoplastic transformation but also for progression of a transformed clone into clinical cancer. That is, the changes that arise abnormally frequently in BS cells very probably are precisely the ones responsible for these processes in other people. In BS, these changes take place spontaneously; in others they may also be spontaneous—very possibly this is the usual situation in human cancer—or they may be the effects of mutational agents either produced internally during normal cell metabolism or received from the environment.

The reader will note that the inherited mutations responsible for the phenotype BS are in a category different from those that arise at the loci mutated, for example, in retinoblastoma, Wilms tumor, and familial polyposis coli. Those loci when mutated become so-called cancer genes and represent one step of many in cancer's initiation and progression. In contrast, homozygosity for mutation at *BLM* constitutes a mutator genotype. As far as is known, mutation at *BLM* is not itself of significance as a step in cancer initiation or progression. In BS cells the mutations that must occur for clinical cancer to emerge were not inherited but are just far more likely to arise spontaneously than in cells of other people—because BS is a mutator phenotype. It also is noteworthy that in BS, every cell in the body capable of further division is at the high risk of neoplastic transformation.

Thus, the basis for the predisposition to cancer in BS doubtless is the remarkably excessive genomic instability featured by BS cells. However, as noted earlier, immunodeficiency is an important feature of BS. Quite conceivably it contributes to the cancer proneness. Its role in progression, however, is difficult to determine in BS because of the major role played by mutation.

GENOMIC INSTABILITY

When the chromosomes are examined microscopically in BS cells dividing in culture, an abundance of gaps, breaks, and structurally rearranged chromosomes is found.[7] However, the difference from normal is quantitative, and similar lesions in the chromosomes are

Table 15-3 The First 100 Cancers Recorded in the Bloom's Syndrome Registry, showing the Age Groups at Time of Diagnosis

Class and Type	Age Group 0–10	11–20	21–30	31–40	41–50	Total
Rare tumors* (n = 5)						
Medulloblastoma	1					1
Wilms tumor	2					2
Osteogenic sarcoma	1	1				2
Leukemia, acute (n = 22)						
Lymphocytic	4	2	1			7
Myelogenous	1	1	3	1		6
Biphenotypic		1		1		2
Other or unspecified	1	3	2	1		7
Lymphoma (n = 22)						
Non-Hodgkin	4	6	6	3	1	20
Hodgkin disease		2				2
Carcinoma (n = 51)						
Skin		2	3	3		8
Auditory canal, external			1	1		2
Tongue, posterior			1	1	2	4
Esophagus, squamous				3		3
Esophagus, adeno					1	1
Stomach			1	1		2
Colon						
Cecum, ascending			1	2		3
Hepatic flexure, transverse		1		2	1	4
Descending, sigmoid, rectum			1	5		6
Tonsil				1		1
Larynx; epiglottis			2	1		3
Lung				1		1
Uterus						
Cervix		1	3			4
Corpus					1	1
Breast			1	5	1	7
Metastatic, primary site unknown			1			1
Totals	14	20	27	32	7	100

*A meningioma was diagnosed at age 9 in one registered individual. Two Wilms tumors and a retinoblastoma diagnosed at 5 months, 22 months, and 2 years of age, respectively are known to have occurred in children with BS who are known to the Registry, but not officially registered.

present in untreated cells from other people, although much less frequently. The two most characteristic cytogenetic abnormalities (1 and 2 below) are the result of a strikingly increased tendency in BS somatic cells for exchange to take place between the DNA strands, probably at the time they replicate during the S phase of the cell-division cycle:

1. The exchanges may be between a chromatid of each of the two homologues of a chromosome pair (e.g., between the two Nos. 1, or the two Nos. 19), the points of exchange being at seemingly homologous regions of the chromatids involved. Following such an interchange, the lesion detectable microscopically at metaphase is a symmetrical, four-armed configuration—a quadriradial, or QR—composed of the pair of chromosomes between which the interchange had taken place (Fig. 15-3). Or,

2. The exchanges may be intrachromasomal, between the two sister chromatids of one chromosome. The consequence of these exchanges also are microscopically visible in appropriately treated cells—SCEs (sister-chromatid exchanges) (Fig. 15-3A). In cells from non-BS individuals, a mean of fewer than 10 SCEs/metaphase is found; in striking contrast, BS cells characteristically have from 50 to 100/metaphase, depending on the type cell examined but always highest in blood lymphocytes in short-term culture.

Submicroscopic mutations also are increased in BS. BS cells taken directly from the circulating blood can be shown to have a dramatic increase over normal in the number of mutations they have accumulated at the two loci that have been studied extensively in humans, namely, the locus on the X chromosome coding for the enzyme HPRT and the glycophorin A locus on chromosome No. 4 that determines the MN blood type (reviewed in ref. 4). The types of mutations that have been detected are many, and include specifically somatic crossing-over.[13] These mutation analyses indicate that the hypermutability of BS somatic cells exists in vivo as well as in vitro. Other evidence of the genomic instability of BS cells, at least in vitro, is excessive mutation at regions of the genome composed of repeat sequences.[14]

Explanation for the Clinical Features

Again, spontaneous mutations arise more frequently than normal in the genome of a cell that itself is mutant at both of its BS loci. The mutations that arise in the somatic cells of a person with BS are of various types and affect many, probably all, regions of the genome. Many of the mutations will be lethal to the cell in which they arise, either via a lethal biochemical imbalance or by inducing apoptosis. Therefore, the leading hypothesis to explain the small but normally proportioned body in BS is excessive cell death. The mutations—and the excessive cell death—presumably occur in all cell lineages throughout both pre- and postnatal development. (Endocrinological studies have failed to provide any explanation for the restriction on growth.) By this hypothesis, the various tissues and organs of the person with BS are constituted of fewer cells than normal.

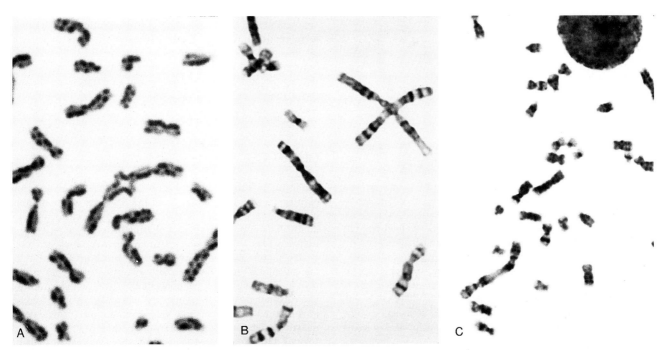

FIG. 15-3 *A. A portion of a Bloom syndrome lymphocyte metaphase. The cell had been cultured in BrdU-containing medium to make possible the differential staining (light or dark) of sister chromatids; alternating regions of light and dark staining signify exchanges between sister chromatids (SCEs). The number of SCEs in cells from normal persons averages <10/metaphase, whereas BS lymphocytes show (as here) 60 to 90/metaphase or more; a greatly elevated SCE frequency is diagnostic of BS. Also present in this cell is a quadriradial configuration (QR), the result of an interchange between chromatids of the No. 1 chromosomes. QRs affecting homologous regions of the homologous chromosomes are present in approximately 1% of BS blood T lymphocytes, but they also are found on rare occasions in cells from healthy persons without BS. Both QRs and SCEs can be induced in* normal cells by exposure to certain DNA-damaging agents, as in (*B*); BS cells, even with an elevated constitutional number of such lesions, show an excessive response to such agents. *B*. G-banded metaphase chromosomes showing a QR, the result of a chromatid interchange at the proximal portions of the long arms of the No. 1 chromosomes. The cell, from a healthy person without BS, had been exposed in vitro to mitomycin C several hours before it entered mitosis. QRs of this type are present in excessive number in untreated cells from persons with BS. *C*. G-banded metaphase chromosomes of a BS lymphocyte showing a telomere association, presumably the result of a chromatid interchange [equivalent to those that resulted in the QRs in (*A*) and (*B*)] that had taken place near the ends of the short arms of the No. 1 chromosomes. (Figure reprinted with permission from reference 4.)

However, among those myriad mutations that are not cell-lethals, some by chance would affect growth-controlling and proto-oncogene loci. This hypothesis explains the frequent emergence of neoplasia in different cell types at various anatomic sites in BS (as discussed more extensively earlier).

Some mutations presumably also would be at loci crucial in determining normal development, in which case localized anatomical defects might result, and as already pointed out minor anomalies are somewhat increased in incidence in BS. It may be significant that major anatomical defects are not increased in BS, possibly indicating that somatic mutation does not play an important etiological role in such in man.

The basis of the pigmentary disturbance in BS is plausibly explained by heritable mutations that arise during development in somatic cell lineages concerned with the determination of the melanin content of the skin. Somatic crossing-over in particular, which is excessive in BS, is the type of mutation that would explain adjacent, localized hyper- and hypopigmented areas. These lesions very possibly are equivalent to the "twin spots" of classical experimental *Drosophila* genetics.

Thus, the clinical analysis of BS is in essence the analysis of the consequences on human development of mutations of various types that will have been arising excessively in somatic cells throughout life, probably at all regions of the genome and in all tissues. It is possible, of course, that at least some of the clinical features of BS are attributable not to somatic mutation but in some completely obscure way to the absence from the cell of the nuclear protein encoded by the *BLM* gene itself (see below), in the same sense that clotting is disturbed in hemophilia. Nevertheless, with the exception of the sun-sensitive facial lesion and the predisposition to diabetes, the predominating features of BS as well as its less constant and even sporadic features can plausibly be attributed to the remarkable hypermutability that obtains in various proliferating lineages of cells when they lack a normal *BLM* gene.

DIAGNOSIS

Any cell type that can be brought into mitosis by the cytogeneticist can be employed to rule a clinical diagnosis of BS in or out. Blood lymphocytes stimulated to enter cell-division cycling by phytohemagglutinin are the most used, but freshly aspirated bone marrow cells or long-term cultures of skin fibroblasts or embryonic/fetal cells also can be examined. The two most valuable indicators of BS are (1) the demonstration of the symmetrical QR interchange configuration in untreated cells in metaphase and (2) the greatly increased number of SCEs in cells allowed to pass two cell-division cycles in medium containing BrdU (Fig. 15-3).

BS is the only disorder that features an increased rate of SCE. Therefore, an SCE analysis is indicated in any child or adult with unexplained growth deficiency (i.e., BS should be included in the differential diagnosis), regardless of whether the facial skin lesion characteristic of BS is present or not.

BS should be considered whenever severe intrauterine growth deficiency is encountered and cannot be explained, especially if the deficiency extends into infancy and childhood. Also, BS might well be considered in small but well-proportioned children or adults with a sun-sensitive, erythematous skin lesion limited to the face even if their growth deficiency is of only moderate degree. Correspondingly, a normal birth weight and postnatal length/height not less than the third percentile for normals militates strongly against the diagnosis BS.

Although surveys have not as yet been carried out, so that the value there of SCE screening is unknown, an SCE analysis very possibly will occasionally identify persons with BS in the following groups of individuals if abnormally small size also is present, even when the characteristic skin lesion is lacking:

1. Persons with excessive numbers of cafe-au-lait spots, usually accompanied by hypopigmented spots;

2. Persons with unexplained immunodeficiency;

3. Children or adults with an unexplained restriction on intelligence;

4. Persons in whom diabetes mellitus develops later than the usual age of onset of Type I and earlier than that of Type II;

5. Infertile men with abnormally small testes for which no explanation can be found, and possibly in short women with an exceptionally early onset of menopause;

6. Children or adults who develop clinical neoplasia. As stated earlier, it is unknown how valuable a routine SCE analysis would be for unusually small persons who develop cancer but who lack a facial lesion; however, in the Registry, 7 of the 71 individuals with BS who have developed cancer were recognized to have BS only at the time or after a cancer was diagnosed. Only then was the significance of their small size, unusual facies, or facial skin lesion recognized by physicians who knew of BS.

BS doubtless is underdiagnosed. Many cases of it long remain in diagnostic wastebaskets such as idiopathic "intrauterine growth retardation," "primordial dwarfism," and "failure to thrive" unless an SCE analysis fortuitously is requested by an informed physician. Other cases erroneously are considered to have some rare disorder other than BS, whereas still others are simply believed to have an undescribed condition. For example, misdiagnosing BS as Russell-Silver dwarfism is particularly common: 10 of the 168 persons with proven BS in the Bloom's Syndrome Registry were thought possibly or definitely to be Russell-Silver dwarfs until cytogenetic study provided the correct diagnosis.

GENETICS

Clinical BS is the phenotype that results from the inheritance from each parent of a mutation at *BLM*, the BS locus in chromosome band 15q26.1.[15] Mutation(s) at *BLM* appear to segregate in most if not all human populations, but in all, BS is very rare. Only in Ashkenazi Jews is mutation at *BLM* known to have reached a relatively high frequency; a survey of BS in Israel in 1977 suggested that more than 1 in 110 Ashkenazi Jews carry *blm^Ash* (a provisional term for the mutation in that population). The recent identification of a 6-bp deletion and 7-bp insertion in exon 10 of *BLM* (see below) referred to as *blm^Ash* now will permit a more accurate determination of the frequency of carriers in that major subgroup of Jewry.* The two mutated loci in any given individual with BS may be identical—homozygous—and this is assumed to be the case when either that person's parents are consanguineous or they both are Ashkenazi Jews; in those two situations the mutations at *BLM* on the two chromosome Nos. 15 are identical by virtue of their descent from a common ancestor who was a carrier of a BS mutation.[15,16] In addition to homozygosity, however, two unlike mutations sometimes are inherited and are responsible for BS, so-

---

*An unreported survey conducted recently in collaboration with the Department of Medical Genetics, Mt. Sinai Hospital Medical School, New York City, sets the number at 1 in 107.

called compound heterozygosity. The phenotype BS seems to be the same regardless of whether the mutant *BLM* loci are or are not inherited from a common ancestor. (As will become apparent below, the vast majority of the many BS-associated mutations at *BLM* that we are detecting are essentially knockout for the BLM protein product.)

The carrier of a BS mutation, an individual ordinarily identified only after having become the parent of a child with BS, is normally developed and healthy. Molecular isolation of *BLM* now does provide another means of heterozygote detection among other relatives of persons with BS, as well as in the population at large.[17,18] The risk of other children with BS is 1 in 4 after an affected child has been born to a union of proven heterozygotes. Pregnancies at risk can be monitored by sonography, cytogenetics, molecular haplotyping, or direct determination of whether a mutation is present on one, both, or neither of the chromosome Nos. 15.

MOLECULAR GENETICS OF BLM

Diverse and complex enzymatic systems exist in the cell that carry out the fundamental processes of the replication and transmission of the genetic material from cell generation to cell generation. To ensure their fidelity, these systems incorporate proofreading capacities of the DNA polymerases and replication machinery, mechanisms that allow DNA replication to bypass damaged DNA (translesion synthesis), repair enzymes that recognize damaged DNA and either repair the damage directly or recruit other enzymes to carry that out, proteins that signal to the cell the presence of DNA damage and that prevent the cell's traversing its cycle prior to repair, and systems that package and condense the chromatin and that ensure the proper segregation of the chromosomes at mitosis. These systems maintain genomic stability and act to prevent errors that might lead on the one hand to cell death or on the other to abnormal, unregulated cellular proliferation.

Genetically determined defects in the systems that maintain genomic stability and ensure fidelity of replication have been identified in many model organisms, and also in the human. In human genetics, genomic instability first was recognized through microscopic observation of chromosomal abnormalities—chromosome breakage—in cultured cells from individuals with certain rare syndromes, first Bloom syndrome, then Fanconi anemia, ataxia-telangiectasia, the Nijmegan breakage syndrome, Werner syndrome and xeroderma pigmentosum (the last only after ultraviolet light irradiation). In all of these syndromes, the cytogenetic abnormalities are accompanied by an increase in the rate of spontaneous somatic mutations and, or, mutagen-induced mutations. This hypermutability provides an explanation for the predisposition to various types of cancers, a feature shared by all these syndromes. These clinical entities along with several others that lack

chromosomal breakage (e.g., the Li-Fraumeni syndrome and Lynch syndromes I and II) but that are characterized by some form of genomic instability at the molecular level all fall under the rubric somatic mutational disorders.

The chromosome abnormalities observed in BS cells noted earlier pointed to a defect in some fundamental process of DNA metabolism that helps maintain genomic stability. Retarded replication-fork progression, abnormal replicational intermediates, and the absence of defects in known DNA-repair systems implicated a disturbance of the process of DNA replication itself.[4] Biochemical studies of a number of enzymes participating in replication and repair revealed abnormalities in the enzymatic activities of DNA ligase I, topoisomerase II in *Brd*U-treated cells, uracil DNA glycosylase, O[6]-methylguanine methyltransferase, N-methylpurine DNA glycosylase, and superoxide dismutase. However, none of these abnormalities, though often demonstrable, identified the primary defect in BS; they appear to be phenotypic consequences of the BS mutation. Because the identification of the primary defect promised to reveal an important element in nucleic acid metabolism, a positional cloning strategy was undertaken to isolate *BLM*—as result of which previously unknown protein in mammalian cells has been identified.

Localization of *BLM* to 15q26.1[15]

The first step in the positional cloning effort to isolate the gene was to identify linkages between *BLM* and mapped polymorphic markers. A limited amount of evidence from cell hybridization studies had suggested that BS is a single-gene disorder.[19] Introduction of a normal human chromosome 15 by microcell-mediated chromosome transfer was shown to correct toward normal the high-SCE phenotype of a BS cell line.[20] Subsequently, homozygosity mapping demonstrated tight linkage between *BLM* and *FES*[15]; *FES* had been localized by *in situ* hybridization to 15q26.1. Linkage in most of these families was detected thereafter at five additional highly polymorphic DNA markers that flank *FES* (depicted in Fig. 15-4). Homozygosity mapping permitted assignment of *BLM* to a 2-cM interval that includes *FES*.

Founder Effect in Ashkenazi Jews with Bloom Syndrome[3,16]

As mentioned earlier, BS is more common in the Ashkenazi Jewish population than in any other known.[3] Several of the polymorphic microsatellite loci found to be tightly linked to *BLM* by homozygosity mapping were genotyped in affected and unaffected individuals from the Ashkenazi Jewish population. A striking allele association between blm[Ash] and one of the six alleles at *FES*, specifically allele C3, and between blm[Ash] and two related alleles of

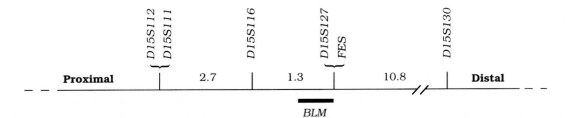

FIG. 15-4 Map positions of six highly polymorphic DNA markers on chromosome 15 tightly linked to BLM. The loci shown above the line representing chromosome 15 were employed in homozygosity mapping (genetic map distances in cM). Braced loci have not been sep-

arated by recombinational analysis. FES and D15S127 are separated by 30 kb (see Fig. 15-6). The location of BLM is represented by the thick line between DNA markers FES/D15S127 and D15S116.

the CA-repeat locus *D15S127* (a locus that is 30 kb proximal to *FES*), specifically alleles 145 bp and 147 bp, was detected in Ashkenazi Jews with BS.[16] (The association of *blm^Ash* with two alleles rather than one at *D15S127* probably results from recurrent mutation at *D15S127* producing toggling between the 145–147 bp alleles.)

This linkage disequilibrium confirmed the linkage results from homozygosity mapping and is strong support for a founder-effect hypothesis to explain the increased incidence of BS in the Ashkenazim relative to other populations: By one historical model, a chromosome bearing *blm^Ash* in the genome of a postulated founder individual was carried into Eastern Europe several centuries ago as the Ashkenazi Jewish population was forming; subsequently, *blm^Ash* and its flanking chromosomal segments increased in frequency in this population as result of genetic drift. In other words, today Ashkenazi Jews with BS inherit their mutated *BLM* gene identical by descent from a common ancestor who lived as many as 30 generations ago, making the parents of such individuals distant cousins. Definitive evidence for the founder-effect hypothesis has been obtained by mutational analysis of the mutated *BLM* in the majority of Ashkenazi Jewish persons ever diagnosed with BS (presented below).

Evidence for Allelic Heterogeneity at *BLM*[21]

A strikingly elevated SCE rate is uniquely characteristic of BS cells and is present in all cell types examined. This includes mitogen-stimulated blood T and B lymphocytes in short-term cultures, Epstein-Barr virus-transformed lymphocytes in long-term culture, cells from the bone marrow in short-term culture, cultured diploid fibroblasts, including fibroblasts from skin, amniotic fluid, chorionic villi, and surgical specimens, and aneuploid SV40-transformed fibroblasts in long-term culture. All persons with BS have high-SCE cells. However, an important and until recently unexplained exception was recognized two decades

ago: a small number of blood lymphocytes with a normal SCE rate circulate in the blood in a minority of persons with clinical BS. This enigmatic high-SCE/low-SCE mosaicism was investigated by comparing its incidence in subpopulations of persons with BS sorted according to whether or not *BLM* was known to have been inherited identical by descent. A striking negative correlation emerged[21]: In persons with BS whose parents share a common ancestor, the case in persons born to either consanguineous or two Ashkenazi Jewish parents (approximately half the BS families), a population of low-SCE cells almost never is found; conversely, the mosaicism occurs almost exclusively in persons with BS whose parents are not known to share a common ancestor. Because those who share a common ancestor predominantly inherit the identical mutation at *BLM*, the negative correlation was interpreted to mean that emergence of low-SCE cells in BS depends in some way on the pre-existence of compound heterozygosity, that is, on having two different mutated *BLM* alleles. A corollary to this is that BS is genetically heterogeneous. That multiple mutations are present at *BLM* has been confirmed now by mutational analysis of *BLM* in different persons with BS (below, Table 15-4).

Somatic Intragenic Recombination[22]

The population cytogenetic data just summarized[21] indicated that high-SCE/low-SCE mosaic persons have to be compound heterozygotes. The requirement of compound heterozygosity plus the high rate of homologous recombination taking place in BS somatic cells compared to normal cells suggested that a specific form of crossing-over, namely, intragenic recombination, explains the mosaicism in some BS persons. Crossing-over between the paternally derived and the maternally derived mutated sites within *BLM* could generate a functionally wild-type *BLM* that corrects the high-SCE phenotype of the BS cell (Fig. 15–5). By this model, the newly generated functionally wild-type gene on

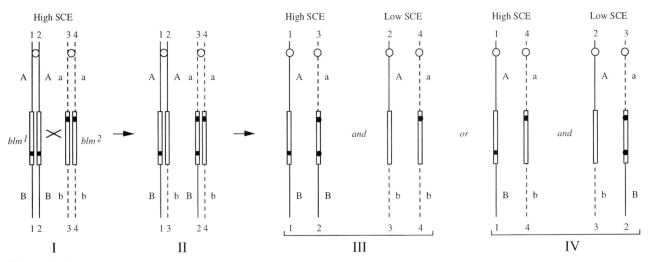

FIG. 15-5 *Model to generate a wild-type* BLM *locus via somatic intragenic recombination: I. The two pairs of sister chromatids of the homologous chromosome 15s in a G2 somatic cell of a BS compound heterozygote* (blm¹/blm²) *are numbered 1-1 to 4-4. Each of the two mutations in* BLM *(the hatched rectangle), represented by black dots, one inherited from each parent, is at a different site in the gene. Flanking markers proximal to and distal to the mutated loci are heterozygous A/a and B/b. II. After homologous interchange between chromatids 2-2 and 3-3 at a point between the sites of mutation within* BLM *(the X in I), a wild-type gene is reconstituted on chromatid 2-3 that corrects to normal the high-SCE phenotype of BS cells. Simultaneously, the distal marker b becomes associated with the wild-type gene on chromatid 2-3. III and IV. By segregational events at mitosis, two pairs of daughter cells are possible. If chro-* matids 2-3 and 4-4 co-segregate to the same daughter cell, the distal marker becomes homozygous b/b (the diagram on the right side of III). On the other hand, if chromatid 2-3 and 3-2 cosegregate, the distal marker remains heterozygous b/B (the diagram on the right side of IV). The proximal marker remains heterozygous A/a in both cases. In the sister cells, segregation of chromatids 1-1 and 3-2 (the diagram on the left side of III) or of chromatids 1-1 and 4-4 (the diagram on the left side of IV) do not give rise to a low-SCE phenotype. (*Note:* Cells of heterozygous carriers of a mutation at BLM, viz. blm/BLM parents of persons with BS, display a low-SCE rate.) (Figure reprinted from Ellis NA, Lennon DJ, Proytcheva M, Alhadeff B, Henderson EE, German J: Somatic intragenic recombination within the mutated locus BLM can correct the high-SCE phenotype of Bloom syndrome cells. *Am J Hum Genet* 57:1019, 1995.)

one chromosome No. 15 can segregate at mitosis with either the nonrecombinant chromatid of the other chromosome No. 15—allele losses distal to *BLM* then ensue (reduction to homozygosity)—or with the recombinant chromatid that now carries a doubly mutant *BLM*—allele losses distal to *BLM* do not ensue.

Evidence supporting the intragenic recombination model was obtained by genotype analysis of 12 loci syntenic with *BLM*—six proximal to it and six distal to it—in 11 persons who exhibited the high-SCE/low-SCE mosaicism.[22] In 5 of the 11 persons, polymorphic loci on chromosome 15q distal to *BLM* that were heterozygous in their high-SCE cells had become homozygous in their low-SCE cells, whereas loci proximal to *BLM* that were heterozygous on 15q had remained heterozygous. In the remaining six persons, loci both proximal and distal to *BLM* that were heterozygous in their high-SCE cells had remained heterozygous in their low-SCE cells. These observations indicate that intragenic recombination between the two different mutated alleles at *BLM* is a mechanism that can generate a functionally wild-type *BLM* gene (Fig. 15-5). Thus, the low-SCE lymphocytes present in the blood of mosaic persons are the progeny of a somatic stem cell in which such an intragenic recombinational event had occurred.

Isolation and Molecular Analysis of *BLM**

The availability of low-SCE cell lines in which somatic intragenic recombination had led to reduction to homozygosity at loci distal

but not proximal to *BLM*[22] provided an efficient strategy to determine the exact location of *BLM*. The objective became to identify (1) the most proximal polymorphic locus that was constitutionally heterozygous and that had been reduced to homozygosity in the low-SCE cell lines and (2) the most distal polymorphic locus that had remained constitutionally heterozygous in them. *BLM* would have to be in the short interval defined by the reduced and the unreduced heterozygous markers. The power of this approach, termed *somatic crossover-point (SCP) mapping,* would be limited only by the density of polymorphic loci available in the immediate vicinity of the gene.

As mentioned earlier, *BLM* had been localized by homozygosity mapping to a 2-cM interval flanking *FES*. A 2-Mb YAC and P1 contig encompassing *FES* was constructed and the required closely spaced polymorphic DNA markers in the contig were identified.[23] BLM then could be assigned by SCP mapping to an interval in this contig of only 250 kb in size, one bounded by the polymorphic loci *D15S1108* and *D15S127* (Fig. 15-6). Then the cosmid clone 905 present in the 250-kb interval was used to isolate a 849-bp clone from a fibroblast cDNA library by direct selection. By hybridization and RT-PCR techniques, this cDNA clone was used to isolate many additional cDNAs from fibroblast, lymphoblastoid,

*Work both published (reviewed in reference 18) and in progress in the authors' laboratory will be mentioned in this and the subsequent section of this chapter. Construction of the physical map of *BLM* region[23] and the identification of mutations in *BLM* by the SSCP analysis[17] were collaborative works of the laboratory of Joanna Groden (University of Cincinnati) and ours.

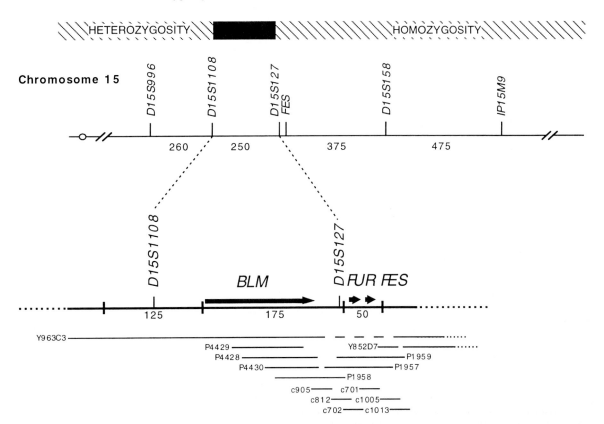

FIG. 15-6 SCP mapping of *BLM*. Genetic map of the *BLM* region of 15q. On the upper horizontal line, the order and distances (shown in kb) between the polymorphic microsatellite loci were estimated by long-range-restriction mapping.[23] The distance between *D15S127* and *FES* (not indicated) was determined to be 30 kb by restriction enzyme mapping of a cosmid contig (see the following). Vertical lines indicate the position of the marker loci, and the circle represents the centromere. The interval between loci *D15S1108* and *D15S127* is expanded below the map. Vertical lines intersecting mark the unmethylated CpG-rich regions identified by long-range restriction mapping, and arrows indicate the direction of transcription of three genes in the region. Certain YACs, P1s, and cosmids (Y, P, and c, respectively) from the contig are depicted by horizontal lines underneath the map.[23] Dashes on the YAC lines indicate internal deletions. At the top of the figure, the horizontal cross-hatched bars indicate regions proximal to *BLM* that had become homozygous. The minimal region to which *BLM* was thus assigned by SCP mapping is represented in black. (Figure reprinted slightly modified from Ellis NA, Groden J, Ye T-Z, Straughen J, Lennon DJ, Ciocci S, Proytcheva M, German J: The Bloom's syndrome gene product is homologous to RecQ helicases. *Cell* 83:655, 1995.)

and HeLa cells. A 4,437-bp cDNA sequence, referred to as H1-5′ was defined that contained a long open reading frame that encoded a 1,417 amino acid protein. By Southern blot analysis of genomic DNA and of sequences cloned in YACs, P1s, and cosmids, H1-5′ sequences hybridized to single-copy sequences spanning about 100 kb of the genome. A 4.5-kb transcript was identified by Northern blot analysis of total RNAs prepared from fibroblast, lymphoblastoid, and HeLa cells proliferating in vitro. Electrophoretic abnormalities were detected in RNA transcripts present in cell lines derived from seven unrelated persons with BS, suggesting that the transcripts were produced by mutant *BLM* genes.

Analysis of H1-5′ sequences amplified by RT-PCR using a single-stranded conformation polymorphism (SSCP) assay, an RNAse cleavage assay (Ambion), or both has disclosed 14 unique mutations in 20 persons with BS out of just the 25 persons examined so far (Table 15-4). Three of the mutations are putative missense substitutions, six are nonsense mutations, two are frameshift mutations, two are exon-skipping mutations, and one is a gross deletion detectable by Southern blot analysis. Ten of the mutations lead to premature translational chain termination; the open reading frame is maintained in the three missense mutations and in one of the exon-skipping mutations. In this exon-skipping mutation the

Table 15-4 *BLM* Mutations Identified in Persons with Bloom Syndrome (August 31, 1996)[a]

Identification[b]	Ancestry	Zygosity of the Mutation[c]	Nucleotide Change[d]	Protein Change[e]
		Missense mutations		
139(ViKre)[f]	Mixed European	Heterozygous	A2089G	Q627R
31(CaDe)[f]	Dutch	Heterozygous	A2089G	Q672R
40(DoRoe)[f]	Mixed European	Heterozygous	G2776A	C901Y[g]
113(DaDem)	Italian	Homozygous	G3238C	C1055S
		Nonsense mutations		
97(AsOk)	Japanese	Homozygous	631delCAA	S186X
112(NaSch)	Mixed European	Heterozygous	A888T	K272X
98(RoMo)[f]	Mixed European	Heterozygous	A1164T	R364X
81(MaGrou)	French Canadian	Homozygous	C1858A	S595X
11(IaTh)[f]	Mixed European	Heterozygous	C2007T	Q645X
61(DoHop)	Mixed European	Homozygous	C2007T	Q645X
NR1(ErBor)[f]	Mixed European	Heterozygous	C2007T	Q645X
NR8(KeSol)[f]	Mixed European	Heterozygous	C2007T	Q645X
51(KeMc)	Mixed European	Homozygous	C2172T	Q700X
		Frameshift mutations		
93(YoYa)[f]	Japanese	Heterozygous	1610insA	514-1-X
15(MaRo)	Ashkenazi Jewish	Homozygous	2281delATCTGAinsTAGATTC	735-4-X
42(RaFr)	Ashkenazi Jewish	Homozygous	2281delATCTGAinsTAGATTC	735-4-X
107(MyAsa)	Ashkenazi/Sephardi Jewish	Homozygous	2281delATCTGAinsTAGATTC	735-4-X
NR2(CrSpe)	Ashkenazi Jewish	Homozygous	2281delATCTGAinsTAGATTC	735-4-X
126(BrNa)	Ashkenazi/Sephardi Jewish	Heterozygous	2281delATCTGAinsTAGATTC	735-4-X
		Exon-skipping mutations		
126(BrNa)	Askenazi/Sephardic	Heterozygous	Skips exon 2[h]	
112(NaSch)	Mixed European	Heterozygous	Skips exon 6[i]	
		Gross deletion		
92(VaBia)	Italian	Homozygous	Skips exons 11 and 12[j]	

[a] Mutation screening has been carried out on 25 persons with BS from whom cell lines were available. Total RNA was prepared by using Trizol (Gibco BRL). Mutations in the RNA product of *BLM* were detected by RT-PCR followed by single-stranded conformation polymorphism (SSCP) analysis (17), by an RNase cleavage assay (unpublished observations) marketed by Ambion, or both techniques. The mutations were then identified by direct sequencing of PCR-amplified cDNA.

[b] Bloom's Syndrome Registry designations. Five unrelated persons with BS were examined in whom mutations had yet to be determined, namely, 22(ElHa), 30(MaKa), 59(FrFit), 65(AnPa), and 140(DrKas).

[c] In all persons studied except 92(VaBia), 93(YoYa), 112(NaSch), 126(BrNa), and the Ashkenazi Jews, zygosity of the mutation was ascertained by analysis of the cDNA. However, homozygosity is implicated by autozygosity at *BLM* (21), the consequence of parental consanguinity or of inheritance of *BLM* from a recent common ancestor, as is the case in Ashkenazi Jews with BS, and by observation of homozygosity of polymorphic DNA markers at loci tightly linked to BLM (16). Zygosity of *BLM* mutations has been confirmed at the level of genomic DNA in 92(VaBia) whose deletion in *BLM* was confirmed by Southern blot analysis, in 93(YoYa), 112(NaSch), and 126(BrNa) whose mutations were sequenced in genomic DNA, and in Ashkenazi Jews with BS for whom a PCR-based restriction enzyme assay has been used (unpublished observations). By "heterozygous," we mean compound heterozygosity.

[d] The nucleotide positions are as identified in the *BLM* cDNA H1-5′ (17). Standard nomenclature has been used to indicate the genetic alteration in the gene.

[e] Number of amino acids starting from the first in-frame ATG found in the *BLM* cDNA (17). An X indicates a stop codon. The amino acid that is changed appears before the codon number. The effect of a frameshift is shown by first indicating the number of BLM amino acid residues that are incorporated followed by the number of out-of-frame residues that are incorporated until a stop codon is reached.

[f] In this heterozygote, the other mutated *BLM* allele has yet to be determined.

[g] This missense mutation formally could be a polymorphism.

[h] An RT-PCR product with a smaller-than-normal size was detected by agarose gel electrophoresis. Sequencing of the abnormal cDNA fragment identified a deletion of exon 2, nucleotides 71 to 172. Sequence analysis of genomic DNA amplified with oligonucleotide primers flanking exon 2 revealed a G-to-T transversion in the 5′ splice site (GT to TT). Splicing out of exon 2 removes the initiator methionine for BLM. Use by the ribosome of the next downstream ATG would result in the generation of a small out-of-frame peptide.

[i] An RT-PCR product with a smaller-than-normal size was detected by agarose gel electrophoresis. Sequencing of the abnormal cDNA fragment identified a deletion of exon 6, nucleotides 1162 to 1294. Sequence analysis of genomic DNA amplified with oligonucleotide primers flanking exon 6 revealed a G-to-A transition in the 3′ splice site (AG to AA). Splicing out of exons 5 and 7 results in the addition of 4 out-of-frame amino acids followed by premature termination.

[j] The mutation present in 92(VaBia) was assigned incorrectly in reference 17 as a G to C at nucleotide position 2596. Subsequently, a deletion of exons 11 and 12—nucleotides 2382 to 2629 in the BLM cDNA—was detected by RT-PCR analysis, and its existence was confirmed in genomic DNA by Southern blot analysis as an approximately 750-bp deletion. Splicing of exons 10 and 13 results in addition of 1 out-of-frame amino acid followed by premature termination.

initiator AUG is not present in the cDNA; the next downstream AUG is out of frame, resulting in failure to produce normal BLM product. From mutation searching, three conclusions can be drawn: (1) The discovery of mutations in the H1-5′ sequence in persons with BS proves that the gene is in fact *BLM*. (2) The fact that multiple mutations exist in the gene confirmed the existence of allelic heterogeneity at BLM. (3) The identification of ten premature translation termination mutations many of which were homozygous in persons with BS demonstrates that (a) loss of function of the BLM protein is the major underlying cause of the syndrome and (b) that "knock-out" mutation at *BLM* is not cell-lethal.[17] In addition, because mutations in *BLM* have been detected in nearly all persons with BS examined, the clinical entity is defined at the molecular level by *BLM* mutation; BS-causing mutations at loci other than *BLM* apparently do not exist, or they are very rare.

Transfection of wild-type *BLM* cDNA into BS cells in culture brings the high-SCE phenotype of these cells towards normal. This observation confirmed that the H1-5′ sequence is derived from *BLM*. Transfection of *BLM* provides an experimental system in which polymorphic base pairs in *BLM* can be to distinguished from bona fide BS-causing missense mutations. This analysis has confirmed that both the Q672R and the C1055S mutations in fact cause BS. Altered *BLM* genes can now be introduced into BS cells to analyze structure-function relationships of BLM.

The frameshift mutation at nucleotide 2281 was detected in five persons with Ashkenazi Jewish ancestry. This mutation introduces a *Bst*NI site that can be detected by restriction enzyme digestion in DNA amplified by PCR of cDNA or genomic DNA. Fifty-one of the 52 chromosomes derived from Ashkenazi Jewish persons with BS that have been examined contain this *Bst*NI site, and therefore contain this specific frameshift mutation. This evidence confirms the hypothesis that founder effect was responsible for the elevated frequency of BS in the Ashkenazi Jewish population. The recent identification of a nonsense mutation at nucleotide 2007 in the *BLM* cDNA in four unrelated persons of mixed non-Jewish European ancestry (see Table 15-4) indicates similarly that founder effect is occurring in other populations but on a much smaller scale than in the Ashkenazi Jewish population.

The *BLM* Gene Product

Homology searching of amino acid sequence databases revealed that the 1417 peptide encoded by the H1-5′ sequence is homologous to the RecQ helicases (Fig. 15-7), a subfamily of DExH box-containing DNA and RNA helicases.[18] The RecQ helicases are part of a larger group of proteins that contain seven amino acid motifs present in most DNA and RNA helicases[18]. RecQ and a human protein isolated from HeLa cells called RECQL (for RecQ-like)

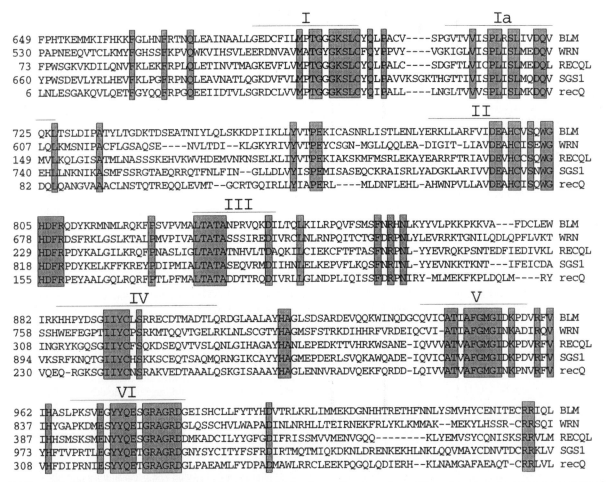

FIG. 15-7 Alignment of the amino acid sequences in the domains containing the seven helicase motifs of all the RecQ helicases known except a gene identified in the nematode by DNA sequencing. Sequence alignments were performed by the Megalign computer program (DNAStar). Numbers at left indicate the amino acid positions in each peptide, and gene product names are at the right. Identities present in all five proteins are boxed. Overlined sequences mark the seven helicase motifs in the helicase domain. The DExH box is in helicase motif II. (Figure reprinted with permission from reference 18.)

exhibit DNA-dependent ATPase and DNA strand-displacement activities that identify them as DNA helicases. These observations strongly suggest that BLM is a DNA helicase.

The recent addition of two other members (Fig. 15-7) to this subfamily has generated considerable interest: (1) the product of the yeast gene *SGS1* (for *slow growth suppresser*), which was first identified by a mutation that suppressed the slow-growth phenotype of yeast containing mutations in the topoisomerase 3 gene,[24] and (2) the gene product encoded in the Werner syndrome gene, *WRN*, which was identified by positional cloning.[25] Both of these products have certain important similarities to *BLM*. Besides the 42–44% amino acid identity across the regions of the proteins that contain the seven conserved helicase motifs, the BLM, WRN, and SGS1 proteins are similar in length and contain highly negatively charged N-terminal regions (the first 650 residues) and highly positively charged C-terminal regions (the last 350 residues). Such similarities in overall structure have raised the possibility that these proteins play related or similar roles in DNA metabolism.

An antibody to the N-terminal part of the BLM protein has been raised, and a protein with an apparent molecular weight of 180 kD has been identified by Western blot analysis of fibroblast, lymphoblastoid, and HeLa cells. By indirect immunofluorescence performed on fibroblast and lymphoblastoid cells, BLM protein is localized to the nucleus, staining in a focal distribution similar to that of many other nuclear antigens associated with DNA metabolism. BLM protein is absent in cells from persons with BS, confirming its identity as BLM.

MANAGEMENT

Growth

A means of increasing growth in BS is unknown—and is not to be found if the hypothesis of excessive cell death secondary to the abnormal number of somatic mutations that arise throughout development is the correct explanation for the restriction on size.

Babies and young children with BS are notoriously poor eaters, and the course normally followed is to set nutritious food before them, supplement it with a multiple vitamin preparation, and just let the child eat as his body dictates through appetite. Coercion to eat is of no avail, and, on the contrary, undue attention from the family would sometimes seem to have undesirable psychological effects. Nonvolitional feeding of infants with BS by, for example, surgically placed intragastric feeding tubes, is under investigation in a few centers, and some promising results are being obtained in the four children so treated. As stated earlier, if the presently unexplained restriction on learning and the adult-onset diabetes are on a nutritional basis, such a simple measure could be valuable in BS.

Growth hormone production in BS when estimated usually is found in the normal to low-normal range. A few affected persons have been treated with growth hormone, usually without much effect. (Why a few males with BS have reached 5 feet or slightly more without any specific treatment is unknown.) Although more information on the possibly beneficial effect of growth hormone with respect to final body size in BS is desirable, reports of cancer that has arisen during or following its administration, including in BS, commonly deter trials.

The Skin

The facial skin lesion of BS is controlled best by avoidance of the sun and the regular use of a hat or bonnet and sun-screening ointments. Especially advisable may be measures to limit sun exposure

in the first few years of life, judging from the observation that in most cases the severity of the skin lesion appears to be established at that time.

Cancer

Although knowledge of the cancer proneness of BS naturally is distressing to an affected family, the information can be lifesaving. Here it is withheld from neither affected adults nor the parents of affected children. Families and patients handle this information well if it is presented to them appropriately by the physician or geneticist in charge, that is, in comprehensible and useful terms. It can be presented in the context of the already great frequency of cancer in the general population and then supplemented by an explanation of the basis for the inordinate increase and its prematurity in the person with BS. That the risk, although always more than in other people, is relatively much less at the early ages can be explained, as well as the shift of type toward carcinoma after adulthood is reached.[12] The potential value such knowledge of cancer proneness provides to an affected person can be emphasized, and some idea of practical and effective surveillance programs to be instituted at different ages can be provided; that is, the physician who makes the diagnosis also, in lieu of treatment in the usual sense, offers a modus operandi.

Until the prognosis of leukemia if diagnosed and treated in its earliest stages can be shown to be better than treatment initiated after the disease becomes symptomatic, periodic hematological surveillance of children with BS is not recommended. However, for adults with BS, close and long-term contact with an internist or clinic knowledgeable about BS is highly advisable. An unusual degree of attention then will be paid to symptoms that in other persons might properly be ignored but that in BS will permit early diagnosis of carcinoma where surgical excision still provides the best chance of cure. (Among symptoms and signs that already have led to early diagnosis of cancer in persons in the Registry—sometimes but unfortunately not always life-saving—are the following: hoarseness [laryngeal carcinoma]; pain in the side of the throat [posterior lingual carcinoma]; mild dysphagia [esophageal carcinoma]; red blood staining in the feces [carcinoma of the lower large bowel]; a lump in the breast palpable by the patient; a positive Papanicolaou smear [cervical carcinoma-in-situ]; lower abdominal pain [uterine adenocarcinoma]; unexplained recurring abdominal discomfort [pelvic lymphoma; adenocarcinoma of the colon]; intussusception [lymphoma of the small bowel]; and, abrupt onset of convulsions [meningioma] or headache [medulloblastoma].) After the age of 20, annual visits with the internist are mandatory, with at least annual screening for carcinoma of the breast, cervix, and colon.

In the treatment of the cancers that arise in persons with BS, consideration is essential of the hypersensitivity such persons have to many of the DNA-damaging chemicals in standard regimens of therapy. Several persons with BS have shown severe destruction of bowel mucosa and bone marrow, and this can be lethal. Although specific recommendations of dosage of chemotherapeutic agents in BS cannot be given, doses approximately half the standard dose of the DNA-damaging agents have usually been tolerated, and in several have proven adequate for apparent cure. Ionizing irradiation has been tolerated normally in the usual dosage.

The "management" of a person with BS is not to be viewed by his physician as of little value just because normal body size cannot be prescribed for nor cancer prevented. Knowledge of the correct diagnosis and then an understanding of the condition is of inestimable value to parents of affected persons. Also, the affected individual benefits both physically and emotionally when in the hands of one who knows the correct diagnosis, understands well the syndrome itself, and is able to communicate both appropriately and wisely accurate information about the syndrome, including its important complications.

CONCLUDING COMMENT

In BS, important observations have emerged from the study of a clinical condition so rare that it has not qualified for coverage in standard textbooks of pediatrics or medicine. It is a condition described just four decades ago by an astute dermatologist who had an interest in rare and unusual disorders, and who believed in publishing so that others could know what he had observed. The things learned subsequently about BS have, quite naturally, depended on technical advances. Thus, cytogenetic techniques permitted the discovery that somatic crossing-over occurs in mammalian cells. Cytogenetic observation of BS cells and long-term contact with affected individuals also provided *some of the earliest and clearest evidence that chromosome mutation is a cause of human cancers.* Most recently, recombinant DNA technologies applied to the BS problem have brought to light a protein not previously known to exist in mammalian cells. With the tentative identification of BLM as a protein intricately involved in DNA metabolism, but one that is not lethal when missing from the nucleus, the BS gene becomes a valuable experimental tool for investigating previously completely obscure nuclear mechanisms by which the genetic material is manipulated. The BLM helicase clearly plays an important role: the major consequence for the cell of absence of the normal function of the *BLM* gene product is an unacceptably high rate of mutation, including hyper-recombination. The isolation of *BLM* opens, of course, a way to understand the genomic instability that characterizes BS cells themselves, but, more important, to help identify and characterize normal cellular systems whose function is to maintain the integrity of the genome in somatic cells.

REFERENCES

1. German J: Bloom's syndrome. I. Genetical and clinical observations in the first twenty-seven patients. *Am J Hum Genet* **21**:196, 1969.
2. German J: Bloom's syndrome. II. The prototype of genetic disorders predisposing to chromosome instability and cancer, in German J (ed): *Chromosomes and Cancer.* New York, John Wiley and Sons, 1974, p. 601.
3. German J: Bloom's syndrome. VIII. Review of clinical and genetic aspects, in Goodman RM, Motulsky AG (eds): *Genetic Diseases among Ashkenazi Jews.* New York, Raven Press, 1979, p. 121.
4. German J: Bloom syndrome: A mendelian prototype of somatic mutational disease. *Medicine* **72**:393, 1993.
5. German J: Bloom's syndrome, in Genodermatoses with Malignant Potential, in Cohen PR, Kurzrock R (eds): *Dermatologic Clinics,* vol 13. Philadelphia, W.B. Saunders, 1995, p. 7.
6. German J: Genes which increase chromosomal instability in somatic cells and predispose to cancer, in Steinberg AG, Bearn AG (eds): *Progress in Medical Genetics,* vol. VIII. New York, Grune & Stratton, 1972, p. 61.
7. Ray JH, German J: The cytogenetics of the "chromosome-breakage syndromes," in German J (ed): *Chromosome Mutation and Neoplasia.* New York, Alan R. Liss, 1983, p. 135.
8. German J: Bloom's syndrome XVII. A genetic disorder that displays the consequences of excessive somatic mutation, in Bonne-Tamir B, Adam A (eds): *Genetic Diversity among Jews.* New York, Oxford University Press, 1992, p. 129.
9. German J, Passarge E: Bloom's syndrome. XIII. Report from the Registry for 1987. *Clin Genet* **35**:57, 1989.
10. German J: Bloom's syndrome and the immune system, in Bjorkander J, Fasth A (eds): Proceedings, 7th Meeting, European Society of Immunodeficiencies, Goteborg, 6-9 June 1996, International Congress Series, Elsevier Science, Amsterdam (in press).
11. Bloom D: Congenital telangiectatic erythema resembling lupus erythematosus in dwarfs. *Am J Dis Child* **88**:754, 1954.
12. German J: Bloom's syndrome. XX. The first 100 cancers. *Cancer Genet Cytogenet,* submitted.
13. Groden J, Nakamura Y, German J: Molecular evidence that homologous recombination occurs in proliferating human somatic cells. *Proc Natl Acad Sci USA* **87**:4315, 1990.
14. Groden J, German J: Bloom's syndrome. XVIII. Hypermutability of a tandem-repeat locus. *Hum Genet* **90**:360, 1992.
15. German J, Roe AM, Leppert M, Ellis NA: Bloom syndrome: An analysis of consanguineous families assigns the locus mutated to chromosome band 15q26.1. *Proc Natl Acad Sci USA* **91**:6669, 1994.
16. Ellis NA, Roe AM, Kozloski J, Proytcheva M, Falk C, German J: Linkage disequilibrium between the FES, D15S127, and *BLM* loci in Ashkenazi Jews with Bloom's syndrome. *Am J Hum Genet* **55**:453, 1994.
17. Ellis NA, Groden J, Ye T-Z, Straughen J, Lennon DJ, Ciocci S, Proytcheva M, German J: The Bloom's syndrome gene product is homologous to RecQ helicases. *Cell* **83**:655, 1995.
18. Ellis NA, German J: Molecular genetics of Bloom's syndrome. *Hum Molec Genet* **5**:1457, 1996.
19. Weksberg R, Smith C, Anson-Cartwright L, Maloney K: Bloom syndrome: A single complementation group defines patients of diverse ethnic origin. *Am J Hum Genet* **42**:816, 1988.
20. McDaniel LD, Schultz RA: Elevated sister chromatid exchange phenotype of Bloom syndrome cells is complemented by human chromosome 15. *Proc Natl Acad Sci USA* **89**:7968, 1992.
21. German J, Ellis NA, Proytcheva M: Bloom's syndrome. XIX. Cytogenetic and population evidence for genetic heterogeneity. *Clin Genet* **49**:223, 1996.
22. Ellis NA, Lennon DJ, Proytcheva M, Alhadeff B, Henderson EE, German J: Somatic intragenic recombination within the mutated locus *BLM* can correct the high-SCE phenotype of Bloom syndrome cells. *Am J Hum Genet* **57**:1019, 1995.
23. Straughen J, Ciocci S, Ye T-Z, Lennon DN, Proytcheva M, Goodfellow P, German J, Ellis NA, Groden J: Physical mapping of the Bloom's syndrome region by the identification of YAC and P1 clones from human chromosome 15 band q26.1. *Genomics* **33**:118, 1996.
24. Gangloff S, McDonald JP, Bendixen C, Arthur L, Rothstein R: The yeast type I topoisomerase top3 interacts with Sgs1, a DNA helicase homolog: a potential eukaryotic reverse gyrase. *Mol Cell Biol* **14**:8391, 1994.
25. Yu C-E, Oshima J, Fu Y-H, Wijsman EM, Hisama F, Alisch R, Matthews S, Nakura J, Miki T, Ouais S, Marin GM, Mulligan J, Schellenberg GD: Positional cloning of the Werner's syndrome gene. *Science* **272**:258, 1996.

Variable Expressivity

A recent analysis of congenital malformations among siblings with FA revealed that there is both interfamilial and intrafamilial phenotypic variation in the specific types of congenital malformations among affected siblings.[5] Fifty-three sibships composed of 120 siblings were analyzed. Even the two sets of monozygotic (MZ) twins described in his report were phenotypically discordant. In MZ twin pair 1, the fetuses were examined after pregnancy termination as a result of prenatal diagnosis performed because of the presence of two prior affected siblings in the pedigree. Twin A had a bifid thumb, whereas twin B had no physical stigmata of FA. The proband in this sibship had duodenal atresia, whereas the other affected sib had no congenital abnormalities. In MZ twin pair 2, 15-year-old girls with FA, twin A had unilateral absence of the radius, bilateral absent thumbs, and an absent right clavicle. Twin B had a bifid right thumb, a hypoplastic left thumb, and an absent left clavicle. However, the analysis showed that the occurrence of malformations among FA siblings is nonrandom; siblings usually were concordant for the presence or absence of multiple congenital malformations. Also, an analysis of hematologic abnormalities in FA demonstrated a concordance in the findings in sibships; the age at detection of hematologic abnormalities in probands and siblings was correlated ($p = 0006$).[40] To explain the clinical heterogeneity in FA, it has been postulated that the phenotypic features of an affected individual depend on the specific FA muation, somatic DNA instability, other genes, and environmental factors. Thus, FA may be caused by genes that directly or indirectly affect morphogenesis.

DIAGNOSTIC CRITERIA

Crosslinker Hypersensitivity

Diagnosis of FA on the basis of clinical manifestations often is difficult and unreliable owing to the considerable overlap of the FA phenotype with those of a variety of genetic and nongenetic diseases. Schroeder et al. first suggested the use of spontaneous chromosomal breakage as a cellular market for FA; however, longitudinal studies of chromosome instability in FA patients have shown a wide variation in the frequency of baseline breakage within the same individual, ranging from no breakage to high levels.[6,41] Numerous studies of the sensitivity of FA cells to a variety of DNA crosslinking agents have been performed over the past 27 years.[7,8,12,13,16,42–44] Hypersensitivity of FA cells to the clastogenic (chromosome-breaking) effect of crosslinking agents provides a unique cellular marker for the disorder. Comparative studies have led to the choice of DEB as the agent most widely used for FA diagnosis.[16,45] Extensive experience with the DEB test has demonstrated the sensitivity, specificity, and reproducibility of the re-

Table 16-1 Summary of Major Congenital Malformations Observed in IFAR Patients

Abnormality	All FA Patients, percent
Radial ray	49.1
Other skeletal	21.6
Renal and urinary tract	33.8
Male genital	19.7
Gastrointestinal	14.3
Heart	13.2
Hearing loss	11.3
Central nervous system	7.7

sults.[13,16] Crosslinker hypersensitivity can be used to identify preanemic patients as well as patients with aplastic anemia or leukemia who may or may not have the physical stigmata associated with FA (Tables 16-1 through 16-6 and Figs. 16-1 and 16-2).

Clinical Features

The International Fanconi Anemia Registry. More than 800 cases of FA have been reported in varying detail in the literature, and these cases have been reviewed by Young and Alter.[4] The cases in the literature, particularly those reported before the present decade, were made when aplastic anemia or leukemia developed in individuals with characteristic physical abnormalities; thus, reviews in the literature are biased toward the most severe clinical cases. The literature also contains cases diagnosed on the basis of physical manifestations alone, without confirmation by DEB testing; some of these cases are now known to be misdiagnosed. The International Fanconi Anemia Registry (IFAR) was established at the Rockefeller University in 1982 to collect clinical, genetic, and hematologic information from a large number of FA patients in order to study the full spectrum of clinical features of the disease.[46] The primary source of case material for the IFAR is physician reporting. Once a potential case is identified, an IFAR questionnaire form is completed by the referring physician, and copies of laboratory reports and other patient records are obtained with the consent of the patient or guardian. Diagnosis of FA is confirmed by study of chromosomal breakage induced by DEB or another crosslinking agent. Clinical information from the IFAR has been analyzed for phenotypic features and hematologic abnormalities, and the results have been reported in the literature.[3,11,13,40,47] The purpose of some of these reports was to address the need for earlier diagnosis of FA by increasing the awareness of clinicians of the complete phenotypic spectrum of the syndrome. Currently, there are over 600 patients in the IFAR with a diagnosis of FA confirmed in the United States. Large numbers of subjects and long follow-up make this database unique compared to literature re-

Table 16-2 Radial Ray Abnormalities in IFAR Patients

Bilateral Radial Ray Defect	Unilateral Radial Ray Defect
Absent radii and thumbs	Absent radius and thumb
Absent radius and bilateral thumb abnormality	Hypoplastic radius and thumb abnormality
Hypoplastic radii and bilateral thumb abnormality	Absent thumb
Bilateral absent thumbs	Hypoplastic thumb
Bilateral hypoplastic thumbs	Bifid thumb
Unilateral absent thumb, contralateral abnormal thumb	Other
Unilateral hypoplastic thumb, contralateral abnormal thumb	
Other	

Table 16-3 Other Skeletal Malformations Reported in IFAR Patients

Abnormality	All FA Patients, percent
Congenital hip	6.6
Vertebral	3.2
Scoliosis	3.2
Rib	3.0
Clubfoot	1.4
Sacral agenesis (hypoplasia)	1.1
Perthes disease	1.1
Sprengel deformity	1.1
Genu valgum	0.8
Leg length discrepancy	0.5
Kyphosis	0.5
Spina bifida	0.3
Navicular aplasia	0.3
Brachydactyly	0.3
Arachnodactyly	0.3
Metacarpal (other than first)	0.3
Craniosynostosis	0.3
Humeral abnormality	0.3
Short toes	0.3
Upper thoracic spine	0.3

Table 16-4 Gastrointestinal Malformations Reported in IFAR Patients

Abnormality	All FA Patients, percent
Anorectal	5.1
Duodenal atresia	4.6
Tracheoesophageal fistula	3.5
Esophageal atresia	1.4
Annular pancreas	1.4
Intestinal malrotation	1.1
Intestinal obstruction	1.1
Duodenal web	0.5
Biliary atresia	0.3
Foregut duplication cyst	0.3

Table 16-5 Central Nervous System Abnormalities Reported in IFAR Patients

Abnormality	All FA Patients, percent
Hydrocephalus or ventriculomegaly	4.6
Absent septum pellucidum, corpus callosum	1.4
Neural tube defect	0.8
Migration defect	0.8
Arnold-Chiari Malformation	0.5
Moyamoya	0.5
Single ventricle	0.3

provides a check on the accuracy of data reporting. Summaries of the phenotypic features and hematologic manifestations of FA presented here are taken from the IFAR. Tables 16-1 through 16-6 and Figs. 16-1 through 16-3 show some of the clinical features manifested by the FA patients examined.

Growth Parameters. FA is associated with abnormal growth parameters both prenatally and postnatally. Short stature is a well-recognized feature of the syndrome; the mean stature of FA patients in the IFAR is near the fifth percentile. However, although patients with FA often are shorter than the general population and shorter than their expected heights, most of these individuals are not extremely short. Weight and head circumference are also often less than the fifth percentile. Some children with FA have reduced growth hormone responsiveness and hypothyroidism, which may further compromise their growth. A significant number of FA patients also exhibit highly elevated levels of insulin with a high insulin:glucose ratio on oral glucose tolerance testing, implying insulin resistance.[48] We suggest endocrine evaluation in all FA children, since correction of growth hormone or thyroid hormone deficiency may improve the final height outcome.

Major Congenital Malformations. In a survey of the clinical findings obtained from the IFAR, a variety of congenital malformations associated with FA have been described. A review of these data indicated that the FA phenotype is more variable than was previously recognized. Gastrointestinal, central nervous system, and skeletal malformations in FA patients, previously not included as part of the FA phenotype, were observed.[11] Major congenital malformations reported in IFAR patients are summarized in Tables 16-1 through 16-5. This analysis showed that most FA patients with congenital malformations are not diagnosed until after the onset of hematologic abnormalities; delayed diagnosis might be due

ports. However, there are potential limitations, such as selective reporting and incompleteness and inaccuracy of data reporting. Approximately 10 percent of the patients were examined at the Rockefeller University Hospital or affiliated institutions, which

Table 16-6 Minor Anomalies and Mild Malformations Reported in IFAR Patients

Abnormality	Specific Types
Skin pigmentation	Café-au-lait spots, hyperpigmentation, hypopigmentation
Eye	Short palpebral fissures (microphthalmia), almond-shaped palpebral fissures, hypertelorism, hypotelorism, epicanthal folds
Nose	Flattened nasal bridge, nasal pit
Ear, minor	Low set, protruding, minor helix abnormality
Oral cavity	Arched palate, geographic tongue, thin upper lip
Face	Triangular face, facial asymmetry, facial flattening
Neck	Webbing of neck, low hairline
Hand	Thenar hypoplasia, clinodactyly of fifth digit, syndactyly of fingers, hyperextensible thumbs, arachnodactyly, contractures
Foot	Syndactyly of toes, wide space between first and second toes, pes planus, hypoplastic toenails
Prominent forehead	
Other	Sacral dimple, frontal hair upsweep, chest asymmetry, pectus excavatum

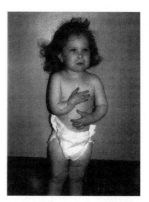

FIG. 16-1 A 2-year-old male of Ashkenazi Jewish ancestry who demonstrates physical features associated with Fanconi anemia. The photograph was taken after surgery on his hands. Before the surgery, the right hand exhibited a hypoplastic radius and absent thumb, whereas the left hand had a hypoplastic thumb. The patient exhibits growth retardation, dysmorphic facial features, microphthalmia, microcephaly, and café-au-lait spots; he also has a kidney abnormality, undescended testes, and a small penis. This patient is homozygous for the IVS4 +4 A>T mutation in FAC.

to lack of physician awareness of the phenotypic spectrum of FA. From a developmental standpoint, it is interesting that radial ray abnormalities in FA patients can be bilateral or unilateral (Table 16-2). Even patients with bilateral abnormalities usually exhibit asymmetry, with their limbs having different specific anomalies (Table 16-2 and Fig. 16-1).[13]

Minor Malformations. Approximately one-third of FA patients do not manifest congenital malformations (Fig. 16-2).[11] In these patients the diagnosis of FA generally is made only after a patient presents with clinical symptoms of hematologic dysfunction; the mean age of diagnosis in this group is considerably older than that for FA patients with malformations. FA patients without congenital malformations frequently have alterations in growth parameters, with height, weight, or head circumference below the fifth percentile. Other very common findings in these patients are skin pigmentation abnormalities and/or microphthalmia. Minor anomalies and mild malformations reported among FA patients lacking major malformations are listed in Table 16-6.[47] It is noteworthy that many FA patients have distinctive facial characteristics, including microphthalmia and small facial size (Fig. 16-3). Increased awareness of the facial anomalies as well as the complete spectrum of

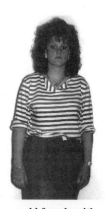

FIG. 16-2 A 17-year-old female with normal phenotypic features. She was diagnosed with FA at age 12 on the basis of hematologic abnormalities and a positive DEB test. She also exhibited short stature and café au lait spots. She died at age 21 of AML. This patient is the product of a consanguineous marriage and was homozygous for the Q13X mutation in exon 1 of FAC.

minor malformations in FA by clinicians should allow an earlier diagnosis to be made in patients without congenital anomalies.

Fertility. Older females have irregular menses, and menopause usually starts during the fourth decade. Fifteen percent of females cited in the literature or reported to the IFAR who reached at least 16 years of age and were not receiving androgen therapy had at least one pregnancy.[4,49] Thus, pregnancy can occur in FA, although it often is associated with complications such as progression of bone marrow failure and preeclampsia. Genital malformations and hypoplastic gonads are common findings in males with FA (Table 16-1).[50] There are extremely few reported cases of affected males having offspring.[51] Results of semen analysis on several males in the IFAR showed abnormal spermatogenesis, with very low sperm counts.

Hematologic Manifestations. An analysis of hematologic data from 388 patients with FA reported to the IFAR showed that hematologic abnormalities were detected in 332 persons at a median age of 7 years (range, birth to 31 years).[40] Actuarial risk of developing a hematologic abnormalities by 40 years of age was 98 percent; actuarial risk of death from hematologic causes was 81 percent by 40 years of age. Initial hematologic findings were diverse; thrombocytopenia associated with an elevated HbF and macrocytosis usually proceeded the onset of anemia or neutropenia. In some cases, patients presented with MDS or AML without a prior diagnosis of aplastic anemia. Thrombocytopenia and pancytopenia often were associated with decreased bone marrow (BM) cellularity. Actuarial risk of clonal cytogenetic abnormalities during BM failure was 67 percent by 30 years of age. Fifty-nine patients developed MDS and/or AML; actuarial risk of MDS and/or AML by 40 years of age was 52 percent.

In a recent study of genotype-phenotype correlations in FA-C patients, it was shown that the *FAC* genotype affects clinical outcome and allows division of these patients into three groups: (1) patients with the IVS4 mutation ($n = 26$), (2) patients with at least one exon 14 mutation (R548X or L554P) ($n = 16$), and (3) patients with at least one exon 1 mutation (322delG or Q13X) and no known exon 14 mutation ($n = 17$).[52] Individuals with IVS4 or exon 14 mutations had a significantly earlier onset of hematologic abnormalities and poorer survival compared to exon 1 patients and to the non-FA-C IFAR population. Sixteen of the 59 FA-C patients (27 percent) have developed AML. The incidence of leukemia in each of the FA-C subgroups ranges from 19 to 37 percent. The median age at diagnosis of leukemia is younger in the IVS4 and exon 14 groups compared with the exon 1 group (10.8 and 15.9 years versus 21.9 years). Twenty-eight of the 59 FA-C patients have died. Leukemia was the cause of death in 13 of those 28 (46 percent). Three patients with a history of leukemia have survived; one patient was recently diagnosed, and two are in remission after BMT.

These data indicate an extraordinarily high risk of bone marrow failure and AML in persons with FA and underscore the potential use of FA as a model of bone marrow failure and leukemia development.

Nonhematologic Malignancies. Patients with FA have an increased cancer predisposition. In addition to the extraordinarily high frequency of AML in FA patients (actuarial risk of 52 percent for the development of MDS and/or AML by 40 years of age),[40] FA patients have been reported to exhibit malignancies of a variety of organ systems, most commonly gastrointestinal and gynecologic (Table 16-7).[4] The high incidence of nonhematologic malignancy in FA patients is especially striking because of the predicted early death from hematologic causes associated with the syndrome (median estimated survival is 23 years; actuarial risk of death from

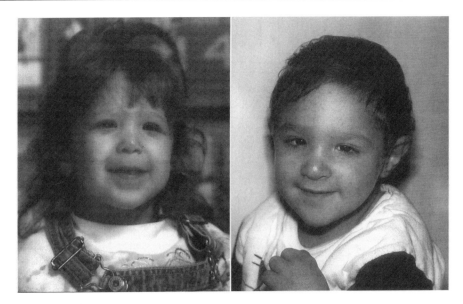

FIG. 16-3 Two unrelated FA patients exhibiting typical facial features of FA. Note microphthalmia and elfinlike facies. These patients are of Ashkenazi Jewish ancestry and are homozygous for the IVS4 +4 A>T mutation in FAC, but similar facial features frequently are seen in genetically diverse FA patients.

hematologic causes is 81 percent by 40 years of age). Thus patients are unusually young when they develop cancer, and the incidence of malignancy probably would be considerably higher if patients had a longer life expectancy. Most of the nonhematologic tumors in FA patients are squamous cell carcinomas. Liver tumors, mostly hepatocellular carcinomas, are also common in FA. Most of these tumors occur in patients who have been treated with androgen therapy for bone marrow failure. Discontinuation of androgens may lead to resolution of the liver tumors.[4]

GENETIC HETEROGENEITY

Complementation Groups

The hypersensitivity of FA cells to crosslinking agents has been used to assess the complementation of the cellular defect in somatic cell hybrids. Successful complementation is considered indicative of the existence of various genes causing FA, as has been previously performed for XP through the analysis of heterokaryons.[53] The most successful approach has involved the use of Epstein-Barr virus-immortalized lymphoblastoid cell lines.

Table 16-7 Nonhematologic Malignancies in FA Patients

Type	Specific Variety	No.
Oropharygeal	Gingiva, tongue, jaw, mandible, pharynx	17
Gastrointestinal	Esophagus, stomach, anus, colon	13
Gynecologic	Vulva, cervix, breast	9
Central nervous system	Medulloblastoma, astrocytoma	5
Other	Skin, renal, bronchial, lymphoma	6

SOURCE: Adapted from Young NS, Alter BP: Clinical features of Fanconi's anemia, in Young NS, Alter BP (eds): *Aplastic Anemia Acquired and Inherited.* Philadelphia, Saunders, 1994, p 275. Eight hundred FA patients reported in the literature are reviewed. Cancers exclude leukemia and liver tumors. The latter tumors are associated with androgen therapy.

Such studies have revealed an extensive degree of genetic heterogeneity. In the first systematic study lymphoblastoid cell lines from seven unrelated FA patients were investigated.[18] A hprt-ouab^R derivative of one of these cell lines (HSC72) was used as a universal fusion partner in hybridizations with the other cell lines, allowing selective outgrowth of hybrids in culture medium containing hypoxanthine-aminopterin-thymidine (HAT) plus ouabain. MMC sensitivity versus resistance of the hybrids was used as a criterion for complementation. Two groups of cell lines could be distinguished among the seven studied: three that failed to complement the reference cell line HSC72 in fusion hybrids (termed A) and three that fully complemented the defect (termed B or non-A). The correction of the drug sensitivity phenotype was confirmed by the analysis of both spontaneous and MMC-induced chromosomal breakage.

The three non-A cell lines subsequently were marked with dominant drug resistance markers that were introduced by stable transfection with plasmids conferring hygromycin or neomycin resistance and allowed the selection of fusion hybrids generated from combinations of these cell lines. Since all possible combinations yielded crosslinker-resistant hybrids, each non-A cell line apparently represented a separate complementation group: FA-B, FA-C, and FA-D.[17] Recently, this analysis was taken a step further by means of the generation of doubly marked derivatives of the three non-A cell lines and analysis of complementation after fusion with cell lines from another 13 FA patients.[19] All cell lines except one failed to complement only one reference group cell line and therefore could be classified as belonging to an existing group. Mutation screening in four patients who had been assigned to the C group by complementation analysis revealed mutations in *FAC*, supporting the validity of the complementation analysis.

A single cell line (EUFA130) derived from a patient of Turkish ancestry complemented all four existing groups and therefore represented a fifth complementation group, FA-E. Since multiple patients have now been assigned to this group, the question arises whether further heterogeneity exists within this group, since the FA-E group is currently defined only as being different from groups A through D.[54] Genetic marking of at least one FA-E cell line will be required to allow selection of fusion hybrids to be generated with the other cell lines currently assigned to the E group.

One Gene per Group?

Complementation groups usually are considered to represent distinct disease genes. However, in another autosomal recessive chromosomal instability disorder, ataxia-telangiectasia, this assumption has not been borne out, since mutations were found in a single gene (*ATM*) in patients previously assigned to four different complementation groups.[55] For FA, however, at least three complementation groups (A, C, and D) must represent distinct genes on the basis of their separate positions in the human genetic map. The first FA gene isolated by expression cloning methodology (*FAC*) mapped to chromosome 9q22.3 by in situ hybridization, whereas different map positions were recently established for *FAA* and *FAD*.[17] *FAA* was mapped by linkage of the disease in FA families classified as FA-A on the basis of complementation studies to microsatellite markers positioned close to the telomere of chromosome 16.[56] A consortium of investigators used a panel of nine FA families classified as FA-A by complementation analysis to map the FAA locus to 16q24.3. A genomewide search using microsatellite markers led to the initial linkage to D16S520. More refined analysis, including other FA families, led to a lod score of 8.01 at $\theta = 0.00$ to marker D16S305. This finding was independently replicated by the results of a genomewide scan using homozygosity mapping to identify genes causing FA.[57] This study was performed using 23 inbred families from the IFAR. Complementation studies were not performed in these patients, but families known to belong to FA-C were excluded from the family set. Significant genetic heterogeneity ($p = 0.0013$) was shown with marker D16S520 (maximum hold score $= 6.08$; $\alpha = 0.66$). Simultaneous search analysis suggested several additional chromosomal regions that were not the locations for FA-C and FA-D that could account for a small fraction of FA in the family set, but sample size was insufficient to provide statistical significance. Fine genetic mapping using multipoint linkage analysis with a test of heterogeneity showed Zmax $= 27.16$, $\theta = 0.00$, $\alpha = 0.73$ at D16S303, the most telomeric marker on chromosome 16q. The mapping panel for this study included 50 multiplex or consanguineous families from the IFAR selected only on the basis of being non-group C.[58]

Microcell-mediated chromosome transfer was used to map the *FAD* gene to the short arm of chromosome 3, 3p22-26.[59] These data suggest that for FA the one group = one gene concept does seem to hold up.[60] Results from the complementation studies thus strongly suggest that at least five distinct genes, when defective, can cause FA.

Relative Prevalence of Complementation Groups

Cell fusion studies are a time-consuming and labor-intensive means of determining the genetic subtype of FA patients. Consequently, only a limited number of patients have been analyzed by functional complementation analysis, and the results may well be biased depending on the different ethnic backgrounds of the patients analyzed. The figures reported in a recent cumulative European/U.S./Canadian survey based on 47 patients indicate 66 percent to be group A, 4.3 percent as B, 12.7 percent as C, 4.3 percent as D, and 12.7 percent as group E (Table 12-8). Results of a fine mapping study based on a racially and ethnically diverse mapping panel of 50 non-C IFAR families indicated that 73 percent of these families were in group A.[58] This result is based on the fraction of families showing linkage to marker D16S303, the most telomeric marker on chromosome 16q, which is known be very close to the location of *FAA* on the physical map.[28] Since approximately 15 percent of IFAR patients are in group C, FA-A accounts for about 62 percent of patients in the IFAR.

Table 16-8 The Five Known FA Complementation Groups

Group	Prototype Cell Line	Ref.	Estimated Relative Prevalence, percent[54,60]
FA-A	HSC72	18	66.0
FA-B	HSC230	17	4.3
FA-C	HSC536	17	12.7
FA-D	HSC62	17	4.3
FA-E*	EUFA130	19	12.7

*Potentially heterogeneous.

It is clear that different populations may have widely different pictures. The IVS4 +4 A>T splice site mutation in *FAC* is responsible for most cases of FA in the Ashkenazi Jewish population.[21,22] In a study of over 3000 Jewish individuals, primarily of Ashkenazi descent, the frequency of IVS4 carriers was shown to be 1 in 89.[39] The high carrier frequency of the IVS4 mutation places FA-C in the group of so-called Jewish genetic diseases, which includes Tay-Sachs, Gaucher, and Canavan diseases, among others. With a carrier frequency > 1 percent and simple testing available, the IVS4 mutation merits inclusion in the battery of tests routinely provided to the Jewish population. Group C also is relatively prevalent among Dutch patients, mainly exhibiting the exon 1 frameshift 322delG, whereas group A is the prevalent complementation group represented in Italy as well as in the Afrikaans-speaking population of South Afria.[54,56,61] However, 22 unrelated patients in Germany, all five currently known complementation groups were found; 13 patients belong to group A, and 6 to group E.[54] We are virtually ignorant about complementation groups in the relatively large Asian populations, even though FA has been encountered in people of Chinese, Korean, Japanese, and Indian ancestry (Auerbach, unpublished IFAR data). Once the genes for the different complementation groups have been identified, the relative prevalences of the groups in different parts of the world can begin to be estimated through mutation screening methods.

THE BASIC DEFECT IN FA

Defining the basic defect in FA has been complicated by the extensive genetic heterogeneity present in the disease. The bulk of the biochemical literature has been derived from the analysis of unclassified FA cell lines. If the fundamental defect is different in the various complementation groups, this could lead to the inadvertent analysis of two or more basic defects simultaneously. This may explain some of the difficulties encountered by different laboratories in reproducing each other's results. At present, hypotheses to account for the pleiotropic FA phenotype postulate abnormalities in DNA repair, oxygen metabolism, growth factor homeostasis, and cell cycle regulation.[23–25,33]

DNA Repair

FA has been considered a DNA repair disorder in which the defects lie in the repair of DNA crosslinks, thus explaining the increased sensitivity of FA cells to DNA crosslinking agents, hypomutability, and increased frequency of forming deletions.[62–67] Defects in DNA repair would cause abnormal cell replication in hematopoietic, osteogenic, and other cells and would lead to the developmental defects. However, biochemical studies of DNA repair defects in FA cells have been inconclusive or contradictory.[23,24] This may represent the confounding effect of studying cells from different complementation groups or the fact that repair deficiencies may be secondary to the primary (proximate) basic defect. The most convincing evidence for a DNA repair defect is in FA-A, where cell extracts are defective in incising crosslinked DNA and have lower amounts of a protein that binds to interstrand crosslinks.[68,69] In contrast, in FA-C it has been suggested that the defect lies in the initial induction of crosslinks, not in the subsequent repair phase.[70]

Oxygen Toxicity

In has been suggested that the FA phenotype may arise from defects in oxygen metabolism.[71] This would explain the sensitivity of the growth of FA cells to ambient oxygen, which is reflected in increased chromosomal aberrations and as accumulation of cells in the G2 phase of the cell cycle.[72–74] The increased sensitivity to oxygen could be due either to increased production of toxic intermediates (e.g., free radicals) or to their decreased removal.[75–77] The sensitivity of FA cells to DNA crosslinking agents is explained as resulting from aberrant handling of reactive metabolities produced during intracellular activation.[71] The increased sensitivity to ambient oxygen could also affect the growth of FA cells in vivo, including those in the hematopoietic cell lineages. However, introduction of FAC cDNA into FA-C lymphoblasts does not alter their oxygen sensitivity.[78] This result is consistent with the view that the oxygen sensitivity is a secondary feature of the basic defect, since SV40-transformed FA fibroblasts are not oxygen-sensitive but still retain their hypersensitivity to DNA crosslinkers.[79]

Growth Factor Homeostasis

The nearly universal bone marrow failure and the high incidence of congenital malformations in FA patients have led to suggestions that the FA genes function directly in cellular growth and/or differentiation.[25,80,81] Antisense oligonucleotides complementary to FAC mRNA inhibit the in vitro clonal growth of normal erythroid and granulocyte-macrophage progenitor cells, even in the presence of exogenous growth factors.[82] Similarly, peripheral blood CD34+ cells isolated from an FA-C patient and transduced with a recombinant adeno-associated virus containing the FAC cDNA exhibit a 5- to 10-fold increase in the number of progenitor colonies formed in vitro.[83] FA fibroblasts grow slower and senesce more rapidly than do matched controls and demonstrate ultrastructural and physiologic changes characteristic of cells from aged individuals.[9,84,85] The FA gene products may play a role in regulating the levels of growth factors, many of which act in both hematopoiesis and osteogenesis.[86] Addition of IL-6 to FA lymphoblast cultures reduces the sensitivity of those cells to MMC and DEB and decreases the number of chromosomal breaks.[87] Increased amounts of tumor necrosis factor-α (TNFα) have been reported in FA cell cultures and in patient serum samples, and anti-TNF alpha antibodies partially correct the chromosomal fragility of FA cells.[87–89]

Cell Cycle Regulation/Apoptosis

The basic defect may directly cause the known abnormalities of cell cycle regulation seen in FA cells.[90] More specifically, it has been suggested that FA cells may be defective in apoptosis, or programmed cell death, implicated in the G2 arrest and death of cells treated with DNA crosslinking agents.[91,92] The high variability of the FA phenotype, including lack of concordance between identical twins, suggests that the FA gene products may function in a cel-

lular process such as apoptosis.[5] Such a relationship is also implied by the involvement of apoptosis in hematopoiesis and in embryonic development, that is, formation of the forelimb, which is abnormal in many FA patients.[93,94] The role of FAC in apoptosis has been investigated by various groups and is discussed in more detail below.

The primary defects in FA probably involve one (or more) of the previously mentioned biologic systems. The FA gene products could function as separate steps in the same pathway (e.g., growth factor homeostasis) or could be in different pathways (some in DNA repair and others in oxygen metabolism), or all products could be part of a multiprotein complex involved in one pathway (e.g., DNA repair). Each of these models would be expected to lead to a set of similar phenotypes in the various patients. Not much is known about the pathways that are implicated in FA. For example, many proteins are known to affect apoptosis and interactions with stress responses, but the specific steps are unclear. Thus, the link between specific cellular processes and the (defective) role of the FA genes needs to be specified.

IDENTIFICATION OF THE FA GENES

In view of the difficulties in defining the basic defect in FA through biochemical analysis of FA cells, various groups have attempted to clone the defective genes directly. The first approach used to identify the FA genes involved correcting the MMC sensitivity of FA cells by introducing genomic DNA from normal cells (marker rescue) and then isolating the complementing DNA. This procedure has been used to isolate the normal human version of several mutant genes in UV- and MMC-sensitive Chinese hamster ovary (CHO) cells.[53] The genes so identified are called *ERCC* (*excision repair cross-complementing*) and are the human homologues of the mutant CHO genes. They show similarities to bacterial and yeast repair genes, suggesting their direct role in similar processes in mammalian cells.[95–99] Several of these genes were subsequently shown to be equivalent to XP genes.[101] With respect to FA, partial complementation of the MMC-sensitive phenotype of both FA-A and FA-D cells using mouse DNA was reported, but these initial studies did not lead to the identification of an FA gene.[102–105]

A further approach to identifying the FA genes has involved searching for an equivalent mutation in a biologic system more amenable to genetic analysis. In XP, somatic cell hybridization was used to determine the relationship between UV-sensitive CHO cell lines and XP complementation groups.[106] Although no CHO homologue to FA is known, a mutant V79 hamster cell line (VH4) has been isolated that corresponds to FA-A cells on the basis of cellular complementation.[107,108] Although attempts are under way to clone the human homologue of the VH4 defective gene by means of genomic transfer experiments, this approach may no longer be necessary given the recent identification of *FAA* (see below). FA-A and VH4 cells appear to have a mitochondrial nuclease activity with an abnormal pH profile. This phenotype behaves as a recessive trait, since it is not observed in heterozygous cells or in tetraploid complemented cells and is similar to that of *Drosophila mus308* mutants.[109–111] These flies have increased sensitivity to nitrogen mustard, chromosome instability, and failure to recover semiconservative DNA replication after exposure to the drug, all features of FA-A cells.[112–114] Although on the basis of these results the *mus308* gene has been considered a potential homologue to *FAA*, the recently identified sequences are not similar.[27,28,115] It is still possible, however, that *mus308* corresponds to one of the other FA genes, a possibility that can be tested experimentally.

To overcome the disadvantages of the described methods for the cloning of FA genes, a cDNA expression cloning procedure was adapted and successfully used to initially clone the gene defective in FA-C cells (*FAC*) and, more recently, *FAA*.

Cloning of *FAC*

The cDNA expression system uses the pREP4 vector, based on the regulatory sequences of the Epstein-Barr virus that allow it to function as an episomal shuttle vector between bacterial and human cells.[116] A cDNA library constructed in pREP4 was used to clone a set of cDNAs that specifically complemented the MMC and DEB sensitivity of FA-C cells.[26] After transfection of the cDNA library into HSC536 (FA-C) cells and selection in MMC and/or DEB, the low-molecular-weight DNA was isolated from populations of growing cells. Eight candidate cDNAs were detected in the various pools and were tested individually for their ability to specifically complement the cellular defect of FA-C cells. A set of complementing cDNAs was identified that coded for the same predicted ORF. Alternate forms of the cDNA contain three alternative 3′ UTRs, each terminated by a consensus polyadenylation signal, in combination with one of two 5′ UTRs. The 5′ UTRs reflect the presence of alternative transcriptional start sites spliced to a common downstream exon, since they all possess suitable splice donor sites only at the 3′ end.[26,117,118] The murine, rat, and bovine cDNAs also are characterized by multiple 3′ UTRs.[119,120] Their significance is not known. The FA-C cells used in the selection of the FAC cDNA carry a mutation predicted to produce an L554P substitution that inactivates the cDNA.[26,121] The second mutant allele of this cell line leads to a deletion of 327 bp that eliminates all putative ATG start codons, leading to a nonfunctional transcript.[122] *FAC* was localized to 9q22.3 by in situ hybridization.[17] The mapping of *FAC* was confirmed by genetic analysis of known FA-C patients.[20,21] Analysis of these patients led to the identification of frameshift, splicing, amino acid substitutions, and chain termination mutations. In some cases (e.g., IVS4 +4 A>T) no protein is detected, whereas in others (e.g., L554P) a protein of normal size is seen.[20,21,123,124] Thus, a variety of protein modifications lead to the FA phenotype, suggesting that all alterations abrogate *FAC* function. Figure 12-4 summarizes known mutations and polymorphic sequence variations in *FAC*.

Features of FAC

The *FAC* coding region contains 14 exons and leads to a predicted protein of 558 amino acids.[26] The noncoding 5′ exons, now called -1, -1a, and -1b, have suitable splice signals as their 3′ ends but not at their 5′ ends.[26,117,118] The region upstream of exon -1 has promoter activity in transfection assays using a luciferase reporter gene.[118] All 17 exons have been mapped to phages isolated from a genomic library; the minimum size of *FAC* is 150 kb, since two introns are not completely defined.[125] The 3′ terminal half of the mouse gene was isolated as a step toward the development of the *Fac⁻/⁻* mouse model; the human and mouse genes are strikingly similar in this region.[126] The mouse ORF shows 79 percent amino acid similarity to the human.[119] The mouse and rat genes have been mapped, the former in close proximity to the flexed-tail locus.[127]

Function of FAC

The predicted structure of FAC (and Fac) does not resemble that of any known protein. The protein is found in the cytoplasm, arguing against a direct role in DNA repair.[123,128] The predicted ORF codes for a 63-kDa protein (558 amino acids) with a preponderance of hydrophobic amino acids but no predicted transmembrane domains.[26] In vitro transcription and translation of the cDNA produce a protein with an apparent molecular weight of 60 kDa, and a protein of similar size is immunoprecipitated from lymphoblasts or transfected cells using anti-FAC antibodies.[116,123,128] The predicted protein has no obvious nuclear localization motifs and, as determined by immunofluorescence and subcellular fractionation, appears to be primarily cytoplasmic.[123,128] Targeting of FAC to the nucleus renders it incapable of correcting the MMC sensitivity of FA-C cells.[71] Immunoprecipitation of FAC from cell extracts has identified a set of associated cytoplasmic proteins of approximately 70, 50, and 30 kDa.[129] The existence of FAC-binding proteins is also supported by the fact that overexpression of the L554P mutant protein in normal cells leads to an FA-like phenotype, suggesting that the presence of elevated levels of an inactive mutant protein sequesters other proteins.[124] The 50-kDa protein appears to be an amino truncated form of FAC that reinitiates at amino acid 55.[22] No functional motifs have been identified within the protein that could serve as clues to its biologic role.[26] Comparison of the primary sequences of the human, mouse, rat, and bovine proteins does not reveal, apart from putative phosphorylation sites, any obvious regions of higher homology, thus precluding identification of more instructive functional domains.[120] The FA cellular phenotype of increased sensitivity to MMC can be re-created by introducing *FAC* antisense oligonucleotides into wild-type cells, suggesting that FAC plays a direct role in protecting cells against the cytotoxic and clastogenic action of this compound.[82]

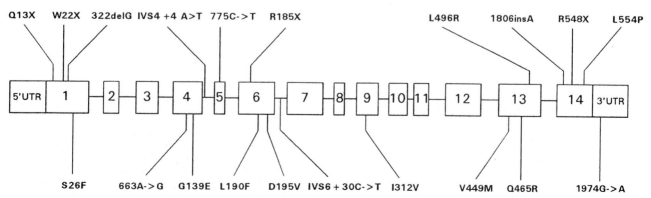

FIG. 16-4 Nucleotide sequence changes in the *FAC* gene. A schematic diagram of the 14 coding exons of the gene is provided, with the pathogenic mutations shown above and polymorphisms shown below the diagram.[161] Data are from Refs. 20, 21, 26, and 161–166.

The cytoplasmic localization of FAC has led to studies aimed at determining whether the protein has a function in apoptosis. Initial studies have focused on the possible role of FAC in MMC-mediated apoptosis. Results suggest that FA-C cells may have a generalized defect in apoptosis that is mediated by treatment with MMC or gamma radiation and may involve a failure to induce p53, although conflicting results regarding p53 have been reported.[130–132] Human MO7e and mouse 32D cells expressing *FAC* constitutively show a significant delay in cell death compared to the neomycin controls after IL-3 deprivation.[133–135] Thus, *FAC* appears to play a role in the apoptotic pathway of hematopoietic cells, a role consistent with its cytoplasmic localization as well as its increased expression in hematopoietic precursors.[136] A hypothesis that could explain these observations is that the normal role of FAC is to modulate the apoptosis that may occur during normal fluctuation of growth factors levels in the marrow microenvironment.[93] More hemopoietic cells will die in FA-C patients than in normal individuals, and with time, this will lead to hematopoietic failure. The high susceptibility of FAC patients to AML remains to be explained.

Patterns of FAC and Fac Expression

The analysis of gene expression can yield two essential pieces of information about gene function: the sites and levels where the gene functions and the mechanisms that mediate expression. In the case of FA-C, the pleiotropic phenotype of patients and the presence of three putative transcription start sites of the gene point to complex regulation.[26,117,118] Both the human and mouse genes are expressed ubiquitously at low levels in adult tissues.[26,119] Analysis of Fac expression, using PCR-derived cDNA libraries from single hemopoietic cells, shows that higher levels of expression can be detected in less differentiated (multilineage progenitors) than in more differentiated cells (single lineage progenitors).[136] During mouse embryogenesis Fac expression is high in undifferentiated mesenchymal cells 8 to 10 days p.c. Starting at 13 days, expression becomes restricted to regions with rapidly replicating chondro- and osteoprogenitors (e.g., perichondrium), a pattern that persists to later stages (15 to 19.5 days), except in regions where differentiation has taken place (e.g., hypertrophic chondrocytes of the epiphyseal growth plate). As bone development proceeds, expression is seen in osteogenic and hematopoietic cells in the zone of calcification.[137]

Cloning of FAA

FAA was cloned by two parallel approaches. One was essentially the same as that used to clone *FAC*.[26] HSC72 (FA-A) cells were transfected and selected in hygromycin and MMC. A surviving cell population was obtained that exhibited a wild-type level of resistance to MMC and was fully cross-resistant to DEB and *cis*-diamminedichloroplatinum(II). Only one clone was identified that corrected crosslinker hypersensitivity of FA-A cells, but not of FA-C cells. Screening of a bacterial artificial chromosome library with the cDNA yielded a positive clone that was used to localize the gene by fluorescence in situ hybridization; a signal was observed at the telomere of chromosome 16q, which is the genetic map location established for *FAA*, thus strengthening the candidacy of this cDNA.[56] To obtain further proof of the identity of the candidate cDNA, cell lines from FA patients classified as FA-A by complementation analysis were screened for mutations in this gene. Various sequence variations were encountered in patients from different ancestral backgrounds; these variations were likely to be

pathogenic on the basis of their severity and their segregation with the disease in three informative multiplex families. These data confirmed that the cDNA indeed represented the FAA gene.[27]

The alternative approach used was positional cloning. Subsequent to the mapping of the FA-A locus to 16q24.3, a consortium was established with the objective of cloning the *FAA* gene as well as a putative breast cancer tumor suppressor gene that maps to the same region of chromosome 16q.[56,57] The candidate region of 16q24.3 was narrowed by further linkage studies and by allelic association analysis. The preliminary physical map of the critical region was developed by screening a gridded chromosome 16 cosmid library with sequence tagged sites and expressed sequence tags. An integrated cosmid contig of about 650 kb was obtained. The cosmids were used for exon trapping and direct selection of cDNAs. Products obtained from the direct selection were used to probe high-density gridded cDNA clones, resulting in the identification of a clone that contained a poly(A) tail and was located at the 3′ end of a candidate gene. An overlapping cDNA clone was then identified; together these two clones gave a combined sequence of 2.3 kb. Exon trapping identified potential additional exons, which were used to extend the sequence by RT-PCR and to screen cDNA libraries for larger clones. One of these was found to be partially deleted in an Italian FA-A patient and was investigated in more detail as a candidate for the *FAA* gene. Several additional mutations, all of which would be expected to disrupt the function of the protein, were observed in FA-A patients of various ethnic origins.[28] The sequence of this putative FAA cDNA was found to be virtually identical to the cDNA isolated from an expression library, as described previously.

ANIMAL MODELS FOR FA-C

Mouse models of human disease can be useful in a variety of studies, including the development of novel therapies. Flexed-tailed mice have been considered as possible models for FA-C, since the *f* locus is positioned close to *Fac*.[127] However, flexed-tail mice do not have an increased sensitivity to MMC.[138] Either the flexed-tail mouse is not mutated at the *Fac* locus or the mutation is mild. Since no natural mouse mutations in the *Fac* locus are known, a murine model must be developed experimentally. Homologous recombination in embryonic stem (ES) cells has been used to target the endogenous *Fac* locus with the consequent removal of exon 8 or exon 9.[139,140] These cells have been used to derive strains of mice (*Fac*$^{-/-}$) in which no active Fac protein is produced. The mutant mice show the characteristic FA sensitivity to DNA crosslinking agents but do not demonstrate any morphologic phenotypes or hematopoietic failure to 1 year of age.

In addition to the cellular sensitivity to DNA crosslinking agents, the principal phenotype of *Fac*$^{-/-}$ mice is markedly decreased fertility of both male and female animals.[139,140] This phenotype appears to be a more severe version of similar complications seen in FA patients (see "Fertility," above). Male mice have testicular atrophy, degeneration of seminiferous tubules, low numbers of mature sperm, and epithelial sloughing in the epididymis. These results suggest that *Fac* plays a role in sperm maturation. Females cannot carry embryos beyond days 9 to 10 of gestation. Analysis of a small number of *Fac*$^{-/-}$ females shows ovarian hypoplasia and/or abnormal decidua, suggesting that the defect is physiologic. The mild hematologic and morphologic phenotype of *Fac*$^{-/-}$ mice perhaps is surprising given the abundant levels of *Fac* expression during embryogenesis, especially in early mesenchyme and zones of endochondral ossification and in early hematopoietic progenitors. Nonetheless, these FA-C mouse models promise to be useful in helping us understand the in vivo role of Fac as well as in testing new therapies.

DIAGNOSIS AND TREATMENT

The DEB Test

The clinical variability in FA is so great that diagnosis must be based on a laboratory test that measures the sensitivity of cells to chromosomal breakage induced by crosslinking agents.[13,16] Comparative studies have led to the choice of DEB as the agent most widely used for FA diagnosis because of reports of false positive and false negative diagnoses when other agents are used. It is recommended that patients have a peripheral blood sample tested at birth if they have congenital malformations known to be associated with FA.[11] All sibs of FA patients also should be screened routinely, because a lack of concordance of phenotype in affected siblings makes clinical diagnosis unreliable even within sibships.[5] Peripheral blood is the preferred tissue for the diagnosis of FA, as the sample is easy to obtain and work with and the results of the analysis of crosslinker-induced chromosome breakage can be obtained within 3 to 4 days. Data from DEB testing indicate that there is great variability in the degree of hypersensitivity in FA patients, although there is no overlap with the normal range (Figs. 16-5).[13] Approximately 10 percent of patients with a positive crosslinker test appear to have two populations of lymphocytes; the majority of crosslinker-treated cells examined have no chromosomal breakage, whereas the remainder exhibit the high number of breaks and exchanges typical of FA patients.[13] Interestingly, there is no correlation between the degree of crosslinker hypersensitivity and the presence or absence of birth defects in FA patients.

The chromosomal breakage test also can be applied to the study of fetal cells obtained by chorionic villus sampling (CVS), amniocentesis (AFC), or percutaneous umbilical blood sampling (PUBS).[14,15] Prenatal testing for FA in North American pregnancies with a known 1 in 4 recurrence risk (in couples who have had a previously affected child) tested from 1978 through August 1996 are as follows: 79 CVS, 67 AFC, 146 total (28 FA, 118 normal). These results are consistent with the expected ratio. Results from CVS sometimes are uncertain; in these cases it is recommended that PUBS be performed to clarify the diagnosis. The protocols used for both prenatal and postnatal diagnosis of FA using the

DEB test are described in detail in *Current Protocols in Human Genetics.*[141]

Hematologic Mosaicism

Two sets of observations suggest that a proportion of FA patients may exhibit hematologic mosaicism. First, two cell types are occasionally detected in chromosomal breakage tests of crosslinker-treated PHA-stimulated peripheral blood lymphocytes, one demonstrating an FA phenotype and the other demonstrating a normal one.[13,142] In addition, lymphoblastoid cell lines derived from FA patients may be DEB/MMC-resistant.[143] Apparently, in a proportion of blood cells from such mosaic patients the disease phenotype has reverted to normal. The origin of such a reversion in an MMC-resistant lymphoblastoid cell line from a female FA-C patient has recently been determined. This patient was compound heterozygous for two frameshift mutations, one in exon 1 (322delG) and the other in exon 14 (1806insA). Becuase of mitotic recombination in the phenotypically reverted cells, both mutations are now present in the same allele, whereas the other one has lost its mutation.[144] This phenomenon has also been described in lymphoblast lines from patients with Bloom syndrome and has been correlated with a presumed hyperrecombination phenotype of Bloom syndrome cells.[145] Although the clinical significance of this type of mosaicism in lymphoid cells is unclear, FA patients with sustained mosaicism may benefit from having phenotypically reverted cells. If such an event occurred in a hematopoietic stem cell, it might provide the capability of normal hematopoiesis and ultimately lead to improvement in the patient's hematologic condition. Several examples of patients with mosaicism who had unusually mild or no hematologic symptoms have been seen[145] (Auerbach, unpublished IFAR data). Thus, hematopoietic mosaicism may serve as a natural model for gene therapeutic intervention to improve hematopoiesis in FA patients. However, most patients in IFAR who manifested lymphocyte mosaicism developed severe hematologic disease. Further studies will be necessary to elucidate the diagnostic and clinical implications of mosaicism in FA.

Treatment

Transplantation with hematopoietic stem cells from bone marrow or umbilical cord blood currently offers the only possibility for a

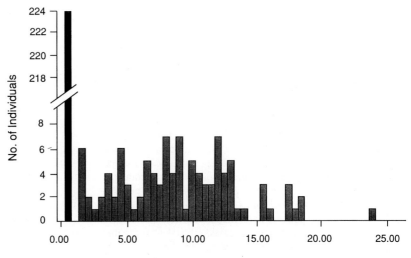

FIG. 16-5 DEB-induced chromosomal breakage in peripheral blood lymphocytes from patients studied at Rockefeller University. Solid bar = DEB-insensitive (non-FA) patients; hatched bars = DEB-sensitive (FA) patients. There is no overlap in the range for the two groups when data are expressed as mean chromosome breaks per cell. Note heterogeneity in the degree of hypersensitivity of FA patients. (*From Ref. 13.*)

cure for bone marrow failure in FA patients as well as a possible cure or prevention of leukemia. Treatment with androgens provide improvement in peripheral blood counts in about 50 percent of FA patients treated, but even patients who exhibit a good response usually become refractory to this treatment in time and eventually require blood cell and platelet transfusions to maintain adequate peripheral blood counts. Complications of androgen therapy include liver toxicity and liver tumors, virilization, and acne. Treatment with hematopoietic growth factors may provide improvement in white blood counts but generally does not result in significant improvement in red blood cell or platelet counts. The use of gene therapy for treatment of FAC currently is under investigation in a phase I clinical trial at the National Institutes of Health. In this approach, hematopoietic progenitor cells from an FAC patient are collected by aphoresis, transduced ex vivo with an retroviral vector containing a normal FAC cDNA, and reinfused into the patient.[146] The aim of this approach is to provide hematopoietic reconstitution with a genetically normalized pool of stem cells. Unfortunately, current methods of targeting retroviral vectors to primitive human stem cells are extremely inefficient. There is no evidence of a long-term cure for any genetic disease achieved by this method; thus, it seems unlikely that gene therapy will provide a cure for FA in the near future.

Early experience with BMT for FA showed a poor outcome that was primarily due to regimen-related toxicity; the use of a specially designed pretransplant conditioning protocol that considers the hypersensitivity of FA cells to DNA crosslinking agents including cyclophosphamide greatly improved the results of transplantation in patients with an unaffected HLA-identical sibling available as a donor.[147-150] Recent analysis of 151 HLA-matched sibling transplants for FA from the multicenter International Bone Marrow Registry (IBMTR) and 18 HLA-matched sibling transplants for FA from Cincinnati shows that increased survival is associated with younger age, less severe hematologic disease, and absence of malignant transformation.[151,152] Experience has indicated that many families will pursue future pregnancies in hopes of having a nonaffected HLA-matched sibling to provide a source of hematopoietic stem cells for transplantation.[153] Although the results of unrelated bone marrow transplants are inferior to those using an HLA-matched sibling, such transplants may be the only option for a patient with severe hematrologic disease or evidence of malignant transformation.[151,154]

In vitro studies have shown that there are a sufficient number of stem/progenitor cells in cord blood for hematopoietic reconstitution; this has led to the use of umbilical cord blood in place of bone marrow as a source of transplantable cells.[155] To test whether umbilical cord blood from an HLA-identical sibling could be used for transplantation, one would first need to harvest the cord blood at the birth of an individual known to be histocompatible and not affected with hematopoietic disease. Cord blood was used successfully for the first time in a clinical trial in 1988 to treat a patient affected with FA.[156,157] Subsequently, the Placental Blood Program was established at the New York Blood Center in 1992 to test the feasibility of using banked placental blood from unrelated donors for transplantation.[158] The results of phase I clinical trials using both matched and mismatched (up to three mismatched antigens with high resolution typing) unrelated donor umbilical cord blood from the Placental Blood Program for transplantation have shown that this source of transplantable hematopoietic stem cells has a high probability of donor engraftment and a low risk of severe acute graft-versus-host disease.[159,160] Several FA patients were included in these trials. Since most FA patients do not have a matched sibling or unrelated donor for transplantation, the availability of an alterative source of stem cells for hematopoietic reconstitution may be a breakthrough in the treatment of this disease.

ACKNOWLEDGMENTS

We gratefully acknowledge the contribution of the many physicians who referred patients to the IFAR and the students, fellows, and collaborators who have contributed to research in Fanconi anemia. Most of all we acknowledge the fortitude and commitment of patients with FA and their families for their continuous support of FA research.

Work in the laboratory of ADA was supported in part by grant HL 32987 from the National Institute of Health, by the Fanconi Anemia Research Fund, Inc. (FARF), and by General Clinical Research Center grant RR00102 from the National Institutes of Health to the Rockefeller University Hospital. Work in the laboratory of MB was supported by grants from NIH (HL 50131), the Medical Research Council of Canada, the National Cancer Institute of Canada, the Genetic Diseases Network (Canada), and private donations. Work in the laboratory of HJ was supported by the Dutch Cancer Society, the European Cancer Centre, Amsterdam, the Commission of the European Union (contract PL 931562), and FARF and FA patient support organizations in Italy, France, Germany, and the Netherlands.

REFERENCES

1. Fanconi G: Familial constitutional panmyelocytopathy, Fanconi's anemia (F.A.): I. Clinical aspects. *Semin Hematol* **4**:233, 1967.
2. Swift M: Fanconi's anemia in the genetics of neoplasia. *Nature* **230**:370, 1971.
3. Auerbach AD, Allen RG: Leukemia and preleukemia in Fanconi anemia patients: A review of the literature and report of the International Fanconi Anemia Registry. *Cancer Genet Cytogenet* **51**:1, 1991.
4. Young NS, Alter BP: Clinial features of Fanconi's anemia, in Young NS, Alter BP (eds): *Aplastic Anemia Acquired and Inherited*, Philadelphia, Saunders, 1994, p 275.
5. Giampietro PF, Verlander PC, Maschan A, Davis JG, Auerbach AD: Fanconi anemia: A model for somatic gene mutation during development. *Am J Med Genet* **52**:36, 1994.
6. Schroeder TM, Anschultz F, Knoff A: Spontane Chromosomenaberrationen bei familiarer Panmyelopathie. *Humangenetik* **1**:194, 1964.
7. Saaki MS, Tonomura A: A high susceptibility of Fanconi's anemia to chromosome breakage by DNA cross-linking agents. *Cancer Res* **33**:1829, 1973.
8. Auerbach AD, Wolman SR: Susceptibility of Fanconi's anaemia fibroblasts to chromosome damage by carcinogens. *Nature* **261**:494, 1976.
9. Weksberg R, Buchwald B, Sargent P, Thompson MW, Siminovitch L: Specific cellular defects in patients with Fanconi anemia. *J Cell Physiol* **101**:311, 1979.
10. Glanz A, Fraser FC: Spectrum of anomalies in Fanconi anaemia. *J Med Genet* **19**:412, 1982.
11. Giampietro PF, Adler-Brecher B, Verlander PC, Pavlakis SG, Davis JG, Auerbach AD: The need for more accurate and timely diagnosis in Fanconi anemia: A report from the International Fanconi Anemia Registry. *Pediatrics* **91**:1116, 1993.
12. Auerbach AD, Adler B, Chaganti RSK: Prenatal and postnatal diagnosis and carrier detection of Fanconi anemia by a cytogenetic method. *Pediatrics* **67**:128, 1981.
13. Auerbach AD, Rogatko A, Schroeder-Kurth TM: International Fanconi Anemia Registry: Relation of clinical symptoms to diepoxybutane sensitivity. *Blood* **73**:391, 1989.
14. Auerbach AD, Sagi M, Adler B: Fanconi anemia: Prenatal diagnosis in 30 fetuses at risk. *Pediatrics* **76**:794, 1985.
15. Auerbach AD, Zhang M, Ghosh R, Pergament E, Verlinsky Y, Nicholas H, Bot EJ: Clastogen-induced chromosomal breakage as a marker for first trimester prenatal diagnosis of Fanconi anemia. *Hum Genet* **73**:86, 1986.
16. Auerbach AD: Fanconi anemia diagnosis and the diepoxybutane (DEB) test (editorial). *Exp Hematol* **21**:731, 1993.

17. Strathdee CA, Duncan AMV, Buchwald M: Evidence for at least four Fanconi anemia genes including *FACC* on chromosome 9. *Nature Genet* 1:196, 1992.
18. Duckworth-Rysiecki G, Toji L, Ng J, Clarke C, Buchwald M: Characterization of a Simian virus 40-transformed Fanconi anemia fibroblast cell line. *Mutat Res* 166:207, 1986.
19. Joenje H, Lo Ten Foe JR, Ostra AB, van Berkel CGM, Rooimans MA, Schroeder-Kurth T, Wdner R-D, Gillies JJP, Buchwald M, Arwert F: Classification of Fanconi anemia patients by complementation analysis: Evidence for a fifth genetic subtype. *Blood* 86:2156, 1995.
20. Verlander PC, Lin JD, Udono MU, Zhang Q, Gibson RA, Mathew CG, Auerbach AD: Mutation analysis of the Fanconi anemia gene *FACC*. *Am J Hum Genet* 54:595, 1994.
21. Whitney MA, Saito H, Jakobs PM, Gibson RA, Moses RE, Grompe MA: A common mutation in the *FACC* gene causes Fanconi anaemia in Ashkenazi-Jewish individuals. *Nature Genet* 4:202, 1993.
22. Yamashita T, Wu N, Kupfer G, Corless C, Joenje H, Grompe M, D'Andrea AD: The clinical variability of Fanconi anemia (type C) results from expression of an amino terminal truncated Fanconi anemia complementation group C polypeptide with partial activity. *Blood* 87:4424, 1996.
23. Strathdee CA, Buchwald M: Molecular and cellular biology of Fanconi anemia. *Am J Pediatr Hematol Oncol* 14:177, 1992.
24. Dos Santos CC, Gavish H, Buchwald M: Fanconi anemia revisited: Old ideas and new advances. *Stem Cell* 12:142, 1994.
25. Liu JM, Buchwald M, Walsh CE, Young NS; Fanconi anemia and novel strategies for therapy. *Blood* 84:3995, 1994.
26. Strathdee CA, Gavish H, Shannon W, Buchwald M: Cloning of cDNAs for Fanconi anaemia by functional complementation. *Nature* 356:763, 1992.
27. Lo Ten Foe, JR, Rooimans MA, Bosnoyan-Collins L, Alon N, Wijker M, Parker L, Lightfoot J, Cheng NC, van Berkel CGM, Strunk MHP, Gille JJP, Kruyt FAE, Pronk JC, Arwert F, Buchwald M, Joenje H: A cDNA for the major Fanconi anemia gene, *FAA*. *Nature Genet* 14:320, 1996.
28. The Fanconi Anaemia Breast Cancer Consortium: Positional cloning of the Fanconi anaemia group A gene. *Nat Genet* (submitted).
29. Schroeder-Kurth TM, Auerbach AD, Obe G: *Fanconi Anemia: Clinical, Cytogenetic and Experimental Aspects*. Heidelberg, Springer-Verlag, 1989.
30. Joenje H, Mathew C, Gluckman E: Fanconi anemia research: current status and prospects. *Eur J Cancer* 31A:268, 1995.
31. Auerbach AD: Fanconi anemia. *Dematol Clin* 13:41, 1995.
32. Alter BP; Fanconi anemia: Current concepts. *Am J Pediatr Hematol Oncol* 14:170, 1992.
33. Gordon-Smith EC, Rutherford TR: Fanconi anemia: Constitutional aplastic anemia. *Semin Hematol* 28:104, 1991.
34. Fanconi G: Familäare infantile perniziosaartige Anämie (pernizioses Blutbild und Konstitution). *Jahrb Kinderh* 117:257, 1927.
35. Estren S, Dameshek W: Familial hypoplastic anemia of childhood: Report of eight cases in two families with beneficial effect of splenectomy in one case. *Am J Dis Child* 73:671, 1947.
36. Dallapiccola B, Alimena G, Brinchi V, Isacchi G, Gandini E: Absence of chromosome heterogeneity between classical Fanconi's anemia and the Estren Dameshek type. *Cancer Genet Cytogent* 2:349, 1980.
37. Macdougall LG, Greeff MC, Rosendorff J, Bernstein R: Fanconi anemia in black African children. *Am J Med Genet* 36:408, 1990.
38. Rosendorff J, Bernstein R, Macdougall L, Jenkins T: Fanconi anemia: Another disease of unusually high prevalence in the Afrikaans population in South Africa. *Am J Med Genet* 2:793, 1987.
39. Verlander PC, Kaporis A, Liu Q, Zhang Q, Seligsohn U, Auerbach AD: Carrier frequency of the IVS4 +4 A>T mutation of the Fanconi anemia gene FAC in the Ashkenazi Jewish population. *Blood* 86:4034, 1995.
40. Butturini A, Gale RP, Verlander PC, Adler-Brecher B, Gillio AP, Auerbach AD: Hematologic abnormalities in Fanconi anemia: An International Fanconi Anemia Registry study. *Blood* 84:1650, 1994.
41. Schroder TM, Tilgen D, Kruger J, Vogel F: Formal genetics of Fanconi's anemia. *Hum Genet* 32:257, 1976.
42. Schuler D, Kiss A, Fabian F: Chromosomal peculiarities and in vitro examinations in Fanconi's anaemia. *Humangenetik* 7:314, 1969.
43. Cervenka J, Arthur D, Yasis C: Mitomycin C test for diagnostic differentiation of idiopathic aplastic anemia and Fanconi anemia. *Pediatrics* 67:119, 1981.
44. Poll EHA, Arwert F, Joenje H, Eriksson AW: Cytogenetic toxicity of antitumor platinum compounds in Fanconi's anemia. *Hum Genet* 61:228, 1982.
45. Schroeder-Kurth TM, Zhu TH, Hong Y, Westphal I: Variation in cellular sensitivities among Fanconi anemia patients, non-Fanconi anemia patients, their parents and siblings, and control probands, in Schroder-Kurth TM, Auerbach AD, Obe G (eds): *Fanconi Anemia: Clinical, Cytogenetic and Experimental Aspects*. Heidelberg, Springer-Verlag, 1989, p 105.
46. Auerbach AD, Rogatko A, Schroder TM: International Fanconi Anemia Registry (IFAR): First report, in Schroeder TM, Auerbach AD, Obe G (eds): *Fanconi Anemia, Clinical Cytogenetic and Experimental Aspects*. Heidelberg, Springer-Verlag, 1989, p 3.
47. Giampietro PF, Verlander PC, Davis JG, Auerbach AD: Diagnosis of Fanconi anemia in patients without congenital malformations: An International Fanconi Anemia Registry Study. *Am J Med Genet* 68:58, 1997.
48. Huma Z, Auerbach AD, Verlander PC, Giampietro PF, Gertner JM: Endocrinological outcome of children with Fanconi anemia (submitted).
49. Alter BP, Frissora CL, Halperin DS, Freedman MH, Chitkara U, Alvarez E, Lynch L, Adler-Brecher B, Auerbach AD: Fanconi's anemia and pregnancy. *Br J Haematol* 77:410, 1991.
50. Bargman GJ, Shahidi NT, Gilbert EF, Opitz JM: Studies of malformation syndromes of man: XLVII. Disappearance of spermatogonia in the Fanconi anemia syndrome. *Eur J Pediatr* 125:162, 1977.
51. Liu JM, Auerbach AD, Young NS: Fanconi anemia presenting unexpectedly in an adult kindred with no dysmorphic features. *Am J Med* 91:555, 1991.
52. Gillio AP, Verlander PC, Batish SD, Giampietro PF, Auerbach AD: Phenotypic consequences of mutations in the Fanconi anemia *FAC* gene: An International Fanconi Anemia Registry study. *Blood* 90:58, 1997.
53. Thompson LH: Properties and applications of human DNA repair genes. *Mutat Res* 247:213, 1991.
54. Joenje H, for EUFAR: Fanconi anemia complementation groups in German and the Netherlands. *Hum Genet* 97:280, 1996.
55. Savitsky K, Bar-Shira A, Gilad S, Rotman G, Ziv Y, Vanagaite L, Tagle DA, Smith S, Uziel T, Sfez S, Ashkenazi M, Pecker I, Frydman M, Harnik R, Patanjali SR, Simmons A, Clines GA, Sartiel A, Gatti RA, Chessa L, Sanal O, Lavin MF, Jaspers NGJ, Taylor MR, Arlett CF, Miki T, Weissman SM, Lovett M, Collins FS, Shiloh Y: A single ataxia telangiectasia gene with a product similar to P1-2 kinase. *Science* 268:1749, 1995.
56. Pronk JC, Gibson RA, Savoia A, Wijker M, Morgan NV, Melchionda S, Ford D, Temtamy S, Ortega JJ, Jansen S, Havenga C, Cohn RI, de Ravel TJ, Roberts I, Westerveld A, Easton DF, Joenje H, Mathew CG, Arwert F: Localisation of the Fanconi anaemia complementation group A gene to chromosome 16q24.3. *Nat Genet* 11:338, 1995.
57. Gschwend M, Levran O, Kruglyak L, Ranade K, Verlander PC, Shen S, Faure S, Weissenbach J, Altay C, Lander ES, Auerbach AD, Botstein D: A locus for Fanconi anemia on 16q determined by homozygosity of mapping. *Am J Hum Genet* 59:377, 1996.
58. Levran O, Fann C, Erlich T, Ott J, Auerbach AD: Linkage analysis of Fanconi anemia: Refinement of the FAA locus at 16q24.3. *Am J Hum Genet* 59:A225, 1996.
59. Whitney M, Thayer M, Reifsteck C, Olson S, Smith L, Jakobs PM, Leach R, Naylor S, Joenje H, Grompe M: Microcell mediated chromosome transfer maps the Fanconi anemia group D gene to chromosome 3p. *Nat Genet* 11:341, 1995.
60. Buchwald M: Complementation groups: One or more per gene? *Nat Genet* 11:228, 1995.
61. Savoia A, Zatterale A, Del Principe D, Joenje H: Fanconi anemia in Italy: High prevalence of complementation group A in two geographic cluster. *Hum Genet* 97:599, 1996.
62. Setlow RB: Repair deficient human disorders and cancer. *Nature* 271:713, 1978.
63. Ishida R, Buchwald M: Susceptibility of Fanconi's anemia lymphoblasts to DNA cross-linking and alkylating agents. *Cancer Res* 42:4000, 1982.
64. Fujiwara Y, Tatsumi M, Sasaki MS: Cross-link repair in human cells and its possible defect in Fanconi's anemia cells. *J Mol Biol* 113:635, 1977.
65. Papadopoulo D, Guillouf C, Mohnrenweiser H, Moustacchi E: Hypomutability in Fanconi anemia cells is associated with increased deletion frequency at the HPRT locus. *Proc Natl Acad Sci USA* 87:8383, 1990.
66. Guillouf C, Laquerbe A, Moustacchi E, Papadopoulo D: Mutagenic processing of psoralen monoadducts differ in normal and Fanconi anemia cells. *Mutagenesis* 8:355, 1993.
67. Laquerbe A, Moustacchi E, Fuscoe JC, Papadopoulo D: The molecular mechanism underlying formation of deletions in Fanconi anemia

cells may involve a site-specific recombination. *Proc Natl Acad Sci USA* **92**:831, 1995.

68. Lambert MW, Tsongalis GJ, Lambert WC, Hang B, Parrish DD: Defective DNA endonuclease activities in Fanconi's anemia, complementation group A, cells. *Mutat Res* **273**:57, 1992.
69. Hang B, Yeung AT, Lambert MW: A damage-recognition protein which binds to DNA containing interstrand cross-links is absent or defective in Fanconi anemia, complementation group A, cells. *Nucleic Acids Res* **21**:4187, 1993.
70. Youssoufian H: Cytoplasmic localization of FAC is essential for the correction of a pre-repair defect in Fanconi anemia group C cells. *J Clin Inv* **97**:2003, 1996.
71. Joenje H, Gille JJP: Oxygen metabolism and chromosomal breakage, in Schroeder-Kurth TM, Auerbach AD, Obe G (eds); *Fanconi Anemia: Clinical, Cytogenetic and Experimental Aspects.* Berlin, Springer-Verlag, 1989, p 174.
72. Schindler D, Hoehn H: Fanconi anemia mutation causes cellular susceptibility to ambient oxygen. *Am J Human Genet* **43**:429, 1988.
73. Joenje H, Arwert F, Eriksson AW, de Koning J, Oostra AB: Oxygen-dependence of chromosomal aberrations in Fanconi's anemia. *Nature* **290**:142, 1981.
74. Poot M, Gross O, Epe B, Pflaum M, Hoehn H: Cell cycle defect in connection with oxygen and iron sensitivity in Fanconi anemia lymphoblastoid cells. *Exp Cell Res* **222**:262, 1996.
75. Korkina LG, Samochatova EV, Maschan AA, Suslova TB, Cheremisina ZP, Afanasev IB: Release of active oxygen radicals by leukocytes of Fanconi anemia patients. *J Leukoc Biol* **52**:357, 1992.
76. Gille JJP, Wortelboer HM, Joenje H: Antioxidant status of Fanconi anemia fibroblasts. *Hum Genet* **77**:28, 1987.
77. Porfirio B, Ambroso G, Giannella G, Isacchi G, Dallapiccola B: Partial correction of chromosome instability in Fanconi anemia by desferrioxamine. *Hum Genet* **83**:49, 1989.
78. Joenje H, Youssoufian H, Kruyt FAE, dos Santos CC, Wevrick R, Buchwald M: Expression of the Fanconi anemia gene *FAC* in human cell lines: Lack of effect of oxygen tension. *Blood Cells Mol Dis* **21**:182, 1995.
79. Saito H, Hammond AT, Moses RE: Hypersensitivity to oxygen is a uniform and secondary defect in Fanconi anemia cells. *Mutat Res* **294**:255, 1993.
80. Chaganti RSK, Houldsworth J: Fanconi anemia: A pleiotropic mutation with multiple cellular and developmental abnormalities. *Ann Genet* **34**:206, 1991.
81. Rosselli F, Sanceau J, Wietzerbin J, Moustacchi E: Abnormal lymphokine production: A novel feature of the genetic disease Fanconi anemia. *Hum Genet* **89**:42, 1992.
82. Segal GM, Magenis RE, Brown M, Keeble W, Smith TD, Heinrich MC, Bagby GC: Repression of Fanconi anemia gene (FACC) inhibits growth of hematopoietic progenitor cells. *J Clin Invest* **94**:846, 1994.
83. Walsh CE, Nienhuis AW, Samuski RJ, Brown MG, Miller JL, Young NS, Liu JM: Phenotypic correction of Fanconi anemia in human hematopoietic cells with a recombinant adeno-associated virus vector. *J Clin Invest* **94**:1440, 1994.
84. Elmore E, Swift M: Growth of cultured cells from patients with Fanconi anemia. *J Cell Physiol* **87**:229, 1975.
85. Willingale-Theune J, Schweiger M, Hirsh-Kauffman M, Meek AE, Paulin-Levasseur M, Traub P: Ultrastructure of Fanconi anemia fibroblasts. *J Cell Sci* **93**:651, 1989.
86. Centrella M, McCarthy TL, Canalis E: Growth factors and cytokines, In Hall BK (ed): *Bone.* Boca Raton, FL, CRC Press, vol 4: *Bone Metabolism and Mineralization,* 1992, p 47.
87. Bagnara GP, Bonsi L, Strippoli P, Ramenghi U, Timeus F, Bonifazi F, Bonafe M, Tonelli R, Bubola G, Brizzi MF, Vitale L, Paolucci G, Pegoraro L, Gabutti V: Production of interleukin 6, leukemia inhibitory factor and granulocyte-macrophage colony stimulating factor by peripheral blood mononuclear cells in Fanconi's anemia. *Stem Cells* **11**(suppl 2):137, 1993.
88. Rosselli F, Sanceau J, Gluckman E, Wietzerbin J, Moustacchi E: Abnormal lymphokine production: A novel feature of the genetic disease Fanconi anemia: II. *In vitro* and *in vivo* spontaneous production of tumor necrosis factor alpha. *Blood* **84**:1216, 1994.
89. Schultz JC, Shahidi NT: Tumor necrosis factor alpha overproduction in Fanconi's anemia. *Am J Hematol* **42**:196, 1993.
90. Kubbies M, Schindler D, Hoehn H, Schinzel A, Rabinovitch PS: Endogenous blockage and delay of the chromosome cycle despite normal recruitment and growth phase explain poor proliferation and frequent endomitosis. *Am J Hum Genet* **37**:1022, 1985.
91. Raff MC: Social controls on cell survival and cell death. *Nature* **356**:397, 1992.
92. Sorensen CM, Barry MA, Eastman A: Analysis of events associated with cell cycle arrest at G2 phase and cell death induced by cisplatin. *J Natl Cancer Inst* **82**:749, 1990.
93. Koury MJ: Programmed cell death (apoptosis) in hematopoiesis. *Exp Hematol* **20**:391, 1992.
94. Jiang H, Kocklar DM: Induction of tissue transglutamine and apoptosis by retinoic acid in the limb bud. *Teratology* **46**:333, 1992.
95. van Duim M, de Wit J, Odjik H, Westerveld A, Yasui A, Koken MHM, Hoeijmakers, JHJ, Bootsma D: Molecular characterization of the human excision repair gene ERCC-1: cDNA cloning and amino acid homology with the yeast repair gene RAD6. *Proc Natl Acad Sci USA* **88**:8865, 1991.
96. Westerveld A, Hoeijmakers JHJ, van Duin M, de Wit J, Odjik H, Pastink A, Wood RD, Bootsma D: Molecular cloning of a human DNA repair gene. *Nature* **310**:425, 1984.
97. Weber CA, Salazar EP, Sterwart SA, Thompson LH: Molecular cloning and biological characterization of a human gene, *ERCC2,* that corrects the nucleotide excision repair defect in CHO UV5 cells. *Mol Cell Biol* **8**:1137, 1988.
98. Wevrick R, Buchwald M: Mammalian DNA-repair genes. *Curr Opin Gen Dev* **3**:470, 1993.
99. Mudgett JS, MacInnes MA: Isolation of the functional human excision repair gene ERCC5 by intercosmid recombination. *Genomics* **8**:623, 1990.
100. Diatloff-Zito C, Rosselli F, Heddle J, Moustacchi E: Partial complementation of the Fanconi anemia defect upon transfection by heterologous DNA. *Hum Genet* **86**:151, 1990.
101. Giavazzi R, Kartner N, Hart IR: Expression of cell-surface P-glycoprotein by an adryamycin-resistant murine fibrosarcoma. *Cancer Res* **45**:4091, 1983.
102. Moustacchi E, Guillouf C, Fraser D, Rosselli F, Diatloff-Zito C, Papadopoulo D: Fanconi's anemia: Genetic and molecular aspects of the defect. *Nouv Rev Fr Hematol* **32**:387, 1990.
103. Dulhanty AM, Rubin JS, Whitmore GF: Complementation of the DNA-repair defect in a CHO mutant cell line by human DNA that lacks highly abundant repetitive sequences. *Mutat Res* **194**:207, 1988.
104. Buchwald M, Clarke C: DNA-mediated transfer of a human gene that confers resistance to mitomycin C. *J Cell Phys* **148**:472, 1991.
105. Diatloff-Zito C, Duchaud E, Viegas-Piquignot E, Fraser D, Moustacchi E: Identification and chromosomal localization of a DNA fragment implicated in the partial correction of the Fanconi anemia group D cellular defect. *Mutat Res* **307**:33, 1994.
106. Thompson LH, Mooney CL, Brookman KW: Genetic complementation between UV-sensitive CHO mutants and xeroderma pigmentosum fibroblasts. *Mutat Res* **150**:423, 1985.
107. Zdzienicka MZ, Arwert F, Neuteboom I, Rooimans M, Simons JWIM: The chinese hamster V79 cell mutant VH-4 is phenotypically like Fanconi anemia cells. *Som Cell Mol Genet* **16**:575, 1990.
108. Arwert F, Rooimans MA, Westerveld A, Simons JWIM, Zdzienicka MZ: The chinese hamster cell mutant V-H4 is homologous to Fanconi anemia (complementation group A). *Cytogenet Cell Genet* **56**:23, 1990.
109. Sakaguchi K, Harris PV, Ryan C, Buchwald M, Boyd JB: Alteration of a nuclease in Fanconi anemia. *Mutat Res* **255**:31, 1991.
110. Sakaguchi K, Zdzienicka MZ, Harris PV, Boyd JB: Nuclease modifications in Chinese hamster cells hypersensitive to DNA cross-linking agents—a model for Fanconi anemia. *Mutat Res* **274**:11, 1992.
111. Boyd JB, Sakaguchi K, Harris PV: The *mus308* mutants of Drosophila exhibit hypersensitivity to DNA cross-linking agents and are defective in a deoxyribonuclease. *Genetics* **125**:813, 1990.
112. Boyd JB, Golino MD, Shaw KES, Osgood CJ, Green MM: Third-chromosome mutagen-sensitive mutants of *Drosophila melanogaster. Genetics* **97**:607, 1981.
113. Schroeder TM, Anschutz F, Knopp A: Spontane chromosomenaberrationen bei familiarer panmyelopathie. *Hum Genet* **1**:194, 1964.
114. Moustacchi E, Diatloff-Zito C: DNA semi-conservative synthesis in normal and Fanconi anemia fibroblasts following treatment with 8-methoxypsoralen and near ultraviolet light or with X-rays. *Hum Genet* **70**:236, 1985.
115. Harris PV, Mazina OM, Leonhardt EA, Cass RB, Boyd JB, Burtis KC: Molecular cloning of *Drosophila mus308,* a gene involved in DNA cross-link repair with homology to prokaryotic DNA polymerase I genes. *Mol Cell Biol* **10**:5764, 1996.

116. Groger RK, Morrow DM, Tykocinski ML: Directional antisense and sense cDNA cloning using Epstein-Barr virus episomal expression vectors. *Gene* **81**:285, 1989.

117. Parker L: Analysis of the 5′ end of human *FAC*. M.Sc. thesis, University of Toronto, 1995.

118. Savoia A, Centra M, Lanzano L, de Cillis GP, Zelante L, Buchwald M: Characterization of the 5′ region of the Fanconi anemia group C gene. *Hum Mol Genet* **4**:1231, 1995.

119. Wevrick R, Clarke CA, Buchwald M: Cloning and analysis of the murine Fanconi anemia group C cDNA. *Hum Mol Genet* **2**:655, 1993.

120. Wong JCY: Cross-species analysis of the Fanconi anemia group C cDNA. M.Sc. thesis, University of Toronto, 1996.

121. Gavish H, dos Santos CC, Buchwald M: Leu554-Pro substitution completely abolishes complementing activity of the Fanconi anemia (FACC) protein. *Hum Mol Genet* **2**:123, 1993.

122. Parker L, dos Santos C, Buchwald M: A mutation (delta 327) in the Fanconi anemia group C gene generates a novel transcript lacking the first two coding exons *Hum Mutat* (in press).

123. Yamashita T, Barber DL, Zhu Y, Wu N, D'Andrea AD: The Fanconi anemia polypeptide FACC is localized to the cytoplasm. *Proc Natl Acad Sci USA* **91**:6712, 1994.

124. Youssoufian H, Li Y, Martin ME, Buchwald M: Induction of Fanconi anemia cellular phenotype in human 293 cells by overexpression of a mutant *FAC* allele. *J Clin Invest* **97**:957, 1996.

125. Savoia A, Centra M, Ianzano L, Zelante Z, Buchwald M: Genomic structure of Fanconi anemia complementation C (*FAC*) gene polymorphisms. *Mol Cell Probes* **10**:213, 1996.

126. Chen M, Tomkins D, Auerbach W, McKerlie C, Youssoufian H, Liu L, Gan O, Carreau Buchwald M: Inactivation of *Fac* in mice produces inducible chromosomal instability and reduced fertility reminiscent of Fanconi anemia. *Nat Genet* **12**:448, 1996.

127. Wevrick R, Barke JE, Nadeau JH, Szpirer C, Buchwald M: Mapping of the murine and rat *Facc* genes and assessment of flexed-tail as a candidate mouse homolog of Fanconi anemia group C. *Mammal Gen* **4**:440, 1993.

128. Youssoufina H: Localization of Fanconi anemia C protein to the cytoplasm of mammalian cells. *Proc Natl Acad Sci USA* **91**:7975, 1994.

129. Youssoufian H, Auerbach AD, Verlander PC, Steimle V, Mach B: Identification of cytosolic proteins that bind to the Fanconi anemia polypeptide FACC in vitro: Evidence of a multimeric complex. *J Biol Chem* **270**:9876, 1995.

130. Kruyt FA, Dijkmans LM, van den Berg TK, Joenje H: Fanconi anemia genes act to suppress a cross-linker-inducible p53-independent apoptosis pathway in lymphoblast cell lines. *Blood* **87**:938, 1996.

131. Rosselli F, Ridet A, Soussi T, Duchaud E, Alapetite C, Moustacchi E: p53-dependent pathway of radio-induced apoptosis is altered in Fanconi anemia. *Oncogene* **10**:9, 1995.

132. Kupfer GM, D'Andrea AD: The effect of the Fanconi anemia polypeptide, FAC, upon p53 induction and G2 checkpoint regulation. *Blood* **88**:1019, 1996.

133. Avanzi GC, Lista P, Giovinazzo B, Miniero R, Sagli G, Benetton G, Coda R, Cattoretti G, Pegoraro L: Selective growth response to IL-3 of a human leukaemic cell line with megakaryoblastic features. *Br J Hematol* **69**:359, 1988.

134. Metcalf D: Multi-CSF-dependent colony formation by cells of a murine hematopoietic cell line: Specificity and action of multi-CSF. *Blood* **65**:357, 1985.

135. Cumming RC, Liu JM, Youssoufian H, Buchwald M: Suppression of apoptosis in hematopoietic factor-dependent cell lines by expression of the FAC gene. *Blood* **88**:4558, 1996.

136. Brady G, Billia F, Knox J, Hoang T, Kirsh IR, Voura E, Hawley R, Cumming R, Buchwald M, Siminovitch K, Miyamoto N, Boehmelt G, Iscove NN: Analysis of gene expression in a complex differentiation hierarchy by global amplification of cDNA from single cells. *Curr Biol* **5**:909, 1995.

137. Krasnoshtein F, Buchwald M: Development expression of the *Fac* gene correlates with congenital defects in Fanconi anemia patients. *Hum Mol Genet* **5**:85, 1996.

138. Urlando C, Krasnoshtein F, Heddle JA, Buchwald M: Assessment of the flexed-tail mouse as a possible model for Fanconi anemia: Analysis of mitomycin C-induced micronuclei. *Mutat Res* **370**:99, 1996.

139. Chen M, Tomkins D, Auerbach W, McKerlie C, Youssoufian H, Liu L, Gan O, Carreau M, Auerbach A, Groves T, Guidos CJ, Freedman MH, Cross J, Percy DH, Dick JE, Joyner AL, Buchwald M: Inactivation of *Fac* in mice produces inducible chromosomal instability and

140. Whitney MA, Royle G, Low MJ, Kelly MA, Axthelm MK, Reifsteck C, Olson S, Braun RE, Heinrich MC, Rathbun RK, Babgy GC, Grompe M: Germ cell defects and hematopoietic hypersensitivity to gamma-interferon in mice with a targeted disruption of the Fanconi anemia C gene. *Blood* **88**:49, 1996.

141. Auerbach AD: Diagnosis of Fanconi anemia by diepoxybutane analysis, in Dracopoli NC, Haines JL, Korf BR, Moir DT, Morton CC, Seidman CE, Seidman JG, Smith DR (eds): *Current Protocols in Human Genetics.* New York, Current Protocols, 1994, p 8.7.1.

142. Kwee ML, Poll EHA, van de Kamp JJP, De Koning H, Eriksson AW, Joenje H: Unusual response to bifunctional alkylating agent in a case of Fanconi anemia. *Hum Genet* **64**:384, 1983.

143. Auerbach AD, Koorse RE, Ghosh R, Venkatraj VS, Zhang M, Chiorazzi N: Complementation studies in Fanconi anemia, in Schroder TM, Auerbach AD, Obe G (eds): *Fanconi Anemia, Clinical, Cytogenetic and Experimental Aspects.* Heidelberg, Springer-Verlag, 1989, p 213.

144. Lo Ten Foe JR, Kwee ML, Rooimans, MA, Oostra AB, Veerman AJP, Pauli RM, Shahidi NT, Dokal I, Roberts I, Altay C, Gluckman E, Gibson RA, Mathew C, Arwert F, Joenje H: Reversion of the cellular disease phenotype in Fanconi anemia: molecular basis and clinical significance. *Eur J Hum Genet* **5**:137–148, 1997.

145. Ellis NA, Lennon DJ, Proytcheva M, Alhadeff B, Henderson EE, German J: Somatic intragenic recombination within the mutated locus BLM can correct the high sister-chromatid exchange phenotype of Bloom syndrome cells. *Am J Hum Genet* **57**:994, 1995.

146. Walsh CE, Grompe M, Vanin E, Buchwald M, Young NS, Nienhuis AW, Liu JM: A functionally active retrovirus vector for gene therapy in Fanconi anemia group C. *Blood* **84**:453, 1994.

147. Gluckman E, Devergie A, Schaison G, Bussel A, Berger R, Sohier J, Bernard J: Bone marrow transplantation in Fanconi anemia. *Br J Haematol* **45**:557, 1980.

148. Berger R, Bernheim A, Gluckman E, Gisselbrecht C: In vitro effect of cyclophosphamide metabolites on chromosomes of Fanconi anaemia patients. *Br J Haematol* **45**:565, 1980.

149. Auerbach AD, Adler B, O'Reilly RJ, Kirkpatrick D, Chaganti RSK: Effect of procarbazine and cyclophosphamide on chromosome breakage in Fanconi anemia cells: Relevance to bone marrow transplantation. *Cancer Genet Cytogent* **9**:25, 1983.

150. Gluckman E, Devergie A, Dutreix J: Bone marrow transplantation for Fanconi's anemia, in Schroder-Kurth TM, Auerback AD, Obe G (eds): *Fanconi Anemia: Clinical, Cytogenetic and Experimental Aspects.* Berlin, Springer-Verlag, 1989, p 60.

151. Gluckman E, Auerbach AD, Horowitz MM, Sobocinski KA, Ash RC, Bortin MM, Butturini A, Camitta BM, Champlin RE, Friedrich W, Good RA, Gordon-Smith EC, Harris RE, Klein JP, Ortega JJ, Pasquini R, Ramsay NKC, Speck B, Vowels MR, Zhang M-J, Gale RP: Bone marrow transplantation for Fanconi anemia. *Blood* **86**:2856, 1995.

152. Kohli-Kumar M, Morris C, DeLaat C, Sambrano J, Masterson M, Mueller R, Shahidi NT, Yanik G, Desantes K, Friedman DJ, Auerbach AD, Harris RE: Bone marrow transplantation in Fanconi anemia using matched sibling donors. *Blood* **94**:2050, 1994.

153. Auerbach AD: Umbilical cord blood transplants for genetic disease: Diagnostic and ethical issues in fetal studies. *Blood Cells* **20**:303, 1994.

154. Davies SM, Kahn S, Wagner JE, Arthur DC, Auerbach AD, Ramsay NKC, Weisdorf DJ: Unrelated donor bone marrow transplantation for Fanconi anemia. *Bone Marrow Transplant* **17**:43, 1996.

155. Broxmeyer HE, Douglas GW, Hangoc G, Cooper S, Bard J, English D, Arny M, Boyse EA: Human umbilical cord blood as a potential source of transplantable hematopoietic stem/progenitor cells. *Proc Natl Acad Sci USA* **86**:3828, 1989.

156. Gluckman E, Broxmeyer HE, Auerbach AD, Friedman HS, Douglas GW, Devergie A, Esperou H, Thierry D, Socie G, Lehn P, Cooper S, English D, Kurtzberg J, Bard J, Boyse EA: Hematopoietic reconstitution in a patient with Fanconi's anemia by means of umbilical-cord blood from an HLA-identical sibling. *N Engl J Med* **321**:1174, 1989.

157. Kohli-Kumar M, Harris RE, Broxmeyer HE, Shahidi N, Auerbach AD: Cord blood transplant in Fanconi anemia. *Br J Haematol* **85**:419, 1993.

158. Rubinstein P, Rosenfield RE, Adamson JW, Stevens CE: Stored placental blood for unrelated bone marrow reconstitution. *Blood* **81**:1679, 1993.

159. Kurtzberg J, Laughlin M, Graham ML, Smith C, Olson JF, Halperin E, Ciocci G, Carrier C, Stevens CE, Rubinstein P: Placental blood as

a source for hematopoietic stem cells for transplantation into unrelated recipients. *N Engl J Med* **335**:157, 1996.

160. Wagner JE, Rosenthal J, Sweetman R, Shu XO, Davies SM, Ramsay NKC, McGlave PB, Sender L, Cairo MS: Successful transplantation of HLA-matched and HLA-mismatched umbilical cord blood from unrelated donors: Analysis of engraftment and acute graft-versus-host disease. *Blood* **88**:795, 1996.

161. Gibson RA, Buchwald M, Roberts RG, Mathew CG: Characterization of the exon structure of the Fanconi anemia group C gene by vectorette PCR. *Hum Mol Genet* **2**:35, 1993.

162. Gibson RA, Hajianpoujr A, Murer-Orlando M, Buchwald M, Mathew CG: A nonsense mutation and exon skipping in the Fanconi anemia group C gene. *Hum Mol Genet* **2**:797, 1993.

163. Gibson RA, Morgan NV, Goldstein LH, Pearson IC, Kesterton IP, Foot NJ, Jansen S, Havenga C, Pearson T, de Ravel TJ, Cohn RJ, Marques IM, Dokal I, Roberts I, March J, Ball S, Milner RD, Llerena JC Jr, Samochatova E, Mohan SP, Vasudevan P, Birjandi F, Hajianpour A, Murer-Orlando M, Mathew CG: Novel mutations and polymorphisms in the Fanconi anemia group C gene. *Hum Mutat* **8**:140, 1996.

164. Lo Ten Foe JR, Rooimans MA, Joenje H, Arwert F: A novel frameshift mutation (1806insA) in exon 14 of the Fanconi anemia C gene, FAC. *Hum Mutat* **7**:264, 1996.

165. Lo Ten Foe JR, Barel MT, Tuss P, Digweed M, Arwert F, Joenje H: Sequence variations in the Fanconi anaemia gene, FAC: pathogenicity of 1806insA and R548X and recognition of D195V as a polymorphic variant. *Hum Genet* **98**:522, 1996.

166. Lo Ten Foe JR, Kruyt FAE, Zweekhorst MBM, Pals G, Gibson RA, Mathew CG, Joenje H, Arwert F: Exon 6 skipping in the Fanconi anemia C gene associated with a nonsense/missense mutation (775C → T) in exon 5. *Hum Mutat* (in press).

CHAPTER 17

Hereditary Nonpolyposis Colorectal Cancer*

C. Richard Boland

1. Hereditary non-polyposis colorectal cancer (HNPCC) is a relatively common autosomal dominant disorder affecting one in 200–1,000 individuals. It is characterized by an increased incidence of cancers of the colon, endometrium, ovary, stomach, and some other (but not all) epithelial organs. Patients with HNPCC have a very high risk of developing colorectal cancer (approximately 80%) and women have increased incidences of endometrial cancer (estimated) to be 20–43% lifetime risk).

2. There is no premorbid phenotype in HNPCC. Unlike familial adenomatous polyposis, affected individuals do not develop large numbers of premalignant lesions of the colon or other affected sites. The diagnosis must be made by family history or genetic testing. A rare subset of HNPCC is Muir-Torre syndrome, which includes sebaceous gland tumors and keratoacanthomas of the skin.

3. HNPCC is due to a germline mutation in one of the DNA mismatch repair genes. The phenotype of the heterozygous state is apparently normal. When a somatic mutation inactivates the wild-type allele of the DNA mismatch repair gene, the tissue develops a hypermutable phenotype, which accelerates multi-step carcinogenesis.

4. The four known HNPCC genes and their chromosomal locations are: hMSH2 (2p), hMLH1 (3p), hPMS2 (7p), and hPMS1 (2q). Germline mutations in any of these four genes appear to produce the same disease. No locus has been found for many HNPCC families.

5. Expression of the DNA mismatch repair gene hMSH2 is preferentially expressed in the proliferative portion of the colonic crypt, and is regulated throughout the cell cycle. Loss of both alleles of hMSH2 or hMLH1 results in complete loss of DNA mismatch repair activity, and the hypermutable phenotype.

6. Although HNPCC accounts for approximately 3% of all colorectal cancers, 15–20% of all colorectal cancers have microsatellite instability (MIN) similar to that seen in HNPCC, and another 15–20% have a minor form of MIN.

7. Genes containing repetitive DNA sequences (microsatellites) are targets for inactivation in tumors with MIN. The type II transforming growth factor-β receptor is the prototype gene which is mutated in these tumors.

8. The diagnosis of HNPCC is initially suspected on the basis of multiple, early-onset cancers of specific organs in the family history, and may be confirmed by genetic diagnosis. hMSH2 and hMLH1 appear to account for at least half of all HNPCC families. There are no "hot spots" in either of these genes, however the frequent occurrence of premature truncating mutations makes the in vitro transcription/ translation assay useful for screening purposes.

9. Cancer mortality may be significantly reduced by appropriate intervention. Screening colonoscopy should be undertaken every two years. Some patients may elect prophylactic removal of the colon, uterus, and ovaries, which will substantially improve survival. No pharmacological intervention is known to be effective in this disease.

INTRODUCTION

Colorectal cancer is a fairly common disease of Western populations with a typical onset at about age 70 years. The international epidemiology of this disease suggests that environmental factors, probably dietary, are the most important influences for the high prevalence of this disease in certain countries.[1] Woven into the epidemiological fabric for colorectal cancer is an important influence of genetic factors. Individuals who have relatives with colorectal neoplasia (i.e., either cancers or adenomatous polyps) have an increased risk for these tumors themselves, which will appear earlier in life.[2–4]

The most readily distinguished form of familial risk is the autosomal dominant genetic disease familial adenomatous polyposis (FAP). This disease has a distinctive phenotypic syndrome characterized by a large number of precursor adenomatous polyps in the colon, and occurs in about 1 in 10,000 births[1]. This is completely unrelated to the more common autosomal dominant colon cancer syndrome termed hereditary nonpolyposis colorectal cancer (HNPCC). This disease has no antecedent clinical phenotype until a cancer develops, and was a controversial entity until the biological basis of this disease was discovered in 1993.[5–8] Patients with HNPCC are at increased risk for cancers of the colon, en-

*This work was supported by Grant RO1-72851 and The Research Service of the Department of Veterans Affairs.

dometrium, ovary, stomach, urinary tract, brain, and other, but not all, epithelial organs.[9–12] The mean age to develop colorectal cancer is in the early to mid-40s, however, many tumors occur in the 20s, and even in teenagers. Although population-based surveys have not been completed, HNPCC may be the most common form of familial predisposition to cancer.[13–22]

The hereditary aspects of colon cancer are complex. The age-adjusted relative risk of developing colorectal cancer in individuals with an affected first degree relative is 1.72 compared to those without a family history. This risk rises to 2.75 when there are two or more affected first-degree relatives, and the relative risk increases as the family history occurs in younger relatives, reaching 5.37 when the affected sibs are 30–44 years.[3] Similarly, the relative risk for colorectal cancer is 1.78 for the first-degree relatives of patients with adenomatous polyps. The relative risk rises to 2.59 when the sib is less than 60 years old, and 3.25 when a sib and parent are both affected.[4] This modest increase in risk, which worsens with increasing familial involvement and earlier age tumors, cannot be attributed solely to HNPCC. In all likelihood, several genetic risk factors play a partial role, as do dietary and other environmental influences. The challenge in defining HNPCC families has been to recognize the disease in the face of a large background incidence of colorectal cancer, and the occasional clusters of sporadic tumors in families.

The historical roots of HNPCC can be traced back to the end of the nineteenth century when a University of Michigan pathologist, A. S. Warthin, recognized a cluster of cancers in the family of his seamstress.[23,24] His patient's family was large, and has been reported five times during the twentieth century, serving as the prototype for HNPCC.[25–29] Following this lead, Lynch documented family histories on this and other families, and by the 1970s it became clear that the medical histories of several large families strongly suggested the involvement of an autosomal dominant disease that gave rise to early onset cancers with a predisposition for proximal colonic involvement, and cancers in certain other organs.[29–32]

Prior to the identification of the genes for this disease, ascertainment was limited by the need for large families with a high degree of involvement. Two different subsets of families were identified. Lynch syndrome I (or site-specific familial colorectal cancer) was attached to those families that only manifested colorectal cancers. Lynch syndrome II (or cancer family syndrome) was assigned to families that also had tumors of other organs, principally of the female genital tract.[31] Over time, it has emerged that these are not distinct syndromes that can be assigned to separate genetic loci or unique mutations.

To cope with the uncertainties surrounding HNPCC, the International Collaborative Group on Hereditary Non-Polyposis Colorectal Cancer convened in 1991 to develop clinical criteria to standardize the study of this disease.[33] The Amsterdam Criteria are listed in Table 17-1, but appear to be overly restrictive, and do not take into account the possibility of later-onset variants, or the implications of noncolonic tumors. Not all HNPCC families, diagnosed genetically, meet the Amsterdam criteria.

Table 17-1 Amsterdam Criteria For HNPCC

1. At least three affected relatives with verified colorectal cancer
2. At lease one is a first-degree relative of the other two
3. FAP is excluded
4. At least two successive generations affected
5. One colon cancer at <50 years of age

SOURCE: Vasen HFA, Mecklin JP, Khan PM, et al: The International Collaborative Group on Hereditary Non-polyposis Colorectal Cancer. *Dis Colon Rect* **34**: 424–425, 1991.

HNPCC has attracted interest not only because of its impact in clinical medicine; the genetic basis of this disease has led to the understanding of a unique pathogenetic mechanism for tumor development. The history surrounding the identification of the HNPCC genes and the unique type of genomic instability associated with these tumors has been reviewed in detail elsewhere.[24]

CLINICAL MANIFESTATIONS OF HNPCC

HNPCC is an autosomal dominantly inherited genetic disease characterized by an increased risk for cancers of the colon, rectum, and a number of other organs (see Table 17-2). These tumors often occur at uncharacteristically early ages. Colorectal cancer is the predominant feature of the syndrome, and occurs in an estimated 80% of all gene carriers. Sixty to seventy percent of the tumors occur proximal to the splenic flexure.[23] There is an increased risk of synchronous and metachronous tumors of the colon, rectum, and other organs. There appears to be no increase in risk for cancer of the lung, breast, prostate, bladder, bone marrow, larynx, or brain.[12] The intestinal tract is most commonly affected, but multiple adenomatous polyposis, such as those seen in FAP, do not occur. Although the incidence of adenomatous polyps may be slightly increased in HNPCC patients,[34,35] the number of patients studied remains small, and this may not, in itself, explain the greatly increased incidence of carcinomas. It has been suggested that a higher rate of progression from adenoma to carcinoma is the major factor accounting for the cancer predisposition in HNPCC (*see* Table 17-3).

The prevalence of HNPCC in the general population is unknown. This is complicated by the fact that there is a 5–6% lifetime prevalence of colorectal cancer in North America. Various estimates of prevalence have been attempted, as listed in Table 13-4.[15–20,36] The apparent incidence of HNPCC families will be higher if one selects for colon cancer patients with early onset tumors. The apparent proportion of families with HNPCC (based upon a history of multiple cancers in the family) is approximately 3–4% of all colorectal cancers (with one remarkable outlier study from Finland.)[18] These estimates predict an HNPCC prevalence in the population of approximately 2/1,000 persons; however, this is probably an underestimate because of limitations in family size (which limits recognition), historical recall (which is inaccurate), penetrance (which is undetermined), and involvement of organs other than the colon (which have not been considered in these studies). A more realistic estimate for the frequency of HNPCC in the general population may be much higher, but probably is less than some early estimates of 1/200.

The diagnosis of HNPCC usually is made by considering the family history. Even a single first-degree relative who develops a colorectal or endometrial cancer at a very young age raises this possibility. A subset of HNPCC families has a constellation of findings termed the Muir-Torre Syndrome.[37,38] This syndrome consists of all of the features of HNPCC plus sebaceous gland tumors (adenomas, epitheliomas, and carcinomas), and keratoacanthomas. The latter is a keratin-filled skin tumor that occurs in sun-exposed areas. Basal and squamous cell carcinomas also occur in Muir-Torre Syndrome. Although these skin tumors are unusual manifestations of HNPCC, this diagnosis should be considered in any patient who has more than one skin tumor of this variety. The genetic loci responsible for Muir-Torre syndrome are the same as those that occur in other HNPCC families.[39,40]

The pathological features of colorectal neoplasms in HNPCC are somewhat unique.[23,41,42,43] As mentioned, the tumors occur at early ages, and most are in the proximal colon. Using typical pathological criteria 37% of colorectal cancers in HNPCC will be

Table 17-2 Cancers in HNPCC

Cancer Site	Lifetime Risk	Relative Risk[9]	Median Age[9]
Colon and Rectum	80% by age 70 (estimate)	—	46
Endometrium	20% by age 70 [113]	—	46
Stomach	—	4.1	54
Ovary	—	3.5	40
Small Intestine	—	25	53
Hepatobiliary System	—	4.9	66
Kidney	—	3.2	66
Ureter	—	22	56

No apparent *increase* in risk: breast, lung, prostate, bladder, skin, marrow, larynx, brain.

classified as poorly differentiated,[23] which would suggest that the tumors would behave aggressively. Contrary to this, colorectal cancers in HNPCC have a better outcome than sporadic tumors matched for stage.[23] Colorectal cancers in HNPCC are significantly more likely to be diploid or near-diploid compared to sporadic tumors.[44,45] In one flow cytometry study, 68% of HNPCC cancers were diploid, and 90% were diploid or near diploid with a DNA index less than 1.27.[45] Over 35% of colorectal cancers in HNPCC are mucinous carcinomas.[23] These pathological features may increase one's suspicion of HNPCC when they are found in familial clusters of cancer (Fig. 17-1).

HNPCC GENES

hMSH2—The First HNPCC Gene

The discovery of the HNPCC genes is an interesting story of excellent basic science research, fierce competition among several labs interested in the problem, and in some instances, unusual good fortune.[24] It had been proposed by Loeb in the 1980s that a hypermutable phenotype would be necessary to account for all of the mutations that seemed to be present in most cancers.[46,47] No mechanism was available to account for this at that time.

In 1993, three laboratories working independently reported that an unusual form of somatic mutation occurred in 12–15% of colorectal cancers. The mutations were insertions or deletions of simple repetitive elements that make up microsatellite sequences (see below). Each laboratory added to the interpretation. One group used an arbitrarily primed polymerase chain reaction (PCR) looking for genomic amplifications or deletions that might be present in colorectal cancers.[48] In this study, they noted that 12% of colorectal cancers harbored somatic deletions that altered the lengths of the microsatellite sequences. Their approach permitted them to estimate that affected tumors carried more than 10^5 of these types of mutations. They also noted that tumors with these "ubiquitous somatic mutations at simple repetitive sequences" had unique features that made them distinct from most colorectal cancers, and proposed that this represented a novel form of carcinogenesis.[49]

Another group, also looking for genetic losses at tumor suppressor gene loci using PCR-based amplification of microsatellite sequences, recognized that microsatellite instability (MIN) was significantly correlated with tumors of the proximal colon. MIN was inversely related with loss of heterozygosity on chromosomes 5q, 17p, and 18q, and positively correlated with improved patient survival. This group proposed that 28% of colorectal cancers developed through this unique mechanism of genomic instability.[50]

Table 17-3 Adenomatous Polyps of the Colon in HNPCC (clinical diagnoses of HNPCC)

3A. Lanspa et al., Nebraska patients[34]

	HNPCC Patients* (N=44, mean age 42.4)	Control Patients (N=88, mean age 44.4)
Adenomatous polyps	30% (13/44)	11% (10/88)
Proximal colonic adenomas	18% (8/44)	1% (1/88)
Multiple colonic adenomas	20% (9/44)	4% (4/88)

3B. Jass et al., New Zealand patients[35]

	HNPCC Patients	Age-matched Autopsy Controls
Men, <50 years old	30% (3/10)[1]	5% (2/42)
Women, <50 years old	44% (4/9)[2]	5% (1/21)
Men, 50–69 years old	66% (2/3)	36% (16/44)
Women, 50–69 years old	100% (1/1)	12% (1/8)
Men >70 years old	none available	46% (13/28)
Women >70 years old	none available	33% (5/15)

[1]p = 0.015 vs. controls (by χ^2)
[2]p = 0.0075 vs. controls (by χ^2)
*Patients judged clinically to be possible gene carriers, but not documented genetically; probably represents 50% risk of gene carriage.

Table 17-4 Frequency of HNPCC

Ascertainment Method	Age Limit	Locale	Proportion of Families Estimated to be HNPCC (%)	Reference
Record Search	70	Finland	3.8	15
Patient Recall	None	Italy	3.9	16
Death Certificates	None	UK	4.0	17
Record Search	50	Finland	30.0	18
Record Search	55	Ireland	6.0	19
Patient Recall	50	Canada	3.1	20

NOTE: All estimates are based on family histories (not genetic diagnoses), and required ≥3 family members with colorectal cancer. These probably are underestimates (see text).
SOURCE: Lynch HT, Smyrk TC, Watson P, et al: Genetics, natural history, tumor spectrum, and pathology of Hereditary Nonpolyposis Colorectal Cancer, an updated review. *Gastroenterology* 104: 1535–1549, 1993.

A third group, representing a multinational collaboration, performed a genome-wide search for a genetic locus of HNPCC. Using two large kindreds, one such locus was mapped to 2p 15-16.[51] Microsatellite markers had been used to map the locus. Pursuing the hypothesis that the HNPCC gene would be a tumor suppressor gene, they looked for loss of heterozygosity in the tumors, using the microsatellites as targets. Instead, they found insertion or deletion mutations at the repetitive sequences, which they termed the replicative error (RER) phenotype.[52] All three groups brought unique insights to bear on the issue, and together they illuminated for the first time the nature of HNPCC, and discovered a novel mechanism for carcinogenesis.

The next step forward in solving the HNPCC riddle came unexpectedly from laboratories focused on yeast genetics who had not previously ventured into human genetics, let alone hereditary colon cancer. The characteristic mutational pattern published in the autoradiograms used to resolve the amplified microsatellites by the three groups described above resembled the mutational pattern seen in bacteria and yeast that had lost genes required for DNA mismatch repair (Fig. 17–2). The microbial DNA mismatch repair systems were complex, and involved several genes of the Mut HLS mismatch repair pathway.[53,54] The system, which consists of several proteins working together in a complex, repairs errors in DNA replication that occur during S phase that result in single base pair mismatches or mispaired loops that occur at repetitive sequences such as microsatellites. Strand et al. demonstrated that mutations in three yeast genes involved in DNA mismatch repair (PMS1, MLH and MSH2) led to 100-700 fold increases in mutations at poly(GT) sequences, and based upon what had been reported in colorectal cancer, specifically suggested that these genes might be the loci sought by those studying HNPCC.[55] In a remarkably short period of time, investigating groups led by Kolodner[56] and Vogelstein[57] reported that a human MutS homolog (hMSH2[1]) could be found on chromosome 2p. Germline mutations of this gene in HNPCC families demonstrated that it was responsible for the disease.[57] hMSH2 was the second homologue found in

the human genome related to the bacterial MutS or yMHS gene. Subsequently, at least eight human homologues of the MutS genes have been found.

The genetics of HNPCC are somewhat complex, but follow the paradigms of other tumor suppressor genes. HNPCC is inherited as an autosomal dominant characteristic when an inactivating germline mutation occurs in hMSH2, or certain other DNA mismatch repair genes. Resultingly, every somatic cell carries one inactivated copy and one wild-type copy of the mismatch repair gene. With certain notable exceptions,[58] the phenotype at the cellular level or for the individual is normal, but susceptible to loss of the wild-type allele in a target tissue,[59] which results in a hypermutable phenotype (MIN or RER as described earlier). The hypermutable cell then is susceptible to the accumulation of mutations at a greatly accelerated rate, which may then result in clonal expansion and the neoplastic phenotype. Thus, a germline mutation at hMSH2 leaves the individual susceptible to the development of hypermutability, which then leads to other mutations responsible for a cancer. There is not yet a suitable explanation for why specific organs are at selective risk to develop cancer. Certain germline mutations appear to have a dominant negative effect, in which heterozygous cells themselves are hypermutable.[58] In this instance, mismatch repair deficiency may be detected in phenotypically normal cells.

Other HNPCC Genes: *hMLH1*, *hPMS1* and *hPMS2*

Shortly after the first HNPCC locus was mapped to 2p, a second HNPCC locus was mapped to 3p in a Scandinavian kindred.[60] Based on the paradigm that led from 2p to hMSH2, these same two groups turned their attention to the MutL gene of *E. coli* (and the yeast MutL homologue). This research led to three human homologues, now termed hMLH1, hPMS1, and hPMS2, located on 3p, 2q, and 7p.[61-63] The characteristics of the four known HNPCC loci are listed in Table 17-5.

Table 17-5 The HNPCC Genes[55,56,60,61,62,64,74]

HNPCC Gene	Chromosomal Location	*E. coli* Homologue	cDNA Size	Genomic Structure	Protein
hMSH2	2p 15–16	MutS	2727 bp	16 exons (over 73 kb)	106 kD
hMLH1	3p 21	MutL	2268 bp	19 exons (over 58 kb)	85 kD
hPMS1	2q 31	MutL	2795 bp	—	—
hPMS2	7p 22	MutL	2586 bp	15 exons (over 16 kb)	96kD

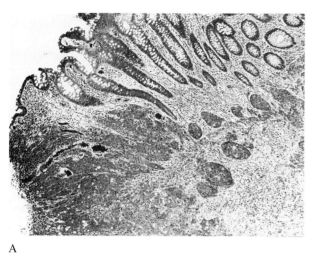

A

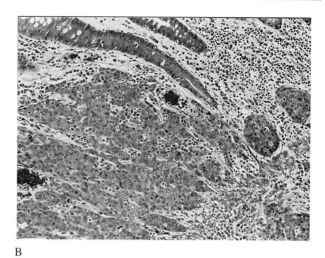

B

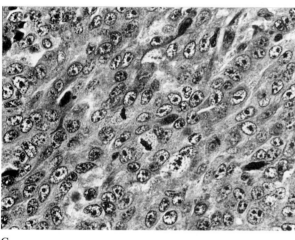

C

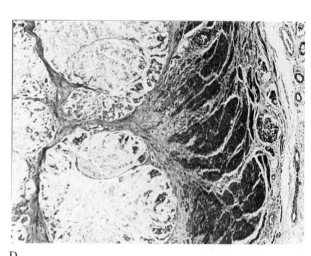

D

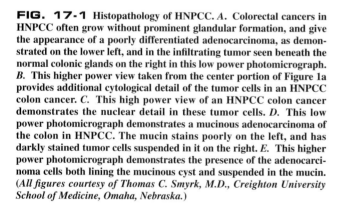

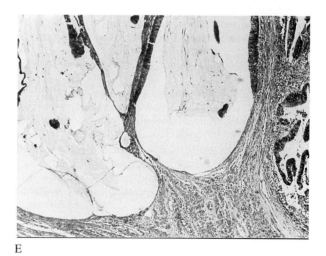

E

FIG. 17-1 Histopathology of HNPCC. *A.* Colorectal cancers in HNPCC often grow without prominent glandular formation, and give the appearance of a poorly differentiated adenocarcinoma, as demonstrated on the lower left, and in the infiltrating tumor seen beneath the normal colonic glands on the right in this low power photomicrograph. *B.* This higher power view taken from the center portion of Figure 1a provides additional cytological detail of the tumor cells in an HNPCC colon cancer. *C.* This high power view of an HNPCC colon cancer demonstrates the nuclear detail in these tumor cells. *D.* This low power photomicrograph demonstrates a mucinous adenocarcinoma of the colon in HNPCC. The mucin stains poorly on the left, and has darkly stained tumor cells suspended in it on the right. *E.* This higher power photomicrograph demonstrates the presence of the adenocarcinoma cells both lining the mucinous cyst and suspended in the mucin. (*All figures courtesy of Thomas C. Smyrk, M.D., Creighton University School of Medicine, Omaha, Nebraska.*)

The identification of the DNA mismatch repair genes and linking them to HNPCC families led to a sharp increase in interest in the field and the identification of numerous families with inactivating germline mutations. hMSH2 and hMLH1 account for the majority of families with HNPCC, and in roughly equal proportions.[64–66] Smaller numbers of families have HNPCC on the basis of mutations and hPMS2, and only one family has been found with a germline mutation in hPMS1.[63] The relative distribution of families with each of these germline mutations is listed in Table 17-6.

CELLULAR AND MOLECULAR BIOLOGY OF HNPCC

It is necessary to become familiar with the DNA mismatch repair system to fully understand the implications of HNPCC. Cancers develop in HNPCC when the DNA mismatch repair system fails. As described, DNA mismatch repair requires the concerted action of several proteins. Loss of any component of the system will inactivate, to some degree, the repair system.

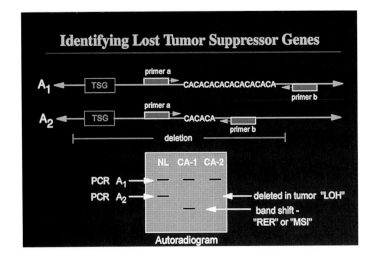

FIG. 17-2 Autoradiogram demonstrating microsatellite instability. A repetitive and polymorphic DNA sequence (microsatellite) is amplified by the polymerase chain reaction (PCR), and the normal tissue, if informative, provides two amplicons. In the case of microsatellite instability, the length of the pcr product changes. In the case of "loss of heterozygosity," one of the pcr products is deleted from the autoradiogram.

The DNA mismatch repair system is schematically illustrated in Figure 17-3.[67–70] During the synthesis of a new strand of DNA, many of the replication errors are immediately corrected by the 3' to 5' exonuclease activity of DNA polymerase. This reduces replication errors to approximately 1 per 10^{12} base pairs. It is estimated that 99.9% of the mutations that escape this proofreading activity are repaired by the mismatch repair system, particularly including single base pair mismatches, and loop-outs of unpaired bases, which tend to occur at repetitive sequences such as microsatellites. A newly synthesized mispair will deform the double helix of DNA, creating a physical aberration. The deformed DNA strand is recognized and bound by a complex made up of a heterodimer of hMSH2 and hMSH6 (hMSH6 initially was called the GT binding protein, or GTBP).[71] There is evidence that other proteins may substitute for MSH6 in forming the recognition complex (the hMSH2 and hMSH6 heteroduplex is termed hMutSα)[72], which may produce variability in the affinity for various types of mismatches.

After the recognition complex binds to a DNA mismatch, the repair system must identify which of the two DNA strands represents the original template and which is the newly synthesized, and therefore erroneous, strand. This is achieved by the recruitment of a second heterodimer, made up of hMLH1 and hPMS2 (called hMUTLα), which binds to the DNA mispair-hMutSα complex, and identifies the newly synthesized DNA strand by virtue of gaps that remain between newly synthesized Okazaki segments. In lower organisms, newly synthesized strands are recognized by the transient absence of methylation; it is not known whether this mechanism also participates in the human mismatch repair system. The repair system also requires the activity of several other enzymes, including helicase II, DNA pol III holoenzyme, DNA ligase, single-stranded DNA-binding pro-

tein, and several other DNA exonucleases. The DNA mismatch repair system excises the newly synthesized strand from the point of its recognition (presumably the gap) back to the mismatch, and then fully resynthesizes it.[53,54,69,70] This process is also known as long patch excision, which distinguishes it from another system (short patch excision) that repairs different types of DNA damage.

Our understanding of the DNA mismatch repair system began with studies in *E. coli* and the MutHLS system. In yeast, six MutS homologues (yMSH1, yMSH2, yMSH3, yMSH4, yMSH5 and yMSH6), and four MutL homologues (yPMS1, yMLH1, yMLH2, and yMLH3) have been identified.[53,72] yMSH2, yPMS1, and yMLH1 mutant strains of *Saccharomyces cerevisiae* undergo destabilization of microsatellite sequences during replication, as do the MutL and MutS mutants of *E. coli*. The human DNA mismatch repair system probably is more complex, but at the time of this writing, mutations in only four of the involved genes can give rise to HNPCC, and certain other genes that participate in mismatch repair, such as hMSH6 (GTBP), have never been linked to HNPCC.

The genomic instability at microsatellite sequences was the initial lead that DNA mismatch repair was inactivated in HNPCC tumors. The phenotype for these cells is normal. A second, somatic event occurs that results in loss of these second or wild-type alleles, attenuating or inactivating the DNA mismatch repair system.[59] Inactivation of both alleles results in the hypermutable phenotype. The hMSH2 protein appears to be a principal element for recognition of DNA mismatches. In yeast, the heterodimeric complex composed of MSH2 and another MutS homologue (MSH6 or MSH3) probably recognizes mismatches and initiates the repair process. In humans, it is clear that MSH6 and MSH2 form an active complex (hMutSα), but the role of MSH3 is not yet known. Dimers of hMSH2 and hMSH3 are termed hMutSβ. Data in yeast suggest that heterogeneity of the paired proteins may mediate the specificity of the DNA errors that can be recognized.[72] There are likely to be additional human mismatch repair proteins involved in the recognition of different types of DNA aberrations.[73]

Another issue that remains unclear is whether there is heterogeneity in the hMutLα complex that can further modify the repair system. Several hPMS2 related genes have been found on chromosome 7, the functions of which remains unknown,[74] and these are potential candidates for additional participants in human DNA mismatch repair.

The hMSH2 gene gives rise to a M_r106,000 protein that may be found immunohistochemically in the nucleus of a variety of tissues. In the intestinal tract, hMSH2 expression is limited to the replicating compartment of the crypt unit.[75,76] Both benign and ma-

Table 17-6 Distribution of Families with HNPCC Germline Mutations

HNPCC Gene	Frequency/Proportion of Families (%)xt
hMSH2	31
hMLH1	33
hPMS1	rare (one family)
hPMS2	4
GTBP (hMSH6)	0
Undetermined locus	32

SOURCE: From Ref. 64 with permission.

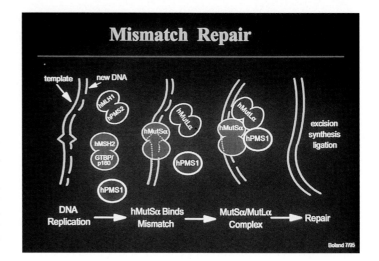

FIG. 17-3 DNA mismatch repair. During new strand synthesis, DNA polymerase may create mismatches or loop-outs, which deform the DNA double helix. The newly synthesized strand transiently has gaps. The hMUTSα complex (made up of hMSH2, or hMSH6 or hMSH3, in the case of hMutSβ) recognizes the mismatch and binds to it. The hMutL binds to the DNA mismatch–hMutSα complex in order to discriminate the strand containing the error, hMutLα is made up of hMLH1 and hPMS2. The role of hPMS1 is not yet determined. The mismatch complex accomplishes long patch excision, resynthesis, and ligation.

lignant colorectal tumors express hMSH2 protein throughout the neoplastic tissue. Tumors from patients with germline mutations in hMSH2 do not express the protein, consistent with the two-hit mechanism of gene inactivation.[76] In cultured cells, expression of the hMSH2 protein is regulated based on progression through the cell cycle. Levels remain relatively low in resting cells, but are induced when progression through the cell cycle towards mitosis is induced.[77]

THE PATHOPHYSIOLOGY OF HNPCC TUMORS

Most sporadic colorectal cancers develop through a mechanism that involves loss of relatively large chromosomal segments, which is thought to represent the deletion of wild-type tumor suppressor genes from the nucleus.[78] A proportion of sporadic colorectal cancers (perhaps 15%), and all HNPCC-related cancers, progress through a different mechanism, one that involves MIN. MIN is correlated inversely with loss of heterozygosity of chromosomes 5q, 17p, and 18q.[50] In sporadic colorectal cancers, over half show mutations in the K-*ras* oncogene. One group has reported that K-*ras* mutations are unusual in tumors with MIN,[49] however, the data here are conflicting. The initial work in this area indicated that mutations at K-*ras*, apc, and p53 were at least as common in HNPCC colon cancers as sporadic ones.[52] A failure to microdissect the neoplastic tissue from infiltrating stroma or inflammatory cells (which can be considerable in these tumors) would lead to a systematic underestimate of cancer-associated mutations. It is probably the case that HNPCC tumors specifically, and MIN tumors in general, have an excess of mutations at microsatellites and single nucleotides, and are relatively less likely to be aneuploid. Colorectal tumors with the MIN phenotype are also more likely to be exophytic, larger, look poorly differentiated, show focal or predominant mucin production, and show an intense Crohn's-like lymphoid reaction.[79]

The genomic instability seen at microsatellites in human colorectal neoplasms is an early event, and can be found in the adenomatous polyps which serve as precursors to cancer in HNPCC.[80] Although MIN has been described in phenotypically normal human lymphocytes in unusual instances,[58] the mucosa in the colons from most patients with HNPCC does not show this abnormality.[81] The adenomatous polyps associated with sporadic tumors with MIN, or those in HNPCC, also have MIN, unlike sporadic adenomas, which rarely do.[80,82] The proportion of microsatellite loci that

are mutated increases with progression from adenoma to carcinoma in both instances.[82,83]

In one series of cancers from patients with HNPCC, 95% showed the MIN phenotype, regardless of stage. In contrast, this type of genomic instability was found in only 3% of early sporadic tumors (i.e., adenomas or intramucosal carcinomas), and 13–24% of sporadic invasive cancers. This latter group showed MIN in 35% of the liver metastases, suggesting that loss of the mismatch repair system may play a role in tumor progression.[84]

One survey reported that 16% of sporadic colorectal cancers, and 86% of colorectal cancers from HNPCC patients had MIN, including all patients in which a germline mutation in hMSH2 was found. This lesion was present in only 3% of 33 sporadic colorectal adenomas, but in 57% of 14 adenomas associated with HNPCC. In addition, MIN was present in all of the extracolonic cancers derived from HNPCC patients.[85] Although MIN has been described in phenotypically normal lymphocytes in patients with certain germline mutations in a DNA mismatch repair gene,[58] the normal-appearing mucosa in the colons with HNPCC does not show this abnormality.[81]

MIN IN NON-HNPCC TUMORS

MIN was first described in colorectal cancers not selected on the basis of a suspicion for HNPCC. Depending on the criteria used, 12–28% of colorectal cancers have MIN.[49,50,52] MIN is neither characteristic of colorectal cancer, limited to tumors of this organ, nor limited to HNPCC. MIN can be found in gastric cancers, endometrial cancers, ovarian tumors, urinary bladder tumors, non–small-cell lung cancers, small-cell lung cancers, breast cancers, and other tumors. In some instances, inactivation of a DNA mismatch repair gene can be found, but this is not always the case. In some colon cancers, MIN can be found in association with loss of heterozygosity at one of the DNA mismatch repair gene loci.[59] In the overwhelming majority of instances, there are no germline mutations at any of the known HNPCC loci when MIN is found.

The presence of the hypermutable phenotype unrelated to the type of genomic instability seen with tumor progression in sporadic colorectal cancers (i.e., that manifested by widespread loss of heterozygosity) led to speculation that a distinct molecular pathway was responsible for HNPCC and related tumors. An increased rate of mutation at the *hprt* locus was found in colorectal cancer cell lines that had MIN.[86] Interestingly, inactivating mutations were found in the type II transforming growth factor (TGF)-

β receptor (called RII) in colon cancer cells with MIN.[87] These mutations all occurred in microsatellite sequences in an expressed portion of the RII. The mutations occurred in short repeated sequences that were characteristic of what one would anticipate after a loss of the DNA mismatch repair system. In each instance, the mutation induced a frame shift, loss of the RII transcript expression, and a failure to bind or respond to the TGFβ ligand. This is of particular importance because the TGFβ system inhibits the growth of colonic epithelial cells, and loss of this system in tumors with MIN represents a critical escape from growth control. Similar inactivating mutations in the RII gene have been found in gastric cancer cell lines and resected gastric carcinoma specimens; the mutations usually occur in a coding polyadenine tract.[88] It appears that inactivating mutations in growth regulating genes may be a key mechanism by which tumors with MIN become neoplastic.

Inactivation of the DNA mismatch repair system is associated with increased resistance to DNA alkylation, which is toxic to wild-type cells.[89] Restoration of the DNA mismatch repair system in a colon cancer cell line defective at the hMLH1 locus increases sensitivity to DNA damage, and restores the G2/M cell cycle check point.[90,91] The DNA mismatch repair system also is required for transcription-coupled DNA repair.[92] These findings imply additional growth advantages for tumor cells defective in DNA mismatch repair, since the G2/M check point may be bypassed in these cells, and an additional level of mutation repair is lost. Evidence is accumulating that DNA mismatch repair-defective cells may be relatively resistant to cytotoxic chemotherapy used to treat cancer.[91,93,94,95] Cell lines have been identified that are deficient for each of the major human DNA mismatch repair genes, which provide valuable models for study.[96]

Mice deficient in DNA mismatch repair genes have been developed using knockout techniques. Somewhat surprisingly, MSH2-deficient mice have a seemingly normal embryonic development, but have a very high risk for developing lymphomas at an early age. Tissues from these animals have a mutator phenotype, are relatively tolerant to methylation damage, and it was initially reported that they may not spontaneously develop tumors of the colon or other sites characteristic of HNPCC.[97] However, it was reported subsequently that MSH2 deficient mice will develop a 70% incidence of intestinal neoplasms (mostly small intestinal) by age 6 months, that 7% develop keratoacanthoma-like skin lesions, and all die by 1 year.[98] Knockout mice who have no MLH1 genes have the MIN phenotype, have no DNA mismatch repair activity in cell extracts, and are sterile because of defective spermatogenesis.[99,100] MLH1-deficient spermatocytes show numerous prematurely separated chromosomes and meiotic pachytene arrest. Male mice defective at the PMS2 locus have abnormal chromosome synapses in meiosis, and are highly prone to the development of sarcomas and lymphomas.[101] None of the knockout mice or the heterozygotes of these model develop a syndrome that closely resembles HNPCC.

MIN and Neoplasia in Ulcerative Colitis

MIN commonly is seen in cancers associated with ulcerative colitis, as well as the dysplasias that antedate these tumors.[102] An intronic polymorphism in the hMSH2 gene is more common in patients who develop colitis-associated neoplasia than in control patients with or without colitis.[103] Moreover, MIN may be found in the non-neoplastic colonic mucosa from patients with chronic ulcerative colitis.[104] It has not yet been confirmed whether inactivation of the DNA mismatch repair system is an essential part of tumor development in chronic inflammation.

THE DIAGNOSIS AND MANAGEMENT OF HNPCC

Identification of the role of the DNA mismatch repair system in the genesis of HNPCC provided a breakthrough in the premorbid diagnosis of the disease. Although many more proteins participate in the DNA mismatch repair system, only three of the genes appear to commonly account for HNPCC: hMSH2, hMLH1, and hPMS2 (Table 17-6).

Insight into the pathophysiology and genetic basis of HNPCC have provided multiple strategies for making this diagnosis. It is possible to screen for HNPCC by observing MIN in a tumor specimen. Although 92% of HNPCC-associated colon cancers have MIN,[65] it is likely that only a minority of tumors with MIN come from HNPCC families.[105] Direct sequencing of the DNA mismatch repair genes is a possible strategy to make the diagnosis of HNPCC, but the number and size of the genes make this clinically impractical. Knowledge of the critical loci for HNPCC makes linkage analysis a possible approach, but multiple affected family members must be available for testing, and the diagnostic power is limited.[106] The large fraction of inactivating germline mutations in hMSH2 that result in a truncated protein suggest that the use of an in vitro transcription/translation assay may be clinically useful. This latter approach provided a positive test in about half of patients who met the Amsterdam criteria for HNPCC.[107]

Direct sequencing of the exons in hMSH2 and hMLH1 is the most straightforward approach to diagnosis. At this time, the full spectrum of disease-producing germline mutations and innocuous polymorphisms has not been catalogued, which may complicate the interpretation of DNA sequence data. Analyses based upon harvesting RNA from lymphocytes is complicated by the observation that both hMSH2 and hMLH1 may undergo alternative splicing that will generate different messages and proteins, which may complicate interpretation.[108–110] Unfortunately, the range of germline mutations in hMSH2 and hMLH1 is wide, and includes insertions, deletions, nonsense mutations, and missense mutation.[65] A list of published mutations at these two loci is listed in Tables 17-7 and 17-8.[110] These considerations make screening for a germline diagnosis in HNPCC a daunting undertaking. Nonetheless, when a mutation is correctly identified in a family, direct sequencing or in vitro transcription/translation will be highly reliable for other at-risk members of that family. In some instances, founding mutations may be responsible for a large proportion of familial colon cancer in a specific geographic region with a relatively immobile population.[112,113]

Finding the germline mutation in an individual family has several implications. First, it permits the physician and genetic counselor to increase the certainty with which a diagnosis is made. Half of those at risk will be informed that they did not inherit a high risk for cancer, and half will be informed with certainty of their risks, for which a surveillance program may be initiated.

The lifetime risk for cancer in HNPCC can only be estimated at this time. Cumulative risk for colorectal cancer has been estimated at 78%, and endometrial cancer has been estimated at 20% in one study[114] and 43% for women in another study from Finland (Fig. 17-4).[115] Patients with HNPCC must be identified because of the extremely high risk for metachronous cancers after successful treatment of the index tumor.[115] Patients with hMLH1-associated HNPCC have a significantly better survival rate when compared with patients with sporadic colorectal cancers (Fig. 17-5).[116] It is unknown whether this observation is generally applicable to all hMLH1 and hMSH2-associated HNPCC families.

Once HNPCC patients are identified, a screening program consisting of colonoscopy or barium enema and sigmoidoscopy significantly reduces the rate of tumor development and death in patients with HNPCC (Fig. 17-6).[117] The observation that a screening

Table 17-7 *hMSH2*

Exon/ Intron	Codon	Mutation	No. of kindreds*	Predicted Protein Change
[5' end]		Deletion of the 5' of the gene	1	Mutated protein absent
3	129–130	2 bp deletion	1	Frameshift[†]
4	252	CAG to TAG	1	Gln252 to stop[†]
5	280	1 bp (T) insertion	1	Frameshift[†]
5	288	CAG to TAG	1	Gln288 to stop[†]
5	270–271	4 bp (CTGT) Deletion	1	Frameshift[†]
intron 5		Splice donor site (A to T at -3)	8, Anglo-Saxon[‡]	In-frame deletion of exon 5[†]
6	322	GGC to GAC	1	Gly322 to Asp
6	339–340	2 bp (AA) deletion	1	Frameshift[†]
[7]		Deletion Exon 7 (transcript)	1	Out-of-frame deletion exon 7[†]
7	359	Ins. of 173 bp at codon 359	1	Frameshift[†]
7	376	2 bp (TA) insertion	1	Frameshift[†]
7	380–381	1 bp (T) deletion	1	Frameshift[†]
7	383	CGA to TGA	1	Arg383 to stop[†]
7	406	CGA to TGA	1	Arg406 to stop[†]
intron 7		Splice donor site (G to C at -1)	1	Out-of-frame deletion exon 7[†]
8	458	TTA to TGA	1	Leu458 to stop[†]
[8]		Del. Exons 8–15 (transcript)	1	Out-of-frame del. of exons 8–15[†]
8	429	CAG to TAG	1	Gln429 to stop[†]
9	481–482	1 bp (A) insertion	1	Frameshift[†]
10	532	1 bp (G) insertion	1	Frameshift[†]
12	596	3 bp (AAT) deletion	3	In-frame deletion of Asn
12	621	CGA to TGA	1	Arg621 to stop[†]
12	601	CAG to TAG	2 (1,Muir-Torre)	Gln601 to stop[†]
12	622	CCA to CTA	1	Pro622 to Leu substitution
12	639	CAT to TAT	1	His639 to Tyr substitution
12	639	CAT to TAT	1	*(Out-of-frame del. of codons 638–669[†])*
12	662	2 bp (AG) deletion	1 (Muir-Torre)	Frameshift[†]
[13]		Deletion Exon 13 (transcript ¶)	2	Out-of-frame deletion of exon 13[†]
14	782–783	1 bp (C) deletion	1	Frameshift[†]
intron 15		Splice donor site (G to T at -1)	2	Out-of-frame deletion of exon 15[†]

*Not all the kindreds reported fulfilled the Amsterdam criteria for HNPCC diagnosis
‡This *hMSH2* founder mutation was found in three families from North America, all of whom report Anglo-Saxon heritage
†Mutations resulting in a premature truncation, or shortening of the hMSH2 protein, that may be detected by IVTT
¶It was recently reported that this alteration may represent an alternatively spliced variant in the population

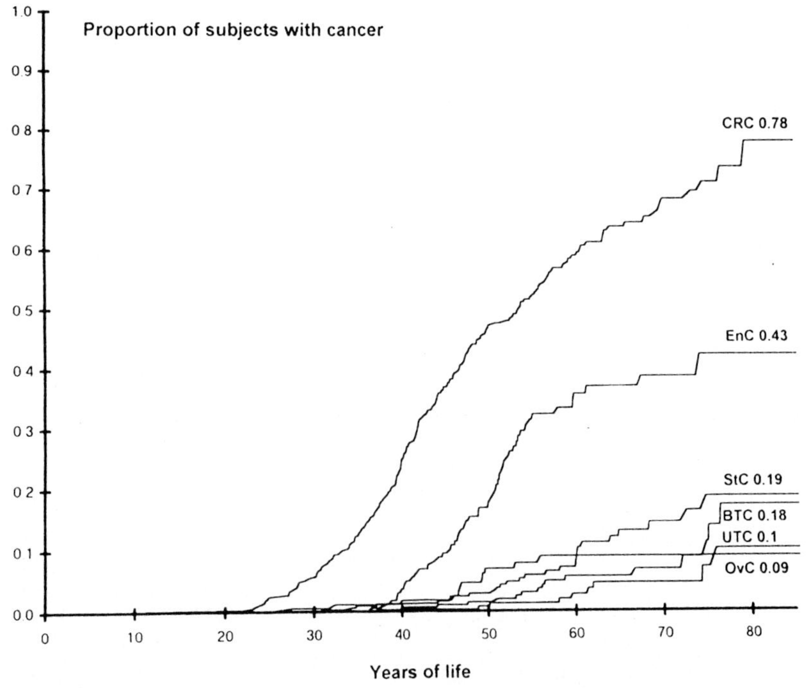

FIG. 17-4 Cancer-risk in HNPCC. Cumulative lifetime risks for the six most common cancer types among 293 putative HNPCC gene carriers. CRC = colorectal cancer; EnC = endometrial cancer (females only); StC = stomach cancer; BTC = biliary tract cancer; UTC = urinary tract cancer; OvC = ovarian cancer (females only) (*from reference 115, with permission*).

Table 17-8 *hMLH1*

Exon/Intron	Codon	Mutation	No. of kindreds*	Predicted Protein Change
1	35	ATG to AGG	1	Met35 to Arg substitution
2	62	CAA to TAA	1	Gln62 to stop†
2	44	TCC to TTC	1	Ser44 to Phe substitution
2	67	GGG to AGG	1	Gly67 to Arg substitution
2	68	ATC to AAC	1	Ile68 to Asn substitution
intron 2		Splice acceptor site (A to G at -2)	1	In-frame deletion exon 3†
4	117	ACG to ATG	2	Thr117 to Met substitution
4	117	ACG to AGG	1	Thr117 to Arg substitution
intron 5		Splice acceptor site (G to A at -1)	5, Finnish‡	Out-of-frame deletion of exon 6†
intron 6		Splice acceptor site (A to G at -2)	1	Out-of-frame deletion exon 7†
intron 7		Splice acceptor site (A to G at -2)	1	Out-of-frame deletion exon 8†
8 and 9	226	CAG to TGA (*transcript*)	1	Arg226 to stop†
8 and 9	226	CGA to CAA	1	Arg226 to Gln substitution
8 and 9	226	CGA to CTA	1	Arg226 to Leu substitution
intron 8		Splice donor site (del. G at -1)	1	Out-of-frame deletion exon 8†
intron 8		Splice acc. site (del. TA at -3 & -2)	1	Out-of-frame del. exon 9–10†
intron 9		Splice donor site (ins. T at -3)	1	Out-of-frame del. exon 9–10†
intron 9		Splice donor site (T to A at -2)	1	Out-of-frame deletion exon 9†
intron 9		Splice acc. site (G to C at -1)	1	Out-of-frame deletion exon 10†
11	307–308	Insertion of GC	1	Frameshift†
11	326	GTT to GCT	2	Val326 to Ala
11	336	Deletion of G	1	Frameshift†
[12]		Deletion Exon 12 (*transcript*)	2	Out-of-frame Deletion of exon 12†
[13]		Deletion Exon 13 (*transcript*)	2	Out-of-frame Deletion of exon 13†
13	506	GTT to GCT	1	Val506 to Ala
13	519	Insert. of T before codon 519	1	Frameshift†
13	470–471	Deletion of AAAG	1	Frameshift†
14	542	CAG to CTG	1	Gln542 to Leu
15	574	CTC to GTC	1	Leu574 to Pro
[15]		Deletion Exon 15 (*transcript*)	1	Out-of-frame Deletion exon 15†
intron 15		Splice donor site (G to A at -1)	1	Out-of-frame Deletion exon 15†
intron 15		Splice acceptor site (A to T at -2)	1	In-frame Deletion exon 16†
intr 15-16		Del. Ex.16, and part of in. 15 and 16	14, Finnish‡	In-frame Deletion exon 16†
16	593–594	Deletion of AG	1	Frameshift†
16	628	Deletion of TT (*transcript*)	1	Frameshift†
16	578	GAG to GGG	1	Glu578 to Gly substitution
16	582	CTC to GTC	1	Leu582 to Val substitution
16	586	Insertion of G	2	Frameshift†
16	616–618	Deletion of AAG	4	In-frame del. of a Lys at 616–618
16	618	AAA to ACG	1	Lys618 to Thr substitution
16	632	GAG to GAA	2	In-frame Deletion exon 16†
16	632	1 bp (G) Deletion	1	Frameshift†
intron 18		Splice donor site (G to A at -1)	1	In-frame Deletion exon 18†
intron 18		Splice acceptor site (A to T at -2)	1	In-frame-Deletion exon 19†
19	712	TGG to TAG	1	Trp712 to stop†
19	727–728	4 bp (CACA) del. (*transcript*)	1	Frameshift (longer product)
19	755–756	TGTT insertion	2	Frameshift (longer product)

*Not all the kindreds reported fulfilled the Amsterdam criteria for HNPCC diagnosis

†Mutations resulting in a premature truncation, or shortening of the *hMLH1* protein, that may be detected by IVTT

‡Mutation involving Exon 6 of *hMLH1* is called *"Finnish mutation2"*; mutation involving Exon 16 of *hMLH1* is called *"Finnish mutation 1"*

program actually lowered the colorectal cancer incidence rates in family members with HNPCC suggests that the adenomatous polyps in this disease may be more prone to malignant transformation than adenomas in the general population, and that their removal is an important part of a prevention program.

When a young individual (i.e., <45 years of age) develops colorectal cancer, this raises the concern that the patient and patient's relatives are at increased risk for HNPCC. One study suggested that the relative risk for colorectal cancer in the close relatives of such patients is increased fivefold and may be even higher for female relatives.[119] MIN is significantly more likely to occur in the colorectal cancers of young patients, and can be found in 58% of

patients under 35 years of age, even when the family history does not suggest HNPCC.[120] Even in such patients, less than half will have detectable germline mutations in the known DNA mismatch repair genes.

The following approach might be followed to identify HNPCC. A careful family history should be taken in all patients who develop a cancer. A full pedigree should be drawn, and critical information should include all relatives who develop tumors, the organs affected, the age of first cancer, the occurrence of multiple cancers, and the ages reached by individuals who did not develop cancer. When the Amsterdam criteria are met (Table 17-1), HNPCC is very likely. Under these circumstances, the in vitro transcription/

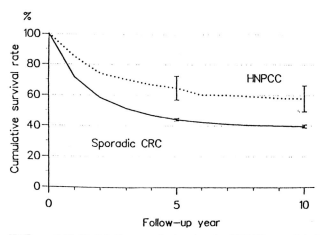

FIG. 17-5 Relative survival rates in hMLH1-associated HNPCC. The cumulative relative survival rates (with 95% confidence intervals) in 175 patients with HNPCC-related colorectal cancers compared with 14,086 patients with sporadic colorectal cancers (*from reference 115, with permission*).

translation assay for premature truncating mutations in hMSH2 or hMLH1 will provide a diagnosis in about half of families.[107] When available, tumor tissue can be valuable. Microsatellite analysis may be performed from paraffin-embedded tissues. Patients with HNPCC are likely to have microsatellite alterations at multiple loci. If no MIN is found, the likelihood of HNPCC is reduced substantially. Sporadic colorectal cancers are common, and phenocopies may occur in some families; if such a tumor were analyzed, it may not show MIN, and provide misleading information. Direct sequencing of the DNA mismatch repair genes may provide important information, but some mutations will be ambiguous, and difficult to interpret.

Although the rodent models suggest that inactivation of each of the DNA mismatch repair genes is associated with a unique phenotype, there is little information suggesting that any gene or specific type of mutation produces a unique phenotype in human populations. One study has suggested that minor variations in noncolorectal cancers may be found between hMSH2 and hMLH1 families.[121] The Muir-Torre syndrome has been attributed to different MSH2 mutations.[122,123] Of interest, not all kindreds with the mutations found in some Muir-Torre syndrome families will necessarily develop the characteristic skin tumors.[123]

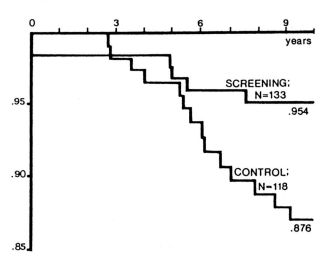

FIG. 17-6 Impact of screening on survival in HNPCC. Cumulative proportions of subjects free of colorectal cancers in HNPCC. Patients who were screened had significantly better survivals than control subjects, who were not screened (P = 0.03) (*from reference 115, with permission*).

TREATMENT OF HNPCC

When an HNPCC patient presents with an invasive cancer, the appropriate treatment is to perform a subtotal colectomy with an ileosigmoid or ileorectal anastamosis. The increased risk for tumor development in the rest of the colon mandates aggressive surgical treatment, but the ability to screen the rectum for recurrent disease makes a total proctocolectomy unnecessary. If a patient should present with an invasive rectal cancer, a total proctocolectomy may be required.

Patients who are identified in the presymptomatic stage by genetic testing should be informed that their lifetime risk of colorectal cancer is probably 80–90% and that surveillance colonoscopy every 3 years can significantly reduce morbidity and mortality.[117] The occurrence of interval cancers in patients who have undergone surveillance at 2- to 3-year intervals has prompted some to argue for more aggressive surveillance, perhaps on an annual basis, because of the unique natural history of these tumors.[124] The age of onset of tumors can be variable within an HNPCC family, leading to the misperception of a skipped generation, which should be taken into account when treating families.[125] In the same vein, a retrospective study has indicated that in only 40% of patients was a family history available that suggested HNPCC when it was actually encountered.[126] In such families, the presence of a villous adenoma in a young patient should heighten the clinical suspicion for HNPCC, and perhaps such a lesion should be interpreted with the same implications as a cancer.[35]

There are no known medical treatments for patients with HNPCC. Aspirin may play an important protective effect against the development of sporadic colorectal cancer; however, its impact on HNPCC is unknown. No other interventions other than diagnostic screening and prophylactic surgery have been demonstrated to have a beneficial effect in this disease.

REFERENCES

1. Boland CR: Neoplasia of the Gastrointestinal Tract, in Yamada T (ed): *Textbook of Gastroenterology* 2d ed. Philadelphia, Lippincott, 1995, pp. 578–595.
2. Cannon-Albright LA, Skomick MH, Bishop DT, et al: Common inheritance of colonic adenomatous polyps and associated colorectal cancers. *N Engl J Med* **319**:533–537, 1988.
3. Fuchs CS, Giovannucci EL, Colditz GA, et al: A prospective study of family history and the risk of colorectal cancer. *N Engl J Med* **331**:1669–1674, 1994.
4. Winawer SJ, Zauber AG, Gerdes H, et al: Risk of colorectal cancer in the families of patients with adenomatous polyps. The National Polyp Study Workgroup. *N Engl J Med* **334**:82–87, 1996.
5. Ionov Y, Peinado MA, Malkhosyan S, et al: Ubiquitous somatic mutations in simple repeated sequences reveal a new mechanism for colonic carcinogenesis. *Nature* **363**:558–561, 1993.
6. Thibodeau SN, Bren G, Schaid D: Microsatellite instability in cancer of the proximal colon. *Science* **260**:816–819, 1993.
7. Peltomaki P, Aaltonen LA, Sistonen P, et al: Genetic mapping of a locus predisposing to human colorectal cancer. *Science* **260**:810–812, 1993.
8. Aaltonen LA, Peltomaki P, Leach FS, et al: Clues to the pathogenesis of familial colorectal cancer. *Science* **260**:812–816, 1993.
9. Lynch HT, Lanspa S, Smyrk T, Boman B, Watson P, and Lynch J: Hereditary nonpolyposis colorectal cancer (Lynch Syndromes I & II): Genetics, pathology, natural history, and cancer control, Part I. *Cancer Genet Cytogenet* **53**:143–160, 1991.
10. Lynch HT, Ens J, Lynch JF, et al: Tumor variation in three extended Lynch syndrome II kindreds. *Am J Gastroenterol* **83**: 74–747, 1988.
11. Vasen HFA, Offerhaus GJA, den Hartog Jager FCA, et al: The tumor spectrum in hereditary non-polyposis colorectal cancer: a study of 24 kindreds in the Netherlands. *Int J Cancer* **46**:31–34, 1990.

12. Watson P, Lynch HT: Extracolonic cancer in hereditary nonpolyposis colorectal cancer. *Cancer* **71**:677–685, 1993.

13. St. John DJB, McDermott FT, Hopper J: Cancer risk in relatives of patients with common colorectal cancer. *Ann Int Med* **118**:785, 1993.

14. Houlston RS, Murday V, Harocopos C, et al: Screening and genetic counselling for relatives of patients with colorectal cancer in a family cancer clinic. *Br Med J* **301**:18–25, 1990.

15. Mecklin J-P, Jarvinen JH, Aukee S, et al: Screening for colorectal carcinoma in cancer family syndrome kindreds. *Scand J Gastroent* **22**:449–453, 1987.

16. Ponz de Leon M, Sassatelli R, Sacchetti C, et al: Familial aggregation of tumors in the three year experience of a population-based colorectal cancer registry. *Cancer Res* **49**:4344–4348, 1989.

17. Stephenson BM, Finan PJ, Gascoyne J, et al: Frequency of familial colorectal cancer. *Br J Surg* **78**:1162–1166, 1991.

18. Mecklin J-P: Frequency of hereditary colorectal cancer. *Gastroenterology* **93**:1021–1025, 1987.

19. Kee F, Collins BJ: How prevalent is cancer family syndrome? *Gut* **32**:309–312, 1991.

20. Westlake PJ, Bryant HE, Huchcroft SA, et al: Frequency of hereditary nonpolyposis colorectal cancer in southern Alberta. *Dig Dis Sci* **36**:1441–1447, 1991.

21. Kee F, Collins BJ: Families at risk of colorectal cancer: who are they? *Gut* **33**:787–790, 1992.

22. Mecklin J-P, Jarvinen HJ, Peltokallio P: Cancer family syndrome: Genetic analysis of 22 Finnish kindreds. *Gastroenterology* **90**:328–333, 1986.

23. Lynch HT, Smyrk TC, Watson P, et al: Genetics, natural history, tumor spectrum, and pathology of hereditary nonpolyposis colorectal cancer: An updated review. *Gastroenterology* **104**:1535–1549, 1993.

24. Marra G and Boland CR: Hereditary nonpolyposis colorectal cancer (HNPCC): The syndrome, the genes, and an historical perspective. *J Natl Cancer Inst* **87**:1114–1125, 1995.

25. Warthin AS; Heredity with reference to carcinoma. *Arch Intern Med* **12**:546–555, 1913.

26. Warthin AS; The further study of a cancer family. *J Cancer Res* **9**:279–286, 1925.

27. Warthin AS; Heredity of carcinoma in man. *Ann Int Med* **4**:681–696, 1931.

28. Hauser IJ, Weller CV: A further report on the cancer family of Warthin. *Am J Cancer* **27**:434–444, 1936.

29. Lynch HT, Krush AJ: Cancer family "G" revisited: 1895–1970. *Cancer* **27**:1505–1511, 1971.

30. Lynch HT, Shaw MW, Magnuson CW, et al: Hereditary factors in two large midwestern kindreds. *Arch Intern Med* **117**:206–212, 1966.

31. Boland CR, Troncale FJ: Familial colonic cancer in the absence of antecedent polyposis. *Ann Intern Med* **100**:700–701, 1984.

32. Boland CR: Familial colonic cancer syndromes. *West J Med* **139**:351–359, 1983.

33. Vasen HFA, Mecklin J-P, Khan PM, et al: The International Collaborative Group on Hereditary Non-polyposis Colorectal Cancer. *Dis Colon Rect* **34**:424–425, 1991.

34. Lanspa ST, Lynch HT, Smyrk TC, et al: Colorectal adenomas in the Lynch syndromes—results of a colonoscopy screening program. *Gastroenterology* **98**:1117–1122, 1990.

35. Jass JR, Stewart SM: Evolution of hereditary non-polyposis colorectal cancer. *Gut* **33**:783–786, 1992.

36. Mecklin J-P, Jarvinen HJ, Aukee S, Elomaa I, Karajalainen K: Screening for colorectal carcinoma in Cancer Family Syndrome kindreds. *Scand J Gastroent* **22**:449–453, 1987.

37. Lynch HT, Lynch PM, Pester J, et al: The Cancer Family Syndrome: Rare cutaneous phenotypic linkage of Torre's syndrome. *Arch Intern Med* **141**:607–611, 1980.

38. Lynch HT, Fusaro RM, Roberts L, et al: Muir-Torre syndrome in several members of a family with a varient of cancer family syndrome. *Br J Derm* **113**:295–301, 1985.

39. Honchel R, Halling KC, Schaid DJ, et al: Microsatellite instability in Muir-Torre syndrome. *Cancer Res* **54**:1159–1163, 1994.

40. Kolodner RD, Hall NR, Lipford J, et al: Structure of the human MSH2 locus and analysis of two Muir-Torre kindreds for msh2 mutations. *Genomics* **24**:516, 1994.

41. Kee F, Patterson CC, Collins BJ, et al: Histologic characteristics and outcome of familial non-polyposis colorectal cancer. *Scand J Gastroenterol* **26**:419–424, 1991.

42. Jass Jr, Smyrk TC, Stewart SM, et al: Pathology of Hereditary Non-Polyposis Colorectal Cancer. *Anticancer Res* **14**:1631–1634, 1994.

43. Mecklin J-P, Sipponen P, Jarvinen HJ: Histopathology of colorectal carcinomas and adenomas in Cancer Family Syndrome. *Dis Colon Rectum* **29**:849–853, 1986.

44. Frei JV: hereditary nonpolyposis colorectal cancer (Lynch syndrome II). Diploid malignancies with prolonged survival. *Cancer* **69**:1108–1111, 1992.

45. Kouri M, Laasonen A, Mecklin J-P, et al: Diploid predominance in hereditary nonpolyposis colorectal carcinoma evaluated by flow cytometry. *Cancer* **65**:1825–1829, 1990.

46. Loeb LA: Mutator phenotype may be required for multistage carcinogenesis. *Cancer Res* **51**:3075–3079, 1991.

47. Loeb LA: Microsatellite instability: marker of a mutator phenotype in cancer. *Cancer Res* **54**:5059–5063, 1994.

48. Peinado MA, Malkhosyan S, Velazquez, et al: Isolation and characterization of allelic losses and gains in colorectal tumors by arbitrarily primed polymerase chain reaction. *Proc Natl Acad Sci USA* **89**:10065, 1992.

49. Ionov Y, Peinado MA, Malkhosyan S, et al: Ubiquitous somatic mutations in simple repeated sequences reveal a new mechanism for colonic carcinogenesis. *Nature* **363**:558, 1993.

50. Thibodeau SN, Bren G, Schaid D: Microsatellite instability in cancer of the proximal colon. *Science* **260**:816, 1993.

51. Peltomaki P, Aaltonen LA, Sistonen P, et al: Genetic mapping of a locus predisposing to human colorectal cancer. *Science* **260**:810, 1993.

52. Aaltonen LA, Peltomaki P, Leach FS, et al: Clues to the pathogenesis of familial colorectal cancer. *Science* **260**:812, 1993.

53. Fishel R, Kolodner RD: Identification of mismatch repair genes and their role in the development of cancer. *Curr Opinion Genet Dev* **5**:382–395, 1995.

54. Kolodner RD: Mismatch repair: mechanisms and relationship to cancer susceptibility. *TIBS* **20**:397–401, 1995.

55. Strand M, Prolla TA, Liskay RM, Petes TD. Destabilization of tracts of simple repetitive DNA in yeast by mutations affecting DNA mismatch repair. *Nature* **365**:274–276, 1993.

56. Fishel R, Lescoe MK, Rao MRS, et al: The human mutator gene homolog *MSH2* and its association with hereditary nonpolyposis colon cancer. *Cell* **75**:1027–1038, 1993.

57. Leach FS, Nicolaides NC, Papadopoulos N, et al: Mutations of a *mutS* homolog in hereditary nonpolyposis colorectal cancer. *Cell* **75**:1215–1225, 1993.

58. Parsons R, Li G-M, Longley M, et al: Mismatch repair deficiency in phenotypically normal human cells. *Science* **268**:738, 1995.

59. Hemminki A, Peltomaki P, Mecklin J-K: Loss of the wild type *MLH1* gene is a feature of hereditary nonpolyposis colorectal cancer. *Nat Genet* **8**:405–410, 1994.

60. Limblom A, Tannergard P, Werelius B, et al: Genetic mapping of a second locus predisposing to hereditary non-polyposis colon cancer. *Nat Genet* **5**:279–282, 1993.

61. Bronner CE, Baker SM, Morrison PT, et al: Mutation in the DNA mismatch repair gene homologue *hMLH1* is associated with hereditary non-polyposis colon cancer. *Nature* **368**:258–261, 1994.

62. Papadopoulos N, Nicolaides NC, Wei YF, et al: Mutation of a *mutL* homolog in hereditary colon cancer. *Science* **263**:1625–1629, 1994.

63. Nicolaides NC, Papadopoulos N, Liu B, et al: Mutations of two *PMS* homologues in hereditary nonpolyposis colon cancer. *Nature* **371**:75–80, 1994.

64. Liu B, Nicolaides NC, Markowitz S, et al: Mismatch repair gene defects in sporadic colorectal cancers with microsatellite instability. *Nat Genet* **9**:48–55, 1995.

65. Liu B, Parsons R, Papadopoulos N, et al: Analysis of mismatch repair genes in hereditary non-polyposis colorectal cancer. *Nat Med* **2**:169, 1996.

66. Luce MC, Marra G, Chauhan DP, et al: *In vitro* transcription/translation assay for the screening of hMLH1 and hMSH2 mutations in familial colon cancer. *Gastroenterology* **109**:1368, 1995.

67. Cooper DL, Lahue RS, Modrich P: Methyl-directed mismatch repair is bidirectional. *J Biol Chem* **268**:11823, 1993.

68. Kunkel TA: Misalignment-mediated DNA synthesis errors. *Biochemistry* **29**:8003, 1990.

69. Modrich P: Mechanisms and biological effects of mismatch repair. *Annu Rev Genet* **25**:229–253, 1991.

70. Sancar A: DNA Repair in Humans. *Annu Rev Genet* **29**:69–105, 1995.
71. Drummond JT, Li G-M, Longley MJ, et al: Isolation of an hMSH2-p160 heterodimer that restores DNA mismatch repair to tumor cells. *Science* **268**:1909, 1995.
72. Marsischky GT, Filosi N, Kane MF, et al: Redundancy of *Saccharomyces cerevisiae* MSH3 and MSH6 in MSH2-dependent mismatch repair. *Genes Dev* **10**:407, 1996.
73. Umar A, Boyer JC, Kunkel TA: DNA loop repair by human cell extracts. *Science* **266**:814, 1994.
74. Nicolaides NC, Carter KC, Shell BK, et al: Genomic organization of the human *PMS2* gene family. *Genomics* **30**:195–206, 1995.
75. Wilson TM, Ewel A, Duguid JR, et al: Differential cellular expression of the human MSH2 repair enzyme in small and large intestine. *Cancer Res* **55**:5146–5150, 1995.
76. Leach FS, Polyak K, Burrell M, et al: Expression of the human mismatch repair gene hMSH2 in normal and neoplastic tissues. *Cancer Res* **56**:235–240, 1996.
77. Marra G, Chang Lin C, Laghi L, Chauhan DP, Young D, and Boland CR: Cell cycle dependent expression of the human Mut S homolog 2 (hMSH2) gene (in press, *Oncogene*, 1996).
78. Fearon ER, Vogelstein B: A genetic model for colorectal tumorigenesis. *Cell* **61**:759–767, 1990.
79. Kim H, Jen J, Vogelstein B, et al: Clinical and pathological characteristics of sporadic colorectal carcinomas with DNA replication errors in microsatellite sequences. *AJ Pathol* **145**:148–156, 1994.
80. Shibata D, Peinado MA, Ionov Y, et al: Genomic instability in repeated sequences is an early somatic event in colorectal tumorigenesis that persists after transformation. *Nat Genet* **6**:273, 1994.
81. Williams GT, Geraghty JM, Campbell F, et al: Normal colonic mucosa in hereditary non-polyposis colorectal cancer shows no generalised increase in somatic mutation. *Br J Cancer* **71**:1077–1080, 1995.
82. Jacoby RF, Marshall DJ, Kailas S, et al: Genetic instability associated with adenoma to carcinoma progression in hereditary colon cancer. *Gastroenterology* **109**:73–82, 1995.
83. Shibata D, Navidi W, Salovaara R, et al: Somatic microsatellite mutations as molecular tumor clocks. *Nat Med* **2**:676–681, 1996.
84. Konishi M, Kikuchi-Yanoshita R, Tanaka K, et al: Molecular nature of colon tumors in hereditary nonpolyposis colon cancer, familial polyposis, and sporadic colon cancer. *Gastroenterology* **111**:307–317, 1996.
85. Aaltonen LA, Peltomaki P, Mecklin J-P, et al: Replication errors in benign and malignant tumors from hereditary nonpolyposis colorectal cancer patients. *Cancer Res* **54**:1645, 1994.
86. Eshleman JR, Lang EZ, Bowerfind GK, et al: Increased mutation rate at the *hprt* locus accompanies microsatellite instability in colon cancer. *Oncogene* **10**:33–37, 1995.
87. Markowitz S, Wang J, Myeroff L, et al: Inactivation of the type II TFG-β receptor in colon cancer cells with microsatellite instability. *Science* **268**:1336, 1995.
88. Myeroff LL, Parsons R, Kim SJ, et al: A transforming growth factor β receptor type II gene mutation common in colon and gastric but rare in endometrial cancers with microsatellite instability. *Cancer Res* **55**:5545–5547, 1995.
89. White RL, Fox MS: Genetic consequences of transfection with heteroduplex bacteriophage lambda DNA. *Mol Gen Genet* **141**:163–171, 1975.
90. Koi M, Umar A, Chauhan DP, et al: Human chromosome 3 corrects mismatch repair deficiency and microsatellite instability and reduces N-methyl-N′nitro-N-nitrosoguanidine tolerance in human colon tumor cells with homozygous hMLH1 mutation. *Cancer Res* **54**:4308–4312, 1994.
91. Hawn MT, Umar A, Carethers JM, et al: Evidence for a connection between the mismatch repair system and the G2 cell cycle checkpoint. *Cancer Res* **55**:3721–3725, 1995.
92. Mellon I, Rajpal DK, Koi M, et al: Transcription-coupled nucleotide excision repair deficiency associated with mutations in human mismatch repair genes. *Science* **272**:557–560, 1996.
93. Carethers JM, Koi M, Hawn ML, et al: In vitro effect of 5-fluorouracil on cells with and without proficiency in DNA mismatch repair. *Gastroenterology* **108**:A454, 1995.
94. Aebi S, Kurdi-Haidar B, Gordon R, et al: Loss of DNA mismatch repair in acquired resistance to cisplatin. *Cancer Res* **56**:3087–3090, 1996
95. Duckett DR, Drummond JT, Murchie AIH, et al: Human MutSα recognizes damaged DNA base pairs containing 0⁶-methylthymine, or the cisplatin-d(GpG) adduct. *Proc Natl Acad Sci USA* **93**:6443–6447, 1996.
96. Boyer JC, Umar A, Risinger JI, et al: Microsatellite instability, mismatch repair deficiency, and genetic defects in human cancer cell lines. *Cancer Res* **55**:6063–6070, 1995.
97. de Wind N, Dekker M, Berns A, et al: Inactivation of the mouse *Msh2* gene results in mismatch repair deficiency, methylation tolerance, hyperrecombination, and predisposition to cancer. *Cell* **82**:321, 1995.
98. Reitmair AH, Redston M, Cai JC, et al: Spontaneous carcinomas and skin neoplasms in Msh2-deficient mice. *Cancer Res* **56**:3842–3849, 1996.
99. Edelmann W, Cohen PE, Kane M, et al: Meiotic pachytene arrest in MLH1-deficient Mice. *Cell* **85**:1125–1134, 1996.
100. Baker SM, Plug AW, Prolla TA, et al: Involvement of mouse Mlh1 in DNA mismatch repair and meiotic crossing over. *Nat Genet* **13**:336–342, 1996.
101. Baker SM, Bronner CE, Zhang L, et al: Male mice defective in the DNA mismatch repair gene PMS2 exhibit abnormal chromosome synapsis in meiosis. *Cell* **82**:309–319, 1995.
102. Suzuki H, Harpaz N, Tarmin L, et al: Microsatellite instability in ulcerative colitis-associated colorectal dysplasias and cancers. *Cancer Res* **54**:4841–4844, 1994.
103. Brentnall TA, Rubin CE, Crispin DA, et al: A germline substitution in the human MSH2 gene is associated with cancer and high grade dysplasia in ulcerative colitis. *Gastroenterology* **109**:151–155, 1995.
104. Brentnall TA, Crispin DA, Bronner MP, et al: Microsatellite instability is present in non-neoplastic mucosa from patients with long-standing ulcerative colitis. *Cancer Res* **56**:1237–1240, 1996.
105. Samowitz WS, Slattery ML, and Kerber RA: Microsatellite instability in human colonic cancer is not a useful clinical indicator of familial colorectal cancer. *Gastroenterology* **109**:1765–1771, 1995.
106. Froggatt NJ, Koch J, Davies R, et al: Genetic linkage analysis in hereditary non-polyposis colon cancer syndrome. *J Med Genet* **32**:352–357, 1995.
107. Luce MC, Marra G, Chauhan DP, et al: In vitro transcription/translation assay for the screening of hMLH1 and hMSH2 mutations in familial colon cancer. *Gastroenterology* **109**:1368–1374, 1995.
108. Hall NR, Taylor GR, Finan PJ, et al: Intron splice acceptor site sequence variation in the hereditary non-polyposis colorectal cancer gene hMSH2. *Eur J Cancer* **30**A:1550–1552, 1994.
109. Charbonnier F, Martin C, Scotte M, et al: Alternative splicing of MLH1 messenger RNA in human normal cells. *Cancer Res* **55**:1839–1841, 1995.
110. Xia L, Shen W, Ritacca F, et al: A truncated hMSH2 transcript occurs as a common variant in the population: Implications for genetic diagnosis. *Cancer Res* **56**:2289–2292.
111. Marra G, and Boland CR: DNA repair and colorectal cancer, in Colorectal Neoplasia, Part I: The Scientific Basis for Current Management, G*astroenterology Clinics of North America*, Philadelphia, W.B. Saunders, **25**:4 (in press, 1996).
112. Lahti MN, Sistonen P, Mecklin JP, et al: Close linkage to chromosome 3p and conservation of ancestral founding haplotype in hereditary nonpolyposis colorectal cancer families. *Proc Natl Acad Sci USA* **91**:6054–6058, 1994.
113. Lahti MN, Kristo P, Nicolaides NC, et al: Founding mutations and Alu-mediated recombination in hereditary colon cancer. *Nat Med* **1**:1203–1206, 1995.
114. Watson P, Vasen HFA, Mecklin JP, et al: The risk of endometrial cancer in hereditary nonpolyposis colorectal cancer. *Am J Med* **96**:516–520, 1994.
115. Aarnio M, Mecklin JP, Aaltonen LA, et al: Life-time risk of different cancers in hereditary non-polyposis colorectal cancer (HNPCC) syndrome. *Int J Cancer* **64**:430–433, 1995.
116. Sankila R, Aaltonen La, Jarvinen HJ, et al: Better survival rates in patients with MLH1-associated hereditary colorectal cancer. *Gastroenterology* **110**:682–687, 1996.
117. Jarvinen HJ, Mecklin JP, and Sistonen P: Screening reduces colorectal cancer rate in families with hereditary nonpolyposis colorectal cancer. *Gastroenterology* **108**:1405–1411, 1995.
118. Ahlquist D: Aggressive polyps in hereditary nonpolyposis colorectal cancer: Targets for screening. *Gastroenterology* **108**:1590–1591, 1995.

119. Hall NR, Finan PJ, Ward B, et al: Genetic susceptibility to colorectal cancer in patients under 45 years of age. *Br J Surg* **81**:1485–1489, 1994.

120. Liu B, Farrington SM, Petersen GM, et al: Genetic instability occurs in the majority of young patients with colorectal cancer. *Nat Med* **1**:348–352, 1995.

121. Vasen HFA, Wijnen JT, Menko FH, et al: Cancer risk in families with hereditary nonpolyposis colorectal cancer diagnosed by mutation analysis. *Gastroenterology* **110**:1020–1027, 1996.

122. Kolodner RD, Hall NR, Lipford J, et al: Structure of the human MSH2 locus and analysis of two Muir-Torre kindreds for msh2 mutations. *Genomics* **24**:516–526, 1994.

123. Liu B, Parsons RE, Hamilton SR, et al: *hMSH2* Mutations in hereditary nonpolyposis colorectal cancer kindreds. *Cancer Res* **54**: 4590–4594, 1994.

124. Vasen HFA, Nagengast FM, Khan PM: Interval cancers in hereditary non-polyposis colorectal cancer (Lynch syndrome). *Lancet* **345**: 1183–1184, 1995.

125. Menko FH, Te Meerman GJ, Sampson JR: Variable age of onset in hereditary nonpolyposis colorectal cancer: Clinical implications. *Gastroenterology* **104**:946–949, 1993.

126. Mecklin JP, Jarvinen HJ: Clinical features of colorectal carcinoma in cancer family syndrome. *Dis Colon Rect* **29**:160–164, 1986.

CHAPTER 18

Werner Syndrome

Gerard D. Schellenberg ▪ Tetsuro Miki ▪ Chang-En Yu ▪ Jun Nakura

1. Werner syndrome (WS) is a rare autosomal recessive disorder that is observed in many different ethnic groups. Prevalence estimates range from 1 to 22,000 to 1 in 1,000,000. All cases of WS appear to be inherited and to result from mutations at a single locus.

2. WS is characterized clinically by the premature appearance of cataracts, scleroderma-like skin pathology, short stature, graying hair and hair loss, and a general appearance of premature aging. Other, more variable features include adult-onset diabetes mellitus, hypogonadism, osteoporosis, osteosclerosis, soft-tissue calcification, hyperkeratosis, ulcers on the feet and ankles, premature vascular disease, elevated rates of some neoplasms, a hoarse high-pitched voice, and flat feet. Subjects often appear 20 to 30 years older than their chronologic age. Thus, WS may be a model disease for accelerated aging. The mean age at death is 47 years, with the leading cause being neoplasia, followed by myocardial infarcts and cerebral vascular incidents.

3. WS subjects are at increased risk for a variety of neoplasms. This increased risk results primarily from an increase in non-epithelial-derived cancers and is not an across-the-board elevation in all common cancers. Soft-tissue sarcomas, osteosarcomas, melanomas, and thyroid cancer are the predominant forms of cancer observed.

4. The gene for WS (*WRN*) is located on chromosome 8p12 and was recently identified by positional cloning methods. The *WRN* gene encodes a 1432-amino acid protein (WRN-H), which shows homology to the superfamily of DExH box DNA and RNA helicases; WRN-H has the seven motifs found in this class of protein, including the ATP-binding site and a Mg^{2+}-binding motif. Outside the helicase domain, WRN-H does not show homology to other known genes.

5. Mutations have been identified in the *WRN* gene in all WS subjects studied. All the mutations identified result in a nonsense mutation or a frameshift, leading to a predicted truncated protein product. One splice-junction mutation is found in 60 percent of Japanese WS subjects.

6. The function of WRN-H is not known. WS is a genomic instability syndrome with elevated rates of chromosomal translocation and deletions and an elevated somatic cell mutation rate. This mutator phenotype does not result from a defect in any known DNA repair system. Thus, WRN-H probably is not a component of a known DNA repair system. A dysfunctional *WRN* gene may result in the generation of mutations by an unknown mechanism rather than failure to repair DNA damage. DNA-synthesis abnormalities and DNA ligation may also be abnormal in WS cells. The role of the defective WRN-H in WS remains to be determined.

Werner syndrome (WS) is a rare autosomal recessive disease that was initially described in 1904 by Otto Werner in his doctoral thesis.[1,2] As a medical student in an ophthalmologic clinic, Werner described a family with two brothers and two sisters, ages 31, 36, 38, and 40 years, with bilateral cataracts, sclerodermal skin changes, hyperkeratosis, and ulcers on the feet and ankles. He observed that one 36-year-old gave "the impression of extreme senility," thus hinting in this early work at the potential connection between WS and accelerated aging.[2] In 1934, Oppenheimer and Kugel[3] extended the description of the disease and gave it the eponym *Werner's syndrome*. Thannhauser, in a classic article published in 1945, described many of the clinical features now associated with WS.[4]

The WS phenotype is complex, age-dependent, and variable (Figs. 18-1 and 18-2). Affected subjects are typically normal

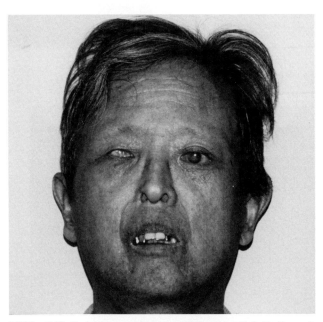

FIG. 18-1 A 51-year-old Japanese WS patient (definite diagnosis by the criteria in Table 18-3) with a known *WRN* mutation.

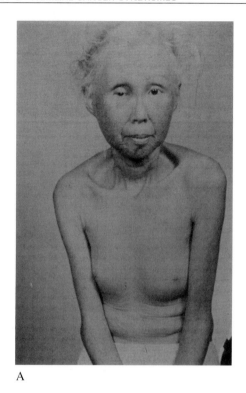

A

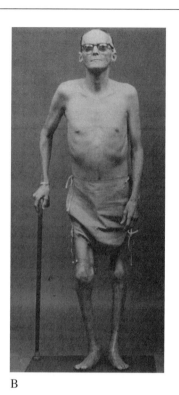

B

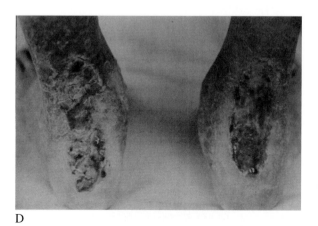

C

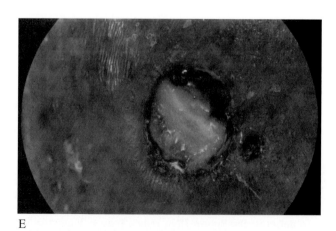

D

E

FIG. 18-2 *A.* A 48-year-old Japanese woman with WS (case 1 in Epstein et al.[6]). *B.* A 51-year-old Caucasian man with WS. Subject has typical thin limbs with normal trunk with scleroderma-like skin atro-phy of the lower legs and feet. *C.* Skin atrophy of the feet and ankles. *D.* and *E.* Ulcers on the ankles.

throughout childhood and early adolescence, with the only symptoms being growth retardation occurring at or near puberty. Beginning in the second and third decades of life, graying and loss of hair begin, and scleroderma-like changes occur typically on the face, legs, and feet. In the fourth and subsequent decades, WS individuals develop many of the diseases which are common in the elderly, including arteriosclerotic vascular disease, neoplasms, diabetes mellitus, osteoporosis, and bilateral cataracts (for reviews of the clinical features of WS, see Refs. 4 through 9). WS individuals often are described as having a "senile" appearance and typically look 20 to 30 years older than their true chronologic age.

Over the past 20 to 30 years, the biochemistry, cell biology, and genetics of WS have been studied intensively. The vigor with which this disorder has been pursued is not based on its importance to public health, since WS is quite rare. The appearance of premature aging has led to the proposal that WS is a partial model of accelerated human aging.[10] Parallels between WS and aging are also based on in vitro studies of cell growth potential. In fibroblasts from normal subjects, the number of doublings a culture is capable of before senescence occurs is inversely proportional to the age of the donor, cultures from children have a cumulative cell-doubling capacity of approximately 50 divisions, while cultures from elderly donors are capable of only 30 to 40 divisions.[7,11] In contrast, WS fibroblasts have a very limited potential for division, with a mean cumulative doubling of only 12.4.[7,12] Thus, WS has been studied in the hope WS also may provide clues to how aging processes contribute to susceptibility to some of the common diseases of old age.

Another feature of WS which has generated substantial interest is the fact that WS subjects have an elevated risk for a wide variety of cancers[13] and that WS cells exhibit genomic instability. Genomic instability has been demonstrated both in vitro and in vivo as an elevated somatic cell mutation rate,[14–17] as well as increased rates of apparently random chromosomal breakage, deletions, and rearrangements.[18–23] A number of other inherited disorders also exhibit the combination of genomic instability and elevated cancer risks (see Chaps. 13, 14, 15, and 17 for discussions of xeroderma pigmentosum, ataxia-telangiectasia, Bloom syndrome, and hereditary nonpolyposis colorectal cancer, respectively). The study of Li-Fraumeni syndrome (Chap. 20), a rare inherited disorder characterized by familial aggregation of a variety of primary cancers,[24] led to the characterization of P53 as a critical factor in cell cycle control and monitoring of DNA damage and repair. The study of WS and other inherited cancer-susceptibility disorders may provide additional clues to the mechanisms of cancer development.

In the past year, positional cloning methods have been used to identify the gene responsible for WS[25] (the *WRN* gene). This gene encodes a predicted protein with substantial homology to a super-family of enzymes termed helicases, which unwind double-stranded RNA or DNA into single strands. Now that the *WRN* gene has been identified, it should be possible to design experimental approaches to directly address questions concerning the relationship of WS to aging and age-related disease processes.

CLINICAL ASPECTS OF WERNER SYNDROME

Prevalence

Prevalence estimates for WS are difficult to obtain because the disorder is extremely rare, a fact which makes case finding difficult. In addition, since the appearance of the full phenotypic spectrum of WS is not complete until the third and fourth decades of life (average age at diagnosis is 38.7 years[6]), younger subjects may be missed. Two methods have been used to generate prevalence and gene-frequency estimates. The first is simple case counting in defined populations. This method depends on case identification by community physicians. Since WS is rare and many physicians may not be familiar with the disorder, underdiagnosis may result and the true prevalence may be underestimated. Also, the number of cases actually identified is typically small, making the estimates inaccurate. The second method for estimating prevalence is based on comparing consanguinity rates in the parents of WS subjects to estimates of consanguinity rates in the general population.[26,27] This method depends on accurate estimates of consanguinity in the general population. Consanguinity rates are difficult to measure and may vary even within an ethnic group or country, depending on whether the cases come from rural or urban settings.[28] Case-counting methods have yielded estimates ranging from 1 in 95,000 to 1 in 455,000 (Table 18-1), corresponding to allele frequencies of 0.0032 and 0.0015, respectively.[5,29] Prevalence estimates based on consanguinity rates range from 1 in 22,000 to 1 in 1,000,000, corresponding to allele frequencies of 0.0067 and 0.001, respectively.[5,6,29] Now that the gene has been cloned, populations can be screened directly for specific mutations[25] and direct measurements of carrier frequencies can be obtained. In a preliminary study, 178 Japanese control subjects were screened for the most common Japanese WS mutation (mutation 4 in Table 18-2) by direct DNA sequencing. This mutation appears to account for 60 percent of all Japanese WS cases. A single heterozygote was identified, yielding an allele frequency of 0.0027 with a 95 percent upper confidence limit of 0.008.[25] Since this mutation appears to account for 60 percent (18 of 30) of the WS cases studied, the allele frequency for all WS alleles should be approximately 0.0045, This frequency estimate is within the range of estimates (0.001 to 0.0067) obtained by the methods described above. Additional studies with a larger sample are needed to establish reliable allele frequency estimates for WS mutations.

Fraction of Werner Syndrome That is Due to Inherited Factors

There is no evidence that WS is genetically or etiologically heterogeneous. The genetic mapping studies discussed below suggest that the WS trait in different ethnic groups is caused by the same locus on chromosome 8.[30,31] Subsequent identification of the gene has permitted mutational analysis; to date, mutations in this gene, either in the homozygous state or as compound heterozygotes, have been identified in all the patients studied.[32,33] Thus, all WS appears to be

Table 18-1 Estimates of Prevalence Rates for WS

Population	Case-Counting Based Estimates	Consanguinity-Based Estimates	Reference
Caucasian (Sardinian)	1/95,000 to 1/203,000	1/93,000 to 1/455,000	29
Japanese	1/300,000 to 1/500,000	1/22,000 to 1/370,000	5
Mostly Caucasian		1/45,000 to 1/1,000,000	6

Table 18-2 Summary of *WRN* Mutations

Mutation	Codon	Exon	Type of Mutation	Nucleotide Sequence	Comment	Predicted Protein Length (aa)
None	—	—	—	—	—	1432
1	1165	30	Substitution	CAG (Gln) to **T**AG (terminator)	Nonsense	1164
2	1305	33	Substitution	CGA (Arg) to **T**GA (terminator)	Nonsense	1304
3	1230–1273	32	4-bp deletion	**gtag-AC**AG to gt-AG	4-bp deletion at splice-donor site	1247
4	1047–1078	26	Substitution	tag-GGT to ta**c**-GGT	Substitution at splice-donor site	1060

inherited. No WS phenocopies have been documented. The existence of new mutations on a heterozygous background cannot be ruled out. While a subject's environment may influence the expression of various components of the WS phenotype, there is no evidence that there is sporadic WS induced by environmental factors.

Diagnostic Criteria

There are no generally accepted standard diagnostic criteria for WS, although several have been used in research. The clinical picture of WS has been developed from case studies of subjects who are frequently in their thirties or forties. Since an early diagnosis usually is not possible, the onset of features such as growth cessation and graying of the hair is estimated retrospectively, depends on the subject's recollections, and may not be precise. Further, cohorts of WS subjects have not been followed longitudinally until death with subsequent autopsies; thus estimates of late-onset features such as vascular disease, diabetes mellitus, and neoplasms may be too low. Estimates of the prevalence of a particular feature can vary considerably. For example, estimates of the percentage of WS patients with vascular disease vary from 25 percent[6] to 100 percent.[29] This variability may reflect the ages of the patient groups studied, different environmental influences (e.g., diet), or differing genetic backgrounds in different ethnic groups. Despite the limitations of the data collected, the clinical description of WS discussed below is remarkably consistent across the large numbers of WS cases which have been described in the literature. The reader is referred to Epstein et al.[6] for an excellent detailed description of the clinical and pathologic findings in a large number of WS subjects.

Two different criteria for diagnosis have been used in research on WS. The criteria used by Nakura et al.[32] (Table 18-3) consist of six primary features found in most WS subjects and an additional nine symptoms that are found less consistently. A diagnosis of "definite" requires all six cardinal symptoms (number 6, when available) and two of the less frequent features. "Probable" WS requires the first three cardinal signs and any two others. One limitation of these criteria is that hyaluronic acid analysis is not routinely available. Also, while parental consanguinity is a useful indicator of recessive inheritance, the majority of Caucasian subjects (64 percent[6]) and many Japanese subjects (20 to 32 percent[34,35]) are not from consanguineous families. Goto and coworkers[30] used a similar set of criteria (Table 18-4), and a diagnosis of WS requires that a subject have three of the four major symptom groups.

Features Found in Most Patients

Cataracts. Perhaps the most constant feature of WS is cataracts (Fig. 18-1), which have been reported to be present in 94 to 100 percent of the subjects studied (Table 18-3).[6,7,35] Cataracts typically appear in the third decade of life. In different case-review studies, the observed mean age at appearance was between 23 years[35] and 30 years.[6] Cataracts are usually bilateral, though they may be at different stages of development in each eye, and are typically indistinguishable from those seen in elderly subjects (see Ref. 6 for a detailed review of ocular pathologies).

Dermatologic Pathology. By the second decade of life most WS subjects have skin with a scleroderma-like appearance. The skin is tight, shiny, and smooth as a result of both dermal atrophy and loss of underlying connective tissue, muscle, and subcutaneous fat tissue.[4,6,34,45] Sites of abnormal skin include the upper and lower limbs; the ankles and feet are particularly severely affected. Atrophy of facial tissues results in the typical "birdlike" appearance with a sharp nose but relatively full cheeks. Hyperkeratosis also occurs, often resulting in ulcers on the feet and ankles. Ulceration can be severe (Fig. 18-2), causing gangrene; amputation is sometimes required. Other skin abnormalities include general hyperpigmentation, areas of hypopigmentation, telangiectasia (36 percent of subjects), nail deformity (42 percent of subjects), and in general thin, dry skin.

Stature and Habitus. Short stature is another feature typical of WS and is observed in most subjects (86 to 100 percent[34,35]). In Japanese subjects, males range in height from 137 to 161 cm (mean, 151 to 152 cm) and females range from 122 to 151 cm (mean, 131.7 to 144.2 cm). Non-Japanese (primarily Caucasian[6]) subjects are somewhat taller, with reported means of 157 cm (5 ft 1 in.) and 146 cm (4 ft 9 1/2 in.) for males and females, respectively. Growth arrest appears during early adolescence (between 10 and 20 years) and appears to result from the lack of a growth spurt at puberty. The short stature is accompanied by low body weight. While many body features are proportional to the subject's size, a consistent feature is thin limbs with a stocky trunk, which are observed in 76 to 100 percent of the subjects studied.[34,35] Muscle atrophy in the limbs is consistently observed. Despite the short stature, thyroid-stimulating hormone and growth hormone levels appear to be normal in adults.[35]

Graying and Loss of Hair. The hair of WS subjects often begins to turn gray in late adolescence, although gray hair can appear as early as 5 years of age.[6,34,35] This feature is perhaps one of the earliest symptoms (Table 18-3). With time, the hair often becomes completely white. Loss of scalp and eyebrow hair and loss of eyelashes occur along with graying of the hair. The combination of the sparse gray or white hair and the dermal atrophy described above gives WS subjects the physical appearance of someone 20 to 30 years older than their chronologic age.

Table 18-3 Signs of WS

Feature	Mean Age of Onset (years)	Onset Range (years)	Number of Patients Affected (%)
Cardinal Signs			
1. Bilateral cataracts	23–30	10–46	94–100
2. Dermatological pathology (tight skin, atrophic skin, pigmentary alterations, ulceration, hyperkeratosis, regional subcutaneous atrophy), characteristic "bird" facies.	23, 25	5–42	86–100
3. Short stature	13	10–20	86–100
4. Consanguinity (3d cousin or greater) or affected sibling	N.A.	N.A.	68
5. Premature graying and/or thinning of scalp hair	20–21	5–42	80–100
6. Positive hyaluronic acid test	N.A.D.	N.A.D.	100
Further Signs and Symptoms			
1. Diabetes mellitus	30–34[6,104,35]	10–55	44–67*
2. Hypogonadism (secondary sexual underdevelopment, diminished fertility, testicular or ovarian atrophy)		N.A.	N.A.
3. Osteoporosis	N.A.D.	N.A.D.	33–100
4. Osteosclerosis of distal phalanges of fingers and/or toes (X-ray diagnosis)	N.A.D.	N.A.D.	N.A.D.
5. Soft tissue calcification	N.A.D.	N.A.D.	25–53
6. Premature atherosclerosis (e.g., history of myocardial infarction)	N.A.D.	N.A.D.	25–100
7. Mesenchymal neoplasms, rare neoplasms, or multiple neoplasms	N.A.D.	20–64†	N.A.D.
8. Voice changes (high-pitched squeaky or hoarse voice)	21–27	10–40	50–100
9. Flat feet		N.A.D.	N.A.D.

*Percent affected given includes subjects with impaired glucose tolerance.
†Range given is for all cancers.
N.A.D. = no available data; N.A. = not applicable.
Note: Diagnostic criteria are reproduced from Nakura et al.[32] (with permission from *Genomics*) and categories are as follows: Definite, all cardinal signs (number 6 when available) and any two others; probable, the first three cardinal signs and any two others; possible, either cataracts or dermatological alterations and any four others; exclusion, onset of signs and symptoms before adolescence (except short stature) or a negative hyaluronic acids test.
Data on prevalence estimates of symptoms and onset means are primarily from several case-report summaries.[6,29,35–39] as summarized by Tollefsbol and Cohen.[7]

Excess Urinary Hyaluronic Acid. Excess hyaluronic acid (HA) in WS subjects' urine has been repeatedly observed.[34–39] Urinary HA was first identified in the analysis of urine for the connective-tissue breakdown product acid glycosaminoglycans. While acid glycosaminoglycan levels were normal, HA was high. HA levels are also elevated in Hutchinson-Gilford syndrome (progeria),[36] an-

other disorder often mentioned as an accelerated aging disorder. HA is absent or is present in low levels in normal subjects.[40]

Features Found in a Subset of Patients

The following signs and symptoms are observed in a subset of patients. As was discussed above, the frequencies of some of these features may represent underestimates. In terms of morbidity and mortality, vascular disease and cancers are the most important; cancers, followed by myocardial and cerebrovascular accidents, are the most common causes of premature death (the average age at death for all causes is 47 years[6]).

Table 18-4 WS Diagnostic Criteria of Goto*

1. Characteristic habitus and stature	Short stature
	Low body weight
	Thin limbs with a stocky trunk
	Beak-shaped nose
2. Premature senescence	Birdlike appearance
	Loss of hair
	Skin hyperpigmentation
	Hoarse voice
	Diffuse arteriosclerosis
	Juvenile bilateral cataracts
	Osteoporosis
3. Scleroderma-like skin changes	Atrophic skin and muscle
	Hyperkeratosis
	Telangiectasia
	Tight skin over the bones of the feet
	Skin ulcers
	Localized calcification
4. Endocrine abnormalities	Diabetes mellitus
	Hypogonadism

*A diagnosis of WS requires three of the four criteria listed in the table.
SOURCE: Adapted from Goto et al.[30]

Hypogonadism. Secondary sexual underdevelopment is a fairly common finding in WS subjects, occurring in 66 percent[35] to 96 percent[29] of the subjects studied. In males, small genitalia and sparse pubic hair are common though not universal. WS women have poorly developed genitalia with small uteruses. In about half the women studied, breasts were small, atrophic, or underdeveloped.[6] Both men and women with hypogonadism have had children, though fertility is reduced. The onset of menses ranged from 9 to 20 years (mean, 13.9 years; $n = 35$). Menstruation frequently ceases prematurely (18 to 45 years, mean = 33 years) before menopause.[6]

Osteoporosis and Soft-Tissue Calcification. Osteoporosis is observed in a subset of WS subjects, often occurring most dramatically in the lower limbs, feet, and ankles and to a less extent in the upper limbs and spine. The rest of the trunk and the skull typically show less severe or no osteoporosis. In case series of Japanese and

Caucasian subjects who were typically about 40 years of age, 33 to 41 percent of subjects showed evidence of loss of bone mass. The exception to this observed prevalence was a study of WS in Sardinians in which all subjects ($n = 6$) showed osteoporosis.[29] Soft-tissue calcification is observed in WS often around the Achilles tendon and the knee and elbow tendons and in the ligaments and tissues surrounding these areas. Soft-tissue calcification of the hands and feet was also observed.

Diabetes Mellitus. A diabetic tendency is observed in 44 to 67 percent of WS subjects.[6,7,34,35,41] In one study of oral glucose tolerance, 55 percent were categorized as having diabetes mellitus and another 22 percent had impaired glucose tolerance. Fasting glucose levels are elevated in only a subset of cases with abnormal glucose tolerance tests, indicating that in WS, diabetes is mild; symptoms of polyuria, polydipsia, pruritus, and weight loss are rarely found.[6] Hyperglycemia is typically treated by dietary restriction. Complications typical of diabetes (nephropathy, retinopathy, and neuropathy) have not been reported for WS. Since some WS subjects show no diabetic tendencies, factors other than mutations in the *WRN* gene must contribute to the appearance of diabetes in these subjects.

Vascular Disease. Premature generalized vascular disease is a common feature in WS. Between 70 and 90 percent of patients show hypercholesterolemia and hypertriglyceridemia,[9,42,43] and most were classified (WHO criteria) as type IIb hyperlipidemia. Vascular calcification is observed, most frequently in the legs and feet. Clinical evidence of vascular disease was reported in 25 to 100 percent of WS subjects (average, 42 percent); the symptoms were abnormal electrocardiograms, congestive heart failure, angina, and infarction. In one autopsy series, all the subjects exhibited atherosclerosis beyond that expected for normals of the same age.[6] Calcification of coronary arteries and of the leaflets or rings of the mitral and/or aortic valves occurs in some subjects.

Neoplasia. WS subjects have an elevated risk of developing a wide variety of carcinomas and sarcomas.[6,13,23,24] The reported case histories of a large number of Japanese and Caucasian WS subjects have been comprehensively reviewed with respect to the prevalence of cancers.[13] In WS patients there was an overrepresentation of nonepithelial cancer, the ratio of epithelial to nonepithelial cancer was 1:1 versus 10:1 in the general population.[45] The most common cancers in the Japanese WS subjects were soft-tissue sarcomas, osteosarcomas, melanomas, and thyroid carcinomas; together, these accounted for 57 percent of cancers in WS patients versus 2 percent in the general Japanese population. Conservative estimates based on the incidence rates of these cancers in the general population and an estimated population of 5000 WS subjects in Japan (probably a considerable overestimate) suggest that the incidence of soft-tissue sarcomas is at least 20-fold higher in WS patients than in the general Japanese population. Acral lentiginous melanoma of the feet and nasal mucosa, the predominant form of melanoma observed in Japanese WS subjects, is extremely rare in Japan (0.16 cases per 100,000 people per year).[46] The osteosarcomas were also in excess of expected rates, with an unusual age distribution; 12 of the 13 cases observed occurred between the ages of 35 and 64 years, unlike the typical occurrence in the general population, where the incidence of osteosarcomas is highest in late adolescence. The thyroid carcinomas observed included both papillary (8 of 21 cases) and follicular carcinomas (10 of 21 cases). While papillary thyroid carcinomas are relatively common among the Japanese, follicular carcinomas are less common[47,48] and are proportionally in excess in WS subjects. In addition to the cancers mentioned above, a strikingly wide spectrum of isolated cases of other carcinomas is observed in WS. Benign meningiomas may be common in WS; in a case series of 147 neoplasias reported by Goto and coworkers,[13] there were 15 benign meningiomas. Whether this represents an elevated frequency among WS patients is not known.

The elevation in cancer incidence in WS is not simply an increase in all forms of neoplasms but rather a selective increase in some relatively rare cancers. Thus, WS is not an exact mimic of aging in terms of neoplasms. Consciously missing from the spectrum of cancers elevated in WS are some of the common epithelial malignancies, particularly prostate cancer, which in normal populations is very common in elderly men.

Central Nervous System. The central nervous system appears to be spared in most WS subjects.[6,49] Single cases of extensive cerebral atrophy[50] and a case of spastic paraparesis with polyneuropathy have been reported. Also, for a limited number of subjects, mild senile dementia and other mental disorders have been reported in 21 percent of the subjects studied.[35] Neuropathologic data are limited; analysis of two intellectually normal WS subjects, 51 and 57 years of age, did not reveal evidence of the Alzheimer disease-type changes (senile plaques and neurofibrillary tangles) typically associated with normal aging.[52] Additional work using more sensitive methods (e.g., antibodies to the Aβ protein and tau, the principal components of Alzheimer-type amyloid and neurofibrillary tangles, respectively) are needed to determine whether age-associated changes are found in the central nervous system of WS subjects.

Other Clinical Features of Werner Syndrome. In addition to the symptoms listed above, a subset (percent affected) of WS subjects have the following findings: flat feet (92 percent), irregular teeth (42 percent), hyperreflexia (79 percent), and a hoarse, high-pitched voice (83 percent; mean age of onset 21 to 27 years) caused by thickening and ulceration of the vocal cords.[4–7,9,34,35]

THE WERNER SYNDROME GENE

Pattern of Inheritance

The first cases of WS reported by Otto Werner in 1904 were familial, and subsequently numerous pedigrees with multiple affected sibs were described. The parents of WS subjects are rarely affected, though several pedigrees with parent-child WS pairs have been reported.[5,9] Thannhauser in 1945 suggested that the inheritance of WS is recessive because of the high rate of consanguinity in the families of WS patients.[4] Elevated rates of consanguinity in WS case series have been consistently observed in studies of both Japanese and Caucasians. Another line of evidence that WS is recessive is provided by the results of segregation analysis. In a study of WS pedigrees by Epstein et al.,[6] estimates of the percentage of affected offspring produced by unaffected parents range from 17.9 ± 2.5 percent to 26.5 ± 3.2 percent, depending on the method used to correct for ascertainment bias. These estimates are close to the 25 percent value expected for a recessively inherited disease. Thus, WS is clearly a recessively inherited disorder, a conclusion subsequently supported by mutational analysis of WS subjects.[25] WS is found equally in both sexes, and there does not appear to be a birth-order effect.[6]

GENETIC LOCALIZATION OF THE WERNER SYNDROME GENE

By the end of the 1980s extensive in vitro biochemical and biologic studies had been performed, but the primary defect responsible for WS has not been identified. Fortunately, genetic mapping methods and resources had been sufficiently developed by that time[53,54] that localization of disease loci for inherited disorders was highly feasible provided that a sufficient number of families could be identified.

Homozygosity Mapping

The genetic mapping of most inherited diseases has involved the use of multigeneration families with multiple affected subjects available for sampling. In these pedigrees, cosegregation of polymorphic marker alleles with the disease phenotype can be used to identify genetic markers in the vicinity of the target gene. For WS, few multiplex families suitable for mapping studies were available. Therefore, to obtain a pedigree collection with sufficient power to localize and eventually clone the WS gene, families were included which consisted of a single affected individual who was the offspring of a consanguineous marriage. (Parents from these families were rarely available.) In this approach, which is called homozygosity mapping,[55,56] only the affected individual from an inbred family needs to be sampled (Fig. 18-3). Since the disease allele comes from the same original chromosome, closely flanking polymorphic markers will come from the same parental chromosome and will be identical (homozygous) in the affected subject. In the region of the disease gene. WS subjects should exhibit excess homozygosity relative to outbred controls. Data from both consanguineous and outbred pedigrees can be analyzed together by using conventional maximum-likelihood methods. The extent to which the region of homozygosity surrounding the disease locus is conserved is determined by the number of recombination events occurring in the meioses between the pedigree founder and the affected subject. The use of affected subjects from consanguineous pedigrees is highly efficient; for example, if one samples a single case from a first-cousin marriage, recombination events from five different meioses can be evaluated (Fig. 18-3).

Two factors can confound homozygosity mapping, particularly when fine-scale localization of a gene is attempted. The first factor is that both copies of the disease locus, and thus the surrounding markers, do not necessarily come from the single founder at the top of the pedigree. For example, there are three places in the first-cousin pedigree shown in Fig. 18-3 (open arrows) where a carrier could introduce a second copy of the disease allele. Thus, there is a chance that the affected offspring of a consanguineous marriage will not be homozygous (not identical by descent) for the markers flanking the disease locus. The second confounding factor is that the genetic marker loci that are used to detect homozygosity can mutate, resulting in the generation of a new allele. The result is heterozygosity at a marker for which both copies were from the same great-grandparental chromosome. The short tandem repeat polymorphism (STRP) markers commonly used for mapping studies are particularly prone to new mutations.[57] Since only the affected subject is typically available, heterozygosity by mutation cannot be distinguished from heterozygosity resulting from recombination.

Localization of the *WRN* Locus

The *WRN* locus was initially localized by using a combination of 8 outbred families and 13 consanguineous pedigrees, all from Japan.[30] A large number of markers were genotyped, spanning much of the genome, and the data were analyzed by conventional maximum-likelihood methods; markers at 8p11.1-21.1 (Fig. 18-4) showed significant cosegregation with the WS phenotype. This localization was confirmed by heterozygosity mapping methods using primarily single affected subjects from a series of Japanese

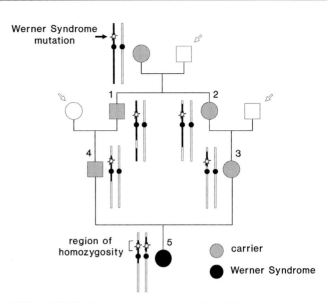

FIG. 18-3 First-cousin marriage pedigree illustrating homozygosity mapping. Chromosome pairs illustrate the narrowing of the region of homozygosity by recombination. Open arrows show where a second copy of the mutated gene can enter the pedigree. Numbers 1 through 5 indicate the five meioses of the pedigree.

consanguineous families.[31] Significant positive-linkage results were also obtained with a panel of nine non-Japanese WS subjects who were primarily Caucasians.[32]

Initial mapping studies placed the *WRN* locus in a broad region from D8S137 to ANK1,[30–32,58,59] an interval spanning 16.6 cM[60,61] (Fig. 18-4). Assignment of the *WRN* locus to this interval was based both on observed recombinants and on multipoint analysis.[32] Marker D8S339 was the closest marker showing the least recombination with WS. The D8S137-ANK1 interval contained relatively few known genes, which included heregulin (HRB), fibroblast growth factor receptor 1 (FGFR1), and DNA polymerase-β. FGFR1 and HRG were excluded by recombination events between these genes and WS in affected subjects. The *pol*-β gene was excluded by DNA sequence analysis (no mutations were found[62]) and by radiation hybrid mapping, which placed the gene outside the D8S137-ANK1 region.[61]

High-Resolution Mapping of the *WRN* Gene

Fine mapping of the *WRN* locus became possible when STRP markers in linkage disequilibrium with WS were identified.[63] The first marker found that showed linkage disequilibrium with WS was at the glutathione reductase (*GSR*) gene. *GSR* had previously been assigned to chromosome 8 by somatic cell hybrid mapping but had not been mapped to a specific region of the chromosome.[64] During the process of mapping *GSR* as a candidate gene, two STRP loci were identified in a cosmid clone containing the gene; in a group of 17 Japanese subjects, both *GSR* markers had alleles which showed significant evidence ($p <0.0025–0.001$) of linkage disequilibrium with the *WRN* gene.[63] Subsequent analysis of other markers in the region demonstrated that D8S339 was also in disequilibrium with *WRN* in the same group of families, an observation confirmed in other studies.[65] *GSR* and D8S339 were subsequently found to be separated by approximately 200 kb (Fig. 18-5). Other markers flanking *GSR* and D8S339, including the clusters D8S131/D8S137 and D8S278/D8S87/D8S259/D8S283, were not in linkage disequilibrium with *WRN*.

To refine the location of the *WRN* gene, chromosome walking methods were used to clone DNA flanking D8S339/GSR. A YAC

Chromosome 8

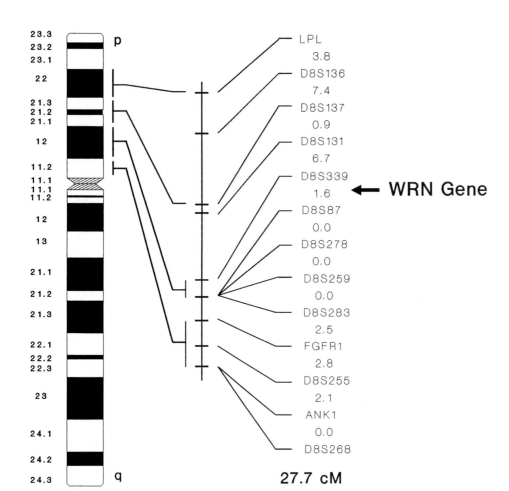

FIG. 18-4 *Genetic map of the WRN region of chromosome 8. Genetic distances are sex-equal and are given in centimorgans (cM). The total length of the map is given at the bottom. (From Oshima et al.[61] Used by permission of Genomics.)*

contig was constructed, using *GSR* as a starting point, and the contig was used as a source of cloned DNA for the identification of an additional 18 additional STRP loci (Fig. 18-5).[66–68] Genotype data from these markers were used in three different approaches in an attempt to narrow the WRN region. First, the markers were used to define recombinants in WS pedigrees. Definitive recombinants were identified at D8S2194/D8S2192 and at D8S2186. Second, the markers were tested for linkage disequilibrium to identify the boundaries of the region of linkage disequilibrium. In Japanese kindreds, markers D8S2196 and D8S2162 and many markers in between were in linkage disequilibrium with *WRN*, while D8S2194/D8S2192 and D8S2186 as well as more distant flanking markers (D8S131/D8S137 and D8S278/D8S259/D8S87/D8S283) were not.[69,70] Third, because markers in this region are in disequilibrium with *WRN*, many of subjects studied are presumed to be descendants of a common ancestor and thus should share a definable common haplotype. The genotype data from markers spanning the region were used to define a common ancestral haplotype and determine where ancestral recombinants had disrupted that haplotype.[63,70] The combined approach using these three methods yielded an interval of approximately 1.2 megabase (Mb) which contained the *WRN* gene.

Positional Cloning of the *WRN* Gene

The *WRN* gene was identified by positional cloning methods,[25] with the effort focused on the 1.2-Mb region indicated by the

above genetic studies. The YAC contig was converted to P1 clones, which are less prone to deletion and rearrangement artifacts. The P1 clones were used as a source of DNA to identify genes in the region, using exon trapping,[71,72] cDNA selection methods (hybridization of cDNA libraries to YAC and P1 clones[73,74]), and DNA sequence analysis (comparison of DNA sequence to the DNA sequence databases of known genes and potential expressed sequence-tagged sites[75]). Each of these methods yielded gene fragments which were then used to isolate full-length cDNA clones for each gene in the *WRN* region. Each gene was screened for mutations by reverse-transcriptase PCR methods or direct DNA sequence analysis of genomic DNA. A total of 10 genes were characterized and screened for mutations before the *WRN* gene was identified. These were *GSR*, protein phosphatase 2 catalytic subunit β (PPP2CB), general transcription factor IIEβ (GTF2E2), a β-tubullin pseudogene 1 (TUBBP1), and six previously unidentified genes of unknown function.

The *WRN* gene was initially identified as a match between the genomic DNA of a P1 and 245-bp sequence in the expressed sequence-tagged database.[25] This short sequence was used to identify a 5.2-kb full-length cDNA clone which encodes a predicted protein of 1432 amino acids. The same gene was also identified by exon trapping.[71,72] Comparison of the DNA sequence to known genes revealed a striking homology to genes in the superfamily of DNA and RNA helicases (Fig. 18-6). Thus, WS joins a list of inherited disorders caused by mutations in helicase genes. These disorders are xeroderma pigmentosum, complementation groups B[76] and D (helicases ERCC2 and ERCC3, respectively[77–81]), trichoth-

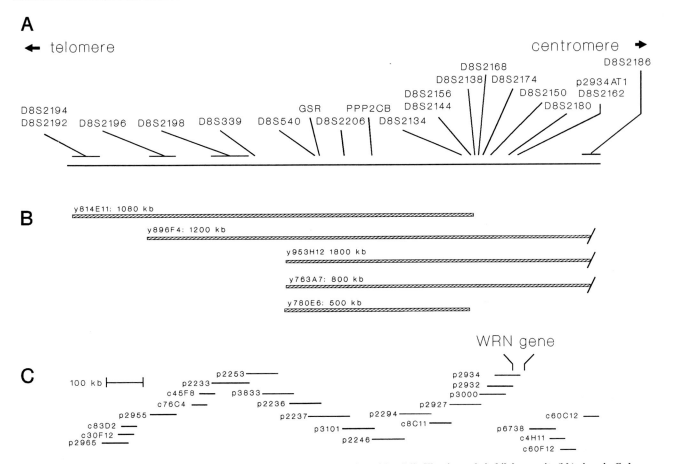

FIG. 18-5 Genetic markers, YACs, P1, and cosmid clones used in the positional cloning of the *WRN* gene. *A.* STRP loci; *B,* YAC clones; *C,* P1 clones (beginning with a "p") and cosmid clones (begin-ning with a "c"). The size scale in kilobase units (kb) given in *C* also applies to *A* and *B.* *(Reproduced from Yu et al.[68] Used by permission of Genomics.)*

iodystrophy (ERCC2[82,83]), Cockayne syndrome (helicase ERCC6,[84]), Bloom syndrome,[85] and X chromosome-linked α-tha-lassemia mental retardation syndrome.[86,87]

Mutational Analysis of the *WRN* Gene

During initial characterization of the gene, four mutations were identified in the 3′ end (Table 18-2).[25] Two (mutations 1 and 2) were single base substitution nonsense mutations which are pre-dicted to result in truncated proteins of 1164 and 1060, compared to 1432 for the normal protein product. Mutation 3 is a 4-bp dele-tion spanning an intron-exon splice junction (5′ acceptor site). The resulting mRNA does not lack the adjacent exon but rather uses a new splice acceptor site 4 bp 3′ to the original site. This mutation was observed in a single family from Syria. The result is a frameshift and a corresponding truncated protein product. The fourth mutation is a single base-pair substitution at a splice junc-tion which abolishes the site and results in skipping of the exon, a frameshift, and a resulting truncated protein (Fig. 18-6).

The first four mutations identified were in the 3′ end of the gene, and all leave the helicase consensus domain intact. This bias resulted from the 3′ being available for mutational analysis first. Since the helicase region contains the ATPase region of the protein and presumably is the enzymatic component of the helicase, 3′-truncated proteins could still retain DNA/RNA-unwinding activity.

To screen the middle and the 5′ end of the gene, the genomic structure of *WRN* was determined. The gene consists of 35 exons with the coding region beginning in the second exon[33] and spans a genomic region of at least 100 kb, although the actual size of the

gene is unknown. Five additional mutations were identified in the remainder of the gene. Two additional nonsense mutations and a splice-junction mutation were identified. Another mutation is a 1-bp deletion that results in a frameshift and a premature stop codon. The fifth mutation is a large genomic deletion (>15 kb) which probably occurred by a recombination event between two highly homologous Alu elements which are separated by 15 kb. Two of these mutations result in predicted truncated protein prod-ucts which do not contain the helicase domains. All mutations iden-tified to date result in a predicted truncated protein product, and no missense mutations have been identified in WS subjects. There is no indication that the severity of the disease correlates with the type of mutation observed. Identification of any phenotype–genotype relationships will require additional work.

Origins of *WRN* Mutations

The existence of a common Japanese founder was confirmed by mutational analysis. Among Japanese subjects, 60 percent had the same mutation (mutation 4). Most of these subjects had the 141-bp allele at *GSR* which was overrepresented in WS cases compared to controls (frequency, 0.40 and 0.07, respectively) and was therefore responsible for the linkage disequilibrium observed at *GSR*. Fur-ther, for two highly polymorphic STRP loci within the *WRN* gene [D8S2162 and p2934AT1 (Fig. 18-5)], haplotypes were identical for all mutation 2 carriers tested. Mutation 2 and a nonsense muta-tion in the 5′ end of the gene were observed in both Japanese and Caucasian subjects. For both mutations, different haplotypes for STRP markers within the *WRN* gene were observed, indicating an

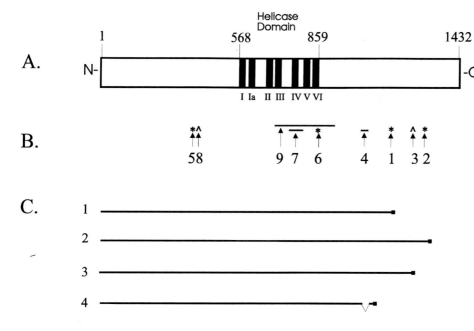

FIG. 18-6 The Werner syndrome helicase. *A.* Schematic diagram of WRN-H with the seven helicase motifs (I–VI) shown as solid bars. *B.* WS mutations: * = nonsense mutation; ^ = frameshift caused by a single base-pair deletion; gray lines = genomic deletions or exons skipped because of splice junction mutations. *C.* The predicted proteins from cDNA containing mutations 1–4. For 4, the break indicates a skipped exon.

independent origin.[33] However, a common founder cannot be completely excluded, since intragenic recombination or mutations at the STRP loci cannot be excluded.

Function of the *WRN* Gene Product. The predicted *WRN* gene product (WRN-H) is a member of a superfamily of DExH box DNA and RNA helicases. These DNA and RNA unwinding proteins share a common structure of seven motifs (I, Ia, II, III, IV, V, and VI) ranging in size from approximately 15 to 25 amino acids.[88] Motif I contains a nucleotide-binding site, and motif II has the DExH sequence of an Mg^{2+}-binding site (DEAH in the *WRN* gene); these sites presumably participate in the hydrolysis of ATP which occurs as the enzyme unwinds a helix. WRN-H shows homology to these seven motifs in helicases from a wide variety of organisms, including *Escherichia coli* (recQ), *Saccharomyces cerevisiae* (SgS1), *Caenorhabditis elegans* (F18C5C), and humans (RECQL).[25] The region of shared homology is in the center of WRN-H, spanning amino acids 540 to 963. The sequences in between the seven motifs are not conserved, although the spacing between motifs is highly conserved.

The amino terminal (amino acids 1–539) and C-terminal (amino acids 964–1432) of WRN-H are not homologous to other helicases or to other known proteins. The amino terminal end is highly acidic, containing 109 glutamate or aspartate residues, including one segment with 14 acidic residues in a stretch of 19 amino acids. Other than the helicase domain, the WRN-H amino acid sequence does not yield clues to the function of this protein. The homology between the predicted protein and other helicases strongly suggests that WRN-H is a functional helicase, although additional work is needed to demonstrate that the protein can unwind DNA or RNA.

The *WRN* Protein and Werner Syndrome

The normal function of WRN-H is unknown. It could function to unwind DNA during replication, repair, transcription, or any number of other transactions requiring duplex unwinding. Other helicases function as part of multiprotein complexes. For example, ERCC2 and ERCC3, which are defective in xeroderma pigmentosum, are part of the RNA polymerase II basal transcription factor (TFIIH).[89] ERCC6, the helicase defective in Cockayne syndrome group B subjects, interacts with the product of the CSA gene, which is mutated in Cockayne

syndrome group A subjects.[90] CSA in turn interacts with TFIIH. Thus, the Cockayne syndrome helicase may also interact with TFIIH. By analogy to these other helicases, WRN-H may interact with other proteins in a complex to perform its normal function in DNA metabolism. Since the N-terminal and C-terminal ends of each of these helicases are unique, presumably protein–protein interactions are dependent on the nonhelicase segments of the protein. Isolation of the other proteins which complex with WRN-H will be critical to understanding the function of this helicase.

Previous studies of the biology of WS have yielded limited information on the potential function of WRN-H. Two different lines of evidence indicate that WS cells have a mutator phenotype. First, both in vitro and in vivo studies demonstrate an elevated mutation rate using the hypoxanthine phosphoribosyltransferase gene as a reporter locus.[14–17] Characterization of the types of mutations which occur in WS cells indicates that the proportion of deletion mutations is elevated. These deletions may occur by nonhomologous recombination, since sequences of the deletions are not homologous.[17] The second indication of genomic instability is the elevated rate of random chromosomal rearrangements in WS cells, again observed both in vitro and in vivo.[18–23]

The WS mutator phenotype could result from a repair defect. For xeroderma pigmentosum and Cockayne syndrome, helicase defects result in faulty nucleotide excision repair and strand-specific transcription-coupled repair, respectively. However, for WS, no defect in DNA repair has been reproducibly demonstrated. Unscheduled DNA synthesis[91–93] and post-UV irradiation cell survival[94] are not defective in WS cells, and there is no increased sensitivity to a variety of DNA-damaging agents, including bleomycin, *cis*-dichlorodiamine platinum, diepoxybutane, isonicotinic acid hydrazide, and methyl methanesulfonate.[93–97] Sister-chromatid exchange is not elevated in WS cells, with or without treatment with clastogens.[96,98] However, there may be a DNA repair system that was not detected in the work cited above.

While no DNA repair defect has been detected, several other alterations in DNA metabolism have been reported. In DNA synthesis, reduced chain-elongation rates[91] and increased distances between synthesis initiation sites[99,100] have been reported. This reduced rate of DNA synthesis could be responsible for the prolonged S phase observed in WS cells. DNA ligation may be abnormal in WS cells.[99,101] While the rate of ligation is not altered, the accuracy of ligation events is reduced,[102,103] suggesting a possible mechanism for generating mutations. Elevated rates of homologous recombination also have been reported.[104] Whether the WRN helicase defect is directly responsible for any of these alterations in DNA handling remains to be determined. The primary mechanism by which defective helicase mutations give rise to the WS phenotype also remains to be determined.

IMPLICATIONS OF IDENTIFICATION OF THE *WRN* GENE FOR DIAGNOSIS

The diagnosis of WS can now potentially be definitively confirmed by mutational analysis of the *WRN* gene; WS subjects should be either homozygous or compound heterozygotes for mutations in this gene. In work to date, mutations have been identified in all subjects studied, including some with diagnoses of "probable" and "possible."[33] The mutational analysis confirms the usefulness of the clinical criteria outlined in Tables 18-3 and 18-4. The principal advantage of mutational analysis is that the diagnosis can be made at a young age, when WS is first suspected. In contrast, the mean age at diagnosis using clinical criteria is 37 years, because in some patients some of the defining symptoms do not develop until the third and fourth decades of life. Screening the *WRN* gene for mutations in Japanese subjects is simplified because one mutation accounts for 60 percent of the WS cases and two others make up an additional 33 percent. In Caucasians, it is not known what the frequencies of the different WS mutations are. Since the gene has 34 coding exons, complete analysis of the entire gene for a subject is expensive. The development of an in vitro protein truncation assay for WS should facilitate mutation detection. Because WS is such a rare disorder, it is unlikely that mutation screening will become universally available.

ACKNOWLEDGMENTS

We thank Thomas D. Bird, Mary T. Ersek, and Raymond J. Monnat for reading the text before publication. We also thank Charles J. Epstein for making some of the photographs available. This work was funded in part by grant RO1 AG12019 (GDS) from the National Institute on Aging. We also thank the WS subjects who participated in the research described here.

REFERENCES

1. Werner CWO: Udber kataract in Verbindung mit Sclerodermie. Doctoral dissertation, Kiel, Schmidt & Klarnig, West Germany, 1904.
2. Werner O (trans. H Hoehn): On cataract in conjunction with sclerodema. *Adv Exp Med Biol* **190**:1, 1985.
3. Oppenheimer BS, Kugel VH: Werner's syndrome, a heredofamilial disorder with scleroderma, bilateral juvenile cataracts, precocioius graying of the hair and endocrine stigmatization. *Trans Assoc Am Phys* **49**:358, 1934.
4. Thannhauser SJ: Werner's syndrome (progeria of the adult) and Rothmund's syndrome: Two types of closely related heredofamilial atrophic dermatoses with juvenile cataracts and endocrine features: A critical study with five new cases. *Ann Intern Med* **23**:559, 1945.
5. Goto M, Tanimoto K, Horiuchi Y, Sasazuki T: Family analysis of Werner's syndrome: A survey of 42 Japanese families with a review of the literature. *Clin Genet* **19**:8, 1981.
6. Epstein CJ, Martin GM, Schultz A, Motulsky AG: Werner's syndrome: A review of its symptomatology, natural history, pathologic features, genetics, and relationship to the natural aging process. *Medicine* **45**:177, 1966.
7. Tollefsbol TO, Cohen HJ: Werner's syndrome: An underdiagnosed disorder resembling premature aging. *Age* **7**:75, 1984.
8. Jacobson HG, Rifkin H, Zucker D: Werner's syndrome: A clinical entity. *Radiology* **74**:373, 1960.
9. Zucker-Franklin D, Rifkin H, Jacobson HG: Werner's syndrome: An analysis of ten cases. *Geriatrics* **23**:123, 1968.
10. Martin GM: Genetic syndromes in man with potential relevance to the pathobiology of aging. *Birth Defects* **14**:5, 1978.
11. Hayflick L: The limited in vitro lifetime of human diploid cell strains. *Exp Cell Res* **37**:614, 1965.
12. Martin GM, Sprague CA, Epstein CJ: Replicative life-span of cultivated human cells. *Lab Invest* **23**:86, 1970.
13. Goto M, Miller RW, Ishikawa Y, Sugano H: Excess of rare cancers in Werner syndrome (adult progeria). *Epidemiol Biomarkers Prevent* **5**:239, 1996.
14. Fukuchi K, Tanaka K, Nakura J, Kumahara Y, uchida T, Okada Y: Elevated spontaneous mutation rate in SV40 Werner syndrome fibroblast cell lines. *Somat Cell Molec Genet* **11**:303, 1985.
15. Fukuchi K, Martin GM, Monnat RJ: Mutator phenotype of Werner syndrome is characterized by extensive deletions. *Proc Natl Acad Sci USA* **86**:5893, 1989.
16. Fukuchi K, Tanaka K, Kumahara Y, Maramo K, Pride M, Martin GM, Monnet RJ: Increased frequency of 6/thioguanine peripheral blood lymphocytes in Werner syndrome patients. *Hum Genet* **84**:249, 1990.
17. Monnat RJ, Hackmann AFM, Chiaverotti TA: Nucleotide sequence analysis of human hypoxanthine phosphoribosyltransferase (HPRT) gene deletions. *Genomics* **13**:777, 1992.
18. Hoehn H, Bryant EM, Au K, Norwood TH, Boman H, Martin GM: Variegated translocation mosaicism in human skin fibroblast cultures. *Cytogenet Cell Genet* **15**:282, 1975.
19. Salk D, Hoehn H, Martin GM: Cytogenetics of Werner's syndrome cultured in skin fibroblasts: Variegated translocation mosaicism. *Hum Genet* **62**:16, 1982.
20. Salk D: Werner's syndrome: A review of recent research with an analysis of connective tissue metabolism, growth control of cultured cells, and chromosomal aberrations. *Hum Genet* **62**:1, 1982.
21. Salk D, Au K, Hoehn H, Martin GM: Cytogenetics of Werner's syndrome cultured skin fibroblasts: Variegated translocation mosaicism. *Cytogenet Cell Genet* **30**:92, 1981.
22. Scappaticci S, Cerimele D, Fraccaro M: Clonal structural chromosomal rearrangements in primary fibroblast cultures and in lymphocytes of patients with Werner's syndrome. *Hum Genet* **62**:16, 1982.
23. Salk D, Au K, Hoehn H, Martin GM: Cytogenetic aspects of Werner syndrome. *Adv Exp Med Biol* **190**:541, 1985.
24. Li FP, Fraumeni JF, Mulvihill JJ, Blattner WA, Dreyfus MG, Tucker MA, Miller RW: A cancer family syndrome in twenty-four kindreds. *Cancer Res* **48**:5358, 1988.
25. Yu CE, Oshima J, Fu YH, Wijsman EM, Hisama F, Alisch R, Matthews S, Nakura J, Miki T, Ouais S, Martin M, Mulligan J, Schellenberg GD: Positional cloning of the Werner's Syndrome gene. *Science* **272**:258, 1996.
26. Barrai I, Mi MP, Morton NE, Yasuda N: Estimation of prevalence under incomplete selection. *Am J Hum Genet* **17**:221, 1965.
27. Dahlberg G: Methods for population genetics. *Am J Biol* **25**:90, 1950.
28. Neal JV, Kodani MB, Brewer R, Anderson RC: The incidence of consanguineous matings in Japan: Remarks on the estimation of comparative gene frequencies and the expected rate of induced recessive mutations. *Am J Hum Genet* **1**:156, 1949.
29. Cerimele D, Cotton F, Scappaticci S, Rabbiosi G, Borroni G, Sanna E, Zei G, Fraccaro M: High prevalence of Werner's syndrome in Sardinia: Description of six patients and estimates of the gene frequency. *Hum Genet* **62**:25, 1982.
30. Goto M, Weber J, Woods K, Drayna D: Genetic linkage of Werner's syndrome to five markers on chromosome 8. *Nature* **355**:735, 1992.
31. Schellenberg GD, Martin GM, Wijsman EM, Nakura J, Miki T, Ogihara T: Homozygosity mapping and Werner's syndrome. *Lancet* **339**:1002, 1992.
32. Nakura J, Wijsman EM, Miki T, Kamino K, Yu CE, Oshima J, Fukuchi K, Weber JL, Piussan C, Saida T, Ogihara T, Martin GM, Schellenberg GD: Homozygosity mapping of the Werner syndrome locus (WRN). *Genomics* **23**:600, 1994.
33. Yu CE, Oshima J, Wijsman EM, Nakura J, Miki T, Puissan C, Matthews S, Fu Y-H, Mulligan J, Martin GM, Schellenberg GD: Werner's syndrome collaborative group: Mutations in the consensus

helicase domains of the Werner's syndrome gene. *Am J Hum Genet* **60**:330, 1997.

34. Goto M, Horiuchi Y, Tanimoto K, Ishii T, Nakashima H: Werner's syndrome: Analysis of 15 cases with a review of the Japanese literature. *J Am Geriatr Soc* **26**:341, 1978.

35. Murata K, Nakashima H: Werner's syndrome: Twenty-four cases with a review of the Japanese medical literature. *J Am Geriatr Soc* **30**:303, 1982.

36. Kieras FJ, Brown WT, Houck GE, Zebrower M: Elevation of urinary hyaluronic acid in Werner's syndrome and progeria. *Biochem Med Metab Biol* **36**:276, 1986.

37. Tokunaga M, Futami T, Wakamatsu E, Endo M, Yosizawa Z: Werner's syndrome as "hyaluronuria." *Clin Chim Acta* **62**:89, 1975.

38. Goto M, Murata K: Urinary excretion of macromolecular acidic glycosaminoglycans in Werner's syndrome. *Clin Chim Acta* **85**:101, 1978.

39. Murata K: Urinary acidic glycosaminoglycans in Werner's syndrome. *Experimentia* **38**:313, 1982.

40. Varada DP, Cifonelli JA, Dorfman A: The acid mucopolysaccharides in normal urine. *Biochem Biophys Acta* **141**:103, 1967.

41. Imura H, Nakao Y, Kuzuya H, Okamoto M, Okamoto M, Yamada K: Clinical, endocrine and metabolic aspects of the Werner syndrome compared with those of normal aging. *Adv Exp Med Biol* **190**:171, 1985.

42. Mori S, Yokote K, Morisaki N, Saito Y, Yoshida S: Inheritable abnormal lipoprotein metabolism in Werner's syndrome similar to familial hypercholesterolemia. *Eur J Clin Invest* **20**:137, 1990.

43. Goto M, Kato Y: Hypercoagulable state indicates an additional risk factor for atherosclerosis in Werner's syndrome. *Thromb Haemost* **73**:576, 1995.

44. Sato K, Goto M, Nishioka K, Arima K, Hori N, Yamashita N, Fujimoto Y, Nanko H, Olwawa K, Ohara K: Werner's syndrome associated with malignancies: Five cases with a survey of case histories in Japan. *Gerontology* **34**:212, 1988.

45. Miller RW, Myers MH: Age distribution of epithelial and non-epithelial cancers. *Lancet* **2**:1250, 1983.

46. Elwood JM: Epidemiology and control of melanoma in white populations and in Japan. *J Invest Dermatol* **92**:214, 1989.

47. Sampson RJ, Key CR, Buncher CR, Iijima S: Thyroid carcinoma at autopsy in Hiroshima and Nagasaki: I. Prevalence of thyroid cancer at autopsy. *JAMA* **209**:65, 1969.

48. Correa P, Chen VW: Endocrine gland cancer. *Cancer* **75**:338, 1995.

49. Postiglione A, Soricelli A, Covelli EM, Iazzetta N, Ruocco A, Milan G, Santoro L, Alfano B, Brunetti A: Premature aging in Werner's syndrome spares the central nervous system. *Neurobiol Aging* **17**:325, 1996.

50. Kakigi R, Endo C, Neshige R, Kohno H, Kuroda Y: Accelerated aging in the brain in Werner's syndrome. *Neurology* **42**:922, 1992.

51. Umehara F, Abe M, Nagawa M, Izumo S, Arimura K, Matsumuro K, Osame M: Werner's syndrome associated with spastic paraparesis and peripheral neuropathy. *Neurology* **43**:1252, 1993.

52. Sumi SM: Neuropathology of the Werner syndrome. *Adv Exp Med Biol* **190**:215, 1985.

53. Weissenbach J, Gyapay G, Dib C, Vignal A, Morissette J, Millasseau P, Vaysseix G, Lathrop M: A second generation linkage map of the human genome. *Nature* **359**:794, 1993.

54. NIH/CEPH Collaborative Mapping Group: A comprehensive genetic linkage map of the human genome. *Science* **258**:148, 1992.

55. Lander ES, Botstein D: Homozygosity mapping: A way to map human recessive traits with the DNA of inbred children. *Science* **236**:1567, 1987.

56. Smith CAB: Detection of linkage in human genetics. *J R Stat Soc B* **15**:153, 1953.

57. Weber JL, Wong C: Mutation of human short tandem repeats. *Hum Mol Genet* **2**:1123, 1993.

58. Ye L, Nakura J, Mitsuda N, Fujioka Y, Kamino K, Ohta T, Jinno Y, Niikawa N, Miki T, Ogihara T: Genetic association between chromosome 8 microsatellite (MS8-134) and Werner syndrome (WRN): Chromosome microdissection and homozygosity mapping. *Genomics* **28**:566, 1995.

59. Thomas W, Rubenstein M, Goto M, Drayna D: A genetic analysis of the Werner syndrome region on human chromosome 8p. *Genomics* **16**:685, 1993.

60. Tomfohrde J, Wood S, Schertzer M, Wagner MJ, Wells DE, Parrish J, Sadler LA, Blanton SH, Daiger SP, Wang ZY, Wilkie PJ, Weber JL: Human chromosome linkage map based on short tandem repeat polymorphisms: Effect of genotyping errors. *Genomics* **14**:144, 1992.

61. Oshima J, Yu CE, Boehnke M, Weber JL, Edelhoff S, Wagner MJ, Wells DE, Wood S, Disteche CM, Martin GM, Schellenberg GD: Integrated mapping analysis of the Werner syndrome region of chromosome 8. *Genomics* **23**:100, 1994.

62. Chang M, Burmer GC, Sweasy J, Loeb LA, Edelhoff S, Disteche CM, Yu CE, Anderson L, Oshima J, Nakura J, Miki T, Kamino K, Ogihara T, Schellenberg GD, Martin GM: Evidence against DNA polymerase beta as a candidate gene for Werner syndrome. *Hum Genet* **93**:507, 1994.

63. Yu C, Oshima J, Goddard KAB, Miki T, Nakura J, Ogihara T, Fraccaro M, Piussan C. Martin GM, Schellenberg GD, Wijsman EM: Linkage disequilibrium and haplotype studies of chromosome 8p 11.1.1 markers and Werner's syndrome. *Am J Hum Genet* **55**:356, 1994.

64. Tutic M, Lu X, Schirmer RH, Werner D: Cloning and sequencing of mammalian glutathione reductase cDNA. *Eur J Biochem* **188**:523, 1990.

65. Kihara K, Nakura J, Ye L, Mitsuda N, Kamino K, Zhao Y, Fujioka Y, Miki T, Ogihara T: Carrier detection of Werner's syndrome using a microsatellite that exhibits linkage disequilibrium with the Werner's syndrome locus. *Jpn J Hum Genet* **39**:403, 1994.

66. Ye L, Nakura J, Mitsuda N: A highly polymorphic dinucleotide repeat at the D8S1222 locus. *Jpn J Hum Genet* **40**:287, 1995.

67. Nakura J, Ye L, Kihara K, Yamagata H, Mamino K, Nakamura Y, Miki T, Ogihara T: Two dinucleotide repeat polymorphisms at the D8S1442 and D8S1443 loci. *Jpn J Hum Genet* **40**:281, 1995.

68. Yu CE, Oshima J, Hisama F, Matthews S, Trask BJ, Schellenberg GD: A YAC, P1 and cosmid contig and 17 new polymorphic markers for the Werner's syndrome region at 8p12. *Genomics* **35**:431, 1996.

69. Goddard KAB, Yu CE, Oshima J, Miki T, Nakura J, Piussan C, Martin GM, Schellenberg GD, Wijsman EM: International Werner's syndrome collaborative group: Toward localization of the Werner syndrome gene by linkage disequilibrium and ancestral haplotyping: Lessons learned from analysis of 35 chromosome 8p11.1.1 markers. *Am J Hum Genet* **58**:1286, 1996.

70. Nakura J, Miki T, Ye L, Mitsuda N, Zhao Y, Kihara K, Yu CE, Oshima J, Fukuchi K, Wijsman EM, Schellenberg GD, Martin GM, Murano S, Hashimoto K, Fujiwara Y, Ogihara T: Narrowing the position of the Werner syndrome locus by homozygosity analysis: Extension of homozygosity analysis. *Genomics* **36**:130, 1996.

71. Buckler AJ, Chang DD, Graw SL, Brook J, Haber DA, Sharp PA, Housman DE: Exon amplification: A strategy to isolate mammalian genes based on RNA splicing. *Proc Natl Acad Sci USA* **88**:4005, 1991.

72. Church DM, Stotler CJ, Rutter JL, Murrell JR, Trofatter JA, Buckler AJ: Isolation of genes from complex sources of mammalian genomic DNA using exon amplification. *Nat Genet* **6**:98, 1994.

73. Parimoo S, Kolluri R, Weissman S: cDNA selection from total yeast DNA containing YACs. *Nucleic Acids Res* **21**:4422, 1993.

74. Parimoo S, Patanjali SR, Shukla H, Chaplin D, Weissman SM: cDNA selection: Efficient PCR approach for the selection of cDNAs encoded in large chromosomal DNA fragments. *Proc Natl Acad Sci USA* **87**:3166, 1991.

75. Altschul SF, Gish W, Miller W, Myers EW, Lipman DJ: Basic local alignment search tool. *J Mol Biol* **215**:403, 1990.

76. Weeda G, van Ham RCA, Vermeulen W, Bootsma D, van der Eb AJ, Hoeijmakers JHJ: A presumed DNA helicase encoded by ERCC is involved in the human repair disorders xeroderma pigmentosa and Cockayne's syndrome. *Cell* **62**:777, 1990.

77. Broughton BC, Thompson AF, Harcourt SA, Vermeulen W, Hoeijmakers JHJ, Botta E, Stefanini M, King MD, Weber CA, Cole J, Arlett CF, Lehmann AR: Molecular and cellular analysis of the DNA repair defect in a patient in xeroderma pigmentosum complementation group D who has the clinical features of xeroderma pigmentosum and Cockayne syndrome. *Am J Hum Genet* **56**:167, 1995.

78. Flejter WL, McDaniel LD, Johns D, Friedberg EC, Schultz RA: Correction of xeroderma pigmentosum complementation group D mutant cell phenotypes by chromosome and gene transfer: Involvement of the human ERCC2 DNA repair gene. *Proc Natl Acad Sci USA* **89**:261, 1992.

79. Frederick GD, Amirkhan RH, Schultz RA, Friedberg EC: Structural and mutational analysis of the xeroderma pimentosum group D (XPD) gene. *Hum Mol Genet* **3**:1783, 1994.

80. Takayama K, Salazar EP, Broughton BC, Lehmann AR, Sarasin A, Thompson LH, Weber CA: Defects in the DNA repair and transcription gene ERCC2(XPD) in trichothiodystrophy. *Am J Hum Genet* **58**:263, 1996.

81. Sung P, Bailly V, Weber C, Thompson LH, Prakash L, Prakash S: Human xeroderma pigmentosum group D gene encodes a DNA helicase. *Nature* **365**:852, 1993.

82. Broughton BC, Steingrimsdottir H, Weber CA, Lehmann AR: Mutations in the xeroderma pigmentosum group D DNA repair/transcription gene in patients with trichothiodystrophy. *Nat Genet* **7**:189, 1994.

83. Takayama K, Salazar EP, Broughton BC, Lehmann AR, Sarasin A, Thompson LH, Weber CA: Defects in the DNA repair and transcription gene ERCC2(XPD) in trichothiodystrophy. *Am J Hum Genet* **58**:263, 1996.

84. Troelstra C, van Gool A, Wit JD, Vermeulen W, Bootsma D, Hoeijmakers JHJ: ERCC6, a member of a subfamily of putative helicases, is involved in Cockayne's syndrome and preferential repair of active genes. *Cell* **71**:939, 1992.

85. Ellis NA, Groden J, Ye TZ, Straughen J, Lennon DJ, Ciocci S, Proytcheva M, German J: The Bloom's syndrome gene product is homologous to RecQ helicases. *Cell* **83**:655, 1995.

86. Stayton CL, Dabovic B, Gulisano M, Gecz J, Broccoli V, Giovanazzi S, Bossolasco M, Monaco L, Rastan S, Boncinelli EE, Bianchi M, Consalez GG: Cloning and characterization of a new human Xq13 gene, encoding a putative helicase. *Hum Mol Genet* **3**:1957, 1994.

87. Ion A, Telvi L, Chaussain JL, Galacteros F, Valayer J, Fellous M, McElreavey K: A novel mutation in the putative DNA helicase XH2 is responsible for male-to-female sex reversal associated with an atypical form of the ATR syndrome. *Am J Hum Genet* **58**:1185, 1996.

88. Gorbalenya AE, Koonin EV, Donchenko AP, Blinov VM: Two related superfamilies of putative helicases involved in replication, repair and expression of DNA and RNA genomes. *Nucleic Acids Res* **17**:4713, 1989.

89. Schaeffer L, Roy R, Humbert S, Moncollin V, Vermeulen W, Hoeijmakers JHJ, Chambon P, Egly JM: DNA repair helicase: A component of BTF2 (TFIIH) basic transcription factor. *Science* **260**:58, 1993.

90. Henning KA, Li L, Iyer N, McDaniel LD, Reagan MS, Legerski R, Schultz RA, Stefanini M, Lehmann AR, Mayne LV, Friedberg EC: The Cockayne syndrome group A gene encodes a WD repeat protein that interacts with CBS protein and a subunit of RNA polymerase II TFIIH. *Cell* **82**:555, 1995.

91. Fujiwara Y, Higashikawa T, Tatsumi M: A retarded rate of DNA replication and normal level of DNA repair in Werner's syndrome fibroblast cultures. *J Cell Physiol* **92**:365, 1977.

92. Higashikawa T, Fujiwara Y: Normal level of unscheduled DNA synthesis in Werner's syndrome fibroblasts in culture. *Exp Cell Res* **113**:438, 1978.

93. Stefanini M, Scappaticci S, Lagomarsini P, Borroni G, Berardesca E, Nuzzo F: Chromosome instability in lymphocytes from a patient with Werner's syndrome is not associated with DNA repair defects. *Mutat Res* **219**:179, 1989.

94. Saito H, Moses RE: Immortalization of Werner syndrome and progeria fibroblasts. *Exp Cell Res* **192**:373, 1991.

95. Arlett CF, Harcourt SA: Survey of radiosensitivity in a variety of human cell strains. *Cancer Res* **40**:926, 1980.

96. Gebhart E, Schnizel M, Ruprecht KW: Cytogenetic studies using various clastogens in two patients with Werner syndrome and control individuals. *Hum Genet* **70**:324, 1985.

97. Gebhart E, Bauer R, Raub U, Schinzel M, Ruprecht KW, Jonas JB: Spontaneous and induced chromosomal instability in Werner syndrome. *Hum Genet* **80**:135, 1988.

98. Gawkrodger DJ, Priestley GC, Vijayalamix, Ross JA, Narcisi P, Hunter JAA: Werner's syndrome. *Arch Dermatol* **121**:636, 1985.

99. Takeuchi F, Hanaoka F, Goto M, Akaoka I, Hori T, Yamada M, Miyamoto T: Altered frequency of initiation sites of DNA replication in Werner's syndrome cells. *Hum Genet* **60**:365, 1982.

100. Hanaoka F, Takeuchi F, Matsumura T, Goto M, Miyamoto T, Tamada M: Decrease in the average size of replicons in a Werner syndrome cell line by a simian virus 40 infection. *Exp Cell Res* **144**:463, 1983.

101. Poot M, Hoehn H, Runger TM, Martin GM: Impaired S-phase transit of Werner syndrome cells expressed in lymphoblastoid cell lines. *Exp Cell Res* **202**:267, 1992.

102. Runger TM, Sobotta P, Dekant B, Moller K, Bauer C, Kraemer KH: In vivo assessment of DNA ligation efficiency and fidelity in cells from patients with Franconi's anemia and other cancer-prone hereditary disorders. *Toxicol Lett* **67**:309, 1993.

103. Runger TM, Bauer C, Dekant B, Moller K, Sobotta P, Czemy C, Poot M, Martin GM: Hypermutable ligation of plasmid DNA ends in cells from patients with Werner syndrome. *J Invest Dermatol* **102**:45, 1994.

104. Cheng RZ, Murano S, Kurz B, Shmookler Reis RJS: Homologous recombination is elevated in some Werner-like syndromes but not during normal or in vitro senescence of mammalian cells. *Mutat Res* **237**:259, 1990.

DEFECTS IN GATEKEEPERS

CHAPTER 19

Retinoblastoma

**Irene F. Newsham ▪ Theodora Hadjistilianou ▪
Webster K. Cavenee**

1. Retinoblastoma is the most common intraocular malignancy in children, with a worldwide incidence between 1 in 13,500 and 1 in 25,000 live births. The presenting signs and symptoms include leukokoria, strabismus, low-vision orbital cellulitis, unilateral mydriasis, and heterochromia. The disease can be unifocal or multifocal and unilateral or bilateral. The average age of diagnosis is 12 months for bilateral and 18 months for unilateral cases, and 90 percent of affected individuals are diagnosed before age 3 years. Unusual manifestations of this disease include late-onset retinoblastoma, 13q-deletion syndrome, retinoma, trilateral retinoblastoma, and second-site primary tumors, including osteosarcoma, Ewing sarcoma, leukemia, and lymphoma.

2. Early diagnosis and treatment are of primary importance in the survival of retinoblastoma patients. A variety of diagnostic approaches are used, including computed tomography (CT), magnetic resonance imaging (MRI), ultrasonography, and fine-needle aspiration biopsy (FNAB). Each has different advantages, and when used in combination, they can establish the proper disease classification. Effective methods for the treatment of retinoblastoma tumors include enucleation, external-beam irradiation, episcleral plaques, xenon arc and argon laser photocoagulation, cryotherapy, and chemotherapy. The choice of treatment depends on several factors, such as multifocal or unifocal disease, site and size of the tumor, diffuse or focal vitreous seeding, age at diagnosis, and histopathologic findings.

3. Retinoblastoma has served as the prototypic example of a genetic predisposition to cancer. It is estimated that 60 percent of cases are nonhereditary and unilateral, 15 percent are hereditary and unilateral, and 25 percent are hereditary and bilateral. A model encompassing these findings suggests a requirement for as few as two stochastic mutational events for tumor formation. The first of these events can be inherited through the germ line or can be somatically acquired, whereas the second occurs somatically in either case and leads to a tumor that is doubly defective at the retinoblastoma locus. Cytogenetic analyses have demonstrated the involvement of a genetic alteration in a gene for negative growth regulation at chromosome band 13q14. This model has been tested and confirmed using restriction-fragment-length polymorphisms (RFLP) for loci on chromosome 13. These studies have shown that the second wild-type retinoblastoma allele may be lost by several somatic mutational mechanisms, including mitotic nondisjunction with loss of the wild-type chromosome, mitotic nondisjunction with duplication of the mutant chromosome, mitotic recombination between the *RB1* locus and the centromere, and other regionalized events, such as deletion and point mutation.

4. The 200-kb genomic locus for *RB1* has been isolated, and its exon/intron structure has been characterized. Current molecular technology has allowed the identification of a variety of aberrations in this locus in retinoblastoma patients and their tumors at the DNA, RNA, and protein levels. *RB1* alterations also have been detected in a variety of clinically related second-site primary tumors and nonrelated tumors, including osteosarcoma, breast carcinoma, and small-cell lung carcinoma. The ability to detect mutations in *RB1* coupled with the isolation of polymorphic sequences within the gene locus, has further extended the prenatal risk assessment for this pediatric tumor.

5. The *RB1* locus is transcribed into a 4.7-kb mRNA with a corresponding protein product of 110 kd that is ubiquitously expressed in normal human and rat tissues, including brain, kidney, ovary, spleen, liver, placenta, and retina. The p110^{RB} protein is differentially phosphorylated, and the unphosphorylated form is found predominantly in the G1 stage of the cell cycle, with an initial phosphorylation occurring at the G1/S boundary. This protein can be physically complexed with a number of viral and cellular proteins. SV40 large T antigen, adenovirus E1A protein, and papillomavirus E7 protein all contain conserved regions which are required for binding with the p110^{RB} protein. The same regions appear to be necessary for the transforming function of the viral proteins.

6. Intracellular proteins whose function is mediated by the retinoblastoma protein have been isolated from complexes formed in vitro using pRB "pocket-binding" affinity chromatography columns against different cell lysates. Transcription factors DRTF and E2F have been isolated, and their physical and functional relationships to the retinoblastoma protein have been assessed. Other cellular proteins identified in these complexes include cyclin D1, p16, and the RB-like proteins p107 and p130. Interestingly, the complexing of these factors to p110^{RB} has also been shown to oscillate in a cell cycle-dependent manner, thereby linking the tumor-suppressing function of the retinoblastoma protein with transcriptional regulation.

CLINICAL ASPECTS AND TREATMENT OF RETINOBLASTOMA

Epidemiology

Retinoblastoma is the most common intraocular malignancy in children. In 1964, Francois[1] reported an incidence varying from 1 in 34,000 to 1 in 14,000 births and noted a steady increase in the frequency of occurrence of the tumor between 1927 and 1960. A number of studies support this finding and indicate a worldwide incidence of 1 in 3500 to 1 in 25,000, with no significant difference between the sexes or races.[2–9] An apparent mortality rate for blacks 2.5 times greater than that for whites has been reported but seems to be attributable to delays in diagnosis rather than a higher disease incidence.[10] In general, there seems to be little correlation of disease incidence with geographic location. However, in some populations (e.g., Jamaicans, Nigerians, Haitians)[11] apparently higher incidence rates have been observed for what appears to be the unilateral sporadic form of retinoblastoma; this may suggest an environmental modification of the probability of tumor formation.[12]

Presenting Signs and Symptoms

Differential Diagnosis In the majority of cases, the first sign at presentation is the characteristic cat's-eye reflex, which is usually noted by the child's parents or pediatrician. This white, pink-white, or yellow-white pupillary reflex, termed leukokoria, results from replacement of the vitreous by the tumor or by a tumor growing in the macula[13,14] (Fig. 19-1). Another common symptom, strabismus (exotropia or esotropia), can occur alone when small macular tumors interfere with vision or can be associated with leukokoria. It is not uncommon to find after an accurate patient history is taken that strabismus has occurred some months before leukokoria.

Less frequent presenting signs for retinoblastoma are red painful eye with secondary glaucoma, low-vision orbital cellulitis, unilateral mydriasis, and heterochromia.[15] Sometimes the tumor can be difficult to differentiate from a variety of simulating lesions, such as persistent hyperplastic primary vitreous, retrolental fibroplasia, Coats disease, toxocara canis infection, retinal dysplasia, and chronic retinal detachment.[16,17] In 265 patients with pseudoretinoblastoma, persistent hyperplastic primary vitreous, followed by retrolental fibroplasia and posterior cataract, was the most common simulating condition.[18] Of 136 children with suspected retinoblastoma reported to the Ocular Oncology Service of the Wills Eye Hospital in Philadelphia between 1974 and 1978, 60 had retinoblastoma and 76 had simulating lesions, the most frequent being ocular toxocariasis (26 percent), persistent hyperplastic primary vitreous (20 percent), and Coats disease (16 percent). Despite these complications, most simulating lesions can be distinguished through modern diagnostic methods (described later in this chapter) or after a careful history of the family and the affected child.[16,17,19]

A complete workup for such a patient includes an ophthalmologic examination; a systemic, pediatric, and radiographic evaluation; and more recently genetic studies (Table 19-1).[17,19,20] At fundus examination, the disease can be unifocal or multifocal; in bilateral cases, usually one eye is in a more advanced stage, while the contralateral eye has one or more tumor foci (Fig. 19-1B). Furthermore, fundus examination of the first-degree relatives may also document the presence of a retinoma or a regressed retinoblastoma and indicate a potential hereditary basis for the tumor.

The average age at diagnosis is 12 months for bilateral retinoblastoma and 18 months for unilateral cases, with 90 percent of the patients diagnosed before age 3. Several factors may influence the time of diagnosis and therapy,[21,22] including (1) ignorance

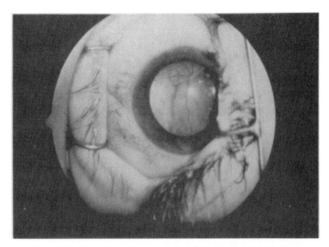

A

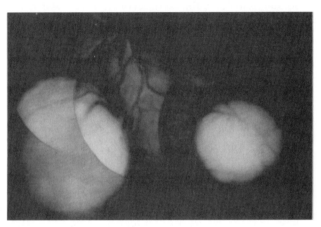

B

FIG. 19-1 Presenting signs of retinoblastoma. *A.* Leukokoria: exophytic retinoblastoma, overlying retinal detachment, clear lens, and visible retinal blood vessels. *B.* Multifocal retinoblastoma. *(Courtesy of R. Frezzotti, M.D., Director of the Institute of Ophthalmological Sciences, University of Siena, Italy.)*

of the revealing signs, (2) difficulty in ophthalmoscopic examination (age of the patient, level of transparency of the media, full mydriasis, and scleral indentation), (3) socioeconomic situation, (4) unusual clinical manifestations, and (5) multiple consultants.

Unusual Clinical Manifestations

Late Retinoblastoma. It is an exceptional instance when retinoblastoma presents after the age of 7, and the older the child, the more unusual the first signs of the disease. These unusual manifestations include orbital cellulitis and edema of the lids; hypopion, hyphema, iris heterochromia, and keratitis (anterior segment); and vitreous opacification, retinal cysts, vitreous hemorrhage, and endophthalmitis (posterior segment).[23] Atypical uveitis in an older child, particularly if associated with secondary glaucoma and a poor response to corticosteroids, may be the first manifestation of a late retinoblastoma[24] (Fig. 19-2A). Repetitive diagnostic anterior chamber paracentesis may yield negative results.[23] Among 618 cases of retinoblastoma in older children, 41 (6.6 percent) were misdiagnosed as primary ocular inflammations.[25]

Sometimes retinoblastoma can resemble a panophthalmitis, which is frequently seen as a reaction to a necrotic uveal melanoma.[26] Pseudohypopion as a result of retinoblastoma cells settled in the anterior chamber is another rare sign of the disease (Fig. 19-2B). A diffuse, infiltrating retinoblastoma can present with

Table 19-1 Clinical and Laboratory Assessment for Retinoblastoma Patients

Ophthalmologic examination

Binocular indirect ophthalmoscopy with scleral
  indentation (child, parents, siblings, relatives)
Site and dimensions of the tumor(s)
Necrosis, calcification
Degree of vascularization, hemorrhage
Vitreous "seeding"
Retinal detachment
Fundus photography and drawing of the lesion(s)
Slit-lamp examination
Pseudohypopion, hyphema
Corneal and lens transparency
Rubeosis iris
Corneal diameter (buphthalmos)
Pupil, anisocoria
Tonometry
Ecography (calcification, biometry)
Aqueous and vitreous cytology and enzymology—
  fine-needle aspiration biopsy
Systemic examination
Radiographic examination
  Skull x-ray
  Computed tomography (orbits and brain with and without
    contrast enhancement)
  Magnetic resonance imaging (orbits and brain)
Pediatric examination
  Bone marrow biopsy
  Lumbar puncture (cerebrospinal fluid examination)
  Serologic tests (toxocara)
  Neurologic evaluation
  Electroencephalogram
Genetic studies
  Esterase D
  High-resolution chromosome analysis—karyotyping
  DNA analysis of blood and tumor tissues

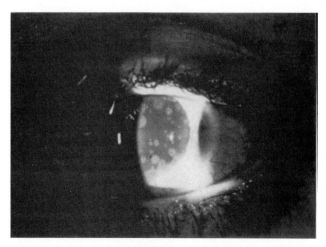

A

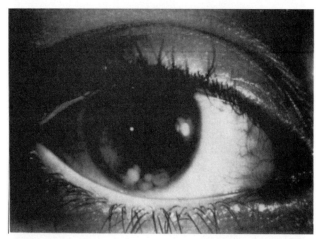

B

FIG. 19-2 Unusual manifestations of retinoblastoma. *A.* Pseudo-uveitis in retinoblastoma. *B.* Nodules at the pupillary margin and pseudohypopion caused by a retinoblastoma. *(Courtesy of R. Frezzotti, M.D., Director of the Institute of Ophthalmological Sciences, University of Siena, Italy.)*

a hypopion or a severe anterior uveitis.[27,28] The term *diffuse infiltrated retinoblastoma* has been used to describe a form of the tumor in which no well-defined exophytic or endophytic mass is evident. This retinoblastoma pattern frequently produces aqueous and vitreous seeding, particularly in older children,[27,29–32] and seems to have a low potential for malignancy, although there is still controversy on this point.[27,28] Furthermore, cystic retinoblastoma, presumably a variant of the diffuse infiltrating type, tends to simulate uveitis and presents with clinically visible cysts.[33,34]

Associated Clinical Abnormalities

13Q-Deletion Syndrome The 13Q-deletion syndrome includes sporadic retinoblastoma in association with moderate growth and mental retardation, a broad prominent nasal bridge, a short nose, ear abnormalities, and muscular hypotonia.[35,36] Niebuhr and Ottosen also reported seven cases of retinoblastoma associated with systemic abnormalities (mental retardation, microcephaly, genital malformations, and ear abnormalities) in a review of 13q deletions and 13 ring chromosomes.[37] Such a karyotypic analysis prompted by the presentation of dysmorphic features can facilitate early detection of a deletion in the long arm of chromosome 13. Subsequent ophthalmoscopic examination can identify the retinoblastoma at an earlier stage.[38]

Retinoma. The term *retinoma* has been used to denote a benign tumor of retinocytic origin. Although the origins of this entity are

obscure, it has been proposed that it arises from a mutation in the retinoblastoma susceptibility gene in a well-differentiated retinocyte and leads to a hyperplastic nodule of differentiated cells.[39] Retinomas are composed of apparently benign cells that show photoreceptor differentiation with no evidence of necrosis or mitotic activity but with numerous rosettes.[40] Characteristically, retinomas have at least two of the following characteristics: irregular translucent retinal mass, calcification, and pigment epithelium migration and proliferation (Fig. 19-3A). Histopathologic and immunohistochemical studies suggest that retinomas are primary benign tumors, not regressed retinoblastomas. Malignant transformation of retinomas is quite rare, although some cases have been reported, notably a 7-year-old girl who developed an undifferentiated retinoblastoma 3 years after the diagnosis of a retinoma.[41,42]

Various physiologic conditions [including reduced blood supply and necrosis, calcium (as an inhibitor of tumor growth), and host immune defense mechanisms] could be implicated in the spontaneous regression of retinoblastoma (Fig. 19-3B). Often, bulbi with intraocular calcification are the final physical embodiment of a spontaneously regressed retinoblastoma.[43] These phthisis bulbi can be attributed to tumor necrosis after ocular ischemia but cannot explain the retinoma, since the vascular supply in these lesions is intact.[44] On the basis of the available data, it appears that the term *regressed retinoblastoma* should be reserved to describe

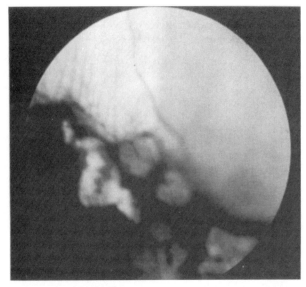

A

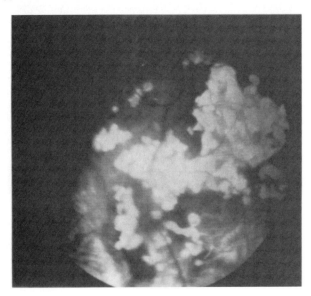

B

FIG. 19-3 Abnormalities associated with retinoblastoma. *A.
Retinoma: translucent retinal mass and pigment epithelium migration
and proliferation. B. Spontaneously regressed retinoblastoma. (Courtesy of R. Frezzotti, M.D., Director of the Institute of Ophthalmological
Sciences, University of Siena, Italy.)*

shrunken, calcified, phthisical eyes, whereas *retinoma* should be
used to refer to nonprogressive retinal lesions that are highly associated with retinoblastoma but lack a malignant pattern.[45]

Trilateral Retinoblastoma. Bader and coauthors[46] coined the term
trilateral retinoblastoma to describe the association between bilateral retinoblastoma and midline brain tumors, usually in the pineal
region. Similar observations had been reported by Jensen and
Miller[10] and Jakobiec, et al.,[47] and had suggested that involvement
of the pineal gland (third eye) represents a further point of origin
for multicentric retinoblastoma rather than a second primary tumor.[48] In patients with hereditary retinoblastoma, both the pineal
and the retina may contain susceptible cells. Since these pineal tumors may be indistinguishable from well-differentiated retinoblastomas, they are also called ectopic retinoblastomas.[46] It is possible
that pineal tumors have been misinterpreted as intracranial spread
of retinoblastoma,[49] whereas the advent of CT scanning and MRI

has facilitated more accurate diagnoses. This is clinically important, since an ectopic intracranial retinoblastoma requires adequate
therapy to the whole neuraxis as well as high-dose equivalent radiotherapy to the primary tumor. Intrathecal therapy with
methotrexate should also be considered.[50]

Second Malignant Tumors. The term *second site primary malignant tumor* refers to nonmetastatic tumors arising in disease-free
patients successfully treated for the initial disease. Some of the tumors found in association with retinoblastoma include osteosarcoma, fibrosarcoma, chondrosarcoma, epithelial malignant tumors,
Ewing sarcoma, leukemia, lymphoma, melanoma, brain tumors,
and pinealoblastoma. These second tumors have been classified
into five groups[51]: (1) tumors appearing in the irradiated area, (2)
tumors appearing outside and remote from the irradiated area, (3)
tumors in patients not receiving radiotherapy, (4) tumors that cannot be characterized as primary or metastases, and (5) tumors appearing in members of retinoblastoma families who are free of
retinal tumors.

Reese, Merriam, and Martin[52] reported the first two cases of
second tumors in 55 retinoblastoma patients treated with external
radiation and surgery. These patients presented with a maxillary
sinus sarcoma and a rhabdomyosarcoma of the temporal muscle.
A similar case of mixed-cell fibrosarcoma has been reported by
Frezzotti and Guerra.[53] A causal relationship between radiation
therapy and secondary tumors has been suggested.[54–56] However,
from the reported series of cases, two important observations have
emerged: (1) The great majority of children in whom second
neoplasms developed had suffered bilateral retinoblastoma, and
(2) the incidence of second neoplasms in this group of children
was similar whether or not they received radiation. These conclusions have been supported by studies that have reported the incidence of second nonocular tumors and analyzed the effect of radiation therapy. Osteogenic sarcomas have been the most common
second site neoplasms in all the published series. Derkinderen,[57]
Lueder,[58] Draper,[59] and their colleagues found low rates of development of second tumors and are in agreement that the incidence
increases with radiation therapy. Abramson et al. reported the incidence of second tumors in patients with hereditary retinoblastoma
and found a frequency of 20 percent at 10 years, 50 percent at 20
years, and 90 percent at 30 years after diagnosis.[60] Somewhat
lower rates have been recorded by other authors. For example, in a
series of 215 bilateral retinoblastomas, second tumors developed
in 4.4 percent of the patients during the first 10 years of follow-up,
in 18.3 percent after 20 years, and in 26.1 percent after 30 years.[61]

Histopathology

Retinoblastoma occurs either as an intraocular mass between the
choroid and the retina (exophytic) or as a bulge from the retina toward vitreous (endophytic). However, most of the advanced tumors examined showed both patterns of growth. Retinoblastoma
rarely spreads superficially (1 percent), forming no mass and invading the whole retina (diffuse infiltrating retinoblastoma).

The tumor is histologically characterized by the presence of
rosettes and fleurettes, which are believed to represent maturation
and differentiation of the neoplastic cells. Rosettes are spherical
structures (circular in section) constituted by uniform cuboidal or
short columnar cells arranged in an orderly fashion around a small
round lumen (Flexner-Wintersteiner rosette) or without any lumen
(Homer-Right rosette). The latter type can often be found in other
neuroectodermal tumors, such as medulloblastomas. Fleurettes are
arranged in the opposite way, with short and thin stromal axes surrounded by fairly differentiated neoplastic cells with the apical part
facing the externum, resembling the shape of a flower (Fig.

19-4*A*). Often the tumor appears highly necrotic, with the surviving cells positioned around blood vessels, creating structures called pseudorosettes. Calcified foci can be found in areas of necrosis, as can debris from nucleic acids, giving rise to basophilic vessel walls.[62,63]

A retinoblastoma tumor is capable of spreading outside the bulb through the eye coats, invading the choroid and the sclera. It is the invasion of this highly vascularized choroid that represents an effective vehicle for distant metastasis (Fig. 19-5*B*), and such choroid invasion is directly correlated with a poor prognosis. Invasion also can involve the optic nerve and meningeal space, providing access to the central nervous system. Growth patterns and other histologic parameters (such as pseudorosettes, necrosis, and calcification), although necessary for the identification of the tumor itself, do not seem to offer much information in regard to the prognosis. The degree of differentiation and the number of mitoses show a weak correlation with the prognosis; however, stronger relationships exist with invasion of the choroid and sclera. In particular, progressive invasion of the eye coats, even in the horizontal plane, is highly informative in determining the prognosis.[64,65]

Diagnosis

Since many of the symptoms described above are clearly not specific to retinoblastoma and since early surgical or conservative treatment is of primary importance in the survival of these patients, it is imperative to confirm these impressions by examination. There are a variety of diagnostic tools available for this, including CT, MRI, ultrasonography, and FNAB. The application and advantages of each procedure are briefly discussed below.

Computed Tomography and Magnetic Resonance Imaging CT is a valuable adjunct in the differential diagnosis, staging, and treatment of retinoblastoma.[66,67] Intraocular calcification in children under 3 years of age is highly suggestive of a retinoblastoma. Some studies have reported that the degree of calcification appeared to depend on tumor size, with the smallest tumor showing calcification 8 mm in diameter and 4 mm in thickness[68,69] (Fig. 19-5*A*). However, in children more than 3 years of age confusion may arise from some simulating lesions, including retinal astrocytoma, retrolental fibroplasia, toxocariasis, and optic-nerve-head drusen, which can also produce calcifications.[68–70] Thus, CT is often coupled with MRI to better detect subtle scleral invasion, infiltrative spread along the optic nerve, subarachnoid seeding, or

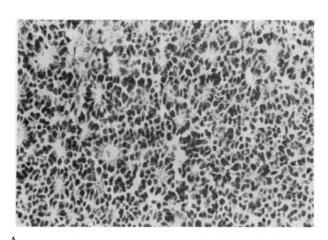

A

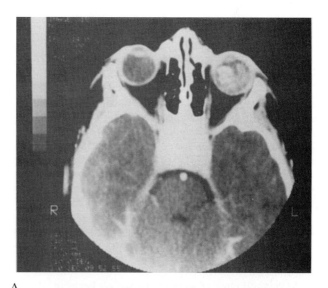

A

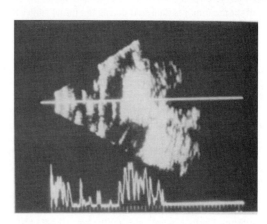

B

FIG. 19-5 Diagnostic tools for retinoblastoma. *A.* CT scan: retinoblastoma filling the whole vitreous cavity with typical calcifications *(Courtesy of C. Venturi, M.D., Department of Neuroradiology, University of Siena, Italy)*. *B.* B scan technique. The echogram shows a lesion with an irregular oval shape and dense acoustic tissue. High attenuation of ultrasound is occurring, with the shadowing of the echoes coming from the orbital tissue. The tumor has developed in the vitreous and occupies it almost entirely. *(Courtesy of E. Motolese, M.D., Institute of Ophthalmological Sciences, University of Siena, Italy.)*

B

FIG. 19-4 Histopathology of retinoblastoma. *A.* A well-differentiated retinoblastoma showing rosettes and fleurettes (hematoxylin-eosin, 100). *B.* Low-differentiated retinoblastoma infiltrating the choroid and sclera (hematoxylin-eosin, 100). *(Courtesy of P. Toti, M.D., Institute of Anatomic Pathology, University of Siena, Italy.)*

involvement of the central nervous system through direct tumor extension or by metastasis.[71] Furthermore, MRI appears to be more sensitive in the differential diagnosis of lesions simulating retinoblastoma[70,72,73] and in the evaluation of the degree of tumor differentiation.[74]

The role of both CT and MRI in staging and therapy is of great importance in accurately determining extraocular disease such as intracranial metastasis, retrobulbar spread, orbital recurrence, and secondary tumors, and it is often on the basis of these diagnostic results that further treatment (radiotherapy and/or chemotherapy) is planned. Still, subtle optic nerve involvement cannot be predicted reliably.[68] By using CT as a diagnostic tool, Danziger and Price[75] proposed the division of retinoblastoma cases into three groups, in which grade I tumors are high-density masses with calcification in any part of the eyeball, grade II tumors are high-density masses involving the optic nerve and orbital soft tissue but with rare calcifications, and grade III tumors are intracranial or extraorbital high-density masses showing marked contrast enhancement. These classifications further aid in the determination of appropriate therapeutic measures.

Ultrasonography. Ultrasonography is another diagnostic technique that can distinguish the type of growth for retinoblastoma and related tumor types. Endophytic and exophytic growths show variations in the ultrasonographic context of both A and B scanning techniques.

B Scan Technique. In the case of an endophytic growth, the retinoblastoma appears as a single or, more often a multiple lesion on the retinal plane. The tumors are monolobate or multilobate and have a roundish or irregular oval shape, with dense acoustics and variable homogeneity (Fig. 19-5B). A discrete attenuation of the ultrasound occurs, with the shadowing of the echoes coming from the orbital tissue. The attenuation is considerable if, as is often the case, areas of calcification are found inside the tumor mass.[76] The tumor itself may develop within the vitreous chamber and occupy it almost entirely, and at times areas of pseudocysts may be found in front of and/or in the context of the neoplastic mass, thus making it difficult to recognize the lesion.[77] Nevertheless, the attenuation of the ultrasound is considerable.

With the exophytic growth, the diagnosis is harder to establish, especially if the tumor is analyzed during the initial stage. It is easily confused, in fact, with the high echogenic portion of the sclera, while no significant evidence of it appears on the retinal plane. The only significant noticeable sign is a certain attenuation of the ultrasound coming from the orbital tissue, with a display on the echogram that simulates the acoustic shadow of the optic nerve but does not resemble it in topography and size.[77]

A Scan Technique. In the case of an endophytic tumor growth, a standardized A scan tracing shows an opening peak that appears at high or medium reflectivity but is never maximal. This is the case because the internal retinal surface is considerably compromised and heterogeneous, thus attenuating the contrast that exists at the vitreous–retinal interface level. The opening peak can be maximal, however, if the tumor has an exophytic growth as long as the layer of the limiting internal membrane and the nerve fibers are not disintegrated by the growth of the tumor.[77,78]

In the opposite case, a peak at high reflectivity found during a subsequent checkup may reveal a peritumorous satellite area, even f small and confined, rather than an opening peak of the tumor. The internal structure of the tumor usually appears quite regular at medium-high reflectivity and at medium reflectivity in the case of a retinoblastoma with no calcifications.[77] Vitreous activity with the absence of seeding is minor in retinoblastoma before photocoagulation, while afterward it is possible to find juxtalesional vitreous

echoes at medium reflectivity and sometimes areas of peritumorous retinal fissions.[79]

Invasion of the sclera entails the loss of its homogeneity as an acoustic interface and causes a decrease in the reflectivity of the closing scleral peak that may be mistaken for the retinal echoes of the same tumor. This represents an important ultrasonographic sign which can determine the margins and posterior borders of the lesion. In the A and B scanning methods, the calcifications are characteristically evident even when the amplitude appears reduced. Furthermore, suspicion of invasion of the optic nerve is indicated by the presence in the nervous tissue of an ultrasonographic tracing that reproduces the features of a retinoblastoma in an A scan.

Fine-Needle Aspiration Biopsy The cytologic approach to the study of retinoblastoma has become particularly relevant as the techniques for obtaining tumor material have improved. Specimens from the posterior chamber can be obtained by using vitrectomy techniques in addition to anterior chamber paracentesis for cytologic and enzymologic evaluation of the aqueous. Aqueous and vitreous aspiration for cytologic studies may be useful in differentiating retinoblastoma from the previously described simulating conditions.

The use of fine-needle biopsy in ophthalmology, originally introduced by Schyberg for the diagnosis of orbital tumors, was utilized in the diagnosis of intraocular neoplasms by Jakobiec et al.[80] and extended to the diagnosis of intraocular and extraocular retinoblastoma by Char and Miller.[81] This approach is not recommended as a routine procedure for retinoblastoma and generally is reserved for children who present with unusual manifestations or for differentiating an orbital recurrence of retinoblastoma from a second malignant neoplasm.[81] A limbar approach is used for anterior segment tumors, whereas a via pars plana approach after opening of the conjunctiva, scleral diathermy, and 1.5-mm sclerotomy is used for posterior tumors.[82,83] Complications that may occur with the use of fine-needle biopsy include intraocular hemorrhage, retinal detachment, and recurrence in the orbit or along the intraocular needle tract. Although tumoral-cell seedings within the scleral needle tracks after biopsy are controversial,[84,85] this possibility suggests that fine-needle biopsy be limited to patients who present diagnostic uncertainties. These patients include older children with suspected retinoblastoma and rather atypical findings and children with orbital masses who previously have been treated for retinoblastoma.[86–88]

Therapy

If a retinoblastoma or a related ocular tumor is discovered at an early stage and diagnostic tools have appropriately classified the type, there are several current and effective methods for treatment, including enucleation, external-beam irradiation, episcleral plaques, xenon arc and argon laser photocoagulation, cryotherapy, and chemotherapy. The choice of treatment depends on several factors, such as (1) multifocal or unifocal disease, (2) site and size of the tumor, (3) diffuse or focal vitreous seeding, (4) age of the child, and (5) histopathologic findings. Therefore, an appropriate therapeutic approach greatly depends on accurate staging of the disease.

Staging and Classification. The most widely used staging system for retinoblastoma, proposed by Reese and Ellsworth,[89] is based on the ophthalmoscopic evaluation of the tumor extension and generally is limited to patients with intraocular retinoblastoma. This system was extended by Pratt to include intraocular and extraocular extension of the disease.[90] Another system is based on an accurate evaluation of the histopathologic findings.[91] Most recently, a pretreatment TNM classification has been introduced that also addresses the importance of visual acuity in addition to patient survival and ocular extension.[92] Table 19-2 presents the different criteria for these classification systems.

Enucleation Enucleation is the standard treatment in unilateral cases and for the more severely affected eye in bilateral ones. An attempt to save the eye is worthwhile only when there is hope for useful vision and no risk of a systemic prognosis.[93] Generally there are several major indications that call for the nonconservative removal of the diseased eye. These tumor characteristics include (1) a large mass involving more than 50 percent of the retina associated with retinal detachment, (2) a buphthalmic painful eye, (3) a phthisical eye (in bilateral cases), and (4) unsuccessful conservative treatment (radiotherapy with or without chemotherapy and photocoagulation). Regardless of which of the various enucleation techniques is used, the procedure should be performed with the least trauma possible for the patient while avoiding scleral perforation, and at least 10 mm of the optic nerve should be resected.[94] Af-

ter enucleation, the use of an implant is recommended not only for cosmetic reasons but also to stimulate orbital growth. Usually a conformer is used for 2 to 3 days directly after surgery, followed by a temporary insert prosthesis (about 1 week after enucleation) after complete healing of the surgical incision.[13]

External Irradiation Retinoblastoma is a highly radiosensitive tumor, and the first attempt at its treatment with x-rays occurred in 1903.[95] External-beam irradiation, utilizing gamma rays from a linear accelerator, is now the most commonly used treatment for intraocular and orbital disease. This technique is indicated when (1) in unilateral retinoblastoma cases there is a large tumor not involving the macula and optic nerve, (2) in bilateral retinoblastoma cases with advanced tumors in both eyes or in the remaining eye when multiple tumors or diffuse vitreous seeding is present, and (3) in orbital tissue where histopathologic studies of the enucleated eye and optic nerve document an invasion of the optic nerve, scleral invasion, or orbital recurrence.[13]

The goal of external irradiation in retinoblastoma is to sterilize the entire retina and vitreous of malignant cells with the best possi-

Table 19-2 Classification Systems for Retinoblastoma

Reese-Ellsworth Classification	Pratt Classification	Standard Classification	TNM Classification
Group I: very favorable prognosis A. Solitary tumor less than 4 dd* in size at or behind the equator B. Multiple tumors, none more than 4 dd in size, at or behind the equator	I: Tumor (unifocal or multifocal) confined to the retina A. Occupying 1 quadrant or less B. Occupying 2 quadrants or less C. Occupying more than 50 percent of the retinal surface	Stage I: lesions amenable to local therapy Stage II: lesions unsuitable for conservative local therapy but still confined to the eye—subdivisions based on histologic assessment of the eye	T1: tumors or tumors 10 dd or less in largest diameter T1a: macula not involved T1b: macula involved T2: tumor or tumors larger than 10 dd involving up to half the retina
Group II: favorable prognosis A. Solitary lesion 4–10 dd at or behind the equator B. Multiple lesions 4–10 dd at or behind the equator	II: Tumor (unifocal or multifocal) confined to the globe A. With vitreous seeding B. Extending to optic nerve head C. Extending to choroid D. Extending to choroid and optic nerve head E. Extending to emissaries	N0: no invasion of the optic nerve N1: invastion up to or into the lamina cribrosa N2: invasion beyond the lamina cribrosa resection line free N3: optic nerve involved up to the resection line	T2a: macula not involved T2b: macula involved T3: tumor or tumors involving more than half the retina T4: extraretinal or orbital extension
Group III: doubtful prognosis A. Any lesion anterior to the equator B. Solitary tumor larger than 10 dd behind the equator	III: Extraocular extension of tumor (regional) A. Extending beyond cut end of optic nerve (including subarachnoid extention) B. Extending through sclera into orbital contents	C0: no choroidal invasion C1: superficial involvement of the choroid up to half its thickness C2: full-thickness choroidal invasion	T4a: invasion of optic nerve T4b: invasion of choroidea, corpus ciliare, iris, or anterior chamber T4c: scleral involvement T4d: two or more of a–c
Group IV: unfavorable prognosis A. Multiple tumors, some larger than 10 dd B. Any lesion extending anteriorly to the ora serrata	C. Extending to choroid and beyond cut end of optic nerve (including subarachnoid extension) D. Extending through sclera into orbital contents and beyond cut end of optic nerve (including subarachnoid extension)	C3: scleral invasion, including tumor in the emissary vessels C4: extrascleral invasion	N: regional lymph nodes NX: minimum requirements to assess the regional lymph nodes cannot be met N0: no evidence of regional lymph node involvement
Group V: very unfavorable prognosis A. Massive tumors involving over 50 percent of the retina B. Vitreous seeding	IV: Distant metastases A. Extending through optic nerve to brain B. Blood-borne metastases to soft tissue and bone C. Bone-marrow metastases	Stage III: local spread beyond the eye without hematogenous metastases 1. Orbital tumors 2. Preauricular or cervical nodes 3. Central nervous system disease Stage IV: hematogenous metastases	N1: evidence of involvement of regional lymph nodes M: distant metastases M0: no evidence of distant metastases M1: evidence of distant metastases (can be subdivided according to the organs involved)

*dd = disk diameter; 1 dd = 1.6 mm.

ble visual prognosis. A dose generally considered to be optimally therapeutic is 4000 rad fractionated into about 20 doses over a 3- to 4-week period. At the Utrecht Retinoblastoma Center, a highly accurate irradiation method has been developed,[96] based on the temporal approach, which ensures precise delivery of a uniform radiation dose to the whole retina or vitreous with maximal sparing of the lens. Accurate positioning of the collimated field is obtained by magnetic fixation of the eye to the beam-defining collimator by a low-vacuum contact lens. Since the eye is fixed in the isocenter of the accelerator, rotation of the gantry directs the beam. Other centers have adopted this technique and have confirmed the extreme precision and sharp beam profile that can be obtained.[97,98]

Four regression patterns after radiation for retinoblastoma have been described by Reese and Ellsworth,[99] and Buys et al.[101] These patterns are described as follows: type I: characterized by calcification, marked alterations of the retinal pigment epithelium, and the cottage cheese aspect; type II: the tumor is shrunken in size and adopts a gray, translucent appearance (fish flesh); type III: a combination of the patterns seen for types I and II; type IV: represented by the typical pattern after cobalt-plaque treatment, with complete destruction of the tumor and choroid; the white scar represents the sclera underlying the tumor.

Buys et al. found that the most common type of regression at the first evaluation was type III (43.8 percent). However, after a minimum of 7 years, a decrease in this pattern was found (from 43.8 to 36 percent). It was also reported that the type II patterns can turn into any one of the other types over a number of years. Furthermore, a correlation seems to exist between the size of the tumor and the regression pattern.[101]

As with most procedures, complications can arise after external irradiation. They are divided into immediate, usually reversible complications and late, usually irreversible complications. The most severe complications are growth retardation of the orbital region, dry-eye syndrome caused by the reduced or absent lacrimal secretion, radiation cataract, iris atrophy, vascular changes, and retinal exudates (radiation retinopathy).[102]

Episcleral Plaques. The use of radon seed brachytherapy for the conservative treatment of retinoblastoma was introduced in 1929. In 1948 Stallard developed radioactive applicators using radium, and these applications were later modified to use ^{60}Co. Later techniques expanded to include ^{125}Ie, ^{192}Ir, and ^{106}Ru eye plaques, which are now all used routinely in the focal treatment of the disease.[103] Many treatment centers have a preference for ^{125}I plaques, since orbital tissues can be shielded with a gold plaque carrier, ridge plaques can limit the spread of radiation to the nerve and foveal region, and there is less radiation exposure for the patient and the assisting staff.[104] Regardless of the type used, the episcleral plaque technique is highly advantageous compared with other forms of therapy because the procedure time is short while the dose of irradiation is delivered directly to the tumor, minimizing radiation effects to the extraocular structures.

The use of radioactive scleral plaques as a primary treatment is particularly successful for medium-size tumors no greater than 12 mm in diameter and more than 3 mm from the optic disk or macula.[105] Scleral plaques are also useful as a secondary treatment for recurrent or new tumors which are impossible to control using photo- or cryocoagulation. The regression patterns seen after plaque treatment appear to be identical to those described for external-beam irradiation (types I, II, and III). However, a type IV radiation regression pattern characterized by complete destruction of the tumor choroid and all vessels, leaving a white scleral patch, has been observed only after cobalt plaque treatment.[100]

Photocoagulation. In 1955, Meyer-Schwickerath developed a photocoagulation technique using a xenon arc in which retinoblas-

tomas are surrounded by a ring of coagulation placed in the normal retina before the tumor tissue itself is treated.[106] The experience of others[104,107–110] suggests that the success of photocoagulation is due to the destruction of the retinal blood supply, not to its effect on the tumor itself or on the underlying choroid. The best results have occurred with tumors up to 4 to 5 disk diameters in size, with an elevation of 4 diopters,[111,112] although tumors up to 6 or more disk diameters have also been treated successfully in this way.[107,108] Indications, contraindications, and results of photocoagulation appear to be disparate. There are different opinions regarding the size, elevation, site, and clinical conditions in which retinoblastoma should be treated with photocoagulation.[109] Photocoagulation has been suggested as a primary approach for small and moderate retinoblastomas posterior to the equator and for the treatment of recurrent or new tumors after external radiotherapy or radioactive plaques.[108] Photocoagulation is not appropriate when tumors lie directly on the optic nerve or when there is vitreous seeding.

Complications arising from the use of photocoagulation may include occasional retinal hemorrhage, retinal traction, retinal folds, macular distortion, iris damage, corneal edema, and/or cataract (caused by inadvertent iris heating or energy absorption by preexisting opacities). The regression patterns observed after photocoagulation treatment depend on the size and elevation of the tumor (Fig. 19-6). Furthermore, it appears that vascularization of the tumor can influence sensitivity to xenon photocoagulation.[107] After photocoagulation, small tumors appear as a flat avascular pigmented scar. Larger tumors may present marked coarctation, reduced vascularization, and a translucent gray appearance similar to that described as fish flesh. However, both of these regression patterns closely resemble those of types I and II after radiotherapy.

Cryocoagulation. Cryotherapy[113] for retinoblastoma can be used as a primary or supplementary treatment after other conservative therapeutic attempts and can be effective in clinical situations involving new or recurrent tumors after irradiation therapy or in tumors anterior to the equator in eyes that have not been treated.[114] Cryotherapy can be successful on tumors up to 3.5 mm in diameter and 2.0 mm in thickness, but more than one treatment may be necessary.[115]

Vitreous base tumors are very rarely cured with cryocoagulation alone.[116] Localization of the tumor is obtained by indentation with a cryoprobe under indirect ophthalmoscopy. Tumors are frozen with applications of $-80°C$ for 30 to 60 s, and the treatment is typically repeated three times.[117] Cryotherapy destroys the tumor by direct intracellular and intravascular formation of microcrystals. The most frequent complications after cryotherapy are conjunctival and lid edema.

Chemotherapy. To date, chemotherapy has played only a secondary role in the treatment of retinoblastoma, since good control can be achieved with more local treatment. There is also a relative paucity of randomized studies on the efficacy of chemotherapy compared with other therapeutic procedures, and this is further complicated by a lack of suitable markers for the detection of minimal residual disease.[57,59,60,118] The first to use a chemotherapeutic agent in retinoblastoma treatment was Kupfer, who obtained partial regression of a retinal tumor mass by using nitrogen mustard.[119] After this preliminary experience, other antitumor drugs, especially vincristine and cyclophosphamide, were used alone or in combination in several situations, such as in association with radiotherapy for advanced disease [120,121] to reduce the mortality caused by micrometastatic disease [120–127] and with locally advanced disease or distant metastasis.[128–130] Especially in the last group of patients, sequential chemotherapy protocols or courses of intensive chemotherapy followed by autologous bone marrow transplantation have given encouraging results. Despite these achievements,

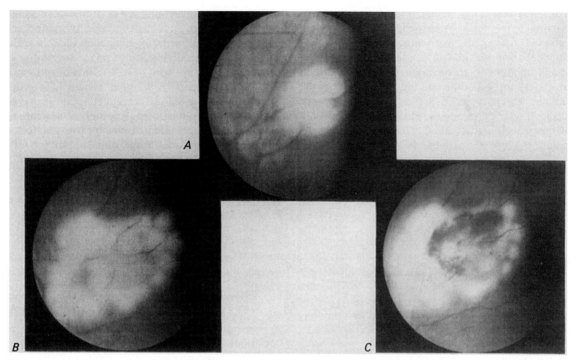

FIG. 19-6 Regression patterns for retinoblastoma after photocoagulation. *A.* A small retinoblastoma. *B.* After indirect xenon-arc photocoagulation. *C.* After direct xenon-arc photocoagulation. *(Courtesy of R. Frezzotti, M.D., Director of the Institute of Ophthalmological Sciences, University of Siena, Italy.)*

the role of antiblastic chemotherapy in the treatment of retinoblastoma remains controversial, and the only generally accepted indications for it are orbital or metastatic disease, trilateral retinoblastoma, and salvage therapy for relapses in the residual eye. More controversial indications include shrinkage of the neoplastic mass, optic nerve infiltration beyond the lamina cribrosa, and choroidal infiltration (whole thickness and/or ciliary body invasion) with or without optic nerve involvement up to the lamina cribrosa. This mode of therapy still awaits homogeneous staging and therapeutic criteria to evaluate its general efficacy.[131,132]

THE GENETICS OF RETINOBLASTOMA

Retinoblastoma has served as the prototypic example of the genetic predisposition to cancer.[133] Although the majority of tumors occur with no preceding family history, the inherited form of the disease has been extensively documented.[134–136] The familial disease is transmitted, with few exceptions, as a typical Mendelian autosomal dominant trait with virtually full penetrance. It has been estimated from epidemiologic data[137] that about 60 percent of cases are nonhereditary and unilateral, 15 percent are hereditary and unilateral, and 25 percent are hereditary and bilateral.

Although there are examples of apparent nonpenetrance among antecedent or collateral relatives of familial retinoblastoma patients, among descendants of such patients penetrance is nearly complete.[137] There have been a few pedigrees reported in which the disease seems to have truly skipped a generation, in other words being transmitted from grandparent to grandchild via an unaffected parent. Retrospective analysis of families of retinoblastoma probands have yielded several examples of presumed obligate carriers who did not develop the disease. Examination of a number of retinoblastoma pedigrees[15,135–139] showed apparent nonpenetrance in 52 of 128 families either through multiply affected sibships with both parents unaffected or through other affected relatives (such as cousins and aunts) with unaffected intervening relatives. In contrast, when pooled data from published sources were used to determine the segregation ratio among the offspring of familial retinoblastoma patients, it was observed that bilaterally affected parents had 49 percent affected offspring, as is expected for a dominantly inherited disease with complete penetrance, whereas unilaterally affected parents had 42 percent affected offspring, indicating some lack of penetrance.[139] These data were relevant to the proposal of a host resistance model by which heritable resistance factors to a predisposing gene are minimal in bilaterally affected individuals, intermediate in unilaterally affected individuals, and maximal in unaffected carriers.[139]

One proposed model[133,137] encompasses the observations that familial cases are generally multifocal and bilateral whereas sporadic cases typically present with unilateral unifocal disease of later diagnosis. According to the model, as few as two stochastic mutational events are required for tumor formation, the first of which can be inherited through the germ line (in heritable cases) or can occur somatically in individual retinal cells (in nonheritable cases). The second event occurs somatically in either case and leads to tumor formation in each doubly defective retinal cell. This empirically based hypothesis has been supported by direct experimental scrutiny using molecular genetic approaches.

Cytogenetics

The involvement of genetic alteration in the first step of this pathway of oncogenesis has been supported by cytogenetic analysis which have shown that a small proportion of patients carry a microscopically visible deletion of one chromosome 13 homologue in all their constitutional cells. Since the first such report[140] more than 30 deletions have been described occurring in a small percentage of retinoblastoma cases[141–143]; the common region of overlap of such deletions is chromosome 13, band q14.[144,145] An example of such a deletion of one constitutional chromosome 13 homologue is illustrated in Fig. 19-7. In the context of the two-hit

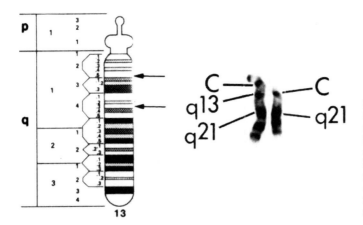

FIG. 19-7 Chromosome 13 deletion in constitutional cells from a patient with retinoblastoma. The idiogram of chromosome 13 to the left indicates the two breakpoints (arrows) of the interstitial deletion. To the right is a G-banded partial karyotype with the normal homologue on the left (centromere, C, bands q13 and q21 indicated) and the deleted homologue on the right (centromere and q21 band indicated). Note that only one chromosome homologue is altered. Hence, this aberration may represent the first and predisposing event in the child. *(Courtesy of David Ledbetter, Baylor College of Medicine, Houston.)*

model, such deletions could act as the first hit and, when they are germinal, could confer the risk of tumor formation in an autosomal dominant manner. Evidence that the same locus is involved in retinoblastoma cases that lack an apparent chromosomal deletion was provided through the demonstration of tight genetic linkage between the retinoblastoma and esterase D loci,[146] the latter being a moderately polymorphic isozymic enzyme whose encoding locus also maps to 13q14.[147]

Furthermore, cytogenetic analysis have provided important information concerning the occasional occurrence of apparent nonpenetrance in some retinoblastoma families. A large kindred has been reported in which unilateral retinoblastoma was transmitted by a number of unaffected individuals. Each affected individual carried the same constitutional deletion involving 13q14, whereas the unaffected carriers had a balanced insertional translocation involving the same region.[148] This and other related reports of chromosomal translocations, inversions, or deletions in transmitting parents[148,150] provide a clear biologic basis for segregation distortion without invoking nonpenetrance. In addition, two reports describe individuals who carry a constitutional deletion involving 13q14 but have no signs of retinoblastoma at age 5[151] or 25 years.[152] Whether a significant proportion of unaffected carriers can be accounted for by such mechanisms remains to be demonstrated. Another theoretical explanation for isolated multiply affected sibships with unaffected parents is parental mosaicism. Chromosomal mosaicism for deletions involving 13q14 was reported in lymphocytes from 5 to 50 sporadic retinoblastoma patients[153] in one series. In these cases a significant proportion of retinal cells must have carried the deletion; alternatively, if relatively few retinoblasts carried the deletion, an individual could be at low risk for expressing the disease but at high risk for its transmission. The increasing resolution of cytogenetic technology and the use of DNA probes for loci in the immediate vicinity of the retinoblastoma locus (gene symbol *RB1*) have also allowed the detection of more subtle genomic rearrangements that were undetectable previously and have shed light on individuals carrying nonpenetrant mutations in the retinoblastoma susceptibility locus (see below).

The presence of 13q14 deletion in patients without mental retardation or major anomalies[154] and in familial cases in which transmission might appear to be autosomal dominant[155] suggests that high-resolution chromosome analysis should be done in all patients with retinoblastoma. When a deletion is found in a proband, parental studies should be considered to rule out deletion, insertional translocation, or mosaicism.

Molecular Genetics

Specific predictions of the nature of the second tumor-eliciting event in the two-step model on oncogenesis[133,137] have been pro-

posed[156]: (1) The autosomal dominant hereditary form of retinoblastoma, in the absence of a gross chromosomal deletion, involves the same genetic locus that is involved in cases showing large deletions of chromosome 13. Thus, the first step in the pathway toward tumorigenesis in these cases is a submicroscopic mutational event at the *RB1* locus. (2) The same genetic change which has occurred as a germ-line mutation in hereditary retinoblastoma occurs as a somatic genetic alteration of the *RB1* locus in a retinal cell in nonhereditary retinoblastoma. (3) The second step in tumorigenesis in both heritable and nonhereditary retinoblastoma involves somatic alteration of the normal allele at the *RB1* locus in such a way that the mutant allele is unmasked. Thus, the first mutation in this process, although it may be inherited as an autosomal dominant trait at the organism level, is in fact a recessive defect in the individual retinal cell.

The model which arises from these considerations is shown in Fig. 19-8, outlining specific chromosomal mechanisms which should allow phenotypic expression of a recessive germinal mutation of the *RB1* locus (Fig. 19-8*a*). This aberration is inherited by an individual who thus carries such a mutation in all somatic as well as germ-line cells (Fig.19-8*b*). Any additional event that results in homozygosity or hemizygosity for the mutant allele (that is, the *RB1* locus is mutant on both chromosome 13 homologues) will result in a tumor clone. Several chromosomal mechanisms can be imagined in this process: (1) mitotic nondisjunction with loss of the wild-type chromosome (Fig. 19-8*c*), resulting in hemizygosity at all loci on chromosome 13, (2) mitotic nondisjunction with duplication of the mutant chromosome (Fig. 19-8*d*), resulting in homozygosity at all loci on the chromosome, (3) mitotic recombination (Fig. 19-8*e*) between the *RB1* locus encoding the mutant allele and the centromere, resulting in heterozygosity at loci in the proximal region and homozygosity throughout the rest of the chromosome, including the *RB1* locus, (4) several other more regionalized events such as gene conversion (Fig. 19-8*f*), deletion (Fig. 19-8*g*), or mutation (Fig. 19-8*h*). Both nonheritable and hereditary retinoblastoma could arise through the appearance of homozygosity at the *RB1* locus, the difference being two somatic events in the former instance and one germinal event and one somatic event in the latter instance.

The approach that has been taken to examine these hypotheses relies on the variability of DNA sequences among humans, which results in inherited differences in restriction-endonuclease recognition sites. In this approach, segments of the human genome are isolated in recombinant DNA form, and the loci homologous to these probe segments are tested for their encompassing restriction-endonuclease recognition sequences, which vary between unrelated individuals. Two types of such variation have been defined. The first and most abundant results from simple base-pair changes within the recognition-site sequence for a particular restriction endonuclease and yields alleles of greater (when the effect of the mu-

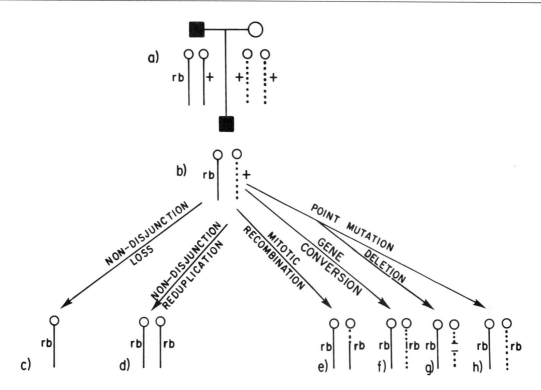

FIG. 19-8 Chromosomal mechanisms that could reveal recessive mutations. In this example, an affected male (a) who carries a recessive defect at the *RB1* locus on chromosome 13, designated rb, in all his cells mates with a genotypically wild-type, +, female. One of their children (b) inherits the defective chromosome 13 from his father and so is rb/+ at the *RB1* locus in all his cells. A tumor in his retinal cells may develop by eliminating the dominant wild-type allele at the *RB1* locus by the mechanisms required to effect the tumor cell genotype shown schematically in c to h. *(Reprinted by permission from Cavenee et al., Nature, vol. 305, p. 779, copyright 1983, Macmillan Journals, Limited.)*

tation is loss of a site) or lesser (when the effect of the mutation is gain of a site) length.[157] The second type results from the insertion or deletion of varying numbers of blocks of like DNA sequence into or out of the genomic locus.[158] Practically, the net result is the observation of two alleles at the locus encompassing a site change (presence or absence of the site) or numerous alleles at a locus subject to insertion or deletion of larger segments of DNA, respectively. In either case, however, any given individual will reveal only two alleles at the locus, one from the paternally derived chromosome and one from the maternally derived homologue. In all cases examined to date these types of markers have been shown to behave in family studies in the manner that would be predicted for simple Mendelian codominant alleles. Recombinant DNA probes for loci mapped along the length of human chromosome 13 have been isolated, characterized,[159,160] and used in multilocus analysis to detect alterations in the somatic genotypes of tumors compared with the germ-line genotype of the individuals harboring these tumors.[156,161,162] A reasonably large series of retinoblastoma cases has been examined in this manner; examples are illustrated in Figs. 15-9 and 10.

Nondisjunction and Duplication. The mechanism depicted in Fig. 19-8*D* in which, together with the nondisjunctional loss of the wild-type chromosome, the mutant chromosome is duplicated, would be difficult to detect cytogenetically or by quantitation of esterase D activity. However, with the use of codominant DNA markers, these events were detected as a loss of one allele at each informative locus on the chromosome. The patient described in Fig. 19-9 was found to be heterozygous at the ESD locus and showed no visible abnormality of either chromosome 13. An examination of tumor tissue from this individual again showed no abnormalities of chromosome 13 except that in addition to the expected two copies of the chromosome, another copy was present as a translocation involving chromosomes 13 and 14. However, the

tumor cells exhibited only one of the two isozymic types of the esterase D enzyme—the allele from the father. It was proposed[163] that this resulted from somatic inactivation of the maternally derived allele of the ESD locus on one homologue of chromosome 13.

Constitutional and tumor cells derived from this patient were tested with seven recombinant DNA probes. Three of the probes revealed heterozygosity in the germ-line tissue: p9A7, which maps in the region 13q22-qter, and pHU26 and pHU10, both of which map in the region 13q12-q22. In each of these cases (Fig. 19-9*A* to *C*), although both codominant alleles were present in the germ line, only one allele at each locus was present in the tumor, and this allele was derived in each case from the chromosome 13 inherited from the father. A reasonable interpretation of these results is diagrammed in Fig. 19-9*D*. Rather than somatic inactivation of the ESD locus on one chromosome 13 homologue, these data are consistent with the complete loss of the entire maternally derived chromosome accompanied by duplication of the paternally derived chromosome. It is likely that this chromosome carried a *de novo* germinal mutation, since the father showed no evidence of retinoblastoma but the subject was bilaterally affected. It is also possible that one or two of the chromosomes 13 in the tumor were derived by mitotic exchange between the wild-type mutant chromosomes (as diagrammed in Fig. 19-8*E*) so that an original mutant chromosome and a recombinant chromosome (or two) were maintained. If this had happened, the point of interchange must have been proximal to the region detected by the most proximal marker locus, since all the markers, including esterase D (which maps to 13q14), show reduction to homozygosity in the tumor.

Mitotic Recombination. Another possible mechanism by which part of a pair of chromosomes may become homozygous, although not previously observed in humans, is illustrated in Fig. 19-8*E*. A somatic, or mitotic, recombination between the mutant and wild-type chromosome homologues, with subsequent segregation, can result in a cell that maintains heterozygosity at loci proximal to the breakpoint of the recombinational event but shows homozygosity at loci distal to such a breakpoint. An instance of this mechanism was presented in patient Rb-412.[156] The germ-line cells from this person had been determined to be heterozygous at the ESD locus as well as heterozygous for a quinacrine-staining satellite heteromorphism on the short arm of chromosome 13. An examination of the tumor cells derived from this patient showed the presence of both types of satellite staining but only one isozymic form of esterase D. A reasonable interpretation of these data[162] was that both chromosomes 13 were present in their entirety in the Rb-412 tumor and that a somatic inactivation of one of the isozymic forms of esterase D had occurred during tumor formation. Alternatively, a mitotic recombination event occurring between the centromere and the ESD locus, as was described above, could generate chromosomes consistent with these results. Germ-line and tumor genotypes of this patient were examined at chromosome 13 loci defined by seven DNA probes (Fig. 19-10). Three of the markers were heterozygous in skin fibroblasts from Rb-412: p1E8, which maps distal to 13q22; p9D11, which maps at 13q22; and p7F12, which maps between the *RB1* locus and the centromere. The tumor tissue from this patient showed a loss of one allele at the 9D11 and 1E8

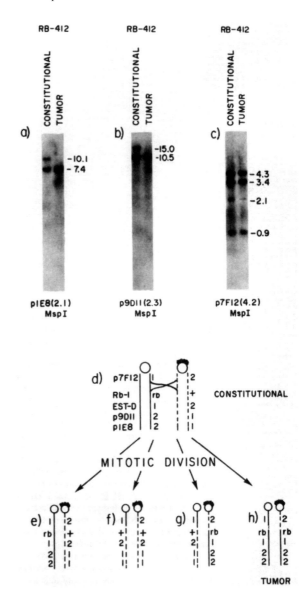

FIG. 19-10 Homozygosity effected by a mitotic recombination event. *A.* The pattern obtained when the hybridization probe was p1E8, which is homologous to a locus on chromosome 13 mapping between band q22 and the terminus of the long arm. *B.* Results obtained when the hybridization probe was p9D11, which is homologous to a locus on chromosome 13 mapping to band q22. *C.* Results obtained with the hybridization probe p7F12, which is homologous to a locus on chromosome 13 mapping between bands q12 and q14. *D.* Schematic diagram showing inferred haplotypes on each chromosome derived from karyology, esterase D determinations, and these data. The cap on the chromosome homologues represented by the dashed lines denotes a fluorescent-staining heterochromatic region. In this figure the point of crossover must lie between the *RB1* and *7F12* loci and is shown occurring between chromatids of the chromosome 13 homologue at the four-strand stage of mitotic chromosome replication. *E–H.* Schematic diagram of the four possible combinations of wild-type and recombinant homologues. Possibilities *E* to *G* result in a phenotypically wild-type cell. The allelic data shown in *H* corresponds to the experimental data and results in homozygosity for the mutant (rb) allele at the *RB1* locus. *(Reprinted by permission from Cavenee et al., Nature, vol, 305, p. 781, copyright 1983, Macmillan Journals, Limited.)*

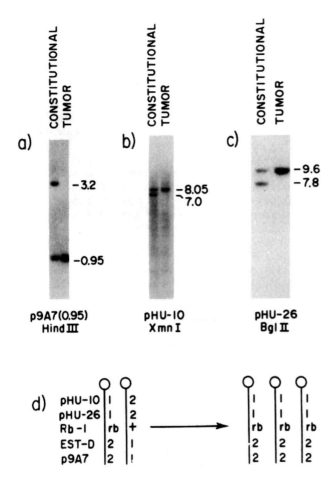

FIG. 19-9 Homozygosity effected by segregation of one chromosome 13 homologue with duplication of the remaining one. *A.* Results obtained when HindIII-digested DNA was hybridized to p9A7, which contains an insert homologous to a locus on chromosome 13 mapping between band q22 and the terminus of the long arm. *B.* The pattern obtained when XmnI-digested DNA was hybridized to the insert fragment derived from the plasmid pHU10, which is homologous to a locus on chromosome 13 mapping between bands q12 and q22. *C.* The pattern obtained when BgIII-digested DNA was hybridized to the insert fragment isolated from the plasmid pHU26, which is homologous to a locus on chromosome 13 mapping between bands q12 and q22. *D.* A schematic diagram incorporating these data with previous analysis of the esterase D alleles present and the karyotype of the two samples from patient Rb-409. *(Reprinted by permission from Cavenee et al., Nature, vol. 305, p. 780, copyright 1983, Macmillan Journals, Limited.)*

loci, whereas the 7F12 locus remained heterozygous (Fig. 19-10C). An interpretation of these results, taken together with the satellite heteromorphism and esterase D data described above, is illustrated in Fig. 19-10D and suggests that a recombination event took place between the mutant and wild-type chromosomes 13 in the cell that gave rise to the tumor. The crossover point was between the 7F12 and the *RB1* loci, and each locus distal to the *RB1* locus became homozygous. Between *RB1* and the terminus of the short arm, however, two markers maintained both the maternal and paternal haplotypes.

Data similar to those shown in Figs. 19-9 and 19-10 have been obtained in more than 75 percent of the retinoblastoma tumors examined. They provide experimental support for the proposed recessive model of oncogenesis,[133,137,156] by which predisposing mutations are revealed by elimination of the homologous wild-type locus through chromosomal segregation or recombination rather than simple point mutation. The supposition that it was the chromosome 13 homologue carrying the wild-type *RB1* allele that was lost during the process of tumorigenesis was tested by comparing constitutional and tumor genotypes of patients with familial retinoblastoma.

The model described in Fig. 19-8 demands that the chromosomes 13 remaining in the tumors of such children be derived from the affected parent. The analysis[163] of one such case, KS2H, is shown in Fig. 19-11. This child was constitutionally heterozygous at the HU26 locus. His retinoblastoma tumor tissue (Rb-KS2H) showed only the longer allele at this locus. His unaffected parent, KS2C, was constitutionally heterozygous at this locus, while his affected parent, KS2F, was homozygous for the longer allele. Therefore, the proband must have inherited the shorter allele at the locus from his unaffected parent, and it was this chromosome that was lost in the tumor. The chromosome remaining in the tumor was inherited from his affected parent and must be the one carrying the initial predisposing mutation at *RB1*. In this family, the proband inherited the predisposition to retinoblastoma from his father, KS2F, who had inherited it from his mother, KS2G (Fig. 19-11B). He obtained the shorter allele from his unaffected mother and the longer allele from his affected father. It is the latter chromosome that must contain the mutant *RB1* locus, and it was this chromosome which was retained in the child's tumor. Corroborating evidence of this interpretation was obtained by examining genotypic combinations at other loci on chromosome 13 in other members of the family. Assignment of the alleles at each of these loci, in combination with those for HU26, and a consideration of the allelic combinations from the grandparents (KS2A, KS2B, and KS2G), parents (KS2C and KS2F), child (KS2H), and child's tumor (Rb-KS2H) made it possible to infer chromosomal haplotypes (Fig. 19-11B). The proband (KS2H) inherited a nonrecombinant

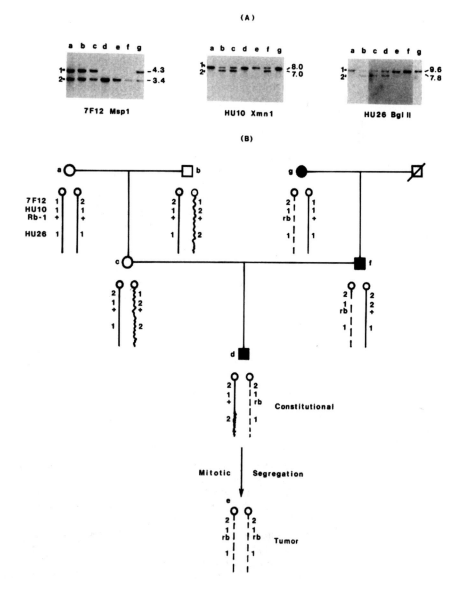

FIG. 19-11 Loss of germ-line heterozygosity in a hereditary retinoblastoma tumor. *A.* DNA was isolated from peripheral blood leukocytes from each of the indicated individuals and from a primary tumor biopsy from the proband, KS2H. The DNA was digested with the indicated restriction endonucleases, separated by electrophoresis through 0.8 % agarose gels, transferred to nylon membranes, and hybridized to the indicated probes homologous to loci on human chromosome 13. The family members are designated: (a) KS2A, (b) KS2B, (c) KS2C, (d) KS2H, (e) Rb-KS2H (tumor), (f) KS2F, and (g) KS2g. *B.* Pedigree Rb-KS2 and inferred chromosome 13 haplotypes at the 7F12, HU10, *RB1*, and HU26 loci. Filled symbols = individuals with retinoblastoma; dashed line = nonrecombinant chromosome; straight and wavy lines = recombinant chromosome. *(Reprinted by permission from Cavenee et al., Science 228:501, 26 April 1985, copyright 1985, American Association for the Advancement of Science.)*

chromosome from his paternal grandmother (KS2G) through his father (KS2F) and a recombinant chromosome from his mother (KS2C). It appears that the chromosome retained in the tumor (Rb-KS2H) was inherited from his affected grandmother (KS2G) through his affected father (KS2F). In other inherited cases examined, the prediction that the chromosome 13 derived from the affected parent would be retained in the tumor has also been confirmed.

It is noteworthy that although the unmasking of predisposing mutations at the RB1 locus occurs in mechanistically similar ways in sporadic and heritable retinoblastoma patients, only the later carry the initial mutation in each of their cells. Patients with heritable disease also seem to be at greatly increased risk for the development of second-site primary tumors, particularly osteogenic sarcoma.[164] A testable corollary of the model outlined above is that this high propensity is not merely fortuitous but is genetically determined by the predisposing *RB1* mutation. This notion of pathogenetic causality in the clinical association between these two rare tumor types was tested by determining the constitutional and osteosarcoma genotypes at RFLP loci on chromosome 13. The data indicated that osteosarcomas arising in retinoblastoma patients had become homozygous specifically around the chromosomal region carrying the *RB1* locus.[165] Furthermore, the same chromosomal mechanisms eliciting losses of constitutional heterozygosity were observed in sporadic osteosarcomas, suggesting a genetic similarity in pathogenetic causality. These findings are of obvious relevance to the interpretation of human mixed-cancer families, as they suggest differential expression of a single pleiotropic mutation in the etiology of clinically associated cancer of different histologic types.

A likely explanation for the association between retinoblastoma and osteosarcoma is that both tumors arise subsequent to chromosomal mechanisms which unmask recessive mutations. This may involve either one common locus that is involved in normal regulation of differentiation of both tissues or separate loci that are located closely within chromosome region 13q14. In either case, germ-line deletions of the retinoblastoma locus may also affect the osteosarcoma locus. Deletions are likely to be an important form of predisposing mutations at the *RB1* locus, since a considerable fraction of bilateral retinoblastoma patients carry visible constitutional chromosome deletions[141–143] and submicroscopic deletions have been detected by reduction of esterase D activity.[147]

These epidemiologic, genetic, cytogenetic, and molecular genetic studies provided data with which to make specific predictions about the nature of the *RB1* locus that have been useful in its molecular isolation. First, any candidate gene should map to the 13q14.1 region of the genome. Second, by analogy with other human diseases, such as Duchenne muscular dystrophy,[166] chronic granulomatous disease,[167] and several of the hemoglobinopathies, at least a proportion of mutations at the *RB1* locus should be submicroscopic deletions. Third, a comparison of normal and tumor tissues from heritable cases should show hemizygous aberrancy in the former and homozygous defects in the latter. Fourth, even in the absence of detectable genomic alterations, defects in the mRNA transcribed from the locus or the protein products translated from the mRNA should be detected in tumors.

To provide DNA probes for landmark locations within 13q14, metaphase chromosomes 13 were sorted using a fluorescence-activated cell sorter, and portions of this were used in the derivation of a chromosome-enriched recombinant DNA library.[168] Several unique sequence probes were isolated from this library, and their physical location were determined by in situ hybridization to metaphase chromosomes and by determining hybridization dosage in normal cells from retinoblastoma patients with cytogenetically visible deletions of chromosome 13. One such probe, termed H3-8, was localized to the region 13q14.1, thus fulfilling the first crite-

rion listed above.[169] When this probe was used to determine the genomic organization of its cognate locus in retinoblastoma tumors, 2 of 37 showed hybridization patterns consistent with homozygous deletion,[170] thus fulfilling the second criterion. In addition, these deletions were shown to arise either germinally or somatically in bilateral or unilateral disease, respectively,[170] thereby fulfilling the third criterion. The H3-8 probe was used to isolate larger overlapping segments of DNA, and a unique sequence subfragment of one of these segments was used as a hybridization probe to determine the genomic organization of the approximately 200-kb locus and the transcription pattern of its 4.7-kb mRNA in tumor and normal tissues. Several provocative findings arose. First, deletions that were entirely contained within the locus were observed in some cases. Further characterization of the complete *RB1* genomic sequence[171] allowed a rigorous and complete cataloging of the different mutations that affect the gene in retinoblastoma tumors. Simple Southern blot hybridizations have identified submicroscopic deletions involving various regions of the gene in up to 40 percent of tumor tissues or constitutional cells from individuals affected by retinoblastoma.[169,170,172–174] Application of the polymerase chain reaction amplification technique coupled with DNA sequencing and RNase protection assays has increased the proportion of retinoblastomas with measurable *RB1* locus alterations by detecting subtle exonic and intronic base changes.[175,176] Figure 19-12 schematically represents some of the characterized retinoblastoma mutations.

The extensive size of the genomic locus has made complete sequence analysis of *RB1* alleles a labor-intensive approach, and so alterations at the transcription level have been pursued to increase the sensitivity of detection of mutations in the locus. When transcription patterns were first analyzed in tumor tissue, no apparent RNA transcript was detected in retinoblastomas or osteosarcomas, although normal-size mRNA was present in retinal cells and several other tissue types (see "Biochemical Characterization of the Retinoblastoma Gene Product" below). These results have been extended by several other groups,[177,178] and transcripts of aberrant size have been identified in tumors previously shown to contain normal genomic structure, thus fulfilling the last criterion listed above. Investigations of *RB1* gene alterations at both the DNA and RNA levels cumulatively reveal a strong correlative relationship between lack of the *RB1* gene product and the appearance of retinoblastoma tumors. In addition, both DNA and RNA alterations appear to be common in both sporadic and heritable disease, as would be expected from the genetic model discussed earlier.

In addition to cancers such as osteosarcoma, that are clinically related to retinoblastoma, other tumors have been found to have aberrancies of the retinoblastoma gene. The involvement of *RB1* in these tumors is inferred from alterations in the gene structure itself or as loss of heterozygosity for DNA markers in the 13q14 region surrounding the *RB1* gene. Some examples of such alterations found in osteosarcomas and breast carcinomas are shown in Fig. 19-12. Molecular analysis of small-cell lung carcinomas have revealed *RB1* structural abnormalities in approximately 15 percent of cases,[179] and loss of heterozygosity for chromosome 13 has been detected in about 25 percent of breast cancers and their derived cell lines analyzed to date.[180,181] A more detailed analysis of the involvement of loss of heterozygosity for chromosome 13 in tumors has been compiled[182] and clearly shows that not all tumors result from direct or indirect alteration of the *RB1* locus. However, the cumulative data suggest that *RB1* is pleiotropically active, and subsets of tumors may share a common pathogenetic mechanism which results from unmasking mutations that affect the tumor-suppressing function of *RB1*.

The observations described above satisfy all the physical criteria for the identity of the *RB1* locus as a tumor-suppressor gene. As in all cases of "reverse genetics," however, proof of this requires

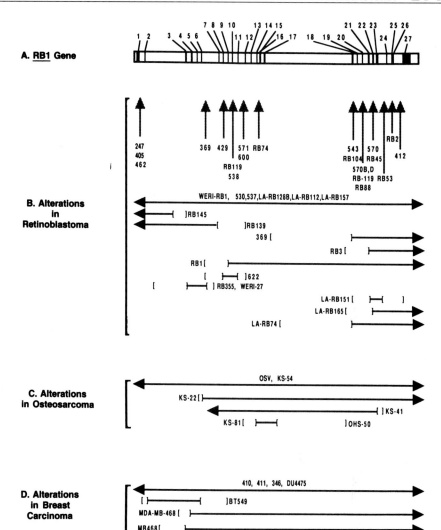

FIG. 19-12 Genomic alteration in the *RB1* gene for retinoblastoma and associated tumors. *RB1* gene alterations are designated as they appeared in their respective primary references. ↔ -complete deletion of the *RB1* locus; []→, ←[], and [] — [] = partial deletion of the *RB1* locus, where one or both deletion endpoints occur within the bracketed area in the genomic sequence. Vertical hatched arrows indicate the position of small deletions/point mutations characterized by PCR/DNA sequencing or RNase protection assays. *(Reprinted by permission from Gennett and Cavenee, Brain Pathology 1:25-32, copyright 1990, ISN Journals.)*

biochemical and functional analysis. The nature of this gene and the effect its elimination has on oncogenesis rely on the cell biologic and biochemical approaches described below. Its isolation alone, however, constitutes a powerful example of the reverse genetics approach to gene identification through physical and genetic mapping.

Genetic Complementation   The genetic model requiring sequential inactivating mutations and structural evidence in its support suggests that retinoblastoma and its genetically associated tumors arise through loss of function of the *RB1* locus. One prediction of this line of reasoning is that the replacement of wild-type *RB1* function into cells which lack that function should have normalizing effects on at least parts of the tumorigenic phenotype. This has been directly addressed through the introduction of the wild-type gene into retinoblastoma (the WERI-Rb27 line) and osteosarcoma (the SaOS-2 line) cells through recombinant retroviral vector transfer and assessment of morphology, growth rate, or tumorigenic capability.[183]

Neither type of cell was affected in any capacity after infection by the vector carrying an irrelevant luciferase (Lux) gene. However, after the introduction of the vector carrying the Rb cDNA, two separate morphologies were apparent in the affected populations: One was flattened and greatly enlarged and represented 90 to 95 percent of the population, while the remainder was composed of small cells and mimicked uninfected cells. This suggested that these two RB+-reconstituted cell lines differed from the RB- parental lines in their morphology and cell division rates, which

correlated with the presence of the expression of wild-type RB. Subcutaneous injection of Lux- and TB+-reconstituted cells into nude mice resulted in palpable tumors only in those injected with Lux-infected cells, indicating that induction of wild-type p110RB protein expression was capable of suppressing tumorigenicity in both retinoblastomas and osteosarcomas. Similar suppression of tumorigenicity has been demonstrated after the introduction of these retroviral RB+ vectors into bladder[184] and prostate[185] carcinoma cells, although the effect of reconstituted RB expression on their morphology and growth rate was less dramatic.

There is also evidence that the location of injection may create environments that are more or less suited for tumor growth. In fact, some cancer cells incapable of forming tumors when injected subcutaneously are able to do so when grafted into the anterior chamber of the rodent eye.[186] When retinoblastoma cells used in the retroviral reconstitution experiments were assayed in this site,[187] the malignant WERI-Rb27 parental line formed tumors 40 days after inoculations of 10^3 to 10^4 cells (compared to the 10^7 cells required in subcutaneous injections). Also, 11 of 14 RB+-reconstituted clones were unable to form tumors. Evaluation of the levels of pp110RB showed that they resulted from the growth of a small fraction of uninfected parental cells such that the tumor cells were unable to express the RB1 protein. All this suggests that pp110RB can function to suppress the tumorigenic phenotype in retinoblastoma cell lines, as predicted by the model.

Other experiments with the breast cancer cell line MDA-468-S4 and retinoblastoma cell lines WERI-*RB1* and Y79 have provided less support for the tumor-suppressing ability of p110RB.[188]

In these studies, expression of exogenous p110RB did not alter growth rate or cloning efficiency in the breast cancer cell line, whereas reintroduction of Rb into both RB cell lines reduced colony formation but had no effect on morphology, growth rate, or tumorigenicity. In clear contrast to the studies described above, the reconstituted retinoblastoma cell line formed intraocular tumors with the same efficiency as did the RB⁻ parental cell lines. These tumors, formed in the anterior chamber of the eye, were excised from the mice and expanded in culture. All the tumor cells recovered showed expression of p110RB at levels similar to those of the original parental clones, indicating that tumor formation was not due to loss of function of the transferred *RB1* gene. These experiments suggest that tumorigenesis is not deterred by replacement of a normal *RB1* allele or expression of RB in homozygously RB-defective cells. Certainly, this confusing situation and the role of p110RB in the tumorigenic process require further exploration.

Prenatal Diagnosis

Advantage has been taken of the increasingly precise molecular elucidation of genomic alterations in retinoblastoma tumors to provide conceptual and methodologic approaches to the assignment of disease risk.[189,190] These methods are either indirect and linkage-based[189] or direct[190] in their detection of genetic defects.

The first approach used polymorphic restriction-fragment-length alleles as linkage markers to deduce genotypes at the *RB1* locus in the children of retinoblastoma gene carriers. This method takes advantage of neutral DNA sequence variation in the popula-

tion, which results in the variable presence of bacterial restriction-endonuclease recognition sites at loci on chromosome 13. This approach had three major limitations. First, most of the loci identified by RFLP[159,160] were genetically distant from the *RB1* locus,[191] and consequently, the reliability of the method was reduced by the occurrence of meiotic recombination. Second, the population frequencies of alleles of these loci were such that only a fraction of families were informative. Third, the method required an affected parent and a first child to define the haplotypic phase. Therefore, analysis was restricted to nuclear families in which informative allelic combinations could be discerned at loci flanking the *RB1* locus.

The family described in Fig. 19-13 illustrates how parental haplotypes of chromosome 13 can be deduced through the analysis of the parents and an affected first child. In this example, the first child (II-1) inherited the predisposition for retinoblastoma (Fig. 19-13B) and the longer alleles at the 7F12 and 9D11 loci (Fig. 19-13A) from his affected father. The fetus (II-2), however, inherited the alternative chromosome 13, which carried the shorter alleles at the 7F12 and 9D11 loci. Since the 7F12 and 9D11 loci flank the *RB1* locus at recombination distances of approximately 12 and 30 percent, respectively, the fetus will have inherited the predisposition for retinoblastoma only if two meiotic crossovers occurred between these two loci. The risk estimate for the development of retinoblastoma by this child arises from the conjoint probability of two such crossing-over events. Since the parental haplotype was inferred from the first child, these risk estimates must also consider crossovers in both children, giving a joint probability of 84 percent that retinoblastoma will not develop in the second child. At age 8

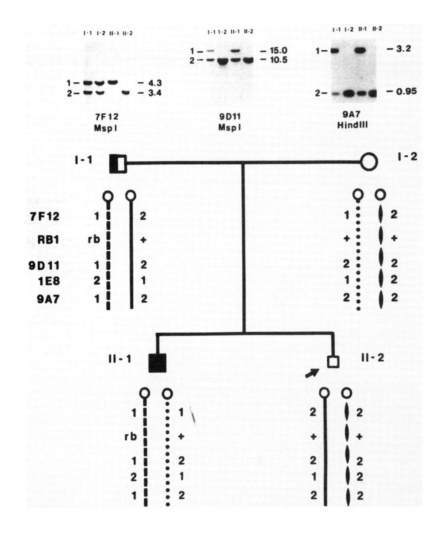

FIG. 19-13 Pedigree of a familial retinoblastoma case that shows no evidence of meiotic recombination. Closed symbols = bilaterally affected family members; half-closed symbols = unilaterally affected members; open symbols = unaffected members. Arrows indicate the family member for whom diagnosis before illness was performed; the indications of the presence or absence of disease are based on subjects' status at their most recent ophthalmic examination. Inferred alleles at the retinoblastoma (*RB1*) locus are designated rb for a mutant allele and + for a wild-type allele. The circles with vertical lines below them that are shown under each family-member symbol represent the member's two constitutional chromosome 13 homologues. The numbers beside each chromosome symbol represent the allelic form of each locus. The vertical order of loci within each family is the same as that shown under the symbol for its I-1 member. The data illustrate the power of information about a first child in discriminating which chromosome a second child has inherited from the affected parent. (*Reprinted from Cavenee et al., New England Journal of Medicine, vol. 314, pp. 1201–1207, 1986, by permission.*)

years this child showed no signs of the disease, in accordance with this prediction.

There were several major limitations to this initial approach. First, chromosome 13 haplotypes could not be determined in the carrier parent unless there was either one affected grandparent or one previously affected child or unless the first unaffected child had passed the age for development of retinoblastoma (which is 7 years or more). Second, there was a chance that gene carriers would remain unaffected because of the somewhat less than absolute penetrance of these predisposing mutations. Third, relatively few and incompletely informative markers for chromosome 13 had been isolated, and these markers were not for the most part tightly linked to the *RB1* locus. This resulted in risk estimates that were much less precise than desired and allowed only a very few clinical decisions to be based solely on these analyses. Most of these limitations could be minimized if several highly informative and closely linked markers were isolated. The isolation of a cDNA for the closely linked gene esterase D[192,193] allowed an RFLP with better allele frequencies than the protein polymorphism at the same locus. Clearly, the most desirable situation in this regard is the ability to determine the gene defect directly in individual retinoblastoma cases. This is particularly important in counseling families with a single case of bilateral retinoblastoma, since in most instances linkage-based analysis can be used only if there is more than one affected family member. There was a similar need for direct determination of mutations of the *RB1* locus in cases of sporadic unilateral retinoblastoma; such patients constitute more than 50 percent of all retinoblastoma cases, and about 10 percent of them carry germline mutations.

The isolation of the retinoblastoma susceptibility gene has allowed these goals to be reached, since, as was previously mentioned, the predictive value of RFLP analysis increases in direct proportion to the proximity of informative marker loci to the disease locus. Intragenic polymorphisms are of course the best of this class, and so far five independent intragenic RFLPs have been described.[194] Four of these polymorphisms were due to restriction site alterations for *KpnI*, *XbaI*, *MboII*, and *TthIII*, and a fifth was due to length variability in the number of tandem repeats of a 50-bp sequence that resulted in eight distinct alleles. The inheritance pattern of these polymorphisms in 13 families with heritable retinoblastoma showed cosegregation of alleles with the disease locus. Furthermore, because of their location within the gene itself, inference errors arising from undetected meiotic recombination within the gene are much reduced in comparison with even the nearest flanking polymorphic probe. As more sequence data have become available, these intragenic polymorphisms have been adapted from standard Southern protocols to PCR amplification methods.[195–197]

These modern approaches to risk assessment may still be complicated somewhat by parental bias in the origin of *RB1* mutations. Evidence has been provided that paternal gametogenesis confers a higher mutation rate on the *RB1* locus.[198,199] The examination of sporadic bilateral retinoblastoma cases showed that disease arises subsequent to a new germ-line mutation in the paternal allele, followed by somatic alteration or loss of the maternally derived wild-type allele in 13 of 14 cases. In contrast, the examination of sporadic unilateral retinoblastoma tumors showed that only 4 of 10 unilateral tumors retained the allele derived from the father. This suggests that mutations in the *RB1* locus occur more commonly during spermatogenesis or that the paternal chromosome in the early embryo is at a higher risk for mutation. Similar analysis of 13 sporadic osteosarcomas showed that 12 were preferentially mutated in the paternal allele.[200] Considering the clinical association between heritable retinoblastoma and second-site primary tumors such as osteosarcoma, the mechanisms which result in germ-line

mutations in retinoblastoma probably are also responsible for producing sporadic related diseases.

Genomic imprinting is one mechanism that might explain the unusual imbalance in mutation and retention of the paternal allele of specific retinoblastomas and related tumors. This is a process, described as epigenetic allele inavtivation, that is dependent on the gamete of origin.[201] Imprinted alleles may act as mutated alleles but differ from mutations in the classical sense in that they show a preference for inheritance from only one sex. Consistent with this is the analysis of polymorphic markers on chromosome 13q in parents of patients with sporadic retinoblastoma, which showed that three of three bilateral tumors retained the paternal chromosome (in accordance with previous studies) and that seven of eight unilateral tumors also did so.[202] The discrepancy between the parental biases shown in this report and those discussed above may be explained by the imprinting process being superimposed on the genetic background of the patient.

Although the pattern of inheritance for retinoblastoma suggests 90 percent penetrance,[203] cases of transmitted, nonpenetrant mutations of the *RB1* locus have been described (see the section on molecular genetics, above), and these asymptomatic mutations may have an impact on the accuracy of DNA diagnostics. DNA analysis at the level afforded by current technologies offers the possibility of discriminating in unaffected offspring noncarriers from asymptomatic carriers of a nonpenetrant mutation. For example, screening of the *RB1* coding structure using exon-by-exon single-stranded conformation polymorphism (SSCP) analysis utilizes the sequence-dependent migration of single-stranded DNA through gel matrices. Such experiments have revealed abnormalities in exon 20 as well as in the promoter region of *RB1*.[204,205] The former were determined to be single-base changes resulting in amino acid substitutions. The discovery of these alterations suggests that they might serve to reduce the functional efficiency of the retinoblastoma gene product rather than ablate its suppressing ability altogether. It is interesting to note that these studies may suggest the potential existence of different sets of functional mutations in retinoblastoma—and that these groups may in turn define differentially functioning regions of the gene product itself. Such predictions require a full characterization of the biochemical role of the retinoblastoma gene product in both normal and tumorigenic cells.

BIOCHEMICAL CHARACTERIZATION OF THE RETINOBLASTOMA GENE PRODUCT

After the documentation of the types of mutations and rearrangements of the *RB1* locus in retinoblastomas and other tumors, an understanding of their significance required an understanding of the normal biologic and biochemical function of the protein that locus encoded. The impetus and basis for this was the prior determination of the genomic structure for *RB1* and the isolation and sequencing of its 4.7-kb mRNA described above. Analysis of the tissue specificity of *RB1* mRNA expression showed ubiquitous presence in normal human and rat tissues, including brain, kidney, ovary, spleen, liver, placenta, and retina. This surprising result was augmented by the demonstration that genomic DNA sequences homologous to human *RB1* cDNA were present in a variety of organisms. The sequences were measurably divergent among vertebrate, with homology decreasing as a function of the distance from humans along the evolutionary tree.[177] Thus, although the tumors elicited by inherited mutations of the *RB1* locus are relatively narrow in type, its broad tissue expression and species conservation suggested a common and potentially pivotal role in the growth or differentiation of cell types of a variety of ontogenies. Moreover, these observations raise the possibility of interaction of the *RB1* gene or its product with others to provide tissue specificity.

The Retinoblastoma Protein

Sequence analysis of an initial cDNA clone provided a great deal of predictive information about the nature and features of the *RB1* protein product[177]: it was 816 amino acids in length, had an estimated molecule mass of 94 kDa, and contained 10 dispersed potential glycosylation sites and a leucine zipper (indicated by the presence of periodic leucine residues every seventh position in an alpha helix,[206] which is thought to be important for dimerization of proteins) within exon 20. Furthermore, the region containing amino acids 663 to 716 contains 14 prolines among its 54 residues; such proline-rich regions have been observed in the nuclear oncogenes, c-*myc* and c-*myb*.[207] The subsequent isolation of several full-length 4.7-kb cDNA clones[172] showed that the initial size estimate of 94 kDa was based on a sequence missing 236 of the 5'-most amino acids, whereas the full-length sequence resulted in a predicted protein of about 110 kDa with the same structural motifs inferred from the first analysis.

Transcriptional analysis of the gene identified three potential sites of initiation at nucleotide positions +1, +44, and +51.[208] Deletion analysis of the 5' RB gene sequences indicated that the region between nucleotides −154 and +186 possessed promoter function, with a critical initiating subregion of nucleotides +13 to +183. Identified enhancer-like sequences included interferon-responsive elements, heat-shock elements, and three Sp1 transcription-factor-binding regions at nucleotides −291, +76, and +123.[209]

These transcriptional and translational features led to the suggestion that the *RB1* gene product might be a nucleic acid-binding protein which exerts its tumor-suppressor activity through the regulation of transcription of a variety of cellular proteins. In 1987, Lee and coworkers[210] prepared rabbit antiserums against a trpE-RB fusion protein and purified an anti-RB antibody that precipitated a protein of 110,000 to 114,000 daltons. These reagents led to the uncovering of several other interesting features. First, there was no evidence of glycosylation despite such potential sites in the sequence. Second, subcellular fractionation of ^{35}S-methionine-labeled cells into nuclear, cytoplasmic, and membrane fractions showed that 85 percent of the RB1 protein resided in the nucleus, a location which was further substantiated by immunohistochemical staining with the anti-RB antibody. In fact, the RB protein was shown to be retained on and eluted from single-stranded DNA cellulose columns. Third, when cells were metabolically labeled with ^{32}P-phosphoric acid, the anti-RB antibody immunoprecipitated ^{32}P-labeled protein which was shown to be identical to the RB protein (pp110^{RB}). Finally, analyses of pp110^{RB} expression and its phosphorylation have led to insights into the mechanisms by which it exerts its effects in normal cells and more general ideas about how tumor cells can bypass controls on their proliferation.

Involvement of pp110^{RB} in the Cell Cycle

Phosphorylation of pp110^{RB} The process of cell proliferation can be subdivided into discrete stages of quiescence (G0), preparation for DNA replication (G1), DNA duplication (S), preparation for mitosis (G2), and actual cell division (M). The traverse of a cell from the G0/G1 through mitosis (M) stages is designated as one cell cycle. Much of what is known about the events which positively and negatively regulate the intricate pathways of this cycle have been deciphered using cell division cycle (cdc) mutants in

yeast.[211] The genetics and biochemistry of these mutants have led to a reasonably detailed view of the complex steps which in combination control the nuclear and cytoplasmic events involved in normal cell proliferation. A great deal of evidence has been accumulated showing that cells of a variety of types require a substantial lag time to progress through a number of substages within G1, regardless of whether the cycling arises from stimulation out of the quiescent G0 stage or from the completion of a previous cell cycle. It is during these substages of G1 that proliferation and cellular differentiation are initiated and controlled, and it appears that the switches for entry into or exit from G1 are the main determinants of postembryonic cell proliferation.[212] Thus, it seems quite reasonable to propose that genes with tumor-suppressor function, such as *RB1*, may function as negative control elements in the process. Further, it may be that the inactivation of such a gene allows defective cells to traverse the stages of the cell cycle under conditions of growth that would be insufficient for the proliferation of normal cells.[211,213]

One way to achieve functional inactivation of the *RB1* gene is to mutate it in such a way that the synthesis of p110^{RB} is reduced or its degradation is increased. This was tested by determining the steady-state amount of p110^{RB} protein in the different phases of the cell cycle[214] through fluorescent staining of cellular p110^{RB} and DNA in conjunction with flow cytometry. The results showed that the amount of p110^{RB} per cell increased as cells progressed through the cell cycle such that cells in later G2/M stages immediately before cell division contained approximately twice as much p110^{RB} as cells entering G1. Further, p110^{RB} had an invariant half-life of about 10 h, and pulse labeling of synchronized cells showed that p110^{RB} was synthesized in both quiescent and proliferative phases. These data suggested that the antiproliferative activity of the protein is not regulated in normal cells at the transcriptional level or the translational level.

The first indication that posttranslational modification of the RB protein is involved in cell cycle control was provided by the uncovering of a correlation in several cell types between cell cycle stage and the phosphorylation state of the protein.[214,215] Cell lysates prepared from quiescent or cycling cells (human umbilical vein endothelial cells, primary T lymphocytes, cells of a human breast cancer, and HeLa cells) showed an apparent size shift from p110^{RB} in the quiescent cells to pp112-114RB in proliferating cells (Fig. 19-14). Treatment of the latter lysates with potato acid phosphatase reduced the more slowly migrating protein species (p112-p114^{RB}) to the same mobility as the p110^{RB} species, suggesting that the former were actually multiply phosphorylated forms of the latter protein species.

The timing of the p110^{RB} to pp112-114RB transition was concurrent with the initiation of incorporation of radioactive thymidine into cellular DNA. Quantitation of the relative abundance of the higher-molecular-weight phosphorylated proteins to their nascent protein products showed that G1 (resting) cells had a 10:1 p110^{RB}:pp112-114RB ratio while G2/M (cycling) cells had a 1:1 ratio. After mitosis and cell division, the ratio returned to 10:1.[216] Regardless of the enzymatic mechanism involved, it is clear that phase-specific phosphorylation and dephosphorylation of the RB protein occurs during the cell cycle and proliferation. Mapping tryptic phosphopeptides of the human protein showed that the phosphorylation was on serine and threonine but not tyrosine residues, suggesting the possibility of cell cycle regulation by serine/threonine protein kinases.[217] One candidate is cdc2, a protein kinase that is known to be important in yeast at the G1/S and G2/M phases[218] and has been isolated in a protein complex that is capable of activating DNA synthesis in G1 cell extracts.[219] Lin et al.[217] found that human cdc2 phosphorylates each of the tryptic p110^{RB} phosphopeptides in vitro and in vivo, and the consensus target sequence for cdc2 phosphorylation[220] (Basic/Polar-Ser/Thr-Pro-X-

Basic) occurs eight times within the p110[RB] protein. Together these studies strongly suggest that human cdc2 is involved in regulating the cell cycle phosphorylation of p110[RB] protein. It is also possible that other cdc2-like kinases exist in the cell and play a role in the process as well.

Changes in the phosphorylation state of the RB protein also have been linked to cellular differentiation. Unlike proliferating cells, which actively cycle and divide, terminally differentiated cells cease normal cellular division and are shunted into a G0/G1 quiescent-like state. The effects of the induction of cellular differentiation on the phosphorylation status of p110[RB] have been analyzed in several leukemic cell lines which could be induced to differentiate after treatment with phorbol esters or retinoic acid. Monoblastic U937 and HL-60 showed a marked dephosphorylation of p110[RB] after differentiation,[221,222] and similar treatment of other partially responsive cells led to a coordinate level of p110[RB] phosphorylation. These experiments have led to several models for the function played by phosphorylation of p110[RB] in G0/G1.[223] The first is that p110[RB] regulates a cellular block which prevents exit from G1 by blocking the initiation of DNA synthesis. Phosphorylation of p110[RB] would render it inactive, thereby releasing the cell from its negative regulation and allowing the cell to progress through a full cell cycle. An alternative model depicts the dephosphorylation of RB as a subcellular event which communicates the

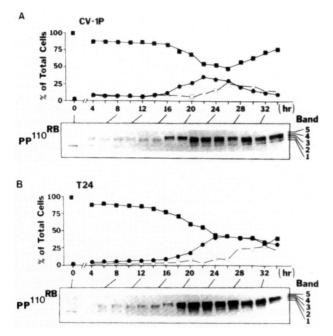

FIG. 19-14 Oscillation of phosphorylation of the p110[RB] protein during the different stages of the cell cycle. CV-1P cells (*A*) and T24 cells (*B*) were synchronized in G0/G1 by density arrest and then allowed to enter the cell cycle by sparsely replating cells in fresh medium. Equal numbers of cells were seeded into about 50 culture dishes (3 × 10⁶ cells per dish) and were allowed to grow to time points of 18 to 34 h. One entire plate was harvested for each lane on the Western blot. A second batch of dishes (1.5 × 10⁶ cells per dish) was plated 16 h later than the first and was harvested for hours 2 to 16. Again, each lane contained cells from one plate. At 2-h intervals after replating, cells were collected for cell cycle distribution analysis and RB protein determination. The percentage of cells in G1 (filled squares), S (filled circles), and G2/M (open squares) at each indicated time was determined by flow cytometry. RB protein was analyzed by immunoprecipitation followed by immunoblotting; five RB bands could be distinguished. The sudden change in signal intensity in CV-1P and T24 cells is due both to a decrease in the number of cells seeded for hours 2 to 16 and to random variability in the counting of different batches. *(Reprinted by permission from Chen et al., Cell, vol. 58, pp. 1193–1198, copyright 1989, Cell Press.)*

precise time for cell cycle exit (i.e., from M to G1/G0). As such, dephosphorylation may be part of a signaling pathway in which intracellular or extracellular factors switch G1 cells into the quiescent stage (G0). One relevant addition to the cell cycle stage effect of p110[RB] is the recent demonstration that it undergoes three separate rounds of phosphorylation in T lymphocytes stimulated to proliferate with the mitogen phytohemagglutin A.[224] The first occurs in middle to late G1, as was described earlier, the second during S phase, and the third in G2/M. Since these modifications occur at different locations on the protein, it is possible that p110[RB] actually has several different proliferation-controlling functions. The complexity of function that phosphorylation of p110[RB] produces at the cellular level is further enhanced by more recent demonstrations that this protein can be physically complexed with a number of viral and cellular proteins.

Cyclin D1, p16, and pp110   Recent developments in our understanding of the components of the cell cycle have strengthened the central role the Rb protein plays in growth regulation. One of the most important checkpoints in mammalian cells in late G1, deemed the restriction point, has many positive and negative controllers, including pp110. These key controllers include cyclins (A, D1-3, E, etc.) cyclin-dependent kinases (cdk2, 4, 6, etc,), and cyclin-dependent kinase inhibitors (p16, p15, etc.).[225] At the biochemical level, the kinase complexes of cyclin D1–cdk4 or cdk6 promote progression through late G1 by phosphorylating the retinoblastoma protein product. The Rb phosphorylation described above can be negatively regulated by cdk4/6I or p16INK/CDKN2 (henceforth referred to as p16) (Fig. 19-15). Thus, it appears that the normal biochemical pathway that regulates progression through G1 can be disrupted by abnormalities targeted at any one of these specific components. As discussed at length throughout this chapter, pRb itself can be inactivated by mutation, deletion, methylation, and viral sequestration (see the viral oncoproteins section, below).

In addition, cell cycle components such as cyclin D1, whose encoding locus resides at 11q13, can be amplified or rearranged and overexpressed in tumor cells.[225–227] D-type cyclins and their associated cdks (4 and 6) are able to bind to pp110 through an N-terminal LXCXE motif.[228–230] In fact, Rb[230] and E2F[231] are the only known substrates for cycD/Cdk4 complexes in vitro, and this complex phosphorylates most of the sites in vivo on the retinoblastoma protein. Their interaction is strengthened by their apparent involvement in a negative feedback loop where hypophosphorylated Rb seems to stimulate cyclin D1 transcription, and D1 and D1/cdk4 complexes are down-regulated in Rb-deficient cells[231–234] (Fig. 19-15).

Negative regulators active at the G1/S boundary such as the cdk inhibitors can also be altered in tumors. One such inhibitor, p16, appears to function normally by down-modulating the phosphorylating activity of its target kinases cdk4[235] and cdk6[236] by binding in competition with cyclin D1. p16 has been found deleted, mutated, or silenced by promoter methylation in a majority of tumor cell lines[237–241] and in a variety of tumors,[242–248] albeit in a much smaller fraction. p16 is elevated in cells that lack functional Rb, suggesting that Rb may suppress p16 expression,[249,250] the reciprocal of what is found for Rb and cyclin D1. This speaks to the positive (cyclin D1) and negative (p16) regulatory roles displayed by each of these cell cycle components and suggests that the pleiotropic tissue specificity of the tumors in which *RB1* inactivation occurs may be at the fundamental level of governing cell growth. It further suggests that the cyclin D1–cdk4–p16 pathway operates upstream of pRB, as both the G1-accelerating function of cyclin D1–ckd4 and growth suppression by p16 require functional pRB.

The inverse correlation and reciprocity of function between cell cycle controllers and Rb are clearly demonstrated in adult small-

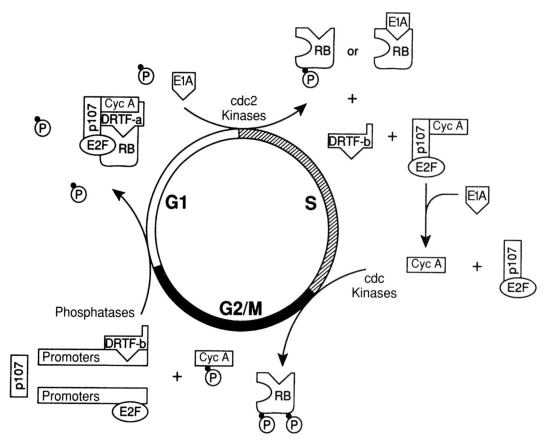

FIG. 19-15 Cell-cycle-dependent binding of cellular proteins to p110^{RB}. The cell-cycle stage-dependent complexing and dissociation of cellular proteins are schematically represented. DRTF and E2F are transcription factors that have been shown to bind to p110^{RB} at the G1 stage of the cell cycle. On phosphorylation of the protein at the G1/S boundary, these transcriptional factors are released from the complex. Phosphorylation of p110^{RB} appears to be controlled by a family of cdc kinases that are active at both the G1/S and G2/M boundaries. E1A has also been shown to bind p110^{RB}, thereby dissociating DRTF and E2F from the G1 complex in much the same manner as occurs when p110^{RB} is phosphorylated. At the completion of the cell cycle, phosphatases dephosphorylate p110^{RB}, thus allowing the protein to sequester E2F and DRTF back into their inactive complexed forms. Cyc A = cyclin A.

cell lung carcinomas (SCLCs) and non-small-cell lung carcinomas (NSCLCs). The Rb gene has been shown to be a common target for somatic mutations.[179] The frequency of absent or aberrant Rb protein expression for these tumors is 90 percent (SCLC) and 15 percent (NSCLC).[251] Several recent studies have examined the loss of p16 gene expression in these tumor types and have found a striking inverse correlation. The absence of p16 was a rare event in SCLC,[252,253] with 80 to 100 percent of cell lines and primary tumors displaying a p16+/pRb-phenotype. In contrast, the majority of NSCLCs (67 to 100 percent) analyzed lacked detectable p16 protein, rendering them p16-/Rb+.[252–254] In one study,[252] cyclin D1 was observed to be overexpressed in most cell lines, suggesting that this alteration may be a common early event in both lung tumor subtypes. However, this controversial model of the role of cyclin D1 as the earliest mutational event has not been substantiated in other studies examining lung[255] or esophageal carcinomas.[226] Nonetheless, the data clearly demonstrate that the p16-Rb pathway is inactivated in both SCLC and NSCLC at a very high frequency but that the targets of the inactivating mutational events are distinct, depending on the subtype of lung tumor analyzed.

pp110^{RB} Protein Complexes

Viral Oncoproteins At about the same time the oscillation of pp110^{RB} phosphorylation within the cell cycle was being uncovered, an unexpected link between this negative growth regulator and the cellular transforming capacities of the viral oncoproteins of polyomaviruses (SV40), adenoviruses (Ad-2 and AD-5), and papillomaviruses (HPV-16) was reported. Each of these DNA tumor viruses encodes a set of proteins, some of which are capable of disrupting the normal regulation of cellular proliferation, leading to in vitro transformation of cells and establishment of the tumorigenic phenotype. For example, the E1A protein of oncogenic adenoviruses is capable of immortalizing primary cells and mediating transcription, negatively and positively, for both viral and cellular genes.[256] Furthermore, the E1A of infected cells can be coimmunoprecipitated with a set of host-cell proteins of various molecular weights. The large T oncoprotein of SV40 is a nuclear phosphoprotein of 708 amino acids which is necessary for cellular transformation by the virus.[257] It typically functions in concert with the SV40 small t protein product but, when expressed at high levels, can perform all the functions required for transformation. Finally, the protein product of the E7 open reading frame of human papillomaviruses of types associated with progressive cervical neoplasia is also capable of immortalizing cells in vitro.[258] The functional similarities between these oncoproteins are also mirrored to some extent in their amino acid sequences and predicted higher-order structures. For example, deletion and mutation studies have shown that small segments of the SV40 T protein (between residues 105 and 114)[259,260] or the E1A protein (between residues 121 and 139)[261] are required for transforming capacity; these regions are structurally homologous. Comparisons of the amino acid sequences of E7 and E1A revealed a similar relationship between the NH$_2$ terminus of E7 and the two conserved regions in E1A.[262] These similarities have led to the prediction that these regions may bind cellular proteins that actively participate in and/or cooperate with the transforming properties of large T, E1A, and E7.[206]

Several lines of evidence point to the retinoblastoma gene product as one such cellular protein. As was mentioned above, earlier studies had shown the E1A protein to be complexed with a variety of cellular proteins, and one of these proteins had a molecular mass of about 110 kDa.[263] Using various monoclonal antibodies raised against large T, E1A, and p110RB as well as polyclonal antibodies raised against E7, in vitro immunoprecipitation from cell lysates showed coprecipitation of the p110RB with each of the oncoproteins from a variety of cell lines transformed by viral infection or their normal counterparts.[264–266] The presence of p110RB in these complexes was further confirmed by the demonstration of the expected protein fragments generated by partial proteolysis using staphylococcus V8 protease.

The extent to which these associations represented functional relationships in which both partners are active participants in a common regulatory pathway has also been documented. The analysis of a series of mutant species of large T and E1A proteins revealed that mutations affecting the sequences necessary for transformation also affected the ability of the oncoprotein to form complexes with p110RB.[259,260,265,267] Examples of the effect mutations of large T have on p110RB binding are shown in Fig. 19-16. Since one function of these viral oncoproteins appears to be the creation of a cellular environment that is permissive for DNA synthesis, it may be that one of their modes of action involves sequestration of the antiproliferative p110RB such that viral infection re-

leases the cell from its negative regulation by RB, allowing it to inappropriately or more frequently enter S phase. An examination of the data derived from immunoprecipitations with large T showed that lysates from ^{32}P-labeled cells contained phosphorylated T but not phosphorylated pp110RB.[268] An RB species did, however, coprecipitate with the anti-T antibody and was shown by densitometric analysis of gel electrophoresis patterns to be p110RB, the unphosphorylated form. This protein species was the only form of p110RB consistently bound to T, even though immunoprecipitation of the same lysates with an anti-RB antibody demonstrated the simultaneous existence of the other phosphorylated forms, that is, p112-114RB. Binding of large T to the unphosphorylated form held true for a stably SV40-transformed derivative of the cells used in the previous experiments, indicating that viral transformation does not alter the overall state of RB protein phosphorylation. These studies also showed that newly synthesized T did not immediately bind to p110RB, and this led to the hypothesis that the structure of T must change in some way to facilitate its successful heterologous binding. In fact, when large T from synchronized ^{35}S-labeled cell lysates was examined by surose gradients, it was determined that newly synthesized large T proteins existed as monomers and over the course of the cell cycle gradually oligomerized[268]; only after oligomerization was the oncoprotein capable of binding to p110RB. This is supported by the SV40 mutant 5080 (Fig. 19-16) that carries a Pro$_{584}$-Leu substitution, which renders it transformation-deficient[270] and inefficient for oligomerization[271]; it also fails to coprecipitate with the RB protein.[269] It is possible that such oligomer-forming behavior is a process by which large T can bind to more than one protein involved in cellular growth regulation. It is tanta-

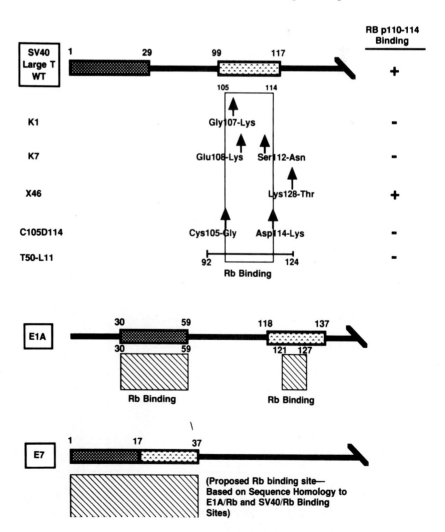

FIG. 19-16 Binding sites for the retinoblastoma protein in SV40 large T antigen, advenovirus E1A, and papillomavirus E7 proteins. The sequences of several SV40 large T mutants are shown with their corresponding p110RB-binding properties; + = T antigen was capable of complexing with the retinoblastoma protein; – = complex formation was abolished by the mutation. Regions in E1A and E7 necessary for binding p110RB assessed by similar mutational analyses are also depicted.

lizing to note that regions of E1A and T involved in binding p110^RB also interact with at least one cellular protein, p107.[272,273] Whatever the reason for the multiple oncoproteins binding to p110^RB, the data together support a model in which the unphosphorylated form of RB (p110^RB) is the species active in growth suppression. It would follow, then, that binding by E1A, E7, or large T would serve to inactivate the growth suppression normally exerted by pRB. Further, in the absence of viral infection, it is the phosphorylation of the RB protein that serves to override growth suppression and allows cell division to take place.

Retinoblastoma Protein Binding Sites Binding of viral oncoproteins to p110^RB and the subsequent release of these infected cells from negative growth control suggested that there may be cellular proteins with analogous properties. These proteins might be sequestered by p110^RB and be maintained in an inactivated form until phosphorylation of p110^RB makes them available for proliferation or transcriptional/translational uses. To determine the regions in the *RB* gene that are required for binding of the viral oncoproteins and potentially other cellular regulatory proteins, a systematic series of deletion mutants were generated in the p110^RB coding regions.[274,275] Polypeptide products generated through in vitro protein synthesis systems were analyzed for their ability to bind and coimmunoprecipitate SV40 large T or E1A. The data showed two distinct noncontiguous regions in p110^RB necessary for complexing with these oncoproteins; these regions included amino acid residues 393 to 572 and residues 646 to 772. It was further determined that a spacer region of undefined length between these two blocks was required to maintain this binding integrity.

Comparison of these binding regions with many of the naturally occurring RB mutations revealed striking similarities. The mutations displayed in Fig. 19-17 are naturally occurring examples from retinoblastomas as well as other tumors commonly found to be mutated for *RB1* (see the discussion above). Each of these mutants was in some way affected in a region essential for the binding of E1A and large T. The absence of p110^RB binding, using mutant proteins of cells from bladder carcinoma,[276] small-cell-lung carcinoma,[277] prostate carcinoma,[278] and osteosarcoma[279] has been confirmed by in vitro immunoprecipitation experiments. This is strong

evidence that the regions that normally bind to viral transforming proteins are also involved in naturally mutated RB proteins in tumorigenic cells.

Cellular Binding Proteins The viral oncoprotein binding data suggested the existence of intracellular proteins whose function is mediated by binding to the RB protein or whose binding mediates the function of the RB protein itself. Several approaches have been used to search for these putative cellular components, and each has been in some way based on complementarity to the viral oncoprotein binding regions. One line of experimentation involved screening a human lung fibroblast cDNA expression library with a 60-kDa recombinant RB protein. This analysis identified two individual cDNAs—RBP-1 and RBP-2280—whose products bound specifically to antimouse pRB monoclonal antibodies, although neither cross-hybridized with the other. Northern analyses of lung mRNA revealed 5.2- and 4.3-kb transcripts homologous to RBP-1, whereas RBP-2 detected a 6.0-kb transcript. DNA sequencing of these cDNAs indicated no homologies to known protein sequences except that each contained a 10-amino acid motif that mimicked the p110^RB binding domain.

A second approach utilized in vitro immunoprecipitation techniques. For these experiments, excess free p110^RB was added to drive the reaction equilibrium toward complex formation with subsequent coprecipitation of these RB complexes with anti-RB antibodies.[280-281] A 56-kDa pRB fusion protein containing both regions necessary for the binding of T antigen to the C terminus stochiometrically precipitated a 46-kDa protein from HeLa cells. Competition studies with large T antigen and the addition of p56 kDa RB protein containing deletion/insertion mutations indicate that this 46-kDa cellular protein is directly associated with the recombinant p56 kDa RB protein through its T-binding domains.

The most successful approach to date for isolating cellular RB complexing proteins involves generating glutathione-S-transferase pRB fusion proteins, which then are used as protein affinity chromatography agents against different cell lysates. The pRB portion of these proteins contains the minimal conserved region required for binding of SV40 large T and adenovirus E1A oncoproteins. When cellular lysates of the retinoblastoma cell line WERI-Rb27

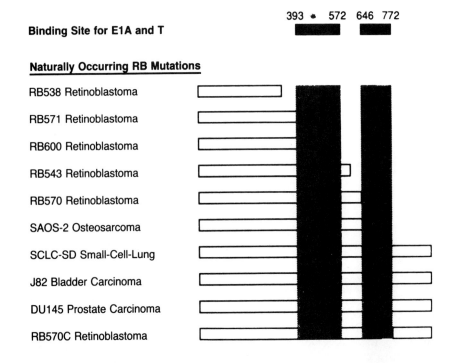

Binding Site for E1A and T

393 ● 572 646 772

Naturally Occurring RB Mutations

RB538 Retinoblastoma
RB571 Retinoblastoma
RB600 Retinoblastoma
RB543 Retinoblastoma
RB570 Retinoblastoma
SAOS-2 Osteosarcoma
SCLC-SD Small-Cell-Lung
J82 Bladder Carcinoma
DU145 Prostate Carcinoma
RB570C Retinoblastoma

FIG. 19-17 Comparison of binding sites of EB to E1A/SV40 T antigen with naturally occurring *RB1* mutations. This comparison includes *RB1* mutations characterized in retinoblastoma, osteosarcoma, bladder carcinoma, and prostate carcinoma cells. The solid boxes at the top of the figure represent the regions of RB essential for binding to E1A and SV40 T antigen. The stippled regions indicate the positions of the binding regions relative to the RB sequences present in the naturally occurring mutants (open boxes). Amino acid sequences that are essential for binding to E1A and SV40 T are absent in each mutant. *(Reprinted by permission from Hu et al., EMBO J 9(4):1147–1155, copyright 1990, Oxford University Press.)*

were passed over affinity columns of fusion proteins that included regions of RB necessary for SV40 T-antigen binding, several cellular proteins ranging in size from 25 to 146 kDa were retained.[282] Similar-sized proteins could be separated from extracts of a variety of tumor cell lines. Each of the proteins was found primarily in the cellular nucleus, and at least one, of 68 to 72 kDa, displayed apparently S-phase-dependent binding behavior.

The function of the proteins isolated in each of these ways became clear through analyses of their physical relationship to p105^{RB} and their effect on cellular transcription. DRTF is a sequence-specific transcription factor found in different forms (DRTF-b or DRTF-a) as embryonal carcinoma stem cells differentiate.[283,284] DRTF-b migrates faster than does DRTF-a in band-shift assays, suggesting that the DRTF-b complex is missing one or more protein components found in DRTF-a. To determine whether this transcription factor interacted with the tumor-suppressor RB product p110^{RB}, E1A protein was added to cell lysates of the embryonic stem-cell line F9. Using band-shift binding assays, it was shown that E1A sequestered a protein from the DRTF-a complex, creating the DRTF-b form, an effect dependent on the E1A-conserved regions 1 and 2 that were previously determined to be necessary for transformation. Monoclonal antibodies to RB produced a similar shift from DRTF-a to DRTF-b, leading to the conclusion that p110^{RB} is part of the DRTF transcription complex and providing a link between tumor-suppressor activity and control of gene transcription.

Since E1A affected the complexing of p110^{RB} into DRTF, E1A-associated proteins were analyzed to see if they were part of the same complex. One such protein, cyclin A, like p110^{RB}, varies in mass amount during the mitotic phase of the cell cycle. The addition of an anti-cyclin A antibody to DRTF complexes caused a disruption of the RB-containing DRTF-a complex but not the RB-deficient DRTF-b complex.[285] Furthermore, the RB-deficient DRTF-b complex could complex with p110^{RB} only when cyclin A was added, thus indicating that cyclin A facilitated the sequestering of RB into the DRTF complex. A consideration of the binding characteristics of DRTF, RB, and cyclin A in light of the cell cycle regulation of the latter two suggests that DRTF has an important cell-specific role in regulating the transcription of genes whose protein products are required for progression through the cell cycle (Fig. 19-15). Such coordinated behavior could provide a molecular mechanism by which viral and cellular transforming oncoproteins might act in part to sequester RB from DRTF-a. This would have the effect of freeing the transcriptionally active DRTF-b form, which is no longer under the negative regulation of p110^{RB}.

These experiments show that Rb probably functions in growth control and differentiation through interactions with a variety of cellular proteins. Other interacting proteins in this category include RIZ[286], Myo D[287], c-Abl[288], MDM2[289], and E2F[286–289] (described below). The transcriptional activators hBRG1/hBRM have also been functionally linked with pRB. hBRG1 (human brahma-related gene 1 protein) and its family member hBRM are the mammalian homologues of the yeast SNF2/SWI2 transcriptional activator and the Drosophila brahma protein. These proteins are thought to restructure chromatin and facilitate the function of specific transcription factors. All share a domain that is also found in many nuclear proteins, such as the E1A-binding protein p300.[290] hBRG1 interacts only with hypophosphorylated pp110^{RB} through the same LXCXE motif found in other pRB-interacting proteins described in this chapter.[291] This suggests that these transcriptional activators are rendered nonfunctional in G1 by their association with pRB and are released upon phosphorylation of the retinoblastoma protein.

E2F is another sequence-specific transcription factor that was initially identified as a cellular factor involved in the regulation of the adenovirus early E2 gene by the E1A protein. Using a glu-

tathione-S-transferase protein fused to the 379 to 792 binding domain residues of p110^{RB} and a degenerate mixture of 62-bp DNA oligonucleotides, Chittenden et al.[292] attempted to determine whether any pRB pocket-binding cellular protein had sequence-specific DNA-binding activity. After several rounds of enrichment, two oligonucleotides were found to be the major components in the selected population. More than 80 percent of the sequenced oligonucleotides shared a class 1 consensus sequence of TTTG-GCGGG, while 15 percent contained a class 2 ATTTGCGCGGG consensus sequence. Comparison of these with other known sequence-binding sites uncovered a strong similarity to the binding site of E2F (TTTCGCGC). One interpretation of this study is that E2F binds specifically to the p110^{RB} product. Isolation of two cDNAs encoding E2F or E2F-like proteins (one of which corresponds to RBP-1, as was discussed earlier)[293,294] should provide the reagents needed to test this hypothesis.

Further studies determined that E2F was associated with the unphosphorylated form of p110^{RB} present in the G1 phase of the cell cycle near the G1-S border.[295,296] This behavior is consistent with the recruitment of unphosphorylated p110^{RB} into the DRTF complex and suggests that E2F can play a role in transcription or regulation, either alone or in concert with other proteins in the DRTF factor. Furthermore, as E2F is released upon entry into S phase, it can be found complexed with cyclin A; an E2F–cyclin A complex may be cooperatively released upon phosphorylation of p110^{RB} in the S phase of the cell cycle. The function of the RB/E2F in G1 phase transition is becoming more clearly defined. The complex is active in silencing the E1A promoter when bound to an E2F binding site.[297] In this form, RB/E2F inhibits the function of other promoter elements, such as enhancers, thereby causing transcription to cease. On phosphorylation of p110^{RB} or addition of E1A, E2F is released and becomes a positive transcriptional element. Thus, positive and negative regulation of transcription is linked not only to E2F but also to the phosphorylation cycle of the retinoblastoma-suppressor gene. All these experiments are consistent with a model in which p110^{RB} controls the transcription of genes which contain E2F sites in their promoters, are cyclically expressed in relation to the cell cycle, and are important for cell proliferation.

pp110^{RB} Protein Family Members An intriguing aspect of the E2F studies described above is the independent association of E2F with both cyclin A and p110^{RB}, even though neither of the latter two contains known structural similarities. Isolation of a retinoblastoma-like protein, p107, has shed light on this confusing phenomenon.[298] Anti-p107 antibodies precipitated p107 together with a few other cellular proteins, the most abundant being cyclin A and another being E2F. The demonstration that this p107 protein is a component of the E2F–cyclin A complex provided the structural basis for its binding behavior. It appears that p107 mediates the indirect binding of E2F to cyclin A, and this explains how E2F can bind the structurally dissimilar p110^{RB} and cyclin A proteins.

Another member of this family of proteins, p130, was recently isolated, increasing the complexity of this growth regulation pathway. p130 shares 50 percent identity with p107 and has homology to pp110^{RB} in the pocket-binding domain.[299] Several studies show that this is the same p130 protein found associated with adenovirus E1A.[300,301] Both p107 and p130 bind to the viral oncoproteins and share the spacer region between the two subunits of the pocket-binding domain. This spacer region mediates their interaction with cyclins A and E.[302–303] Since these pRb-related proteins can bind to E2F[300], they also exhibit growth-suppressing properties similar to those seen with pRB.[303] Interestingly, p130 has been mapped to the long arm of chromosome 16, in a region known to undergo allelic deletion and translocation in another pediatric cancer, Wilms' tumor.[304–306] This suggests that these Rb-related family members should be studied further for mutations in adult tumors not altered for either Rb or p16 and examined for their potential role as tumor-suppressor genes in the fashion described above for the retinoblastoma gene.

Retinoblastoma Mouse Models

The retinoblastoma genotypes and related phenotypes described throughout this chapter paint a somewhat paradoxic picture of the function of *RB1*. The p110[RB] protein seems to play a central role in the regulation of the cell cycle activity common to all cells, yet germ-line mutations in *RB1* predispose individuals to a very specific spectrum of tumors. Thus, it remains unclear whether p110[RB] serves solely as a barrier against specific tumorigenesis or actually plays an important role in normal cellular development. One approach which has been undertaken to resolve and define these issues for *RB1* involves the generation and analysis of animal models such as homozygous mutant (Rb–/–) knockout or transgenic mice. By creating mouse embryonic stem cell lines manipulated genetically to a null status at the *RB1* locus and fusing these cell lines with normal blastocyst-stage mouse embryos, mice heterozygous for the mutant Rb allele (Rb+/–) are generated. These predisposed heterozygous mice can be observed for signs of increased tumor incidence and phenotypic abnormalities as well as backcrossed to generate homozygous Rb–/– progeny whose development and tumor profiles should help define the role *RB1* in the normal cell.

Several Rb–/– mice have been engineered with insertional mutations in the regions of exons 3–4[305] and exon 20.[306] Observations of these mice and the progeny of their backcrosses were strikingly similar and unexpected. Most notable was the absence of any retinoblastomas or retinomas in the over 200 Rb +/– mice observed. These mice are genotypically equivalent to humans who inherit a mutated *RB1* allele and are inevitably diagnosed, at greater than 90 percent penetrance, with retinoblastoma tumors. This systemic difference is further exemplified by the high incidence of brain tumors[306] and pituitary adenocarcinomas[305] exhibited in these Rb +/– animals after 8 to 10 months of observation. Molecular analysis of these tumors reveals loss of the remaining wild-type Rb allele, providing evidence that the two-hit hypothesis described in this chapter for humans also holds for these heterozygous mouse tissues.

Backcrosses of Rb +/– mice did not produce the expected 25 percent Rb –/– progeny. In fact these Rb –/– embryos were not viable past approximately 13 days of gestation,[305,306] precluding the ability to study pRb[110] function in normal development. However chimeric animals partially composed of Rb-deficient cells were viable and showed a widespread contribution of these mutant cells to all adult tissues and normal development of most tissues, including the retina and erythrocytes.[307] This indicates that Rb function is not required for the differentiation of cells in many adult tissues. When nonviable Rb–/– embryos were examined pathologically, significant defects in the brain and blood-forming tissues were discovered. There was massive cell death in the central nervous system tissues which was highest in the hindbrain. An apparent block in hepatic erythoropoiesis most likely accounts for the observation that 65 to 90 percent of red blood cells remain nucleated.

The results from these mouse models do little to solve the Rb paradox but suggest that there may be fundamental systemic differences in the function of pRb in mouse and human tissues. Despite these discrepancies, it is clear that Rb does not play a critical role in regulating cell division or cell differentiation up to the thirteenth day of gestation of the mouse. One explanation for the lack of retinoblastoma tumors in Rb +/– animals is that the population of susceptible target cells in the relatively small mouse eye is be-

low the threshold required for tumorigenesis to occur. However, retinoblastomas have been observed in transgenic mice expressing SV40 T antigen (see viral oncoprotein section, above).[308] Thus, there may be a requirement for additional genetic alterations to occur for retinoblastoma tumors to appear in the mouse. Alternatively, in the absence of Rb expression, an Rb-related protein such as p107 or p130 (see the Rb protein family member section, above) might provide an analogous function in most tissues, preempting a role for p110[RB] in tumorigenesis in the mouse.

Rb –/– cells isolated from early viable embryos provide a source for a variety of cell types that can be used to look in more detail at the function of Rb at the cellular level. Most important these cells do not possess the multitude of other genetic lesions present in most human tumor cell genomes which might confuse or mask the precise role the pRb loss plays in tumorigenesis. Preliminary observations on Rb–/– fibroblasts show a shorter G1 phase of the cell cycle and a smaller cell size than in the wild type.[309] In addition, although most cell cycle-regulated genes analyzed show no temporal or quantitative differences, cyclin E is derepressed earlier in G1 than is the case in wild-type cells. Cyclin E, found associated with cdk2, is one of the components responsible for phosphorylating pRb in late G1.[225] Further studies utilizing a number of other tissue types as well as cells from doubly Rb and p53 mutant mice[310–313] will no doubt add to our understanding of the role Rb plays in normal cellular function as well as how it cooperates with other cellular oncogenes and tumor suppressor genes with which it shares cellular control pathways.

ACKNOWLEDGMENTS

The authors are grateful to Prof. R. Frezzotti for his support and constructive criticisms and Dr. E. Motolese and Dr. G. Addabbo for assistance with sections of this review. Thanks also to Ms. C. Mallia for secretarial assistance. The work cited in this review was partly supported by a National Research Council (Italy) grant on retinoblastoma, #9000111.

REFERENCES

1. Francois J: Recent data on the heredity of retinoblastoma, in Boniuk M (ed): *Ocular and Adnexal Tumors*. St. Louis, Mosby, 1964.
2. Beck K, Jensen OA: Bilateral retinoblastoma in Denmark. *Arch Ophthalmol* **39**:561, 1961.
3. Hemmes GF, Tfsdscar J, Francois J: in Boniuk M (ed): *Ocular and Adnexal Tumors*. St. Louis, Mosby, 1964, p 123.
4. Albert DM, Lahav M, Lesser R, Craft J: Recent observations regarding retinoblastoma. *Trans Ophthal Mol Soc UK* **94**:909, 1974.
5. Berkow RL, Freshman JK: Retinoblastoma in Navajo Indian Children. *Am J Dis Child* **137**:137, 1983.
6. Devesa SA: The incidence of retinoblastoma. *Am J Ophthalmol* **80**:263, 1975.
7. Sanders BM, Draper GJ, Kingston JE: Retinoblastoma in Great Britain 1969–80: Incidence, treatment, and survival. *Br J Ophthalmol* **75**:567, 1988.
8. Matsunaga E: Genetic epidemiology of retinoblastoma, in Lynch HP III, Hirayama T (eds): *Genetic Epidemiology of Cancer*. Boca Raton, FL, CRC, 1987, p 119.
9. Mahoney MC, Burnett WS, Majerovics A, Tanenbaum H: The epidemiology of ophthalmic malignancies in New York State. *Ophthalmology* **97**:1143, 1990.
10. Jensen RD, Miller RW: Retinoblastoma: Epidemiologic characteristics. *N Engl J Med* **285**:307, 1971.
11. Bras G, Cole H, Ashmeade-Dyer A, Walter DC: Report on 151 childhood malignancies observed in Jamaica. *J Natl Cancer Inst* **43**:417, 1969.

12. Parkin DM, Stiller CA, Draper GJ, Bieber C: The international incidence of childhood cancer. *Int J Cancer* **42**:511, 1988.

13. Frezzotti R, Bardelli AM, Fois A, Lasorella G, Acquaviva A, Hadjistilianou T, Bernardini C: Retinoblastoma: Terapie conservative del retinoblastoma, in Frezzotti R (ed): *Patologie Clinica e Terapia delle malattie dell' Orbita.* Ralazione 65° Congresso S.O.I., Siena 5–8, 1985, p 405.

14. Senft S, Al-Kaft A, Bergquist G, Jaafar M, Nasr A, Hidayat A, Sackey K, Cothier E: Retinoblastoma: The Saudi Arabian experience. *Ophthalmol Paed Genet* **9**(2):115, 1988.

15. Ellsworth RM: The practical management of retinoblastoma. *Trans Am Ophthalmol Soc* **67**:461, 1969.

16. Francois J: Differential diagnosis of leukocoria in children. *Ann Aphthalmol* **10**:1375, 1978.

17. Shields JA, Augsburger JJ: Current approaches to the diagnosis and management of retinoblastoma. *Surv Ophthalmol* **25**:347, 1981.

18. Howard GM, Ellsworth RM: Differential diagnosis of retinoblastoma: A statistical study of 500 children. *Am J Ophthalmol* **60**:610, 1965.

19. Balmer A, Gailloud CL, Uffer S, Munier F, Pescia G: Retinoblastome et pseudoretinoblastome: Etude diagnostique. *Klin Mbl Augenheilk* **192**:589, 1988.

20. Murphree L, Rother C: Retinoblastoma, in Ryan SR (ed): *Retina.* St. Louis, Mosby, 1989, p 515.

21. Balmer A, Gaillaud C: Retinoblastoma: Diagnosis and treatment. *Dev Ophthalmol* **7**:36, 1983.

22. Haik GB, Siedlecki A, Ellsworth RM, Sturgis-Buckhait L: Documented delays in the diagnosis of retinoblastoma. *Ann Ophthalmol* **17**:731, 1985.

23. Binder PS: Unusual manifestations of retinoblastoma. *Am J Ophthalmol* **77**(5):674, 1974.

24. Richards WW: Retinoblastoma simulating uveitis. *Am J Ophthalmol* **65**(3):427, 1968.

25. Stafford W, Yanoff M, Parnell BL: Retinoblastoma initially misdiagnosed as primary ocular inflammation. *Arch Ophthalmol* **82**:771, 1969.

26. Rozansky VM: A necrotic retinoblastoma simulating panophthalmitis. *Surv Ophthalmol* **9**:381, 1964.

27. Morgan G: Diffuse infiltrating retinoblastoma. *Br J Ophthalmol* **55**:600, 1971.

28. Garner A, Kanski JJ, Kinnear F: Retinoblastoma: Report of a case with minimal retinal involvement but massive anterior segment spread. *Br J Ophthalmol* **71**:858, 1987.

29. Schofield PB: Diffuse infiltrating retinoblastoma. *Br J Ophthalmol* **44**:35, 1960.

30. Nicholson DH, Norton EWD: Diffuse infiltrating retinoblastoma. *Trans Am Ophthalmol Soc* **78**:265, 1980.

31. Shields JA, Shields CL, Eagle RC, Blair CJ: Spontaneous pseudohypopon secondary to diffuse infiltrating retinoblastoma. *Arch Ophthalmol* **106**:1301, 1988.

32. Shields CL, Shields JA, Shah P: Retinoblastoma in older children. *Ophthalmology* **98**:395, 1991.

33. Ginsberg J, Spaulding A, Asburg T: Cystic retinoblastoma. *Am J Ophthalmol* **80**(5):930, 1975.

34. Ohnishi Y, Yamana Y, Minei M, Yoshitomi F: Snowball opacity in retinoblastoma. *Jpn J Ophthalmol* **26**: 159, 1982.

35. Allderdice PW, Davis JG, Miller OJ: The 13q-deletion syndrome. *Am J Hum Genet* **21**:499, 1969.

36. Francke U, King F: Sporadic bilateral retinoblastoma and 13q- chromosome deletion. *Med Pediatr Oncol* **2**:379, 1976.

37. Niebuhr E, Ottosen J: Ring chromosome D(13) associated with multiple congenital malformations. *Ann Genet* **16**:157, 1973.

38. Seidman DJ, Shields JA, Augsburger JJ, Nelson LB, Lee ML, Sciorra LJ: Early diagnosis of retinoblastoma based on dysmorphic features and karyotype analysis. *Ophthalmology* **94**:663, 1987.

39. Gallie BL, Ellsworth RM, Abramson DH, Phillips RA: Retinoma: Spontaneous regression of retinoblastoma or benign manifestation of the mutation. *Br J Cancer* **45**:513, 1982.

40. Margo C, Hidayat CA, Kopelman J, Zimmerman LE: Retinocytoma: A benign variant of retinoblastoma. *Arch Ophthalmol* **101**:1519, 1983.

41. Eagle RC, Shields JA, Donoso L, Milner RS: Malignant transformation of spontaneously regressed retinoblastoma, retinoma/retinocytoma variant. *Ophthalmology* **96**:1389, 1989.

42. Abramson DH: Retinoma, retinocytoma, and the retinoblastoma gene (editorial). *Arch Ophthalmol* **101**:1517, 1983.

43. Khodadoust AA, Roozitalab HM, Smith RE, Green WR: Spontaneous regression of retinoblastoma. *Surv Ophthalmol* **21**:467, 1977.

44. Aaby AA, Price RL, Zakov ZN: Spontaneously regressing retinoblastoma, retinoma or retinoblastoma group O. *Am J Ophthalmol* **96**:315, 1983.

45. Gallie BL, Phillips RA, Ellsworth RM, Abramson DH: Significance of retinoma and phthisis bulbi for retinoblastoma. *Ophthalmology* **89**:1393, 1982.

46. Bader JL, Miller RN, Meadows AT, Zimmerman LE, Champion LAA, Voute PA: Trilateral retinoblastoma. *Lancet* **582**:8194, 1980.

47. Jakobiec FA, Tso M, Zimmerman LE, Danis P: Retinoblastoma and intracranial malignancy. *Cancer* **39**:2048, 1977.

48. Dudgeon J, Lee WR: The trilateral retinoblastoma syndrome. *Trans Ophthalmol Soc UK* **103**:523, 1983.

49. Zimmerman LE, Burns RP, Wankum G, Tully R, Esterly JA: Trilateral retinoblastoma: Ectopic intracranial retinoblastoma associated with bilateral retinoblastoma. *Paediatr Ophthalmol Strabismus* **19**(6):320, 1982.

50. Kingston JE, Plowman PN, Hungerford JL: Ectopic intracranial retinoblastoma in childhood. *Br J Ophthalmol* **69**:742, 1985.

51. Francois J, De Sutter E, Coppieters R, De Bie S: Late extraocular tumors in retinoblastoma survivors. *Ophthalmologica (Basel)* **181**:93, 1980.

52. Reese AB, Merriam GR, Martin HE: Treatment of bilateral retinoblastoma by irradiation and surgery: Report on 15 years results. *Am J Ophthalmol* **32**:175, 1949.

53. Frezzotti R, Guerra R: Sarcoma following irradiated retinoblastoma. *Arch Ophthalmol* **70**:471, 1963.

54. Forrest AW: Tumors following radiation about the eye. *Trans Am Acad Ophthalmol Otolaryngol* **65**:694, 1961.

55. Soloway HB: Radiation induced neoplasms following curative therapy for retinoblastoma. *Cancer* **19**:1984, 1966.

56. Sagerman RH, Cassady R, Tretter P, Ellsworth R: Radiation induced neoplasia following external beam therapy for children with retinoblastoma. *Am J Roentgenol Radium Ther Mucl Med* **105**:529, 1969.

57. Derkinderen DJ, Koten JW, Wolterbeek R, Beemer FA, Tan KE, Den Otter W: Non ocular cancer in hereditary retinoblastoma survivors and relatives. *Ophthalmic Paediatr Genet* **8**:23, 1987.

58. Leuder GT, Judisch GF, O'Gorman TW: Second non ocular tumors in survivors of heritable retinoblastoma. *Arch Ophthalmol* **104**:372, 1986.

59. Draper GJ, Sanders BM, Kingston JE: Second primary neoplasms in patients with retinoblastoma. *Br J Cancer* **53**:661, 1986.

60. Abramson DH, Ellsworth RM, Kitchin FD, Tung G: Second non-ocular tumors in retinoblastoma survivors: Are they radiation-induced? *Ophthalmology* **91**:1351, 1984.

61. Roarty JD, McLean IW, Zimmerman LE: Incidence of second neoplasms in patients with bilateral retinoblastoma. *Ophthalmology* **95**:1583, 1988.

62. Sang DN, Albert DM: Retinoblastoma: Clinical and histopathologic features. *Hum Pathol* **13**:133, 1982.

63. Brown DH: The clinicopathology of retinoblastoma. *Am J Ophthalmol* **97**:189, 1984.

64. Tosi P, Cintorino P, Toti V, Ninfo V, Montesco MC, Frezzotti R, Radjistilianou T, Acquaviva A, Barbini P: Histopathological evaluation for the prognosis of retinoblastoma. *Ophthalmic Paediatr Genet* **10**:173, 1987.

65. Kopelman JE, McLean IW, Rosenberg SH: Multivariate analysis of risk factors of metastasis in retinoblastoma treated by enucleation. *Ophthalmology* **94**:371, 1987.

66. Goldberg L, Danziger A: Computer tomographic scanning in the management of retinoblastoma. *Am J Ophthalmol* **84**(3):380, 1977.

67. De Nicola M, Salvolini V: La risonanza magnetica nucleare e la tomografia assiale computerizzata nel retinoblastoma, in *Tumori intraoculari.* International Symposium Intraocular Tumors. Palermo, Medical Books, 1990, p 43.

68. Char DH, Hedges TR, Norman D: Retinoblastoma: CT diagnosis. *Ophthalmology* **91**:1347, 1984.

69. Arrigg PG, Hedges RT, Char DH: Computed tomography in the diagnosis of retinoblastoma. *Br J Ophthalmol* **67**:558, 1983.

70. Mafee MF, Goldberg MF, Greenwald MJ, Schulman J, Malmed A, Flanders AE: Retinoblastoma and simulating lesions: Role of CT and MR imaging. *Radiol Clin North Am* **25**(4):667, 1987.

71. Schulman JA, Peyman G, Mafee MF, Laurence L, Bauman AE, Goldman A: The use of magnetic resonance imaging in the evaluation of retinoblastoma. *J Pediatr Ophthalmol Strabismus* **23**:144, 1986.

72. Mafee MF, Goldberg MF, Cohen SB, Gotsis ED, Safran M, Chekuri L, Raofi B: Magnetic resonance imaging versus computed tomogra-

phy of leukocoric eyes and use of in vitro proton magnetic resonance spectroscopy of retinoblastoma. *Ophthalmology* **96**:965, 1989.

73. Haik BG, Saint Louis L, Smith ME, Ellsworth RM, Abramson DH, Cahill P, Deck M, Coleman DJ: Magnetic resonance imaging in the evaluation of leukocoria. *Ophthalmology* **92**:1143, 1985.

74. Benhamou E, Borges J, Tso MOM: Magnetic resonance imaging in retinoblastoma and retinocytoma: A case report. *J Paediatr Ophthalmol Strabismus* **26**:276, 1989.

75. Danziger A, Price HI: CT findings in retinoblastoma. *Am J Radiol* **133**:695, 1979.

76. Coleman DJ, Lizzi FC, Jack PL: *Ultrasonography of the Eye and Orbit.* Philadelphia, Lea & Febiger, 1977, p 209.

77. Sampaolesi R, Zacrate J: Errors in the diagnosis of retinoblastoma, in *Ultrasound in Ophthalmology.* Proceedings of the 11th S.I.D.U.O. Congress. Kluwer Academic, 1986, p 189.

78. Ossolning KC: *Proceedings of the 10th Course and Workshop on Clinical Echo-Ophthalmology.* Vienna, December 12–15, 1973.

79. Motolese E, Addabbo G: Diagnosi ecografica delle neoplasie oculari. Atti Convegno interdisciplinare problemi oculari nell'infanzia. Siena 14-15 ottobre, 1988. *Boll Ocul* **68**(5), Bologna, Cappelli, 1989.

80. Jakobiec FA, Coleman DJ, Chattock A, Smith M: Ultrasonically guided needle biopsy and cytologic diagnosis of solid intraocular tumors. *Ophthalmology* **86**:1662, 1979.

81. Char DH, Miller TR: Fine needle biopsy in retinoblastoma. *Am J Ophthalmol* **97**:686, 1984.

82. Shields JA: Diagnostic approaches to intraocular tumors, in *Diagnosis and Management of Intraocular Tumors.* St. Louis, Mosby, 1983.

83. Midena E, Segato T, Piermarocchi S, Boccato P: Fine needle aspiration biopsy in ophthalmology. *Surv Ophthalmol* **29**:410, 1985.

84. Augsburger JJ, Shields JA, Folberg R, Lang W, O'Hara BJ, Claricci J: Fine needle aspiration biopsy in the diagnosis of intraocular cancer. *Ophthalmology* **92**:39, 1985.

85. Karcioglu ZA, Gordon R, Karcioglu G: Tumor seeding in ocular fine needle aspiration biopsy. *Ophthalmology* **92**:1763, 1985.

86. Frezzotti R, Tosi P, Bardelli AM, Cintorino M, Hadjistilianou T: Cytologic diagnosis of retinoblastoma. *Proceedings I International Symposium on Ophthalmic Cytology,* Parma, Italy, October 9, 1987.

87. Arora R, Betharia SM: Fine needle aspiration of paediatric orbital tumors. *Orbit* **7**(2):115, 1988.

88. Frezzotti R, Hadjistilianou T, Greco G, Bartolomei A, Pannini S, Minacci C, Disanto A, Cintorino M: L'agobiopsia (FNAB) nella diagnosi differenziale delle neoplasie oculari ed orbitarie. *Atti LXIX Congresso S.O.I.* Rome, Oct. 12–15, 1989.

89. Reese AM, Ellsworth RM: Management of retinoblastoma. *Ann NY Acad Sci* **114**:958, 1964.

90. Pratt CB: Management of malignant solid tumors in children. *Pediatr Clin North Am* **19**(4):1141, 1972.

91. Stannard C, Lipper S, Sealy R, Sevel D: Retinoblastoma: Correlation of invasion of the optic nerve and choroid with prognosis and metastases. *Br J Ophthalmol* **63**:560, 1979.

92. Rosengren B, Monge OR, Flage T: Proposal of new pretreatment clinical TNM-classification of retinoblastoma. *Acta Oncol* **28**(4):547, 1989.

93. Shields JA, Shields CL, Sivalingam V: Decreasing frequency of enucleation in patients with retinoblastoma. *Am J Ophthalmol* **108**:185, 1989.

94. Ellsworth RM: Orbital retinoblastoma. *Trans Am Ophthalmol Soc* **72**:79, 1974.

95. Hilgartner HL: Report of a case of double glioma treated with X-ray. *Tex J Med* **18**:322, 1903.

96. Schipper J: An accurate and simple method for megavoltage radiation therapy of retinoblastoma. *Radiothes Oncol* **1**:31, 1983.

97. Harnett AN, Hungerford J, Lambert G, Hirst A, Darlinson R, Hart B, Trodd TC, Plowman P: Modern lateral external beam (lens sparing) radiotherapy for retinoblastoma. *Ophthalmic Paediatr Genet* **8**(1):53, 1987.

98. McCormick B, Ellsworth RM, Abramson DH: Results of external beam radiation for children with retinoblastoma: A comparison of two techniques. *J Pediatr Ophthalmol* **26**:239, 1989.

99. Reese AB, Ellsworth RM: The evaluation and current concept of retinoblastoma therapy. *Trans Am Acad Ophthalmol Otolaryngol* **67**:164, 1963.

100. Buys RJ, Abramson DH, Ellsworth RM, Haik B: Radiation regression patterns after colbalt plaque insertion for retinoblastoma. *Arch Ophthalmol* **101**:1206, 1983.

101. Abramson DH, Gerardi CM, Ellsworth RM, McCormick B, Sussman D, Turner L: Radiation regression patterns in treated retinoblastoma:

7 to 21 years later. *J Paediatr Ophthalmol Strabismus* **28**(2):108, 1991.

102. MacFaul PA, Bedford MA: Ocular complications after therapeutic irradiation. *Br J Ophthalmol* **54**:237, 1970.

103. Lommatzch PK: Die Anwendung von Betastrahlen mit 106 Ur/106 Rh Applikatoren bei dei Behandlung des Retinoblastomas. *Klin Monatsbl Augenheilkd* **156**:662, 1970.

104. Char DH: Retinoblastoma therapy, in *Clinical Ocular Oncology.* New York, Churchill Livingstone, 1989, p 207.

105. Shields J, Giblin ME, Shields C, Macroe AM, Karlsson V: Episcleral plaque radiotherapy for retinoblastoma. *Ophthalmology* **96**:530, 1989.

106. Meyer-Schwickerath G: The preservation of vision by treatment of intraocular tumors with light coagulation. *Arch Ophthalmol* **66**:458, 1961.

107. Frezzotti R, Hadjistilianou T: Is retinoblastoma vascularization a prognostic factor for xenon photocoagulation and for radiosensitivity? *Orbit* **7**(2):101, 1988.

108. Hadjistilianou T, Greco G, Frezzotti R: Photocoagulation therapy of retinoblastoma. *Orbit* **9**(4):283, 1990.

109. Abramson DH: The focal treatment of retinoblastoma with emphasis on xenon arc photocoagulation. *Acta Ophthalmol* **67**(suppl 194):6, 1989.

110. Shields JA, Shields CL, Parsons H, Giblin ME: The role of photocoagulation in the management of retinoblastoma. *Arch Ophthalmol* **108**:205, 1990.

111. Hopping W, Meyer-Schwickerath G: Light coagulation treatment in retinoblastoma, in Boniuk M (ed): *Ocular and Adnexal Tumors.* St. Louis, Mosby, 1964.

112. Hopping W, Schmitt G: The treatment of retinoblastoma. *Mod Probl Ophthalmol* **13**:106, 1977.

113. Lincoff H, McLean J, Long R: The cryosurgical treatment of intraocular tumors. *Am J Ophthalmol* **63**:389, 1967.

114. Abramson DH, Ellsworth RM, Rozakis GW: Cryotherapy for retinoblastoma. *Arch Ophthalmol* **100**:1253, 1982.

115. Shields JA, Parson H, Shields CL, Giblin ME: The role of cryotherapy in the management of retinoblastoma. *Am J Ophthalmol* **108**:260, 1989.

116. Molteno ACB, Griffiths JS, Marcus PB, Van Der Watt JJ: Retinoblastoma treated by freezing. *Br J Ophthalmol* **55**:492, 1971.

117. Rubin ML: Cryopexy for retinoblastoma. *Am J Ophthalmol* **66**:870, 1968.

118. White L: The role of chemotherapy in the treatment of retinoblastoma. *Retina* **3**:194, 1983.

119. Kupfer C: Retinoblastoma treated with intravenous nitrogen mustard. *Am J Ophthalmol* **36**:1721, 1953.

120. Haye C, Schlienger B: La chimiotherapie des tumers de la retine. *Bull Mem Soc Franc Ophthalmol* **92**:119, 1980.

121. Zucher JM, Lemercier N, Schlienger P, Marguilis E, Haye C: Chemotherapeutic conservative management in twenty-three patients with locally extended bilateral retinoblastoma. *Eur J Clin Oncol* **10**:1, 1982.

122. Wolff JA, Boesel CP, Dyment PG, Ellsworth RM, Gallie B, Hammond D, Leiken SL, Maurer HS, Tretter PK, Wara WM: Treatment of retinoblastoma. A preliminary report. *Int Cong Series* **570**:364, 1981.

123. Pratt CB: Management of malignant solid tumors in children. *Pediatr Clin North Am* **19**(4):1141, 1972.

124. Howarth C, Meyer D, Hustu O, Johnson WW, Shanks E, Pratt C: Stage-related combined modality treatment of retinoblastoma. *Cancer* **45**:851, 1980.

125. Acquaviva A, Barberi L, Bernardini C, D'Ambrosio A, Lasorella G: Medical therapy in retinoblastoma in children. *J Neurosurg Sci* **26**(1):49, 1982.

126. Zelter M, Gonzales G, Schwartz L, Gallo G, Schvartzman, Damel A, Sackmann MF: Treatment of retinoblastoma: Results obtained from a prospective study of 51 patients. *Cancer* **61**:153, 1988.

127. Akiyama K, Iwasaki M, Amemiya T, Yanai M: Chemotherapy for retinoblastoma. *Ophthalmic Paediatr Genet* **10**(2):111, 1988.

128. Pratt CB, Kun LE: Response of orbital and central nervous system metastases of retinoblastoma following treatment with cyclophosphamide/doxorubicin. *Pediatr Hematol Oncol* **4**:125, 1987.

129. Hungerford J, Kingston J, Plowman N: Orbital recurrence of retinoblastoma. *Ophthalmic Paediatr Genet* **8**:63, 1987.

130. Saarinen UM, Sariola N, Hovi L: Recurrent disseminated retinoblastoma treated by high-dose chemotherapy, total body irradiation, and autologous bone marrow resuce. *Am J Hematol Oncol* **13**(4):315, 1991.

131. White L: Chemotherapy in retinoblastoma: Current status and future directions. *Am J Pediatr Hematol Oncol* **13**(2):189, 1991.

132. White L: Chemotherapy in retinoblastoma: Where do we go from here? *Ophthalmic Paediat Genet* **12**(3):115, 1991.

133. Hethcote HW, Knudson AGIR: Model for the incidence of embryonal cancers: Application to retinoblastoma. *Proc Natl Acad Sci USA* **75**:2453, 1978.

134. Falls HF, Neel JV: Genetics of retinoblastoma. *Arch Ophthalmol* **151**:197, 1951.

135. Schappert-Kimmiiser J, Hemmes GD, Nijiland R: The heredity of retinoblastoma. *Ophthalmologica* **151**:197, 1966.

136. Vogel F: Neue untersuchunger zur genetik des retinoblastoms. *Z Menschl Vereh Konstit Lehre* **34**:205, 1957.

137. Knudson AGJR: Mutation and cancer: Statistical study of retinoblastoma. *Proc Natl Acad Sci USA* **68**:820, 1971.

138. Macklin MT: A study of retinoblastoma in Ohio. *Am J Hum Genet* **12**:1, 1960.

139. Matsunaga E: Hereditary retinoblastoma: Delayed mutation or host resistance? *Am J Hum Genet* **30**:406, 1978.

140. Lele KP, Penrose LS, Stallard HB: Chromosome deletion in a case of retinoblastoma. *Ann Hum Genet* **27**:171, 1963.

141. Chaum E, Ellsworth RM, Abramsom DH, Haik BG, Kitchin FD, Chaganti RSK: Cytogenetic analysis of retinoblastoma: Evidence for multifocal origin and in vivo gene amplification. *Cytogenet Cell Genet* **38**:82, 1984.

142. Turleau C, de Grouchy U, Chavin-Coi IN F, Junien C, Seger J, Schieinger P, Leblanc A, Haye C: Cytogenetic forms of retinoblastoma: Their incidence in a survey of 66 patients. *Cancer Genet Cytogenet* **16**:321, 1985.

143. Squire J, Gallie BL, Phillips RA: A detailed analysis of chromosomal changes inheritable and non-heritable retinoblastoma. *Hum Genet* **70**:291, 1985.

144. Francke U: Retinoblastoma and chromosome 13. *Cytogenet Cell Genet* **16**:131, 1976.

145. Ward P, Packman S, Loughman W, Sparkes M, Sparkes RS, McMahon A, Gregory T, Ablin A: Location of the retinoblastoma susceptibility gene(s) and the human esterase D locus. *J Med Genet* **21**:92, 1984.

146. Sparkes RS, Murphree AL, Lingua RW, Sparkes MC, Field LL, Funderburk SJ, Benedict WF: Gene for hereditary retinoblastoma assigned to human chromosome 13 by linkage analysis to esterase D. *Science* **219**:971, 1983.

147. Sparkes RS, Sparkes MC, Wilson MG, Towner JW, Benedict WF, Murphree AL, Yunis JJ: Regional assignment of genes for esterase D and retinoblastoma to chromosome band 13q14. *Science* **208**:1042, 1980.

148. Strong LC, Riccardi VM, Ferrell RD, Sparkes RS: Familial retinoblastoma and chromosome 13 deletion transmitted via an insertional translocation. *Science* **213**:1501, 1981.

149. Sparkes RS, Muller H, Klisak I: Retinoblastoma with 13q-chromosomal deletion associated with maternal paracentric inversion of 13q. *Science* **203**:1027, 1979.

150. Riccardi VM, Hittner HM, Francke U, Pippin S, Holmquist GP, Kretzer FL, Ferrell R: Partial triplication and deletion of 13q: Study of a family presenting with bilateral retinoblastoma. *Clin Genet* **15**:332, 1979.

151. Warburton D, Anyane-Yeboa K, Taterka P: Deletion of 13q14 without retinoblastoma: A case of non-penetrance. *Am J Hum Genet* **39**:A137, 1986.

152. Wilson WG, Carter BT, Conway BP, Atkin JF, Watson BA, Sparkes RS: Variable manifestations of deletion (13)(q14.1-q14.3) in two generations. *Am J Hum Genet* **39**:A47, 1986.

153. Motegi T: High rate of detection of 13q14 deletion mosaicism among retinoblastoma patients (using more extensive methods). *Hum Genet* **61**:95, 1982.

154. Wilson WG, Campochiaro PA, Conway BP, Sudduth KW, Watson BA, Sparkes RS: Deletion (13)(q14.1-q14.3) in two generations: Variability of ocular manifestations and definition of the phenotype. *Am J Med Genet* **28**:675, 1987.

155. Fukushima Y, Kuroki Y, Ito T, Kondo I, Nishigaki I: Familial retinoblastoma (mother and son) with 13q14 deletion. *Hum Genet* **77**:104, 1987.

156. Cavenee WK, Dryja TP, Phillips RA, Benedict WF, Godbout R, Gallie BL, Murphree AL, Strong LC, White RL: Expression of recessive alleles by chromosomal mechanisms in retinoblastoma. *Nature* **305**:779, 1983.

157. Barker D, Schaefer M, White RL: Restriction sites containing CpG show a higher frequency of polymorphism in human DNA. *Cell* **36**:131, 1984.

158. Wyman AR, White RL: A highly polymorphic locus in human DNA. *Proc Natl Acad Sci USA* **77**:6754, 1980.

159. Cavenee WK, Leach RJ, Mohandas T, Pearson P, White RL: Isolation and regional localization of DNA segments revealing polymorphic loci from human chromosome 13. *Am J Hum Genet* **36**:10, 1984.

160. Dryja TP, Rapaport JM, Weichselbaum R, Bruns GAP: Chromosome 13 restriction fragment length polymorphisms. *Hum Genet* **65**:320, 1984.

161. Dryja TP, Cavenee WK, White RL, Rapaport JM, Peterson R, Albert DM, Bruns GAP: Homozygosity of chromosome 13 in retinoblastoma. *N Engl J Med* **310**:550, 1984.

162. Godbout R, Dryja TP, Squire JA, Gallie BL, Phillips RA: Somatic inactivation of genes on chromosome 13 is a common event in retinoblastoma. *Nature* **304**:550, 1983.

163. Cavenee WK, Hansen MF, Nordenskjold M, Kock E, Maumenee I, Squire JA, Phillips RA, Gallie BL: Genetic origin of mutations predisposing to retinoblastoma. *Science* **228**:501, 1985.

164. Abramson DH, Ellsworth RM, Kitchin FD, Tung G: Second nonocular tumors in retinoblastoma survivors: Are they radiation-induced? *Ophthalmology* **99**:1351, 1984.

165. Hansen MF, Koufos A, Gallie BL, Phillips RA, Fodstad O, Brogger A, Gedde-Dahl T, Cavenee WK: Osteosarcoma and retinoblastoma: A shared chromosomal mechanism revealing recessive predisposition. *Proc Natl Acad Sci USA* **82**:6216, 1985.

166. Monaco AP, Bertelson CJ, Middlesworth W, Colletti C-A, Aldridge J, Fischbeck KH, Bartlett R, Pericak-Vance MA, Roses AD, Kunkel LM: Detection of deletions spanning the Duchenne muscular dystrophy locus using a tightly linked DNA segment. *Nature* **316**:842, 1985.

167. Royer-Pokora B, Kunkel LM, Monaco AP, Goff SC, Newburger PE, Baehner PL, Cole FS, Curnutte JT, Orkin SH: Cloning the gene for an inherited human disorder—chronic granulomatous disease—on the basis of its chromosomal location. *Nature* **322**:32, 1986.

168. Lalande M, Dryja TP, Schreck RR, Shipley J, Flint A, Latt SA: Isolation of human chromosome 13-specific DNA sequences cloned from flow sorted chromosomes and potentially linked to the retinoblastoma locus. *Cancer Genet Cytogenet* **13**:283, 1984.

169. Lalande M, Donlon T, Petersen RA, Lieberparb R, Manter S, Latt SA: Molecular detection and differentiation of deletions in band 13q14 in human retinoblastoma. *Cancer Genet Cytogenet* **23**151, 1986.

170. Dryja TP, Rapoport JM, Joyce JM, Petersen RA: Molecular detection of deletions involving band q14 of chromosome 13 in retinoblastomas. *Proc Natl Acad Sci USA* **83**7391, 1986.

171. Bookstein R, Lee EY-HP, To H, Young L-J, Sey T, Hayes R, Friedmann T, Lee W-H: Human retinoblastoma susceptibility gene: Genomic organization and analysis of heterozygous intragenic deletion mutants. *Proc Natl Acad Sci USA* **85**:2210, 1988.

172. Friend SH, Bernards R, Rogelj S, Weinberg RA, Rapoport JM, Albert DM, Dryja TP: A human DNA segment with properties of the gene that predisposes to retinoblastoma and osteosarcoma. *Nature* **323**:643, 1986.

173. Fung Y-KT, Murphree A, Tang A, Qian J, Hinrichs S, Benedict W: Structural evidence for the authenticity of the human retinoblastoma gene. *Science* **236**:1657, 1987.

174. Horsthemke B, Gregor V, Barnert H, Hopping W, Passarge E: Detection of submicroscopic deletions and a DNA polymorphism at the retinoblastoma locus. *Hum Genet* **76**:257, 1987.

175. Dunn J, Phillips R, Zhu X, Becker A, Gallie B: Mutations in the *RB1* gene and their effect on transcription. *Mol Cell Biol* **9**:4596, 1989.

176. Yandell D, Campbell T, Dayton S, Petersen R, Walton D, Little J, McConkie-Rosell A, Buckley E, Dryja T: Oncogenic point mutations in the human retinoblastoma gene: Their application to genetic counseling. *N Engl J Med* **321**:1639, 1989.

177. Lee W-H, Bookstein R, Hong F, Young L-J, Shew J-Y, Lee EY-HP: Human retinoblastoma susceptibility gene: Cloning, identification, and sequence. *Science* **235**:1394, 1987.

178. Horowitz J, Park S-H, Bogenmann E, Cheng J-C, Yandell D, Kaye F, Minna J, Dryja T, Weinberg R: Frequent inactivation of the retinoblastoma anti-oncogene is restricted to a subset of human tumor cells. Proc Natl Acad Sci USA **87**:2775, 1990.

179. Harbour J, Lai S-L, Whang-Peng J, Gazdar A, Minna J, Kaye F: Abnormalities in structure and expression of the human retinoblastoma gene in SCLC. *Science* **242**:263, 1988.

180. Tang A, Varley J, Chakroborty S, Murphree A, Fung Y-KT: Structural rearrangement of the retinoblastoma gene in human breast carcinoma. *Science* **242**:263, 1988.

181. Bookstein R, Lee EY-HP, Peccei A, Lee W-H: Human retinoblastoma gene: Long-range mapping and analysis of its deletion in a breast cancer cell line. *Mol Cell Biol* **9**:1628, 1989.

182. Seizinger B, Klinger H, Junien C, Nakamura Y, Lebeau M, Cavenee W, Emanual B, Ponder B, Naylor S, Mitelman R, Louis D, Menon A, Newsham I, Decker J, Laelbing M, Henry IV, Deimling A: Report of the committee on chromosome and gene loss in human neoplasia. *Cytogenet Cell Genet* **58**:1080, 1991.

183. Huang H-JS, Yee J-K, Shew J-Y, Chen P-L, Bookstein R, Friedmann T, Lee EY-HP, Lee W-H: Suppression of the neoplastic phenotype b y replacement of the RB gene in human cancer cells. *Science* **242**:1563, 1988.

184. Takahashi R, Hashimoto T, Xu H-J, Matsui T, Mikki T, Bigo-Marshall H, Aaronson S, Benedict W: The retinoblastoma gene functions as a growth and tumor suppressor in human bladder carcinoma cells. *Proc Natl Acad Sci USA* **88**:5257, 1991.

185. Bookstein R, Shew J-Y, Chen P-L, Scully P, Lee W-H: Suppression of tumorigenicity of human prostate carcinoma cells by replacing a mutated RB gene. *Science* **247**:712, 1990.

186. Niederkorn J, Streilein J, Shaddock J: Deviant immune responses to allogeneic tumors injected intracamerally and subcutaneously in mice. *Invest Ophthalmol Vis Sci* **20**:355, 1981.

187. Madreperla S, Whittum-Hudson J, Prendergast R, Chen P-L, Lee W-H: Intraocular tumor suppression of retinoblastoma gene-reconstituted retinoblastoma cells. *Cancer Res* **51**:6381, 1991.

188. Muncaster M, Cohen B, Phillips R, Gallie B: Failure of *RB1* to reverse the malignant phenotype of human tumor cell lines. *Cancer Res* **52**:654, 1992.

189. Cavenee WK, Murphree AL, Shull MS, Benedict WF, Sparkes RS, Kock E, Nordenskjold M: Prediction of familial predisposition to retinoblastoma. *N Engl J Med* **314**:1201, 1986.

190. Horsthemke B, Barnert HJ, Greger V, Passarge E, Hopping W: Early diagnosis in hereditary retinoblastoma by detection of molecular deletions at gene locus. *Lancet* **28**:511, 1987.

191. Leppert M, Cavenee W, Callahan P, Holm T, O'Connell P, Thompson K, Lathrop GM, Lalouel J-M, White R: A primary genetic map of chromosome 13q. *Am J Hum Genet* **39**:425, 1986.

192. Lee EY-HP, Lee WH: Molecular cloning of the human esterase D gene, a genetic marker for retinoblastoma. *Proc Natl Acad Sci USA* **83**:6337, 1986.

193. Squire J, Dryja TP, Dunn J, Goddard A, Hoffman T, Musarella M, Willard HF, Becker AJ, Gallie BL, Phillips RA: Cloning of the esterase D gene: A polymorphic probe closely linked to the retinoblastoma locus on chromosome 13. *Proc Natl Acad Sci USA* **83**:6573, 1986.

194. Wiggs J, Nordenskjold M, Yandell D, Rapaport J, Grondin V, Janson M, Werelius B, Peterson R, Craft A, Riedel K, Liberfarb R, Walton D, Wilson W, Dryja TP: Prediction of risk of hereditary retinoblastoma using DNA polymorphisms within the retinoblastoma gene. *N Engl J Med* **318**:151, 1988.

195. Vaughn G, Toguchida J, McGee T, Dryja T: PCR detection of the TthIII 1 RFLP within the retinoblastoma locus by PCR. *Nucleic Acids Res* **18**:4965, 1990.

196. McGee T, Cowley G, Yandell D, Dryja T: Detection of the Xba I RFLP within the retinoblastoma locus by PCR. *Nucleic Acids Res* **18**:207, 1990.

197. Scharf S, Bowcock A, McClure G, Klitz W, Yandell D, Erlich H: Amplification and characterization of the retinoblastoma gene VNTR by PCR. *Am J Hum Genet* **50**:371, 1992.

198. Dryja T, Mukai S, Petersen R, Rapaport J, Walton D, Yandell D: Parental origin of mutations of the retinoblastoma gene. *Nature* **339**:556, 1989.

199. Zhu X, Dunn J, Phillips R, Goddard A, Paton K, Becker A, Gallie B: Preferential germline mutation of the paternal allele in retinoblastoma. *Nature* **340**:313, 1989.

200. Toguchida J, Ishizaki K, Sasaki M, Hakamura Y, Ikenaga M, Kato M, Sugimot M, Kotoura Y, Yamamuro T: Preferential mutation of paternally derived RB gene as the initial event in sporadic osteosarcoma. *Nature* **338**:156, 1989.

201. Sapeinza C: Genome imprinting and dominance modification. *Ann NY Acad Sci* **564**:24, 1989.

202. Leach R, Magewu N, Buckley J, Benedict W, Rother C, Murphree A, Griegels, Rajewsky M, Jones P: Preferential retention of paternal alleles in human retinoblastoma: Evidence for genomic imprinting. *Cell Growth Diff* **1**:401, 1990.

203. Vogel W: Genetics of retinoblastoma. *Hum Genet* **52**:1, 1979.

204. Onadim Z, Hogg A, Baird P, Cowell J: Oncogenic point mutations in exon 20 of the *RB1* gene in families showing incomplete penetrance and mild expression of the retinoblastoma phenotype. *Proc Natl Acad Sci USA* **89**:6177, 1992.

205. Sakai T, Ohtani N, McGee T, Robbins P, Dryja T: Oncogenic germline mutations in Sp1 and ATF sites in the human retinoblastoma gene. *Nature* **353**:83, 1991.

206. Landshulz WH, Johnson PF, McKnight SL: The leucine zipper: A hypothetical structure common to a new class of DNA binding proteins. *Science* **240**:1759, 1988.

207. Patthy L: Evolution of the proteases of blood coagulation and fibrinolysis by assembly from modules. *Cell* **41**:657, 1985.

208. Hong FD, Huang H-JS, To H, Young L-JS, Oro A, Bookstein R, Lee EY-HP, Lee W-H: Structure of the human retinoblastoma gene. *Proc Natl Acad Sci USA* **86**:5502, 1989.

209. Jones NC, Rigby PWJ, Ziff EB: Trans-acting protein factors and the regulation of eukaryotic transcription: Lessons from studies on DNA tumor viruses. *Gene Dev* **2**:267, 1988.

210. Lee W-H, Shew J-Y, Hong FD, Sery TW, Donoso LA, Young L-J, Bookstein R, Lee EY-HP: The retinoblastoma susceptibility gene encodes a nuclear phosphorprotein associated with DNA binding activity. *Nature* **329**:642, 1987.

211. Cross F, Weintraub H, Roberts J: Simple and complex cell cycles. *Annu Rev Cell Biol* **5**:341, 1989.

212. Pardee AB: G₁ events and regulation of cell proliferation. *Science* **246**:605, 1989.

213. Pardee AB: Molecules involved in proliferation of normal and cancer cells: Presidential address. *Cancer Res* **47**:1488, 1987.

214. Mihara K, Cao X-R, Yen A, Chandler S, Driscoll B, Murphree AL, T-ang A, Fung Y-KT: Cell cycle-dependent regulation of phosphorylation of the human retinoblastoma gene product. *Science* **246**:1300, 1989.

215. Decaprio JA, Ludlow JW, Lynch D, Furukawa Y, Griffin J, Liwnica-Worms H, Huang C-M, Livingston DM: The product of the retinoblastoma susceptibility gene has properties of a cell cycle regulatory element. *Cell* **58**:1085, 1989.

216. Buchkovich K, Duffy LA, Harlow E: The retinoblastoma protein is phosphorylated during specific phases of the cell cycle. *Cell* **58**:1097, 1989.

217. Lin BT-Y, Gruenwald S, Morla AO, Lee W-H, Wang JYJ: Retinoblastoma cancer suppressor gene product is a substrate of the cell cycle regulator cdc2 kinase. *EMBO J* **10**:857, 1991.

218. Nurse P, Thuriaux P, Nasmyth K: Genetic control of the cell division cycle in the fission yeast Schizosaccharomyces pombe. *Mol Gen Genet* **146**:167, 1976.

219. D'Urso G, Marraccino RL, Marshak DR, Roberts JM: Cell cycle control of DNA replication by a homologue from human cells of the p34c-src protein kinase. *Science* **250**:786, 1990.

220. Shenoy S, Choi J-K, Bagrodia S, Copeland TD, Maller JL, Shalloway D: Purified maturation promoting factor phosphorylates pp60c-src at the sites phosphorylated during fibroblast mitosis. *Cell* **57**:763, 1989.

221. Chen P-L, Scully P, Shew J-Y, Wang JYJ, Lee W-H: Phosphorylation of the retinoblastoma gene product is modulated during the cell cycle and cellular differentiation. *Cell* **58**:1193, 1989.

222. Furukawa Y, Decaprio JA, Freedman A, Kanakura Y, Nakamura M, Ernst TJ, Livingston DM, Griffin JD: Expression and state of phosphorylation of the retinoblastoma susceptibility gene product in cycling and noncycling human hematopoietic cells. *Proc Natl Acad Sci USA* **87**:2770, 1990.

223. Cooper JA, Whyte P: RB and the cell cycle: Entrance or exit? *Cell* **58**:1009, 1989.

224. Decaprio JA, Furukawa Y, Ajchenbaum F, Griffin JD, Livingston DM: The retinoblastoma-susceptibility gene product becomes phosphorylated in multiple stages during cell cycle entry and progression. *Proc Natl Acad Sci USA* **89**:1795, 1992.

225. Hunter T, Pines J: Cyclins and cancer: II. Cyclin D and CDK inhibitors come of age. *Cell* **79**:573, 1994.

226. Jinag W, Kahn SM, Tomita N, Zhang Y-J, Lu SH, Weinstein IB: Amplification and expression of the human cyclin D gene in esophageal cancer. *Cancer Res* **52**:2980, 1992.

227. Motokura T, Arnold A: Cyclins and oncogenesis. *Biochim Biophys Acta* **1155**:63, 1993.

228. Dowdy SF, Hinds PW, Louie K, Reed S, Arnold A, Weinberg RA: Physical interaction of the retinoblastoma protein with human D cyclins. *Cell* **73**:499, 1993.

229. Ewen ME, Sluss HK, Sherr CJ, Matshushime H, Kato J, Livingston DM: Functional interactions of the retinoblastoma protein with mammalian D-type cyclins. *Cell* **73**:487, 1993.

230. Kato J, Matsushime H, Hiebert SW, Ewen ME, Sherr CJ: Direct binding of cyclin D to the retinoblastoma gene product (pRb) and pRb phosphorylation by the cyclin D-dependent kinase CDK4. *Gene Dev* **7**:331, 1993.

231. Fagan R, Flint KJ, Jones N: Phosphorylation of E2F-1 modulates its interaction with the retinoblastoma gene product and the adenoviral E4 19 kDa protein. *Cell* **78**:799, 1994.

232. Bates S, Parry D, Bonetta L, Vousden K, Dickson C, Peters G: Absence of cyclin D/cdk complexes in cells lacking functional retinoblastoma protein. *Oncogene* **9**:1633, 1994.

233. Mller H, Lukas J, Schneider A, Warthoe P, Bartek J, Ellers M, Strasu M: Cyclin D1 expression is regulated by the retinoblastoma protein. *Proc Natl Acad Sci USA* **91**:2945, 1994.

234. Tam SW, Theodoras AM, Shay JW, Draetta GF, Pagano M: Differential expression and regulation of cyclin D1 protein in normal and tumor human cells: Association with Cdk4 is required for Cyclin D1 function in G1 progression. *Oncogene* **9**:2663, 1994.

235. Serrano M, Hannon GJ, Beach D: A new regulatory motif in cell-cycle control causing specific inhibition of cyclin D/CDK4. *Nature* **366**:704, 1993.

236. Hannon GI, Beach D: p15INK4B is a potential effector of TGF-B-induced cell cycle arrest. *Nature* **371**:257, 1994.

237. Kamb A, Gruis NA, Weaver-Feldhaus J, Lie Q, Harshman K, Tavtigian SV, Stockert E, Day RSI, Johnson BE, Skolnick MH: A cell cycle regulator potentially in volved in genesis of many tumor types. *Science* **264**:436, 1994.

238. Nobori T, Miura K, Wu DJ, Lois A, Takabayashi K, Carson DA: Deletions of the cyclin-dependent kinase-4 inhibitor gene in multiple human cancers. *Nature* **368**:753, 1994.

239. Merlo A, Herman JG, Mao L, Lee DJ, Gabrielson E, Burger PC, Baylin SB, Sidransky D: 5′ CpG island methylation is associated with transcriptional silencing of the tumour suppressor p16/CDKN2/MTS1 in human cancers. *Nat Med* **1**:686, 1995.

240. Costello JF, Berger MS, Huang H-JS, Cavenee WK: Silencing of p16/CDKN2 expression in human gliomas by methylation and chromatin condensation. *Cancer Res* **56**:2405, 1996.

241. Arap W, Kishikawa R, Furnari FB, Cavenee WK, Huang H-JS: Replacement of the p16/CDKN2 gene suppresses human glioma cell growth. *Cancer Res* **55**:1351, 1995.

242. Bonetta L: Open questions on p16. *Nature* **370**:180, 1994.

243. Cairns P, Mao L, Merlo A, Lee DJ, Schwab D, Eby Y, Tokino K, van der Riet P, Blaugrund JE, Sidransky D: Rates of p16 (MTS1) mutations in primary tumors with 9p loss. *Science* **265**:415, 1994.

244. Kamp A, Liu Q, Harshman K, Tavtigian S: Rates of p16 (MTS1) mutations in primary tumors with 9p loss. *Science* **265**:416, 1994.

245. Spruck CHI, Gonzalex-Sulueta M, Shibata A, Simoneay AR, Lin M-F, Gonzales F, Tsai YC, Jones PA: p16 gene in uncultured tumours. *Nature* **370**:183, 1994.

246. He J, Olson JJ, James CD: Lack of p16INK4 or retinoblastoma protein (pRb) or amplification-associated overexpression of cdk4 is observed in distinct subsets of malignant glial tumors and cell lines. *Cancer Res* **55**:4833, 1995.

247. Mori T, Miura K, Aoki T, Nishihara T, Mori S, Nakamura M: Frequent somatic mutation of MTS1/CDK4 (multiple tumor suppressor/cyclin-dependent kinase 4 inhibitor) gene in esophageal squamous cell carcinoma. *Cancer Res* **54**:3396, 1994.

248. Caldas C, Hahn SA, da Costa LT, Redston MS, Schutte M, Seymour AB, Weinstein CK, Hruban RH, Yeo CJ, Kern SE: Frequent somatic mutations and homozygous deletions of the p16 (MTS1) gene in pancreatic adenocarcinoma. *Nat Genet* **8**:27, 1994.

249. Parry D, Bates S, Mann DJ, Peters G: Lack of cyclin D/Cdk complexes in RB-negative cells correlates with high levels of p16INK4/MTS1 tumour suppressor gene product. *EMBO J* **14**:503, 1995.

250. Li Y, Nichols MA, Shay JW, Xiong Y: Transcriptional repression of the D-type cyclin-dependent linases inhibitor p16 by the retinoblastoma susceptibility gene product, pRb. *Cancer Res* **54**:6078, 1994.

251. Shimizu E, Coxon A, Otterson GA, Steinberg SM, Kratzke RA, Kim YW, Fedorko J, Oie H, Johnson B, Mulsine JL, Minna JD, Gazdar AF, Kaye FJ: *Oncogene* **9**:2441, 1994.

252. Shapiro GI, Edwards CD, Kobzik L, Godleski J, Richars W, Sugarbaker DJ, Rollins BJ: Reciprocal Rb inactivation and p16INK4 expression in primary lung cancers and cell lines. *Cancer Res* **55**:505, 1995.

253. Otterson GA, Kratzke RA, Coxon A, Kim YW, Kaye FJ: Absence of p16INK4 protein is restricted to the subset of lung cancer lines that retains wild-type RB. *Oncogene* **9**:3375, 1994.

254. Sakaguchi M, Fuji Y, Hirabayashi H, Yoon H-E, Komoto Y, Oue T, Kusafuka T, Okada A, Matsuda H: Inversely correlated expression of p16 and Rb protein in non-small cell lung cancers: An immunohistochemical study. *Int J Cancer* **65**:442, 1996.

255. Schauer IE, Siriwardana S, Langan TA, Sclarani RA: Cyclin Da overexpression vs. retinoblastoma inactivation: Implications for growth control evasion in non-small cell and small cell lung cancer. *Proc Natl Acad Sci USA* **91**:7827, 1994.

256. Berk A: Adenovirus promoters and E1A transactivation. *Annu Rev Genet* **20**:45, 1986.

257. Livingston DM, Bradley MK: Review: The simian virus 40 large T antigen—a lot packed into a little. *Mol Biol Med* **4**:63, 1987.

258. Zur Hausen H, Schneider A, in Howley PM, Salzman MP (eds): *The Papovaviridae*, vol 2: *The Papillomaviruses*. New York, Plenum, 1987, pp 245–263.

259. Cherington V, Brown M, Paucha E, St. Louis J, Spiegelman BM, Roberts TM: Separation of simian virus 40 large T-antigen-transforming and origin-binding functions from the ability to block differentiation. *Mol Cell Biol* **8**:1380, 1988.

260. Clayton CE, Murphy D, Lovett M, Rigby PWJ: A fragment of the SV40 T-antigen gene transforms. *Nature* **299**:59, 1982.

261. Whyte P, Ruley HE, Harlow E: Two regions of the adenovirus early region 1A proteins are required for transformation. *J Virol* **62**257, 1988.

262. Phelps WC, Yee CL, Munger K, Howley PM: The human papilloma type 16 E7 gene encodes transactivation and transformation functions similar to those of adenovirus E1A. *Cell* **53**:539, 1988.

263. Harlow E, Whyte P, Franza BR Jr, Schley C: Association of adenovirus early-region 1A proteins with cellular polypeptides. *Mol Cell Biol* **6**:1579, 1986.

264. Whyte P, Buchkovich KJ, Horowitz JM, Friend SH, Raybuck M, Weinberg RA, Harlow E: Association between an oncogene and an antioncogene: The adenovirus E1A proteins bind to the retinoblastoma gene product. *Nature* **234**:124, 1988.

265. Decaprio JA, Ludlow JW, Figge J, Shew J-Y, Huang C-M, Lee W-H, Marsilio E, Paucha E, Livingston DM: SV40 large tumor antigen forms a specific complex with the product of the retinoblastoma susceptibility gene. *Cell* **54**:275, 1988.

266. Dyson N, Howley PM, Munger K, Harlow E: The human papilloma virus-16 E7 oncoprotein is able to bind to the retinoblastoma gene product. *Science* **243**:934, 1989.

267. Kalderon D, Smith AE: In vitro mutagenesis of a putative DNA binding domain of SV40 large T. *Virology* **139**:109, 1984.

268. Ludlow JW, Decaprio JA, Huang C-M, Lee W-H, Paucha E, Livingston DM: SV40 large T antigen binds perferentially to an under-phosphorylated member of the retinoblastoma susceptibility gene product family. *Cell* **56**:57, 1989.

269. Ludlow JW, Shon J, Pipas JM, Livingston DM, Decaprip JA: The retinoblastoma susceptibility gene product undergoes cell cycle-dependent dephosphorylation and binding to and release from SV40 large T. *Cell* **60**:387, 1990.

270. Peden KWC, Srinivasan A, Parber JM, Pipas JM: Mutants with changes within or near a hydrophobic region of simian virus 40 large tumor antigen are defective for binding cellular protein p53. *Virology* **168**:13, 1989.

271. Tack LC, Cartwright CA, Wright JH, Eckhard W, Peden KWC, Srinivasan A, Pipas JM: Properties of a simian virus 40 mutant T antigen substituted in the hydrophobic region: Defective ATP-ase and oligomerization activities and altered phosphorylation accompany an inability to complex with cellular p53. *J Virol* **63**:3362, 1989.

272. Dyson N, Buchovich K, Whyte P, Harlow E: The cellular 107K protein that binds to adenovirus E1A also associates with the large T antigens of SV40 and JC virus. *Cell* **58**:249, 1989.

273. Ewen ME, Ludlow JW, Marsilio E, Decaprio JA, Millikan RC, Cheng SH, Paucha E, Livingston DM: An N-terminal transformation-governing sequence of SV40 large T antigen contributes to the binding of both p110^RB and a second cellular protein, p120. *Cell* **58**:257, 1989.

274. Hu Q, Dyson N, Harlow E: The regions of the retinoblastoma protein needed for binding to adenovirus E1A or SV40 large T antigen are common sites for mutations. *EMBO J* **9**(4):1147, 1990.

275. Huang S, Wang N-P, Tseng BY, Lee W-H, Lee EH-YP: Two distinct and frequently mutated regions of retinoblastoma protein are required for binding to SV40 T antigen. *EMBO J* **9**(6):1815, 1990.

276. Horowitz J, Yandell DW, Park S-H, Canning S, Whyte P, Buchkovich K, Harlow E, Weinberg RA, Dryja TP: Point mutational inactivation of the retinoblastoma antioncogene. *Science* 243:937, 1989.

277. Shew J-Y, Ling N, Yang X, Fodstad O, Lee W-H: Antibodies detecting abnormalities of the retinoblastoma susceptibility gene product (pp110^RB) in osteosarcomas and synovial sarcomas. *Oncogene Res* 4:205, 1989.

278. Bookstein R, Shew J-Y, Chen P-L, Scully P, Lee W-H: Suppression of tumorigenicity of human prostate carcinoma cells by replacing a mutated RB gene. *Science* 247:712, 1990.

279. Shew J-Y, Lin BT-Y, Chen P-L, Tseng BY, Yang-Feng TL, Lee W-H: C-terminal truncation of the retinoblastoma gene product leads to functional inactivation. *Proc Natl Acad Sci USA* 87:6, 1990.

280. Defeo-Jones D, Huang PS, Jones RE, Haskell KM, Vuocolo GA, Hanobik MG, Huber HE, Oliff A: Cloning of cDNAs for cellular proteins that bind to the retinoblastoma gene product. *Nature* 352:251, 1991.

281. Huang S, Lee W-H, Lee EY-HP: A cellular protein that competes with SV40 T antigen for binding to the retinoblastoma gene product. *Nature* 350:160, 1991.

282. Kaelin WG, Pallas DC, Decaprio JA, Kaye FJ, Livingston DM: Identification of cellular proteins that can interact specifically with the T/E1A-binding region of the retinoblastoma gene product. *Cell* 64:521, 1991.

283. Partridge JF, Lathangue NB: A developmentally regulated and tissue-dependent transcription factor complexes with the retinoblastoma gene product. *EMBO J* 10:3819, 1991.

284. Bandara LR, Lathangue NB: Adenovirus E1A prevents the retinoblastoma gene product from complexing with a cellular transcription factor. *Nature* 351:494, 1991.

285. Bandara LR, Adamczewski JP, Hunt T, Lathangue NB: Cyclin A and the retinoblastoma gene product complex with a common transcription factor. *Nature* 352:249, 1991.

286. Buyse IM, Shao G, Huang S: The retinoblastoma protein binds to RIZ, a zinc-finger protein that shares an epotope with the adenovirus E1A protein. *Proc Natl Acad Sci USA* 92:4467, 1995.

287. Gu W, Schneider JW, Condorelli G, Kaushal S, Mahdavi V, Nadal-Ginard B: Interaction of myogenic factors and the retinoblastoma protein mediates muscle cell commitment and differentiation. *Cell* 72:309, 1993.

288. Welch PJ, Wang JYJ: Abrogations of retinoblastoma protein function by c-Abl through tyrosine kinase-dependent and -independent mechanisms. *Mol Cell Biol* 15:5542, 1995.

289. Xiao Z-X, Chen J, Levine AJ, Modjtahedi N, Xing J, Sellers WR, Livingston DM: Interaction between the retinoblastoma protein and the oncoprotein MDM2. *Nature (London)* 375:694, 1995.

290. Eckner R, Ewen ME, Newsome D, Gerdes M, DeCaprio JA, Lawrence JB, Lingston DM: Molecular cloning and functional analysis of the adenovirus E1A-associated 300-kD protein (p300) reveals a protein with properties of a transcriptional adaptor. *Gene Dev* 8:869, 1994.

291. Strober BE, Dunaief JL, Sushovan G, Goff SP: Functional interactions between the hBRM/hBRG1 transcriptional activators and the pRB family of proteins. *Mol Cell Biol* 16:1576, 1996.

292. Chittenden T, Livingston DM, Kaelin WG: The T/E1A-binding domain of the retinoblastoma product can interact selectively with a sequence-specific DNA-binding protein. *Cell* 65:1073, 1991.

293. Helin K, Lees JA, Vidal M, Dyson N, Harlow E, Fattaey A: A cDNA encoding a pRB-binding protein with properties of the transcription factor E2F. *Cell* 70:337, 1992.

294. Kaelin WG, Krek W, Sellers WR, Decaprio JA, Ajchenbaum F, Fuchs CS, Chittenden T, Li Y, Farnham PJ, Blanar MA, Livingston DM,

295. Flemington EK: Expression cloning of a cDNA encoding a retinoblastoma-binding protein with E2F-like properties. *Cell* 70:351, 1992.

295. Chellappan SP, Hiebert S, Mudry JM, Horowitz JM, Nevins JR: The E2F transcription factor is a cellular target for the RB protein. *Cell* 65:1053, 1991.

296. Bagchi S, Weinmann R, Raychaudhuri P: The retinoblastoma protein copurifies with E2F-I, and E1A-regulated inhibitor of the transcription factor E2F. *Cell* 65:1063, 1991.

297. Weintraub SJ, Prater CA, Dean DC: Retinoblastoma protein switches the E2F site from positive to negative element. *Nature* 358:259, 1992.

298. Ewen ME, Xing Y, Lawrence JB, Livingston DM: Molecular cloning, chromosomal mapping, and expression of the cDNA for p107, a retinoblastoma gene product-related protein. *Cell* 66:1155, 1991.

299. Hannon GJ, Demetrick D, Beach D: Isolation of the Rb-related p130 through its interaction with CDK2 and cyclins. *Gene Dev* 7:2378, 1993.

300. Cobrinik D, Whyte P, Peeper DS, Jacks T, Weinberg RA: Cell cycle-specific association of E2F with the p130 E1A-binding protein. *Gene Dev* 7:2392, 1993.

301. Li Y, Graham C, Lacy S, Duncan AMV, Whyte P: The adenovirus E1A-associated 130-kD protein is encoded by a member of the retinoblastoma gene family and physically interacts with cyclins A and E. *Gene Dev* 7:2366, 1993.

302. Ewen ME, Faha B, Harlow D, Livingston D: Interaction of p107 with cyclin A independent of complex formation with viral oncoproteins. *Science* 255:85, 1992.

303. Zhu L, van der Heuvel K, Fattaey A, Ewen M, Livingston D, Dyson N, Harlow E: Inhibition of cell proliferation by p107, a relative of the retinoblastoma protein. *Gene Dev* 7:1111, 1993.

304. Maw MA, Grundy PE, Millow LJ, Eccles MR, Dunn RS, Smith PJ, Feinberg AP, Law DJ, Paterson MC, Telzerow PE: A third Wilms' tumor locus on chromosome 16q. *Cancer Res* 52:3094, 1992.

305. Slater RM, Mannens MM: Cytogenetics and molecular genetics of Wilms' tumor of childhood. *Cancer Genet Cytogenet* 61:111, 1992.

306. Newsham I, Röhrborn-Kindler A, Daub D, Cavenee WK: A constitutional BWS-related t(11;16) chromosome translocation occurring in the same region of chromosome 16 implicated in Wilms' tumors. *Gene Chrom Cancer* 12:1, 1995.

307. Jacks T, Faxeli A, Schmitt EM, Bronson RT, Goodell MA, Weinberg RA: Effects of an Rb mutation in the mouse. *Nature* 359:295, 1992.

308. Lee EY-HP, Chang CY, Hu N, Wang Y-CJ, Lai C-C, Herrup K, Lee W-H, Bradley A: Mice deficient for Rb are nonviable and show defects in neurogenesis and haematopoiesis. *Nature* 359:288, 1992.

309. Williams BO, Schmitt EM, Remington L, Bronson RT, Albert DM, Weinberg RA, Jacks T: Extensive contribution of Rb-deficient cells to adult chimeric mice with limited histopathological consequences. *EMBO J* 13:4251, 1994.

310. Windle JJ, Albert DM, O'Brien JM, Marcus DM, Disteche CM, Bernards, Mellon PL: Retinoblastoma in transgenic mice. *Nature* 343:665, 1990.

311. Herrera RE, Sah VP, Williams BO, Makela TP, Weinberg RA, Jacks T: Altered cell cycle kinetics, gene expression, and G1 restriction point regulation in Rb-deficient fibroblasts. *Mol Cell Biol* 16:2402, 1996.

312. Harvey M, Vogel H, Lee EY-HP, Bradley A, Donehower LA: Mice deficient in both p53 and Rb develop tumors primarily of endocrine origin. *Cancer Res* 55:1146, 1995.

313. Williams BO, Remington L, Albert DM, Mukai S, Bronson RT, Jacks T: Cooperative tumorigenic effects of germline mutations in Rb and p53. *Nat Genet* 7:480, 1994.

CHAPTER 20

The Li-Fraumeni Syndrome

David Malkin

1. The Li-Fraumeni syndrome (LFS) is a rare autosomal dominantly inherited disorder. It is characterized by the diagnosis of bone or soft-tissue sarcoma at an early age in an individual who has one first-degree relative with early-onset cancer and a second close relative with early-onset cancer or sarcoma diagnosed at any age.

2. Families in which the classic phenotype of the syndrome is not expressed completely are termed Li-Fraumeni syndrome-like (LFS-L) and are represented by many different features. Common to all these families is the occurrence of a variety of cancers of a distinct histopathologic type.

3. Germ-line alterations of the p53 tumor-suppressor gene located on chromosome 17p13 have been observed in the majority of LFS families and in a proportion of LFS-L families. This gene encodes a 53-kD nuclear phosphoprotein that is composed of 393 amino acids. Genetic alterations primarily result from base-pair substitutions that result in missense mutations. These changes are among the most frequently observed genetic abnormalities in human cancer. Somatic inactivation of p53 occurs through base-pair substitutions or binding to other cellular proteins or to certain DNA tumor virus proteins.

4. The p53 protein binds specific DNA sequences and appears to be a transcription factor that may regulate the expression of other growth regulatory genes in a positive or negative manner. The antiproliferative effect of wild-type p53 is exerted at a checkpoint control site before G1/S of the cell cycle, with G2/M and the mitotic spindle being other potential targets. p53 mediates apoptosis and plays an important role in modulating the cellular response to DNA damage induced by UV irradiation or γ-irradiation and certain chemotherapeutic agents.

5. p53 mutations are not observed in all classic LFS families. Germ-line p53 mutations are seen in a small number of patients and families with cancer phenotypes that only superficially resemble LFS. Other mechanisms of p53 inactivation may occur in some clinical settings, and other genes involved in cell cycle regulation may be altered in p53 wild-type families.

6. Mouse models of p53 deficiency have been created. These p53 knockouts exhibit an increased rate of development of a spectrum of tumors, including lymphomas and sarcomas. Transgenic p53 mice have been generated that have a tumor phenotype distinct from that of the p53-deficient animals. Mice heterozygous for a deleted p53 allele exhibit an intermediate phenotype in that the rate of tumor formation is slower than that of the p53-null animals yet faster than that of wild-type littermates. These mice have been used as in vivo models to analyze p53 function and dysfunction in the setting of interventions with chemotherapy, radiation therapy, or teratogenic agents.

7. Predictive genetic testing for carriers of mutant p53 is available in research settings in a few centers. The interpretation of results with respect to diagnostic capabilities and options for therapeutic intervention is under scrutiny. The value of such screening is tempered by the need to evaluate risk counseling issues, the need for informed consent, and regulations on testing.

Studies of hereditary cancer clusters have led to the identification of genes critical to both carcinogenesis and normal development. The Li-Fraumeni family cancer syndrome (LFS) is a rare but important familial cancer syndrome that represents the paradigm of human cancer predisposition to multiple childhood- and adult-onset neoplasms. Before the identification of a specific genetic defect that was inherited in a significant proportion of LFS families, it could not be definitely established that such a diverse spectrum of tumors could result from the alteration of a specific gene as a presumptive initiating event. The span of time from the initial clinical description of a family with this constellation of tumors to the identification of germ-line alterations of the p53 tumor-suppressor gene in many families was 20 years. The realization of a genetic link resulted from expertise in classic genetic epidemiology and the molecular biology of sporadic tumorigenesis and in many ways represented the realization of the development of the now burgeoning field of molecular epidemiology. The link between an extremely rare clinical phenotype (LFS) with alterations of perhaps the most commonly altered gene in human cancer (p53) points out the value of studying rare genetic phenotypes. These studies have led to a more clear understanding of the role p53 plays in cell cycle control as well as to a cloudier picture of the way in which the LFS phenotype is derived in the absence of p53 alterations. The generation of mouse models of deficient p53 has provided an opportunity to study not only the tumorigenic effects of this genotype but also the potential results of therapeutic, carcinogenic, and teratogenic interventions in tissues harboring an altered p53 allele.

In addition to expanding our knowledge of cell cycle control, the study of these LFS families formed the early foundations on which recommendations and guidelines could be established to develop and monitor genetic testing programs for predisposition to both early- and late-onset disease. The models developed for other genetic diseases have been helpful as guides, but the unique imprecise nature of human carcinogenesis and the p53–LFS association require complex interactions between several disciplines.

At the time of this writing, the genetics of LFS are still being established and the complex roles of p53 are being elucidated. A vast literature has been generated about this gene, and characterizations of its roles in clinical genetics and clinical medicine are relatively early in their development. Future editions of this textbook will surely clarify the relationship between the LFS phenotype and the variable genotype.

CLINICAL ASPECTS OF THE LI-FRAUMENI SYNDROME

Historical Perspective

In 1969, Li and Fraumeni reported the results of a retrospective survey of 280 medical records and 418 death certificates of childhood rhabdomyosarcoma patients diagnosed in the United States.[1,2] Five families were identified in whom siblings or cousins had been diagnosed with a childhood sarcoma. A high concentration of cancers of diverse types was observed on the ancestral line of one parent in each family. The most frequent of these cancers were soft-tissue sarcomas, early-onset breast cancers, and other early-onset cancers. In fact, three of the mothers of the index children had developed breast cancer before 30 years of age. Other frequently occurring tumors included acute leukemias; brain tumors; and carcinoma of the lung, pancreas, and skin in first- and second-degree relatives and adrenocortical carcinoma in siblings. By making assumptions about family size, the authors estimated that among this series of childhood probands, considerably less than one pair of affected siblings would have been expected by chance. The occurrence of cancer in both a parent and a child in these families suggested the possibility of vertical transmission of an oncogenic agent through generations of genetically susceptible individuals.[1] Although it was implied, inherited predisposition on an exclusively genetic basis was not directly implicated.

Within the first few years after these initial reports, several other phenotypically similar families were described in which unusual clusterings of cancers were observed.[3–6] In particular, Lynch and colleagues, in describing these pedigrees, coined the term *SBLA syndrome*: the letters represented what the authors considered the principal component tumors: sarcoma (S), breast and brain cancer (B), leukemia, lung, and laryngeal cancer (L), and adrenocortical carcinoma (A).[7] Although this terminology was initially prevalent, the syndrome is now more commonly known as the Li-Fraumeni syndrome.

It was suggested from the original reports that the familial occurrence of neoplasms originating at discordant sites might represent a counterpart of the tendency for a single individual to develop multiple primary tumors.[1,2] In fact, subsequent epidemiologic studies have confirmed that the neoplasms in LFS tend to develop in children and young adults, often as multiple primary cancers in affected individuals.[8] These studies also provided evidence to indicate that genetic predisposition is a primary causative factor. A follow-up study of the original four families found that over a 12-year period, 10 of the 31 surviving family members had developed 16 additional cancers, in comparison with less than 1 expected from general population rates.[9] These 16 malignancies were of the same types that had originally been observed and included five breast cancers, four soft-tissue sarcomas, and two central nervous system tumors. Even after exclusion of the sarcomas that had arisen in the radiation fields of previous tumors, the remaining number of cancers still represented a significant excess above the expected (12 observed, 0.5 expected). Furthermore, 12 of these 16 cancers (pri-

marily sarcomas and breast carcinomas) occurred in family members who had survived their original cancers. The high frequency of second cancers with the same histopathologic diagnosis as types originally described in these families supported the argument in favor of genetic predisposition.

Defining the Classic Li-Fraumeni Syndrome

Ascertainment biases have complicated the interpretation of the original description and subsequent reports of LFS kindreds. These biases develop from the preferential attention given to the most dramatically affected kindreds, the possibility of chance occurrence of cancer in rare families (phenocopies), the uncertainty of the prevalence of the syndrome in the general population, and uncertainties in defining the spectrum of cancers in the syndrome and ultimately in characterizing the penetrance of the predisposing gene or genes.[10] The first attempt to formulate a "definition" of the syndrome was presented by Li and colleagues in 1988, based on a prospective analysis of the characteristic component tumors and other detailed information on 24 kindreds.[11] To be eligible for this study, each kindred was required to conform to the following criteria: (1) a bone or soft-tissue sarcoma diagnosed under 45 years of age in an individual who was then designated the proband, (2) one first-degree relative of the proband with cancer diagnosed before 45 years of age, and (3) one first- or second-degree relative of the proband in the same lineage with cancer before age 45 years or sarcoma diagnosed at any age.

These criteria have until recently found wide acceptance as a clinical definition of the syndrome, and families that adhere to these criteria have been referred to as having "classic" LFS. Such a family is illustrated in Fig. 20-1. This extensive study revealed continued expression of the dominantly inherited syndrome among young family members. Within the 24 families, 151 blood relatives had developed cancer, and of these cancers, 119 (79 percent) were diagnosed before the age of 45, compared with 10 percent of all cancers in this age range in the general population. Of note, excess occurrences were predominantly confined over time to the six previously described cancer types: breast carcinomas,

Li-Fraumeni Syndrome "Classic" Pedigree

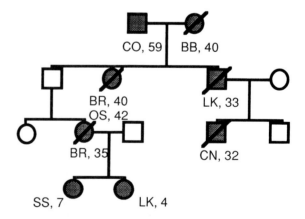

FIG. 20-1 Classic Li-Fraumeni syndrome pedigree. Notable features include the presence of a sarcoma before age 45 years and at least two first-degree relatives with cancer before age 45. In addition, multiple primary tumors occur in an affected member. Note should also be made of the presence of tumors less typical of the component neoplasms of LFS. The pattern of inheritance best fits an autosomal dominant model. BB = bilateral breast cancer; BR = breast cancer; CN = brain tumor; CO = colon cancer; LK = leukemia; SS = soft-tissue sarcoma; OS = osteosarcoma.

soft-tissue sarcomas, osteosarcomas, leukemias, brain tumors, and adrenocortical carcinomas. Adenocortical carcinomas were confined to children under 14 years of age. Multiple primary tumors occurred in 15 family members, with the second and subsequent cancers also representing the principal tumor types. The analysis failed to implicate any additional tumors as components of the syndrome. However, subsequent analysis of many families at several major centers as well as in relatively isolated settings has identified cases that resemble the "classic" syndrome yet, in lacking one particular criterion or being associated with other, less frequently observed cancers, fail to meet the most stringent interpretation of the definition.[12–16] Several tumors are now considered to be associated with LFS, including germ-cell tumors,[17] melanoma,[17,18] and prostate and pancreatic cancer.[19] Families with these component tumors have been referred to as extended LFS.[20] A reevaluation of the component tumors of classic LFS is currently being performed through the efforts of the Third Workshop on Collaborative, Interdisciplinary Studies of p53 and Li-Fraumeni Syndrome.

Defining Li-Fraumeni Syndrome-Like Families

Several families have been identified which demonstrate the clustering of tumors seen in typical extended LFS families but do not conform to the classic definition. These families have been defined in more than one way, reflecting the confusion arising from the lack of a definitive causative association in all cases. Eeles and colleagues have defined Li-Fraumeni-syndrome-like (LFS-L) as the clustering of two different tumors seen in extended LFS in individuals who are first- or second-degree relatives with respect to each other and are affected at any age.[20] Birch et al. have suggested that an age restriction of under 60 years be imposed[16] because estimates of age-specific cancer risk in classic LFS are elevated up to but not beyond this point.[10] Further molecular epidemiologic studies are required to clarify the distinction between LFS and LFS-L and to determine the importance of perceived or actual differences.

GENETIC ASPECTS OF LI-FRAUMENI SYNDROME

Classic Genetic Analysis

Williams and Strong[21] and Lustbader and colleagues[13] performed segregation analyses in hospital-based series of survivors of childhood soft-tissue sarcoma patients. Among the first-degree relatives of children in the series, 34 cancers occured (21 expected), with the excess being predominantly breast cancers and sarcomas diagnosed at a young age. The relatives at the most elevated risk were those of children with soft-tissue sarcomas diagnosed at young ages, with sarcomas of embryonal histologic subtype, and with multiple primary sarcomas.[12,19,21] It became evident that the cancer distribution in the families was most compatible with a rare autosomal dominant gene, the gene frequency being equal to 0.00002, or 1 in 50,000. The penetrance was estimated to be almost 50 percent by 30 years and 90 percent by 60 years of age.[21] This point becomes significant for any potential revisions to the original classic definition in that the age limot for tumor occurrence has been increased from 45, as established in 1988, to the current 60 years, as recommended by participants in the Third Workshop on Collaborative, Interdisciplinary Studies of p53 and Li-Fraumeni Syndrome in 1996 (in preparation). The relative risk of developing cancer in children who carried the gene or genes

was estimated to be 100 times the background rate. Although the age-specific penetrance was somewhat higher in females, this phenomenon was thought to be due to the occurrence of breast cancer. Maternal and paternal lineages appear to contribute equally to the evidence favoring a dominant gene.[13] These calculations have generally held up to the test of time, even as the genetic etiology of the syndrome has become apparent. Nevertheless, in spite of the careful phenotypic and statistical study of the syndrome, it became clear that the identification of a defective gene or genes conferring a predisposition in carriers within these families would assist in clarifying the definition of the syndrome.

Searching for an Etiologic "Agent"

Early attempts to isolate the LFS-gene or genes were hampered by a variety of factors. The rarity, ambiguity of definition, and infrequent recognition of the syndrome, along with the high mortality among affected family members, significantly reduced the number of available informative tissue and blood samples. Cancers occurring in relatives who were not gene carriers were not histopathologically distinct from cancers in gene carriers. Consistent constitutional karyotypic alterations do not occur in these families, precluding a specific chromosomal site on which to focus a search for the responsible gene. Precancerous conditions such as benign adenomas and associated phenotypic malformations are not characteristic of LFS families and therefore cannot be used to map genes in the same fashion that the presence of aniridia (absence of the iris) was useful in the localization of the Wilms' tumor gene (*WT1*) to chromosome 11p13.[22–24]

Early cytogenetic, immunologic, serologic, and other attempts to determine the biologic basis of LFS were largely uninformative.[25] A report of two families suggested an association of HLA tissue type B12 with the disorder,[6] yet no follow-up of this observation is available. Studies of fibroblast cell lines from affected members of one family showed reduced cell killing by graded doses of ionizing radiation, and apparent activation of the c-*raf*-1 oncogene was reported in one of these lines.[26] However, fibroblasts from other families have demonstrated a normal cytotoxic response.[27] More recently, normal skin fibroblasts derived from affected LFS patients have been shown to exhibit features consistent with immortalization in the absence of stimulation by exogenous oncogenic or viral factors.[28] These features of altered morphology, aneuploidy, anchorage-independent growth, and an extended life span in culture appeared to occur spontaneously.[29] Furthermore, these spontaneously immortalized cells have also been shown to form tumors in nude mice when transformed by an activated Ha-*ras* oncogene,[30] perhaps suggesting that alterations in other genes, including the tumor-suppressor genes, enhance susceptibility to *ras*-induced transformation.

MOLECULAR BIOLOGY OF p53

The p53 Tumor-Suppressor Gene

Comparisons between the frequencies of familial tumors, in particular retinoblastoma and Wilms' tumor,[31–33] and their sporadic counterparts led Knudson et al. to suggest that the familial forms of some cancers could be explained by the inheritance of constitutional mutations in growth-limiting genes. The resulting inactivation of these genes could facilitate cellular transformation.[34] Inactivations of these growth-limiting, or tumor-suppressor, genes result from mutations in both alleles or a mutation in one allele followed by a loss of or reduction to homozygosity in the second as well as functional or structural alterations of the transcribed message or protein product. Mutant tumor suppressor genes may be found in either germ cells or somatic cells. In germ cells they arise spontaneously in the gamete or are transmitted from generation to generation within a family.

Alterations of the p53 tumor-suppressor gene and its encoded protein are the most frequently encountered genetic events in human malignancy.[35-38] The human gene, located on the short arm of human chromosome 17 band 13,[39] is approximately 20 kilobases (kb) in length, yields a 2.8-kb mRNA transcript, and encodes a 53-kD nuclear phosphoprotein[40] composed of 393 amino acids. The gene contains 11 exons, only the first of which is noncoding. Analysis of the nucleotide and amino acid sequences demonstrates five evolutionarily conserved domains from Xenopus to human.[41] Attempts to identify p53-like genes in invertebrates such as sea urchins, yeast, worms, and Drosophila have been unsuccessful. The conserved regions are regarded as being essential for the normal function of the wild-type protein. The first conserved domain is contained within the noncoding exon 1; the other four are encompassed by codons 129–146, 171–179, 234–260, and 270–287 in exons 4, 5, 7, and 8, respectively (Fig. 20-2).[41] Several properties of the p53 protein are indicated by the presence of two DNA-binding domains,[42] two SV40 large tumor-antigen (T-Ag) binding sites,[43,44] a nuclear localization signal,[45] an oligomerization domain,[46,47] and several phosphorylation sites.[48]

The p53 protein was initially identified in SV40-transformed cells, where it was thought to be a transformation-specific protein, or tumor antigen, because of its apparent interaction with the large T antigen of the SV40 virus.[40,49] This virus, which is found in monkeys, is a member of the polyomavirus family. These viruses encode viral T-antigen proteins, which are synthesized immediately after infection. The proteins are responsible for the loss of cell growth control that is induced by the virus both in vitro and in vivo. Transfection assays in rat fibroblast NIH 3T3 cells initially suggested that p53 was an oncogene as it was capable of immortalizing these cells by itself or of transforming them in conjunction with the *ras* oncogene.[50-52] It was subsequently demonstrated that only mutant forms of p53 conferred these biologic properties, while the wild-type protein actually suppressed transformation.[53] Analysis of two colorectal tumors demonstrated allelic deletions of chromosome 17p and expressed high levels of p53 mRNA from the remaining allele. The second allele was shown to harbor a point mutation that changed a valine to alanine at residue 143 in

one tumor and changed arginine to histidine at codon 175 in the other.[53a] These observations provided a practical illustration of the Knudson two-hit hypothesis and were subsequently extended by the demonstration of a variety of amino acid substitutions in several different tumor types.[53b] These exciting reports, coupled with the fact that the introduction of wild-type p53 protein blocks the growth of many transformed cells,[54,55] suggest that the normal funtion of p53 is in fact that of a growth suppressor.[56]

The p53 protein consists of five primary structural regions (Fig. 20-2). First, an acidic N terminus acts as a transcriptional activating domain if placed in apposition to DNA through the DNA-binding domain. Second, the internal highly conserved hydrophobic proline-rich region appears to be important in maintaining the overall structural integrity of the protein. Third, the DNA-binding region between amio acid residues 120 and 290 recognizes a DNA sequence motif containing two contiguous or closely spaced monomers $5'$-(purine)3C(A/T)(A/T)G-(pyrimidine)3-$3'$.[56a,57] Fourth, the highly charged basic region at the C terminus is required for the formation of homologous p53 tetrameric complexes.[58] Fifth, a nuclear transport sequence spanning codons 316 to 325 aids the protein's localization into the nucleus.[59] p53 is multiply phosphorylated by at least four protein kinases, with two sites being at the N terminus, which is phosphorylated by a casein kinase I-like enzyme[60] and DNA-dependent protein kinase.[61] The other phosphorylation sites are at the C terminus, at position 315, phosphorylated by p34[cdc2] kinase, and CKII at condon 392, phosphorylated by casein kinase II.[62] The latter enzyme phosphorylates many substrates, including both transcription factors and DNA-binding proteins. The casein kinase II site also acts as a binding site for a ribosomal RNA moiety. These structural features all support the cell cycle control role of p53 activity (see below).

The p53 protein binds specific DNA sequences and appears to be a transcription factor that may regulate the expression of other growth regulatory genes in a positive or negative manner.[63,64] The introduction of wild-type p53 protein into a variety of tranformed cell types inhibits their growth, most likely by blocking progression of cells through the cell cycle late in the G1 phase of cell replication at a checkpoint control site before G1/S.[65-68] Recent evidence also suggests that the antiproliferative effect of p53 may involve cell cycle regulation at the G2/M restriction point.[69-72] Cells lacking wild-type p53 display an attenuated G2 checkpoint response. The addition of methylxanthines such as caffeine, which are known to disrupt cell cycle arrest at the G2 checkpoint, leads to increased sensitivity of cultured cells to both radio- and chemotherapy.[73,74] Because cells lacking functional p53 have already lost the ability to arrest in G1, the loss of the G2 checkpoint seems to have an additive effect. This observation implies that p53-negative tumor cells may be more responsive to a combination of DNA-damaging agents and agents that abrogate the G2 checkpoint. As a component of a spindle checkpoint, p53 may ensure the maintenance of diploidy during cell cycle progression.[75] p53 may actively participate in maintaining genomic stability through regulation of centrosome duplication or as a monitor that limits centrosome overproduction.[76] Although p53 may not play a major role in the S-phase recombinational events leading to sister chromatid formation,[77] suggesting that conversion of radiation damage to chromatin lesions is independent of p53, the time to peak levels of chromosomal damage is shorter in p53-deficient cells. This observation is consistent with kinetic differences based on specific p53 genotypes. These kinetic differences also have been observed in p53-deficient LFS-derived lymphocytes.[78]

Other functions of p53 are suggested by experiments demonstrating that reentry of resting cells into the cell cycle can be blocked by the introduction of anti-p53 antibodies or antisense p53 cDNA fragments.[79,80] p53 may potentiate cell differentiation in this manner. Early work suggested that wild-type p53 could be

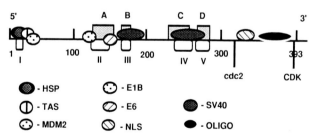

FIG. 20-2 Structural features of the p53 gene and its encoded protein. The gene encodes a 53-kDa nuclear phosphoprotein. The 393 amino acids are spread over 11 exons. The transcription activation site (TAS), heat shock protein binding site (HSP), SV40 large T antigen binding sites (SV40), nuclear localization signal (NLS), oligomerization domain (OLIGO), and phosphorylation sites (P) all identify potential functional regions. The five evolutionarily conserved domains (HCD I–V) correspond closely to the regions most frequently mutated in sporadic cancer [hotspot regions (HSR A–D)]. Sites of binding of the extracellular E1B 55-kDa protein of adenovirus type 5 (E1B) and the E6 gene product of human papillomavirus type 16 and 18 (E6) are also indicated, as is the position of the MDM2 gene product binding site (MDM2).

involved in restricting precursor cell populations by mediating apoptosis, or programmed cell death, in the absence of appropriate differentiation or proliferation signals.[81,82] In p53-deficient thymocytes, substantial resistance to apoptotic induction by radiation was observed compared with wild-type littermates.[83,84] These observations were corroborated in solid tumors in nude mice subjected to radiation or chemotherapy.[85] Strikingly, acquired resistance could be induced by repeated low doses of radiation, with acquired p53 mutations being observed in 50 percent of tumors. The relative degree of radioresistance and apoptosis seems to be cell type-specific, for in colorectal carcinoma cells lines and head and neck squamous-cell cancer cell lines lacking functional p53,[86,87] significant differences in response compared to wild-type counterparts could not be demonstrated.

As was suggested above, cells that either lack p53 gene expression or overexpress mutant p53 do not exhibit G1 arrest. The fidelity of DNA repair during cell cycle arrest may play a role in the capacity of cells to tolerate radiation injury and therefore have an impact on radiation sensitivity. It has been reported in this context that p53 may play a role in the cellular response to γ-radiation damage, ultraviolet light, or certain chemotherapeutic drugs through inhibition of DNA synthesis[84,85,88–93] after DNA damage and thereby provide a cell cycle "checkpoint."[94,95] This response is particularly effective in the setting of double-strand DNA breaks. The in vitro effect has been observed in vivo in SCID mice carrying xenografts treated with either adriamycin or γ-irradiation.[96]

Transcriptional targets of p53 include *mdm-2*, a gene which is commonly amplified in human sarcomas and is involved in a negative regulatory system that terminates a cell's response to DNA damage.[97,98] Other targets include a cyclin of unknown function called cyclin G1[99]; Bax, a promoter of apoptosis[100]; GADD45, a DNA repair protein[101]; and p21[CIP1/WAF1], a multifunctional regulatory and the best candidate to date for the control of cell cycle arrest.[102–104] The abundant increases in p53 protein expression induced by ionizing radiation lead to the transcription of p21[CIP1/WAF1]. This inhibits cyclin-dependent kinase activity, which is in turn required for entry into S phase and DNA replication. Furthermore, p21[CIP1/WAF1] also binds and inhibits a subunit of DNA polymerase called PCNA (poliferating cell nuclear antigen) directly,[105] thereby blocking DNA replication.

GADD45 is also induced by stresses that arrest cell growth or agents that induce DNA damage. Like p21[CIP1/WAF1], GADD45 has been shown to bind PCNA to induce excision repair of damaged DNA by a poorly understood mechanism.[106] p53 also binds ERCCC3, an excision repair molecule that recognizes and removes damaged DNA segments.[107] Taken together, these observations suggest that p53 may inhibit DNA replication through p21 while simulating DNA repair through GADD45 or ERCC3 simultaneously.

Structural analysis of the p53 core-DNA cocrystal using x-ray diffraction,[108] as well as the oligomerization domain using multidimensional NMR spectroscopy,[109,109a] suggests that several highly conserved amino acid residues within the central core form actual contacts at the minor or major grooves of the DNA helix. Furthermore, each monomeric unit of p53 interacts with another subunit; the resulting dimer in turn interacts with another dimer, forming a four-helix bundle or p53 tetramer. It is believed that this cooperative binding greatly facilitates interactions with p53 response elements.[110]

Inactivation of p53 function occurs via several mechanisms. The occurrence of missense mutations, deletions, or nonsense mutations of the gene prevents the protein from oligomerizing and forming tetrameric complexes that can bind specific DNA sequences.[111] In fact, representative mutants from each of the four mutation hotspot regions (Fig. 20-2) have been tested for binding to p53-binding sites in vitro and for activation of p53-binding site

reporter gene expression in vivo and in vitro. All mutants lose the ability to bind p53-binding sites and therefore cannot activate expression of adjacent reporter genes.[56,112–114] Some mutations alter the conformation of the p53 protein, exposing epitopes that may alter certain functional properties. Because these properties are found in only a fraction of p53 mutants, they are unlikely to be central to p53 function. Nevertheless, the possibility remains that subtle genetic changes induce conformational alterations that affect the structure of functionally important domains distant from the mutation sites.[111] Conformational changes of a mutant molecule also can affect wild-type molecules complexed with the mutant form within tetramers, preventing the complex from binding to DNA and transcriptionally activating reporter genes.[112,114,115] In fact, the vast majority of p53 mutations are missense in nature,[116] accounting for upward of 85 percent of reported gene alterations. This observation is in stark contrast to many other genes in which variably sized deletions, alterations, or splice site defects are reported.

Inactivation of the p53 protein through binding of other cellular proteins also may prevent normal binding and thus prevent transcriptional activation.[117,118] Some of the DNA tumor virus genes, including SV40 T antigen, the E1B gene of adenovirus, and the E6 gene of human papillomavirus, encode proteins that bind to p53. In cells that coexpress one of these viral oncoproteins along with p53, expression of p53-inducible reporter genes cannot be activated.[118] This inhibition of expression may be critical for viral replication and/or cell transformation. Disruption of normal p53 function may also be altered by alteration of *mdm-2*, a cellular gene that was originally identified by virtue of its amplification in a spontaneously transformed mouse cell line.[97,98,117,119] The Mdm-2 gene product binds to p53, resulting in inhibition of the ability of p53 to transactivate genes adjacent to p53-binding sites. At least in human sarcomas, the amplification of *Mdm-2* may lead to consequent overexpression of Mdm-2, which probably interferes with p53 activity.[97,120] Finally, p53 interactions with other tumor-suppressor genes have been observed. Interaction with the Wilms' tumor gene (*WT1*) in transfected cells modulates the ability of each protein to transactivate its targets.[121] Coincident mutations in p53 and the retinoblastoma susceptibility gene (*RB1*) cooperate in transformation of certain cell types in mice.[122,123]

Therefore, although the precise functions of p53 are not clear, models have been proposed to account for the many observations summarized above.[94,124] In a cell with normal p53, levels of the protein rise in response to DNA damage mediated by pRB1,[125] and the cell arrests before the G1/S transition. At this point, genomic repair or apoptosis ensues, with the mechanism being determined by the transforming oncoprotein or oncoproteins. In cells in which the p53 pathway has been inactivated by gene mutations or by host or viral oncoprotein interactions, G1 arrest does not occur and damaged DNA is replicated. During mitosis, the presence of damaged DNA results in mutation, aneuploidy, mitotic failure, and cell death. p53 alterations are necessary but not sufficient for the ultimate cancer that arises from these malignant clones, as other genetic events are clearly required.

Patient Mutations: Li-Fraumeni Syndrome

Inactivating mutations of the p53 gene and disruptions of the p53 protein have been associated with some fraction of virtually every sporadically occurring malignancy. Included among these are osteosarcomas,[126] soft-tissue sarcomas,[127] rhabdomyosarcomas,[128] leukemias,[129,130] brain tumors,[131] and carcinomas of the lung[132] and breast.[133] Together, these tumors account for more than two-thirds of the cancers in selected series of LFS families[2,11,134] (Fig. 20-3).

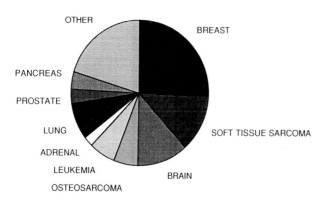

FIG. 20-3 Relative incidence of tumor types by age in 24 Li-Fraumeni syndrome families. The frequencies are confounded by the means of ascertainment, in this case through the proband, who has a sarcoma and who was therefore excluded from the tabulations. (*Adapted from Garber et al.*[10])

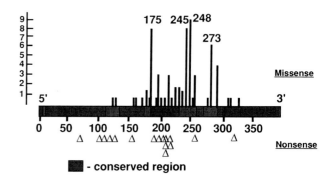

Location of Human Germline *p53* Mutations

■ - conserved region

FIG. 20-4 Sites and frequency of reported human germ-line p53 mutations. The horizontal axis represents the codon number; the vertical axis indicates the number of reported mutations. Missense mutations are designated above the p53 cartoon, while nonsense mutations are seen below the cartoon. It is noteworthy that the four most frequently cited amino acid residues are at codons 175, 245, 248, and 282—not dissimilar to acquired mutations.

Transgenic mice that overexpress mutant alleles of the p53 gene in the presence of two wild-type alleles produce offspring with a high incidence of osteosarcoma, lung adenocarcinoma, lymphoma, and rhabdomyosarcoma.[135]

Based on these observations, five LFS families were studied to determine whether p53 played any role in the occurrence of cancer in affected family members. Base-pair mutations were identified in the germ line of affected members in each of the five families studied.[136] These missense mutations were all found within one highly conserved region of the gene, affecting codons 245, 248 (two families), 252, and 258 of the p53 gene. In fact, subsequent analysis of one of the families revealed the codon 252 change to be artifactual; a 2-bp deletion was identified at codon 184 in exon 5.[137] This observation raises concerns with respect to the application of research technology in gene analysis to the clinical setting, as will be discussed below. Tumors in affected individuals that were tested had lost the remaining wild-type allele.[136] Furthermore, analysis of one of these families, using a highly polymorphic DNA sequence telomeric of p53, confirmed the cosegregation of the abnormal p53 allele with the polymorphism. Unaffected members could be identified as gene carriers, suggesting that they might be at risk of developing cancer at a later date. After this initial report, a sixth classic LFS family was reported with another constitutional mutation in the same region as the previously identified ones.[137] In this family, however, one affected member was not a carrier of the mutant gene, suggesting that the mechanism of tumor formation in this individual did not involve p53. The apparent clustering of germ-line p53 mutations in a short span of 14 codons within a highly conserved domain initially sparked much speculation about its possible significance, with suggestions that germ-line mutations may be restricted and that other mutations may be lethal in this context.[138] However, extensive analysis of other classic LFS families and subsequently several clinical scenarios of LFS-L phenotypes demonstrated the wide spectrum of germ-line p53 mutations that were not dissimilar to those observed in soradic tumors (Fig. 20-4).

Several families that fit the operative definition of LFS have been studied. Isolated families with germ-line p53 mutations have been reported.[139,140] However, one study of eight families from the Manchester registry in England suggested that mutations of the p53 gene would not be found in all classic LFS families.[141] Only two of these families were initially shown to carry germ-line mutations when only exon 7 was examined. Further analysis of other exons has still demonstrated the apparent absence of mutations within exons 5 to 8 in some of these families.[142] Ongoing studies suggest that not all classic LFS families have detectable germ-line mutations of the p53 gene. In one quite typical Li-Fraumeni kin-

dred, although no p53 gene mutations were identified, overexpression of wild-type 53 was observed, suggesting that the biologically or biochemically altered protein yielded a similar phenotype to the mutant gene, perhaps by one of the several mechanisms described above.[143] Evidence from several studies conducted in the United States, France, and the United Kingdom[16,144,145] suggests that the actual frequency of germ-line p53 mutations in classic LFS families is somewhere between 50 and 70 percent. In the French series, germ-line p53 mutations were particularly associated with families in which a young child was affected with rhabdomyosarcoma, while in the U.K. series the mutations appeared to be associated with families that included children with rhabdomyosarcoma and/or adrenocortical carcinoma. It is likely that as the clinical definition is expanded, the rate of germ-line p53 mutations observed will increase.

The lack of 100 percent concordance between p53 mutations and the classic phenotype may be explained in several ways. It is possible that posttranslational p53 alterations, as described previously,[143,146] occur more frequently than has been found to date. Recently, mutations outside the most commonly cited hotspot regions have been identified, particularly in the oligomerization domain.[146a] Presumably, more of these types of mutations will be discovered as these regions of the gene are more extensively analyzed. Evidence for endogenous promoter defects leading to aberrant expression of the p53 message has been sought with inconclusive success. Complete p53 deletion, the effects of modifier genes, or alterations of other genes that may influence the phenotype generated by the presence of a specific germ-line p53 alteration have also been postulated. In spite of these gaps, the high frequency of germ-line p53 mutations in LFS families and the tight association of tumor formation in p53-deficient mice (see below) confirm a causal association of germ-line p53 alterations and cancer predisposition.

Patient Mutations: Non-Li-Fraumeni Syndrome

As DNA screening techniques improved, it became possible to analyze large populations of patients for constitutional abnormalities of the p53 gene. Several recent studies have demonstrated that certain groups of "high-risk" patients and their families carry germ-line p53 mutations that presumably predispose them to the development of their respective malignancies. Germ-line p53 mutations may be inherited from a parent who is healthy at the time when cancer is diagnosed in the child. Numerous studies of non-LFS patients and families have helped characterize the genetic heterogeneity of the p53 carrier state.

A striking feature of LFS kindreds is the high frequency, approaching 50 percent, of affected members who develop multiple primary neoplasms.[9] One multicenter study demonstrated germ-line mutations of the p53 tumor-suppressor gene in leukocyte DNA from 4 of 59 patients (6.8 percent) who had survived second cancers but did not have family histories compatible with LFS.[147] Although one mutation at codon 248 in exon 7 was identical to that previously implicated in LFS,[136] three other mutations at codons 273, 282, and 325 had not been previously reported in the germ line. In addition to implicating codons outside the classically defined conserved regions of the p53 gene, this study demonstrated the occurrence of germ-line p53 mutations in patients with cancers not commonly represented among LFS component tumors. These included non-Hodgkin's lymphoma, colon and gastric carcinoma, and neuroblastoma. A subsequent analysis of four patients with multifocal osteosarcoma and no family history of cancer demonstrated one apparently *de novo* germ-line p53 mutation.[148] A similar analysis of patients with multifocal glioma demonstrated a very high frequency of germ-line p53 mutations, although several of these individuals had family histories consistent with LFS or LFS-L.[148a] This observation suggests that other cancer patients who present with multiple nonfamilial tumors carry germ-line p53 mutations.

An extensive analysis of 196 patients with malignant sarcomas was reported along with the second tumor study cited above.[149] Exons 2 through 11 were screened, thereby encompassing the complete coding region of the gene as well as less frequently evaluated regions. Eight of these 196 (4 percent) harbored germ-line p53 muations, and five of the eight mutations were identified in patients from families with a high incidence of cancer. Both missense and nonsense germ-line mutations were found. The nonsense mutations arose as a result of a single-base frameshift mutation involving an insertion in two cases, a two-base deletion in one case, and the direct creation of a stop codon in one case. All occurred in codons outside the conserved domains (codons 71–72, 151–152, and 209–210), and all presumably yield a truncated p53 protein. Novel mutations, as well as the passage of a mutant allele for generations in at least one family, were also observed. In these cases, as in the previously described study, the affected individual presented a history that was not entirely consistent with LFS. This study also confirmed the observation of neutral polymorphisms within the p53 sequence that must be carefully evaluated to rule out their disease-associated potential. One of these, at codon 213 in exon 6 (a nonconserved region), has been frequently identified in sporadic tumors.[116,127] Finally, this study pointed out the vagaries of the clinical definition of LFS in that one family with definitive germ-line inheritance of p53 mutations had an excess of gastric carcinoma, a tumor that is thought to be rare in the operative definition of the syndrome. However, this family is from Japan, a country with a significantly higher incidence of gastric carcinoma than exists in North American or European populations. Other factors, both genetic and environmental, may influence the types of tumors that arise in patients who are carriers of the same p53 germ-line mutations.

Although sarcomas and multiple primary cancers in affected patients constitute the most consistent characteristic features of the LFS phenotype, certain other cancers are also commonly represented. Among these, early-onset breast cancer is most frequently encountered. However, little is known about the frequency of germ-line p53 mutations in breast cancer patients outside families with classic LFS. Using a hydroxylamine mismatch base-pair technique, five families with early-onset breast cancer were screened for constitutional mutations in all 11 exons

of the p53 gene.[150] No mutations were identified in these families, suggesting that p53 probably did not play a significant role in the genesis of hereditary early-onset breast cancer. These observations are also supported by another study that screened 25 breast cancer families in which no germ-line mutations of the gene were found in exons 5 through 9.[151] Nevertheless, in a third study, 1 of 67 unselected breast cancer patients and 1 of 40 early-onset breast cancer patients were found to be carriers of mutant p53.[152] The mutation found in the unselected patient was at codon 181 (exon 5). The patient's pedigree showed a strong family history of cancer, although it did not quite fit the classic definition of LFS, as the relative with sarcoma was 47 years old (i.e., older than 45) at the time of diagnosis. In addition, studies of other family members as well as functional studies of the mutant gene suggest that this codon 181 mutation may be functionally silent and may not impart any increased cancer risk.[153] By contrast, the mutation found in the early-onset breast cancer patient was at codon 245, a highly conserved amino acid. The identical mutation was identified in the patient's mother, who also had breast cancer. These findings suggest that germ-line p53 mutations occur rarely in early-onset breast cancer outside of LFS families and are corroborated by similar results reported elsewhere.[154] It is clear that other genetic e responsible for the genesis of this familial cancer clustering. In fact, two genes for early-onset hereditary breast cancer have been isolated, *BRCA1* and *BRCA2*, and intense efforts are in progress to fully characterize the mutational spectrum, genotype-phenotype correlation, and clinical implications of these genes.

Initial surveys of patients ascertained solely by the presence of a neoplasm that is a component tumor of LFS have yielded interesting observations. Adrenocortical carcinoma (ADCC) occurs rarely in the pediatric cancer population.[155] However, in LFS kindreds it is not uncommon to encounter at least one affected individual with this tumor.[11,16] Analysis of five patients with ADCC demonstrated inherited germ-line p53 mutations in three.[156] Each of the families had cancer constellations that were consistent with LFS. In a survey of children with apparently sporadic adrenocortical carcinoma, 3 of 6 (50 percent) harbored germ-line p53 mutations, and in one the alteration was demonstrated to be inherited from the child's mother, who subsequently developed breast cancer.[157]

Two studies of childhood sarcoma patients confirmed the presence of germ-line p53 mutations in a small fraction of those who lacked striking family histories of cancer. Among 235 children with osteosarcoma, 7 (3 percent) were found to carry mutations, and 3 of these 7 lacked a family history of cancer.[158] A similar survey of 33 childhood rhabdomyosarcoma patients identified 3 (9 percent) with germ-line p53 mutations.[159] Although no association between the presence of mutations and histopathologic subtype or tumor grade was noted, it was of interest that the average age at onset of the tumors in children carrying germ-line p53 mutations was lower than that of children with wild-type p53 ($p = 0.06$), suggesting that the biologic nature of the tumors may be different.

A screen of primary lymphoblasts from 25 pediatric patients with acute lymphoblastic leukemia identified p53 mutations in 4, one of whom was shown to harbor the mutation (in exon 8) in the remission marrow, suggesting its germ-line origin.[160] The proband's family history was consistent with LFS. An analysis of primary lymphoblasts in affected members of 10 familial leukemia pedigrees identified two families in which nonhereditary p53 alterations were present.[161] These included a 2-bp deletion in exon 6 in one and a codon 248 missense mutation in the other. Therefore, although leukemia represents a common component tumor of LFS, it appears that germ-line mutations of p53 in primary leukemia patients are rare events. However, it is possible that when such alterations do exist in the germ line, they are potentially associated with an increased risk of secondary acute myelogenous leukemia related to prior treatment of the primary cancer with topoisomerase inhibitors.[162]

Most published germ-line p53 mutations occur in the conserved regions of the gene and are missense in nature. There are no obvious differences in the mutation types or sites between LFS and LFS-L families. Approximately 75 percent are transitions, and the majority of these occur at CpG dinucleotides (Table 20-1). Transversions and occasional base-pair deletions or insertions have also been described. Three examples of intronic mutations have been reported. A novel germ-line p53 splice-acceptor site mutation was found in a family that closely resembles the breast-ovarian cancer syndrome and in which the proband had a choroid plexus carcinoma.[163] This mutation, involving a single-base substitution in intron 5, results in deletion of exon 6 and creation of a frameshift leading to a premature stop codon in exon 7 that is thought to yield significant disruptions of the message. Another report identified a point mutation in the splice donor site of intron 4, leading to an aberrant larger transcript that could be detected in both tumor and constitutional DNA.[164] The third example is somewhat more unusual in that the mutation, detected in intron 5, consisted of a deletion of an 11-bp sequence that involved a region of splicing recognition. Like the first example, this deletion resulted in deletion of exon 6 and a premature stop codon in exon 7.[165] All three pedigrees resembled LSF but were more consistent with the LFS-L phenotype.

Whether specific germ-line p53 mutations are more penetrant and are associated with different cancer phenotypes has not been resolved. Studies of possible correlations between mutation type and cancer phenotype are limited by the relative lack of fully characterized families. Furthermore, the influence of external factors on the development of malignancy in carriers is also unknown. One would expect that exposure to occupational or environmental carcinogens will contribute to the precise determination of cancer type and age at onset. At least superficially, however, it does not appear that the pattern of germ-line alterations of p53 differs significantly from that of somatic mutations. Perhaps as more genotype-phenotype studies are performed, a distinctive pattern will emerge.

The studies described above clearly demonstrate that patients with germ-line p53 mutations cannot be identified soley by a review of the family's history of cancer. The method by which the proband was ascertained will influence the frequency of carriers in the study population (Table 20-2). It has been shown that germ-line p53 mutations may be inherited from a parent who has no clinical evidence of cancer at the time the disease is diagnosed in the child. A tumor may arise in a child before one does in the parent as a result of the presumed stochastic acquisition of one or more additional genetic abnormalities in the cell that give rise to the malignant clone. Multicenter studies are in progress to determine the frequency of germ-line p53 mutations in patients afflicted with other component tumors of LFS. These, as well as studies of non-LFS cancer-prone families, will help characterize the genetic heterogeniety of the p53 carrier status.

Table 20-1 Types of p53 Mutations Found in the Germ Line

Mutation	Li-Fraumeni Syndrome, %	Li-Fraumeni-Like Syndrome, %
Missense	70	84
Transition	81	67
Transversion	19	33
CpG site	69	4
Nonsense	4	4
Insertion/deletion	26	12

Table 20-2 Estimated Frequency of Germ-Line p53 Mutations in Specific Cancer Patients and Families

Clinical Phenotype	Mutation Frequency, %
LFS and ADCC	75–100
LFS	50–85
LFS variant	10–30
Multisite cancer (non-LFS)	0–20
Sporadic ADCC	40–70
Sporadic rhabdomyosarcoma	5–15
Osteosarcoma	1–10
Second neoplasms	5–15
Early-onset breast cancer	<1

Molecular Genetic Approaches to Li-Fraumeni Syndrome Patients

As both the biologic and biochemical characteristics of p53 have been elucidated, it has also been important to attempt to establish the functional significance of germ-line p53 mutations and the structural features of the corresponding mutant p53 proteins. In addition, before associating a germ-line p53 mutation with the development of cancer, one must carefully determine its functional significance. In one particularly extensive analysis, seven distinct p53 mutations identified from LFS families were studied.[153] Oligonucleotide-directed mutagenesis of the p53 cDNA was performed to generate mutant clones that could then be subcloned into expression vectors for transfection assays. The structural properties of the germ-line p53 mutants showed a high degree of variability. However, with the exception of one mutant, at codon 181, none of the germ-line mutants retained all the structural features of the wild-type protein. Six of seven missense mutations disrupted the growth inhibitory properties and structure of the wild-type p53 protein. One mutation, at codon 181, was not recognized by the antibody PAb 240, which recognizes an epitope specific for a mutant conformation,[166] and did not appear to alter the ability to suppress cell growth when transfected into Saos-2 osteosarcoma cells. Genetic analysis of this mutation demonstrated that it was not always associated with the development of cancer in the family from which it was derived. The mutation was not present in a member of the kindred who had developed two cancers, and the codon 181 mutant gene, not the normal allele, was somatically lost in tumor tissue from a cancer in another relative. It thus became apparent that certain germ-line mutations of p53 might change the amino acid sequence in a conserved domain yet not be associated with an increased cancer risk.[153]

The functional significance of heterozygous germ-line mutations in members of LFS families has also been examined through the expression of the mutant p53 allele in normal skin fibroblasts.[167] It was observed that both normal and mutant p53 RNA are expressed at low levels. In contrast to the transfection studies, the normal skin fibroblasts provide a system in which both wild-type and mutant p53 alleles are naturally expressed at similarly low levels without potentially interfering dosage effects. Based on the studies demonstrating that mutant p53 may inactivate the transcriptional activity of the wild-type protein, it has been postulated that direct analysis of the transcriptional activity of p53 expressed in fibroblasts or lymphocytes should permit the detection of inactivating germ-line mutations.[168] Using a short-term biologic assay in which p53 cDNA was amplified from cells and cloned into a eukaryotic expression vector that was then transfected with a reporter plasmid for the transcriptional activity of p53 into Saos-2 cells lacking p53, analysis of transcriptional activation could be performed. This assay demonstrated transcriptional activity in two of five and three of five clones from two LFS patients, respectively, indicating the presence of both wild-type and mutant p53 in these cells. The rapidity and apparent sensitivity of this assay suggest that it may be valuable as a functional screen. Yet another functional assay has been described that takes advantage of the fact that plasmids can be generated by homologous recombination in vivo in the yeast *S. cerevisiae*.[169] By this method, p53 is tested for its ability to activate transcription from a promoter containing p53 binding sites in these yeast. Cotransformation of a p53 PCR product and a cut promoter-containing plasmid results in repair of the plasmid with the PCR product in vivo and constitutive expression of full-length human p53 protein in the yeast. Clones that have repaired the plasmid are selected on media lacking leucine, and subsequent screening for histidine prototrophy identifies colonies that contain transcriptionally active p53.[169] This assay has the advantage of being rapid (less than 5 days) and having few steps, although it does assume that cancer-causing mutations of p53 are defective in transactivation. Subsequent improvements in the efficiency of this assay have increased the spectrum of mutants, including temperature-sensitive forms that can be functionally evaluated.[170]

The combined value of appropriate multiple functional assays, standard DNA sequence analysis, and careful evaluation of the inheritance pattern of a potential mutation cannot be overestimated in conferring a significant level of confidence to the clinical relevance of a germ-line p53 gene sequence alteration with respect to the patient's disease or the risk to unaffected relatives.

Animal Models

Transgenic animals that carry distinct deregulated oncogenes develop tumors that appear to be cell-type-specific. Because of difficulties in studying the effects of the genetic defects and potential interventions in humans, the development of mouse models that reflect the human genotype provides formidable tools with which to study the role of natural germ-line p53 mutations in carcinogenesis and perhaps to develop treatment regimens. To better study p53 in vivo, several mouse models have been created that either lack functional p53 or express dominant-negative mutant alleles that inhibit wild-type p53 function. These animals have been used to study the interactions of p53 with other cell cycle regulatory elements that function in a p53-dependent or -independent manner. Furthermore, studies of both germ-line and somatic alterations in p53 in mice have greatly enhanced our understanding of the pathobiologic role of this gene in carcinogenesis.

The first attempt to determine the in vivo role of p53 in neoplasia involved generating p53 transgenic mice that carry transgenes encoding for a p53 protein that differs from wild-type p53 either by a [193]Arg→Pro or by a [135]Ala→Val substitution.[135] The transgenes are under the transcriptional control of the endogenous promoter, and the mice carry the normal wild-type p53 complement. Thus, they weakly resemble the human p53 genotype, although neither mutation has been implicated in LFS. The transgene was expressed in a wide range of tissues, yet tumors (primarily osteosarcomas, lymphomas, and adenocarcinomas of the lung) occur in only 20 percent of the mice, suggesting the presence of intrinsic tissue-specific differences. These mice provided a model with which to analyze the interactions of genetic and environmental factors in influencing cancer predisposition. For example, upon infection of the p53 transgenics with the polychemia-inducing strain of Friend leukemia virus (FV-P), the animals progressed to the late stage of erythroleukemia more rapidly than did normal mice.[171] In addition, Friend leukemic cell lines derived from the p53 transgenic mice overproduce mutant p53 protein and demonstrate a high rate of rearrangement of the *ets*-related *Spi*-1 oncogene, as had been previously reported in similar lines derived

from nontransgenic animals. Thus, p53 appears to play a rate-limiting role in the progression of the disease, with its mutant form present as an early even that accelerates neoplastic transformation. This transgenic model in fact contributed to the hypothesis that the tumor spectrum in LFS may arise from the transmission of a mutant p53 gene (Fig. 20-5).

Because p53 is implicated in cell cycle control, it was proposed that this protein may be essential for normal embryonic development.[172] Although p53 is virtually ubiquitously expressed in murine tissues, its relatively short half-life of 20 min (wild-type conformation) yields generally low total protein levels. The amount of p53 mRNA expressed in developing mouse embryos reaches a maximum at 9 to 11 days, after which levels fall markedly.[173] Homologous recombination has been used in mouse embryonic stem (ES) cells to derive null alleles of p53.[172,174,175] Two models have been developed from the replacement with a neo[r] cassette of exons 2 through 6 of the gene.[174,175] The third model includes an insertion of a *pol*II promoter-driven neo[r] cassette into exon 5, together with a deletion of 350 nucleotides of intron 4 and 106 nucleotides of exon 5.[172] None of the p53[−/−] mice express detectable intact or truncated mRNA or protein. The mutant p53 allele has been established in the germ line of chimeric mice with mixed inbred (C57Bl/6 × 129/Sv),[172,175] pure 129/Sv,[176] or 129/O1a[174,176] backgrounds. In all these situations, spontaneous development of different tumor types, principally lymphomas and sarcomas, occurred in more than 75 percent of the animals before 6 months of age. In heterozygotes (p53[+/−]), tumor development, predominantly sarcoma, is delayed. Nevertheless, by 18 months of age, approximately 50 percent have developed neoplasms. Interestingly, multiple primary tumors have been noted in approximately 30 percent of the tumor-bearing p53[−/−] mice. In all mouse backgrounds, virtually none of the p53[+/+] animals had developed tumors by 18 months of age.

The importance of genetic background in influencing specific tumor type is best exemplified by the occurrence of unusual cancers, including pineoblastomas and islet-cell tumors, in p53[−/−] mice crossed with mice heterozygous for an *RB1* mutation in exon 3 of that gene.[122,123] In addition to these unusual tumor phenotypes, these mice had decreased viability and demonstrated other uncharacteristic pathologies, including bronchial epithelial hyperplasia and retinal dysplasia. Interestingly, in this situation the mechanism by which the *RB1* allele was knocked out may be significant in the cancer phenotype that is derived from the intercross. Deletion of exon 20 of *RB1* when crossed with p53[−/−] animals yields animals with a variety of endocrine tumors, including

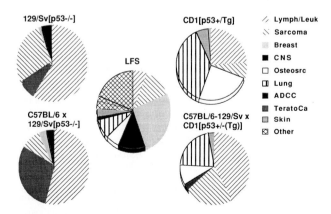

FIG. 20-5 Spectrum of tumors in p53 mouse models compared with the human LFS phenotype. Not all tumors are represented; rather, those most frequently encountered with the category "other" contain isolated reports within specific mouse models. The particular mouse strain and the p53 genotype are indicated above each pie.

pituitary adenomas, medullary carcinoma of the thyroid, and parathyroid carcinomas, in addition to the previously mentioned islet-cell tumors.[123] Surprisingly, no pineoblastomas are found. In both intercross models, the accumulation of abnormal genetic events results in an increased rate of tumorigenesis. Thus, as the number of null alleles of each tumor-suppressor gene is increased, the age at onset decreases and the rate of tumorigenesis increases.

The relative lack of strain-to-strain variability in the p53-null-induced phenotype suggests that the p53 genotype is important in dictating phenotype. Evidence from other genetic crosses supports this premise. For example, adenomatous polyposis coli (APC)-mutant (Min) mice develop bowel adenomas with malignant potential. This malignant phenotype demonstrates great strain-to-strain variability, and in fact the development of malignant tumors is accelerated and modified when they are outbred to different genetic backgrounds, in particular to one carrying a modifier of *Min* termed *Mom*-1.[177] It is likely that similar or other variations of the p53-null-induced phenotype can be induced in a like manner by the interaction of modifier genes that play a role in the development of p53-induced tumors.

The interaction of genetic events in early embryonic development has been facilitated by the use of p53-null animals. As was described earlier, amplification of the *mdm*-2 gene product is thought to represent an alternative mechanism for preventing p53 function in tumor development. Recently, it was shown that Mdm-2-null mice are not viable, being embryonically lethal near the time of implantation.[178] However, when mice heterozygous for *mdm*-2 were crossed with those heterozygous for p53, viable progeny homozygous for both p53 and *mdm*-2 were obtained.[178,179] These observations suggest that a critical in vivo function of Mdm-2 is the negative regulation of p53 activity.

Provocative studies have tested whether the tumorigenic activity of a mutant p53 allele is altered by the presence or absence of wild-type p53 in vivo. Mice carrying the ^{135}Ala→Val mutant transgene were crossed with p53-deficient mice.[180] The mutant p53-Tg accelerated tumor formation in p53$^{+/-}$ but not p53$^{-/-}$ mice, suggesting that this loss-of-function mutation had a dominant negative effect with respect to tumor incidence and cell growth rates. Although the tumor spectrum was similar in transgenic and non-transgenic mice, the transgenice mice showed a predisposition to lung adenocarcinomas. Thus, a given p53 alteration may have distinct tissue specificity with respect to its tumorigenic potential. It will ultimately be of interest to extend this approach to other alleles that behave differently in vivo or in vitro. At least one group[181] is trying to establish mouse models to study tumor-derived p53 mutants in vivo that would establish a more precise model of LFS and clarify the role played by point mutant forms of altered p53 as distinct from the null genotype.

In some strains, p53$^{-/-}$ mice become colonized with pathogens, suggesting that p53 deficiency may be associated with a poorer prognosis after infection with common low-virulence organisms or viruses.[175] In all strains, the p53$^{-/-}$ state is compatible with normal murine development, although the yield of p53$^{-/-}$ offspring from heterozygous crosses varies from 16.6 to 23 percent.[172,175] This apparent increase in fetal loss has been correlated in part by demonstration of fetal exencephaly in a subset of animals,[182] yet it does not mirror the human counterpart in that fetal loss is not characteristic of human LFS families.[183] This may in fact be related to the fact that humans harboring p53 mutations are heterozygous, whereas the mice are homozygously deleted of p53 alleles. Thus, the presence of one wild-type p53 allele in a human may be sufficient to ensure fetal viability.

p53-deficient mice are more sensitive to the effects of certain carcinogenic agents.[184] Mice exposed to dimethylnitrosamine (DMN) developed liver hemangiosarcomas more rapidly than did similarly treated p53$^{+/+}$ animals.[184] p53$^{-/-}$ mice treated with an

initiator, dimethylbenzanthracene (DMBA), and a promoter, 12-O-tetradecanoyl-phorbol-13-acetate (TPA), showed a more rapid rate of malignant progression of skin papillomas to carcinomas compared to their p53$^{+/+}$ counterparts. These studies help distinguish whether p53 mutations play rate-limiting or tissue-specific roles in the tumor progression pathway.

p53-deficient mice have been utilized to evaluate the effects of environmental factors on both tumorigenesis and development. p53-deficient and transgenic mice exposed to sublethal doses of γ-irradiation develop tumors, predominantly sarcomas, earlier than do untreated animals.[92,93] This susceptibility is associated with a twofold increase in the accumulation of radiation-induced double-strand DNA breaks compared to what is seen in p53$^{+/+}$ animals. Using p53-transgenic mice, it has been demonstrated that the presence of p53 mutations does not alter the latency period of chronic ultraviolet B-induced squamous-cell carcinoma but does significantly increase the number of tumors and the propensity for multiple tumor formation.[185] Although p53 protein was undetectable in the keratinocytes of the untreated mice, it was elevated in 93 percent of skin tumors derived from the treated animals. These studies confirm that p53 prevents the accumulation of cells sustaining radiation- or chemically induced DNA damage.

It has been demonstrated that caloric restriction inhibits the development of spontaneous lymphoma in C57BL/6 mice.[186] Such treatment of p53$^{-/-}$ mice modulates spontaneous tumorigenesis, delaying the onset of tumor formation by a median of 16 weeks in ad libitum fed mice and 25 weeks in calorie-restricted animals.[187] It is thought that dietary pertubations can influence the outcome of a genomic liability such as the accelerated tumorigenesis demonstrated in p53-deficient mice. Given the important role of p53 in cell cycle control, a p53-deficient state would be expected to deregulate the differentiation and development and yield aberrant morphogenesis and embryonic lethality. In fact, studies of the effects of the teratogen and DNA-damaging carcinogen benzo[a]pyrene[188] and the anticonvulsant and teratogenic drug phenytoin[189] on pregnant p53-deficient mice demonstrated a twofold to fourfold increase in the incidence of in utero fetal resorption (death), teratogenicity, and postpartum lethality over p53$^{+/+}$ controls. These observations provide substantial support for the embryoprotective role of p53.

The cumulative data from these studies indicate that loss or alterations of p53 may accelerate prior tumor predisposition, that the rate and spectrum of development of some cancers may be strain-dependent, and that normal murine development is possible even in the absence of p53. Certain similarities exist between the various p53 mouse models and LFS families in that a p53-related transformation pathway leads to development of a wide spectrum of cancers. Inheritance of one mutant and one wild-type p53 allele in affected members of LFS families is more analogous to the p53$^{+/-}$ or p53-Tg mice that developed tumors at a relatively slower rate. However, none of these animal models presents a completely accurate reflection of the LFS genotype in that the vast majority of documented human germ-line p53 mutations are missense in nature, with less than 10 percent being nonfunctional. Although the transgenic mice carry point mutations, the ^{135}Ala and ^{193}Arg mutations have not been reported in the human germ line. Although null alleles are valuable tools, their effects reflect the complete absence of gene function, a phenomenon that is not generally observed in the human syndrome. Changes at the nucleotide level would represent a more exact model and are being developed. Finally, although the tumor spectrum in current p53-altered mice is highly variable, none of these mice spontaneously mimic the human phenotype in its preponderance of sarcomas and breast cancer, except when the animals are radiated. Furthermore, the lymphomas predominant in mice are seen only rarely in LFS. Although these differences could be species-dependent, it is reasonable to suspect that specific mutations influence tumor development and yield a more accurate human phenotype. This hypothesis is substantiated by the recent studies of p53-null crosses exemplifying the in vivo role of p53 in distinct pathways of cell cycle control. The *Mdm*-2-null mouse which results in an early embryonic lethal phenotype is rescued by deletion of p53 in that double-homozygous null mice are viable. A shift in tumor phenotype resulting from cooperativity of mutations is demonstrated in the intercrosses of Min mice and p53-deficient mice, highlighting the striking tissue-specific differences in the tumor-suppressor effects of p53.[190] Mice which overexpress a c-*myc* transgene stochastically develop clonal tumors—a relatively low incidence of T-cell lymphomas.[191] Lymphoma development is dramatically accelerated by the synergistic activity of the p53-null mutation in intercrosses,[192] while no significant increase in tumor incidence was seen in *myc* mice carrying a single function p53 allele. These studies, although making a strong case for the biochemical and functional interactions of p53 with other genes crucial to tumor formation, also leave the way open to the analysis of similar synergistic effects that might be observed with a spectrum of p53 point mutations yielding disrupted p53 function rather than the null allele that yields no function whatsoever. The tumors derived from these mice, carrying point mutations, will most closely resemble spontaneous tumors that can be studied for biochemical interactions and response to therapy. It also will be possible to evaluate in vivo the effect of coexistence of mutant and wild-type p53 and the functional influence of one on the other.

Laboratory Science Meets Clinical Practice

Several important issues exist as a result of the identification of germ-line mutations of the p53 tumor-suppressor gene in rare cancer-prone families. These include ethical concerns about predictive testing in unaffected members of LFS and LFS-L families, selection of patients to be tested, and selection of practical and accurate laboratory techniques to definitively identify p53 mutations. In addition, the development of pilot testing programs and evaluation of the roles of interventions based on testing results have to be considered.

For several reasons, p53 testing is still not believed to be appropriate for the general population, particularly in light of the demonstrably low carrier rate. Even in the general cancer population, the prevalence of germ-line p53 mutations will be a fraction of 1 percent. Although the sensitivity and specificity of screening methods have improved with the advent of automated DNA sequence analysis and functional assays, both false positive and false negative results have been noted.

Even within the high-risk population, problems are apparent. It is unclear why the same germ-line p53 mutation can give rise to different cancer phenotypes, and it is not clear if in families that do not have classic LFS the cancer risks from p53 mutation are as high as they are in LFS.[20] Because 85 percent of all missense mutations described in the germ line occur in exons 5, 7, and 8 of the gene, predictive testing must include those regions. However, most centers are now sequencing the entire coding region of p53 as well as the flanking splice-acceptor sites to increase the likelihood of identifying less common alterations.

Recommendations for multicenter research studies that incorporate a multidisciplinary approach to surveying, screening, and testing were established in 1992[193] and are being updated. These initial recommendations, although specifically addressing p53 testing in LFS, could be applied to a number of other cancer-predisposition gene testing programs. In fact, both the American Society of Clinical Oncology[194] and the American Society of Human Genetics[195] have developed policy statements that include brief reference to p53 testing. Although the interpretation of who should be tested remains open, certain common recommendations are stated, including the necessity that cancer risk counseling be part of the mission of clinical oncologists, the need for informed consent, formats for regulation of genetic testing, and continued efforts to address research issues.

The component malignancies of LFS are for the most part exceedingly difficult to cure, whith the possible exception of early-detected breast cancer, childhood acute lymphoblastic leukemia, and rare germ-cell tumors of the testis. Although the prognosis for component solid tumors improves with earlier stage at diagnosis, only mammographic screening for breast cancer has been shown to reduce mortality.[196] Its efficacy under age 50 (the predominant risk in LFS) is disputed. Furthermore, the potential theoretical risk of repeated low-dose radiation from such screening methods to tissue that harbors altered p53 has not been carefully scrutinized in this setting. Chemopreventive trials are under way, but the rarity of the germ-line mutatnt p53 carrier state makes studies of these patients impractical.

Despite the many drawbacks of predictive testing for p53 at this time, the possibility of reducing the marked loss of human potential resulting from the death of a child or young adult makes further pilot research efforts worthwhile. To this end, further studies of the role of p53 in the development of human cancer, the development of more accurate testing techniques, and the development of novel animal models will continue to be important.

REFERENCES

1. Li FP, Fraumeni JF Jr: Soft tissue sarcomas breast cancer and other neoplasms: A familial cancer syndrome? *Ann Intern Med* **71**:747, 1969.
2. Li FP, Fraumeni JF Jr: Rhabdomyosarcoma in children: Epidemiologic study and identification of a familial cancer syndrome. *J Natl Cancer Inst* **43**:1365, 1969.
3. Bottomley RH, Trainer AL, Condit PT: Chromosome studies in a cancer family. *Cancer* **28**:519, 1971.
4. Lynch HT, Krush AJ, Harlan WL, Sharp EA: Association of soft tissue sarcoma, leukemia, and brain tumours in families affected with breast cancer. *Am J Surg* **39**:199, 1973.
5. Blattner WA, McGuire DB, Mulvihill JJ, Lampkin BC, Hananian J, Fraumeni JF Jr: Genealogy of cancer in a family. *JAMA* **241**:259, 1979.
6. Pearson ADJ, Craft AW, Ratcliffe JM, Birch JM, Morris-Jonese PH, Roberts DF: Two families with the Li-Fraumeni cancer family syndrome. *J Med Genet* **19**:362, 1982.
7. Lynch HT, Mulcahy GM, Harris RE, Guirgis HA, Lynch JF: Genetic and pathologic findings in a kindred with hereditary sarcoma, breast cancer, brain tumours, leukemia, lung, laryngeal, and adrenal cortical carcinoma. *Cancer* **41**:2055, 1978.
8. Draper GJ, Sanders BM, Kingston JE: Second primary neoplasms in patients with retinoblastoma. *Br J Cancer* **53**:661, 1986.
9. Li FP, Fraumeni JF Jr: Prospective study of a family cancer syndrome. *JAMA* **247**:2692, 1982.
10. Garber JE, Goldstein AM, Kantor AF, Dreyfus MG, Fraumeni JF Jr, Li FP: Follow-up study of twenty-four families with Li-Fraumeni syndrome. *Cancer Res* **51**:6094, 1991.
11. Li FP, Fraumeni JF Jr, Mulvihill JJ, Blattner WA, Dreyfus MG, Tucker MA, Miller RW: A cancer family syndrome in twenty-four kindreds. *Cancer Res* **48**:5358, 1988.
12. Birch JM, Hartley AL, Blair V, et al: Cancer in the families of children with soft tissue sarcoma. *Cancer* **66**:2239, 1990.
13. Lustbader Ed, Williams WR, Bondy ML, Strom S, Strong LC: Segregation analysis of cancer in families of childhood soft-tissue sarcoma patients. *Am J Hum Genet* **51**:344, 1992.
14. Hartley AL, Birch JM, Kelsey AM, Marsden HB, Harris M, Teare MD: Malignant melanoma in families of children with osteosar-

coma, chondrosarcoma and adrenal cortical carcinoma. *J Med Genet* **24**:664, 1987.

15. Hartley AL, Birch JM, Tricker K, Wallace SA, Kelsey AM, Harris M, Morris Jones PH: Wilms tumour in the Li-Fraumeni cancer family syndrome. *Cancer Genet Cytogenet* **67**:133, 1993.

16. Birch JM, Hartley AL, Tricker KJ, et al: Prevalence and diversity of constitutional mutations in the p53 gene among 21 Li-Fraumeni families. *Cancer Res* **54**:1298, 1994.

17. Hartley AL, Birch JM, Kelsey AM, Marsden HB, Harris M, Teare MD: Are germ cell tumours part of the Li-Fraumeni cancer family syndrome? *Cancer Genet Cytogenet* **42**:221, 1989.

18. Garber JE, Liepman MK, Gelles EJ, Corson JM, Antman KH: Melanoma and soft tissue sarcoma in seven patients. *Cancer* **66**:2432, 1990.

19. Strong LC, Stine M, Norsted TL: Cancer in survivors of childhood soft tissue sarcoma and their relatives. *J Natl Cancer Inst* **79**:1213, 1987.

20. Eeles RA: Germ line mutations in the p53 gene, in Ponder BAJ, Cavenee WK, Solomon E (eds): *Cancer Surveys, vol 25: Genetics and Cancer: A Second Look.* Cold Spring Harbor, NY, Cold Spring Harbor Laboratory Press, 1995, p 101.

21. Williams WR, Strong LC: Genetic epidemiology of soft tissue sarcomas in children, in Muller H, Weber W (eds); *Familial Cancer.* 1st International Research Conference on Familial Cancer. Basel, Karger, 1985, p 151.

22. Call KM, Glaser T, Ito CY, Buckler AJ, Pelletier J, Haber DA, Rose EA, Kral A, Yeger H, Lewis WH, Jones C, Housman DE: Isolation and characterization of a zinc finger polypeptide gene at the human chromosome 11 Wilms tumour locus. *Cell* **60**:509, 1990.

23. Gessler M, Poustka A, Cavenee W, Neve RL, Orkin SH, Bruns GAP: Homozygous deletion in Wilms tumors of a zinc-finger identified by chromosome jumping. *Nature* **343**:774, 1990.

24. Huang A, Campbell CE, Bonetta L, McAndrews-Hill MS, Coppes MJ, Williams BRG: Tissue, developmental, and tumor-specific expression of divergent transcripts in Wilms tumour. *Science* **250**:991, 1990.

25. Li FP: Cancer families: Human models of susceptibility to neoplasia. *Cancer Res* **48**:5381, 1988.

26. Bech-Hansen NT, Sell BM, Lampkin BC, Blattner WA, McKeen EA, Fraumeni JF Jr, Paterson MC: Transmission of in vitro radioresistance in a cancer-prone family. *Lancet* **1**:1135, 1981.

27. Chang EH, Pirollo KF, Zou ZQ, Cheung HY, Lawler EL, Garner R, White E, Bernstein WB, Fraumeni JF Jr, Blattner WA: Oncogenes in radioresistant, noncancerous skin fibroblasts from a cancer-prone family. *Science* **237**:1036, 1987.

28. Little JB, Nove J, Dahlberg WK, Troilo P, Nichols WW, Strong LC: Normal cytotoxic response of skin fibroblasts from patients with Li-Fraumeni cancer syndrome to DNA-damaging agents in vitro. *Cancer Res* **47**:4229, 1987.

29. Bischoff FZ, Strong LC, Yim SO, Pratt DR, Siciliano MJ, Giovanella BC, Tainsky MA: Tumorigenic transformation of spontaneously immortalized fibroblasts from patients with a familial cancer syndrome. *Oncogene* **7**:183, 1991.

30. Bischoff FZ, Yim SO, Pathak S, Grant G, Siciliano MJ, Giovanella BC, Strong LC, Tainsky MA: Spontaneous abnormalities in normal fibroblasts from patients with Li-Fraumeni cancer syndrome: Aneuploidy and immortalization. *Cancer Res* **50**:3234, 1990.

31. Knudson AG: Mutation and cancer: Statistical study of retinoblastoma. *Proc Natl Acad Sci USA* **68**:820, 1971.

32. Knudson AG, Strong LC: Mutation and cancer: A model for Wilms tumour of the kidney. *J Natl Cancer Inst* **48**:313, 1972.

33. Knudson AG, Strong LC, Anderson DE; Hereditary cancer in man. *Prog Med Genet* **9**:13, 1973.

34. Comings DE: A general theory of carcinogenesis. *Proc Natl Acad Sci USA* **70**:3324, 1973.

35. Caron de Fromentel C, Soussi T: TP53 suppressor gene: A model for investigating human mutagenesis. *Gene Chromos Cancer* **4**:1, 1992.

36. Harris CC: p53: At the crossroads of molecular carcinogenesis and risk assessment. *Science* **262**:1980, 1993.

37. Harris CC, Hollstein M: Clinical implications of the p53 tumor suppressor gene. *N Engl J Med* **329**:1318, 1993.

38. Hollstein M, Sidransky D, Vogelstein B, Harris CC: p53 mutations in human cancers. *Science* **253**:49, 1991.

39. McBride OW, Merry D, Givol D: The gene for human p53 cellular tumor antigen is located on chromosome 17 short arm (17p13). *Proc Natl Acad Sci USA* **83**:130, 1986.

40. Lane DP, Crawford LV: T antigen is bound to a host protein in SV40-transformed cells. *Nature* **278**:261, 1979.

41. Soussi T, Caron de Fromentel C, May P: Structural aspects of the p53 protein in relation to gene evolution. *Oncogene* **5**:945, 1990.

42. Foord OS, Bhattacharya P, Reich Z, Rotter V: A DNA binding domain is contained in the C-terminus of wild-type p53 protein. *Nucleic Acids Res* **19**:5191, 1991.

43. Fields S, Jang SK: Presence of a potent transcription activating sequence in the p53 protein. *Science* **249**:1046, 1990.

44. Jenkins JR, Rudge K, Currie GA: Cellular immortalization by a cDNA clone encoding the transformation associated phosphoprotein p53. *Nature* **312**:651, 1984.

45. Addison C, Jenkins JR, Sturzbecher H-W: The p53 nuclear localization signal is structurally linked to a p34cdc2 kinase motif. *Oncogene* **5**:423, 1990.

46. Milner J, Medcalf EA: Cotranslation of activated mutant p53 with wild-type drives the wild-type p53 protein into the mutant conformation. *Cell* **65**:765, 1991.

47. Stenger JE, Mayr GA, Mann K, Tegtmeyer P: Formation of stable p53 homotetramers and multiples of tetramers. *Mol Carcinogen* **5**:102, 1992.

48. Meek DW, Eckhart W: Phosphorylation of p53 in normal and simian virus 40-transformed NIH 3T3 cells. *Mol Cell Biol* **8**:461, 1988.

49. Linzer DIH, Levine AJ: Characterization of a 54K dalton cellular antigen present in SV40 transformed cells and uninfected embryonal carcinoma cells. *Cell* **17**:43, 1979.

50. Eliyahu D, Michalovitz D, Eliyahu S, Pinhasi-Kimhi O, Oren M: Wild-type p53 can inhibit oncogene-mediated focus formation. *Proc Natl Acad Sci USA* **86**:8763, 1984.

51. Jenkins JR, Chumakov P, Addison C, Sturzbecher HW, Wode-Evans A: Two distinct regions of the murine p53 primary amino acid sequence are implicated in stable complex formation within simian virus 40 antigen. *J Virol* **62**:3903, 1988.

52. Rovinski B, Benchimol S: Immortalisation of rat embryo fibroblasts by the cellular p53 oncogene. *Oncogene* **2**:445, 1988.

53. Hinds PW, Finlay CA, Levine AJ: Mutation is required to activate the p53 gene for cooperation with the ras oncogene and transformation. *J Virol* **63**:739, 1989.

53a. Baker SJ, Fearon ER, Nigro JM, Hamilton SR, Preisinger AC, Jessup JM, vanTuinen P, Ledbetter DH, Barker DF, Nakamura Y, White R, Vogelstein B: Chromosome 17 deletions and p53 gene mutations in colorectal carcinomas. *Science* **244**:217, 1989.

53b. Nigro JM, Baker SJ, Preisinger AC, Jessup JM, Hostetter R, Cleary K, Bigner SH, Davidson N, Baylin S, Devilee P, Glover T, Collins FS, Weston A, Modali R, Harris CC, Vogelstein B: Mutations in the p53 gene occur in diverse human tumor types. *Nature* **342**:705, 1989.

54. Baker SJ, Markowitz K, Fearon ER, Wilson JKV, Vogelstein B: Suppression of human colorectal carcinoma cell growth by wild-type p53. *Science* **249**:1912, 1990.

55. Diller L, Kassel J, Nelson CE, Gryka MA, Litwack G, Gebhardt MA, Friend SH: p53 functions as a cell cycle control protein in osteosarcomas. *Mol Cell Biol* **10**:5772, 1990.

56. Levine AJ, Momand J, Finlay CA: The p53 tumor suppressor gene. *Nature* **351**:453, 1991.

56a. El-Deiry WS, Kern SE, Pientenpol JA, Kinzler KW, Vogelstein B: Definition of a consensus binding site for p53. *Nat Genet* **1**:45, 1992.

57. Funk WD, Park DT, Karas RH, Wright WE, Shay JW: A transcriptionally active DNA-binding site for p53 protein complexes. *Mol Cell Biol* **12**:2866, 1992.

58. Iwabuchi K, Li B, Bartel P, Fields S: Use of the two-hybrid system to identify the domain of p53 involved in oligomerization. *Oncogene* **8**:1693, 1993.

59. Shaulsky G, Goldfinger N, Ben-Zeev A, Rotter V: Nuclear accumulation of p53 protein is mediated by several nuclear localization signals and plays a role in tumorigenesis. *Mol Cell Biol* **10**:6565, 1990.

60. Milne DM, Palmer RH, Campbell DG, Meek DW: Phosphorylation of the p53 tumor-suppressor protein at three N terminal sites by a novel casein kinase I-like enzyme. *Oncogene* **7**:1316, 1992.

61. Lees-Milner SP, Chen Y, Anderson CW: Human cells contain a DNA-activated protein kinase that phosphorylates simian virus 40 T-antigen, mouse p53, and the human Ku autoantigen. *Mol Cell Biol* **9**:3982, 1990.

62. Meek DW, Simon S, Kikkawa U, Eckhart W: The p53 tumor suppressor proteins is phosphorylated at serine 389 by casein kinase II. *EMBO J* **9**:3253, 1990.

63. Finlay CA, Hinds PW, Levine AJ: The p53 proto-oncogene can act as a suppressor of transformation. *Cell* **57**:1083, 1989.

64. Vogelstein B, Kinzler KW: p53 function and dysfunction. *Cell* **70**:523, 1992.

65. Mercer WE, Shields MT, Lin D, Appella E, Ullrich SJ: Growth suppression induced by wild-type p53 protein is accompanied by selective down-regulation of proliferating cell-nuclear antigen expression. *Proc Natl Acad Sci USA* **88**:1958, 1991.

66. Baker SJ, Markowitz K, Fearon ER, Wilson JKV, Vogelstein B: Suppression of human colorectal carcinoma cell growth by wild-type p53. *Science* **249**:1912, 1990.

67. Diller L, Kassel J, Nelson CE, Gryka MA, Litwack G, Gebhardt MA, Friend SH: p53 functions as a cell cycle control protein in osteosarcomas. *Mol Cell Biol* **10**:5772, 1990.

68. Michalovitz D, Halevy O, Oren M: Conditional inhibition of transformation and of cell proliferation by a temperature-sensitive mutant of p53. *Cell* **62**:671, 1990.

69. Paules RS, Levedakou EN, Wilson SJ, Innes CL, Rhodes N, Tlsty TD, Galloway DA, Donehower LA, Tainsky MA, Kaufmann WK: Defective G2 checkpoint function in cells from individuals with familial cancer syndrome. *Cancer Res* **55**:1763, 1995.

70. Guillof C, Rosselli F, Krisnaraju K, Moustacchi E, Hoffmann B, Liebermann DA: p53 involvement in control of G2 exit of the cell cycle: Role in DNA damage-induced apoptosis. *Oncogene* **10**:2263, 1995.

71. Stewart N, Hicks GG, Paraskevas F, Mowat M: Evidence for a second cell cycle block at G2/M by p53. *Oncogene* **10**:109, 1995.

72. Wang Y, Prives C: Increased and altered DNA binding of human p53 by S and G2/M but not G1 cyclin-dependent kinases. *Nature* **376**:88, 1995.

73. Fan S, Smith MK, Rivet DJ, Duba D, Zhan Q, Kohn K, Fornace AJ, O'Connor PM: Disruption of p53 function sensitizes breast cancer MCF-7 cells to cisplatin and pentoxifylline. *Cancer Res* **55**:1649, 1995.

74. Powell SN, DeFrank JS, Connell P, Eogen M, Preffer F, Dombkowski D, Tang W, Friend S: Differential sensitivity of p53(−) and p53(+) cells to caffeine-induced radiosensitization and override of G2 delay. *Cancer Res* **55**:1643, 1995.

75. Cross SM, Sanchez CA, Morgan CA, Schimke MK, Ramel S, Idzerda RL, Raskind WH, Reid BJ: A p53-dependent mouse spindle checkpoint. *Science* **267**:1353, 1995.

76. Fukasawa K, Choi T, Kuriyama R, Rulong S, Vande Woude GF: Abnormal centrosome amplification in the absence of p53. *Science* **271**:1744, 1996.

77. Bouffler SD, Kemp CJ, Balmain A, Cox R: Spontaneous and ionizing radiation-induced chromosomal abnormalities in p53-deficient mice. *Cancer Res* **5**:3883, 1995.

78. Parshad R, Price FM, Pirollo KF, Chang EH, Sandford KK: Cytogenetic responses to G2 phase X-irradiation in relation to DNA repair and radiosensitivity in cancer prone family with Li-Fraumeni syndrome. *Radiat Res* **136**:236, 1993.

79. Funk WD, Park DT, Karas RH, Wright WE, Shay JW: A transcriptionally active DNA-binding site for p53 protein complexes. *Mol Cell Biol* **12**:2866, 1992.

80. Eliyahu D, Raz A, Gruss P, Givol D, Oren M: Participants of p53 cellular tumor antigen in transformation of normal embryonic cells. *Nature* **312**:646, 1984.

81. Yonish-Rouach E, Resnitzky D, Lotem J, Sachs L, Kimchi A, Oren M: Wild-type p53 induces apoptosis of myeloid leukemic cells that is inhibited by interleukin-6. *Nature* **352**:345, 1991.

82. Shaw P, Bovey R, Tardy S, Sahli R, Sordat B, Costa J: Induction of apoptosis by wild-type p53 in a human colon tumor-derived cell line. *Proc Natl Acad Sci USA* **89**:4495, 1992.

83. Clarke AR, Purdie CA, Harrison DJ, Morris RG, Bird CC, Hooper ML, Wyllie AH: Thymocyte apoptosis induced by p53-dependent and independent pathways. *Nature* **362**:849, 1993.

84. Lowe SW, Schmitt EM, Smith SW, Osborne BA, Jacks T: p53 is required for radiation-induced apoptosis in mouse thymocytes. *Nature* **362**:847, 1993.

85. Lowe SW, Ruley HE, Jacks T, Housman DE: p53-dependent apoptosis modulates the cytotoxicity of anticancer agents. *Cell* **74**:957, 1993.

86. Slichenmeyer WJ, Nelson WG, Slebos RJ, Kastan MB: Loss of a p53-associated G1 checkpoint does not decrease cell survival following DNA damage. *Cancer Res* **53**:4164, 1993.

87. Brachman DG, Beckett M, Graves D, Haraf D, Vokes E, Weichselbaum RR: p53 mutation does not correlate with radiosensitivity in 24 head and neck cancer cell lines. *Cancer Res* **53**:3667, 1993.

88. Maltzman W, Czyzk L: UV irradiation stimulates levels of p53 cellular tumor antigen in nontransformed mouse cells. *Mol Cell Biol* **4**:1689, 1984.

89. Kuerbitz SJ, Beverly SP, Walsh WV, Kastan MB: Wild-type p53 is a cell cycle checkpoint determinant following irradiation. *Proc Natl Acad Sci USA* **89**:7491, 1992.

90. Kastan MB, Onyekwere O, Sidransky D, Vogelstein B, Craig RW: Participation of p53 protein in the cellular response to DNA damage. *Cancer Res* **51**:6304, 1991.

91. Yamaizumi M, Sugano T: UV-induced nuclear accumulation of p53 is evoked through DNA damage of actively transcribed genes independent of the cell cycle. *Oncogene* **9**:2775, 1994.

92. Lee JM, Abrhamson JLA, Kandel R, Donehower LA, Bernstein A: Susceptibility to radiation-carcinogenesis and accumulation of chromosomal breakage in p53-deficient mice. *Oncogene* **9**:3731, 1994.

93. Lee JM, Bernstein A: p53 mutations increase resistance to ionizing radiation. *Proc Natl Acad Sci USA* **90**:5742, 1993.

94. Lane DP: p53, guardian of the genome. *Nature* **358**:15, 1992.

95. Zambetti GP, Levine AJ: A comparison of the biological activities of wild-type and mutant p53. *FASEB J* **7**:855, 1993.

96. Lowe LW, Bodis B, McCarthy A, Remington LH, Ruley E, Fisher D, Housman DE, Jacks T: p53 can determine the efficacy of cancer therapy in vitro. *Science* **266**:807, 1994.

97. Barak Y, Juven T, Haffner R, Oren M: mdm-2 expression is induced by wild-type p53 activity. *EMBO J* **12**:461, 1993.

98. Wu X, Bayle H, Olson D, Levine AJ: The p53-mdm2 autoregulatory feedback loop. *Gene Dev* **7**:1126, 1993.

99. Okamoto K, Beach D: Cyclin G is a transcriptional target of the tumor suppressor protein p53. *EMBO J* **13**:4816, 1994.

100. Myashita T, Reed TC: Tumor suppressor p53 is a direct transcriptional activator of the numan bax gene. *Cell* **80**:293, 1995.

101. Kastan MB, Zhan Q, El-Deiry WS, Carrier F, Jacks T, Walsh WV, Plunkett BS, Vogelstein B, Fornace AJ; A mammalian cell cycle checkpoint pathway utilizing p53 and GADD45 is defective in ataxia-telangiectasia. *Cell* **71**:587, 1992.

102. Harper JW, Adami GR, Wei N, Keyomarsi K, Elledge SJ: The p21 Cdk-interacting protein Cip1 is a potent inhibitor of G1 cyclin-dependent kinases. *Cell* **75**:805, 1993.

103. Xiong Y, Hannon GJ, Zhang H, Casso D, Kobayashi R, Beach D: p21 is a universal inhibitor of cylcin kinases. *Nature* **366**:701, 1993.

104. Gu Y, Turck CW, Morgan DO: Inhibition of CDK2 activity in vivo by an associated 20K regulatory subunit. *Nature* **366**:707, 1993.

105. Pines J: p21 inhibits cyclin shock. *Nature* **369**:520, 1994.

106. Smith ML, Chen I-T, Zhan Q, Bae I, Chen C-Y, Glimer TM, Kastan MB, O'Connor PM, Fornace AJ Jr: Interaction of the p53-regulated protein GADD45 with proliferating cell nuclear antigen. *Science* **266**:1376, 1994.

107. Wang XW, Forrester K, Yeh H, Feitelson MA, Gu JR, Harris CC: Hepatitis B virus X protein inhibits p53 sequence-specific DNA binding, transcriptional activity, and association with transcription factor ERCC3. *Proc Natl Acad Sci USA* **91**:2230, 1994.

108. Cho Y, Gorina S, Jeffrey PD, Pavletich NP: Crystal structure of a p53 tumor suppressor-DNA complex: Understanding tumorigenic mutations. *Science* **265**:346, 1994.

109. Clore GM, Omichinski JF, Sakaguchi K, Zambrano N, Sakamoto H, Appella E, Gronenborn AM: High-resolution structure of the oligomerization domain of p53 by multidimensional NMR. *Science* **265**:386, 1994.

109a. Lee W, Harvey TS, Yin Y, Yau P, Litchfield D, Arrowsmith CH: Solution structure of the tetrameric minimum transforming domain of p53. *Struct Biol* **1**:877, 1994.

110. Prives C: How loops, β sheets, and α helices help us to understand p53. *Cell* **78**:543, 1994.

111. Vogelstein B, Kinzler KW: X-rays strike p53 again. *Nature* **370**:174, 1994.

112. Farmer G, Bargonetti J, Zhu H, Friedman P, Prywes R, Prives C: Wild-type p53 activates transcription in vitro. *Nature* **358**:83, 1992.

113. Kern SE, Kinzler KW, Bruskin A, Jarosz D, Friedman P, Prives C, Vogelstein B: Identification of p53 as a sequence-specific DNA-binding protein. *Science* **252**:1708, 1991.

114. Kern SE, Pientenpol JA, Thiagalingam S, Seymour A, Kinzler KW, Vogelstein B: Oncogenic forms of p53 inhibit p53-regulated gene expression. *Science* **256**:827, 1992.

115. Milner J, Medcalf EA: Cotranslation of activated mutant p53 with wild-type p53 protein drives the wild-type p53 protein into the mutant conformation. *Cell* **65**:765, 1991.

116. Cariello NF, Cui L, Beroud C, Soussi T: Database and software for the analysis of mutations in the human p53 gene. *Cancer Res* **54**:4454, 1994.

117. Momand J, Zambetti GP, Olson DC, George D, Levine AJ: The mdm-2 oncogene product forms a complex with the p53 protein and inhibits p53-mediated transactivation. *Cell* **69**:1237, 1992.

118. Sheffner M, Werness BA, Huibregste JM, Levine AJ, Howley PM: The E6 oncoprotein encoded by human papillomavirus types 16 and 18 promotes the degradation of p53. *Cell* **63**:1129, 1990.

119. Fakharzadeh SS, Trusko SP, George DL: Tumorigenic potential associated with enhanced expression of a gene that is amplified in a mouse tumor cell line. *EMBO J* **10**:1565, 1991.

120. Oliner JD, Kinzler KW, Meltzer PS, George DL, Vogelstein B: Amplification of a gene encoding a p53-associated protein in human sarcomas. *Nature* **358**:80, 1992.

121. Maheswaran S, Park S, Bernard A, Morris JF, Rauscher FJ, Hill DE, Haber DA: Physical and functional interaction between WT1 and p53 proteins. *Proc Natl Acad Sci USA* **90**:5100, 1993.

122. Williams BO, Remington L, Albert DM, Mukai S, Bronson RT, Jacks T: Cooperative tumorigenic effects of germ line mutations in Rb and p53 proteins. *Nat Genet* **7**:480, 1994.

123. Harvey M, Vogel H, Lee EYHP, Bradley A, Donehower LA: Mice deficient in both p53 and Rb develop tumors primarily of endocrine origin. *Cancer Res* **55**:1146, 1995.

124. Shimamura A, Fisher DE: p53 in life and death. *Clin Cancer Res* **2**:435, 1996.

125. Hansen R, Reddel R, Braithwaite A: The transforming oncoproteins determine the mechanism by which p53 suppresses cell transformation: pRB-mediated growth arrest or apoptosis. *Oncogene* **11**:2535, 1995.

126. Miller CW, Aslo A, Tsay C, Slamon D, Ishizaki K, Toguchida J: Frequency and structure of p53 rearrangements in human osteosarcoma. *Cancer Res* **50**:7950, 1990.

127. Toguchida J, Yamaguchi T, Ritchie B, Beauchamp RL, Dayton SH, et al: Mutation spectrum of the p53 gene in bone and soft tissue sarcomas. *Cancer Res* **52**:6194, 1992.

128. Felix CA, Kappel CC, Mitsudomi T, Nau MM, Tsokos M, et al: Frequency and diversity of p53 mutations in childhood rhabdomyosarcoma. *Cancer Res* **52**:2243, 1992.

129. Slingerland JM, Minden MD, Benchimol S: Mutation of the p53-gene in human myelogenous leukemia. *Blood* **77**:1500, 1991.

130. Prococimer M, Rotter V: Structure and function of p53 in normal cells and their aberrations in cancer cells: Projection of the hematologic cell lineages. *Blood* **84**:2391, 1994.

131. Mashiyama S, Murakami Y, Yoshimoto T, Sekiya T, Hayashi K: Detection of p53 gene mutations in human brain tumors by single-strand conformation polymorphism analysis of polymerase chain reaction products. *Oncogene* **6**:1313, 1991.

132. Takahashi T, Nan MM, Chiba I, Buchhagen DL, Minna JD: p53: A frequent target for genetic abnormalities in lung cancer. *Science* **246**:491, 1989.

133. Osborne RJ, Merlo GR, Mitsudomi T, Venesio T, Liscia DS, et al: Mutations in the p53 gene in primary human breast cancers. *Cancer Res* **51**:6194, 1991.

134. Malkin D: p53 and the Li-Fraumeni syndrome. *Biochem Biophys Acta* **1198**:197, 1994.

135. Laviguer A, Maltby V, Mock D, Rossant J, Pawson T, Bernstein A: High incidence of lung, bone, and lymphoid tumors in transgenic mice overexpressing mutant alleles of the p53 oncogene. *Mol Cell Biol* **9**:3982, 1989.

136. Malkin D, Li FP, Strong LC, Fraumeni JF Jr, Nelson CE, Kim DH, Kassel J, Gryka MA, Bischoff FZ, Tainsky MA, Friend SH: Germ line p53 mutations ina familial syndrome of breast cancer, sarcomas, and other neoplasms. *Science* **250**:1233, 1990.

137. Malkin D, Friend SH: Correction: A Li-Fraumeni syndrome mutation. *Science* **259**:878, 1993.

137a. Srivastava S, Zou Z, Pirollo K, Blattner W, Chang EH: Germ line transmission of a mutated p53 gene in a cancer-prone family with Li-Fraumeni syndrome. *Nature* **348**:747, 1990.

138. Vogelstein B: A deadly inheritance. *Nature* **348**:681, 1990.

139. Law JC, Strong LC, Chidambaram A, Ferrell RE: A germ line mutation in exon 5 of the p53 gene in an extended cancer family. *Cancer Res* **51**:6385, 1991.

140. Metzger AK, Sheffield VC, Duyk G, Daneshuar L, Edwards MSB, Cogen PH: Identification of a germ line mutation in the p53 gene in a patient with intracranial ependymoma. *Proc Natl Acad Sci USA* **88**:7825, 1991.

141. Santibanez-Koref MF, Birch JM, Hartley AL, Morris-Jones PH, Craft AW, et al: p53 germ line mutations in Li-Fraumeni syndrome. *Lancet* **338**:1490, 1991.

142. Birch JM: Germ line mutations in the p53 tumor suppressor gene: Scientific, clinical and ethical challenges. *Br J Cancer* **66**:424, 1992.

143. Barnes DM, Hanby AM, Gillett CE, Mohammed S, Hodson S, Bobrow LG, Leigh IM, Purkis T, MacGEoch C, Spur AM, Bartek J, Vojtesek B, Picksley SM, Lane DP: Abnormal expression of wild-type p53 protein in normal cells of a cancer family patient. *Lancet* **340**:259, 1992.

144. Frebourg T, Barbier N, Yan Y-X, Garber JE, Dreyfus M, Fraumeni JF Jr, Li FP, Friend SH: Germ line p53 mutations in 15 families with Li-Fraumeni syndrome. *Am J Hum Genet* **56**:608, 1995.

145. Brugieres L, Gardes M, Moutou C, Chompret A, Meresse V, et al: Screening for germ line p53 mutations in children with malignant tumor and a family history of cancer. *Cancer Res* **53**:452, 1993.

146. Birch JM, Heighway J, Teare MD, Kelsey AM, Hartley AL, Tricker KJ, Crowther D, Lane DP, Santibanez-Koref MF: Linkage studies in a Li-Fraumeni family with increased expression of p53 protein but no germ line mutation in p53. *Br J Cancer* **70**:1176, 1994.

146a. Varley JM, McGown G, Thorncroft M, Cochrane S, Morrison P, Woll P, Kelsey AM, Mitchell ELD, Boyle J, Birch JM, Evans DGR: A previously undescribed mutation within the tetramerization domain of TP53 in a family with Li-Fraumeni syndrome. *Oncogene* **12**:2437, 1996.

147. Malkin D, Jolly KW, Barbier N, Look AT, Friend SH, Gebhardt MC, Andersen TI, Borresen A-L, Li FP, Strong LC: Germ line mutations of the p53 tumor suppressor gene in children and young adults with second malignant neoplasms. *N Engl J Med* **326**:1309, 1992.

148. Iavarone A, Mattay KK, Steinkirchner TM, Israel MA: Germ line and somatic p53 gene mutations in multifocal osteogenic sarcoma. *Proc Natl Acad Sci USA* **89**:4207, 1992.

148a. Kyritsis AP, Bondy ML, Xiao M, Berman EL, Cunningham JE, Lee PS, Levin VA, Saya H: Germ line p53 gene mutations in subsets of glioma patients. *J Natl Cancer Inst* **86**:344, 1994.

149. Toguchida J, Yamaguchi T, Dayton SH, Beauchamp RL, Herrera GE, Ishizaki K, Yamamuro T, Meyers PA, Little JB, Sasaki MS, Weichselbaum RR, Yandell DW: Prevalence and spectrum of germ line mutations of the p53 gene among patients with sarcoma. *N Engl J Med* **326**:1301, 1992.

150. Prosser J, Elder PA, Condie A, MacFayden I, Steel CM, Evans HJ: Mutations in p53 do not account for heritable breast cancer: A study in five affected families. *Br J Cancer* **63**:181, 1991.

151. Warren W, Eeles RA, Ponder BAJ, Easton DF, Averill D, Ponder MA, Anderson K, Evans AM, DeMars R, Love R, Dundas S, Stratton MR, Trowbridge P, Cooper CS, Peto J: No evidence for germ line mutations in exons 5–9 of the p53 gene in 25 breast cancer families. *Oncogene* **7**:1043, 1992.

152. Borresen A-L, Andersen TI, Garber J, Barbier N, Thorlacius S, Eyfjord J, Ottestad L, Smith-Sorensen B, Hovig E, Malkin D, Friend SH: Screening for germ line TP53 mutations in breast cancer patients. *Cancer Res* **52**:3234, 1992.

153. Frebourg T, Barbier N, Kassel J, Ng YS, Romero P, Friend SH: A functional screen for germ line p53 mutations based on transcriptional activation. *Cancer Res* **52**:6976, 1992.

154. Sidransky D, Tokino T, Helzlsouer K, Zehnbauer B, Rausch G, Shelton B, Prestigiacomo L, Vogelstein B, Davidson N: Inherited p53 gene mutations in breast cancer. *Cancer Res* **52**:2984, 1992.

155. Loriaux DL, Cutler GB Jr: Diseases of the adrenal glands, in Kohler PO (ed): *Clinical Endocrinology*. New York, Wiley, 1986, p 157.

156. Sameshima Y, Tsunematsu Y, Watanabe S, Tsukamoto T, Kawaha K, et al: Detection of novel germ line p53 mutations in diverse cancer prone families identified by selecting patients with childhood adrenocortical carcinoma. *J Natl Cancer Inst* **84**:703, 1992.

157. Wagner J, Portwine C, Rabin K, Leclerc J-M, Narod SA, Malkin D: High frequency of germ line p53 mutations in childhood adrenocortical cancer. *J Natl Cancer Inst* **86**:1707, 1994.

158. McIntyre JF, Smith-Sorensen B, Friend SH, Kassel J, Borresen A-L, Yan YX, Russo C, Sato J, Barbier N, Miser J, Malkin D, Gebhardt MC: *J Clin Oncol* **12**:925, 1994.

159. Diller L, Sexsmith E, Gottlieb A, Li FP, Malkin D: Germ line p53 mutations are frequently detected in young children with rhabdomyosarcoma. *J Clin Invest* **95**:1606, 1995.

160. Felix CA, Nau MM, Takahashi T, Mitsudomi T, Chiba I, Poplack DG, Reaman GH, Cole DE, Letterio JJ, Whang-Peng J, Knutsen T, Minna JD: Hereditary and acquired p53 mutations in childhood acute lymphoblastic leukemia. *J Clin Invest* **89**:640, 1992.

161. Felix CA, D'Amico D, Mitsudomi T, Nau MM, Li FP, Fraumeni JF Jr, Cole DE, McCalla J, Reaman GH, Whang-Peng J, Knutsen T, Minna JD, Poplack DG: Absence of hereditary p53 mutations in 10 familial leukemia pedigrees. *J Clin Invest* **90**:653, 1992.

162. Felix CA, Hosler MR, Provisor D, Salhany K, Sexsmith EA, Slater DJ, Cheung NKV, Winick NJ, Strauss EA, Heyn R, Lange BJ, Malkin D: The p53 gene in pediatric therapy-related leukemia and myelodysplasia. *Blood* **10**:1996.

163. Jolly KW, Malkin D, Douglass EC, Brown TF, Sinclair AE, Look, AT: Splice-site mutation of the p53 gene in a family with hereditary breast-ovarian cancer. *Oncogene* **9**:97, 1994.

164. Warneford SG, Wilton LJ, Townsend ML, Rowe PB, Reddell RR, Dalla-Pozza L, Symonds G: Germ line splicing mutation of the p53 gene in a cancer-prone family. *Cell Growth Differ* **3**:839, 1992.

165. Felix CA, Strauss EA, D'Amico D, Tsokos M, Winter S, Mitsudomi T, Nau MM, Brown DL, Leahey AM, Horowitz ME, Poplack DG, Costin D, Minna JD: A novel germ line p53 splicing mutation in a pediatric patient with a second malignant neoplasm. *Oncogene* **8**:1203, 1993.

166. Gannon JV, Greaves R, Iggo R, Lane DP: Activating mutations in p53 produce common conformation effects: A monoclonal antibody specific for the mutant form. *EMBO J* **9**:1591, 1990.

167. Srivastava S, Tong YA, Devadas K, Zou A-Q, Sykes VW, Chang EW: Detection of both mutant and wild-type p53 protein in normal skin fibroblasts and demonstration of a shared second hit on p53 in diverse tumors from a cancer-prone family with Li-Fraumeni syndrome. *Oncogene* **7**:987, 1992.

168. Frebourg T, Kassel J, Lam KT, Gryka MA, Barbier N, Andersen TI, Borresen A-L, Friend SH: Germ line mutations of the p53 tumor suppressor gene in patients with high risk for cancer inactivate the p53 protein. *Proc Natl Acad Sci USA* **89**:6413, 1992.

169. Ishioka C, Frebourg T, Yan Y-X, Vidal M, Friend SH, Schmidt S, Iggo R: Screening patients for heterozygous p53 mutations using a functional assay in yeast. *Nat Genet* **5**:124, 1993.

170. Flaman JM, Frebourg T, Moreau V, Charbonnier F, Martin C, Chappuis P, Sappino AP, Limacher IM, Bron L, Benhatter J: A simple p53 functional assay for screening cell lines, blood and tumors. *Proc Natl Acad Sci USA* **92**:3963, 1995.

171. Lavigueur A, Bernstein A: p53 transgenic mice: Accelerated erythroleukemia induction by Friend virus. *Oncogene* **6**:2197, 1991.

172. Donehower LA, Harvey M, Slagle BL, McArthur MJ, Montgomery CA, Butel J, Bradley A: Mice deficient for p53 are developmentally normal but susceptible to spontaneous tumors. *Nature* **356**:215, 1992.

173. Rogel A, Popliker M, Webb C, Oren M: p53 cellular tumor antigen: Analysis of mRNA levels in normal cell adult tissues, embryos, and tumors. *Mol Cell Biol* **5**:2851, 1985.

174. Purdie CA, Harrison DJ, Peter A, Dobbie L, White S, Howie SEM, Salter DM, Bird CC, Wyllie AH, Hooper ML, Clarke AR: Tumor incidence, spectrum and ploidy in mice with a large deletion in the p53 gene. *Oncogene* **9**:603, 1994.

175. Jacks T, Remington L, Williams BO, Schmitt EM, Halachmi S, Bronson RT, Weinberg RA: Tumor spectrum analysis in p53 mutant mice. *Current Biol* **4**:1, 1994.

176. Harvey M, McArthur MJ, Montgomery CA Jr, Bradley A, Donehower LA: Genetic background alters the spectrum of tumors that develop in p53-deficient mice. *FASEB J* **7**:849, 1993.

177. Dietrich WF, Lander ES, Smith JS, Moser AR, Gould KA, Luongo C, Borenstein N, Dove W: *Cell* **75**:631, 1993.

178. Montes de Oca Luna R, Wagner DS, Lozano G: Rescue of embryonic lethality in mdm-2-deficient mice by deletion of p53. *Nature* **378**:203, 1995.

179. Jones SN, Roe AE, Donehower LA, Bradley A: Rescue of embryonic lethality in Mdm-2-deficient mice by absence of p53. *Nature* **378**:206, 1995.

180. Harvey M, Vogel H, Morris D, Bradley A, Bernstein A, Donehower LA: A mutant p53 transgene accelerates tumor development in heterozygous but not nullizygous p53-deficient mice. *Nat Genet* **9**:305, 1995.

181. Liu G, Montes de Oca Luna R, Lozano G: Establishing mouse models to study tumor derived p53 mutants in vivo: Cancer genetics and tumor suppressor genes. *Cold Spring Harbor Lab Meeting* **172**:1996.

182. Sah VP, Attardi LD, Mulligan GJ, Williams BO, Bronson RT, Jacks T: A subset of p53-deficient embryos exhibit exencephaly. *Nat Genet* **7**:480, 1994.

183. Hartley AL, Birch JM, Blair V, Kelsey AM, Morris-Jones PH: Fetal loss and infant deaths in families of children with soft-tissue sarcoma. *Int J Cancer* **56**:646, 1994.

184. Harvey M, McArthur MJ, Montgomery CA Jr, Butel JS, Bradley A, Donehower LA: Spontaneous and carcinogen-induced tumorigenesis in p53-deficient mice. *Nat Genet* **5**:225, 1993.

185. Li G, Ho VC, Berean K, Tron VA: Ultraviolet radiation induction of squamous cell carcinomas in p53 transgenic mice. *Cancer Res* **55**:2070, 1995.

186. Koizumi A, Tsudada M, Wada Y, Masuda H, Weindruch R: *J Nutr* **122**:1446, 1992.

187. Hursting SD, Perkins SN, Phang JM: Calorie restriction delays spontaneous tumorigenesis in p53-knockout transgenic mice. *Proc Natl Acad Sci USA* **91**:7036, 1994.

188. Nicol CJ, Harrison ML, Laposa RR, Gimelshtein IL, Wells PG: A teratologic suppressor role for p53 in benzo[a]pyrene-treated transgenic p53-deficient mice. *Nat Genet* **10**:181, 1995.

189. Laposa RR, Chan KC, Wiley MJ, Wells PG: Evidence for DNA damage and teratological suppressor genes in the initiation of and resistance to chemical teratogenesis: phenytoin teratogenicity in p53-deficient mice. *Toxicologist* **15**:161, 1995.

190. Clarke AR, Cummings MC, Harrison DJ: Interaction between murine germ line mutations in p53 and APC predisposes to pancreatic neoplasia but not to increased intestinal malignancy. *Oncogene* **11**:1913, 1995.

191. Stewart M: *Int J Cancer* **53**:1023, 1993.

192. Blyth K, Terry A, O'Hara M, Baxter EW, Campbell M, Stewart M, Donehower LA, Onions De, Neil JC, Cameron ER: Synergy between a human c-myc transgene and p53 null genotype in murine thymic lymphomas: Contrasting effects of homozygous and heterozygous p53 loss. *Oncogene* **10**:1717, 1995.

193. Li FP, Garber JE, Friend SH, Strong LC, Patenaude AF, Juengst ET, Reilly PR, Corea P, Fraumeni JF Jr: Recommendations on predictive testing for germ line p53 mutations among cancer-prone individuals. *J Natl Cancer Inst* **84**:1156, 1992.

194. American Society of Clinical Oncology: Statement of the American Society of Clinical Oncology: Genetic testing for cancer susceptibility. *J Clin Oncol* **14**:1730, 1996.

195. American Society of Human Genetics: Statements of the American Society of Human Genetics on genetic testing for breast and ovarian cancer predisposition. *Am J Hum Genet* **55**:i, 1994.

196. Shapiro S: Determining the efficacy of breast cancer screening. *Cancer* **63**:1873, 1989.

CHAPTER 21

Wilms Tumor

Daniel A. Haber

1. Wilms tumor is a pediatric kidney cancer that can arise sporadically or in children with congenital syndromes confering genetic susceptibility. In addition, some 10% of children with Wilms tumor present with bilateral cancers, evidence of a predisposing genetic lesion.

2. The genetic loci associated with the development of Wilms tumor have been identified by analysis of gross karyotype abnormalities in children with Wilms-associated syndromes, as well as by molecular analyses of DNA losses in tumor specimens. A genetic locus on chromosome 11, band p13 has been linked to Wilms tumor arising in the context of aniridia and abnormalities of genito-urinary development (e.g., WAGR syndrome). A second locus on chromosome 11, band p15 is associated with hemi-hypertrophy (e.g., Beckwith-Wiedemann syndrome) and predisposition to Wilms tumor and other pediatric neoplasms. A third Wilms locus has recently been mapped to chromosome 17q12-21.

3. The WT1 gene, mapping within the 11p13 genetic locus, was isolated in 1990. It encodes a transcription factor whose expression is strictly developmentally regulated in the normal kidney. Like the fetal kidney cells from which they appear to originate, most Wilms tumors express high levels of WT1 protein. However, in a fraction of Wilms tumors, WT1 is either deleted or mutated to an inactive form, consistent with its characterization as a tumor suppressor gene. Reintroduction of wild-type WT1 into a Wilms tumor cell line with an aberrant endogenous WT1 transcript results in inhibition of cell growth.

4. Inactivation of WT1 in one germline allele confers a high degree of susceptibility to Wilms tumor, which is triggered by loss of the second WT1 allele in somatic tissues. Hemizygosity for WT1 in the germline also results in a variable degree of developmental abnormalities in the genito-urinary tract, more prominent in males than in females. Moreover, specific point mutations within the DNA binding domain of WT1 result in a dominant negative phenotype, characterized by severe abnormalities in sexual and renal development (Denys-Drash syndrome). In the mouse, hemizygous inactivation of WT1 is not associated with genitourinary defects or tumor predisposition. However, homozygous inactivation of WT1 leads to failure of renal and gonadal development, as well as to malformations of the heart and diaphragm.

5. The protein encoded by WT1 belongs to a class of zinc-binding transcription factors, with multiple variants produced by alternative splicing. The four zinc finger domains of WT1 recognize GC-rich DNA target sequences, an effect that is modulated by the variable insertion of three amino acids (KTS) between zinc fingers 3 and 4. WT1 appears to function as a transcriptional repressor, although physiologically-relevant target genes remain to be defined. Potential protein interactors include another tumor suuupprressor gene product, p53, whose function is modulated by WT1. Inducible expression of WT1 in tissue culture cells triggers apoptosis, associated with repression of the epidermal growth factor receptor and induction of the cyclin-dependent kinase inhibitor p21. Dimerization of WT1 may contribute to the dominant negative phenotype displayed by mutants with a disrupted DNA binding domain. Characterization of the normal pathways involved in WT1 function and of any potential interactions with other Wilms tumor genes may lead to a better understanding of normal kidney development and tumorigenesis.

Wilms tumor or nephroblastoma is a pediatric kidney cancer that can present either as a sporadic case or in the setting of genetic predisposition. Both epidemiologic studies of tumor incidence and early genetic studies pointed to the presence of one or more genes whose loss was associated with tumor development. The isolation of the first of these genes, WT1, has led to the discovery of a tumor suppressor gene, encoding a transcription factor with a striking kidney-specific pattern of expression. Mutations in WT1 have been linked both to the formation of Wilms tumor and to a range of developmental abnormalities in genito-urinary development. The characterization of this gene and the ongoing search for the other Wilms tumor genes provide a key to understanding the basis of normal kidney development and in tumorigenesis.

HISTOLOGY

The histological characteristics of Wilms tumor are complex, consistent with its classification as a primitive, multilineage malignancy of renal stem cells.[1] The classic description is that of a "triphasic" tumor, including blastemal, epithelial and stromal components (see Figure 21-1). All of these components are thought to be derived from the malignant stem cell, although genetic evidence of shared lineage has not been demonstrated. Wilms tumors can vary in the predominance of one histologic component over the others, and some tumors show evidence of further multilineage differentiation, with the presence of muscle or neural elements.

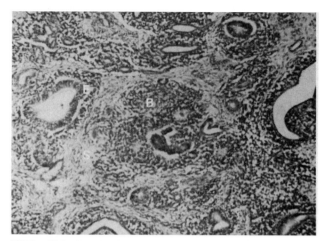

FIG. 21-1 Wilms tumor histology. The classic triphasic histologic pattern includes areas of primitive blastemal cells (B), epithelial cells (E), and stromal cell components (S). Tumors can also contain areas of further differentiation along muscle and rarely neural lineages. Expression of the WT1 tumor suppressor gene appears restricted to the epithelial and blastemal components of Wilms tumors. *(Photomicrograph (hematoxylin and eosin stain) provided by Dr. Nancy Harris, Department of Pathology, Massachusetts General Hospital, Boston, Massachusetts).*

Clinical prognosis does not appear to be affected by the histologic appearance of the tumors, with the exception of anaplastic variants that have a more aggressive course.[2] Tumors with triphasic histology characteristic of Wilms tumor may arise outside the kidney. Such "extrarenal" Wilms tumors have been reported from a number of sites, primarily the pelvis and abdomen.[3] Although Wilms tumor is primarily a cancer of children under 5 years of age, it has also been reported in young adults. The histology of these tumors is similar to that of classic Wilms tumor seen in young children, leading to the suggestion that they arise from a small number of renal stem cells that have persisted into adulthood.

The relationship between Wilms tumor and normal renal development is best illustrated by the persistent nephrogenic rests seen within the normal kidney of children with Wilms tumor.[4,5] These lesions, also called precursor lesions, persistent metanephric blastema, nephroblastomatosis or nodular renal blastema are comprised of primitive blastemal cells with varying degrees of differentiation. They are usually less than 1 cm in diameter, but rarely can become massive, compressing the normal kidney and mistaken for a genuine tumor. Although foci of Wilms tumor can arise within a large nephrogenic rest, the precursor lesions themselves do not appear to be malignant and some have been shown to regress when followed noninvasively. Nephrogenic rests are present in the normal kidney at birth, but are rarely found after 1 year of age. In contrast, virtually all children with genetic susceptibility to Wilms tumor have one or more such lesions within otherwise normal kidney. In these children, nephrogenic rests may represent the effect of a constitutional mutation predisposing to abnormal renal development, the first step toward the formation of Wilms tumor. In support of this notion is the observation that nephrogenic rests located in the periphery of a renal lobe, so-called "perilobar rests," are found more frequently in the kidneys of children whose genetic susceptibility to Wilms tumor is associated with the locus on chromosome 11p15. Nephrogenic rests located within the renal lobe, known as "intralobar rests" are smaller and less well defined histologically, and are seen more commonly in the kidneys of children with evidence of a genetic lesion at the chromosome 11p13 locus.[5] However, even in the absence of genetic predisposition, some 30% of children with apparently sporadic Wilms tumor have nephrogenic rests within the normal surrounding kidney. Molecu-

lar evidence indicates that these nephrogenic rests harbor the same mutation in WT1 as that found in the accompanying Wilms tumor, suggesting that both the tumor and the precursor lesion are derived from the same renal stem cell in which the tumor suppressor gene was mutated.[6]

CLINICAL FEATURES

Nephroblastosis was first described in 1899 by a German physician, Max Wilms, as a uniformaly fatal cancer of children. With the use of modern multimodality therapy, the treatment of Wilms tumor has advanced dramatically, with a reported cure rate of 90% by the National Wilms' Tumor Study Group.[7] Wilms tumor usually arises by age 5, with equal incidence between sexes and among different ethnic groups. In children with genetic susceptibility, the age of incidence is usually under 2, and frequent screening by renal ultrasound is recommended. The usual presenting feature is that of an abdominal mass, with an adrenal malignancy such as neuroblastoma as the main differential diagnostic consideration. Initial preoperative evaluation is directed at excluding the presence of pulmonary metastases, local spread into the inferior vena cava, or involvement of draining lymph nodes. The surgical management of Wilms tumor calls for skill and experience, requiring the resection of the affected kidney, exploration of the inferior vena cave and lymph node dissection. Of utmost importance is the examination of the contralateral kidney for any synchronous tumor. The occurence of bilateral tumors in some 10% of cases is an indication of genetic susceptibility to Wilms tumor, but it cannot be excluded by a negative family history or the absence of associated congenital abnormalities. Most children with bilateral tumors have no prior evidence of genetic risk, and genetic studies to date have indicated that most of these children may harbor *de novo* germline mutations.[8,9] In the presence of bilateral Wilms tumors, most surgeons will perform a full nephrectomy on the side with the larger tumor and a partial nephrectomy on the other side, attempting to preserve as much renal function as possible.

Postoperative treatment of Wilms tumor with chemotherapy and radiation therapy is evolving as multi-institutional groups adjust the recommended regimens so as to improve the effectiveness and lower the toxicity of treatment.[10] Most children who fit into favorable prognostic groups based on tumor histology and stage are treated with chemotherapy including actinomycin D and vincristine. Radiation therapy in addition to chemotherapy is reserved for patients with anaplastic tumors or cancers of advanced stage. Wilms tumor appears to be very sensitive to chemotherapy drugs and even patients with advanced metastatic disease have an excellent cure rate. The incidence of secondary malignancies in children cured of Wilms tumor is low and appears to be treatment-related, consisting primarily of soft tissue sarcomas arising within the radiation field and acute leukemia attributed to the use of alkylating agents and radiation therapy.[11] Genetic predisposition to Wilms' tumor is only rarely associated with susceptibility to other tumor types, such as gonadoblastoma in Denys-Drash syndrome or adrenal carcinoma and hepatocellular carcinoma in Beckwith-Wiedemann syndrome. In the absence of such congenital syndromes, the great majority of children treated for Wilms tumor are fertile when they reach reproductive age, and the risk of Wilms tumor arising in their offspring has been found to be very low.[12]

THE KNUDSON MODEL IN WILMS TUMOR

Much of the conceptual basis for the genetic study of tumor suppressor genes was laid by Knudson in a series of epidemiologic studies of retinoblastoma, Wilms tumor and neuroblastoma.[13-15] These childhood tumors are remarkable in that 10–30% of affected children present with bilateral or multicentric cancers. Bilateral tumors have an age of onset that is one to two years earlier than that of unilateral cancers, and in the case of the eye tumor retinoblastoma, they are often associated with a positive family history. By comparing the incidence of unilateral versus bilateral retinoblastomas in patients with a positive family history, Knudson found that the data fit the Poisson distribution for a single rare event. Thus, these individuals, who had inherited one genetic mutation, only required one additional "genetic hit" in the target tissues to develop a tumor (see Fig. 21-2). Given the number of target cells at risk for the second hit, multiple tumors are common and they tend to arise early in life. In contrast, in the absence of genetic predisposition, two rare independent events are required for tumor formation, hence a low incidence of tumors, which are unilateral and which present at a later age. In addition to the difference in the mean age of tumor development between inherited and sporadic cases, the rate of decline in the incidence of new tumors is also predicted by the Knudson "two-hit" model. In genetically predisposed individuals, the age of onset declines exponentially, consistent with the exponential rate of differentiation of susceptible nephroblasts. In contrast, in sporadic cases, a more delayed decline in the incidence of new tumors is noted, suggesting that the second genetic lesion is dependent on the variable timing of the initial mutation.

The predictions of the Knudson model were first confirmed by the cloning of the retinoblastoma susceptibility gene, RB1.[16-18] Indeed, the two genetic hits represent the inactivation of the two alleles of this tumor suppressor gene.[19-22] The first hit appears to be most commonly a mutation or small deletion which is found in the germline of predisposed individuals, or in somatic tissues in sporadic cases. Loss of the second allele, which represents the second hit, is most commonly seen as a wholesale loss of a chromosome or a chromosomal recombinational event in somatic tissues. Such large chromosomal losses may be more frequent than the initial point mutation, but are only tolerated in the heterozygous state, explaining their prevalence as second rather than first hits. They have proven to be of critical importance in molecular mapping studies of tumor suppressor genes such as those responsible for retinoblastoma and Wilms tumor, since the loss of surrounding restriction fragment length polymorphisms (RFLP) points to the presence of a critical genetic locus.[23]

The epidemiology of Wilms tumor shares a number of features with that of retinoblastoma. Bilateral tumors are noted in 5–10% of cases, and as predicted by the Knudson model, these present at an earlier age than unilateral cases.[14,24,25] However, familial Wilms tumor is rare, estimated at <1% of cases. Based on the number of bilateral tumors, the mathematical model proposed by Knudson and Strong predicts that some 30% of children have a genetic predisposition to Wilms tumor. In the majority of cases, this genetic susceptibility appears to represent a *de novo* germline mutation, rather than a transmitted parental gene. In this context, it is of interest that in most Wilms tumors that show allelic DNA losses involving the 11p13 genetic locus, the lost allele (representing the second hit) is of maternal origin. These observations suggest that the initial mutation is likely to occur in the paternal germ cells during spermatogenesis.

Another distinction between retinoblastoma and Wilms tumor is the presence of a phenotype conferred by a single mutated allele. Individuals with a germline mutation in RB1 who fail to develop a tumor during the first few years of life have no detectable ocular abnormalities as adults, suggesting that hemizygosity for RB1 is phenotypically silent. In contrast, children with hemizygous deletions involving the 11p13 Wilms tumor locus (WAGR syndrome) have developmental abnormalities of the genito-urinary tract as well as nephrogenic rests within both kidneys.[26,27] Since nephrogenic rests consist of a proliferation of primitive blastemal cells, their presence may increase the size of the target cell population, thus enhancing the probability of a second genetic hit. The number of genetic lesions important in the development of Wilms tumor may in fact be greater than two. The Knudson model, based on the statistics of "hit kinetics," has proved to be accurate in predicting the number of genetic events that are rate limiting. However, genetic events that are necessary for malignant transformation but that are more frequent or that are dependent on these initial "hits" will not be detected by such an analysis. At least three genetic loci have been implicated in the initial events in Wilms tumorigenesis, and tumor specimens have been shown to have a number of additional chromosomal abnormalities that may have a role in tumor progression. The isolation of the first of these genes and the characterization of the genetic lesions that contribute to the development of Wilms tumor have provided an initial appreciation for the genetic complexity of this malignancy.[28]

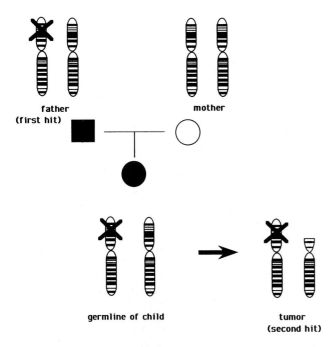

FIG. 21-2 Schematic representation of the Knudson model. Based on epidemiologic analyses of the age of incidence and number of tumors observed in children with genetic predisposition versus those with sporadic tumors, Knudson and Strong[12-14] predicted that two *rate limiting* "hits" are required for tumorigenesis. This hypothesis has evolved with the detection of allelic losses in tumors, and the concept of recessive oncogenes or tumor suppressor genes.[18,22] Thus, a mutation present either in the germline or in the germ cells of a parent constitutes the first hit. The child born with such a mutation in the germline requires only one additional hit in the target tissue to trigger tumorigenesis. The relatively high frequency of this second hit explains the early age of onset of tumors and the fact that they are often bilateral. In contrast, a child without a germline mutation requires two independent rare events within the target tissue, in order to achieve two rate limiting hits. The low probability of two independent mutations at the same locus explains the later onset of tumors in sporadic cases and the fact that they are unilateral. In most cases of Wilms tumor, the initial hit results from a point mutation or a small deletion within the target tumor suppressor gene, while the second hit consists of a gross chromosomal deletion or non-disjunction event. These large chromosomal events can be identified by the loss of restriction fragment length polymorphisms (RFLP) in the affected locus (so-called loss of heterozygosity), thus providing a clue to the presence of a tumor suppressor gene.

In the figure: father (first hit); mother; germline of child; tumor (second hit)

GENETIC LOCI ASSOCIATED WITH WILMS TUMOR

The identification of the major genetic loci associated with the development of Wilms tumor has resulted from studies of both germline and tumor material, using karyotype analysis, genetic linkage and molecular genetic studies, as well as clinical observations on patients with congenital abnormalities. Two distinct genetic loci have been mapped to the short arm of chromosome 11 (Table 21-1), while a third locus on chromosome 17q has been implicated in some familial cases .

Chromosome 11p13 Locus

The first linkage of Wilms tumor susceptibility to a chromosomal locus was derived from a clinical observation. In 1964, Miller and coworkers noted a higher than expected incidence of Wilms tumor in children with aniridia, a rare eye abnormality consisting of malformation or absence of the iris.[29] While Wilms tumor arises in 1 in 10, 000 children and aniridia occurs in 1 in 70, 000 children, aniridia is noted in 1 in 70 children with Wilms tumor and this tumor develops in 1 in 3 children with aniridia. As would be expected from the Knudson model, children with aniridia who develop a Wilms tumor have a high incidence of bilateral tumors, consistent with the presence of a predisposing germline lesion. This lesion is most clearly evident in children with a constellation of symptoms that includes aniridia, developmental abnormalities of the genito-urinary tract (such as hypospadia, undescended testes, renal hypoplasia or ureteral atresia) and mental retardation.[26,27] Children with this so-called WAGR syndrome (an acronym for <u>W</u>ilms, <u>A</u>nirida, <u>G</u>enito-urinary defects, mental <u>R</u>etardation) were found to have a gross cytogenetic deletion within band 13 of the short arm of chromosome 11[30,31] (Figure 21-3). This discovery was the first to link a gene conferring susceptibility to Wilms tumor to a genetic locus. The complex congenital abnormalities of children with WAGR syndrome results from a deletion which affects a number of adjacent genes, a so-called contiguous gene syndrome (see Figure 21-4). The aniridia locus was distinguished from the Wilms tumor locus by the existence of patients with an 11p13 chromosome translocation who suffered from aniridia without developing Wilms tumor.[32,33] Aniridia is now known to result from a hemizygous deletion of a homeobox gene, Pax 6.[34] The genito-urinary defects associated with WAGR syndrome are variable in their severity and appear to

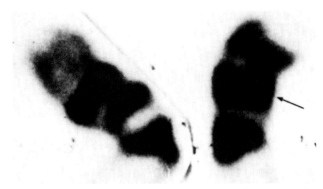

FIG. 21-3 Cytogenetic abnormality in WAGR syndrome. One of the two chromosomes 11 in the germline of a child with WAGR syndrome contains a deletion within band p13 (arrow). This large hemizygous deletion, encompassing a number of contiguous genes, leads to a >50% probability of developing Wilms tumor, abnormal development of the iris (aniridia), abnormalities of genito-urinary development and mental retardation.

result from hemizygosity for the Wilms tumor gene itself (see below). The etiology of the mental retardation is still unclear.

The involvement of the chromosome 11p13 locus in Wilms tumor development was also evidenced by molecular analysis of tumor specimens. Chromosome abnormalities in Wilms tumor specimens are complex, but frequently involve the short arm of chromosome 11.[35–38] More precise molecular studies, involving the use of polymorphic DNA markers were used to demonstrate loss of heterozygosity on chromosome 11p.[39–42] This represents the loss of gross chromosomal fragments or recombinational events resulting in the loss of the second allele of a putative tumor suppressor gene (the second genetic hit). The loss of heterozygosity at chromosome 11p13 that results from such mechanisms usually extends to the telomere, spanning the 11p15 locus. It can therefore be difficult to distinguish involvement of the two Wilms loci on the short arm of chromosome 11, but cases in which a more limited loss of DNA affects each locus in isolation have confirmed the independence of these two genetic loci.[43,44]

Chromosome 11p15

Like the 11p13 Wilms tumor locus, the 11p15 locus has been implicated both by genetic susceptibility studies and by allelic losses in tumor specimens.[39–46] However, the genetic mechanisms underlying the effects of the 11p15 locus appear to be more com-

Table 21-1 Summary of the Two Major Congenital Syndromes Associated with Increased Susceptibility to Wilms Tumor*

	WAGR Syndrome	Beckwith-Wiedemann Syndrome
Chromosomal locus	11p13	11p15
Tumor-suppressor gene	WT1	Unknown
Wilms tumor incidence	<50%	<5%
Associated features	Aniridia	Macroglossia
	Genitourinary defects	Organomegaly/hemihypertrophy
		Umbilical hernia
	Mental retardation	Neonatal hypoglycemia
		Additional tumors
		Adrenocortical carcinoma
		Hepatoblastoma

*The WAGR syndrome results from a hemizygous chromosomal deletion within the chromosome 11p13 locus, affecting the WT1 and aniridia genes. Beckwith-Wiedemann syndrome results from an abnormality in the 11p15 locus that may involve gene dosage as well as parental imprinting. The gene responsible for this syndrome and for the associated risk of developing Wilms tumor has not been identified.

chromosome band 11p13:

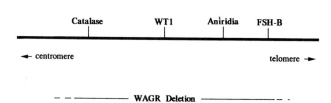

FIG. 21-4 Schematic map of the WAGR region. The 11p13 chromosomal deletion in children with WAGR syndrome is flanked on the centromeric side by the gene encoding catalase and on the telomeric side by the gene for the B subunit of follicle stimulating hormone. Within the deletion are located the Wilms tumor susceptibility gene WT1 and the anirida gene.

plex, involving genomic imprinting and unequal duplication of parental chromosomes. Increased susceptibility to Wilms tumor was noted by Wiedemann and by Beckwith in a syndrome which now bears their name.[47,48] Beckwith-Wiedemann syndrome consists of abnormally enlarged organs particularly the tongue and abdominal viscera, which can result in an umbilical hernia. Soft tissues can also be enlarged with one side more affected than the other, resulting in hemi-hypertrophy of the body. Neonatal hypoglycemia is also evident in more serious cases. Pediatric neoplasms are seen in 7.5% of children with Beckwith-Wiedemann syndrome, a far lower incidence than that in patients with WAGR syndrome, and these tumors include adrenocortical carcinoma and hepatoblastoma as well as Wilms tumor. The true penetrance of Beckwith-Wiedemann syndrome is difficult to ascertain, since the different manifestations of the syndrome can be quite variable, often rendering the clinical diagnosis uncertain.[49,50]

The association of Beckwith-Wiedemann syndrome with the chromosome 11p15 locus is based on genetic linkage studies in the rare families in which the condition is inherited,[51,52] as well as gross cytogenetic abnormalities in the germline of some sporadically affected individuals.[53,54] Abnormal karyotypes in such patients most frequently consist of a duplication of chromosome band 11p15, although in two cases, a ring chromosome has been reported.[55] The role of genetic imprinting in Beckwith-Wiedemann syndrome is suggested by a number of unusual observations. In the familial syndrome, the disease appears to be more severe when the affected chromosome is transmitted by the mother, rather than the father.[56] In contrast, in cases where trisomy for 11p15 is present, the duplicated chromosome is invariably of paternal origin.[57] Finally, molecular

studies have shown that in some cases of Beckwith-Wiedemann syndrome, affected children are diploid for 11p15, but have inherited two copies of the paternal chromosome and no maternal chromosome—so-called "uniparental isodisomy."[58,59] One possible explanation for these unusual genetic abnormalities may be that they can lead to differences in the dosage of a critically regulated gene (Figure 21-5). If such a gene were imprinted and expressed only from the paternal allele, duplication of the paternal chromosome, either in the form of uniparental isodisomy or partial 11p15 trisomy would then lead to a two-fold overexpression. In familial transmission of Beckwith-Wiedemann syndrome, a mutation resulting in increased expression of this gene would be expected to have a greater impact if it arose on the imprinted maternal allele than in the already expressed paternal allele.

The Wilms tumor gene at the 11p15 locus remains to be identified, but a number of candidate genes are of particular interest. The insulin-like growth factor II (IGF II) gene encodes an embryonic growth factor whose expression in most tissues is derived solely from the paternally derived allele. Inactivation of one allele of IGF II in the mouse germline results in small-sized offspring if the disrupted gene is transmitted by the father, but has no effect if transmitted by the mother.[60,61] Thus, the organomegaly associated with Beckwith-Wiedemann syndrome could be attributed to the doubling of IGF II expression levels caused by duplication of actively transcribed paternal allele.[62,63] The potential role of IGF II in Beckwith-Wiedemann syndrome is supported by the observation that some affected children show constitutional loss of imprinting of this gene (ie. expression from both alleles), without evidence of gross chromosomal alterations.[64, 65] Furthermore, sporadic Wilms tumors have high expression of IGF II,[66,67] and some tumors also show loss or relaxation of imprinting,[68,69] suggesting that this growth factor may also contribute directly to tumorigenesis. However, two other candidate genes at chromosome 11p15 have recently been reported. The cyclin dependent kinase inhibitor p57 is also imprinted,[70] and inactivating mutations in the expressed paternal allele have been detected in the germline of two children with Beckwith-Wiedemann syndrome.[71] These observations suggest that the overgrowth syndrome may result from loss of growth inhibition by p57, although additional genetic events would presumably be required to explain the chromosomal evidence for increased paternal gene copy number. A third gene at chromosome 11p15, H19, has also been implicated in Wilms tumorigenesis. H19 encodes an abundant transcript lacking an open reading frame, suggesting that it functions as RNA.[72] Transfection studies have shown that it suppresses tumor formation in nude mice, with-

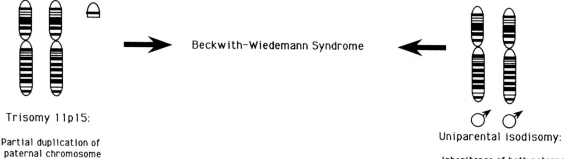

FIG. 21-5 Genetic mechanisms underlying Beckwith-Wiedemann syndrome. Beckwith-Wiedemann syndrome (hemihypertrophy, organomegaly, neonatal hypoglycemia and susceptibility to Wilms tumor, adrenocortecal carcinoma and hepatoblastoma) can be inherited and has been linked to chromosome 11p15 by studies of large pedigrees. In sporadic cases, gross chromosome abnormalities in the germline of affected children have also implicated chromosome 11p15 and have suggested that genomic imprinting may play a role in the syndrome. In

some cases, RFLP analysis has shown that affected children have inherited two copies of the paternal chromosomes 11, and neither of the maternal chromosomes 11.[57,58] In other cases, a partial duplication of the paternal 11p15 chromosomal fragment results in trisomy for this genetic locus.[52] These observations are consistent with a mechanism whereby the maternal allele is silent or "imprinted" and the syndrome results from the increased gene dosage caused by the presence of two paternal alleles.

out affecting in vitro growth properties.[73] Of particular interest is the observation that H19 and IGF II share regulatory sequences, with a reciprocal pattern of imprinting. Thus, H19 is expressed from the maternally-derived allele,[72] and expression would be lost in children who inherit two copies of the paternally-derived chromosome 11.

The association between the 11p15 chromosomal locus and Wilms tumor is supported by the increased incidence of this tumor in children with Beckwith-Wiedemann syndrome. However, molecular genetic analyses of Wilms tumor specimen have demonstrated allelic losses that affect 11p15, but spare the 11p13 genetic locus.[43,45] These allelic losses are usually indicative of gene deletion or "loss of function" events, which are difficult to reconcile with the apparent increased gene dosage mechanism commonly invoked for Beckwith-Wiedemann syndrome. It is therefore possible that the 11p15 Beckwith-Wiedemann and Wilms tumor locus contains multiple genes, disrupted by different genetic mechanisms. Molecular studies have also suggested that both the 11p13 and 11p15 Wilms tumor genes can contribute to tumorigenesis within the same tumor, based on cases in which distinct allelic losses are seen at both of these loci.[45,74] Unlike the WT1 gene isolated from the Wilms tumor locus on chromosome 11p13 which appears to be specifically involved in kidney development and tumorigenesis (see below), the putative gene(s) residing at chromosome locus 11p15 has been linked to a number of different tumor types. In addition to adrenocortical carcinoma, Wilms tumor and hepatoblastoma that are associated with Beckwith-Wiedemann syndrome, somatic allelic losses at 11p15 have been reported in breast cancer, lung cancer and acute myelogenous leukemia.[75,76]

Familial Wilms Tumor

Familial transmission of susceptibility to Wilms tumor is rare, estimated at less than 1% of cases.[14,25] Thus, the majority of children with evidence of genetic susceptibility appear to have *de novo* germline mutations. The 11p13 Wilms tumor gene WT1 has been implicated in a few familial cases of children with bilateral tumors or genitourinary defects.[8,9] However, in three large pedigrees of familial Wilms tumor, genetic linkage analysis has excluded chromosome 11.[77-79] Recently, analysis of a Canadian Wilms tumor kindred, remarkable for the relatively late onset of tumors and the absence of associated genitourinary defects, has indicated genetic linkage to chromosome 17q12-22.[80]

THE WT1 GENE AT CHROMOSOME 11P13

Identification and characterization of WT1

The isolation of the 11p13 Wilms tumor gene resulted from the analysis of patients with chromosomal deletions and translocations as well as the generation of human-hamster cell hybrids containing defined segments of chromosome 11p13.[81-86] These studies provided detailed maps of the WAGR region within chromosome 11p13, flanked on the centromeric side by the gene encoding catalase[87,88] and on the telomeric side by the gene for the b subunit of follicle stimulating hormone[89-92] (see Figure 21-4). The WT1 gene was isolated within the smallest region of overlap among chromosomal deletions.[93,94]

WT1 encodes a protein migrating at 55kD, with two regions of recognizable homology that indicate it functions as a transcription factor (Figure 21-6). The carboxy terminus contains four "zinc finger" domains, loop structures of amino acids that each contain two regularly spaced cysteines and histidines, bind to zinc ions and mediate recognition of a specific DNA sequence.[95] The amino terminus of WT1 is rich in prolines and glutamines, a feature shared by the transactivation domains of some transcription factors.[96] Two alternative splices are present within the WT1 transcript, resulting in four distinct mRNA species that are expressed in constant proportion to each other.[97] Alternative splice I, inserted within the amino terminus of WT1, encodes 17 amino acids including five serines and one threonine, potential sites for protein phosphorylation. Alternative splice II encodes three amino acids (lysine, threonine, serine, or "KTS") that disrupt the critical spacing between the third and fourth zinc finger domains. In the absence of alternative splice II, the WT1 zinc finger domains share extensive homology with the Early Growth Response gene (EGR 1, also known as NGFIA, Krox 24, Zif 268)[98] and recognize the EGR1 DNA binding consensus sequence.[89] WT1 protein also recognizes a TC-rich sequence[100,101] and binding site selection experiments have identified the sequence 5'-GCGTGGGAGT-3' as a potential higher affinity binding site.[102] In transient transfection experiments using promoter reporter constructs, WT1 functions as a repressor of transcription.[103] This effect, combined with the ability of WT1 to bind the GC-rich sequences present in many promoters have led to the identification of many potential WT1 target genes.[104] These have included EGR1,[99] IGF II,[105] platelet-derived growth factor-A (PDGF-A),[106,107] IGF receptor,[108,109] epidermal growth factor receptor (EGFR),[101] c-myc and bcl2,[110] retinoic acid receptor α,[111] Pax 2,[112] transforming growth factor β,[113] among many others. However, with the possible exception of EGFR,[101] IGF II[114] and

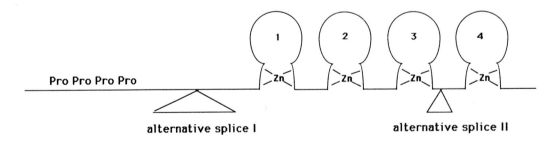

FIG. 21-6 Functional domains of the WT1 gene product. The predicted polypeptide encoded by WT1 contains two functional domains: The carboxy terminus contains four "zinc fingers" of the cysteine-histidine class, which constitute the DNA binding domain of WT1. This domain has a high degree of homology with that of the early growth response (EGR) Gene 1 and it confers a similar DNA binding specificity. The amino terminus of WT1 is rich in prolines (Pro) and con-stitutes the transactivation domain of WT1. This domain appears to be capable of suppressing the transcription of genes that are potential targets of WT1. Two alternative splices are variably inserted in the WT1 transcript, resulting in the presence of four distinct mRNA species. The function of alternative splice I is unknown, while insertion of alternative splice II disrupts the linker between zinc fingers 3 and 4 and alters the DNA binding specificity of the encoded protein.

IGFR,[109] none of these WT1-regulated promoters are correlated with regulation of endogenous genes by WT1. Thus, a level of target specificity may be evident with native promoters that is not observed in transient transfection assays. Interpretation of transient transfection experiments is futher confounded by evidence that WT1 can function as an activator as well as a repressor of transcription, depending upon cellular and promoter context, and even upon the choice of expression vector.[115–117]

Insertion of alternative splice II (KTS) abolishes binding of WT1 to the GC-rich promoters.[99] An alternative DNA binding sequence has been proposed,[118] but no potential targets have been identified. The WT1(+KTS) isoform accounts for ~80% of the cellular WT1 transcript,[97] suggesting that it makes an important contribution to the function of this tumor suppressor. Recently, WT1(+KTS) has been shown to associate with subnuclear clusters, in contrast to WT1(−KTS) which is diffusely localized in the nucleus.[119,120] Colocalization and coimmunoprecipitation studies have suggested that WT1(+KTS) is associated with small nucleoriboproteins (snRNPs), implying a potential role in pre-mRNA splicing.[119] However, the subnuclear clusters containing WT1(+KTS) are distinct from interchromatin granules containing the essential splicing factor SC35, that are thought to constitute assembly sites for the cellular splicing machinery.[120] Thus, the identity of WT1-associated subnuclear clusters is uncertain, and the relationship between WT1 and the pre-mRNA splicing machinery remains to be defined. In addition to alternative splicing, WT1 is phosphorylated in vivo, although the physiological consequences of this protein modification are unknown.[121]

Expression of WT1 during kidney development

WT1 is normally expressed in a small number of tissues, primarily those of the developing genitourinary tract.[122,123] This expression pattern is in marked contrast to the ubiquitously expressed tumor suppressor genes RB or p53, and may provide insight into the normal role of WT1 in cellular growth and differentiation. In the mouse kidney, WT1 expression is detectable by day 8 of gestation, rising to peak sharply around birth, and then rapidly declining to low adult levels by day 17.[123] In humans, WT1 expression has been reported to be high in 20 week kidney, and barely detectable in the adult organ.[74] Within the developing kidney, specific structures have been shown by in situ RNA hybridization to express WT1, including the condensed mesenchyme, renal vesicle and glomerular epithelium[122] (Figure 21-7). The transient expression pattern of WT1 in these early kidney structures is consistent with a gene that is critical during a defined period in normal kidney development (Figure 21-8). Disruption of this gene by a mutation may thus lead to uncontrolled proliferation of the early renal progenitor cells that are characteristic of Wilms tumor.

WT1 is also expressed in other specific cell types, such as the Sertoli cells of the testis, granulosa cells of the ovary, muscle cells of the uterus, stromal cells of the spleen, and mesothelial cells of the pericardial, pleural and peritoneal lining.[124-126] The WT1 pattern of expression in these tissues differs from that seen in the kidney, with persistent high levels of expression in adult organs. Expression of WT1 is also noted in acute leukemia cells, although the normal hematopoietic counterparts that express WT1 have not been identified. In addition to Wilms tumors, WT1 mutations have been reported in mesothelioma and leukemia.[126,127] However, with the exception of one case of gonadoblastoma,[128] individuals with a germline WT1 mutation do not have an increased incidence of tumors from tissues other than kidney. This suggests that the role played by WT1 in these tissues is not "rate-limiting" for tumorigenesis as it appears to be in the kidney.[28]

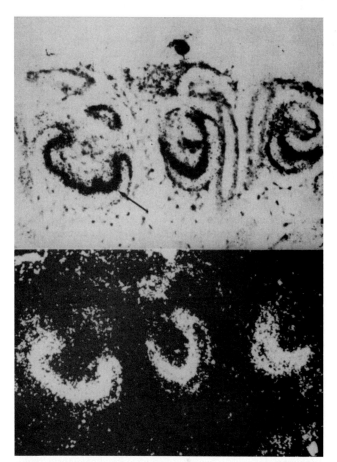

FIG. 21-7 Localization of WT1 mRNA expression in the developing kidney. Analysis of 20-week human kidney by *in situ* hybridization with the WT1 probe. Light phase (upper panel) and dark phase (lower panel) photomicrographs are shown to demonstrate the hybridization signal and the structures within the developing kidney that express WT1 mRNA. The "S-shaped body" is a precursor of the renal glomerulus, whose inner surface demonstrates high levels of WT1 mRNA expression (arrow). *(Photomicrograph kindly provided by Dr. Nic Hastie, Medical Research Council, Edinburgh, UK.)*

Inactivation of WT1 in the germline and in Wilms tumors

Germline mutations in one WT1 allele have been documented in children with bilateral Wilms tumors, consistent with the predictions of Knudson and Strong.[8,9] The germline mutation results either from a *de novo* event or, rarely, from familial transmission. Tumor specimens from these children confirm loss of the remaining wild-type WT1 allele, evidence of the "second hit." However, unlike retinoblastoma in which the initial germline mutation is phenotypically silent, a heterozygous WT1 mutation in the germline may result in dramatic developmental abnormalities. Mutations that result in a premature termination result in a phenotype that is similar to that of WAGR patients, bearing a hemizygous deletion of WT1.[9] This consists of variable severity of genitourinary abnormalities (undescended testes, abnormal urethral meatus, malformed kidneys), that are more severe in boys than in girls. This observation suggests that WT1 itself is the gene responsible for the genitourinary defects seen in children with WAGR syndrome. However, children with specific germline mutations that affect the WT1 DNA binding domains develop a far more severe constellation of genitourinary abnormalities, known as Denys-Drash syndrome.[128] These children have gross abnormalities of sexual development, resulting in pseudohermaphroditism and mesangial sclerosis of the kidney, leading to renal failure within

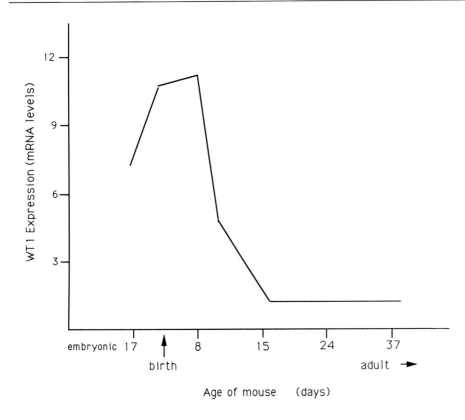

FIG. 21-8 Time course of WT1 expression in the mouse kidney. Schematic representation of WT1 mRNA levels in the mouse kidney assayed by Northern blot. WT1 expression is detectable at the earliest embryonic time point, peaks about the time of birth and then rapidly declines to adult levels.[95] In human kidney, WT1 is expressed at high levels at 20 weeks, and is no longer detectable in the adult organ.[66,94] Other tissues with high WT1 mRNA levels, such as the gonads, do not show this dramatic pattern of expression. Instead, WT1 expression increases during fetal development and remains high in the adult tissue.[96]

the first years of life. These observations suggest that expression of WT1 proteins with altered DNA binding domains can exert a "dominant negative" effect that disrupts normal genitourinary development to a far greater extent than simple reduction in gene dosage seen in WAGR syndrome.

Most Wilms tumors express high levels of WT1 mRNA and protein, consistent with their apparent cells of origin in the fetal kidney. By *in situ* RNA hybridization, WT1 expression has been localized to the epithelial and blastemal histological components within the tumor.[122] While in most Wilms tumors the WT1 transcript appears to be grossly intact, in ~10% of cases, deletions and point mutations within the gene have been identified[74, 129–133] (Figure 17-9). These mutations identify WT1 as the target of gene inactivation events at the chromosome 11p13 locus, and confirm its characterization as a tumor suppressor gene. The majority of WT1 mutations reported in Wilms tumors are homozygous, resulting from an initial point mutation in one allele, followed by loss of the second allele through a gross chromosomal event. However, some tumors have been found to express a single mutated WT1 allele, along with the remaining wild-type allele.[74,131] These observations have suggested that specific types of mutations, particularly those involving the DNA binding domain of WT1, may act as "dominant negative" mutations, in effect suppressing the function of the coexpressed wild-type allele.[134,135] A potential mechanism of action for such dominant negative mutations has been defined in vitro. WT1 dimerizes through the amino terminus domain, and mutants with an altered DNA binding domain abrogate the transactivational properties of wild-type WT1.[120,136,137] These mutants physically associate with subnuclear clusters and recruit transcriptionally active WT1(-KTS), in effect achieving an apparent intranuclear sequestration of the wild-type protein.[120]

In addition to mutational inactivation, unusual mechanisms of disrupting WT1 function contribute to Wilms tumor. An in-frame deletion of WT1 exon 2, within the transactivation domain is observed in ~10% of primary Wilms tumor specimens.[138] This splicing abnormality is not associated with a mutation in flanking

exon-intron junctions, but it is observed together with omission of alternative splice II (WT1 exon 5), suggesting a gene-specific abnormality in pre-mRNA processing. The encoded protein, WT1-del2, is a potent transcriptional activator, capable of antagonizing transcriptional repression of promoter reporters by wild-tpe WT1.[138] Another unusual disruption of WT1 occurs in a rare pediatric sarcoma, desmoplastic small round cell tumor (DSRT), which is characterized by a chromosomal translocation fusing the potent transactivation domain of the Ewing Sarcoma gene EWS to zinc fingers 2-4 of WT1.[139,140] These two transactivating variants of WT1, together with two Wilms tumor-associated point mutations that also convert WT1 into a potent transactivator,[126,141] provide strong genetic evidence for the physiological importance of transcriptional repression by wild-type WT1. They also raise the possibility that specific target genes might be repressed by wild-type WT1 and induced by these transforming WT1 variants.

In addition to abnormalities in pre-mRNA splicing, RNA editing has been reported in WT1.[142] The altered amino acid, within the transactivation domain of WT1 appears to result in subtle change in transactivational activity. The RNA edited WT1 transcripts constitute a fraction of the mRNA in rat kidney, but their role in Wilms tumor development is unknown.

Inactivation of WT1 in the mouse and animal models of Wilms tumor

WT1 is highly conserved in the mouse, both in terms of nucleotide conservation and pattern of tissue and developmental expression.[123] However, the genetic consequences of WT1 inactivation differ between human and mouse, particularly with respect to tumorigenesis. The small eye mouse mutation[143,144] is homologous to the aniridia phenotype in humans, and involves the Pax6 gene on mouse chromosome 2, which is syntenic with human chromosome band 11p13. One variant of the mouse mutation, so-called Sey/Dey,

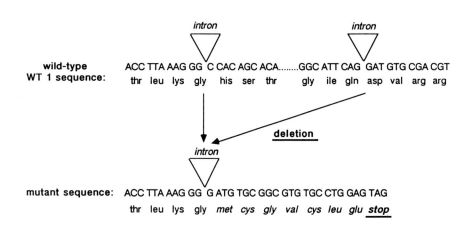

FIG. 21-9 Presence of inactivating mutations within the WT1 transcript. A subset of Wilms tumors contain inactivated copies of WT1, consistent with its characterization as a tumor suppressor gene. Gross deletions of WT1 appear to be rare, but small internal deletions or mutations can be found by nucleotide sequence analysis using the polymerase chain reaction (PCR). In this example,[7] a fragment of genomic DNA encoding an entire exon (flanked by two introns) has been deleted. The WT1 transcript in this Wilms tumor is the product of abnormal splicing, joining together the exons on either side of the deletion. The abnormal splice junction results in a frameshift, leading to seven novel amino acids (italics) followed by premature chain termination caused by a stop codon.

includes small eyes, a small body size and a white belly patch. The Sey/Dey mutation results from a hemizygous chromosomal deletion analogous to the WAGR deletion in humans, including hemizygosity for the mouse WT1 gene.[123,145] Homozygosity for the Sey/Dey allele is an embryonic lethal, but heterozygous mice have no detectable abnormalities of genito-urinary development, nor do they appear to have an increased risk of renal tumors. These observations have been confirmed in WT1-hemizygous mice generated by homologous recombination.[146] This apparent discrepancy between the effect of hemizygosity for WT1 in mouse and man raises a number of interesting questions. WT1 pathways in the mouse may involve a greater functional redundancy or genetic safeguards than humans, confering protection against malignant transformation in a somatic kidney cell, following loss of the remaining wild-type allele. Alternatively, the small number of target cells in the mouse kidney may reduce the probability of the second genetic hit. Finally, an intriguing genetic observation is that the two Wilms tumor loci that share the short arm of human chromosome 11 are separated in the mouse, with 11p13 syntenic with mouse chromosome 2 while 11p15 maps to mouse chromosome 7.[145] Thus, whereas a single chromosomal recombinational event is sufficient to cause loss of both genes in humans, two separate genetic events would be required in the mouse. While the mouse appears to be a reluctant Wilms tumor model, nephroblastomas do arise in the rat. The best studied models are nephroblastomas that arise either spontaneously or following transplacental treatment with the chemical carcinogen n-ethylnitrosourea or X-irradiation.[147-149] Point mutations in WT1 have been observed in some rat nephroblastomas,[150] implying that its inactivation contributes to tumorigenesis.

In contrast to the WT1-hemizygous mice, homozygous inactivation of WT1 has profound developmental consequences. WT1-null mice die at embryonic day 11.[146] The precise cause of death is uncertain, but gross cardiac and diaphragmatic defects appear to be implicated. WT1 is expressed in the mesothelial lining of these organs,[125,126] suggesting a potential developmental role. Of particular interest, WT1-null mice fail to develop either kidneys or gonads. Developmental arrest in the gonads precedes the sexually-undifferentiated stage, implicating WT1 in a very early step in gonadogenesis. The arrest in kidney differentiation precedes the induction of mesoderm by the ureteric bud, and mesenchymal tissue from WT1-null mice is resistant to exogenous induction signals.[146] Histological analysis of nephrogenic tissue from WT1-null mice reveals widespread apoptosis of blastemal stem cells. The role of WT1 in kidney development thus appears to involve a survival and potentially a permissive function for differentiating stem cells. The stage of peak WT1 expression which accompanies the differentiation of glomeruli is not reached in WT1-null mice, consistent with

a developmental arrest at the first developmental stage requiring WT1 expression.

Functional properties of WT1

Reconstitution of WT1 function in models of kidney differentiation remains to be achieved. However, a number of different functional properties are evident in cultured cell lines. Stable transfection of wild-type WT1 into a Wilms tumor cell line results in growth inhibition.[138] Inducible expression of the WT1(−KTS) isoform triggers apoptosis in osteosarcoma cell lines.[101] This effect is associated with transcriptional repression of the epidermal growth factor receptor (EGFR) and inhibition of endogenous EGFR synthesis, and it is abrogated by constitutive expression of EGFR. Thus, in these cells, inhibition of a growth factor pathway contributes to WT1-mediated cell death. Unlike other transcription factors whose overexpression triggers apoptosis, the ability of WT1 to induce cell death is independent of p53, indicating that it is not the result of conflicting growth-regulating signals, but rather a direct effect of WT1.[101] Expression of high levels of WT1 also leads to G1 phase cell cycle arrest.[151] This effect is associated with induction of the cyclin-dependent kinase inhibitor p21, and it is also independent of p53, another tumor suppressor known to induce p21 expression.[152] Increased p21 mRNA expression rapidly follows the inducible expression of WT1 protein, but direct regulation of the p21 promoter by WT1 has not been demonstrated. As in other developmental pathways, the combination of apoptotic signals and p21 induction may contribute to cellular differentiation.[153,154]

In addition to its growth inhibiting properties, WT1 also demonstrates the ability to inhibit apoptosis, specifically that mediated by p53.[155] WT1 and p53 proteins are coimmunoprecipitated from Wilms tumor specimens and developing rat kidney, and expression of WT1 leads to stabilization of wild-type p53 and modulation of its transactivational properties,[116,155] in addition to inhibition of apoptosis. Inhibition of p53-mediated cell death is observed in cells expressing low levels of WT1, consistent with the anti-apoptotic role of WT1 in renal stem cells that has been postulated by analysis of WT1-null mice. The ability of WT1 to stabilize and partially inactivate p53 is of particular interest, given that the majority of sporadic Wilms tumors contain wild-type WT1 and express high steady state levels of wild-type p53,[156,157] unlike many tumor types in which p53 is stabilized by inactivating mutations. Mutational inactivation of p53 in Wilms tumor is associated with the rare anaplastic variant,[158] which displays resistance to chemotherapy and an adverse prognosis.

CONCLUDING REMARKS

Wilms tumor is a genetically complex embryonic tumor, whose histological appearance is consistent with arrested differentiation of renal stem cells. The identification of the first Wilms tumor suppressor gene, WT1, has revealed a transcriptional regulator that is required for early kidney differentiation, but whose inactivation, presumably at a later stage of kidney development, results in Wilms tumor. Further characterization of this gene and isolation of additional Wilms tumor genes will provide geater understanding of the link between normal differentiation in the kidney and malignant transformation.

REFERENCES

1. Bennington J Beckwith J: Tumors of the kidney, renal pelvis and ureter. *in Atlas of Tumor Pathology,* series 2, fascile 12. Washington, DC, Armed Forces Institute of Pathology, 1975.
2. Breslow N, Churchill F, Nesmith B, Thomas P, Beckwith J, Othersen H, D'Angio G: Clinicopathologic features and prognosis for Wilms' tumor patients with metastases at dignosis. *Cancer* **58**: 2501, 1986.
3. Coppes M, Wilson P, Weitzman S: Extrarenal Wilms' tumor: staging, treatment and prognosis. *J Clin Oncol* **9**:167, 1991.
4. Bove K, McAdams A: The nephroblastomatosis complex and its relationship to Wilms' tumor: a clinicopathologic treatise. *Perspect Pediatr Pathol* **3**:185, 1976.
5. Beckwith J, Kiviat N, Bonadio J: Nephrogenic rests, nephroblastomatosis, and the pathogenesis of Wilms' tumor. *Ped Pathol* **10**:1, 1989.
6. Park S, Bernard A, Bove K, Sens D, Hazen-Martin D, Garvin A, Haber D: Inactivation of WT1 in nephrogenic rests, genetic precursors to Wilms' tumour. *Nature Genetics* **5**:363, 1993.
7. National Wilms Tumor Study Committee: Wilms' tumor: status report, 1990. *J Clin Oncol* **9**:877, 1990.
8. Huff V, Miwa H, Haber D, Call K, Housman D, Strong L, Saunders G: Evidence for WT1 as a Wilms tumor (WT) gene: intragenic germinal deletion in bilateral WT. *Am J Hum Genet* **48**:997, 1991.
9. Pelletier J, Bruening W, Li F, Haber D, Glaser T, Housman D: WT1 mutations contribute to abnormal genital system development and hereditary Wilms' tumour. *Nature* **353**:431, 1991.
10. Grundy P, Breslow N, Green D, Sharples K, Evans A, D'Angio G: Prognostic factors for children with recurrent Wilms' tumor: results from the second and third National Wilms' Tumor Study. *J Clin Oncol* **7**:638, 1989.
11. Bryd R, Levine A: Late treatment of Wilms' tumor. *in: Clinical and Biological Manifestations,* eds. C. Pochedly and E.S. Baum. New York, Elsevier **19**:347, 1984.
12. Li F, Gimbrere K, Gelber R, Sallan S, Flamant F, Green D, Heyn R, Meadows A: Outcome of pregnancy in survivors of Wilms' tumor. *JAMA* **257**:216, 1987.
13. Knudson A: Mutation and cancer: statistical study of retinoblastoma. *Proc Natl Acad Sci USA* **68**:820, 1971.
14. Knudson A, Strong L: Mutation and cancer: a model for Wilms tumor of the kidney. *J Natl Cancer Inst* **48**:313, 1972.
15. Knudson A , Strong L: Mutation and cancer: neuroblastoma and pheochromocytoma. *Am J Hum Genet* **24**:514, 1972.
16. Friend S, Bernards R, Rogelj S, Weinberg R, Rapaport J, Albert D, Dryja T: A human DNA segment with properties of the gene that predisposes to retinoblastoma and osteosarcoma. *Nature* **323**:643, 1986.
17. Lee W, Bookstein R, Hong F, Young L, Shew J, Lee E: Human retinoblastoma susceptibility gene: cloning, identification, and sequence. *Science* **235**:1394, 1987.
18. Fung Y, Murphree A, T'Ang A, Ouian J, Hinrichs S, Benedict W: Structural evidence for the authenticity of the retinoblastoma tumor susceptibility gene. *Science* **236**:1657, 1987.
19. Comings D: A general theory of carcinogenesis. *Proc Natl Acad Sci USA* **70**:3324, 1973.
20. Knudson A: Hereditary cancer, oncogenes, and antioncogenes. *Cancer Res* **45**:1437, 1985.
21. Dunn J, Philips R, Becker A, Gallie B: Identification of germline and somatic mutations affecting the retinoblastoma gene. *Science* **241**:1797, 1988.
22. Yandell D, Campbell T, Dayton S, Petersen R, Walton D, Little J, McConkie-Rosell A, Buckley, E Dryja T: Oncogenic point mutations in the human retinoblastoma gene: their application to genetic counselling. *N Engl J Med* **321**:1689, 1989.
23. Cavenee W, Dryja T, Phillips R, Benedict W, Godbout R, Gallie B, Murphree A, Strong L, White R: Expression of recessive alleles by chromosomal mechanisms in retinoblastoma. *Nature* **305**:779, 1983.
24. Matsunaga E: Genetics of Wilms' tumor. *Hum Genet* **57**:231, 1981.
25. Cochran W, Froggatt P: Bjilateral nephroblastoma in two sisters. *J Urol* **97**:216, 1967.
26. Pendergrass T: Congenital anomalies in children with Wilms' tumor, a new survey. *Cancer* **37**:403, 1976.
27. Breslow N, Beckwith J: Epidemiological features of Wilms' tumor: results of the National Wilms' Tumor Study. *J Natl Cancer Inst* **68**:429, 1982.
28. Haber D, Housman D: Rate-limiting steps: the genetics of pediatric cancers. *Cell* **64**:5, 1991.
29. Miller R, Fraumeni J, Manning M: Association of Wilms' tumor with aniridia, hemihypertrophy and other congenital malformations. *N Eng J Med* **270**:922, 1964.
30. Riccardi V, Sujansky E, Smith A, Francke U: Chromosomal imbalance in the aniridia-Wilms' tumor association: 11p interstitial deletion. *Pediatrics* **61**:604, 1978.
31. Francke U, Holmes L, Atkins L, Riccardi V: Aniridia-Wilms' tumor association: evidence for specific deletion of 11p13. *Cytogenet Cell Genet* **24**:185, 1979.
32. Simola K, Knuutila S, Kaitila I, Pirkola A, Pohja P: Familial aniridia and translocation t(4;11)(q22;p13) without Wilms' tumor. *Hum Genet* **63**:158, 1983.
33. Moore J, Hyman S, Antonarakis S, Mules E, Thomas F: Familial isolated aniridia associated with a translocation involving chromosomes 11 and 22 (t(11;22)(p13;q12.20)). *Hum Genet* **72**:297, 1986.
34. Ton C, Hirronen M, Miwa H, Weil M, Monaghan P, Jordan T, vanHeyningen V, Hastie N, Meigers-Heijboer H, Drechsler M, Royer-Pokora B, Collins F, Swaroop A, Strong LC, Saunders GF: Positional cloning and characterization of a paired box- and homeobox-containing gene from the aniridia region. *Cell* **67**:1059, 1991.
35. Kondo K, Chilcote R, Maurer H, Rowley J: Chromosome abnormalities in tumor cells from patients with sporadic Wilms' tumor. *Cancer Res* **44**:5376, 1984.
36. Douglass E, Wilimas J, Green A, Look A: Abnormalities of chromsomes 1 and 11 in Wilms' tumor. *Cancer Genet Cytogenet* **14**:331, 1985.
37. Solis V, Pritchard J, Cowell J: Cytogenetic changes in Wilms' tumors. *Cancer Genet Cytogenet* **34**:223, 1988.
38. Wang-Wuu S, Soukup S, Bove K, Gotwals B, Lampkin B: Chromosome analysis of 31 Wilms tumors. *Cancer Res* **50**:2786, 1990.
39. Fearon E, Vogelstein B, Feinberg A: Somatic deletion and dupication of genes on chromosome 11 in Wilms' tumours. *Nature* **309**:176, 1984.
40. Koufos A, Hansen M, Lampkin B, Workman M, Copeland N, Jenkins N, Cavenee W: Loss of alleles at loci on human chromosome 11 during genesis of Wilms' tumour. *Nature* **309**:170, 1984.
41. Orkin S, Goldman D, Sallan S: Development of homozygosity for chromosome 11p markers in Wilms' tumour. *Nature* **309**:172, 1984.
42. Reeve A, Housiaux P, Gardner R, Chewing W, Grindley R, Millow L: Loss of a Harvey ras allele in sporadic Wilms' tumour. *Nature* **309**:174, 1984.
43. Mannens M, Slater R, Heyting C, Bliek J, Kraker Jd, Coad N, Pagter-Holthuizen P, Pearson P: Molecular nature of genetic changes resulting in loss of heterozygosity of chromosome 11 in Wilms' tumor. *Hum Genet* **81**:41, 1988.
44. Glaser T, Jones C, Douglass E, Housman D: Consitutional and somatic mutations of chromosome 11p in Wilms' tumor. 253, 1989.
45. Henry I, Jeanpierre M, Couillin P, Barichard F, Serre J, Journel H, Lamouroux A, Turleau C, Grouchy J, Junien C: Molecular definition of the 11p15.5 region involved in Beckwith-Wiedemann syndrome and probably in predisposition to adrenocortical carcinoma. *Hum Genet* **81**:273, 1989.
46. Reeve A, Sih S, Raizis A, Feinberg A: Loss of allelic heterozygosity at a second locus on chromosome 11 in sporadic Wilms' tumor cells. *Mol Cell Biol* **9**:1799, 1989.
47. Wiedemann H: Complexe malformatif familial avec hernie ombilicale et macroglossie—Un syndrome nouveau? *J Genet Hum* **13**:223, 1964.
48. Beckwith J: Macroglossia, omphalocele, adrenal cytomegaly, gigantism and hyperplastic visceromegaly. *Birth Defects* **5**:188, 1969.

49. Sotelo-Avila C, Gonzalez-Crussi F, Fowler J: Complete and incomplete forms of Beckwith-Wiedemann syndrome: their oncogenic potential. *J Ped* **96**:47, 1980.

50. Wiedemann H: Tumor and hemihypertrophy associated with Wiedemann-Beckwith's syndrome. *Eur J Ped* **141**:129, 1983.

51. Koufos A, Grundy P, Morgan K, Aleck K, Hadro T, Lampkin B, Kalbakji A Cavenee W: Familial Wiedemann-Beckwith syndrome and a second Wilms' tumor locus both map to qqp15.5. *Am J Hum Genet* **44**:711, 1989.

52. Ping J, Reeve A, Law D, Young M, Boehnke M, Feinberg A: Genetic linkage of Beckwith-Wiedemann syndrome to 11p15. *Am J Hum Genet* **23**:165, 1989.

53. Waziri M, Patil S, Hanson J Bartley S: Abnormality of chromosome 11 in patients with features of Beckwith-Wiedemann syndrome. *J Pediatr* **102**:873, 1983.

54. Turleau C, Grouchy J, Nihoul-Fekete C, Chavin-Colin F Junien C: Del 11p13/nephroblastoma without aniridia. *Hum Genet* **67**:455, 1984.

55. Romain D, Gebbie O, Parfitt R, Columbano-Green L, Smythe R, Chapman C, Kerr A: Two cases of ring chromosome 11. *J Med Genet* **20**:380, 1983.

56. Niikawa N, Ishikiriyama S, Takahashi S, Inagawa A, Tonoki H, Ohta Y, Hase N, Kamei T, Kajii T: The Widemann-Beckwith syndrome: Pedigree studies on five families with evidence for autosomal dominant inheritance with variable expressivity. *Am J Med Genet* **24**:41, 1986.

57. Brown K, Williams J, Maitland N, Mott M: Genomic imprinting and the Beckwith-Wiedemann syndrome. *Am J Hum Genet* **46**:1000, 1990.

58. Henry I, Bonaiti-Pellie C, Chehensse V, Beldjord C, Schwartz C, Utermann G, Junien C: Uniparental paternal disomy in a genetic cancer-predisposing syndrome. *Nature* **351**:665, 1991.

59. Grundy P, Telzerow P, Haber D, Li F, Paterson M, Garber J: Chromosome 11 uniparental isodisomy in a child with hemihypertrophy and embryonal neoplasms. *Lancet* 1992.

60. DeChiara T, Efstradiadis A, Robertson E: A growth-deficiency phenotype in heterozygous mice carrying an insulin-like growth factor II gene disrupted by targeting. *Nature* **345**:78, 1990.

61. DeChiara T, Roberson E, Efstradiatis A: Parental imprinting of the mouse insulin-like growth factor I gene. *Cell* **64**:849, 1991.

62. Giannoukakis N, Deal C, Paquette J, Goodyer C, Polychronakos C: Parental genomic imprinting of the human IGF2 gene. *Nature Genetics* **4**:98, 1993.

63. Ohlsson R, Nystrom A, Pfeifer-Ohlsson S, Tohonen V, Hedborg F, Schofield P, Flam F, Ekstrom T: IGF2 is parentally imprinted during human embryogenesis and in the Beckwith-Wiedemann syndrome. *Nature Genetics* **4**:94, 1993.

64. Weksberg R, Shen D, Fei Y, Song Q, Squire J: Disruption of insulin-like growth factor 2 imprinting in Beckwith-Wiedemann syndrome. *Nature Genetics* **5**:143, 1993.

65. Ogawa O, Becroft D, Morison I, Ecles M, Skeen J, Mauger D, Reeve A: Constitutional relaxation of insulin-like growth factor II gene imprinting associated with Wilms' tumour and gigantism. *Nature Genetics* **5**:408, 1993.

66. Reeve A, Eccles M, Wilkins R, Bell G, Millow L: Expression of insulin-like growth factor-II transcripts in Wilms' tumour. *Nature* **317**:258, 1985.

67. Scott J, Cowell J, Roberson M, Priestly L, Wadey R, Hopkins B, Pritchard J, Bell G, Rall L, Graham C, Knott T: Insulin like growth factor-II gene expression in Wilms' tumor and embryonic tissues. *Nature* **317**:260, 1985.

68. Rainier S, Johnson L, Dobry C, Ping A, Grundy P, Feinberg A: Relaxation of imprinted genes in human cancer. *Nature* **362**:747, 1993.

69. Ogawa O, Eccles M, Szeto J, McNoe L, Yun K, Maw M, Smith P, Reeve A: Relaxation of insulin-like growth factor II gene imprinting implicated in Wilms' tumour. *Nature* **362**:749, 1993.

70. Matuoka S, Thompson J, Edwards M, Barletta J, Grundy P, Kalikin L, Harper J, Elledge S, Feinberg A: Imprinting of the gene encoding a human cyclin-dependent kinase inhibitor, p57^{KIP2}, on chromosome 11p15. *Proc Natl Acad Sci USA* **93**:3026, 1996.

71. Hatada I, Ohashi H, Fukushima Y, Kaneko Y, Inoue M, Komoto Y, Okada A, Ohishi S, Nabetani A, Morisaki H, Nakayama M, Niikawa N, Mukai T: An imprinted gene p57^{KP2} is mutated in Beckwith-Wiedemann syndrome. *Nature Genet* **14**:171, 1996.

72. Bartolomei M, Zemel S, Tilghman S: Parental imprinting of the mouse H19 gene. *Nature* **351**:153, 1991.

73. Hao Y, Crenshaw T, Moulton T, Newcomb E, Tycko B: Tumour-suppressor activity of H19 RNA. *Nature* **365**:764, 1993.

74. Haber D, Buckler A, Glaser T, Call K, Pelletier J, Sohn R, Douglass E Housman D. An internal deletion within an 11p13 zinc finger gene contributes to the development of Wilms' tumor. *Cell* **61**:1257, 1990.

75. Weston A, Willey J, Modali R, Sugimura H, McDowell E, Resau J, Light B, Haugen A, Mann D, Trump B, Harris C: Differential DNA sequence deletions from chromosomes 3,11,13, and 17 in squamous-cell carcinoma, large-cell carcinoma and adenocarcinoma of the lung. *Proc Natl Acad Sci USA* **86**:5099, 1989.

76. Ahuja H, Foti A, Zhou D, Cline M: Analysis of proto-oncogenes in acute myeloid leukemia: loss of heterozygosity for the Ha-ras gene. *Blood* **75**:819, 1990.

77. Huff V, Compton D, Chao L, Strong L, Geiser C, Saunders G: Lack of linkage of familial Wilms' tumour to chromosomal band 11p13. *Nature* **336**:377, 1988.

78. Grundy P, Koufos A, Morgan K, Li F, Meadows A, Cavenee W: Familial predisposition to Wilms' tumour does not map to the short arm of chromosome 11. *Nature* **336**:374, 1988.

79. Schwartz C, Haber D, Stanton V, Strong L, Skolnick M, Housman D: Familial predisposition to Wilms tumor does not segregate with the WT1 gene. *Genomics* **10**:927, 1991.

80. Rahman N, Arbour A, Tonin P, Renshaw J, Pelletier J, Baruchel S, Pritchard-Jones K, Stratton M, Narod S: Evidence for a familial Wilms' tumour gene (FWT1) on chromosome 17q12-21. *Nature Genet* **13**:461, 1996.

81. Glaser T, Jones C, Call K, Lewis W, Bruns G, Junien C, Waziri M, Housman D: Mapping the WAGR region of chromosome 11p: somatic cell hybrids provide a fine-structure map. *Cytogen Cell Genet* **46**:620, 1987.

82. Glaser T, Rose E, Morse H, Housman D, Jones C: A panel of irradiation-reduced hybrids selectively retaining human chromosome 11p13: their structure and use to purify the WAGR gene complex. *Genomics* **6**:48, 1990.

83. Porteous D, Bickmore W, Christie S, Boyd P, Cranston G, Fletcher J, Gosden J, Rout D, Seawright A, Simola K, van Heyningen V, Hastie N: HRAS1 selected chromosome transfer generates markers that colocalize aniridia- and genitourinary dysplasia-associated translocation breakpoints and the Wilms' tumor gene within 11p13. *Proc Natl Acad Sci USA* **84**:5355, 1987.

84. Davis L, Byers M, Fukushima Y, Quin S, Nowak N, Scoggin C, Shows T: Four new DNA markers are assigned to the WAGR region of 11p13: Isolation and regional assignment of 112 chromosome 11 anonymous DNA segments. *Genomics* **3**:264, 1988.

85. Couillin P, Azoulay M, Henry I, Ravise N, Grisard M, Jeanpierre C, Barichard F, Metezeau F, Chandelier J, Lewis W, van Heyningen V, Junien C: Characterization of a panel of somatic cell hybrids for subregional mapping along 11p and within band 11p13. Subdivision of the WAGR complex region. *Hum Genet* **82**:171, 1989.

86. Gessler M, Thomas G, Couillin P, Junien C, McGillvray B, Hayden M, Jaschek G, Bruns G: A deletion map of the WAGR region of chromosome 11. *American Journal of Human Genetics* **44**:486, 1989.

87. Junien C, Turleau C, Grouchy Jd, Said R, Rethore M, Tenconi R, Dufier J: Regional assignment of catalase (CAT) gene to band 11p13. Association with the aniridia-Wilms' tumor-gonadoblastoma (WAGR) complex. *AN Genet* **23**:165, 1980.

88. van Heyningen V, Boyd P, Seaqright A, Fletcher J, Fantes J, Buckton K, Spowart G, Porteous D, Hill R, Newton M, Hastie N: Molecular analysis of chromosome 11 deletions in aniridia-Wilms' tumor syndrome. *Proc Natl Acad Sci USA* **82**:8592, 1985.

89. Glaser T, Lewis W, Bruns G, Watkins P, Rogler C, Shows T, Powers V, Willard H, Goguen J, Simola K, Housman D:The B-subunit of follicle-stimulating hormone is deleted in patients with aniridia and Wilms' tumour, allowing a further definition of the WAGR locus. *Nature* **321**:882, 1986.

90. Compton D, Weil M, Jones C, Riccardi V, Strong L, Saunders G:Long range physical map of the Wilms' tumor-aniridia region on human chromosome 11. *Cell* **55**:827, 1988.

91. Gessler M, Bruns G: A physical map around the WAGR complex on the short arm of chromosome 11. *Genomics* **5**:43, 1989.

92. Rose E, Glaser T, Jones C, Smith C, Lewis W, Call C, Minden M, Champagne E, Boncetta L, Yeger H, Housman D: Complete physical map of the WAGR region of 11p13 localizes a candidate Wilms' tumor gene. *Cell* **60**:495, 1990.

93. Call K, Glaser T, Ito C, Buckler A, Pelletier J, Haber D, Rose E, Kral A, Yeger H, Lewis W, Jones C, Housman D: Isolation and characteri-

zation of a zinc finger polypeptide gene t the human chromosome 11 Wilms' tumor locus. *Cell* **60**:509, 1990.

94. Gessler M, Poustka A, Cavenee W, Neve R, Orkin S, Bruns G: Homozygous deletion in Wilms tumours of a zinc-finger gene identified by chromosome jumping. *Nature* **343**:774, 1990.

95. Evans R, Hollenberg S: Zinc figners: gilt by association. *Cell* **52**:1, 1988.

96. Mitchell P, Tijan R:Transcriptional regulation in mammalian cells by sequence-specific DNA binding proteins. *Science* **245**:371, 1989.

97. Haber D, Sohn R, Buckler A, Pelletier J, Call K, Housman D: Alternative splicing and genomic structure of the Wilms tumor gene WT1. *Proc Natl Acad Sci USA* **88**:9618, 1991.

98. Sukhatme V, Cao X, Chang L, Tsai-Morris C, Stamenkovich D, Ferreira P, Cohen D, Edwards S, Shows T, Curran T, LeBeau M, Adamson E: A zinc finger encoding gene coregulated with c-fos during growth and differentiation and after cellular depolarization. *Cell* **53**:37, 1988.

99. Rauscher F, Morris J, Tournay O, Cook D, Curran T: Binding of the Wilms' tumor locus zinc finger protein to the EGR-1 consensus sequence. *Science* **250**:1259, 1990.

100. Wang Z, Qiu Q, Enger K, Deuel T: A second transcriptionally active DNA-binding site for the Wilms tumor gene product, WT1. *Proc Natl Acad Sci USA* **90**:8896, 1993.

101. Englert C, Hou X, Maheswaran S, Bennett P, Ngwu C, Re G, Garvin A, Rosner M, Haber D: WT1 suppresses synthesis of the epidermal growth factor receptor and induces apoptosis. *EMBO J* **14**:4662, 1995.

102. Nakagama H, Heinrich G, Pelletier J, Housman D: Sequence and structural requirements for high-affinity binding by the WT1 gene product. *Mol Cell Biol* **15**:1489, 1995.

103. Madden S, Cook D, Morris J, Gashler A, Sukhatme V, Rauscher III F: Transcriptional repression mediated by the WT1 Wilms tumor gene product. *Science* **253**:1550, 1991.

104. Rauscher III F: The WT1 Wilms tumor gene product: a developmentally regulated transcription factor in the kidney that functions as a tumor suppressor. *FASEB J* **7**:896, 1993.

105. Drummond I, Badden S, Rohwer-Nutter P, Bell G, Sukhatme V, Rauscher III F: Repression of the insulin-like growth factor II gene by the Wilms tumor suppressor WT1. *Science* **257**:674, 1992.

106. Gashler A, Bonthron D, Madden S, Rauscher III F, Collins T, Sukhatme V: Human platelet-derived growth factor A chain is transcriptionally repressed by the Wilms tumor suppressor WT1. *Proc Natl Acad Sci USA* **89**:10984, 1992.

107. Wang Z, Madden S, Deuel T, Rauscher III F: The Wilms' tumor gene product, WT1, represses transcription of the platelet-derived growth factor A-chain gene. *J Biol Chem* **267**:21999, 1992.

108. Werner H, Re G, Drummond I, Sukhatme V, Rauscher III F, Sens D, Garvin A, Le Roith D,Roberts Jr C: Increased expression of the insulin-like growth factor I receptor gene IGF1R in Wilms tumor is correlated with modulation of IGF1R promoter activity by the WT1 Wilms tumor gene product. *Proc Natl Acad Sci USA* **90**:5828, 1993.

109. Werner H, Shen-Orr Z, RauscherIII F, Morris J, Toberts C, LeRoith D: Inhhibition of cellular proliferation by the Wilms' tumor suppressor WT1 is associated with supperession of insulin-like growth factor I receptor gene expression. *Mol Cell Biol* **15**:3516, 1995.

110. Hewitt S, Hamada S, McDonnell T, Rauscher III F, Saunders G: Regulation of the proto-oncogenes bcl-2 and c-myc by the Wilms' tumor suppressor gene WT1. *Cancer Research* **55**:5386, 1995.

111. Goodyer P, Dehbi M, Torban E, Bruening W, Pelletier J: Repression of the retinoic acid receptor-a gene by the Wilms' tumor suppressor gene product, wt1. *Oncogene* **10**:1125, 1995.

112. Ryan G, Steele-Perkins V, Morris J, Rauscher III F: Repression of Pax-2 by WT1 during normal kidney development. *Development* **121**:867, 1995.

113. Dey B, Sukhatme V, Roberts A, Sporn M, Rauscher III F, Kim S: repression of the transforming growth factor b1 gene by the Wilms tumor suppressor WT1 gene product. *Mol. Endocrinol.* **8**:595, 1994.

114. Nichols K, Re G, Yan Y, Garvin A, Haber D: WT1 induces expression of insulin-like growth factor 2 in Wilms' tumor cells. *Cancer Res* **55**:4540, 1995.

115. Wang Z-Y, Qiu Q-Q, Deuel T: The Wilms' tumor gene product WT1 activates or suppresses transcription through separate functional domains. *J Biol Chem* **268**:9172, 1993.

116. Maheswaran S, Park S, Bernard A, Morris J, Rauscher III F, Hill D, Haber D: Physical and functional interction between WT1 and p53 proteins. *Proc Natl Acad Sci USA* **90**:5100, 1993.

117. Reddy J, Hosono S, Licht J: The transcriptional effect of WT1 is modulated by choice of expression vector. *J Biol Chem* **270**:29976, 1995.

118. Bickmore W, Oghene K, Little M, Seawright A, van Heyningen V, Hastie N: Modulation of DNA binding specificity by alternative splicing of the Wilms tumor wt1 gene transcript. *Science* **257**:235, 1992.

119. Larsson S, Charlieu J, Miyagawa K, Engelkamp D, Rassoutzadegan M, Ross A, Cuzin F, van Heyningen V, Hastie N: Subnuclear localization of WT1 in splicing or transcription factor domains is regulated by alternative splicing. *Cell* **81**:391, 1995.

120. Englert C, Vidal M, Maheswaran S, Ge Y, Ezzell R, Isselbacher K, Haber D: Truncated WT1 mutants alter the subnuclear localization of the wild-type protein. *Proc Natl Acad Sci USA* **92**:11960, 1995.

121. Ye Y, Raychaudhuri B, Gurney A, Campbell C, Williams B: Regulation of WT1 by phosphorylation: inhibition of DNA binding, alteration of transcriptional activity and cellular translocation. *EMBO J* **15**:5606, 1996.

122. Pritchard-Jones K, Fleming S, Davidson D, Bickmore W, Porteous D, Gosden C, Bard J, Buckler A, Pelletier J, Housman D, van Heyningen V, Hastie N: The candidate Wilms' tumour gene is involved in genitourinary development. *Nature* **346**:194, 1990.

123. Buckler A, Pelletier J, Haber D, Glaser T, Housman D: Isolation, characterization, and expression of the murine Wilms' tumor gene (WT1) during kidney development. *Mol Cell Biol* **11**:1707, 1991.

124. Pelletier J, Schalling M, Buckler A, Rogers A, Haber D, Housman D: Expression of the Wilms' tumor gene WT1in the murine urogenital system. *Genes & Dev* **5**:1345, 1991.

125. Armstrong J, Pritchard-Jones K, Bickmore W, Hastie N, Bard J: The expression of the Wilms' tumor gene, WT1, in the developing mammalian embryo. *Mechanisms of Development* **40**:85, 1992.

126. Park S, Schalling M, Bernard A, Maheswaran S, Shipley G, Roberts D, Fletcher J, Shipman R, Rheinwald J, Demetri G, Griffin J, Minden M, Housman D, Haber D: The Wilms tumour gene WT1 is expressed in murine mesoderm-derived tissues and mutated in a human mesothelioma. *Nature Genetics* **4**:415, 1993.

127. King-Underwood L, Renshaw J, Pritchard-Jones K: Mutations in the Wilms' tumor gene WT1 in leukemias. *Blood* **87**:2171, 1996.

128. Pelletier J, Bruening W, Kashtan C, Mauer S, Manivel J, Striegel J, Houghton D, Junien C, Habib R, Fouser L, Fine R, Silverman B, Haber D, Housman D: Germline mutations in the Wilms' tumor suppressor gene are associated with abnormal urogenital development in Denys-Drash syndrome. *Cell* **67**:437, 1991.

129. Ton C, Huff V, Call K, Cohn S, Strong L, Housman D, Saunders G: Smallest region of overlap in Wilms' tumor deletions uniquely implicates an 11p13 zinc finger gene as the disease locus. *Genomics* **10**:293, 1991.

130. Cowell J, Wadey R, Haber D, Call K, Housman D, Prichard J: Structural rearrangements of the WT1 gene in Wilms' tumor cells. *Oncogene* **6**:595, 1991.

131. Little M, Prosser J, Condie A, Smith P,van Heyningen V, Hastie N: Zinc finger point mutations within the WT1 gene in Wilms tumor patients. *Proc Natl Acad Sci USA* **89**:4791, 1992.

132. Coppes M, Liefers G, Paul P, Yeger H, Williams B: Homozygous somatic WT1 point mutations in sporadic unilateral Wilms tumor. *Proc Natl Acad Sci USA* **90**:1416, 1993.

133. Varanasi R, Bardeesy N, Gharemani M, Petruzzi M-J, Nowak N, Adam M, Grundy P, Shows T, Pelletier J: Fine structure analysis of the WT1 gene in sporadic Wilms tumors. *Proc Natl Acad Sci USA* **91**:3554, 1994.

134. Herskowitz I. Functional inactivation of genes by dominant negative mutations. *Nature* **329**:219, 1987.

135. Haber D, Timmers H, Pelletier J, Sharp P, Housman D: A dominant mutation in the Wilms tumor gene WT1 cooperates with the viral oncogene E1A in transformation of primary kidney cells. *Proc Natl Acad Sci USA* **89**:6010, 1992.

136. Reddy J, Morris J, Wang J, English M, Haber D, Shi Y, Licht J: WT1-mediated transcriptional activation is inhibited by dominant negative mutant proteins. *J Biol Chem* **270**:10878, 1995.

137. Moffett P, Bruening W, Nakagama H, Bardeesy N, Housman D, Housman D, Pelletier J: Antagonism of WT1 activity by protein self-association. *Proc Natl Acad Sci USA* **92**:11105, 1995.

138. Haber D, Park S, Maheswaran S, Englert C, Re G, Hazen-Martin D, Sens D, Garvin A: WT1-mediated growth suppression of Wilms tumor cells expressing a WT1 splicing variant. *Science* **262**:2057, 1993.

139. Ladanyi M, Gerald W: Fusion of the EWS and WT1 genes in the desmoplastic small round cell tumor. *Cancer Res* **54**:2837, 1994.

140. Gerald W, Rosai J, Ladanyi M: Characterization of the genomic break-point and chimeric transcripts in the EWS-WT1 gene fusion of desmoplastic small round cell tumor. *Proc Natl Acad Sci USA* **92**:1028, 1995.

141. Park S, Tomlinson G, Nisen P, Haber D: Altered trans-activational properties of a mutated WT1 gene product in a WAGR-associated Wilms' tumor. *Cancer Research* **53**:4757, 1993.

142. Sharma P, Bowman M, Madden S, RauscherIII F, Sukumar S: RNA editing in the Wilms' tumor susceptibility gene, WT1. *Genes Dev* **8**:720, 1994.

143. Theiler K, Varnum D, Stevens L: Development of Dickie's small eye, a mutation in the house mouse. *Anat. Embryol* **155**:81, 1978.

144. Hogan B, Horsburgh G, Cohen J, Hetherington C, Fisher G, Lyon M: Small eyes (Sey): a homozygous lethal mutation on chromosome 2 which affects the differentiation of both lens and nasal placodes in the mouse. *J Embryol Exp Morph* **97**:95, 1986.

145. Glaser T, Lane J, Housman D: A mouse model of the Aniridia-Wilms' tumor deletion syndrome. *Science* **250**:823, 1990.

146. Kreidberg J, Sariola H, Loring J, Maeda M, Pelletier J, Housman D, Jaenisch R: WT1 is required for early kidney development. *Cell* **74**:679, 1993.

147. Hasgekar N, Pendse A, Lalitha V: Rat renal mesenchymal tumor as an experimental model for human congenital mesoblastic nephroma. *Ped Pathol* **9**: 131, 1989.

148. Ohaki Y: Renal tumors induced transplacentally in the rat by N-ethylnitrosourea. *Ped Pathol* **9**:19, 1989.

149. Deshpande R, Hasgekar N, Chitale A, Lalitha V: Rar renal mesenchymal tumor as an experimental model for human congenital mesoblastic nephroma: II Cmparative pathology. *Ped Pathol* **9**:141, 1989.

150. Sharma P, Bowman M, Yu B, Sukumar S: A rodent model for Wilms tumors: embryonal kidney neoplasms induced by N-nitros-N'-methylurea. *Proc Natl Acad Sci USA* **91**:9931, 1994.

151. Kudoh T, Ishidate T, Moriyama M, Toyoshima K, Akiyama T: G1 phase arrest induced by Wilms tumor protein WT1 is abrogated by cyclin/CDK complexes. *Proc Natl Acad Sci USA* **92**:4517, 1995.

152. Englert C, Maheswara S, Garvin AJ, Kreidberg J, Haber D: Induction of p21 by the Wilms tumor suppressor gene WT1. *Cancer Res*, in press, 1997.

153. Sherr C, Roberts R: Inhibitors of mammalian G1 cyclin-dependent kinases. *Genes & Dev.* **9**:1149, 1995.

154. Wang J, Walsh K: Resistance to apoptosis conferred by cdk inhibitors during myocyte differentiation. *Science* **273**:359, 1996.

155. Maheswaran S, Englert C, Bennett P, Heinrich G, Haber D: The WT1 gene product stabilizes p53 and inhibits p53-mediated apoptosis. *Genes & Dev* **9**:2143, 1995.

156. Lemoine N, Hughes C, Cowell J: Aberrant expression of the tumour suppressor gene p53 is very frequent in Wilms' tumours. *J Pathol* **168**:237, 1992.

157. Malkin D, Sexsmith E, Yeger H, Williams B, Coppes M: Mutations of the p53 tumor suppressor gene occur infrequently in Wilms' tumor. *Cancer Research* **54**:2077, 1994.

158. Bardeesy N, Falkoff D, Petruzzi M, Nowak N, Zabel B, Adam M, Aguiar M, Grundy P, Shows T, Pelletier J: Anaplastic Wilms' tumour, a subtype displaying poor prognosis, harbours p53 gene mutations. *Nature Genet* **7**:91, 1994.

CHAPTER 22

Neurofibromatosis Type 1

David H. Gutmann ▪ Francis S. Collins

1. Von Recklinghausen neurofibromatosis, or neurofibromatosis type 1 (NF1), is a common autosomal dominant disorder that affects one in 3000 individuals. It is characterized clinically by the finding of two or more of the following: café au lait spots, neurofibromas, freckling in non-sun-exposed areas, optic glioma, Lisch nodules, distinctive bony lesions, and a first-degree relative with NF1. Less common manifestations include short stature and macrocephaly. NF1 patients can also have learning disabilities, seizures, scoliosis, hypertension, plexiform neurofibromas, or pheochromocytomas.

2. There is a high spontaneous mutation rate in NF1, with 30 to 50 percent of cases representing new mutations. Although the penetrance of NF1 is essentially 100 percent, NF1 tends to show variable expressivity in that there is a wide range of clinical severity and complications in patients within the same family, who all presumably carry the same mutation.

3. Syndromes related to NF1 include neurofibromatosis type 2 (bilateral vestibular neurofibromatosis), segmental NF, spinal NF, Watson syndrome, and neurofibromatosis–Noonan syndrome.

4. The gene for NF1 was identified by positional cloning and resides on chromosome 17q11.2. This gene has an open reading frame of 8454 nucleotides and spans approximately 300,000 nucleotides of genomic DNA. The messenger RNA is 11,000 to 13,000 nucleotides and is detectable at varying levels in all tissues examined. Germ-line mutations in the *NF1* gene have been found in affected patients and range from large (megabase) deletions to missense and nonsense mutations.

5. The protein product of the *NF1* locus (neurofibromin) is 2818 amino acids and is expressed as a 250-kDa protein in brain, spleen, kidney, testis, and thymus. This protein has structural and functional similarity to a family of GTPase-activating proteins (GAPs) that down-regulates a cellular proto-oncogene, p21-*ras*. *ras* has been implicated in the control of cell growth and differentiation, and the ability of neurofibromin to down-regulate p21-*ras* suggests that the loss of neurofibromin may lead to uncontrolled cell growth or tumor formation. Subcellular localization and biochemical purification experiments have demonstrated that neurofibromin is associated with cytoplasmic microtubules.

6. Somatic mutations in the *NF1* gene that result in an absence of neurofibromin expression have been described for a variety of tumor types. Loss of neurofibromin in neurofibrosarcomas derived from NF1 patients results in increased p21-*ras* activation and presumably tumor formation. Neurofibromin expression is also absent in non-NF1 patients' tumors, including metastatic malignant melanomas and neuroblastomas. The loss of neurofibromin in malignancy supports the notion that neurofibromin is a tumor-suppressor gene product.

7. The diagnosis of neurofibromatosis is based largely on clinical criteria despite progress in defining the molecular genetics of the disorder. Treatment of patients with NF1 is directed at education and genetic counseling, early detection of malignancy, and surveillance for the appearance of complications of NF1.

Von Recklinghausen neurofibromatosis, or neurofibromatosis type 1 (NF1), is one of the most common autosomal dominant disorders in humans, afflicting all ethnic groups, both sexes, and all age groups. It is more common than Duchenne muscular dystrophy and Huntington disease combined and has a greater prevalence in the western world than does cystic fibrosis. Yet NF1 has received far less attention in the public eye and the medical literature than have these other single-gene disorders. Among the multitude of reasons for this decreased visibility, three seem to stand out: (1) The pleiotropic and variable manifestations of NF1 affect many different organ systems and thus lead to the involvement of a multitude of subspecialists in the care of these patients. However, until recently no single specialist or subspecialist had considered NF1 a disease of major concern. Now this role has been taken on by medical geneticists. (2) Until very recently, NF1 lacked a firm biologic basis, and investigations into its pathogenesis were more descriptive than definitive. In the absence of a biologic hypothesis for the basic defect, very little attention was given to this disorder by basic scientists. (3) It is a tragic reality that many patients with NF1 are at least to some degree disfigured. In a society that often values physical beauty more than strength of character, such individuals have been discriminated against, either overtly or subtly, and often have responded by remaining in the background. There have been few poster children for von Recklinghausen neurofibromatosis, no telethons, and very little public sympathy. The learning disabilities suffered by many individuals with NF1 have further inhibited their ability to achieve positions of power, wealth, and influence.

All these circumstances are undergoing a turnaround. The founding of the National Neurofibromatosis Foundation (NNFF) in America in 1978, LINK (Let's Increase Neurofibromatosis Knowledge) in 1982 and the International Neurofibromatosis Association in 1992 signifies a new determination of NF1 sufferers and their families to increase public awareness of the disease, support research, and reach out to each other in support groups. The clinical care of NF patients, previously fragmented and poorly coordinated, has been greatly improved over the past 15 years by the establishment of a large number of NF specialty clinics, which are now present in most major medical centers. The directors of such clinics are usually pediatricians, internists, neurologists, or geneticists, and the clinics offer diagnosis, counseling, and regular evaluation of affected individuals for complications of the disease and coordinated access to subspecialists when the need arises. Such clinics, initially arising out of the pioneering efforts of Vincent Riccardi at Baylor, have provided a wealth of information about the natural history of the disease and corrected a number of misconceptions.

From the scientific point of view, the identification of the *NF1* gene by a positional cloning strategy[1-3] and the recognition that the protein product is a participant in p21-*ras*-mediated growth control[4-7] have catapulted NF1 into the scientific spotlight, resulting in the recruitment of a significant number of basic scientists into research on this disorder who previously would not have paid it much mind. Thus, the complexion of NF1 has changed dramatically over the past 15 years, and it now seems highly appropriate to include a chapter on this disorder in this textbook.

There are three recent excellent books[8-10] on neurofibromatosis, with particular emphasis on the clinical aspects. No attempt will be made here to duplicate those sources and the wealth of clinical detail they provide; the interested reader is referred to those sources as well as to the classic monograph of Crowe, Schull, and Neel.[11] Furthermore, no coverage of neurofibromatosis type 2 (NF2, formerly referred to as central neurofibromatosis or bilateral vestibular neurofibromatosis) will be attempted.[12,13]

CLINICAL ASPECTS OF NEUROFIBROMATOSIS TYPE 1

Historical Perspective

Scattered descriptions of cases that almost certainly represent NF1, sometimes even including drawings, can be found through many centuries of medical writing.[14,15] While other writers had previously focused on the skin tumors and occasionally had noted the familial nature of the disorder, it was von Recklinghausen in 1882 who gave the disease its first full description, including the recognition that the tumors arose from the fibrous tissue surrounding small nerves, leading to his designation of these tumors as neurofibromas.[16] The autosomal dominant inheritance pattern was defined early in the twentieth century.[17] A crucial diagnostic element, the iris nodule, was defined by the Viennese ophthalmologist Lisch in 1937,[18] although the true significance and usefulness of this observation have come to general attention only in the past decade.[19,20]

The landmark study of Crowe, Schull, and Neel[11] brought together for the first time all the salient clinical features of NF1, including the high incidence, the high spontaneous mutation rate, the usefulness of the café au lait spot as a diagnostic feature, and the recognition of the wide range of complications that can occur. Other important large-scale studies of the disease include those of Borberg[21] (followed up 35 years later by Sorenson et al.[22]), Carey et al.,[23] Riccardi,[9,24] and Huson et al.[25-27] While none of these studies is completely devoid of bias of ascertainment, together they provide a wealth of information about this pleiotropic disease.

Incidence

Because NF1 often is not diagnosed at birth, especially if the case is a new mutation, true birth incidence rates are difficult to obtain. Population surveys in the United States,[11] Russia,[28] Denmark,[29] and Wales[26] (Table 22-1) have resulted in an estimate of disease prevalence of approximately 1 in 2500 to 1 in 5000. A lower estimate of 1 in 7800 is provided by the Russian study, but this almost certainly represents an underestimate. When underascertainment and increased mortality are considered, the true birth incidence of NF1 is probably about 1 in 3000. There is no evidence that this frequency varies among ethnic groups. This is expected for a disorder with such a high percentage of spontaneous mutations.

Diagnostic Criteria

Despite opinions to the contrary in the medical literature, the diagnosis of NF1 usually is not difficult or controversial when performed by an experienced clinician. In 1987, the National Institutes of Health (NIH) convened a consensus panel to define diagnostic criteria for NF1, and the list that resulted (Table 22-2) reflects extensive clinical experience and only rarely leads to a false positive diagnosis.[30] The same panel also set out the distinguishing features between NF1 and NF2 (see below), ending many decades of confusion about these two disorders, which are now known to be completely distinct, both genetically and clinically.

The diagnostic criteria listed in Table 22-2 do not eliminate the occurrence of certain clinical dilemmas, however. A frequent dilemma is the identification of a child under 4 years of age with six or more café au lait spots, no family history, and no other manifestations of NF1. According to the NIH criteria, this is insufficient evidence to make a diagnosis of NF1, but such children must be followed for the appearance of other manifestations. Most of these children will eventually turn out to have NF1. This is one situation in which a molecular diagnostic test to identify a gene mutation would be of considerable utility.

Table 22-1 Estimates of Prevalence and Mutation Rate of NF1

Methods of Study (Year)	Ascertainment	Prevalence	Mutation Rate
Crowe et al. (1956)	Surveys of admissions at general hospital and state mental institutions	1/2500–3000	$1.4–2.6 \times 10^{-4}$
Sergeyev (1975)	Population sample of 16-year-old Russian youths	1/7800	$4.4–4.9 \times 10^{-5}$
Samuelsson and Axelson (1981)	Population-based	1/4600	4.3×10.5^{-5}
Huson et al. (1989)	Population-based	1/2500–4950	$3.1–10.5 \times 10^{-5}$

Table 22-2 Diagnostic Criteria for NF1

Two or more of the following

Six or more café-au-lait spots
  1.5 cm or larger in postpubertal individuals
  0.5 cm or larger in prepubertal individuals
Two or more neurofibromas of any type or
  one or more plexiform neurofibromas
Freckling of armpits or groin
Optic glioma (tumor of the optic pathway)
Two or more Lisch nodules (benign iris hamartomas)
A distinctive bony lesion
Dysplasia of the sphenoid bone
Dysplasia or thinning of long bone cortex
First-degree relative with NF1

DEFINING FEATURES PRESENT IN MOST PATIENTS

Café au Lait Spots

The café au lait spot (Fig. 22-1), a flat, evenly pigmented macule, usually is not apparent at birth but becomes visible during the first year of life.

While up to 25 percent of the normal population will have one to three café au lait spots,[31] the presence of six or more is highly suspicious for NF1[11] if the size criteria listed in Table 22-2 are closely followed. Melanocytes within a café au lait spot have an increased number of macromelanosomes,[32] al-

though this is not diagnostic for NF1. The café au lait spots tend to fade in later life and may be difficult or impossible to identify in elderly individuals.

Peripheral Neurofibromas

Peripheral neurofibromas are soft fleshy tumors (Figs. 22-1 and 22-2) that are usually not present in childhood but make their appearance slightly before or during adolescence.[9] They tend to increase in size and number with age, although the rate can be extremely variable. Some females affected with NF1 note an increase in the rate of progression during pregnancy, suggesting that these tumors may be hormone-responsive. Pathologically, these lesions are made up of a mixture of cell types, including Schwann cells, fibroblasts, mast cells, and vascular elements.[33]

A subset of patients can have firmer and sometimes painful neurofibromas along the course of peripheral nerves. These neurofibromas can be quite difficult to manage surgically. Even more challenging are the spinal neurofibromas arising from dorsal nerve roots, which can lead to pain and neurologic compromise.

Freckling

The occurrence of freckles in axilla, groin, and intertriginous areas was first pointed out by Crowe,[34] and is a useful diagnostic feature. Such freckling is not apparent at birth but often appears during childhood. The occurrence of such freckling in the inflammatory areas and other skin folds[35] is a curious observation that suggests that these lesions are modulated by the local environment.

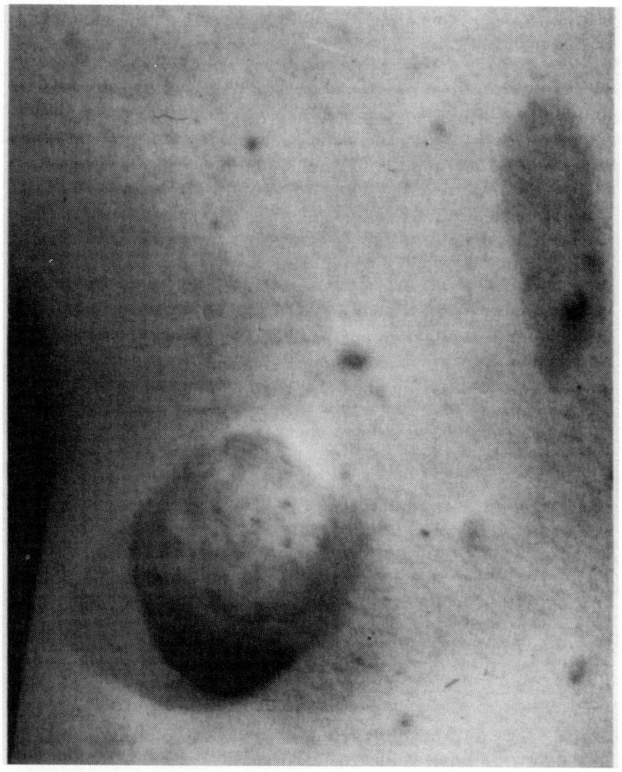

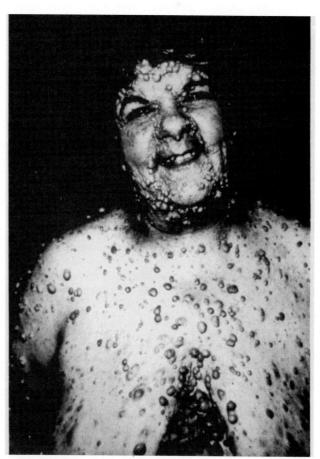

FIG. 22-1 Typical neurofibroma and a café au lait spot on the skin of an adult with NF1.

FIG. 22-2 An older individual with NF1, demonstrating extensive involvement on the skin surface with peripheral neurofibromas.

Lisch Nodules

Raised, often pigmented nodules of the iris, pathologically representing hamartomas, are now called Lisch nodules (Fig. 22-3) and represent an extremely important diagnostic feature of NF1.[19,20] Like café au lait spots and freckling, Lisch nodules never result in significant disease but can be helpful in establishing the diagnosis. While they can be seen with simple lighting in individuals with light irises, a slit-lamp examination is usually essential to be certain of their presence and to distinguish them from iris nevi.

Time Course

The defining features of NF1 described above, while somewhat variable in appearance, tend to follow the pattern shown in Fig. 22-4. As implied by the figure, it is unusual for an individual with NF1 to reach adolescence without having amply satisfied the diagnostic criteria in Table 22-2.

COMMON BUT NONDIAGNOSTIC AND NONMORBID FEATURES

While not considered specific enough for inclusion in the list of diagnostic criteria, macrocephaly[25] and short stature[24] are common accompaniments of NF1. The macrocephaly reflects concomitant megalencephaly. Careful studies of adult height suggest that individuals with NF1 are on average about 3 in. shorter than predicted by their family backgrounds.[9,25] With both of these circumstances, it is important not to overlook other, more significant causes. For instance, aqueductal stenosis leading to hydrocephalus is a known but uncommon complication of NF1 that requires surgical intervention.[36] Similarly, growth failure can occasionally arise as a result of hypothalamic involvement by optic glioma.

VARIABLE BUT SIGNIFICANT COMPLICATIONS

The defining features of NF1 listed in Table 22-2 are found in most affected patients and, while often associated with significant cos-

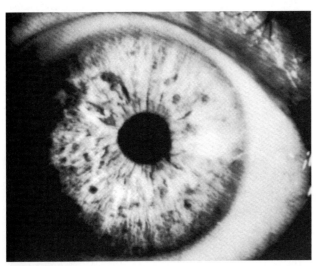

FIG. 22-3 Typical Lisch nodules (hamartomas) of the iris in an adult with NF1.

metic concerns related to neurofibroma growth, usually are not life-threatening. A range of other complications which are quite variable from one patient to the next can be more serious. Approximately one-third of patients with NF1 suffer from one or more of these serious complications during their lifetimes (Fig. 22-5).

Learning Disability

Frank mental retardation (IQ less than 70) is uncommon in NF1. Recent molecular information indicates that such patients are much more likely to have the disease because of a large deletion that removes the entire *NF1* gene and considerable flanking DNA.[37] Presumable, other nearby genes are also reduced to hemizygosity by the deletion in these patients and contribute to the retardation.

Although retardation in uncommon, standard IQ testing reveals a downward shift of performance scores by 5 to 10 IQ points in affected individuals.[35] Approximately 40 to 60 percent of all individuals with NF1 have learning disabilities. Analysis of the specific behavioral phenotype in children with NF1 has demonstrated a higher incidence of minor signs of neurologic impairment (motor abnormalities involving balance and gait), lower IQ scores, and poor performance on tasks involving nonverbal learning. In addition, children with NF1 often exhibit areas of increased T_2 signal intensity on magnetic resonance imaging of the brain. It has been suggested that children with such areas (unidentified bright objects, or UBOs) have significantly lower IQ and language scores, with impaired visual motor integration and coordination.[38] Although this hypothesis is intriguing, it has not been confirmed in all studies examining this association. UBOs are most commonly seen in the basal ganglia, cerebellum, brainstem, and subcortical white matter regions. In one pathologic study, these hyperintense foci corresponded to areas of vacuolar and spongiotic change with fluid-filled vacuoles surrounded by infiltrating astrocytes.[39] Recent studies have demonstrated increased neurofibromin expression in activated astrocytes both in vivo and in vitro, suggesting that reduced *NF1* gene expression may alter the normal astrogliotic response in the brain.[40,41] Intervention is highly warranted if the above problems emerge, and all children with NF1 should be followed closely for developmental progress and subjected to a thorough educational evaluation at age 3 or 4 if there is any indication of significant delay.

Plexiform Neurofibromas

A plexiform neurofibroma is a much more complex, usually congenital (though often not immediately visible) lesion that may diffusely involve nerve, muscle, connective tissue, vascular elements, and overlying skin.[35] Such lesions, which occur in approximately 10 percent of affected individuals, commonly lead to overgrowth of surrounding tissues during childhood and in their most severe form can lead to massive distortion of the face or an extremity (Fig. 22-6). When these lesions occur around the orbit, they are often associated with sphenoid wing dysplasia, and the tumor may extend inside the cranial vault, accompanied by pulsating exophthalmos.[9] Severe plexiform lesions are almost invariably apparent by age 4 or 5, and so it is possible to reassure older individuals without plexiform lesions that they are not at significant risk for the development of this particularly troubling and disfiguring complication.

Malignancy

The frequency of malignancy in NF1 is difficult to discern accurately, as most series reflect a referral bias and therefore overesti-

Frequency
of
Finding
100%
50%
0%
>6 CAL'S
Lisch
nodules
Freckling
Neurofibromas
Birth
5
10
15
20
50
Age

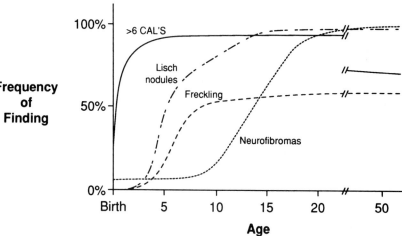

FIG. 22-4 Typical time course of appearance of the major clinical features of NF1. CAL = café au lait spots.

mate the occurrence of this complication.[42] Nonetheless, there is clearly an increased risk of specific cancers in NF1, amounting to perhaps 2 to 5 percent of affected individuals.[9,23,25,29,43]

A particularly aggressive and often fatal malignancy is the neurofibrosarcoma, or malignant peripheral nerve sheath tumor (MPNST), which commonly arises in a plexiform neurofibroma in a young adult. Often the first symptom is pain, which should always prompt rapid investigation in an individual with a plexiform lesion. These malignancies are relatively resistant to chemotherapy and radiation.[44]

Complication
Severe head and neck PNFS 1·2%*
Severe pseudoarthrosis 2·1%
Severe retardation 0·8%
Learning difficulties 5·6%
Min. retardation 24·2%
Mod. retardation 2·4%
Scoliosis 5·2%
PNFs (except*) 25·5%
Optic glioma 0·7% +
Aqueduct stenosis 2·1%
Rhabdomyosarcoma 1·5%
Peripheral nerve malignancy 1·5%
CNS Tumours, other than+ 0·7-1·5%
Renal artery stenosis 2·1%
Spinal NFS 2·1%
Gastrointestinal NFS 2·1%
Endocrine tumours 3·1%
Epilepsy 4·2%
0
5
10
15
20
25
30
'Lifelong' risk
Age (years)

FIG. 22-5 Age range of presentation and frequency of major NF1 complications. PNF = plexiform neurofibroma; NFS = neurofibrosarcoma. (*From Huson et al.*[27] *Used by permission.*)

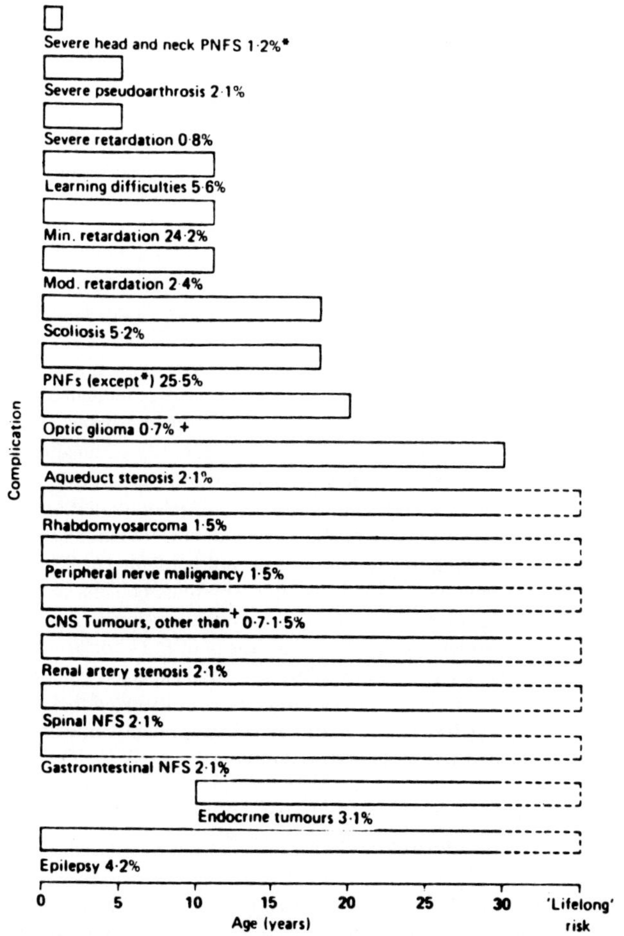

A second strongly associated tumor is optic glioma. MRI scanning of affected children with NF1 has revealed radiographic evidence of optic nerve or optic chiasm enlargement in up to 15 to 20 percent of patients,[45,46] but the vast majority of these patients have normal vision and never become symptomatic. In fact, there is evi-

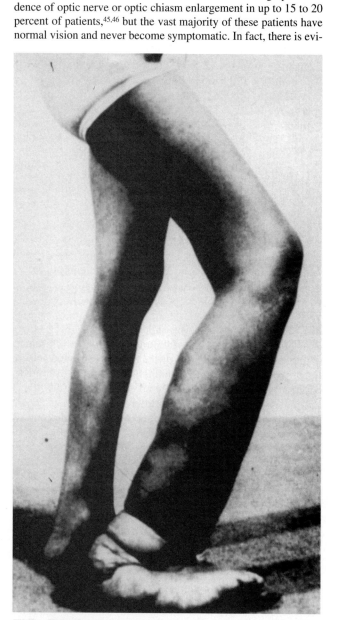

FIG. 22-6 Massive plexiform neurofibroma of the lower extremity in an adolescent with NF1.

dence that many of these lesions regress with age. A small subgroup, however, presents with progressive visual loss associated with an expanding lesion. While this occurs only in a minority of patients with NF1, all series of juvenile optic glioma are heavily populated with children with NF1, and the discovery of this tumor should certainly prompt a close examination for other features of the disease.

While the risk of other malignancies of the nervous system is less impressive, there appears to be a moderately increased risk of central nervous system tumors, especially astrocytomas.[33] Pheochromocytoma is commonly quoted as a complication of NF1 but is in fact quite uncommon in this population.[11,42,43]

Seizures

A seizure disorder will develop in approximately 5 percent of patients with NF1, and the onset can occur at any time.[9] While occasionally a definable intracranial tumor will be found to be at fault, usually no cause can be defined. In this regard, the recent advent of MRI scanning has uncovered MRI inhomogeneities in the brains of many children with NF1 on T_2-weighted images. These UBOs are of uncertain etiology and generally should not be interpreted as clinically significant.[47] There is some evidence that they tend to disappear with age, and it is not correct, on the basis of current evidence, to refer to them as hamartomas.

Scoliosis

Vertebral defects, including scalloping from dural ectasia,[48] are extremely common in NF1, and approximately 10 percent of affected individuals have scoliosis during late childhood and adolescence.[9] This can in some instances be severe enough to require bracing and/or surgery and may or may not be associated with local neurofibroma formation.

Pseudarthrosis

A peculiar and uncommon complication which defies the classification of NF1 as a disorder purely of the neural crest is the involvement of long bones. This often is noted first as bowing, particularly of the tibia, in young children. This may progress to thinning of the cortex, pathologic fracture, and severe difficulties with nonunion of the fragments. This process may go on to form a pseudarthrosis, or false joint, leaving the limb severely compromised. The pathologic basis of this unusual process is unknown.

Hypertension

Hypertension is extremely common in adults with NF1, affecting perhaps one-third of these patients.[24] In general, this proves to be essential hypertension with no underlying cause, but the new development of hypertension should always raise the possibility of renal artery stenosis, which is particularly common in children,[49] or pheochromocytoma, which occasionally occurs in adults with NF1 (see above).

Miscellaneous Complications

Frequent but less well understood problems associated with neurofibromatosis include headache, which can be bothersome but usually not disabling. The new onset of headache should always

trigger evaluation for an intracranial tumor, but many patients experience lifelong stable headache patterns with no identifiable etiology. Generalized itching or itching localized to newly developing neurofibromas is reported by many individuals.[9] Similarly, constipation seems to be a frequent concomitant of the disease, especially in patients who have plexiform neurofibromas in the pelvic area.[50] These complications may interfere with autonomic innervation of the colon and produce both bowel and bladder problems.

GENETIC ASPECTS OF NF1

Inheritance Pattern

Preiser and Davenport[17] surveyed the literature in 1918 and concluded that approximately 50 percent of the children of individuals affected with NF1 were also afflicted, regardless of sex. They noted numerous examples of male-to-male transmission, concluding that the disease follows an autosomal dominant pattern of inheritance. In 1981, Hall suggested that the sex of the affected parent might have an impact on the severity of the disease,[51,52] a phenomenon we would now ascribe to parental imprinting.[53] In that study, children of affected mothers tended to be slightly more severely affected than did children of affected fathers. Subsequent careful analyses of this issue have failed to confirm this maternal effect,[23,54,55] although a very modest effect would be difficult to exclude with such variability of the disease.

Mutation Rate

All large series indicate after careful examination that 30 to 50 percent of patients with NF1 do not have an affected parent.[11,29,55] Such individuals presumably represent spontaneous mutations. With the cloning of the *NF1* gene, several examples have now been documented of *de novo* alterations in the *NF1* gene in such individuals (see below). Given that NF1 is a common disease and that so many of its sufferers have new mutations, one cannot escape the conclusion that the mutation rate for this locus is unusually high. In fact, calculations of this frequency (Table 22-1) indicate a mutation rate of approximately 10^{-4} per allele per generation. Evidence based on linkage analysis has indicated that the vast majority of new mutations arise from the paternal allele,[56,57] indicating that these mutations apparently occur during spermatogenesis. Whether they are meiotic or mitotic errors has not been determined, although mitotic errors are suggested by the absence of a significant paternal age effect in new mutation cases.

With such a high mutation rate, it would be predicted that the reproductive fitness of individuals with NF1 must be significantly reduced in order for the disease to be present at an equilibrium frequency. The Welsh study[55] found a fitness of 0.31 for affected males and 0.60 for affected females (1.0 is the expected value). A large proportion of the reduced fertility can be attributed to a failure of affected individuals to marry, which presumably reflects the psychosocial consequences of the condition.

Penetrance

The penetrance of NF1 is essentially 100 percent in individuals who have reached adulthood and have been subjected to careful examination by an experienced physician, including a slit-lamp examination. Rare cases of normal parents giving rise to two affected children have been described[58] and could be examples of germ-line mosaicism in one of the parents, although the possibility of independent spontaneous mutations cannot be excluded until molecular studies are carried out in such patients. The importance of careful examination of both parents before giving genetic counseling cannot be overemphasized, however. There are numerous reports of circumstances in which one of the parents was sufficiently mildly affected to be unaware of his or her diagnosis.

Variable Expressivity

NF1 is a classic example of the tendency for autosomal dominant conditions to show variable expressivity, which can at times be dramatic in NF1. Even the more constant defining features of the disease are subject to considerable heterogeneity when considered closely. It has been known for some time that large families with multiple afflicted individuals are likely to demonstrate a wide range of severity and complications, and the variability within a family of significant size is similar to the variability seen in comparisons of different families. This indicates that the specific germline mutation at the *NF1* locus does not accurately predict the phenotype in a specific individual, since all affected individuals in the same family carry the same mutation.

To distinguish between genetic influences and environmental and/or chance influences, Easton and coworkers[59] examined a series of monozygotic twins concordant for NF1 and compared them with other pairs of first-degree affected relatives. There was a significant correlation in the number of café au lait spots and neurofibromas between identical twins, with a lower but significant correlation in first-degree relatives and almost no correlation between more distant relatives. This suggests that these features are controlled by other genetic influences but that the specific mutation in the *NF1* gene itself plays a minor role. Optic glioma, scoliosis, epilepsy, and learning disability were concordant in twin pairs, but plexiform neurofibromas were not. Furthermore, there was no indication that the presence of one complication predicted the occurrence of another except for the fact that neurofibrosarcoma has been commonly observed to occur almost exclusively in individuals with plexiform neurofibromas.

Related Syndromes

NF1 has been described in the literature in association with almost every imaginable disorder, but most of these reports appear to represent the coincidental occurrence of two unrelated conditions. A classification scheme proposed by Riccardi and Eichner[9] divides the neurofibromatoses into eight syndromes, but this scheme has not found wide application because of the blurred boundaries between several categories. A full discussion of variant syndromes is beyond the scope of this chapter, but a few of the most relevant conditions will be mentioned below.

Neurofibromatosis Type 2. Type 2 neurofibromatosis, formerly designated central neurofibromatosis or bilateral vestibular neurofibromatosis, is now appreciated to be distinct, both clinically and genetically, from NF1.[60,61] The *NF2* gene has been mapped to chromosome 22 and was identified in 1993.[12,13] Individuals with NF2 often have a small number of café au lait spots (rarely more than six) and may have one or two peripheral neurofibromas but usually not more. They occasionally have Lisch nodules.[62] Ophthalmologic evaluation is extremely useful because of the presence of posterior subcapsular cataracts in a sizable proportion of these patients.[63] The hallmark of NF2 is the development of bilateral eighth cranial nerve tumors, properly called vestibular schwannomas rather than acoustic neuromas, in 95 percent of these patients

by age 30 years.[60] Inheritance is autosomal dominant. Other tumors of cranial and cervical nerve roots are common, and management presents great challenges for neurosurgeons and otolaryngologists. Past statements that acoustic neuroma is a complication of NF1 are almost certainly due to the confusion between these two entities; since more careful definitions of the two disorders have been applied, there has been no indication that individuals with NF1 have an increased risk of eighth cranial nerve tumors compared with the general population. NF2 is much less common than NF1, affecting approximately 1 in 50,000 individuals.

Segmental NF1. Occasionally individuals are encountered who have features of NF1 limited to one segment of the body.[64] These features may include café au lait spots, freckling, and peripheral or plexiform neurofibromas, and Lisch nodules may be seen in an individual who has that segment of the body affected. Such individuals invariably have normal parents but on rare occasions can have a child with classic NF1.[65] There is strong circumstantial evidence that these cases represent somatic mutation of the *NF1* gene early in embryogenesis, so that derivatives of that mutant line display the features of NF1. If the mosaicism involves the germ line, the disease can then be transmitted. Recently, germ-line mosaicism for an *NF1* gene mutation was found in a clinically unaffected father of a child with new-onset NF1.[66] In addition, somatic mosaicism for an *NF1* gene deletion was detected in an individual with NF1.[67] Analysis of cases of segmental NF1 probably will demonstrate similar somatic mosaicism.

Watson Syndrome. A variant of NF1 that appears to breed true in certain families involves multiple café au lait spots, dull intelligence, short stature, pulmonary valvular stenosis, and only a small number of neurofibromas.[68] Reevaluation of these families has indicated they also have Lisch nodules, further contributing to the blurring of these two phenotypes. In fact, molecular analyses have demonstrated that in at least two families that appear to fall into the category of Watson syndrome, deletions are present in the *NF1* gene. Currently there appears to be no distinguishing aspect between the deletions causing Watson syndrome and those associated with more classic NF1.

Neurofibromatosis–Noonan Syndrome. The occurrence of features reminiscent of Noonan syndrome in patients with neurofibromatosis has been noted for some time,[69] raising the question of whether these could be overlapping syndromes or even could be due to deletion of adjacent genes. In most of these families, however, individuals with clear-cut Noonan syndrome represent only a proportion of those affected with NF1, and some of the features associated with Noonan syndrome (such as pectus excavatum, mild hypertelorism, and short stature) are frequently observed in NF1.[70] A linkage study of autosomal dominant Noonan syndrome occurring in the absence of NF1 has indicated no linkage to markers in the *NF1* region of chromosome 17, casting into doubt any notion that Noonan syndrome, at least in the aggregate, could be due to a mutation in a gene closely adjacent to NF1. At least one family with neurofibromatosis–Noonan syndrome (NFNS) has been found to harbor a deletion in the *NF1* gene, but the fact that very large deletions removing flanking regions on either side of *NF1* do not consistently result in NFNS casts further doubt on the adjacent gene theory. The most appropriate synthesis of the data at the present time indicates that the phenotype of NF1 can include features that overlap with those described in Noonan syndrome, but these disorders are probably genetically distinct.

Spinal Neurofibromatosis. Rare families have been identified with a predominance of spinal tumors and relatively few peripheral neurofibromas. A linkage study has indicated that one such family appears to be linked to NF1 whereas another does not, implying locus heterogeneity for this set of conditions.[71]

MOLECULAR BIOLOGY OF THE *NF1* GENE

Cloning of the *NF1* Gene

Since no information was available on the structure or function of the *NF1* gene product before the 1980s, the only feasible approach available to identify the gene was positional cloning.[72] The isolation of the gene for von Recklinghausen neurofibromatosis began with an international collaboration to assemble linkage data in families with NF1. By early 1987, this worldwide effort made possible the construction of an exclusion map that narrowed the candidate chromosomes to a handful.[73] Examination of these selected chromosomes with RFLP markers culminated in the establishment of linkage of NF1 to the pericentromeric region of chromosome 17 in the late spring of 1987.[73-76] No linkage disequilibrium was ever found. One of the linked markers was an anonymous probe called pA10-41, and another was the gene for nerve growth factor receptor (17q12-22).[77] The linkage of NF1 with the nerve growth factor (NGF) receptor gene was exciting because of the role of NGF in neural crest tissue development. Further analysis using RFLP markers, however, excluded the NGF receptor gene as a candidate for the *NF1* gene, as numerous crossover events were identified.[78]

An intense genetic mapping effort resulted in the establishment of a multipoint linkage map constructed from data assembled by the NF1 collaborative group (Fig. 22-7). This map represented the outcome of the study of 142 families with over 700 affected individuals and narrowed the distance between flanking probes and the *NF1* gene to 3 cM, or about 3 million bp.[79] Candidate genes in this interval, such as the *erb*A1 and *erb*B2 proto-oncogenes, were sub-

sequently excluded as candidate genes for NF1 by the identification of recombinants.

The discovery of two patients with NF1 and balanced translocations involving the long arm of chromosome 17 dramatically accelerated the process. These two NF1 patients had reciprocal translocations, one between chromosomes 1p34.3 and 17q11.2 and the other between chromosomes 17q11.2 and 22q11.2.[80-84] Support for the notion that these translocations disrupt the *NF1* gene was provided by the fact that one breakpoint in each of the translocations involved 17q11.2, precisely where the *NF1* gene had been mapped by linkage analysis.

The identification of translocation breakpoints permitted analysis of the genetic region by physical mapping techniques and bridged the gap between linkage mapping and physical mapping.[85] Using restriction enzymes that recognize rare restriction sites in DNA, one could search for an anomalously migrating DNA fragment resulting from the disruption of this region by the translocations. To identify the translocation breakpoints by physical mapping, markers capable of visualizing these areas had to be generated. Using a series of chromosome 17-specific *Not*I-linking clones tested against a somatic-cell hybrid mapping panel, a clone termed 17L1A was identified that detected abnormalities by pulsed-field gel electrophoresis in the 1;17 translocation patient and her affected offspring (Fig. 22-8). The presence of abnormal fragments provided conclusive evidence that the translocation breakpoints map near the 17L1A clone.

The use of cosmid libraries to look for abnormal fragments on pulsed-field gel electrophoresis provided an additional clone, called 1F10, which detected abnormal fragments in both translocation patients. These two cloned probes were then shown to reside on the same 600-kb DNA fragment and bracketed the two translocations. This narrowed the interval in which the *NF1* gene must reside to 600 kb of DNA.[83] Of interest was the fact that 17L1A represented a CpG island, a hypomethylated region often associated with five regulatory sequences of active genes.

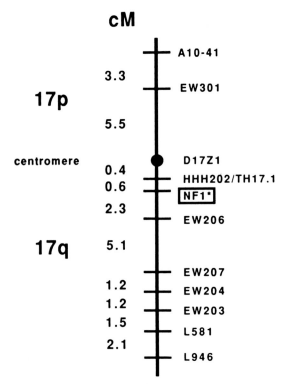

FIG. 22-7 Linkage map for chromosome 17 demonstrating the position of the *NF1* locus relative to other DNA markers linked to the disease. The map distance of the various markers is represented in centimorgans (cM).

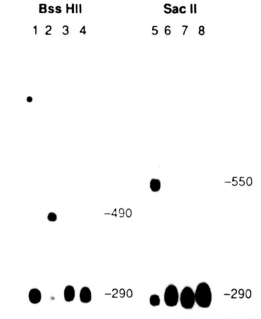

FIG. 22-8 Pulsed-field gel analysis with probe 17L1A in an NF1 patient with [1;17] translocation. Genomic DNA is digested with a rare-cutting restriction enzyme (either BssHII or SacII), separated by pulsed-field gel electrophoresis, and probed with 17L1A. The DNA source in each lane is 1 and 8, patients with NF1; 2 and 5, a patient with a 1;17 translocation has a unique band not seen in the other DNA samples, indicating the presence of a rearrangement of the DNA in the region near the *NF1* gene in this patient. (*Adapted from Fountain et al.*[80] *Used by permission.*)

The construction of a physical map of the region around the *NF1* gene laid the groundwork for identifying candidate cDNA transcripts. Using a combination of jump library clones, yeast artificial chromosome probes, and cosmids, candidate cDNA transcripts were identified. Unexpectedly, however, the first candidate gene came from another route: By comparison with a syntenic region on mouse chromosome 11, the mouse *evi2* gene, which is involved in virally induced murine leukemia, was found to map between these two breakpoints.[86–88] Cloning of the human *EVI2A* gene excluded it as a candidate for the *NF1* gene in that neither translocation actually interrupted the gene and no mutations were found in it in other patients with NF1.[89] A second candidate gene, *EVI2B* similar to *EVI2A*, was identified but also was excluded as a potential candidate.[88] The third candidate gene, *OMGP* (oligodendrocyte myelin glycoprotein), which was exciting because of its almost exclusive expression in Schwann cells and oligodendrocytes, also failed to satisfy the criteria for an *NF1* gene candidate, as no mutations could be identified in this gene in NF1 patients.[90,91]

The fourth candidate gene was much larger and was cloned and shown to be the *NF1* gene in several ways.[1–3] First, the transcript crossed both translocation breakpoints and would therefore be interrupted in these unique NF1 patients.[1–3] Second, more subtle mutations were identified in patients with NF1 that would alter the coding potential of this candidate transcript.[2] These included a patient with a *de novo* 400-nucleotide insertion that produced an abnormally large fragment on Southern blot analysis using the NF1 cDNA as a probe and another patient with a nonsense mutation.[92] These mutations provided conclusive evidence that the correct gene had been found.

The *NF1* gene has an open reading frame of nearly 9 kb and spans approximately 300 kb of genomic DNA (Fig. 22-9).[93] The messenger RNA has been estimated to be 11 to 13 kb and has been detected in all tissues examined by RT-PCR and Northern blot

analysis. At least 57 exons have been identified with three additional alternatively spliced exons (see "Identification of *NF1* Gene Product," below). The three previous candidate genes were all found embedded in one large intron and were transcribed from the opposite strand from the *NF1* gene.[89] The predicted protein has 2818 amino acids and a molecular weight of 327 kDa.[94] Analysis of the amino acid sequence failed to reveal any nuclear localization signals or transmembrane domains, suggesting that the gene product resides in the cytoplasm. Comparison of the gene to other previously identified coding sequences revealed unexpected sequence similarity between the *NF1* gene product and a family of GTPase-activating proteins (GAPs) (see "Neurofibromin as a GTPase-activating Protein," below).[4] Analyses of homologous genes from mouse, chicken, hamster, and Drosophila species demonstrate striking species conservation and underscore the fundamental importance of this gene.[95–98]

Further analysis of the genomic organization of the *NF1* gene demonstrated that the promoter of this gene resides within a CpG-rich region; this is consistent with the observation that most active eukaryotic gene promoters are contained within CpG islands.[99] During the construction of a yeast artificial chromosome contig containing the entire *NF1* gene, other homologous loci were found by low-stringency hybridization on Southern blot.[100,101] These loci were determined by a hybrid mapping panel and fluorescent in situ hybridization to reside on chromosomes 14, 15, and 22. At least two loci were found on chromosome 14. These homologous loci apparently represent unprocessed pseudogenes in that their coding sequences contain frameshift, nonsense, and missense mutations. However, these loci also may represent mutation reservoirs that can be crossed into the *NF1* locus on chromosome 17 by interchromosomal gene conversion. This phenomenon could potentially contribute to the high rate of mutation in NF1.

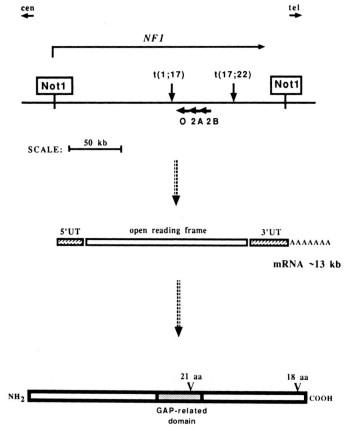

FIG. 22-9 The genetic organization of the *NF1* locus. The genomic structure of the *NF1* locus demonstrates the location of the two *Not*I restriction sites separated by 1300 kb. The initiation codon is located upstream of the centromeric *Not*I site and is positioned within a CpG-rich area. The position of the two translocation breakpoints [t(1;17) and t(17;22)] described in two patients with NF1 and their interruption of the *NF1* gene are illustrated. Three genes (O for OMgP, 2A for *EVI2A*, and 2B for *EVI2B*) are embedded within one intron on the opposite strand from the *NF1* gene. The mRNA for *NF1* is 11 to 13 kb and has an open reading frame of 8454 nucleotides with at least 2 kb of 3′ untranslated sequence. Translation of this open reading frame predicts a protein of 2818 amino acids with an estimated molecular weight of 327 kDa. Sequence similarity between a central 300- to 400-amino acid region of the *NF1* gene product, neurofibromin, and a family of GTPase-activating proteins (GAPs) is illustrated by the GAP-related domain. The location of the two alternatively spliced isoforms is denoted by the 21-amino acid insertion into the GAP-related domain and the 18-amino acid insertion in the C terminus of neurofibromin.

Patient Mutations

Analysis of NF1 patients for mutations is still in its infancy and is hampered by the large size of the gene. Approximately 20 mutations have been studied in some detail. Five types of *NF1* gene mutations have been described to date in patients with NF1: (1) Translocations have been described in two patients with NF1 and were described earlier in this chapter. These balanced translocations provided some of the first clues to the precise physical location of the *NF1* gene on chromosome 17. (2) Megabase deletions have been reported in patients with NF1.[37] These deletions extend well beyond the *NF1* gene and may include other genes on chromosome 17q11.2. These patients manifest typical NF1 but also have significant mental retardation. (3) Large internal deletions entirely contained within the *NF1* gene have been reported in patients with NF1. One of these deletions removed 90 kb of DNA encompassing the 5′ portion of the *NF1* gene, while the other deleted 40 kb of *NF1* DNA.[102] The phenotypes of these patients were indistinguishable from those of classic NF1 patients. (4) Small rearrangements within the *NF1* gene have been described. One of these rearrangements involved the insertion of a human *Alu* repeat in the intron between two *NF1* exons, resulting in abnormal mRNA splicing and premature termination of the *NF1* mRNA coding sequence.[92] (5) Many point mutations have been described in patients with NF1.[2] These mutations include the creation of stop codons, missense mutations, and frameshift mutations. One of these missense mutations involves a nonconservative substitution at codon 1423 within the NF1-GAP-related domain (NF1GRD).[103] This mutation, when expressed in insect Sf9 cells, results in a reduced ability of the NF1GRD to accelerate the hydrolysis of *ras*-GTP and perhaps altered *NF1* gene product, termed neurofibromin, function. This mutation has also been observed in anaplastic astrocytomas and colonic adenocarcinomas. Thus far, there does not appear to be a hotspot for mutation within the *NF1* gene, as all these mutations are randomly distributed throughout the *NF1* coding sequences.[104] To this end, the phenotypes of patients with all the above mutation types (except megabase deletions) are likely to be similar in that they all result in the loss of a functional protein. The fact that mutations all result in a loss of *NF1* protein function is consistent with the notion of *NF1* as a tumor-suppressor gene.

The tumor-suppressor mechanism suggests that loss of both copies of the *NF1* gene would culminate in a transformed or neoplastic phenotype.[105-108] In this hypothesis, affected individuals would inherit one mutated *NF1* gene from their parents (or as a new mutation), but neurofibromas or neurofibrosarcomas would develop only when the second gene became nonfunctional as a result of somatic mutation. This set of events is termed the Knudson hypothesis and was first elegantly demonstrated for retinoblastoma.[109,110] In patients with retinoblastoma, all somatic cells contain the germ-line inherited mutation in one of the retinoblastoma genes. Retinoblastomas arise as a result of the loss of the second copy of the retinoblastoma gene in retinal cells.

Occasionally, the second somatic mutation in the tumor can be detected by Southern blot analysis. In white blood cells from patients with NF1, the DNA may be heterozygous for a particular DNA marker polymorphism on chromosome 17, but when tumor cells develop, the remaining wild-type gene is lost, eliminating that particular allele (Fig. 22-10). This is termed loss of heterozygosity and is taken as proof that a second somatic event has occurred which results in the loss of the one remaining *NF1* gene. Interpretation of these data for chromosome 17 are confounded by the frequent loss of heterozygosity for markers near the p53 gene on chromosome 17p as well.[111] Loss of heterozygosity centered at the *NF1* locus has been observed in selected tumors from some patients with NF1, supporting the notion that *NF1* is a tumor-suppressor gene and that the manifestations of the disease result from somatic

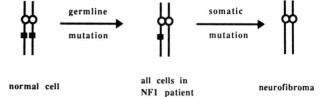

FIG. 22-10 Illustration of loss of heterozygosity in NF1. A given DNA marker polymorphism, denoted by the filled squares, is present in a normal *NF1* chromosome 17. A germ-line mutation found in all cells in an NF1 patient would alter the *NF1* gene to result in the loss of one of the DNA markers. Because the patient has one normal chromosome 17 DNA polymorphism and one mutated chromosome 17 DNA polymorphism, the patient is said to be heterozygous with respect to that DNA marker. Mutation of the one remaining normal *NF1* gene in a tumor results in the loss of both copies of the gene and the loss of heterozygosity with respect to that DNA marker polymorphism.

loss of the second *NF1* gene copy. A tumor in a NF1 patient has been found to display loss of heterozygosity for chromosome 17 markers but in addition demonstrates a large deletion in the *NF1* gene in tumor cell but not white blood cell DNA.[112] This supports the notion that a second hit occurs in the *NF1* gene during the development of neurofibrosarcomas in patients with NF1.

Mutations in the *NF1* gene have been described in other tumor types, including malignant melanomas, neuroblastomas, pheochromocytomas, and neurofibrosarcomas.[113,114] Examination of a series of malignant melanoma cell lines derived from metastatic foci demonstrated reduced or absent neurofibromin expression in up to 25 percent of tumors.[115,116] Similar examination of neuroblastomas revealed that *NF1* mRNA and neurofibromin expression is reduced in up to 30 percent of neuroblastomas.[116,117] Similarly, three neurofibrosarcomas derived from NF1 patients demonstrated elevated levels of *ras*-GTP and nearly undetectable levels of neurofibromin, suggesting a relationship between lack of neurofibromin expression and unregulated *ras* in these cells (see below).[118,119] Abnormalities at the DNA level have been reported for pheochromocytomas from NF1 patients.[120] Examination of these fresh tumors demonstrated loss of neurofibromin expression in six of six pheochromocytomas as well as one adrenal cortical tumor from patients with NF1.[121] It is likely that examination of other tumors will uncover alterations in neurofibromin expression that are consistent with its proposed role as a tumor-suppressor gene product. Consistent with the proposed role of neurofibromin as a negative growth regulator, tumors from patients with and without NF1 have been examined for alterations in *NF1* gene expression. The hallmark of NF1 is the neurofibroma, a benign tumor composed predominantly of Schwann cells, fibroblasts and, to a lesser extent, mast cells. It has been presumed that the cellular defect in the neurofibroma results from abnormal Schwann cell function secondary to loss of neurofibromin function. Malignancies in NF1 are believed to result from the constitutional inactivation of one *NF1* gene followed by a number of somatic events, including inactivation of the other *NF1* allele. Although loss of the normal allele has been proved for the malignant nerve sheath tumor (neurofibrosarcoma),[112] it had not been evaluated in the etiology of the benign neurofibroma. Recent work has demonstrated loss of heterozygosity in 22 neurofibromas from five unrelated NF1 patients.[122] In eight of these tumors, somatic deletions involving the wild-type *NF1* gene could be demonstrated, indicating that inactivation of the normal *NF1* gene is associated with the development of the neurofibroma. In related studies on Schwann cells derived from the dorsal root ganglia of neurofibromin-deficient mice, abnormalities in Schwann cell proliferation and high levels of activated p21-*ras* were observed, as would be predicted by loss of neurofibromin GAP function.[123] In addition, these neurofibromin-deficient

Schwann cells had abnormal proliferative responses to neuronal contact. Additional studies have also demonstrated abnormalities in fibroblasts derived from neurofibromin-deficient mouse embryos.[124] These results collectively suggest that defects in both the Schwann cells and the fibroblasts may contribute to the development of the benign neurofibroma.

Children with NF1 are at increased risk for the development of malignant myeloid disorders. Although myeloid disorders are an uncommon complication of NF1 in childhood, NF1 constitutes as many as 10 percent of the spontaneous cases of myeloid proliferative disorders in children. Examination of bone marrow samples from children with NF1 in whom malignant myeloid disorders developed demonstrated loss of heterozygosity at the NF1 locus.[125] In each case, the mutant NF1 allele was inherited from the parent with NF1 and the normal allele was deleted in the myeloid leukemic cells. These results are consistent with the hypothesis that loss of neurofibromin expression predisposes myeloid cells to leukemic transformation. Mice heterozygous for a germ-line NF1 mutation also develop myeloid leukemias with loss of the wild-type NF1 allele in the leukemic cells.[126] Analysis of these myeloid leukemic cells with loss of neurofibromin expression demonstrates an exaggerated and prolonged increase in p21-ras activation in response to granulocyte macrophage colony stimulating factor (GM-CSF). This increased sensitivity to GM-CSF reflects abnormal p21-ras signaling which probably leads to chronic clonal hyperproliferation and malignant transformation. Primary leukemic cells from children with NF1 also show an exaggerated increase in p21-ras activity in response to GM-CSF.[127]

Additional support for the hypothesis that neurofibromin functions to suppress growth by regulating ras derives from experiments on the ability of one of these neurofibrosarcoma cell lines (ST88-14) to grow in soft agar.[128] Whereas ST88-14 cells form colonies in soft agar, ST88-14 cells treated with pharmacologic agents that block ras function fail to grow in soft agar. These results argue that neurofibromin loss leads to increased ras activity, which in turn is partly responsible for the abnormal growth properties of these tumor cells.

Animal Models

The search for spontaneous animal models of NF1 was initially disappointing. Three early models of NF1 were reported. In the bicolor damselfish, spontaneous neurofibromas and hyperpigmented spots develop, but the disorder appears to be transmissible, and these tumors tend to be more invasive and malignant than human neurofibromas.[129] One murine model was reported as resulting from the overexpression of the HTLV-I tat gene in mice.[130] Neurofibroma-like tumors developed in the offspring. However, other phenotypic features of NF1 were absent, and the neurofibromas lacked Schwann cells, unlike human NF1 neurofibromas. Similarly, the relationship between HTLV-I and human NF1 is unclear, since there is no increased incidence of HTLV-I exposure or infection in NF1 patients.[131] The third model of NF1 was achieved by injecting N-nitroso-N-ethylurea into pregnant Syrian golden hamsters.[98,132] The progeny develop neurofibromas histologically identical to those observed in NF1 patients as well as pigmented lesions similar to café au lait spots. However, these hamsters also have Wilms' tumors and other malignancies not typically seen in NF1 patients. Recently, point mutations in the neu proto-oncogene were identified in these hamster tumors. No mutations have been identified to date in the hamster NF1 gene by Southern or western blot analysis.[132]

In an effort to develop a mouse model for neurofibromatosis, mice were generated that carried a null mutation at the murine NF1 locus using gene targeting in embryonic stem cells.[133,134] Heterozy-gous mutant mice containing one mutant NF1 and one wild-type allele are phenotypically normal without evidence of neurofibromas, pigmentary, or Lisch nodules. However, 75 percent of heterozygous mice succumb to tumors within 27 months compared with 15 percent of wild type animals.[138] In addition to developing the tumor type seen in older wild-type mice, heterozygote NF1 mice develop certain tumor types characteristic of human NF1. One animal developed a neurofibrosarcoma at 21 months of age, and 12 developed adrenal tumors at 15 to 28 months. Nine of the adrenal tumors were pheochromocytomas. Examination of these tumors demonstrated loss of the wild-type NF1 allele and evidence of reduction to homozygosity for the NF1 gene in the tumor DNA. These data support the hypothesis that the loss of NF1 gene function contributes to the development of tumors.

The breeding of heterozygous knockout animals to yield mice in which both copies of the NF1 gene were disrupted by homologous recombination (homozygous knockout mice) produced embryos that died in utero from generalized tissue edema.[133,134] Examination of the heart in these mice at embryonic day 12.5 demonstrates a double-outlet right ventricle defect resulting from a failure of the aorta and pulmonary artery to separate. Double-outlet right ventricles have been observed in developing chicks in which the neural crest cells migrating to form elements of the cardiac vasculature are ablated. These results suggest that neurofibromin may be critical for the function of these neural crest-derived cells, although other mechanisms are possible. In addition to the cardiac vessel defect, the skeletal musculature is hypoplastic relative to normal mouse embryos. The existence of a muscle-specific isoform of the NF1 gene and the observation that neurofibromin expression is increased in skeletal and cardiac muscle during embryonic development argue that neurofibromin also may be critical for normal muscle differentiation.[135,136] Additionally, examination of the sympathetic ganglia in these homozygous mutant mice demonstrates hyperplasia and an increased mitotic index.[137] These neurons also exhibit a reduced requirement for exogenous survival factors (neurotrophins), arguing that loss of neurofibromin may drive some cells to proliferate even in the absence of survival factors.

Identification of the NF1 Gene Product

The protein product of the NF1 locus has been identified. Using antibodies generated against fusion proteins and synthetic peptides, a unique 250-kDa protein is identifiable in all cell lines examined.[138-142] This NF1-GAP-related protein was originally termed NF1GRP to underscore its relationship to mammalian GAP and the yeast IRA1 and IRA2 genes (see below).[4,140] The NNFF consortium agreed to call this protein product neurofibromin. This protein was localized to the cytoplasm by differential centrifugation, glycerol gradients, and indirect immunofluorescence.[138,143] The difference between the predicted (327 kDa) and the observed (250 kDa) molecular weights results from anomalous migration in SDS-PAGE, not from posttranslational modifications (Gutmann DH: unpublished results). Expression of the full-length cDNA in insect cells produces a protein that migrates at 250 kDa.[144] Similarly, antibodies directed against both N- and C-terminal epitopes all recognize the same 250-kDa protein.[145]

The tissue distribution of neurofibromin is somewhat controversial in that the mRNA appears to be present at some level in all tissues.[1] Initial examination of whole-cell homogenates from mouse and rat tissues suggested that neurofibromin was also ubiquitously expressed.[140] Subsequent analysis by western blotting, immunoprecipitation, and immunohistochemistry demonstrated that the highest levels of expression are in the brain, spleen, kidney, testis, and thymus[98,139] (Gutmann DH: unpublished data). Immunohistochemical analysis of tissue sections from human and rodent tissues demonstrates prominent nervous system expression of neurofibromin.[98,138,139] Neurofibromin can be detected in the dendritic processes of central nervous system neurons (pyramidal neurons in cortical layers 2 and 5 and cerebellar Purkinje cells), peripheral nervous system neuronal axons, nonmyelinating Schwann cells, oligodendrocytes, and dorsal-root ganglia but not, astrocytes, microglia, and myelinating Schwann cells.[139,146] Neurofibromin expression is expressed in reactive astrocytes.[147] There does not appear to be abundant expression in lung, muscle, intestine, heart, or skin.

The expression of neurofibromin during embryogenesis is being studied in the avian and rodent systems. Preliminary results suggest that neurofibromin is expressed in the developing brain and spinal cord.[96,97] This pattern of expression could potentially account for the described learning disabilities previously unattributable to a purely neural crest-derived tissue disorder. Neurofibromin expression appears to rise dramatically after day 10 of mouse development. In the rat, neurofibromin is ubiquitously expressed from day 10 through day 16, after which it becomes increased in spinal cord and brain.[148] At this time, neurofibromin can be found in skeletal muscle, skin, lung, adrenal cortex, and cartilage. By postnatal day 6, the distribution of neurofibromin is identical to that seen in adults. These data, combined with the observation that homozygous mouse *NF1* gene knockouts exhibit developmental arrest and death around embryonic day 13, suggest that events occurring during this time interval depend heavily on the proper expression of neurofibromin. Future studies directed at understanding these events will provide insights into the pathogenesis of NF1.

Neurofibromin as a GTPase-Activating Protein

As was mentioned above, analysis of the amino acid sequence of the *NF1* gene product revealed sequence similarity between a small portion of the gene and a family of GAPs.[4,149–154] These proteins, both in mammals and in yeast, appear to regulate the GTP state of the cellular p21-*ras* proto-oncogene.[155,156] GAP molecules accelerate the hydrolysis of p21-*ras*-GTP to p21-*ras*-GDP, converting the proto-oncogene from the active form to the inactive form.[153,157] Although the effector of p21-*ras* in mammalian cells is unknown, in yeast, p21-*ras* is important in cAMP regulation.[155,158,159] This sequence similarity was supported by functional studies in mammalian cells and yeast, suggesting that the NF1GRD can act as a GAP molecule in vitro and in vivo.[5–7,160,161] Recent experiments also have demonstrated that the full-length neurofibromin molecule has GAP-like activity.[118,119,144]

It is exciting to postulate that neurofibromin functions as a tumor-suppressor gene product by down-regulating the normal function of the p21-*ras* proto-oncogene (Fig. 22-11). Previous studies demonstrated that p21-*ras* functions as part of a tyrosine kinase signal transduction pathway involving receptor tyrosine kinases such as epidermal, nerve, and platelet-derived growth factors (EGF, NGF, and PDGF) receptors.[162–164] Support for the involvement of p21-*ras* in such pathways derives from a large number of experiments in a wide variety of signal transduction systems. First, overexpression of the active form of p21-*ras* (v-*ras*) results in neurite extension in a rat pheochromocytoma cell line (PC12) similar to that observed with NGF treatment.[165,166] This effect can be reversed by injecting PC12 cells with antibodies against p21-*ras*.[167] There is conflicting data regarding the existence of a separate p21-*ras*-independent pathway that also culminates in neurite extension.[168] Second, overexpression of activated p21-*ras* can induce morphologic transformation of fibroblast cell lines and unlimited cell proliferation.[169,170] Third, some fibroblast cell lines can be induced to differentiate into adipocytes with overexpression of activated p21-*ras*.[171] Fourth, p21-*ras* is associated with surface immunoglobulin capping as part of a signal transduction (antigen presentation) pathway in B lymphocytes.[172,173]

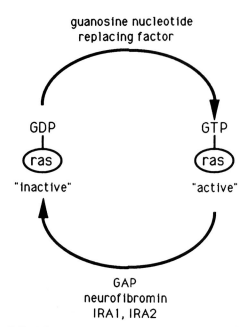

FIG. 22-11 The p21-*ras* cycle of activation and inactivation by GAP-related proteins. p21-*ras* is inactive in the GDP-bound state and is converted to an active GTP-bound state by guanosine nucleotide-replacing proteins that substitute GTP for GDP. Interaction of GAP-like proteins with p21-*ras* accelerates the conversion of p21-*ras*-GTP to p21-*ras*-GDP by increasing the intrinsic GTPase activity of p21-*ras* and converting p21-*ras* to the inactive GDP-bound form. In resting cells, the majority of p21-*ras* is inactive and in the GDP-bound form.

GAP molecules such as mammalian GAP and the yeast IRA1 and IRA2 proteins may serve to regulate p21-*ras*-mediated growth and differentiation pathways by maintaining p21-*ras* in the inactive GDP-bound state. This model is supported by studies that demonstrate that stimulation of tyrosine kinase receptors such as the EGF and PDGF receptors results in phosphorylation of mammalian GAP on tyrosine residues and inactivation of its GTPase-activating properties.[163,174,175] This inactivation would lead to increased p21-*ras* in the active GTP-bound state and to unregulated cell proliferation in the case of EGF and PDGF. The role of GAP in NGF receptor signal transduction pathways leading to cell differentiation and neurite extension is less well understood. By analogy, it is appealing to suggest that inactivation of neurofibromin as a result of mutation results in higher levels of p21-*ras*-GTP within affected cells and unlimited cell proliferation, leading to the formation of neurofibromas or neurofibrosarcomas. As was stated previously, examination of three neurofibrosarcomas demonstrated dramatically reduced expression of neurofibromin and elevated p21-*ras*-GTP levels.[118,119] Neurofibromin is phosphorylated on serine and threonine residues in response to EGF and PDGF stimulation but not on tyrosine residues and therefore must involve a pathway distinct from the tyrosine phosphorylation cascade that acts on mammalian GAP.[176,177]

Recent studies have suggested that neurofibromin may suppress cell growth through mechanisms unrelated to *ras* regulation. In NIH3T3 fibroblasts, overexpression of the *NF1* tumor-suppressor gene resulted in a threefold reduction in cell growth without any changes in *ras* activity.[178] Similarly, overexpression of full-length neurofibromin in a human colon carcinoma cell line resulted in reduced tumor growth in nude mice. In these experiments, the growth-suppressor activity of neurofibromin resulted from neurofibromin interfering with *ras* activation of raf.[179,180] Finally, *ras* activity can regulate neurofibromin expression.[41] This finding suggests either that neurofibromin is a critical regulator of *ras* in some cells or that neurofibromin may be stimulated by *ras* activation to perform some other function or functions within cells.

Further work will be required to distinguish between these not mutually exclusive possibilities.

Neurofibromin Associates with Cytoplasmic Microtubules

Subcellular localization of neurofibromin demonstrated an association with cytoplasmic microtubules by indirect immunofluorescence and biochemical purification.[143,145,181] Previously described proteins that associate with microtubules (MAPs) fall into three classes based on their molecular weights: MAP1 (250 kDa), MAP2 (250 kDa), and tau (35 to 65 kDa).[182–185] Some of these proteins are involved in the stabilization of microtubules through bundling, a process in which the tight association of microtubule filaments is facilitated.[186,187] Other MAP molecules actively promote microtubule movement, and some are involved in microtubule-mediated intracytoplasmic transport.[188] Subpopulations of microtubules are implicated in signal transduction pathways involving neurotransmitters and surface receptors.[189]

Biochemical properties of MAP molecules include GTP and temperature-dependent microtubule association, dissociation from microtubules by ion-exchange chromatography, improved association with taxol treatment, and coimmunoprecipitation with tubulin.[190–195] These properties have been observed with neurofibromin and indicate that there are specific interactions between neurofibromin and microtubules. Studies have also demonstrated that tubulin can partially inhibit the GAP activity of neurofibromin, an effect that is reversed with antitubulin antibodies.[144] In addition, a 20-amino acid sequence is found in neurofibromin that is shared with two other MAP molecules (MAP2 and tau) and has been reported to be a serine phosphorylation sequence that is important in regulating tau association with microtubules.[143,196] Phosphorylation of tau on that serine residue results in a conformational change and dissociation from the microtubules.

The finding that neurofibromin associates with microtubules does not mean that neurofibromin is a MAP. Intracytoplasmic or-

ganelles copurify with microtubules in a manner analogous to MAP molecules, yet these organelles would not be considered MAP molecules since they lack a role in stabilizing or facilitating microtubule-mediated functions. Further examination of the biochemical and physical nature of this association is necessary before neurofibromin can be assigned as a member of the MAP family.

The discovery that neurofibromin is a GAP-like molecule that associates with microtubules suggests several hypotheses to explain its function in cell growth and differentiation (Fig. 22-12). One model, which fits the upstream view of p21–ras–GAP interactions, envisions that neurofibromin is regulated by serine/threonine kinases.[197,198] Neurofibromin would be active as a GAP while associated with microtubules, keeping p21-ras in the inactive form and inhibiting cell division. After phosphorylation, neurofibromin would dissociate from the microtubules and its GAP activity would be reduced or altered. Alternatively, neurofibromin could be compartmentalized in the microtubule compartment (perhaps performing some other function) until it is required for the control of p21-ras. Phosphorylation of neurofibromin on critical serine residues would release it from the microtubules to interact with p21-ras. Support for this alternative model is provided by experiments that have failed to demonstrate any alteration of GAP activity after neurofibromin phosphorylation in vitro. Similarly, the interaction of neurofibromin with microtubules may actually reduce its GAP activity, as suggested by recent experiments,[144] and its dissociation from the microtubules may allow neurofibromin to associate with and down-regulate p21-ras. Of interest is the finding that the same domain of neurofibromin, the GAP-related domain, is the portion of neurofibromin required for microtubule association, suggesting a direct relationship between neurofibromin, p21-ras regulation, and microtubule association.[143,144,199] Further studies have demonstrated the involvement of neurofibromin in a B-lymphocyte signal transduction pathway involving microtubules and p21-ras. In this system, neurofibromin and p21-ras colocalize during immunoglobulin receptor internalization and neurofibromin is rapidly phosphorylated.[177] A second model, which falls into the category of a downstream hypothesis for p21–ras–GAP interac-

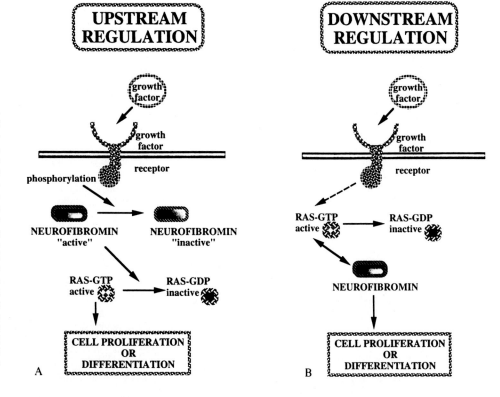

FIG. 22-12 Upstream versus downstream models of p21–ras–neurofibromin interactions. *A.* In the upstream model, stimulation of appropriate cells expressing growth factor receptors leads to an inactivation of neurofibromin, perhaps through phosphorylation cascades. Inactivation of neurofibromin releases p21-ras from its down-regulation, allowing p21-ras to predominate in the active GTP-bound form and signal other intracellular proteins to culminate in cell proliferation or differentiation. *B.* The downstream model on the other hand envisions p21-ras as a regulator of neurofibromin and states that it transmits a signal via neurofibromin and p21-ras to culminate in cell proliferation or differentiation. For more detail, refer to the text.

tion, is that neurofibromin is induced by the process of p21-*ras*-GTP to p21-*ras*-GDP conversion to transmit a signal through its influence on microtubule organization. Further investigations will be required to refute or support either of these two not mutually exclusive hypotheses unequivocally.

Neurofibromin Isoforms

Several isoforms of neurofibromin have been identified that arise from alternative splicing.[2,94] The first inserts 21 amino acids within the NF1GRD. This type 2 isoform is expressed in tissues different from those in which type 1 neurofibromin is expressed, and may be regulated by brain-specific differentiation events.[200] It is expressed in many species, including chickens.[201] The type 2 isoform is the predominant mRNA species after week 22 of human fetal development and can be induced in a neuroblastoma cell line by retinoic acid treatment.[200] Similar induction of type 2 neurofibromin expression is observed during Schwann cell differentiations as reflected by an increase in *NF1* mRNA and neurofibromin levels as well as a switch from type 1 to type 2 NF1 mRNA in Schwann cells stimulated to differentiate in response to treatments that increase intracellular AMP.[201,202] In addition, *NF1* isoform expression is altered during mouse embryogenesis, with type 2 NF1 mRNA expressed before embryonic day 10 and type 1 *NF1* mRNA predominating thereafter.[203] Studies in yeast demonstrate that this isoform also has GAP-like catalytic activity, although moderately reduced from that observed with native type 1 neurofibromin.[201] Whether this isoform can associate with cytoplasmic microtubules is being investigated.

A second, less well-characterized isoform has been identified near the C terminus of the protein and results from an 18-amino acid insertion.[2,94] This isoform is detected on the RNA level predominantly in muscle. It is expressed in cardiac muscle (both fetal and adult), skeletal muscle, and some smooth muscle tissues.[204] Little or no expression is found in brain, spleen, or kidney. The expression of an isoform of *NF1* in muscle is intriguing in light of a small number of patients with NF1 and cardiac disease.[205,206] In addition, it recently was demonstrated that neurofibromin expression increases while p21-*ras* activity decreases in myoblasts stimulated to differentiate in vitro.[136] Similarly, neurofibromin is transiently expressed in developing myotomes during murine and chick embryonic development.[96,97,148] The relationship between the muscle expression of this isoform and the clinical manifestations of NF1 remains unelucidated.

Recently, an additional isoform of the *NF1* gene was identified which is expressed predominantly in the brain.[207] This alternatively spliced isoform containing exon 9a is enriched in human and rodent cerebral cortex, where its expression correlates with cortical neuron maturation both in vitro and in vivo.[208] The finding of a brain-specific *NF1* isoform suggests that neurofibromin may play unique roles during central nervous system development.

Biologic Properties of Neurofibromas

Both plexiform and cutaneous neurofibromas can arise from any nerve throughout the body and at any time, including embryonically. Neurofibromas tend to grow more rapidly during pregnancy and puberty, implying some hormone sensitivity.[209,210] Neurofibromas grow as a mixed population of cells that includes fibroblasts, mast cells, Schwann cells, axons, perineural cells, and endothelial cells.[209-215] The clonal nature of neurofibromas is controversial and has not been resolved conclusively.[216,217]

Neurofibromas have been found to contain mitogens that stimulate Schwann cell and fibroblast proliferation.[218,219] One study using purified Schwann cells from neurofibromas demonstrated that these NF1 Schwann cells promoted angiogenesis and could invade chicks' chorioallantoic membranes.[220] These results suggest that neurofibroma Schwann cells are intrinsically different from normal Schwann cells. NF1 fibroblasts have also been examined for evidence of abnormal growth characteristics. Although many of these studies have been difficult to reproduce, it has been suggested that NF1 fibroblasts are more sensitive to ionizing radiation and have an increased rate of transformation by Kirsten murine sarcoma viruses.[221-224]

Diagnosis and Treatment

Conventional Treatment of NF1 Patients. The treatment of patients affected with NF1 often requires the expertise of many medical and surgical subspecialists coordinated by one physician or a team of physicians familiar with NF1.[225] For this reason, we advocate the establishment of neurofibromatosis clinics staffed by physicians who regularly see NF1 patients and are familiar with the diagnosis, management, and complications of the disorder. Closely affiliated with the clinic should be a diverse collection of other physicians and health care providers with subspecialties in given areas of medicine or surgery. These persons include ophthalmologists, neurologists, plastic surgeons, neurosurgeons, otolaryngologists, psychiatrists, social workers, child psychologists, orthopedic surgeons, dermatologists, and oncologists. The role of an NF clinic is not only to provide coordinated care from a centralized caregiver familiar with NF1 but also to provide up-to-date information to patients and their families about the disease through regular communication via NNFF-sponsored newsletters and scientific symposia.

The approach to a new patient suspected of having NF1 involves careful history taking and examination. Before the clinic appointment, it is helpful for a genetic counselor to contact the patient to review the patient's clinical features and family history. Often this phone call will precipitate further investigation on the part of the patient and family members in an attempt to determine which other family members have features consistent with NF1. A careful exploration of the family may uncover relatives with subtle features of NF1; this is particularly true in light of its variable expressivity. Hospital records, autopsy reports, and surgical pathology reports should also be requested.

Once the patient arrives in the clinic, he or she should be examined thoroughly by one of the NF1 physicians. A careful cutaneous examination is performed to look for palpable neurofibromas, axillary or inguinal freckling, and café au lait spots. The café au lait spots can be better visualized under a Woods lamp. The number of pigmented lesions and their greatest diameters are recorded. An ophthalmologic examination with attention to measurement of visual acuity is important to rule out symptomatic optic glioma. In individuals beyond the age of 7 to 8, inspection of the iris should reveal Lisch nodules, especially in patients with light-colored irises. If Lisch nodules are not appreciated and diagnostic criteria for NF1 have not been met, referral to an opthalmologist for a slit-lamp evaluation is made. During a general physical examination, attention is focused on the detection of any curvature of the spine, especially in young children. Severe cases are referred to an orthopedic surgeon. In addition, inspection of the long bones of the upper and lower extremities is warranted in young children to exclude bowing and thinning of the cortices of these bones and prevent the formation of pseudarthroses. Suspicious bones are examined by plain x-rays, and affected patients are referred to an orthopedic surgeon knowledgeable about the bracing and management of this problem. In children, height, weight, and head circumference are noted during each visit and are charted to evaluate a child's growth curve. Inspection of the face and fingers is done to look for facial dysmorphisms or dermatoglyphics suggestive of disorders besides NF1. In addition, blood pressure should be measured during each visit. We recommend routine general medical appointments spaced 6 months after each visit to the NF1 clinic to allow for blood pressure determinations twice a year. Any abnormal rise in blood pressure always warrants further investigation for renal artery stenosis or pheochromocytoma. Patients should be questioned about headache (location, frequency, and character) and bowel or bladder difficulties to screen for deep neurofibromatous involvement of splanchnic nerves.

A screening neurologic examination should be performed during each visit, with special attention to visual acuity, visual fields, and funduscopic evaluation. We strongly advocate the limited and directed use of brain imaging studies and do not obtain them unless there is a change in the symptoms or in the neurologic examination. The limited use of brain imaging studies is based on the low yield of these studies in detecting asymptomatic lesions that require treatment as well as the high likelihood of finding a high-intensity lesion on T_2-weighted MRI. These high-intensity lesions are sometimes referred to as UBOs and can be seen in upward of 60 percent of these children. Their clinical significance is uncertain, and their detection often raises unnecessary concern on the part of both the family and the physician.

During the evaluation attention is also paid to the social history. In children, school performance is a good reflection of overall learning ability. Formal evaluation of IQ by the school district is recommended early (age 3 to 4) to identify children with learning disabilities. Early detection and aggressive intervention appear to be beneficial in NF1 patients. We encourage families to communicate regularly with the school and to obtain physical, speech, and occupational therapy as appropriate.

Patients with NF1 are seen on a yearly basis in the clinic, during which time they are educated about new information regarding the disease; a forum is provided for a discussion of their concerns and questions. In addition, patients are monitored for the development of new complications, and new family members are evaluated for signs of NF1. The removal of neurofibromas that are particularly large or cosmetically distressing or that rub on clothing straps is coordinated with a plastic surgeon. Otherwise, we encourage patients not to have multiple neurofibromas removed solely for cosmetic reasons, since they can grow back in these areas after surgery.

An integral part of the diagnosis and care of NF1 patients involves the genetic counselor. In our clinic, genetic counselors explain in detail the pattern of inheritance of NF1 (autosomal dominant), its penetrance (essentially 100 percent by 5 years of age), and its variable expressivity. Education is provided, and common misconceptions regarding the disease are dispelled. The emotional impact of NF1 on the patient as well as the other family members is addressed. Families are also given information about support group resources. Explanations of the natural history of the disorder, its behavior during puberty and pregnancy, and its unpredictability are explored. Prenatal counseling is provided for the parents and sibs of affected patients. Prenatal testing when appropriate is offered to families in which linkage analysis is informative (see below).

Molecular Genetic Approaches to NF1 Patients. With the entire *NF1* gene cloned and the protein identified, it is now theoretically possible to study gene mutations in patients with NF1. The approaches taken to screen for mutations involve a combination of DNA, RNA, and protein analysis. However, given the large size of the gene and the heterogeneity of the mutations, the search for causative mutations is quite labor-intensive. In the years since the

cloning of the full-length *NF1* gene, only a handful of mutations have been characterized owing to the arduous task of screening 60 exons for DNA alterations. Therefore, routine clinical application of DNA analysis in the diagnosis of NF1 is not yet a reality. In families in which the clinical diagnosis is certain, multiple members are affected, and closely linked polymorphic markers are informative, linkage analysis using closely spaced markers or microsatellite repeat sequences remains the most practical application of DNA diagnostics.[226]

It is possible that mutations in different regions and/or domains of the *NF1* gene will produce different phenotypes, as has been demonstrated for mutations within the dystrophin gene. As was true with the dystrophin gene, in which other related but distinct disorders were caused by mutations within the same gene, it is important to study neurologic disorders with abnormalities similar to those found in NF1 for alterations in the *NF1* gene.

To date, it has not been possible to provide diagnostic information by surveying for alterations at the protein level. No anomalously migrating protein species have been observed, as was noted for Becker muscular dystrophy. It appears that all the mutations described so far result in a lack of neurofibromin expression as opposed to a smaller or larger protein product. Theoretically, an assay capable of distinguishing 100 percent levels from 50 percent levels of neurofibromin could detect most affected individuals (since most mutations would be null at the protein level). This requires a level of reliable quantification that has not been achieved, however.

NF1 remains a clinical diagnosis. Using the diagnostic criteria established in the NIH consensus statement, the diagnosis of NF1 can confidently be made in the vast majority of individuals. For selected individuals desiring prenatal diagnosis, genetic testing and counseling can be provided. In families with two or more affected individuals with NF1, linkage analysis can be performed. Recently, a commercial test for *NF1* gene mutations was developed which relies on a protein truncation assay.[227] With this technique, RNA from white blood cells is reverse transcribed and converted into overlapping *NF1* cDNA fragments in vitro. Neurofibromin proteins from individuals with NF1 that are larger or smaller than the predicted fragment sizes are then used to direct the search for the underlying *NF1* gene mutation. The advantage of this system is the speed with which mutations can potentially be identified. However, it is unclear at this point whether this test will identify a significant portion of *NF1* gene mutations in individuals with NF1 to warrant more widespread use.

The cloning of the *NF1* gene has opened the door to a more complete understanding of NF1 pathobiology with the eventual goal of designing specific, nonsurgical treatments for affected patients. The finding of elevated p21-*ras*-GTP levels in tumors from NF1 patients suggests that drug therapies directed at up-regulating neurofibromin GAP activity or down-regulating p21-*ras* activity may have a beneficial effect on the growth of neurofibromas. A number of groups have been studying the lipid sensitivity of neurofibromin GAP activity in vitro and have found that specific lipids preferentially alter neurofibromin GAP activity as opposed to mammalian p120-GAP catalytic activity.[160,228-230] The discovery of a compound capable of up-regulating or replacing neurofibromin may prove to be a useful therapy in the future.

Similarly, drugs that interfere with p21-*ras* activity, such as pharmaceutical agents that block farnesylation, a reaction necessary for p21-*ras* membrane localization, may have therapeutic potential in NF1.[231,232,233] Farnesylation-blocking agents have been shown to inhibit the mitogenic effects of growth factors and the tumorigenic properties of neuroblastoma cells. More useful therapies may involve drugs that inhibit farnesyl transferase (the addition of farnesyl groups to the p21-*ras* protein) rather than lovastatin and compactin, which are HMG-CoA reductase inhibitors that block farnesyl synthesis. Further study of these and related drugs may uncover useful therapies for NF1 patients.

ACKNOWLEDGMENTS

We thank the members of our neurofibromatosis research group, past and present, especially Drs. Lone Andersen, Steve Doran, Jane Fountain, R. Todd Geist, Paula Gregory, Douglas Marchuk, Anna Mitchell, Margaret Wallace, and Susan Wilson-Gunn. We also thank our collaborators elsewhere, including Drs. Roymarie Ballester, Dafna Bar-Sagi, Mark Boguski, Gideon Bollag, Dennis Choi, Jeff DeClue, Julian Downward, Ab Guha, Chung Hsu, Tyler Jacks, Richard Jove, David Louis, Douglas Lowy, Frank McCormick, Lynn Rutkowski, Gihan Tennekoon, and Michael Wigler. We also thank numerous members of the NF1 research community for providing preprints of manuscripts and are particularly grateful to Dr. Susan Huson for supplying drafts of several chapters on the clinical manifestations of NF1. Nancy North provided expert assistance in the preparation of this manuscript.

REFERENCES

1. Wallace MR, Marchuk DA, Anderson LB, Letcher R, Odeh HM, Saulino AM, Fountain JW, Brereton A, Nicholson J, Mitchell AL, Brownstein BH, Collins FS: Type 1 neurofibromatosis gene: Identification of a large transcript disrupted in three NF1 patients. *Science* **249**:181, 1990.
2. Cawthon RM, Weiss R, Xu G, Viskochil D, Culver M, Stevens J, Robertson M, Dunn D, Gesteland R, O'Connell P, White R: A major segment of the neurofibromatosis type 1 gene: cDNA sequence, genomic structure, and point mutations. *Cell* **62**:193, 1990.
3. Viskochil D, Buchberg AM, Xu G, Cawthon RM, Stevens J, Wolff RK, Culver M, Carey JC, Copeland NG, Jenkins NA, White R, O'Connell P: Deletions and a translocation interrupt a cloned gene at the neurofibromatosis type 1 locus. *Cell* **62**:187, 1990.
4. Xu G, O'Connell P, Viskochil D, Cawthon R, Robertson M, Culver M, Dunn D, Stevens J, Gesteland R, White R, Weiss R: The neurofibromatosis type 1 gene encodes a protein related to GAP. *Cell* **62**:599, 1990.
5. Xu G, Lin B, Tanaka K, Dunn D, Wood D, Gesteland R, White R, Weiss R, Tamanoi F: The catalytic domain of the neurofibromatosis type 1 gene product stimulates *ras* GTPase and complements ira mutants of *S. cerevisiae. Cell* **63**:835, 1990.
6. Martin GA, Viskochil D, Bollag G, McCabe PC, Crosier WJ, Haubruck H, Conroy L, Clark R, O'Connell P, Cawthon RM, Innis MA, McCormick F: The GAP-related domain of the neurofibromatosis type 1 gene product interacts with *ras* p21. *Cell* **63**:843, 1990.
7. Ballester R, Marchuk DA, Boguski M, Saulino AM, Letcher R, Wigler M, Collins FS: The *NF1* locus encodes a protein functionally related to mammalian GAP and yeast IRA proteins. *Cell* **63**:851, 1990.
8. Huson SM, Hughes RAC: *The Neurofibromatoses: A Pathogenetic and Clinical Overview.* London, Chapman and Hall, 1994.
9. Riccardi VM, Eichner JE: *Neurofibromatosis: Phenotype, Natural History and Pathogenesis*, 2d ed. Baltimore, Johns Hopkins University Press, 1992.
10. Korf BR, Carey JC: Molecular genetics of neurofibromatosis, in Rubenstein AE, Korf BR (ed): *Neurofibromatosis: A Handbook for Patients, Families, and Health-Care Professionals.* New York, Thieme, 1990, p. 178.
11. Crowe FW, Schull WJ, Neel JV: *A Clinical, Pathological and Genetic Study of Multiple Neurofibromatosis.* Springfield, IL, Charles C Thomas, 1956.
12. Trofatter JA, MacCollin MM, Rutter JL, Murrell JR, Duyao MP, Parry DM, Eldridge R, Kley N, Menon AG, Pulaski K, Haase VH, Ambrose CM, Munroe E, Bove C, Haines JL, Martuzza RL, MacDonald ME, Seizinger DR, Short MP, Buckler AJ, Gusella JF: A

13. Rouleau GA, Merel P, Lutchman M, Sanson M, Zucman J, Marineau C, Hoang-Zuan K, Demczuk S, Desmaze C, Plougastel B, Pulst SM, Lenoir G, Bijlsma E, Fashold R, Dumanski J, de Jong P, Parry D, Eldridge R, Aurias A, Delattre O, Thomas G: Alteration in a new gene encoding a putative membrane-organizing protein causes neurofibromatosis type 2. *Nature* **363**:515, 1993.
14. Zanca A: Antique illustrations of neurofibromatosis. *Int J Dermatol* **19**:55, 1980.
15. Hecht F: Recognition of neurofibromatosis before von Recklinghausen. *Neurofibromatosis* **2**:180, 1989.
16. Von Recklinghausen FD: *Ueber die multiplen fibrome der Hautund inhre beziehung zu den multiplen neuromen.* Berlin, Hirschwald, 1882.
17. Preiser SA, Davenport CB: Multiple neurofibromatosis (von Recklinghausen disease) and its inheritance. *Am J Med Sci* **156**:507, 1918.
18. Lisch K: Ueber beteiligung der augen, insbesondere das vorkommen von irisknotchen bei der neurofibromatose (Recklinghausen). *Augenheilkde* **93**:137, 1937.
19. Lewis RA, Riccardi VM: Von Recklinghausen neurofibromatosis: Incidence of iris hamartomata. *Ophthalmology* **88**:348, 1981.
20. Lubs M-LE, Bauer MS, Formas ME, Djokic B: Lisch nodules in neurofibromatosis type 1. *N Engl J Med* **324**:1264, 1991.
21. Borberg A: Clinical and genetic investigations into tuberous sclerosis and Recklinghausen's neurofibromatosis. *Acta Psychiatr Neurol Suppl* **71**:1, 1951.
22. Sorenson SA, Mulvhill JT, Nielsen A: Longterm follow up of von Recklinghausen neurofibromatosis: Survival and malignant neoplasms. *N Engl J Med* **314**:1010, 1986.
23. Carey JC, Laub JM, Hall BD: Penetrance and variability in neurofibromatosis: A genetic study of 60 families. *Birth Defects* **15**(5B):271, 1979.
24. Riccardi VM: Von Recklinghausen neurofibromatosis. *N Engl J Med* **305**:1617, 1981.
25. Huson SM, Harper PS, Compston DAS: Von Recklinghausen neurofibromatosis: A clinical and population study in south east Wales. *Brain* **111**:1535, 1988.
26. Huson SM, Compston DAS, Harper PS, Clark P: A genetic study of von Recklinghausen neurofibromatosis in south east Wales: I. Prevalence, fitness, mutation rate, and effect of parental transmission on severity. *J Med Genet* **26**:704, 1989.
27. Huson SM, Compston DAS, Harper PS: A genetic study of von Recklinghausen neurofibromatosis in south east Wales: II. Guidelines for genetic counselling. *J Med Genet* **26**:712, 1989.
28. Sergeyev AS: On the mutation rate of neurofibromatosis. *Hum Genet* **28**:129, 1975.
29. Samuelsson B, Axelsson R: Neurofibromatosis: A clinical and genetic study of 96 cases in Gothenburg, Sweden. *Acta Derm Venereol Suppl (Stockh)* **95**:67, 1981.
30. NIH Consensus Development Conference: Neurofibromatosis statement. *Arch Neurol* **45**:575, 1988.
31. Burwell RG, James NJ, Johnston DI: Café au lait spots in school children. *Arch Dis Child* **57**:631, 1982.
32. Benedict PH, Szabo G, Fitzpatrick TB, Sinesi SJ: Melanotic macules in Albright s syndrome and in neurofibromatosis. *JAMA* **205**:72, 1968.
33. Lott IT, Richardson EP Jr: Neuropathological findings and the biology of neurofibromatosis. *Adv Neurol* **28**:23, 1981.
34. Crowe FW: Axillary freckling as a diagnostic aid in neurofibromatosis. *Ann Intern Med* **61**:1142, 1964.
35. Riccardi VM, Eichner JE: *Neurofibromatosis: Phenotype, Natural History, and Pathogenesis.* Baltimore, Johns Hopkins University Press, 1986.
36. Horwich A, Riccardi VM, Francke V: Brief clinical report: Aqueductal stenosis leading to hydrocephalus, an unusual manifestation of neurofibromatosis. *Am J Med Genet* **14**:577, 1983.
37. Kayes LM, Riccardi VM, Burke W, Bennett RL, Stephens K: Large de novo DNA deletion in a patient with sporadic neurofibromatosis, mental retardation and dysmorphism. *J Med Genet* **29**:686, 1992.
38. North K, Joy P, Yuille D, Cocks N, Mobbs E, Hutchiins P, McHugh K, de Silva M: Specific learning disability in children with neurofibromatosis type 1: Significance of MRI abnormalities. *Neurology* **44**:878, 1994.
39. DiPaolo DP, Zimmerman RA, Rorke LB, Zackai EH, Bilaniuk LT, Yachnis AT: Neurofibromatosis type 1: Pathologic substrate of high signal intensity foci in the brain. *Radiology* **195**:721, 1995.

40. Giordano MJ, Mahadeo DK, He YY, Geist RT, Hsu C, Gutmann DH: Increased expression of the neurofibromatosis 1 (NF1) gene product, neurofibromin, in astrocytes in response to cerebral ischemia. *J Neuroscience Res* **43**:246, 1996.

41. Gutmann DH, Giordano MJ, Mahadeo DK, Lau N, Silbergeld D, Guha A: Increased neurofibromatosis 1 gene expression in astrocytic tumors: Positive regulation by p21-*ras*. *Oncogene* **12**:2121, 1996.

42. Brasfield RD, Das Gupta TK: Von Recklinghausen's disease: A clinicopathological study. *Ann Surg* **175**:86, 1972.

43. Hope DG, Mulvhill JJ: Malignancy in neurofibromatosis. *Adv Neurol* **29**:33, 1981.

44. Thomas JE, Piepgras DG, Scheithauer BW, Onofrio BM, Shives TC: Neurogenic tumors of the sciatic nerve: A clinicopathologic study of 35 cases. *Mayo Clin Proc* **58**:640, 1983.

45. Lewis RA, Gerson LP, Axelsson KA, Riccardi VM, Whitford RP: Von Recklinghausen neurofibromatosis: II. Incidence of optic gliomata. *Ophthalmology* **91**:929, 1984.

46. Listernick R, Charrow J, Greewald MJ, Esterly NA: Optic gliomas in children with neurofibromatosis type 1. *J Pediatr* **114**:788, 1989.

47. Duffner PK, Cohen ME, Seidel FG, Shucard DW: The significance of MRI abnormalities in children with neurofibromatosis. *Neurology* **39**:373, 1989.

48. Holt JF: Neurofibromatosis in children. *AJR* **130**:615, 1978.

49. Daniels SR, Loggie JM, McEnery PT, Towbin RB: Clinical spectrum of intrinsic renovascular hypertension in children. *Pediatrics* **80**:698, 1993.

50. Hochberg FH, Dasilva AB, Galdabini J, Richardson EP Jr: Gastrointestinal involvement in von Recklinghausen's neurofibromatosis. *Neurology* **24**:1144, 1974.

51. Hall JG: Possible maternal and hormonal factors in neurofibromatosis. *Adv Neurol* **29**:125, 1981.

52. Miller M, Hall JG: Possible maternal effect on severity of neurofibromatosis. *Lancet* **2**:1071, 1978.

53. Hall JG: Genomic imprinting: Review and relevance of genetic diseases. *Am J Hum Genet* **46**:857, 1990.

54. Riccardi VM, Wald JS: Discounting an adverse maternal effect on severity of neurofibromatosis. *Pediatrics* **79**:386, 1987.

55. Huson SM, Clark D, Compston DAS, Harper PS: A genetic study of von Recklinghausen's neurofibromatosis in south east Wales: I. Prevalance, fitness, mutation rate and effect of parental transmission on severity. *J Med Genet* **26**:704, 1989.

56. Jadayel D, Fain P, Upadhyaya M, Ponder MA, Huson SM, Carey J, Fryer A, Mathew CGP, Barker DF, Ponder BAJ: Paternal origin of new mutations in von Recklinghausen neurofibromatosis. *Nature* **343**:558, 1990.

57. Stephens K, Kayes L, Riccardi VM, Rising M, Sybert VP, Pagon RA: Preferential mutation of the neurofibromatosis type 1 gene in paternally-derived chromosomes. *Hum Genet* **88**:279, 1992.

58. Riccardi VM, Lewis RA: Penetrance of von Recklinghausen neurofibromatosis: A distinction between predecessors and descendents. *Am J Hum Genet* **42**:284, 1988.

59. Easton DF, Ponder MA, Huson SM, Ponder BAJ: An analysis of variation in expression of neurofibromatosis (NF) type (NF1): Evidence for modifying genes. *Am J Hum Genet* **53**:305, 1993.

60. Eldridge R: Central neurofibromatosis with bilateral acoustic neuroma. *Adv Neurol* **29**:57, 1981.

61. Martuza RL, Eldridge R: Neurofibromatosis 2 (bilateral acoustic neurofibromatosis). *N Engl J Med* **318**:684, 1988.

62. Charles SJ, Moore AT, Yates JRW, Ferguson-Smith MA: Lisch nodules in neurofibromatosis type 2. *Arch Ophthalmol* **107**:1571, 1989.

63. Kaiser-Kupfer MI, Freidlin V, Datiles MB: The association of posterior capsular lens opacity with bilateral acoustic neuromas in patients with neurofibromatosis. *Arch Ophthalmol* **107**:541, 1989.

64. Trattner A, David M, Hodak E, Ben-David E, Sandbank M: Segmental neurofibromatosis. *J Am Acad Dermatol* **23**:866, 1990.

65. Rubenstein AE, Bader JL, Aron AA, Wallace S: Familial transmission of segmental neurofibromatosis. *Neurology* **33** (suppl 2):76, 1983.

66. Lazaro C, Ravella A, Gaona A, Volpini V, Estivill X: Neurofibromatosis type 1 due to germline mosaicism in a clinically normal father. *N Engl J Med* **33**:1403, 1994.

67. Colman SD, Rasmussen SA, Ho VT, Abernathy CR, Wallace MR: Somatic mosaicism in a patient with neurofibromatosis type 1. *Am J Hum Genet* **58**:484, 1996.

68. Allanson JE, Upadhyaya M, Watson GH, Parington M, Mackenzie A, MacLeod R, Safarazi M, Broadhead W, Harper PS: Watson syndrome: Is it a subtype of type 1 NF? *J Med Genet* **28**:752, 1991.

69. Opitz JM, Weaver DD:L The neurofibromatosis-Noonan syndrome. *Am J Med Genet* **21**:477, 1985.

70. Stern HJ, Saal HM, Fain PR, Golgar DE, Rosenbaum KN, Barher DF: Clinical reliability of type 1 neurofibromatosis: Is there a NF-Noonan syndrome? *J Med Genet* **29**:184, 1992.

71. Pulst S-M, Riccardi VM, Fain P, Korenberg JR: Familial spinal neurofibromatosis: Clinical and DNA linkage analysis. *Neurology* **41**:1923, 1991.

72. Collins FS: Positional cloning: Let's not call it reverse anymore. *Nat Genet* **1**:3, 1992.

73. Barker D, Wright E, Nguyen K, Cannon L, Fain P, Goldgar D, Bishop DT, Carey J, Kivlin J, Willard H, Nakamura Y, O'Connell P, Leppert M, White RL, Skolnick M: A genomic search for linkage of neurofibromatosis to RFLPs. *J Med Genet* **24**:536, 1987.

74. Diehl SR, Boehnke M, Erickson RP, Baxter AB, Bruce MA, Lieberman JL, Platt DJ, Ploughman LM, Seiler KA, Sweet AM, Collins FS: Linkage analysis of von Recklinghausen neurofibromatosis to DNA markers on chromosome 17. *Genomics* **1**:361, 1987.

75. Seizinger BR, Rouleau GA, Lane AH, Farmer G, Ozelius LJ, Haines JL, Parry DM, Korf BR, Pericak-Vance MA, Faryniarz AG, Hobbs WJ, Iannazzi JA, Roy JC, Menon A, Bader JL, Spence MA, Chao MV, Mulvihill JJ, Roses AD, Martuza RL, Breakefield XO, Conneally PM, Gusella JF: Linkage analysis in von Recklinghausen neurofibromatosis (NF1) with DNA markers for chromosome 17. *Genomics* **1**:346, 1987.

76. Skolnick MH, Ponder B, Seizinger B: Linkage of NF1 to 12 chromosome 17 markers: A summary of eight concurrent reports. *Genomics* **1**:382, 1987.

77. Seizinger BR, Rouleau GA, Ozelius LJ, Lane AH, Faryniarz AG, Chao MV, Huson S, Korf BR, Parry DM, Pericak-Vance MA, Collins FS, Hobbs WJ, Falcone BG, Iannazzi JA, Roy JC, St. George-Hyslop PH, Tanzi RE, Bothwell MA, Upadhyaya M, Harper P, Goldstein AE, Hoover DL, Bader JL, Spence MA, Mulvihill JJ, Aylsworth AS, Vance JM, Rossenwasser GOD, Gaskell PC, Roses AD, Martuza RL, Breakefield XO, Gusella JF: Genetic linkage of von Recklinghausen neurofibromatosis to the nerve growth factor receptor gene. *Cell* **49**:589, 1987.

78. Darby JK, Feder J, Selby M, Riccardi V, Ferrel R, Siao D, Goslin K, Rutter W, Shooter EM, Cavilli-Sforza LL: A discordant sibship analysis between beta-NGF and neurofibromatosis. *Am J Hum Genet* **37**:52, 1985.

79. Goldgar DE, Green P, Parry DM, Mulvihill JJ: Multipoint linkage analysis in neurofibromatosis type 1: An international collaboration. *Am J Hum Genet* **44**:6, 1989.

80. Fountain JW, Wallace MR, Bruce MA, Seizinger BR, Menon AG, Gusella JF, Michels VV, Schmidt MA, Dewald GW, Collins FS: Physical mapping of a translocation breakpoint in neurofibromatosis. *Science* **244**:1085, 1989.

81. Ledbetter DH, Rich DC, O'Connell P, Leppert M, Carey JC: Precise localization of NF1 to 17q11.2 by balanced translocation. *Am J Hum Genet* **44**:20, 1989.

82. Menon AG, Ledbetter DH, Rich DC, Seizinger BR, Rouleau GA, Michels VV, Schmidt MA, Dewald G, DallaTorre CM, Haines JL, Gusella JF: Characterization of a translocation within the von Recklinghausen neurofibromatosis region of chromosome 17. *Genomics* **5**:245, 1989.

83. O'Connell P, Leach R, Cawthon RM, Culver M, Stevens J, Viskochil D, Fournier REK, Rich DC, Ledbetter DH, White R: Two NF1 translocations map within a 600-kilobase segment of 17q11.2. *Science* **244**:1087, 1989.

84. Schmidt MA, Michels VV, Dewald GW: Cases of neurofibromatosis with rearrangements of chromosome 17 involving band 17q11.2. *Am J Med Genet* **28**:771, 1987.

85. Fountain JW, Wallace MR, Brereton AB, O'Connell P, White RL, Rich DC, Ledbetter DH, Leach RJ, Fournier REK, Menon AG, Gusella JF, Barker D, Stephens K, Collins FS: Physical mapping of the von Recklinghausen neurofibromatosis region on chromosome 17. *Am J Hum Genet* **44**:58, 1989.

86. Buchberg AM, Bedigian HG, Taylor BA, Brownell E, Ihle JN, Nagata S, Jenkins NA, Copeland NG: Localization of evi-2 to chromosome 11: Linkage to other proto-oncogene and growth factor loci using interspecific backcross mice. *Oncogene Res* **2**:149, 1989.

87. Cawthon RM, Anderson LB, Buchberg AM, Xu G, O'Connell P, Viskochil D, Weiss RB, Wallace MR, Marchuk DA, Culver M, Stevens J, Jenkins NA, Copeland NG, White R: cDNA sequence and genomic structure of *EVI2B*, a gene lying within an intron of the neurofibromatosis type 1 gene. *Genomics* **9**:446, 1991.

88. O'Connell P, Viskochil D, Buchberg AM, Fountain J, Cawthon RM, Culver M, Stevens J, Rich DC, Ledbetter DH, Wallace M, Carey JC, Jenkins NA, Copeland NG, Collins FS, White R: The human homolog of murine *evi2* lies between two von Recklinghausen neurofibromatosis translocations. *Genomics* 7:547, 1990.

89. Cawthon RM, O'Connell P, Buchberg AM, Viskochil D, Weiss RB, Culver M, Stevens J, Jenkins NA, Copeland NG, White R: Identification and characterization of transcripts from the neurofibromatosis 1 region: The sequence and genomic structure of *EVI2* and mapping of other transcripts. *Genomics* 7:555, 1990.

90. Mikol DD, Gulcher JR, Stefansson K: The oligodendrocyte-myelin glycoprotein belongs to a distinct family of proteins and contains the HNK-1 carbohydrate. *J Cell Biol* 110:471, 1990.

91. Viskochil D, Cawthon R, O'Connell P, Xu G, Stevens J, Culver M, Carey J, White R: The gene encoding the oligodendrocyte-myelin glycoprotein is embedded within the neurofibromatosis type 1 gene. *Mol Cell Biol* 11:906, 1991.

92. Wallace MR, Anderson LB, Saulino AM, Gregory P, Glover T, Collins FS: A de novo insertion mutation causing neurofibromatosis type 1. *Nature* 353:864, 1991.

93. Li Y, O'Connell P, Breidenbach HH, Cawthon R, Stevens J, Xu G, Neil S, Robertson M, White R, Viskochil D: Genomic organization of the neurofibromatosis 1 gene (NF1). *Genomics* 25:9, 1995.

94. Marchuk DA, Saulino AM, Tavakkol R, Swaroop M, Wallace MR, Andersen LB, Mitchell AL, Gutmann DH, Boguski M, Collins FS: cDNA cloning of the type 1 neurofibromatosis gene: Complete sequence of the NF1 gene product. *Genomics* 11:931, 1991.

95. Buchberg AM, Cleveland LS, Jenkins NA, Copeland NG: Sequence homology shared by neurofibromatosis type 1 gene and IRA1 and IRA2 negative regulators of the *RAS* cyclic AMP pathway. *Nature* 347:291, 1990.

96. Kavka AL, Chan SW, Hellen K, Yu H, Gutmann DH, Barabld KF: Expression of avian neurofibromatosis (aNF1) message and protein in neural crest cells (in preparation).

97. Stocker KM, Baizer L, Coston T, Sherman L, Ciment G: Regulated expression of neurofibromin in migrating neural crest cells of avian embryos. *J Neurobiol* 27:535, 1995.

98. Nakamura T, Nemoto T, Arai M, Kasuga T, Gutmann DH, Collins FS, Ishikawa T: Specific expression of the neurofibromatosis type 1 (NF1) gene in hamster Schwann cell. *Am J Pathol* 144:549, 1994.

99. Bird AP: CpG-rich islands and the function of DNA methylation. *Nature* 321:209, 1986.

100. Legius E, Marchuk DA, Hall BK, Andersen LB, Wallace MR, Collins FS, Glover TW: NF1-related locus on chromosome 15. *Genomics* 13:1316, 1993.

101. Marchuk DA, Tavakkol R, Wallace MR, Brownstein BH, Taillon-Miller P, Fong C-T, Legius E, Andersen LB, Glover TW, Collins FS: A yeast artificial chromosome contig encompassing the type 1 neurofibromatosis gene. *Genomics* 13:372, 1992.

102. Upadhyaya M, Cheryson A, Broadhead W, Fryer A, Shaw DJ, Huson S, Wallace MR, Andersen LB, Marchuk DA, Viskochil D, Black D, O'Connell P, Collins FS, Harper PS: A 90 kb DNA deletion associated with neurofibromatosis type 1. *J Med Genet* 27:738, 1990.

103. Li Y, Bollag G, Clark R, Stevens J, Conroy L, Fults D, Ward K, Friedman E, Samowitz W, Robertson M, Bradley P, McCormick F, White R, Cawthon R: Somatic mutations in the neurofibromatosis 1 gene in human tumors. *Cell* 69:275, 1993.

104. Upadhyaya M: Analysis of mutations at the neurofibromatosis 1 (NF1) locus. *Hum Mol Genet* 1:735, 1992.

105. Marshall CJ: Tumor suppressor genes. *Cell* 64:313, 1991.

106. Sager R: Tumor suppressor genes: The puzzle and the promise. *Science* 246:1406, 1989.

107. Weinberg RA: Tumor suppressor genes. *Science* 254:1138, 1991.

108. Stanbridge EJ: Human tumor suppressor genes. *Annu Rev Genet* 24:615, 1990.

109. Knudson AG: Mutation and cancer: Statistical study of retinoblastoma. *Proc Natl Acad Sci USA* 68:820, 1971.

110. Knudson AG: Hereditary cancer, oncogenes, and antioncogenes. *Cancer Res* 45:1437, 1985.

111. Menon AG, Anderson KM, Riccardi VM, Chung RY, Whaley JM, Yandell DW, Farmer GE, Freiman RM, Lee JK, Li FP, Barker DF, Ledbetter DH, Kleider A, Martuza RL, Gusella JF, Seizinger BR: Chromosome 17p deletions and p53 gene mutation associated with the formation of malignant neurofibrosarcomas in von Recklinghausen neurofibromatosis. *Proc Natl Acad Sci USA* 87:5435, 1990.

112. Legius E, Marchuk DA, Collins FS, Glover TW: Somatic depletion of neurofibromatosis type 1 gene in a neurofibrosarcoma supports a tumor suppressor gene hypothesis. *Nature Genet* 3:122, 1993.

113. Glover TW, Stein CK, Legius E, Andersen LB, Brereton A, Johnson S: Molecular and cytogenetic analysis of tumors in von Recklinghausen neurofibromatosis. *Gene Chrom Cancer* 3:62, 1991.

114. Seizinger BR: NF1: A prevalent cause of tumorigenesis in human cancers. *Nat Genet* 3:97, 1993.

115. Andersen LB, Fountain JW, Gutmann DH, Tarle SA, Glover TW, Dracopoli NC, Housman DE, Collins FS: Mutations in the neurofibromatosis 1 gene in sporadic malignant melanomas. *Nat Genet* 3:118, 1993.

116. Johnson MR, Look AT, DeClue JE, Valentine MB, Lowy DR: Inactivation of the NF1 gene in human melanoma and neuroblastoma cell lines without impaired regulation of GTP-*ras*. *Proc Natl Acad Sci USA* 90:5539, 1993.

117. The I, Murthy AE, Hannigan GE, Jacoby LB, Menon AG, Gusella JF, Bernards A: Neurofibromatosis type 1 gene mutations in neuroblastoma. *Nat Genet* 3:62, 1993.

118. DeClue JE, Papageorge AG, Fletcher J, Diehl SR, Ratner N, Vass WC, Lowy DR: Abnormal regulation of mammalian p21*ras* contributes to malignant tumor growth in von Recklinghausen (type 1) neurofibromatosis. *Cell* 69:265, 1992.

119. Basu TN, Gutmann DH, Fletcher JA, Glover TW, Collins FS, Downward J: Aberrant regulation of *ras* proteins in tumor cells from type 1 neurofibromatosis patients. *Nature* 356:713, 1992.

120. Xu W, Mulligan LM, Ponder MA, Liu L, Smith BA, Mathew CGP, Ponder BAJ: Loss of *NF1* alleles in phaeochromocytomas from patients with type 1 neurofibromatosis. *Gene Chrom Cancer* 4:337, 1992.

121. Gutmann DH, Cole JL, Stone WJ, Ponder BAJ, Collins FS: Loss of neurofibromin in adrenal gland tumors from patients with neurofibromatosis type 1. *Gene Chrom Cancer* 10:55–58, 1994.

122. Colman SD, Williams CA, Wallace MR: Benign neurofibromas in type 1 neurofibromatosis (NF1) show somatic deletions of the *NF1* gene. *Nat Genet* 11:90, 1995.

123. Kim HA, Rosenbaum T, Marchionni MA, Ratner N, DeClue JE: Schwann cells from neurofibromin-deficient mice exhibit activation of p21-*ras*, inhibition of cell proliferation and morphological changes. *Oncogene* 11:324, 1995.

124. Rosenbaum T, Boissy YL, Kombrinck K, Brannan CI, Jenkins NA, Copeland NG, Ratner NA: Neurofibromin-deficient fibroblasts fail to form perineurium in vitro. *Development* 121:3583, 1995.

125. Shannon KM, O'Connell P, Martin GA, Paderanga D, Olson K, Kinndorf P, McCormick F: Loss of normal *NF1* allele from the bone marrow of children with type 1 neurofibromatosis and malignant myeloid disorders. *N Engl J Med* 330:597, 1994.

126. Largaespada DA, Brannan CI, Jenkins NA, Copeland NG: NF1 deficiency causes *ras*-mediated granulocyte/macrophage colony stimulating factor hypersensitivity and chronic myeloid leukemia. *Nat Genet* 12:137, 1996.

127. Bollag G, Clapp DW, Shih S, Adler F, Zhang YY, Thompson P, Lange BJ, Freedman MH, McCormick F, Jacks T, Shannon K: Loss of NF1 results in activation of the *Ras* signaling pathway and leads to abberant growth in haematopoietic cells. *Nat Genet* 12:144, 1996.

128. Yan N, Ricca C, Fletcher J, Glover T, Seizinger BR, Manne V: Farnesyltransferase inhibitors block the neurofibromatosis type 1 (NF1) malignant phenotype. *Cancer Res* 55:3569, 1995.

129. Schmale MC, Hensley GT, Udey LR: Neurofibromatosis in the bicolor damselfish as a model of von Recklinghausen neurofibromatosis. *Ann NY Acad Sci* 486:386, 1986.

130. Hinrichs SH, Nerenberg M, Reynolds RK, Khoury G, Jay G: A transgenic mouse model for human neurofibromatosis. *Science* 237:1340, 1987.

131. Nerenberg MI, Minor T, Nagashima K, Takebayashi K, Akai K, Wiley CA, Riccardi VM: Absence of association of HTLV-1 infection with type 1 neurofibromatosis in the United States or Japan. *Neurology* 41:1687, 1991.

132. Nakamura T, Hara M, Kasuga T: Transplacental induction of peripheral nervous tumor in the Syrian golden hamster by *N*-nitroso-*N*-ethylurea. *Am J Pathol* 135:251, 1989.

133. Jacks T, Shih TS, Schmitt EM, Bronson RT, Bernards A, Weinberg RA: Tumor predisposition in mice heterozygous for a targeted mutation in NF1. *Nat Genet* 7:353, 1994.

134. Brannan CI, Perkins AS, Vogel KS, Ratner N, Nordlund ML, Reid SW, Buchberg AM, Jenkins NA, Parada LF, Copeland NG: Targeted disruption of the neurofibromatosis type-1 gene leads to developmen-

tal abnormalities in heart and various neural crest-derived tissues. *Gene Dev* **8**:1019, 1994.

135. Gutmann DH, Andersen LB, Cole JL, Swaroop M, Collins FS: An alternatively spliced mRNA in the carboxy terminus of the neurofibromatosis type 1 (NF1) gene is expressed in muscle. *Hum Mol Genet* **2**:989, 1993.

136. Gutmann DH, Cole JL, Collins FS: Modulation of neurofibromatosis type 1 (NF1) gene expression during in vitro myoblast differentiation. *J Neurosci Res* **37**:398, 1994.

137. Vogel KS, Brannan CI, Jenkins NA, Copeland NG, Parada LF: Loss of neurofibromin results in neurotrophin-independent survival of embryonic sensory and sympathetic neurons. *Cell* **82**:733, 1995.

138. DeClue JE, Cohen BD, Lowy DR: Identification and characterization of the neurofibromatosis type 1 protein product. *Proc Natl Acad Sci USA* **88**:9914, 1991.

139. Daston MM, Scrable H, Nordlund M, Sturbaum AK, Nissen LM, Ratner N: The protein product of the neurofibromatosis type 1 gene is expressed at highest abundance in neurons, Schwann cells, and oligodendrocytes. *Neuron* **8**:415, 1992.

140. Gutmann DH, Wood DL, Collins FS: Identification of the neurofibromatosis type 1 gene product. *Proc Natl Acad Sci USA* **88**:9658, 1991.

141. Hattori S, Ohmi N, Makawa M, Hoshino M, Kawakita M, Nakamura S: Antibody against neurofibromatosis type 1 gene product reacts with a triton-insoluble GTPase activating protein ras p21. *Biochem Biophys Res Commun* **177**:83, 1991.

142. Golubic M, Roudebush M, Dobrowolski S, Wolfman A, Stacey DW: Catalytic properties, tissue, and intracellular distribution of the native neurofibromatosis type 1 protein. *Oncogene* **7**:2151, 1992.

143. Gregory PE, Gutmann DH, Boguski M, Mitchell AM, Parks S, Jacks T, Wood DL, Jove R, Collins FS: The neurofibromatosis type 1 gene product, neurofibromin, associates with microtubules. *Somat Cell Mol Genet* **19**:265, 1993.

144. Bollag G, McCormick F, Clark R: Characterization of full-length neurofibromin: Tubulin inhibits *RAS* GAP activity. *EMBO J* **12**:1923, 1993.

145. Gutmann DH, Collins FS: Recent progress toward understanding the molecular biology of von Recklinghausen neurofibromatosis. *Ann Neurol* **31**:555, 1992.

146. Nordlund M, Gu X, Shipley MT, Ratner N: Neurofibromin is enriched in the endoplasmic reticulum of CNS neurons. *Neuroscience* **13**:1588, 1993.

147. Hewett SJ, Choi DW, Gutmann DH: Expression of the neurofibromatosis 1 (NF1) gene in reactive astrocytes in vitro. *Neuroreport* **6**:1565, 1995.

148. Daston MM, Ratner N: Neurofibromin, a predominantly neuronal GTPase activating protein in the adult, is ubiquitously expressed during development. *Dec Dyn* **19**:216, 1993.

149. Tanaka K, Nakafuku M, Satoh T, Marshall MS, Gibbs JB, Matsumoto K, Kaziro Y, Toh-e A: S. cerevisiae genes *IRA1* and *IRA2* encode proteins that may be functionally equivalent to mammalian ras GTPase activating protein. *Cell* **60**:803, 1990.

150. Tanaka K, Matsumoto K, Toh-e A: *IRA1*, an inhibitory regulator of the *RAS*-cyclic AMP pathway in *Saccharomyces cerevisiae*. *Mol Cell Biol* **9**:757, 1989.

151. Tanaka K, Nakafuku M, Tamanoi F, Kaziro Y, Matsumoto K, Toh-e A: *IRA2*, a second gene of *Saccharomyces cerevisiae* that encodes a protein with a domain homologous to mammalian ras GTPase-activating protein. *Mol Cell Biol* **10**:4303, 1990.

152. Tanaka K, Lin BK, Wood DR, Tamanoi F: *IRA2*, an upstream negative regulator of *RAS* in yeast, is a *RAS* GTPase-activating protein. *Proc Natl Acad Sci USA* **88**:468, 1991.

153. Trahey M, Wong G, Halenbeck R, Rubinfeld B, Martin GA, Ladner M, Long CM, Crosier WJ, Watt K, Koths K, McCormick F: Molecular cloning of two types of GAP complementary DNA from human placenta. *Science* **242**:1697, 1988.

154. Wang Y, Boguski M, Riggs M, Rodgers L, Wigler M: Sar1, a gene from Schizosaccharomyces pombe encoding a GAP-like protein that regulates ras1. *Cell Regul* **2**:253, 1992.

155. Wigler MH: GAPs is understanding ras. *Nature* **346**:696, 1990.

156. Marshall CJ: How does p21 ras transform cells? *Trends Genet* **7**:91, 1991.

157. Adari H, Lowy DR, Willumsen BM, Der CJ, McCormick F: Guanosine triphosphatase activating protein (GAP) interacts with the p21 ras effector binding domain. *Science* **240**:518, 1988.

158. Mitts MR, Bradshaw-Rouse J, Heideman W: Interactions between adenylate cyclase and the yeast GTPase-activating protein *IRA1*. *Mol Cell Biol* **11**:4591, 1991.

159. Broach JR: *RAS* genes in *Saccharomyces cerevisiae*: Signal transduction in search of a pathway. *Trends Genet* **7**:28, 1991.

160. Golubic M. Tanaka K, Dobrowolski S, Wood D, Tsai MH, Marshall M, Tamanoi F, Stacey DW: The GTPase stimulatory activity of the neurofibromatosis type 1 and yeast *IRA2* proteins are inhibited by arachidonic acid. *EMBO J* **10**:2897, 1991.

161. Weismuller L, Wittinghofer A: Expression of the GTPase activating domain of the neurofibromatosis type 1 (NF1) gene in *Escherichia coli* and the role of the conserved lysine residue. *J Biol Chem* **267**:10207, 1992.

162. Kamata T, Feramisco JR: Epidermal growth factor stimulates guanine nucleotide binding activity and phosphorylation of ras oncogene proteins. *Nature* **310**:147, 1984.

163. Moran MF, Polakis P, McCormick F, Pawson T, Ellis C: Protein-tyrosine kinases regulate the phosphorylation, protein interactions, subcellular distribution, and activity of p21^{ras} GTPase-activating protein. *Mol Cell Biol* **11**:1804, 1991.

164. Satoh T, Endo M, Nakafuku M, Akiyama T, Yamamoto T, Kaziro Y: Accumulation of p21 ras-GTP in response to stimulation with epidermal growth factor and oncogene products with tyrosine kinase activity. *Proc Natl Acad Sci USA* **87**:7926, 1990.

165. Bar-Sagi D, Feramisco JR: Microinjection of the ras oncogene protein into PC12 cells induces morphological differentiation. *Cell* **42**:841, 1985.

166. Noda M, Ko M, Ogura A, Liu D-G, Amano T, Takano T, Ikawa Y: Sarcoma viruses carrying ras oncogenes induce differentiation-associated properties in a neuronal cell line. *Nature* **318**:73, 1985.

167. Hagag N, Halegoua S, Viola M: Inhibition of growth factor-induced differentiation of PC12 cells by microinjection of antibody to ras p21. *Nature* **319**:680, 1986.

168. Zhang K, Papageorge AG, Lowy DR: Mechanistic aspect of signalling through ras in NIH3T3 cells. *Science* **257**:671, 1992.

169. Feramisco JR, Clark R, Wong G, Arnheim N, Milley R, McCormick F: Transient reversion of ras oncogene-induced cell transformation by antibodies specific for amino acid 12 of ras protein. *Nature* **314**:639, 1985.

170. Feramisco JR, Gross M, Kamata T, Rosenberg M, Sweet RW: Microinjection of the oncogene form of the human H-*ras* (T-24) protein results in rapid proliferation of quiescent cells. *Cell* **38**:109, 1984.

171. Benito M, Porras A, Nebreda AR, Santos E: Differentiation of 3T3-L1 fibroblasts to adipocytes induces by transfection of ras oncogenes. *Science* **253**:565, 1991.

172. Graziadei L, Raibowol K, Bar-Sagi D: Co-capping of ras proteins with surface immunoglobulins in B lymphocytes. *Nature* **347**:396, 1990.

173. Kaplan S, Bar-Sagi D: Association of p21 ras with cellular polypeptides. *J Biol Chem* **266**:18934, 1991.

174. Downward J, Graves JD, Warne PH, Rayter S, Cantrell DA: Stimulation of p21^{ras} upon T-cell activation. *Nature* **346**:719, 1990.

175. Ellis C, Moran M, McCormick F, Pawson T: Phosphorylation of GAP and GAP-associated proteins by transforming and mitogenic tyrosine kinases. *Nature* **343**:377, 1990.

176. Gutmann DH, Basu TN, Gregory PE, Wood DL, Downward J, Collins FS: The role of the neurofibromatosis type 1 (*NF1*) gene product in growth factor-mediated signal transduction. *Neurology* **42**:A183, 1992.

177. Boyer M, Gutmann DH, Collins F, Bar-Sagi D: Co-capping of neurofibromin, but not GAP, with surface immunoglobulins in B lymphocytes. *Oncogene* **9**:349, 1994.

178. Johnson MR, DeClue JE, Felzmann S, Vass WC, Xu G, White R, Lowy DR: Neurofibromin can inhibit ras-dependent growth by a mechanism independent of its GTPase-accelerating function. *Mol Cell Biol* **14**:641, 1994.

179. Li Y, White R: Suppression of a human colon cancer cell line by introduction of an exogenous *NF1* gene. *Cancer Res* **56**:2872, 1996.

180. Clark GJ, Drugan JK, Terrell RS, Bradham C, Der CJ, Bell RM, Campbell S: Peptides containing a consensus Ras binding sequence from Raf-1 and the GTPase activating protein NF1 inhibit Ras function. *Proc Natl Acad Sci USA* (**93**):1577, 1996.

181. Gutmann DH, Gregory PE, Wood DL, Collins FS: The neurofibromatosis type 1 gene product encodes a signal transduction protein which associates with microtubules. *J Cell Biochem* **16B**:A143, 1992.

182. Cleveland DW: Microtubule mapping. *Cell* **60**:701, 1990.

183. Matus A: Microtubule-associated proteins. *Curr Opin Cell Biol* **2**:10, 1990.

184. Olmsted JB: Microtubule-associated proteins. *Annu Rev Cell Biol* **2**:421, 1986.

185. Wiche G: High-MW microtubule-associated proteins: Properties and functions. *Biochem J* **259**:1, 1989.

186. Obar RA, Collins CA, Hammarback JA, Shpetner HS, Vallee RB: Molecular cloning of the microtubule-associated mechanochemical enzyme dynamin reveals homology with a new family of GTP-binding proteins. *Nature* **347**:256, 1990.

187. Shpetner HS, Vallee RB: Identification of dynamin, a novel mechanochemical enzyme that mediates interactions between microtubules. *Cell* **59**:421, 1989.

188. Van der Bliek AM, Meyerowitz EM: Dynamin-like protein encoded by the Drosophila shibire gene associated with vesicular traffic. *Nature* **351**:411, 1991.

189. Jasmin BJ, Changeux J-P, Cartaud J: Compartmentalization of cold-stable and acetylated microtubules in the subsynaptic domain of chick skeletal muscle fibre. *Nature* **344**:673, 1990.

190. Vallee RB: A taxol-dependent procedure for the isolation of microtubules and microtubule-associated proteins (MAPs). *J Cell Biol* **92**:435, 1982.

191. Vallee RB: Reversible assembly purification of microtubules without assembly-promoting agents and further purification of tubulin, microtubule-associated proteins, and MAP fragments. *Methods Enzymol* **134**:89, 1986.

192. Vallee RB: Molecular characterization of high molecular weight microtubule-associated proteins: Some answers, many questions. *Cell Motil Cytoskeleton* **15**:204, 1990.

193. Vallee RB, Bloom GS, Theurkauf WE: Microtubule-associated proteins: Subunits of the cytomatrix. *Cell Biol* **99**:38, 1984.

194. Vallee RB, Collins CA: Purification of microtubules and microtubule-associated proteins from sea urchin eggs and cultured mammalian cells using taxol, and use of exogenous taxol-stabilized brain microtubules for purifying microtubule-associated proteins. *Methods Enzymol* **134**:116, 1986.

195. Collins CA: Reversible assembly purification of taxol-treated microtubules. *Methods Enzymol* **196**:246, 1991.

196. Steiner B, Mandelkow E-M, Biernat J, Gustke N, Meyer HE, Schmidt B, Mieskes G, Soauling HD, Drechsel D, Kirschner MW, Goedert M, Mandelkow E: Phosphorylation of microtubule-associated protein tau: Identification of the site for calcium-calmodulin dependent kinase and relationship with tau phosphorylation in Alzheimer tangles. *EMBO J* **9**:3539, 1990.

197. Hall A: *ras* and GAP: Who's controlling whom? *Cell* **61**:921, 1990.

198. McCormick F: *ras* GTPase activating protein: Signal transmitter and signal terminator. *Cell* **56**:5, 1989.

199. Mitchell AL, Gutmann DH, Gregory PE, Cole J, Park S, Jove R, Collins FS: Localization of the domain in the neurofibromatosis type 1 protein (neurofibromin) that interacts with microtubules. *Am J Hum Genet* **43**:A62, 1993.

200. Nishi T, Lee PSY, Oka K, Levin VA, Tanase S, Morino Y, Saya H: Differential expression of two types of the neurofibromatosis type 1 (NF1) gene transcripts related to neuronal differentiation. *Oncogene* **6**:1555, 1991.

201. Anderson LB, Ballester R, Marchuk DA, Chang E, Gutmann DH, Saulino AM, Camonis J, Wigner M, Collins FS: A conserved alternative splice in the von Recklinghausen neurofibromatosis (NF1) gene produces two neurofibromin isoforms, both of which have GTPase activating protein ability. *Mol Cell Biol* **13**:487, 1993.

202. Gutmann DH, Tennekoon GI, Cole JL, Collins FS, Rutkowski JL: Modulation of the neurofibromatosis type 1 gene product, neurofibromin, during Schwann cell differentiation. *J Neurosci Res* **36**:216, 1993.

203. Gutmann DH, Cole JL, Collins FS: Expression of the neurofibromatosis type 1 (NF1) gene during mouse embryonic development. *Prog Brain Res* **105**:327, 1995.

204. Gutmann DH, Geist RT, Rose K, Wright DE: Expression of two new protein isoforms of the neurofibromatosis type 1 (NF1) gene product, neurofibromin, in muscle tissues. *Dev Dyn* **202**:302, 1995.

205. Neiman HL, Mena E, Holt JF, Stern AM, Perry BL: Neurofibromatosis and congenital heart disease. *AJR* **122**:146, 1974.

206. Kaufman RL, Hartmann AF, McAlister WH: Congenital heart disease associated with neurofibromatosis. *Birth Defects* **VIII**:92, 1972.

207. Danglot G, Regnier V, Fauvet D, Vassal G, Kujas M, Bernheim A: Neurofibromatosis 1 (NF1) mRNAs expressed in the central nervous system are differentially spliced in the 5' part of the gene. *Hum Mol Gen* **34**:915–920, 1995.

208. Geist RT, Gutmann DH: Expression of a developmentally-regulated neuron-specific isoform of the neurofibromatosis 1 (NF1) gene. *Neurosci Lett* **211**:85–88, 1996.

209. Martuza RL, MacLaughlin DT, Ojemann RG: Specific estradiol binding in schwannomas, meningiomas, and neurofibromas. *Neurosurgery* **9**:665, 1981.

210. Riccardi VM: Growth-promoting factors in neurofibroma crude extracts. *Ann NY Acad Sci* **486**:66, 1986.

211. Peltonen J, Aho H, Rinne UK, Penttinen R: Neurofibromatosis tumor and skin cells in culture. *Acta Neuropathol (Berl)* **61**:275, 1983.

212. Peltonen J, Jaakkola S, Lebwohl M, Renvall S, Risteli L, Virtanen I, Uitto J: Cellular differentiation and expression of matrix genes in type 1 neurofibromatosis. *Lab Invest* **59**:760, 1988.

213. Pintar JE, Sonnenfeld KH, Fisher J, Klein RS, Kreider B: Molecular and immunocytochemical studies of neurofibromas and related cell types. *Ann NY Acad Sci* **486**:96, 1986.

214. Krone W, Jirikowski G, Muhleck O, Kling H, Gall H: Cell culture studies on neurofibromatosis (von Recklinghausen): II. Occurrence of glial cells in primary cultures of peripheral neurofibromas. *Hum Genet* **63**:247, 1983.

215. Krone W, Mao R, Muhleck S, Kling H, Fink T: Cell culture studies on neurofibromatosis (von Recklinghausen): Characterization of cells growing from neurofibromas. *Ann NY Acad Sci* **486**:354, 1986.

216. Fialkow PJ, Sagebiel RW, Gartler SM, Rimoin DL: Multiple cell origin of hereditary neurofibromatosis. *N Engl J Med* **284**:298, 1971.

217. Skuse GR, Kosciolek BA, Rowley PT: The neurofibroma in von Recklinghausen neurofibromatosis has a unicellular origin. *Am J Hum Genet* **49**:600, 1991.

218. Pleasure D, Kreider B, Sobue G, Ross AH, Koprowski H, Sonnenfeld KH, Rubenstein AE: Schwann-like cells cultured from human dermal neurofibromas: Immunohistological identification and response to Schwann cell mitogens. *Ann NY Acad Sci* **486**:227, 1986.

219. Ratner N, Lieberman MA, Riccardi VM, Hong D: Mitogen accumulation in von Recklinghausen neurofibromatosis. *Ann Neurol* **27**:298, 1990.

220. Sheela S, Riccardi VM, Ratner N: Angiogenic and invasive properties of neurofibroma Schwann cells. *J Cell Biol* **111**:645, 1990.

221. Bidot-Lopez P, Frankel JW: Enhanced viral transformation of skin fibroblasts from neurofibromatosis patients. *Ann Clin Lab Sci* **13**:27, 1983.

222. Frankel JW, Bidot P, Kopelovich L: Enhanced sensitivity of skin fibroblasts from neurofibromatosis patients to transformation by the Kirsten murine sarcoma virus. *Ann NY Acad Sci* **486**:403, 1986.

223. Kopelovich L, Rich RF: Enchanced radiotolerance to ionizing radiation is correlated with increased cancer proneness of cultured fibroblasts from precursor states in neurofibromatosis patients. *Cancer Genet Cytogenet* **22**:203, 1986.

224. Woods WG, McKenzie B, Letourneau MA, Byrne TD: Sensitivity of cultured skin fibroblasts from patients with neurofibromatosis to DNA-damaging agents. *Ann NY Acad Sci* **486**:336, 1986.

225. Huson SM: Recent developments in the diagnosis and management of neurofibromatosis. *Arch Dis Child* **64**:745, 1989.

226. Andersen LB, Tarle SA, Marchuk DA, Leguis E, Collins FS: A compound nucleotide repeat in the neurofibromatosis (NF1) gene. *Hum Mol Genet* **2**:1083, 1993.

227. Heim RA, Silvermna LM, Farber RA, Kam-Morgan LNW, Luce MC: Screening for truncated NF1 proteins. *Nat Genet* **8**:218, 1994.

228. Tsai M-H, Yu C-L, Stacey DW: A cytoplasmic protein inhibits the GTPase activity of H-Ras in a phospholipid-dependent manner. *Science* **250**:982, 1990.

229. Gibbs JB: *Ras* C-terminal processing enzymes: New drug targets? *Cell* **65**:1, 1991.

230. Bollag G, McCormick F: Differential regulation of *ras*GAP and neurofibromatosis gene product activities. *Nature* **351**:576, 1991.

231. Chen W-J, Andres DA, Goldstein JL, Brown MS: Cloning and expression of a cDNA encoding the alpha subunit of rat p21ras protein farnesyltransferase. *Proc Natl Acad Sci USA* **88**:11368, 1991.

232. Kinsella BT, Erdman RA, Maltese WA: Posttranslational modification of Ha-*ras* p21 by farnesyl versus geranylgeranyl isoprenoids is determined by the COOH-terminal amino acid. *Proc Natl Acad Sci USA* **88**:8934, 1991.

233. Qiu M-S, Pitts AF, Winters TR, Green SH: *Ras* isoprenylation is required for *ras*-induced but not for NGF-induced neuronal differentiation of PC12 cells. *J Cell Biol* **115**:795, 1991.

CHAPTER 23

Neurofibromatosis Type 2

Mia MacCollin ■ James Gusella

1. **Neurofibromatosis 2 (NF2) is an autosomal dominant disorder that affects approximately 1 in 40,000 individuals. It is characterized by the development of bilateral vestibular schwannomas and other histologically benign intracranial, spinal, and peripheral nerve tumors. The only nontumorous manifestations of NF2 are cataract and retinal hamartoma. NF2 is fully penetrant by age 60 years, or half of all cases represent new mutations.**

2. **Syndromes related to NF2 include sporadic unilateral vestibular schwannoma, mosaic inactivation of the *NF2* gene, schwannomatosis, and multiple meningiomas. NF2 is genetically and clinically distinct from von Recklinghausen disease or neurofibromatosis type 1.**

3. **The gene for NF2 on chromosome 22q was identified by positional cloning. It spans 110 kb with 16 constitutive exons and 1 alternatively spiced exon. The NF2 protein product is a member of the protein 4.1 family of cytoskeleton-associated proteins. These proteins play a critical role in maintaining membrane stability and cell shape by connecting integral membrane proteins to the spectrin–actin lattice of the cytoskeleton.**

4. **A large number of germ-line mutations have been detected in NF2 patients, with the majority predicted to result in gross protein truncation. Detection of somatic alterations in NF2-related tumors has supported the hypothesis that the *NF2* gene acts as a true tumor suppressor in both schwannomas and meningiomas. *NF2* also appears to play a role in the development of mesothelioma, although this tumor is not seen in patients with NF2.**

5. **Diagnosis of NF2 is currently dependent on clinical criteria, although genetic diagnosis may soon be feasible. Treatment of NF2-related tumors remains largely surgical. Advances in hearing augmentation, such as auditory brainstem implants, may improve the quality of life for many patients.**

CLINICAL ASPECTS

Historical Notes and Nomenclature

Neurofibromatosis (NF) was first described by Fredrich Daniel von Recklinghausen in an 1882 monograph.[1,2] In 1902, Henneberg and Koch recognized a clinically distinct form of NF which lacked skin alterations typical of von Recklinghausen disease and included acoustic neuromas.[3] They referred to this distinct disorder as central neurofibromatosis in contrast to the peripheral features of von Recklinghausen disease. In 1915, Bassoe and Nuzum described a patient with bilateral cerebellopontine angle tumors and other central nervous system tumors.[4] In 1930 a family with 38 members who had bilateral cerebellopontine angle tumors transmitted in an autosomal dominant fashion was reported, emphasizing the genetic nature of this disorder.[5] Several subsequent works confirmed that the form of NF characterized by bilateral cerebellopontine angle tumors is a disorder distinct from the more common or peripheral NF.[6–8] Overlapping clinical features, such as multiple spine and skin tumors, continue to cause confusion between these two diseases.[9]

In 1987, a Consensus Development Conference was held at the National Institutes of Health (NIH) to clarify the various clinical types of NF, and 4 years later a second NIH conference was held to evaluate the clinial aspects of acoustic neuroma.[10,11] As a result of these efforts, formal diagnostic criteria were proposed that have improved diagnostic certainty and allowed clinical and molecular genetic studies of phenotypically homogenous groups of patients. The conferees recommended the adoption of the term *neurofibromatosis type 2* (NF2) instead of central, bilateral vestibular, or bilateral acoustic neurofibromatosis. In addition, the term *vestibular schwannoma* was preferred to the previously used *acoustic neuroma* based on the observation that the tumors originate from the vestibular rather than the acoustic branch of the eighth cranial nerve. Finally, the older term *neurilemmoma* has been replaced by *schwannoma* based on work implicating the Schwann cell as the cell of origin in these tumors.[12]

Incidence of Inherited and Sporadic Disease

NF2 is a rare disorder, and because of the wide variety of specialists who manage these patients and the frequent misdiagnoses, its prevalence is difficult to ascertain. Evans et al. found the incidence at birth to be approximately 1 in 40,000 in a population-based study.[13] This makes NF2 approximately 10 times less common than neurofibromatosis type 1 (NF1), which has an incidence of 1 in 3000.[10] In both this work and that of Parry et al., sporadic versus inherited cases were divided evenly.[14] This may reflect a relatively high mutation rate at the *NF2* locus and a low reproductive fitness, especially in severely affected patients.[13] Unilateral vestibular schwannoma, unlike NF2, is a very common disorder, with an incidence of about 1 per 100,000 per year.[11] In two large autopsy series the incidence of occult vestibular schwannoma was even higher

443

(0.82 to 0.87 percent).[15,16] Less than 5 percent of individuals with unilateral vestibular schwannoma eventually develop bilateral disease and NF2.[11,17] Both unilateral vestibular schwannoma and NF2 show no racial, ethnic, or gender predilection.

Diagnostic Criteria

Diagnostic criteria for both NF1 and NF2 have been proposed by the NIH (Table 23-1).[10] Several workers have suggested expansion of these criteria in the hope that diagnosis may be made earlier in patients with multiple features of the disorder but without bilateral vestibular schwannoma.[18,19] Caution must be used in counseling patients on their reproductive and health risks when they do not meet the NIH criteria, since the more liberal criteria have not been validated clinically. When the NIH criteria are applied strictly, it is rare to find an overlap between NF1 and NF2 in a single patient. Nearly all individuals with NF2 eventually develop bilateral vestibular schwannoma, and this alone is enough to diagnose the disorder. In the presence of other cardinal features of NF2, such as a positive family history, or other NF2-related tumors, the diagnosis may be considered in an individual with unilateral vestibular schwannoma on the presumption that bilateral tumors will appear in time. Since the appearance of all NF2-related tumors increases with age, the diagnosis should be strongly suspected in a child of an affected individual who has any manifestation, including a skin tumor alone.[20]

Major Clinical Features of NF2

Vestibular Schwannoma. The occurrence of bilateral vestibular schwannoma is a nearly universal feature of individuals with NF2, and so the diagnosis of NF2 should be reconsidered in any individual without a positive family history who does not have these tumors. Vestibular tumors usually originate within the internal auditory canal, where the eighth nerve lies in close proximity to the facial nerve (Fig. 23-1). Initial symptoms include tinnitus, hearing loss, and balance dysfunction. Significant facial palsy is rare even in large tumors and if present should suggest a facial nerve tumor. Disability is often insidious in onset, although occasionally sudden hearing loss may occur, presumably owing to vascular compromise by the tumor. Patients often report difficulty in using the telephone in one ear or unsteadiness when walking at night or on uneven ground. With time, vestibular tumors extend medially into the cerebellar pontine angle and, if left untreated, cause compression of the brainstem and hydrocephalus. Schwannomas also may develop on other cranial nerves, with sensory nerves more frequently affected than motor nerves.[7,14]

Table 23-1 Diagnostic Criteria for NF2

Bilateral eighth-nerve masses seen with appropriate imaging techniques (e.g., CT or MRI)

    or

A first-degree relative with NF2 and unilateral eighth nerve mass or two of the following

    Neurofibroma

    Meningioma

    Glioma

    Schwannoma

    Juvenile posterior subcapsular lenticular opacity

SOURCE: Adapted from Mulvihill JJ, Parry DM, Sherman JL, Pikus A, Kaiser-Kupfer MI, Eldridge R: NIH conference: Neurofibromatosis 1 (Recklinghausen disease) and neurofibromatosis 2 (bilateral acoustic neurofibromatosis): An update. *Ann Intern Med* **113**:39, 1990.

Meningioma. Approximately half of individuals with NF2 develop meningioma (Fig. 23-2).[14,18] Most of these tumors are intracranial; spinal meningioma is not uncommon, and there is a single report of a cutaneous meningioma.[9] There is no site of predilection for meningioma as there is for schwannoma, although meningioma intermixed with schwannoma is a common and incidental finding when the cerebral pontine angle is explored surgically.[21] Because of the multiplicity and slow growth patterns of these tumors, often it is neither possible nor advisable to remove all meningiomas from an NF2 patient. Therapy should be considered when a tumor causes symptoms resulting from compression or development of edema in the adjacent brain. Special attention is needed for meningiomas in the orbit that may compress the optic nerve and result in visual loss, and meningiomas at the skull base that may cause symptoms of cranial neuropathy, brainstem compression, and hydrocephalus.

Spinal Tumors. Two-thirds or more of NF2 patients develop spinal tumors. This can be one of the most devastating and difficult to manage aspects of this disease (Fig. 23-3).[14,22] The most common spinal tumor is a schwannoma, which often originates within the intravertebral canal on the dorsal root and extends both medially and laterally to form a dumbbell shape. This configuration is identical to that of spinal neurofibromas in NF1 and occasionally may cause diagnostic confusion between the two disorders. Less commonly, patients develop meningiomas of the spinal coverings. Intramedullary tumors, such as astrocytoma and ependymoma, are reported to occur in 5 to 10 percent of all NF2 patients, although 33 percent of severely affected individuals who underwent complete spinal imaging had evidence of intramedullary cord tumors.[14,18,22] Most individuals with spinal cord tumors have multiple tumors (>50 percent in the study of Mautner et al.[20]), and there is no site of predilection for either intra- or extramedullary tumor formation.[22] Although ependymoma in patients without NF2 is optimally treated with complete resection and occasionally with radiotherapy and chemotherapy, it is unclear whether ependymoma in NF2 patients warrants aggressive management.[23,24]

Other Features of NF2. In addition to vestibular schwannoma and spinal schwannoma, NF2 patients are prone to the development of schwannomas along other cranial nerves, in the brachial and lumbar plexuses, and along peripheral nerves. Two-thirds of these patients will develop skin tumors, primarily schwannomas.[14,18] Unlike NF1 patients, it is rare for a single patient to develop more than 10 skin tumors.[14] Two to 4 percent of these individuals develop intracranial or spinal astrocytomas.[14,18] There have been several reports of peripheral neuropathy occurring in the context of NF2, although the pathophysiology of this process is unknown.[14,18,25,26]

The ophthalmologic consequences of NF2 are an underrecognized and important aspect of the disease.[27-29] For example, Bouzas et al. studied 54 NF2 patients and found that one-third had decreased visual acuity in one or both eyes, directly or indirectly related to the diagnosis.[28] Posterior subcapsular lens opacity progressing to actual cataract is the most common ocular finding (Fig. 23-4). Lens opacities may appear before vestibular schwannoma in at-risk children.[20] Retinal hamartoma and epiretinal membrane are seen in up to one-third of these patients, making indirect ophthalmoscopy mandatory in the evaluation of NF2 patients. Finally, the neuro-ophthalmologic consequences of intracranial and intraorbital tumors may result in decreased visual acuity and diplopia. Since all NF2 patients are also at risk for hearing loss, early recognition of visual impairment from any of these causes is extremely important.

Features Not Associated with NF2. Because NF2 is uncommon and since diagnostic confusion continues to exist, it is worth noting several features associated with NF1 that are not increased in the NF2 population. NF2 patients do not have the associated cognitive

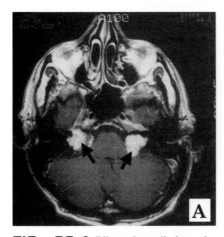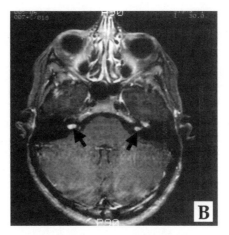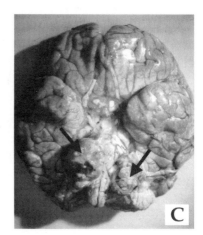

FIG. 23-1 Bilateral vestibular schwannoma. *A.* Axial T$_1$-weighted contrast-enhanced image of the skull base in a 45-year-old man with NF2. Very large multilobulated tumors with extracannicular extension are seen (arrows). *B.* Similar MRI of the patient's presymp-

tomatic nephew. Small enhancing masses are seen in both internal auditory canals. *C.* Gross pathologic view of the skull base; arrows point to tumors in the cerebellar pontine angles (*Photo courtesy of Dr. David Louis, Neuropathology Department, Massachusetts General Hospital.*)

problems, including mental retardation and learning disability, that NF1 patients have, nor do they have significant numbers of Lisch nodules. The schwannomas of NF2 rarely, if ever, transform to neurofibrosarcomas, and the overall incidence of malignant tumors in the NF2 population is probably not increased over that in the general population. Approximately half of NF2-affected individuals have small numbers of café au lait macules.[14,18] Since 10 percent of the general population also has one or two of these macules, this finding has limited diagnostic value.[30,31] NF2 patients do not have significant numbers of café au lait macules (six or more over 15 mm in greatest diameter in postpubertal persons), although their skin is more frequently scrutinized, perhaps leading to this misconception.[10]

Clinical Course

In a large population-based study, the average age of the onset of symptoms among NF2 patients was 21 years, with a range of 2 to 52 years.[18] Similar findings were reported by Parry et al., who reported an average age at onset of symptoms of 20

years and a range of 7 to 70 years.[14] Most patients present with symptoms referable to compression of the eighth cranial nerve, including deafness, tinnitus, and balance dysfunction. Other presenting problems may include facial weakness, visual impairment, and painful skin tumors. Headache and seizure are distinctly uncommon modes of presentation. In the case of deafness, the inability to use a phone in one ear is often an important clue, as it is the only test of unilateral hearing that normally occurs in everyday life. Unfortunately, the study of Parry et al. documented an 8-year lag between age at first symptom and diagnosis, underscoring the need for increased clinical recognition of this disorder.[14] Recognition of NF2 in the pediatric population is an especially critical area, as NF2 is classically thought of as an adult disease. Skin tumors and ocular findings, which often are not prominent in an older patient, may be important clues in the pediatric range.[10]

The clinical course of NF2 is extremely variable and depends on tumor burden, surgical management, and complications. A small number of NF2 patients develop only vestibular schwannoma with disability primarily related to the seventh and eighth cranial nerves. More commonly, patients exhibit a progressive deterioration with

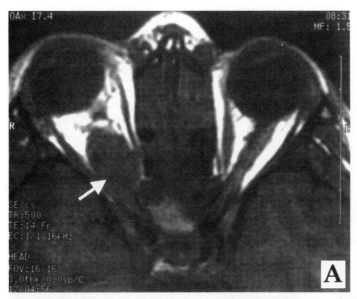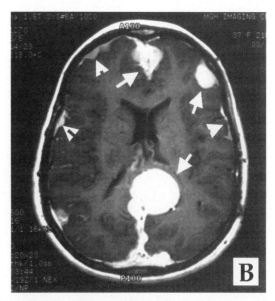

FIG. 23-2 Radiographic appearance of an intracranial meningioma in NF2. *A.* Orbital mass in a child with NF2. Orbital tumors in children may be confused with optic glioma; the latter tumor is seen in

NF1 but not NF2. T$_1$-weighted, MRI. *B.* Multiple discrete lesions (arrows) and diffuse enhancement (arrowheads) suggestive of meningiomatosis in an adult.

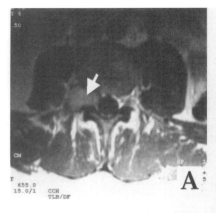
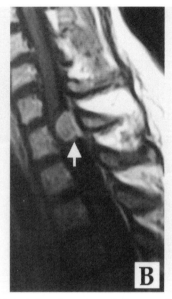
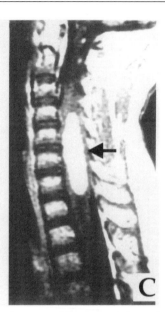

FIG. 23-3 Spinal cord tumors associated with NF2. *A.* A dorsal root schwannoma that has assumed a "dumbbell" configuration. *B.* A meningioma in the thoracic spine of a child (arrow). *C.* An in-tramedullary cervical spine tumor. Biopsy revealed ependymoma, although the radiographic appearance also is consistent with astrocytoma. T$_1$-weighted contrast enhanced MRIs.

loss of hearing, ambulation, and sight along with chronic pain caused by the tumor burden. Although the spectrum of NF2 among affected individuals is quite wide, there is some intrafamilial homogeneity that may be helpful in the counseling and management of patients with a positive family history. The course of NF2 is most likely minimally affected by gender or pregnancy.[32,33]

The average age at death in the NF2 population has been reported to be 36 years; in the same study, actuarial survival after diagnosis was 15 years.[18] It is important to realize that several factors may affect this figure in the near future. Early recognition of the disease, both clinically and by presymptomatic diagnosis of at-risk offspring, allows diagnosis of tumors at an earlier and presumably more surgically approachable stage.[34] Improvements in imaging techniques have allowed the detection of smaller tumors and better preoperative assessment of anatomy.[35] Finally, the advances in surgical techniques described below certainly will improve outcome.[36]

Related Syndromes

Unilateral Vestibular Schwannoma. Sporadic unilateral vestibular schwannoma is a common tumor in the general population, accounting for 5 to 10 percent of all intracranial tumors and the vast majority of cerebral pontine angle tumors.[37] Less than 5 percent of individuals with vestibular schwannoma develop bilateral tumors, and the probability of doing so is critically dependent on the age at which the tumor is detected (Fig. 23-5).[17] For those under age 25, the development of a unilateral vestibular schwannoma should prompt a careful evaluation for other features of the disease. Conversely, there is little rationale for screening persons 55 and over with unilateral vestibular schwannoma for NF2. The offspring of persons with unilateral vestibular schwannoma alone do not have an increased incidence of either NF2 or unilateral vestibular schwannoma.

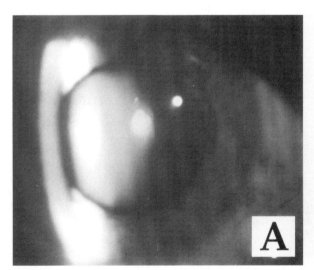
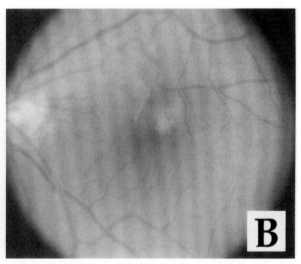

FIG. 23-4 Ocular findings in NF2. *A.* Slit-lamp photograph revealing posterior capsular cataract. *B.* Fundus photograph revealing an epiretinal membrane near the macula. (*Courtesy of Dr. Muriel Kaiser, National Eye Institute.*)

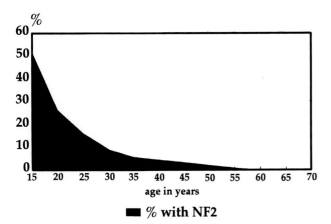

%

60
50
40
30
20
10
0

15 20 25 30 35 40 45 50 55 60 65 70

age in years

■ % with NF2

FIG. 23-5 Age-specific risk of having NF2 on presenting with vestibular schwannoma. (*From Evans et al.,[17] by permission of The Journal of Laryngology and Otology.*)

Mosaicism in the *NF2* Gene. Several individuals with segmental manifestations of NF1 have been described and characterized as having somatic mosaicism for *NF1* gene mutation.[38] There is at least one report of molecularly confirmed somatic mosaicism for an inactivating mutation of the *NF2* gene, and the affected individual had a notably milder phenotype compared to others with a similar mutation.[39] Other reports of clinically suspected mosaicism have been made in individuals with unilateral vestibular schwannoma and multiple other ipsilateral tumors.[32] Germ-line mosaicism has also been reported, resulting in affected siblings carrying an identical *NF2* gene mutation with clinically normal parents in whom the mutation could not be detected in lymphoblast DNA.[40] It remains unclear whether persons with somatic mosaicism carry any genetic risk for bearing affected offspring (i.e., if somatic mosaicism may coexist with germ-line mosaicism).

Recognition of mosaic individuals may be problematic, as they may not have bilateral vestibular schwannomas and genetic analysis in peripheral tissues such as lymphocytes may not reveal the underlying mutation. Mosaicism should be considered in any individual with unilateral vestibular schwannoma and other NF2-related tumors, especially if the tumors are anatomically localized. Molecular genetic analysis of resected tumor material may be a viable alternative to analysis of peripheral tissues for a definitive diagnosis of mosaicism. Germ-line mosaicism for *NF2* mutations appears to be sufficiently rare to make screening of the siblings of an affected individual with normal parents unnecessary.

Schwannomatosis. Schwannomatosis is defined as multiple pathologically proven schwannomas without vestibular schwannoma diagnostic of NF2.[41] Previous terms for this condition have included *multiple neurilemmomas, agminated neurilemmomas, multiple schwannomas,* and *neurilemmomatosis.* Schwannomatosis appears to be a clinically distinct entity from NF1 and NF2. Persons with schwannomatosis may develop intracranial, spinal nerve root, or peripheral tumors; like persons with NF2, they do not develop malignancy. In one-third of all reported cases, schwannomatosis patients have had anatomically localized tumors suggestive of segmental disease.[41–43] There are few cases of familial involvement with schwannomatosis in which autosomal dominant inheritance with highly variable expressivity and incomplete penetrance is seen. Although schwannomatosis appears to be a tumor-suppressor gene syndrome, it is unclear if it is due to an aberration in the NF1, NF2, or an unknown transcript.

Multiple Meningiomas. Although many patients with NF2 develop multiple meningiomas, the appearance of meningiomas rarely predates that of vestibular schwannoma in a single patient. Rare instances of families with multiple meningiomas without vestibular schwannoma segregating as an autosomal dominant trait have been reported.[44] Recently, a genetic linkage analysis of one such family showed that the trait segregates separately from the *NF2* gene, implicating a second meningioma locus that may function as a tumor suppressor in this disorder.[45] This result is supported by the data presented below, which implicate a non-*NF2* gene in approximately half of all sporadic meningiomas. Multiple meningiomas in a patient without a family history may more commonly be due to noncontiguous spread of a single tumor.[46] Presumably the latter condition carries no genetic risk to offspring. Because sporadic meningioma is classically a tumor of older adults, the finding of a single meningioma in an individual under age 25 years should prompt an evaluation for an underlying genetic condition.[17]

Histopathology

The tumors of NF2 are derived from Schwann cells, meningeal cells, and glial cells and are inevitably histologically benign. Vestibular schwannomas from NF2 patients have several pathologic differences from those which occur sporadically. About 40 percent of vestibular tumors from NF2 patients have a lobular pattern that is uncommon in sporadic tumors.[21] Intermixture of meningioma with vestibular schwannoma in NF2 patients is not uncommon.[21] NF2-associated vestibular schwannomas have been reported to be more invasive of the eighth cranial nerve and to have a higher proportion of dividing cells.[47,48] Meningiomas from patients with NF2 have been reported to be predominantly fibroblastic, although a more recent report revealed equal numbers of fibroblastic and meningothelial tumors.[12,49] No histologic differences between glial tumors in NF2 and those in sporadic cases have been reported.[49]

GENETIC ASPECTS OF NF2

Historical Aspects

Early studies on the pathogenetic mechanisms underlying NF2 revealed that NF2-related tumors often lost large stretches of chromosome 22.[50–52] This finding not only suggested that the *NF2* gene is on chromosome 22 but also supported the hypothesis that it is a classic tumor suppressor.[53] In conjunction with these initial investigations on tumors, studies were made of a large NF2-affected kindred by the method of linkage analysis.[54] This genetic linkage approach confirmed the position of *NF2* on chromosome 22 and refined its localization to band 22q12. Further work with tumor material and other affected kindreds narrowed the critical region on chromosome 22 to approximately 6 mb.[55]

In 1992 a single affected individual was identified who, along with her affected daughter, carried a 30-kb deletion recognizable with the probe neurofilament heavy chain and the rare cutting enzyme *Not*I (Fig. 23-6).[58] Taking this patient's deleted region as a target, the transcribed sequences within this area were isolated by using the method of exon trapping. Subsequent identification of cDNA using these exons as probes revealed that the predicted protein carried especially high homology to the 4.1 family of cytoskeletal-associated proteins. Because of this homology, the putative protein product has been named *merlin* (for moezin-ezrin-radixin-like protein); alternatively, *schwannomin* has been suggested to reflect the role of this protein in the prevention of the development of schwannomas.[56]

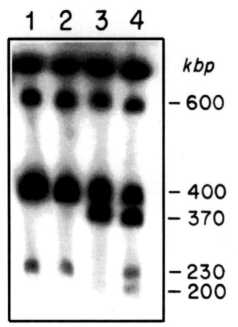

FIG. 23-6 Pulsed-field gel analysis of lymphoblast DNA from NF2 patients. DNA in agarose blocks was digested with the rare cutting restriction enzyme *Not*I, subjected to electrophoresis, blotted, and hybridized to a radiolabeled neurofilament heavy chain probe. Lane 1: unrelated NF2 patient. Lane 2: unaffected individual. Lane 3: affected daughter. Lane 4: affected mother. (*From Trofatter et al.,*[55] *by permission of Cell.*)

Clinical Genetics

NF2 shows autosomal dominant transmission with full penetrance by age 60.[14,18] In two studies a parent of origin effect on severity was observed, with the mean age in paternally inherited cases being 24 years and that in maternally inherited cases being 18 years.[6,18] Subsequent work has not confirmed this disparity, which may reflect a difference in the reproductive fitness of severely affected males versus females.[14] There is a marked degree of heterogeneity in NF2, and several authors have divided the disease into clinical subtypes. The mild, or Gardner, subtype is characterized

by the onset of symptoms in the third decade or later, few associated brain or spinal tumors, and survival into the sixth decade. The severe, or Wishart, subtype involves onset before age 25, rapid clinical progression, multiple intracranial and spinal tumors, and death in the third or fourth decade. The existence of a third subtype (Lee-Abbott) with variable age at hearing loss, cataract, and early age at death has not been confirmed.[14,18,57] The manifestations and clinical subtype of NF2 usually are similar within members of a family.[14,18,40] Despite the clinical heterogeneity of NF2, there is no evidence of genetic heterogeneity as is seen in other tumor-suppressor gene syndromes, such as tuberous sclerosis complex.[58] All series have shown that half of affected individuals do not have an affected parent; *de novo* alteration in the *NF2* gene has been documented in several of these individuals.[40,59]

Function of the NF2 Protein Product

The *NF2* gene spans 110 kilobases and includes 16 constitutive exons and 1 alternatively spliced exon.[55,56] NF2 is widely expressed, producing mRNAs in three different size ranges of approximately 7, 4.4, and 2.6 kb.[55,60] Two major alternative forms of the NF2 protein product exist. Isoform 1 is a protein of 595 amino acids produced from exons 1 through 15 and exon 17. The presence of the alternatively spliced exon 16 alters the C terminus of the protein, replacing 16 amino acids with 11 novel residues in isoform 2. Additional alternative splices predicting other minor species have also been described.[61,62] The *NF2* gene is highly conserved through evolution, as the mouse protein is 98 percent identical to human NF2, and the mouse *NF2* gene, which maps to chromosome 11 in a region of synteny conservation with 22q, is similarly alternatively spliced.[63,64]

The NF2 protein product is a member of the protein 4.1 family of cytoskeleton-associated proteins (Fig. 23-7). The proteins of this family include protein 4.1 itself, talin, ezrin, radixin, moesin, and several protein tyrosine phosphatases. All family members have a homologous domain of approximately 270 amino acids at the N terminus.[65] In the NF2 protein and its close relatives, this domain is followed by a long alpha-helical segment and a charged C-terminal domain. Protein 4.1, the best studied member of the family, plays a critical role in maintaining membrane stability and cell

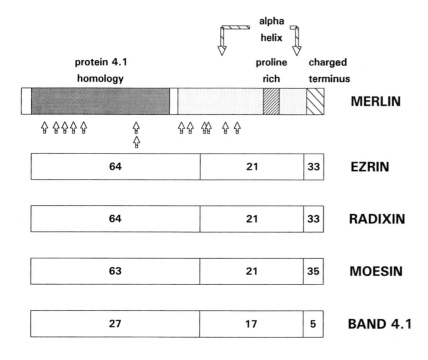

FIG. 23-7 ERM proteins related to NF2. This schematic diagram depicts the domains of the NF2 protein, which include a region of homology in the amino terminal half that defines membership in the protein 4.1 family, a long alpha-helical domain, and a charged carboxyl terminus. Arrows below the diagram indicate the relative location of 13 NF2 frame-preserving mutations involving either missense change or a codon deletion. These changes have been found in schwannomas, meningiomas, colon carcinomas, and NF2 patients. Comparable diagrams are shown for the ERM proteins and protein 4.1, dividing the proteins into three regions on the basis of their degree of amino acid identity with the NF2 protein product. The percentage amino acid identity is shown within each region. (*By permission of Current Biology, Current Opinion in Genetics and Develop 6:87, 1996.*)

shape in the erythrocyte by connecting integral membrane proteins, glycophorin, and the anion channel to be spectrin–actin lattice of the cytoskeleton. Protein 4.1 is the only other family member in which disease-causing mutation is known (see Chap. 115 in Scriver et al: *MMBID*, 7/e.).

The ERM proteins (ezrin, radixin, moesin), to which the NF2 protein is most closely related, share 70 to 75 percent amino acid identity with each other and are located in actin-rich surface projections such as microvilli, filopodia, membrane ruffles, lamellipodia in migrating cells, neuronal growth cones, and mitotic cleavage furrows. The NF2 protein is 45 to 46 percent identical to the ERMs with a common structural pattern except for the two different charged carboxy termini produced by alternative splicing. Both isoforms localize preferentially to the motile regions of cultured cells, such as the leading or ruffling edges, where they colocalize with F-actin. Where it has been tested, the NF2 protein does not colocalize with ezrin or moesin, suggesting a membrane–cytoskeleton linker function that is distinguishable from the ERM proteins.[66] A function of the NF2 protein in the motile regions of the cell suggests that schwannomas and meningiomas may form when the appropriate cell loses the ability to accurately regulate cell movement, shape, or communication, leading to a loss of growth control.

Germ-Line Mutations

Studies aimed at identifying germ-line mutations in NF2 patients by RT-PCR of mRNA, the protein truncation method, or scanning exons amplified from genomic DNA have met with great success.[55,56,59,67–69] In at least two studies, exon scanning was shown to detect mutation in two-thirds of the individuals studied.[40,59] Small numbers of patients have been reported to have gene deletions detected by Southern blot or flanking microsatellite analysis.[55,70–72] A wide variety of mutations have been identified in all NF2 exons except for exons 16 and 17. The vast majority of the alterations predict truncation of the protein product as a result of the introduction of a stop codon, a frameshift with premature termination, or a splicing alteration, supporting the view that loss of the protein's normal function is crucial to the development of tumors.[70–72] C to T transitions in CGA codons causing nonsense mutations are an especially common occurrence.[73] Less than 10 percent of detected mutations involve in-frame deletions and missense mutations, indicating that alteration of particular functional domains can abolish the NF2 tumor-suppressor activity.[74] No frequent polymorphisms, even in codon wobble positions, have been reported in the *NF2* gene.

The previously noted intrafamilial homogeneity in NF2 suggested a correlation between the highly variable phenotype of the disease and the underlying genotype. Several studies have supported this hypothesis in considering mild versus severe disease. Missense mutations in exons 7, 11, and 15 have been associated with mild disease.[68,69,74] Nonsense mutations have been associated with severe disease regardless of their position within the gene; an especially severe and homogeneous phenotype has been associated with a specific nonsense mutation in exon 6.[68,69,73,75,76] A notable exception to this rule is a patient with a nonsense mutation in exon 2 who became symptomatic at age 41 years and was not diagnosed with NF2 until age 49 years.[39] Somatic mosaicism was felt to be present on the basis of molecular analysis of lymphocyte DNA, which may explain this patient's mild phenotype. Frameshift mutations involving insertion or deletion of base pairs in several exons also have been associated with severe disease.[68,69,75] Splice site mutation has been associated with both mild and severe disease.[68,75] Interestingly, large deletions of the *NF2* gene have been associated with a mild phenotype.[70,71] This is in contradistinction to large deletions at the *NF1* locus, which produce a severe phenotype.[77]

A more detailed analysis of the effects of genotype on phenotype was reported recently.[40] Clinical information on 47 patients from 21 families with 20 different germ-line mutations, including age at onset and diagnosis, number of meningiomas, spinal and skin tumors, and the presence of cataracts and retinal abnormalities, was compared to the underlying genotype (Table 23-2). When each patient was considered as an independent random event, the patients with nonsense or frameshift mutations had more manifestations consistent with severe disease (earlier ages at onset and diagnosis and a higher frequency and number of tumors) than did patients with splice site mutations. However, when the family was the unit of comparison, statistically significant differences between the two groups were observed only for the age variables. This suggests that intrafamilial variability in the frequency and number of neural tumors was sufficient to decrease the strength of the correlation between genotype and phenotype. It is interesting that among this group of patients retinal abnormalities (hamartomas and epiretinal membranes) occurred only in relatives in five families with nonsense mutations; this may represent a new genotype/phenotype correlation.

These investigators did not identify mutations in 11 other NF2 families, most of which had clinical findings at the mild end of the spectrum. These mutations may be in unscreened regions of the introns and untranslated regulatory elements; they also could include large deletions that were not identified through exon scanning. These observations may have an impact on the types of mutation screening that will be needed in the future for presymptomatic diagnosis, since patients with mild phenotypes may be more likely to seek molecular diagnostic services than are those with severe manifestations.

Somatic Mutations

A number of studies have looked at somatic mutations in the *NF2* gene in resected tumor tissues from both NF2-affected and NF2-unaffected individuals. Mutations found in tumor material but not in normal tissue from the same individual are essential in confirming that *NF2* behaves like other well-documented tumor-suppressor genes.[53] In a study of 38 sporadic and *NF2*-derived schwannomas, Jacoby et al. found 25 somatic mutations affecting expression

Table 23-2 Relationship of Phenotypic Variables to Underlying Mutation Type*

	Total	Nonsense	Splice	Unfound
Mean age at onset (years)	19	12	22	24
Mean age at diagnosis (years)	27	20	33	29
Mean age at hearing loss (years)	24	20	28	24
Meningioma (%)	55	85	50	24
Spinal tumor (%)	67	89	57	46
Skin tumor (%)	70	90	44	71
Retinal hamartoma/ epiretinal membrane (%)	17	45	0	0
Families (*n*)	31	13	7	11
Individuals (*n*)	53	20	16	17

*Patients with nonsense mutations have a more severe phenotype than do those with splice site mutations and appear to be particularly disposed to retinal pathology. Individuals in whom no mutation can be detected by exon scanning have the mildest phenotype.
SOURCE: Adapted from Parry D, MacCollin M, Kaiser-Kupfer M, Pulaski K, Nicholson HS, Bolesta M, Eldridge R, Gusella J: Germline mutations in the neurofibromatosis 2 (NF2) gene: Correlations with disease severity and retinal abnormalities. *Am J Hum Genet* **59**:529, 1996.

of the merlin protein.[78] All 25 mutations involved gross truncation with nonsense, frameshift, or splice site alteration. Deletion was an especially common mechanism of mutation, with over half the mutations (14 of 25) involving the removal of 1 to 34 base pairs. As would be expected, many of these tumors (16 of 38) also showed loss of polymorphic markers on chromosome 22, indicating large deletions of that chromosome. Similar results have been reported in a follow-up study by the same group and by several other groups.[79–85] No differences have been reported between mutations detected in vestibular and nonvestibular tumors or between tumors derived from NF2 patients and sporadic tumors. These studies support the hypothesis that the *NF2* gene is the major tumor suppressor for schwannoma.

Analysis of meningiomas, the second most common tumor type in NF2, has revealed slightly different results. Wellenreuther et al., in a comprehensive analysis of 70 sporadic meningiomas, identified 43 mutations in 41 tumors.[86] Similar to the results in schwannoma, only 1 of the 43 involved a nontruncating event. Mutational events were much more common in tumors that had lost heterozygosity for chromosome 22, supporting the hypothesis that *NF2* is the meningioma locus on chromosome 22. These authors found that *NF2* mutations occurred much more frequently in specific pathologic subtypes of meningiomas. These and other studies suggest that *NF2* is a tumor suppressor for meningioma but that another protein or proteins not on chromosome 22 may also fill this role.[83,84,87]

Analysis of ependymomas has shown involvement to a lesser degree, with only one tumor in eight carrying a mutation in the *NF2* gene.[88] Perhaps more important, the same authors analyzed a cohort of 30 astrocytomas and found no alterations. This result is important because it supports the hypothesis that these alterations are truly causative and specific, not a secondary effect of tumorigenesis in general.

Loss of heterozygosity has also been observed for chromosome 22q markers in many different types of tumors that are not characteristic of NF2.[89] Screening for mutations that affect the *NF2* gene in such tumors has yielded mixed results. Only a handful of putative mutations of the *NF2* gene have been found in malignant melanoma, breast adenocarcinoma, and colon cancer, and none have been seen in ovarian carcinoma or hepatocellular carcinoma.[90–93] Two recent reports demonstrate a high rate of *NF2* mutation in malignant mesothelioma, suggesting that loss of *NF2* may be important in the progression of this aggressive mesodermal tumor type.[94,95] Thus, *NF2* appears to play an important, if not primary, role in the proliferation of some cells beyond those giving rise to the nervous system tumors of NF2.

DIAGNOSIS AND TREATMENT

Diagnosis of NF2 is based on the NIH clinical criteria (Table 23-1). A careful clinical examination with special attention to a dermatologic evaluation, the neurologic symptomatology, and a slit-lamp examination to evaluate possible retinal or lenticular manifestations are mandatory. Initial radiographic evaluation of a patient known or suspected to have NF2 should include a cranial MRI scan with and without gadolinium enhancement. Small intracanalicular tumors may not be seen on standard 5-mm slice thickness through the posterior fossa. Optimal evaluation includes 3-mm cuts overlapping by 1.5 mm on both axial and coronal views through the internal auditory canals.[35] Large vestibular schwannomas (>2 cm) and meningiomas may be visualized by computer tomography (CT). In general, however, CT is obscured by bony artifact in the region of the internal auditory canal and skull base and cannot substitute for MRI. Audiologic evaluation including brain-

stem auditory evoked response (BAER) may rarely reveal a functional deficit in a nerve in which no enhancement is visible. BAER also may be useful in defining the baseline functional impact of an otherwise presymptomatic tumor. Spinal MRI may be helpful in defining asymptomatic tumors; it is mandatory in individuals with unexplained neurologic symptoms or signs.[22]

Increasingly, presymptomatic genetic testing may supplant clinical testing for individuals at risk for NF2.[34,96–98] Because NF2 is a fully penetrant disease and because the age of onset shows homogeneity within families, such testing probably is useful only for the children of an at-risk individual. The age at testing will depend on the attitude of the family toward presymptomatic surgery and the severity of disease in the family. Genetic testing may be done on the basis of linkage when there is more than one affected family member or on the basis of mutational analysis of a known affected individual. Because no mutation can be detected in at least one-third of individuals with typical NF2, mutational analysis is not useful for confirming or excluding a suspected diagnosis.

Therapy for vestibular schwannoma remains primarily surgical.[35,36,99,100] Close neurologic monitoring is mandatory for determining the timing of surgical intervention. Small vestibular tumors (<1.5 mm) which are completely intercanalicular, often may be completely resected with preservation of both hearing and facial function.[35,36] Larger tumors probably are best managed expectantly, with debulking or decompression carried out when brainstem compression or increasing facial and/or hearing function ensues.[36] Other cranial and spinal tumors, including meningiomas, other cranial nerve schwannomas, and ependymomas, should be monitored for symptomatology; these tumors are very slow growing, and intervention on a minimally functionally active tumor may produce disability years before it would occur otherwise. Facial nerve reconstruction may be very important for patients who find facial palsy more debilitating than hearing loss.[36,101]

Stereotactic radiosurgery, most commonly with the gamma knife, has been offered as an alternative to surgery in selected patients with vestibular schwannomas.[102,103] Radiation therapy for other NF2-associated tumors should be carefully considered since radiation exposure may induce, accelerate, or transform tumors in a patient with an inactivated tumor-suppressor gene. Of special concern is the recent observation that in an international survey of malignancy in NF2 patients, two of four individuals had previously received radiation therapy in the area in which the malignancy developed.[104]

There is currently no medical therapy available for NF2 patients. Various agents, including progesterone inhibitors, and antiangiogenesis factors have shown promising results in cell culture and animal models.[105–107] Management of patients with vestibular tumors should include counseling on the often insidious problems with balance they may encounter. Drowning or near drowning owing to underwater disorientation is an especially important consideration.[6]

Hearing and speech augmentation and preservation play an important role in the management of NF2 patients. All these patients and their families should be referred to audiologists to receive training in optimization of hearing and speech production. Lip-reading skills may be enhanced by teaching, and sign language often may be more effectively acquired before the patient loses hearing. Hearing aids may be helpful early in the course of the disease. Rarely, patients who have had a vascular insult to the cochlea but otherwise are without nerve damage may benefit from a cochlear implant.[108] An alternative technology for placement of a cochlear implant-type electrode proximal to the nerve in the lateral recess of the fourth ventricle recently was developed by the House Ear Institute in Los Angeles.[109,110] Initial results with this device in 24 adult deafened NF2 patients have been extremely promising.[111]

Resources for Patients with NF

Diagnosis, evaluation, and treatment of complex patients with NF are best done in an NF center with experience in the multiple complications and delicate management of this disease.[17,32] Such multidisciplinary clinics are now available in most major medical centers and are accredited by the National Neurofibromatosis Foundation (NNFF) in New York City. Both the NNFF and Neurofibromatosis, Inc. (Lanham, MD), publish newsletters and maintain a network of local support chapters that are invaluable resources for patient and family education and support.

REFERENCES

1. Von Recklinghausen F: *Ueber die multiplen Fibrome der Haut und ihre Beziehung zu den Multiplen Neuromen.* Berlin, Hirschwald, 1882.
2. Crump TT: Translation of case reports in Ueber die multiplen Fibrome der Haut und ihre Beziehung zu den multiplen Neuromen by F.V. Recklinghausen. *Adv Neurol* 29:259, 1981.
3. Henneberg R, Koch M: Ueber centrale Neurofibromatose und die Geschwulste des Kleinhirnbruckenwinkels (Acusticus-neurome). *Arch Psychiatrie* 36:251, 1902.
4. Bassoe P, Nuzum F: Report of a case of central and peripheral neurofibromatosis. *J Nerv Ment Dis* 42:785, 1915.
5. Gardner WJ, Frazier CH: Bilateral acoustic neurofibromas: A clinical study and field survey of a family of five generations with bilateral deafness in thirty-eight members. *Arch Neurol Psychiatr* 23:266, 1930.
6. Kanter WR, Eldridge R, Fabricant R, Allen JC, Koerber T: Central neurofibromatosis with bilateral acoustic neuroma: Genetic, clinical and biochemical distinctions from peripheral neurofibromatosis. *Neurology* 30:851, 1980.
7. Martuza RL, Eldridge R: Neurofibromatosis 2 (bilateral acoustic neurofibromatosis). *N Engl J Med* 318:684, 1988.
8. Riccardi VM: *Neurofibromatosis: Phenotype, Natural History, and Pathogenesis,* 2d ed. Baltimore, Johns Hopkins University Press, 1992, p 224.
9. Argenyi ZB, Thieberg MD, Hayes CM, Whitaker DC: Primary cutaneous meningioma associated with von Recklinghausen's disease. *J Cutan Pathol* 21:549, 1994.
10. Mulvihill JJ, Parry DM, Sherman JL, Pikus A, Kaiser-Kupfer MI, Eldridge R: NIH conference: Neurofibromatosis 1 (Recklinghausen disease) and neurofibromatosis 2 (bilateral acoustic neurofibromatosis): An update. *Ann Intern Med* 113:39, 1990.
11. Eldridge R, Parry DM: Summary: Vesticular schwannoma (acoustic neuroma): Consensus Development Conference. *Neurosurgery* 30:961, 1992.
12. Russell D, Rubinstein L: *Pathology of Tumors of the Nervous System,* 5th ed. Baltimore, Williams & Wilkins, 1989.
13. Evans DG, Huson SM, Donnai D, Neary W, Blair V, Teare D, Newton V, Strachan T, Ramsden R, Harris R: A genetic study of type 2 neurofibromatosis in the United Kingdom: I. Prevalence, mutation rate, fitness and confirmation of maternal transmission effect on severity. *J Med Genet* 29:841, 1992.
14. Parry DM, Eldridge R, Kaiser-Kupfer MI, Bouzas E, Pikus A, Patronas N: Neurofibromatosis 2 (NF2): Clinical characteristics of 63 affected individuals and clinical evidence for heterogeneity. *Am J Med Genet* 52:450, 1994.
15. Leonard J, Talbot M: Asymptomatic acoustic neurilemoma. *Arch Otolaryngol* 91:117, 1970.
16. Stewart T, Liland J, Schuknecht H: Occult schwannoma of the vestibular nerve. *Arch Otolaryngol* 101:91, 1975.
17. Evans DGR, Ramsden R, Huson SM, Harris R, Lye R, King T: Type 2 neurofibromatosis: The need for supraregional care? *J Laryngol Otol* 107:401, 1993.
18. Evans DGR, Huson SM, Donnai D, Neary W, Blair V, Newton V, Harris R: A clinical study of type 2 neurofibromatosis. *Q J Med* 304:603, 1992.
19. Mautner VF, Lindenau M, Koppen J, Hazim W, Kluwe L: Type 2 neurofibromatosis without acoustic neuroma [German]. *Zentralbl Neurochirurgie* 56:83, 1995.
20. Mautner VF, Tatagiba M, Guthoff R, Samii M, Pulst SM: Neurofibromatosis 2 in the pediatric age group. *Neurosurgery* 33:92, 1993.
21. Sobel R, Wang Y: Vestibular (acoustic) schwannomas: Histological features in neurofibromatosis 2 and in unilateral cases. *J Neuropathol Exp Neurol* 52:106, 1993.
22. Mautner VF, Tatagiba M, Lindenau M, Funsterer C, Pulst SM, Kluwe L, Zanella F: Spinal tumors in patients with neurofibromatosis type 2: MR imaging study of frequency, multiplicity, and variety. *AJR* 165:951, 1995.
23. McCormick P, Torres R, Post K, Stein B: Intramedullary ependymoma of the spinal cord. *J Neurosurg* 72:523, 1990.
24. Epstein FJ, Farmer JP, Freed D: Adult intramedullary spinal cord ependymoma: The result of surgery in 38 patients. *J Neurosurg* 79:204, 1993.
25. Thomas PK, King RHM, Chiang TR, Scaravilli F, Sharma AK, Downie AW: Neurofibromatosis neuropathy. *Muscle Nerve* 13:93, 1990.
26. Kilpatrick T, Hjorth R, Gonzales MF: A case of neurofibromatosis 2 presenting with a mononeuritis multiplex. *J Neurol Neurosurg Psychiatry* 55:391, 1992.
27. Kaiser-Kupfer M, Freidlin V, Datiles M, Edwards P, Sherman J, Parry D, McCain L, Eldridge R: The association of posterior capsular lens opacities with bilateral acoustic neuromas in patients with neurofibromatosis type 2. *Arch Ophthalmol* 107:541, 1989.
28. Bouzas E, Parry D, Eldridge R, Kaiser-Kupfer M: Visual impairment in patients with neurofibromatosis 2. *Neurology* 43:622, 1993.
29. Ragge N, Baser M, Klein J, Nechiporuk A, Sainz J, Pulst SM, Riccardi V: Ocular abnormalities in neurofibromatosis 2. *Am J Ophthalmol* 20:634, 1995.
30. Crowe FW, Schull WJ: Diagnostic importance of the cafe au lait spot in neurofibromatosis. *Arch Intern Med* 91:758, 1953.
31. Kopf AW, Levine LJ, Rigel DS, Friedman RJ, Levenstein M: Prevalence of congenital-nevus-like nevi, nevi spili and cafe au lait spots. *Arch Dermatol* 121:766, 1985.
32. Short MP, Martuza RL, Huson SM: Neurofibromatosis 2: Clinical features, genetic counselling and management issues, in Huson SM, Hughes RAC (eds): *The Neurofibromatoses: A Pathogenetic and Clinical Overview.* London, Chapman and Hall, 1994, p 414.
33. Short MP, Bove C, MacCollin M, Mohney T, Ramesh V, Terenzio A, Gusella J: Gender differences in neurofibromatosis, type 2. *Neurology* 4(suppl 2):A159, 1994.
34. Harsh G, MacCollin M, McKenna M, Nadol J, Ojemann R, Short MP: Molecular genetic screening for children at risk of neurofibromatosis 2. *Arch Otolaryngol Head Neck Surg* 121:590, 1995.
35. Briggs R, Brackmann D, Baser M, Hitselberg W: Comprehensive management of bilateral acoustic neuromas. *Arch Otolaryngol Head Neck Surg* 120:1307, 1994.
36. Ojemann RG: Management of acoustic neuromas (vestibular schwannomas). *Clin Neurosurg* 40:489, 1993.
37. Bruce J, Fetell M: Tumors of the skull and cranial nerves, in Rowland LP (ed): *Merritt's Textbook of Neurology,* 9th ed. Baltimore, Williams & Wilkins, 1995, p 320.
38. Moss C, Green SH: What is segmental neurofibromatosis? *Br J Dermatol* 130:106, 1994.
39. Bourn D, Carter SA, Evans DGR, Goodship J, Coakham H, Strachan T: A mutation in the neurofibromatosis type 2 tumor-suppressor gene, giving rise to widely different clinical phenotypes in two unrelated individuals. *Am J Hum Genet* 55:69, 1994.
40. Parry D, MacCollin M, Kaiser-Kupfer M, Pulaski K, Nicholson HS, Bolesta M, Eldridge R, Gusella J: Germline mutations in the neurofibromatosis 2 (NF2) gene: Correlations with disease severity and retinal abnormalities. *Am J Hum Genet* 59:529, 1996.
41. MacCollin M, Woodfin W, Kronn D, Short MP: Schwannomatosis: A clinical and pathologic study. *Neurology* 46:1072, 1996.
42. Berger T, Lapins N, Engel M: Agminated neurilemomas. *J Am Acad Dermatol* 17:891, 1987.
43. Buenger K, Porter N, Dozier S, Wagner R: Localized multiple neurilemmoma of the lower extremity. *Cutis* 51:36, 1993.
44. Sieb JP, Pulst SM, Buch A: Familial CNS tumors. *J Neurol* 239:343, 1992.
45. Pulst SM, Rouleau G, Marineau C, Fain P, Sieb J: Familial meningioma is not allelic to neurofibromatosis 2. *Neurology* 43:2096, 1993.
46. Von Deimling A, Kraus J, Stangl A, Wellenreuther R, Lenartz D, Schramm J, Louis D, Ramesh V, Gusella J, Wiestler O: Evidence of subarachnoid spread in the development of multiple meningiomas. *Brain Pathol* 5:11, 1995.

47. Jaaskelainin J, Paetau A, Pyykko I, Blomstedt G, Palva T, Troupp H: Interface between the facial nerve and large acoustic neurinomas: Immunohistochemical study of the cleavage plane in NF2 and non-NF2 cases. *J Neurosurg* **870**:541, 1993.

48. Aguiar P, Tatagiba M, Samii M, Dankoweit-Timpe E, Ostertag H: The comparison between the growth fraction of bilateral vestibular schwannomas in neurofibromatosis 2 (NF2) and unilateral vestibular schwannomas using the monoclonal antibody MIB 1. *Acta Neurochir (Wien)* **134**:40, 1995.

49. Louis D, Ramesh V, Gusella J: Neuropathology and molecular genetics of neurofibromatosis 2 and related tumors. *Brain Pathol* **5**;163, 1995.

50. Seizinger B, Martuza R, Gusella J: Loss of genes on chromosome 22 in tumorigenesis of human acoustic neuroma. *Nature* **322**:644, 1986.

51. Seizinger B, de la Monte S, Atkins L, Gusella J, Martuza R: Molecular genetic approach to human meningioma: Loss of genes on chromosome 22. *Proc Natl Acad Sci USA* **68**:820, 1971.

54. Rouleau GA, Wertelecki W, Haines JL, Hobbs W, Trofatter J, Seizinger B, Martuza R, Supermeau D, Conneally P, Gusella J: Genetic linkage of bilateral acoustic neurofibromatosis to a DNA marker on chromosome 22. *Nature* **329**:246, 1987.

55. Trofatter J, MacCollin M, Rutter J, Murrell J, Duyao M, Parry D, Eldridge R, Kley N, Menon A, Pulaski K, Haase V, Ambrose C, Munroe D, Bove C, Haines J, Martuza R, MacDonald M, Seizinger B, Short MP, Buckler A, Gusella J: A novel Moesin-, Ezrin-, Radixin-like gene is a candidate for the neurofibromatosis 2 tumor suppressor. *Cell* **72**:791, 1993.

56. Rouleau G, Merel P, Lutchman M, Sanson M, Zucman J, Marineau C, Hoang-Xuan K, Demczuk S, Desmaze C, Plougastel B, Pulst S, Lenoir G, Bijisma E, Rashold R, Dumanski J, de Jong P, Parry D, Eldridge R, Aurias A, Delattre O, Thomas G: Alteration in a new gene encoding a positive membrane-organizing protein causes neuro-fibromatosis type 2. *Nature* **363**:515, 1993.

57. Lee DK, Abbott ML: Familial central nervous system neoplasia: Case report of a family with von Recklinghausen's neurofibromatosis. *Arch Neurol* **20**:154, 1969.

58. Narod S, Parry D, Parboosingh J, Lenoir G, Ruttledge M, Fischer G, Eldridge R, Martuza R, Frontali M, Haines J, Gusella J, Rouleau G: Neurofibromatosis type 2 appears to be a genetically homogeneous disease. *Am J Hum Genet* **51**:486, 1992.

59. MacCollin M, Ramesh V, Jacoby L, Louis D, Rubio MP, Pulaski K, Trofatter J, Short MP, Bove C, Eldridge R, Parry D, Gusella J: Mutational analysis of patients with neurofibromatosis 2. *Am J Hum Genet* **55**:314, 1994.

60. Gutmann DH, Wright DE, Geist R, Snider W: Expression of the neurofibromatosis 2 (NF2) gene isoforms during rat embryonic development. *Hum Mol Genet* **4**:471, 1995.

61. Pykett M, Murphy M, Harnish P, George D: The neurofibromatosis 2 (NF2) tumor suppressor gene encodes multiple alternatively spliced transcripts. *Hum Mol Genet* **3**:559, 1994.

62. Hitotsumatsu T, Kitamoto T, Iwaki T, Fukui M, Tateishi J: An exon 8 spliced out transcript of the neurofibromatosis 2 gene is constitutively expressed in various human tissues. *J Biochem (Tokyo)* **116**:1205, 1994.

63. Haase V, Trofatter J, MacCollin M, Tarttelin E, Gusella J, Ramesh V: The murine NF2 homologue encodes a highly conserved merlin protein with alternative forms. *Hum Mol Genet* **3**:407, 1994.

64. Hara T, Bianchi A, Seizinger B, Kley N: Molecular cloning and characterization of alternatively spliced transcripts of the mouse neurofibromatosis 2 gene. *Cancer Res* **54**:330, 1994.

65. Arpin M, Algrain M, Louvard D: Membrane-actin microfilament connections: An increasing diversity of players related to band 4.1. *Curr Opin Cell Biol* **6**:136, 1994.

66. Gonzalez-Agosti C, Xu L, Pinney D, Beauchamp R, Hobbs W, Gusella J, Ramesh V: The merlin tumor suppressor localizes preferentially in membrane ruffles. *Oncogene* **13**:1239, 1996.

67. Pulaski K, Pettingell W, MacCollin M, Gusella J: Mutational analysis of NF2 by in vitro expression assay. *Am J Hum Genet* **55**:1383, 1994.

68. Merel P, Hoang-Xuan K, Sanson M, Bijlsma E, Rouleu G, Laurent-Puig P, Pulst S, Baser M, Lenoir G, Sterkers J, Philippon J, Resche F, Mautner V, Fischer G, Hulsebos T, Aurias A, Delattre O, Thomas G: Screening for germ-line mutations in the NF2 gene. *Genes Chrom Cancer* **12**:117, 1995.

69. Bourn D, Carter S, Mason S, Evans DGR, Strachan T: Germline mutations in the neurofibromatosis type 2 tumour suppressor gene. *Hum Mol Genet* **3**:813, 1994.

70. Watson C, Gaunt L, Evans G, Patel K, Harris R, Strachan T: A disease-associated germline deletion maps the type 2 neurofibromatosis (NF2) gene between the Ewing sarcoma region and the leukaemia inhibitory factor locus. *Hum Mol Genet* **2**:701, 1993.

71. Kluwe L, Pulst S, Koppen J, Matner VP: A 163-bp deletion at the C-terminus of the schwannomin gene associated with variable phenotypes of neurofibromatosis type 2. *Hum Genet* **95**:443, 1995.

72. Sanson M, Marineau C, Desmaze C, Lutchman M, Ruttledge M, Baron C, Narod S, Delattre O, Lenoir G, Thomas G, Aurias A, Rouleau G: Germline deletion in a neurofibromatosis type 2 kindred inactivates the NF2 gene and a candidate meningioma locus. *Hum Mol Genet* **2**:1215, 1993.

73. Sainz J, Figueroa K, Baser M, Mautner VF, Pulst SM: High frequency of nonsense mutations in the NF2 gene caused by C to T transitions in five CGA codons. *Hum Mol Genet* **4**:137, 1995.

74. MacCollin M, Mohney T, Trofatter J, Wertelecki W, Ramesh V, Gusella J: DNA diagnosis of neurofibromatosis 2: Altered coding sequence of the merlin tumor suppressor in an extended pedigree. *JAMA* **270**:2316, 1993.

75. Ruttledge M, Andermann A, Phelan C, Claudio J, Han F, Chretien N, Rangaratnam S, MacCollin M, Short MP, parry D, Michels V, Riccardi V, Weksberg R, Kitamura K, Bradburn J, Hall B, Propping P, Rouleau G: Type of mutation in the neurofibromatosis type 2 gene (NF2) frequently determines severity of disease. *Am J Hum Genet* **59**:331, 1996.

76. MacCollin M, Braverman N, Viskochil D, Ruttledge M, Davis K, Ojemann R, Gusella J, Parry D: A point mutation associated with a severe phenotype of neurofibromatosis 2. *Ann Neurol* **40**:440, 1996.

77. Kayes L, Burke W, Riccardi V, Bennett R, Ehrlich P, Rubenstein A, Stephens K: Deletions spanning the neurofibromatosis 1 gene: Identification and phenotype of five patients. *Am J Hum Genet* **54**:424, 1994.

78. Jacoby LJ, MacCollin M, Louis D, Mohney T, Rubio MP, Pulaski K, Trofatter J, Kley N, Seizinger B, Ramesh V, Gusella J: Exon scanning for mutation of the NF2 gene in schwannomas. *Hum Mol Genet* **3**:413, 1994.

79. Jacoby L, MacCollin M, Barone R, Ramesh V, Gusella J: Frequency and distribution of NF2 mutations in schwannomas. *Genes Chromosom Cancer* **17**:45, 1996.

80. Biljlsma E, Merel P, Bosch A, Westerveld A, Delatre O, Thomas G, Hulsebos T: Analysis of mutations in the SCh gene in schwannomas. *Genes Chromosom Cancer* **11**:7, 1994.

81. Twist E, Ruttledge M, Rousseau M, Sanson M, Papi L, Merel P, Delattre O, Thomas G, Rouleau G: The neurofibromatosis type 2 gene is inactivated in schwannomas. *Hum Mol Genet* **3**:147, 1994.

82. Sainz J, Huynh D, Figueroa K, Ragge N, Baser M, Pulst SM: Mutations of the neurofibromatosis type 2 gene and lack of the gene product in vestibular schwannomas. *Hum Mol Genet* **3**:885, 1994.

83. Deprez RHL, Bianchi A, Groen N, Seizinger B, Hagemeijer A, van Drunen E, Bootsma D, Koper J, Avezaat C, Kley N, Zwarthoff E: Frequent NF2 gene transcript mutations in sporadic meningiomas and vestibular schwannomas. *Am J Hum Genet* **54**:1022, 1994.

84. Merel P, Hoang-Xuan K, Sanson A, Moreau-Aubry EK, Bijlsma C, Lazaro JP, Moisan F, Resche I, Nishisho X, Estivill JY, Delattre M, Poisson C, Theillet T, Hulsebos T, Delattre O, Thomas G: Predominant occurrence of somatic mutations of the NF2 gene in meningiomas and schwannomas. *Genes Chromosom Cancer* **13**:211, 1995.

85. Welling DB, Guida M, Goll F, Pearl DK, Glasscock ME, Pappas DG, Linthicum F, Roberts D, Thomas P: Mutational spectrum in the neurofibromatosis type 2 gene in sporadic and familial schwannomas. *Hum Genet* **98**:189, 1996.

86. Wellenreuther R, Kraus J, Lenartz D, Menon A, Schramm J, Louis D, Ramesh V, Gusella J, Wiestler O, von Deimling A: Analysis of the neurofibromatosis 2 gene reveals molecular variants of meningioma. *Am J Pathol* **146**:827, 1995.

87. Ruttledge M, Sarrazin J, Rangaratnam S, Phelan C, Twist E, Merel P, Delattre O, Thomas G, Nordenskjold M, Collins VP, Dumanski JP, Rouleau G: Evidence for the complete inactivation of the NF2 gene in the majority of sporadic meningiomas. *Nat Genet* **6**:180, 1994.

88. Rubio MP, Correa K, Ramesh V, MacCollin M, Jacoby L, von Deimling A, Gusella J, Louis D: Analysis of the neurofibromatosis 2 gene in human ependymomas and astrocytomas. *Cancer Res* **54**:45, 1994.

89. Seizinger BR, Klinger HP, Junien C, Nakamura Y, Le Beau M, Cavenee W, Emanuel B, Ponder B, Naylor S, Mitelman F, Louis D, Menon A, Newsham I, Decker J, Kaelbling M, Henry I, von Deimling A: Reports of the committee on chromosome and gene loss in human neoplasia. *Cytogenet Cell Genet* **58**:1080, 1991.

90. Krakawa H, Hayashi N, Nagase H, Ogawa M, Nakamura Y: Alternative splicing of the NF2 gene and its mutation analysis of breast and colorectal cancers. *Hum Mol Genet* 3:565, 1994.
91. Bianchi AB, Hara T, Ramesh V, Gao J, Klein-Szanto AJ, Morin F, Menon AG, Trofatter JA, Gusella JF, Seizinger B, Kley N: Mutations in transcript isoforms of the neurofibromatosis 2 gene in multiple human tumour types. *Nat Genet* 6:185, 1994.
92. Englefield P, Foulkes W, Campbell I: Loss of heterozygosity on chromosome 22 in ovarian carcinoma is distal to and is not accompanied by mutations in NF2 at 22112. *Br J Cancer* 70:905, 1994.
93. Kanai Y, Tsuda H, Oda T, Sakamoto M, Hirohashi S: Analysis of the neurofibromatosis 2 gene in human breast and hepatocellular carcinomas. *Jpn J Clin Oncol* 25:1, 1995.
94. Sekido Y, Pass H, Bader S, Mew D, Christman M, Gazdar A, Minna J: Neurofibromatosis type 2 (NF2) gene is somatically mutated in mesothelioma but not in lung cancer. *Cancer Res* 55:1227, 1995.
95. Bianchi AB, Mitsunaga S, Cheng J, Klein W, Jhanwar S, Seizinger B, Kley N, Klein-Szanto A, Testa J: High frequency of inactivating mutations in the neurofibromatosis type 2 gene (NF2) in primary malignant mesotheliomas. *Proc Natl Acad Sci USA* 92:10854, 1995.
96. Ruttledge M, Narod S, Dumanski J, Parry D, Eldridge R, Wertelecki W, Parboosingh J, Faucher M, Lenoir G, Collins V, Nordenskjold M, Rouleau G: Presymptomatic diagnosis for neurofibromatosis 2 with chromosome 22 markers. *Neurology* 43:1753, 1993.
97. Sainio M, Strachan T, Blomstedt G, Salonen O, Setala K, Palotie A, Palo J, Pyykko I, Peltonen L, Jaaskelainen J: Presymptomatic DNA and MRI diagnosis of neurofibromatosis 2 with mild clinical course in an extended pedigree. *Neurology* 45:1314, 1995.
98. Bijlsma EK, Merel P, Fleury P, van Asperen C, Westerveld A, Delattre O, Thomas G, Hulsebos T: Family with neurofibromatosis type 2 and autosomal dominant hearing loss: Identification of carriers of the mutated NF2 gene. *Hum Genet* 96:1, 1995.
99. Nadol J, Chiong C, Ojemann R, McKenna M, Martuza R, Montgomery W, Levine R, Ronner S, Glynn R: Preservation of hearing and facial nerve function in resection of acoustic neuroma. *Laryngoscope* 102:1153, 1992.
100. Miyamoto R, Campbell R, Fritsch M, Lochmueller G: Preservation of hearing in neurofibromatosis 2. *Otolaryngol Head Neck Surg* 103:619, 1990.
101. Tatagiba M, Matthies C, Samii M: Facial nerve reconstruction in neurofibromatosis 2. *Acta Neurochir (Wien)* 126:72, 1994.
102. Linskey M, Lunsford D, Flickinger J: Tumor control after stereotactic radiosurgery in neurofibromatosis patients with bilateral acoustic tumors. *Neurosurgery* 31:829, 1992.
103. Lunsford LD, Linskey M: Stereotactic radiosurgery in the treatment of patients with acoustic tumors. *Otol Clin North Am* 25:471, 1992.
104. Baser M, MacCollin M, Sujansky E, Evans DGR, Rubenstein A: Malignant nervous system tumors in patients with neurofibromatosis 2. Presented at the 1996 FASEB summer research conference on neurofibromatosis, Snowmass, CO, June 29, 1996.
105. Matsuda Y, Kawamoto K, Kiya K, Kurisu K, Sugiyama K, Uozumi T: Antitumor effects of antiprogesterones on human meningioma cells in vitro and in vivo. *J Neurosurg* 80:527, 1994.
106. Lamberts S, Tanghe H, Avezaat C, Braakman R, Wijngaarde R, Koper J, de Jong FH: Mifepristone (RU 486) treatment of meningiomas. *J Neurol Neurosurg Psychiatry* 55:486, 1992.
107. Takamiya Y, Friedlander R, Brem H, Malick A, Martuza R: Inhibition of angiogenesis and growth of human nerve-sheath tumors by AGM-1470. *J Neurosurg* 78:470, 1993.
108. Hoffman R, Kohan D, Cohen N: Cochlear implants in the management of bilateral acoustic neuromas. *Am J Otol* 13:525, 1992.
109. Brackmann D, Hitselberger W, Nelson R, Moore J, Waring M, Portillo F, Shannon R, Telischi F: Auditory brainstem implant: I. Issues in surgical implantation. *Otolaryngol Head Neck Surg* 108:624, 1993.
110. Shannon R, Fayad J, Moore J, Lo W, Otto S, Nelson R, O'Leary M: Auditory brainstem implant: II. Postsurgical issues and performance. *Otolaryngol Head Neck Surg* 108:634, 1993.
111. Staller S, Otto S, Menapace C: Clinical trials of the auditory brainstem implant. *Audiol Today* 7:9, 1995.

CHAPTER 24

Renal Carcinoma

W. Marston Linehan ▪ Richard D. Klausner

1. Renal carcinoma appears in both a sporadic form and a hereditary form. Eighty-five percent of sporadic renal carcinomas are of the clear-cell histologic type, 5 to 10 percent are papillary renal carcinomas, and the remainder are rare histologic types such as chromophobe and collecting duct renal carcinomas.

2. The most well-characterized form of hereditary renal carcinoma is von Hippel-Lindau (VHL) syndrome. VHL is a hereditary cancer syndrome in which affected individuals are at risk to develop tumors in a number of organs, including the kidneys, cerebellum, spine, eye, inner ear, adrenal glands, and pancreas. VHL families are categorized as VHL type I (without pheochromocytoma) or VHL type II (with pheochromocytoma).

3. The *VHL* gene, which has the characteristics of a tumor-suppressor gene, has been identified on the short arm of chromosome 3. The *VHL* gene has three exons and encodes a protein of 213 amino acids. Both copies of the gene are inactivated in tumors in VHL patients: mutation in the inherited allele and loss of the wild-type allele. *VHL* gene mutation analysis provides a method for the early diagnosis of VHL in asymptomatic individuals or in clinical situations, such as hereditary pheochromocytoma, in which the diagnosis is in doubt. VHL manifestations often occur in childhood; testing early in life is recommended so that appropriate intervention can be instituted. There is a marked genotype/phenotype correlation between *VHL* gene mutation and the manifestation of VHL; VHL type II families are characterized by missense mutations of the *VHL* gene. There is a hotspot for VHL type II at a single codon in the 5′ end of exon 3 of the *VHL* gene.

4. Inactivation of both copies of the *VHL* gene is an early event in clear-cell renal carcinoma, in which a high percentage of *VHL* gene mutations and LOH have been detected. *VHL* gene mutations, including nucleotide insertions, deletions, substitutions, and nonsense mutations, have been found in each of the three exons. Neither *VHL* gene mutation nor VHL LOH is found in papillary renal carcinoma. A molecular genetic classification of renal carcinoma—clear-cell versus papillary—has been proposed, with clear-cell renal carcinoma characterized by *VHL* gene mutation. *VHL* gene mutations have been detected in DNA extracted from formalin-fixed material and tissue aspirates, providing a potentially useful diagnostic tool. Somatic *VHL* gene mutations have been detected in sporadic tumors from other organs affected in VHL, including cerebellar hemangioblas-

toma and epididymal cystadenoma. With the exception of rare reports, VHL is not mutated or implicated in other sporadic cancers, such as lung carcinomas, breast carcinoma, and ovarian cancer.

5. The VHL suppressor gene product has begun to be characterized. VHL forms a stable trimolecular complex with two subunits of the highly conserved heterotrimeric transcription elongation factor elongin (SIII). Elongin is composed of three subunits: A, B, and C. Elongin A is required to inhibit the processing of RNA pol II, allowing cell processivity of transcription. Elongin B enhances the assembly of elongin C to either elongin A or VHL. VHL and elongin A compete for binding to B and C via a short shared sequence motif. This sequence, which is found in the third exon of *VHL*, is highly mutated in both VHL and sporadic renal cell carcinoma, and these loss-of-function *VHL* mutations are associated with loss of assembly of VHL with the B and C subunits. While VHL can competitively inhibit the assembly of a functional ABC transcription elongation factor, it is not clear that inhibition of transcription elongation is the mode of action of VHL. The VHL protein has been found both in the nucleus and in the cytosol of transiently transfected cells. There is a tightly regulated, cell density-dependent transport of VHL into and/or out of the nucleus. In densely grown cells, the VHL signal appears predominantly in the cytoplasm, whereas in sparse cultures, most of the signal is detected in the nucleus. Immunofluorescence studies of mutant VHL protein revealed that the C-terminal region of the VHL protein is required for localization to or retention in the cytosol. In exon 1 deletion mutants, the protein remains predominantly in the cytosol under both sparse and confluent conditions.

6. Sporadic clear-cell renal carcinomas are characterized by a high degree of neoangiogenesis; angiogenesis is also a striking feature in the clinical manifestations of VHL. Both clear-cell renal carcinoma and cerebellar hemangioblastoma are characterized by a marked elevation in the expression of vascular endothelial growth factor (VEGF). The increased expression of VEGF is reversed in renal carcinoma cells by the reintroduction of the wild-type *VHL* gene. This reversal is blocked by either anoxia or low serum conditions, suggesting that VHL may play a role in the normal regulated induction of angiogenesis. This critical gene is one of the first identified targets of VHL function.

7. Hereditary papillary renal cell carcinoma (HPRC) is a hereditary cancer syndrome in which affected individuals

are at risk to develop bilateral, multifocal papillary renal cell carcinoma. This syndrome, which has an autosomal dominant inheritance pattern, is distinct from other hereditary renal carcinomas. HPRC does not link to chromosome 3, and there are no germ-line *VHL* gene mutations.

Renal carcinoma, the most common cancer in the kidney, affects nearly 28,000 Americans annually and is associated with over 12,000 deaths per year.[1] Renal carcinoma, which accounts for approximately 3 percent of adult cancers, most commonly occurs in adults between the ages of 50 and 70; however, it has been reported in children as young as 3 years.[2] The clear-cell type (or a variant) accounts for 80 to 85 percent of renal carcinomas. Little is known about the etiology of renal cancer, although a number of environmental, hormonal, and cellular factors have been studied. Renal carcinoma has been increasing at a rate of approximately 2 percent per year and affects males twice as frequently as females.[3] There is a strong correlation with cigarette smoking and an increased incidence of renal cancer among leather workers and workers exposed to asbestos.[4-7] There is an increased incidence of renal carcinoma in patients with end-stage renal disease, and this is particularly notable in patients who have acquired cystic disease.[8,9] The risk to end-stage renal patients with cystic changes on dialysis of developing renal cell carcinoma has been estimated to be 30 times higher than that in the general population.[10] Five to 10 percent of renal carcinomas are of the papillary histologic type.[11,12] The remaining tumors are made up of rare histologic types such as chromophobe and collecting duct renal carcinomas.

Renal carcinoma occurs in both hereditary and nonhereditary, sporadic forms. Estimates from case-control studies suggest that up to 4 percent of renal carcinoma may be hereditary on the basis of family history.[3] There are three forms of hereditary renal cell carcinoma (Table 24-1). One is hereditary clear-cell renal carcinoma (HCRC), in which 50 percent of the offspring of an affected individual are likely to develop renal carcinoma.[13,14] A second form is that associated with von Hippel-Lindau (VHL) syndrome, in which affected individuals develop tumors in a number of organs, including the kidneys.[3,15] A third form is hereditary papillary renal carcinoma (HPRC).[16,17] While patients with sporadic renal carcinoma are likely to develop a solitary renal tumor between the ages of 50 and 70, patients with hereditary renal cell carcinoma tend to develop multifocal early-onset renal carcinoma.[3]

LOCATION OF THE CLEAR-CELL RENAL CARCINOMA GENE: CHROMOSOME 3

An initial indication of the location of a renal carcinoma gene came from the studies of Cohen et al., who in 1979 reported a family with an autosomal dominant inheritance pattern of bilateral, multifocal renal carcinoma.[13] Affected individuals in this kindred were characterized by a balanced germ-line translocation from chromosome 3 to chromosome 8. Subsequently, Pathak reported a renal cell carcinoma family with a chromosome 3 to chromosome 11 translocation,[18] and in 1989 Kovaks et al. described a family carrying a constitutional translocation (3;6)(p13;q25.1) in which

affected individuals developed multiple, bilateral early-onset renal carcinoma.[19]

These and other findings led to genetic studies of chromosome 3 in nonhereditary renal cell carcinoma. When renal carcinoma was evaluated for loss of heterozygosity (LOH) on chromosome 3 by RFLP analysis (Fig. 24-1), consistent loss of a segment of the short arm of chromosome 3 was detected in tumor tissue from patients with sporadic, nonhereditary clear-cell renal carcinoma.[20-28] Cytogenetic analysis of sporadic renal cell carcinoma confirmed these findings.[23,28-30] Loss of a segment of chromosome 3 was found to be a consistent feature of the common form of renal carcinoma—clear-cell renal carcinoma—but not of papillary renal carcinoma.[21,31-34] In a detailed analysis of 60 tumors, Anglard et al. detected LOH in nearly 90 percent of clear-cell renal carcinomas and defined by deletion analysis (Fig. 24-2) an area of minimal deletion in the 3p21-26 region of chromosome 3.[21] As this region was too large to study by the conventional cloning methods available at the time, investigators turned to the hereditary form of renal cell carcinoma associated with VHL to search for the kidney cancer gene.

VON HIPPEL-LINDAU

VHL is a hereditary cancer syndrome in which affected individuals are at risk to develop tumors in a number of organs, including the kidneys. In the early 1860s, ophthalmologists' reports began to describe angiomatous lesions of the retina that were associated with blindness and occasionally were associated with similar cerebellar lesions.[35] In 1894 Collins described angiomas which appeared in

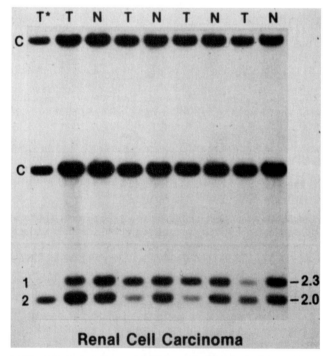

FIG. 24-1 RFLP analysis of sporadic renal cell carcinoma tumors (T) and corresponding normal tissue (N) with a probe for the chromosome 3p DNF 15S2 locus. 1 and 2 indicate the two polymorphic chromosome 3p alleles; C indicates a constant band. The bands on the lower part of the figure represent the 2.3- and 2.0-kb alleles, one of which is lost in the tumors indicated. The residual bands represent the presence of normal lymphocytes; the lane marked T* indicates a renal tumor grown in an immunodeficient mouse. (*From Zbar et al.[20]*)

Table 24-1 Hereditary Forms of Renal Carcinoma

1. Hereditary clear-cell renal carcinoma	(HCRC)
2. Von Hippel-Lindau	(VHL)
3. Hereditary papillary renal carcinoma	(HPRC)

CHROMOSOME 3 DELETION MAP: SPORADIC RENAL CELL CARCINOMA

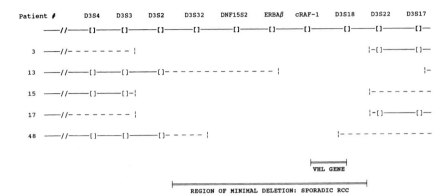

FIG. 24-2 Deletion map showing the area of minimal deletion on chromosome 3p in sporadic renal cell carcinoma. Analysis of the genotypes identified the locus in the telomeric portion of chromosome 3p bounded by the markers D3S2 and D3S22 as the region of a potential renal cell carcinoma disease gene. *(From Anglard et al.[21])*

the retinas of two siblings.[36] Von Hippel, a German ophthalmologist, first recognized that there was a hereditary component to the retinal angiomas.[37] The Swedish ophthalmologist Lindau determined that the retinal angiomas and cerebellar hemangioblastomas together were part of the familial syndrome that bears his name.[38] Although subsequent clinical reports of small families confirmed the association of the retinal angiomas, CNS hemangioblastomas, renal tumors and cysts, epididymal cystadenomas, pancreatic cysts and tumors, and pheochromocytomas,[35] it was not until 1964 that Melmon and Rosen codified the term *von Hippel-Lindau* with a definitive article in which a large family with these diverse manifestations (Table 24-2) was characterized.[39]

VHL is estimated to occur in 1 in 36,000 live births; inheritance of the gene follows an autosomal dominant pattern with 80 to 90 percent penetrance but with highly varied expressivity.[15] The age at onset of VHL is variable and depends on (1) which asymptomatic lesions are sought and (2) the expression within the family. The retinal angiomas are generally the earliest lesions to detect, followed by CNS and spinal hemangiomas. The mean age at diagnosis of retinal hemangiomas is 25 years (range, 1 to 67 years); for CNS hemangioblastoma it is 30 years (11 to 78 years), and for renal cell carcinoma, it is 37 years (16 to 67 years).[35] In kindreds with pheochromocytoma (VHL type II), pheochromocytoma is often detected before other manifestations and can appear before age 10.

Renal Manifestations of VHL

Renal cell carcinoma occurs in 28 to 45 percent of individuals affected with VHL. Affected individuals may develop renal cysts, renal cysts lined with renal cell carcinomas, or solid renal cell carcinomas. Although the renal tumors often are detected when they are small and are confined to the kidney, these tumors are malignant and can metastasize (Fig. 24-3). Poston et al.[40] characterized the findings after renal surgery in 161 lesions from 12 patients with VHL and renal cell carcinoma. Pathologic evaluation revealed 45 solid lesions, 41 of which were renal cell carcinomas, and 116 cys-

Table 24-2 Von Hippel-Lindau Manifestations

Bilateral, multifocal clear-cell renal carcinoma
Bilateral, multifocal renal cysts
Cerebellar and spinal hemangioblastoma
Endolymphatic sac tumors (ELSTs)
Retinal angioma
Pancreatic cysts, microcystic adenomas, islet-cell tumors
Pheochromocytoma
Epididymal cystadenoma

tic lesions, 25 of which were malignant. Of 66 malignant lesions, 35 (53 percent) contained cells with only clear-cell cytologic features; 30 (46 percent) were composed of predominantly clear cells with scattered granular cells. A single malignant lesion (1.5 percent) was found to have sarcomatoid renal cell carcinoma with clear and granular cells. This study established the clear-cell cytologic feature as the primary finding in renal lesions in VHL patients.[40] When Walther et al.[41] examined in detail grossly normal renal parenchyma from 16 VHL patients, microscopic renal cystic

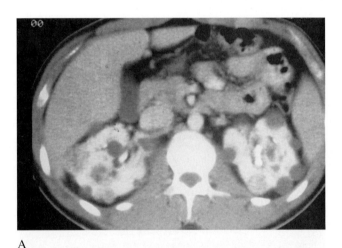

A

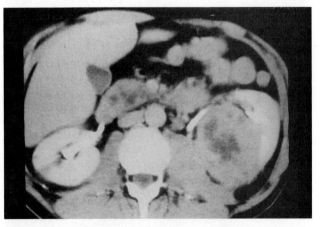

B

FIG. 24-3 *A.* Abdominal CT of a VHL patient reveals bilateral, multifocal renal carcinomas and cysts. *B.* Abdominal CT of a VHL patient reveals a large renal mass which had spread to the lungs.

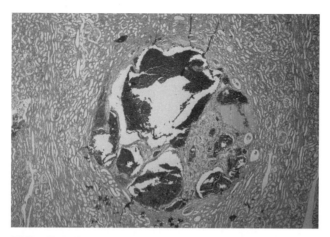

FIG. 24-4 A microscopic focus of renal cell carcinoma detected in grossly "normal" renal tissue from a VHL patient.

and solid neoplasms containing only clear-cell cytologic features were found (Fig. 20-4). The extrapolated number of lesions in the average kidney, represented at the mean age of 37 years, was estimated as 1100 nonmalignant cysts with a clear-cell lining and 600 clear-cell neoplasms.[41]

For the detection of even small renal lesions in VHL, computer tomography (CT) and ultrasound are the preferred techniques.[35,42,43] Treatment of renal cell carcinoma involves parenchymal-sparing surgery whenever possible.[44–48] Intraoperative ultrasound may be used to identify solid as well as cystic lesions to be removed surgically.[49,50] The prevalence of microscopic renal carcinoma makes it likely that tumors will reappear; the goal of surgery is to maintain renal function as long as possible while reducing the risk of metastases. A serial CT study of the natural history of renal lesions in VHL patients revealed that there is a wide variation in the growth rates of renal lesions.[51] Although clinicians often recommend surgery when solid renal lesions reach the size of 2.5 to 3 cm, the role of surgical resection in the management of VHL-associated renal carcinoma, that is, whether survival can be extended or quality of life enhanced by aggressive screening and early detection programs, remains to be determined.

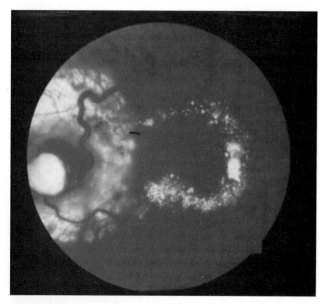

FIG. 24-5 Retinal lesion in a VHL patient showing the hypervascular retinal angioma that characterizes VHL.

Retinal Angioma

Retinal angiomas are often the first manifestation of VHL (Fig. 24-5). Fifty-eight to 60 percent of affected VHL patients will develop these benign vascular tumors of the retina. The histologic pattern of the ocular manifestation is strikingly similar to that of clear-cell renal cell carcinoma and cerebellar hemangioblastoma. These tumors can be multifocal, bilateral, and recurrent. While the mean age at diagnosis is reported to be 25 years, these tumors can occur in infants. Although retinal angiomas are nonmalignant, these tumors can cause glaucoma, cataracts, retinal detachment, and blindness. It is critical that at-risk individuals have a thorough ophthalmologic examination. This examination often includes tonometry, fluorescein angioscopy, and indirect ophthalmoscopy. Periodic ophthalmologic evaluation is a part of the management of VHL patients. Treatment of retinal angiomas often consists of laser therapy. An aggressive approach to the screening and treatment of eye lesions in VHL patients often results in successful long-term preservation of vision. Many clinicians recommend initiation of ophthalmologic screening at an early age (1 year) so that preservation of vision can be maintained.[15]

CNS Hemangioblastoma

CNS hemangioblastomas occur in 60 to 65 percent of affected VHL individuals and can cause increased intracranial pressure, obstructive hydrocephalus, hemorrhage, and death. The hemangioblastomas are characterized by three cell types: endothelial cells, stromal cells, and pericytes. These vascular tumors form channels and caverns and can organize into a vascular mural nodule within a fluid-filled cyst. The cells in the CNS tumors are remarkably similar to those seen in clear-cell renal carcinomas, as well as epididymal cystadenomas. There is marked hypertrophy of the afferent and efferent vessels in the cerebellar and spinal tumors; the gross appearance of these tumors can be that of a mass of blood vessels. VHL-associated CNS hemangioblastomas occur most often in the spine and cerebellum as well as in the brain stem at the craniocervical junction. These tumors occasionally occur above the tentorium.[15,52] Hemangioblastoma can occur in the pituitary, although this is an uncommon occurrence. The number of CNS lesions, as well as the number of renal and pancreatic lesions, is often underestimated by radiographic imaging studies.

Although the mean age at diagnosis of CNS hemangioblastoma in VHL patients is 29 years, these tumors can occur in children. Symptoms can include headache, nausea, broad-based gait, and vertigo. Signs include papilledema, dysmetria, ataxia, slurred speech, and nystagmus; focal weakness may be an indication of a spinal lesion. Diagnosis of CNS hemangioblastoma is done by T$_1$-weighted MRI (Fig. 24-6) of both the head and the spine.[15,52] Treatment most often consists of surgical removal. Surgical selection is often complicated in VHL patients. The decision to recommend surgery relates to the size, number, and location of tumors and the presence of associated findings such as syringomyelia and hydrocephalus. More studies will be needed to determine whether quality of life can be enhanced or survival can be extended by early CNS tumor detection and aggressive genetic and clinical screening programs.[52] Focused radiation therapy with the "gamma knife" is sometimes utilized, although its role in the management of CNS hemangioblastoma remains to be determined.

Pheochromocytoma

Pheochromocytoma has been reported to occur in 18 percent of affected individuals.[15] There is a marked clustering of pheochromo-

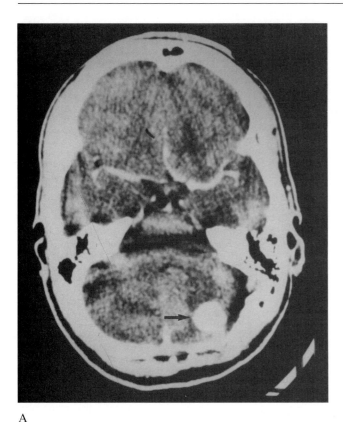

A

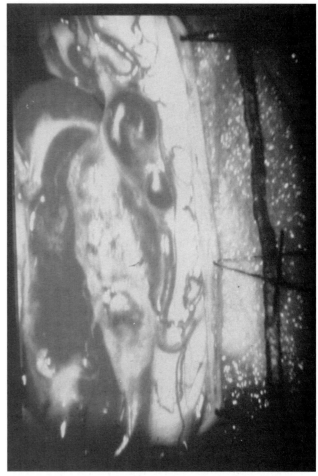

B

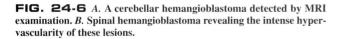

FIG. 24-6 *A*. A cerebellar hemangioblastoma detected by MRI examination. *B*. Spinal hemangioblastoma revealing the intense hypervascularity of these lesions.

cytoma in certain families, and this is now known as a distinct subtype of VHL: VHL type II. The pheochromocytoma can be bilateral, multifocal, and extraadrenal and can become malignant. Symptoms of pheochromocytoma in VHL patients include paroxysmal or sustained hypertension, episodic sweating, palpitations, headaches, and anxiety attacks and are due to the release of the catecholamines epinephrine and norepinephrine. Blood pressure can increase to levels that cause fatal cerebral hemorrhage or acute myocardial infarction. Unsuspected pheochromocytoma can be particularly ominous in a patient who has a cerebellar hemangioblastoma, is pregnant, or is undergoing surgical resection of a CNS, renal or pancreatic lesion.

Abdominal CT scanning, which often is performed during the initial screening of VHL patients, frequently provides the initial detection of VHL-associated pheochromocytoma (Fig. 24-7). MRI scanning is a particularly useful method for making the diagnosis. If there is a suspicion that a patient may have an extraadrenal pheochromocytoma (Fig. 24-8), ^{131}I-MIBG (metaiodobenzylguanidine) scintigraphy may be recommended.[53] The diagnosis of pheochromocytoma is made by demonstrating elevated levels of catecholamines and/or their metabolites in the urine or blood. Evaluation of VHL patients includes measurement of serum and blood catecholamines, most often epinephrine, norepinephrine, and metanephrine. The clonidine suppression and/or glucagon stimulation tests may aid in making the diagnosis of an indeterminate or potentially nonfunctioning adrenal mass lesion.[54,55] The treatment of pheochromocytoma consists of surgical resection of tumors that are functioning or are larger than 5 cm. Treatment of bilateral pheochromocytoma may require the surgical removal of both glands. Because the removal of both adrenal glands requires

that the patient be on lifetime replacement therapy, some physicians perform partial adrenalectomies to preserve functioning adrenal tissue. While this has the potential advantage of preserving adrenal function, such patients need careful monitoring for recurrent pheochromocytoma. The addition of laparoscopic adrenalectomy has added another, potentially less invasive method for the management of VHL-associated tumors.[54,56] Detection and treatment of functioning pheochromocytomas are important. Undetected pheochromocytomas are life-threatening and have led to the deaths of VHL patients. The role of the treatment of occult, nonfunctioning pheochromocytomas is under study.

Pancreatic Manifestations of von Hippel-Lindau

VHL-associated pancreatic lesions include pancreatic cysts, serous microcystic adenomas, and islet-cell tumors (Fig. 24-9). Pancreatic cysts are the most common manifestations; however, the frequency depends on the individual family being studied. The reported frequency of pancreatic cysts in VHL patients varies from 0 percent in two large families[57,58] to 93 percent in others.[59] Pancreatic cysts usually appear in the 20- to 40-year age group; however, they have been detected in patients as young as 15 years of age. The cysts appear throughout the body of the pancreas with no localization to a particular site. Epithelium-lined collections of serous fluid produce the cysts, which vary in size from 7 mm to over 10 cm. A serous cystadenoma (or microcystic adenoma) contains multiple macroscopic and microscopic cysts which are separated by thickened walls of stroma arranged in a stellate pattern with a central

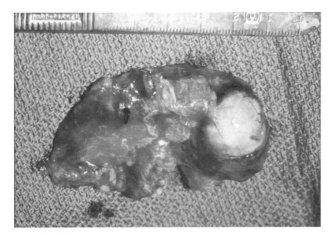

A

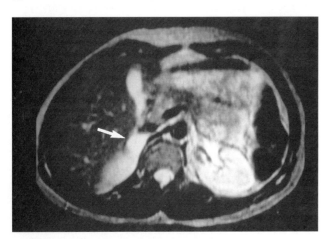

B

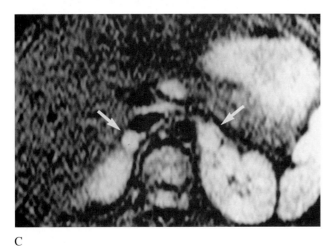

C

FIG. 24-7 *A.* **Adrenal gland removed at surgery with a large pheochromocytoma on the left side of the gland (right side of image).** *B, C.* **Abdominal CT imaging reveals a solitary right-sided pheochromocytoma (lower left). In another patient abdominal MRI reveals the presence of bilateral pheochromocytomas in a 12-year-old boy (upper right).**

nidus, which can be scarlike or calcified.[35] Pancreatic cysts are most often asymptomatic. Symptoms can be caused by biliary obstruction or can be associated with such diffuse disease that pancreatic insufficiency results and steatorrhea and diarrhea occur. Obstruction is managed by the placement of biliary stents; pancreatic insufficiency is managed by enzyme replacement. Rarely, cys-

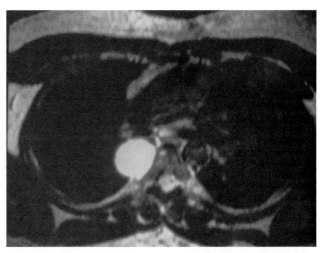

FIG. 24-8 MRI showing an extraadrenal pheochromocytoma.

tic enlargement is associated with so much local pain or early satiety that percutaneous drainage is required.[35]

Pancreatic islet-cell tumors occur in VHL patients, apparently independently of pancreatic cystic disease. These tumors, which are of neural origin, are composed of nests of polygonal cells with vesicular nuclei. Like VHL-associated renal tumors and CNS and retinal tumors, pancreatic islet-cell tumors are markedly vascular. While most are slow-growing and asymptomatic, pancreatic islet-cell tumors can grow rapidly or metastasize. Diagnosis of islet-cell tumors is made by CT, where the tumor appears as a characteristically intensely enhancing lesion. Although the standard treatment of growing islet-cell tumors is surgical resection, the decision to recommend surgery for the management of VHL-associated islet-cell tumors is complicated. While advanced islet-cell tumors are life-threatening and can invade locally and metastasize, the role of surgical resection in prolonging survival and improving the quality of life remains to be determined.

Papillary Cystadenoma of the Epididymis and Broad Ligament

Papillary cystadenoma of the epididymis can be unilateral or bilateral and are present in 10 to 26 percent of affected VHL males. These

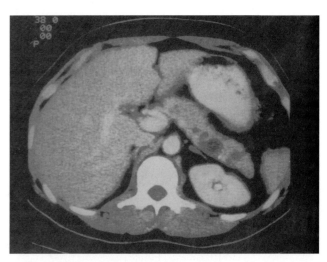

FIG. 24-9 Abdominal imaging reveals pancreatic cysts and islet-cell tumors in a VHL patient.

benign tumors, which can involve the spermatic cord, are most often found in the globus major of the epididymis. The lesions, which are typically 2 to 3 cm in size, can reach 5 cm. The histology of these tumors resembles that of renal and pancreatic cysts and endolymphatic sac tumors. The epididymal cysts are lined by clear cells that contain glycogen and fat with papillary and tubular structures and a surrounding collagenous pseudocapsule.[35] These tumors do not have malignant potential, and treatment is most often conservative. Rarely a symptomatic epididymal cystadenoma will require surgery. A lesion that has a histologic appearance similar to that of epididymal cystadenoma occurs in the broad ligament, the embryologically analogous structure in women.[35,60]

Endolymphatic Sac Tumors

A more recently appreciated manifestation of VHL is the presence of a tumor in the inner ear, an endolymphatic sac tumor (ELST) (Fig. 24-10). Lying between the dura of the posterior fossa, the endolymphatic sac is located at the end of the endolymphatic sac canal.[35] Although the prevalence and clinical characteristics of endolymphatic sac tumors in VHL patients have only recently been characterized,[35a] it has been estimated that up to 10 percent of VHL patients may have ELST. ELST is a low-grade malignancy with a papillary histologic growth pattern. Although a metastatic ELST has not been reported, this tumor can invade locally and be associated with hearing damage or facial paresis. Evaluation of VHL patients for ELST involves imaging with high-resolution CT and MRI through the inner ear. Audiologic evaluation is used for assessment of hearing and cochlear function. Significant audiologic abnormalities may be detected in up to 50 percent of VHL patients. The possibility exists that there are two components, one neoplastic and the other neurologic, to the otologic manifestations of VHL. It is not known if these two aspects of VHL are related. Early detection of the endolymphatic sac tumors is possible with MRI and CT of the internal auditory canal

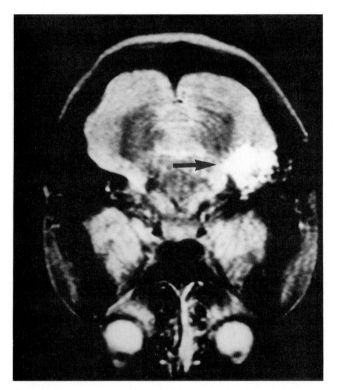

A

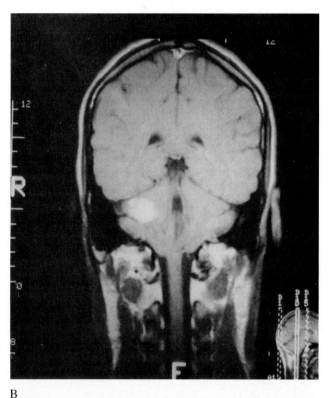

B

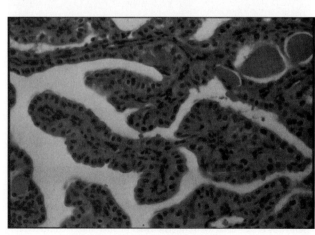

C

FIG. 24-10 *A, B.* Imaging studies reveal endolymphatic sac tumors (ELSTs) in VHL patients. Histologically, this tumor is a low-grade papillary neoplasm which invades locally but has low potential to metastasize.

(IAC). The role of early surgical intervention to preserve hearing remains to be determined.[35]

THE *VHL* GENE: CHARACTERISTICS OF A TUMOR-SUPPRESSOR GENE

To determine whether the genetics of VHL fit Knudson's two-hit hypothesis of a tumor-suppressor gene, Tory et al.[61] evaluated renal cell carcinoma, pheochromocytoma, spinal hemangioblastoma, and cerebellar hemangioblastoma in VHL patients. Multiple renal cell carcinomas, pheochromocytomas, and spinal and cerebellar hemangioblastomas from VHL patients showed loss of the wild-type chromosome 3p allele, demonstrating that both copies of the *VHL* gene were inactivated in VHL tumor tissue.[61] To assess for the earliest abnormalities in the renal manifestations of VHL, Lubensky et al.[62] performed a detailed analysis of chromosome 3p LOH in microdissected renal lesions from VHL patients by PCR-SSCP analysis (Fig. 24-11). Two benign cysts, five atypical cysts, five microscopic renal cell carcinomas in situ, five single cell-lined cysts, and two microscopic renal cell carcinomas and seven macroscopic renal cell carcinomas were evaluated. Twenty-five of 26 renal lesions had (1) nonrandom allelic loss at the *VHL* gene locus with loss of the wild-type allele and (2) retention of the inherited, mutated *VHL* allele.[62] Although clinical, radiologic, and pathologic data have suggested that benign and atypical renal lesions may represent the precursors of renal cell carcinoma in VHL patients, the finding of LOH of the *VHL* gene as an early event suggests that atypical and benign clear-cell cysts may represent early stages in the development and progression of renal cell carcinoma in VHL patients.[62]

THE *VHL* GENE IS LOCALIZED TO CHROMOSOME 3

In 1988 Seizinger et al.[63] localized the *VHL* gene to a locus in the telomeric region of the short arm of chromosome 3, in the region of the *cRAF1* oncogene at 3p25. To further characterize the *VHL* gene locus, Lerman et al. isolated a collection of 2000 lambda phage-carrying single-copy DNA fragments which were ordered as RFLP markers for the construction of a fine linkage map spanning the distal portion of chromosome 3p and encompassing the *VHL* locus.[64] These markers made the localization and subsequent identification of the *VHL* gene possible. When Hosoe et al. and Richards et al. performed multipoint linkage analysis (Fig. 24-12) with chromosome 3p markers in VHL families, the gene locus was determined to be in a 4-cM interval between *cRAF1* and *D3S18*, an anonymous marker at 3p25.5[65,66]

Presymptomatic Diagnosis of von Hippel-Lindau by DNA Polymorphism Analysis

With flanking DNA markers available, Glenn et al.[67] compared the results of DNA linkage analysis with those of a comprehensive clinical screening examination. Forty-three individuals at risk for developing VHL were informative with polymorphic markers. In 42 of 43 at-risk individuals, polymorphism analysis accurately identified individuals carrying the *VHL* gene among asymptomatic family members.[67] All nine of the at-risk individuals predicted to carry the *VHL* gene were found on clinical examination to have evidence of occult manifestations; no clinical evidence of VHL was detected in 32 of 33 of the at-risk individuals predicted to carry the wild-type allele of the *VHL* gene.[67] The single patient who was classified clinically as having VHL who was not predicted by linkage analysis to carry the *VHL* gene was a 42-year-old at-risk female who was found to have a solid renal mass. When the mass was surgically removed, a small focus of clear-cell renal cell carcinoma was found. When the *VHL* gene was later identified

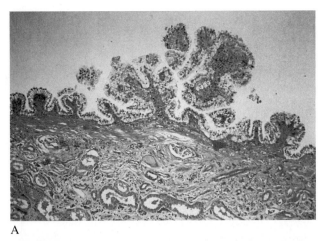

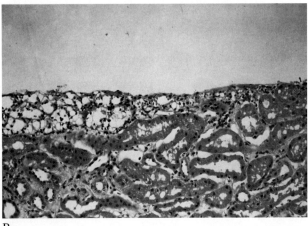

FIG. 24-11 Histology of early renal lesions in a VHL patient. Lubensky et al.[62] detected *VHL* gene LOH in microdissected material in 25 of 26 renal lesions, including lesions such as renal cell carcinoma (top) and atypical cysts lined by two to three layers of clear epithelial cells.

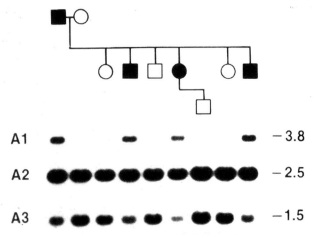

FIG. 24-12 Linkage analysis demonstrating cosegregation of the A1 allele of the chromosome 3p marker *D3S18* with VHL. The darkened boxes represent individuals affected with VHL. (*From Hosoe et al.[65]*)

and the mutation in this kindred was determined, this patient was found not to carry a germ-line VHL mutation. A somatic *VHL* gene mutation was, however, subsequently found in her tumor,[68] which, as would be predicted, was different from that identified in her affected siblings. She was an example of a "phenocopy," that is, an individual who is found to have a tumor in a target organ in a hereditary cancer syndrome but does not carry the *VHL* gene.[67]

Genotypic Homogeneity/Phenotypic Heterogeneity in Von Hippel-Lindau Syndrome

To further localize the *VHL* gene, over 100 VHL families from North America were evaluated. Different patterns of VHL manifestation appeared among these families. In the initial genetic studies, one large family was identified whose *VHL* phenotype was markedly distinct from that of typical VHL. Whereas pheochromocytoma normally is identified in 18 percent of affected VHL individuals, in this kindred 57 percent (27 of 47) of affected family members were found to have pheochromocytoma. Four of 47 affected family members had spinal or cerebellar hemangioblastomas; none of the affected family members had renal cell carcinoma (0 of 47) or pancreatic cysts (0 of 24).[67,69] The clinical findings were confirmed by genetic analysis. The family linked to *RAF1* and *D3S18,* markers that have been shown to be linked to typical VHL. Subsequently, a number of families have been characterized with this pattern of VHL, that is, with pheochromocytomas. These findings formed the initial basis for the classification of VHL (Table 24-3) kindreds as VHL type I (VHL without pheochromocytomas) or type II (with pheochromocytomas).

Identification of the *VHL* Gene

Once the *VHL* gene was localized to the 3p25 locus, the area was covered with overlapping yeast artificial chromosomes (YACs) and cosmid-phage contigs.[70] A critical step in the identification of the gene occurred when Yao et al.[70a] identified overlapping germ-line deletions in three unrelated VHL patients during the construction of a long-range (2.5-Mb) restriction map of the regions surrounding the *VHL* gene. A cosmid (cosmid 11) was identified that mapped to the smallest nested deletion. Two candidate cDNAs, denoted g7 and g6, were isolated from a 1GT11 teratocarcinoma library screened by conserved sequences in cosmid 11. As previous studies had determined that there is genotypic homogeneity in VHL, the *VHL* gene was considered to be at a single locus. G6 was found to be an unlikely candidate, as no mutations were detected there in 120 unrelated VHL patients. When inactivating mutations were searched for in constitutional DNA derived from 221 unrelated VHL patients by Southern blot analysis, aberrant bands ranging in size from 4 to 25 kb were detected in 28 of the 221 VHL kindreds. SSCP analysis identified inactivating mutations that segregated with VHL in three families. These findings (Fig. 24-13) indicated that g7 is the VHL tumor-suppressor gene.[70] *VHL* gene expression has been detected in all human tissues tested; the 6- and 6.5-kb transcripts probably represent alternatively spliced forms of

g7 mRNA. The human *VHL* gene, which has three exons, encodes a protein of 213 amino acids.

Genotype/Phenotype Correlations

Clinical heterogeneity is a feature of VHL. To determine the relationship between *VHL* gene mutations and the clinical manifestation of the VHL, Chen et al.[71] searched for *VHL* gene mutations in 114 families (Fig. 24-14). Mutations, including microdeletions/insertions, nonsense mutations, deletions, and/or missense mutations, were detected in 75 percent of the families (85 of 114). Mutations were detected in each of the three exons, clustering in the 3' end of exon 1 and the 5' end of exon 3. There were a small number of mutations in exon 2. While 56 percent of the mutations associated with VHL type I mutations were deletions, nonsense mutations, or microdeletions/insertions, 96 percent of the mutations in VHL type II (VHL with pheochromocytoma) kindreds were found to be missense mutations. There was also a clustering of VHL type II mutations in a small region in the 5' end of exon 3 of the *VHL* gene; mutation in codon 238 accounted for 43 percent of the VHL type II mutations.[71] Subsequent studies have confirmed the association of missense mutations with VHL type II families. Brauch et al.[72] identified a missense mutation at nucleotide 505 (T to C) in 14 VHL type II families from the Black Forest region of Germany. This mutation had previously been identified in two VHL type II families living in Pennsylvania (the kindred described in the section on phenotypic heterogeneity, above). Haplotype analysis among the 100 patients with the nucleotide 505 mutation indicated a founder effect.[72] A nucleotide 547 missense mutation has also been described in a large VHL family with pheochromocytoma with no members affected with renal cell carcinoma.[73] Similar mutation patterns have been detected in families from Europe [74,75] and Japan.[76-78]

Hereditary forms of pheochromocytoma can be found in association with VHL, multiple endocrine neoplasia type 2 (MEN 2), and neurofibromatosis type 1. Families with multiple pheochromocytomas in which there is uncertainty about the diagnosis are candidates for *VHL* gene mutation analysis.[72,74,75,77-80] For example, the abdominal imaging studies in Fig. 24-15 are from an 11-year-old boy with pheochromocytoma whose mother had had a pheochromocytoma removed when she was 11 years of age and whose uncle had died at age 9 with severe hypertension. The clinical impression had previously been that this family was affected with either MEN 2 or "familial pheochromocytoma."

When the child's mother underwent abdominal imaging (Fig. 24-16A, B), she was found to have a pancreatic mass, which was removed surgically and found to be an islet-cell tumor. Germ-line *VHL* gene mutation analysis was performed, and a nucleotide 595 (leucine-phenylalanine) missense mutation was detected, confirming the diagnosis of VHL type II.

When a 25-year-old female from a pheochromocytoma family (six other members had been diagnosed with pheochromocytoma) was evaluated, a retroperitoneal mass was detected (Fig. 24-17A, B). She was found to have malignant pheochromocytoma with pulmonary metastases. Germ-line *VHL* mutation analysis revealing a missense mutation in exon 2 confirmed the diagnosis of VHL type II.

Mutations of the *VHL* Tumor-Suppressor Gene in Renal Carcinoma

To evaluate the role of VHL in the origin of sporadic, nonhereditary renal cell carcinoma, Gnarra et al.[68] searched for a *VHL* gene mutation in tumors from 108 patients with both localized and advanced renal cell carcinoma. LOH of the *VHL* gene was detected in 98 per-

Table 24-3 Classification of VHL

Type I	VHL without pheochromocytoma
Type II	VHL with pheochromocytoma
Type IIA	Pheochromocytoma, CNS hemangioblastomas, and retinal angiomas
Type IIB	VHL IIA plus pancreatic involvement and renal manifestations (tumors, cysts)

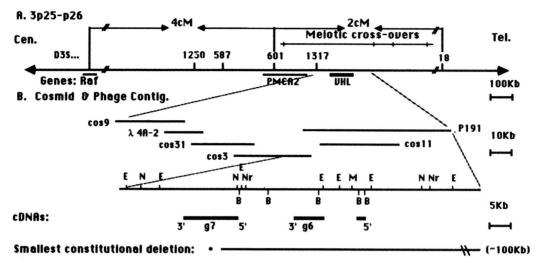

FIG. 24-13 Physical and genetic map encompassing the *VHL* gene locus on chromosome 3p. The *VHL* locus was determined by meiotic mapping and multipoint linkage analysis. The nested deletions identified in the germ-line DNA of the three unrelated VHL patients[123] were shown under the map. *(From Latif et al.[70])*

cent of clear-cell renal carcinomas; *VHL* mutations were identified in 57 percent of the samples (Fig. 24-19A). Mutations, including nucleotide deletions, substitutions, insertions, and nonsense mutations, were found in each of the three exons. The presence of splice site mutations that would eliminate the translation of exon 2 and the high percentage of mutations (45 percent) involving exon 2 indicated that exon 2 may contain an important function of the protein.[3,68] The detection of somatic *VHL* mutation in small, clinically localized renal cell carcinomas (<2 cm) suggests that inactivation of this gene is an early event in renal carcinogenesis.[81] When 119 tumors from 11 different tissues were evaluated, no additional somatic *VHL* gene mutations were detected. Neither chromosome 3 LOH nor *VHL* gene mutations were detected in tumor tissue from patients with papillary renal carcinoma (Fig. 24-19B). *VHL* gene mutations have been identified in clear-cell renal carcinomas in Japan,[82] Europe,[83–85] and North America.[79]

When tumor tissues from patients with hereditary renal carcinoma characterized by 3;8 translocation[13] were analyzed for *VHL*

mutations,[68,86] two of four tumors were found to have mutations of the wild-type *VHL* gene. In this kindred it is the inherited derivative chromosome 8 carrying the portion of chromosome 3 distal to the breakpoint that is deleted in the kidney tumors and the normal chromosome 3 that is retained.[14] The wild-type *VHL* allele was found to be mutated in the tumors, demonstrating a mechanism of clear-cell renal carcinoma tumorigenesis in the chromosome (3;8) translocation family that involves the loss of both copies of the *VHL* gene.[68,86] The association of *VHL* gene mutation and clear-cell renal carcinoma in three independent clinical entities—(1) sporadic clear-cell renal carcinoma, (2) clear-cell renal carcinoma associated with VHL, and (3) clear-cell renal carcinoma associated with 3:8 translocation hereditary clear-cell renal carcinoma—demonstrates the inactivation of the *VHL* gene is a critical event in clear-cell renal carcinoma.

Detection of *VHL* gene inactivation in clear-cell renal carcinoma but not in papillary renal carcinoma supports the proposal of a molecular genetic classification of renal carcinoma—papillary

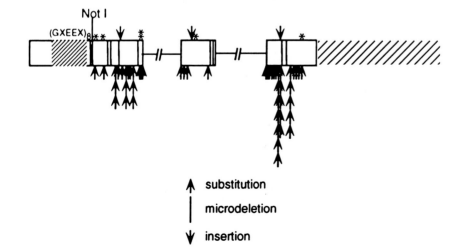

FIG. 24-14 *VHL* gene germ-line mutation distribution in VHL kindreds. The boxes indicate cloned exons. The 3' UTR and the exon 1 pentameric acidic repeat are indicated by cross-hatching. *(From Chen et al.[71])*

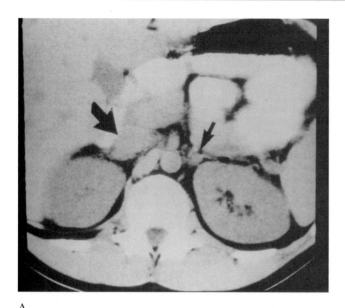

A

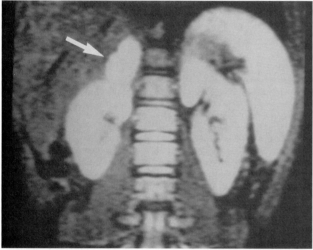

B

FIG. 24-15 Abdominal CT *(A)* and abdominal MRI *(B)* reveal the presence of pheochromocytoma in a 11-year-old child found to have a mutation of the *VHL* gene.

Silencing the *VHL* Gene by DNA Methylation

Herman et al.[92] demonstrated another potential mechanism for inactivation of the *VHL* gene in clear-cell renal carcinoma by showing hypermethylation of the normally unmethylated CpG island in the 5' region of the gene. The hypermethylation was observed in 5 of 26 (19 percent) clear-cell renal carcinomas evaluated. In four of the tumors, one copy of the *VHL* gene was lost; the fifth retained two heavily methylated *VHL* alleles. One of the five tumors had a missense mutation in addition to hypermethylation of the single remaining allele; the other four tumors with *VHL* hypermethylation had no detectable mutations. None of the five tumors expressed the *VHL* gene. When one of the renal cell carcinoma cell lines with a hypermethylated (and silent) *VHL* gene was treated with 5-aza-2'-deoxycytidine, the *VHL* gene was reexpressed. While the extent of hypermethylation of the *VHL* gene in a larger series of tumors and the potential role of agents such as 5-aza-2'-deoxycytidine remain to be determined, this study provides an additional mechanism for inactivation of the *VHL* gene in clear-cell renal carcinoma.[92]

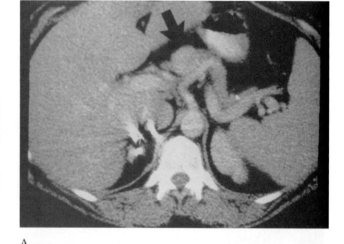

A

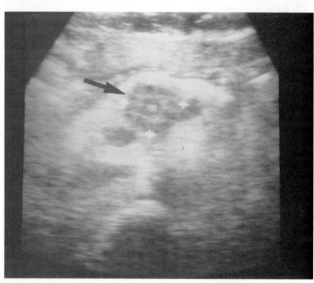

B

FIG. 24-16 Abdominal CT *(A)* reveals a pancreatic lesion in a woman whose 9-year-old child was found to have a pheochromocytoma. Abdominal ultrasound *(B)* confirmed that the pancreatic lesion is solid. The mass was removed surgically and was found to be an islet-cell tumor.

versus clear-cell renal carcinoma—with clear-cell renal carcinoma being characterized by inactivation of the *VHL* gene (Fig. 24-19).

The microdissection techniques for archival DNA[87] provide a method for the detection of *VHL* gene mutations in paraffin-embedded material[88] which may furnish clinicians with improved strategies for both diagnosis[89] and classification of renal tumors. Similar methods applied to aspirate cytology may allow improved clarification of whether an indeterminate mass in a kidney or another organ is a clear-cell renal carcinoma.

VHL gene mutations were detected when the sporadic forms of other tumors that appear in VHL patients were analyzed. Kanno et al.[90] detected abnormal *VHL* gene SSCP patterns in 7 of 13 sporadic hemangioblastomas, 3 of which were characterized by direct sequencing. Somatic mutations in the three tumors included two missense mutations and one microdeletion, one in exon 1 and two in exon 2.[90] Gilcrease et al. detected a somatic *VHL* gene mutation in one of two sporadic cystadenomas of the epididymis.[91] *VHL* gene mutations appear to play a role in tumorigenesis in a subset of sporadic epididymal cystadenomas and CNS hemangioblastomas.

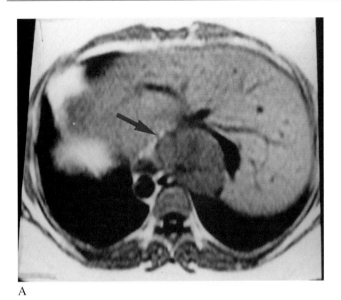

A

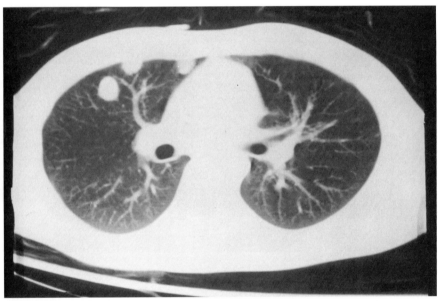

B

FIG. 24-17 Abdominal CT (top) reveals a retroperitoneal mass in a 24-year-old female who had had two previous surgical resections of pheochromocytoma. Lung CT revealed the presence of metastatic foci in the chest. *VHL* gene analysis revealed a mutation in exon 2 of the *VHL* gene, confirming the diagnosis of VHL.

Characterization of the *VHL* Suppressor Gene Product

When the *VHL* gene was identified, the deduced amino acid sequence predicted no significant homology to other proteins. No functional or structural motifs that could provide insight into function of the VHL protein were found. In order to characterize the *VHL* gene product, Duan et al. identified the homologous rat gene, which encodes a 185-amino acid protein with 88 percent sequence identity to the 213-amino acid human *VHL* gene product.[93] When epitope-tagged human and rat proteins were introduced into cell lines and examined by immunofluorescence microscopy, a variety of patterns were observed. The VHL protein was found to be localized to the nucleus and the cytosol but not to the cell surface. Both the human and the rat proteins coimmunoprecipitated a similar set of other protein bands, including bands at 16 and 9 kDa and a group of bands migrating between 50 and 70 kDa.

A large percentage of both sporadic and hereditary *VHL* gene mutations include missense mutations in the protein. When cDNA constructs containing naturally occurring *VHL* point mutations were tested for coimmunoprecipitation, a number of the mutants

appeared to assemble poorly, if at all, with the 16- and 9-kDa proteins.[93] Notable among those which failed to associate with p16 and p9 were proteins with the arginine to glutamine or the arginine to tryptophan mutation at amino acid 167. These mutations correspond to a VHL type II germ-line mutation hotspot.[71,94] The Trp-117 mutant had diminished but detectable association with the p16 and p9 proteins. However, the Tyr-98 mutants, from a VHL type II kindred, formed complexes that were identical to the wild type. The loss of binding to specific proteins by naturally occurring inactivating mutants suggests the functional importance of these complexes and indicates that mutations in different domains of the VHL protein may play a role in determining organ-specific tumorigenesis.[71,94]

VHL Associates with Two Transcription Elongation Proteins

The finding that the heterotrimer consisting of *VHL* and the two proteins of 9kDa and 16 kDa did not form when the VHL protein contained certain naturally occurring missense mutations led to studies

Sporadic renal carcinoma *VHL* mutations

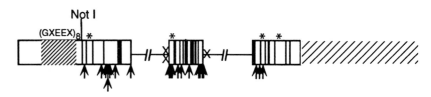

↑ substitution

| microdeletion

↓ insertion

X splice site

* nonsense

FIG. 24-18 *VHL gene mutation distribution in sporadic clear-cell renal carcinoma. The boxes indicate cloned exons. The 3′ UTR and the exon 1 pentameric acidic repeat are indicated by cross-hatching. (From Gnarra et al.[68])*

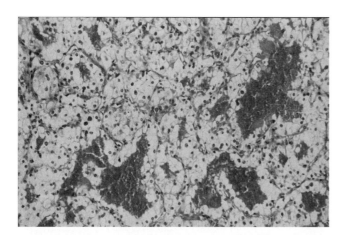

A

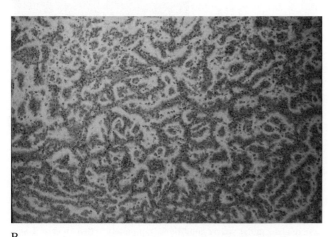

B

FIG. 24-19 Somatic *VHL* gene mutations and LOH are characteristic of clear-cell renal carcinoma *(A)* but are not found in papillary renal carcinoma *(B)*.

to identify these proteins. When the p9 band was sequenced,[95] it was found to match a sequence in elongin C, a 112-amino acid protein that had been found to be a subunit of the heterotrimeric transcription elongation factor elongin (SIII).[96] When p16 underwent se-

quence analysis, a peptide from p16 showed identity to a sequence in elongin B.[95,97] Elongin (SIII) is a heterotrimeric complex consisting of two regulatory subunits (B and C) and a transcriptionally active subunit (elongin A) (Fig. 24-20). The elongin (SIII) complex has been shown to activate transcriptional elongation by mammalian RNA polymerase II by suppressing the transient pausing of the polymerase at sites within the transcription units.[98] The VHL protein, which does not bind with the transcriptionally active subunit of the elongin (SIII) complex, elongin A, tightly and specifically binds to elongins B and C and can prevent their assembly to the transcriptionally active subunit of the elongin (SIII) complex, elongin A.[95] The finding that the cellular transcription factor elongin (SIII) is a functional target of the VHL protein and that point-mutant derivatives, corresponding to naturally occurring *VHL* missense mutations,

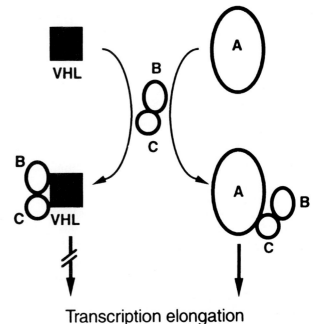

Transcription elongation

FIG. 24-20 A model for the interaction between elongin (SIII) and *VHL*. Elongin A forms a heterotrimeric complex with elongins B and C and activates transcription elongation by RNA pol II. *VHL* binds elongins B and C and inhibits the elongin ABC complex activation of transcriptional elongation. *(From Duan et al.[95])*

inhibit this interaction suggested that the tumor-suppression function of the VHL protein may be related to its ability to inhibit transcriptional elongation.[95,99]

A potential locus for *VHL* elongin B/C binding has been described by Kibel et al.[99] Aso et al. detected significant sequence homology between residues 547 and 560 of elongin A and *VHL* residues 155 to 167.[100] Kibel et al. determined that peptides in *VHL* residues 157 to 172 fail to inhibit *VHL*–elongins B and C binding, while wild-type residues block the interaction.[100] This region is frequently mutated in sporadic clear-cell renal carcinoma and in the germ lines of VHL patients; it is the region of the amino acid 167 hotspot.[94]

The VHL Gene Product Forms a Stable Complex with Human CUL-2, a Member of the Cdc53 Family of Proteins. Pause et al. have recently shown that Hs-CUL-2, a member of the cullin multigene family, specifically associated with the trimeric pVHL-elongin B-C (VBC) complex in vivo and in vitro.[95] The yeast Hs-CUL-2 homolog, Cdc53, has been shown to be a part of the complex that targets cell cycle proteins for ubiquitin-mediated proteolytic degradation. Hs-CUL-2, which may be required for VHL function, is considered to be potentially a partner in the VHL tumor suppressor gene pathway. The finding is that Hs-Cul-2 forms a complex with pVHL-elongin B-C cell cycle regulation as a potential target for the VHL gene pathway.[95a]

Posttranscriptional Regulation of Vascular Endothelial Growth Factor mRNA by the *VHL* Product

Sporadic clear-cell renal carcinomas are characterized by a high degree of neoangiogenesis. Angiogenesis is also a striking feature in the clinical manifestations of VHL. VHL renal tumors, spinal and cerebellar hemangioblastomas, retinal angiomas, islet-cell tumors, and epididymal cystadenomas are markedly hypervascular. A number of polypeptide growth factors have been implicated in the migration, proliferation, and differentiation of vascular endothelial cells, including vascular endothelial growth factor (VEGF). VEGF, which normally is expressed in the brain, kidney, and other tissues, is markedly elevated in renal carcinomas as well as sporadic and VHL-associated CNS hemangioblastomas.[101–106] When the effect of *VHL* on VEGF was evaluated, introduction of the wild-type *VHL* gene into renal carcinoma cells with *VHL* mutations resulted in decreased VEGF mRNA expression.[101,107] Renal cell carcinoma (RCC) cell lines express high levels of VEGF mRNA and protein. In normal cells, VEGF expression is regulated by multiple factors, including hypoxia, which is an inducer of VEGF mRNA levels. RCC cell lines show constitutively high levels of VEGF mRNA in both normoxic and hypoxic cells. Introduction of a wild-type, but not a mutant, *VHL* gene into these RCC cells reconstitutes the hypoxia-regulated expression of VEGF mRNA and inhibits VEGF expression under normoxic conditions. An analogous effect is seen in these cells in response to serum deprivation. Only in cells expressing wild-type *VHL* is VEGF expression suppressed in 10% serum and induced with serum deprivation. Surprisingly, *VHL* overexpression affected neither VEGF transcription initiation nor VEGF elongation, suggesting that *VHL* regulates VEGF at a posttranscriptional level. Determination of the mechanism of *VHL*-mediated regulation of VEGF and related genes should lead to significant advances in our understanding of the mechanism of tumorigenesis in VHL and sporadic RCC. Interestingly, wild-type *VHL* repressed the normoxic expression of other hypoxia-induced genes, such as the glucose transporter GLUT1 and the platelet-derived growth factor B chain (PDGF-B).[107]

Determinants of Nuclear/Cytoplasmic Localization of the *VHL* Gene Product

Critical to an understanding of the function of the *VHL* gene is determination of its location in the cell and the factors that regulate its transport. The VHL protein was shown by Duan et al. to be present in both the nucleus and the cytoplasm.[93] To define the determinants of *VHL* localization, Lee et al. showed that there is a tightly regulated, cell-density-dependent transport of *VHL* into and/or out of the nucleus.[108] When cells expressing an epitope-tagged (FLAG) VHL protein were plated in sparse conditions, most of the protein was detected in the cytoplasm. In densely grown cells, the VHL protein is found in the cytoplasm. Immunofluorescence studies of mutant VHL protein revealed that the C-terminal region of the VHL protein is required for localization to, or retention in, the cytosol. When a frameshift mutant, which removes all of exon 3, was examined, VHL was present only in the nucleus in most of the cells grown in both sparse and confluent conditions. In contrast, when the entire exon 1 was deleted, the protein remained predominantly in the cytosol under both sparse and confluent conditions (Fig. 24-21).[108] The factors associated with sparse and confluent conditions that determine localization of the VHL protein have not been identified. Understanding these factors as well as the genetic determinants of *VHL* localization should provide significant insights into the function of the *VHL* gene and show how inactivation of this gene results in the manifestations that appear in VHL and in sporadic clear-cell renal carcinoma.

PAPILLARY RENAL CARCINOMA

Five to 10 percent of sporadic renal carcinomas are of the papillary histologic type.[3,11,68] Papillary renal carcinoma is significantly less hypervascular and tends to be of lower grade than clear-cell renal carcinoma. The clinical course of papillary renal carcinoma may be more indolent than that of clear-cell renal carcinoma.[109,110] Sporadic papillary renal carcinoma frequently appears as bilateral, multifocal disease; multiple tumor nodules and areas of atypical hyperplastic growth may appear throughout the kidney.[111,112] Whether the presence of multifocal, bilateral papillary renal carcinoma is primarily due to genetic events, is secondary to an agent

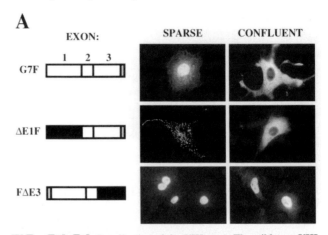

FIG. 24-21 Localization of the *VHL* gene. The wild-type VHL protein is found predominantly in the cytoplasm when transiently transfected COS-7 cells are grown under confluent conditions and in the nucleus under sparse conditions (top panel). When an exon 1 deletion mutant is analyzed, immunofluorescence localizes the protein to the cytoplasm in both sparse and confluent cells. When an exon 3 deletion mutant is introduced into the COS-7 cells, there is striking localization, predominantly to the nucleus, in both the sparse and the confluent conditions. *(From Lee et al.[108])*

such as a renotrophic virus, or results from exposure to environmental factors is not known.

Most common among the cytogenetic changes that have been described in tumor tissue from patients with papillary renal carcinoma are those involving trisomy of chromosomes 7, 10, and 17.[33,111,113] More recently, a consistent t(X;1)(p11.2;q21) translocation in papillary RCC was described as a feature in at least some papillary renal carcinomas.[114–116] Whether the t(X;1) translocation represents a distinct subtype of papillary RCC is under study.

HEREDITARY PAPILLARY RENAL CELL CARCINOMA

Multigenerational kindreds in which the members are affected with papillary RCC have been described by Zbar et al.[16,17] Affected family members in these kindreds develop multiple tumors of varying size in both kidneys. The gross appearance of the kidneys from affected family members is striking; multiple tumors of varying size appear in both kidneys (Fig. 24-22). This disorder has an autosomal dominant inheritance pattern and is distinct from other forms of hereditary renal carcinoma, such as VHL. While VHL renal tumors are uniformly of the clear-cell histologic type, HPRC tumors are exclusively papillary.[16] HPRC does not link to chromosome 3, and *VHL* mutations are not found in the germ line.[16]

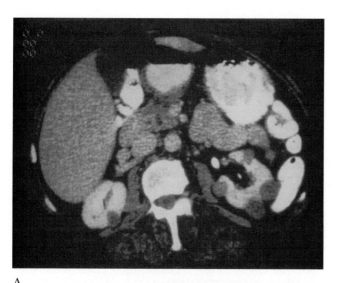

A

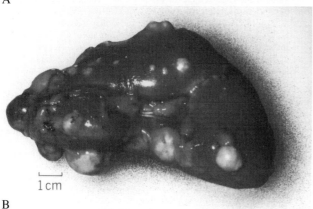

1 cm

B

FIG. 24-22 A kidney from an affected individual in a hereditary papillary renal carcinoma kindred showing multifocal papillary renal carcinomas. *(From Zbar et al.[16])*

Schmidt et al. have recently found that the HPRC gene is located at chromosome 7q31.1-34. Missense mutations in the tyrosine kinase domain of the *MET* gene (located in the chromosome 7q area of interest) have been found in the germline of affected members of HPRC kindreds. These results suggest that germline gain-of-function mutations of the *MET* gene are likely to be associated with the papillary renal tumorigenesis observed in affected HPRC individuals.[16a]

PROSPECTUS

Genetics

There are three forms of hereditary renal carcinoma: VHL, HCRC, and HPRC. VHL is characterized by mutation of the *VHL* gene. Currently, *VHL* gene mutation can be detected in 75 to 90 percent of VHL families. As advanced mutation detection methods are developed (FISH-based deletion analysis, analysis of the 3'UTR promoter, etc.), the mutation detection percentage should increase. VHL has been categorized as type I and type II, with type II families being characterized by the presence of pheochromocytoma. Nearly all type II families carry a missense mutation, and there is a VHL type II hotspot in exon 3 of the *VHL* gene. Studies in progress will determine whether there are genotype/phenotype correlations with other VHL-associated tumors, such as CNS hemangioblastomas, pancreatic tumors, and ELSTs.

The role of genetic and clinical screening programs in the management of individuals at risk for a multisystem hereditary cancer syndrome such as VHL is complex. Unlike some syndromes, in which testing is not routinely performed in at-risk individuals under the age of 18 because medical intervention is not required, in individuals at risk for VHL, germ-line mutation testing is recommended at an early age. Early intervention can often be of significant benefit to affected VHL patients, particularly those with retinal, adrenal, and CNS lesions. Retinal angiomas, which can occur in very young children, are bilateral and multifocal and can cause early loss of vision which eventually may lead to blindness. Treatment with laser therapy can preserve vision and decrease the morbidity of VHL-associated retinal angiomas. Pheochromocytoma and CNS hemangioblastomas can appear before the age of 10. Occult pheochromocytoma can be lethal, and early detection of functioning pheochromocytomas is critical. While the benefit of detection of an occult functioning pheochromocytoma is clear, the benefit of detection and treatment of occult, nonfunctioning pheochromocytomas is not known. In some patients occult CNS hemangioblastomas also can have significant morbidity, including stroke, paralysis, and death. However, longitudinal studies will be needed to determine whether aggressive screening for CNS lesions will enhance quality of life or increase survival.

The role of early diagnosis of VHL-associated renal, pancreatic, and endolymphatic sac tumors is less well defined. Greater understanding of the natural history of these VHL manifestations will be required in determining the most appropriate management of patients with these malignancies. At present there is no consensus about which patients with VHL-associated renal carcinomas are best treated with surgical resection. RCC can spread in asymptomatic individuals, and advanced renal carcinoma has been reported as the direct cause of death in one-third of VHL patients.[15,117] Thus, physicians managing these patients often recommend removal of the tumors when they have reached a certain size, such as 2.5 to 3 cm. The clinical rationale is that removal of tumors of this size may reduce the incidence of metastasis while preserving quality of life. VHL-associated pancreatic islet-cell tumors are malignant lesions which can become metastatic. Surgical resection is often recommended to prevent metastasis; however, prospective trials will be required to define the role of surgery in the management of these tumors. The ELSTs represent a similar clinical challenge. These tumors can have profound manifestations in VHL patients. Patients with ELSTs may lose total hearing in an ear within a matter of 3 to 4 days. Trials are in progress to determine whether early surgical intervention will preserve hearing in VHL patients with ELST.

When tumors from other organs affected by VHL, such as sporadic cerebellar hemangioblastoma and epididymal cystadenoma, have been analyzed, mutations have been found. Further studies of these tumors as well as other sporadic tumors from organs affected in VHL (such as pancreatic tumors, ELSTs, retinal angiomas, and pheochromocytomas) will be required to determine the role of *VHL* gene inactivation in these neoplasms.

Papillary Renal Carcinoma

Linkage analysis is under way in HPRC families; identification of the gene for this autosomal dominant disease should be straightforward. Subsequent studies will determine the role of this gene in sporadic papillary renal carcinoma. Much remains to be learned about the genetics and subtypes of papillary renal carcinoma. At present it appears that there may be two subtypes of sporadic papillary renal carcinoma; one is characterized by a t(X;1) translocation. Little is known about the factors associated with the development of multifocal, bilateral sporadic papillary renal carcinoma. The genetic or environmental features that characterize individuals with bilateral, multifocal papillary renal carcinoma with no apparent hereditary feature (no parents, siblings, or offspring involved) remain to be determined.

A number of kindreds have been evaluated in which multiple members (two to six) have clear-cell renal carcinoma. Whether these findings are coincidental, are the result of an undetermined combination of genetic and environmental factors, or are an example of complex genetics is not known.

Diagnosis

VHL gene mutation analysis is now an integral aspect of the diagnosis of VHL and the screening of at-risk asymptomatic individuals. Predictions about which types of tumors will appear are possible in some instances, particularly in VHL type II kindreds. Germ-line *VHL* gene mutation analysis is likely to be useful in kindreds with "familial pheochromocytoma" or those with clinical manifestations of MEN 2 in which the diagnosis is in doubt.

VHL gene mutation analysis may be useful in assisting in the diagnosis of an indeterminate renal mass or an extrarenal mass in a patient with clear-cell kidney cancer.

Patients who present with advanced renal carcinoma have 8 to 15 percent 2-year survival. Those who are diagnosed with early stage renal carcinoma have 95 percent 5-year survival. It is possible that detection of an inactivated *VHL* gene will aid in the early diagnosis of clear-cell renal carcinoma. Cancer cells, including renal carcinoma cells, may circulate years in advance of the clinical detection of metastasis.[118–121] It is possible that the detection of a mutated *VHL* gene in the urine or in circulating cells will provide a method for early diagnosis of this disease.

Prevention and Treatment

It is hoped that an understanding of the molecular mechanisms of cancer will lead to the development of new strategies for preven-

tion and treatment. Although the VHL protein has been shown to inhibit transcription elongation in vitro, the role of this protein in vivo remains to be determined. VHL binding to elongins B and C has been localized to a small region of the 5′ end of exon 3.[122] This locus accounts for 30 to 40 percent of naturally occurring germ-line *VHL* mutations. Identification of other proteins which associate with the VHL protein should lead to significantly greater understanding of the function of this gene and show how inactivation of the gene leads to VHL and clear-cell kidney cancer. The finding that sporadic renal carcinoma and VHL-associated renal and CNS tumors produce high levels of VEGF and that introduction of the wild-type *VHL* gene leads to decreased expression of VEGF and related proteins[101,122] raises the question of whether antiangiogenesis therapy can be of benefit. Ultimately, it is hoped that knowledge of the mechanism of the *VHL* gene and other genes involved in renal carcinoma will lead to the development of targeted methods for early diagnosis, prevention, and treatment of diseases such as sporadic and hereditary renal carcinoma.

ACKNOWLEDGMENT

We gratefully acknowledge the work of our many collaborators and colleagues whose studies are discussed here.

REFERENCES

1. Boring CC, Squires TS, Tong T: Cancer statistics. *CA Cancer J Clin* **44**:7, 1994.
2. Linehan WM, Shipley W, Parkinson D: Cancer of the kidney and ureter, in DeVita VT, Hellman S, Rosenberg SA (eds): *Cancer: Principles and Practice of Oncology.* Philadelphia, Lippincott, 1996, p 19.
3. Linehan WM, Lerman MI, Zbar B: Identification of the VHL gene: Its role in renal carcinoma. *JAMA* **273**:564, 1995.
4. Malker HR, Malker BK, McLaughlin JK, Blot WJ: Kidney cancer among leather workers. *Lancet* **1**:56, 1984.
5. Maclure M: Asbestos and renal adenocarcinoma: A case-control study. *Environ Res* **42**:353, 1987.
6. Maclure M, Willett W: A case-control study of diet and risk of renal adenocarcinoma. *Epidemiology* **1**:430, 1990.
7. Yu MC, Mack TM, Hanisch R, Cicioni C, Henderson BE: Cigarette smoking, obesity, diuretic use, and coffee consumption as risk factors for renal cell carcinoma. *JNCI* **77**:351, 1986.
8. Chung-Park M, Parveen T, Lam M: Acquired cystic disease of the kidneys and renal cell carcinoma in chronic renal insufficiency without dialysis treatment. *Nephron* **53**:157, 1989.
9. Matson MA, Cohen EP: Acquired cystic kidney disease: Occurrence, prevalence, and renal cancers. *Medicine (Baltimore)* **69**:217, 1990.
10. Brennan JF, Stilmant MM, Babayan RK, Siroky MB: Acquired renal cystic disease: implications for the urologist. *BR J Urol* **67**:342, 1991.
11. Kovacs G, Ishikawa I: High incidence of papillary renal cell tumours in patients on chronic haemodialysis. *Histopathology* **22**:135, 1993.
12. Bard RH, Lord B, Fromowitz F: Papillary adenocarcinoma of kidney. *Urology* **XIX**:16, 1982.
13. Cohen AJ, Li FP, Berg S, Marchetto DJ, Tsai S, Jacobs SC, Brown RS: Hereditary renal-cell carcinoma associated with chromosomal translocation. *N Engl J Med* **301**:592, 1979.
14. Li FP, Decker H, Zbar B, Stanton VP, Kovacs G, Seizinger BR, Aburantani H, Sandberg AA, Berg S, Hosoe S, Brown RS: Clinical and genetic studies of renal cell carcinomas in family with a constitutional chromosome 3;8 translocation. Genetics of familial renal carcinoma. *Ann Intern Med* **118**:106, 1993.
15. Glenn GM, Choyke PL, Zbar B, Linehan WM: Von Hippel-Lindau disease: Clinical review and molecular genetics, in Anderson EE (ed): *Problems in Urologic Surgery: Benign and Malignant Tumors of the Kidney.* Philadelphia, Lippincott, 1990, p 312.

16. Zbar B, Tory K, Merino M, Schmidt L, Glenn G, Choyke P, Walther MM, Lerman M, Linehan WM: Hereditary papillary renal cell carcinoma. *J Urol* **151**:561, 1994.

16a. Schmidt L, Duh F, Chen F, Kishida T, Glenn G, Choyke P, Scherer SW, Zhuang Z, Lubensky I, Dean M, Allikmets R, Chidambaram A, Bergerheim UR, Feltis TJ, Casadevall C, Zamarron A, Bernues M, Richard S, Lips CJM, Walther MM, Tsui L, Geil L, Orcutt ML, Stackhouse T, Lipan J, Slife L, Brauch H, Decker J, Niehans G, Hughson MD, Moch H, Storkel S, Lerman MI, Linehan WM, and Zbar B: Germline and somatic mutations in the tyrosine kinase domain of the MET proto-oncogene in papillary renal carcinomas. *Nature Genetics* **16**(May):68–73, 1997.

17. Zbar B, Glenn G, Lubensky IA, Choyke P, Magnusson G, Bergerheim U, Pettersson S, Amin M, Hurley K, Linehan WM: Hereditary papillary renal cell carcinoma: Clinical studies in 10 families. *J Urol* **153**:907, 1995.

18. Pathak S, Strong LC, Ferrell RE, Trindade A: Familial renal cell carcinoma with 3:11 chromosome translocation limited to tumor cells. *Science* **217**:939, 1982.

19. Kovacs, G, Brusa P, de Riese W: Tissue-specific expression of a constitutional 3;6 translocation: Development of multiple bilateral renal-cell carcinomas. *Int J Cancer* **43**:422, 1989.

20. Zbar B, Brauch H, Talmadge C, Linehan WM: Loss of alleles of loci on the short arm of chromosome 3 in renal cell carcinoma. *Nature* **327**:721, 1987.

21. Anglard P, Brauch TH, Weiss GH, Latif F, Merino MJ, Lerman MI, Zbar B, Linehan WM: Molecular analysis of genetic changes in the origin and development of renal cell carcinoma. *Cancer Res* **51**:1071, 1991.

22. Szucs S, Muller-Brechlin R, DeRiese W, Kovacs G: Deletion 3p: The only chromosome loss in a primary renal cell carcinoma. *Cancer Genet Cytogenet* **26**:369, 1987.

23. Kovacs G, Erlandsson R, Boldog F, Ingvarsson S, Muller-Brechlin R, Klein G, Sumegi J: Consistent chromosome 3p deletion and loss of heterozygosity in renal cell carcinoma. *Proc Natl Acad Sci USA* **85**:1571, 1988.

24. Linehan WM, Miller E, Anglard P, Merino M, Zbar B: Improved detection of allele loss in renal cell carcinomas after removal of leukocytes by immunologic selection. *JNCI* **81**:287, 1989.

25. Boldog F, Arheden K, Imreh S, Strombeck B, Szekely L, Erlandsson R, Marcsek Z, Sumegi J, Mitelman F, Klein G: Involvement of 3p deletions in sporadic and hereditary forms of renal cell carcinoma. *Genes Chromosom Cancer* **3**:403, 1991.

26. Morita R, Ishikawa J, Tsutsumi M, Hikiji K, Tsukada Y, Kamidono S, Maeda S, Nakamura Y: Allelotype of renal cell carcinoma. *Cancer Res* **51**:820, 1991.

27. Ogawa O, Kakehi Y, Ogawa K, Koshiba M, Sugiyama T, Yoshida O: Allelic loss at chromosome 3p characterizes clear cell phenotype of renal cell carcinoma. *Cancer Res* **51**:949, 1991.

28. Presti JC, Rao PH, Chen Q, Reuter VE, Li FP, Fair WR, Jhanwar SC: Histopathological, cytogenetic, and molecular characterization of renal cortical tumors. *Cancer Res* **51**:1544, 1991.

29. Yoshida HA, Ohyashiki K, Ochi H, Gibas Z, Pontes JE, Prout GR, Huben R, Sandberg AA: Cytogenetic studies of tumor tissue from patients with nonfamilial renal cell carcinoma. *Cancer Res* **46**:2139, 1986.

30. Carroll PR, Murty VVS, Reuter V, Jhanwar S, Fair WR, Whitemore WF, Chaganti RSK: Abnormalities of chromosome region 3p12-14 characterize clear cell renal carcinoma. *Cancer Genet Cytogenet* **26**:253, 1987.

31. Kovacs G, Wilkens L, Papp T, de Riese W: Differentiation between papillary and nonpapillary renal cell carcinomas by DNA analysis. *JNCI* **81**:527, 1989.

32. Kovacs G: Papillary renal cell carcinoma: A morphologic and cytogenetic study of 11 cases. *Am J Pathol* **134**:27, 1989.

33. Kovacs G, Fuzesi L, Emanual A, Kung HF: Cytogenetics of papillary renal cell tumors. *Genes Chromosom Cancer* **3**:249, 1991.

34. Anglard P, Trahan E, Liu S, Latif F, Merino M, Lerman M, Zbar B, Linehan WM: Molecular and cellular characterization of human renal cell carcinoma cell lines. *Cancer Res* **52**:348, 1992.

35. Choyke, PL, Glenn GM, Walther MM, Patronas NJ, Linehan WM, Zbar BZ: Von Hippel Lindau disease: Genetic, clinical and imaging features. *Radiology* **194**:629, 1995.

35a. Manski TJ, Heffner DK, Glenn GM, Patronas NJ, Pikus AT, Katz D, Lebovics R, Sledjeski K, Choyke PL, Zbar B, Linehan WM, Oldfield EH: Endolymphatic sac tumors: A source of morbid hearing loss in von Hippel-Lindau disease. *JAMA* **277**:1461, 1997.

36. Collins ET: Two cases, brother and sister, with peculiar vascular new growth, probably primarily retinal, affecting both eyes. *Trans Ophthalmol Soc UK* **14**:141, 1894.

37. Von Hippel E: Uber eine sehr seltene erkrankrung der netzhaut. *Klinische Boebachtungen Arch Ophthalmol* **59**:83, 1904.

38. Lindau A: Studien uber kleinhirncysten bau: pathogenese und beziehungen zur angiomatous retinae. *Acta Pathol Microbiol Scand Suppl* **1**:1, 1926.

39. Melmon KL, Rosen SW: Lindau's disease: Review of the literature and study of a large kindred. *Am J Med* **36**:595, 1964.

40. Poston CD, Jaffe GS, Lubensky IA, Solomon D, Zbar B, Linehan WM, Walther MM: Characterization of the renal pathology of a familial form of renal cell carcinoma associated with von Hippel-Lindau disease: Clinical and molecular genetic implications. *J Urol* **153**:22, 1995.

41. Walther MM, Lubensky IA, Venzon D, Zbar B, Linehan WM: Prevalence of microscopic lesions in grossly normal renal parenchyma from patients with von Hippel-Lindau disease, sporadic renal cell carcinoma and no renal disease: Clinical implications. *J Urol* **154**:2010, 1995.

42. Choyke PL, Filling-Katz MR, Shawker TH, Gorin MB, Travis WD, Chang R, Seizinger BR, Dwyer AJ, Linehan WM: Von Hippel-Lindau disease: Radiologic screening for visceral manifestations. *Radiology* **174**:815, 1990.

43. Jamis-Dow CA, Choyke PL, Jennings SB, Linehan WM, Thakore KN, Walther MM: Small (<3 cm) renal masses: Detection with CT versus US and pathologic correlation. *Radiology* **198**:785, 1996.

44. Pearson JC, Weiss J, Tanagho EA: A plea for conservation of kidney in renal adenocarcinoma associated with von Hippel-Lindau disease. *J Urol* **124**:910, 1980.

45. Palmer JM, Swanson DA: Conservative surgery in solitary and bilateral renal carcinoma: indications and technical considerations. *J Urol* **120**:113, 1987.

46. Frydenberg M, Malek RS, Zincke H: Conservative renal surgery for renal cell carcinoma in von Hippel-Lindau's disease. *J Urol* **194**:461, 1993.

47. Walther MM, Choyke PL, Weiss G, Manolatos C, Long J, Reiter R, Alexander RB, Linehan WM: Parenchymal sparing surgery in patients with hereditary renal cell carcinoma. *J Urol* **153**:913, 1995.

48. Walther MM, Thompson N, Linehan WM: Enucleation procedures in patients with multiple hereditary renal tumors. *World J Urol* **13**:248, 1995.

49. Walther MM, Choyke PL, Hayes W, Shawker TH, Thakore K, Alexander RB, Linehan WM: Evaluation of color doppler intraoperative ultrasound in parenchymal sparing renal surgery. *J Urol* **152**:1984, 1995.

50. Marshall FF, Holdford SS, Hamper UM: Intraoperative sonography of renal tumors. *J Urol* **148**:1393, 1992.

51. Choyke PL, Glenn G, Walther MM, Zbar B, Weiss GH, Alexander RB, Hayes WS, Long JP, Thakore KN, Linehan WM: The natural history of renal lesions in von Hippel-Lindau Disease: A serial CT study in 28 patients. *AJR* **159**:1229, 1992.

52 Filling-Katz MR, Choyke PL, Oldfield E, Charnas L, Patronas NJ, Glenn GM, Gorin MB, Morgan JK, Linehan WM, Seizinger BR, Zbar B: Central nervous system involvement in von Hippel Lindau disease. *Neurology* **41**:41, 1991.

53. Maurea S, Cuocolo A, Reynolds JC, Tumeh SS, Begley MG, Linehan WM, Norton JA, Walther MM, Keiser HR, NEumann RD: Iodine-313-metaiodobenzylguanidine scientigraphy in preoperative and postoperative evaluation of paragangliomas: Comparison with CT and MRI. *J Nucl Med* **34**:173, 1993.

54. Keiser HR, Doppman JL, Robertson CN, Linehan WM, Averbuch SC: Daignosis, localization and management of pheochromocytoma, in Lack EE (ed): *Pathology of the Adrenal Gland.* New York, Churchill Linvingston, 1990, p 237.

55. Bouck NP, Polverini PJ: Identification of a new inhibitor of neovascularization controlled by a tumor suppressor gene. *J Northwestern U Cancer Center* **1**:4, 1990.

56. Perry RR, Keiser HJ, Norton JA, Wall RT, Robertson CN, Travis W, Pass HI, Walther MM, Lineham WM: Surgical management of pheochromocytoma with the use of metyrosine. *Ann Surg* **212**:621, 1990.

57. Green JS, Bowmer MI, Johnson GJ: Von Hippel-Lindau disease in a Newfoundland kindred. *Can Med Assoc J* **134**:133, 1986.

58. Seizinger BR: Von Hippel Lindau disease: A model system for the isolation of tumor suppressor genes associated with the primary genetic mechanisms of cancer. *Adv Nephrol Necker Hisp* **23**:29, 1994.

59. Neumann HPH: Basic criteria for clinical diagnosis and genetic counselling in von Hippel-Lindau syndrome. *Vasa* **16**:220, 1987.

60. Karsdorp N, Elderson A, Wittebol-Post D: Von Hippel Lindau disease: New strategies in early detection and treatment. *Am J Med* **97**:158, 1994.

61. Tory K, Brauch H, Linehan WM, Barba D, Oldfiend E, Filling-Katz M, Seizinger B, Nakamura Y, White R, Marshall FF, Lerman MI, Zbar B: Specific genetic change in tumors associated with von Hippel-Lindau disease. *JNCI* **81**:1097, 1989.

62. Lubensky IA, Gnarra JR, Bertheau P, Walther MM, Linehan WM, Zhuang Z: Allelic deletions of the VHL gene detected in multiple microscopic clear cell renal lesions in von Hippel-Lindau disease patients. *Am J Pathol* **149**:2089, 1996.

63. Seizinger BR, Rouleau GA, Ozelius LJ, Lane AH, Farmer GE, Lamiell JM, Haines J, Yuen JW, Collins D, Majoor-Krakauer D, et al: Von Hippel-Lindau disease maps to the region of chromosome 3 associated with renal cell carcinoma. *Nature* **332**:268, 1988.

64. Lerman MI, Latif F, Glenn GM, Daniel LN, Brauch H, Hosoe S, Hampsch K, Delisio J, Orcutt M, McBride OW, Grzeschik K, Takahashi T, Minna J, Anglard P, Linehan WM, Zbar B: Isolation and regional localization of a large collection (2,000) of single copy DNA fragments on human chromosome 3 for mapping and cloning tumor suppressor genes. *Hum Genet* **86**:567, 1991.

65. Hosoe S, Brauch H, Latif F, Glenn G, Daniel L, Bale S, Choyke P, Gorin M, Oldfield E, Berman A, Goodman J, Orcutt ML, Hampsch K, Delisio J, Modi W, McBride W, Anglard P, Weiss G, Walther MM, Linehan WM, Lerman MI, Zbar B: Localization of the von Hippel-Lindau disease gene to a small region of chromosome 3. *Genomics* **8**:634, 1990.

66. Richards FM, Maher ER, Latif F, Phipps ME, Tory K, Lush M, Croseey PA, Oostra B, Gustavson KH, Green J, Turner G, Yates JRW, Linehan WM, Affara NA, Lerman M, Zbar B, Ferguson-Smith MA: Detailed genetic mapping of the von Hippel-Lindau disease tumour suppressor gene. *J Med Genet* **30**:104, 1993.

67. Glenn GM, Linehan WM, Hosoe S, Latif F, Yao M, Choyke P, Gorin MB, Chew E, Oldfield E, Manolatos C, Orcutt ML, McClellan MW, Weiss GH, Tory K, Jensson O, Lerman MI, Zbar B: Screening for von Hippel-Lindau disease by DNA-polymorphism analysis. *JAMA* **267**:1226, 1992.

68. Gnarra JR, Tory K, Weng Y, Schmidt L, Wei MH, Li H, Latif F, Liu S, Chen F, Duh F, Lubensky IA, Duan R, Florence C, Pozzatti R, Walther MM, Bander NH, Grossman HB, Brauch H, Pomer S, Brooks JD, Issacs WB, Lerman MI, Zbar B, Linehan WM: Mutation of the VHL tumour suppressor gene in renal carcinoma. *Nat Genet* **7**:85, 1994.

69. Glenn GM, Daniel LN, Choyke P, Linehan WM, Oldfield E, Gorin M, Hosoe S, Latif F, Weiss G, Walther M, Lerman MI, Zbar B: Von Hippel-Lindau disease: Distinct phenotypes suggest more than one mutant allele at the VHL locus. *Hum Genet* **87**:207, 1991.

70. Latif F, Tory K, Gnarra J, Yao M, Duh F, Orcutt ML, Stackhouse T, Kuzmin I, Modi W, Geil L, Schmidt L, Zhou F, Li H, Wei MH, Glenn G, Richards FM, Crossey PA, Ferguson-Smith MA, Le Paslier D, Chumakov I, Cohen D, Chinault CA, Maher ER, Linehan WM, Zbar B, Lerman MI: Identification of the von Hippel-Lindau disease tumor suppressor gene. *Science* **260**:1317, 1993.

70a. Yao M, Latif F, Kuzmin I, Stackhouse T, Zhou FW, Tory K, Orcutt ML, Duh FM, Richards F, Maher E, La Forgia S, Huebner K, Le Pasilier D, Linehan WM, Lerman M, Zbar B: Von Hippel-Lindau disease: Identification of deletion mutations by pulsed field gel electrophoresis. *Hum Genet* **92**:605, 1993.

71. Chen F, Kishida T, Yao M, Hustad T, Glavac D, Dean M, Gnarra JR, Orcutt ML, Duh FM, Glenn G, Green J, Hsia YE, Lamiell J, Li H, Wei MH, Schmidt L, Tory K, Kuzmin I, Stackhouse T, Latif F, Linehan WM, Lerman M, Zbar B: Germline mutations in the von Hippel-Lindau disease tumor suppressor gene: correlation with phenotype. *Hum Mutat* **5**:66, 1995.

72. Brauch H, Kishida T, Glavac D, Chen F, Pausch F, Hofler H, Latif F, Lerman MI, Zbar B, Neumann HPH: Von Hippel Lindau (VHL) disease with pheochromocytoma in the Black Forest region of Germany: Evidence for a founder effect. *Hum Genet* **95**:551, 1995.

73. Tisherman SE, Tisherman BG, Tisherman SA, Dunmire S, Levey GS, Mulvihill JJ: Three-decade investigation of familial pheochromocytoma. *Arch Intern Med* **153**:2550, 1993.

74. Crossey PA, Eng C, Ginalska-Malinowska M, Lennard TW, Wheeler DC, Ponder BA, Maher ER: Molecular genetic diagnosis of von Hippel-Lindau disease in familial phaeochromocytoma. *J Med Genet* **32**:335, 1995.

75. Neumann HP, Eng C, Mulligan LM, Glavac D, Zauner I, Ponder BA, Crossey PA, Maher ER, Brauch H: Consequences of direct genetic testing for germline mutathions in the clinical management of families with multiple endocrine neoplasia, type II [see comments]. *JAMA* **274**:1149, 1995.

76. Kanno H, Shuin T, Kondo K, Ito S, Hosaka M, Torigoe S, Fujii S, Tanaka Y, Yamamoto I, Kim I, Yao M: Molecular genetic diagnosis of von Hippel-Lindau disease: Analysis of five Japanese families. *Jpn J Cancer Res* **87**:423, 1996.

77. Shuin T, Kondo K, Kaneko S, Sakai N, Yao M, Hosaka M, Kanno H, Ito S, Yamamoto I: Results of mutation analyses of von Hippel-Lindau disease gene in Japanese patients: Comparison with results in United States and United Kingdom. *Hinyokika Kiyo* **41**:703, 1995.

78. Clinical Research Group for VHL in Japan: Germline mutations in the von Hippel-Lindau disease (VHL) gene in Japanese VHL. *Hum Mol Genet* **4**:2233, 1995.

79. Whaley JM, Naglich J, Gelbert L, Hsia YE, Lamiell JM, Green JS, Collins D, Neumann PH, Laidlaw J, Li FP, Klein-Szanto AJP, Seizinger BR, Kley N: Germ-line mutations in the von Hippel-Lindau tumor-suppressor gene are similar to von Hippel-Lindau aberrations in sporadic renal cell carcinoma. *Am J Hum Genet* **55**:1092, 1994.

80. Gross DJ, Avishai N, Meiner V, Filon D, Zbar B, Abeliovich D: Familial pheochromocytoma associated with a novel mutation in the von Hippel-Lindau gene. *J Clin Endocrinol Metab* **81**:147, 1996.

81. Knudson AG: VHL gene mutation and clear-cell renal carcinomas. *Cancer J* **1**:180, 1995.

82. Shuin T, Kondo K, Torigoe S, Kishida T, Kubota Y, Hosaka M, Nagashima Y, Kitamura H, Latif F, Zbar B, Lerman MI, Yao M: Frequent somatic mutations and loss of heterozygosity of the von Hippel-Lindau tumor suppressor gene in primary human renal cell carcinomas. *Cancer Res* **54**:2852, 1994.

83. Crossey PA, Richards FM, Foster K, Green JS, Prowse A, Latif F, Lerman MI, Zbar B, Affara NA, Ferguson-Smith MA, Maher ER: Identification of intragenic mutations in the von Hippel-Lindau disease tumor suppressor gene and correlation with disease phenotype. *Hum Mol Genet* **3**:1303, 1994.

84. Foster K, Prowse A, van den Berg A, Fleming S, Hulsbeek MM, Crossey PA, Richards FM, Cairns P, Affara NA, Ferguson-Smith MA: Somatic mutations of the von Hippel-Lindau disease tumour suppressor gene in non-familial clear cell renal carcinoma. *Hum Mol Genet* **3**:2169, 1994.

85. Bailly M, Bain C, Favrot MC, Ozturk M: Somatic mutations of von Hippel-Lindau (VHL tumor-suppressor gene in European kidney cancers. *Int J Cancer* **63**:660, 1995.

86. Schmidt L, Li F, Brown RS, Berg S, Chen F, Wei MH, Tory K, Lerman MI, Zbar B: Mechanism of tumorigenesis of renal carcinomas associated with the constitutional chromosome 3;8 translocation. *Cancer J* **1**:191, 1995.

87. Zhuang Z, Bertheau P, Emmert-Buck MR, Liotta LA, Gnarra J, Linehan WM, Lubensky IA: A microdissection technique for archival DNA analysis of specific cell populations in lesions <1 mm in size. *Am J Pathol* **146**:620, 1995.

88. Zhuang Z, Gnarra JR, Dudley CF, Zbar B, Linehan WM, Lubensky IA: Detection of von Hippel-Lindau disease gene mutations in paraffin-embedded sporadic renal cell carcinoma specimens. *Mod Pathol* **9**:838, 1996.

89. Long JP, Anglard P, Gnarra JR, Walther MM, Merino MJ, Liu S, Lerman MI, Zbar B, Linehan WM: The use of molecular genetic analysis in the diagnosis of renal cell carcinoma. *World J Urol* **12**:69, 1994.

90. Kanno H, Kondo K, Ito S, Yamamoto I, Fujii S, Torigoe S, Sakai N, Masahiko H, Shuin T, Yao M: Somatic mutations of the von Hippel-Lindau tumor suppressor gene in sporadic central nervous system hemangioblastomas. *Cancer Res* **54**:4845, 1994.

91. Gilcrease MZ, Schmidt L, Zbar B, Truong L, Rutledge M, Wheeler TM: Somatic von Hippel-Lindau mutation in clear cell papillary cystadenoma of the epididymis. *Hum Pathol* **26**:1341, 1995.

92. Herman JG, Latif F, Weng Y, Lerman MI, Zbar B, Liu S, Samid D, Duan DR, Gnarra JR, Linehan WM, Baylin SB: Silencing of the VHL tumor suppressor gene by DNA methylation in renal carcinoma. *Proc Natl Acad Sci USA* **91**:9700, 1994.

93. Duan DR, Humphrey JS, Chen DYT, Weng Y, Sukegawa J, Lee S, Gnarra JR, Linehan WM, Klausner RD: Characterization of the VHL

tumor suppressor gene product: Localization, complkex formation and the effect of natural inactivating mutations. *Proc Natl Acad Sci USA* **92**:6459, 1995.

94. Gnarra JR, Duan DR, Weng Y, Humphrey JS, Chen DYT, Lee S, Pause A, Dudley CF, Latif F, Kuzmin I, Schmidt L, Duh FM, Stackhouse T, Chen F, Kishida T, Wei MH, Lerman MI, Zbar B, Klausner RD, Linehan WM: Molecular cloning of the von Hippel-Lindau tumor suppressor gene and its role in renal carcinoma. *Biochim Biophys Acta* **1242**:201, 1996.

95. Duan DR, Pause A, Burgess WH, Aso T, Chen DYT, Garret KP, Conaway RC, Conaway JW, Linehan WM, Klausner RD: Inhibition of transcription elongation by the VHL tumor suppressor protein. *Science* **269**:1402, 1995.

95a. Pause A, Lee S, Worrell RA, Chen DYT, Burgess WH, Linehan WM, Klausner RD: The von Hippel-Lindau tumor-suppressor gene product forms a stable complex with human CUL-2, a member of the Cdc53 family of proteins. *Proc Natl Acad Sci USA* **94**:2156, 1997.

96. Garrett KP, Tan S, Bradsher JN, Lane WS, Conaway JW, Conaway RC: Molecular cloning of an essential subunit of RNA polymerase II elongation factor SIII. *Proc Natl Acad Sci USA* **91**:5237, 1994.

97. Garrett KP, Aso T, Bradsher JN, Foundling SI, Lane WS, Conaway RC, Conaway JW: Positive regulation of general transcription factor SIII by a tailed ubiquitin homolog. *Proc Natl Acad Sci USA* **92**:7172, 1995.

98. Aso T, Lane WS, Conaway JW, Conaway RC: Elongin (SIII): A multisubunit regulator of elongation by RNA polymerase II. *Science* **269**:1439, 1995.

99. Kibel A, Iliopoulos O, DeCaprio JA, Kaelin WG Jr:Binding of the von Hippel-Lindau tumor suppressor protein to Elongin B and C [see comments]. *Science* **269**:1444, 1995.

100. Aso T, Lane WS, Conaway JW, Conaway RC: Elongin (SIII): a multisubunit regulator of elongation by RNA polymerase II [see comments]. *Science* **269**:1439, 1995.

101. Gnarra J, Zhou S, Merrill MJ, Wagner J, Krumm A, Papavassiliou E, Oldfield E, Klausner RD, Linehan WM: Post-transcriptional regulation of vascular endothelial growth factor mRNA by the VHL tumor suppressor gene product. *Proc Natl Acad Sci USA* **93**:10589, 1996.

102. Siemeister G, Weindel K, Mohrs K, Barleon B, Martiny-Baron G, Marme D: Reversion of deregulated expression of vascular endothelial growth factor in human renal carcinoma cells by von Hippel-Lindau tumor suppressor protein. *Cancer Res* **56**:2299, 1996.

103. Berger DP, Herbstritt L, Dengler WA, Marme D, Mertelsmann R, Fiebig HH: Vascular endothelial growth factor (VEGF) mRNA expression in human tumor models of different histologies. *Ann Oncol* **6**:817, 1995.

104. Takahashi A, Sasaki H, Kim SJ, Tobisu K, Kakizoe T, Tsukamoto T, Kumamoto Y, Sugimura T, Terada M: Markedly increased amounts of messenger RNAs for vascular endothelial growth factor and placenta growth factor in renal cell carcinoma associated with angiogenesis. *Cancer Res* **54**:4233, 1994.

105. Sato K, Terada K, Sugiyama T, Takahashi S, Saito M, Moriyama M, Kakinuma H, Suzuki Y, Kato M, Kato T: Frequent overexpression of vascular endothelial growth factor gene in human renal cell carcinoma. *Tohuku J Exp Med* **173**:355, 1994.

106. Wizigmann-Voos S, Breier G, Risau W, Plate KH: Up-regulation of vascular endothelial growth factor and its receptors in von Hippel-Lindau disease-associated and sporadic hemangioblastomas. *Cancer Res* **55**:1358, 1995.

107. Iliopoulos O, Jiang C, Levy AP, Kaelin WG, Goldberg MA: Negative regulation of hypoxia-inducible genes by the von Hippel-Lindau protein. *Proc Natl Acad Sci USA* **93**:10595, 1996.

108. Lee S, Chen DYT, Humphrey JS, Gnarra JR, Linehan WM, Klausner RD: Nuclear/cytoplasmic localization of the VHL tumor suppressor gene product is determined by cell density. *Proc Natl Acad Sci USA* **93**:1770, 1996.

109. Mydlo JH, Bard RH: Analysis of papillary renal adenocarcinoma. *Urology* **XXX**:529, 1987.

110. Boczko S, Fromowitz FB, Bard RH: Papillary adenocarcinoma of kidney. *Urology* **XIV**:491, 1979.

111. Kovacs G: Papillary renal cell carcinoma: A morphologic and cytogenetic study of 11 cases. *Am J Pathol* **134**:27, 1989.

112. Kovacs G, Hoene E: Multifocal renal cell carcinoma: A cytogenetic study. *Virchows Arch A Pahtol Anat Histopathol* **412**:79, 1987.

113. Hughson MD, Johnson LD, Silva FG, Kovacs G: Nonpapillary and papillary renal cell carcinoma: A cytogenetic and phenotypic study. *Mod Pathol* **6**:449, 1993.

114. Shipley JM, Birdsall S, Clark J, Crew J, Gill S, Linehan WM, Gnarra J, Fisher S, Craig IW, Cooper CS: Mapping the X chromosome breakpoint in two papillary renal cell carcinoma cell lines with a t(X;1)(p11.2;q21.2) and the first report of a female case. *Cytogenet Cell Genet* **71**:280, 1995.

115. Suijkerbuijk RF, Meloni AM, Sinke RJ, de Leeuw B, Wilbrink M, Janssen HAP, Geraghty MT, Monaco AP, Sandberg AA, Geurts van Kessel A: Identification of a yeast artificial chromosome that spans the human papillary renal cell carcinoma-associated t(X;1) breakpoint in Xp11.2. *Cancer Genet Cytogenet* **71**:164, 1993.

116. Meloni AM, Dobbs RM, Pontes JE, Sandberg AA: Translocation (X;1) in papillary renal cell carcinoma: A new cytogenetic subtype. *Cancer Genet Cytogenet* **65**:1, 1993.

117. Horton WA, Wong V, Eldridge R: Von Hippel-Lindau disease: Clinical and pathological manifestations in nine families with 50 affected members. *Arch Intern Med* **136**:769, 1976.

118. Pontes JE, Pescatori E, Connelly R, Hashimura T, Tubbs R: Circulating cancer cells in renal-cell carcinoma. *Prog Clin Biol Res* **348**:1, 1990.

119. Liotta LA, Kleineman J, Seidel GM: Quantitative relationships of intravascular tumor cells, tumor vessels and pulmonary metastasis following tumor implantation. *Cancer Res* **34**:997, 1974.

120. Buttler TP, Gullino PM: Quantitation of cell shedding into efferent blood of mammary adenocarcinoma. *Cancer Res* **35**:512, 1975.

121. Moreno JG, Croce CM, Fischer R, Monne M, Vihko P, Mulholland SG, Gomella LG: Dectection of hematogenous micrometastasis in patients with prostate cancer. *Cancer Res* **52**:6110, 1992.

122. Kibel A, Iliopoulos O, DeCaprio JA, Kaelin WG: Binding of the von Hippel-Lindau tumor suppressor protein to elongin B and C. *Science* **269**:1444, 1995.

123. Yao M, Latif F, Kuzmin I, Stackhouse T, Zhou FW, Tory K, Orcutt ML, Duh FM, Richards F, Maher E, La Forgia S, Huebner K, Le Pasilier D, Linehan WM, Lerman M, Zbar B: Von Hippel-Lindau disease: Identification of deletion mutations by pulsed field gel electrophoresis. *Hum Genet* **92**:605, 1993.

CHAPTER 25

Multiple Endocrine Neoplasia Type 2

B.A.J. Ponder

1. Multiple endocrine neoplasia type 2 (MEN 2) is an uncommon autosomal disorder of tumor formation and developmental abnormalities which affects about 1 in 30,000 individuals. It is characterized by the occurrence of C-cell tumors of the thyroid [medullary thyroid carcinoma (MTC)], often in association with tumors of the adrenal medulla (pheochromocytoma) and parathyroid hyperplasia or adenoma. Developmental abnormalities, which occur in a minority of cases, principally affect the autonomic nerve plexuses of the intestine. The thyroid "C" cells, adrenal medulla, and intestinal autonomic plexuses but not the parathyroid glands are derived from neural ectoderm.

2. Distinct clinical subtypes of MEN 2 are defined by the combination of tissues affected and the presence or absence of developmental abnormalities. In MEN 2A, thyroid C cells, adrenal medulla, and parathyroids may all be involved but developmental abnormalities are rare. In FMTC (familial MTC), only thyroid C-cell tumors are seen; there are no developmental abnormalities. In MEN 2B, thyroid C cells and adrenal medullary tumors are common but parathyroid abnormality is uncommon; there are constant developmental abnormalities involving hyperplasia of the intestinal autonomic nerve plexuses and disorganized growth of peripheral nerve axons in the lips, oral mucosa, and conjunctiva, giving rise to a characteristic facies. The onset of thyroid and adrenal tumors in MEN 2B tends to occur early, and their behavior may be more aggressive.

3. The gene for MEN 2 was identified by positional cloning. It lies on chromosome 10q11.2. This gene, *ret,* is a previously known receptor tyrosine kinase. Mutations in *ret* in MEN 2A and FMTC result in constitutive activation of the receptor; in MEN 2B, the extent of activation is unclear but the substrate specificity of the tyrosine kinase is altered. There are clear correlations between specific mutations in *ret* and the phenotypes which result. Loss of activity mutations in *ret* results in Hirschsprung disease of the colon and rectum (HSCR), in which there is an absence of intestinal autonomic nerve plexuses, in distinction to the hyperplasia in MEN 2B. In a few families, MEN 2A and HSCR coexist, apparently as a result of the same *ret* mutation; the mechanism for this is not understood. *ret* is unusual among tumor predisposing genes in that MEN 2 mutations result in gain of function: it is not a tumor-suppressor gene.

4. The tumors characteristic of MEN 2 also occur in a nonhereditary form. Somatic mutations of *ret* are found in these tumors, but almost all are of the same type as the germ-line mutations characteristic of MEN 2B, which alter the substrate specificity of the tyrosine kinase. This may imply that *ret* mutations of the type seen in MEN 2A and FMTC, which result in activation of a normal tyrosine kinase domain, are effective in tumorigenesis only during a restricted period in development.

5. MEN 2 is a good example of an inherited cancer syndrome in which screening of family members leads to early diagnosis and effective treatment by thyroidectomy and adrenalectomy. Since each of the tissues involved in tumor formation secretes a characteristic product (calcitonin, adrenaline, parathyroid hormone), biochemical monitoring of family members at risk provides a sensitive means of early detection. This can now be refined by predictive genetic testing for the characteristic *ret* mutations.

INTRODUCTION: THE MULTIPLE ENDOCRINE NEOPLASIA SYNDROMES

Multiple endocrine neoplasia (MEN) is characterized by the occurrence of tumors which involve two or more endocrine glands in a single patient or in close relatives. There are two types of MEN syndrome,[1] with distinct patterns of tissue involvement (Table 25-1). MEN 1 (sometimes called Werner syndrome[1–3]) includes tumors of parathyroid, pituitary, and pancreatic islet cells and less frequently adrenocortical, carcinoid, and multiple lipomatous tumors.[4–6] MEN 1 is dominantly inherited; the predisposing locus has been mapped by linkage to chromosome 11q13,[7] but at the time of this writing, the gene has not been identified. There is no evidence to suggest genetic heterogeneity. MEN 2 (sometimes called Sipple syndrome and previously called MEA II or MEN II, although MEN 2 is now preferred) includes tumors of the thyroid C cells and adrenal medulla and hyperplasia or adenoma of the parathyroids.[8–10] There also may be various developmental abnormalities, which are described below. The predisposing gene for MEN 2 is *ret,* a receptor tyrosine kinase which maps to chromosome 10q11.2. The great majority of MEN 2 families have detectable mutations in *ret,* but a few are unaccounted for,[11] and genetic heterogeneity remains a possibility.[12]

Patients have occasionally been described as having tumors which are a combination of those associated with MEN 1 and MEN 2, for example, pituitary tumors and pheochromocytoma. It is unclear whether these are more than chance occurrences[13] and

Table 25-1 Endocrine Involvement in the MEN Syndromes

MEN 1	MEN 2
Parathyroid	Thyroid C cells
Anterior pituitary	Adrenal medulla
Pancreatic islets	Parathyroid
Adrenal cortex	

whether there is an additional MEN "overlap" syndrome. A spectrum of endocrine tumors which overlaps that of MEN 1 and MEN 2 is seen in some inbred strains of rats[14,15] and in transgenic mice homozygous for loss of activity of the retinoblastoma gene, which have been reported to develop thyroid C-cell and pituitary tumors. The human MEN 1 and MEN 2 syndromes are genetically and almost always clinically distinct. Familial pheochromocytomas occur in two other human inherited cancer syndromes: von Hippel-Lindau syndrome (Chap. 24) and neurofibromatosis type 1 (Chap. 22).

CLINICAL ASPECTS OF MEN 2

Three clinical types of MEN 2 [MEN 2A, MEN 2B, and familial medullary thyroid carcinoma (FMTC)] are distinguished by the combination of tissues involved (Table 25-2).[16–18]

The Component Tumors of MEN 2

As in the other inherited cancer syndromes, each of the component tumors of MEN 2 also has a nonhereditary counterpart.

Medullary Thyroid Carcinoma. The characteristic tumor of MEN 2 is the medullary thyroid carcinoma (MTC), which is derived from the C cells of the thyroid. These are malignant tumors, metastasizing usually at a stage when the primary tumor is 5 to 10 mm in diameter, at first locally within the neck and then to distant sites.[19,20] The C cells and the tumors derived from them secrete the hormone calcitonin. This provides a valuable marker for early diagnosis and for following the later course of disease.[21] There is no obvious syndrome of calcitonin overproduction.

Pheochromocytoma. The tumor derived from the adrenal medulla is the pheochromocytoma. Generally these tumors are nonmalignant, at least until they are of large size.[22] They commonly secrete adrenaline and noradrenaline, which if undetected can lead to fatal hypertensive episodes, especially in situations such as general anesthesia and childbirth.

Parathyroid. The parathyroid abnormalities in MEN 2 are benign, either hyperplasia or the formation of true benign adenomas.[23] Parathyroid involvement is often clinically silent but may present with symptomatic hypercalcemia or renal stones.

The Clinical Types of MEN 2 Syndromes

MEN 2A

Clinical Features. MEN 2A is the most common type, accounting for about 65 percent of families that could be classified in a recent international survey of *ret* mutations in MEN 2 families.[11] The penetrance of *ret* mutations in MEN 2A is incomplete.[24] About 70 percent of gene carriers develop symptomatic disease within their lifetimes, with MTC as the usual first manifestation. Almost all gene carriers can, however, be detected by biochemical screening for MTC by age 40 (Fig. 25-1; see below). On average, about 50 percent of gene carriers will develop pheochromocytoma and perhaps 5 to 10 percent will develop symptomatic parathyroid disease, but the pattern varies considerably both between and within families.[24] Some of the variation between families can be attributed to different mutant *ret* alleles (see below); the contribution of genetic background, environment, and chance to within-family variation has not been elucidated.

Incidence. The incidence of MEN 2A has not been documented accurately. An attempt to identify all new cases of MTC (hereditary and nonhereditary) in a 2-year period in the United Kingdom, using ascertainment from cancer registries and requests for calcitonin estimations from regional assay laboratories, suggested an overall incidence of about 1 per 1 million per year.[25] Wide variations in the number of registrations between different registries suggested, however, that the data might not be very accurate. It generally is assumed that 20 to 25 percent of MTCs are heritable. This figure is not based on a systematic population-based study but derives largely from two observations: In early clinical studies, about 15 percent of consecutive cases of MTC had an evident family history[19,20,26]; in later series in which families of apparently isolated cases were investigated further by more careful history taking or by genetic or biochemical screening, up to 10 percent showed familial involvement.[27,28] Together, these figures add up to about 20 to 25 new cases of MEN 2 (all types) per year in the United Kingdom (population 55 million).

New Mutations. Some apparently sporadic cases of MTC are new mutations to the hereditary disease. The frequency is not precisely known. There are a few documented cases,[29] and MEN 2 mutations occur on many different haplotypes, indicating separate origins.[30] However, many MEN 2A families have been traced back through several generations, suggesting that founder mutations are not un-

Table 25-2 Patterns of Tissue Involvement in the MEN 2 Syndromes

	MEN 2A	MEN 2B	FMTC
Thyroid C cells	Tumor	Tumor	Tumor
Adrenal medulla	Tumor	Tumor	Not involved
Parathyroid	Hyperplasia/benign tumor	Not involved	Not involved
Enteric ganglia	Normal*	Hyperplasia	Normal
Other developmental abnormalities	None	Various†	None

*Usually there is no abnormality of enteric ganglia in MEN 2A, but a few families have been described in which there is absence of ganglia from a variable length of the intestine in some individuals.
†Includes musculoskeletal abnormalities and others; see text.

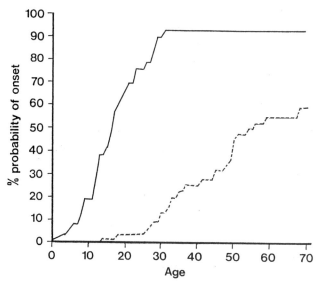

FIG. 25-1 Age-related probability of detection of disease in MEN 2A. Shown is the probability that an individual with the gene for MEN 2A will have presented to medical attention (dotted line) or be detectable by a pentagastrin stimulation test (solid line) by a given age. *(Reproduced with permission from Easton et al. Am J Hum Genet 44:208–215, 1989. Published by University of Chicago Press.)*

common. This contrasts with MEN 2B, where new mutations are more usual.[31]

Clinical Variants. No developmental abnormalities are known to be consistently associated with MEN 2A. There are, however, two clinical variants. A small number of families have been described in which several individuals have an itchy skin lesion in the interscapular area with histologic features of lichen amyloidosis.[32,33] A dermatomal distribution in one family[33] suggested a neurologic basis for the lesion, but this remains unsubstantiated. Several families have been described in which there is cosegregation of MEN 2A (or FMTC) and Hirschsprung disease of the colon and rectum (HSCR), with individuals having both phenotypes.[34–37] This is a surprising and intriguing observation, because the *ret* mutations in MEN 2 are thought to result in activation of the gene, whereas those typical of HSCR are associated with loss of activity. It is almost certainly significant that each of the MEN 2/HSCR families described to date has one of two specific *ret* mutations (see below).

Familial MTC

Clinical Features and Definition. The term *familial MTC* (FMTC) denotes families in which MTC is the only abnormality. The original evidence for a separate category of site-specific MTC came from two large kindreds in the United States in which there were multiple cases of MTC but no evidence, either clinically or on biochemical screening, of adrenal or parathyroid involvement.[18] A particular feature of these families was the late onset and low mortality of the tumors. There were no developmental abnormalities. The categorization of FMTC as a distinct variety of MEN 2 was justifiable in this extensive kindred and has subsequently received support from mutational analysis of the *ret* gene which indicates that the spectrum of mutations in families designated as having FMTC is indeed different from (although overlapping) that described in MEN 2A.[11] Nevertheless, the inconstant occurrence of adrenal or parathyroid involvement in MEN 2A families clearly leads to a difficulty in the classification of small families in which MTC is the only feature: Is the family truly FMTC or a MEN 2A family in which by chance the adrenal or parathyroid components have not yet manifested? As more data are collected, it may be

possible to classify families with respect to risks of different tumors on the basis of the *ret* mutation which is present (see below). For the present, however, an arbitrary definition has been generally adopted: to qualify as FMTC a family should have at least four individuals with proven MTC and no clinical or biochemical evidence of an adrenal or parathyroid abnormality either in the affected members or in available first-degree relatives.[38] Families which fail to meet these criteria either because there are fewer affected cases or because clinical or biochemical data are not available are assigned to an "MEN 2—other" or undefined category. Clinical impressions as well as the results of *ret* mutation analysis indicate that FMTC is less common than MEN 2A.

MEN 2B

Clinical Features. MEN 2B is probably the least common variety of MEN 2 but is the most clearly distinct. MTC and pheochromocytoma are common as in MEN 2A but tend to present at a younger age (18 years and 24 years for MTC and pheochromocytoma in MEN 2B compared to 38 years for MTC in MEN 2A) (EuroMEN collaboration: unpublished data).[39] Parathyroid involvement in MEN 2B is rare or absent.[22] The main distinguishing features of MEN 2B are the consistent developmental abnormalities.[17,40–46] A characteristic facies (Fig. 25-2) with thick blubbery lips, nodules on the anterior tongue and the conjunctivae, and thickening of the corneal nerves visible on ophthalmologic examination results from disorganized growth of axons, leading to thickening and irregularity of peripheral nerves.[40,41] (Note, however, that the corneal nerve thickening may be difficult to score.[42]) Hyperplasia of the intrinsic autonomic ganglia in the wall of the intes-

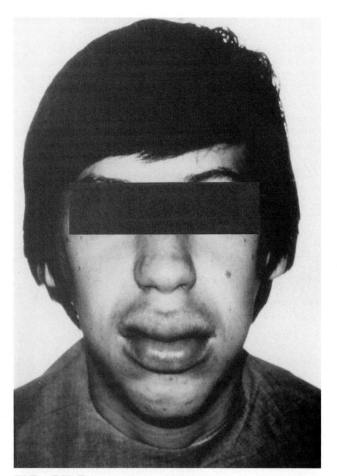

FIG. 25-2 Typical facies of MEN 2B showing the prominent "blubbery" lips caused by neuroma tissue.

tine leads to disordered gut motility,[43] which commonly presents in infancy or childhood as failure to thrive, or alternating episodes of constipation and diarrhea. These abnormalities can be recognized on rectal biopsy. A generalized hypotonia ("floppy baby") has been described in newborn infants.[44] There may be a variety of skeletal abnormalities, including pes cavus, slipped femoral epiphyses, pectus excavatum, and bifid ribs[45] and a general abnormality of body shape with features resembling those of Marfan syndrome but without the aortic, palatal, or lens abnormalities. Delayed puberty has been noted in a few girls with MEN 2B; the mechanism is unclear. Impotence in men is neurologic in origin.

New Mutations. The earlier onset of tumors and the developmental abnormalities presumably confer a reproductive disadvantage. As a result, perhaps one-half of all MEN 2B cases result from new mutations.[31] As in retinoblastoma and neurofibromatosis type 1, new mutations occur predominantly on the chromosome from the male parent.[46] It has been suggested that the sex of the transmitting parent also may affect the probability that the disease will manifest in a male or a female child, with an excess of affected female children among the offspring of transmitting males.[46] An interesting commentary on these findings was written by Sapienza.[47]

Differences between Hereditary and Nonhereditary Tumors: Multifocal Hyperplasia

The histologic appearances of the fully developed MTC, pheochromocytoma, or parathyroid adenomas of MEN 2 patients are indistinguishable from those of nonhereditary cases. However, just as familial cancers at any site are commonly multiple and associated with multiple preneoplastic changes in the target tissue, in the MEN 2 syndromes there are multiple foci of hyperplasia in the target tissues before the development of overt tumors[48,49] (Fig. 25-3). This may provide a histologic basis for recognition of an isolated case as being of the hereditary type and provides the basis for biochemical screening to detect the increased amounts of calcitonin or catecholamines produced by the hyperplastic C cells and adrenal medulla.[21] The biochemical test for C-cell hyperplasia (see "Biochemical Screening," below) is made more sensitive by the use of a stimulus (usually intravenous pentagastrin or calcium) that causes the C cells to release stored calcitonin into the circulation. Measurement of calcitonin levels before and after the stimulus provides an indication of C-cell mass. The test is sufficiently sensitive to detect C-cell hyperplasia before the stage of progression to

invasive tumor, and surgery based on presymptomatic calcitonin screening is likely to be curative.[21]

Other Causes of C-Cell Hyperplasia. It is important to note that although it is a useful indication of hereditary disease, C-cell hyperplasia may not be completely specific for MEN 2. Increased C-cell numbers (although possibly in a different histologic pattern) have been described in autopsy samples from the general population,[50–52] and there are several well-documented instances in which members of MEN 2 families have had thyroidectomy on the basis of increased calcitonin levels on screening and the thyroid histology has been reported as C-cell hyperplasia but subsequent genetic testing has shown them not to have inherited the familial MEN 2 mutation.[53,54] There may be genetic or nongenetic influences on C-cell mass independent of the MEN 2 mutation that complicate the assessment of C-cell hyperplasia.

Diagnostic Criteria for MEN 2

Failure to Recognize Hereditary Disease. A recent survey for the Royal College of Physicians in the United Kingdom[25] showed that the diagnosis of MEN 2 often is missed. The possibility of hereditary disease in an apparently isolated case of MTC is discounted or not pursued with sufficient vigor.

Part of the problem may stem from terminology. An isolated case of MTC is often referred to as "sporadic." "Sporadic" in turn is often incorrectly used to signify "nonhereditary," and so clinicians may come to regard any isolated case as nonhereditary. In fact, of course, a "sporadic" case may be hereditary, lacking a family history because the phenotype was not manifest in immediate relatives (MEN 2 is incompletely penetrant; Fig. 25-1), because the history has been poorly taken or because the case is a new mutation (particularly common in MEN 2B, and in such cases the diagnosis should be signaled by the associated phenotype) (Fig. 25-2).

Evaluation of an Apparently Sporadic Case. Guidelines for estimating the probability that an apparently isolated patient presenting with MTC at a given age is in fact hereditary are given by Ponder et al.[55] An apparently sporadic case of MTC, pheochromocytoma, or parathyroid disease should be evaluated carefully for the possibility of MEN 2, first by taking a detailed family history (with special attention to possible indications of the MEN 2 syndrome—goiter, possible hypertensive sudden death, renal stones) and second by evaluation of the surgical specimen for evidence of multifocal hyperplasia.

GENETIC LOCI

Genetic Loci Involved in Germ-Line Mutations in MEN 2

The great majority of MEN 2 families show linkage to chromosome 10q11.2 and have demonstrable mutations in *ret*[11] (Table 25-3). Around 15 percent of FMTC families and families were fewer than four cases of MTC (in the MEN 2—other category) have not been found to have *ret* mutations,[11] even though in some of these families the known coding region of *ret* has been carefully examined. This raises the possibility that another locus may be involved which predisposes primarily to MTC, possibly with low penetrance.[12] There have been occasional reports of "MTC only" families in which there is evidence against linkage on chromosome 10q, but the linkage results have relied on C-cell hyperplasia as the

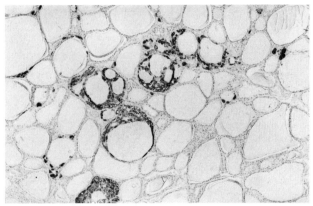

FIG. 25-3 C-cell hyperplasia in MEN 2A thyroid. Prominent groups of C cells are demonstrated by immunochemistry for calcitonin among the thyroid follicles which are unstained. *(Photograph courtesy of Dr. G. Thomas.)*

Table 25-3 Percentages of MEN 2 Families with Different Phenotypes in Which *ret* Mutations Have Been Detected

Phenotype	No. Families	Mutation +ve (%)	Mutation −ve (%)
MEN 2A			
MTC, pheochromocytoma, PTH	94	91 (97)	3 (3)
MTC, pheochromocytoma, no PTH	96	95 (99)	1 (1)
MTC, PTH, no pheochromocytoma	13	13 (100)	0 (0)
MEN 2B	79	75 (95)	4 (5)
FMTC*	34	30 (88)	4 (12)
Other MTC*	161	136 (85)	25 (15)
Total	477	440 (92)	37 (8)

*See text.

SOURCE: Data from the International RET Mutation Consortium (submitted).

MEN 2 phenotype. Because C-cell hyperplasia can be a difficult phenotype to define,[50–54] it is uncertain how these results should be interpreted.

Genetic Loci Involved in Somatic Mutations

Loss of heterozygosity (LOH) studies show a low level of chromosomal instability in MTC and pheochromocytomas. Mulligan et al,[56] in a systematic search, identified six chromosomal regions which showed a frequency of LOH of 10 percent or more in a combined series of MTC and pheochromocytoma: 1p, 3p, 3q, 11p, 13, and 22. There were no clear differences between sporadic and familial tumors. Losses are rarely seen at the *ret* locus on chromosome 10q. Chromosome 1p is the most frequently involved in both MTC and pheochromocytoma.[56,57] In almost all cases, the entire chromosome arm is lost. This is not associated with isochromosome 1q formation.[56] A localized region of loss at 1p32 was reported[57] but appears not to be a consistent finding in other studies. No mutations have been identified in candidate genes lying within the regions of LOH.

SPECIFIC GENES

ret is the only gene known to be involved in the inherited predisposition to MEN 2 and the only gene known to cause a predisposition to MTC. Germ-line mutations in other genes may predispose to pheochromocytoma in von Hippel-Lindau (VHL) syndrome (Chap. 24) and neurofibromatosis type 1 (Chap. 22). It is not clear whether there is an additional syndrome of site-specific pheochromocytoma or whether all these families will fall within VHL. Germ-line mutations in the gene for MEN 1 (yet to be identified) predispose to parathyroid tumors.[4–6]

Mutations of *ret* in MEN 2

Identification of *ret* as a Proto-Oncogene. The *ret* proto-oncogene is a cell-surface glycoprotein that is a member of the receptor tyrosine kinase (RTK) family.[58] The name *ret* is an acronym for "rearranged during transfection," reflecting the original identification of *ret* as a chimeric oncogene formed by rearrangement during transfection assays using DNA from human lymphomas and gastric tumors.[59] Three different rearranged versions of *ret* have since been described in vivo, specifically in papillary thyroid carcinomas (which arise from thyroid follicular epithelial cells and are therefore distinct from the C-cell–derived MTC).[60–62] These rearranged versions are termed *ret* PTC-1, -2, and -3. In each case, the effect of the rearrangement, which occurs as a somatic event, is to fuse the tyrosine kinase region of *ret* with different activating sequences that are expressed in thyroid epithelial cells. The fused activating genes contribute a new N-terminal portion to the *ret* protein which is capable of dimerization, leading to activation of the tyrosine kinase domain independent of any ligand. Mutations of the *ret*-PTC type are not seen in MEN 2-related tumors.

Identification of *ret* in MEN 2. *ret* lay in the region for the MEN 2 locus defined by linkage analysis and was therefore a candidate gene.[63,64] At that time, *ret* was known as a proto-oncogene, whereas all the tumor predisposing genes identified to that point acted as suppressor genes. The plausibility of *ret* as a candidate was, however, strengthened by the first reports that the *ret* knockout mouse had a phenotype which resembled HSCR[65] and the known association of MEN 2 and HSCR in some families. Mutation analysis of *ret* in MEN 2 families revealed mutations in the extracellular domain of the gene in MEN 2A and FMTC[66–68] and subsequently in the tyrosine kinase domain in MEN 2B.[69–71]

ret Structure. The coding sequence consists of 21 exons in a genomic sequence of approximately 55 kb.[72,73] The protein exists in three main 3′ alternatively spliced forms of 1072 to 1114 amino acids.[74] There is a cleavable signal sequence of 28 amino acids; an extracellular domain, which is glycosylated, has a conserved[75,76] cysteine-rich region close to the cell membrane and a region of cadherin homology further out[77]; a transmembrane domain; and a tyrosine kinase domain with a short interkinase region of 27 amino acids (Fig. 25-4). Further details of the structure are given in Refs. 72–74 and 78–80.

A Ligand for the ret Receptor. A ligand for *ret* was recently identified.[81–85] This is glial-derived neurotropic factor (GDNF), which was already known as a tropic factor for dopaminergic neurons,[81] but acting through an unknown receptor. Once again, the phenotype of a transgenic knockout mouse provided the clue.[82,83] This phenotype had several features in common with the *ret* knockout mice, suggesting GDNF as a possible *ret* ligand. This was rapidly confirmed.[84] Uniquely for a tyrosine kinase receptor, it was found that the interaction of GDNF with *ret* was not direct but required a second protein, termed GDNFRα, bound to the cell membrane through a lipid linkage.[84,85] At present, nothing has been published in detail about the expression of these proteins in relation to the tissues involved in MEN 2, or about mutations in the genes that encode them. It remains possible that there are *ret* ligands besides GDNF.

Germ-Line ret Mutations in MEN 2. A summary of the mutations is given in Table 25-3 and Fig. 25-4. All MEN 2 germ-line

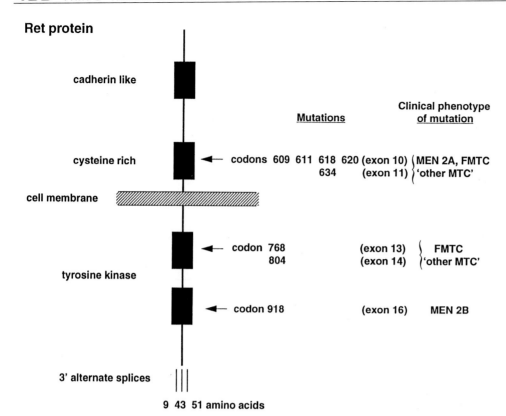

Ret protein

cadherin like

cysteine rich

cell membrane

tyrosine kinase

3' alternate splices

9 43 51 amino acids

Mutations

Clinical phenotype
of mutation

codons 609 611 618 620 (exon 10) MEN 2A, FMTC
634   (exon 11) 'other MTC'

codon 768   (exon 13) FMTC
804   (exon 14) 'other MTC'

codon 918   (exon 16) MEN 2B

FIG. 25-4 The main features of the protein encoded by the *ret* proto-oncogene, and the sites of the mutations in the different clinical varieties of MEN 2.

mutations so far identified are point mutations that lead to amino acid substitution.

Mutations in MEN 2A and FMTC. The majority of mutations in MEN 2A and FMTC lie in one of five cysteine codons in the cysteine-rich region of the extracellular domain[11,38] and result in substitution of the cysteine by another amino acid. A few mutations in families with MTC have been found in exons 13 and 14 of the intracellular domain[86,87] (Figs. 25-4 and 25-5). Figure 25-5 shows clearly that there is a correlation between the codon involved in the mutation and the MEN 2 phenotype.[11] In families with MEN 2A with both pheochromocytoma and parathyroid involvement, almost all the mutations are in codon 634; in MEN 2A families lacking pheochromocytoma and in FMTC, codons 609, 611, 618, and 620 are more frequently involved. This correlation is highly significant; 160 of 186 families with at least one proven case of pheochromocytoma have mutations in codon 634, compared with 18 of 43 families with no evidence of pheochromocytoma (p <0.0001).[11] There may also be an effect not only of the position of the cysteine codon but of the particular amino acid substitution

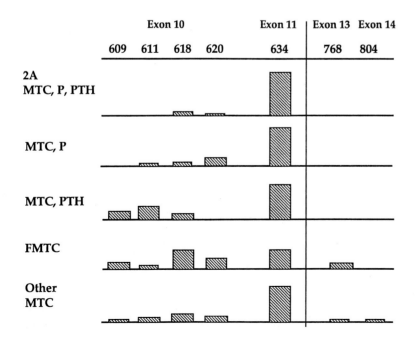

	Exon 10				Exon 11	Exon 13	Exon 14
	609	611	618	620	634	768	804
2A MTC, P, PTH							
MTC, P							
MTC, PTH							
FMTC							
Other MTC							

FIG. 25-5 Proportion of mutations in different codons of *ret* in different phenotypic subtypes of MEN 2A, FMTC, and other MTC families. Based on data from the International Ret Mutation Consortium summarized in Table 25-3.

involved. Mutations at codon 634 seen in MEN 2 include all the possible amino acid substitutions allowed by the coding sequence. The most common changes are cysteine to arginine (C634R; TGC→CGC) and cysteine to tyrosine (C634Y; TGC→TAC), which may reflect the known frequency of T→C and G→A changes rather than the particular biologic significance of these substitutions. Nevertheless, it is intriguing that while C634R was present in 88 of 169 MEN 2A families with a codon 634 mutation, none of 9 FMTC families with a codon 634 mutation had this change.[11] Furthermore, Mulligan et al.[38] found a highly significant association between the C634R mutation, compared to all other 634 mutations, and the presence in the family of parathyroid disease. This, however, awaits replication in an independent study.[11] Four families (three meeting the criteria for FMTC and one "other") have been identified with a glu→asp mutation in codon 768 (exon 13),[86,87] and two families with MTC have been placed in the "other" category with a leu→val mutation in codon 804 (exon 14).[86] Thus, mutations in this region of the intracellular domain seem to be specifically associated with MTC rather than with pheochromocytoma or parathyroid disease.

Mutations in MEN 2B. Eighty-two of 86 MEN 2B families reported to date have an identical mutation: methionine→threonine in codon 918 of exon 16.[11,69-71,88] Each of the four families lacking this mutation has typical and well-documented phenotypic features, and in two, the entire coding sequence of the *ret* gene has been sequenced and no abnormality has been found[89] (unpublished data).

Mutations in Families with MEN 2 and HSCR. Each of the six families reported has a mutation in either cys 618 or cys 620.[33,37,90] No other mutation has been found after careful examination of the remainder of the gene in these families, and so the conclusion must be that the same mutation can result in apparently contrasting phenotypes in the same individual. Families with HSCR alone with no evidence of MEN 2 have also been reported to have missense mutations in cysteine codons 609 and 620.[35,36]

Expression of ret in Development. Three of the tissues principally involved in MEN 2—thyroid C cells, adrenal medulla, and intestinal autonomic ganglia—are derived from neural ectoderm.[91] The parathyroids are derived from the endoderm of the third and fourth pharyngeal pouches. The lineage relationships between C cells and other cells of neuroectodermal origin are still unclear, but the origin of C cells from vagal neural crest and the biochemical similarities with enteric neurons[92] suggest they share a common precursor with enteric neurons and ultimately with the sympathoadrenal progenitor which is the precursor of chromaffin cells and sympathetic neurons.[93]

In situ hybridization studies during mouse and rat development show that *ret* is expressed in the neural crest-derived cells which migrate from the region of the hindbrain into the posterior pharyngeal arches and from there to form the thyroid C cells and the vagal neural crest which gives rise to the intestinal autonomic nerves.[94,95] *ret* is also expressed in migrating cells derived from the trunk neural crest as they coalesce alongside the aorta to form the sympathetic ganglia and the chromaffin cells which will form the adrenal medulla and in the endoderm of the pharyngeal pouches which give rise to the parathyroids.[94,96] The expression of *ret* is therefore consistent with a role in the development and differentiation of the tissues which are involved in MEN 2. It is perhaps surprising that *ret* homozygous knockout mice appear at birth to have absent intestinal autonomic ganglia but normal C cells and adrenal medulla.[65] The mice die at this stage, probably of respiratory or kidney failure resulting from other developmental defects, and so the possible role of *ret* expression in postnatal development cannot

be assessed. However, the tentative conclusion must be that while disordered *ret* expression can lead to tumor formation, normal *ret* expression is not necessary for C-cell or adrenal medullary development up to the time of birth. A caveat is that while the C cells and adrenal medulla may appear grossly normal, the development of the cells might have been perturbed in some way that is not readily apparent. There is a further possibility, with some evidence to support it, that the C-cell population is heterogeneous, with only some C cells expressing *ret*.[95,97] It might be, therefore, that the C cells which are seen in the knockout mice are only one component of the population, with the other component being absent.

In the later stages of embryogenesis in the mouse and in rodent and human thyroid and adrenal medullas after birth, there appears to be only weak and patchy expression of *ret* by the criteria of in situ hybridization and immunohistochemistry.[95,97] In most MTCs and pheochromocytomas, by contrast, *ret* is expressed at high levels.[98,99] At present nothing is known about the role of *ret* in C-cell or adrenal medullary development or in the adult glands. The mechanism and significance of the apparent increase in the expression in tumors are uncertain but may in part have a trivial explanation in terms of stabilization of the *ret* mRNA or protein as a result of the mutation.[100]

Function of ret at the Cellular Level. *ret* is an RTK. Binding of ligand results in dimerization of the receptor, activation of the tyrosine kinase, and initiation of onward signaling pathways.[101] Evidence is slowly accumulating,[102-106] but there is no coherent picture of the signaling events which follow *ret* activation. Analysis is complicated by the three 3' alternative splice forms of *ret*, which might be predicted from the sequence context of their tyrosines to differ in the affinity with which they bind different signaling molecules and may therefore signal through different pathways, and by the likelihood (supported by some evidence)[106] that the pathways of signaling are specific for different cell types, which implies that studies should be done in cells which resemble as closely as possible those involved in MEN 2.

Consequences of ret Mutations. Transfection experiments[101,104] have shown that both the MEN 2A (cys 634 arg) and the MEN 2B (met 918 thr) mutations lead to activation of *ret* tyrosine kinase. The evidence is of two types: (1) biologic, in which transfection of mutant but not wild-type *ret* induces transformation of NIH 3T3 cells and differentiation of rat PC12 (pheochromocytoma) cells, and (2) biochemical, in which the *ret* protein becomes phosphorylated on tyrosine and acquires tyrosine kinase activity against added substrates.

Extracellular Domain Cysteine Mutations. The cysteine mutations activate *ret* by inducing covalent dimerization (Fig. 25-6).[101,104,107,108] In view of the genotype–phenotype correlations observed with mutations of different cysteine codons, it would be of interest to compare the activities of the different mutants in transfection assays and confirm that they cause activation by a similar covalent dimerization. No such studies have been reported.

The Met 918 Thr MEN 2B Mutation. This mutation has proved to be of considerable interest, because its effect is to convert the substrate specificity of the *ret* tyrosine kinase from that typical of an RTK to that typical of a cytoplasmic tyrosine kinase.

Residue 918 is predicted from modeling studies to lie at the base of a pocket in the protein that is involved in substrate binding.[58,69] The substitution of threonine for methionine is predicted to alter the dimensions of the pocket and thus the substrate specificity. Tyrosine kinases fall into two classes: RTKs and cytoplasmic tyrosine kinases. Almost all RTKs have methionine at the equivalent position to codon 918, whereas almost all cytoplasmic

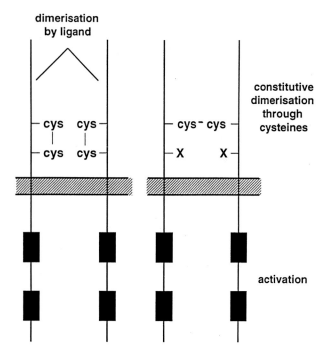

FIG. 25-6 Constitutive activation of *ret* as a result of mutation of a cysteine in the extracellular domain.

tyrosine kinases have threonine (Fig. 25-7).[58] Songyang et al.[109] used degenerate peptide libraries to demonstrate that whereas RTKs prefer hydrophobic amino acids at positions +1 and +3 downstream of the target tyrosine in their substrate, cytoplasmic tyrosine kinases prefer a hydrophilic residue at +1 and a hydrophobic residue at +3. These different amino acid contexts flanking the tyrosine provide different preferred substrates for different groups of SH2 domains on signaling molecules and hence the possibility of different pathways of downstream signaling.

When wild-type (equivalent to MEN 2A) and MEN 2B *ret* tyrosine kinases were compared for their ability to phosphorylate model substrates, a clear shift toward the specificity characteristic of a cytoplasmic tyrosine kinase was seen with the MEN 2B mutation.[109] The inference that the MEN 2B mutation has altered the pathway of downstream signaling is supported by the observation that activated MEN 2B *ret* differs from activated wild-type *ret* both in the pattern of tyrosine phosphorylation of the *ret* protein itself[110] and in the patterns of tyrosine phosphorylations seen in cell extracts.[104]

The MEN 2B mutation does not lead to covalent dimerization of *ret*.[104] It remains unresolved whether it also leads to activation of the receptor through an intramolecular mechanism.[101,104]

The 768 and 804 Mutations. The glu 768 asp mutation[86,87] involves a residue that is highly conserved in different RTKs. Modeling suggests a possible effect both on ATP binding and on substrate specificity, each of which is being tested experimentally. The

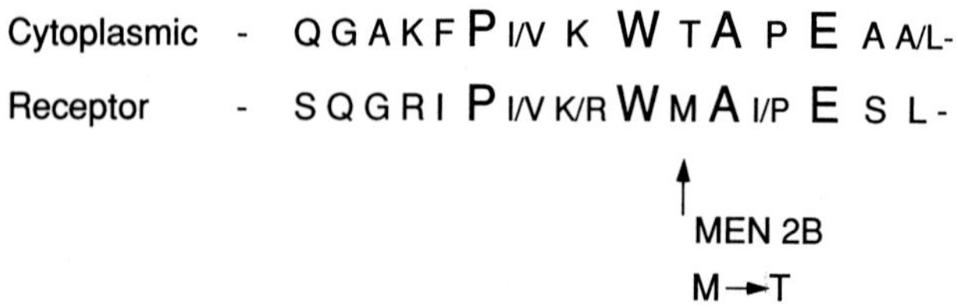

Cytoplasmic - Q G A K F P I/V K W T A P E A A/L-

Receptor - S Q G R I P I/V K/R W M A I/P E S L-

↑
MEN 2B
M → T

FIG. 25-7 Amino acid sequence of consensus receptor and cytoplasmic tyrosine kinases in the substrate binding region of Hanks domain VIII, showing the mutation characteristic of MEN 2B.

val 804 leu mutation[86] also affects a conserved residue, but no modeling studies have been reported.

Genes Involved in Somatic Mutations

The genetic events in the progression of MEN 2 tumors and in the initiation and progression of the related nonhereditary tumors are largely unknown. Baylin et al.[111] showed that the tumors are clonal. Several candidate oncogenes have been screened for mutations or altered expression (N-*ras*, Ha-*ras*, N-*myc*, c-*myc*, 1-*myc*, c-*mos*, β nerve growth factor, and the low-affinity nerve growth factor receptor).[112,113] Apart from one report of overexpression of N-*myc* in 6 of 21 MTCs analyzed by in situ hybridization,[114] all the studies were negative.

The role of mutations of *ret* in sporadic tumors is of some interest. In the inherited cancer syndromes, nonhereditary tumors often have mutations in the same gene that shows germ-line mutations in hereditary cases. In MEN 2 this is partly true, with an interesting twist. Among 157 apparently sporadic MTCs in the literature, 39 percent are reported to have a somatic mutation in *ret* codon 918 (the MEN 2B mutation), but mutations of the cysteine codons characteristic of MEN 2A and FMTC are rare, on the order of 1 to 3 percent.[28,67,115] Somatic mutations in the intracellular domain are seen a little more frequently: codon 768 in 4 of 72 sporadic MTCs[87,116] (Eng et al., unpublished) and codon 883 in exon 15 in 4 of 111 MTCs[116,117] (Eng et al., unpublished). In pheochromocytomas, the picture is slightly different. Six of 112 (5 percent) sporadic pheochromocytomas had a mutation in *ret* codon 918,[118,119] 2 of 112 had proven somatic mutations of codon 634,[119,120] and a further 3 tumors have been reported with novel somatic mutations affecting the 3′ splice acceptor site of exon 9, codons 632 through 633, and codon 925.[118,121] None of 32 non-MEN 2-associated parathyroid lesions was found to have *ret* mutations.[122]

Detailed study of codon 918 mutations in sporadic MTCs by PCR analysis of microdissected portions of primary tumors and metastases has shown that the tumors are most often mosaic for the mutation; that is, there are mutant and nonmutant clones, implying that the 918 mutation is not the initiating event in formation of sporadic MTC.[123] One tumor was found to have different areas with codon 918 and codon 883 mutations. Mosaicism for codon 918 mutation was also found in two of three MEN 2A tumors studied, in which a germ-line codon 634 was also present.

Synthesis: Speculation on How *ret* Mutations Result in Tumor Formation

Carlson et al.[124] showed that induction of raf-1 signaling in TT cells (an MTC cell line bearing a codon 634 mutation)[125] results in both differentiation and silencing of *ret* expression. Possibly, during development, C cells move from a "predetermined" to a terminally differentiated state in which *ret* expression is reduced and the potential for proliferation is lost.[124] Inappropriate continued activation of *ret* by a cysteine mutation might override the differentiation program, allowing continued proliferation and the hyperplasias seen in MEN 2. In this scheme, the effects of mutations in the different cysteine codons might depend on the degree of activation that resulted. The combined HSCR/MEN 2 phenotype occasionally seen with mutations of cys 618 and cys 620 might (speculatively) be a result of the 618/620 mutations causing inappropriate activation of *ret* sufficient to result in tumor formation but insufficient to sustain the development of enteric neurons: If these mutations also impaired ligand binding, any reinforcement of *ret* activation by that means would be reduced. The lack of developmental abnormalities in MEN 2A and FMTC compared to MEN 2B might be the case because although the timing of *ret* signaling is inappropriate, the pathways of signaling are normal. Similarly, the preponderance of MEN 2B-type somatic mutations in tumors could occur because once they are past a certain stage of differentiation and development, thyroid C cells and adrenal medullary cells are no longer susceptible to transformation by increased *ret* activity alone but are susceptible to the altered pathways of signaling induced by the MEN 2B mutation. The lack of parathyroid involvement in MEN 2B might be the case either because the MEN 2B-specific signaling pathways are not present in parathyroid cells or because the MEN 2B mutations, unlike MEN 2A, still retain partial dependence on ligand binding for activity, and the ligand may not be present in parathyroid tissue. Evidence is not available to test any of these alternatives.

Implications for Diagnosis

Biochemical Screening. Regular screening by biochemical testing and imaging, followed by surgery where necessary, has been shown to be effective in preventing mortality and morbidity in MEN 2 families.[21,126–128]

In families with MEN 2A or FMTC, it is generally recommended that screening be started at about 4 to 5 years of age, continued annually until about age 20, and then possibly (this is controversial) continued at rather wider intervals until age 35. Screening should consist of measurement of plasma calcitonin after stimulation with intravenous pentagastrin, calcium, or both combined[21,127,128]; blood pressure measurement; urinary or plasma catecholamines; possibly imaging of the adrenals; and serum calcium levels. Thyroid surgery should consist of total thyroidectomy and central node dissection with conservation of normal parathyroid in situ or autotransplantation to the forearm.[129] It is controversial whether after the detection of a unilateral adrenal abnormality one or both adrenals should be removed.[130] The risks of serious problems from pheochromocytoma developing subsequently in the remaining adrenal must be balanced against the inconvenience and possible dangers of life after adrenalectomy and hormone replacement. Current opinion generally favors bilateral adrenalectomy. There is no consensus about screening for MEN 2B. Because of the sometimes early development and aggressive nature of the thyroid tumor, screening for MTC in the child or a known MEN 2B patient probably should start by age 1 year.[131,132] Normal calcitonin levels may be high in infants, and screening results may be difficult to interpret. In this situation, some clinicians have advocated thyroidectomy on the basis of the MEN 2B phenotype alone. Greater certainty can now be provided by DNA testing for the MEN 2B mutation.

Although generally effective, biochemical screening has several problems. The stimulated calcitonin tests are somewhat unpleasant, and compliance is not always good. Occasional false positive results have been obtained, and results on successive tests which fluctuate at and just above the normal level are common and a frequent cause of anxiety to physicians and family members. Finally, there is the problem of whether to initiate a program of screening for the families of apparently sporadic cases of one of the MEN 2 component tumors. Although many physicians are reluctant to burden a family with these tests, not following such a screening program will inevitably lead to missing some opportunities for early diagnosis.

DNA Testing. The number of distinct *ret* mutations which occur in MEN 2 is small. One of these mutations can be detected in over 90 percent of cases. DNA testing is therefore relatively simple and is now in routine clinical use.[53]

In a family known to have MEN 2 in which the causative mutation can be identified, DNA testing of unaffected family members at risk will eliminate those who do not have the mutation from the need for biochemical screening and simplify the decision to have surgery in those whose screening results are equivocal. Increasingly, opinion is moving toward a recommendation for thyroidectomy in childhood on the basis of DNA testing alone, without waiting for biochemical testing to show abnormalities indicative of C-cell hyperplasia. This may seen surprising given that the chances of presentation with symptomatic disease in MEN 2A are only on the order of 50 percent by age 50[24] and that a good biochemical screen for early disease is available. It probably reflects a mixture of concern about continued compliance with the biochemical screening and the possibility that equivocation over borderline results may lead to surgery being carried out too late; there is also the view that thyroidectomy even in young children has low morbidity and that the best thing for the child and family is to deal with the problem and put it behind them. Because of the lower probability of adrenal disease and the much greater morbidity of adrenalectomy, prophylactic removal of the adrenals is not advised except when there is evidence of abnormality.

The genotype/phenotype correlations outlined above[11] may provide some indication of the probability of adrenal or parathyroid involvement, but the data are too few and the overlaps too great to recommend that mutation data be used to exclude families from adrenal or parathyroid screening.

DNA Testing in an Apparently Sporadic Case. DNA testing plays an important role in determining which apparently sporadic cases have heritable disease. All apparently sporadic cases of MTC should be offered DNA testing. If the patient is dead, normal or tumor tissues from pathology specimens may be tested. The limited range of mutations makes this technically feasible in most cases, and since MEN 2A-type mutations rarely occur as somatic events, they can be interpreted as probably germ line in origin even if they are found in tumor (the same does not, of course, apply to MEN 2B mutations). If there is no family history on careful review and no evidence of C-cell hyperplasia on the thyroidectomy specimen, the probability of hereditary disease will vary according to the age at diagnosis of the index case but is almost certainly well below 10 percent.[27,55] In this case, failure to find a mutation in exons 10, 11, 13, 14, and 16 of *ret* excludes MEN 2A with >99 percent probability[11] and, if there is no abnormal phenotype, MEN 2B as well. The residual probability of FMTC or "MTC only" familial disease is a little higher, since up to 15 percent of such families have no detectable *ret* mutation, but it is still probably below 2 percent. It remains a matter of clinical judgment, according to the circumstances and perceptions of each family, whether to pursue biochemical screening of family members at these levels of risk. On the one hand, one does not wish to lose any possibility of early diagnosis and treatment of a potentially lethal and unpleasant cancer (but possibly the FMTC, which is most likely to be missed, could be treated satisfactorily at clinical presentation); on the other hand, one does not want to run the risk of unnecessarily "medicalizing" a family over a period of many years.

Direct mutation testing of unselected cases of apparently sporadic pheochromocytomas suggests that roughly 5 percent may carry a *ret* mutation and that another 5 percent will have a VHL mutation[119] (Chap. 24). Mutation screening of apparently sporadic cases of pheochromocytoma for MEN 2A and VHL mutations is probably worthwhile. The incidence of occult MEN 2 among apparently sporadic cases of parathyroid hyperplasia and adenoma appears to be low,[122] and unless there are other suggestive features, DNA screening probably is not justified.

ACKNOWLEDGMENTS

B.A.J. Ponder is a Gibb Fellow of the Cancer Research Campaign [CRC].

REFERENCES

1. Thakker RV, Ponder BAJ: Multiple endocrine neoplasia. *Clin Endocrinol Metab* **2**:1031, 1988.
2. Thakker RV: Multiple endocrine neoplasia type 1, in Grossman A (ed): *Clinical Endocrinology*. Oxford, Blackwell, 1992, p 597.
3. Werner P: Multiple endocrine adenomatosis: Multiple hormone producing tumours: A familial syndrome. *Clin Gastroenterol* **3**:671, 1974.
4. Marx SJ, Vinik AI, Santen RJ, Floyd JC, Mills JL, Green J: Multiple endocrine neoplasia type 1: Assessment of laboratory tests to screen for the gene in a large kindred. *Medicine (Baltimore)* **65**:226, 1986.
5. Vasen HFA, Lamers CBHW, Lips CJM: Screening for multiple endocrine neoplasia syndrome type 1: A study of 11 kindreds in the Netherlands. *Arch Intern Med* **149**:2717, 1989.
6. Trump D, Farren B, Wooding C, Pang JT, Besser GM, Buchanan KD, Edwards CR, Heath DA, Jackson CE, Jansen S, Lips K, Monson JP, O'Halloran D, Sampson J, Shalet SM, Wheeler MH, Zink A, Thakker RV: Clinical studies of multiple endocrine neoplasia type 1 (MEN 1). *Q J Med* **89**:653, 1996.
7. Larsson C, Skogseld B, Oberg K. Nakamura Y, Nordenskjold M: Multiple endocrine neoplasia type 1 gene maps to chromosome 11 and is lost in insulinoma. *Nature* **332**:85, 1988.
8. Smith DP, Ponder BAJ: The MEN 2 syndromes and the role of the ret protooncogene. *Adv Cancer Res* **70**:199, 1996.
9. Schimke RN: Genetic aspects of multiple endocrine neoplasia. *Annu Rev Med* **35**:25, 1984.
10. Cancer WG, Wells SA: Multiple endocrine neoplasia type 2A. *Curr Probl Surg* **XXII**:7, 1985.
11. Eng C, Clayton D, Schuffenecker I, et al.: The relationship between specific net protooncogene mutations and disease phenotype in multiple endocrine neoplasia type 2: International RET Mutation Consortium. *JAMA* **276**:1575, 1996.
12. Nelkin BD, De Bustros AC, Mabrey M, Baylin SB: The molecular biology of medullary thyroid carcinoma. *JAMA* **261**:3130, 1989.
13. Schimke RN: Multiple endocrine neoplasia: How many syndromes? *Am J Med Genet* **37**:375, 1990.
14. DeLellis RA, Nunnemacher G, Bitman WR, Gagel RF, Tashjian AH, Blount M, Wolfe HJ: C-cell hyperplasia and medullary thyroid carcinoma in the rat. *Lab Invest* **40**:140, 1979.
15. Sass B, Rabstein LS, Madison R, Nims AM, Peters RL, Kelloff GJ: Evidence of spontaneous neoplasms in F344 rats throughout the natural life-span. *JNCI* **54**:1449, 1975.
16. Schimke KN, Hartmann WH, Prout TE, Rimoin DL: Syndrome of bilateral pheochromocytoma, medullary thyroid carcinoma and multiple neuromas. *N Engl J Med* **279**:1, 1968.
17. Khairi MRA, Dexter RN, Burzynoki NJ, Johnson CC Jr: Mucosal neuroma, pheochromocytoma and medullary thyroid carcinoma: Multiple endocrine neoplasia type 3. *Medicine (Baltimore)* **54**:89, 1975.
18. Farndon JR, Leight GS, Dilley WG, Baylin SB, Smallridge RC, Harrison TC, Wells SA Jr: Familial medullary thyroid carcinoma without associated endocrinopathies; a distinct clinical entity. *Br J Surg* **73**:278, 1986.
19. Chong GC, Beaths OH, Sizemore GW, Woolmer LH: Medullary carcinoma of the thyroid gland. *Cancer* **35**:695, 1975.
20. Saad MF, Ordonez NG, Rashid RK, Guido JJ, Hill CS Jr, Hickey RC, Samaan NA: Medullary carcinoma of the thyroid: A study of the clinical features and prognostic factors in 161 patients. *Medicine (Baltimore)* **63**:319, 1984.
21. Gagel RF, Tashjian AH, Cummings T, Papathanasopoulos N, Kaplan MM, Delellis RA, Wolfe HJ, Reichlin S: The clinical outcome of prospective screening for multiple endocrine neoplasia type 2A. *N Engl J Med* **318**:478, 1988.
22. Dralle H, Schurmeyer TH, Kotzerke TH, Kemnitz J, Crosse H, von zur Muhlen A: Surgical aspects of familial phaeochromocytoma. *Hormone Metab Res Suppl Series* **21**:34, 1989.
23. Van Heerden JA, Kent RB, Sizeman GW, Grant CS, ReMine WH: Primary hyperparathyroidism in patients with multiple endocrine neoplasia syndromes. *Arch Surg* **118**:533, 1983.
24. Easton DF, Ponder MA, Cummings T, Gagel RF, Hansen HH, Reichlin S, Tashjian AH Jr, Telenius-Berg M, Ponder BAJ: The clinical and age-at-onset distribution for the MEN 2 syndrome. *Am J Hum Genet* **44**:208, 1989.
25. Harris R, Williamson P: Confidential enquiry into counselling for genetic disorders. *J R Coll Physi Lond* **30**:316, 1991.
26. Sizemore GW, Carney JA, Hunter H II: Epidemiology of medullary carcinoma of the thyroid gland: A 5-year experience (1971–1976). *Surg Clin North Am* **57**:633, 1977.
27. Ponder BAJ, Finer M, Coffey R, Harmer CL, Maisey M, Ormerod MG, Pembrey ME, Ponder MA, Rosswick P, Shalet S: Family screening in medullary thyroid carcinoma presenting without a family history. *Q J Med* **252**:299, 1986.
28. Eng C, Mulligan LM, Smith DP, Healey CS, Frilling A, Raue F, Neumann HPH, Pfragner R, Behmel A, Lorenzo MJ, Stonehouse TJ, Ponder MA, Ponder BAJ: Mutation of the RET pro-oncogene in sporadic medullary thyroid carcinoma. *Genes Chromosom Cancer* **12**:209, 1995.
29. Mulligan LM, Eng C, Healey CS, Ponder MA, Feldman CL, Li P, Jackson CE, Ponder BAJ: A *de novo* mutation of the RET proto-oncogene in a patient with MEN 2A. *Hum Mol Genet* **3**:1007, 1994.
30. Narod SA, Lavone MF, Morgan K, Calmettes C, Solbol H, Goodfellow PJ, Lenoir GM: Genetic analysis of 24 French families with multiple endocrine neoplasia type 2A. *Am J Hum Genet* **51**:469, 1992.
31. Norum RA, Lafreniere RC, O'Neal LW, Nikolai TF, Delaney JP, Sisson JC, Sobol H: Linkage of the multiple endocrine neoplasia type 2B gene (MEN 2B) to chromosome 10 markers linked to MEN 2A. *Genomics* **8**:313, 1990.
32. Gagel RF, Levy ML, Donovan DT, Alford BR, Wheeler T, Tschen JA: Multiple endocrine neoplasia type 2A associated with cutaneous lichen amyloidosis. *Ann Intern Med* **111**:802, 1989.
33. Chabre O, Labat F, Berthod F, Jarel V, Bachelot Y: Cutaneous lesions associated with multiple endocrine neoplasia type 2A: Lichen amyloidosis or notalgia paresthetica? *Henry Ford Hosp Med J* **40**:245, 1992.
34. Verdy M, Weber AM, Roy CC, Morin CL, Cadotte M, Brochu P: Hirschsprung's disease in a family with multiple endocrine neoplasia type 2. *J Paediatr Gastroenterol Nutr* **1**:603, 1982.
35. Mulligan LM, Eng C, Attie T, Lyonnet S, Marsh DJ, Hyland VJ, Robinson BG, Frilling A, Verellen-Dumoulin C, Safar A, Venter DJ, Munnich A, Ponder BAJ: Diverse phenotypes associated with exon 10 mutations of the RET proto-oncogene. *Hum Mol Genet* **3**:2163, 1994.
36. Angrist M, Bolk S, Thiel B, Puffenberger EG, Hofstra RM, Buys CHCM, Cass DT, Chakravarti A: Mutation analysis of the RET receptor tyrosine kinase in Hirschsprung's disease. *Hum Mol Genet* **4**:821, 1995.
37. Borst MJ, van Camp JM, Peacock ML, Decker RA: Mutation analysis of multiple endocrine neoplasia type 2A associated with Hirschsprung disease. *Surgery* **117**:386, 1995.
38. Mulligan LM, Eng C, Healey CS, Clayton D, Kwok JBJ, Gardner E, Ponder MA, Frilling A, Jackson CE, Lehnert H, Neumann HPH, Thibodeau SN, Ponder BAJ: Specific mutations of the RET proto-oncogene are related to disease phenotype in MEN 2A and FMTC. *Nat Genet* **6**:70, 1994.
39. Vasen HFA, Kruseman ACN, Berkel H: Multiple endocrine neoplasia syndrome type 2: the value of screening and central registration: A study of 15 kindreds in the Netherlands. *Am J Med* **83**:487, 1987.
40. Dyck PJ, Carney A, Sizemore GW: Multiple endocrine neoplasia type 2B: Phenotype recognition. *Ann Neurol* **6**:302, 1979.
41. Khalil MK, Lorenzetti DWC: Eye manifestations in medullary carcinoma of the thyroid. *Br J Ophthalmol* **64**:789, 1980.
42. Kinoshita S, Tanaki F, Ohasi Y, Ikeda M, Takai S: Incidence of prominent corneal nerves in multiple endocrine neoplasia type 2A. *Am J Ophthalmol* **111**:307, 1991.
43. Carney JA, Go VLW, Sizemore GW, Hayles AB: Alimentary-tract ganglioneuromatosis: A major component of the syndrome of multiple endocrine neoplasia, type 2B. *N Engl J Med* **295**:1287, 1976.
44. Fryns JP, Chrzanowska K: Mucosal neuromata syndrome (MEN type IIb (III)). *J Med Genet* **25**:703, 1988.
45. Carney JA, Bianco AJ, Sizeman GW, Hayles AB: Multiple endocrine neoplasia with skeletal manifestations. *J Bone Joint Surg* **63A**:405, 1981.

46. Carlson KM, Bracamontes J, Jackson CE, Clark R, Lacroix A, Wells SA Jr, Goodfellow PJ: Parent of origin effects in multiple endocrine neoplasia type 2B. *Am J Hum Genet* **55**:1076, 1994.
47. Sapienza C: Parental origin effects, genomic imprinting and sex-ratio distortion: Double or nothing? *Am J Hum Genet* **55**:1073, 1994.
48. Wolfe HJ, Melvin KEW, Cervi-Skinner SJ: C cell hyperplasia preceding medullary thyroid carcinoma. *N Engl J Med* **289**:437, 1973.
49. Block MA, Jackson CE, Greenawald KA, Yott JB, Tashjian AH: Clinical characteristics distinguishing hereditary from medullary thyroid carcinoma. *Arch Surg* **115**:142, 1980.
50. O'Toole K, Genoglio-Prieser C, Pushparag N: Endocrine changes associated with the aging process: III. Effect of age on the number of calcitonin immunoreactive cells in the thyroid gland. *Hum Pathol* **16**:991, 1985.
51. Gibson WGH, Peng TC, Croker BP: C cell nodules in adult human thyroid: A common autopsy finding. *Am J Clin Pathol* **75**:347, 1981.
52. Gibson WGH, Peng TC, Croker BP: Age-associated C-cell hyperplasia in the human thyroid. *Am J Pathol* **106**:388, 1982.
53. Lips CJM, Landsvater RM, Hoppener JWM, Geerdink RA, Blijham G, Jansen-Schillhorn van Veen JM, van Gils APG, de Wit MJ, Zewald RA, Berends MJH, Beemer FA: Brouwers-Smalbraak J, Jansen RPM, Ploos van Amstel HK, van Vroonhoven TJMV, Vroom TM: Clinical screening as compared with DNA analysis in families with multiple endocrine neoplasia type 2A. *N Engl J Med* **331**:828, 1994.
54. Wolfe HJ, Kaplan M, Cummings T, Ponder BAJ, Ponder M, Gardner G, Papi L, Reichlin S: Re-evaluation of histologic ceriteria for C cell hyperplasia in MEN 2A using genetic recombinant markers. *Henry Ford Hosp J Med* **40**:312, 1992.
55. Ponder BAJ, Ponder MA, Coffey R, Pembrey ME, Gagel RP, Telenius-Berg M, Semple P, Easton DF: Risk estimation and screening in families of patients with medullary thyroid carcinoma. *Lancet* **i**:397, 1988.
56. Mulligan LM, Gardner E, Smith BA, Mathew CGP, Ponder BAJ: Genetic events in tumor initiation and progression in multiple endocrine neoplasia. *Genes Chromosom Cancer* **6**:166, 1993.
57. Moley JF, Brother MB, Fong CT, White PS, Baylin SB, Nelkin B, Wells SA, Brodeur GM: Consistent association of 1p loss of heterozygosity with phaeochromocytomas from patients with multiple endocrine neoplasia type 2 syndromes. *Cancer Res* **52**:770, 1992.
58. Hanks SK, Quinn AM, Hunter T: The protein kinase family: Conserved features and deduced phylogeny of the catalytic domain. *Science* **241**:42, 1988.
59. Takahashi M, Cooper GM: RET fusion protein encodes a fusion protein homologous to tyrosine kinases. *Mol Cell Biol* **7**:1378, 1987.
60. Grieco M, Santoro M, Berlingieri MT, Melillo RM, Donghi R, Bonzgarzone I. Pierotti MA, Della Porta G, Fusco A, Vecchio G: PTC is a novel rearranged form of the RET proto-oncogene and is frequently expressed *in vivo* in human papillary thyroid carcinomas. *Cell* **60**:557, 1990.
61. Bongarzone I, Monzini N, Borrello MG, Carcano C, Ferraresi G, Arighi E, Mondellini P, Della Porta G, Pierotti MA: Molecular characterisation of a thyroid fusion-sapecific transforming sequence formed by the fusion of *ret* tyrosine kinase and the regulatory subunit R1 of cyclic AMP-dependent protein kinase A. *Mol Cell Biol* **13**:358, 1993.
62. Santoro M, Dathan NA, Berlingieri MT, Bongarzone I, Paulin C, Grieco M, Pierotti MA, Vecchio G, Fusco A: Molecular characterisation of RET/PTC3, a novel rearranged version of the RET protooncogene in a human papillary thyroid carcinoma. *Oncogene* **9**:509, 1994.
63. Gardner E, Mullian LM, Eng C, Healey CS, Kwok JAJ, Ponder MA, Ponder BAJ: Haplotype analysis of MEN 2 mutations. *Hum Mol Genet* **3**:1771, 1994.
64. Mole SE, Mulligan LM, Healey CS, Ponder BAJ, Tunnacliffe A: Localisation of the gene for multiple endocrine neoplasia type 2A to a 480 kb region in chromosome band 10q11.2. *Hum Mol Genet* **2**:247, 1993.
65. Schuchardt A, D'Agati V, Larrson-Blomberg L, Constantini F, Pachnis V: The c-ret receptor tyrosine kinase gene is required for the development of the kidney and the enteric nervous systrem. *Nature* **367**:380, 1994.
66. Mulligan LM, Kwok JBJ, Healey CS, Elsdon M, Eng C, Gardner E, Love DR, Mole SE, Moore JK, Papi L, Ponder MA, telenius H, Tunnacliffe A, Ponder BAJ: Germ-line mutations of the RET proto-oncogene in multiple endocrine neoplasia type 2A. *Nature* **363**:458, 1993.
67. Donis-Keller H, Dou S, Chi D, Carlson KM, Toshima K. Lairmore TC, Howe JR, Moley JF, Goodfellow P, Wells SA Jr: Mutations in the

68. Schuffenecker I, Billaud M, Calender A, Chambe B, Ginet N, Calmettes C, Modigliani E, Lenior GM, the GETC: RET proto-oncogene mutations in French MEN 2A and FMTC families. *Hum Mol Genet* **3**:1939, 1994.
69. Carlson KM, Dou S, Chi D, Scavarda N, Toshima K, Jackson CE, Wells SA, Goodfellow PJ, Donis-Keller H: Single missense mutation in the tyrosine kinase catalytic domain of the RET protoncogene is associated with multiple endocrine neoplasia type 2B. *Proc Natl Acad Sci USA* **91**:1579, 1994.
70. Eng C, Smith DP, Mulligan LM, Nagai MA, Healey CS, Ponder MA, Gardner E, Scheumann GFW, Jackson CE, Tunnacliffe A, Ponder BAJ: Point mutation within the tyrosine kinase domain of the RET proto-oncogene in multiple endocrine neoplasia type 2B and related sporadic tumours. *Hum Mol Genet* **3**:237, 1994.
71. Hofstra RMW, Landsvater RM, Ceccherini I, Stulp RP, Stelwagen T, Luo Y, Pasini B, Hoppener JWM, Ploos van Amstel HK, Romeo G, Lips CJM, Buys CHCM: A mutation in the RET proto-oncogene associated with multiple endocrine neoplasia type 2B and sporadic medullary thyroid carcinoma. *Nature* **367**:375, 1994.
72. Ceccherini I, Hofstra RMW, Luo Y, Stulp RP, Barone V, Stelwagen T, Bocciardi R, Nijveen H, Bolino A, Seri M, Ronchetto P, Pasimi B, Bozzano M, Buys CHCM, Romeo G: DNA polymorphisms and conditions for SSCP analysis of the 20 exons of the ret proto-oncogene. *Oncogene* **9**:3025, 1994.
73. Kwok JBJ, Gardner E, Warner JP, Ponder BAJ, Mulligan LM: Structural analysis of the human ret proto-oncogene using exon trapping. *Oncogene* **8**:2575, 1993.
74. Myers SM, Eng C, Ponder BAJ, Mulligan LM: Characterisation of ret protooncogene 3' splicing variants and polyadenylation sites: A novel C terminus for ret. *Oncogene* **11**:2039, 1995.
75. Iwamoto I. Taniguchi M, Asai N, Ohkusu K, Nakashima I, Takahashi M: cDNA cloning of mouse ret proto-oncogene and its sequence similarity to the cadherin superfamily. *Oncogene* **8**:1087, 1993.
76. Sugaya R, Ishimaru S, Hosoya T, Saigo K. Emori Y: A Drosophila homology of human protooncogene ret transiently expressed in embryonic neuronal precursor cells including neuroblast and CNS cells. *Mech Dev* **45**:139, 1994.
77. Schneider R: The human protooncogene ret: A communicative cadherin? *Trends Biochem Sci* **17**:468, 1992.
78. Lorenzo MJ, Eng C, Mulligan LM, Stonehouse TJ, Healey CS, Ponder BAJ, Smith DP: Multiple mRNA isoforms of the human ret protooncogene generated by alternate splicing. *Oncogene* **10**:1377, 1995.
79. Takahashi M, Buma Y, Iwamoto T, Iwaguma Y, Ikeda H, Hiai H: Cloning and expression of the ret protooncogene encoding a tyrosine kinase with two potential transmembrane domains. *Oncogene* **3**:571, 1988.
80. Asai N, Iwashita T, Matsumama M, Takahashi M: Mechanism of activation of the ret protooncogene by multiple endocrine neoplasia type 2A mutations. *Mol Cell Biol* **15**:1613, 1995.
81. Liu LF-H, Doherty DH, Uke JD, Behtash S, Collins F: GDNF: A glial cell line-derived neurotrophic factor for mid-brain doperminergic neurons. *Science* **260**:1130, 1993.
82. Sanchez MP, Silos-Santiago I. Frisen J, He B, Lira SA, Barbacid M: Renal agenesis and the absence of enteric neurons in mice lacking GDNF. *Nature* **382**:70, 1996.
83. Pichel JG, Shen L, Sheng HZ, Granholm A-C, Drago J, Grinberg A, Lee EJ, Huang SP, Scarma M, Hoffer BJ, Sariola H, Westphal H: Defects in enteric innervation and kidney development in mice lacking GDNF. *Nature* **382**:73, 1996.
84. Treanor JS, Goodman L, de Sauvage F, Stone DM, Poulsen KT, Beck CD, Gray C, Armanini MP, Pollock RA, Heft F, Phillips HJ, Goddard A, Moore MW, Buj-Bello A, Davies AM, Asai N, Takahashi M, Vandlen R, Hewerson CE, Rosenthal A: Characterisation of a multicomponent receptor for GDNF. *Nature* **382**:80, 1996.
85. Jing S, Wen D, Yu Y, Holst PL, Luo Y, Fang M, Tamir R, Antonio L, Hu Z, Cupples R, Louis J-C, Hu S, Altrock B, Fox FM: GDNF-induced activation of the ret protein tyrosine kinase is mediated by GDNF-a, a novel receptor for GDNF. *Cell* **85**:1113, 1996.
86. Bolino A, Schuffenecker I, Luo Y, Seri M, Silengo M, Tocco T, Chabrier G, Houdent C, Murat A, Schlumberger M, Tourniaire J, Lenoir GM, Romeo G: RET mutations in exons 13 and 14 of FMTC patients. *Oncogene* **10**:2415, 1995.

RET proto-oncogene are associated with MEN 2A and FMTC. *Hum Mol Genet* **2**:851, 1993.

87. Eng C, Smith DP, Mulligan LM, Healey CS, Zvelebil MJ, Stonehouse TJ, Ponder MA, Jackson CE, WAterfield MD, Ponder BAJ: A novel point mutation in the tyrosine kinase domain of the RET protooncogene in sporadic medullary thyroid carcinoma and in a family with FMTC. *Oncogene* 10:509, 1995.

88. Rossel M, Schuffenecker I, Schlumberger M, Bonnardel C, Modigliani E, Gardet P, Navarro J, Luo Y, Romeo G, Lenoir G, Billaud M: Detection of a germ line mutation at codon-918 of the ret protooncogene in French MEN 2B families. *Hum Genet* 95:403, 1995.

89. Toogood AA, Eng C, Smith DP, Ponder BAJ, Shalet SM: No mutation at codon 918 of the ret gene in a family with multiple endocrine neoplasia type 2B. *Clin Endocrinol* 43:759, 1995.

90. Landsvater RM, Jansen RPM, Hofstra RMW, Buys CHCM, Lips CJM, Ploos van Amstel HK: Mutation analysis of the ret protooncogene in Dutch families with MEN 2 and FMTC. *Hum Genet* 97:11, 1996.

91. Le Douarin N: *The Neural Crest.* Cambridge, UK, Cambridge University Press, 1982.

92. Tamir H, Liu K-P, PLayette RF, Hsuing S-C, Adlersberg M, Nurez EA, Gershon MD: *J Neurosci* 9:1199, 1989.

93. Anderson DJ: Molecular control of cell fate in the neural crest: The sympathoadrenal lineage. *Annu Rev Neurosci* 16:129, 1993.

94. Pachnis V, Maukoo B, Constantini F: Expression of the c-ret protooncogene during mouse embryogenesis. *Development* 119:1005, 1993.

95. Tsuzuki T, Takahashi M, Asai N, Iwashita T, Matsuyene M, Asai J: Spatial and temporal expressio of the ret proto-oncogene product in embryonic, infant and adult rat tissues. *Oncogene* 10:191, 1995.

96. Van der Geer P, Wiley S, Lai VK-M, Olivier JP, Gish GD, Stephens R, Kaplan D, Shoelson S, Pawson T: A conserved amino terminal shc domain binds to glycophosphotyrosine motifs in activated receptors and phosphopeptides. *Curr Biol* 5:404, 1995.

97. Durbec PL, Larsson-Blomberg WB, Schuchardt A, Constantini P, Pachnis V: Common origin and developmental dependence on c-ret of subsets of enteric and sympathetic neuroblasts. *Development* 122:349, 1996.

98. Fabien N, Paulin C, Santoro M, Berger B, Grieco M: The ret protooncogene is expressed in normal human parafollicular thyroid cells. *Int J Oncol* 4:623, 1994.

99. Santoro M, Rosati R, Grieco M, Berlinger M, D'Amato GLC, de Franciscis V, Fusco A: The ret proto-oncogene is consistently expressed in human pheochromocytoma and thyroid medullary carcinomas. *Oncogene* 5:1595, 1990.

100. Miya A, Yamamoto M, Morimoto H, Tanaka N, Shin E, Karakawa K, Toyoshima K, Ishikaza Y, Mori T, Takai S-I: Expression of the ret proto-oncogene in human medullary thyroid carcinomas and pheochromocytomas of MEN 2A. *Henry Ford Hosp Med J* 40:215, 1992.

101. Pawson T, Schlessinger J: SH2 and SH3 domains. *Curr Biol* 3:434, 1993.

102. Borrello MG, Pelicci G, Arighi E, De Filippis L, Greco A, Bongarzone I, Rizzetti MG, Pelicci PG, Pierotti MA: The oncogenic versions of the Ret and Trk tyrosine kinases bind Shc and Grb2 adaptor proteins. *Oncogene* 9:1661, 1994.

103. Santoro M, Wong WT, Aroca P, Santos E, Matoskova B, Grieco M, Fusco A, Di Fiore PP: An epidermal growth factor receptor/ret chimera generates mitogenic and transforming signals: Evidence for a ret-specific signalling pathway. *Mol Cell Biol* 14:663, 1994.

104. Pandey A, Duan H, Di Fiore PP, Dixit VM: The ret receptor protein tyrosine kinase associates with the SH2-containing adapter protein Grb10. *J Biol Chem* 270:21461, 1995.

105. Santoro M, Carlomagno F, Romanova A, Bottaro DlP, Dathan NA, Grieco M, Fusco A, Vecchio G, Matoskova B, Kraus MH, De Fiore PP: Activation of RET as a dominant transforming gene by germ line mutations of MEN 2A and MEN 2B. *Science* 267:381, 1995.

106. Iwashita T, Asai N, Murakami H, Matsuyama M, Takahashi M: Identification of tyrosine residues that are essential for transforming activity of the ret proto-oncogene with MEN 2A or MEN 2B mutation. *Oncogene* 12:481, 1996.

107. Van Weering DHJ, Medema JP, van Puijenbroek A, Burgering BMT, Baas PD, Bos JL: Ret receptor tyrosine kinase activates extracellular signal regulated kinase Z in SK-N-Mc cells. *Oncogene* 11:2207, 1995.

108. Wada M, Asai N, Tsuzuki T, Maruyama S, Ohiwa M, Imai T, Funahashi H, Takagi H, Takshashi M: Detection of ret homodimers in MEN 2A associated phaeochromocytomas. *Biochem Biophys Res Commun* 218:606, 1996.

109. Songyang Z, Carraway KL III, Eck MJ, Harrison SC, Feldman RA, Mohammadi M, Schlessinger J, Hubbard SR, Smith DP, Eng C, Lorenzo MJ, Ponder BAJ, Mayer BJ, Cantley LC: Catalytic specificity of protein-tyrosine kinases is critical for selective signalling. *Nature* 373:539, 1995.

110. Liu X, Vega QC, Decker RA, PLandey A, Worby CA, Dixon JE: Oncogenic RET receptors display different autophosphorylation sites and substrate binding specificities. *J Biol Chem* 271:5309, 1996.

111. Baylin SB, Gann DS, Hsu SH: Clonal origin of inherited medullary thyroid carcinoma and phaeochromocytoma. *Science* 193:321, 1976.

112. Moley JF, Brother MB, Wells SA, Spengler BA, Bredler JL, Brodeur GM: Low frequency of ras gene mutations in neuroblastomas, phaeochromocytomas and medullary thyroid cancers. *Cancer Res* 51:1596, 1991.

113. Moley JF, Wallin GK, Brother MB, Kim M, Wells SA Jr, Brodeur GM: Oncogene and growth factor expression in MEN 2 and related tumours. *Henry Ford Hosp Med J* 40:284, 1992.

114. Boultwood J, Wyllie FS, Williams GD, Wynford Thomas D: N-myc expression in neoplasia of human thyroid C cells. *Cancer Res* 48:4073, 1988.

115. Zedenius J, Wallin G, Hamberger B, Nordenskjold M, Weber G, Larsson C: Somatic and MEN2A de novo mutations identified in the ret protooncogene by screening of sporadic MTCs. *Hum Mol Genet* 3:1259, 1994.

116. Marsh DJ, Andrew SD, Learoyd DL, Pojer R, Eng C, Robinson BG: Deletion-insertion mutations encompassing RET codon 634 is associated with medullary thyroid carcinoma. *Hum Mutat* (in press).

117. Dou S, Chi D, Carlson KM, Moley JA, Wells SA Jr, Donis-Keller H: RET proto-oncogene mutations associated with sporadic cases of medullary thyroid carcinoma. Fifth International Workshop on Multiple Endocrine Neoplasia, 1994, p 3 Karolinska Inst, Stockholm, Sweden.

118. Beldjord C, Desclaux-Arramond F, Raffin-Sanson M, Corvol J-C, De Keyzer Y, Luton J-P, Plouin P-F, Bertagna X: The ret protooncogene in sporadic phaeochromocytomas: Frequent MEN 2-like mutations and new molecular defects. *J Clin Endocrinol Metab* 80:2063, 1995.

119. Eng C, Crossey PA, Mulligan LM, Healey CS, Houghton C, Prowse A, Chew SL, Dahia PLM, O'Riordan JLH, Toledo SPA, Smith DP, Maher ER, Ponder BAJ: Mutations of the ret protooncogene and the Von Hippel Lindau disease tumour suppressor gene in sporadic and syndromic phaeochromocytoma. *J Med Genet* 32:934, 1995.

120. Komminoth P, Kunz EK, Matias-Guiu X, Hiort O, Christensen G, Colomer A, Rother J, Heitz PU: Analysis of ret protooncogene point mutations distinguishes heritable from non-heritable thyroid carcinomas. *Cancer* 76:479, 1995.

121. Lindor NM, Honchel R, Khosla S, Thibodeau SN: Mutations in the ret plrotooncogene in sporadic phaeochromocytomas. *J Clin Endocrinol Metab* 80:627, 1995.

122. Padberg BC, Schroder S, Jochum W, Kastendieck H, Roth J, Heitz PU, Komminoth P: Absence of ret protooncogene point mutations in sporadic hyperplastic and neoplastic lesions of the parathyroid gland. *Am J Pathol* 147:1600, 1995.

123. Eng C, Mulligan LM, Healey CS, Houghton C, Frilling A, Raue F, Thomas GA, Ponder BAJ: Heterogeneous mutation of the RET protooncogene in subpopulations of medullary thyroid carcinoma. *Cancer Res* 56:2167, 1996.

124. Carson EB, McMahon M, Baylin SB, Nelkin BD: Ret gene silencing is associated with Raf-1-induced medullary thyroid carcinoma cell differentiation. *Cancer Res* 55:2048, 1995.

125. Carlomagno F, Salvatore D, Santoro M, de Franciscis V, Quadro L, Panariello L, Colantuoni V, Fusco A: Point mutation of the RET proto-oncogene in the TT human medullary thyroid carcinoma cell line. *Biochem Biophys Res Commun* 207:1022, 1995.

126. Ponder BAJ: Medullary carcinoma of the thyroid, in Peckham M, Pinedo, Veronesi U (eds): *Oxford Textbook of Oncology*, vol 2. Oxford, UK, Oxford Medical Publications, 1996, p 2110.

127. Telenius-Berg M, Berg B, Hamberger B: Impact of screening on prognosis in the multiple endocrine neoplasia type 2 syndromes: Natural history and treatment results in 105 patients. *Henry Ford Hosp Med J* 32:225, 1984.

128. Wells SA, Baylin SB, Leight GS, Dale JK, Dilley WG, Farndon JR: The importance of early diagnosis in patients with hereditary medullary thyroid carcinoma. *Ann Surg* 195:595, 1982.

129. Malletta LE, Blewins T, Jordan PM, Noon GP: Autogenous parathyroid grafts for generalized primary parathyroid hyperplasia: Contrasting outcome in sporadic hyperplasia versus multiple endocrine neoplasia type 1. *Surgery* **101**:738, 1987.

130. Jansson S, Tisell LE, Fjalling M, Lindberg S, Jacobson L, Zacharison BF: Early diagnosis of and surgical strategy for adrenal medullary disease in MEN II gene carriers. *Surgery* **103**:11, 1988.

131. Vasen HFA, van der Feltz M, Raue F, Kruseman AN, Koppeschaar HPF, Pieters G, Seif FJ, Blum WF, Lips CJM: The natural course of multiple endocrine neoplasia type IIb. *Arch Intern Med* **251**:1250, 1992.

132. Samaan NA, Draznin MB, Halpin RE, Bloss RS, Hawkins E, Lewis RA: Multiple endocrine syndrome type IIb in early childhood. *Cancer* **68**:1832, 1991.

CHAPTER 26

Multiple Endocrine Neoplasia Type 1

Stephen J. Marx

1. **Multiple endocrine neoplasia type 1 (MEN1) is an autosomal dominant disorder with endocrine tumors of the parathyroids, the g.i.–endocrine tissues, and the anterior pituitary. Additional associations include foregut carcinoid, facial angiofibromas, and lipomas.**

2. **Most of the tumors are benign and produce symptoms and signs by oversecreting hormones (parathyroid hormone, gastrin, prolactin, etc.). Associated gastrinomas and carcinoid tumors have a high malignant potential.**

3. **The commonest endocrinopathy is primary hyperparathyroidism with several features different from features in sporadic parathyroid adenoma. Hyperparathyroidism in MEN1 is expressed early, 50% of gene carriers express it by age 25. Most MEN1 cases have multiple parathyroid tumors. Hyperparathyroidism can exacerbate the simultaneous Zollinger-Ellison syndrome in MEN1.**

4. **MEN1 is likely a tumor suppressor gene since most MEN1 tumors show loss of heterozygosity (LOH) affecting the normal allele at 11q13, the *MEN1* locus.**

5. **MEN1-associated tumors, when they occur on a sporadic basis, frequently show LOH at 11q13. This suggests indirectly that the MEN1 gene contributes to many sporadic tumors.**

6. **The MEN1 gene was isolated by positional cloning. The encoded protein, "menin," has no signature domains pointing to known interactions. Its function is not known.**

7. **MEN1 mutations have been found in over 90% of MEN1 families and in a similar fraction of cases with sporadic MEN1. Most mutations predict truncation of the protein and are thus likely to cause loss of function. This supports menin's predicted function as a tumor suppressor.**

DEFINITIONS AND HISTORY

Multiple endocrine neoplasia is a broad term that encompasses many distinct disorders. Literally interpreted, it includes all cases and families with endocrine neoplasia in more than one tissue type. Thus it includes cases with two coincidental endocrine neoplasms such as parathyroid adenoma and pituitary microadenoma, and it can include cases with a neoplasm that stimulates another tumor, such as pancreatic islet tumor secreting GHRH, that causes pituitary hyperplasia.

Within this broad definition, multiple endocrine neoplasia type 1 (MEN1) and multiple endocrine neoplasia type 2 (MEN2) stand out as occurring repeatedly in sporadic cases and also within families. The main endocrine expressions of MEN1 are parathyroid tumor, gastro-intestinal endocrine tumors, anterior pituitary tumor, and foregut carcinoid tumor. Nonendocrine expressions include lipoma, facial angiofibroma, and collagenoma (Table 26-1).

The first description of a case with MEN1 is generally attributed to Erdheim.[1] He reported in 1903 the autopsy of a patient with acromegaly, pituitary adenoma, and four enlarged parathyroids. Familial transmission of MEN1 was recognized in 1953–54 by Moldawar[2,3] and Wermer.[4] Subsequently Wermer's syndrome has been an eponym for MEN1. With delineation of gastrinoma[5–7] and prolactinoma[8,9] as clinical entities in 1955 and 1971 respectively, they were almost simultaneously recognized as components of MEN1. In the 1970s and 1980s knowledge about MEN1 advanced with the development of new and improved radioimmunoassays for hormones and other peptides. During these times, features of MEN1 also changed with advances in pharmacology,

Table 26-1 Summary features of multiple endocrine neoplasia type 1 with estimated average penetrance (in parentheses) among cases expressing the *MEN1* gene.

Endocrine features	Non-endocrine features
Primary hyperparathyroidism (90%)	Facial angiofibromas (85%)
Entero-pancreatic	Lipomas (30%)
Gastrinoma (40%)	Collagenomas (70%)
Insulinoma (10%)	
Pancreatic polypeptide or	
nonfunctioning (10%)	
Other—glucagonoma, VIPoma,	
somatostatinoma, etc. (2%)	
Foregut Carcinoid	
Thymic carcinoid (2%)	
Bronchial carcinoid (2%)	
Gastric enterochromaffin-like	
tumor (5%)	
Anterior pituitary	
Prolactinoma (15%)	
Other—growth hormone/prolactin,	
growth hormone, ACTS, etc. (5%)	
Nonsecreting (2%)	

such as acid secretion-blocking drugs for Zollinger-Ellison syndrome[10-13] and dopamine agonists for prolactinoma.[14] Important advances were also made, beginning with total gastrectomy for Zollinger-Ellison syndrome in 1961,[5] with improved pituitary microsurgery, and with use of intraoperative ultrasound to image multiple tumors of pancreas or parathyroids.[15,16]

The genetic etiology for MEN1 has been only recently clarified. Larsson et al. showed in 1988 that the *MEN1* gene was likely a tumor suppressor gene, based on MEN1 tumors showing loss of the normal allele from chromosome 11 MEN1 in tumors.[17] At the same time they reported tight genetic linkage of MEN1 to the *PYGM* locus at 11q13. The *MEN1* gene was cloned in 1997.[18]

CLINICAL ASPECTS

Prevalence

There are no population-based studies of the prevalence of MEN1. Autopsy series have estimated a prevalence of 2.5 per thousand.[19,20] However, biochemical tests have suggested prevalence of 0.01–0.175 per thousand.[21-24]

An alternate estimate can be derived from the fraction of MEN1 among cases with evaluation for single tissue endocrine tumor. Primary hyperparathyroidism is likely to be the main source of MEN1 case ascertainment; the fraction of MEN1 among primary hyperparathyroidism is estimated at 1–18%.[25] The cause for this variable fraction is not known but selection bias is likely. The true fraction is probably 2–3%; this, combined with a population annual incidence of 0.5 per 1,000 for primary hyperparathyroidism,[26] gives an estimate of MEN1 annual incidence of 0.15 per thousand.

Among patients with Zollinger-Ellison syndrome, the prevalence of MEN1 has been 16–38%, much higher than that of MEN1 among sporadic primary hyperparathyroidism.[24,27,28] Among patients with pituitary tumor, the prevalence of MEN1 has been 2.7–3%.[29,30]

Fraction Due to Inherited Factors vs Sporadic Cases

The majority of cases of MEN1 are probably inherited. In a British series, there were 36 sporadic cases versus 220 familial cases among 62 families.[31] In our series (Marx et al. unpublished) there are 40 sporadic cases versus approximately 450 familial cases in 65 families. "Sporadic" cases, of course, may have hereditary MEN1 that has not been recognized.

Diagnostic Criteria

Similar broad diagnostic criteria have been informally used by most groups.[18,31] MEN1 is defined as a case with endocrine tumor (not necessarily simultaneous) in two of the major three tissue systems (parathyroid, g.i.–endocrine, and anterior pituitary). That is to say, carcinoid tumor, lipoma, facial angiofibroma, and other features (Table 26-1) have not traditionally been used for ascertainment. Familial MEN1 is defined as a family that includes at least one case of MEN1 and at least one first degree relative with endocrine tumor in one of the three principal MEN1-associated tissues. It is understood that these criteria will encompass several disorders that are not caused by the *MEN1* gene.

Expressions of MEN1 by Tissue System

Benign and Malignant Neoplasia. An essential feature of MEN1 is that its main expressions are guided by the hormone(s) that are oversecreted. Thus, MEN1 is expressed mainly as hyperparathyroidism, Zollinger-Ellison syndrome, and hyperprolactinemia. The neoplasms in general are small and benign. Only the pituitary tumor, and much less commonly a pancreatic islet tumor, can produce clinical signs through a local mass effect. At the same time MEN1 is a genuine familial cancer syndrome. Gastrinomas, thymic carcinoid, and bronchial carcinoid all are common expressions of MEN1 with a high malignant potential. Some less common expressions (see below) also have malignant potential.

Parathyroid Gland

Primary Hyperparathyroidism as the Commonest Endocrinopathy in MEN1. Primary hyperparathyroidism is the commonest endocrine expression of MEN1[32-36] with 87–100% prevalence among carriers expressing any endocrinopathy (Table 26-1). Among obligate carriers of the *MEN1* gene, approximately 90% will express primary hyperparathyroidism by age 50,[31,37] rare carriers do not express the trait at any age. The prevalences for other endocrinopathies vary widely, depending largely on the methods to test the tissue.

Primary Hyperparathyroidism in MEN1 Differs from in Sporadic Hyperparathyroidism Cases. Most features of primary hyperparathyroidism in MEN1 are similar to those in sporadic primary hyperparathyroidism.[31,38-40] These include a long early asymptomatic stage, generally low morbidity, and rapid amelioration after parathyroidectomy. Typical symptoms and signs include weakness, kidney stone, and back pain. Hypercalcemic crisis[41] or parathyroid cancer[42] is extremely rare. However, the hyperparathyroidism in MEN1 also has important differences from that in sporadic cases (Table 26-2).

Primary hyperparathyroidism begins earlier in MEN1 with 50% of carriers expressing this by age 18–25,[36,37] with recognition as early as age 4.[36] Clinically important primary hyperparathyroidism in MEN1 is rare before age 15. The female: male gender ratio is 1.0 in MEN1 versus 3.0 in sporadic hyperparathyroidism. Primary hyperparathyroidism can exacerbate Zollinger-Ellison (Z.-E.) syndrome (see below) in MEN1 (Figure 26-1). This can influence a decision towards parathyroid surgery for this criterion which is not relevant in sporadic hyperparathyroidism. On the other hand, because of excellent stomach acid control by antisecretory drugs, concommitant Z.-E. syndrome is usually not a sole indication for parathyroid surgery.

Parathyroid gland clinical biology differs in MEN1 and sporadic cases. In sporadic cases there is usually a single parathyroid tumor. In MEN1, multiple glands are usually enlarged, and the enlargement is highly asymmetric.[43,44] Surgical outcomes differ in MEN1 from outcome in sporadic cases. Because of the multiplicity of tumors and the associated occurrence of occasional tumor in unusual location, postoperative persistence of hyperparathyroidism in MEN1 can be 40–60% with inexperienced surgeons[45] and as high as 10% with experienced surgeons.[44-46] The desire to identify all four parathyroid glands and to remove all but part of one results in an increased rate of postoperative hypoparathyroidism, as high as 30%.[44,46,47] While rare in sporadic cases,[48] in MEN1 postoperative late recurrent primary hypoparathyroidism reaches very high rates with time, 50% after 12 years.[45]

Gastro-Intestinal Tissues

Overview. G-I endocrine tumors develop at younger ages in MEN1 than in sporadic cases. The G-I endocrine tumors in MEN1

Table 26-2 Distinguishing features among three categories of primary hyperparathyroidism.

Feature	Sporadic adenoma(s)	Multiple endocrine neoplasia type 1	Familial hypocalciuric hypercalcemia
Percent of hyperparathyroid	94	2	2
Heredity	Sporadic	Autos. dom.	Autos. dom.
Hypercalcemia onset age (yr)	50–60	15–25	0 (at birth)
Sex ratio (F:M)	3:1	1:1	1:1
Calcium in urine	High	High	Normal to low
PTH in serum	High	High	Normal (15% high)
Endocr. tumors outside parathyr.	No	Often	No
Parathyr. glands pathology	Adenoma, often one	Adenoma, multiple	Hyperplasia, mild
Surgical result*			
Immed cure (%)	95%	92%	Below 5%
Persistence (%)	5%	8%	Above 95%
Hypopara (%)	2%	5%	2%
Late recur (%)	2%	Above 50%	NA†

*Surgical results are for cases with appropriate preoperative evaluation and with an experienced parathyroid surgeon. Hypoparathyroidism is considered a "cure."

†B NA = Not applicable, since virtually no operations lead to transient normocalcemia in familial hypocalciuric hypercalcemia.

are usually multiple. Though primary hyperparathyroidism is usually present when the G-I endocrine tumor expresses itself, in a small fraction of cases Zollinger-Ellison syndrome or insulinoma can be expressed first.[49] The G-I endocrine tumors in MEN1 usually present with symptoms of hormone release, rather than symptoms of tumor expansion or metastasis.[50,51] In fact such tumors may be too small to be imaged.[50]

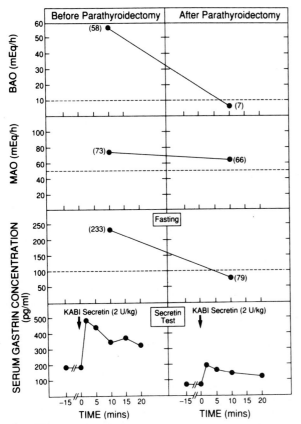

FIG. 26-1 The gastrin-gastric acid axis in a case of MEN1 with Zollinger-Ellison syndrome before and after normalization of serum calcium through parathyroidectomy. Successful parathyroidectomy caused remission in typical expressions of gastrinoma. Panels show basal acid output (BAO), maximal acid output after pentagrastrin (MAO), and gastrin fasting or after intravenous secretin. Dashed lines are upper limits of normal (53).

Hormone Oversecretion and Storage in Tumors. Among the G.I.-endocrine tumors in MEN1, gastrinoma is expressed most commonly at up to 54%.[41,50–52] Insulinoma is expressed second most commonly in FMEN1, as often as 21%.[41,50] Glucagonoma, VIPoma, GRIFoma, intestinal carcinoid, gastric enterochromaffin like cell tumor (ECLoma) and somatostatinoma each have been much less frequent. Furthermore, MEN1 patients can express more than one G.I. endocrine tumor. Conversely, MEN1 occurs in approximately 20% of cases with Z.E. syndrome, 4% with insulinoma, and 33% with GRFoma.[53] Nonfunctional endocrine tumors are a major component of MEN1. Though only one tumor may hypersecrete a hormone and cause symptoms and signs, typically there are many associated pancreatic islet tumors. While these might synthesize hormonal peptides, they do not oversecrete them. Still they have the potential to cause subsequent oversecretion and/or cancer.[54]

Histologic evaluations of the MEN1 pancreas from surgical specimens have shown multiple tumors in about 50%,[55,56] but diffuse micronodules (diameter <0.5 cm) have been found in all.[55] There is disagreement about whether or not there are important components of diffuse islet hyperplasia or nesidioblastosis (islets budding from ducts). The rate of positivity of immunostaining in 201 macro or micronodules was pancreatic peptide (26%), glucagon (24%), insulin (23%), gastrin (4%), and no hormone (18%) (48); that study was done before recognition of the frequent extrapancreatic locations of gastrinomas in MEN1.[50,55]

Gastrinoma. Zollinger-Ellison syndrome is a symptom complex resulting from gastrinomas. Gastrinomas originate in the pancreatic islets or proximal duodenum.[6,57–59] The initial syndrome was the triad of (a) non-beta islet cell tumor of the pancreas, (b) gastric acid hypersecretion, and (c) severe peptic ulcers of the stomach and small intestine. With increasing awareness of the disease and with ready availability of acid blocking drugs, the disease is now seen in milder and different forms (see below).[51,52,60] All the usual features of Zollinger-Ellison syndrome result from gastrin's ability to stimulate secretion of acid from the stomach.

Gastrinomas in sporadic and familial MEN1 are mostly in the "gastrinoma triangle," the duodenum or pacreatic head.[50–52,61–64] This location contrasts with sporadic gastrinomas, of which 40–80% occurs in the pancreas.[52,58,62,63,65] Furthermore, while most sporadic gastrinomas are solitary and large, those in MEN1 are multiple, small, and submucosal.[57] MEN1 gastrinoma versus sporadic has been suggested to have lesser[52,58,66] or similar malignancy.[52,58,67,68] Apparently milder malignancy can result from earlier ascertainment; however, it is clear that metastatic gastrinoma can occur,[52,58,69] and it can dominate clinical management.[70]

Most gastrinomas in MEN1 occur after age 40.[31,50,52,58] Occasionally Zollinger-Ellison syndrome is the earliest expression of MEN1,[49] but it has not occurred during childhood in MEN1.

Abdominal pain is the commonest symptom, and symptoms of g.i. reflux occur in up to two thirds of cases. Some patients do not show these symptoms despite high acid output.[53] Diarrhea can be associated; in 10–30% of cases it is the sole symptom or sign. The diarrhea is a direct consequence of acid oversecretion with associated (a) high fluid secretion into bowel, (b) inactivation of pancreatic enzymes, and (c) mucosal ulceration.[51,52,69,71,72] Whereas atypical ulcer location was once common in Zollinger-Ellison syndrome, current practices recognize ulcers in locations similar to idiopathic peptic disease.[51,52]

Gastrinoma should be evaluated in any MEN1 patient with symptoms listed above. Furthermore, fasting gastrin should be measured periodically in a symptomatic MEN1 cases above age 40. The most useful tests for diagnosis are acid output, fasting gastrin, and stimulated gastrin. Because of widespread availability, endoscopy is often used as a substitute for acid measurements.

The upper limit for basal acid output (BAO) in the absence of acid-reducing surgery is 15 mEq/h for both genders.[51,52,73] This criterion alone is insufficient for diagnosis. There are many false positives (such as some cases of idiopathic peptic disease, a much commoner disorder)[51,52] and some false negatives (exemplified by the post-parathyroidectomy state)[74] (Figure 26-1). Maximal acid output (MAO) after subcutaneous pentagastrin (6 µg/kg) correlates with parietal cell mass.[51,52,61] However the variability of this response and of the BAO/MAO ratio give them little diagnostic use.[51,52,69,71] Unfortunately, gastric acid output measurements are not widely available. Documentation of fasting gastric pH above 3.0 in a patient not taking acid blocking medications can exclude Zollinger-Ellison syndrome. In a case with hypergastrinemia, this can establish hypo- or achlorhydria (Table 26-3).

The clinical diagnosis of gastrinoma is dependent upon documentation of dysregulated hypersecretion of gastrin. Virtually all cases have high fasting gastrin.[75,76] With the widespread use of acid-blocking drugs, drug-induced hypergastrinemia has become the most common condition to exclude[77] (Table 26-3). Another consideration is hypochlorhydria, which is very common among patients with sporadic primary hyperparathyroidism (another state concentrated among women beyond age 50). Another consideration, specific to MEN1, is the interaction of gastrinoma and hyperparathyroidism. Zollinger-Ellison syndrome can be diminished or even enter remission after successful parathyroidectomy (Figure 26-1).[77] However, it is not known if parathyroidectomy slows the growth of the gastrinomas.

Two separate gastrin measurements should be made as values can fluctuate. Most cases of Z.-E. syndrome show a gastrin above 1000 pg/ml, more than 10-fold above normal. With gastric acid below 3.0, the diagnosis is established. When the diagnosis is uncertain, provocative testing should be done. Stimulants have included secretin, calcium infusion, and a standardized meal. The most effective stimulus is secretin. An abnormal response is a positive change of serum gastrin greater than 200 pg/ml.[51,52,78]

Once the diagnosis has been established, management must combine acid control, which may be accomplished pharmacologically, and tumor evaluation. The mainstay of tumor evaluation is imaging with radioactive octreotide. This agent is effective in distinguishing local from metastatic gastrinoma.[79–81]

Insulinoma. Insulinoma is expressed in 10–20% of cases of FMEN1.[34,82] Mean age of onset is younger in MEN1 than in sporadic cases (age 29 vs 45).[31] Though they are associated with multiple islet tumors, their high surgical cure rate suggests that (a) the insulinoma syndrome in MEN1 usually results from one hypersecreting adenoma and (b) that adenoma is usually large and often the largest islet tumor in that patient.[83–86]

Commonest expression of insulinoma is neuroglycopenia, often worst on fasting and relieved by eating sweets. Once suspected, hypoglycemia should be documented during symptoms and during fasting. Other possible etiologies should be excluded including prescribed medications, surreptitious use of hypoglycemic agents, wasting, hypoadrenalism, and growth hormone deficiency (in children). The most reliable test is a supervised fast. Most cases show hypoglycemia (sugar <40 mg/dl) and symptoms by 48 hours, but apparently negative tests should be carried to 72 hours. Glucose, insulin, C-peptide, and proinsulin fraction should be measured at the time of hypoglycemia.[87] The single most useful test is an insulin concentration above 6 µU/ml at the time of hypoglycemia. This establishes insulin mediation of hypoglycemia; however, it does not exclude surreptitious use of insulin or sulfonylureas or hypoglycemia caused by antibodies against the insulin receptor.

Treatment of insulinoma in MEN1 is surgery. Insulinoma in MEN1 is usually benign. Approximately 15% of MEN1 insulinomas recur late after surgery; this could reflect malignancy, an independent tumor or, incomplete resection of the primary. Because of the frequent association with multiple non-functioning islet tumors, it is desirable to identify the approximate location of insulin hypersecretion before resection. This can be done most effectively by selective arteriography with calcium infusion.[88] Transhepatic venous sampling has high yield, but it is not widely available and it has substantial potential for morbidity.[89] Individual tumors are often small and are best localized with intraoperative ultrasound.[15,90] Noninvasive imaging methods, including octreotide, have low sensitivity for insulinoma, based on experience with sporadic insulinoma.[89]

Glucagonoma. Glucagonomas are islet tumors, causing a syndrome of a specific dermatitis, weight loss, glucose intolerance, and anemia.[92–94] The rash is termed migratory necrolytic erythema.[95,96] Glucagonoma is rare in MEN1 (~3%), and glucagonoma patients rarely have MEN1. Most cases occur after age 40. They are usually pancreatic body or tail, large at presentation[92,97] with 50–80% showing metastases at presentation.[93,94] Glucose intolerance characteristically predates recognition of gluca-

Table 26-3 Causes of fasting hypergastrinemia.

With deficient gastric acid production	With gastric acid production
Medications	Retained gastric antrum syndrome
Histamine H_2-receptor antagonists	Small bowel resection
Blockers of stomach acid pump	Chronic gastric outlet obstruction
Chronic renal failure	Antral G-cell hyperplasia or hyperfunction
Atrophic gastritis (includes pernicious anemia)	Gastrinoma
Postvagotomy/gastric resection	

gonoma by 5 years.[94] Glucose intolerance in MEN1 is more often idiopathic or secondary to Cushing's syndrome.

VIPoma. VIPomas are g.i.–endocrine tumors that oversecrete VIP. They cause severe watery diarrhea ("pancreatic cholera," a misnomer), hypokalemia, and hypochlorhydria.[98–102] It is sometimes called Verner-Morrison syndrome and sometimes called WDHA syndrome for *w*atery *d*iarrhea, *h*ypokalemia, and *a*chlorhydria. Over 80% are in the pancreas,[103,104] but several occur in intestinal carcinoid or pheochromocytoma.[105] In children (age 2–4), the tumor is usually an extrapancreatic ganglioneuroma or ganglioneuroblastoma[104] and is not associated with MEN1. Just as glucagonomas, VIPomas in adults present usually after age 40 and are usually large and metastatic. Associated hypercalcemia in up to 50% of cases may be caused by tumor secretion of parathyroid hormone-related peptide but this must be distinguished from associated primary hyperparathyroidism in MEN1.

GRFoma. Growth hormone releasing factor (GRF) can be oversecreted by a tumor, a GRFoma. This is a rare tumor that stimulates the pituitary to release excessive growth hormone.[106,107] Approximately one third of GRFomas are associated with MEN1 (excluding their downstream stimulation of the pituitary).[108–110] GRFomas occur in the lung (53%), pancreas (30%), or small intestine (10%). They are often large and metastatic at presentation.[108,111] GHRH is a 44 amino acid peptide. Its oversecretion results in somatotroph hyperplasia and growth hormone excess. Most cases of growth hormone excess (with or without MEN1) are caused by primary tumor of the pituitary. GRFoma is diagnosed by finding growth hormone excess and high blood levels of GHRH.

Somatostatinoma. Somatostatin-secreting tumor causes a syndrome of mild diabetes mellitus, gall bladder disease, weight loss and anemia.[112,113] There is a frequent association of this rare tumor with MEN1 or with MEN2, but its prevalence in an MEN1 population seems very low. Most somatostatinomas are in the pancreatic head.[114,115] Fewer are in the proximal duodenum or ampulla of Vater. At presentation most are large and metastatic. Commonly somatostatin is the "second" hormone secreted by a tumor.[115] Somatostatin is a 14 amino acid peptide with multiple inhibitory effects on the GI tract. It inhibits release of many hormones, including insulin, gastrin, and growth hormone. It decreases stomach acid secretion, decreases bile flow and gall bladder contractility, it decreases pancreatic enzyme and fluid secretion, it decreases absorption of lipid, D-xylose, vitamin B_{12}, and folate.[116] All these actions contribute to its presentations.

PPomas and Nonfunctional Pancreatic Endocrine Tumors. PPomas are pancreatic tumors that oversecrete pancreatic polypeptide but do not cause a recognizable syndrome.[83,117–120]. Nonfunctional tumors, may overproduce a peptide, but do not secrete enough to cause a recognizable syndrome.[50,83,114,118] These tumors, if they cause symptoms, do so by local growth or by metastatic growth. They are probably the commonest tumors in MEN1.[41,54,72,119] But because most do not cause symptoms, this has received limited evaluation.[54] The finding of multiple pancreatic islet tumors is a strong predictor of MEN1.[55,56] If these tumors cause symptoms, these tumors are usually in the pancreatic head, large, and malignant.

Carcinoid Tumor of Foregut

Bronchus or Thymus Carcinoid. Carcinoid tumors occur in derivatives of foregut, midgut, or hindgut. Carcinoid tumor in MEN1 is in foregut derivatives (bronchi, thymus, stomach, pancreas,

duodenum).[121] This contrasts with sporadic carcinoid which is predominantly hindgut in origin.[122] Unlike the equal sex distribution of sporadic bronchial carcinoid, that in MEN1 is 4:1 female predominant. Thymic carcinoids are 90% male in sporadic cases and in MEN1.[123]

Common presentations of carcinoid are through mass effect or incidental to chest imaging or thymectomy (for primary hyperparathyroidism in MEN1). Carcinoid tumors of the bronchus or thymus rarely cause the carcinoid syndrome or secrete serotonin. They occasionally secrete histamine which is converted to 5-hydroxyindoleacetic acid and measurable in urine. Occasionally they cause an atypical carcinoid syndrome with facial flushing, lacrimation, headache, and bronchoconstriction; the biochemical cause is not known. Bronchial and thymic carcinoid can oversecrete endocrine peptides including ACTH,[124,125] GHRH,[126] calcitonin and others. Sporadic carcinoid tumors are often malignant, and this has been found also in thymic carcinoid in MEN1.[123]

Gastric ECLomas. Histamine-secreting enterochromaffin-like cells (ECL cells) are prominent among the endocrine cells of the human gastric oxyntic mucosa. In sporadic cases they produce tumors unrelated to hypergastrinemia. In MEN1, ECLomas are associated with hypergastrinemia.[127–129] It is thought that hypergastrinemia is associated with ECL cell stimulation. This has been seen in animal models and in pernicious anemia. However, ECLomas are uncommon in association with sporadic gastrinoma.[58,127,128] Gastric ECLomas have no associated hormonal syndrome, and their natural history is unknown. They have recently been recognized in up to 15% of MEN1 cases incidental to endoscopies for gastrinoma.[130]

G.I. Tract Carcinoid Tumor. Carcinoid tumors are structurally indistinguishable from other enteropancreatic tumors; thus, the term carcinoid tumor has been applied to all of these tumors.[50,58] Carcinoid of the midgut or hindgut is common in the general population but rare in MEN1. In fact, there seems to be no real association of these latter carcinoids with MEN1. Carcinoid of the terminal ileum often metastasizes to the liver, secretes serotonin, and causes the carcinoid syndrome.[51,122,130.5]

Carcinoid Tumor Syndrome. Carcinoid tumors can secrete a variety of bioactive peptides and small molecules.[51,122,130.5] Carcinoid tumor syndrome is a complex thought to result from these products. It includes episodes of flushing, diarrhea, abdominal cramping, wheezing, dyspnea, and palpitations. Blood pressure falls rather than rises. It usually arises when midgut carcinoid tumor metastasizes to the liver. It can arise from bronchial carcinoid without metastases. Most foregut carcinoids in MEN1 do not produce this syndrome.

Anterior Pituitary Tumor. Symptoms and signs of pituitary tumor are evident in 10–30% of MEN1 cases. The symptoms and signs of pituitary tumor have similar age, sex, and hormone distributions to those in tumors not associated with MEN1.[31,35] The sex ratio favors women because the majority of tumors are prolactinomas (40–75%) with approximately 10% secreting prolactin and growth hormone, 10% growth hormone only, and 5% ACTH.[131] Oversecretion of LH/FSH or TSH are less common. 5% are hormone non-secreting and important as they present by mass effect (hypopituitarism, pituitary apoplexy, visual compromise).

Aside from mass effect, prolactinoma is recognized as galactorrhea amenorrhea, and/or infertility in women. Hypogonadism may occur in men. Biochemical diagnosis depends on fasting prolactin above 300 ng/ml. Milder elevations occur too but are hard to distinguish from loss of inhibition through stalk compression.

Imaging is a useful supplement for diagnosis. Excellent images can be obtained with gadolinium-enhanced magnetic resonance imaging. As for prolactinoma, the features of other hormone secreting tumors are similar in MEN1 and sporadic cases.

Other Tissue Features of MEN1

Thyroid Neoplasms. Thyroid adenoma has long been recognized as an occasional association in MEN1,[33] but no detailed analysis has established a significant connection.

Primary Adrenocortical Neoplasms. Rare cases of MEN1 have shown hypercortisolism or hyperaldosteronism.[33,132] One analysis of adrenal cortical enlargement in MEN1 indicated frequent silent enlargement.[132,133] Adrenal cancer has been reported.[133,134]

Lipoma. While a common neoplasm, lipoma seems especially common in MEN1 at 20–30% of cases.[135] They may occur anywhere, single or multiple. Large visceral lipomas can be noted by imaging or at laparotomy.

Skin Lesions. One survey of 32 MEN1 cases showed multiple facial angiofibromas in 88%.[135] These were clinically and histologically identical to the lesions in tuberous sclerosis. Confetti-like hypopigmented macules (6%) and multiple gingival papules (6%) were another finding that had previously been associated with tuberous sclerosis. Other unusual findings included collagenomas in 72%.

Intrafamilial Homogeneity of MEN1

Prolactinoma Variant. One or two unusual expressions of MEN1 sometimes occur in a small kindred. These may be random events. Typically, large kindreds are essential for efforts to recognize an unusual phenotype. Even then, atypical methods of ascertainment are one potential source of bias. Three large MEN1 kindreds (9–83 affected members) have shown high frequency of prolactinoma (35–65%) but low frequency of gastrinoma (2.5–11%).[136–139] The largest family has also shown 14% carcinoid tumors.[140]

In an extraordinarily large MEN1 pedigree from Tasmania, prolactinoma was found commonly (50%) in 2 branches but uncommonly in others. Though gastrinoma was not included in the analysis, the observations were used to suggest that the "prolactinoma phenotype" required a second mutation other than that causing MEN1.[141]

Other Variants of MEN1.

Hyperparathyroidism Variant. Several kindreds, reported initially as isolated familial hyperparathyroidism, subsequently expressed features of MEN1.[34] However, one large kindred showed only minimal features of MEN1 on followup,[34,142] and another showed likely linkage to 11q13 with lod score of 2.1.[143] There are also types of familial primary hyperparathyroidism not caused by the MEN1 gene (see below).

Insulinoma Variant. Several MEN1 kindreds showed disproportional prevalence of insulinoma with little gastrinoma.[34,36]

Acromegaly Variant. In one kindred, two brothers and an uncle showed acromegaly.[144] Haplotype analysis showed the same 11q13 haplotype in all 3 and in their unaffected father. Tumor LOH analyses in the children showed that two tumors had 11q13 LOH affecting the allele from the unaffected mother. This kindred

does not meet the definition of MEN1 but seems likely an expression of germline mutation in the *MEN1* gene.

Cancer Variant. Most gastrinomas are multiple in MEN1.[57] A high, though undetermined, fraction have metastasized by the time they cause symptoms. In some kindreds gastrinomas have seemed particularly aggressive.[36] This question requires additional study.

Treatment of MEN1

Treatment of the multiple expressions of MEN1 is not covered here. Suffice it to say that treatment can be complex and expensive. In general, each hormone oversecreting tumor must be handled as an independent disorder requiring pharmacologic or surgical management.[145] Mild expressions (such as mild hyperparathyroidism) may only require periodic monitoring while malignant expressions may prove refractory to most measures.

DIFFERENTIAL DIAGNOSIS

As pleiomorphic as it is, MEN1 has a potentially long list of conditions that must be distinguished from it. Conditions to be covered here are those that are the most relevant clinically and also those that may have special relevance with regard to metabolic pathway disturbed.

Sporadic Multiple Endocrine Neoplasia

Any combination of endocrine neoplasia in more than one tissue is multiple endocrine neoplasia. Some such cases, might be expressions of MEN1 germline mutation.

Pancreatic islet tumors can cause secondary endocrine tumors, when the primary tumor secretes "ectopically" ACTH[146,147] or growth hormone releasing hormone.[148]

Many reports, based on single cases, are probably random coincidences.[149] There has been an association between primary hyperparathyroidism and nonmedullary thyroid cancer,[150,151] perhaps independent of the association attributable to radiation (see below). There have been other endocrine tumors with prolactinoma[152–155] or with acromegaly.[156,157] Some of the more intriguing cases have combined components of MEN1 and MEN2 within a single patient.[158–171]

A relation between radiation and thyroid neoplasia has been long recognized.[172,173] More recently a relation between radiation and parathyroid neoplasia has also been recognized. Parathyroid and thyroid neoplasia, when they coexist, are often a consequence of prior radiation exposure.[173–183] The thyroid neoplasms may be uni- or multifocal and benign or malignant; the parathyroid tumors are almost always benign and sometimes multiple.

The McCune-Albright syndrome is a complex of polyostotic fibrous dysplasia, cafe-au-lait skin pigmentation and any among the following endocrine disorders: sexual precocity, hyperthyroidism, gigantism, growth hormone oversecretion, and adrenal hyperfunction.[184] This is caused by an activating mutation in Gs-alpha, a subunit of the stimulatory G-protein involved in signal transduction.[185] The mutation is apparently lethal in the germ line but it can occur early in ontogeny so that the carrier is chimeric. The mutation appears to cause tumor in tissues where overproduction of cyclic AMP leads to cell proliferation.[184]

Familial Endocrine Neoplasia

Disorders Affecting Multiple Endocrine Organs

Multiple Endocrine Neoplasia Type 2. MEN2[187] consists of neoplasms of thyroid C-cells, adrenal medulla, and parathyroid. A distinct variant, MEN2b has low penetrance for parathyroid tumors but has ganglioneuromas, submucosal neuromas, and a marfanoid habitus. MEN2 is caused by mutation of the *ret* gene on chromosome 10. It encodes the catalytic subunit of a membrane bound tyrosine kinase whose normal ligand is glial cell derived growth factor. The mutations in MEN2 are in focused regions of the *ret* gene, and all are believed to be activating mutations. Because MEN2 rarely presents as hyperparathyroidism alone, MEN2 is not difficult to distinguish from MEN1.

Carney Syndrome. Carney syndrome is a rare autosomal dominant complex of myxomas (cardiac, cutaneous, and breast), pigmented skin lesions, and endocrine tumors.[188,189] The endocrinopathies include pigmented bilateral adrenal lesions, acromegaly, and sertoli or leydig cell tumor of testis.[190] The disorder is usually linked to 2p.[191]

Von Hippel-Lindau Disease. This disorder is characterized by hemangioblastoma of the CNS, retinal angiomatosis, renal cell carcinoma, visceral cysts and pheochromocytoma.[192] Pancreatic cysts and pancreatic islet cell tumors are associated. The islet cell tumors occur in 10%. They are usually nonfunctional and can be benign or malignant. Patients with this disease also rarely show other endocrine tumor such as carcinoid, prolactinoma, and medullary thyroid cancer.[193] The *vhl* gene functions by a tumor suppressor gene mechanism, is at 3p, and has been cloned.[194] It encodes a protein that interacts with several other proteins important in the cell cycle.[195]

Neurofibromatosis Type 1. Neurofibromatosis type 1 causes neural disturbances including cafe-au-lait spots, neurofibromas, benign and malignant tumors of the nervous system, Lisch nodules of the iris, and mental retardation.[196] Pheochromocytoma occurs in about 1%. Hyperparathyroidism, usually single adenoma, has been associated at least 11 times.[197] Rare associations include duodenal somatostatinoma,[198] adrenocortical adenoma.[199,200] The *nf1* gene is on 17q, functions as a tumor suppressor, and has been cloned.[201] It encodes a protein, neurofibromin, with GTPase activating protein (GAP)-like domain that downregulates GTP-bound ras.

Disorders Affecting One Endocrine Organ

Familial Hypocalciuric Hypercalcemia. The hereditary disorder most often requiring differentiation from MEN1 is familial hypocalciuric hyperclcemia (FHH), also termed familial benign hypercalcemia. This is an autosomal dominant form of hypercalcemia with a prevalence similar to that of MEN1. Features which distinguish it from MEN1 are highlighted above (Table 26-2).[202] In FHH, hypercalcemia is present at birth, and its level remains stable throughout life. In FHH urine calcium is usually in the normal range; as a result, there is no increased incidence of calcium urolithiasis. The most useful diagnostic index in hypercalcemic patients is the ratio of calcium clearance over creatinine clearance. Values in FHH are below 0.01 while those in typical primary hy-

perparathyroidism are above. PTH values are typically normal in FHH.[203] The parathyroid glands are normal to minimally enlarged, and subtotal parathyroidectomy is followed by persistent hypercalcemia in FHH. FHH is usually or always a disturbance in calcium recognition by the parathyroid cell and perhaps the renal tubular cell. Most familial cases are linked to 3q and can be attributed to mutations in a parathyroid cell surface calcium-sensing receptor.[204] Occasional cases are linked to 19p or other loci.[205,206] FHH cases with homozygous mutation at 3q express extremely severe neonatal primary hyperparathyroidism with severe enlargement of all parathyroid glands.[207,208]

Familial Hyperparathyroidism and Jaw Tumors. Several families have been described with parathyroid tumors and jaw tumors.[209] The parathyroid tumors sometimes have a micro- or macrocystic appearance.[210] Parathyroid cancer has occurred also in many of these families. Other features clearly associated in one large family are Wilms tumor and nephroblastoma.[211] Seven of these families have shown linkage to 1q21-32, and there was LOH about this locus in renal hamartomas but not in parathyroid tumors.[211,212]

Two large families with autosomal dominant hyperparathyroidism plus parathyroid cancer[213,214] might express this disorder but have not been tested for linkage to 1q.

Familial Hyperparathyroidism. Isolated familial hyperparathyroidism has been described in many, mostly small kindreds. Some undoubtedly have MEN1,[34] others have FHH, while others have different disorders. Most have been consistent with autosomal dominant transmission, with one showing a recessive mode.[215] Unusual features in some families have been early age of onset, severe hypercalcemia, and occasionally tumor of one parathyroid gland.[216,217] In one report, 3 or 4 tumors representing different kindreds, showed LOH at 13q, raising the possibility of germ line mutation in a tumor suppressor gene in that region.[218]

Familial Pancreatic Islet Tumors. There are two reports of familial insulinoma without other endocrinopathy.[219,220] In each kindred, this was seen in a father and a daughter.

Familial Pituitary Tumors. Acromegaly alone has been seen in several families.[144,221–225] Haplotype and tumor LOH studies in one family suggested that the tumor might be an expression of MEN1 germline mutation.[144] Four families have had prolactinomas in first degree relatives.[226]

Familial Carcinoid Tumors. Occasionally carcinoid tumors show familial clustering independent of MEN1.[227–231] The tumors have been in the terminal ileum or appendix (five families) or in the duodenum (one family).

CELLULAR EXPRESSIONS OF MEN1

MEN1 Growth Factor

A growth factor was detected in MEN1 plasma when incubated with cultured parathyroid cells.[232–235] High levels were independent of age among adults.[236] Preliminary data pointed to high levels even in young, asymptomatic MEN1 gene carriers.[237] This growth factor shared many features with FGF-2 or basic fibroblast growth factor including size, immunologic epitopes, and reactivity towards endothelium.[238,239] The FGF family is small, but all members are potent mitogens.[240] The MEN1 growth activity could be tumor-derived. However, parathyroid tumors have apparently been excluded as the source.[235] Pituitary tumor is a possible source since the circulating growth activity falls after treatment of pituitary tumors by surgery or medication.[241]

Any role for a circulating growth factor in MEN1 remains unknown. It could be an unimportant byproduct of the neoplastic process. It could be an autocrine or paracrine factor that escapes into the circulation. It could be a circulating factor that acts on one or more target tissues to help initiate the neoplastic process. Since the *MEN1* gene is a tumor suppressor, it was recognized that the MEN1 growth factor could not be the product of this gene. However, it remains possible that overexpression of the MEN1 growth factor is an early consequence of inactivation of one or both copies of the MEN1 gene.

Chromosomal Instability

Several studies have suggested increased frequency of chromosomal breakage in MEN1. Cultured lymphocytes in FMEN1 showed increased frequency of gaps and chromatid-type abnormalities.[242] Lymphocytes also showed increased chromosomal breakage.[243] Lastly, another group found that cultured lymphocytes and cultured fibroblasts from FMEN1 cases showed increased chromosomal instability.[243.5]

GENETIC LOCI

Hereditary Patterns

Genetic Linkage

Near Homogeneity. Larsson first reported genetic linkage of MEN1 in four Swedish kindreds to *PYGM* (muscle phosphorylase locus) at 11q13 in 1988.[17] This was confirmed in a single large American kindred, with MEN1 linked to *INT-2* at 11q13.[244] Subsequently many MEN1 kindreds have shown similar linkage to several probes at 11q13. The kindreds have been in Japan,[245] Asia,[246] Finland,[247] North America,[248] plus England, France, Tasmania, and Sweden.[249] A workshop-based survey of 87 families (including many of those cited above), suggested that the trait was linked to 11q13 in all kindreds evaluated to that point.[250]

Prolactinoma Variant. The largest kindred with the prolactinoma variant of MEN1 is located almost solely in Newfoundland, Canada. That variant has been termed MEN1$_{Burin}$, after the Burin Peninsula where most live.[137] Linkage of MEN1 to 11q13 was demonstrated in that kindred.[251] Furthermore, a common founder for the four apparently separate families with MEN1$_{Burin}$ was suggested by finding linkage to the same allele of *PYGM* in each family.

Locus Heterogeneity. Subsequently one large kindred meeting the criteria of MEN1 provided evidence for locus heterogeneity, since their MEN1 trait was not linked to 11q13.[252] That kindred had several features that would be unusual for MEN1. In generation 1 there was a case of primary hyperparathyroidism. In generation 2 there were (a) a case with acromegaly, (b) a case with acromegaly and possible hyperparathyroidism, and (c) as asymptomatic carrier. In generation 3 there was a case with prolactinoma. Screening suggested that other members might express the trait in mild forms. Linkage analysis of affected cases excluded 11q13.

Rare Situations

Twins. MEN1 was described in a pair of identical twins. Their disease expressions differed though not strikingly.[253] At age 25 both had hyperparathyroidism and prolactinoma. One also had gastrinoma and Cushing's disease. Undoubtedly other twins have been seen in the accumulated experience. The stochastic nature of the tumors makes inter-individual variability likely.

Homozygotes. A sibship was reported in which apparently unrelated parents each were likely heterozygotes for MEN1.[254] Linkage analysis suggested that two of three siblings were homozgotes (double heterozygotes) for MEN1. Their features of MEN1 were not unusually severe, though both (a male and a female) had unexplained infertility. Another sibship includes two parents with the MEN1$_{Burin}$, prolactinoma variant of MEN1.[137] They had two children. One seemed unaffected, and a daughter expressed galactorrhea at 23 (presumed prolactinoma) and died at age 30 of an invasive thymic carcinoid without expressing hyperparathyroidism. Her MEN1 allele status was not known.

Sporadic MEN1

There have been many case reports of sporadic MEN1 cases.[33] Some have two, three or more features of MEN1. Many such reports represent coincidental occurrence of two common diseases, such as parathyroid adenoma and prolactinoma. Many others, however, are likely expressions of the *MEN1* gene (see below, *MEN1* germline mutations among sporadic cases).

Endocrine tumor in a single tissue system is also a predictable expression of the *MEN1* gene. This has not been possible to test until the *MEN1* gene had been isolated. In the near future *MEN1* mutation will be explored in sporadic primary hyperparathyroidism (particularly that caused by multiple parathyroid tumors), sporadic Zollinger-Ellison syndrome, and sporadic pituitary tumor.

11q13 Loss of Heterozygosity

MEN1 Tumors and Tissues

Tumors. Larsson reported loss of alleles from the copy of chromosome 11, inherited from the unaffected parent, in two MEN1 insulinomas.[17] This led to their prediction that the *MEN1* gene would be a tumor suppressor gene or function by a sequential gene inactivation mechanism ("two-hit hypothesis").[255,256] Subsequently, depending on the probes used, loss of heterozygosity has been shown to be frequent in MEN1 tumors of the parathyroids,[257–262] approaching 100% of tumors following microdissection.[263,264] 11q13 LOH has also been found in 85% of nongastrinoma pancreatic islet tumors[265] and in 40% of gastrinomas.[265] Fewer MEN1 tumors of pituitary, carcinoid, and lipoma have been tested, but approximately 50% of each type show 11q13 LOH.[266] Adrenal cortex shows generally silent bilateral enlargement in about a third of MEN1 cases; 11q13 LOH was not found.[132]

Even within MEN1, inactivation of both copies of the *MEN1* gene is not necessarily sufficient for tumor development. A study of MEN1 tumors has suggested involvement of other oncogenes. In particular there was 1p LOH in 21% of MEN1 parathyroids.[267] There has been no extensive survey to determine the full extent of other genes that may cooperate in development of these neoplasms.

Angiofibroma. Three MEN1 angiofibromas did not show 11q13 LOH.[266] It is notable that two angiofibromas in tuberous sclerosis also did not show LOH at either of the two TSC disease loci.[268] Both diseases are associated with tumors that show LOH, but it is not clear that the angiofibromas are neoplasms. On the other hand, if they are neoplasms, they may have a large stromal/fibrous component, and the neoplastic component may not have been sufficiently cleared from normal tissue admixture to allow LOH to be recognized. 11q13 LOH was also not found in an angiomyolipoma and in an esophageal leiomyoma in MEN1.[266]

Sporadic Tumors

Endocrine Tumors. In general sporadic tumors have shown a lower frequency of 11q13 LOH than the same tumors in MEN1, suggesting that mutation of the *MEN1* gene may contribute often to these sporadic tumors and also that other oncogenes play an even more important role than in MEN1.[269] Twenty to sixty percent of sporadic parathyroid tumors show 11q13 LOH.[218,257,259,261] 11q13 LOH has been found in 19% of sporadic insulinoma[265] and in 45% of sporadic gastrinoma, this latter being a similar incidence to that in MEN1 gastrinoma in the same study.[265] Analyses on smaller numbers of sporadic islet tumors have found similar frequencies of 11q13 LOH.[259,270] Sporadic pituitary tumors have shown variable LOH, perhaps relating to the quality of the tissue and of the probes available: 3% (selectively high LOH for prolactinoma?),[259] 33% in somatotropinomas,[271] 15–30% similarly distributed among 88 nonfunctioning, growth hormone, prolactin, and ACTH.[272] One large analysis found approximately 30% 11q13 LOH in invasive pituitary tumors versus 3% in noninvasive.[273] The highest rate of 11q13 LOH among sporadic tumors has been reported at 78% among carcinoids.[274] In this series, 11q13 LOH was found similarly in carcinoids of foregut, midgut, and hindgut. One report found 14% 11q13 LOH in benign and malignant follicular tumors of the thyroid but not in papillary tumors.[275] Thirty-five percent of aldosteronomas showed 11q13 LOH.[276]

Uremic Parathyroids. Renal failure causes a multifactorial enlargement of the parthyroid glands (secondary hyperparathyroidism). Occasionally, the process becomes sufficiently dysregulated as to resist suppression and occasionally to cause hypercalcemia (tertiary hyperparathyroidism). In either secondary or tertiary hyperparathyroidism, occasionally surgical removal of portions of the parathyroids is the best treatment. Three studies of these abnormal tissues have found that they sometimes contain monoclonal components.[218,277,278] 11q13 LOH was found in 0–16%.

Non-Endocrine tumors. 11q13 LOH has been found in several tumors without known relation to MEN1. This includes in situ and invasive breast cancer[279,280] and cervical cancer.[281,282]

MEN1 GENE

Method of Discovery

Positional Candidates. The search for the *MEN1* gene was accelerated by Larsson's finding that it was linked to 11q13 and that it was likely to be a tumor suppressor gene, since MEN1 tumors showed LOH about this locus.[17] In the ensuing years, the candidate interval was gradually narrowed somewhat by identifying kindred members with important meiotic recombinations between *MEN1* and nearby loci.[248,249,283] In addition, several "positional candidate" genes,[284] which had been mapped to this interval, were tested for mutations and excluded as the *MEN1* gene, including *FAU*,[285] *phospholipase C beta*,[286] and *REL A*.[187] In retrospect, it is evident that testing of positional candidates could not have uncovered the *MEN1* gene at that time.

Positional Cloning. Identification of the *MEN1* gene was achieved by positional cloning, with a combination of methods.[18] In short, these methods were (a) assemble a large contig of overlapping cloned DNA including new polymorphic markers, (b) narrow the candidate interval using recombinant cases and 11q13 LOH, (c) identify candidate genes by many approaches, ultimately from genomic sequence, and (d) search for mutations in candidate genes by dideoxyfingerprinting analysis of MEN1 probands (Figure 26-2).

A contig, overlapping DNA, cloned in YACs, BACs, PACs, P1s, and cosmids, was assembled to assure coverage of 2.8 mil-

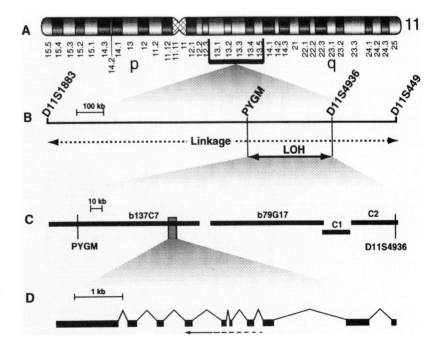

FIG. 26-2 Steps in positional cloning of the *MEN1* gene. (A) Initial linkage to chromosome 11q13 was followed by (B) finer mapping by meiotic recombination and yet finer mapping by loss of heterozygosity analyses in tumors. (C) Nearly complete bacterial clone coverage was achieved across the most likely interval. Shotgun DNA sequencing revealed 8 candidate genes. (D) One of these candidates had mutations in 14 *MEN1* probands among a testing panel of 15 probands (18).

lion bases encompassing the *MEN1* gene. Thirty-three candidate genes were identified in this interval. New polymorphic probes were developed to help narrow the interval through linkage and LOH analyses.[265,283]

The candidate interval was narrowed with analysis of LOH in tumors together with newly developed polymorphic probes. Some 200 tumors were analyzed, mostly from familial MEN1 but some from sporadic cases.[263,265,288] Because PCR reactions with tumor DNA sometimes gave confusing results (unexpected retention of two alleles within a larger zone of allelic loss) attributable to admixture with nontumor DNA, most tumors were microdissected with pipettes or with laser assistance.[264,280]

The minimal candidate interval from meiotic recombinations was between *D11S1883* and *D11S449* (Figure 26-2). However four tumors allowed a shift of the centromeric border to *PYGM*, and one tumor moved the telomeric border centromerically to *DS11S4936*. Thus the size of the candidate interval had been narrowed from 3,000 kb based on meiotic recombination down to only 300 kb based on LOH.

Genomic sequence for most of the 300 kb interval in the final steps of the search was obtained by shotgun sequencing of two BACs and by obtaining additional cosmid sequences available publicly. This sequence was used to identify eight genes in the minimal interval. Seven genes were initially matched through computer software to publicly available ESTs (expressed sequence tags), and one gene was found from a computer software prediction of introns and exons.

Mutation Testing with a Panel of MEN1 Probands. Full length cDNA of a candidate transcript was isolated and sequenced. The intron/exon boundaries were determined from comparing the cDNAs and genomic sequences. Candidate genes were tested for mutations, using a panel of probands from 15 MEN1 kindreds. Mutations were screened by dideoxyfingerprinting, a method that combines features of dideoxy chain termination sequencing and single strand conformation polymorphism.[290]

Most genes showed occasional polymorphisms (present in normals and MEN1 probands). Only one anonymous gene showed many mutations. Mutations of this anonymous gene were identified in 14 of the 15 MEN1 probands. The mutations were present in other family members and not in 142 normal chromosomes. Most mutations were nonsense/stop codons or frameshifts; a few were missense mutations or inframe deletions. These mutations, specific for MEN1, established the identification of the *MEN1* gene.

Germline *MEN1* Mutations

Frequency in MEN1 Families. Germline mutations in the open reading frame of the *MEN1* gene were found in members of 47 of 50 MEN1 kindreds from North America[291] (Figure 26-3). Among the three probands without mutation, one kindred had a lod score of 3.25 at 11q13. Germline mutation was not evaluated in the 5′, 3′, or intronic portions of the *MEN1* gene. Thus, it is apparent that all or most families with typical MEN1 do have germline mutation in this gene.

Frequency Among Sporadic Cases. Only one group or sporadic cases has been evaluated for frequency of *MEN1* germline mutation. This is the group with sporadic MEN1, defined as endocrine tumor in two or more of the main MEN1-related tissues. Among eight cases meeting this criterion, *MEN1* mutation was identified in seven, a prevalence similar to that among the probands of MEN1 kindreds in the same study.[291] All eight cases had multiple parathyroid tumors. This re-emphasizes the relation of this feature to MEN1 and the likelihood that a sporadic MEN1 case with solitary parathyroid adenoma may have a lower chance of an *MEN1* germline mutation. One of these seven was shown to have a new *MEN1* mutation. There were neither sufficient information or sufficient first degree relatives available to test this in other cases. Other conditions that might have a substantial fraction of mutations are sporadic gastrinoma and sporadic primary parathyroid hyperplasia.

Repeating *MEN1* Germline Mutations. Eight mutations occurred more than one time among 50 North American MEN1 kindreds.[291] The most common ones occurred 6 (512delC) and 5 (416delC) times. Haplotype analysis indicated that several kindreds in the two large clusters must share a common ancestor (Emmert Buck MR unpub). In addition a different repeating mutation (R460X) arose twice independently, because the families had different haplotypes.[291]

Genotype-Phenotype Correlations. Only one type of feature within MEN1 families has been analyzed to uncover a characteristic mutation pattern. Three kindreds with the prolactinoma variant of MEN1 were tested. Two kindreds had germline *MEN1* mutations (R460X and Y312X). The third did not have a mutation identified but showed tight linkage to 11q13 (lod score 3.25), suggesting that it has a mutation in an untested portion of the *MEN1* gene.

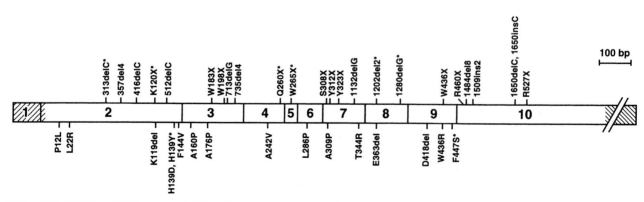

FIG. 26-3 Unique MEN1 mutations in 32 families and in 8 sporadic cases (with asterisk (*)). MEN1 message is diagramed with exons numbered; untranslated regions are cross-hatched. 13 frameshift mutations and 11 nonsense (stop codons) mutations are shown above the diagram. Three in-frame deletions and 13 missense mutations are shown below. Eight mutations were encountered more than once among families (291).

The identified mutations showed no recognizable difference from other *MEN1* mutations.[291] Thus, no explanation for the prolactinoma variant could be recognized from type of *MEN1* mutation. Other explanations for such a phenotype could include other polymorphism in *MEN1,* linked feature in a neighboring gene, *MEN1* mutation occurring in a predisposing background, and unrecognized observer bias.

Families With Possible MEN1 Phenocopies

Familial Hyperparathyroidism. Familial hyperparathyroidism has been shown sometimes to be an expression of MEN1.[34] An analysis of five families indicated *MEN1* mutation in none.[291] The features in these kindreds making MEN1 less likely were advanced age in most members; features against familial hypocalciuric hypercalcemia were that each proband had multiple parathyroid tumors and hypercalciuria.

Other Phenocopies Without MEN1 Mutation. The MEN1 trait in at least one family was not linked to 11q13.[252] The possibility of a phenocopy not caused by *MEN1* mutation should be evaluated in that and other kindreds.

Sporadic *MEN1* Mutations

The roles of the *MEN1* gene in sporadic tumors are under active study. Mutation of the *MEN1* gene has been implicated in 20% of sporadic parathyroid adenomas,[291a] 33% of sporadic gastrinoma,[91] and 17% of sporadic insulinoma.[91] It is likely that it will be implicated through mutation or other inactivation mechanisms in additional fractions of these neoplasms and in other neoplasms.

Functions of the MENI Gene

The function of the *MEN1* gene is not known.[18] The gene is approximately 9,000 bases with a message of 2,800 bases. Across 10 exons, it encodes a protein, named "menin," that is 610 amino acids long. The protein is highly homologous to the mouse menin (Guru SC unpublished), but it does not have other known homologies in humans or other species. The predicted sequence does not have clearly identifiable domains such as a signal sequence, transmembrane domain(s), or nuclear localization signal.

There is only modest information that can be derived from the identified mutations.[291] In particular the missense mutations are not clustered and thus do not highlight a particularly critical region. The converse interpretation is that missense mutation at various loci can compromise the molecule. Most of the mutations (frameshifts and stops) are, in fact, likely to abolish protein function. This supports predictions that *MEN1* is a tumor suppressor gene.

IMPLICATIONS FOR DIAGNOSIS

Periodic Biochemical Testing

For Diagnosis of MEN1. The standard of care has been that members of MEN1 kindreds undergo periodic biochemical testing. Recent recommendations have been to begin this testing at age 15[37] or as early as age 8.[31] The latter is based on the earliest recognized age for important signs. Parameters for testing must be dictated by cost and local availability. An optimal panel could consist of ion-

ized calcium, parathyroid hormone, and prolactin. Such a panel should be repeated approximately every two years. Any patient who does not convert to a positive test by age 30 has far reduced (about 10%) likelihood of being a gene carrier. But testing should be continued at longer intervals indefinitely, since no maximal age for conversion to a positive test has been determined.

For Followup of MEN1. Patients with established MEN1 should undergo periodic testing for expression of new endocrinopathies and for recurrence of treated endocrinopathies. Monitoring and treatment of recognized hormone excess states is beyond this topic. Even more so than for diagnostic testing, testing of known carriers must depend on cost and availability (Table 26-4). Sometimes symptoms, such as ulcer or hypoglycemia, will present before an abnormality is found by biochemical testing.

Genetic Linkage Testing

Until the recent isolation of the *MEN1* gene, genetic linkage was the only method to establish that the trait in a family was linked to 11q13 and to make a highly confident genetic diagnosis in an asymptomatic member of an MEN1 family.[250,247] After MEN1 gene discovery, genetic linkage analysis will have limited applications. The most clearcut use will be in the unusual MEN1 family with no *MEN1* mutation identified. There, linkage analysis might establish if the disease is linked to 11q13 or not. In one study *MEN1* mutation could not be found in 3 of 50 probands; only one of those families was large, and a significant lod score of 3.25 was established between *MEN1* and 11 q13.[291]

Interpretation of Mutation Testing

The full implications of *MEN1* mutation testing are uncertain since limited data are available.[18,291] By dideoxyfingerprinting and cycle sequencing, germline mutation was recognizable in 47 of 50 families. This implies that virtually every MEN1 family has a mutation in the *MEN1* gene. The implication is that robust *MEN1* germline mutation testing is possible, and this can be applied to families and sporadic cases.

It is not known what sorts of *MEN1* mutations will be found in tumor tissues. They may or may not be similar to the germline mutations already identified.

Availability of *MEN1* Germline Mutation Testing

The mutations are spread over 10 exons, and 40 different mutations were found among 50 probands and 11 sporadic cases.[291] Though some mutations repeated as often as 6 times, there will clearly be many additional mutations and no hotspots seem likely to serve as a general shortcut to mutation detection. Furthermore, the relatively high fraction with missense mutations or inframe deletion mutations predict that, even if the messages are ex-

Table 26-4 A typical panel of tests for periodic monitoring of a patient with MEN1.

Parathyroids	G.I. Endocrine
Ionized calcium (annually)	Fasting sugar and gastrin (annually)
PTH (annually)	CAT scan (q five yrs; needs more evaluation)
Pituitary	
Prolactin (annually)	
Sella MRI (q10 yrs)	

pressed, a protein truncation type assay would fail to recognize about 30% of mutations.

Currently available methods (cycle sequencing alone or with dideoxy fingerprinting or with single strand conformer polymorphism) are likely to yield similarly high diagnostic yield under carefully controlled conditions. It is likely that these will be developed by academic centers. It is not clear if there will be sufficient demand to lead to commercial development as well.

Cases for Possible *MEN1* Mutation Testing

Several cases have rather clear justification for *MEN1* mutation testing.

- First would be an affected member in an MEN1 family that has not previously had a member tested. Testing can establish the diagnosis and also assist in possible development of an inexpensive test for other members, such as based upon a specific restriction digest or based upon hybridization to allele specific oligonucleotides.
- Second would be a likely affected member of an MEN1 family, concerned for confirmation of mutational status.
- Third, would be the unaffected adults in an MEN1 family. Those without mutation would be freed from the recommendation to undergo regular biochemical screening (Table 26-4).
- Fourth, would be unaffected children in an MEN1 family. It is difficult to predict the highly unusual circumstances that might warrant such testing. In general children should not receive testing that will not have a major effect on their immediate care. Such testing deprives them of their right to decide as an adult whether to undergo such testing.

Issues for Genetic Counseling

The issues to consider for counseling are, in general, covered in detail in this chapter. Several additional points can be made. MEN1 generally does not have major effects on fertility. Primary hyperparathyroidism in a mother is considered a risk factor for pregnancy complications.[292] However, the mild hyperparathyroidism that is common in MEN1 rarely leads to complications for mother or child. Prolactinoma can clearly impair fertility in women or men, and it should be monitored during pregnancy. Most women (and men) with prolactinoma are able to conceive when treated with a dopamine agonist.[293] A patient education manual is available on the international communications web at http://www.NIDDK.NIH.GOV.[294]

REFERENCES

1. Erdheim J: Zur normalen und pathologischen histologie der glandula throidea, parathyroidea, und hypophysis. *Beitr Z Path Anat* **33**:158, 1903.
2. Moldawer MP: Case records of the Massachusetts General Hospital, case 39501. *N Engl J Med* **249**:990, 1953.
3. Moldawer MP, Nardi GL, Raker JW: Concomitance of multiple adenomas of the parathyroids and pancreatic islet cells with tumor of the pituitary a syndrome with familial incidence. *Am J Med Sc* **228**:190, 1954.
4. Wermer P: Genetic aspects of adenomatosis of endocrine glands. *Am J Med* **16**:363, 1954.
5. Schmid JR, Labhart A, Rossier PH: Relationship of multiple endocrine adenomas to the syndrome of ulcerogenic islet cell adeno-

6. mas (Zollinger-Ellison). Occurrence of both syndromes in one family. *Am J Med* **31**:343, 1961.
6. Zollinger RM, Ellison EH: Primary peptic ulceration of the jejunum associated with islet cell tumors of the pancreas. *Ann Surg* **142**:709, 1955.
7. Gregory RH, Tracy HJ, French JM, Sircus W: Extraction of a gastrin-like substance from a pancreatic tumor in a case of Zollinger-Ellison syndrome. *Lancet I* 1040, 1960.
8. Lewis UJ, Singh RN, Seavey BK: Human prolactin: isolation and some properties. *Biochem Biophys Res Commun* **44**:1169, 1971.
9. Malarkey WB: Prolactin and the diagnosis of pituitary tumors. *Ann Rev Med* **30**:249, 1979.
10. Howard JM, Chremos AN, Collen MJ: Famotidine, a new potent long acting histamine H2-receptor antagonist: comparison with cimetidine and ranitidine in the treatment of Zollinger-Ellison syndrome. *Gastroenterology* **188**:1026, 1985.
11. Metz DC, Pisegna JR, Fishbeyn VA, Benya RV, Jensen RT: Control of gastric acid hypersecretion in the management of patients with Zollinger-Ellison syndrome. *World J Surg* **17**:468, 1993.
12. Frucht H, Maton PN, Jensen RT: Use of omeprazole in patients with Zollinger-Ellison syndrome. *Dig Dis Sci* **36**:394, 1991.
13. Maton PN, Vinayek R, Frucht H: Long term efficacy and safety of omeprazole in patients with Zollinger-Ellison syndrome. *Gastroenterology* **97**:827, 1989.
14. Bevan John S, Webster Jonathan, Burke Christopher W, Scanlon Maurice F: Dopamine agonists and pituitary tumor shrinkage. *Endocrine Reviews* **13**:220, 1992.
15. Norton JA, Cromack DT, Shawker TH. Intraoperative ultrasonographic localization of islet cell tumors: a prospective comparison to palpation. *Ann Surg* **207**:160, 1988.
16. Norton JA, Shawker TH, Jones BL, et al. Intraoperative ultrasound and reoperative parathyroid surgery: an initial evaluation. *World J Surg* **10**:631, 1986.
17. Larsson C, Skogseid B, Oberg K, Nakamura Y, Nordenskjold M: Multiple endocrine neoplasia type 1 gene maps to chromosome 11 and is lost in insulinoma. *Nature* **332**:85, 1988.
18. Chandrasekharappa SC, Guru SC, Manickam P, Olufemi S-E, Collins FS, Emmert-Buck MR, Debelenko LV, Zhyang Z, Lubensky IA, Liotta LA, Crabtree JS, Wang Y, Roe BA, Weisemann J, Boguski MS, Agarwal SK, Kester MB, Kim YS, Heppner C, Dong Q, Spiegel AM, Burns AL, Marx SJ: Positional cloning of the gene for multiple endocrine neoplasia type 1. *Science* **276**:404, 1997.
19. Lipps CJM, Vassen HFA, Lamers CBWH: Berdjis, C.C.: Polyglandular syndrome: II. Multiple endocrine adenomas in man. A report of 5 cases and a review of the literature. *Oncologia* **15**:288, 1962.
20. Lips CJM, Vasen HFA, Lamers CBHW: Multiple endocrine neoplasia syndromes. *CRC Cri Rev* **2**:117, 1984.
21. Eberle F, Grun R: Multiple Endocrine Neoplasia, type I (MEN1). *Ergeb Inn Med* **46**:76, 1981.
22. Oberg K, Skogseid B, Eriksson B: Multiple endocrine neoplasia type 1 (MEN-1): clinical, biochemical and genetical investigations. *Acta Oncologia* **28**:383, 1989.
23. Betts JB, O'Malley BP, Rosenthal FD: Hyperparathyroidism: a prerequisite for Zollinger-Ellison syndrome in multiple endocrine adenomatosis type 1. *A J Med* **193**:69, 1980.
24. Watson RGP, Johnston CF, O'Hare MMT, et al: The frequency of gastrointestinal endocrine tumors in a well defined population–Northern Ireland. *Quarterly Journal of Medicine* **72**:647, 1985.
25. Brandi ML, Marx SJ, Aurbach GD, Fitzpatrick LA: Familial multiple endocrine neoplasia type I: A new look at pathophysiology. *Endocrine Rev* **8**:391, 1987.
26. Heath Hunter III, Hodgson Stephen, Kennedy Margaret A: Primary hyperparathyroidism: incidence, morbidity, and potential economic impact in a community. *N Engl J Med* **302**:189, 1980.
27. Bardram L, Stage JG: Frequency of endocrine disorders in patients with the Zollinger-Ellison syndrome. A collective surgical experience. *Scand J Gastroenterol* **20**:233, 1985.
28. Farley DR, van Heerden JA, Grant CS, Miller LJ, Ilstrup DM: The Zollinger-Ellison syndrome. A collective surgical experience. *Ann Surg* **215**:561, 1992.
29. Schaaf L, Gerschner M, Geissler W, Eckert B, Seif FJ, Usadel KH: The importance of multiple endocrine neoplasia syndromes in differential diagnosis. *Klin Wochenschr* **68**:669, 1990.
30. Scheithauer BW, Laws ER Jr, Kovacs K, Horvath E, Randall RV, Carney JA: Pituitary adenomas of the multiple endocrine neoplasia type I syndrome. *Semin Diagn Pathol* **4**:205, 1987.

31. Trump D, Farren B, Wooding C, Pang JT, Besser GM, Buchanan KD, Edwards CR, Heath DA, Jackson CE, Jansen S, Lips K, Monson JP, O'Halloran D, Sampson J, Shalet SM, Wheeler MH, Zink A, and Thakker RV: Clinical studies of multiple endocrine neoplasia type 1 (MEN1). *Q J Med* **89**:563, 1996.

32. Majewski JT, Wilson SD: The MEA-I syndrome: an all or none phenomenon? *Surgery* **86**:475, 1979.

33. Ballard HS, Frame B, Hartsock RJ: Familial multiple endocrine adenoma-peptic ulcer complex. *A J Med* **43**:481, 1964.

34. Marx SJ, Spiegel AM, Levine MA, et al. Familial hypocalciuric hypercalcemia: the relation to primary parathyroid hyperplasia. *N Engl J Med* **307**:416, 1982.

35. Vasen HFA, Lamers CBHW, Lips CJM: Screening for multiple endocrine neoplasia syndrome type I. *Arch Intern Med* **149**:2717, 1989.

36. Skogseid B, Eriksson B, Lundqvist G: Multiple endocrine neoplasia type 1: a 10-year prospective screening study in four kindreds. *J Clin Endocrinol Metab* **73**:281, 1991.

37. Marx SJ, Vinik AI, Santen RJ, Floyd JC, Jr, Mills JL, Green J: Multiple endocrine neoplasia type I: assessment of laboratory tests to screen for the gene in a large kindred. *Medicine* **65**:226, 1986.

38. Samaan NA, Ovais S, Ordonez NG, Choksi UA, Selvin RV, Hickey RC: Multiple endocrine syndrome type 1. Clinical laboratory findings, and management in five families. *Cancer* **64**:741, 1989.

39. Lamers C, Froeling PGAM: Clinical significance of hyperparathyroidism in familial multiple endocrine adenomatosis type I (MEA I). *Am J Med* **66**:422, 1979.

40. Betts JB, O'Malley BP, Rosenthal FD: Hyperparathyroidism: a prerequisite for Zollinger-Ellison syndrome in multiple endocrine adenomatosis type 1-report of a further family and a review of the literature. *Quarterly J of Med* **73**:69, 1980.

41. Eberle F, Grun R: Multiple endocrine neoplasia, type I (MEN I), in Frick P, Harnack G-A, Kochsiek K, Martini GA, Prade A (eds): *Advances in Internal Medicine and Pediatrics*. Berlin Heidelberg, New York, Springer-Verlag; 77, 1981.

42. Shepherd JJ: Latent familial multiple endocrine neoplasia in Tasmania. *Medical Journal of Australia* **142**:395, 1985.

43. Marx SJ, Menczel J, Campbell G, Aurbach GD, Spiegel AM, Norton JA: Heterogeneous size of the parathyroid glands in familial multiple endocrine neoplasia type 1. *Clin Endorcinol* **35**:521, 1991.

44. Hellman P, Skogseid B, Juhlin C, Akerstrom G, Rastad J: Findings and long-term result of parathyroid surgery in multiple endocrine neoplasia type 1. *World J Surg* **16**:718, 1992.

45. Rizzoli R, Green J III, Marx SJ: Primary hyperparathyroidism in familial multiple endocrine neoplasia type I. *American Journal of Medicine* **78**:468, 1985.

46. Prinz RA, Gamvros OI, Sellu D, Lynn JA: Subtotal parathyroidectomy for primary chief cell hyperplasia of the multiple endocrine neoplasia type I syndrome. *Ann Surg* **193**:26, 1981.

47. van Heerden JA, Kent III RB, Sizemore GW, Grant CS, ReMine WH: Primary hyperparathyroidism in patients with multiple endocrine neoplasia syndromes. *Arch Surg* **118**:533, 1983.

48. Rudberg C, Akerstrom G, Palmer M, et al: Later results of operation for primary hyperparathyroidism in 441 patients. *Surgery* **99**:643, 1986.

49. Benya RV, Metz DC, Venzon DJ, Fishbeyn VA, Strader DB, Orbuch M, Jensen RT: Zollinger-Ellison syndrome can be the initial endocrine manifestation in patients with multiple endocrine neoplasia-type I. *Am J Med* **5**:436, 1994.

50. Norton JA, Levin B, Jensen RT: Principles and Practice of Oncology, in DeVita VT, Hellman S, Rosenberg SA (eds): *Cancer*. Philadelphia, Lippincott J.B.; 1335, 1993.

51. Metz DC, Jensen RT: Endocrine tumors of the pancreas. In: *Bockus gastroenterology*. Haubrich WB, Berk F, Schaffner JE, eds. Philadelphia: WB Saunders, 1993.

52. Jensen RT, Gardner JD: Gastrinoma. In Go VLW, Brooks FP, DiMagno EP (eds): *The Exocrine Pancreas*. New York, Raven Press, 1993.

53. Metz DC, Jensen RT, Bale A, Skarulis MC, Eastman RC, Nieman L, Norton JA, Friedman E, Larsson C, Amorosi A, Brandi ML, Marx SJ: Multiple endocrine neoplasia type 1: clinical features and management. In The Parathyroids. Ed. Bilezekian JP, Levine MA & Marcus R. Raven Press, 591, 1994.

54. Skogseid B, Oberg K, Eriksson B, Juhlin C, Grandberg D, Akerstrom G, Rastad J: Surgery for asymptomatic pancreatic lesion in multiple endocrine neoplasia type I. *World J Surg* **7**:872, 1996.

55. Kloppel G, Sillemar S, Stamm B, Hacki WH, Heitz PN: Pancreatic lesions and hormonal profile in pancreatic tumors in multiple endocrine neoplasia type I. *Cancer* **57**:1824, 1986.

56. Thompson NW, Lloyd RU, Nishiyama RH: MEN-1 pancreas: A histological and immunohistochemical study. *World J Surg* **8**:561, 1984.

57. Pipeleers-Marichial M, Somers G, Willems G: Gastrinomas in the duodenum of patients with multiple endocrine neoplasia type 1 and the Zollinger-Ellison syndrome. *N Engl J Med* **322**:723, 1990.

58. Jensen RT, Gardner JD: Zollinger-Ellison syndrome: clinical presentation, pathology, diagnosis and treatment, in Dannenberg A, Zakim D (eds): *Peptic Ulcer and Other Acid-Related Diseases*. New York, Academic Research Association; 117, 1991.

59. Norton JA, Doppman JL, Jensen RT: Curative resection in Zollinger-Ellison syndrome: results of a 10 year prospective study. *Ann Surg* **215**:8, 1992.

60. Ruszniewski P, Podevin P, Cadiot G, Marmuse JP, Mignon M, Vissuzaine C, Bonfils S, Lehy T: Clinical anatomical, and evolutive features of patients with the Zollinger-Ellison syndrome combined with type I multiple endocrine neoplasia. *Pancreas* **8**:295, 1993.

61. Neuburger P, Lewin M, Bonfils S: Parietal and chief cell population in four cases of the Zollinger-Ellison syndrome. *Gastroenterology* **63**:937, 1972.

62. Norton JA, Doppman JL, Collen MJ: Prospective study of gastrinoma localization and resection in patients with Zollinger-Ellison syndrome. *Ann Surg* **204**:468, 1986.

63. Stabile BE, Morrow DJ, Passaro E Jr.: The gastrinoma triangle: operative implications. *Am J Surg* **147**:25, 1984.

64. Norton JA, Jensen RT: Unresolved issues in the management of patients with Zollinger-Ellison syndrome. *World J Surg* **15**:151, 1991.

65. Zollinger RM, Ellison EH, Fabri PJ, Johnson J, Sparks J, Carey LC: Primary peptic ulceration of the jejunum associated with islet cell tumors: twenty-five year appraisal. *Ann Surg* **192**:422, 1980.

66. Oberg K, Skogseid B, Eriksson B: Multiple endocrine neoplasia type 1 (MEN-1). *Acta Oncologia* **28**(3):383, 1989.

67. Zollinger RM: Gastrinoma factors influencing prognosis. *Surgery* **97**:49, 1985.

68. Podevin P, Ruszniewski P, Mignon M: Management of multiple endocrine neoplasia type 1 (MEN 1) in Zollinger-Ellison syndrome. *Gastrenterology* **98**:A230, 1990.

69. Jensen RT, Gardner JD, Raufman J-P: Zollinger-Ellison syndrome: Current concepts and management. *Ann Intern Med* **98**:59, 1983.

70. Weber HC, Venzon DJ, Lin JT, Fishbein VA, Orbuch M, Strader DB, Gibril F, Metz DC, Fraker DL, Norton JA, Jensen RT: Determinants of metastatic rate and survival in patients with Zollinger-Ellison syndrome: A prospective long-term study. *Gastroenterology* **108**:1637, 1995.

71. Isenberg JI, Walsh JH, Grossman MI: Zollinger-Ellison syndrome. *Gastroenterology* **65**:140, 1973.

72. Shimoda SS, Saunders DR, Rubin C: The Zollinger-Ellison syndrome with steatorrhea: Mechanisms of fat and vitamin B12 malabsorption. *Gastroenterology* **55**:705, 1968.

73. Feldman M: Gastric secretion, in Sleisenger MH, Fordtran JS (eds): *Gastrointestinal Disease*. Philadelphia, WB Saunders; 541, 1983.

74. Norton JA, Cornelius MJ, Doppman JL: Effect of parathyroidectomy in patients with hyperparathyroidism and multiple endocrine neoplasia type I. *Surgery* **102**:958, 1987.

75. Yonda RJ, Ostroff JW, Ashbaugh CD, Guis MS, Goldberg HI: Zollinger-Ellison syndrome with a normal screening gastrin level. *Dig Dis Sci* **34**:1929, 1989.

76. Wolfe MM, Jensen RT: Zollinger-Ellison syndrome. *N Engl J Med* **317**:1200, 1987.

77. Metz DC, Pisegna JR, Fishbeyn VA, Benya RV, Jensen RT: Current maintenance doses of omeprazole in Zollinger-Ellison syndrome are too high. *Gastroenterology* **103**:1498, 1992.

78. Frucht H, Howard JM, Slaff JE: Secretin and calcium provocative tests in patients with Zollinger-Ellison syndrome: A prospective study. *Ann Intern Med* **111**:713, 1989.

79. Krenning EP, Kwekkeboom DJ, Oei HY, deJong RJB, Dop FJ, Reubi JC, Lambers SWJ: Somatostatin-receptor scintigraphy in gastroenteropancreatic tumors. *Ann NY Acad Sci* **733**:416, 1994.

80. Gibril F, Reynolds JC, Doppman JL, Chen CC, Venzon DJ, Termanini B, Weber HC, Stewart CA, Jensen RT: Somatostatin receptor scientigraphy: A prospective study of its sensitivity compared

to other imaging modalities in detecting primary and metastatic gastrinomas. *Ann Intern Med* **125**:26, 1996.

81. Termanini B, Gibril F, Reynolds JC, Doppman JL, Chen CC, Sutliffe VE, Jensen RT: Value of somatostatin receptor scintigraphy: a prospective study in gastrinoma of its effect on clinical management. *Gastroenterol* **112**:335, 1997.

82. Galbut DL, Markowitz AM: Insulinoma: diagnosis, surgical management and long term followup. Review of 41 cases. *Am J Surg* **139**:682, 1980.

83. Eckhauser FE, Cheung PS, Vinik A, Strodel WE, Lloyd R, Thompson NW: Nonfunctioning malignant neuroendocrine tumors of the pancreas. *Surgery* **100**:978, 1986.

84. Rasbach DA, van Heerden JA, Telander RL, Grant CS, Carney A: Surgical management of hyperinsulinism in the multiple endocrine neoplasia type 1 syndrome. *Arch Surg* **123**:584, 1985.

85. Pasieka JL, McLoed MK, Thompson NW, Burney RE: Surgical approach to insulinomas. Assessing the need for preoperative localization. *Arch Surg* **127**:442, 1992.

86. van Heerden JA, Edis AJ, Service FJ: Surgical aspects of insulinomas. *Ann Surg* **189**:677, 1992.

87. Eastman RC, Kahn CR: Hypoglycemia, in Moore WT, Eastman EC (eds): *Diagnostic Endrocrinology*. Toronto, BC Decker; 183, 1990.

88. Doppman JL, Miller DL, Chang R: Insulinomas: localization with selective intrarterial injection of calcium. *Radiology* **178**:237, 1991.

89. Doherty GM, Doppman JL, Shawker TH, et al: Results of a propective strategy to diagnose, localize and resect insulinomas. *Surgery* **110**:989, 1991.

90. Grant CS, van Heerden JA, Charboneau JW, James EM, Reading CC: Insulinoma: the value of intraoperative ultrasonography. *Arch Surg* **123**:843, 1988.

91. Zhuang Z, Vortmeyer AO, Pack S, Huang S, Pham TA, Wang C, Park WS, Agarwal SK, Debelenko LV, Kester MB, Guru SC, Manickam P, Olufemi SE, Yu F, Heppner C, Skarulis MC, Venzon DJ, Emmert-Buck MR, Spiegel AM, Chandrasekharappa SC, Collins FS, Burns AL, Marx SJ, Jensen RT, Liotta LA, Lubensky IA: Somatic mutations of the MEN1 tumor suppressor gene in sporadic gastrinomas and insulinomas. *Canc Res* (in press).

92. Boden G: Glucagonomas and insulinomas. *Gastroenterol Clin North Am* **18**:831, 1989.

93. Leichter SB: Clinical and metabolic aspects of glucagonoma. *Medicine* **59**:100, 1980.

94. Guillausseau PJ, Guillausseau C, Villet R: Les glucagonomas. Aspect Cliniques biologiques, Anatomo-pathologiques et therapeutiques (Revue général de 130 cas). *Gastroenterol Clin Biol* **6**:1029, 1982.

95. Wilkinson DS: Necrolytic migratory erythema with carcinoma of the pancreas. *Trans St John's Hosp Dermatol Soc* **59**:244, 1973.

96. Mallison CN, Bloom SR, Warin AP: A glucagonoma syndrome. *Lancet* **2**:1, 1974.

97. Holst JJ: Hormone producing tumors of the gastrointestinal tract, in Cohen S, Soloway RD (eds): *Glucago-producing tumors*. New York, Churchill Livingstone; 57, 1985.

98. Verner JV, Morrison AB: Endocrine pancreatic ilset disease with diarrhea: Report of a case due to diffuse hyperplasia of non beta islet tissue with a review of 54 additional cases. *Arch Intern Med* **133**:492, 1974.

99. Matsumoto KK, Peter JB, Schultze RG: Watery diarrhea and hypokalemia associated with pancreatic islet cell adenoma. *Gastroenterology* **50**:231, 1966.

100. Mekhjian H, O'Dorisio TM: VIPoma syndrome. *Sem Oncoloby* **14**:282, 1987.

101. Kane MG, D'Dorisio TM, Krejs GJ: Production of secretory diarrhea by intravenous infusion of vasoactive intestinal peptide. *N Engl J Med* **309**:1482, 1983.

102. Namihara Y, Achord JL, Subramony C: Multiple endocrine neoplasia, type 1, with pancreatic cholera. *Am J Gastroenterol* **82**:794–797, 1987.

103. Welbourn RB, Wood SM, Polak JM, Bloom SR: Pancreatic endocrine tumors, in Bloom SR, Polak JM (eds): *Gut Hormones*. New York, Churchill-Livingstone; 547, 1981.

104. Long RG, Bryant MG, Mitchell SJ, Adrian TE, Polak JM, Bloom SR: Clinicopathological study of pancreatic and ganglioneuroblastoma tumors secreting vasoactive intestinal polypeptide (Vipomas). *Brit Med J* **282**:1767, 1981.

105. Capella C, Polak JM, Butta R: Morphologic patterns and diagnostic criteria of VIP-producing endocrine tumors. A histologic, histo-

chemical, ultrastructural and biochemical study of 32 cases. *Cancer* **52**:1860, 1983.

106. Rivier J, Spress J, Thorner M, Vale W: Characterization of a growth-hormone releasing factor from a human pancreatic islet cell tumor. *Nature* **300**:276, 1982.

107. Thorner M, Perryman RI, Cronin MJ: Somatotroph hyperplasia. *J Clin Invest* **70**:965, 1982.

108. Sano T, Asa SL, Kovacs K: Growth hormone releasing-producing tumors: clinical, biochemical and morphological manifestations. *Endocrine Rev* **9**:357, 1988.

109. Asa SL, Singer W, Kovacs K, et al: Pancreatic endocrine tumour producing growth hormone-releasing hormone associated with multiple endocrine neoplasia type I syndrome. *Acta Endocrinologica* **115**:331, 1987.

110. Barkan AL, Shenker Y, Grekin RJ: Acromeglay from ectopic GHRH secretion by malignant carcinoid tumor: successful treatment with long-acting somatostain analogue SMS. *Cancer* **61**:221, 1986.

111. Sano T, Yamasaki R, Saito H: Growth hormone releasing hormone (GHRH)—secreting pancreatic tumor in a patient with multiple endocrine neoplasia type 1. *Am J Surg Pathol* **11**:810, 1987.

112. Larsson LI, Hirsch MA, Holst JJ: Pancreatic somatostatinoma clinical features and physiologic implications. *Lancet* **1**:666, 1977.

113. Ganda OP, Weir GC, Soeldner JS: Somatostatinoma: A somatostatin-containing tumor of the endocrine pancreas. *N Engl J Med* **296**:963, 1977.

114. Vinik AI, Strodel WE, Eckhauser FE, Moattari AR, Lloyd R: Somatostatinomas, Ppomas and Neurotensinomas. *Seminars Oncol* **14**:263, 1987.

115. Boden G, Shimoyama R: Hormone-producing tumors of the gastrointestinal tract, in Cohen S, Soloway RD (eds): *Somatostatinoma*. New York, Churchill Livingstone; 85, 1985.

116. Yamada T, Chiha T: The gastrointestinal system, in Makhlouf GM (ed): Somatostatin, Section 6, Handbook of Physiology. Bethesda, MD. *Am. Physiol Soc* 431, 1979.

117. Kent RB, van Heerden JA, Weiland LH: Nonfunctioning islet cell tumors. *Ann Surg* **193**:185, 1981.

118. O'Dorisio TM, Vinik AI: Pancreatic polypeptide and mixed peptide-producing tumors of the gastrointestinal tract, in Cohen S, Soloway RD (eds): *Contemporary Issues in Gastroenterology*. Edinburgh, Churchill Livingstone; 117, 1984.

119. Takahashi H, Nakano K. Adachi Y: Multiple nonfunctional pancreatic islet cell tumor in multiple endocrine neoplasia type 1; a case report. *Acta Pathol Jpn* **38**:667, 1988.

120. Heitz PU, Kasper M, Polak JM, Kloppel G: Pancreatic endocrine tumors: immunocytochemical analysis of 125 tumors. *Hum Pathol* **13**:163, 1982.

121. Duh Q-Y: Carcinoids associated with multiple endocrine neoplasia syndromes. *Am J Surg* **154**:142, 1987.

122. Godwin JD: Carcinoid tumors. An analysis of 2837 cases. *Cancer* **36**:560, 1975.

123. Teh BT, McArdle J, Chan SP, Menon J, Hartley L, Pullan P, Ho J, Khir A, Wilkinson S, Larsson C, Cameron D, Shepherd J: Clinicopathologic studies of thymic carcinoids in multiple endocrine neoplasia type 1. *Medicine* **76**:21, 1997.

124. Pass HI, Doppman JL, Nieman L: Management of the ectopic ACTH syndrome due to thoracic carcinoids. *Ann Thorac Surg* **50**:52, 1990.

125. Doppman JL, Pass HI, Nieman LK: Detection of ACTH-producing bronchial carcinoid tumors: MR imaging vs CT. *Am J Roentgenol* **156**:39–43, 1991.

126. Glikson M, Gil-Ad I, Calun E, Dresner R: Acromegaly due to ectopic growth hormone-releasing hormone secretion by a bronchial carcinoid tumour. Dynamic hormonal responses to various stimuli. *Acta Endocrinol* (Copenh) **125**:366, 1991.

127. Maton PN, Dayal Y: Clinical implication of hypergastrinemia. In *Peptic ulcer and other acid-related diseases*. Dannenberg A, Zakim D, eds. New York: Academic Research Association, 213, 1993.

128. Frucht H, Maton PN, Jensen RT: Use of omeprazole in patients with Zollinger-Ellison syndrome. *N Engl J Med* **322**:723, 1990.

129. Jensen RT: Gastrinoma as a model for prolonged hypergastrinemia In: Gastrin (Walsh JH Ed). New York, Raven Press, 1993.

130. Benya RV, Metz DC, Hijazi YM, Fishbeyn VA, Pisegna JR, Jensen RT: Fine needle aspiration cytology for the evaluation of submucosal nodules in patients with Zollinger-Ellison sndrome. *Am J Gastroenterol* **88**:258, 1993.

130.5. Thompson GB, van Heerden JA, Martin JK, Scutt AJ, Ilstrup DM, Carney JA. Carcinoma of the gastrointestinal tract: presentation, management, and prognosis. *Surgery* 98:1054, 1985.

131. Scheithauer BW, Laws ER Jr, Kovacs K, Horvath E, Randall RV, Carney JA: Pituitary adenomas of the multiple endocrine neoplasia type I syndrome. *Seminars in Diagnostic Pathology* 4:205, 1987.

132. Skogseid B, Larsson C, Lindgran PG, et al.: Clinical and genetic features of adrenocortical lesions in multiple endocrine neoplasia type 1. *J Clin Endorcrinol Metab* 75:76, 1992.

133. Skogseid B, Rastad J, Gobl A, Larsson C, Backlin K, Juhlin C, Akerstrom G, Oberg K: Adrenal lesion in multiple endocrine neoplasia type 1. *Surgery* 118:1077, 1995.

134. Houdelette P, Chagnon A, Dumotier J, Marthan E: Corticosurrenalome malin dans le cadre d'un syndrome de Wermer. *J Chir (Paris)* 126:385, 1989.

135. Darling TN, Skarulis MC, Steinberg SM, Marx SJ, Spiegel AM, Turner M: Multiple facial angiofibromas and collagenomas in patients with multiple endocrine neoplasia type 1. *Arch Dermatol* 133:853, 1997.

136. Hershon KS, Kelly WA, Shaw CM, Schwartz R, Bierman EL: Prolactinomas as part of the multiple endocrine neoplastic syndrome type 1. *American Journal of Medicine* 74:713, 1983.

137. Farid NR, Buehler S, Russell NA, Maroun FB, Allerdice P, Smyth HS: Prolactinomas in familial multiple endocrine neoplasia syndrome type 1. *American Journal of Medicine* 69:874, 1980.

138. Bear JC, Urbina RB, Fahey JF, Farid NR: Variant multiple endocrine neoplasia I (MEN I-Burin): further studies and non-linkage to HLA-1. *Hum Hered* 35:15, 1985.

139. Marx SJ, Powell D, Shimkin PM, et al.: Familial hyperparathyroidism. Mild hypercalcemia in at least nine members of a kindred. *Ann Intern Med* 78:371, 1973.

140. Green JS: Development implementation and evaluation of clinical and genetic screening programs for hereditary tumor syndromes. Ph.D. thesis, Memorial University, Newfoundland, Canada. 1995.

141. Burgess JR, Shepherd JJ, Parameswaran V, Hoffman L, Greenaway TM: Prolactinomas in a large kindred with multiple endocrine neoplasia type 1: Clinical features and inheritance pattern. *J Clin Endocrinol Metab* 81:1841, 1996.

142. Goldsmith RE, Sizemore GW, Chen I, Zalme E, Altemeier WA: Familial hyperparathyroidism description of a large kindred with physiologic observations and a review of the literature. *Ann Intern Med* 842:36, 1976.

143. Kassem M, Zhang X, Brask S, Ericksen EF, Mosekilde L, Kruse TA: Familial isolated primary hyperparathyroidism. *Clin Endocrinol* 41:415, 1994.

144. Yamada S, Yoshimoto K, Sano T, Takada K, Itakura M, Usui M, Teramoto A: Inactivation of the tumor suppressor gene on 11q13 in brothers with familial acrogigantism without multiple endocrine neoplasia type 1. *Clin Endocrinol Metab* 82:239, 1997.

145. Arnold A, Brown MF, Urena P, Gaz RD, Sarfati E, Drueke TB: Monoclonality of parthyroid tumors in chronic renal failure and in primary parathyroid hyperplasia. *J Clin Invest* 95:2047, 1995.

146. Maton PN, Gardner JD, Jensen RT: Cushing's syndrome in patients with Zollinger-Ellison syndrome. *N Engl J Med* 315:1, 1986.

147. Kloppel G, Heitz PU: Pancreatic endocrine tumors. *Path Res Pract* 183:155–175, 1988.

148. Melmed S, Ezrin C, Kovacs K, Goodman RS, Frohman LA: Acromegaly due to secretion of growth hormone by an ectopic pancreatic islet-cell tumor. *N Engl J Med* 312:9, 1986.

149. Schimke RN: Multiple endocrine adenomatosis syndrome. *Adv Intern Med* 21:249, 1976.

150. Calcatera TC, Paglia D: the coexistence of parathyroid adenoma and thyroid carcinoma. *The Laryngoscope* 89:1166, 1979.

151. Simpson RJ, Moss J, Jr: Parathyroid adenoma and nonmedullary thyroid carcinoma association. *Otolaryngoly Head & Neck Surgery* 101:584, 1989.

152. Doumith R, Gennes JL, Cabane JP, Zygelman N: Pituitary prolactinoma, adrenal aldosterone producing adenoma, gastric schwannoma and clonic polyadenomas: a possible variant of multiple endocrine neoplasia (MEN) type 1. *Acta Endocrinol* 100:189, 1982.

153. Holland OB, Gomez-Sanchez CE, Kem DC, Weiberger MH, Kramer NJ, Higgins JR: Evidence against prolactin stimulation of aldosterone in normal subjects and in patients with primary hyperaldosteronism, including a patient with primary hyperaldosteronismn and prolactin producing pituitary macroadenoma. *J Clin Endocrinol Metab* 45:1064, 1977.

154. Blumenkopf B, Boekelheide K: Neck paraganglinoma with a pituitary adenoma. Case Report. *J Neurosurg* 57:426, 1982.

155. Nelson DR, Stachura ME, Dunlap DB: Case report: Illeal carcinoid tumor complicated by retroperitoneal fibrosis and prolactinoma. *Am J Med Sc* 296:129, 1988.

156. Barzilay J, Heatley GJ, Cushing GW: Benign and malignant tumors in patients with acromegaly. *Arch Intern Med* 151:1629, 1991.

157. Anderson RJ, Lufkin EG, Sizemore GW, Carney JA, Sheps SG, Silliman YE: Acromegaly and pituitary adenoma with pheochromocytoma: a variant of multiple endocrine neoplasia. *Clin Endocrinol* 14:605, 1981.

158. Morris JA, Tymms DJ: Oat cell carcinoma, pheochromocytoma and carcinoid tumors—Multiple APUD neoplasia—A case report. *J Pathol* 131:107, 1980.

159. Steiner AL, Goodman AD, Powers SR: A study of a kindred with pheochromocytoma, medullary thyroid carcinoma, hyperparathyroidism and Cushing's disease: Multiple endocrine neoplasia type 2. *Medicine* 47:371, 1968.

160. Farhi F, Dikman SH, Lawson W, Cobin RH, Zak FG: Paragangliomatosis associated with multiple endocrine adenomas. *Arch Pathol Lab Med* 100:495, 1976.

161. Hansen OP, Hansen M, Hansen HH, Rose B. Multiple endocrine adenomatosis of the mixed type. *Acta Med Scand* 200:327, 1976.

162. Boden G, Owen OE: Familial hyperglucagonemia. An autosomal dominant disorder. *N Engl J Med* 296:534, 1977.

163. Cameron D, Spiro HM, Lansberg L: Zollinger-Ellison syndrome with multiple endocrine adenomatosis type II. *N Engl J Med* 299:152, 1978.

164. Janson KL, Roberts JA, Varela M: Multiple endocrine adenomatosis. In support of the common origin theories. *J Urol* 119:161, 1978.

165. Alberts MW, McMeekin JO, George JM: Mixed multiple endocrine neoplasia syndromes. *JAMA* 244:1236, 1980.

166. Cusick JF, Ho KC, Hagen TC, Kun LE: Granular-cell pituicytoma associated with multiple endocrine neoplasia type 2. *J Neurosurg* 56:594, 1982.

167. Manning GS, Stevens KA, Stock JL: Multiple endocrine neoplasia type 1. Association with marfanoid habitus, optic atrophy, and other abnormalities. *Arch Intern Med* 143:2315, 1983.

168. Bertnard JH, Ritz P, Reznik Y, Grollier G, Potier JC, Evrad C, Mahoudeau JA: Sipple's syndrome associated with a large prolactinoma. *Clin Endocrinol* 27:607, 1987.

169. Jerkins TW, Sacks HS, O'Dorisio TM, Tuttle S, Solomon SS: Medullary carcinoma of the thyroid, pancreatic nesidioblastosis and microadenosis, and pancreatic polypeptide hypersecretion: a new association and clinical and hormonal response to a long-acting somatostatin analog. *J Clin Endocrinol Metab* 64:1313, 1987.

170. Maton PN, Norton JA, Nieman LK, Doppman JL, Jensen RT: Multiple endocrine neoplasia type II with Zollinger-Ellison syndrome caused by a solitary pancreatic gastrinoma. *JAMA* 262:535, 1989.

171. Reschini E, Catania A, Airaghi L, Manfredi MG, Crosignani PG: Scintigraphic study of extra-adrenal ganglioneuroma in a patient with overlap between multiple endocrine neoplasia types 1 and 2. *Clin Nucl Med* 17:573, 1992.

172. Modan B, Baidatz D, Mart H, Steinitz R, Levin SG: Radiation-induced head and neck tumors. *Lancet I* 277, 1975.

173. Schneider AB, Shore-Freedman E, Weinstein RA: Radiation-induced thyroid and other head and neck tumors: Occurrence of multiple tumors and analysis of risk factors. *J Clin Endcrinol Metab* 63:107, 1986.

174. Rosen IB, Strawbridge HG, Bain J: A case hyperparathyroidism associated with radiation of the head and neck area. *Cancer* 36:1111, 1975.

175. Tisell LE, Carlsson S, Lindberg S, Ragnhult I: Autonomous hyperparathyroidism. A possible late complication of neck radiotherapy. *Acta Chir Scand* 142:889, 1976.

176. Christensson T: Familial hyperparathyroidism. *Ann Intern Med* 85:614, 1976.

177. Hedman I, Hansson G, Lundberg LM, Tisell LE: A clinical evaluation of radiation-induced hyperparathyroidism based on 148 surgically treated patients. *World J Surg* 8:96, 1984.

178. Christmas TJ, Chapple CR, Noble JG, Milroy EJG, Cowie AGA: Hyperparathyroidism after neck irradiation. *Br J Surg* 75:873, 1988.

179. Fujiwara S, Spoto R, Ezaki HAB, et al.: Hyperparathyroidism among atomic bomb survivors in Hiroshima. *Radiation Res* 130:372, 1992.

180. Printz RA, Paloyan E, Lawrence AM, Pickleman JR, Braithwaite S, Brooks MH: Radiation-associated hyperparathyroidism: A new syndrome? *Surgery* **822**:276, 1977.

181. Tisell LE, Hansson G, Lindberg S, Ragnhult I: Hyperparathyroidism in persons treated with X-rays for tuberculous cervical adenitis. *Cancer* **40**:846, 1977.

182. Cohen J, Gierlowski TC, Schneider AB: A prospective study of hyperparathyroidism in individuals exposed to radiation in childhood. *JAMA* **264**:581, 1990.

183. Katz A, Braunstein GD: Clinical, biochemical and pathologic features of radiation-associated hyperparathyroidism. *Arch Intern Med* **143**:79, 1983.

184. Weinstein LS: Other skeletal diseases of G proteins—McClune-Albright syndrome. In *Principles of Bone Biology*, eds. Bilezikian J, Raisz L, and Rodan G. Academic Press, 877, 1996.

185. Weinstein LS, Shenker A, Gejman PV, Merino MJ, Friedman E, Spiegel AM: Activating mutations of the stimulatory G protein in the McCune-Albright syndrome. *N Engl J Med* **325**:1688, 1991.

186. Landis CA, Masters SB, Spada A, Pace AM, Bourne HR, Vallar L: GTPase inhibiting mutations activate the subunit of Gs and stimulate adenylyl cyclase in human pituitary tumors. *Nature* **340**:692, 1989.

187. Ponder B: Multiple endocrine neoplasia. *Metabolic & Molecular Bases of inherited disease* CD-ROM: McGraw Hill Pub. Version I, 1997.

188. Schweitzer-Cagianut M, Froesch ER, Hedinger C: Familial Cushing's syndrome with primary adrenocortical microadenomatosis (primary adrenocortical nodular dysplasia). *Acta Endorcinol* (Copenh) **94**:529, 1980.

189. Carney JA, Gordon H, Carpenter PC, Shenoy BV, Go VLW: The complex of myxomas, spotty pigmentation and endocrine overactivity. *Medicine* **64**:270, 1985.

190. Banik S, Hasleton PS, Lyon RL: An unusual variant of multiple endocrine neoplasia syndrome: a case report. *Histopathology* **8**:135, 1984.

191. Stratakis CA, Carney JA, Lin JP, Papaniccolaou DA, Karl M, Kastner DL, Pras E, Chrousos GP: Carney complex, a familial multiple neoplasia and lentiginosis syndrome. Analysis of 11 kindreds and linkage to the short arm of chromosome 2. *J Clin Invest* **97**:699, 1996.

192. Linehan WM and Klausner R: Von-Hippel-Lindau syndrome. *Metabolic & Molecular Bases of inherited disease* CD-ROM: McGraw Hill Pub. Version I, 1997.

193. Neumann HPH: Basic criteria for clinical diagnosis and genetic counseling in von-Hippel Lindau syndrome. *J Vasc Dis* **16**:220, 1987.

194. Latif F, Tory K, Gnara J et al.: Identification of the von-Hipple-Lindau disease tumor suppressor gene. *Science* **260**:1317, 1993.

195. Pause A, Lee S, Worrell RA, Chen DY, Burgess WH, Linehan WM, Klausner RD: the von Hippel-Landau tumor-suppressor gene product forms a stable complex with human CUL-2, a member of the Cdc53 family of proteins. *Proc Natl Acad Sci USA* **94**:2156, 1997.

196. Guttman GH, Collins FS: Von Recklinghausen neurofibromatosis. *Metabolic & Molecular Bases of inherited disease* CD-ROM: McGraw Hill Pub. Version I, 1997.

197. Weinstein RS, Harris RL: Hypercalcemic hyperparathyroidism and hypophosphatemic osteomalacia complicating neurofibromatosis. *Calcif Tissue Int* **46**:261, 1990.

198. Swinburn BA, Yeong ML, Lane MR, Nicholson GI, Holdaway IM: Neurofibromatosis associated with somatostatinoma: a report of two patients. *Clin Endocrinol* **28**:353, 1988.

199. Sartori P, Symons JC, Taylor NF, Grant OB: Adrenal cortical adenoma in a 13 year old girl with neurofibromatosis. *Acta Paediatr Scand* **78**:476, 1989.

200. DeAngelis LM, Kelleher MB, Kalmon DP, Fetell MR: Multiple paragangliomatosis in neurofibromatosis: a new neuroendocrine neoplasia. *Neurology* **37**:129, 1987.

201. Cawthon RM, Weiss R, Xu C, et al.: A major segment of the Neurofibromatosis type 1 gene: cDNA sequence, genomic structure, and point mutations. *Cell* **62**:193, 1990.

202. Marx SJ, Attie M, Levine MA, Spiegel AM, Downs RW, Jr, Lasker RD: The hypocalciuric or benign variant of familial hypercalcemia: clinical and biochemical features in fifteen kindreds. *Medicine* **60**:397, 1981.

203. Firek AF, Kao PC, Heath H III: Plasma intact parathyroid hormone (PTH) and PTH-related peptide in familial benign hypercalcemia:

204. Greater responsiveness to endogenous PTH than in primary hyperparathyroidism. *J Clin Endo Metab* **72**:541, 1991.

204. Brown EM, Pollak M, Seidman CE, Seidman JG, Chou YHW, Riccardi D, Herbert SC: Calcium-ion-sensing cell-surface receptors. *N Engl J Med* **333**:234, 1995.

205. Heath H III, Jackson CE, Otterud B, Leppert MF: Genetic linkage analysis in familial benign (hypocalciuric) hypercalcemia: evidence for locus heterogeneity. *Am J Hum Genet* **53**:193, 1993.

206. Trump D, Whyte MP, Wooding C, Pang JT, Pearce SHS, Kocher DV, Thakker RV: Linkage studies in a kindred from Oklahoma, with familial benign (hypocalciuric) hypercalcaemia (FBH) and developmental elevations in serum parathyroid hormone levels, indicate a third locus for FBH. *Hum Genet* **96**:183, 1995.

207. Pollack MR, Chou YHW, Marx SJ, et al.: Familial hypocalciuric hypercalcemia and neonatal severe hyperparathyroidism: effects of mutant gene dosage on phenotype. *J Clin Invest* **93**:1108, 1994.

208. Pearse SHR, Trump D, Wooding C, Besser GM, Hew SL, Grant DB, Heath DA, Hughes IA, Paterson CR, Whyte MP, Thakker RV: Calcium-sensing receptor mutations in familial benign hypercemia and neonatal hyperparathyroidism. *J Clin Invest* **96**:2683, 1995.

209. Jackson CE, Norum RA, Boyd SB, Talpos GB, Wilson SD, Taggart T, Mallette LE: Hereditary hyperparathyroidism and multiple ossifying jaw fibromas: a clinically and genetically distinct syndrome. *Surgery* **108**:1006, 1990.

210. Mallette LE, Malini S, Rappaport MP, Kirkland JL: Familial cystic parathyroid adenomatosis. *Ann Int Med* **107**:54, 1987.

211. Teh BT, Farnebo F, Kristoffersson U, Sundelin B, Cardinal J, Axelson R, Yap A, Epstein M, Heath H III, Cameron D, Larsson C: Autosomal dominant primary hyperparathyroidism and jaw tumor syndrome associated with renal hamartomas and cystic kidney disease: linkage to 1q21-q32 and loss of the wild type allele in renal hamartomas. *J Clin Endocrinol Metab* **81**:4204, 1996.

212. Szabo J, Heath B, Hill VM, Jackson CE, Zarbo RJ, Mallette LE, Chew SL, Besser GM, Thakker RV, Huff V, Leppert MF, Heath H III: Hereditary hyperparathyroidism—jaw tmor syndrome: the endocrine tumor gene HRPT2 maps to chromosome 1q21-q31. *Am J Hum Genet* **56**:944, 1995.

213. Wassif WS, Moniz CF, Friedman E, Wong S, Weber G, Nordenskjold M, Peters TJ, Larsson C: Familial isolated hyperparathyroidism: A distinct genetic entity with an increased risk of parathyroid cancer. *J Clin Endocrinol Metab* **77**:1485, 1993.

214. Streeten E, Weinstein LS, Norton JA, Mulvihill JJ, White B, Friedman E, Jaffe G, Brandi ML, Stewart K, Zimering MB, Spiegel AM, Aurbach GD, Marx SJ: Studies in a kindred with parathyroid carcinoma. *J Clin Endocrinol Metab* **75**:362, 1992.

215. Law WM Jr, Hodgson S, Heath H III: Autosomal recessive inheritance of familial hyperparathyroidism. *N Engl J Med* **309**:650, 1983.

216. Allo M, Thompson NW: Familial hyperparathyroidism caused by solitary adenomas. *Surgery* **92**:486, 1982.

217. Huang SM, Duh O-Y, Shaver J, Siperstein AE, Kraimp JL, Clark OH: Familial hyperparathyroidism without multiple endocrine neoplasia. *World J Surg* **21**:22, 1997.

218. Farnebo F, Teh B, Dotzenrath C, Wassif WS, Svensson A, White I, Betz R, Goretzki P, Sandelin K, Farnebo LO, Larsson C: Differential loss of heterozygosity in familial, sporadic, and uremic hyperparathyroidism. *Hum Genet* **99**:342, 1997.

219. Tragl KH, Mayr WR: Familial islet cell adenomatosis. *Lancet I* 426, 1977.

220. Maioli M, Cicarese M, Pacifico A, et al.: Familial insulinoma: description of two cases. *Acta Diabetol* **29**:38, 1992.

221. Kinnamon JEC: Heredity and symptoms in acromegaly. *Acta Otolaryngol* **82**:230, 1976.

222. Kurisaka M, Takei Y, Tsubokawa T, Motiyasu N: Growth hormone-secreting pituitary adenoma in uniovular twin brothers: case report. *Neurosurgey* **8**:226, 1981.

223. Jones MK, Evans PJ, Jopnes IR, Thomas JP: Familial acromegaly. *Clin Endocrinol (Oxf)* **20**:355, 1984.

224. Abbassioun K, Fatourechi V, Amirjamshidi A, Meibodi NA: Familial acromegaly with pituitary adenoma. Report of three affected siblings. *J Neurosurg* **64**:510, 1986.

225. Pestell RG, Alford FP, Best JD: Familial acromegaly. *Acta Endocrinol* (Copenh) **121**:286, 1989.

226. Berezin M, Karasik A: Familial prolactinoma. *Clin Endoc* **42**:483, 1995.

227. Eschbach JW, Rinaldo JA: Metastatic carcinoid: A familial occurrence. *Ann Intern Med* **57**:647, 1962.

228. Anderson RE: A familial instance of appendiceal carcinoid tumors. *Am J Surg* **111**:738, 1966.

229. Wale RJ, William JA, Veeley AH: Familial occurrence in carcinoid tumors. *Aust NZ J Surg* **53**:325, 1983.

230. Moertel CG, Dockerty MB: Familial occurrence of metastizing carcinoid tumors. *Ann Intern Med* **78**:389, 1973.

231. Yeatman TJ, Sharp JV, Kimura AK: Can susceptibility to carcinoid tumors be inherited? *Cancer* **63**:390, 1989.

232. Brandi ML, Fitzpatrick LA, Coon HG, Aurbach GD. Bovine parathyroid cells: cultures maintained for more than 140 population doublings. *Proc Natl Acad Sci USA* **83**:1709, 1986.

233. Sakaguchi K, Santora A, Zimering M, Curcio F, Aurbach GD, Brandi ML: Functional epithelial cell line cloned from rat parathyroid glands. *Proc Natl Acad Sci USA* **84**:3269, 1987.

234. Brandi ML, Ornberg R, Sakaguchi K, et al.: Establishment and characterization of a clonal line of parathyroid endothelial cells. *FASEB J* **4**:3152, 1990.

235. Brandi ML, Aurbach GD, Fitzpatrick LA: Parathyroid mitogenic activity in plasma from patients with familial multiple endocrine neoplasia type 1. *N Engl J Med* **314**:1287, 1985.

236. Marx SJ, Sakagucki K, Green J, Aurbach GD, Brandi ML: Mitogenic activity on parathyroid cells in plasma from members of a large kindred with multiple endocrine neoplasia type 1. *J Clin Endocrinol Metab* **67**:149, 1988.

237. Friedman E, Larsson C, Amorosi A, Brandi ML, Bale A, Metz D, Jensen RT, Skarulis M, Eastman RC, Nieman L, Norton JA, Marx SJ: Multiple endocrine neoplasia type 1: pathology pathophysiology, and differential diagnosis. In *The Parathyroids* eds. Bilezekian JP, Levine MA & Marcus R. Raven Press, 647, 1994.

238. Zimering MB, Brandi ML, DeGrange DA, et al.: Circulating fibroblast growth factor-like substance in familial multiple endocrine neoplasia type 1. *J Clin Endocrinol Metab* **70**:149, 1990.

239. Bikelavi A, Klein S, Pintucci G, Rifkin DB: Biological roles of fibroblast growth factor-2. *Endocr Rev* **18**:26, 1997.

240. Brem H, Klagsbrun M. The role of fibroblast growth factors and related oncogenes in tumor growth. *Cancer Treat Res* **63**:211, 1992.

241. Zimering MB, Katsumata N, Sato Y, Brandi ML, Aurbach GD, Marx SJ, Friesen HG: Increased basic fibroblast growth factor in plasma from multiple endocrine neoplasia type 1: relation to pituitary tumor. *J Clin Endocrinol Metab* **76**:1182, 1993.

242. Gustavsson KH, Jansson R, Oberg K: Chromosomal breakage in multiple endocrine adenomatosis (type 1 and II). *Clin Genet* **23**:143, 1983.

243. Benson L, Gustavson KH, Rastad J, Akerstrom G, Oberg K, Ljunghall S: Cytogenetical investigations in patient with primary hyperparathyroidism and multiple endocrine neoplasia type 1. *Hereditas* **108**:227, 1988.

243.5. Scappaticci S, Maraschio P, Del Ciotto N, Fossati GS, Zonta A, Fraccarp M: Chromosome abnormalities in lymphocytes and fibroblasts of subjects with multiple endocrine neoplasia type 1. *Cancer Genet Cytogenet* **52**:85, 1991.

244. Bale SJ, Bale AE, Stewart K, Dachowski L, McBride OW, Glaser T, Green JE III, Mulvihill JJ, Brandi ML, Sakaguchi K, Aurbach GD, Marx SJ: Linkage analysis of multiple endocrine neoplasia type 1 with int-2 and other markers on chromosome 11. *Genomics* **4**:320, 1989.

245. Sakurai A, Katai M, Itakura Y, Nakajima K, Baba K, and Hashizume K: Genetic screening in hereditary multiple endocrine neoplasia type 1: Absence of a founder effect among Japanese families. *Jpn J Cancer Res* **87**:985, 1996.

246. Teh BT, Hii SI, David R, Parameswaran V, Grimmond S, Walters MK, Tan TT, Nancarrow DJ, Chan SP, Mennon J, Larsson C, Zaini A, Khalid AK, Shepherd JJ, Cameron DP, Hayward NK: Multiple endocrine neoplasia type (MEN1) in two Asian families. *Hum Genet* **94**:468, 1994.

247. Kytola S, Leisti J, Winqvist R, Salmela P: Improved carrier testing for multiple endocrine neoplasia, type 1, using new microsatellite-type DNA markers. *Hum Genet* **96**:449, 1995.

248. Smith CM, Wells SA, Gerhard DS: Mapping eight new polymorphisms in 11q13 in the vicinity of multiple endocrine neoplasia type 1: identification of a new distal recombinant. *Hum Genet* **96**:377, 1995.

249. Courseaux A, Grosgeorge J, Gaudray P, Pannett AAJ, Forbes SA, Williamson C, Bassett D, Thakker RV, Teh BT, Farnebo F, Shepherd J, Skogseid B, Larsson C, Giraud S, Zhang CX, Salandre J, Calender A: Definition of the minimal MEN1 candidate area based on a 5-Mb integrated map of proximal 11q13. *Genomics* **37**:354, 1996.

250. Larsson C, Calender A, Grimmond S, Giraud S, Hayward NK, Teh BT, Farnebo F: Molecular tools for presymptomatic testing in multiple endocrine neoplasia type 1. *J Intern Med* **2328**:239, 1995.

251. Petty EM, Green JS, Marx SJ, Taggart RT, Farid N, Bale AE: Mapping the gene for hereditary hyperparathyroidism and prolactinoma (MEN1-Burin) to chromosome 11q: evidence for a founder effect in patients from Newfoundland. *Am J Hum Genet* **54**:1060, 1994.

252. Stock JL, Warth MR, Teh BT, Coderre JA, Overdorf JH, Baumann G, Hintz RL, Hartman ML, Seizinger BR, Larsson C, Aronin N: A kindred with a variant of multiple endocrine neoplasia type 1 demonstrating frequent expression of pituitary tumors but not linked to the multiple endocrine neoplasia type 1 locus at chromosome region 11q13. *J Clin Endocrinol Metab* **82**:486, 1997.

253. Bahn RS, Scheithauer BW, van Heerden JA, Laws ER Jr, Horvath E, Gharib H: Nonidentical expressions of multiple endocrine neoplasia type 1 in identical twins. *Mayo Clin Proc* **61**:689, 1986.

254. Brandi ML, Weber G, Svensson A, Falchetti A, Tonelli F, Castello R, Furlani L, Scappaticci S, Fraccaro M, Larsson C: Homozygotes for the autosomal dominant neoplasia syndrome (MEN1). *Am J Hum Genet* **53**:1167, 1993.

255. de Mars R: Published Discussion. *23rd Annual Symposium of Fundamental Cancer Research* Williams & Wilkins: 105. (Abstract), 1969.

256. Knudson AG: Mutation and cancer: Statistical study of retinoblastoma. *Proc Natl Acad Sci USA* **68**:820, 1971.

257. Friedman E, Sakaguchi K, Bale AE, et al.: Clonality of parathyroid tumors in familial multiple endocrine neoplasia type 1. *N Engl J Med* **321**:213, 1989.

258. Thakker RV, Bouloux P, Wooding C, et al.: Association of parathyroid tumors in multiple endocrine neoplasia type 1 with loss of alleles on chromosome 11. *N Engl J Med* **321**:218, 1989.

259. Bystrom C, Larsson C, Blomberg C, et al.: Localization of the MEN 1 gene to a small region within chromosome 11q13 by deletion mapping in tumors. *Proc Natl Acad Sci USA* **87**:1968, 1990.

260. Radford DM, Ashley SM, Wells SA, Gerhard DS: Loss of heterozygosity of markers on chromosome 11 in tumors from patients with multiple endocrine neoplasia syndrome type 1. *Cancer Res* **50**:6529, 1990.

261. Friedman E, DeMarco L, Gejman PV, et al.: Allelic loss from chromosome 11 in parathyroid tumors. *Cancer Res* **525**:6804, 1992.

262. Morelli A, Falchetti A, Amorosi A, Tonelli F, Bearzi I, Ranaldi R, Tomassetti P, Brandi ML: Clonal analysis by chromsome 11 microsatellite-PCR of microdissected parathyroid tumors from MEN1 patients. *Biochem Biophys Res Comm* **227**:736, 1996.

263. Lubensky IA, Debelenko LV, Zhuang Z, Emmert-Buck MR, Dong Q, Chandrasekharappa SC, Guru SC, Manickam P, Olufemi SE, Marx SJ, Spiegel AM, Collins FS, Liotta LA: Allelic deletions in chromosome 11q13 in multiple tumors from individual MEN1 patients. *Canc Res* **56**:5272, 1996.

264. Zhuang Z, Bertheau P, Emmert-Buck MR, Liotta LA, Gnarra J, Linehan WM, Lubensky IA: A microdissection technique for archival DNA analysis of specific cell populations in lesions <1 mm in size. *Am J Pathol* **146**:620, 1995.

265. Debelenko LV, Zhuang Z, Emmert-Buck MR, Chandrasekharappa SC, Manickam P, Guru SC, Marx SJ, Spiegel AM, Collins FS, Jensen RT, Liotta LA, Lubensky IA: Allelic deletions on chromosome 11q13 in MEN1-associated and sporadic duodenal gastrinomas and pancreatic endocrine tumors. *Canc Res* **157**:2238, 1997.

266. Dong Q, Debelenko L, Chandrasekharappa S, Emmert-Buck MR, Zhuang Z, Guru SC, Manickam P, Skarulis M, Lubensky IA, Liotta LA, Collins FS, Marx SJ, Spiegel AM. Loss of heterozygosity at 11q13: analysis of pituitary tumors, lung carcinoids, lipomas, and other uncommon tumors in familial multiple endocrine neoplasia type 1. *J Clin Endocrinol Metab* **82**:1416, 1997.

267. Williamson C, Pannett A, Pang JT, McCarthy M, Sherppard MN, Monson JP, Clayton RN, Thakker RV: Localisation of a tumour suppressor gene causing endocrine tumours to a four centimorgan region on chromosome 1. Program and Abstracts Endo Soc. 961 (abstract), 1996.

268. Henske EP, Scheithauer BW, Short MP, Wollmann R, Nahmias J, Hornigold N. Slegtenhorst M, Welsh CT, Kwiatkowski DJ: Allelic

loss is frequent in tuberous sclerosis kidney lesions but rare in brain lesions. *Am J Human Genet* **59**:400, 1996.

269. Tahara H, Smith AP, Gaz RD, Cryns VL, Arnold A: Genomic localization of novel candidate tumor suppressor gene loci in human parathyroid adenomas. *Canc Res* **56**:599, 1996.

270. Eubanks PJ, Sawicki MP, Samara GJ, Gratti R, Nakamura Y, Tsao D, Johnson C, Hurwitz M, Wan YJ, Passaro E: Putative tumor-suppressor gene on chromosome 11 is important in sporadic endocrine tumor formation. *Am J Surg* **167**:180, 1994.

271. Thakker RV, Pook MA, Wooding C, Boscaro M, Scanarini M, Clayton RN: Association of somatotrophinomas with loss of alleles on chromsome 11 and with gsp mutations. *J Clin Invest* **91**:2815, 1993.

272. Boggild MD, Jenkinson S, Pistorello M, Boscaro M, Scanarini M, McTernan P, Perrett CW, Thakker RV, Clayton RN: Molecular genetic studies of sporadic pituitary tumors. *J Clin Endocrinol Metab* **78**:387, 1994.

273. Bates AS, Farrell WE, Bicknell EJ, McNicol AM, Talbots AJ, Broome JC, Perrett CW, Thakker RV, Clayton RN: Allelic deletion in pituitary adenomas reflects aggressive biological activity and has potential value as a prognostic marker. *J Clin Endocrinol Metab* **82**:818, 1997.

274. Jakobovitz O, Devora N, DeMarco L, Barbosa AJA, Simoni FB, Rechavi G, Friedman E: Carcinoid tumors frequently display genetic abnormalities involving chromosome 11. *J Clin Endocrinol Metab* **81**:3164, 1996.

275. Matsuo K, Tang SH, Fagin JA: Allelotype of human thyroid tumors: loss of chromosome 11q13 sequences in follicular neoplasms. *Mol Endocrinol* **5**:1873, 1991.

276. Iida A, Blake K, Tunny T, Klemm S, Stowasser M, Hayward N, Gordon R, Nakamura Y, Imai TK: Allelic losses on chromosome band 11q13 in aldosterone-producing adrenal tumors. *Genes Chromosomes Canc* **12**:73, 1995.

277. Falchetti A, Bale AE, Amorosi A, Bordi C, Cicci P, Bandini S, Marx SJ, Brandi ML: Progression of uremic hyperparathyroidism involves allelic loss on chromosome 11. *J Clin Endocrinol Metab* **76**:139, 1993.

278. Arnold A, Brown MF, Urena P, Gaz RD, Sarfati E, Drueke TB: Monoclonality of parathyroid tumors in chronic renal failure and in primary parathyroid hyperplasia. *J Clin Invest* **95**:2047, 1995.

279. Zhuang Z, Merino MJ, Chuaqui R, Liotta LA, Emmert-Buck MR: Identical allelic loss on chromosome 11q13 in microdissected in situ and invasive human breast cancer. *Canc Res* **55**:467, 1995.

280. Chuaqui RF, Zhuang Z, Emmert-Buck MR, Liotta LA, Merino MJ: Analysis of loss of heterozygosity on chromosome 11q13 in atypical ductal hyperplasia and in situ carcinoma of the breast. *Am J Pathol* **150**:297, 1997.

281. Srivatsan ES, Misra BC, Venugopalan M, Wilczynski SP: Loss of heterozygosity for alleles on chromosome 11 in cervical carcinoma. *Am J Hum Genet* **49**:868, 1991.

282. Popescu NC, Zimonjic DB: Alterations of Chromosome 11q13 in cervical carcinoma cell lines. *Am J Hum Genet* **58**:422, 1996.

283. Debelenko LV, Emmert-Buck MR. Manickam P, Kester MB, Guru SC, DiFranco EM, Olufemi SE, Agarwal SK, Lubensky IA, Zhuang Z, Burns AL, Spiegel AM, Liotta LA, Collins FS, Marx SJ, Chandrasekharappa SC: Haplotype analysis defines a minimal interval for the multiple endocrine neoplasia type 1 (MEN1) gene. *Canc Res* **57**:1039, 1997.

284. Collins FS: Positional cloning moves from perditional to traditional. *Nat Genet* **9**:347, 1995.

285. Kas K, Weber G, Merregaert J, Michiels L. Sandelin K, Skogseid B, Thompson N, Nordenskjold M, Larsson C, Friedman E: Exclusion of FAU as the multiple endocrine neoplasia type 1 (MEN1) gene. *Human Mol Genet* **2**:349, 1993.

286. DeWit MJ, Landsvater RM, Sinke RJ, van Kessel A, Lips CJ, Hoppener JW: Exclusion of the phosphatidylinositol-specific phospholipase C beta 3 (PLC beta 3) gene as candidate for the multiple endocrine neoplasia type 1 (MEN1) gene. *Hum Genet* **99**:133, 1997.

287. Landsvater RM, DeWit MJ, Peterson LF, Sinke RJ, van Kessel AD, Lips CJM, Hoppener JWM: Exclusion of the nuclear factor-kB3 (REL A) gene as candidate for the multiple endocrine neoplasia type (MEN1) gene. *Biochem Molecular Med* **60**:76, 1997.

288. Emmert-Buck MR, Lubensky IA, Dong Q, Manickam P, Guru SC, Kester MB, Olufemi S-E, Agarwal SK, Burns AL, Spiegel AM, Collins FS, Marx SJ, Zhuang Z, Liotta LA, Chandrasekharappa SC, Debelenko LV: Localization of the *MEN1* gene based on tumor LOH analysis. *Canc Res* **57**:1855–58, 1997.

289. Emmert-Buck MR, Bonner RF, Smith PD, Chuaqui RF, Zhuang Z, Goldstein SR, Weiss RA, Liotta LA: Laser capture microdissection. *Science* **274**:998, 1996.

290. Sarkar G, Yoon HS, Sommer SS: Dideoxy fingerprinting (ddF): a rapid and efficient screen for the presence of mutations. *Genomics* **13**:441, 1992.

291. Agarwal SK, Kester MB, Debelenko LV, Heppner C, Emmert-Buck MR, Skarulis MC, Doppman JL, Kim YS, Lubensky IA, Zhuang Z, Green JS, Guru SC, Manickam P, Olufemi SE, Liotta LA, Chandrasekharappa SC, Collins FS, Spiegel AM, Burns AL, Marx SJ: Germline mutations of the MEN1 gene in familial multiple endocrine neoplasia type 1 and related states. *Hum Molec Genet* **7**:1177, 1997.

291a. Heppner C, Kester MB, Agarwal SK, Debelenko LV, Emmert-Buck MR, Guru SC, Manickam P, Olufemi SE, Skarulis MC, Doppman JL, Alexander RH, Kim YS, Saggar SK, Lubensky IA, Zhuang Z, Liotta LA, Chandrasekharappa SC, Collins FS, Spiegel AM, Burns AL, Marx SJ: Somatic mutation of the MEN1 gene in parathyroid tumors. *Nat Genet* **16**:375, 1997.

292. Kohlmeier L, Marcus R: Calcium disorders of pregnancy. *Endocrinol Metab Clin North Am* **1**:15, 1995.

293. Ciccarelli E, Camanni F: Diagnosis and drug therapy of prolactinoma. *Drugs* **51**:954–965, 1996.

294. Marx SJ: Familial multiple endocrine neoplasia type 1. NIH Publication No. 96-3048, 1996.

CHAPTER 27

Malignant Melanoma

Alexander Kamb ■ Meenhard Herlyn

1. Melanoma is one of the more common cancers in the United States and is increasing rapidly in occurrence. Environmental factors, particularly sun exposure, have been strongly implicated in melanoma risks.

2. Accumulated evidence points to a set of genetic changes that underlie the evolution from melanocytes to metastatic melanoma. In addition, a significant proportion of the disease is familial, suggesting that specific genes regulate susceptibility. Study of familial melanoma provides one route to the identification of genes that contribute to all melanomas, including the more common sporadic form.

3. The investigation of somatic lesions in melanoma tumors and cell lines has permitted clinicians and molecular geneticists to focus on defined regions in the genome. Several chromosomal areas have been delineated on the basis of various types of analysis. These regions exhibit loss of heterozygosity (LOH) and in some cases homozygous deletions. The most commonly observed abnormality in melanoma is LOH and homozygous deletion at 9p21. Chromosomal aberrations at 9p21 may occur early in tumor development, although certain results suggest that their ultimate effect may be manifested later.

4. Linkage analysis of melanoma-prone kindreds also identified 9p21 as the site of a potential tumor-suppressor gene involved in melanoma susceptibility. Interestingly, the initial linkage studies were hindered by the use of dysplastic nevi rather than melanoma itself as the phenotypic trait, emphasizing the importance of phenotype definition in linkage analysis. The melanoma susceptibility locus discovered at 9p21, called MLM, is inherited as a dominant allele with penetrance that ranges upward from 50 percent. Its expressivity is highly variable.

5. The identity of MLM has been determined largely through deletion mapping in melanoma cell lines. It encodes a negative growth regulator, p16, the expression of which causes cell cycle arrest. p16 is part of a growth control pathway that involves cyclin-dependent kinases, cyclins, and the retinoblastoma gene product *Rb*. An impressive list of experiments supports a role for p16 not only in melanoma formation but also in the genesis of many other tumors. p16 inactivation may occur in nearly half of all advanced human cancers.

6. Genes other than p16 also play a part in melanoma formation. One of these is cyclin-dependent kinase 4 (cdk4), a target of p16's biochemical inhibitory activity. cdk4 is mutated in some tumors and in the germ line of rare familial melanoma cases. It is only the second germ-line oncogene to be described. Through cdk4 and *Rb*, p16 is tied into the basic cell cycle control apparatus.

7. The identification of genes involved in familial and sporadic melanoma raises the possibility of gene-based tests for cancer predisposition and for the classification of tumors. p16, as the primary genetic element in familial melanoma, is an interesting case study in genetic testing. Technical and economic issues are especially important in this realm. With respect to somatic gene testing, technical concerns are superseded by the pressing need to demonstrate the clinical utility of information about p16 status in tumors. Therapeutic implications of genetic discoveries are not insignificant but remain largely speculative and long-term.

Melanoma is a malignancy that originates from melanocytes, the pigment-producing cells in skin. Melanocytes generate a light-absorbing shield of melanin that protects the skin from damage caused by ultraviolet radiation (UV). They transfer much of this pigment to keratinocytes in the suprabasal skin layers via dendritic connections. It is ironic that melanocytes themselves are among the targets of UV, spurred into malignant growth by the agent they are intended to counter. Melanocytes arise from neural crest-derived progenitors that migrate from the developing central nervous system into the skin and are homogeneously distributed at the junction between the epidermal and dermal layers. Since they are born of colonists themselves, it is perhaps not surprising that melanocytes, when fully transformed, are as aggressive and migratory as any tumor cells. Melanocytes are present in the skin at roughly equal densities in all races.[1] Dark-skinned people do not have more melanocytes; instead, each melanocyte produces on average more melanin pigment than does each melanocyte in light-skinned people. Consequently, individuals differ little in the numbers of precursor cells that can give rise to melanomas.

Several factors have contributed to a heightened awareness of melanoma. People are more conscious of the dangers of sun exposure. Melanoma, like lung cancer, is gaining a reputation as a neoplasm on the rise, a cancer whose incidence is profoundly affected by controllable environmental influences. In addition, the genetic principles that underlie the disease are beginning to emerge.[2]

Melanoma responds poorly to chemical and radiation therapy, and the most effective treatment is surgical excision before the tumor is well advanced.[3] Early detection thus is of paramount importance. Because the skin lesions are relatively easy to spot, frequent examination and prompt treatment are highly successful medical strategies. By contrast, clinical and histologic diagnosis of early lesions remains difficult and controversial. For individuals who have hundreds of moles, diagnosis is especially problematic. Partly because of the efficacy of early detection, genetic analysis of melanoma offers hope as part of a comprehensive plan to limit the morbidity of the disease. Genetic tests may provide the means to assess risk and recognize individuals who require more intensive observation. Although genetic studies in melanoma have lagged somewhat behind those in neoplasms such as colon cancer, the future appears bright in terms of the effort to understand the biology of melanoma, predict its clinical behavior, and eventually discern how to defeat it.[4]

INCIDENCE OF MELANOMA

The overall incidence of melanoma in the United States currently is 37,000 cases per year, placing it significantly below only prostate, breast, lung, and colon cancers in occurrence.[5] The population-averaged lifetime risk of developing melanoma can be as high as 1 in 60 in particular groups; more typically it is 1 in 90.[6,7] This rate of occurrence is increasing rapidly, more so than for any other cancer site except the lung. Since the 1930s, the incidence of melanoma has jumped nearly 20-fold.[7] The reason for this probably is related to the fashion for tanning and outdoor activities. The development of melanoma is strongly influenced by genetic as well as environmental factors, especially exposure to UV.[8] This is dramatically illustrated by epidemiologic studies that relate melanoma incidence to ethnographic and geographic factors. Melanoma is nearly three times more common in the southern latitudes of the United States than in the northern United States.[3] The highest incidence of melanoma occurs in Queensland, Australia, whereas one of the lowest occurs in south India. Both regions have a high degree of sun exposure. The difference is that Australians are largely light-skinned, whereas south Indians are dark-skinned. Thus, the genetics of skin color interact with sunlight exposure to determine the overall rate of melanoma.

DEVELOPMENT OF MELANOMA

Clinical Features

Melanoma presents in a variety of clinically distinct forms: superficial spreading melanoma, lentigo maligna melanoma, acral lentigious melanoma, and nodular melanoma.[3] At least two of these types—lentigo maligna melanoma and superficial spreading melanoma—may exist for several years in a preinvasive state, providing a prolonged window of opportunity for removal. Once the lesion thickens and begins to invade, the prognosis worsens considerably. The survival of melanoma patients correlates strongly with the thickenss of the primary lesion and its degree of invasion into the dermis. If it is clinically localized, the 5-year survival rate is 85 percent.[3]

Often it is useful to classify cells based not on the clinical criteria described above but on a scheme with a more chronologic emphasis. The transition from normal melanocytes to metastatic melanoma occurs in a series of defined stages. Each stage is characterized broadly by changes in morphology and growth properties (Fig. 27-1). The first abnormal state that is recognizably different from the melanocyte is the nevus cell. This cell type differs little in microscopic appearance from a normal melanocyte, yet it can contain random chromosomal abnormalities. The next stage is the premalignant melanoma, often discernible as a raised mole that has

acquired atypical architectural and cytologic features. This premalignant lesion can evolve further into a primary melanoma that is capable of breaking through the dermal layer into the underlying blood vessels. Finally, the most insidious form, metastatic melanoma, arises from the primary lesion. This end stage is invasive and migratory and ultimately, if unchecked, kills the patient. The secondary sites of metastasis include brain, bone, lung, and liver.

Models of Melanoma in Tissue Culture

Specific genetic components are presumed to account for the morphologic features that distinguish the various clinical forms of melanoma. One important goal of melanoma research is to identify genes that influence the phenotype of the tumor. Thus, it is helpful to develop a tractable experimental system in which to study tumor progression. Fortunately, some of the features of melanoma in situ can be reproduced in tissue culture.[9]

Much has been learned about the properties of the different melanoma stages through the study of cells in culture. The overall pattern of melanoma, as in other cancer types, involves progressive loss of dependence on exogenous growth signals as melanocytes evolve toward malignancy (Table 27-1). For example, normal melanocytes placed in culture require phorbol ester, basic fibroblast growth factor, α-melanocyte-stimulating factor, and insulin-like growth factor-1. However, most lines derived from early melanomas no longer require phorbol ester. By the time metastases appear, the cells have lost their dependence on any of these agents and grow rapidly in culture dishes without special serum factors. The behavior of cells in culture which have been established from clinically defined stages of melanoma is presumed to be relevant to the transitions that occur as melanocytes evolve in the body toward metastatic melanoma. Thus, thorough characterization of such cell lines is likely to be of great value in understanding the biology of melanoma.

GENETICS OF MELANOMA

Genetic analysis of melanoma has two aspects: the study of predisposition in melanoma-prone kindreds and the study of somatic genetic alterations that occur as tumors evolve in the body. Both approaches have considerable appeal and, as described below, may converge on the same set of genes important in melanoma development.

Somatic Genetics of Melanoma Tumors

Melanomas, like practically all tumors, progressively accumulate abnormalities in their DNA as they evolve more malignant traits.[10,11] These abnormalities include chromosomal losses, duplications, translocations, and deletions. In addition to cytogenetically detectable aberrations, melanomas incorporate more subtle somatic changes, such as microsatellite variability and point mutations.[12–15] The question of which of these changes are causal in tumorigenesis and which are merely effects of the transformed state is difficult to answer in many cases.

9p21 LOH

One of the most consistent somatic changes in melanomas is the loss of chromosomal material from the short arm of chromosome

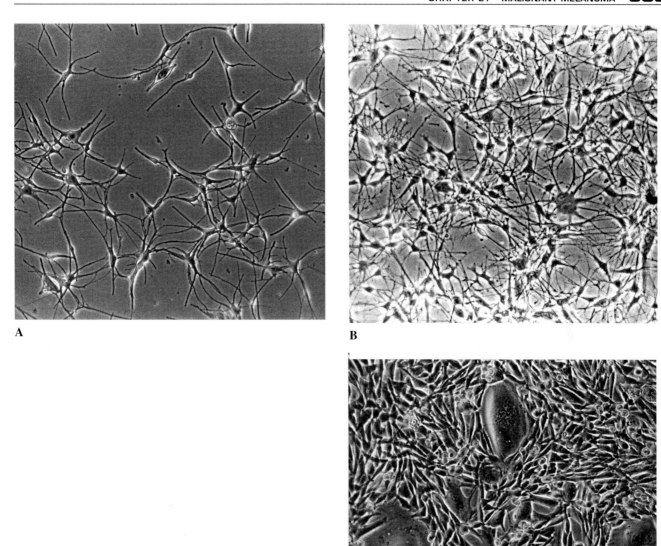

FIG. 27-1 Cells in culture. *A.* Normal melanocytes. *B.* Nevus cells. *C.* Metastatic melanoma cells.

Table 27-1 Culture Characteristics of Normal Melanocytes and Cells from Nonmalignant Primary and Metastatic Melanocytic Lesions

Parameter	Melanocytes	Nevus	Primary Melanoma		Metastatic Melanoma
			Early	Late	
Chromosomal abnormalities	None	None (few random)	(#1, 6, 7, 9) Nonrandom	(#1, 6, 7, 9) Nonrandom	(#1, 6, 7, 9, 11) Nonrandom
Life span (doublings)	Finite (<60)	Finite (<50)	Infinite (>100)	Infinite (>100)	Infinite (>100)
Response to phorbol ester	Stimulation	Stimulation	Inhibition	Inhibition	Inhibition
Growth factor requirements	I, FGF, aMSH, TPA*	Same as melanocytes†	I only	None	None
Growth in soft agar (percent)	<0.001	0.001–3 (average 0.9)	5–10 (average 8)	5–20	5–70 (average 25)
Growth in nude mice (percent)	None	None	80	100	100

*I = insulin; FGF = basic fibroblast growth factor; αMSH = α-melanocyte stimulating hormone. †Cultures are often independent of FGF and/or TPA.

9 (9p).[11,16,17] This cytogenetic abnormality is observed in over half of malignant melanomas. Some studies suggest that the initial change involving loss of heterozygosity (LOH) on 9p is a relatively early event in melanoma development, occurring before the primary lesion matures.[11] More recent work has demonstrated that a large proportion of the 9p abnormalities ultimately are detected as homozygous deletions of 9p21 in advanced malignancies.[18] Whether the homozygous deletions are present at an earlier stage in tumor development remains an open question, although some studies suggest that they may be a later phenomenon.[19] If this is the case, the role of the early LOH lesions in melanoma is unclear. In a subsequent section, the molecular identity of the 9p21 tumor suppressor is discussed.

Other LOH Sites

Chromosomal abnormalities other than 9p LOH have been observed as common features in primary melanoma tumors (Table 27-2).[11] These abnormalities include LOH regions on 3p, 6q, 10q, 11q, and 17p. 3p and 10q losses are detected in tumors <1.5 mm in thickness, suggesting that hypothetical tumor-suppressor loci on these chromosomal arms may be important at earlier stages of melanoma formation. 6q, 11q, and 17p LOH is detected only in more invasive tumors. Homozygous deletions at a specific site on 3p were described recently.[20] These deletions frequently remove a gene termed *FHIT*, suggesting that it may be the relevant tumor-suppressor locus in the region. However, the *FHIT* location on 3p is a fragile site that is prone to rearrangement, and further studies are necessary to establish a causal relationship between *FHIT* inactivation and tumor growth. 17p contains the p53 tumor-suppressor gene, and although point mutations in p53 are relatively uncommon in melanomas, p53 may account for a fraction of 17p LOH.[21,22] Additional regions of abnormality on 1p, 3q, and 17q have been described in melanoma cell lines and metastases.[23–27] 17q contains the metastasis-suppressor gene *NM23* and the *NF1* tumor-suppressor gene, a gene that is found to be mutated in some melanoma cell lines.[27–29]

Kindred Analysis

Apart from skin tone, predisposition to melanoma may be strongly influenced by heredity. As early as 1952, the familial nature of nonocular melanoma was described, and current estimates indicate that 5 to 10 percent of all melanoma cases may have a genetic ba-

Table 27-2 Loss of Heterozygosity in Primary Melanoma Specimens

Chromosome Arm	Percent LOH
1p	5
3p	19
3q	14
6q	31
9p	47
9q	19
10q	31
11q	17
13q	9
17p	16
17q	4
22q	6

SOURCE: Data are taken from Ref. 11. Experiments on each chromosome arm involved 21 to 41 informative samples.

sis.[30,31] This heritable component is inferred from melanoma cases that cluster in specific families. The definition of familiality varies, but typically melanoma patients who have at least one first-degree relative with melanoma are classified as familial cases. For first-degree relatives of melanoma patients, the increased risk is calculated to be 2.0; with a relative under 50 affected, the risk is 6.5.[32,33]

On the basis of the commonly accepted figures, over 90 percent of melanomas are predicted to have a nongenetic, or sporadic, origin, a percentage similar to that reported for cancer sites such as breast and colon. Sporadic melanoma may truly be independent of heredity, arising solely from random wear and tear occurring during a lifetime. Alternatively, it may be caused by multiple genes or weakly penetrant alleles that modify an individual's risk modestly, but in the aggregate, strongly affect the overall incidence of disease in a population.

Dysplastic Nevus Syndrome

During the past few decades numerous families with multiple cases of melanoma have been identified.[34–36] Individuals in many of these kindreds were reported to have unusual numbers of large nevi, and the nevus count on the skin was shown to be a risk factor for melanoma.[37] A variety of pathologic studies suggested that certain nevi could be classified as dysplastic and therefore more likely to produce melanomas.[38,39] These nevi resemble the clinically miniature early superficial spreading melanomas.[3] Such observations gave rise to the notion of a disease, dysplastic nevus syndrome (DNS), characterized by the frequent occurrence of atypical moles and an increased risk of melanoma.

Melanoma Susceptibility Locus

Some DNS/melanoma kindreds served as the basis for genetic linkage analysis in which molecular genetic markers positioned at various places throughout the genome were tested for linkage to DNS and melanoma. Because dysplastic nevi are believed to be precursors to melanomas, initial attempts to determine a genetic basis for melanoma focused on DNS. However, these attempts were hindered by the difficulties of diagnosing and classifying moles. A reported linkage assignment on 1p36 was not reproduced in other families.[40–46] When the phenotype was restricted to melanoma itself, definitive linkage was obtained with markers in 9p21 (Fig. 27-2).[47] This linkage study produced a cumulative lod score (base 10 logarithm of the odds of linkage) of nearly 13, suggesting a probability of linkage in excess of 1 trillion to 1; one large kindred had a lod score of nearly 6. The genetic locus identified by linkage analysis was designated the melanoma susceptibility locus (MLM).

The history of the discovery of MLM is an ideal example of the importance of phenotypic definition to linkage analysis.[48] DNS proved to be an unreliable phenotype that was difficult to diagnose objectively. The use of melanoma itself as the primary phenotypic trait reduced the number of affecteds in the analysis but placed the phenotypic definition on a firm, objective foundation. This definition provided the key to the identification of MLM.

MLM is inherited in a dominant Mendelian fashion; a single defective germ-line copy of the gene predisposes to melanoma. The penetrance of the disease gene (the likelihood that an individual carrier will develop melanoma by age 80) has been estimated at 53 percent using three 9p21-linked kindreds.[49] More recent studies suggest that the penetrance may vary depending on the particular allele and/or the kindreds under consideration. In some kindreds, the penetrance appears to approach 100 percent.[50] As with many other cancer predisposition genes, inheritance of a defective

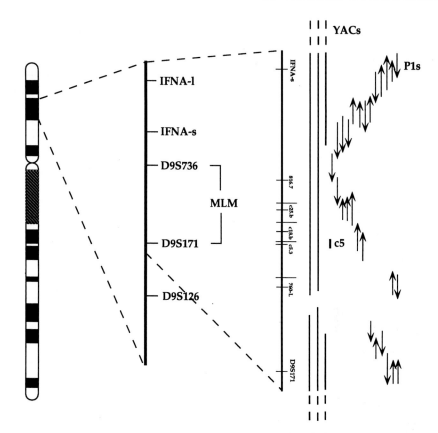

FIG. 27-2 Genetic and physical maps of the 9p21 region containing MLM. A cartoon of human chromosome 9 is shown with the 9p21 region expanded. Shown are five microsatellite markers; MLM maps between D9S736 and D9S171 by recombinant analysis. This region was aligned to a physical map of P1, yeast artificial chromosomes (YACs), and cosmid clones. Several new markers were generated, some of which are shown (e.g., c5.3). In addition, the location of cosmid c5 is shown. This cosmid contains sequences from p15 and p16.

MLM allele increases the probability of melanoma; it does not guarantee illness. For melanoma, the increased lifetime risk caused by inheritance of predisposing MLM alleles is roughly 50-fold. This risk is dependent on the level of sun exposure.[49]

MLM behaves as a classical tumor-suppressor locus. Although the increased risk is dominantly inherited, the mutant locus acts in cells as a recessive. Tumors that arise in MLM gene carriers invariably lose the wild-type chromosome by deletion or nondisjunction.[51] This feature accords with the proposal of Knudson that was based originally on studies of the retinoblastoma (*RB1*) tumor-suppressor gene.[52] In the general case of a tumor-suppressor gene, two hits are required to inactivate the locus, one for the maternal copy and one for the paternal. In familial cancers, one hit occurs through the inheritance of a defective allele. Thus, a single somatic event is necessary to complete the functional inactivation of the locus.

The relationship between nevi and melanoma remains unclear. The role of nevi as melanoma precursors has not been disputed, but the genetic underpinnings of mole incidence and size are unresolved. No simple genetic basis for nevi has been discovered. Nevertheless, MLM may influence mole size and number. A comparison of MLM carriers and noncarriers revealed that carriers had roughly 50 percent more nevi.[49] If real, the phenotypic effect is dominant or codominant, involving the inheritance of a single defective MLM copy. This deduction has implications for the role of MLM in melanocyte biology.

GENES THAT INFLUENCE MELANOMA

p16

After the establishment of melanoma linkage to 9p21 markers, an effort to isolate MLM was undertaken. However, isolation of the gene proceeded largely without recourse to the 9p21-linked kin-

dreds (Fig. 27-2). Instead, cell lines were used as the primary tools for gene localization. Previous work had revealed the presence of melanoma cell lines with large homozygous deletions in 9p21.[16,17] This implied that the genetic locus MLM and a tumor-suppressor locus presumed to underlie the 9p21 deletions might be one and the same. Under this assumption, standard positional cloning methods of recombinant chromosome analysis were bypassed in favor of the simpler strategy of deletion breakpoint localization in cell lines.

In one study, a collection of nearly 100 melanoma cell lines was assembled to identify and map deletion breakpoints in 9p21.[18] Roughly 60 percent of those lines proved to have detectable homozygous deletions, and the deletions clustered around a single site in 9p21 (Fig. 27-3). This site contained two genes, one that encoded the previously identified cyclin-dependent kinase (cdk) inhibitor p16 and a second that subsequently was shown to encode the related cdk inhibitor p15.[53–57] A variety of deletional and DNA sequence-based studies soon pointed to *p16* (also designated P16INK4A, MTS1, and *cdk*N2) as the relevant locus. Inactivating point mutations were found in the p16 coding sequence but not in p15 in cell lines and tumors.[54,58,59] In addition, no homozygous deletions were found that removed p15 but left p16 intact.[60] In contrast, there were several examples of deletions that left p15 intact but selectively removed p16.

Conclusive evidence for the role of *p16* in tumorigenesis was obtained through study of the gene in 9p21-linked families. Linked *p16* sequence variants were found in many, although not all, of these kindreds (Table 27-3).[61–66] Several of the sequence variants obviously were disruptive to the protein, causing truncation of the predicted product, and several other missense changes subsequently were shown to encode defective p16 molecules.[67–69] *p16* germ-line mutations are found rarely in sporadic cases and in familial cases that do not manifest strong signs of 9p21 linkage. For instance, in 38 cases that met the typical definition of familiality but were not part of extended 9p21-linked kindreds, no *p16* muta-

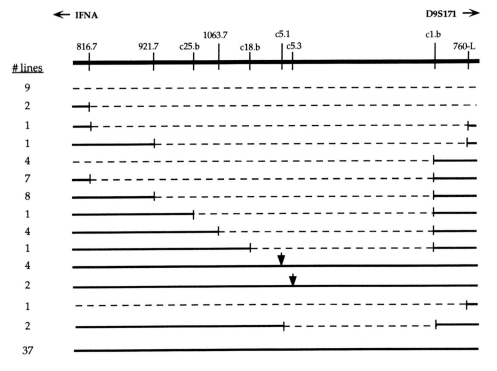

FIG. 27-3 Homozygous deletions in melanoma cell lines. Markers used to detect homozygous deletions are shown above. Melanoma cell lines are grouped into families based on which markers are missing, as indicated by the dashed lines. The two arrows show homozygous deletions that remove a single marker. The number of cell lines per family is listed on the left.

tions were detected.[62] On the basis of such studies, it is likely that *p16* accounts for only a proportion of the total melanoma incidence that is generally considered familial. To date there are no firm estimates for the population frequency of predisposing MLM alleles. Extrapolation from some of the work cited above suggests a frequency in the U.S. population of no more than one in a few thousand.[60,64]

Through remarkable serendipity, two individuals homozygous for a predisposing MLM allele have been identified.[65] Both homozygous persons carry two copies of the same mutant *p16* allele that contains a deletion of 19 bp, an allele that is especially prevalent in melanoma-prone families in Holland. The chance intermarriage of two gene carriers from relatively isolated Dutch villages produced the homozygous individuals. Interestingly, the homozy-

Table 27-3 Parameters Associated with Melanoma-Prone Kindreds and Mutations

Kindred	lod Score	Cases	Cases with Haplotype or Mutation	Mutation	Effect
3346	5.97	21	21	—	—
1771	3.57	12	12	Val126Asp	Missense
3137	1.90	17	16	—	—
1764	1.04	4	4	—	—
3012	0.64	4	4	Gly101Trp	Missense
3006	0.19	6	3	—	—
D4	1.22	6	6	Del(218-237)	Frameshift
2482	1.65	—	—	—	—
377	1.64	—	—	—	—
1016	1.41	6	6	Val126Asp	Missense
1017	1.24	4	4	Gly101Trp	Missense
567	1.08	4	4	Arg58Ter	Stop
479	1.03	5	5	Val126Asp	Missense
2884	0.52	2	2	IVS2+1	Splice
909	0.47	—	—	—	—
2209	0.24	—	—	—	—
928	0.12	4	6	Gly101Trp	Missense
481	0.00	3	3	Gly101Trp	Missense
873	−0.03	2	3	Arg87Pro	Missense
373	−0.34	3	3	Asn71Ser	Missense

NOTE: lod scores for the first five kindreds were calculated for markers between IFNA and D9S171.[62] The lod score for D4 was computed using D9S171.[65] Note that this mutation was misreported in the original work. lod scores for the last 12 kindreds were calculated for IFNA.[61] A number of other studies have reported germ-line p16 mutations that are not listed here.[50,63,66]

gous gene carriers were normal except that one of them developed two primary melanomas by age 15. The other individual, however, lived to age 55 with no melanomas, although she died of an internal adenocarcinoma. It is worth noting that the melanoma patient had numerous nevi, whereas the other carrier was relatively mole-free. The latter individual, however, had offspring, some of whom were classified as DNS cases. These facts demonstrate two important aspects of *p16* function. First, *p16* is not essential for normal development or viability, a conclusion confirmed by the recent demonstration of viable *p16* knockout mice.[70] Second, *p16* mutations have variable expressivity; phenotypic effects may depend on unknown genetic factors as well as environmental factors, including but perhaps not restricted to sun exposure.

The weight of the evidence strongly supports the view that *p16* is MLM. As is the case with many familial tumor suppressors, *p16* germ-line mutations increase cancer risk, whereas *p16* somatic mutations also occur in sporadic tumors during the transition toward malignancy.

p15

A continuing mystery is the existence of kindreds that are definitely 9p21-linked but for which mutations cannot be found in *p16* (Table 27-3).[60,61] These kindreds served as the initial impetus to explore *p15* as a candidate for a second melanoma susceptibility gene on 9p21. *p15* has considerable sequence similarity to *p16* (77 percent at the protein level in humans) and encodes a protein with biochemical behavior nearly identical to that of p16.[56,57] It is located within 20 kb of *p16* on chromosome 9 and probably was derived from *p16* by gene duplication, divergence, and, in the human lineage, a gene conversion event.[71] Both proteins cause growth arrest when overexpressed in certain cell lines and in normal cells.[59,67,72,73] p15 regulation, however, is markedly different from p16 regulation. p15 is induced by TGF-β; p16 is not.[56] This adds further interest to the possible role of *p15* in cancer, since TGF-β is an important regulator of cell growth. Despite the obvious appeal of *p15* as an alternative MLM-like gene, no germ-line mutations have been reported so far in *p15*.[59]

E1β/p19ARF

Another potential candidate for a tumor-suppressor gene is encoded at the *p16* locus, although its role in cancer is obscure (Fig. 27-4). This gene, termed p19ARF or p16E1β, actually overlaps the p16 coding sequence.[74–76] The p16E1β transcript originates from a promotor distinct from the normal *p16* promotor. This second upstream promotor produces a transcript that contains the second and third coding exons of p16 (E2 and E3) but incorporates an alternative first exon (E1β) in place of the normal first exon of *p16* (Fig. 27-3). The reading frame used to encode p16 is closed immedi-

ately upstream of the E1β–E2 junction, suggesting that if this frame were used for translation, a truncated p16 molecule missing the first third of the protein would result. No such protein has been detected in vivo. An alternative reading frame (ORF2), however, potentially encodes a protein of 19 kDa, hence the name P19ARF. This protein bears no homology to any known protein sequence. However, it is conserved between mouse and human.[71,77]

The E1β exon is deleted selectively in several melanoma cell lines, leaving the p16 transcript and protein intact.[74,78] This implies an important role for p16E1β in the tumor-suppressor function of the *p16* locus. No E1β mutations have been observed in the germ lines of familial cases. Moreover, no E1β-specific point mutations have been detected in cell lines or tumors.[74]

Antibodies raised against p19ARF detect a 19-kDa protein in vivo, and overexpression of p19ARF causes cessation of cell growth.[77] However, unlike p16 and other cdk inhibitors, p19ARF does not inhibit cdk4 in vitro. Paradoxically, the level of the E1β transcript increases as quiescent T cells enter the cell cycle.[74] In addition, comparison of human and mouse sequences reveals that the reading frame predicted to encode p19ARF is no more conserved than is the other alternative to the p16 reading frame (ORF3).[71,74] Thus, there is little evidence for evolutionary selective pressure on the p19ARF protein. E1β/p19ARF may represent one of the more bizarre genes in the mammalian genome. It is a member of a complex locus and is transcribed from a separate, independently regulated promotor, overlapping considerably a gene that is translated in a different reading frame, and both genes components of the cell cycle regulatory apparatus.

cdk4

On the heels of the discovery that *p16* germ-line mutations predispose to melanoma, a second melanoma predisposition gene was uncovered. A proportion of melanoma-prone families that are not linked to 9p21 segregate mutations in a gene that encodes one of the targets of p16's inhibitory activity, cdk4.[79] These mutations affect a single site in the p16 coding sequence that renders the molecule resistant to *p16* binding and inhibition. The identical lesion also has been observed as a somatic mutation in a sporadic melanoma.[80] Thus, cdk4 behaves as a proto-oncogene; the mutant form is converted into an overactive growth promotor, an oncogene. This is only the second example of germ-line mutations in a proto-oncogene. The other example is the *ret* proto-oncogene, in which germ-line mutations predispose to the cancer susceptibility syndrome multiple endocrine neoplasia 2A.[81] Based on the observed frequency of mutations, kindreds that segregate *cdk4* mutations may be 10-fold less frequent than *p16* kindreds.

A Growth Control Pathway in Melanocytes

The identification of cdk4 germ-line mutations in melanoma-prone kindreds is exciting for another reason. cdk4, p16, *Rb*, and D cyclins constitute part of a growth control pathway that operates in a variety of, perhaps all, tissues (Fig. 27-5).[82] Several lines of evidence suggest that p16 inhibits cdk4, preventing phosphorylation of Rb protein. Hypophosphorylated Rb binds transcription factors such as members of the E2F family, interfering with their ability to activate the transcription of genes involved in DNA synthesis.[83] Sporadic tumors seldom contain mutations in more than one component of this pathway, an observation that supports the mutually dependent function of the genes.[84–87] In contrast, mutations in p53, although rare in melanoma, occur as frequently in p16+ tumors as in p16− tumors, an indication that p53 and p16 function in separate pathways of growth control.[13] p16, cdk4, and Rb thus play a

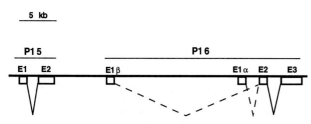

FIG. 27-4 The p26 locus is complex. The relative positions of *p15* coding exons (1 and 2) and *p16* exons are shown. Dashed lines indicate an alternative splice that distinguishes the E1β transcript from the *p16* transcript.

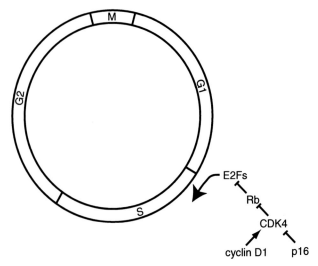

FIG. 27-5 The cell cycle and the p16 growth control pathway. Eukaryotic cell division is broken up into four phases: G1, during which the cell prepares to synthesize DNA; S, the phase of DNA replication; G2, during which the cell prepares for mitosis; and M, the mitotic period. The transition between G1 and S is monitored carefully by the cell. p16, acting through cdk4 and Rb, exercises its control over cell division at this point. Arrows indicate a positive effect; blunt-ended lines, an inhibitory effect.

central role in the regulation of the cell cycle. They may constitute a primary circuit that integrates information relevant in the decision to proceed through the first stages of cell division.

To date, three of the four known components of the pathway have been implicated in hereditary cancer syndromes: *cdk4*, *p16*, and *RB1*. Curiously, *RB1* mutant gene carriers do not suffer from excessive melanoma but suffer from a specific childhood tumor of the eye.[88] Why the phenotype of cdk4 and *p16* mutations differs from the *RB1* mutant phenotype is unclear, but it emphasizes the complexity of the growth control pathways that operate in cells.

The Role of p16 in Cancer

The evidence that *p16* is an important cancer gene is compelling. Germ-line mutations in *p16* increase melanoma risk. Deletions in p16, as well as a smaller number of point mutations, are found in a large percentage of melanomas and many other cancer types.[89] In melanoma tumors and cell lines, the large majority of point mutations that are detected have the hallmarks of UV-induced changes, signs of the link between UV and p16 inactivation in tumors.[58,90,91] Loss of p16 expression owing to methylation has been reported in a variety of cell lines.[92–94] Overexpression of p16 in a range of cell types causes arrest at the G1/S checkpoint in the cell cycle.[67,70,73] Mice in which the *p16* gene has been inactivated by homologous recombination are cancer-prone.[70] p16 functions in vitro as a biochemical inhibitor of cdk4, a protein known to promote passage through the G1/S checkpoint. Taken together, these data leave little room for doubt that p16 plays a key role in a variety of human cancers but do not delineate the precise nature of the role.

p16 and Other cdk Inhibitors

Many other cdk inhibitors have been identified, including p15, p18, p21, p27, and p57.[56,95–102] All, including p16, are expressed in a wide variety of tissues.[74] The biochemical behavior of p16 protein differs little from, for example, that of p15.[56] All cdk inhibitors, when overexpressed in particular cell types, induce cell

cycle arrest, yet p16 appears to be a special case. None of the other genes is mutated at an appreciable frequency in tumors or cell lines.[59,103–105] The physiologic function of p16 that may distinguish it from other cdk inhibitors, rendering it more vulnerable to mutational inactivation, is not obvious.

Attempts to define the physiologic function of p16 in vivo have focused on two general areas: its role in programmed cell death, or apoptosis, and its role in cellular senescence. In one model system, p16 expression correlated with protection from apoptosis, a finding that does not explain why tumor cells would dispense with p16.[106] More germane perhaps, p16-deficient mouse cells are highly sensitive to oncogenic transformation and readily form colonies in culture.[70] This result suggests that loss of p16 expression may contribute to immortalization. Other studies have reported an increase in p16 levels as cells approach senescence, followed by a fall as cells become immortalized.[107–109] On the basis of this correlation, it seems reasonable to propose a role for p16 in suppressing immortalization. To achieve this effect, p16 must work through Rb. Consequently, Rb and the other components of the p16 pathway are implicated as accessory molecules in the control of cellular life span. This proposed role for p16 leaves unexplained the early 9p LOH events in melanoma development.

p16 Mutations and Predisposition to Nonmelanoma Cancers

It is perplexing, given the widespread involvement of p16 in sporadic cancer, that *p16* mutant gene carriers are predisposed only to melanoma. Some studies have suggested an association between pancreatic cancer and melanoma in certain families, but a clear role for MLM in cancers besides melanoma has been difficult to prove.[51,110] A simple explanation may lie in considerations about rate-limiting steps in tumorigenesis. If, as the data begin to suggest, p16 inactivation is a relatively late step in tumor development, its removal may not be rate-limiting in most tumor types. For reasons that are obscure, p16 inactivation may be important at an earlier stage in melanoma formation, or it may be the final brake that is released in cells that suffer an enormous environmental insult in the form of UV exposure and consequent high rates of mutation. It is more complicated, although not impossible, to hypothesize a role for *p16* mutations both early during melanoma formation in nevi and later in the escape from senescence.

GENETICS AND MELANOMA DIAGNOSIS

Germ-Line Testing for Melanoma Susceptibility

With the identification of the major genetic factors underlying hereditary melanoma, *p16* and to a lesser extent *cdk4*, the possibility of germ-line testing for melanoma risk has been realized. Contrary to many other types of genetic testing, a melanoma predisposition screen has certain clear advantages. First, in principle the results of such a test provide valuable information to guide behavior. If an individual tests positive (i.e., carries a high-risk allele), steps can be taken to avoid sun exposure and maintain vigilance for abnormal growths on the skin. Such behavior would not only diminish the chance of melanoma but also facilitate early detection and removal of the lesion, by far the most successful approach to combating the disease. Second, although many independent sequence changes have been described, the *p16* gene is small, consisting of only 158 codons. By contrast, the coding sequences of the breast cancer susceptibility genes *BRCA1* and *BRCA2* are huge, roughly 12 and 25 times the size of *p16*, respectively.[111,112] The relatively small size of *p16* should reduce dramatically the technical difficulties and cost associated with a genetic screen. In the case of *cdk*4, a screen that targets a single codon may be sufficient.[79]

Excitement about the value of a melanoma susceptibility screen is blunted somewhat by other considerations, especially the economic realities of such a test. The combined gene frequency of *p16* and *cdk*4 predisposing alleles is low. Thus, for random population-based screening, the a priori probability of getting a positive result is very low, a disincentive to pay for such a test. In addition, the possibility of missing MLM mutations that fall outside the coding sequence must be considered. Several kindreds that show a strong indication of 9p21 linkage appear to have wild-type *p16* coding regions.[61,62] This suggests that a percentage of *p16* mutations fall outside the coding sequences or that a second *MLM* gene resides in 9p21. A test must detect such mutations or sacrifice informativeness.

The greatest value of a melanoma susceptibility test may apply to individuals at higher risk of melanoma than the majority of the population. This includes people with many moles and people with affected relatives. With roughly 37,000 melanoma cases per year in the United States, such a test might be relevant to over 100,000 people every year. If the criterion of numerous nevi also is used, the number of higher-risk individuals may exceed 1 million. This is a potential market size that may drive the development of a commercial test, but whether a specialized melanoma genetic test could be economically self-sustaining in the short term remains debatable. It may make more sense to provide an MLM test when the costs of such gene-based diagnostic screens are lower or when it becomes part of a larger panel of susceptibility gene tests.

Somatic Gene Testing

An alternative to germ-line p16 and cdk4 testing is afforded by the potential for somatic gene testing in tumors. *p16* is one of the most frequently altered genes in human cancer, inactivated in perhaps half of all advanced tumors.[54] Here economic considerations contribute a strong impetus for test development if certain criteria can be met. First, a slew of technical issues relate to detection of *p16* alterations in cancer cells caused by homozygous deletions, the most common form of *p16* inactivation, methylated DNA, and other somatic changes. Detection of such disparate lesions is a particularly significant problem in tumors that are invariably adulterated by normal somatic cells.[60] Second, the clinical relevance of such a somatic *p16* gene test must be demonstrated firmly. The test must prove useful in the diagnosis or prognosis of cancer. Most desirable would be test results that aid in customization of cancer therapy. Clinical studies that address these issues are critically important. At least one report has detailed the significance of *p16* gene status as a prognostic indicator in childhood acute lymphocytic leukemia.[113] Thus, there is the exciting possibility that *p16* gene tests, as well as tests for many other cancer genes, ultimately may supplement or replace traditional modes of subjective histologic analysis in the classification and treatment of tumors.

GENETICS AND MELANOMA THERAPY

Advances in our understanding of the genetics of melanoma have had little impact on treatment and are not likely to have a rapid effect in the future. The difficulties of translating genetic knowledge into practical therapeutic advances are immense. Here, as in the traditional approach to cancer therapy, the challenge is to achieve specificity. An effective therapeutic agent must target cancer cells

and leave normal cells relatively unharmed. With some of the molecules that regulate melanoma development now in hand, it is at least possible to formulate potential strategies.

Targeting cdk4

Immunotherapy tailored to abnormal cdk4 molecules offers a route to novel melanoma therapy. Indeed, T cells have been identified that recognize tumor cells that harbor mutant cdk4 proteins.[80] One of the weaknesses of this approach, however, is the small number of tumors likely to have sustained cdk4 alterations. Thus, a treatment that targets mutant cdk4 is unlikely to have general success in combating the vast majority of melanomas.

Complementation of Defective *p16* Genes in Tumors

An alternative approach is to devise treatments that rely on *p16*. Because *p16* mutations occur in many tumors besides melanoma, the investment in such a treatment probably would have benefits that extended well beyond melanoma. Once again, however, specificity and delivery are key factors. Simple reintroduction of functional *p16* sequences into tumor cells causes growth arrest.[114,115] However, the sequences also arrest normal cells.[73] Therefore, a strategy that depends on restored expression of *p16* in tumor cells must include either a means for selective delivery of *p16* into tumor cells or a mechanism for regulated expression that permits normal cell growth.

Manipulating the Cell Cycle

Finally, it may be possible to use cell cycle regulators such as p16 to protect normal cells from the ravages of conventional chemo- or radiotherapy. If a method for specific induction of growth arrest in normal cells could be found, a state of temporary arrest could be induced in normal cells that would endow them with resistance to subsequent cytotoxic treatments. This general concept was explored in the past.[116-119] *p16* provides a new molecular tool to study the value of such an approach. At least in one model system, *p16* expression causes reversible cell cycle arrest that protects cells from chemotherapeutic agents.[120] The challenge in this approach is to achieve a general protection of normal tissues by reversible induction of p16 or other regulators. The strategy is attractive because the induction does not need to be selective. Many tumors have lost the function of the p16 growth control pathway either by mutation of *p16* itself or by alteration of downstream components such as cdk4 and *RB1*. Thus, most tumors would not respond to an agent that induces p16 expression by entering a state of arrest. Only normal cells, which maintain the integrity of the p16 pathway, would arrest and be rendered resistant to cytotoxic treatments.

REFERENCES

1. Clark WH: The skin, in Rubin E, Farber JL (eds): *Pathology.* Philadelphia, Lippincott, 1988.
2. Kamb A: Human melanoma genetics. *J Invest Dermatol Symp Proc* **1**:177, 1996.
3. Fitzpatrick TB, Sober AM, Mihm MC Jr: Malignant melanoma of the skin, in Braunwald E, Isselbacher KJ, Petersdorf RG, Wilson JD, Martin JB, Fauci AS (eds): *Principles of Internal Medicine,* 13/e, pp 1595. New York, McGraw-Hill, 1987.

4. Fearon ER, Vogelstein B: A genetic model for colorectal tumorigenesis. *Cell* **61**:759–767, 1990.

5. National Cancer Institute: 1987 Annual Cancer Statistics Review. NIH publication No. 88-2789, 1988 C. *J Natl Cancer Inst* **83**:170, 1991.

6. Sober AJ, Lew RA, Koh HK, Barnhill RL: Epidemiology of cutaneous melanoma. *Dermatol Clin North Am* **9**:617, 1991.

7. Nigel DS, Fridman RJ, Kopf AW: The incidence of malignant melanoma in the United States: Issues as we approach the 21st century. *J Am Acad Dermatol* **34**:839, 1996.

8. Green A, Swerdlow AJ: Epidemiology of melanocytic nevi. *Epidemiol Rev* **11**:204, 1989.

9. Herlyn M: *Molecular and Cellular Biology of Melanoma.* Austin, TX, RG Landes, 1993.

10. Fountain JW, Bale SJ, Housman DE, Dracopoli NC: Genetics of melanoma. *Cancer Surv* **9**:645, 1990.

11. Healy E, Rehman I, Angus B, Rees JL: Loss of heterozygosity in sporadic primary cutaneous melanoma. *Genes Chromosom Cancer* **12**:152, 1995.

12. Walker GJ, Palmer JM, Walters MK, Nancarrow DJ, Hayward NK: Microsatellite instability in melanoma. *Melanoma Res* **4**:267, 1994.

13. Gruis NA, Weaver-Feldhaus J, Liu Q, Frye C, Ecles R, Orlow I, Lacombe L, Ponce-Castoneda V, Lianes E, et al: Genetic evidence in melanoma and bladder cancers that p16 and p53 function in separate pathways of tumor suppression. *Am J Pathol* **146**:1199, 1995.

14. Peris K, Keller G, Chimenti S, Amantea A, Derl H, Hofler H: Microsatellite instability and loss of heterozygosity in melanoma. *J Invest Dermatol* **105**:625, 1995.

15. Quinn AG, Healy E, Rehman I, Sikkink S, Rees JL: Microsatellite instability in human non-melanoma and melanoma skin cancer. *J Invest Dermatol* **104**:309, 1995.

16. Olopade OI, Jenkins R, Linnenbach AJ, et al: Molecular analysis of chromosome 9p deletion in human solid tumors. *Proc Am Assoc Cancer Res* **21**:318, 1990.

17. Fountain JW, Karayiorgou M, Ernstoff MS, Kirkwood JM, Vlock DR, Titus-Ernstoff L, Bouchard B, Vijayasaradhi S, Houghton AN, Lahti J, et al: Homozygous deletions within human chromosome band 9p21 in melanoma. *Proc Natl Acad Sci USA* **89**:10557, 1992.

18. Weaver-Feldhaus J, Gruis NA, Neuhausen S, Le Paslier D, Stockert E, Skolnick MH, Kamb A: Localization of a putative tumor suppressor gene by using homozygous deletions in melanomas. *Proc Natl Acad Sci USA* **91**:7563, 1994.

19. Reed JA, Loganzo F Jr, Shea CR, Walker GJ, Flores JF, Glending JM, Bogdany JK, Shiel MJ, Haluska FG, Fountain JW, Albino AP: Loss of expression of the p16/cyclin-dependent kinase inhibitor 2 tumor suppressor gene in melanocytic lesions correlates with invasive stage of tumor progression. *Cancer Res* **55**:2713, 1995.

20. Sozzi G, Veronese ML, Negrini M, Baffa R, Cotticelli MG, Inoue H, Tornielli S, Pilotti S, De Gregorio L, Pastorino U, Pierotti MA, Ohta M, Huebner K, Croce CM: The FHIT gene 3p14.2 is abnormal in lung cancer. *Cell* **85**:17, 1996.

21. Volkenandt M, Schlegel U, Nanus DM, Albino AP: Mutational analysis of the human 53 gene in malignant melanoma cell lines. *Pigment Cell Res* **4**:35, 1991.

22. Levin DB, Wilson K, Valadares de Amorim G, Webber J, Kenny P, Kusser W: Detection of p53 mutations in benign and dysplastic nevi. *Cancer Res* **55**:4278, 1995.

23. Balaban GB, Herlyn M, Clark WH Jr, Nowell PC: Karyotypic evolution in human malignant melanoma. *Cancer Genet Cytogenet* **19**:113, 1986.

24. Dracopoli ND, Alhadeff B, Houghton AN, Old LJ: Loss of heterozygosity at autosomal and X-linked loci during tumor progression in a patient with melanoma. *Cancer Res* **47**:3995, 1987.

25. Cowan JM, Halaban R, Francke U: Cytogenetic analysis of melanocytes from premalignant nevi and melanomas. *J Natl Cancer Inst* **80**:1159, 1988.

26. Horsman DE, White VA: Cytogenetic analysis of uveal melanoma: Consistent occurrence of monosomy 3 and trisomy 8q. *Cancer* **71**:811, 1993.

27. Andersen LB, Fountain JW, Gutmann DH, Tarle SA, Glover TW, Dracopoli NC, Housman DE, Collins FS: Mutations in the neurofibromatosis 1 gene in sporadic melanoma cell lines. *Nat Genet* **3**:118, 1993.

28. Johnson MR, Look AT, DeClue JE, Valentine MB, Lowy DR: Inactivation of the NF1 gene in human melanoma and neuroblastoma cell lines without impaired regulation of GRP.Ras. *Proc Natl Acad Sci USA* **90**:5539, 1993.

29. Welch DR, Chen P, Miele ME, McGary Ct, Bower JM, Stanbridge EJ, Weissman BE: Microcell-mediated transfer of chromosome 6 into metastatic human C8161 melanoma cells suppresses metastasis but does not inhibit tumorigenicity. *Oncogene* **9**:255, 1994.

30. Cawley EP: Genetic aspects of malignant melanoma. *Arch Dermatol* **65**:440, 1952.

31. Greene MH, Fraumeni JF Jr: The hereditary variant of malignant melanoma, in Clark WH Jr, Goldman LI, Mastrangelo MJ (eds): *Human Malignant Melanoma,* New York, Grune & Stratton, 1979.

32. Wallace DC, Exton LA, McLeod GR: Genetic factor in malignant melanoma. *Cancer* **27**:1262, 1971.

33. Goldgar DE, Easton DF, Cannon-Albright LA, Skolnick MH: A systematic population-based assessment of cancer risk in first degree relatives of cancer probands. *J Natl Cancer Inst* **86**:1600, 1994.

34. Turkington RW: Familial factors in malignant melanoma. *JAMA* **192**:77, 1965.

35. Smith EE, Henley WS, Knox JM, Lane M: Familial melanoma. *Arch Intern Med* **117**:820, 1966.

36. Anderson DE, Smith JL Jr, McBride CM: Hereditary aspects of malignant melanoma. *JAMA* **200**:741, 1967.

37. Swerdlow AJ, English J, Mackie RM, O'Doherty CJ, Hunter JAA, Clark J: Benign nevi associated with high risk of melanoma. *Lancet* **2**:168, 1984.

38. Clark WH, Reimer RR, Greene M, Ainsworth AM, Mastrangelo M: Origin of familial malignant melanomas from heritable melanocyte lesions. *Arch Dermatol* **114**:732, 1978.

39. Lynch HT, Frichot BC, Lynch J: Familial atypical multiple mole melanoma syndrome. *J Med Genet* **15**:352, 1978.

40. Greene MH, Goldin LR, Clark WH, et al: Familial malignant melanoma: Autosomal dominant trait possibly linked to the Rhesus locus. *Proc Natl Acad Sci USA* **80**:6071, 1983.

41. Bale SJ, Dracopoli NC, Tucker MA, Clark WH Jr, Fraser MC, Stanger BZ, Green P, Donis-Keller H, Housman DE, Green MH: Mapping the gene for hereditary cutaneous malignant melanoma-dysplastic nevus to chromosome 1p. *N Engl J Med* **320**:1367, 1986.

42. Van Haeringen A, Bergman W, Nolen MR, van der Kooij-Meijs E, Hendrikse I, Wijnen JT, Khan PM, Klasen EC, Frants RR: Exclusion of the dysplastic nevus syndrome (DNS) locus from the short arm of chromosome 1 by linkage studies in Dutch families. *Genomics* **5**:61, 1989.

43. Cannon-Albright LA, Goldgar De, Wright EC, et al: Evidence against the reported linkage to the cutaneous melanoma-dysplastic naevus syndrome locus to chromosome 1p36. *Am J Hum Genet* **46**:912, 1990.

44. Kefford RF, Salmon J, Shaw HM, Donald JA, McCarthy WH: Hereditary melanoma in Australia: Variable association with dysplastic nevi and absence of genetic linkage to chromosome 1p. *Cancer Genet Cytogenet* **51**:45, 1991.

45. Nancarrow DJ, Palmer JM, Walters MK, Kerr BM, Hofner GJ, Garske L, McLeod GR, Hayward NK: Exclusion of the familial melanoma locus (MLM) from the PND/DIS47 and MYCL1 regions of chromosome arm 1p in 7 Australian pedigrees. *Genomics* **12**:18, 1992.

46. Goldstein AM, Dracopoli NC, Engelstein M, Fraser MC, Clark WH Jr, Tucker MA: Linkage of cutaneous malignant melanoma/dysplastic nevi to chromosome 9p, and evidence for genetic heterogeneity. *Am J Hum Genet* **54**:489, 1994.

47. Cannon-Albright LA, Goldgar DE, Meyer LJ, Lewis CM, Anderson DE, Fountain JW, Hegi ME, Wiseman RW, Petty EM, Bale AE, Olopade OI, Diaz MO, Kwiatkowski DJ, Piepkorn MW, Zone JJ, Skolnick MH: Assignment of a locus for familial melanoma, MLM, to chromosome 9p13-p22. *Science* **258**:1148, 1992.

48. Skolnick MH, Cannon-Albright LA, Kamb A: Genetic predisposition to melanoma. *Eur J Cancer* **30**:1991, 1994.

49. Cannon-Albright LA, Meyer LJ, Goldgar DE, Lewis CM, McWhorter WP, Jost M, Harrison D, Anderson DE, Zone JJ, Skolnick MH: Penetrance and expressivity of the chromosome 9p melanoma susceptibility locus (MLM). *Cancer Res* **54**:6041, 1994.

50. Walker GJ, Hussussian CJ, Flores JF, Glendening JM, Haluska FG, Dracopoli NC, Hayward NK, Fountain JW: Mutations of the CDKN2/p16INK4 gene in Australian melanoma kindreds. *Hum Mol Genet* **4**:1845, 1995.

51. Gruis NA, Sandkuijl LA, van der Velden PA, Bergman W, Frants RR: CDKN2 explains part of the clinical phenotype in Dutch familial atypical multiple-mole melanoma (FAMMM) syndrome families. *Melanoma Res* **5**:169, 1995b.

52. Kundson AG: Mutation and cancer: Statistical study of retinoblastoma. *Proc Natl Acad Sci USA* **68**:820, 1971.
53. Serrano M, Hannon GJ, Beach D: A new regulatory motif in cell-cycle control causing specific inhibition of cyclin D/CDK4. *Nature* **366**:704, 1993.
54. Kamb A, Gruis NA, Weaver-Feldhaus J, Liu Q, Harshman K, Tavtigian SV, Stockert E, Day RS, Johnson BE, Skolnick MH: A cell cycle regulator potentially involved in genesis of many tumor types. *Science* **264**:436, 1994.
55. Nobori T, Miura K, Wu DJ, Lois A, Takabayashi K, Carson DA: Deletions of the cyclin-dependent kinase-4 inhibitor gene in multiple human cancers. *Nature* **368**:753, 1994.
56. Hannon GJ, Beach D: p15 INK4B is a potential effector of TFG-β-induced cell cycle arrest. *Nature* **371**:257, 1994.
57. Jen J, Harper JW, Bigner SH, Bigner DD, Papadopoulos N, Markowitz S, Wilson JKV, Kinzler KW, Vogelstein B: Deletion of p16 and p15 genes in brain tumors. *Cancer Res* **54**:6353, 1994.
58. Liu Q, Neuhausen S, McClure M, Frye C, Weaver-Feldhaus J, Gruis NA, Eddington K, Allalunis-Turner MJ, Skolnick MH, Fujimura FJ, Kamb A: CDKN2 (MTS1) tumor suppressor gene mutations in human tumor cell lines. *Oncogene* **10**:1061, 1995.
59. Stone S, Dayananth P, Jiang P, Weaver-Feldhaus JM, Tavtigian SV, Skolnick MH, Kamb A: Genomic structure, expression, and mutational analysis for the P15 (MTS2) gene. *Oncogene* **11**:987, 1995.
60. Kamb A, Liu Q, Harshman K, Tavtigian SV: Response to rate of p16 (MTS1) mutations in primary tumors with 90 loss. *Science* **265**:416, 1994.
61. Hussussian CJ, Struewing JP, Goldstein AM, Higgins PAT, Ally DS, Sheahan MD, Clark WHJ, Tucker MA, Dracopoli NC: Germline p16 mutations in familial melanoma. *Nat Genet* **8**:15, 1994.
62. Kamb A, Shattuck-Eidens D, Eeles R, Liu Q, Gruis NA, Ding W, Hussey C, Tran T, Miki Y, Weaver-Feldhaus J, McClure M, Aitken JF, Anderson DE, Bergman W, Frants R, Goldgar DE, Green A, MacLennan R, Martin NG, Meyer LJ, Youl P, Zone JJ, Skolnick MH, Cannon-Albright LA: Analysis of the p16 gene (CDKN2) as a candidate for the chromosome 9p melanoma susceptibility locus. *Nat Genet* **8**:22, 1994.
63. Borg A, Johannsson U, Johannsson O, Hakansson S, Westerdahl J, Masback A, Olsson H, Ingvar C: Novel germline p16 mutation in familial malignant melanoma in southern Sweden. *Cancer Res* **56**:2497, 1996.
64. Holland EA, Beaton SC, Becker TM, Grulet OM, Peters BA, Rizos H, Kefford RF, Mann GJ: Analysis of the p16 gene, CDKN2, in 17 Australian melanoma kindreds. *Oncogene* **11**:2289, 1995.
65. Gruis NA, van der Velden PA, Sandkuijl LA, Prins DE, Weaver-Feldhaus J, Kamb A, Bergman W, Frants RR: Homozygotes for CDKN2 (p16) germline mutation in Dutch familial melanoma kindreds. *Nat Genet* **10**:351, 1995.
66. Liu L, Lassam NJU, Slingerland JM, Bailey D, Cole D, Jenkins R, Hogg D: Germline p16INK4A mutation and protein dysfunction in a family with inherited melanoma. *Oncogene* **11**:405, 1995.
67. Koh J, Enders GH, Cynlacht BD, Harlow E: Tumor-derived p16 alleles encoding proteins defective in cell-cycle inhibition. *Nature* **375**:506, 1995.
68. Ranade K, Hussussian CJ, Sikorski RS, Varmus HE, Goldstein AM, Tucker MA, Serrano M, Hannon GJ, Beach D, Dracopoli NC: Mutations associated with familial melanoma impair p16 INK4 function. *Nat Genet* **10**:114, 1995.
69. Yang R, Gombart AF, Serrano M, Koeffler P: Mutational effects on the p16INK4a. *Cancer Res* **55**:2503, 1995.
70. Serrano M, Lee H, Chin L, Cordon-Cardo C, Beach D, DePinho RA: Role of the INK4a locus in tumor suppression and cell mortality. *Cell* **85**:27, 1996.
71. Jiang P, Stone S, Wagner R, Wang S, Dayananth P, Kozak CA, Wold B, Kamb A: Comparative analysis of homo sapiens and mus musculus cyclin-dependent kinase (CDK) inhibitor genes p16 (MTS1) and p15 (MTS2). *J Mol Evol* **41**:795, 1995.
72. Serrano M, Gomez-Lahoz E, DePinho RA, Beach D, Bar-Sagi D: Inhibition of *ras*-induced proliferation and cellular transformation by p16INK4. *Science* **267**:249, 1995.
73. Lukas J, Parry D, Aagaard L, Mann DJ, Bartkova J, Strauss M, Peters G, Bartek J: Retino-blastoma-protein-dependent cell-cycle inhibition by the tumor suppressor p16. *Nature* **375**:503, 1995.
74. Stone S, Jiang P, Dayananth P, Tavtigian SV, Katcher H, Parry D, Peters G, Kamb A: Complex structure and regulation of the P16 (MTS1) locus. *Cancer Res* **55**:2988, 1995.

75. Mao L, Merlo A, Bedi G, Shapiro GI, Edwards CD, Rollins BJ, Sidransky DA: A novel p16 INK4A transcript. *Cancer Res* **55**:2995, 1995.
76. Duro D, Bernard O, Della Valle V, Berger R, Larsen CJ: A new type of p161INK4/MTS1 gene transcript expressed in B-cell malignancies. *Oncogene* **11**:212, 1995.
77. Quelle D, Zindy F, Ashmun RA, Sherr CJ: Alternative reading frames of the INKa tumor suppressor gene encode two unrelated proteins capable of inducing cell cycle arrest. *Cell* **83**:993, 1995.
78. Glendening JM, Flores JF, Wlaker GJ, Stone S, Albino AP, Fountain JW: Homozygous loss of the p15INK4B gene (and not the p16INK4 gene) during tumor progression in a sporadic melanoma patient. *Cancer Res* **55**:5531, 1995.
79. Zuo L, Weger J, Yang Q, Goldstein AM, Tucker MA, Walker GJ, Hayward N, Dracopoli NC: Germline mutations in the p16INK4a binding domain of CDK4 in familial melanoma. *Nat Genet* **12**:97, 1996.
80. Wolfel T, Hauer M, Schneider J, Serrano M, Wolfel C, Klehmann-Hieb E, De Plaen E, Hankeln T, Meyer zum Buschenfelde KH, Beach D: A p16INK4a-insensitive CDK4 mutant targeted by cytolytic T lymphocytes in a human melanoma. *Science* **269**:1281, 1995.
81. Mulligan LM, Kwok JBJ, Healey CS, Elsdon MJ, CE, Gardner E, Love DR, Moore JK, Papi L, Ponder MA, Telenius H, Tunnacliffe A, Ponder BAJ: Germ-line mutations of the RET proto-oncogene in multiple endocrine neoplasia type 2A. *Nature* **363**:774, 1993.
82. Sherr CJ: G1 phase progression: Cycling on cue. *Cell* **79**:551, 1994.
83. Lukas J, Petersen BO, Holm K, Bartek J, Helin K: Deregulated expression of E2F family members induce S-phase entry and overcomes p16INK4A-mediated growth suppression. *Mol Cell Biol* **16**:1047, 1996.
84. He J, Allen JR, Collins VP, Allalunis-Turner MJ, Godbout R, Day RS III, James CD: CDK4 amplification is an alternative mechanism to p16 gene homozygous deletion in glioma cell lines. *Cancer Res* **54**:5804, 1994.
85. Okamoto A, Demetrick DJ, Spillare EA, Hagiwara K, Hussain SP, Bennett WP, Forrester K, Gerwin B, Serrano M, Beach DH, et al: Mutations and altered expression of P16INK4 in human cancer. *Proc Natl Acad Sci USA* **91**:11045, 1994.
86. Otterson GA, Dkatzke RA, Coxon A, Kin YW, Kaye FJ: Absence of p16INK4 protein is restricted to the subset of lung cancer lines that retains wildtype RB. *Oncogene* **9**:3375, 1994.
87. Aagaard L, Lukas J, Bartkova J, Kjerulff AA, Strauss M, Bartek J: Aberrations of p16Ink4 and retinoblastoma tumor-suppressor genes occur in distinct sub-sets of human cancer cell lines. *Int J Cancer* **61**:115, 1995.
88. DeVita VT, Hellman S, Rosenberg SA: *Cancer: Principles and Practice of Oncology.* Philadelphia: Lippincott, 1989.
89. Kamb A: Cell-cycle regulators and cancer. *Trends Genet* **11**:136, 1995.
90. Maestro R, Boiocchi M: Sunlight and melanoma: An answer from MTS1 (p16). *Science* **267**:15, 1995.
91. Pollock PM, Yu F, Qiu L, Parsons PG, Hayward NK: Evidence for u.v. induction of CDKN2 mutations in melanoma cell lines. *Oncogene* **11**:663, 1995.
92. Herman JG, Merlo A, Mao L, Issa JJ-P, Davidson NE, Sidransky D, Baylin SB: Inactivation of the *CDKN2/p16/MTS1* gene is frequently associated with aberrant DNA methylation in all common human cancers. *Cancer Res* **55**:4525, 1995.
93. Merlo A, Herman JG, Mao L, Lee DJ, Gabrielson E, Burger PC, Baylin SB, Sidransky D: 5′ CpG island methylation is associated with transcriptional silencing of the tumour suppressor *p16/CDKN2/MTS1* in human cancers. *Nat Med* **1**:686, 1995.
94. Gonzalez-Zulueta M, Bender CM, Yang AS, Nguyen T, Beart RW, Van Tornout JM, Jones PA: Methylation of the 5′ CpG island of the p16/CDKN2 tumor suppressor gene in normal and transformed human tissues correlates with gene silencing. *Cancer Res* **55**:4531, 1995.
95. El-Deiry WF, Tokino T, Velculescu VE, Levy DB, Parsons R, Trent JM, Lin D, Mercer WE, Kinzler KW, Vogelstein B: WAF1, a potential mediator of p53 tumor suppression. *Cell* **75**:817, 1993.
96. Gu W, Turck CW, Morgan DO: Inhibition of CDK2 activity *in vivo* by an associated 20K regulatory subunit. *Nature* **366**:707, 1993.
97. Harper JW, Adami GR, Wei N, Keyomarsi K, Elledge KK: The p21 Cdk-interacting protein Cip1 is a potent inhibitor of G1 cyclin-dependent kinases. *Cell* **75**:805, 1993.
98. Xiong Y, Hannon GJ, Zhang H, Casso D, Kobayashi R, Beach D: p21 is a universal inhibitor of cyclin kinases. *Nature* **366**:701, 1993.
99. Polyak K, Lee M-H, Bromage HE, Koff A, Roberts JM, Tempst P, Massague J: Cloning of p27Kip1, a cyclin-dependent kinase inhibitor

and a potential mediator of extracellular antimitogenic signals. *Cell* **78**:59, 1994.

100. Toyoshima H, Hunter T: P27, a novel inhibitor of G1 cyclin-Cdk protein kinase activity, is related to p21. *Cell* **78**:67, 1994.

101. Guan K-L, Jenkins CW, Li Y, Nichols MA, Wu X, O'Keefe CL, Matera AG, Xiong Y: Growth suppression by p18, a p16[INK4/MTS1] and p14INK4B/MTS2-related CDK6 inhibitor, correlates with wild-type pRb function. *Genes Dev* **8**:2939, 1994.

102. Lee MH, Reynisdottir I, Massague J: Cloning of p57KIP2, a cyclin-dependent kinase inhibitor with unique domain structure and tissue distribution. *Genes Dev* **9**:639, 1995.

103. Kawamata N, Seriu T, Koeffler HP, Bartram CR: Molecular analysis of the cyclin-dependent kinase inhibitor family: p16(CDKN2/MTS1/INK4A), p18(INK4C) and p27(Kip1) genes in neuroblastomas. *Cancer* **77**:570, 1996.

104. Orlow I, Iavorone A, Crider-Miller SJ, Bonilla F, Latres E, Lee MH, Gerald WL, Massague J, Weissman BE, Cordon-Cardo C: Cyclin-dependent kinase inhibitors p57/KIP2 in soft tissue sarcomas and Wilms tumor. *Cancer Res* **56**:1219, 1996.

105. Rusin MR, Okamoto A, Chorazy M, Czyzewski K, Harasim J, Spillare EA, Hagiwara K, Hussain SP, Xiong Y, Demetrick DJ, Harris CC: Intragenic mutation of the p16(INK4), p15(INK4B) and p18 genes in primary non-small-cell lung cancers. **65**:734, 1996.

106. Wang J, Walsh K: Resistance to apoptosis conferred by Cdk inhibitors during myocyte differentiation. *Science* **273**:359, 1996.

107. Reznikoff CA, Yeager TR, Belair CD, Savelieva E, Puthenveettil JA, Stadler WM: Elevated p16 at senescence and loss of p16 at immortalization in human papillomavirus 16 E6, but not E7, transformed human uroepithelial cells. *Cancer Res* **56**:2886, 1996.

108. Hara E, Smith R, Parry D, Tahara H, Stone S, Peters G: Regulation of p16/CDKN2 expression and its implications for cell immortalization and senescence. *Mol Cell Biol* **16**:859, 1986.

109. Rogan EM, Bryan TM, Hukku B, Maclean K, Chang AC, Moy EL, Englezou A, Warneford SG, Dalla-Pozza L, Reddel RR: Alterations in p53 and p16INK4 expression and telomere length during spontaneous immortalization of Li-Fraumeni syndrome fibroblasts. *Mol Cell Biol* **15**:475, 1986.

110. Bergman W, Watson P, de Jong J, Lunch HT, Fusaro RM: Systemic cancer and the FAMMM syndrome. *Br J Cancer* **61**:932, 1990.

111. Miki Y, Swensen J, Shattuck-Eidens D, et al: A strong candidate for the breast and ovarian cancer susceptibility gene BRCA1. *Science* **266**:66, 1994.

112. Tavtigian SV, Simard J, Rommens J: The complete BRCA2 gene and mutations in chromosome 13Q-linked kindreds. *Nat Genet* **12**:1, 1996.

113. Heyman M, Rasool O, Borgonovo Brandter L, et al: Prognostic importance of p15INK4B and p16INK4 gene inactivation in childhood acute lymphocytic leukemia. *J Clin Oncol* **14**:1512, 1996.

114. Jin X, Nguyen D, Zhang WW, Kyritsis AP, Roth JA: Cell cycle arrest and inhibition of tumor cell proliferation by the p16INK4 gene mediated by an adenovirus vector. *Cancer Res* **55**:3250, 1995.

115. Fueyo J, Gomez-Manzano C, Yung WK, Clayman GL, Liu TJ, Bruner J, Levin VA, Kyritsis AP: Adenovirus-mediated p16/CDKN2 gene transfer induces growth arrest and modifies the transformed phenotype of glioma cells. *Oncogene* **12**:103, 1996.

116. Pardee AB, Janes LJ: Selective killing of transformed baby hamster kidney (BHK) cells. *Cell Biol* **72**:4994, 1975.

117. Hartwell LH, Kastan MB: Cell cycle control and cancer. *Science* **266**:1821, 1994.

118. Kohn KW, Jackman J, O'Connor PM: Cell cycle control and cancer chemotherapy. *J Cell Biochem* **54**:440, 1994.

119. Darzynkiewicz Z: Apoptosis in anticancer strategies: Modulation of cell cycle or differentiation. *J Cell Biochem* **58**:151, 1995.

120. Stone S, Dayananth P, Kamb A: Reversible, p16-mediated cell cycle arrest as protection from chemotherapy. *Cancer Res* **56**:3199, 1996.

CHAPTER 28

Cowden Syndrome

Charis Eng ■ Ramon Parsons

1. **Cowden syndrome (CS) is an autosomal dominant disorder characterized by multiple hamartomas, benign disorganized growths, and a risk of breast and thyroid cancer.**

2. **The great majority of tumors, including those of the thyroid and breast, are benign. Up to 10% of affected individuals develop nonmedullary thyroid carcinoma and up to 50% of affected females develop breast cancer.**

3. **The pathognomonic hamartoma is the trichilemmoma, a benign tumor of the infundibulum of the hair follicle.**

4. **The susceptibility gene for CS is likely a tumor suppressor gene as evidenced indirectly by loss of heterozygosity in the *CS* critical interval on 10q22–23 in various CS-related tumors.**

5. **The *CS* gene, *PTEN,* was isolated by a combination of genetic mapping analyses, somatic genetics and a candidate gene approach. *PTEN* located on 10q23.3 encodes a 403-amino acid protein which contains a putative phosphatase signature motif and has sequences homologous to tensin.**

6. **Germline mutations in *PTEN* have been found in four or five CS families. These mutations result in predicted protein truncation or likely loss of function, hence supporting its predicted function as a tumor suppressor.**

Cowden syndrome (CS) [OMIM 158350], named after Rachel Cowden, is an autosomal dominant inherited cancer syndrome characterised by multiple hamartomas involving organ systems derived from all three germ cell layers and a risk of breast and thyroid cancers.[1] Females with CS have been reported to have as high as a 67% risk of fibrocystic disease of the breasts and a 25–50% lifetime risk of developing adenocarcinoma of the breast.[2,3] This maximum lifetime risk exceeds that of the general population in the United States (11%). Furthermore, affected individuals are said to have a 3–10% lifetime risk of developing epithelial thyroid carcinoma[3–5]: this, too, exceeds that of the general population (1%).

The CS susceptibility gene, *PTEN*, is on chromosome sub-band 10q23.3.[6,7]

CLINICAL ASPECTS

Incidence

CS has not been well recognised: as of 1993, there were approximately 160 reported cases in the world literature.[8] From an informal population-based study, the estimated gene frequency is one in a million.[6] Because of frequencies such as this, this syndrome is often listed as rare, but exponents of the field suspect that it is much more common than believed. Because of the variable, protean and often subtle external manifestations of CS, many cases remain undiagnosed[9,10] (Eng, unpublished). Indeed, between two centers in the U.S. dedicated to the study of Cowden syndrome (Dana-Farber Cancer Institute, Boston, and Columbia University Cancer Center, New York), over 70 cases have been ascertained (Eng and Peacocke, unpublished). These cases are not included in those reported prior to 1993. Further, each of the features of CS could occur in the general population as well, thus confounding recognition of this disease. Despite the apparent rarity of CS, the syndrome is worthy of note from both scientific and clinical viewpoints.

Because CS is likely under-diagnosed, a true count of the fraction of isolated cases (defined as no obvious family history) and familial cases (defined as two or more related affected individuals) cannot be performed. From the literature and the experience of both major US CS centers, the majority of CS cases are isolated. As an estimate, perhaps 10–25% of CS cases are familial.

Diagnostic Criteria

Cowden syndrome usually presents by the late 20s. It has variable expression and, probably, an age-related penetrance although the exact penetrance is unknown. By the third decade, 99% of affected individuals would have developed the mucocutaneous stigmata although any of the features could be present already (see Tables 28-1 and 28-2, Figure 28-1). Because the clinical literature on CS consists mostly of reports of the most florid and unusual families or case reports by subspecialists interested in their respective organ systems, the spectrum of component signs is unknown. Despite this, the most commonly reported manifestations are mucocutaneous lesions, thyroid abnormalities, fibrocystic disease and carcinoma of the breast, gastrointestinal hamartomas, multiple, early-onset uterine leiomyoma, macrocephaly (specifically, megencephaly) and mental retardation (Table 28-1).[3–5,11] Pathognomonic mucocutaneous lesions are trichilemmomas and papillomatous papules (Table 28-2, Figure 28-1). Because of the lack of uniform diagnostic criteria for CS prior to 1995, a group of individuals, the International Cowden Consortium, interested in systematically studying this syndrome arrived at a set of consensus operational diagnostic criteria (Table 28-2).

The two most commonly recognized cancers in CS are carcinoma of the breast and thyroid.[3] By contrast, in the general population, lifetime risks for breast and thyroid cancers are approximately 11% (in women), and 1%, respectively. Breast cancer has

Table 28-1 Common Manifestations of Cowden Syndrome

Mucocutaneous lesions (90–100%)
  Trichilemmomas
  Acral keratoses
  Verucoid or papillomatous papules
Thyroid Abnormalities (50–67%)
  Goiter
  Adenoma
  Cancer (3–10%)
Breast Lesions
  Fibroadenomas/Fibrocystic disease (76% of affected females)
  Adenocarcinoma (25–50% of affected females)
Gastrointestinal Lesions (40%)
  Hamartomatous polyps
Macrocephaly (38%)
Genito-urinary Abnormalities (44% of females)
  Uterine leiomyoma (multiple, early onset)

Table 28-2 International Cowden Syndrome Consortium Operational Criteria for the Diagnosis of Cowden Syndrome (Ver. 1996)*

Pathognomonic Criteria
Mucocutanous lesions:
  Trichilemmomas, facial
  Acral keratoses
  Papillomatous papules
  Mucosal lesions
Major Criteria
Breast CA
Thyroid CA, esp. follicular thyroid carcinoma
Macrocephaly (Megalencephaly) (say, ≥97%ile)
Lhermitte-Duclos disease (LDD)
Minor Criteria
Other thyroid lesions (e.g., adenoma or multinodular goiter)
Mental retardation (say, IQ ≤ 75)
GI hamartomas
Fibrocystic disease of the breast
Lipomas
Fibromas
GU tumors (e.g., uterine fibroids) or malformation

Operational Diagnosis in an Individual:
1. Mucocutanous lesions alone if:
  a) there are 6 or more facial papules, of which 3 or more must be trichilemmoma, or
  b) cutaneous facial papules and oral mucosal papillomatosis, or
  c) oral mucosal papillomatosis and acral keratoses, or
  d) palmo plantar keratoses, 6 or more
2. 2 Major criteria but one must include macrocephaly or LDD
3. 1 Major and 3 minor criteria
4. 4 minor criteria

Operational Diagnosis in a Family where One Individual is Diagnostic for Cowden
1. The pathognomonic criterion/ia
2. Any one major criterion with or without minor criteria
3. Two minor criteria

*Operational diagnostic criteria are reviewed and revised on a continuous basis as new clinical information becomes available.

yet to be observed in men with CS. In women with CS, lifetime risk estimates for the development of breast cancer range from 25 to 50%.[3–5,12] The mean age at diagnosis is likely 10 years earlier than breast cancer occurring in the general population.[3,5] Although Rachel Cowden died of breast cancer at the age of 31[1,2] and the earliest recorded age at diagnosis of breast cancer is 14,[3] the great majority of breast cancers are diagnosed after the age of 30–35 (range 14–65).[5]

The lifetime risk for thyroid cancer can be as high as 10% in males and females with CS. Because of small numbers, it is unclear if the age of onset is truly earlier than that of the general population. Histologically, the thyroid cancer is predominantly follicular carcinoma although papillary histology has also been observed[3,4,11] (Eng, unpublished observations). Medullary thyroid carcinoma has yet to be observed in patients with CS.

Benign tumors are also common in CS. Benign tumors or disorders of breast and thyroid are the most frequently noted and likely represent true component features of this syndrome (Table 28-1). Fibroadenomas and fibrocystic disease of the breast are common signs in CS, as are follicular adenomas and multinodular goiter of the thyroid. An unusual central nervous system tumor, cerebellar dysplastic gangliocytoma or Lhermitte-Duclos disease, has only recently been associated with CS.[13,14]

Other malignancies and benign tumors have been reported in patients or families with CS (Tables 28-3 and 28-4). Whether each of these tumors is a true component of CS or whether some are coincidental findings is as yet unknown.

Differential Diagnosis

With the variable expression of Cowden syndrome, this disorder can be considered a great imitator of many syndromes. A few differential diagnoses to consider include neurofibromatosis type 1 (NF 1), basal cell nevus syndrome (Gorlin syndrome), Proteus syndrome, Darier-White disease and Bannayan-Zonana (Ruvalcaba-Myhre-Smith) syndrome. NF 1 is an autosomal dominant inherited cancer syndrome with many features. The only two consistent features are café-au-lait macules and fibromatous tumors of the skin. The plexiform neuroma is highly suggestive of NF 1. The susceptibility gene for this syndrome has been isolated.[15,16] Because of the large size of the gene, direct mutation analysis is still not practical. In informative families, linkage analysis is feasible for predictive testing purposes and is 98% accurate.[17] Basal cell nevus syndrome is an autosomal dominant condition characterized by basal cell nevi, basal cell carcinoma and diverse developmental abnormalities. In addition, affected individuals can develop other tumors and cancers, such as fibromas, hamartomatous gastric polyps and medulloblastomas. However, the dermatologic findings and developmental features in Cowden syndrome and basal cell nevus syndrome are markedly different. For instance, the palmar pits together with the characteristic facies of the latter are never seen in CS. The susceptibility gene for basal cell nevus syndrome has recently been isolated and is the human homolog of the Drosophila *patched* gene, *PTC* on 9q22–31.[18] Linkage analysis and mutation analysis are (technically) possible. However, since it is not known what proportion of patients with this syndrome will actually turn out to have mutations in *PTC*, predictive testing based on mutation analysis alone should be deferred until more data become available. Proteus syndrome could be considered in the differential diagnosis of CS because of the common theme of overgrowth.[19] However, many of the rest of the features of Proteus syndrome, such as the skeletal abnormalities, hemihypertrophy, hypertrophy of the skins of the soles and macrodactyly, are rarely, if ever seen, in CS. Bannayan-Zonana syndrome is probably a group of autosomal dominant disorders characterised by macrocephaly, hamartomas and telangiectasias.[20,21] This may sound quite similar to CS but the dermatologic findings in CS are quite distinct. It is, of course, possible that a subset of Bannayan-Zonana syndrome is actually allelic to CS.

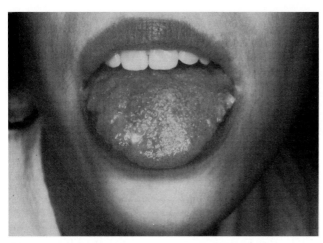

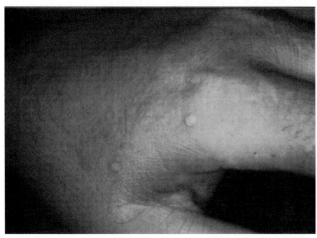

FIG. 28-1 Characteristic mucocutaneous features of Cowden syndrome. *A.* Scrotal tongue comprising papillomatous papules. *B.* Papillomatous papules of the skin.

Finally, Darier-White disease is an autosomal dominant disorder characterised by keratotic, often oozing, papules in the "seborrheic areas" of the skin and sometimes can be confused with CS. Nonetheless, the dermatologic findings of these two syndromes, especially at the microscopic level, are distinct. The susceptibility locus for Darier-White disease has been mapped to 12q23–24.1.[22,23]

Although Peutz-Jeghers syndrome might be initially considered in the differential diagnosis, it can be quickly discarded. The pigmentation of the peroral region in this autosomal dominant hamartoma syndrome is pathognomonic.[24,25] Further, the histology of the hamartomas in Peutz-Jeghers patients is unique. They are unlike the hamartomatous polyps seen in CS and in juvenile polyposis. Clinically, while Peutz-Jeghers polyps are often symptomatic (interssuception, rectal bleeding), CS polyps are rarely so. There is a small but finite subset of juvenile polyposis cases that are noted to have "congenital anomalies."[26] Syndromologists have wondered whether these should truly be considered under the rubric of juvenile polyposis or whether they are really misclassified CS cases or Bannayan-Zonana cases.

Histology

Like other inherited cancer syndromes, multifocality and bilateral involvement is the rule. Hamartomas are the hallmark of CS.

Table 28-3 Reported Malignancies in Patients with Cowden Syndrome

Central nervous system
   Glioblastoma multiforme
Mucocutaneous
   Squamous cell carcinoma
   Basal cell carcinoma
   Malignant melanoma
   Merkel cell carcinoma
Breast
   Adenocarcinoma
Endocrine
   Nonmedullary thyroid carcinoma
Pulmonary
   Non small cell carcinoma
Gastrointestinal
   Colorectal carcinoma
   Hepatocellular carcinoma
   Pancreatic carcinoma
Genitourinary
   Uterine carcinoma
   Ovarian carcinoma
   Transitional cell carcinoma of the bladder
   Renal cell carcinoma
Other
   Liposarcoma

These are classic hamartomas in general, and are benign tumors comprising all the elements of a particular organ but in a disorganized fashion. Of note, the hamartomatous polyps found in this syndrome are different in histomorphology from Peutz-Jeghers polyps, which have a distinct appearance.

With regard to the individual cancers, even of the breast and thyroid, as of mid 1997, there has yet to be a systematic study published. Recently, however, one study has attempted to look at benign and malignant breast pathology in CS patients. Although these are preliminary studies, without true matched controls, it is, to date, the only study that examine breast pathology in a series of CS cases. Breast histopathology from 59 cases belonging to 19 CS women was systematically analysed.[10] Thirty-five specimens had some form of malignant pathology. Of these, 31 (90%) had ductal adenocarcinoma, one tubular carcinoma and one lobular carcinoma-in-situ. Sixteen of the 31 had both invasive and in situ (DCIS) components of ductal carcinoma while 12 had DCIS only and two only invasive adenocarcinoma. Interestingly, it was noted that 19 of these carcinomas appeared to have arisen in the midst of densely fibrotic hamartomatous tissue.

Benign thyroid pathology is more common in CS than malignant. Multinodular goiter and thyroid adenomas are often noted. Follicular thyroid carcinomas are more common than papillary histology.[3,11,12] No systematic studies on thyroid pathology in CS have been performed.

GENETICS

Inheritance patterns in families with CS implicate an autosomal dominant pattern.[3,14] Figure 28-2 is a pedigree of an hypothetical CS family. Expression is variable and true penetrance is unknown, although it is likely to be high and age-related. It is believed by some that the penetrance is 90% by the age of 20.[6] The precise penetrance will be clarified after further study of the susceptibility gene within families and affected individuals.

Table 28-4 Noncutaneous Benign Lesions Reported in
Cowden Syndrome

Nervous system
   Lhermitte-Duclos disease
   Megencephaly
   Glioma
   Meningioma
   Neuroma
   Neurofibroma
   Bridged sella turcica
   Mental retardation
Breast
   Fibrocystic disease
   Fibroadenoma
   Hamartoma
   Gynecomastia of male breast
Thyroid
   Goiter
   Adenoma
   Thyroiditis
   Thyroglossal duct cyst
   Hyperthyroidism
   Hypothyroidism
Gastrointestinal
   Hamartomatous polyposis of entire tract
   Diverticuli of colon and sigmoid
   Ganglioneuroma
   Leiomyoma
   Hepatic hamartoma
Genitourinary
   Female
      Leiomyomas
      Ovarian cysts
      Vaginal and vulvar cysts
      Various developmental anomalies (e.g., duplicated collecting system)
   Male
      Hydrocele
      Varicocele
      Hypoplastic testes
Skeletal
   Craniomegaly
   Adenoid facies
   High arched palate
   Hypoplastic zygoma
   Kyphoscoliosis
   Pectus excavatum
   Bone cysts
   Rudimentary sixth digit
Other
   Hypoplastic vulva
   Atrial septal defect
   Arteriovenous malformations
   Eye cataracts
   Retinal angioid streaks

Cytogenetic and nonsystematic genetic analyses reported prior to 1996 were uninformative with regard to the localization of the CS susceptibility gene and to the nature of the gene.[14,27–29]

Linkage Analysis Localizes *CS* to 10q22-23

A total autosomal genome scan, using dinucleotide repeat markers at 10–20-cM intervals, was performed in 12 classic CS families comprising 40 affected individuals in a collaborative study performed by the International Cowden Syndrome Consortium.[6] Regions containing candidate genes such as *BRCA1*, *BRCA2*, *APC*, *hMSH2*, *hMLH1*,

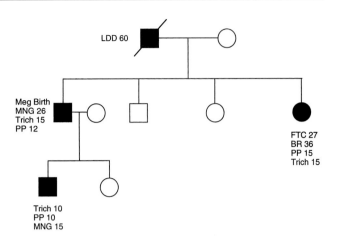

FIG. 28-2 Hypothetical CS family pedigree. LDD Lhermitte-Duclos disease, Meg megencephaly, MNG multinodular goiter, Trich trichilemmoma, PP papillomatous papules, FTC follicular thyroid carcinoma, BR breast adenocarcinoma.

hPMS1/2, *RB1*, *p53*, *p16/MTS1*, *RET* and *ATM* were excluded. Markers in the region of chromosome sub-band 10q22–23 revealed significant evidence for linkage to CS, with Zmax of 8.92 (theta=0.02) for the marker D10S573. Critical recombinants occurred at the markers D10S215 and D10S564, narrowing the region of interest to 5 cM. Despite the clinical variability and diverse ethnic origin of the studied families, no genetic heterogeneity was observed among the 12 families which originated from the US, UK, France and the Netherlands. Further genetic analysis revealed a new recombinant placing the consensus critical interval centromeric of D10S541.[7] Taken together with previous recombinant data, this recombinant helped place the putative gene between the markers D10S215 and D10S541, a region of <1 cM.

Somatic Genetics

Because both benign and malignant thyroid tumors and breast carcinomas are components of CS, loss of heterozygosity (LOH) analysis using markers flanking the putative *CS* locus was performed.[30–32] Approximately 25% of follicular thyroid adenomas and 40–50% of breast adenocarcinomas had LOH in the *CS* region, perhaps arguing that *CS* plays a somatic role in sporadic thyroid and breast neoplasia. If this were true, therefore, the LOH data suggest that the putative *CS* gene could be a tumor suppressor.

PTEN AS CS SUSCEPTIBILITY GENE

Recombinant data, supported by our somatic LOH data, placed the putative *CS* gene in the narrow critical interval between D10S215/S579 and D10S541. A novel candidate tumor suppressor gene *PTEN* lies precisely in this region.

Two groups searching for putative tumor suppressor genes on chromosome sub-band 10q23 independently isolated a novel gene, *PTEN* (= *MMAC1*).[32,33] The group led by Parsons identified homozygous deletions in breast, brain and prostate cancer within the *CS* consensus interval on 10q23. Exon trapping using BAC templates which encompassed the minimal region of deletions was performed to isolate gene(s) within the critical interval. Two exon-trap products appeared to match several unassembled ESTs which revealed an open reading frame (ORF) of 403 amino acids. Thus far, both groups' cDNA clones implicate that the full coding region encompasses 1209 bp. The gene comprises 9 exons and likely spans a genomic distance of over 120 kb.[32,33]

Sequence analysis of the ORF demonstrated a protein tyrosine phosphatase domain and homology to tensin and auxilin.[32,33] Hence, this new gene was dubbed *PTEN* for Phosphatase and Tensin homolog deleted on chromosome Ten. Further examination of the regions of homology revealed that the phosphatase domain of PTEN contained the consensus (I/V)-H-C-X-A-G-X-X-R-(S/T) motif found in all tyrosine phosphatases.[34] The PTEN phosphatase domain shares the closest homologies with that of CDC-14, PRL-1 (phosphatase of regenerating liver) and BVP (baculovirus phosphatase).[32] These phosphatases belong to a sub-class of tyrosine phosphatases called dual-specificity phosphatases which remove phosphate groups from both tyrosine as well as serine and threonine.

The PTEN homology to the amino terminus of tensin and homology is approximately 35% over 160 amino acids[32]522 (Salgia and Eng, unpublished). The phosphatase signature motif lies within this region. In fact, the homologous domains of tensin and auxilin share many amino acid residues with the phosphatase consensus site.[35] Because the signature motifs of tensin and auxilin lack the full complement of residues, it is believed that these two molecules cannot hydrolyse phosphopeptides. However, these proteins may form a pocket capable of binding phosphoprotein substrates. Although the real function of the phosphatase-like domains is unknown, given the current state of knowledge, some believe that these domains can bind phosphopeptides in a manner distinct from PTB and SH2 domains.[35–37]

To determine if *PTEN/MMAC1* is involved in the pathogenesis of sporadic breast, brain, kidney and prostate cancers, cell lines and a few primary tumors were examined for mutations in this gene. Homozygous deletions, insertions, frameshift and nonsense *PTEN* mutations were indeed found in 19/80 glioblastoma, 4/4 prostate cancer, 1/4 kidney cancer and 6/74 breast cancer cell lines, xenografts and primary tumors combined. Somatic mutation of *PTEN* is nearly always accompanied by loss of the wild type allele. From these data, it would appear that mutations in *PTEN* are etiologic for some sporadic breast, prostate, kidney and brain cancers. At least in brain tumors of the glial line, it preliminarily appears that mutation frequency increased with the advanced stage of the tumor: 6/6 somatic mutations were noted in glioblastoma multiforme and 0/3 low grade gliomas.[33] This observation should be confirmed with larger numbers, with other tumor types and with primary tumors. One way or the other, PTEN seems to behave like a classic tumor suppressor.

To determine if germline *PTEN* mutations could be etiologic for CS, the groups led by Eng and Parsons chose five CS families (utilizing 12 affected and 8 unaffected individuals) for analysis.[7] All five met the International Cowden Consortium operational diagnostic criteria for CS as outlined above (Table 28-2). Four of these families have been described before and have been shown to be linked to 10q22–23.[6] The fifth was comprised of two brothers who showed 10q22–23 haplotype sharing, but no further family members are available. In addition, hamartomas from one of these

two brothers and from one member of one of the four 10q-linked families demonstrated LOH in the region between D10S579/S215 and D10S541.[31]

A genomic, PCR-based approach followed by direct sequence analysis, using two different technologies (radioactive double stranded cycle sequencing and fluorophor-based semi-automated sequencing with dye terminator technology) was used.[7] Genomic DNA from affected members of each of the five families was initially amplified using primers specific for *PTEN* exon 5, which contains the putative tyrosine/dual specificity phosphatase signature motif. Three of the five CS families were shown to have germline heterozygous mutations in this exon (Fig. 28-3). Family D was found to have a G to T substitution at codon 157 which resulted in a nonsense mutation within the putative phosphatase domain and immediately after the tyrosine/dual specificity phosphatase signature motif. Two families (2053 and BH) shared an identical missense mutation, G129E, which is a nonconservative amino acid alteration occurring in one of the conserved glycines of the putative tyrosine/dual specificity phosphatase signature motif (see above). The identical mutations did not arise on a similar haplotype, arguing against a founder effect in this instance. *PTEN* mutations segregated with CS within each family. No unaffected family member carried these mutations. Another CS (family C) family had a truncating mutation within exon 7 (Fig. 28-3). In each family, the family-specific germline *PTEN* mutation segregated with disease but not in unaffected family members nor normal controls. No germline mutations have been detected in family 0014 despite sequencing of all 9 exons using a PCR-based approach.

Given these data, *PTEN* is likely the susceptibility gene for CS.

IMPLICATIONS FOR DIAGNOSIS AND PREDICTIVE TESTING

With the identification of *PTEN* as the susceptibility gene for CS and the original linkage studies indicating no genetic heterogeneity, it is theoretically possible to perform direct mutation analysis of *PTEN* for molecular diagnosis of CS. Direct mutation analysis has advantages over linkage analysis as it can be performed even if only one individual is available. However, since the discovery of *PTEN*'s involvement in CS was relatively recent, the actual proportion of isolated and familial cases who carry germline *PTEN* mutations is unknown. If a germline *PTEN* mutation was detected in a previously undiagnosed individual or an individual with an unclear clinical presentation, then the diagnosis becomes obvious. If, however, no germline *PTEN* mutation was found in such an individual, then the result should be considered nondiagnostic. Until the mutation frequency and mutation spectrum of *PTEN* in CS is comprehensively determined, exclusion of a CS diagnosis in a "new" case based on mutation analysis alone should not be done.

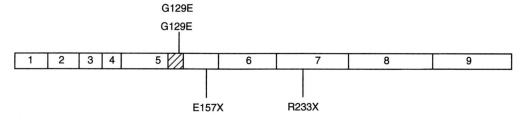

FIG. 28-3 Diagram of *PTEN* showing position and nature of germline mutations in 4 of 5 CS families. Hatched box within exon 5 represents the phosphatase signature motif. (See text for details)

If a family-specific mutation is already known, then screening for that particular mutation in as yet unaffected family members would yield results which are 100% accurate, barring administrative error. If a family-specific mutation cannot be identified in a family which clearly fits the International Cowden Consortium operational diagnostic criteria for CS (e.g., in the case of family 0014 above), then predictive testing based on direct mutation analysis is not possible. However, in the rare instances where the family is large and many affected members are available (as in family 0014), then linkage analysis using makers within and closely flanking *PTEN* (D10S579 or D10S215, AFMa086wg9, D10S541) might be considered.

Note Added in Proof

Germline mutations of *PTEN* have been found in two kindreds with classic Bannayan-Zonana Ruvalcaba-Myhre-Smith syndrome.[38] This suggests that Bannayan-Zonana syndrome is allelic to CS.

GENETIC COUNSELING AND MEDICAL MANAGEMENT

The key to proper genetic counseling in CS is recognition of the syndrome. Families should be counseled as for any autosomal dominant trait with high penetrance. What is unclear, however, is the variability of expression between and within families. We suspect that there are CS families who have nothing but trichilemmomas and therefore, never come to medical attention.

The two most serious, and established, component tumors in CS are breast cancer and nonmedullary thyroid cancer. Patients with CS or those who are at risk for CS should undergo surveillance for these two cancers. Beginning in their teens, these individuals should undergo annual physical examinations paying particular attention to the thyroid examination. Beginning in their mid 20's, women with CS or those at risk for it should be encouraged to perform monthly breast self examinations and to have careful breast examinations during their annual physicals. The value of annual imaging studies is unclear since there are no objective data available. Nonetheless, we usually recommend annual mammography and/or breast ultrasounds performed by skilled individuals in women-at-risk beginning at age 30 or five years earlier than the earliest breast cancer case in the family, whichever is younger. Some women with CS develop severe, sometimes disfiguring, fibroadenomas of the breasts well before age 30. This situation should be treated individually. For example, if the fibroadenomas cause pain or if they make breast cancer surveillance impossible, then some have advocated prophylactic mastectomies.[2]

Whether other tumors are true components of CS is unknown. For now, therefore, surveillance for other organs should follow the American Cancer Society guidelines.

The key to successful management of CS patients and their families is a multi-disciplinary team. There should always be a primary care provider, usually a general internist, who orchestrates the care of such patients, some of whom will need the care of surgeons, gynecologists, dermatologists, oncologists and geneticists at some point.

REFERENCES

1. Lloyd KM, Denis M: Cowden's disease: a possible new symptom complex with multiple system involvement. *Ann Intern Med* **58**:136, 1963.
2. Brownstein MH, Wolf M, Bilowski JB: Cowden's disease. *Cancer* **41**:2393, 1978.
3. Starink TM, van der Veen JPW, Arwert F, de Waal LP, de Lange GG, Gille JJP, Eriksson AW: The Cowden syndrome: a clinical and genetic study in 21 patients. *Clin Genet* **29**:222,1986.
4. Hanssen AMN, Fryns JP: Cowden syndrome. *J Med Genet* **32**:117, 1995.
5. Longy M, Lacombe D: Cowden disease. Report of a family and review. *Ann Genet.* **39**:35, 1996.
6. Nelen MR, Padberg GW, Peeters EAJ, Lin AY, van den Helm B, Frants RR, Coulon V, Goldstein AM, van Reen MMM., Easton DF, Eeles RA, Hodgson S., Mulvihill JJ, Murday VA, Tucker MA, Mariman ECM, Starink TM, Ponder BAJ, Ropers HH, Kremer H., Longy M, and Eng C: Localization of the gene for Cowden disease to 10q22–23. *Nature Genet* **13**:114, 1996.
7. Liaw D, Marsh DJ, Li J., Dahia PLM, Wang SI, Zheng Z, Bose S, Call KM, Tsou HC, Peacocke M, Eng C, and Parsons R: Germline mutations of the *PTEN* gene in Cowden disease, an inherited breast and thyroid cancer syndrome. *Nature Genet* **16**:64, 1997.
8. Lyons CJ, Wilson CR, Horton JC: Association between meningioma and Cowden's disease. *Neurology* **43**:1436, 1993.
9. Haibach H, Burns TW, Carlson HE, Burman KD, and Deftos LJ: Multiple hamartoma syndrome (Cowden's disease) associated with renal cell carcinoma and primary neuroendocrine carcinoma of the skin (Merkel cell carcinoma). *Am J Clin Pathol* **97**:705, 1992.
10. Schrager CA, Schneider D, Gruener AC, Tsou HC, and Peacocke M: Clinical and pathological features of breast disease in Cowden's syndrome: an underrecognised syndrome with an increased risk of breast cancer. *Hum Pathol* (in press).
11. Mallory SB: Cowden syndrome (multiple hamartoma syndrome). *Dermatol Clin* **13**:27, 1995.
12. Eng C: Cowden syndrome. *J Genet Counsel* **6**:181, 1997.
13. Padberg GW, Schot JDL, Vielvoye GJ, Bots GTAM, and de Beer FC: Lhermitte-Duclos disease and Cowden syndrome: a single phakomatosis. *Ann Neurol* **29**:517, 1991.
14. Eng C, Murday V, Seal S, Mohammed S, Hodgson SV, Chaudary MA, Fentiman IS, Ponder BAJ, and Eeles RA: Cowden syndrome and Lhermitte-Duclos disease in a family: a single genetic syndrome with pleiotropy? *J Med Genet* **31**:458, 1994.
15. Viskochil D, Buchberg AM, Xu G, Cawthon RM, Stevens J, Wolff RK, Culver M, Carey JC, Copeland NG, Jenkins NA, White R, and O'Connell P: Deletions and translocation interrupt a cloned gene at the neurofibromatosis type 1 locus. *Cell* **62**:187, 1990.
16. Wallace MR, Marchuk DA, Anderson LB, Letcher R, Oden HM, Saulino AM, Fountain JW, Bereton A, Nicholson J, Mitcehll AL, Brownstein BH, and Collins FS: Type 1 neurofibromatosis gene: identification of a large transcript disrupted in three NF 1 patients. *Science* **249**:181, 1990.
17. Ward K, O'Connell P, Carey J, Leppert M, Jolley S, Plaetke R, Ogden B, White R: Diagnosis of neurofibromatosis 1 by using tightly linked, flankin DNA markers. *Am J Hum Genet* **46**:943, 1990.
18. Johnson RL, Rothman AL, Xie J, Goodrich LV, Bare JW, Bonifas JM, Quinn AG, Myers RM, Cox DR, Epstein EH, and Scott MP: Human homolog of *patched*, a candidate gene for the basal cell nevus syndrome. *Science* **272**:1668, 1996.
19. Gorlin RJ: Proteus syndrome. *J Dysmorphol* **2**:8–9, 1984.
20. Higginbottom MC, Schultz P: The Bannayan syndrome: an autosomal dominant disorder consisting of macrocephaly, lipomas and hemangiomas, and risk for intracranial tumours. *Pediatrics* **69**:632, 1982.
21. Halal F, Silver K: Slowly progressive macrocephaly with hamartomas: a new syndrome? *Am J Med Genet* **33**:182, 1989.
22. Bashir R, Munro CS, Mason S, Stephenson A, Rees JL, Strachan T: Localisation of a gene for Darier's disease. *Hum Mol Genet* **2**:1937, 1993.
23. Craddock N, Dawson E, Burge S, Parfitt L, Mant B, Roberts Q, Daniels J, Gill M, McGuffin P, Powell J, Owen M: The gene for Darier's disease maps to chromosome 12q23–24.1. *Hum Mol Genet* **2**:1941, 1993.
24. Eng C, Blackstone MO: Peutz-Jeghers syndrome. *Med Rounds* **1**:165, 1988.
25. Rustgi AK: Medical progress—hereditary gastrointestinal polyposis and nonpolyposis syndromes. *N Engl J Med* **331**:1694, 1994.
26. Coburn MC, Pricolo VE, DeLuca FG, Bland KI: Malignant potential in intestinal juvenile polyposis syndromes. *Ann Surg Oncol* **2**:386, 1995.
27. Carlson HE, Burns TW, Davenport SL, Luger AM, Spence MA, Sparkes RS, and Orth DN: Cowden disease: gene marker studies and

measurements of epidermal growth factor. *Am J Hum Genet* **38**:908, 1986.

28. Starink TM, van der Veen JP, Goldschmeding R: Decreased natural killer cell activity in Cowden's syndrome [letter]. *J Am Acad Dermatol* **15**:294, 1986.

29. Willard W, Borgen P, Bol R, Tiwari R, Osbourne M: Cowden's disease. A case report with analysis at the molecular level. *Cancer* **69**:2969, 1992.

30. Marsh DJ, Zheng Z, Zedenius J, Kremer H, Padberg GW, Larsson C, Longy M, Eng C: Differential loss of heterozygosity in the region of the Cowden locus within 10q22–23 in follicular thyroid adenomas and carcinomas. *Cancer Res.* **57**:500, 1997.

31. Marsh DJ, Dahia PLM, Coulon V, Zheng Z, Dorion-Bonnet F, Call KM, Little R, Lin AY, Goldstein A, Eeles RA, Hodgson SV, Richarson A-L, Robinson BG, Weber HC, Longy M, Eng C: Allelic imbalance, including deletion of *PTEN/MMAC1,* at the Cowden disease locus on 10q22-23 in hamartomas from patients with Cowden disease and germline *PTEN* mutation. *Genes Chromosomes Cancer* (in press).

32. Li J, Yen C, Liaw D, Podsypanina K, Bose S, Wang S, Puc J, Miliaresis C, Rodgers L, McCombie R, Bigner SH, Giovanella BC, Ittman M, Tycko B, Hibshoosh H, Wigler MH, Parsons R: *PTEN,* a putative protein tyrosine phosphatase gene mutated in human brain, breast and prostate cancer. *Science* **275**:1943, 1997.

33. Steck PA, Pershouse MA, Jasser SA, Yung WKA, Lin H, Ligon AH, Langford LA, Baumgard ML, Hattier T, Davis T, Frye C, Hu R, Swedlund B, Teng DHF, Tavtigian SV: Identification of a candidate tumour suppressor gene, *MMAC1,* at chromosome 10q23.3 that is mutated in multiple advanced cancers. *Nature Genet* **15**:356, 1997.

34. Tonks NK, Neel BG: From form to function: signaling by protein tyrosine phosphatases. *Cell* **87**:365, 1996.

35. Haynie DT, Ponting CP: The N-terminal domains of tensin and auxilin are phosphatase homologues. *Prot Science* **5**:2643, 1996.

36. Jungbluth A, Eckerskorn C, Gerisch G, Lottspeich F, Stocker S, Schweiger A: Stress-induced tyrosine phosphorylation of actin in *Dictyostelium* cells and localization of the phosphorylation site to tyrosine-53 adjacent to the DNaseI binding loop. *FEBS Lett* **375**:87, 1995.

37. Lo SH, Janmey PA, Hartwig JH, Chen LB: Interactions of tensin with actin and identification of its three distinct actin-binding domains. *J Cell Biol* **125**:1067, 1994.

38. Marsh DJ, Dahia PLM, Zheng Z, Liaw D, Parsons R, Gorlin RJ, Eng C: Germline mutations in *PTEN* are present in Bannayan-Zonana syndrome. *Nature Genet* **16**:333, 1997.

CHAPTER 29

Skin Cancer (Gorlin's Syndrome)

Jonathan L. Rees

1. Nonmelanoma skin cancer is the commonest malignancy in many Caucasian populations. Approximately 80% of the tumors are basal cell carcinomas, the majority of the remaining 20% being squamous cell carcinomas. Putative precursor lesions, such as actinic keratoses, are even more common. Basal cell carcinomas and squamous cell carcinomas are readily diagnosed on the basis of clinical appearances and histopathological confirmation. Basal cell carcinomas rarely metastasize and although squamous cell carcinomas have a low rate of metastasis, overall case fatality is low. Surgical therapy or radiotherapy is highly effective.

2. The main environmental cause is ultraviolet radiation and the major genetic influence is through the major physiological adaptation to ultraviolet radiation, namely pigmentation. Studies of coat colour in the mouse suggest that over 100 loci are involved in determining pigmentation, and to date the loci important in accounting for differences in pigmentary characteristics between different human populations are largely unknown. Recently variations in the melanocortin 1 receptor, the receptor for melanocyte stimulating hormone, have been associated with red hair and fair skin in a British population.

3. Familial disorders characterized by a simple Mendelian inheritance pattern probably account for fewer than 1% of all cases of skin cancer. The most common disorder is the nevoid basal cell carcinoma syndrome (Gorlin syndrome), an autosomal dominant disorder, with a prevalence of 1 in 56,000 in a U.K. population. Nevoid basal cell carcinoma syndrome is characterized by multiple basal cell carcinomas, a high incidence of other neoplasms including medulloblastomas, ocular abnormalities, and a variety of developmental abnormalities including odontogenic keratocysts. The gene for nevoid basal cell carcinoma syndrome was mapped by several groups to 9q22-31 and recently identified as the human homologue of the drosophila gene *patched*. Functional characterization of this gene in the human system is awaited but early experiments on its distribution in mouse are consistent with the developmental anomalies seen in patients with the nevoid basal cell carcinoma syndrome. Loss of heterozygosity data is compatible with its role as a tumor suppressor and some developmental anomalies, such as the keratocysts, may also fit the two-hit model. The other developmental anomalies suggest a dosage effect.

4. There is no inherited syndrome principally characterized by an elevated risk of squamous cell carcinoma (increased rates of squamous cell carcinoma and basal cell carcinoma are seen in xeroderma pigmentosa). The Ferguson Smith syndrome (self-healing epitheliomata of Ferguson Smith) is characterized by lesions that clinically and pathologically resemble squamous cell carcinomas but are distinct as they spontaneously involute. On a worldwide basis the syndrome is extremely rare. The Ferguson Smith syndrome maps to the same locus as the nevoid basal cell carcinoma syndrome. It is not known at present whether the two conditions are allelic or caused by separate genes.

5. p53 mutations are common in both basal cell carcinoma and squamous cell carcinoma. Nonmelanoma skin cancers, however, are not a feature of the Li-Fraumeni syndrome. The mutational spectrum in nonmelanoma skin cancer with frequent C→T and CC→TT transitions strongly supports ultraviolet radiation as the relevant mutagen.

6. Although basal cell carcinomas and squamous cell carcinomas show frequent p53 mutation and *ras* mutations have been described in both tumor types, loss of heterozygosity studies show clear differences between the two tumor types. In basal cell carcinomas, which usually are diploid, allelic loss is uncommon and is almost entirely confined to the Gorlin locus on 9q. By contrast in squamous cell carcinoma the fractional allelic loss is 25–30%, with loss of heterozygosity being common on chromosomes 3, 9, 13, and 17. Loss of heterozygosity studies clearly distinguish squamous cell carcinoma from basal cell carcinoma, keratoacanthoma (a regressing form of nonmelanoma skin cancer) and other rarer tumor types, including appendageal tumors.

Based on their underlying biology and clinical behavior skin cancers are usefully classified according to their cell of origin; melanoma from melanocytes or melanocyte precursors (melanoma skin cancer); and nonmealnoma skin cancer (NMSC), the majority of which are derived from the major cell type of the epidermis, the keratinocyte. There are two common types of nonmelanoma skin cancer, basal cell carcinoma (BCC) and (cutaneous) squamous cell carcinoma (SCC). A small number of tumors arise from other cell types of the epidermis or dermis including Merkel cells and endothelial cells, and although they are technically nonmelanoma skin cancers, they have little in common with the keratinocyte-derived cells tumors and will not be discussed further. Melanoma skin cancer is discussed in Chapter 27. Xeroderma pigmentosa is associated with dramatically increased rates of both nonmelanoma skin cancer and melanoma skin cancer and is dealt with in Chapter 13.

Because NMSC have a low case-fatality and often are treated outside the hospital setting, and because some lesions may be treated without histological confirmation, incidence data for NMSC are notoriously unreliable.[1] Nevertheless, for predominantly Caucasian populations in many parts of the world, NMSC is the commonest human malignancy.[1–5] It is estimated that in the United States over three-quarters of a million individuals present with NMSC every year, accounting for over one-third of all incident cancers.[1] Approximately 80% of NMSC are BCC with most of the remaining 20% being SCC. In areas with high ambient ultraviolet radiation and a predominantly Caucasian population, such as Australia, over half the population over the age of 40 have NMSC or cognate lesions.[1,6,8] The relative neglect of serious study of NMSC probably reflects a number of facts most notably the relative ease and success of surgical or other destructive therapy.[9] Although in part this may be attributed to the ease of their detection, their visibility, this is not a complete explanation as melanomas are equally if not more visible and yet show a significant mortality. Recent work has shown that even when keratinocytes have accumulated multiple genetic abnormalities and when by conventional histopathological criteria they show considerable de-differentiation, their clinical behavior is relatively benign in comparison to other epithelial malignancies.[10,11] Given the frequency of NMSC and that ultraviolet radiation, the main cause of NMSC, is the most ubiquitous human carcinogen it is tempting to speculate that evolutionary constraints on keratinocytes make them relatively resistant to the adoption of an aggressive malignant phenotype.

ETIOLOGY

The population contribution of single-gene disorders to NMSC is dwarfed by the influence of ultraviolet radiation. Clinically characterized single gene disorders such as the nevoid basal cell carcinoma syndrome (Gorlin syndrome) and the Ferguson Smith syndrome (self-healing epitheliomata of Ferguson Smith) and other rarer syndromes account for fewer than 1% of incident cases of NMSC. Even in these disorders expressivity is influenced by the biology of the response to ambient ultraviolet radiation. In black skin BCC may be entirely absent in the NBCCS (highlighting the inadequacy of the syndrome name), whereas in countries with high ambient ultraviolet radiation such as Australia, the age of presentation is markedly younger than in more temperate latitudes.[12,15] Despite the small contribution from these characterized Mendelian syndromes, the genetic contribution to NMSC is considerable as can be appreciated by considering the relation between pigmentary status, cancer risk and ultraviolet exposure.[16,17]

Proof of the importance of ultraviolet radiation in the causation of NMSC comes from several sources.[1,16,20] First, both SCC and BCC are most common on sun exposed body sites (although there are differences in body-site distribution between the two tumors, suggesting that other factors may be important or that the quantitative relation with UVR differs between BCC and SCC). Second, the results of *forced* or *voluntary* population migrations, most notably of individuals of Anglo-Saxon origin to Australia, support a role for sun exposure.[1,17] Within genetically homogenous populations tumor rates are inversely proportional to distance from the equator with rates for instance being higher in Brisbane than Melbourne.[17] Third, the mutational spectra of target genes such as p53 directly implicates a role for ultraviolet radiation mutagenesis in NMSC.[21,22] Fourth, NMSC rates are orders of magnitude different

between human populations with different pigmentary characteristics.[23,24] Finally, some, but possibly not all forms of iatrogenically administered ultraviolet radiation cause NMSC.[25,27] It is salutary to remember that the color of one's skin and the ability to tan in response to ultraviolet radiation are largely the result of an evolutionary tradeoff between the need to protect against solar damage in areas of high ambient ultraviolet radiation, and the need to ensure adequate ultraviolet B radiation reaches the basal layer of skin to ensure adequate vitamin D synthesis to avoid metabolic bone disease.[17,28] The genetic basis of these pigmentary differences are likely to be complex, in the mouse over a hundred loci are known to be important in determining coat color, although recent candidate approaches based on the melanocortin 1 receptor may explain the predisposition of those with Celtic ancestry to NMSC.[29,31,32] Although ultraviolet radiation is the major cause of NMSC, other factors are important, including ionizing radiation, chemical carcinogens, and some forms of iatrogenic immunosuppression.[33–36]

BASAL CELL CARCINOMA

Basal cell carcinomas are characteristically indolent small pearly edged lesions with accompanying telangiectasia and an ulcerated centre occurring most commonly on the face or less commonly upper trunk or elsewhere.[34,35,37,39] They are the most common tumor in the United States with over 750,000 incident cases per year.[40] Histologically the tumors show downgrowths of keratinocytes from the epidermis lined by palisades of cells resembling basal cells. There are a number of clinicopathological variants with differences in clinical behavior, although the molecular basis for these differences is unknown and different tumor subtypes may be seen in the same individual. Differentiation with features of eccrine or hair epithelia may occur. Although BCC are invasive and can track down nerves or invade underlying tissues such as bone, metastasis is extremely uncommon (<1:4000) and calls into question the diagnosis.[34,35,41] Destruction of the tumor using a variety of modalities including surgical excision, curetting, and cautery, cryotherapy or radiotherapy is usually curative. Basal cell carcinomas are a central feature of the nevoid basal cell carcinoma syndrome and the Bazex-Dupre-Christol syndrome.

Nevoid Basal Cell Carcinoma Syndrome (OMIM 109400)

NBCCS is inherited as an autosomal dominant trait with a high rate (40%) of new mutation and an estimated incidence in a U.K. population of 1:56,000.[15] Fewer than 0.5% of patients presenting with a BBC will have NBCCS, although the proportion will be higher in subjects presenting with a BCC at an early age or with multiple tumors. Subjects show a characteristic facial appearance, an increased frequency of a number of neoplasms, most notably basal cell carcinomas, odontogenic keratocysts, and a variety of other developmental abnormalities.[15,42,43] Gorlin has recently reviewed the clinical features.[13] Cutaneous signs include the development of multiple (up to several hundred or more) BCC and palmar-plantar pits. BCC occur most commonly on the face, neck, or upper trunk and histologically are identical to sporadic basal cell carcinomas. Tumors commonly appear at or after puberty but presentation appears to be influenced by the amount of ambient ultraviolet radiation and other cutaneous characteristics. In blacks BCC may be uncommon or not seen at all, whereas among whites in Australia the average age of BCC presentation is relatively young.[12,14] Tumors have been reported as early as 2 years of age. BCC do not occur in about 10% of documented cases of NBCCS. The clinical appearance of the lesions is said to be distinctive and may resemble benign cutaneous lesions, including skin tags or seborrhoeic warts or melanocytic nevi.[13] Gorlin reports that before puberty these lesions are harmless and that only a minority change and become aggressive.[13] Palmar or plantar pits occur in over half the cases, more commonly on the hands than feet, and are more common in adults than children. Typically, they are several millimetres across, have a telangiectatic base, and are clinically distinct from the pits seen in Darier's disease. BCC may develop in the base of the pits.

Patients with NBCCS are at increased risk of a number of other neoplasms, benign or malignant, including medulloblastoma (approximately 5%), meningioma, cardiac fibromas, and ovarian sarcomas and fibromas (15%). Patients also show a variety of other developmental defects; multiple odontogenic keratocysts that are often asymptomatic and peak during the second or third decade which occur in up to 85% of subjects; a characteristic facial appearance with frontal and biparietal bulging, prominent supraorbital ridges, and a low occiput and a long mandible; they are often tall with some showing a Marfinoid build; and a variety of skeletal manifestations including bifid ribs, short fourth metacarpals and cortical defects of the long bones. Ophthalmic abnormalities such as squint or cataract are also seen in 25% of cases.[15] Cases with unilateral cutaneous signs have been described.[44] It seems likely that some of the many patients who present with multiple BCC may be form frustes of the NBCCS syndrome.

Genetic Loci Involved in BCC

Mapping of NBCCS by several groups to 9q22–31 and the finding of loss of heterozygosity in up to 70% of sporadic basal cell carcinomas suggests an underlying tumor suppressor gene important in both familial and sporadic BCC.[45,48] Loss of the same wild-type allele in multiple BCC from the same individual with NBCCS is in keeping with this.[49] There is no evidence of genetic heterogeneity. Recently two groups have identified the gene for NBCCS as being the human homologue of the drosophila gene *patched*. Hahn et al. searched a 2-megabase region of 9q22 before characterising PTC, a 23 exon gene spanning 34kb, for mutations in patients with NBCCS.[50,51] Six mutations, consisting of four deletions or insertions resulting in frameshifts, and two point mutations, were identified among a panel of unrelated NBCCS patients, in addition to a frameshift mutation in a new case of NBCCS with no change being found in the phenotypically normal parents. The authors identified two sporadic (nonfamilial) BCC with mutations and loss of the remaining allele, one of them being a CC-TT transition typical of ultraviolet radiation induced mutagenesis. By contrast Johnson et al., having previously cloned the murine PTC cDNA, screened human cDNA libraries for a human homologue that they mapped using radiation hybrids to 9q22.3.[52] The authors identified a three amino acid insertion in a kindred with NBCCS and a 11bp deletion resulting in a premature stop codon in a new incident case of NBCCS (phenotypically normal parents showed wild-type sequence only). One mutation, a C-T transition was found in 12 sporadic BCC cases. Recent results suggest that over one-half of psoradic BCC harbor *patched* mutations.[52a]

Human PTC consists of an open reading of 4242 nucleotides encoding a putative protein of 1296 amino acids, which shows 39% identity and 60% similarity to its Drosophila counterpart.[50,51] Northern blots of various human tissues show the presence of several transcripts that appear differentially expressed.[50,51] In skin, expression as shown by *in situ* hybridization and Northern blots ap-

pears low, although as would be expected from studies in Drosophila where *patched* downregulates its own expression, increased expression is seen in basal cell carcinomas harboring mutant *patched*.[52a] How PTC leads to BCC awaits functional experiments but work in Drosophila, and analogies with other tumor suppressors, suggest clues. In Drosophila PTC is a transmembrane glycoprotein which represses the hedgehog mediated induction of several genes involved in cell-cell communication, including decapentaplegic (*dpp*) (and *ptc* itself). Because Dpp is a member of the TGF-β signaling pathway, and TGF-β is known to play an important signalling role in many epithelia including skin, then it is possible that disturbance of this pathway will lead to increased activity of hedgehog targets. Also thought to be involved in this pathway is *mad*, human homologues of which are known to be involved in colorectal cancer.[53,54] Although the embryonic distribution of human *PTC* is not known, it is possible to correlate many of the features of NBCCS with sites of *ptc* expression in the mouse embryo.[50,51] Whereas some of the abnormalities such as the odontogenic keratocysts may like BCC be explained by a two hit mechanism, the widespread developmental abnormalities suggest a dosage effect and of course fall outside the strict Knudson paradigm for the recessive nature at the cellular level of tumor suppressor genes.[55]

Other Genetic Targets in BCC

Unusually for an epithelial malignancy LOH studies on sporadic BCC show a low frequency of allele loss (at loci other than the NBCCS locus that is lost in up to 70% of BCC), a result in keeping with the usual diploid nature of these tumors.[48,56,58] LOH of 14 or 33% for chromosome arm 1q has been reported, but otherwise LOH appears uncommon, unless it is confined to small areas that have not been examined.[48,56] Interestingly, despite the presence of p53 mutation, LOH of 17p is uncommon but a second inactivating p53 mutation on the remaining allele is common.[48,59,61]

Mutations of p53, ras and a GTPase activating protein have been described in BCC. Abnormal expression of p53 is common in BCC and depending on the antibody and exact immunocytochemical method employed is increased compared with normal skin in upward of 50% of tumors.[61–66] In many instances this increased expression represents overexpression of wild-type sequence.[61] Various studies have reported the presence of p53 mutations in BCC. As with squamous cell carcinoma the mutation spectrum reflects in large part the particular characteristics of UVR mutagenesis with frequent C-T transitions at (dipyrimidine sites) and double CC-TT transitions, with the result that the mutation hot spots differ from those seen in many internal malignancies.[21,22,67,69] The absolute rate of p53 mutation in BCC varies considerably between different studies ranging from 20 to 60%.[59,61,70,74] These differences may be accounted for by small statistical sample sizes, technical factors particularly relating to the difficulties in separating stromal or inflammatory elements in small tumors, but also could conceivably represent genuine differences in molecular epidemiology. The presence of more than one p53 point mutation, one on each allele, perhaps reflects the high ultraviolet radiation mutagenic load skin is exposed to.[61,75]

Ras mutations are common in the murine chemical carcinogenesis model of skin cancer and investigators early on examined human NMCS including BCC for the presence of such changes.[76,77] Activating mutations of ras could be expected based on the known properties and base specificity of ultraviolet radiation induced mutations. As for p53, and possibly for similar reasons, *ras* mutation rates show a wide scatter between 0 and 30%.[70,72,77,83] There is one report of mutations of the GTPase activating protein (which is involved in downregulating *ras* proteins and in signal transduction) in three of 21 BCC.[84] To date there are no studies showing a relation between the presence of specific genetic change to clinical behavior or histological subtype of BCC, nor has a definite precursor lesion been identified, although some authors have identified p53 immunopositive clones harboring p53 mutations close to clinically obvious BCC.[72,74,85] It remains possible that these lesions are precursors of other types of NMSC.[64]

Bazex-Dupre-Christol Syndrome (OMIM 301845)

This is an extremely uncommon X-linked dominant condition characterized by multiple basal cell carcinomas developing in the second and third decade, and follicular atrophoderma present from birth or early childhood.[86–89] Hypotrichosis and other abnormalities may be present. The basal cell carcinomas may resemble those seen in the NBCCS. It has recently been mapped to Xq24–27.[90]

Rombo Syndrome (MIM 180730)

There is one report of this syndrome that was transmitted through four generations consistent with an autosomal dominant trait.[91] Basal cell carcinomas were described together with vermiculate atrophoderma, abnormal eyelashes and eyebrows and in one case trichoepitheliomas.

SQUAMOUS CELL CARCINOMA

SCC are invasive tumors with the ability to metastasize with a histological resemblance to differentiated suprabasal keratinocytes.[4,33,39,92,93] They usually arise on sun exposed skin, grow quicker than basal cell carcinoma, and produce a more indurated untidy keratotic lesion with ulceration. There may be associated signs of ultraviolet radiation damage to skin, including actinic keratoses. Histology shows aberrant differentiation, frequent mitoses and variable degrees of dysplasia. Metastasis rates are between 0.1 and 4% but the overall mortality is low.[4,33,93,95] Cutaneous SCC are less aggressive in their biological behavior than other keratinocyte derived tumors such as those of the oral cavity or cervix, or from SCC of the lip, which are also caused by ultraviolet radiation exposure.[33,93] There is some evidence that SCC arising in the sites of thermal burns or in sites of chronic inflammation may behave more aggressively.[33] Most cutaneous SCC are readily amenable to surgery or radiotherapy.

Whereas there are no clinically identified precursor lesions for BCC, some SCC are thought to arise from actinic keratoses or areas of Bowen's disease (*in situ* carcinoma).[33,96] Actinic keratoses are focal areas of cutaneous dysplasia characterized clinically by redness and scaling that are usually only minimally indurated or show no induration.[96,97] They are usually multiple, and their body site distribution mirrors cumulative ultraviolet radiation exposure being high on the scalps of balding men, face, and backs of hands and lower arms.[97] Epidemiological studies in Australia report a prevalence for actinic keratoses of around 50% over the age of 40, and that the risk of progression from a single AK to a SCC is less than 1:1000 per year.[1,98] One-quarter of actinic keratoses may resolve spontaneously over a 1-year period, whereas approximately half of SCC arise in a pre-existing actinic keratosis, with the other half apparently arising *de novo*.[98,99] Actinic keratoses are at least 15 times commoner than SCC.[1] Sporadic squamous cell carcino-

mas, unlike keratoacanthomas or the epitheliomata of Ferguson Smith, show no significant propensity to clinical regression.[33] There are no single gene disorders that specifically feature squamous cell carcinomas. (Ferguson Smith tumors, although showing certain similarities, are distinct.)

Genetic Change in Squamous Cell Carcinoma

Aneuploidy is common in SCC (unlike BCC) occurring in between 20 and 80% of cases. SCC show distinct patterns of loss of heterozygosity compared with other non cutaneous squamous cell cancers and other skin tumors such as basal cell carcinomas or keratoacanthomas.[58,103,107] Loss of heterozygosity in SCC is especially common on chromosome 3 (25%), 9 (40%) and 17 (40%) with an overall fractional allelic loss of 30%.[11,48] With the exception of chromosome 17 and p53, the identity of the underlying putative tumor suppressor genes for cutaneous SCC are unknown. Loss of 3p is common in other keratinocyte squamous malignancies including oral carcinoma, but the target gene is at present unknown: Studies examining the recently identified FHIT gene have not been reported for skin SCC.[108,109] The target gene(s) underlying LOH on chromosome 9 also is unknown. Current data suggest that the NBCCS or the Ferguson Smith locus is not a primary target in SCC, rather deletion mapping studies suggest an area of 9p that includes p16 and p15.[106,110] Studies examining these genes for mutation have not been reported, nor have other areas of 9p been excluded.[111]

Brash first showed that p53 mutations were common in SCC, but perhaps more importantly showed that the pattern of mutation involving frequent C-T and CC-TT transitions bore the molecular footprint of ultraviolet radiation induced mutagenesis.[21] Ultraviolet radiation can influence the carcinogenic process in number of ways.[17] Ultraviolet radiation is mutagenic, in animal systems can act as a tumor promoter, and there is evidence in animals, if not in humans, that local and systemic immunosuppression induced by ultraviolet may be important in skin carcinogenesis. The finding of ultraviolet radiation-induced mutations was therefore important direct proof of the mutagenic role of ultraviolet radiation in human skin cancer (the increased incidence of SCC in patients with xeroderma pigmentosa could, although perhaps not very convincingly, be attributed to the ultraviolet induced abnormalities of immune function or to effects on tumor promotion). Subsequent studies have in large part confirmed the earlier findings, although not unfamiliarly for studies of genetic change in NMSC the absolute rates of p53 mutation in SCC vary considerably from 10 to over 60%.[21,69,70,83,112,115] These differences may reflect genuine epidemiological differences, technical factors, or statistical sampling errors as most studies are relatively small. There is a suggestion that the type of mutations may vary in different studies. Studies of premalignant lesions such as Bowen's disease and actinic keratoses also show a high rate of p53 mutation.[116,118] It is not known whether preinvasive lesions harboring p53 mutations are more likely to progress to SCC than those without mutation, although given the frequency of nonprogression, even with p53 mutations, the majority of actinic keratoses would be expected to regress or at least not progress. In contrast with BCC, where allelic loss is uncommon, as with many other malignancies, loss of the remaining wild type allele is common in SCC. It remains possible that there are targets other than p53 on chromosome 17.[11]

The timing of p53 mutation during squamous cell cancer development and the role p53 plays in keratinocyte physiology also has been examined.[22,118] Wild-type p53 protein expression is increased in human skin following exposure to even doses of ultraviolet radiation too small to induce erythema.[119,121] Increased expression is seen with ultraviolet A, B and C, although when normalized so that equierythemal doses of erythema are produced, the largest increase is seen for ultraviolet B.[119] The pattern of induction throughout the epidermis is not easily explained on the basis of the known penetration characteristics of the various wavebands of ultraviolet radiation.[119] It is widely assumed that the upregulation of p53 expression in response to ultraviolet radiation is a direct result of DNA damage, although more modest increases are seen following a range of stimuli that are not known to cause DNA damage.[121] The functional significance of the increased expression is not clear. For instance individuals with the Li-Fraumeni syndrome harboring p53 mutations do not show an excess of NMSC nor has photosensitivity been reported in this group of patients. In an attempt to assess the function of p53, Brash and colleagues irradiated mice null for p53 and showed that the number of sunburn cells formed in response to ultraviolet radiation was diminished.[118] (Sunburn cells are defined morphologically, and are thought to represent apoptotic keratinocytes.)[122] They argued that wild-type p53 plays an important role in facilitating apoptosis in response to DNA damage and that loss of this function would allow clonal expansion of mutated clones, thus implicating a role for ultraviolet radiation in mutagenesis and tumor promotion.[22,118] It remains unclear why the increase in p53 expression following ultraviolet B radiation is seen throughout both the proliferative and terminally differentiated compartment, and why sunburn cells are seen only in the terminally differentiated compartment.[119] Interestingly no increase in sunburn cell formation following irradiation has been reported in mice carrying a mutant p53 transgene.[123]

The timing of p53 mutations in the development of SCC also has been studied. Sensitive techniques such as the ligase mediated PCR that do not rely on the presence of a clonally expanded group of cells, have shown that p53 mutations can be identified in normal sun-exposed skin and in irradiated cultured keratinocytes.[124] Clusters of p53 immunopositive cells harboring p53 mutation have also been described close to BCC, and although these could represent BCC precursors, perhaps it is more likely that they are related to squamous cell cancer development.[64,72] It has been suggested that because dissection of different regions of actinic keratoses shows no heterogeneity for p53 mutation then p53 mutation may be the initiating event in SCC development.[118] Given the high proliferative rate of many actinic keratoses this argument is not decisive as other changes may have already occurred. In keeping with this, recent work has shown that in many actinic keratoses increased proliferation, elevated wild-type p53 expression, changes in p21[waf/cip1] expression, and chromosomal loss all occur without or before p53 mutation.[11] There may be many pathways to SCC development, and within certain limits, the order of genetic change may not be critical. The high rate of regression, and the low rate of progression to SCC, raises the possibility that actinic keratoses and SCC are cognate phenomenon, both responses to ultraviolet radiation-induced genetic damage and that the rare apparent progression from an actinic keratoses to a SCC is owing to misdiagnosis of early *in situ* SCC as actinic keratoses.[125,126] The finding of higher rates of genetic change in actinic keratoses than in SCC, although compatible with this, does not provide it, and the hypothesis remains speculative.[11]

As with BCC a number of studies have looked for *ras* mutations in SCC. Although some early studies reported a high frequency of ras mutations (principally of H-*ras* at codon 12), as has been found in studies of other human cancers, later results have qualified earlier work with lower mutation rates being reported. Rates therefore vary from 0 to 46% in different studies.[70,71,77,80,82] There is some evidence that ras mutation rates are higher in some risk groups such as patients with xeroderma pigmentosa than in control tumors.[79,127,128] Definitive studies conducted simultaneously on samples from different populations are required. In addi-

tion to studies of point mutations of *ras* there are reports of alteration in *ras* expression, gene amplification or gene deletion that appear particularly common in tumors occurring on the basis of xeroderma pigmentosa.[79,127]

KERATOACANTHOMA

Keratoacanthomas (KA) are interesting tumors that, although sharing histological and clinical overlap with SCC, are defined by their history of spontaneous regression.[39,129,130] Characteristically keratoacanthomas develop over the course of a few months and show rapid growth resulting in lesions a few centimeters across, with a keratin plug and a cellular shoulder, before regressing leaving a scar. KA show many similarities to SCC, and because the defining feature of a KA is natural regression, in clinical practice where lesions are excised or biopsied differentiation from SCC is often problematic. Keratoacanthomas are distinct from the self-healing epitheliomata of Ferguson Smith.[131]

Given their interesting natural history they have received little serious attention. Various theories have been proposed to account for their regressing course; that they have a viral pathogenesis; that they are follicular tumors and that their growth pattern mimics the hair follicle's anagen and telogen; and that they are SCC that are immunologically rejected by the host.[129,130,132] There are particular diagnostic problems with any analysis of these tumors because the gold standard of distinction between a keratoacanthoma and a SCC relies on natural history which is compromised by removal or biopsy.

Studies conflict as to the frequency of aneuploidy in KA, and whether it is possible to clearly distinguish KA from SCC on the basis of ploidy.[58,102,103] (Although subsequent allelotyping of KA and SCC suggest that differences are likely.) Increases in p53 expression have been described, although definitive studies of mutation rates have not been reported.[70,71,77,80,82] *Ras* mutations have been described in a small number of tumors and an attempt made to link the presence of mutation with regression rather than progression.[136,137] A recent study of loss of heterozygosity in keratoacanthomas showed a low fractional allelic loss based on examination of 26 autosomes of only 1.3% with only sporadic loss seen.[107] This suggests clear differences from squamous cell carcinoma (FAL score of 30%) and make it likely that keratoacanthomas and SCC are different *de novo* rather than keratoacanthomas, being the result of a successful immunological attack of a SCC.[11,48,132] LOH at the Ferguson Smith locus was uncommon.[107]

FERGUSON SMITH SYNDROME (OMIM 132800)

This originally was described in a single individual and the familial nature of the disorder was only recognized later.[131,138,139] It is inherited as an autosomal dominant, has been reported to skip generations, and the largest series all originate from Scotland, with the possibility that they all derive from a single mutation in the late eighteenth century.[139] The incidence is unknown but worldwide the tumors appear exceptionally rare. Clinically the condition is characterized by the presence of recurrent lesions identical to squamous cell carcinomas that develop over a few months, then resolve spontaneously leaving a depressed scar. More than one lesion may present at the same time. Histologically the lesions are well differentiated squamous cell carcinomas rather than keratoacanthomas.[131] (Although many still refer to them as keratoacanthomas, or argue that they are indeed a form of familial keratoacanthoma.) Tumors may present in the second decade but occur more commonly later on in life. Tumors on the face and scalp are common and although most tumors occur on sun-exposed areas, tumors have been reported of the anus and the perineum.[140] There are no associated extracutaneous features, and whilst disabling and destructive with tumors capable of underlying infiltration, they do not usually effect mortality. There are reports of genuine SCC with metastases developing in individuals with the Ferguson Smith syndrome.[131] The disorder may be unilateral.[140]

In studies of 13 British families linkage has been shown to 9q22–31, the same locus as for the NBCCS.[141] Whether the two disorders are allelic or reflect mutations of two different genes is not known but now that the NBCCS gene has been identified as the human homologue of *patched*, this should be resolved quickly. LOH of Ferguson Smith tumors have not been published and it remains possible that the target gene is not a tumor suppressor.

MUIR TORRE SYNDROME (OMIM 158320)

This is best considered part of the Lynch type 2 family cancer syndrome secondary to an underlying defect in mismatch repair.[142–144] It is characterised cutaneously by sebaceous gland tumors, including sebaceous adenomas, sebaceous epitheliomas, and sebaceous carcinomas, and less commonly keratoacanthomas.[145] It is inherited as an autosomal dominant but expressivity is variable.[146] The true incidence is unknown but the author suspects the cutaneous aspects are widely underdiagnosed or misdiagnosed. Replication errors have been demonstrated in the cutaneous tumors including tumors such as actinic keratoses not considered part of the syndrome (replication errors are otherwise uncommon in NMSC).[147,148]

EPIDERMODYSPLASIA VERRUCIFORMIS (OMIM 226400)

This is characterized by the onset in childhood of a combination of plane wart, red plaque, and pityriasis versicolor-like lesions in which a range of human papilloma virus types may be identified, with the development of squamous cell cancers on sun exposed areas later, and depressed cell mediated immunity.[149,150] The mode of inheritance is unclear although the majority of reports favour an autosomal recessive.[149] The condition is extremely rare and apart from identification of new papilloma viruses it has received little genetic attention.[150]

DYSKERATOSIS CONGENITA (OMIM 305000)

Squamous cell cancers of the skin and other epithelia have been reported in this condition, which is characterized by leucoplakia, nail dystrophy, and cutaneous atrophy and pigmentation.[151,152] It is usually an X-linked recessive syndrome, although other patterns of inheritance have been described.[152] The X-linked form has been mapped to Xq28.[153]

APPENDAGEAL TUMORS

Basal cell carcinoma and squamous cell carcinoma aside, there are a large number of different types of epidermal tumors of varying degrees of aggressiveness which on a clinicopathological basis are believed to relate to the pilosebaceous unit or eccrine or apocrine sweat glands.[154,155] They are uncommon in comparison to BCC or SCC, and often are only correctly diagnosed after histological examination. The vast majority of tumors are solitary and occur without any family history. Examination of a range of appendageal tumors for LOH showed a low frequency of LOH at selected loci and failed to find any consistent pattern, a finding perhaps not surprising given their pathological heterogeneity and relatively benign clinical course.[85] Particular familial syndromes that usually are characterized by multiple tumors include Cowden syndrome (multiple hamartoma syndrome, OMIM 158350) an autosomal dominant trait comprising multiple hair follicle tumors, oral papillomas, and breast cancer, which maps to 10q22–23; familial trichoepithelioma (OMIM 132700), which has recently been mapped to 9p; and familial cyclindromatosis (turban tumors, OMIM 123850), which maps to 16q12–q13 and that shows LOH for this locus in the tumors.[131,156,158]

COMPLEX TRAITS AND SKIN CANCER SUSCEPTIBILITY

In numerical terms the contribution of the highly penetrant single gene disorders described earlier to nonmelanoma skin cancer is small, accounting for perhaps fewer than 1% of cases. Nevertheless, the genetic influence on skin cancer development is considerable. Although ultraviolet radiation is viewed as the major environmental cause of NMSC this is in large part only because populations adapted to areas of low ambient ultraviolet radiation have in the relatively recent evolutionary past migrated to areas of high exposure.[17,18] The major genetic determinant of NMSC worldwide therefore is pigmentation (and any other genetic determinants of the cutaneous response to ultraviolet radiation). Blacks have rates of NMSC greater than 50-fold lower than whites, and Japanese who have migrated to areas of higher UVR still show rates four to 12 times lower than those seen in Caucasians (although differences in sun exposure habits cannot be excluded entirely).[23,159,160] Even within Caucasian populations rates vary perhaps fivefold between those with red hair or who tend to burn rather than tan (and who are often red-haired or of Irish or Welsh so-called Celtic ancestry), and those who tan rather than burn from southern Europe.[19,20] Although the genetics of pigmentation appear complex with in the mouse upwards of a 100 loci involved in determining coat color, there are in humans single loci effecting pigmentation that exert considerable effects on skin cancer rates.[29,31] For instance oculocutaneous albinos living in areas of high ambient ultraviolet radiation show dramatically increased risks of NMSC, and without appropriate care and sun avoidance may die from complications of their tumors in early adult life.[159,161] Recently, associations between variants of the melanocortin 1 receptor and the inability to tan and red hair were described in a British population.[32] The melanocortin 1 receptor is the principal receptor for melanocyte stimulating hormone present on melanocytes and genetic analyses in the mouse have shown that melanocyte stimulating hormone controls the switch from the production of pheomelanin (red/yellow melanin) to eumelanin (black/brown melanin), an action antagonized by agouti.[29,31] Although eumelanin is photoprotective, pheomelanin has poor sunscreen activities and actually may generate free radicals in response to UVR.[162,163] Particular alleles of the melanocortin 1 receptor recently have been described to be associated with melanoma and it seems possible that the same may hold for non-melanoma skin cancer.[164]

It is likely that there are a number of other genetic influences on NMSC development of unknown magnitude, including the relation between immunological aspects of cutaneous function and tumor risk.[165,166] Possible associations are between NMSC and glutathione S-transferase GSTM1 polymorphisms, between HLA haplotypes and NMSC, and between NMSC and genetic determinants of susceptibility to the immunosuppressive actions of ultraviolet radiation.[167–170] The influence of differences in DNA repair rates on NMSC is discussed in Chapters 3 and 13.[171,173]

REFERENCES

1. Marks R: An overview of skin cancers: Incidence and causation. *Cancer* 75(Suppl):607, 1995.
2. Gallagher RP, Ma B, McLean DI, Yang CP, Ho V, Carruthers, JA, Warshawski LM: Trends in basal cell carcinoma, squamous cell carcinoma, and melanoma of the skin from 1973 through 1987. *J Am Acad Dermatol* 23:413, 1990.
3. Glass AG, Hoover RN: The emerging epidemic of melanoma and squamous cell skin cancer. *JAMA* 262:2097, 1989.
4. Preston DS, Stern RS: Nonmelanoma cancers of the skin. *N Engl J Med* 327:1649, 1992.
5. Green A: Changing patterns in incidence of nonmelanoma skin cancer. *Epithel Cell Biol* 1:47, 1992.
6. Marks R, Jolley D, Dorevitch AP, Selwood TS: The incidence of non-melanocytic skin cancers in an Australian population: results of a five-year prospective study. *Med J Aust* 150:475, 1989.
7. Marks R, Staples M, Giles GG: Trends in non-melanocytic skin cancer treated in Australia: the second national survey. *Int J Cancer* 53:585, 1993.
8. Kricker A, English DR, Randell PL, Heenan PJ, Clay CD, Delaney TA, Armstrong BK: Skin cancer in Geraldton, Western Australia: a survey of incidence and prevalence. *Med J Aust* 152:399, 1990.
9. Fleming ID, Amonette R, Monaghan T, Fleming MD: Principles of management of basal and squamous cell carcinoma of the skin. *Cancer* 75(Suppl):699, 1995.
10. Rehman I, Quinn AG, Healy E, Rees JL: High frequency of loss of heterozygosity in actinic keratoses, a usually benign disease. *Lancet* 344:788, 1994.
11. Rehman I, Takata M, Wu YY, Rees JL: Genetic change in actinic keratoses. *Oncogene* 12:2483, 1996.
12. Goldstein AM, Pastakia B, DiGiovanna JJ, Poliak S, Santucci S, Kase R, Bale AE, Bale SJ: Clinical findings in two African-American families with the nevoid basal cell carcinoma syndrome (NBCC). *Am J Med Genet* 50:272, 1994.
13. Gorlin RJ: Nevoid basal-cell carcinoma syndrome. *Medicine* 66:98, 1987.
14. Shanley S, Ratcliffe J, Hockey A, Haan E, Oley C, Ravine D, Martin N, Wicking C, and Chenevix-Trench G. Nevoid basal cell carcinoma syndrome: review of 118 affected individuals. *Am J Med Genetics* 50:282, 1994.
15. Evans DG, Ladusans EJ, Rimmer S, Burnell LD, Thakker N, Farndon PA: Complications of the naevoid basal cell carcinoma syndrome: results of a population based study. *J Med Genet* 30:460, 1993.
16. IARC monographs on the evaluation of carcinogenic risks to humans: Solar and ultraviolet radiation. Lyon, France: *IARC* 55:1992.
17. NRPB Board statement on effects of ultraviolet radiation on human health and health effects from ultraviolet radiation. Chilton Didcott, Oxon: *Natl Radiat Prot Bd* 6(2):1995.
18. Kricker A, Armstrong BK, English DR: Sun exposure and non-melanocytic skin cancer. *Cancer Causes Control* 5:367, 1994.
19. Kricker A, Armstrong BK, English DR, Heenan PJ: Pigmentary and cutaneous risk factors for non-melanocytic skin cancer—a case-control study. *Int J Cancer* 48:650, 1991.
20. Urbach F, Rose DB, Bonnem RDH, Bonnem M: Genetic and environmental interactions in skin carcinogenesis in Urbach F, Rose DB, Bonnem RDH, Bonnem M (eds): *Genetic and Environmental Carcinogenesis*. Baltimore, Williams & Wilkins, 1971 pp. 355–371.
21. Brash DE, Rudolph JA, Simon JA, Lin A, McKenna GJ, Baden HP, Halperin AJ, Ponten J: A role for sunlight in skin cancer: UV-induced p53 mutations in squamous cell carcinoma. *Proc Natl Acad Sci USA* 88:10124, 1991.
22. Brash DE, Ziegler A, Jonason AS, Simon JA, Kunula S, Leffel DJ: Sunlight and sunburn in human skin cancer: p53, apoptosis, and tumor promotion. *J Invest Dermatol Symp Proc* 1(S):136S, 1996.
23. Scotto J, Fears TR, Fraumeni JF: Incidence of nonmelanoma skin cancer in the United States. *NIH Pub* 83, 1983.
24. Fleming ID, Barnawell JR, Burlison PE, Rankin JS: Skin cancer in black patients. *Cancer* 35:600, 1975.
25. Stern RS: Risks of cancer associated with long-term exposure to PUVA in humans: current status 1991. *Blood Cells* 18:91; 98, 1992.
26. Stern RS, Laird N: The carcinogenic risk of treatments for severe psoriasis. *Cancer* 73:2759, 1994.
27. Bhate SM, Sharpe GR, Marks JM, Shuster S, Ross WM: Prevalence of skin and other cancers in patients with psoriasis. *Clin Exp Dermatol* 18:401, 1993.
28. Bodmer WF, Cavalli-Sforza LL: Racial Differentiation, in *Genetics, Evolution, and Man*, Ch 19 San Francisco: W.H. Freeman, 1976, pp. 559–604.
29. Jackson IJ: Molecular and developmental genetics of mouse coat color. *Ann Rev Genet* 28:189, 1994.
30. Jackson IJ: Mouse coat colour mutations: a molecular genetic resource which spans the centuries. *BioEssays* 13:439, 1991.
31. Barsh GS: The genetics of pigmentation: from fancy genes to complex traits. *Trends Genet* 12:299, 1996.
32. Valverde P, Healy E, Jackson I, Rees JL, Thody AJ: Variants of the melanocyte-stimulating hormone receptor gene are associated with red hair and fair skin in humans. *Nat Genet* 11:328, 1995.
33. Kwa RE, Campana K, Moy RL: Biology of cutaneous squamous cell carcinoma. *J Am Acad Dermatol* 26:1, 1992.
34. Miller SJ: Biology of basal cell carcinoma(i). *J Am Acad Dermatol* 24:1, 1991.
35. Miller SJ: Biology of basal cell carcinoma (II). *J Am Acad Dermatol* 24:161, 1991.
36. Bouwes Bavinck JM, Vermeer BJ, Claas FHJ, Schegget JT, Van Der Woude FJ: Skin cancer and renal transplantation. *J Nephrol* 7:261, 1994.
37. Lang PJJ, Maize JC: Basal cell carcinoma, in Friedman RJ, Rigel DS, Kopf AW, Harris MN, Baker D (eds): *Cancer of the Skin*. Philadelphia, W.B. Saunders, 1991, pp. 35–73.
38. Mackie RM: Basal cell carcinoma, in *Skin Cancer*, 2nd ed, ch 7, London, Martin Dunitz, 1996, pp. 112–132.
39. Mackie RM: Epidermal skin tumors, in Champion RH, Burton JL, Ebling FJG (eds): *Textbook of Dermatology*. London, Blackwell Scientific, 1992, pp. 1505–1524.
40. Miller DL, Weinstock MA: Nonmelanoma skin cancer in the United States: Incidence. *J Am Acad Dermatol* 30:774, 1994.
41. Lo JS, Snow SN, Reizner GT, Mohs FE, Larson PO, Hruza GJ: Metastatic basal cell carcinoma: report of twelve cases with a review of the literature. *J Am Acad Dermatol* 24:(Pt 1):715, 1991.
42. Gorlin RJ, Goltz RW: Multiple nevoid basal-cell epithelioma, jaw cysts and BIFID rib. *N Engl J Med* 262:908–912, 1960.
43. Bale AE, Gailani MR, Leffell DJ: Nevoid basal cell carcinoma syndrome. *J Invest Dermatol* 103(Suppl.):126S, 1994.
44. Sharpe GR, Cox NH: Unilateral naevoid basal cell carcinoma syndrome: An individually controlled study of fibroblast sensitivity to radiation. *Clin Exp Dermatol* 15:352, 1990.
45. Farndon PA, Mastro RGD, Evans DGR, Kilpatrick MW: Location of gene for Gorlin syndrome. *Lancet* 339:581, 1992.
46. Gailani MR, Bale SJ, Leffel DJ, DiGiovanna JJ, Peck GL, Pollak S, Drum MA, Pastakia B, McBride OW, Kase R, Greene M, Mulvihill JJ, Bale AE: Developmental defects in Gorlin's syndrome related to a putative tumor suppressor gene on chromosome 9. *Cell* 111–117, 1992.
47. Reis A, Kuster W, Linss G, Gebel E, Hamm H, Fuhrmann W, Wolff G, Groth W, Gustafson G, Kuklik M, et al: Localisation of gene for the naevoid basal-cell carcinoma syndrome [letter]. *Lancet* 339:617, 1992.

48. Quinn AG, Sikkink S, Rees JL: Basal cell carcinomas and squamous cell carcinomas show distinct patterns of chromosome loss. *Cancer Res* 54:4756, 1994.

49. Bonifas JM, Bare JW, Kerschmann RL, Epstein EH: Parental origin of chromosome 9q22.3–q31 lost in basal cell carcinomas from basal cell nevus syndrome patients. *Hum Mol Genet* 3:447, 1994.

50. Hahn H, Wicking C, Zaphiropoulos PG, Gailani MR, Shanley S, Chidambaram A, Vorechovsky I, Holmberg E, Unden AB, Gillies S, Negus K, Smyth I, Pressman C, Leffell DJ, Gerrard B, Goldstein AM, Dean M, Toftgard R, Chenevix-Trench G, Wainwright B, Bale AE: Mutations of the human homolog of Drosophila *patched* in the nevoid basal cell carcinoma syndrome. *Cell* 85:841, 1996.

51. Hahn H, Christiansen J, Wicking C, Zaphiropoulos PG, Chidambaram A, Gerard B, Vorechovsky I, Bale AE, Toftgard R, Dean M, Wainwright B: A mammalian *patched* homolog is expressed in target tissues of *sonic hedgehog* and maps to a region associated with developmental abnormalities. *J Biol Chem* 271:12125, 1996.

52. Johnson RL, Rothman AL, Xie JW, Goodrich LV, Bare JW, Bonifas JM, Quinn AG, Myers RM, Cox DR, Epstein EH Jr, Scott MP: Human homolog of *patched*, a candidate gene for the basal cell nevus syndrome. *Science* 272:1668, 1996.

52a. Gailani MR, Stahle-Backdahl M, Leffell DJ, Glynn M, Zaphiropoulos PG, Pressman C, Unden AB, Dean M, Brash DE, Bale AE, Toftgard R: The role of the human homologue of *Drosophila patched* in sporadic basal cell carcinomas. *Nat Genet* 14:78, 1996.

53. Thiagalingam S, Lengauer C, Leach FS, Schutte M, Hahn SA, Overhauser J, Wilson JKV, Markowitz S, Hamilton SR, Kern SE, Kinzler KW, Vogelstein B: Evaluation of candidate tumor suppressor genes on chromosome 18 in colorectal cancers. *Nat Genet* 13:343, 1996.

54. Riggins GJ, Thiagalingam S, Rozenblum E, Weinstein CL, Kern SE, Hamilton SR, Wilson JKV, Markowitz SD, Kinzler KW, Vogelstein B: *Mad*-related genes in the human. *Nat Genet* 13:347, 1996.

55. Levanat S, Gorlin RJ, Fallet S, Johnson DR, Fantasia JE, Bale AE: A two-hit model for developmental defects in Gorlin syndrome. *Nat Genet* 12:85, 1996.

56. Bare JW, Lelbo RV, Epstein EH: Loss of heterozygosity at chromosome 1q22 in basal cell carcinomas and exclusion of the basal cell nevus syndrome gene from this site. *Cancer Res* 52:1494, 1992.

57. Ananthaswamy HN, Applegate LA, Goldberg LH, Bales ES: Deletion of the c-Ha-ras-1 allele in human skin cancers. *Mol Carcinogen* 2:298, 1989.

58. Newton JA, Camplejohn RS, McGibbon DH: A flow cytometric study of the significance of DNA aneuploidy in cutaneous lesions. *Br J Dermatol* 117:169, 1987.

59. Ziegler A, Leffell DJ, Kunala S, Sharma HW, Gailani M, Simon JA, Halperin AJ, Baden HP, Shapiro PE, Bale AE, et al: Mutation hotspots due to sunlight in the p53 gene of nonmelanoma skin cancers. *Proc Natl Acad Sci USA* 90:4216, 1993.

60. van der Riet P, Karp D, Farmer E, Wei Q, Grossman L, Tokino K, Ruppert JM, Sidransky D: Progression of basal cell carcinoma through loss of chromosome 9q and inactivation of a single p53 allele. *Cancer Res* 54:25, 1994.

61. Campbell C, Quinn AG, Angus B, Rees JL: The relation between p53 mutation and p53 immunostaining in nonmelanoma skin cancer. *Br J Dermatol* 129:235, 1993.

62. McGregor JM, Yu CC, Dublin EA, Levison DA, Macdonald DM: Aberrant expression of p53 tumor-suppressor protein in nonmelanoma skin cancer. *Br J Dermatol* 127:463, 1992.

63. McNutt NS, Saenz-Santamaria C, Volkenandt M, Shea CR, Albino AIP: Abnormalities of p53 protein expression in cutaneous disorders. *Arch Dermatol* 130:225, 1994.

64. Rees JL: p53 and the origins of skin cancer. *J Invest Dermatol* 104:883, 1995.

65. Rees JL: Genetic alterations in nonmelanoma skin cancer. *J Invest Dermatol* 103:747, 1994.

66. Ro YS, Cooper PN, Lee JA, Quinn AG, Harrison D, Lane D, Horne CH, Rees JL, Angus B: p53 protein expression in benign and malignant skin tumors. *Br J Dermatol* 128:237, 1993.

67. Hollstein M, Sidransky D, Vogelstein B, Harris CC: p53 mutations in human cancers. *Science* 253:49, 1991.

68. Soussi T: The p53 tumor suppressor gene: a model for molecular epidemiology of human cancer. *Molec Med Tod* 32, 1996.

69. Dumaz N, Stary A, Soussi T, Daya-Grosjean L, Sarasin A: Can we predict solar ultraviolet radiation as the causal event in human tumors by analysing the mutation spectra of the p53 gene? *Mutat Res* 307:375, 1994.

70. Moles JP, Moyret C, Guillot B, Jeanteur P, Guihou J, Theillet C, Basset-Seguin N: p53 gene mutations in human epithelial skin cancers. *Oncogene* 8:583, 1993.

71. Anathaswamy HN, Pierceall WE: Molecular alterations in human skin tumors, in Klein-Szanto AJP, Anderson MW, Barrett JC, Slaga TJ (eds): Comparative Molecular Carcinogenesis. Proceedings of the 5th International Conference on Carcinogenesis and Risk Assessment, held in Austin, Texas, November 22nd, 1991. New York: Wiley-Liss, 1992, pp. 61–84.

72. Urano Y, Asano T, Yoshimoto K, Iwahana H, Kubo Y, Kato S, Sasaki S, Takeuchi N, Uchida N, Nakanishi H, Arase S, Itakura M: Frequent p53 accumulation in the chronically sun-exposed epidermis and clonal expansion of p53 mutant cells in the epidermis adjacent to basal cell carcinoma. *J Invest Dermatol* 104:928, 1995.

73. Rady P, Scinicariello F, Wagner RF, Tyring SK: p53 mutations in basal cell carcinomas. *Cancer Res* 52:3804, 1992.

74. Gailani MR, Leffell DJ, Ziegler A, Gross EG, Brash DE, Bale AE: Relationship between sunlight exposure and a key genetic alteration in basal cell carcinoma. *J Natl Cancer Inst* 88:349, 1996.

75. Ziegler A, Leffell DJ, Kunala S, Sharma HW, Gailani M, Simon JA, Halperin AJ, Baden HP, Shapiro PE, Bale AE, et al: Mutation hotspots due to sunlight in the p53 gene of nonmelanoma skin cancers. *Proc Natl Acad Sci USA* 90:4216, 1993.

76. Burns PA, Bremner R, Balmain A: Genetic changes during mouse skin tumorigenesis. *Environ Health Perspect* 93:41, 1991.

77. Campbell C, Rees JL: The role of ras gene mutations in murine and human skin carcinogenesis. *Skin Cancer* 8:245, 1993.

78. Campbell C, Quinn AG, Rees JL: Codon 12 Harvey-ras mutations are rare events in nonmelanoma human skin cancer. *Br J Dermatol* 128:111, 1993.

79. Suarez HG, Daya-Grosjean L, Schlaifer D, Nardeux P, Renault G, Bos JL, Sarasin A: Activated oncogenes in human skin tumors from a repair-deficient syndrome, xeroderma pigmentosum. *Cancer Res* 49:1223, 1989.

80. Van der Schroeff J, Evers LM, Boot AJM, Bos JL: ras oncogene mutations in basal cell carcinomas and squamous cell carcinomas of human skin. *J Invest Dermatol* 94:423, 1990.

81. Pierceall WE, Goldberg LH, Tainsky MA, Mukhopadhyay T, Ananthaswamy HN: Ras gene mutation and amplification in human nonmelanoma skin cancers. *Mol Carcinogen* 4:196, 1991.

82. Spencer JM, Kakhn SM, Jiang W, DeLeo VA, Weinstein IB: Activated ras genes occur in human actinic keratoses, premalignant precursors to squamous cell carcinomas. *Arch Dermatol* 131:796, 1995.

83. Kubo Y, Urano Y, Yoshimoto K, Iwahana H, Fukuhara K, Arase S, Itakura M: p53 gene mutations in human skin cancers and precancerous lesions: comparison with immunohistochemical analysis. *J Invest Dermatol* 130:440, 1994.

84. Friedman E, Gejman PV, Martin GA, McCormick F: Nonsense mutations in the C-terminal SH2 region of the GTPase activating protein (GAP) gene in human tumors. *Nat Genet* 5:242, 1993.

85. Takata M, Quinn AG, Hashimoto K, Rees JL: Low frequency of loss of heterozygosity at the nevoid basal cell carcinoma locus and other selected loci in appendageal tumors. *J Invest Dermatol* 106:1141, 1996.

86. Bazex A, Dupre A, Christol B: Atrophodermaie folliculaire, proliferations basocellulaires et hypothichose. *Ann Derm Syphiol* 93:241, 1966.

87. Viksnins P, Berlin A: Follicular atrophoderma and basal cell carcinomas: The Bazex syndrome. *Arch Dermatol* 113:948, 1977.

88. Goeteyn M, Geerts ML, Kint A, De Weert J. The Bazex-Dupre-Christol Syndrome. *Arch Dermatol* 130:337, 1994.

89. Kidd A, Carson L, Gregory DW, De Silva D, Holmes J, Dean JCS, Haites N: A Scottish family with Bazex-Dupre-Christol syndrome: Follicular atrophoderma, congenital hypotrichosis, and basal cell carcinoma. *J Med Genet* 33:493, 1996.

90. Vabres P, Lacombe D, Rabinowitz LG, Aubert G, Anderson CE, Taieb A, Bonafe JL, Hors-Cayla MC: The gene for Bazex-Dupre-Christol syndrome maps to chromosome Xq. *J Invest Dermatol* 105:87, 1995.

91. Michaelsson G, Olsson E, Westermark P: The Rombo syndrome: a familial disorder with vermiculate atrophoderma, milia, hypotrichosis, trichoepitheliomas, basal cell carcinomas and peripheral vasodilation with cyanosis. *Acta Dermato-Venereologica* 61:497, 1981.

92. Mackie, RM: Squamous cell carcinoma, in *Skin Cancer*, 2nd ed, ch 8. London, Martin Dunitz, 1996, pp. 133–156.

93. Rowe DE, Carroll RJ, Day CL: Prognostic factors for local recurrence, metastasis, and survival rates in squamous cell carcinoma of the skin, ear, and lip. *J Am Acad Dermatol* **26**:976, 1992.

94. Lund HZ: How often does squamous cell carcinoma of the skin metastasize. *Arch Dermatol* **92**:635, 1965.

95. Moller R, Reymann F, Hou-Jensen K: Metastases in dermatological patients with squamous cell carcinoma. *Arch Dermatol* **115**:703, 1979.

96. Callen JP: Possible precursors to epidermal malignancies, in Friedman RJ, Rigel DS, Kopf AW, Harris MN, Baker D (eds): *Cancer of the Skin*. Philadelphia, W.B. Saunders, 1991, pp. 27–34.

97. Sober AJ, Burstein JM: Precursors to skin cancer. *Cancer* **75**Suppl:645, 1995.

98. Marks R, Rennie G, Selwood TS: Malignant transformation of solar keratoses to squamous cell carcinoma. *Lancet* **i**:795, 1988.

99. Marks R, Foley P, Goodman G, Hage BH, Selwood TS: Spontaneous remission of solar keratoses: the case for conservative management. *Br J Dermatol* **115**:649, 1986.

100. Frentz G, Moller U: Clonal heterogeneity in curetted human epidermal cancers and precancers analysed by flow cytometry and compared with histology. *Br J Dermatol* **109**:173, 1983.

101. Chi H, Kawachi Y, Otsuka F: Xeroderma pigmentosum variant: DNA ploidy analysis of various skin tumors and normal-appearing skin in a patient. *Int J Dermatol* **33**:775, 1994.

102. Herzberg AJ, Kerns BJ, Pollack V, Kinney RB: DNA image cytometry of keratoacanthoma and squamous cell carcinoma. *J Invest Dermatol* **97**:495, 1991.

103. Sktephenson TJ, Cotton DW: Flow cytometric comparison of keratoacanthoma and squamous cell carcinoma [letter]. *Br J Dermatol* **118**:582, 1988.

104. Nawroz H, van der Riet P, Hruban RH, Koch W, Ruppert JM, Sidransky D: Allelotype of head and neck squamous cell carcinoma. *Cancer Res* **54**:1152, 1994.

105. Ah-See KW, Cooke TG, Pickford IR, Soutar D, Balmain A: An allelotype of squamous carcinoma of the head and neck using microsatellite markers. *Cancer Res* **54**:1617, 1994.

106. Quinn AG, Sikkink S, Rees JL: Delineation of two distinct deleted regions on chromosome 9 in human nonmelanoma skin cancers. *Genes Chrom Cancer* **11**:222, 1994.

107. Waring AJ, Takata M, Rehman I, Rees JL: Loss of heterozygosity analysis of keratoacanthoma reveals multiple differences from cutaneous squamous cell carcinoma. *Br J Cancer* **73**:649, 1996.

108. Roz L, Wu CL, Porter S, Scully C, Speight P, Read A, Sloan P, Thakker N: Allelic imbalance on chromosome 3p in oral dysplastic lesions: An early event in oral carcinogenesis. *Cancer Res* **56**:1228, 1996.

109. Ohta M, Inoue H, Cotticelli MG, Kastury K, Baffa R, Palazzo J, Siprashvili Z, Mori M, McCue P, Druck T, Croce CM, Huebner K: The *FHIT* gene, spanning the chromosome 3p14.2 fragile site acid renal carcinoma-associated t(3;8) breakpoint, is abnormal in digestive tract cancers. *Cell* **84**:587, 1996.

110. Quinn AG, Campbell C, Healy E, Rees JL: Chromosome 9 allele loss occurs in both basal and squamous cell carcinomas of the skin. *J Invest Dermatol* **102**:300, 1994.

111. Puig S, Ruiz A, L·zaro C, Castel T, Lynch M, Palou J, Vilalta A, Weissenbach J, Mascaro J-M, Estiville X: Chromosome 9p deletions in cutaneous malignant melanoma tumors: The minimal deleted region involves markers outside the *p16 (CDKN2)* gene. *Am J Hum Genet* **57**:395, 1995.

112. Sato M, Nishigori C, Zghal M, Yagi T, Takebe H: Ultraviolet-specific mutations in p53 gene in skin tumors in xeroderma pigmentosum patients. *Cancer Res* **53**:2944, 1993.

113. Dumaz N, Drougard C, Sarasin A, Daya-Grossjean L: Specific UV-induced mutation spectrum in the p53 gene of skin tumors from DNA-repair-deficient xeroderma pigmentosa patients. *Proc Natl Acad Sci* **90**:10529, 1993.

114. Matsumura Y, Sato M, Nishigori C, Zghal M, Yagi T, Imamura S, Takebe H: High prevalence of mutations in the p53 gene in poorly differentiated squamous cell carcinomas in xeroderma pigmentosum patients. *J Invest Dermatol* **105**:399, 1995.

115. Pierceall WE, Mukhopadhyay T, Goldberg LH, Ananthaswamy HN: Mutations in the p53 tumor suppressor gene in human cutaneous squamous cell carcinomas. *Mol Carcinogen* **4**:445, 1991.

116. Campbell C, Quinn AG, Ro YS, Angus B, Rees JL: p53 mutations are common and early events that precede tumor invasion in squamous cell neoplasia of the skin. *J Invest Dermatol* **100**:746, 1993.

117. Taguchi M, Watanabe S, Yashima K, Murakami Y, Sekiya T, Ikeda S: Aberrations of the tumor suppressor p53 gene and p53 protein in solar keratosis in human skin. *J Invest Dermatol* **103**:500, 1994.

118. Ziegler A, Jonason AS, Leffell DJ, Simon JA, Sharma HW, Kimmelman J, Remington L, Jacks T, Brash DE: Sunburn and p53 in the onset of skin cancer. *Nature* **372**:773, 1994.

119. Campbell C, Quinn AG, Angus B, Farr PM, Rees JL: Wavelength specific patterns of p53 induction in human skin following exposure to UV radiation. *Cancer Res* **53**:2697, 1993.

120. Hall PA, McKee PH, Menage HD, Dover R, Lane DP: High levels of p53 protein in UV-irradiated normal human skin. *Oncogene* **8**:203–207, 1993.

121. Healy E, Reynolds NJ, Smith M, Campbell C, Farr PM, Rees JL: Dissociation between erythema and p53 expression in human skin: Effects of UVB irradiation and skin irritants. *J Invest Dermatol* **103**:493–499, 1994.

122. Young AR: The sunburn cell. *Photodermatology* **4**:127–134, 1987.

123. Li G, Mitchell DL, Ho VC, Reed JC, Tron VA: Deceased DNA repair but normal apoptosis in ultraviolet-irradiated skin of p53-transgenic mice. *Am J Pathol* **148**:1113–1123, 1996.

124. Nakazawa H, English D, Randell PL, Nakazawa K, Martel N, Armstrong BK, Yamasaki H: UV skin cancer: Specific p53 gene mutation in normal skin as a biologically relevant exposure measurement. *Proc Natl Acad Sci USA* **91**:360, 1994.

125. Marks R: Premalignant disease of the epidermis The Parkes Weber lecture 1985. *J Roy Col Phys London* **20**:116, 1986.

126. Harvey I, Shalom D, Marks RM, Frankel SJ: Nonmelanoma skin cancer. *BMJ* **299**:1118, 1989.

127. Daya-Grosjean L, Robert C, Drougard C, Suarez H, Sarasin A: High mutation frequency in ras genes of skin tumors isolated from DNA repair deficient xeroderma pigmentosum patients. *Cancer Res* **53**:1625, 1993.

128. Ishizaki K, Tsujimura T, Nakai M, Nishigori C, Sato K, Katayama S, Kurimura O, Yoshikawa K, Imamura S, Ikenaga M: Infrequent mutation of the *ras* genes in skin tumors of xeroderma pigmentosum patients in Japan. *Int J Cancer* **50**:382, 1992.

129. Straka BF, Grant-Kels JM: Keratoacanthoma, in Friedman RJ, Rigel DS, Kopf AW, Harris MN, Baker D (eds): *Cancer of the Skin*. Philadelphia, W.B. Saunders, 1991, pp. 390–407.

130. Schwartz RA: Keratoacanthoma. *J Am Acad Dermatol* **30**:1, 1994.

131. Mackie, RM: Cancer-associated genodermatoses, in *Skin Cancer*, 2nd ed, ch 4. London: Martin Dunitz, 1996, pp. 30–51.

132. Patel A, Halliday GM, Cooke BE, Barneston RS: Evidence that regression in keratoacanthoma is immunologically mediated: a comparison with squamous cell carcinoma. *Br J Dermatol* **131**:789, 1994.

133. Kerschmann RL, McCalmont TH, LeBoit PE: p53 oncoprotein expression and proliferation index in keratoacanthoma and squamous cell carcinoma. *Arch Dermatol* **130**:181, 1994.

134. Lee Y-S, Teh M: p53 expression in pseudoepitheliomatous hyperplasia, keratoacanthoma, and squamous cell carcinoma of skin. *Cancer* **73**:2317, 1994.

135. Stephenson TJ, Royds J, Silcocks PB, Bleehen SS: Mutant p53 oncogene expression in keratoacanthoma and squamous cell carcinoma. *Br J Dermatol* **127**:566, 1992.

136. Corominas M, Leon J, Kamino H, Cruz-Alverez M, Novick SC, Pellicer A: Oncogene involvement in tumor regression: H-ras activation in the rabbit keratoacanthoma model. *Oncogene* **4**:645, 1991.

137. Corominas M, Kamino H, Leon J, Pellicer A: Oncogene activation in human benign tumors of the skin (keratoacanthomas): is H-ras involved in differentiation as well as proliferation? *Proc Natl Acad Sci USA* **86**:6372, 1989.

138. Ferguson-Smith J: Multiple primary, self-healing epitheliomata of the skin. *Br J Dermatol* **60**:315, 1948.

139. Ferguson-Smith MA, Wallace DC, James ZH, Renwick JH: Multiple self-healing squamous epithelioma. *Birth Defects: Original Article Series* **7**:157, 1971.

140. Rook A, Moffatt JL: Multiple self-healing epitheliomata of Ferguson Smith type. Report of a case of ulilateral distribution. *Arch Dermatol* **525**, 1956.

141. Goudie DR, Yuille MAR, Leversha MA, Furlong RA, Carter NP, Lush MJ, Affara NA, Ferguson-Smith MA: Multiple self healing squamous epitheliomata (ESS1) mapped to chromosome 9q22–q31 in families with common ancestry. *Nat Genet* **3**:165, 1993.

142. Lynch HT, Fusaro RM, Roberts L, Voorhees GJ, Lynch JF: Muir-Torre syndrome in several members of a family with a variant of the cancer family syndrome. *Br J Dermatol* **113**:295, 1985.

143. Papadopoulos N, Nicolaides NC, Wei Y, Ruben SM, Carter KC, Rosen CA, Haseltine WA, Fleischmann RD, Fraser CM, Adams MD, Venter JC, Hamilton SR, Petersen GM, Watson P, Lynch HT, Peltomaki P, Mecklin J, de la Chapelle A, Kinzler KW, Vogelstein B: Mutation of a *mutL* homolog in hereditary colon cancer. *Science* **263**:1625, 1994.

144. Nyström-Lahti M, Parsons R, Sistonen P, Pylkkänen L, Aaltonen LA, Leach FS, Hamilton SR, Watson P, Bronson E, Fusaro R, Cavalieri J, Lynch J, Lanspa S, Smyrk T, Lynch P, Drouhard T, Kinzler KW, Vogelstein B, Lynch HT, de la Chapelle A, Peltomäki P: Mismatch repair genes on chromosomes 2p and 3p account for a major share of hereditary nonpolyposis colorectal cancer families evaluable by linkage. *Am J Hum Genet* **55**:659, 1994.

145. Schwartz RA, Torre DP: The Muir-Torre syndrome: A 25-year retrospect. *J Am Acad Dermatol* **33**:90, 1995.

146. Hall NR, Murday VA, Chapman P, Williams MA, Burn J, Finan PJ, Bishop DT: Genetic linkage in Muir-Torre syndrome to the same chromosomal region as cancer family syndrome. *Eur J Cancer* **30A**:180, 1994.

147. Honchel R, Halling KC, Schaid DJ, Pittelkow M, Thibodeau SN: Microsatellite instability in Muir-Torre syndrome. *Cancer Res* **54**:1159, 1994.

148. Quinn AG, Healy E, Rehman I, Sikkink S, Rees JL: Microsatellite instability in human nonmelanoma and melanoma skin cancer. *J Invest Dermatol* **104**:309, 1995.

149. Jablonska S: Epidermodysplasia verruciformis, in Friedman RJ, Rigel DS, Kopf AW, Harris MN, Baker D (eds): *Cancer of the Skin*. Philadelphia, W.B. Saunders, 1991, pp. 101–116.

150. Majewski S, Jablonska S: Epidermodysplasia verruciformis as a model of human papillomavirus-induced genetic cancer of the skin. *Arch Dermatol* **131**:1312, 1995.

151. Connor JM, Teague RH: Dyskeratosis congenita: Report of a large kindred. *Br J Dermatol* **105**:321, 1981.

152. Davidson HR, Connor JM: Dyskeratosis congenita. *J Med Genet* **25**:843, 1988.

153. Arngrimsson R, Dokal I, Luzzatto L, Connor JM: Dyskeratosis congenita: three additional families show linkage to a locus in Xq28. *J Med Genet* **30**:618, 1993.

154. Hashimoto K: Adnexal carcinomas of the skin, in Friedman RJ, Rigel DS, Kopf AW, Harris MN, Baker D (eds): *Cancer of the Skin*. Philadelphia, W.B. Saunders, 1991, pp. 209–218.

155. Mackie RM: Skin appendage tumors, in *Skin Cancer*, 2nd ed, ch 12. London, Martin Dunitz, 1996, pp. 242–277.

156. Nelen MR, Padberg GW, Peeters EAJ, Lin AY, Van den Helm B, Frants RR, Coulon V, Goldstein AM, Van Reen MMM, Easton DF, Eeles RA, Hodgson S, Mulvihill JJ, Murday VA, Tucker MA, Mariman ECM, Starink TM, Ponder BAJ, Ropers HH, Kremer H, Longy M, Eng C: Localization of the gene for Cowden disease to chromosome `10q22–23. *Nat Genet* **13**:114, 1996.

157. Harada H, Hashimoto K, Ko MSH: The gene for multiple familial trichoepithelioma maps to chromosome 9p21. *J Invest Dermatol* **107**:41, 1996.

158. Biggs PJ, Wooster R, Ford D, Chapman P, Mangion J, Quirk Y, Easton DF, Burn J, Stratton MR: Familial cylindromatosis (turban tumor syndrome) gene localised to chromosome 16q12–q13: Evidence for its role as a tumor suppressor gene. *Nat Genet* **11**:441, 1995.

159. Halder RM, Bridgeman-Shah S: Skin cancer in African Americans. *Cancer* **75**(Suppl):667, 1995.

160. Chuang TY, Reizner GT, Elpern DJ, Stone JL, Farmer ER: Nonmelanoma skin cancer in Japanese ethnic. Hawaiians in Kauai, Hawaii: An incidence report. *J Am Acad Dermatol* **33**:422, 1995.

161. Spritz RA: Molecular genetics of oculocutaneous albinism. *Hum Mol Genet* **3**:Spec No: 1469, 1994.

162. Hill HZ: The function of melanin or six blind people examine an elephant. *Bio Essays* **14**(1):49, 1992.

163. Thody AJ: Skin pigmentation and its regulation, in Priestly GC (ed): *Molecular Aspects of Dermatology*, John Wiley and Sons, 1993, pp. 55–73.

164. Valverde P, Healy E, Sikkink S, Haldane F, Thody AJ, Carrothers A, Jackson IJ, Rees JL: The AspGlu variant of the melanocortin 1 receptor (*MCIR*) is associated with melanoma. *Hum Mol Genet* **5**:1663, 1996.

165. Streilein JW, Taylor JR, Vincek V, Kurimoto I. Shimizu T, Tie C, Golomb C: Immune surveillance and sunlight-induced skin cancer. *Immunol Today* **15**:174, 1994.

166. de Berker D, Ibbotson S, Simpson NB, Matthew JNS, Idle JR, Rees JL: Reduced experimental contact sensitivity in squamous cell but not basal cell carcinomas of the skin. *Lancet* **345**:425, 1995.

167. Heagerty AH, Fitzgerald D, Smith A, Bowers B, Jones P, Fryer AA, Zhao L, Alldersea J, Strange RC: Glutathione S-transferase GSTM1 phenotypes and protection against cutaneous tumors. *Lancet* **343**:266, 1994.

168. Bouwes Bavinck JN, Claas FHJ: The role of HLA molecules in the development of skin cancer. *Hum Immunol* **41**:173, 1994.

169. Czarnecki D, Tait B, Nicholson I. Lewis A: Multiple Nonmelanoma skin cancer: Evidence that different MHC genes are associated with different cancers. *Dermatology* **188**:88, 1994.

170. Streilein JW, Taylor JR, Vincek V, Kurimoto I, Richardson J, Tie C, Medema J-P, Golomb C: Relationship between ultraviolet radiation-induced immunosuppression and carcinogenesis. *J Invest Dermatol* **103**(Suppl):107S, 1994.

171. Wei Q, Matanoski GM, Farmer ER, Hedayati MA, Grossman L: DNA repair and aging in basal cell carcinoma: a molecular epidemiology study. *Proc Natl Acad Sci USA* **90**:1614, 1993.

172. Wei Q, Matanoski GM, Farmer ER, Hedayati MA, Grossman L: DNA repair and susceptibility to basal cell carcinoma: A case-control study. *Am J Epidemiol* **140**:598, 1994.

173. Hall J, English DR, Artuso M, Armstrong BK, Winter M: DNA repair capacity as a risk factor for non-melanocytic skin cancer—a molecular epidemiological study. *Int J Cancer* **58**:179, 1994.

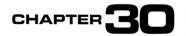

CHAPTER 30

Breast Cancer

Fergus J. Couch ▪ Barbara L. Weber

1. Breast cancer is the most frequently diagnosed cancer in western women and the leading cause of death in U.S. women age 40 to 55. Breast cancer is heterogeneous in its clinical, genetic, and biochemical profile. The large majority of affected women present with a breast mass or mammographic abnormality as the only clinically detectable manifestation of disease, yet approximately 30 percent of women diagnosed with breast cancer go on to develop metastatic disease which is ultimately fatal.

2. Numerous risk factors for the development of breast cancer have been identified. Family history, suggesting an inherited component in the development of some breast cancers, is one of the strongest known risk factors. It is estimated that 15 to 20 percent of women with breast cancer have a family history of the disease, with approximately 5 percent of all breast cancers attributable to dominant susceptibility alleles. Two major breast cancer susceptibility genes (*BRCA1* and *BRCA2*) have been identified; others are being actively sought.

3. Breast cancer may present in a preinvasive form or an invasive form. Treatment depends on the stage at diagnosis, patient age at the time of diagnosis, and the presence or absence of the estrogen receptor in tumor cells. The prognosis is largely dependent on the stage at diagnosis.

4. *BRCA1* is a highly penetrant breast cancer susceptibility gene on chromosome 17q21 that is thought to account for 40 to 50 percent of inherited breast cancers. Families with germ-line mutations in *BRCA1* have an autosomal dominant inheritance pattern of breast cancer as well as an increase incidence of ovarian cancer. The mutation spectrum of *BRCA1* is well defined, and links to cell cycle control and development are becoming evident.

5. *BRCA2* is a highly penetrant breast cancer susceptibility gene on chromosome 13q12-13 that is thought to account for 30 to 40 percent of inherited breast cancers. Families with germ-line mutations in *BRCA2* also have an autosomal dominant inheritance pattern of breast cancer, an increased incidence of ovarian cancer that is less striking that that with BRCA1, and an increased incidence of male breast cancer cases. The mutation spectrum of *BRCA2* is still being defined, and no progress has been made on elucidating *BRCA2* function.

6. Sporadic breast cancers have been studied extensively for molecular changes that may provide clues to etiology, prognosis, and improved treatment approaches. Growth factors and their receptors, intracellular signaling molecules, regulators of cell cycling, adhesion molecules, and proteases have all been shown to be altered in sporadic breast cancer.

INTRODUCTION

Breast cancer is among the most common human cancers, representing 32 percent of all incident cancers in the United States. Currently, more than 180,000 women in the United States and almost 1 million women worldwide are diagnosed with breast cancer every year.[1] Because of the magnitude of the public health problem, the desire to reduce the impact of this disease on American women, and the suitability of breast cancer as a model for the study of the molecular basis of cancer, an increasing number of investigators have focused on this disease in recent years. As a result, tremendous strides have been made in identifying susceptibility genes for breast cancer, defining regions of the human genome that harbor unidentified breast cancer-related genes, and characterizing a number of genes that are somatically altered in sporadic breast cancers. In turn, advances in these areas provide the reagents necessary to translate scientific discoveries into clinical practice as a means of improving the detection, treatment, and ultimately prevention of breast cancer. In an effort to catalogue this large body of knowledge, this chapter provides (1) an overview of the clinical aspects of breast cancer, (2) a detailed description of the two recently isolated breast cancer susceptibility genes, *BRCA1* and *BRCA2*, (3) information on genes which contribute to less common inherited breast cancer syndromes, (4) a summary of the genomic regions thought to harbor unidentified breast cancer-related genes, (5) a synopsis of genes that have been implicated in the development and progression of sporadic breast cancer, and (6) a review of the clinical uses of these genes for predisposition testing, disease detection, prognostication, and therapy selection.

CLINICAL ASPECTS OF BREAST CANCER

Incidence and Mortality

Breast cancer is the leading cause of death for American women between ages 50 and 55.[2] The most recent data suggest that 12 percent of all American women (one in eight) will be diagnosed with breast cancer, and approximately 30 percent of the women diagnosed with breast cancer will die of the disease. Overall there are more than 50,000 deaths from breast cancer every year in the United States alone. Adding to concern is the fact that breast cancer incidence in the United States has been rising steadily since 1930, with an average increase of 1.2 percent per year, as reported by the Connecticut Tumor Registry.[3] The incidence in all ages groups has increased, with the greatest increase occurring in older women.[4] Many investigators have attempted to explain these data, and while it appears that the advent of screening mammography and the aging of the population play a role in the increasing incidence of breast cancer, the increase reflects a real trend, suggesting that environmental or lifestyle changes may be effecting an increase in the number of breast cancers that develop. However, it is important to evaluate the age-adjusted risk for breast cancer, as breast cancer risk rises steeply with age. Data from the National Cancer Institute Surveillance Program indicate that a 35-year-old woman has a risk of 1 in 2500, a 50-year-old woman has a risk of 1 in 50, and it is not until age 85 that risk reaches 1 in 8. Interestingly, while incidence rates have been steadily increasing, mortality rates have remained relatively constant[5] (Fig. 30-1). This constancy in the face of increasing incidence may be explained by better reporting, increases in less aggressive forms of the disease, improved detection strategies, and/or improvements in treatment.

Risk Factors

The search for breast cancer risk factors is based on a desire to explain the rising incidence of breast cancer and an obvious interest in identifying modifiable lifestyle or environmental factors that will reduce the likelihood of developing breast cancer in individual women. The best studied and most significant risk factor is a family history of breast cancer. While shared exposure to another risk factor cannot be excluded, this most commonly represents heritable factors that increase the likelihood of developing breast cancer. The breast cancer susceptibility genes *BRCA1* and *BRCA2* represent the most dramatic examples, but as they probably account for only 15 to 20 percent of the breast cancer that clusters in families,[6] it is clear that other, less penetrant, but more common heritable factors remain to be identified. Relative risk for breast cancer with respect to family history ranges from 1.4 for a woman whose mother was diagnosed with breast cancer after age 60[7,8] to 150 for a 40-year-old woman with an inherited *BRCA1* alteration.[9] Weaker risk factors for breast cancer include early age at menarche (relative risk, 1.2),[10] nulliparity (relative risk, 2.0),[11] and late age at menopause (relative risk, 2.0).[12] Pike and colleagues postulated

that these factors all reflect an increased number of menstrual cycles compared to multiparous women and that this is the underlying risk factor; work on this hypothesis is ongoing.[13] Additionally, terminal differentiation of breast epithelial cells does not occur until the onset of lactation after the completion of a full-term pregnancy. This final stage of differentiation also may confer increased resistance to carcinogens. Radiation exposure is clearly a risk factor, with significant increases in breast cancer observed among atomic bomb survivors (maximum relative risk, 13)[14,15] and in women who received mantle radiation for Hodgkin disease as children (incidence ratio, 75.3).[16] Additional factors that have appeared as risk factors in some but not all studies include bottle feeding as opposed to breast-feeding, alcohol intake greater than two drinks per day, a high-fat diet, prolonged oral contraceptive use, and estrogen replacement therapy.[17,18] Risk factor data are summarized in Table 30-1.

Histology of Breast Cancer

Breast carcinoma arises from the epithelium of the mammary gland, which includes the milk-producing lobules and the ducts that carry milk to the nipple (Fig. 30-2). Malignant transformation of the stromal, vascular, or fatty components of the breast is not included in this definition and is extremely rare. These facts may largely explain why breast size is not a risk factor for breast cancer, as all women have a similar amount of breast epithelium while breast size is determined largely by the amount of stromal and fatty tissue. The transition from normal to malignant breast epithelium has not been as well studied as the parallel changes in colonic epithelium; however, there is increasing evidence the breast epithelium undergoes a transformation from normal to hyperplastic, followed by the appearance of atypia in association with the hyperplasia, ultimately becoming malignant. Malignant cells continue to evolve from noninvasive carcinoma, typified by ductal carcinoma in situ (DCIS), to invasive carcinoma and ultimately to cells with metastatic potential.

Lobular Carcinoma in Situ. Lending confusion to the progression from normal to malignant epithelium is the entity of lobular carcinoma in situ (LCIS), which is not a preinvasive lesion but appears to be a marker of increased risk for the development of invasive cancer. LCIS was not identified as a clinical entity until 1941 and was originally believed to be the precursor lesion of invasive lobular carcinoma. Since its original description, LCIS has been recognized as a purely histologic diagnosis. Clinical diagnosis is

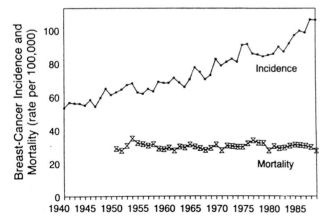

FIG. 30-1 Breast cancer incidence and mortality trends. Incidence of breast cancer in the United States from 1940 to 1985 is indicated by closed circles. Mortality rates, indicated by Xs, have remained fairly constant despite the rising incidence.[5]

Table 30-1 Risk Factors for Breast Cancer

Risk Factor	Risk Category	Relative Risk	Reference
Family history	Mother >60	1.4	7
	Two first-degree relatives	4–6	8
BRCA1/BRCA2 mutation	Carrier	150 (at age 40)	9
Age at menarche	<14	1.3	10
Age at menopause	>55	1.5	12
Parity	No full-term birth	1.9	11
Benign breast disease	Atypical hyperplasia	4.0	18
Radiation	Atomic bomb survivors	13	14,15
	Mantle radiation for Hodgkin disease	75	16

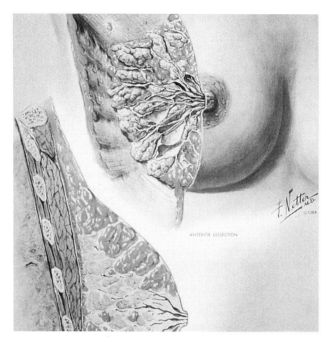

FIG. 30-2 Normal breast architecture. The breast is shown partially dissected from an anterior view (above) and in a sagittal section. Mammary ducts are seen radiating out from the nipple and terminating in milk-producing lobules. Fat and stoma surround and interdigitate with the ductal and lobular structure.[28]

not possible, as LCIS does not form a palpable lesion and therefore cannot be identified on physical examination and is not visible on mammography. Thus, the diagnosis of LCIS always is made as an incidental finding on a breast biopsy obtained for diagnosis of an adjacent lesion. In addition, the incidence of LCIS in the general population is unknown because the nature of the diagnosis precludes studies based on mammographic screening. Evidence that LCIS is a marker lesion and not a true malignant lesion comes from studies demonstrating that it is frequently multicentric and/or bilateral and that the invasive cancer that may develop subsequently is likely to occur distant from the known focus of LCIS and is more often of ductal than lobular histology.[19]

The risk of invasive breast cancer after a diagnosis of LCIS has been the subject of many studies; the series with the longest follow-up was reported by Rosen and colleagues at the Memorial Sloan-Kettering Cancer Institute.[20] In this cohort, followed for a mean of 24 years, 37 percent of the women with LCIS who were not lost to follow-up developed invasive breast cancer; more than half these women developed an invasive lesion at least 15 years after the initial diagnosis of LCIS. When the data were analyzed with the assumption that all the women lost to follow-up remained cancer-free, the percentage of patients developing invasive disease dropped to 31 percent.[20] Because of the substantial risk of invasive carcinoma and the inability to predict where it will occur in the breasts of a women with LCIS, the treatment of LCIS presents a conundrum. Currently patients are offered a choice between frequent mammographic surveillance and bilateral mastectomies. This widely discrepant choice obviously is a difficult one and seems particularly harsh considering the emphasis on breast conservation for the treatment of invasive disease.

Although there has been considerable speculation that LCIS represents a histologic marker of genetic predisposition to breast cancer, recent work suggests that this may not be not the case. In a study of 436 women with familial breast cancer and an equal number of age-matched controls selected randomly from a general hospital, Lakhani and colleagues provided evidence that LCIS was underrepresented in the familial cohort, including the subset of known *BRCA1* and *BRCA2* mutation carriers, compared to the

controls (3 percent versus 6 percent, $p = 0.013$).[21] Data suggest that women with LCIS and a family history of breast cancer may be more likely to develop invasive cancer than are those with LCIS alone[22]: however, no study comparing invasive cancer risk in women with a family history with and without LCIS has been reported. Thus, the question of whether family history and LCIS represent compounding risk factors remains unanswered.

Ductal Carcinoma in Situ. Unlike LCIS, DCIS is considered a true precursor lesion of invasive ductal carcinoma (Fig. 30-3). Historically, patients presented with a palpable breast mass, a nipple discharge, or both. Before the use of mammography, pure DCIS lesions without an invasive component were uncommon, constituting only 1 to 5 percent of all breast cancer cases.[23] Patients were treated with total mastectomy. However, after the widespread dissemination of screening mammography, the clinical picture of DCIS changed radically, with 50 to 60 percent of DCIS being diagnosed solely as a mammographic abnormality and pure DCIS representing more than 30 percent of breast cancers diagnoses by screening mammography.[24] The most common mammographic manifestation of DCIS is clustered microcalcifications.

Information on the risk of progression from DCIS to invasive cancer is limited because until recently patients were treated with total mastectomy. While this is essentially 100 percent effective in preventing disease progression and death, the natural history of the lesion was obscured by the procedure. Estimates from small series of patients inadvertently treated with biopsy alone suggest that 30 to 50 percent of DCIS lesions evolve into invasive cancer within 6 to 10 years of diagnosis.[25,26] In nearly all these patients, the invasive cancer occurred at or near the original biopsy site and was of ductal histology.

As was noted above, historically, treatment of DCIS consisted of mastectomy, and in women with multifocal lesions this is still the treatment of choice. However, when the lesion is localized, recent data suggest that lumpectomy followed by radiation does not compromise survival, allowing breast conservation for women who choose this approach.[27] A large, randomized clinical trial designed to confirm this observation and validate this treatment is being conducted by the National Surgical Adjuvant Breast and Bowel Project (NSABP).

It is clear that DCIS alone or in association with an invasive lesion may be found in women with breast cancer caused by germline mutations in the breast cancer susceptibility gene *BRCA1* or *BRCA2*. However, recent data suggest that the frequency of DCIS may be lower in inherited breast cancers than in age-matched unselected controls.[21] The biologic meaning of this finding is unclear

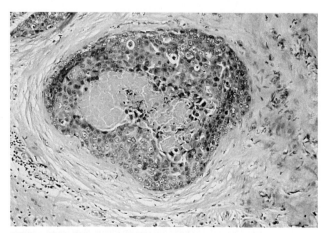

FIG. 30-3 Ductal carcinoma in situ. A focus of comedo-type DCIS is shown stained with hematoxylin-eosin. The malignant cells are wholly contained within the duct and do not invade the surrounding stroma. The central region is filled with necrotic cellular debris.

but could reflect an early transition from noninvasive to invasive breast cancer and/or an invasive tumor with a rapid growth rate. This would result in a lesion where the noninvasive component might be too small be clinically recognizable or where the ratio of invasive to noninvasive cancer in a given lesion makes the detection of the noninvasive component difficult.

Invasive Breast Cancer. Invasive breast cancer may be ductal or lobular in histologic type, and while there are a few distinguishing clinical features, the natural history and treatment of the two lesions are virtually identical. About 80 percent of invasive breast cancers are ductal carcinomas. Infiltrating lobular carcinoma is less common, representing only 5 to 10 percent of breast cancers. The remainder of invasive breast cancer consists of a variety of "special types," including tubular cancer, characterized by prominent tubule

formation; medullary carcinoma, a lesion that appears poorly differentiated under the microscope but is thought to have a more favorable prognosis than other breast cancers[29]; and mucinous (or colloid) carcinoma, characterized by the abundant accumulation of extracellular mucin, bulky tumors, and a good prognosis.[17] Of particular note, approximately 15 percent of invasive carcinomas are not detectable mammographically, particularly invasive lobular carcinomas. The clinical implication of this false negative rate is that mammography alone is not sufficient for the evaluation of a breast mass. In the presence of a palpable breast mass, a negative mammogram should be followed by ultrasound and/or biopsy. A cystic lesion on ultrasound may be presumed benign and aspirated or followed. A solid or complex lesion should be subjected to excisional biopsy. The mammographic and histopathologic appearance of invasive breast cancer is illustrated in Fig. 30-4.

A

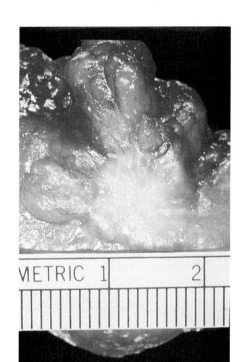

B

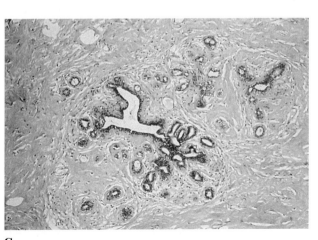

C

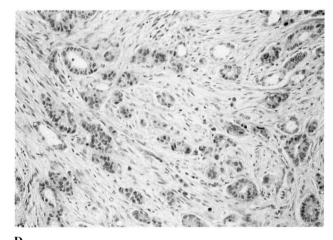

D

FIG. 30-4 Invasive breast cancer. *A.* Mammogram showing a spiculated mass with poorly defined borders that is characteristic of an invasive breast cancer. *B.* Invasive ductal carcinoma gross pathology. An unfixed biopsy specimen illustrates the gross pathologic correlates of the mammogram. The hard, white invasive cancer extends into the breast in all directions, with no defined border and numerous stellate extensions.

C. Normal breast histopathology. The ducts are shown cut in cross section, lined with a single layer of ductal epithelium. The surrounding stroma stains pink in this preparation (hematoxylin-eosin). *D.* Invasive ductal carcinoma histopathology. Malignant epithelial cells are characterized by large pleomorphic nuclei invading the breast stroma individually and in clusters and forming ductlike structures in some cases.

The treatment and prognosis of a woman with breast cancer are strongly influenced by the stage at the time of diagnosis. Multiple staging systems have been proposed, but the most commonly used system is the one adopted by both the American Joint Committee (AJC) and the International Union against Cancer (UICC).[30] This staging system is a detailed TNM (tumor, nodes, metastasis) system but can be summarized as in Table 30-2. Data compiled from several studies with extensive follow-up suggest that 10-year disease-free survival rates for women with invasive breast cancer are approximately 80 percent for women diagnosed with stage I disease, decreasing to 55 percent (stage II), 40 percent (stage III), and 10 percent (stage IV) as the stage at diagnosis increases[31,32] (Fig. 30-5).

As breast cancer is considered a systemic disease at the time of detection, treatment is designed to achieve two distinct goals: (1) local control of the tumor in the breast and the ipsilateral axillary lymph nodes and (2) eradication of clinically occult systemic micrometastases. Local control may be obtained in most cases by mastectomy alone or by lumpectomy (removal of the tumor with histologically negative margins) followed by radiation therapy to the affected breast. Lumpectomy without radiation is associated with a 35 percent local recurrence rate and thus is considered unacceptable[33] and is rarely used. As multiple randomized studies have shown that the breast-conserving approach of lumpectomy and radiation does not compromise survival compared to mastectomy, this therapeutic choice is often left to the individual patient. Relative contraindications to the use of breast conservation are related to the presence of a multicentric or multifocal tumor, extensive DCIS in association with an invasive tumor, or a large tumor (> 5 cm). Large tumors are particularly problematic in a small breast, where the cosmetic result associated with a complete excision may be compromised by the relative amount of tissue that must be removed to obtain clear margins around the tumor. However, the choice of procedure generally is dictated only by personal preference (some patients feel more comfortable with removal of the entire breast despite data supporting the safety of lumpectomy) and convenience (some patients choose mastectomy to avoid 6 to 7 weeks of daily radiotherapy treatments).

Once local control has been achieved by one of the two surgical options discussed above, adjuvant therapy may be used to reduce the likelihood of a systemic recurrence. Often confusing to patients, the decision to use adjuvant chemotherapy is not dictated by the choice of local therapy but by the stage of disease and the menopausal status of the patient. The adjuvant regimens most commonly used include a 3- to 6-month course of chemotherapy and/or a prolonged course of the partial estrogen antagonist tamoxifen. Surgical oophorectomy (removal of both ovaries) performed after local therapy also has been shown to reduce the risk of systemic recurrence in premenopausal patients. While the needs of each patient must be addressed individually, generalizations can be made about the choice of therapy (Table 30-3). First, there is increasing evidence that women with tumors less than 1 cm in diameter, without involved axillary nodes, do not require adjuvant ther-

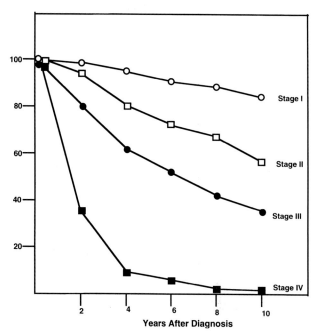

FIG. 30-5 Stage-specific survival for breast cancer. Survival at 2-year intervals is indicated by stage (IUCC). Stage I = open circles; stage II = open squares; stage III = shaded circles; stage IV = shaded squares. (*Adapted from Ref. 31 with permission.*)

apy. The 10-year survival rates for women in this category exceed 90 percent, and the relative benefit derived from adjuvant treatment adds little to this excellent prognosis. In contrast, numerous studies support the use of adjuvant therapy in premenopausal women with tumors greater than 1 cm in diameter regardless of nodal status. In this setting, chemotherapy is associated with the greatest increase in overall survival, with tamoxifen generally being added for women with tumors that appear to be hormonally responsive by virtue of expressing the estrogen receptor (ER). More controversial is the treatment of postmenopausal women, as tamoxifen alone may be of equivalent benefit to chemotherapy, obviating the need for chemotherapy in postmenopausal women with

Table 30-2 AJC and IUCC Staging System for Breast Cancer

Stage 0	Carcinoma in situ
Stage I	Tumor 2 cm, axillary nodes not involved
Stage II	Tumor between 2 and 5 cm and/or involved but mobile axillary lymph nodes
Stage III	Tumor larger than 5 cm and/or fixed axillary lymph nodes; includes inflammatory breast cancer
Stage IV	Distant metastases beyond ipsilateral axillary lymph nodes

NOTE: This table is a condensed summary of the staging system designed to provide a framework with which to interpret survival curves. A detailed schema for use in clinical practice is provided in Ref. 30.

Table 30-3 Adjuvant* Treatment Options for Women with Breast Cancer

Patient Characteristics	Standard Treatment[†]
Premenopausal	
Tumor <1 cm, negative nodes	None
Tumor ≥1 cm, negative nodes	Chemotherapy plus tamoxifen if ER+
Tumor ≥1 cm, positive nodes	Chemotherapy plus amoxifen if ER+
Postmenpausal	
Tumor <1 cm, negative nodes	None
Tumor ≥1 cm, negative nodes, ER+	Tamoxifen or none
Tumor ≥1 cm, negative nodes, ER−	Chemotherapy or none
Tumor ≥1 cm, positive nodes, ER+	Tamoxifen ± chemotherapy
Tumor ≥ cm, positive nodes, ER−	Chemotherapy

*Generally given after adequate surgical therapy.
[†]The standard treatment options listed in this table are generalizations based on multiple studies. In clinical practice, each patient must be evaluated individually and treatment recommendations may vary with the clinical scenario.

ER-positive tumors. Postmenopausal women with ER-negative tumors, without involved axillary nodes, may receive no adjuvant therapy or a course of chemotherapy, depending on a number of variables, including the size and grade of the tumor, as well as the general health status of the patient. Postmenopausal women with involved axillary nodes may receive chemotherapy and/or tamoxifen, depending on their ER status. Chemotherapy may be administered for 3 to 6 months, is given in the outpatient setting, and is generally well tolerated. The most commonly employed regimens include cyclophosphamide and doxorubicin or cyclophosphamide, methotrexate, and 5-fluorouracil. Tamoxifen is self-administered orally and is taken daily for a minimum of 5 years after the diagnosis.

Finally, autologous bone marrow transplantation is an experimental adjuvant therapy approach that may be an option for women with a high risk of systemic relapse. These women generally are defined by the presence of 10 or more involved axillary lymph nodes or the presence of inflammatory breast cancer, a particularly aggressive form of invasive carcinoma that presents clinically with diffuse breast pain, swelling, and redness. Ten-year survival rates for both of these clinical entities are only 15 to 20 percent in the absence of systemic therapy. Conventional-dose chemotherapy, which may improve survival by 10 to 15 percent, is still associated with 10-year recurrence rates of 60 to 65 percent.[34] Autologous bone marrow transplantation for breast cancer was designed as a means of delivering very high doses of chemotherapy that would be fatal in the absence of a method for protecting bone marrow stem cells from the toxic effects of treatment. In this setting, bone marrow cells may be harvested directly from the iliac crest or by pheresis of stem cells from peripheral blood. Stem cells are stored (by freezing) during intensive chemotherapy and reinfused into the patient when the drugs have been cleared. While this approach is promising, the long-term results are not available.

The interventions described above are of clear benefit in reducing the risk of recurrence; nonetheless, overall at least 30 percent of patients with breast cancer will relapse and die of the disease. Metastatic disease (stage IV) may be extremely variable in course. Ten-year survival rates are dismal at 5 to 10 percent,[32] with the median survival for patients with metastatic disease being approximately 18 months. However, while some patients with metastatic breast cancer may succumb within months of a recurrence, others, particularly those with metastases to bone as the only site of disease, may do well with minimally progressive disease for years. Time to recurrence is also extremely variable, as some patients will relapse with aggressive, drug-resistant tumors within weeks of the completion of adjuvant therapy and some patients will have disease-free intervals of up to 30 years before ultimate disease recurrence.

Treatment for metastatic disease must be individualized but may include chemotherapy, hormonal therapy, and palliative radiation therapy. Surgical resection of chest wall recurrences after mastectomy may be indicated in some cases. Unfortunately, treatment of metastatic breast cancer is uniformly considered palliative. The only exception at present may be a subset of patients who achieve complete remission of all clinically detectable tumor with standard chemotherapy and then undergo autologous bone marrow transplantation. While long-term follow-up of large numbers of patients with metastatic breast cancer who have undergone autologous bone marrow transplantation is not available, data from Peter at Duke University suggest that 10 to 15 percent of these patients may attain durable complete remissions.[35]

THE GENETICS OF BREAST CANCER

Breast cancer is a complex and heterogeneous disease caused by interactions of both genetic and nongenetic factors; however, a family history of breast cancer has long been recognized as a significant risk factor. In 1984, Williams and Anders on used segregation analysis to compare various models that might explain the pattern of aggregation of breast cancer in families.[36] They were the first to provide evidence for an autosomal dominant breast cancer susceptibility gene with age-related penetrance. This model was supported in 1988 by Newman and colleagues,[37] and the hypothesis was proved correct in 1994 with the isolation of the susceptibility gene *BRCA1*.[38]

Two high-penetrance breast cancer susceptibility genes have been identified (*BRCA1* and *BRCA2*).[38-40] and a third (*BRCA3*) is being actively sought. Breast cancer in families with germ-line mutations in these genes appears as an autosomal dominant trait, as predicted by previous work. In addition, mutations in several other genes, such as *TP53*, have been identified as rare causes of hereditary breast cancer. Finally, it is very likely that other, lower-penetrance genes are responsible for inherited susceptibility to breast cancer in families in which the incidence of breast cancer is higher than that in the general population but the inheritance pattern does not fit the classic model of Mendelian inheritance.

Familial clustering of breast cancer was first described by physicians in ancient Rome.[41] The first documentation of familial clustering of breast cancer in modern times was published in 1866 by a French surgeon who reported 10 cases of breast cancer in four generations of his wife's family; four other women in this family died as a result of hepatic tumors.[42] Given the strong influence of molecular genetics in medicine in recent years, there is a tendency to assume that familial clustering of disease results from a genetically inherited predisposition. However, other explanations for familial clustering of breast cancer are possible, including (1) geographically limited environmental exposure to carcinogens which might affect an extended family living in close proximity, (2) culturally motivated behavior that alters the risk factor profile, such as age at first live birth and contraceptive choice, and (3) socioeconomic influences that, for example, might result in differing dietary exposures. In addition, multiple complex inherited genetic factors are likely to influence the extent to which a risk factor for breast cancer plays a role in any single individual; such modifying effects are likely to be shared among genetically similar members of an extended family. Nonetheless, while noninherited factors certainly play a role in familial clustering of breast cancer, recent advances have provided unequivocal evidence for the presence of breast cancer susceptibility genes that are directly responsible for 5 to 10 percent of all breast cancers.

Inherited breast cancer has several distinctive clinical features: Age at onset is considerably lower than in sporadic cases, the prevalence of bilateral breast cancer is higher, and the presence of associated tumors in affected individuals is noted in some families. Associated tumors may include ovarian, colon, prostate, and endometrial cancers and sarcomas.[43,44] However, inherited breast cancer does not appear to be distinguished by histologic type, metastatic pattern, or survival characteristics. The study of *BRCA1*, the first major breast cancer susceptibility gene to be identified and isolated,[38,45] has greatly expanded our knowledge of inherited breast cancer, and the study of this and other genes continues at a rapid pace.

BRCA1

Clinical Features of Affected Families. In 1990, chromosome 17q21 was identified as the location of a susceptibility gene for early-onset breast cancer now termed *BRCA1*.[38,45] Linkage between the genetic marker D17S74 on 17q21 and the appearance of ovarian cancer in several large kindreds was subsequently demonstrated.[46] A collaborative study designed to estimate the proportion of breast cancer resulting from *BRCA1* provided an analysis of more than 200 families. These data suggested that breast/ovarian cancer was linked to markers in this region in more than 90 percent of families with apparent autosomal dominant transmission of breast cancer and at least one case of ovarian cancer. Linkage between breast cancer and genetic markers on 17q12-q21 was observed in just 45 percent of families with breast cancer only. However, the percentage of site-specific breast cancer families attributed to *BRCA1* mutations rose to almost 70 percent when the median age of onset of breast cancer in the families was less than 45 years.[9]

As was described above, breast cancer in these families appears as a classic Mendelian trait of autosomal dominant transmission with high penetrance, with approximately 50 percent of the children of carriers developing breast and/or ovarian cancer by age 85. Female mutation carriers are estimated to have an 87 percent lifetime risk of developing breast cancer[9] and a 40 to 60 percent lifetime risk of developing ovarian cancer,[47] as shown in Fig. 30-6. Approximately 20 percent of female *BRCA1* mutation carriers will develop breast cancer by age 40 years, 51 percent by age 50 years, and 87 percent by age 70. *BRCA1* mutation carriers also have an increased incidence of bilateral breast cancer. In a later study of 33 families with evidence of germ-line mutations in *BRCA1* conducted by the Breast Cancer Linkage Consortium, the cumulative risk of developing a second breast cancer was estimated to be 65 percent for mutations carriers who live to age 70.[47] However, these penetrance figures may be overestimates resulting from ascertainment bias; these data were derived from families collected for linkage analysis, and in general only the most severely affected families were collected and studied.

Risk for other cancers may also be increased in the presence of an inherited *BRCA1* mutation. Data published in 1993 from a study of a large Icelandic breast/ovarian cancer family suggested that prostate cancer may also be a component of the *BRCA1* syndrome.[48] The Breast Cancer Linkage Consortium estimated a relative risk of 3.33 for prostate cancer in males thought to carry *BRCA1* germ-line mutations and a relative risk of 4.11 for colon cancer. It is important to note that the excess colon cancer risk reflects the experience of only a few families, suggesting either very low penetrance with regard to colon cancer or a limited number of specific mutations that increase colon cancer risk. No significant

excesses were observed for cancers originating from other anatomic sites.[49] Male breast cancer is only rarely associated with *BRCA1* germ-line mutations.

To determine whether tumors that arise as a result of *BRCA1* mutations have clinical and pathologic characteristics that differ from those of sporadic tumors, Lynch and colleagues analyzed 180 tumors from hereditary breast/ovarian or site-specific breast cancer families.[50] Ninety-eight of the 180 tumors were considered as a subset more likely to result from *BRCA1* mutations on the basis of linkage analysis or the presence of ovarian cancer in the family. Patients in both subgroups were significantly younger than the population average for women with breast cancer. In addition, the "*BRCA1* group" was found to have more aneuploid and more high S-phase tumors, but surprisingly, disease-free survival was longer in this group than in the group thought less likely to have *BRCA1* mutations. Tubular and lobular cancers were less common in the group where the presence of *BRCA1* mutations was suspected. These investigators suggested that *BRCA1* mutations may result in tumors with adverse pathologic indicators but a paradoxically better survival than expected. Unfortunately, this study was performed before it was possible to determine which tumors were actually attributable to *BRCA1* mutations. A subsequent study of the pathobiology of breast cancer associated with *BRCA1* and other hereditary breast cancer genes supported these results.[51] Finally, a significantly increased incidence of high-grade tumors in women with germ-line *BRCA1* mutations has been reported by two groups.[21,52] In general, it appears that *BRCA1*-associated tumors are frequently of high grade; however, the possibility that these tumors are associated with a paradoxically better survival compared with tumors of similarly high grade from patients who are unlikely to have *BRCA1* mutations remains to be proved.

Isolation of *BRCA1*. No information was available on the structure and function of the *BRCA1* gene before its identification in 1994; thus, positional cloning was utilized by several groups in an attempt to isolate the gene. These efforts began in 1990 with the identification of chromosome 17q21 as the location of *BRCA1*. Initial linkage analysis was performed on seven families and yielded a maximum cumulative lod score of 5.98.[45] Few polymorphic genetic markers were available for this region of chromosome 17 at that time, and many of the available markers were of low heterozygosity. Thus, the initial *BRCA1* candidate region spanned a large

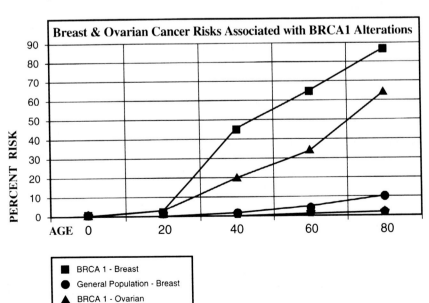

FIG. 30-6 Breast and ovarian cancer risks associated with *BRCA1* mutations. Age-adjusted risk for breast and ovarian cancer risk for *BRCA1* mutation carriers are compared to the general population risk. (*Adapted from Ref. 9 with permission.*)

20-cM region of chromosome 17q12.1-21.3. Several interesting candidate genes, including THRA1 (thyroid hormone receptor-α), RARA (retenoic acid receptor alpha), EDH17B1 and EDH17B2 (17β-estradiol dehydrogenase), NME1 (nm23), and ERBB2 (c-erb-B2), fell within this region (Fig. 30-7).

An intensive genetic mapping effort resulted in the identification of many new polymorphic genetic markers, and the candidate region was rapidly reduced to a 4-cM interval flanked by the markers THRA1 and D17S183.[53,54] High-density genetic maps of the *BRCA1* region were generated by using several of the newly identified markers,[55–57] and the boundaries of the *BRCA1* region were further narrowed by identification of genetic recombinants at D17S857 and D17S78 (a 1- to 1.5-Mb interval).[58,59] This region was later minimally narrowed by the identification of a recombination event with the marker D17S856.[60] Several candidate genes, including THRA1, RARA, ERBB2, NME1, and prohibition (somatically mutated in a number of sporadic breast cancers), were excluded as candidates for *BRCA1* by these recombination events. Furthermore, no mutations were detected in EDH17B1 or EDH17B2 in affected families,[58] resulting in the exclusion of all the previously considered candidate genes.

To facilitate the construction of physical maps of the *BRCA1* region, several framework maps were constructed, including radiation hybrid maps,[61,62] a somatic cell hybrid map,[63] and a fluorescence in situ hybridization (FISH) map.[64] These maps were used to order genomic clones and sequence-tagged sites (STSs) within the *BRCA1* candidate interval. Physical maps of overlapping genomic clones were generated by screening a variety of yeast artificial chromosome (YAC) libraries with STS-based probes. YAC, cosmid, and P1 contigs were generated across the 1.5-Mb *BRCA1* region,[65,66] with gaps in both YAC and cosmid contigs filled by P1 and bacterial artificial chromosome (BAC) clones.[60] Isolation efforts were hampered by the presence of an unstable genomic region in the candidate interval that was ultimately spanned by BAC but never by cosmids, P1s, or YACs.[38]

Transcription maps of the region were generated by using the genomic clones as templates for a variety of gene isolation techniques.[59,65,67–69] Exon amplification,[70] cDNA selection,[71–73] and direct cDNA library screening were all used to isolate cDNA clones from the region. Clones were extended by further cDNA library screening, sequenced, and compared to genetic databases in an attempt to identify function through homology. The region appears to be very gene-rich, with as many as 30 genes identified within the 1- to 1.5-Mb interval. cDNA clones were screened for mutations in affected individuals by single-stranded conformational polymorphism (SSCP) analysis[74] or direct sequencing in an attempt to identify the *BRCA1* gene. In late 1994, this effort culminated with the identification of the *BRCA1* gene by Miki and colleagues.[38]

BRCA1 is a novel gene with 126 bp of homology to a RING finger motif near the 5' end of the gene, suggesting that *BRCA1* may function as a transcription factor. The protein does not display homology to any other known motif or cloned gene. *BRCA1* is composed of 24 exons, with an mRNA that is 7.8 kb in length, and 22 coding exons translating into a protein of 1863 amino acids (Fig. 30-8). The entire gene covers approximately 100 kb of genomic sequence. The structure of *BRCA1* is unusual, with most exons in the expected 100- to 500-bp size but with exon 11 (approximately 3500 bp) constituting approximately 60 percent of the coding region of the gene. The functional or evolutionary significance of this unusual structure is unknown. Exon 4 is thought to be an artifact of the isolation method and is omitted from the gene sequence. *BRCA1* is situated head to head and may share a bidirectional promoter sequence with, 1A1.3B, a homologue of the gene encoding CA-125, an ovarian carcinoma-related serum antigen.[75]

Mutational Spectrum. After the identification of *BRCA1*, more than 300 sequence variations were detected (Fig. 30-8). Initial reports described eight disease-associated mutations within the gene,[38,76] followed shortly afterward by an increasing number of novel mutations.[77–79] Surprisingly, almost all described mutations are germ line, as *BRCA1* mutations are rare in sporadic breast and ovarian tumors,[80–83] suggesting that *BRCA1* coding region mutations play a limited role in the development of sporadic breast cancer. A single individual has been reported to be homozygous for a *BRCA1* mutation, inheriting the same mutation from each parent.[84] This homozygous individual is developmentally normal but was diagnosed with breast cancer at age 32.

A variety of mutation detection techniques have been used to identify *BRCA1* mutations including SSCP,[77,78,85] the protein truncation assay,[86,87] multiplex heteroduplex analysis,[88] and, most commonly, direct sequencing. Details of these mutations are available on the Breast Cancer Information Core (BIC) website: (http://www.nchgr.nih.gov/dir/Intramural_research/Lab_transfer/Bic/index.htm 1). A recent report describing the first 254 sequence variants in the *BRCA1* gene showed that 55 percent of the mutations were located in exon 11 (which contains 62 percent of the gene-coding sequence), suggesting that sequence alterations are scattered evenly throughout *BRCA1*.[89] In this sample set, 52 percent of the mutations were unique, with 87 percent resulting in truncation or absence of the protein product. This number included 196 frameshift and nonsense mutations, 21 splice variants which also

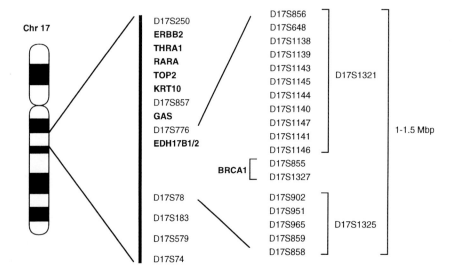

FIG. 30-7 Genetic markers flanking the *BRAC1* locus. Idiogram of chromosome 17 depicting the order of polymorphic markers and candidate genes surrounding the *BRCA1* gene on 17q21. D17S855 and D17S1327 markers are located within *BRCA1*. The position of D17S1321 and D17S1325 relative to the other markers is not known. Genes are shown in boldface.

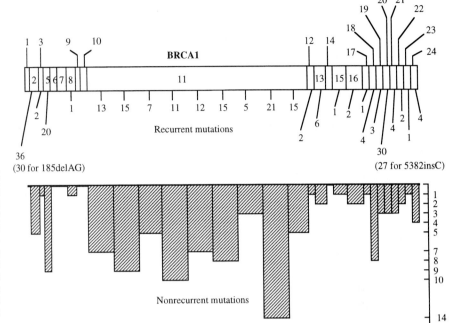

FIG. 30-8 Structure and mutation spectrum of *BRCA1*. The 24 exons of *BRCA1* are represented by vertical lines within the gene; the translation start and stop sites are as indicated. The 5′ region of homology to the RING finger motif found in a family of transcription factors is indicated by a shaded rectangle under the gene. The locations of eight of the most common mutations are indicated above the gene. Exons 1 and 4 do not contain coding sequence; of particular note is the very large exon 11, containing more than half the coding region.

create frameshifts and stop codons in the gene, and 4 ill-defined noncoding region mutations. The remaining sequence variants were nontruncating missense mutations within the *BRCA1* coding sequence. The four noncoding region mutations were inferred from inactivation of transcription of one allele of *BRCA1*.[38,90,91] The specific DNA alterations which result in inactivation of transcription in these samples have not been determined. Serova and colleagues also determined various regions of the *BRCA1* cDNA that when mutated led to complete loss of the allele-specific transcript, presumably as a result of destabilization and degradation of mRNA.[91] Two studies have identified a genotype/phenotype correlation,[90,92] suggesting that mutations in the 5′ half of *BRCA1* predispose to both breast and ovarian cancer, while mutations closer to the 3′ portion of the gene are predominantly associated with site-specific breast cancer. Finally, mutations occurring in two terminal regions of *BRCA1* may be associated with a more severe phenotype, as defined by high tumor grade,[93] suggesting that these two regions may be important in the control of mammary cell growth.

There are several common mutations in the *BRCA1* gene, with the 11 most common mutations accounting for 43 percent of all the mutations. The two most common mutations in *BRCA1* are 185delAG and 5382insC, each accounting for approximately 10 percent of the total.[89] The 185delAG mutation was recently identified as a very common variant in the Ashkenazi Jewish population,[94,95] with a frequency of about 1 in 100 compared to the overall frequency of *BRCA1* mutations in an unselected Caucasian population of about 1 in 1000, suggesting the presence of a founder effect in the Ashkenazi Jewish population. Other *BRCA1* mutations have also been detected in the Jewish population, but at much lower levels.[96] Analysis of germ-line *BRCA1* mutations in Jewish and non-Jewish women with early-onset breast cancer indicated that approximately 21 percent of Jewish women who develop breast cancer before age 40 carry the 185delAG mutation.[97,98] In contrast, *BRCA1* mutation screening in unselected populations suggests that only 10 percent of women with breast cancer under age 35 carry *BRCA1* germ-line mutations.[99]

Some of the disease-associated *BRCA1* mutations are missense changes, but as with most genes, the distinction between missense mutations and neutral polymorphisms is often difficult to determine in the absence of a functional assay. Examples of missense mutations thought to increase susceptibility to breast cancer are

C61G and C64G, which disrupt the sequence encoding the RING finger motif and thus presumably disrupt the function of *BRCA1*. M11 is thought to disrupt the start codon and may prevent translation, but the significance of this mutation remains to be determined.[89] Thirty-five sequence variants within the *BRCA1* gene are thought to be neutral polymorphisms.[89,100]

Molecular Biology of *BRCA1*

BRCA1 does not appear to be a member of a known gene family on the basis of sequence analysis. Southern blotting of human genomic DNA detects a single band, suggesting that only one gene is present in the human genome. Northern blotting of human and mouse tissue with a *BRCA1* probe has been performed by a number of laboratories. Initial reports using a *BRCA1* fragment as a probe described a 7.8-kb RNA and several splice variants formed as a result of alternate splicing at the 5′ end of the transcript,[38] as identified by Brown and colleagues.[101] Subsequent work with a probe representing the complete coding region of *BRCA1* identified several additional transcripts. Three of these variants have been identified as (1) an in-frame deletion of exon 11, (2) a deletion of exon 11 111 bp from the 5′ splice acceptor, and (3) an in-frame deletion of exon 10.[102,103] The functional significance of these isoforms is under investigation.

The murine homologue of *BRCA1* has been characterized by several groups.[104–106] The mouse cDNA sequence predicts a protein of 1812 amino acids, 51 residues shorter than the human cDNA. The human and mouse cDNAs display 58 percent identity and 73 percent similarity at the protein level with perfect conservation in the RING finger domain near the N terminus and high homology in a putative acidic transactivation domain at the C terminus,[104] suggesting that these domains play an important role in *BRCA1* function.

The two regions of 100 percent homology between human and murine *BRCA1* have been studied in detail by several groups. The N-terminal RING finger domain has been extensively screened for a DNA-binding function, with no success reported. Studies of protein–protein interaction by yeast twin-hybrid analysis has resulted in the identification of a *BRCA1* binding protein termed BAP1 (*BRCA1* activator protein-1) (D. Jensen and F. Rauscher, personal communication), but the function of this putative *BRCA1*-binding protein is unknown. Studies of the C-terminal acidic activation domain by a similar method have shown that this region of *BRCA1*, as well as the complete *BRCA1* protein, can function as a coactivator of transcription.[107] Finally, *BRCA1* has a small region of weak homology to a p53 binding site, suggesting that *BRCA1* may interact with p53 to activate the transcription of a variety of genes. Homology between a loosely defined granin consensus sequence and the human and mouse *BRCA1* proteins has been reported,[108] but the functional significance of this finding is controversial.

BRCA1 Gene Regulation. Shortly after the identification of *BRCA1*, the sequence of 1345 bp of genomic DNA proximal to the putative transcription start site was identified.[101] This 1345-bp region was notable for the inclusion of the putative promoters of both the *BRCA1* gene and the *1A1.3B* gene, a homologue of CA-125 encoding a protein of unknown function that is overexpressed in some ovarian tumors. These genes are located head to head, with transcription start sites located 295 bp apart, raising the possibility that sharing of promoters between the two genes acts as a regulatory mechanism. Physical mapping of the *BRCA1* region identified a large duplicated region of 30 kb containing the 5' end of the *BRCA1* gene. This region contains a partial pseudogene of *BRCA1* containing exons 1A, 1B, and 2; the functional *1A1.3B* gene; a 1A1.3B pseudogene containing exons 1A, 1B, and 3; and the functional *BRCA1* gene.[101] A second transcription start site for *BRCA1* also was identified which initiates transcription in an alternative exon 1 located in intron 1. Thus, two promoters for *BRCA1* have been located, separated by approximately 2 kb of genomic DNA. These *BRCA1* promoters contain consensus binding elements for multiple transcription factors including p53 and AP2, although no data are available concerning the functionality of these sites. Little is known about the transcriptional regulation of the *BRCA1* gene, although *BRCA1* mRNA and protein levels have been shown to be altered by some steroid hormones.[109–112] Estrogen and a mixture of estrogen and progesterone increase *BRCA1* RNA and protein levels in human cell lines,[109,110] and RNA levels in animal models (protein levels were not analyzed in this system).[112]

Subcellular Localization of BRCA1 The subcellular localization of *BRCA1* was initially studied by cell fractionation and immunofluorescence of breast cancer cell lines, breast epithelial cell lines, and breast tumor tissue. *BRCA1* was detected in the nucleus of the normal cells and in the cytoplasm or in both the cytoplasm and the nucleus of almost all breast cancer cell lines through the use of three polyclonal *BRCA1* antibodies.[113] Staining of primary cells from pleural effusions and cells in tissues sections also provided evidence that *BRCA1* was located predominantly in the cytoplasm of malignant cells, suggesting that subcellular mislocalization of *BRCA1* may be a mechanism by which *BRCA1* plays a role in the pathogenesis of sporadic breast tumors. However, a similar study performed by Scully and colleagues, using fixed tissue sections and *BRCA1* monoclonal antibodies, demonstrated localization of *BRCA1* to the nucleus in every section analyzed. This group also tested a variety of methods of tissue fixation and determined that technical variation may lead to apparent cytoplasmic localization of *BRCA1*.[114] To add to this confusion, *BRCA1* was noted to have homology to a granin consensus sequence. Granins are proteins that are secreted and modified to form bioactive peptides that act on the cell surface. In studies by Jensen and colleagues, polyclonal antibodies against the last 20 C-terminal amino acids identified a 190-kD protein localized to the cytoplasm, Golgi network, and secretory vesicles.[108] Fractionation studies and confocal imaging supported these results, the latter purportedly identifying the protein they believed to be *BRCA1* being released from a secretory

body on the extracellular surface. Subsequent experiments indicate that the two polyclonal antibodies used by Jensen and colleagues detect *BRCA1* as well as EGF-R and Her-2/neu and that it is the latter two proteins that are detected on the extracellular surface and in the Golgi network.[115] Immunofluorescence studies of *BRCA1* using a variety of *BRCA1* polyclonal and monoclonal antibodies have demonstrated that *BRCA1* transfected into cell lines is localized in the nucleus, while *BRCA1* splice forms or mutants deleted for the consensus nuclear localization signal in exon 11 are located in the cytoplasm.[102] The current consensus is that *BRCA1* is localized to the nucleus in normal cells; however, no consensus has been reached concerning the location of *BRCA1* in cells from breast cancer lines or tumors. Therefore, it is unknown whether aberrant localization of *BRCA1* is a mechanism by which *BRCA1* plays a role in the development of sporadic breast cancer. A functional consensus nuclear localization signal in *BRCA1* exon 11 has been identified,[102] multiple laboratories have replicated the initial observation that *BRCA1* is a nuclear protein, and the controversy is largely resolved.

Tumor-Suppressor Function. Before its isolation, *BRCA1* was predicted to function as a tumor-suppressor gene based on frequent loss of heterozygosity in *BRCA1*-associated tumors, where the deleted allele was invariantly the wild-type allele.[54,116] These data suggested that malignant transformation occurs when both functional copies of *BRCA1* are lost, a pattern indicative of a tumor-suppressor gene. After the isolation of the gene, Thompson and colleagues demonstrated that the presence of antisense oligonucleotides complementary to *BRCA1* RNA significantly increased the growth rate of MCF-7 cells in comparison to untreated cells, indicating that reduction of *BRCA1* RNA levels was associated with an increased growth rate in these cells.[117] Analysis of *BRCA1* RNA levels in tumors also suggested that *BRCA1* was down-regulated in sporadic tumors compared to normal breast epithelium. Subsequent studies using NIH-3T3 fibroblasts indicated that *BRCA1* antisense RNA could reduce native *BRCA1* RNA levels and result in a transformed phenotype in these cells. This group also demonstrated that nontumorigenic NIH-3T3 cells formed tumors in nude mice when treated with antisense *BRCA1* RNA.[118] The growth-inhibitory properties of *BRCA1* were then tested in animal models and cell lines. Retroviral transfer of wild-type *BRCA1* inhibited the growth of two breast cancer cell lines and three ovarian cancer cell lines. Finally, it was demonstrated that the development of MCF-7 tumors in nude mice was inhibited in the presence of wild-type *BRCA1* and unaffected by the presence of mutant *BRCA1*, adding further support to the hypothesis that *BRCA1* functions as a tumor suppressor.[92]

Further study of the role of *BRCA1* in cell growth control has proved difficult because of consistent problems with the development of cell lines stably transfected with wild-type *BRCA1*, as transfected cells die rapidly in culture. Shao and colleagues analyzed this phenomenon and determined that constitutive expression of *BRCA1* results in induction of apoptosis, especially notable in conjunction with serum starvation or calcium ionophore treatment,[119] suggesting that *BRCA1* may play a role in the regulation of apoptosis.

BRCA1 and the Cell Cycle. A connection between *BRCA1* and the cell cycle was originally suggested by studies of breast cancer cell lines treated with estrogen, which demonstrated that *BRCA1* and cyclin A RNA levels increased in parallel in response to the hormone treatment.[109] It is now known that *BRCA1* is a nuclear phosphoprotein that is phosphorylated in a cell-cycle-dependent manner.[120] The greatest expression and phosphorylation of *BRCA1* were observed in the S and M phases of the cell cycle. Cyclin-dependent kinase 2 and cyclin D- and A-associated kinases bind to and phosphorylate *BRCA1*, suggesting that *BRCA1* function may be regulated by cyclin-dependent kinase phosphorylation. Subsequent studies showed that *BRCA1* RNA levels were highest in rapidly growing cells, decreased after growth factor withdrawal, and increased at the G1/S phase boundary in synchronized cells.[110] *BRCA1* RNA levels also were reduced in senescent cells and cells treated with TBE-B, indicating that *BRCA1* expression is sensitive to in vitro growth conditions and may play a role in G1/S phase checkpoint control or merely be up-regulated at this point in the cell cycle in response to cellular messages. Vaughan and colleagues described similar findings and extended their analysis to include *BRCA1* protein levels. In this study, induction of *BRCA1* occurred before the initiation of DNA synthesis at the G1/S boundary.[111] The cumulative data suggest that *BRCA1* plays a role in cell cycle checkpoint control and is regulated by kinases and phosphatases that are known to play a role in the regulation of the cell cycle.

***BRCA1* and Development.**   The first studies of the role of *BRCA1* in development were performed by in situ hybridization of mouse embryos. Whole mount embryos hybridized with mouse *BRCA1* probe indicated that *BRCA1* was widely expressed in many developing tissues, suggesting that *BRCA1* may play a role in tissue development, possibly as a ubiquitous transcription factor.[112] Northern blots of mouse mammary gland RNAs also were used to demonstrate that *BRCA1* was highly expressed in the mouse gland during pregnancy, remaining above pregestational levels at least 4 weeks after postlactational regression of the mammary epithelium. These results suggest that *BRCA1* is involved in cell proliferation in breast epithelial cells and is regulated, at least secondarily, by ovarian hormone changes during pregnancy.

Subsequently, Gowen and colleagues produced mice homozygous for a *BRCA1* null allele. The null allele was generated by the complete deletion of *BRCA1* exon 11 and flanking intron sequences, resulting in embryonic lethality 10 to 13 days after conception.[121] Abnormalities were most evident in the neural tube, with 40 percent of the embryos exhibiting spina bifida and anencephaly. In all homozygous null mice, the neuroepithelium appeared disorganized, with excessive cell growth as well as increased cell death. This report substantiated the work of Marquis and colleagues,[112] suggesting that *BRCA1* plays an important role in early murine development. Hakem and colleagues also reported on the development of homozygous null *BRCA1* mice. The construct used for the generation of these mice was made by targeted deletion of exons 5 and 6, introducing stop codon in all three reading frames. The early truncation of the protein, coupled with deletion of a portion of the RING finger domain, was expected to yield a severely affected phenotype. These homozygous null mice have a phenotype slightly different from that of mice produced by Koller and colleagues and die before day 7.5 of embryogenesis.[122] The death of mutant embryos before gastrulation was postulated to result from failure of the proliferative burst necessary for the development of early germ layers. No increase in apoptosis was detected in these mice, but cell proliferation was reduced. These results again suggest a role for *BRCA1* as a growth activator in early development. Further analysis demonstrated that the absence of *BRCA1* was associated with reduced expression of mdm-2 and cyclin E, while expression of the cyclin-dependent kinase (cdk) inhibitor p21 was dramatically increased. Finally, Liu and colleagues generated a homozygous *BRCA1* null mouse by replacing 186 bp of exon 11 with a neomycin resistance gene, resulting in protein truncation. These homozygous null animals die at 4.5 to 8.5 days of embrogenesis.[123] The embryos fail to form egg cylinders and are unable to

complete gastrulation. Thus, accumulating data increasingly suggest that *BRCA1* plays a role in cell cycle regulation, but how this function is associated with tumor suppression and early embryonic development remains unknown.

BRCA2

Clinical Features of Affected Families.   Initial progress toward the identification of a second breast cancer susceptibility gene came from a linkage analysis of 22 families with multiple cases of early-onset female breast cancer and at least one case of male breast cancer. Twelve of these families also had at least one individual diagnosed with ovarian cancer.[124] All 22 families were analyzed for linkage between breast cancer and genetic markers flanking the *BRCA1* candidate region on chromosome 17. A maximum lod score of -16.63 was obtained, providing strong evidence against linkage to *BRCA1* in these families. This study demonstrated that only a small proportion of breast cancer families with at least one case of male breast cancer were likely to be associated with germ-line mutations in *BRCA1*, arguing strongly for the existence of at least one additional breast cancer susceptibility gene, now known to be *BRCA2*. Shortly after the appearance of this report, a large collaborative group succeeded in identifying linkage in large female and male breast cancer families between polymorphic genetic markers on chromosome 13q12-13 and the disease phenotype.[125] A genomewide linkage search using 15 large breast cancer families located a familial early-onset breast cancer susceptibility gene (*BRCA2*) in a 6-cM region between the markers D13S289 and D13S267, with a maximum total multipoint LOD score of 9.58, 5 cM proximal to D13S260.

BRCA2, which was identified in late 1995, has a cancer risk profile similar but not identical to that of *BRCA1*. Lifetime breast cancer risk to *BRCA2* mutation carriers is estimated to be 85 percent, and lifetime ovarian cancer risk appears to be in the range of 10 to 20 percent. While significantly above the general population risk of 1 percent, *BRCA2*-associated ovarian cancer risk is lower than the 40 to 60 percent lifetime risk of ovarian cancer associated with *BRCA1* mutations (Fig. 30-9). Also in contrast to *BRCA1*, *BRCA2* mutations are associated with a 6 percent lifetime risk of male breast cancer. Although in absolute terms this represents significantly less cancer risk to men than to women, the relative risk represents a similar 100-fold increase over the general population risk. Elevated risks for the development of prostate, pancreatic, colon, and other cancers may be associated with *BRCA2* mutations but remain poorly defined.

Isolation of *BRCA2*.   After the demonstration of the linkage of familial breast cancer to chromosome 13q12-13, several laboratories began evaluating families not linked to *BRCA1* for linkage to this region, particularly those with male breast cancer cases. Icelandic pedigrees with male breast cancer cases were shown to be linked to chromosome 13q12-13, and a common haplotype was identified, suggesting a common founder.[126] Additional reports described recombination events at the markers D13S1444 on the proximal side and D13S310 on the distal side of the *BRCA2* candidate region[127] and narrowing of the centromeric boundary to D13S260.[125] An unexpected addition to the fine mapping of the *BRCA2* region was provided by the identification of a homozygous somatic deletion in a single pancreatic cancer[128] that mapped between D13S260 and D13S171, spanning a region estimated at 250 kb. Despite the uncertainty surrounding the relationship between *BRCA2* and this deletion, the 250-kb region was prioritized for transcription mapping (Fig. 30-10).

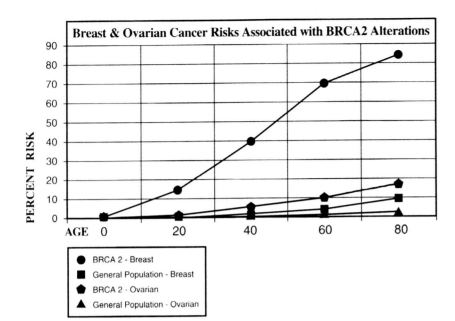

FIG. 30-9 Breast and ovarian cancer risks associated with *BRCA2* mutations. Age-adjusted risk for breast and ovarian cancer for *BRCA2* mutation carriers is compared to general population risk. (*Adapted from Ref. 39 with permission.*)

Several physical maps of the *BRCA2* region were generated by using YACs, PACs, and cosmids.[128] YACs and PACs,[39] YACs and cosmids,[129] and BACs, PACs, and P1s.[127] Contigs were assembled by STS mapping and end-clone hybridization. Using the physical map contigs as templates, exon amplification and direct selection were used to isolate cDNA fragments from the *BRCA2* candidate region.[39,40,127] Gene fragments were assembled into larger cDNA clones, and a total of seven different transcription units with extended and substantial coding potential, two pseudogenes, and at least nine additional short transcription units were identified in a 600-kb region.[127] Six of the seven genes identified had full-length cDNAs greater than 4.0 kb as detected by Northern blotting. At this point in the search for *BRCA2*, sequence data from a 900-kb region thought to contain *BRCA2* were completed by DNA sequencing groups at the Sanger Center and Washington University, and the assembled sequence was released over the Internet, greatly

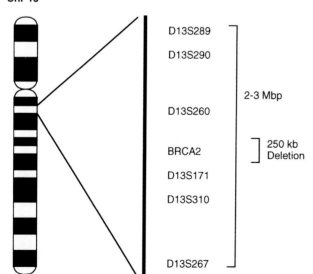

FIG. 30-10 Genetic markers flanking the *BRCA2* locus. Idiogram of chromosome 13 depicting the order of polymorphic markers in the 13q12-13 *BRCA* region. The *BRCA2* gene lies within a 250-kb region homozygously deleted in a single pancreatic cancer.[128]

facilitating this effort. Alignment of cDNAs and screening of the EST database using this sequence allowed identification of additional genes in this region. Mutation screening of these genes, as well as smaller cDNAs and exons, was performed by conformation-sensitive gel electrophoresis (CSGE) and direct sequencing. The culmination of this effort was the identification of a partial sequence of the *BRCA2* gene[39] and six mutations which truncated the putative *BRCA2* protein. Shortly afterward, the complete cDNA sequence of *BRCA2* was published by another collaborative group.[40]

The *BRCA2* cDNA is approximately 11.5 kb in length and is contained within 70 kb of genomic DNA. The coding region is 11.2 kb in length and is composed of 26 exons, with exon 1 forming part of the 5′ untranslated region. Like *BRCA1*, *BRCA2* has a large exon 11 (4.8 kb), and is expressed in most tissues at very low levels, with higher expression in testes.[40] *BRCA2* cDNA has no significant homology to any previously described gene, and the protein contains no previously defined functional domains (Fig. 30-11).

Mutational Spectrum. The mutational spectrum of *BRCA2* is just beginning to be defined. More than 100 *BRCA2* mutations have been defined to date,[39,40,130–136] with a tabulated list available on the BIC website (http//www.nchgr.nih.gov/dir/Intramural_research/Lab_transfer/Bic/index.htm 1). Interestingly, several similarities with *BRCA1* are apparent. First, *BRCA2* mutations span the entire coding region of the gene, adding little information on important functional regions and making mutation screening in this very large gene difficult. No mutation hotspots have been detected. Second, most mutations reported to date are truncating mutations created mainly by small insertions and deletions, again adding little in the way of clues for defining functional regions. Few nonsense mutations have been identified. One particularly interesting mutation is a 126-bp deletion in exon 23 that does not create a frameshift, suggesting that this domain may be important for *BRCA2* function.[130] third, a single mutation, 6174delT, is present at an increased frequency in individuals of Ashkenazi Jewish descent, perhaps in as many as 1 percent of such individuals, as is seen with *BRCA1*.[130,131,137] Finally, few mutations have been identified in the *BRCA2* gene in sporadic breast or ovarian cancers, suggesting that mutations in coding regions in *BRCA2* do not play a role in the pathogenesis of sporadic breast cancer.

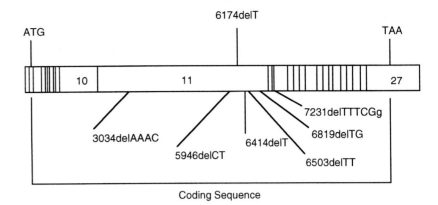

FIG. 30-11 Structure of the *BRCA2* gene. The 27 exons of the *BRCA2* cDNA are shown as sections within the *BRCA2* gene structure. The translation start and stop sites are as indicated. The location of the first six mutations described is indicated below the gene. The common Ashkenazi mutation 6174delT is represented above the gene diagram.

Rare Causes of Inherited Breast Cancer Syndromes

Li-Fraumeni Syndrome. Li-Fraumeni syndrome (LFS), now known to be associated with germ-line mutations in TP53, was first identified as a syndrome in 1969 in a description of four kindreds in which cousins or siblings had childhood soft-tissue sarcomas and other relatives had excessive cancer occurrence.[138] Subsequent epidemiologic efforts resulted in the enumeration of the major component neoplasms, including breast cancer, soft-tissue sarcomas and ostersarcomas, brain tumors, leukemias, and adrenalcortical carcinomas, with several additional tumor types likely to merit inclusion.[139,140] Segregation analysis of families identified through a family member with sarcoma confirmed the autosomal dominant pattern of transmission of cancer susceptibility, with age-specific penetrance functions estimated to reach 90 percent by age 70.[41] Nearly 30 percent of tumors in reported families occur before age 15 years.[140]

The pattern of breast cancer in LFS families is remarkable. Among 24 LFS families currently under study, 44 women have been diagnosed with breast cancer, of whom 77 percent were between ages 22 and 45 years (Li FP, Garber JE, unpublished data). Bilateral disease was documented in 25 percent of these women; 11 percent had additional primary tumors. It has been suggested that males may have later-onset tumors in LFS families because they to not get breast cancer, which is so dramatic among female LFS family members.

As was noted above, in 1990, germ-line mutations were identified in the p53 tumor suppressor gene (TP53) in affected members of LFS families.[142,143] Mutations were clustered in the conserved sequences of the gene (exons 5 through 9), an observation which was thought to increase the significance of these findings. Additional families meeting the classic criteria for the clinical syndrome of LFS have been evaluated for the presence of germ-line alterations in p53. Approximately 50 percent of such carefully defined families have had alterations identified in the p53 gene. While mutations are more frequently identified in hotspots within the conserved sequences, they have been seen throughout the gene.[144–148] p53 genes ostensibly normal by sequencing but abnormal in a functional assay or with regard to expression have also been observed.[149–150]

The prevalence of germ-line TP53 alterations among women diagnosed with breast cancer before age 40 has been estimated at less than 1 percent.[151,152] It is therefore a rare explanation for breast cancer occurrence in the population; nonetheless, p53 mutation screening formed the basis for the first predisposition testing programs for breast cancer susceptibility. However, the technical difficulties of p53 analysis, the low prevalence of TP53 mutations in the general population, and the profound psychological impact of such testing have kept this genetic test from widespread application. The role of TP53 in LFS and breast cancer is discussed further in Chap. 20.

Cowden Disease. Cowden disease, also known as the multiple hamartoma syndrome, is a rare autosomal dominant familial cancer syndrome that is characterized by an increased risk of breast cancer, genodermatosis, and multiple more variable clinical features. The most consistent and characteristic findings are mucocutaneous lesions, including multiple facial trichilemmomas, papillomatosis of the lips and oral mucosa, and acral keratoses. Vitiligo and angiomas also have been reported. The syndrome is inherited in an autosomal dominant mode with variable expressivity and complete penetrance of the dermatologic lesions by age 20.[153]

Benign proliferations in other organ systems are common in patients with Cowden disease, including thyroid goiter and adenomas, gastrointestinal polyps, uterine leiomyomas, and lipomas. Nonmalignant abnormalities of the breast are similarly noted in these patients and include fibroadenomas, fibrocystic lesions, areolar and nipple malformations, and ductal epithelial hyperplasia.[153–155] Central nervous system involvement was only recently recognized and includes megaencephaly, epilepsy, and gangliocytomas of the cerebellum.[156,157] (See Chap. 28.)

A marked increase in breast cancer incidence compared to the general population was observed in a series of recently published cases of Cowden disease.[155] Breast neoplasms occurred in 10 of the 21 female patients; the lesions were bilateral in 4 of these women. Lesions were said to be exclusively intraductal in 2 of the 10 women; however, given the fact that these are true precursor lesions, these intraductal carcinomas are likely to represent a manifestation of the underlying genetic defect. Additional cases of Cowden disease have been published, bringing the number of reported patients to 83, of whom 51 are female.[153] Thus, the total number of women with breast cancer and Cowden disease totals 15 (29 percent), with bilateral invasive tumors in 4 women. As many of the women in these families are still alive and at risk of developing breast cancer, the number of these women with breast cancer is likely to increase, increasing current estimates for the lifetime risk of developing breast cancer in women with this syndrome. However, increased recognition of Cowden disease could continue to disproportionately increase the number of Cowden patients without breast cancer and ultimately reduce estimates of the breast cancer rate. The gene for Cowden disease recently was mapped to chromosome 10q22-23 by linkage analysis of 12 families from four different countries.[158] The maximum two-point LOD score of 8.92 was achieved at D10S573. Multipoint analysis places the gene in a 5-c*M* region between D10S215 and D10S564. Haplotype analysis demonstrated that all 12 families were linked to this locus, indicating that Cowden disease is a single-gene disorder.

Muir-Torre Syndrome. Muir-Torre syndrome, a variant of Lynch syndrome type II, is the eponym given to the association between multiple skin tumors and multiple benign and malignant tumors of the upper and lower gastrointestinal and genitourinary tracts.[159,160] Many of the manifestations are common lesions (basal cell carcinomas, keratoacanthomas, colonic diverticula) which occur at younger ages but in a distribution similar to that in the general population. Inheritance of this syndrome is autosomal dominant, with high penetrance.[160] Females with the syndrome reportedly have an increased risk of breast cancer, particularly after menopause, although lifetime risk has not been calculated.[161] Four genes responsible for inherited forms of colon cancer not associated with polyposis recently were described, including MLH1 and MSH2, PMS1, and PMS2.[162–166] Mutations in these genes are thought to lead to the development of hereditary nonpolyposis colorectal cancer (HNPCC) through loss of the ability to repair damaged DNA, accumulation of replication errors, and genome instability. As various malignancies in Muir-Torre syndrome display microsatellite instability similar to that seen in colon cancer patients with HNPCC, it was postulated that mutations in one or more HNPCC-related genes may be the underlying defect in Muir-Torre syndrome. This observation was recently verified by linkage and mutation analysis demonstrating that mutations in MSH2 predispose to Muir-Torre syndrome.[167,168] A truncating mutation in MLH1 also has been detected in a Muir-Torre syndrome family.[169] Further discussion of the role of MLH1 and MSH2 in carcinogenesis is presented in Chap. 17.

Ataxia-telangiectasia. Ataxia-telangiectasia (AT) is an autosomal recessive disorder that is characterized by cerebellar ataxia, oculocutaneous telangiectasias, radiation hypersensitivity, and an increased incidence of malignancy. Chromosomal fragility and resultant DNA rearrangements are thought to result from the genetic defect which underlies the clinical syndrome of AT. AT is characterized by an autosomal recessive pattern of inheritance, with the complete clinical syndrome occurring only in homozygous individuals. Of note, AT homozygotes, accounting for 3 to 11 live births per million,[70] are estimated to have a risk of cancer which is 60 to 180 times greater than that of the general population,[171]; cancers observed in association with AT include non-Hodgkin lymphoma (nearly 100 percent lifetime risk) and a significant but lower risks of developing breast cancer, ovarian cancer, lymphocytic leukemia, and malignancies of the oral cavity, stomach, pancreas, and bladder. However, breast cancer risk in AT mutation carriers does not approach the risk observed in women with inherited mutations in p53, *BRCA1*, or *BRCA2*. Initially, reports of increased susceptibility to cancer were limited to homozygous AT mutation carriers, who represent approximately 0.2 to 0.7 percent of the general population in the United States.[171] However, a study published in 1987 suggested that AT heterozygotes, who do not display the typical neurologic findings seen in homozygotes, have a fivefold increased incidence of breast cancer.[172] This finding was particularly significant given that AT heterozygotes represent up to 7 percent of the general population[170] and that screening mammography, a source of ionizing radiation, could possibly contribute to the increased breast cancer incidence seen in this population. However, this study has been criticized for methodologic flaws including small sample size, inappropriateness of the control group, and lack of quantitation of radiation exposure. In addition, two groups have analyzed a total of 80 families with evidence for an inherited form of breast cancer for linkage between breast cancer and genetic markers flanking the AT locus on chromosome 11, finding strong evidence against this association.[173,174] Both groups concluded that the contribution of AT mutations to familial breast cancer is likely to be minimal. Nonetheless, as AT results from an alteration in the ability to repair DNA damage, the hypothesis that AT heterozygotes may have a decreased capacity to repair DNA could explain an increased susceptibility to cancer in such individuals. The AT gene (*ATM*) on human chromosome 11q22 has been identified[175] and is described in detail in Chap. 14. On the basis of preliminary work, it appears that heterozygote carriers of ATM mutations are not at significantly increased risk of developing breast cancer.

A summary of the clinical and genetic characteristics of the rare genetic syndromes associated with increased breast cancer risk is presented in Table 30-4.

Other Breast Cancer Susceptibility Loci

A large number of genes have been implicated in breast cancer tumorigenesis through identification of mutations in tumors, and several of these genes are discussed later in this chapter. Two genes, in addition to those described above, have been implicated in familial breast cancer susceptibility by identification of mutations that segregate with the disease in families or by linkage analysis. First, the ER has been suggested as a candidate locus for familial late-onset breast cancer susceptibility.[176] One extended family with eight women with late-onset breast cancer was identified with a single haplotype flanking the ER locus that consistently segregated with the disease, yielding a maximum LOD score of 1.85. The frequent expression of the estrogen receptor in breast cancer is associated with responsiveness to hormonal treatment and a favorable prognosis. Therefore, mutations in the ER might modify the hormonal response in breast epithelium and potentially result in inherited susceptibility to breast cancer. However, no mutations associated with inherited cancer have been identified in the ER, although several somatic mutations have been identified in breast cancer biopsies and established breast cancer cell lines.[177]

Another breast cancer susceptibility locus has been proposed on chromosome 8p12-22,[178] based on linkage analysis of several

Table 30-4 Rare Causes of Inherited Breast Cancer Syndromes

Syndrome	Clinical Manifestations	Genetic Mutation	Mode of Inheritance
Li-Fraumeni syndrome	Breast cancer, sarcoma, brain tumors, leukemia, adrenocortical carcinoma	TP53	Autosomal dominant
Cowden disease	Multiple mucocutaneous lesions, vitiligo, angiomas, benign proliferative disease of multiple organ systems, breast cancer, thyroid cancer, colonic neoplasms	Locus on chromosome 10q22-23	Autosomal dominant
Muir-Torre syndrome	Cancers of the GI tract, skin, GU system and breast (benign and malignant)	*MSH2, MLH1*	Autosomal dominant
Peutz-Jeghers syndrome	Abnormal melanin deposits, GI polyposis, cancers of the GI tract, breast, uterus, ovary, and testis	Unknown	Autosomal dominant
Ataxia-telangectasia	Cerebellar ataxia, oculocutaneous telangectasias, radiation hypersensitivity, leukemia, lymphoma, and numerous solid tumors, including breast	ATM	Autosomal recessive

breast cancer families with polymorphic genetic markers on chromosome 8p. This analysis yielded a maximum LOD score of 2.51 using the polymorphic markers NEFL and D8S259. Several groups have attempted to preproduce this result, with little success. However, the region is thought to harbor tumor-suppressor genes involved in sporadic prostate cancer[179] and sporadic breast tumors,[178] as defined by LOH studies. Studies of male breast tumors identified 83 percent LOH at one marker on chromosome 8p and two distinct regions of loss on chromosome 8p12-21.3 and 8p22.[180] These data suggest that a tumor-suppressor gene functioning as an inherited susceptibility gene may be involved in breast cancer pathogenesis in a small subset of families, especially those with cases of male breast cancer. As whole-genome linkage studies commence in an effort to identify other familial breast cancer susceptibility genes, the 8p12-22 region will be at the forefront as a strong candidate locus.

SOMATIC ALTERATIONS IN BREAST CANCER

Another approach to understanding the pathogenesis of breast cancer is the study of noninherited (sporadic) breast cancers. This is an important complementary approach to the study of germ-line alterations for several reasons. First, the large majority of breast cancers do not arise as a result of inherited mutations in breast cancer susceptibility genes, and sporadic tumors may have fundamental molecular genetic differences. Second, genes that are frequently dysregulated or mutated in sporadic breast cancer are candidate genes for susceptibility loci, as was demonstrated with p53 and LFS. Third, the study of genetic alterations per se, such as mutations, deletions, and amplifications, provides clues to the mechanisms that result in the genomic instability which is inherent in cancer cells. This section provides a summary of chromosomal regions commonly deleted in breast cancer (resulting in loss of heterozygosity) as well as an overview of genes that are mutated or dysregulated in sporadic breast cancers. Some of these genetic alterations have been identified as markers of particularly aggressive tumor behavior, while a few have become potential therapeutic targets. A summary of the genes altered in sporadic breast cancers is in Table 30-5.

Loss of Heterozygosity

Loss of heterozygosity (LOH) has long been associated with the presence of tumor-suppressor genes in DNA because the analysis of many tumors has demonstrated that the wild-type allele of a mutated tumor-suppressor gene is often lost during tumorigenesis. In the case of germ-line mutations in tumor-suppressor genes, as suggested by Knudsen's "two-hit hypothesis,"[181] individuals from "cancer families" inherit an inactivating mutation in one allele of the implicated tumor-suppressor gene in all cells. Therefore, only one somatic event is required to inactivate the remaining copy, making the development of cancer a much more common event than it is in individuals born without the "first hit." The mechanism by which LOH occurs is not known, but the end result is physical deletion of large regions of chromosomes. LOH has been studied in detail in sporadic and familial breast tumors, resulting in the identification of many putative tumor-suppressor loci. A subset of these loci are likely to function as inherited breast cancer susceptibility loci.

The most common regions of LOH in breast cancer are located on chromosomes 17p, 17q, 16q, 13q, 11p, 1p, 3p, and 18q.[182–184]

Table 30-5 Somatic Alterations in Breast Cancer

Gene/Region	Modification	Frequency	Reference
Growth factors and receptors			
EGFR	Overexpression	20–40	201, 202
HER-2/neu	Overexpression	20–40	199, 203, 204
FGF1/FGF4	Overexpression	20–30	216
TGF-α	Overexpression	Not reported	213
Intracellular signaling molecules			
Ha-*ras*	Mutation	5–10	220
c-*src*	Overexpression	50–70	225
Regulators of cell cycle			
TP53	Mutation/ inactivation	30–40	230, 231, 236
RB1	Inactivation	20	244, 245
Cyclin D	Overexpression	35–45	247, 249, 250
TGF-β	Dysregulation	Not reported	257, 259, 261, 262
Adhesion molecules and proteases			
E-cadherin	Reduced/absent expression	60–70	275, 276
P-cadherin	Reduced/absent expression	30	276
Cathepsin D	Overexpression	20–24	287, 288
MMPs	Increased expression	20–80	281, 282
Other genes			
bcl-2	Overexpression	30–45	266, 267
c-*myc*	Amplification	5–20	270, 271
nm23 (NME1)	Decreased expression	Not reported	292, 293

Many other loci have been identified. The 17q LOH region was originally thought to harbor the *BRCA1* gene, but more complete analysis has identified at least three independent regions on chromosome 17q, only one of which contains *BRCA1*.[185–187] LOH also has been associated with the *BRCA2* gene on chromosome 13q12-13. These data demonstrate that the known inherited susceptibility genes are associated with LOH in tumors and that other susceptibility genes might be isolated from other LOH regions.

The 17p LOH region can be divided into two separate loci, one containing TP53 on 17p13.1 and a second more distal region on 17p13.3.[188] Studies of chromosome 1 also have identified multiple regions of loss on 1p13, 1p22, and 1p31.2-32.2.[189] Three regions of LOH have been identified on chromosome 11 at 11p15.5, 11q13, and 11q22-qter with 19 percent, 23 percent, and 37 to 43 percent LOH, respectively, demonstrated in a group of breast tumors. Significant association between LOH on chromosomes 11p15, 17q21, and 3p also has been detected, suggesting that the putative tumor-suppressor genes at these loci may function together in a tumorigenic pathway.[184] LOH has been detected on chromosome 16q22.1 and 16q22.4-qter in a large number of breast tumors[190]; this is of interest, as chromosome 16q is the location of the E-cadherin gene, which has been implicated in sporadic breast cancer. Further discussion of the role of E-cadherin in breast cancer can be found below. Finally, an association has been seen between LOH on chromosome 9p, 3p, and 6q,[191] suggesting the existence of a tumorigenic pathway involving all these loci. Another example of cooperativity between distant loci was reported by Smith and colleagues,[192] who analyzed 133 breast cancers for TP53 mutations and LOH on 13 chromosome arms. In this series, TP53 mutations were strongly associated with LOH at two specific loci: 3p24-26 ($p <0.001$) and 7q31 ($p <0.05$). Surprisingly, there was no association between TP53 mutations and LOH at 17p, the site of the p53 gene, suggesting that breast cancers frequently have only one defective TP53 allele.

Many sites of LOH correspond with the location of known tumor-suppressor genes. Examples include the *DCC* gene on chromosome 18q, with 52 percent LOH in breast tumors,[193] and the *APC* gene on chromosome 5q21.[194] These genes have been screened for mutations in familial breast cancer samples, and none have been identified, seemingly eliminating these LOH regions as candidate loci for inherited susceptibility genes. However, it is possible that tumor-suppressor genes other than *DCC* and *APC* exist in these locations.

Recently, investigators began analyzing atypical ductal hyperplasia, precancerous lesion of the breast, for LOH, which has been demonstrated on chromosomes 16q and 17p in these lesions.[195] Analysis of DCIS, a malignant but noninvasive lesion of the breast, resulted in the identification of LOH on chromosomes 8p, 13q, 16q, 17p, and 17q.[196] These results suggest that known genes such as *BRCA1*, *BRCA2*, and p53 or unknown tumor-suppressor genes in these chromosomal regions are altered as the first steps in breast tumorigenesis and may provide clues to the location of additional breast cancer susceptibility genes. LOH in breast cancer also has been tracked in stages from primary tumors to the onset of metastasis, demonstrating LOH on chromosome 7q31 at all stages,[197] suggesting that LOH of chromosome 7q31 is another early event in breast tumorigenesis.

Growth Factor Receptors

An important class of genes frequently altered in sporadic breast cancer are members of the epidermal growth factor receptor (EGFR) family of growth factor receptors. The members of this family of proto-oncogenes (EGFR, erbB-2 or HER-2/neu, erbB-3, and erbB-4) all share extensive homology and encode transmembrane glycoproteins with tyrosine kinase activity. They become oncogenic through gene amplification or overexpression at the mRNA and protein levels, leading to aberrations in signal transduction pathways and deregulation of cellular proliferation.[198] All the members of this family have been described as overexpressed in breast carcinoma; the most extensively studied receptors, EGFR and erbB-2 are known to be overexpressed in 20 to 40 percent of breast cancers.[199–204]

Recent work has revealed a complex system of interaction between the various members of the EGFR family as well as cross-regulation between growth factor-activated signal transduction pathways and estrogen-responsive pathways. For example, estrogen receptor-positive (ER+) breast cancer cell lines that overexpress erbB-2 demonstrate decreased erbB-2 protein expression in response to treatment with estradiol or EGF.[205] The erbB-2 pathway also has been linked to the *ras* oncogene signal transduction pathway,[206] suggesting that cooperation between various oncogenes may be important in breast tumorigenesis.

Overexpression of erbB-2 has been associated with a less favorable prognosis in patients with breast cancer, particularly in tumors with involvement of axillary lymph nodes.[203,207,208] It also has been reported that overexpression of erbB-2 identifies a subgroup of patients who are more resistant to chemotherapy, and a recent study suggested that higher doses of chemotherapy with regimens containing doxorubicin can in part overcome this effect.[209] In addition, ER+ patients who overexpress erbB-2 are less likely to have a clinically significant response to the estrogen antagonist tamoxifen and have overall shorter survival than do patients with ER+, erbB-2-negative tumors.[210] Finally, evidence is accumulating that

down-regulation of erbB-2 protein levels with monoclonal antibodies or antisense oligonucleotides may be useful therapeutically. p185HER2 monoclonal antibodies have antiproliferative effects in vitro on cells that overexpress erbB-2 and sensitize human breast cancer cells to tumor necrosis factor.[211] In addition, erbB-2 antisense oligonucleotides[212] can inhibit the proliferation of breast cancer cells.

Of note, the well-described growth factor TGF-α is a member of the EGF family and is a ligand for EGFR. Elevated expression of TGF-α has been consistently associated with neoplastic transformation, with transgenic mouse models providing direct evidence for the role of TGF-α in malignant transformation of breast epithelium. In this regard, metallothionein-directed expression of TGF-α in transgenic mice and constitutive TGF-α expression promote uniform epithelial hyperplasia of several organs and induce postlactational secretory mammary adenocarcinomas.[213]

The fibroblast growth factors (FGFs) and their receptors (FGFRs) also are thought to play a role in breast cancer. However, as specific genetic alterations (such as duplication) in FGFs or FGFRs have not been reported in breast tumors, their causal role in breast tumorigenesis is less clear than that of EGFR or HER-2/neu. This large group of proteins may be involved in cell transformation by deregulated activation of a receptor tyrosine kinase through an autocrine mechanism. Acidic FGF (FGF1) and basic FGF (FGF2) initially were identified as heparin-binding growth factors that stimulate the proliferation of vascular endothelium. They are expressed in a number of tumors and have strong angiogenic properties.[214,215] FGF3, initially identified as int-2 because it is activated by the insertion of murine mammary tumor provirus, is associated with the transformation of murine mammary epithelium. At least nine FGFs and four FGFRs have been identified. A recent study of seven of the nine known family members and all four known receptors in a panel of 10 tumor cell lines and 103 breast tumor samples provided evidence for FGF1 and FGF2 expression in almost all samples as well as limited expression of FGF5, FGF6, FGF7, and FGF9, FGF3 was not expressed in any sample; FGF4 and FGF8 were not assayed. FGFR1 and FGFR4 were expressed at high levels in 22 percent and 32 percent of samples, respectively.[216]

Intracellular Signaling Molecules

While it is clear that overexpression and/or mutation of mediators of intracellular signaling play a key role in malignant transformation, relatively little work has focused on the specific role of these molecules in the development of breast cancer. However, recent work suggests that dysregulation of several signaling pathways intersects directly with many breast cancer-related proteins, such as the receptor tyrosine kinases. The proto-oncogene Ha-*ras* is the most extensively studied example of the involvement of signaling pathways in breast cancer development. Additionally, work in the past few years has produced evidence that rare Ha-*ras* alleles are associated with inherited susceptibility to breast cancer.[217] More recent work suggests that these rare alleles may be associated with altered penetrance of the major breast cancer susceptibility gene, *BRCA1*.[218] However, the mechanism underlying this association remains unclear. Some investigators have suggested that the presence of the rare alleles is a marker of genomic instability that predisposes to cancer, while others have suggested that function may be altered by changes in *ras* regulatory regions or that mutations in genes in close physical proximity to the Ha-*ras* locus, which are therefore genetically linked, may be the underlying cause of the increase in cancer susceptibility associated with these alleles.

Experimental models have been used to determine whether chemically induced breast neoplasia is associated with Ha-*ras* changes. Using the spontaneously immortalized but nontransformed breast line MCF10A, loss of one Ha-*ras* allele and induction of a mutation in the remaining allele at the first position of codon 12[219] have been observed after carcinogen exposure. These changes were associated with the ability of these cells to form colonies in soft agar but not with the emergence of tumorigenesis in animals.

There is evidence that while *ras* coding region mutations occur in less than 10 percent of breast cancers, the pathway *ras* services may be deregulated in breast cancer more frequently. Bland and colleagues examined 85 breast cancer specimens with immunohistochemical staining for the presence of multiple oncogene products, including Ha-*ras*, and correlated the results with the clinical outcome.[220] The oncogenes with the strongest prognostic correlation to survival were Ha-*ras* and c-*fos*. Coexpression of c-*myc* and Ha-*ras* with c-*fos* also correlated with an increased likelihood of recurrence and decreased survival. Other studies also suggested cooperativity between Ha-*ras* and both rat c-erbB-2 and human TGF-α[221] in transformation but similarly demonstrated that additional genetic changes are required for a fully tumorigenic phenotype. Finally, a linking has been established between the expression of Ha-*ras* and the appearance of the multidrug resistance phenotype. Transfection of the breast cell line MCF-10A with c-Ha-*ras* and c-erbB-2 results in up-regulation of the *mdr-1* gene (multidrug resistance-1), appearance of the protein product on the cell surface, and the multidrug resistance phenotype.[222] Transfection with either proto-oncogene alone has no effect, strongly suggesting cooperativity. As was noted above, the association between c-erbB-2 expression and breast cancer prognosis has been investigated extensively, and recent work suggests that erbB-2 expression may correlate with Ha-*ras* expression.[223] Interestingly, in this study, if chemotherapy is included in the model, tumors coexpressing Ha-*ras* and c-erbB-2 are less responsive to both chemotherapy and the partial estrogen antagonist tamoxifen.

The signaling pathway involving the proto-oncogene c-*src* also has been linked to genetic alterations in breast cancer. Specifically, the phosphotyrosine residues of receptor tyrosine kinases serve as binding sites for proteins that contain SRC homology 2 (SH2) domains. Using glutathione-*S*-transferase fusion proteins containing the SH2 region, it has been demonstrated that in human breast carcinoma cell lines the SH2 domain binds to activated EGFR and to p185her2/neu. These investigators also have shown that endogenous pp60c-*src* is tightly associated with tyrosine-phosphorylated EGFR, raising the possibility that this association may be an integral part of malignant transformation of breast epithelium.[224] In a related study, protein tyrosine kinase activity was assayed in 72 primary breast cancer specimens; increased activity compared to normal breast tissue was identified in all 72 samples. In this study, at least 70 percent of the cytosolic protein tyrosine kinase activity originated from the presence of the c-*src* oncogene product.[225] Since cytosolic protein tyrosine kinase activity parallels malignancy in breast tumors[226] and since most of this activity is precipitated by anti-*src* antibodies, it appears likely c-*src* plays a significant role in the manifestation of breast cancer.[225]

Regulators of the Cell Cycle

Accumulating evidence indicates that derangements in the protein machinery that normally regulates passage through the cell cycle are critical contributors to uncontrolled cell growth and cancer.[227,228] TP53 (encoding p53) was initially regarded as a tumor-suppressor gene that is deleted or mutated in a large number of human tumors from a variety of tissue types. p53 was known to have DNA-binding and transcriptional activation domains, and more recent work has established that p53 plays a central role in regulating progression through the cell cycle. The strongest link between

TP53 mutations and breast cancer comes from the increased incidence of early-onset breast cancer seen in LFS, the family cancer syndrome caused by germ-line alterations in TP53.[142] Additional evidence for the involvement of TP53 in breast cancer comes from studies demonstrating decreased ability to form tumors in nude mice and reduced capacity for growth in soft agar when wild-type TP53 in a retroviral vector is introduced into breast cancer cell lines with mutated TP53. Alterations in TP53 in breast cancer may be detected by analyzing the coding region for mutations[229,230] or in some cases by using antibody demonstrating aberrant localization or altered levels of p53. TP53 mutations have been detected in 15 to 45 percent of human breast cancer specimens in several studies.[231-234] Of note, several groups have investigated racial differences in the TP53 mutations found in breast cancer. While striking differences between Caucasian and African-American patients in the type and/or frequency of TP53 mutations have not been reported, significantly lower survival rates have been reported in association with TP53 mutations in black patients compared to white patients (four- to fivefold excess death rate, $p = 0.012$).[235]

Interestingly, TP53 mutations do not appear to be evenly distributed among the various histologic types of breast cancer. In one series, 148 human breast cancers were surveyed for TP53 mutations, with mutations identified in 39 percent of medullary cancers and 26 percent of invasive ductal lesions but only 12 percent of invasive lobular cancers. No TP53 mutations were detected in the 19 mucinous and 8 papillary carcinomas examined.[236] In all studies where survival data were available, TP53 mutations were associated with a significantly poorer prognosis. Finally, TP53 mutations have been reported in approximately 15 percent of DCIS lesions.[233]

In addition to mutations, alterations in the subcellular location of p53 have been noted in breast cancer specimens compared to normal breast epithelium. In an analysis of 27 breast cancers, sequestration of p53 in the cytoplasm was demonstrated in 37 percent of the breast cancers analyzed, overexpression of nuclear p53 in another 30 percent of tumors, and complete lack of staining in the remaining 33 percent.[237] While other studies have not found p53 alteration in all samples studied, these data suggest that p53 alterations are among the most common genetic changes found in breast carcinoma.

The relationship between TP53 mutations and the chemoresistance of breast cancer cells was initially suggested by a report hinting that specific mutations in the DNA-binding domain of p53 lead to primary resistance to doxorubicin, one of the most widely used and effective chemotherapeutic agents for breast cancer.[238] In this study, 11 of 63 tumors had mutations in this region. Four of these 11 patients progressed on doxorubicin, as opposed to only 2 of 52 patients without p53 DNA-binding region mutations. Among the patients with p53 DNA-binding-domain mutations who did respond to doxorubicin, most relapsed within 3 months of treatment. Similar data were reported in a second study reporting a smaller benefit from chemotherapy, hormonal therapy, and radiation in patients with tumors harboring TP53 mutations.[239]

The retinoblastoma tumor-suppressor gene (*RB1*) appears to play a role in breast tumorigenesis in at least a proportion of cases; however, *RB1* has not been as well characterized in breast cancer as TP53. Like p53, RB regulates cell cycle progression, with dephosphorylated RB acting to halt cell cycle progression in G1. The link between *RB1* and breast cancer was first suggested by studies demonstrating structural rearrangements and inactivation of *RB1* in breast cancer.[240,241] This observation was followed by work demonstrating that estradiol decreases expression of RB, fueling speculation that estrogen may act as a tumor promoter by decreasing expression of critical tumor-suppressor genes.[242] Further evidence for the role of *RB1* in breast cancer was provided by demonstration that, using retroviral-mediated gene transfer, wild-type *RB1* introduced into breast cancer cells with a known *RB1* mutation results in decreased tumorgenicity in nude mice and a reduction in anchorage-independent growth.[243]

Current estimates suggest that *RB1* may be activated in approximately 20 percent of breast cancers.[244] One group of investigators described the incidence of *RB1* alterations in 96 primary breast cancers and related their findings to patient and tumor characteristics as well as oncogene amplifications and TP53 mutations.[245] In this series, *RB1* alterations were found to occur more frequently in ER+ tumors and less frequently in tumors with her2/neu or c-*myc* amplification. *RB1* alterations were associated with small (<2cm) tumors without axillary node involvement. In contrast, a study of 197 breast cancer specimens using immunohistochemistry to evaluate the expression of *RB1*[246] suggested that loss of *RB1* expression was correlated with the presence of axillary nodal metastasis; however, neither group of investigators was able to demonstrate a correlation with relapse-free or overall survival.

Various cyclins accumulate at different checkpoints and complex with cdks. Binding of a cdk to a specific cyclin partner activates the kinase activity of the cdk, which in turn phosphorylates and activates downstream target proteins that are necessary to propel the cell into the next phase of the cell cycle.[227,228] Overproduction of cyclins and cdks or their presence at an inappropriate time would be expected to cause unregulated cell division. Consequently, these molecules are candidate proto-oncogenes. In one of the first studies of the role of cyclins in breast carcinoma, 20 breast cancer cell lines were assayed for expression of cyclin A, B1, C, D1, D2, D3, and E; increased expression of one or more cyclins was demonstrated in 7 of 20 lines (35 percent). Five of the seven displayed increased expression of cyclin D1. This group also noted cyclin D1 overexpression in 45 percent of 124 primary breast cancers.[247] Cyclin D1, which regulates the G1–S transition, was recently identified as the *PRAD1* oncogene located at chromosome 11q13.[248] Cyclin D1 overexpression appears to be a relatively early event in tumor development.[249,250] Evidence for the early involvement of cyclin D in breast cancer was provided by Steeg and colleagues, who demonstrated cyclin D1 overexpression in early 18 percent of benign breast lesions but in 76 percent of low-grade DCIS, 87 percent of high-grade DCIS, and 83 percent of infiltrating ductal cancers.[251] Induced expression of cyclin D1 in breast cancer cells leads to an increase in the proportion of cells progressing through G1 and removes the requirement for growth factor stimulation normally necessary for completion of the cell cycle.[252] A more recent analysis of cyclin D1-null mutant mice provides an interesting and not unexpected link with mammary development, as these mice do not undergo the massive mammary epithelial proliferation associated with pregnancy despite a normal ovarian hormone response.[254]

The growth inhibitory protein of TGF-β is thought to exert its effect on cell growth through inhibition of cell cycle progression. Because a number of tumorigenic cell lines have lost responsiveness to TGF-β, it is believed to play a role in tumor supression, with malignant transformation being partially dependent on the loss of TGF-β expression or function. The growth inhibitory effects of TGF-β are initiated by binding to cell surface TGF-β receptors. After ligand/receptor binding, multiple molecular targets have been suggested, including down-regulation of c-*myc* and cyclin expression, accumulation of hypophosphorylated RB, and inactivation of cdk2 and cdk4.[255] Work in this area is ongoing, but any one of these effects could potentially result in G1 arrest. Of particular interest in regard to breast cancer, TGF-β is hormonally regulated. Jeng and colleagues demonstrated that TGF-β isoforms are differentially regulated,[256] with TGF-β2 and TGF-β3 levels being suppressed by estrogen, with little effect on TGF-β1 levels. While early work suggested that TGF-β (isoforms not specified) is induced to high levels by the growth inhibitory estrogen antagonist tamoxifen,[257] later work demonstrated that short exposure (6 h) to tamoxifen resulted in a slight decrease in TGF-β1 protein whereas longer exposure had

no effect. Thus, the increase in unfractionated TGF-β in response to tamoxifen probably is due to increases in TGF-β2 and/or TGF-β3.[258] Paradoxically, while TGF-β is a strong growth inhibitor of normal mammary tissue, recent evidence suggests that enhanced TGF-β secretion correlates with aggressive malignant behavior. This was first demonstrated with the growth stimulatory effect of TGF-β1 on the breast cancer cell lines T47D and MCF-7.[259] In support of these studies, the breast cancer cell line MCF-7 transfected with TGF-β1 cDNA formed tumors in ovariectomized mice in the absence of estrogen supplementation, while the parental MCF-7 cells did not.[260] Prominent TGF-β1 expression also has been associated with axillary lymph node metastases ($p = 0.015$), but this association was not found in tumors that expressed both TGF-β1 and TGF-β2.[261] In a study of 50 breast cancers, one group reported that 90 percent expressed TGF-β1, 78 percent expressed TGF-β2, and 94 percent expressed TGF-β3, with 74 percent of the tumors expressing all three isoforms. Expression of all three isoforms was more likely to be associated with lymph node metastases than with the expression of one or two isoforms ($p = 0.025$).[262] However, other studies have not confirmed the usefulness of TGF-β expression as a prognostic factor in breast cancer.[263]

Regulators of Apoptosis

Apoptosis, the genetically programmed process of active (energy-requiring) cell death, is clearly important in understanding both neoplastic transformation and resistance to cytotoxic chemotherapy in breast cancer. Apoptosis can be induced by a variety of stimuli, including withdrawal of growth factors, DNA damage, viral infection, and expression of p53.[264] As emerging evidence suggests that cytotoxic chemotherapy may exert a major effect on cancer cells by inducing apoptosis in response to chemotherapy-induced DNA damage, resistance to chemotherapy in some cases may result from inhibition of the apoptotic response.[265]

The proto-oncogene *bcl-2*, which normally functions to suppress apoptosis in a variety of cell types, has been studied extensively in several human cancers, including breast carcinoma, where it is overexpressed in 30 to 45 percent of cases.[266,267] *bcl-2* expression in human breast tissue varies dramatically throughout the menstrual cycle, suggesting that *bcl-2* regulation is hormone-dependent.[268] Consistent with this hypothesis is the finding that *bcl-2* expression is increased in ER+ tumors and further increases after treatment with tamoxifen.[266] Conversely, *bcl-2* expression is down-regulated in tumors expressing aberrant p53.[269] However, no genetic alterations that would increase *bcl-2* levels have been reported in breast cancers.

c-myc

Numerous investigators have examined the role of the c-*myc* proto-oncogene in breast cancer, with variable results. c-*myc* amplification was examined in 89 Norwegian breast cancer patients without axillary node involvement; amplification was noted in only one tumor.[270] However, another group used immunohistochemical methods to study 206 breast carcinomas and reported nuclear staining in 12 percent and cytoplasmic staining in 95 percent of these tumors. The presence of cytoplasmic staining was associated with increased disease-free survial compared to patients with tumors where c-*myc* was detected in the nucleus.[271] Finally, a study of 42 invasive breast cancers and 11 normal breast tissues suggested that while c-*myc*, as detected by immunohistochemistry, was present in both normal and malignant tissues, the level of expression in tumors was higher than it was in normal breast tissue.[272]

Cell Adhesion Molecules

Normal mammary epithelial cells are arranged in two layers: (1) a luminal epithelium and (2) a basal layer composed of myoepithelial cells and a small number of basal or stem cells. The basal layer is highly proliferative and is in direct contact with the basement membrane. During mammary carcinogenesis, tumor cells must escape normal adhesion mechanisms and traverse the basement membrane to invade surrounding structures. In this setting, interactions between breast carcinoma cells and their microenvironment are important determinants of the growth, invasion, and metastatic potential of tumor cells. In an effort to elucidate these interactions, researchers have investigated cell adhesion mechanism, proteolytic enzymes, and the paracrine stimulation of growth factor receptors.[273]

Several factors participate in the maintenance of normal cell–cell and cell–matrix interactions. Cell–cell interactions are mediated via desmosomes and cadherin-containing junctions. In adult breast tissue, E-cadherin is expressed in normal ductal epithelial cells, and a reduction in E-cadherin expression is being investigated as a possible marker of invasive and metastatic potential. P-cadherin normally is expressed only in embryonal cells and in the basal layer of the adult epithelium. In examining cell–cell interactions, one study of 11 cases of invasive breast carcinoma suggested that in histologically normal areas, myoepithelial cells contain higher levels of cell-matrix adhesion molecules than do luminal epithelial cells.[274] In these normal areas, both myoepithelial and luminal cells have cadherin-containing junctions necessary for cell–cell interactions. In regions containing invasive carcinoma, normal E-cadherin staining was maintained in 10 of 11 cases but α-catenin, the cytoplasmic component of E-cadherin-mediated junctions, was down-regulated or was distributed in an irregular punctate pattern. Similar findings were reported in a study of 26 primary breast carcinomas, in which E-cadherin expression was decreased or lost in 63 percent of cases and α-catenin was reduced or absent in 81 percent of cases.[275,] In this study, all patients with known metastatic disease at the time of biopsy had abnormal α-catenin staining, suggesting a role for α-catenin in maintaining normal cell–cell interactions. In keeping with other studies, expression of both E- and P-cadherin in 57 invasive breast carcinomas was noted to be altered, with reduce E-cadherin expression in 67 percent of tumors and abnormal P-cadherin in the luminal cells of 30 percent of invasive carcinomas.[276] All specimens with abnormal P-cadherin staining were histologic grade III and also revealed decreased E-cadherin expression. Of note, while an earlier study observed P-cadherin expression in lobular carcinomas of all grades,[277] P-cadherin expression in ductal carcinomas has been limited to high-grade lesions. These findings suggest that in some aggressive breast carcinomas, decreased or absent E-cadherin may be replaced by P-cadherin. This association between reduced E-cadherin staining and an aggressive histologic appearance also was noted in 109 patients with invasive ductal carcinomas, with an association between reduced E-cadherin expression and reduced disease-free survival in univariate analysis (5-year DFS = 70 percent in the E-cadherin positive group; DFS = 38 percent in the reduced E-cadherin group; p = 0.027).[278] However, longer follow-up and further validation will be required to determine whether E-cadherin is an independent predictor of disease prognosis.

Matrix Metalloproteinases

Extracellular proteinases are believed to be important in modulating both cell–matrix interactions and the degradation of the basement membrane necessary for invasion and metastasis. The matrix metalloproteinases (MMPs) include the gelatinases MMP-2 (gelatinase A) and MMP-9 (gelatinase B). The gelatinases, which are secreted as zymogens and are activated by cell membrane-associated proteins, have specific activity against type IV collagen, a component of the basement membrane.[279] This collagenase activity, the results of specific inhibition studies, and higher levels of immunostaining in invasive breast cancers (relative to preinvasive cancers) implicate these MMPs in tumor invasiveness.[273,280] Membrane-type metalloproteinase (MT-MMP), another member of the MMP family, has been postulated to be the membrane-associated activator of MMP-2. The inhibitory component of this pathway consists of tissue inhibitors of metalloproteinase (TIMP-1 and 2). TIMPs are believed to exert their inhibitory activity by direct binding with the activated MMPs.

In an analysis of MMP-8, MMP-9, and TIMP-1 expression in breast cancer cells, protein levels were measured in the tumor tissue of 53 breast cancer patients.[281] MMP-8 and MMP-9 appeared to be coordinately regulated, and both were elevated in invasive tumors. However, increased levels of the MMP inhibitor TIMP-1 also were found in association with increased levels of the MMPs. These findings do not support earlier data suggesting that metastatic potential is associated with decreased TIMP-1 expression.

Of great interest is whether these proteases are produced by tumor cells or surrounding "normal" stromal cells and, if they are produced by stromal cells, whether the tumor cells are able to induce the expression of proteases. In an attempt to address this question, in situ hybridization was used to demonstrate that MT-MMP mRNA was expressed exclusively in the stromal cells in 83 of 83 human tumor specimens (including breast) analyzed.[282] In contrast, using an antibody directed against MT-MMP, protein was detected on the surface of invasive carcinoma cells.[283] This apparent discrepancy also has been described for MMP-2, with MMP-2 mRNA detected in tumor fibroblasts but MMP-2 protein detected in carcinoma cells.[284] Taken together with earlier studies suggesting that conditioned media or the membrane fraction from breast carcinoma lines up-regulates the expression of MMP-2 in fibroblasts,[285,286] these findings suggest close interaction between tumor and stromal cells. An unifying hypothesis is that both MT-MMP and MMP-2 are produced in peritumor fibroblasts in response to the paracrine stimulation of carcinoma cells, that MT-MMP may activate MMP-2 on the stromal cell membrane, that the enzymes are secreted into the extracellular matrix, that each binds to the surface of malignant cells, and that one or both enzymes may subsequently be internalized by tumor cells.

Cathepsins

The cathepsins are another class of proteases that may affect the invasive and metastatic potential of malignant cells. These proteins are expressed at low levels in all cells, and once they are autoactivated, they have enzymatic activity against several matrix proteins, including those in the basement membrane. Levels of cathepsin expression in breast cancer have been studied as possible prognostic markers. Cathepsin D expression has been examined by immunostaining of 151 breast carcinomas, with "strong" cathepsin D expression detected in 22 percent of cases, correlating with the nonductal histologic type (p = 0.0243) and metastases at the time of diagnosis (p = 0.0068) but not with tumor size, histologic grade, lymph node metastases, or ER/PR status. On univariate analysis, "strong" cathepsin D staining appeared to predict a significantly worse prognosis (median survival = 40 months in high-cathepsin D group, median survival not yet reached at 140 months of follow-up in low-cathepsin D group; p = 0.047). In multivariate analysis, however, no significant correlation between "strong" cathepsin D staining and prognosis persisted after adjusting for other known prognostic markers.[287] The relationship between cathepsin D and other pathologic features has been investigated in a large series of 1752 primary breast cancer patients. In this study, cathepsin D was associated with tumor size and grade and the presence or absence of nodal metastasis. On multivariate analysis performed on 489 patients from this series, cathepsin D independently predicted relapse-free survival and overall survival.[288] While the reason for the discrepancy between the findings of these two studies is not clear; it may be that the scoring of the intensity of cathepsin D staining as a continuous variable and the larger sample size of later study allowed detection of the prognostic significance of this marker.

Mediators of Metastasis

In addition to the well-characterized cell adhesion molecules and matrix metalloproteases that are thought to play a role in the development of metastatic breast cancer, *NME1* (encoding nm23) is a gene that is difficult to characterize with regard to its normal function and as result of decreased expression.[289] NME1 was initially isolated as a gene which is differentially expressed in melanoma cells with discrepant metastatic potential.[290] The highest level of nm23 expression is seen in cells with low metastatic potential. Shortly after the isolation of *NME1*, data were presented suggesting that *NME1* is differentially expressed in human breast cancers, with low *NME1* mRNA levels found in association with histopathologic indicators of high metastatic potential.[291] These data are supported by studies demonstrating that transfection of *NME1* into human MDA-MB-435 breast carcinoma cells reduces the metastatic potential of these cells when injected into the mammary fat pad of mice. Reduction in metastatic potential was associated with decreased ability of cells to form colonies in soft agar and an altered response to TGF-β.[292] Murine developmental studies also demonstrated a role for nm23 in the functional differentiation of the mammary gland. In this study, *NME1* expression increased with functional differentiation of the mammary gland in nulliparous and pregnant animals.[293] Howlett and colleagues subsequently demonstrated a link between nm23 and human breast epithelial differentiation by using a culture system designed to mimic breast stroma. In this system, transfected breast cancer cell lines that overexpressed nm23 regained several aspects of the normal phenotype, including acinar formation, basement membrane production, and eventual growth arrest.[294] In investigations of the biologic function of NME1, it became clear that this gene is identical to PUF, a factor known to alter *myc* transcription in vitro.[295] However, data suggesting that nm23 can function as a growth inhibitor[294] led to confusion about how nm23 can be both a tumor suppressor and an activator of the proto-oncogene c-*myc*. It is possible that this is due to a tissue-specific effect, as *NME1* expression is increased in aggressive neuroblastomas but is reduced in aggressive breast cancers.[296]

CLINICAL IMPLICATIONS OF BREAST CANCER SUSCEPTIBILITY

As was discussed in this chapter, advances in molecular genetics have provided data that allow risk estimation for women with inherited mutations in dominant cancer susceptibility genes and prognostic determinations for women with sporadic breast cancer. Unfortunately, our ability to make clinically useful interventions on the basis of these data remains limited. Studies which allow an estimation of risk reduction from prophylactic surgical intervention are essentially unavailable, and the science of chemoprevention is in its infancy. There are limited data available to assess the efficacy of enhanced surveillance programs for individuals at high risk of developing breast cancer. Finally, there is little information available about the interaction of multiple risk factors, and so recommendations regarding modification of exposure to hormonal agents or dietary changes in the face of increased breast cancer risk caused by family history may be premature. Thus, in counseling women at increased risk of breast cancer, clinicians rely almost entirely on clinical judgment and the wishes of the women being counseled. Women at increased risk of breast cancer are offered the options of increased surveillance and prophylactic surgery and may be eligible for chemoprevention as part of an approved research protocol.

For women diagnosed with breast cancer, whether inherited or sporadic, prognostic information is most useful when coupled with targeted therapeutic approaches, very few of which exist. Identification of highly aggressive tumors is of little benefit if we have only the standard treatment to offer. The challenge for the future is to learn to use data on the molecular characteristics of an individual tumor to benefit patients and ultimately to prevent the development of breast cancer.

Recommendations for Women with Inherited Susceptibility to Breast Cancer

As was noted above, it is not known whether increased surveillance will reduce breast cancer-related mortality in high-risk women. Furthermore, women from high-risk breast cancer families are well aware that mammography and clinical breast examination may not detect premalignant lesions. In the face of a striking family history and close personal losses, these women may be unconvinced that mammography and clinical breast examination offers the protection they seek. Such women often inquire about prophylactic mastectomy in the absence of other preventive options. There are few data demonstrating the efficacy of prophylactic mastectomy in this setting. Furthermore, there are theoretical considerations that call into question the rationale for prophylactic surgery. Current surgical technique does not allow the complete removal of all breast tissue in a prophylactic total mastectomy. Since a germ-line mutation will be present in all residual breast tissue, individuals may remain at increased risk after surgery. Similarly, prophylactic oophorectomy does not guarantee protection from ovarian carcinoma, since tumors may arise spontaneously in the peritoneal reflection. These uncertainties make it difficult to counsel individuals about the potential benefits of these procedures. Nonetheless, the anxiety faced by women who harbor mutations in a breast cancer susceptibility gene can be overwhelming. Women must be presented with available data and allowed to make decisions which reflect their needs but do not offer a false sense of security.

Current recommendations include breast examination and mammography every 6 to 12 months beginning between ages 25 and 35 for women at increased risk of breast cancer resulting from direct or indirect molecular demonstration of a breast cancer-related genetic mutation.[297] Although no data exist to determine whether an increased frequency of clinical examination and screening mammography in this population reduces mortality, there are preliminary data that *BRCA1*-related tumors may have a faster growth rate than do sporadic tumors.[21] In addition, patient anxiety may be allayed somewhat by offering the option of two mammograms per year. Prophylactic mastectomy may be an option for interested women, who should be provided with information regarding the lack of evidence for or against risk reduction by this procedure.

In women with a documented *BRCA1* mutation, pelvic examinations with transvaginal ultrasound every 6 to 12 months for women under age 40 and/or those still interested in childbearing may be of benefit. Prophylactic oophorectomy at the completion of childbearing or at the time of menopause is recommended by the American College of Obstetrics and Gynecology; however, there is a low but measurable incidence of peritoneal malignancies after oophorectomy which may derive from peritoneal cells which are at similar risk for malignant transformation and are not removed by oophorectomy. It may be prudent for women at increased risk of breast cancer to avoid the use of exogenous estrogens when possible, as no data exist regarding the effect of estrogens on the penetrance of breast cancer susceptibility genes. However, a dilemma arises in that there may be some benefit to taking oral contraceptives to reduce ovarian cancer risk and in that heart disease and osteoporosis are more prevalent in women who do not use estrogen replacement therapy after menopause.

REFERENCES

1. Kelsey JL, Horn-Ross PL: Breast cancer: Magnitude of the problem and descriptive epidemiology. *Epidemiol Rev* **15**:7, 1993.
2. Miller BA: Causes of breast cancer and high risk groups, incidence and demographics, in Harris JR, Hellman S, Henderson IC, Kinne DW (eds): *Breast Diseases*. Philadelphia, Lippincott, 1991, p 119.
3. Miller BA, Feuer EJ, Hankey BF: The increasing incidence of breast cancer since 1982: Relevance of early detection. *Cancer Causes Control* **2**:67, 1991.
4. Glass A, Hoover RN: Changing incidence of breast cancer. *JNCI* **80**:1076, 1988.
5. Holford TR, Roush GC, McKay LA: Trends in female breast cancer in Connecticut and the United States. *J Clin Epidemiol* **44**:29, 1991.
6. Slattery ML, Kerber RA: A comprehensive evaluation of family history and breast cancer risk. *JAMA* **270**:1563, 1993.
7. Colditz GA, Willett WC, Hunter DJ, et al: Family history, age and risk of breast cancer. *JAMA* **270**:338, 1993.
8. Gail MH, Brinton LA, Byar DP, et al: Projecting individualized probabilities of developing breast cancer for white females who are being examined annually. *J Natl Cancer Inst* **81**:1879, 1989.
9. Easton DF, Bishop DT, Ford D, Crockford GP, and the Breast Cancer Linkage Consortium: Genetic linkage analysis in familial breast and ovarian cancer. Results from 214 families. *Am J Hum Genet* **52**:678, 1993.
10. Kampert JB, Whittemore AS, Paffenbarger RS Jr: Combined effect of childbearing, menstrual events, and body size on age-specific breast cancer risk. *Am J Epidemiol* **128**:962, 1988.
11. White E: Projected changes in breast cancer incidence due to the trend toward delayed childbearing. *Am J Public Health* **77**:495, 1987.
12. Trichopoulos D, MacMahon B, Cole P: Menopause and breast cancer risk. *JNCI* **48**:605, 1972.
13. Pike MC, Spicer DV, Dahmoush L, Press MF: Estogens, progesterones, normal breast cell proliferation, and breast cancer risk. *Epidemiol Rev* **15**:17, 1993.
14. Tokunaga M, Land CE, Tokuoka S, Nishimori I. Soda M, Akiba S: Incidence of female breast cancer among atomic bomb survivors, 1950–1985. *Radiat Res* **138**:209, 1994.
15. McGregor H, Land CE, Choi K, Tokuoka S, Liu PI, Wakabayashi T, Beebe CW: Breast cancer incidence among atomic bomb survivors, Hiroshima and Nagasaki, 1950–1969. *J Natl Cancer Inst* **59**:799, 1977.
16. Bhatia S, Robison LL, Oberlin O, Greenberg M, Bunin G, Fossati-Bellani F, Meadows AT: Breast cancer and other second neoplasms after childhood Hodgkin's disease. *N Engl J Med* **334**:791, 1996.
17. Harris JR, Lippman ME, Veronesi U, Willett W: Breast cancer. *N Engl J Med* **327**:319, 1992.
18. DuPont WD, Page DL: Risk factors for breast cancer in women with proliferative breast disease. *N Engl J Med* **312**:146, 1985.
19. Kinne DW: Clinical managment of lobular carcinoma in situ, in Harris JR, Hellman S, Henderson IC, Kinne DW (eds): *Breast Diseases*. Philadelphia, Lippincott, 1991, pp 239–244.
20. Rosen PP, Lieberman PH, Braun DW et al: Lobular carcinoma in situ of the breast. *Am J Surg Pathol* **2**:225, 1978.
21. Lakhani SR, Sloane JP, Gusterson BA, Anderson TJ, et al: Pathology of familial breast cancer: differences between breast cancers in carriers of BRCA1 or BRCA2 mutations and sporadic cases. Lancet **349**:1505, 1997.
22. Haagensen CD, Bodian C, Haagensen DE Jr: *Breast Carcinoma, Risk and Detection*. Philadelphia, Saunders, 1981, p 238.
23. Rosner D, Bedwani RN, Vana J, et al: Noninvasive breast carcinoma: Results of a national surgey by the American College of Surgeons. *Ann Surg* **192**:139, 1980.
24. Baker LH: Breast cancer detection demonstration project: Five year summary report. *CA* **32**:194, 1982.
25. Page DL, Dupont WD, Rogers LW, et al: Intraductal carcinoma of the breast: Follow-up after biopsy only. *Cancer* **49**:751, 1982.
26. Rosen PP, Braun DW, Kinne DW: The clinical significance of pre-invasive breast cancer. *Cancer* **46**:919, 1980.
27. Solin LJ, Recht A, Fourquet A, et al: Ten-year results of breast-conserving surgery and definitive irradiation for intraductal carcinoma (ductal carcinoma in-situ) of the breast. *Cancer* **68**:2337, 1991.
28. Netter FH: *The Ciba Collection of Medical Illustrations*, vol 2: *The Reproductive System*. Rochester NY, Case Hoyt Corporation, 1977, p 245.
29. Fisher ER, Kenney JP, Sass R, Dimitrov NV, Siderits RH, Fisher B: Medullary breast cancer of the breast revisited. *Breast Cancer Res Treat* **50**:23, 1990.
30. American Joint Committee on Cancer. *Manual for Staging for Breast Carcinoma*, 3d ed. Philadephia, Lippincott, 1989.
31. Harris JR: Staging of breast carcinoma, in Harris JR, Hellman S, Henderson IC, Kinne DW (eds): *Breast Diseases*. Philadelphia, Lippincott, 1991, p 330.
32. Clark GM, Sledge GW Jr, Osborne CK, McGuire WL: Survival from first recurrence: Relative importance of prognostic factors in 1015 breast cancer patients. *J Clin Onol* **5**:55, 1987.
33. Fisher B, Anderson S, Redmond C: Relanalysis and results after 12 years follow-up in a randomized clinical trial comparing total mastectomy with lumpectomy with or without irradiation in the treatment of breast cancer. *N Engl J Med* **333**:1456, 1995.
34. Valero V, Buzdar AU, Hortobagyi GN: Locally advanced breast cancer. *Oncologist* **1**:8, 1996.
35. Peters WP: High dose chemotherapy with autologous bone marrow transplantation for the treatment of breast cancer. Yes. *Important Adv Oncol* 215, 1995.
36. Williams WR, Anderson DE: Genetic epidemiology of breast cancer. Segregation and analysis of 200 Danish pedigrees. *Genet Epidemiol* **1**:7, 1984.
37. Newman B, Austin MA, Lee M, King MC: Inheritance of breast cancer: Evidence for autosomal dominant transmission in high risk families. *Proc Natl Acad Sci USA* **85**:3044, 1988.
38. Miki Y, Swensew J, Shattuck-Eidens D, Futreal A, Harshman K, Tavtigian S, et al: A strong candidate for the breast and ovarian cancer susceptibility gene BRCA1. *Science* **266**:66, 1994.
39. Wooster R, Bignell G, Lancaster J, Swift S, Seal S, Mangion J, Collins N, Gregory S, Gumbs C, Micklem G, Barfoot R, Hamoudi R, Patel S, Rice C, Biggs P, Hashim Y, Smith A, Connor F, Arason A, Gudmundsson J, Ficenec D, Kelsell D, Ford D, Tonin P, Bishop DT, Spurr NK, Ponder BAJ, Eeles R, Peto J, Devilee P, Cornelisse C, Lynch H, Narod S, Lenoir G, Egilsson V, Barkadottir RB, Easton DF, Bentley DR, Futreal PA, Ashworth A, Stratton MR: Indentification of the breast cancer susceptibility gene BRCA2. *Nature* **378**:789, 1995.
40. Tavtigian SV, Simard J, Romens J, Couch F, Shattuck-Eidens D, Neuhausen S, et al: The complete BRCA2 gene and mutations in chromosome 13q-linked kindreds. *Nat Genet* **12**:333, 1996.
41. Lynch HT, Guirgis HA, Brodkey F, et al: Genetic heterogeneity and familial carcinoma of the breast. *Surg Gynecol Obstet* **142**:693, 1976.
42. Broca P: *Taite de tumerus*. Paris, Asselin, 1866.
43. Nelson CL, Sellers TA, Rich SS, Potter JD, McGovern PG, Kushi LH: Familial clustering of colon, breast, uterine, and ovarian cancers as assessed by family history. *Genet Epidemiol* **10**:235, 1993.
44. Anderson DE, Badzioch MD: Familial breast cancer risks: Effects of prostate and other cancers. *Cancer* **72**:144, 1993.
45. Hall JM, Lee MK, Newman B, Morrow JE, Anderson LA, Huey B, King MC: Linkage of early onset break cancer to chromosome 17q21. *Science* **250**:1684, 1990.
46. Narod SA, Feuteun J, Lynch HT, Watson P, Conway T, Lynch J, Lenoir GM: Familial breast-ovarian cancer locus on chromosome 17q21-21. *Lancet* **338**:82, 1991.
47. Easton DF, Bishop DT, Ford D, Crockford GP: Breast Cancer Linkage Consortium: Breast and ovarian cancer incidence in BRCA1 mutation carriers. *Lancet* **343**:962, 1994.

48. Aragon A, Barkardottir RB, Egilsson V: Linkage analysis of chromosome 17 markers and breast ovarian cancer in Icelandic families and possible relationship to prostatic cancer. *Am J Hum Genet* **52**:711, 1993.

49. Ford D, Easton DF, Bishop DT, Narod SA, Goldgar DE: Breast Cancer Linkage Consortium: Risk of cancer in BRCA1 mutation carriers. *Lancet* **343**:962, 1994.

50. Lynch HT, Marcus J, Watson P, Page D: Distinctive clinicopathologic features of BRCA1-linked hereditary breast cancer. *Proc ASCO* **13**:56, 1994.

51. Marcus JN, Watson P, Page DL, Narod SA, Lenoir GM, Tonin P, Linder-Stephenson L, Salerno G, Conway TA, Lynch HT: Hereditary breast cancer: Pathobiology, prognosis, and BRCA1 and BRCA2 gene linkage. *Cancer* **77**:697, 1996.

52. Eisinger F, Stoppa-Lyonnet D, Longy M, Kerangeuven F, Noguchi T, Bailly C, Vincet-Saloman A, Jacquemier J, Birnbaum D, Sobol H: Germ line mutation at BRCA1 affects the histoprognostic grade in hereditary breast cancer. *Cancer Res* **56**:471, 1996.

53. Bowcock AM, Anderson LA, Friedman LS, Black DM, Osborne-Lawrence S, Rowell SE, Hall JM et al: THRA1 and D17S183 flank an interval of <4cM for the breast-ovarian cancer gene (BRCA1) on chromosome 17q21. *Am J Hum Genet* **52**:718, 1993.

54. Chamberlain JS, Boehnke M, Frank TS, Kiousis S, Xu J, Guo SW, Hauser ER, Norum RA, Helmbold EA, Markel DS, Keshavari SM, Jackson CE, Calzone K, Garber J, Collins FS, Weber BL: BRCA1 maps proximal to D17S579 on chromosome 17q21 by genetic analysis. *Am J Hum Genet* **52**:792, 1993.

55. Anderson LA, Friedman L, Osborne-Lawrence S, Lynch E, Weissenbach J, Bowcock A, King MC: High density genetic map of the BRCA1 region of chromosome 17q12-q21. *Genomics* **17**:618, 1993.

56. Albertsen H, Plaetke R, Ballard L, Fujimoto E, Connolly J, Lawrence E, Rodriguez P, Robertson M, Bradley P, Milner B, Fuhrman D, Marks A, Sargent R, Cartwright P, Matsunami N, White R: Genetic mapping of the BRCA1 region on chromosome 17q21. *Am J Hum Genet* **54**:516, 1994a.

57. Couch FJ, Kiousis S, Casatilla LH, Xu J, Chandrasekharappa SC, Chamberlain JS, Collins FS, Weber BL: Characterization of 10 new polymorphic dinucleotide repeats and generation of a high density microsatellite-based physical map of the BRCA1 region of chromosome 17q21. *Genomics* **24**:419, 1994.

58. Kelsell DLP, Black DM, Bishop DT, Spurr NK: Genetic analysis of the BRCA1 region in a large breast/ovarian family: Refinement of the minimal region containing BRCA1. *Hum Mol Genet* **2**:1823, 1993.

59. Simard J, Feunteun J, Lenoir G, Tonin P, Normand T, The VL, Vivier A, et al: Genetic mapping of the breast-ovarian cancer syndrome to a small interval on chromosome 17q12-21: Exclusion of candidate genes EDH17B2 and RARA. *Hum Mol Genet* **2**:1193, 1993.

60. Neuhausen SL, Swenson J, Miki Y, Liu Q, Tavtigian S, Shattuck-Eidens D, Kamb A, Hobbs MR, Gingrich J, Shizuya H, Kim UJ, Cochran C, Cutreal AP, Wiseman RW, Lynch HT, Tonin P, Narod S, Cannon-Albright L, Skolnick MH, Goldgard DE: A P1-based physical map of the region from D17S776 to D17S78 containing the breast cancer susceptibility gene BRCA1. *Hum Mol Genet* **3**:1919, 1994.

61. Abel KJ, Boehnke M, Prahalad M, Ho P, Flejter WL, Watkins M, Vanderstoep J, Chandrasekharappa SC, Collins FS, Glover TW, Weber BL: A radiation hybrid map of the BRCA1 region of chromosome 17q12-21. *Genomics* **17**:632, 1993.

62. O'Connell P, Albertsen H, Matsunami N, Taylor T, Hundley JE, Johnson-Pais TL, Reus B, Lawrence E, Ballard L, White R, Leach RJ: A radiation hybrid map of the BRCA1 region. *Am J Hum Genet* **54**:526, 1994.

63. Black DM, Nicolai H, Borrow J, Solomon E: A somatic cell hybrid map of the long arm of human chromosome 17, containing the familial breast cancer locus (BRCA1). *Am J Hum Genet* **52**:702, 1993.

64. Flejter WL, Barcroft CL, Guo S-W, Lynch ED, Boehnke M, Chandrasekharappa S, Hayes S, Collins FS, Weber BL, Glover TW: Multicolor FISH mapping with Alu-PCR-amplified YAC clone DNA determines the order of markers in the BRCA1 region on chromosome 17q12-q21. *Genomics* **17**:624, 1993.

65. Albertsen HM, Smith SA, Mazoyer S, Fujimoto E, Stevens J, Williams B, Rodriguez P, Cropp CS, Slijepcevic P, Carlson M, Robertson M, Bradley P, Lawrence E, Harrington T, Mei Sheng Z, Hoopes R, Stenverg N, Brothman A, Callahan R, Ponder BAJ, White R: A physical map and candidate genes in the BRCA1 region of chromosome 17q12-21. *Nat Genet* **7**:472, 1994.

66. Couch FJ, Castilla LH, Xu J, Abel KJ, Welsch P, King SE, Wong L, Ho PP, Merajver SD, Brody LC, Yin G, Hayes ST, Gieser LM, Flejter

WL, Glover TW, Friedman LS, Lynch ED, Meza JE, King MC, Law DJ, Deaven L, Bowcock AM, Collins FS, Weber FL, Chandrasekharappa SE: A YAC-, P1-, and cosmid-based physical map of the BRCA1 region on chromosome 17q21. *Genomics* **25**:264, 1995.

67. Brody LC, Abel KJ, Castilla LH, Couch FJ, McKinley DR, Yin GY, Hop PP, Merajver SD, Chandrasekharappa SC, Xu J, Cole JE, Struewing JP, Valdes JM, Collins FS, Weber BL: Construction of a transcription map surrounding the BRCA1 locus of human chromosome 17. *Genomics* **25**:238, 1995.

68. Friedman LS, Ostermeyer EA, Lynch ED, Welsch P, Szabo CI, Meza JE, Anderson LA, Dowd P, Lee MK, Rowell SE, Ellison J, Boyd J, King MC: 22 genes from chromosome 17q21: Cloning, sequencing, and characterization of mutations in breast cancer families and tumors. *Genomics* **25**:256, 1995.

69. Osborne Lawrence S, Welsch PL, Spillman M, Chandrasekharappa SC, Gallardo TD, Lovett M, Bowcock AM: Direct selection of expressed sequences within a 1-Mb region flanking BRCA1 on human chromosome 17q21. *Genomics* **25**:256, 1995.

70. Buckler AJ, Chang DD, Graw SL, Brook JD, Haber DA, Sharp PA, Housman DE: Exon amplification: A strategy to isolate mammalian genes based on RNA splicing. *Proc Natl Acad Sci USA* **88**:4005, 1991.

71. Lovett M, Kere J, Hinton LM: Direct selection: A method for the isolation of cDNAs encoded by large genomic regions. *Proc Natl Acad Sci USA* **88**:9628, 1991.

72. Parimoo S, Psantanjali SR, Shukla H, Chaplin DD, Weissman SM: cDNA selection: Efficient PCR approach for the selection of cDNAs encoded in large chromosomal DNA fragments. *Proc Natl Acad Sci USA* **88**:9623, 1991.

73. Tagle DA, Swaroop M, Lovett M, Collins FS: Magnetic bead capture of expressed sequences within large genomic segments. *Nature* **161**:751, 1993.

74. Orita M, Suziki Y, Sekiya T, Hayashi K: Rapid and sensitive detection of point mutations and DNA polymorphisms using the polymerase chain reaction. *Genomics* **5**:874, 1989.

75. Brown MA, Nicolai H, Xu CF, Griffiths BL, Jones KA, Solomon E, Hosking L, Trowsdale J, Black DM, McFarlane R: Regulation of BRCA1. *Nature* **372**:733, 1995.

76. Futreal AP, Liu Q, Shattuck-Eidens D, Cochran C, Harshman K, Tavtigian S, Bennett LM, Haugen-Strano A, Swensen J, Miki Y, Eddington K, McClure M, Frye C, Weaver-Feldhaus J, Ding W, Gholami Z, Soderkvist P, Terry L, Jhanwar S, Berchuk A, Iglehart JD, Marks J, Ballinger DG, Barrett JC, Skolnick MH, Kamb A, Wiseman R: BRCA1 mutations in primary breast and ovarian carcinomas. *Science* **266**:120, 1994.

77. Castilla LH, Couch FJ, Erdos MR, Hoskins KF, Calzone KA, Garber JE, Boyd J, Lubin MD, DeShano ML, Brody LC, Collins FS, Weber BL: Mutations in the BRCA1 gene in families with early-onset breast and ovarian cancer. *Nat Genet* **8**:387, 1994.

78. Friedman LS, Ostermeyer EA, Szabo CI, Dowd P, Lynch ED, Rowell SE, King MC: Confirmation of BRCA1 by analysis of germ line mutations linked to breast and ovarian cancer in ten families. *Nat Genet* **8**:399, 1994.

79. Simard J, Tonin P, Durocher F, Morgan K, Rommens J, Gingras S, Samson C, Leblanc JF, Belanger C, Dion F, Liu Q, Skolnick M, Goldgar D, Shattuck-Eidens D, Labrie F, Narod SA: Common origins of BRCA1 mutations in Canadian breast and ovarian cancer families. *Nat Genet* **8**:392, 1994.

80. Merajver SD, Pham TM, Caduff RF, Chen M, Poy EL, Cooney KA, Weber BL, Collins FS, Johnston C, Frank TS: Somatic mutations in the BRCA1 gene in sporadic ovarian tumors. *Nat Genet* **9**:439, 1995.

81. Hosking L, Trowsdale J, Nicolai H, Solomon E, Foulkes W, Stamp G, Signer E, Jeffreys A: A somatic BRCA1 mutation in an ovarian tumor. *Nat Genet* **9**:343, 1995.

82. Takahashi H, Behbakht K, McGovern PE, Chiu HC, Couch FJ, Weber BL, Friedman LS, King MC, Furusato M, LiVolsi VA, Menzin A, Liu P, Benjamin I, Morgam MA, King SA, Reban BA, Cardonic A, Mikuta JJ, Rubin SC, Boyd J: Mutation analysis of the BRCA1 gene in ovarian cancers. *Cancer Res* **55**:2998, 1995.

83. Matsushima M, Kobayashi K, Emi M, Saito H, Saito J, Suzumori K, Nakamura Y: Mutation analysis of the BRCA1 gene in 76 Japanese ovarian cancer patients: Four germ line mutations, but no evidence of somatic mutation. *Hum Mol Genet* **4**:1953, 1995.

84. Boyd M, Harris F, McFarlane R, Davidson R, Black DM: A human BRCA1 gene knockout. *Nature* **375**:541, 1995.

85. Inoue R, Fukotomi T, Ushijima T, Matsumoto Y, Sugimura T, Nagao M: germ line mutations of BRCA1 in Japanese breast cancer families. *Cancer Res* **55**:3521, 1995.

86. Hogervorst FBL, Cornelis RS, Bout M, van Vliet M, Oosterwiik JC, Olmer R, Bakker B, Klijn JGM, Vasen HFA, Meijers-Heijboer H, Menko FH, Cornelisse CJ, de Dunnen JT, Devilee P, van Ommen GJB: Rapid detection of BRCA1 mutations by the protein truncation test. *Nat Genet* **10**:208, 1995.

87. Plummer SJ, Anton-Culver H, Webster L, Noble B, Liao S, Kennedy A, Belinson J, Casey G: Detection of BRCA1 mutations by the protein truncation test. *Hum Mol Genet* **4**:1989, 1995.

88. Gayther SA, Harrington P, Russell P, Kharkevich G, Garkav T, Sera F, Ponder BAJ: UKCCCR familial ovarian cancer study group: Rapid detection of regionally clustered germ-line BRCA1 mutations by multiplex heteroduplex analysis. *Am J Hum Genet* **58**:451, 1996.

89. Couch FJ, Weber BL: Breast Cancer Information Core: Mutations and polymorphisms in the familial early-onset breast cancer (BRCA1) gene. *Hum Mutat* **8**:8, 1996.

90. Gayther SA, Warren W, Mazoyer S, Russell PA, Harrington PA, Chiano M, Seal S, Hamoudi R, van Rensburg EJ, Dunning AM, Love R, Evans G, Easton D, Clayton D, Stratton MR, Ponder BAJ: Germ line mutations of the BRCA1 gene in breast/ovarian cancer families provide evidence for a genotype/phenotype correlation. *Nat Genet* **10**:208, 1995.

91. Serova O, Montagna M, Torchard D, Narod SA, Tonin P, Sylla B, Lynch HT, Feunten J, Lenoir GM: A high incidence of BRCA1 mutations in 20 breast-ovarian cancer families. *Am J Hum Genet* **58**:42, 1996.

92. Holt JT, Thompson ME, Szabo C, Robinson-Benion C, Arteaga CL, King MC, Jensen RA: Growth retardation and tumour inhibition by BRCA1. *Nat Genet* **12**:298, 1996.

93. Sobol H, Stoppa-Lyonnet D, Bressac-de-Paillerets B, Peyrat JP, Kerangueven F, Nanin N, Noguchi T, Elsinger F, Guinebretier JM, Jacquemier J, Birnbaum D: Truncation at conserved terminal regions of BRCA1 protein is associated with highly proliferating hereditary breast cancers. *Canc Res* **56**:3126, 1996.

94. Tonin P, Serova O, Lenoir G, Lynch HT, Durocher F, Simard J, Morgan K, et al: BRCA1 mutations in Ashkenazi Jewish women. *Am J Hum Genet* **57**:189, 1995.

95. Streuwing JP, Abeliovich D, Peterz T, Avishai N, Kaback MM, Collins FS, Brody LC: The carrier frequency of the BRCA1 185delAG mutation is approximately 1 percent in Ashkenazi Jewish individuals. *Nat Genet* **11**:198, 1995.

96. Berman DB, Wagner-Costalas J, Schultz DC, Lynch HT, Daly M, Godwin AK: Two distinct origins of a common BRCA1 mutation in breast-ovarian cancer families: A genetic study of 15 185delAG mutation kindreds. *Am J Hum Genet* **58**:1166, 1996.

97. Fitzgerald MG, MacDonald DJ, Krainer M, Hooever I, O'Neil E, Unsal H, Silva-Arrieto S, Finkelstein DM, Geer-Romero P, Engelhart C, Sigroi DC, Smith BL, Younger JW, Garber JE, Duda RBN, Mayzel KA, Isselbacher KH, Friend SH, Haber DA: Germ line BRCA1 mutations in Jewish and non-Jewish women with early onset breast cancer. *N Engl J Med* **334**:143, 1996.

98. Offit K, Gilewski T, McGuire P, Schluger A, Hampel H, Brown K, Swensen J, Neuhausen S, Skolnick M, Norton L, Goldgar D: Germ line BRCA1 185delAG mutations in Jewish women with breast cancer. *Lancet* **347**:1643, 1996.

99. Langston AA, Malone KE, Thompson JD, Daling JR, Ostrander EA: BRCA1 mutations in a population-based sample of young women with breast cancer. *N Engl J Med* **334**:137, 1996.

100. Durocher F, Shattuck-Eidens D, McClure M, Labrie L, Skolnick MH, Goldgar DE, Simard JE: Comparison of BRCA1 polymorphisms, rare sequence variants and/or missense mutations in unaffected and breast/ovarian cancer populations. *Hum Mol Genet* **5**:835, 1996.

101. Brown MA, Xu CF, Nicolai H, Griffiths B, Chambers JA, Black D, Solomon E: The 5' end of the BRCA1 gene lies within a duplicated region of human chromosome 17q21. *Cancer Res* **12**:2507, 1996.

102. Thakur S, Zhang HB, Peng Y, Le H, Carroll B, Ward T, Yao J, Farid LM, Couch FJ, Wilson RB, Weber BL: Localization of BRCA1 and a splice variant identifies the nuclear localization signal. *Mol Cell Biol* **17**:444, 1997.

103. Wilson CA, et al: Differential subcellular localization, expression and biological toxicity of BRCA1 and the splice variant BRCA1-delta 11b. *Oncogene* **14**:1, 1997.

104. Abel KJ, Xu J, Yin GY, Lyons RH, Meisler MH, Weber BL: Mouse BRCA1: Localization, sequence analysis and identification of evolutionarily conserved domains. *Hum Mol Genet* **4**:2265, 1995.

105. Bennett LM, Haugen-Strano A, Cochran C, Brownlee HA, Fiedorek FT, Wiseman RW: Isolation of the mouse homologue of BRCA1 and genetic mapping to mouse chromosome 11. *Genomics* **29**:576, 1995.

106. Sharan SK, Wims M, Bradley L: Murine BRCA1: Sequence and significance for human missense mutations. *Hum Mol Genet* **4**:2275, 1995.

107. Chapman MS, Verma IM: Transcriptional activation by BRCA1. *Nature* **382**:678, 1996.

108. Jensen RA, Thompson ME, Jetton TL, Szabo CI, van der Meer R, Helou B, Tonick SR, Page DL, King MC, Holt JT: BRCA1 is secreted and exhibits properties of a granin. *Nat Genet* **12**:303, 1996.

109. Gudas JM, Nguyen H, Li T, Cowan KH: Hormone-dependent regulation of BRCA1 in human breast cancer cells. *Cancer Res* **55**:4561, 1995.

110. Gudas JM, Li T, Nguyen H, Jensen D, Rauscher FJ III, Cowan KH: Cell cycle regulation of BRCA1 messenger RNA in human breast epithelial cells. *Cell Growth Diff* **7**:717, 1996.

111. Vaughn JP, David PL, Jarboe MD, Huper A, Evans C, Wiseman RW, Berchuck A, Iglehart JD, Futreal PA, Marks JR: BRCA1 expression is induced before DNA synthesis in both normal and tumor derived breast cells. *Cell Growth Differ* **7**:711, 1996.

112. Marquis ST, Rajan JV, Wynshaw-Boris A, Xu J, Yin GY, Abel KJ, Weber BL, Chodosh LA: The developmental pattern of BRCA1 expression and modulation by ovarian hormones imples a role in differentiation of the breast and other tissues. *Nat Genet* **11**:17, 1995.

113. Chen Y, Chen CF, Riley DJ, Allred DC, Chen PL, Con Hoff D, Osborne CK, Lee WH: Aberrant subcellular localization of BRCA1 in breast cancer. *Science* **270**:789, 1995.

114. Scully R, Ganesan S, Brown M, DeCaprio JA, Cannistra SA, Feunteun J, Schnitt S, Livingston DM: Localization of BRCA1 in human breast and ovarian cancer cells. *Science* **272**:122, 1996.

115. Wilson CA, Payton MN, Pekar SK, Zhang K, Pacifici RE, Gudas JL, Thukral S, Calzone C, Reese DM, Slamon DI: BRCA1 protein products: Antibody specificity. *Nat Genet* **13**:265, 1996.

116. Smith SA, Easton DF, Evans DGR, Ponder BAJ: Allele losses in the region 17q12-q21 in familial breast and ovarian cancer involve the wild-type chromosome. *Nat Genet* **2**:128, 1992.

117. Thompson ME, Jensen RA, Obermiller PS, Page DL, Holt JT: Decreased expression of BRCA1 accelerates growth and is often present during sporadic breast cancer progression. *Nat Genet* **9**:444, 1995.

118. Rao VN, Shao N, Ahmad M, Shyam E, Reddy P: Antisense RNA to the putative tumor suppressor gene BRCA1 transforms mouse fibroblasts. *Oncogene* **12**:523, 1996.

119. Shao N, Chai YL, Shyam E, Reddy P, Rao VN: Induction of apoptosis by the tumor suppressor protein BRCA1. *Oncogene* **13**:18, 1996.

120. Chen Y, Farmer AA, Jones DC, Chen PL, Lee WH: BRCA1 is a 220-kDa nuclear phosphoprotein that is expressed and phosphorylated in a cell cycle-dependent manner. *Cancer Res* **56**:3168, 1996.

121. Gowen LC, Johnson BL, Latour AM, Sulik KK, Koller BH: BRCA1 deficiency results in early embryonic lethality characterized by neuroepithelial abnormalities. *Nat Genet* **12**:194, 1996.

122. Hakem R, de la Pompa JL, Sirard C, Mo R, Woo M, Hakem A, Reitmair A, Billia F, Firpo E, Hui CC, Roberts J, Rossant J, Mak TW: The tumor suppressor gene BRCA1 is required for embryonic cellular proliferation in the mouse. *Cell* **85**:1009, 1996.

123. Liu CY, Fleskin-Nikitin A, Li S, Zeng Y, Lee WH: Inactivation of the mouse BRCA1 gene leads to failure in the morphogenesis of the egg cylinder in early postimplantation development. *Genes Dev* **10**:1835, 1996.

124. Stratton MR, Ford D, Neuhausen S, Seal S, Wooster R, Friedman LS, King MC, Egilsson V, Devilee P, McManus R, Daly PA, Smyth E, Ponder BAJ, Peto J, Cannon-Albright L, Easton DF, Goldgar DE: Familial male breast cancer is not linked to the BRCA1 locus on chromosome 17q. *Nat Genet* **7**:103, 1994.

125. Wooster R, Neuhausen S, Mangion J, Quirk Y, Ford D, Collins N, et al: Localization of a breast cancer susceptibility gene, BRCA2, to chromosome 13q12-13. *Science* **265**:2088, 1994.

126. Gudmundsson J, Johannesdottir G, Arason A, Berghorsson JT, Ingvarsson S, Egilsson V, Barkardottir RB: Frequent occurrence of BRCA2 linkage in Icelandic breast cancer families and segregation of a common BRCA2 haplotype. *Am J Hum Genet* **58**:749, 1996.

127. Couch FJ, Rommens JM, Neuhausen SL, Belanger C, Dumont M, Abel K, Bell R, Berry S, Bogden R, Cannon-Albright L, Farid L, Frye C, Hattier T, Janecki T, Jiang P, Kehrer R, Leblanc J-F, McArthur-Morrison J, McSweeney D, Miki Y, Peng Y, Samson C, Schroeder M, Snyder SC, Stringfellow M, Stroup C, Swedlund B, Swensen J, Teng D, Thakur S, Tran T, Tranchant M, Welver-Feldhaus J, Wong AKC, Shizuya H, Labrie F, Skolnick MH, Goldgar DE,

Kamb A, Weber BL, Tavtigian SV, Simard J: Generation of an integrated transcription map of the BRCA2 region on chromosome 13q12-q13. *Genomics* **36**:86, 1996.

128. Schutte M, Rozenblum E, Moskaluk CA, Xiaoping G, Shamsul Hoque ATM, Hahn SA, da Costa LT, deJong PJ, Kern SE: An integrated high resolution physical map of the DPC/BRCA2 region at chromosome 13q12. *Cancer Res* **55**:4570, 1995.

129. Fischer SG, Cayanis E, deFatima Bonaldo M, Bowcock AM, Deaven LL, Efelman IS, Gallardo T, Kalachikov S, Lawton L, Longmire JL, Lovett ML, Osbourne-Lawrence S, Rothstein R, Russo JJ, Bento Soares M, Sunjevarici I, Venkatraj VS, Warburton D, Zhang P, Efstratiad A: A high-resolution annotated physcial map of the human chromosome 13q12-13 region containing of the breast cancer susceptibility locus BRCA2. *Proc Natl Acad Sci USA* **93**:690, 1996.

130. Couch FJ, Farid LM, DeShano ML, Tavtigian SV, Calzone KA, Campeau L, Peng Y, Bogden B, Chen Q, Neuhausen S, Shattuck-Eidens D, Godwin AK, Daly M, Radford DM, Sedlacek S, Rommens J, Simard J, Garber J, Merajver S, Weber BL: BRCA2 germ line mutations in male breast cancer cases and breast cancer families. *Nat Genet* **13**:123, 1996.

131. Neuhausen S, Gilewski T, Norton L, Tran T, McGuire P, Swensen J, Hampel H, Borgen P, Brown K, Skolnick M, Shattuck-Eidens D, Jhanwar S, Goldgar D, Offit K: Recurrent BRCA2 6174delT mutations in Ashkenazi Jewish woman affected by breast cancer. *Nat Genet* **13**:126, 1996.

132. Phelan CM, Lancaster JM, Tonin P, Gumbs C, Cochran C, Carter R, Ghadirian P, Perret C, Moslehi R, Dion F, Faucher MC, Dole K, Sarimi S, Foulkes W, Lounis H, Warner E, Goss P, Anderson D, Larsson C, Narod SA, Futreal PA: Mutation analysis of the BRCA2 gene in 9 site-specific breast cancer families. *Nat Genet* **13**:120, 1996.

133. Lancaster JM, Wooster R, Mangion J, Phelan CM, Cochran C, Gumbs C, Seal S, Barfoot R, Collins N, Bignell C, Patel S, Hamoudi R, Larsson C, Wiseman RW, Berchuck A, Iglehart JD, Marks HR, Ashworth A, Stratton MR, Futreal PA: BRCA2 mutations in primary breast and ovarian cancers. *Nat Genet* **13**:238, 1996.

134. Miki Y, Katagiri T, Kasumi F, Yoshimoto T, Nakamura Y: Mutations analysis on the BRCA2 gene in primary breast cancers. *Nat Genet* **13**:245, 1996.

135. Teng DHF, Bogden R, Mitchell J, Baumgard M, Bell R, Berry S, Davis T, Ha PC, Kehrer R, Jammulapati S, Chen Q, Offit K, Skolnick MH, Tavtigian SV, Jhanwar S, Swedlund B, Wong AKC, Kamb A: Low incidence of BRCA2 mutations in breast carcinoma and other cancers. *Nat Genet* **13**:241, 1996.

136. Takahashi H, Chiu HC, Bandera CA, Behbakht K, Liu PC, Couch FJ, Weber BL, LiVolsi VA, Furusato M, Rebane BA, Cardonic A, Benjamin I, Morgan MA, King SA, Mikuta JJ, Rubin SC, Boyd J: Mutations of the BRCA2 gene in ovarian carcinomas. *Cancer Res* **56**:2738, 1996.

137. Tonin P, Weber B, Offit K, Couch F, Rebbeck T, Neuhausen S, Godwin A, Daly M, Wanger J, Berman D, Grana G, Fox E, Kane M, Kolodner R, Haber D, Struewing J, Warner E, Rosen B, Foulkes W, Lerman C, Peshkin O, Lynch HT, Lenoir G, Narod S, Garber J: Frequency of recurrent *BRCA1* and *BRCA2* mutations in Ashkenazi Jewish breast cancer families. *Nature Med* **2**:1179, 1996.

138. Li FP, Fraumeni JF Jr: Soft-tissue sarcomas, breast cancer, and other neoplasms: Familial syndrome? *Ann Intern Med* **71**:747, 1969.

139. Li FP, Fraumeni JF, Mulvihill JJ, Blattner WA, Dreyfus MG, Tucker MA, Miller RW: A cancer family syndrome in 24 kindreds. *Cancer Res* **48**:5358, 1988.

140. Strong LC, Williams WR, Tainsky MA: The Li-Fraumeni syndrome: From clinical epidemiology to molecular genetics. *Am J Epidemiol* **135**:190, 1992.

141. Williams WR, Strong LC: Genetic epidemiology of soft tissue sarcomas in children, in Muller HR, Weber W (eds): *Familial Cancer: First International Research Conference.* Basel, Karger, 1985, pp 151–153.

142. Malkin D, Li FP, Strong LC, Fraumeni JF Jr, Nelson CE, Kim DH, Kassel J, Gryka MA, Bischoff FZ, Tainsky MA, et al: Germ line p53 mutations in a familial syndrome of breast cancer, sarcomas, and other neoplasms. *Science* **250**:1233, 1990.

143. Srivastava S, Zou Z, Pirollo K, Blattner W, Chang EH: Germ line transmission of a mutated p53 gene in a cancer-prone family with Li-Fraumeni syndrome. *Nature* **348**:747, 1991.

144. Law JC, Strong LC, Chidambaram A, Ferell RE: A germ line mutation in exon 5 of the p53 gene in an extended cancer family. *Cancer Res* **51**:6385, 1991.

145. Santibanez-Koref MF, Birch JM, Harley AL, Morris-Jones PH, Craft AH, Eden T, Crowther D, Kelsey AM, Harris M: p53 germ line mutations in Li-Fraumeni syndrome. *Lancet* **338**:1490, 1991.

146. Srivastava S, Tong YA, Devadas K, Zou Z-Q, Sykes VW, Chen Y, Blattner WA, Pirollo K, Chang EH: Detection of both mutant and wild type p53 protein in normal skin fibroblasts and demonstration of a shared second hit on p53 in diverse tumors from a cancer prone family with Li-Fraumeni syndrome. *Oncogene* **7**:987, 1992.

147. Brugieres L, Gardes M, Moutou C, Chompret A, Meresse V, Martin A, Poisson N, Flamant F, Bonaiti-Pellie KC, Lemerle J, Feunteun J: Screening for germ line p53 mutations in children with malignant tumors and a family history of cancer. *Cancer Res* **53**:452, 1993.

148. Sameshima Y, Tsynematsu Y, Watanabe S, Tsukamoto T, Kawa-ha K, Hirata Y, Mizoguchi H, Sugimura T, Terada M, Yokota J: Detection of novel germ-line p53 mutations in diverse cancer-prone families identified by selecting patients with childhood adrenalcortical carcinoma. *JNCI* **84**:703, 1992.

149. Frebourg T, Kassel J, Lam KT, Gryka MA, Barbier N, Andersen TI, Borresen A-L, Friend SH: Germ-line mujtations of the p53 tumor suppressor gene in patients with high risk for cancer inactivate the p53 protein. *Proc Natl Acad Sci USA* **89**:6413, 1992.

150. Barnes DM, Hanby AM, Gillett CE, Mohammed S, Hodgson S, Bobrow LG, Leigh IM, Purkis T, MacGeoch C, Spurr NK, Bartek J, Vojtesek B, Picksley SM, Lane DP: Abnormal expression of wild type p53 protein in normal cells of a cancer family patient. *Lancet* **340**:259, 1992.

151. Sidransky D, Tolino T, Helzlsouer K, Zehnbauer B, Rausch G, Shelton B, Prestigiacomo L, Vogelstein B, Davidson N: Inherited p53 gene mutations in breast cancer. *Cancer Res* **52**:2984, 1992.

152. Borresen A-L, Andersen TI, Garber J, Barbier-Piraux N, Thorlacius S, Eyfjord J, Ottestad L, Smith-Sorensen B, Hovig E, Malkin D, Friend SH: Screening for germ type TP53 mutations in breast cancer patients. *Cancer Res* **52**:3234, 1992.

153. Starink TM: Cowden's disease: Analysis of fourteen new cases. *J Am Acad Dermatol* **11**:1127, 1984.

154. Wood DA, Darling HH: A cancer family manifesting multiple occurrences of bilateral carcinoma of the breast. *Cancer Res* **3**:509, 1943.

155. Brownstein MH, Wolf M, Bikowski JB: Cowden's disease: A cutaneous marker of breast cancer. *Cancer* **41**:2393, 1978.

156. Padberg GW, Schot JDL, Vielvoye GJ, Bots GThAM, de Beer FC: Lhermitte-Duclos disease and Cowden disease: A single phakomatosis. *Ann Neurol* **29**:517, 1991.

157. Eng C, Murday V, Seal S, Mohammed S, Hodgson SC, Chaudary MA, Fentiman IS, Ponder BA, Eeles RA: Cowden syndrome and Lhermitte-Duclos disease in a family: A single genetic syndrome with pleiotropy. *J Med Genet* **31**:458, 1994.

158. Nelen MR, Padberg GW, Peeters EAJ, Lin AY, van den Helm B, Frants RR, Coulon V, Goldstein AM, van Reen MMM, Easton DF, Eeles RA, Hodgson S, Mulvihill JJ, Murday VA, Tucker MA, Mariman ECM, Starink TM, Ponder BAJ, Ropers HH, Kremer H, Longy M, Eng C: Localization of the gene for Cowden disease to chromosome 10q22-23. *Nat Genet* **13**:114, 1996.

159. Muir EG, Yates-Bell AJ, Barlow KA: Multiple primary carcinomata of the colon, duodenum, and larynx associated with keratoacanthomata of the face. *Br J Surg* **54**:191, 1967.

160. Hall NR, Williams AT, Murday VA, Newton JA, Bishop DT: Muir-Torre syndrome: A variant of the cancer family syndrome. *J Med Genet* **31**:627, 1994.

161. Anderson DE: An inherited form of large bowel cancer. *Cancer* **45**:1103, 1980.

162. Papadopoulos N, Nicolaides N, Wei YF, et al: Mutation of mutL homolog in hereditary colon cancer. *Science* **263**:1625, 1994.

163. Bronner EC, Baker SM, Morrison PT, et al: Mutation in the DNA mismatch repair gene homologue hMLH1 is associated with hereditary non-polyposis colon cancer. *Nature* **368**:258, 1994.

164. Fishel R, Lescoe MK, Rao MRS, et al: The human mutator gene homolog MSH2 and its association with hereditary nonpolyposis colon cancer. *Cell* **75**:1027, 1993.

165. Leach FS, Nicolaides N, Papadopoulos N, et al: Mutations of a mutS homolog in hereditary nonpolyposis colon cancer. *Cell* **75**:1215, 1993.

166. Nicolaides NC, Carter, KC, Shell, BK, et al: Genomic organization of the human PMS2 gene family. *Genomics* **30**:195, 1995.

167. Liu B, et al: Analysis of mismatch repair genes in hereditary non-polyposis colorectal cancer patients. *Nat Med* **2**:169, 1996.

168. Kolodner RD, Hall NR, Lipford J, Kane MF, Rao MRS, Morrison P, Wirth L, et al: Structure of the human MHS2 locus and analysis of two Muir-Torre kindreds for MSH2 mutations. *Genomics* **24**:516, 1994.

169. Bapat B, Xia L, Madlensky L, Mitri A, Tonin P, Narod SA, Gallinger S: The genetic basis of Muir-Torre syndrome includes the hMLH1 locus. *Am J Hum Genet* **3**:736, 1996.

170. Swift M, Morrell D, Cromartie E, Chamberlin AR, Skolnick MH, Bishop DT: The incidence and gene frequency of ataxia-telangiectasia in the United States. *Am J Hum Genet* **39**(5):573, 1986.

171. Morrell D, Cromartie E, Swift M: Mortality and cancer incidence in 263 patients with ataxia-telangiectasia. *J Natl Cancer Inst* **77**:89, 1986.

172. Swift M, Morrell D, Massey RB, Chase CL: Incidence of cancer in 161 families affected by ataxia-telangiectasia. *N Engl J Med* **325**:1831, 1987.

173. Cortessis V, Ingles S, Millikan R, Diep A, Gatti RA, Richardson L, Thompson WD, Paganini-Hill A, Sparkes RS, Haile RW: Linkage analysis of DRD2, a marker linked to the ataxia-telangiectasia gene, in 64 families with premenopausal bilateral breast cancer. *Cancer Res* **53**:5083, 1993.

174. Wooster R, Ford D, Mangion J, Ponder BAJ, Peto J, Easton DF, Stratton M: Absence of linkage to the ataxia telangiectasia locus in familial breast cancer. *Hum Genet* **92**:91, 1993.

175. Savitsky K, Bar-Shira A, Gilad S, Rothman G, Ziv Y, Banagaite L, Tagle DA, Smith S, Uziel T, Sfez S, Ashjenazi M, Pecker I, Frydman M, Harnik R, Patanjali SR, Simmons S, Clines GA, Sateil A, Gatti RA, Chessa L, Sanal O, Lavin MF, Jaspers NGJ, Taylor AMR, Arlett CF, Miki T, Weissman SM, Lovett M, Collins FS, Shiloh YS: A single ataxia telangiectasia gene with a product similar to PI-3 kinase. *Science* **268**:1749, 1995.

176. Zuppan P, Hall JM, Lee MK, Pongliktmongkol M, King MC: Possible linkage of the estrogen receptor gene to breast cancer in a family with late-onset disease. *Am J Hum Genet* **48**:1065, 1991.

177. Sluyser M: Mutations in the estrogen receptor gene. *Hum Mutat* **6**:97, 1995.

178. Kerangueven F, Essioux L, Dib A: Noguchi T, Allione F, Geneix J, Longy M, Lidereau R, Eisinger F, Pebusque MJ: Loss of heterozygosity and linkage analysis in breast carcinoma: Indication for a putative third susceptibility gene on the short arm of chromosome 8. *Oncogene* **10**:1023, 1995.

179. Latil A, Baron JC, Cussenot O, Fournier G, Soussi T, Boccon-Gibod L, LeDuc A, Rouesse J, Lidereau R: Genetic alterations in localized prostate cancer: Identification of a common region of deletion on chromosome arm 18q. *Genes Chromosom Cancer* **11**:119, 1994.

180. Chuaqui RF, Sanz-Ortega J, Vocke C, Linehan WM, Sanz-Esponera J, Zhuang J, Emmert-Buck MR, Merino MJ: Loss of heterozygosity on the short arm of chromosome 8 in male breast carcinoma. *Cancer Res* **55**:4995, 1995.

181. Knudson AG: Mutation and cancer: Statistical study of retinoblastoma. *Proc Natl Acad Sci USA* **68**:820, 1971.

182. Callahan R, Cropp C, Merlo GR, Diella F, Venesio T, Lidereau R, Cappa AR, Lisicia DS: Genetic and molecular heterogeneity of breast cancer cells. *Clin Chim Acta* **217**:63, 1993.

183. Cleton-Jansen AM, Moerland EW, Kuipers-Dijkshoorn NJ, Callen DF, Sutherland GR, Hansen B, Devilee P, Cornelisse CJ: At least two different regions are involved in allelic imbalance on chromosome arem 16q in breast cancer. *Genes Chromosom Cancer* **9**:101, 1994.

184. Gudmundsson J, Barkardottir RB, Eirikdottir G, Baldursson T, Arason A, Egilsson V, Ingvarsson S: Loss of heterozygosity at chromosome 11 in breast cancer. Association of prognostic factors with genetic alterations. *Br J Cancer* **72**:696, 1995.

185. Cropp CS, Champeme MH, Lindereau R, Callahan R: Indentification of three regions on chromosome 17q in primary human breast carcinomas which are frequently deleted. *Cancer Res* **53**:5617, 1993.

186. Kirchweger R, Zeillinger R, Schneeberger C, Speiser P, Louason G, Theillet C: Patterns of allele losses suggest the existence of five distinct regions of LOH on chromosome 17 in breast cancer. *Int J Cancer* **56**:193, 1994.

187. Nagai MA, Medeiros AC, Bretani MM, Bretani RR, Marques LA, Mazoyer S, Mulligan LM: Five distinct deleted regions on chromosome 17 defining different subsets of human primary breast tumors. *Oncology* **52**:448, 1995.

188. Cornelis RS, Van Vilet M, Vos CR, Cleton-Jansen M, van de Vijver MJ, Peterse JL, Khan PM, Borreson AL, Cornelisse CJ, Devilee P: Evidence for a gene on 17p13.3, distal to TP53, as a target for allele loss in breast tumors without p53 mutations. *Cancer Res* **54**:4200, 1994.

189. Mathew S, Murty VV, Bosl GJ, Chagnati RS: Loss of heterozygosity identifies multiple sites of allelic deletions on chromosome 1 in human male germ cell tumors. *Cancer Res* **54**:6265, 1994.

190. Dorion-Bonnet F, Mautalen S, Hostein I, Longy M: Allelic imbalance study of 16q in human primary breast carcinomas using microsatellite markers. *Genes Chromosom Cancer* **14**:171, 1995.

191. Eiriksodottir G, Sigurdsson A, Jonasson JG, Agnarsson BA, Sigurdsson H, Gudmundsson J, Bergthorsson JT, Barkardottir RB, Egilsson V, Ingvarsson S: Loss of heterozygosity on chromosome 9 in human breast cancer: Association with clinical variables and genetic changes at other chromosome regions. *Int J Cancer* **64**:378, 1995.

192. Smith HS, Lu Y, Deng G, Martinez O, Krams S, Ljung BM, Thor A, Lagios M: Molecular aspects of early stages of breast cancer progression. *J Cell Biochem* **17G**:144, 1993.

193. Kashiwaba M, Tamura G, Suzuki Y, Maesawa C, Ogasawara S, Sakata K, Satodate R: Epitheial-cadherin gene is not mutated in ductal carcinomas of the breast. *Jpn J Cancer Res* **86**:1054, 1995.

194. Medeiros AC, Nagai MA, Neto MM, Brentani RR: Loss of heterozygosity affecting the APC and MCC genetic loci in patients with primary breast carcinomas. *Cancer Epidemiol Biomarkers Prevent* **3**:331, 1994.

195. Lakahani SR, Collins N, Stratton MR, Sloane JP: Atypical ductal hyperplasia of the breast: Clonal proliferation with loss of heterozygosity on chromosomes 16q and 17p. *J Clin Pathol* **48**:611, 1995.

196. Radford DM, Fair KL, Phillips NJ, Ritter JH, Steinbrueck T, Holt MS, Donis-Keller H: Alleotyping of ductal carcinoma in situe of the breast: Deletion of loci on 8p, 13q, 16q, 17p, and 17q. *Cancer Res* **55**:3399, 1995.

197. Champene MH, Bieche I, Beuzelin M, Lidereay R: Loss of heterozygosity on 7q31 occurs early during breast tumorigenesis. *Genes Chromosom Cancer* **12**:304, 1995.

198. Bacus SS, Zelnick CR, Plowman G, Yarden Y: Expression of the erb-2 family of growth factor receptors and their ligands in breast cancer. *Am J Clin Pathol* **102**:S13, 1994.

199. Slamon DJ, Godolphin W, Jones LA, et al: Studies of the Her-2/neu protooncogene in human breast and ovarian cancer. *Science* **244**:707, 1989.

200. Kraus MH, Issing W, Miki T, et al: Isolation and characterization of ERBB3, a third member of the ERBB/epidermal growth factor receptor family: Evidence for overexpression in a subset of human mammary tumors. *Proc Natl Acad Sci USA* **86**:9193, 1989.

201. Lewis S, Locker A, Todd JH, Bell A, Nicholson R, Elston CW, Blarney RW, Ellis IO: Expression of epidermal growth factor receptor in breast carcinoma. *J Clin Pathol* **43**:385, 1990.

202. Hawkins RA, Kilen E, Whittle IR, Jack WL, Cherry U, Prescott RJ: Epidermal growth factor receptors in intracranial and breast tumors: Their clinical significance. *Br J Cancer* **63**:553, 1990.

203. Paik S, Hazan R, Fisher ER, Sass RE, Fisher B, Redmond C, et al: Pathologic findings from the National Surgical Adjuvant Breast and Bowel Project: Prognostic significance of erbB-2 protein overexpression in primary breast cancer. *J Clin Oncol* **8**:103, 1990.

204. Clark GM, McGuire WL: Follow-up study of HER-2/neu amplification in primary breast cancer. *Cancer Res* **51**:944, 1991.

205. Antoniotti S, Taverna D, Maggiora P, Sapei ML, Hynes NE, DeBartoli M: Oestrogen and epidermal growth factor down-regulate erbB-2 oncogene protein expression in breast cancer cells by different mechanisms. *Br J Cancer* **70**:1095, 1994.

206. Janes PW, Daily RJ, deFazio A, Sutherland RL: Activation of the Ras signalling pathway in human breast cancer cells overexpressing erbB-2. *Oncogene* **9**:3601, 1994.

207. Toikkanen S, Helin H, Isola H, Joensuu H: Prognostic significance of HER-2 oncoprotein expression in breast cancer. A 30-year follow-up. *J Clin Oncol* **10**:1044, 1992.

208. Gusterson BA, Gelber RD, Goldhirsch A, Price KN, Save-Soderborgh J, Anbazhasgan R, et al: Prognostic importance of c-erbB-2 expression in breast cancer. *J Clin Oncol* **10**:1049, 1992.

209. Muss HB, Thor AD, Berry DA, Kute T, Liu ET, Koerner F, et al: c-erbB-2 expression and response to adjuvant therapy in women with node-positive early breast cancer. *N Engl J Med* **330**:1260, 1994.

210. Leitzel K, Teramoto Y, Konrad K, Chichilli VM, Volas G, Grossberg H, Harvey H, Demers L, Lipton A: Elevated serum c-erbB-2 antigen levels and decreased response to hormone therapy of breast cancer. *J Clin Oncol* **13**:1129, 1995.

211. Hudziak RM, Lewis GD, Winget M, Fendly BM, Shewpard HM, Ulrich A: Antisense oligonucleotides may be useful therapeutically. *Mol Cell Biol* **9**:1165, 1989.

212. Colomer R, Lupu R, Bacus SS, Gelmann EP: erbB-2 antisense oligonucleotides inhibit the proliferation of breast carcinoma cells with erbB-2 oncogene amplification. *Br J Cancer* **70**:819, 1994.

213. Sandgren EP, Luetteke NC, Palmiter RD, Brinster RL, Lee DC: Over-expression of TGFα in transgenic mice: induction of epithelial hyperplasia, pancreatic metaplasia, and carcinoma of the breast. *Cell* **61**:1121, 1990.

214. Buick RN, Tannock IF: Properties of malignant cells, in Tannock IF (ed): *The Basic Science of Oncology.* New York, McGraw-Hill, 1992, p 151.

215. Burgess WH, Maciag T: The heparin-binding (fibroblast) growth factor family of proteins. *Annu Rev Biochem* **58**:575, 1989.

216. Penault-Llorca F, Bertucci F, Adelaide J, et al: Expression of FGF and FGFR genes in human breast cancer. *Int J Cancer* **61**:170, 1995.

217. Conway K, Edmiston S, Fried DB, Hulka BS, Garrett PA, Liu ET: Ha-ras rare alleles in breast cancer susceptibility. *Breast Cancer Res Treat* **35**:97, 1995.

218. Phelan CM, Rebbeck TR, Weber BL, Devilee P, Lynch HT, et al: Ovarian cancer risk in BRCA1 carriers is modified by the HRAS1 variable number of tandem repeat (VNTR) locus. *Nat Genet* **12**:309, 1996.

219. Zhang PL, Calaf G, Russo J: Allele loss and point mutation in codons 12 and 61 of the c-Ha-ras oncogene in carcinogen-transformed human breast epithelial cells. *Mol Carcinog* **9**:46, 1994.

220. Bland KI, Konstadoulakis MM, Vezeridis MP, Wanebo HJ: Oncogene protein co-expression: Value of Ha-ras, c-myc, c-fos, and p53 as prognostic discriminants for breast carcinoma. *Ann Surg* **221**:706, 1995.

221. Ciardello F, Gottardis M, Basolo F, Normanno N, Dickson RB, Bianco AR, Salomon DS: Additive effects of c-erb-2, c-Ha-ras, and transforming growth factor-alpha genes on in vitro transformation of human mammary epithelial cells. *Mol Carcinog* **6**:43, 1992.

222. Sabbatini AR, Basolo F, Valentini P, Mattii L, Calcvo S, Fiore L, Ciardello F, Petrini M: Induction of multidrug resistance (MDR) by transfection of MCF-10A cell line with c-Ha-ras and c-erbB-2 oncogenes. *Int J Cancer* **59**:208, 1994.

223. Giai M, Roagna R, Ponzone R, deBortoli M, Dati C, Sismondi P: Prognostic and predictive relevance of c-erB-2 and ras expression in node positive and negative breast cancer. *Anticancer Res* **14**:1441, 1994.

224. Luttrell DK, Lee A, Lansing TJ, Crosby RM, Jung KD, Willard D, Luther M, Rodriguez M, Berman J, Gilmer TM: Involvement of pp60c-src with two major signaling pathways in human breast cancer. *Proc Natl Acad Sci USA* **91**:83, 1994.

225. Ottenhoff-Kalff AE, Rijksen G, van Buerden EA, Hennipman A, Michels AA, Staal GE: Characterization of protein tyrosine kinases from human breast cancer: Involvement of the c-src oncogene product. *Cancer Res* **52**:4773, 1992.

226. Hennipman A, van Oirschot BA, Smits J, Rijksen G, Staal GE: Tyrosine kinase activity in breast cancer, benign breast disease, and normal breast tissue. *Cancer Res* **49**:516, 1989.

227. Hunter T, Pines J: Cyclins and cancer: II Cyclin D and CDK inhibitors come of age. *Cell* **79**:573, 1994.

228. Marx J: How cells cycle toward cancer. *Science* **263**:319, 1994.

229. Hollstein M, Sidransky D, Vogelstein B, Harris CC: p53 mutations in human cancers. *Science* **253**:49, 1991.

230. Borresen AL, Andersen TI, Garber J, et al: Screening for germ line p53 mutations in breast cancer patients. *Cancer Res* **52**:3234, 1992.

231. Deng G, Chen LC, Schott DR, Thor A, Bhargava V, Ljung BM, Chew K, Smith HS: Loss of heterozygosity and p53 gene mutations in breast cancer. *Cancer Res* **54**:499, 1994.

232. Andersen TI, Holm R, Nesland JM, Heimdal KR, Ottestad L, Borresen-AL: Prognostic significance of TP53 alterations in breast carcinoma. *Br J Cancer* **68**:540, 1993.

233. Elledge RM, Fuqua SAW, Clark GM, Pujol P, Allred DC: The role and prognostic significance of p53 gene alterations in breast cancer. *Breast Cancer Res Treat* **27**:95, 1993.

234. Saitoh S, Cunningham J, De Vries EM, McGovern RM, Schroeder JJ, Hartmann A, Blaszyk H, Wold LE, et al: p53 gene mutations in breast cancers in midwestern US women: Null as well as missense-type mutations are associated with poor prognosis. *Oncogene* **9**:2869, 1994.

235. Shiao YH, Chen VW, Scheer WD, Cheng X, Correa P: Racial disparity in the association of p53 gene alterations with breast cancer survival. *Cancer Res* **55**:1485, 1995.

236. Marchetti A, Buttitta F, Pelligrini S, Campani D, Diella F, Cecchetti, Callahan R, Bistocchi M: p53 mutations and histological type of invasive breast carcinoma. *Cancer Res* **53**:4665, 1993.

237. Moll UM, Riou G, Levine AJ: Two distinct mechanisms alter p53 in breast cancer. Mutation and nuclear exclusion. *Proc Natl Acad Sci USA* **87**:5863, 1992.

238. Aas T, Borresen AL, Geisler S, et al: Specific p53 mutations are associated with de novo resistance to doxorubicin in breast cancer patients. *Nat Med* **2**:811, 1996.

239. Bergh J, Norberg T, Sjogren S, Lindgren A, Holmberg L: Complete sequencing of the p53 gene provides prognostic information in breast cancer patients particularly in relation to adjuvant systemic therapy and radiotherapy. *Nat Med* **10**:1029, 1995.

240. T'Ang A, Varley JM, Chakraborty S, Murphree AL, Fung YK: Structural rearrangement of the retinoblastoma gene in human breast carcinoma. *Science* **242**:263, 1988.

241. Lee EY, To H, Shew JY, Bookstein R, Scully P, Lee WH: Inactivation of the retinoblastoma susceptibility gene in human breast cancers. *Science* **241**:218, 1988.

242. Gottardis MM, Saceda M, Garcia-Morales P, Fung YK, Solomon H, Sholler PF, Lippman ME, Martin MB: Regulation of retinoblastoma gene expression in hormone-dependent breast cancer. *Endocrinology* **136**:5659, 1995.

243. Wang NP, To H, Lee WH, Lee EY: Tumor suppressor activity of RB and p53 genes in human breast carcinoma cells. *Oncogene* **8**:279, 1993.

244. Fung YK, T'Ang A: The role of the retinoblastoma gene in breast cancer development. *Cancer Treat Res* **61**:59, 1992.

245. Berns EM, deKlein A, van Putten WL, van Staveren IL, Bootsma A, Klijn JG, Foekens JA: Association between RB-1 gene alterations and factors of favourable prognosis in human breast cancer, without effect on survival. *Int J Cancer* **64**:140, 1995.

246. Sawan A, Randall B, Agnus B, Wright C, Henry JA, Ostrowski J, Hennessy C, Lennard TW, Corbett I, Horne CH: Retinoblastoma and p53 gene expression related to relapse and survival in human breast cancer. An immunohistochemical study. *J Pathol* **168**:23028, 1992.

247. Buckley MF, Sweeney KJE, Hamilton JA, Sini RL, Manning DL, Nicholson RI, deFazio A, et al: Expression and amplification of cyclin genes in human breast cancer. *Oncogene* **8**:2127, 1993.

248. Motokura T, Bloom T, Kim HG, et al: A BCL1-linked candidate oncogene which is rearranged in parathyroid tumors encodes a novel cyclin. *Nature* **350**:512, 1991.

249. Bartokova J, Lukas J, Muller H, Lutzhoft D, Strauss M, Bartek J: Cyclin D1 protein expression and function in human breast cancer. *Int J Cancer* **57**:353, 1994.

250. Zhang SY, Caamano J, Cooper F, Guo X, Klein Szanto JP: Immunohistochemistry of cyclin D1 in human breast cancer. *Am J Clin Pathol* **102**:695, 1994.

251. Weinstat-Saslow D, Merino MJ, Manrow RE, Lawrence JA, Bluth RF, Wittenbel KD, Simpson JF, Page DL, Steeg PS: Overexpression of cyclin D mRNA distinguishes invasive and in situ breast carcinomas from non-malignant lesions. *Nature Med* **12**:1257, 1995.

252. Musgrove EA, Lee CSL, Buckley MF, Sutherland RL: Cyclin D1 induction in breast cancer cells shortens G1 and is sufficient for cells arrested in G1 to complete the cell cycle. *Proc Natl Acad Sci USA* **91**:8022, 1994.

253. Wang TC, Cardiff RD, Zukerberg L, Lees E, Arnold A, Schmidt EV: Mammary hyperplasia and carcinoma in MMTV-cyclin D1 transgenic mice. *Nature* **369**:669, 1994.

254. Sicinski P, Donaher JL, Parker SB, et al: Cyclin D1 provides a link between development and oncogenesis in the retina and breast. *Cell* **82**:621, 1995.

255. Alexandrow MG, Moses HL: Transforming growth factors β and cell cycle regulation. *Cancer Res* **55**:1452, 1995.

256. Jeng MH, ten Dijke P, Iwata KK, Jordan VC: Regulation of the levels of three transforming growth factor beta mRNAs by estrogen and their effect on the proliferation of human breast cancer cells. *Mol Cell Endocrinol* **97**:115, 1993.

257. Knabbe C, Lippman ME, Wakefield LM, Flanders KC, Kasid A, Derynck R, Dickson RB. Evidence that transforming growth factor-β is a hormonally regulated negative growth factor in human breast cancer cells. *Cell* **48**:417, 1987.

258. Perry RR, Kang Y, Greaves BR: Relationship between tamoxifen-induced transforming growth factor beta 1 expression, cytostasis and apoptosis in human breast cancer cells. *Br J Cancer* **72**:1441, 1995.

259. Croxtall JD, Jamil A, Ayub M, Colletta AA, White JO: TGF-β stimulation of endometrial and breast cancer cell growth. *Int J Cancer* **50**:822, 1992.

260. Arteaga CL, Dugger TC, Winnier AR, Forbes JT: Evidence for a positive role of transforming growth factor β in human breast cancer cell tumorigenesis. *J Cell Biochem* **17G**:187, 1993.

261. Walker RA, Dearing SJ, Gallacher B: Relationship of transforming growth factor β1 to extracellular matrix and stromal infiltrates in invasive breast carcinoma. *Br J Cancer* **69**:1160, 1994.

262. MacCallum J, Bartlett JM, Thompson AM, Keen JC, Dixon JM, Miller WR: Expression of transforming growth factor. β mRNA isoforms in human breast cancer. *Br J Cancer* **69**:1006, 1994.

263. Dublin EA, Barnes DM, Wang DY, King RJ, Levison DA: TGFα and TGFβ expression in mammary carcinoma. *J Pathol* **170**:15, 1993.

264. Thompson CB: Apoptosis in the pathogenesis and treatment of disease. *Science* **267**:1456, 1995.

265. Fisher DE: Apoptosis in cancer therapy: Crossing the threshold. *Cell* **78**:539, 1994.

266. Johnston SRD, MacLennan KA, Sacks NPM, Salter J, Smith IE, Doswett M: Modulation of Bcl-2 and Ki-67 expression in oestrogen receptor human breast cancer by tamoxifen. *Eur J Cancer* **30A**:1663, 1994.

267. Joensuu H, Pylkkanen L, Toikkanen S: bcl-2 protein expression and long-term survial in breast cancer. *Am J Pathol* **145**:1191, 1992.

268. Sabourin JC, Martin A, Baruch J, Truc JB, Gompel A, Poitut P: bcl-2 expression in normal breast tissue druing the menstrual cycle. *Int J Cancer* **59**:1, 1994.

269. Haldar S, Negrini M, Monne M, Sabbioni S, Croce CM: Down-regulation of bcl-2 by p53 in breast cancer cells. *Cancer Res* **54**:2095, 1994.

270. Ottestad L, Andersen TI, Nesland JM, Skrede M, Tveit KM, Nustad K, Borresen AL: Amplification of c-erbB-2, int-2, and c-myc genes in node-negative breast carcinomas: Relationship to prognosis. *Acta Oncol* **32**:389, 1993.

271. Pieulainen T, Lipponen P, Aaltomaa S, Eskelinen M, Kosma VM, Syrjanen K: Expression of c-myc proteins in breast cancer as related to established prognostic factors and survival. *Anticancer Res* **15**:959, 1995.

272. Pavelic ZP, Pavelic L, Lower EE, Gapany M, Gapany S, Barker EA, Preisler HD: c-myc, c-erbB-2, and Ki-67 expression in normal breast tissue and in invasive and noninvasive breast carcinoma. *Cancer Res* **52**:2597, 1992.

273. Porter-Jordan K, Lippman ME: Overview of the biologic markers of breast cancer. *Hematol Oncol Clin North Am* **8**:73, 1994.

274. Glukhova M, Koteliansky V, Sastre X, Thiery JP: Adhesion systems in normal breast and in invasive breast carcinoma. *Am J Pathol* **146**:706, 1995.

275. Rimm DL, Sinard JH, Morrow JS: Reduced a-catenin and E-cadherin expression in breast cancer. *Lab Invest* **72**:506, 1996.

276. Palacios J, Benito N, Pizarro A, et al: Anomalous expression of P-cadherin in breast carcinoma. *Am J Pathol* **146**:605, 1995.

277. Rasbridge SA, Gillett CE, Sampson SA, et al: Epithelial (E-) and placental (P-) cell adhesion molecule expression in breast carcinoma. *J Pathol* **169**:245, 1993.

278. Siitonen SM, Kokoene JT, Helin HJ, et al: Reduce E-cadherin expression is associated with invasiveness and unfavorable prognosis in breast cancer. *Am J Clin Pathol* **105**:394, 1996.

279. Stetler-Stevenson WG: Type IV collagenases in tumor invasion and metastasis. *Cancer Metastasis Rev* **9**:289, 1990.

280. Yu M, Sato H, Seiki M, Thompson EW: Complex regulation of membrane-type matrix metalloproteinase expression and matrix metalloproteinase-2 activation by concanavalin A in MDA-MB-231 human breast cancer cells. *Cancer Res* **55**:3272, 1995.

281. Duffy MJ, Blaser J, Duggan C, et al: Assay of matrix metalloproteinase types 8 and 9 by ELISA in human breast cancer. *Br J Cancer* **71**:1025, 1995.

282. Okada A, Bellocq JP, Rouyer N et al: Membrane-type metalloproteinase (MT-MMP) gene is expressed in stromal cells of human colon, breast and head and neck carcinomas. *Proc Natl Acad Sci USA* **92**:2730, 1995.

283. Sato H, Takino T, Okada Y, et al: A matrix metalloproteinase expressed on the surface of invasive tumor cells. *Nature* **370**:61, 1994.

284. Polette M, Gilbert N, Stas I, et al: Gelatinase expression and localization in human breast cancers: An in situ hybridization study and immunohistochemical detection using confocal microscopy. *Virchows Arch* **424**:641, 1994.

285. Ito A, Nakajima Y, Nagase H, et al: Co-culture of human breast adenocarcinoma MCF-7 cells and human dermal fibroblasts enhances the production of matrix metalloproteinases 1, 2 and 3 in fibroblasts. *Br J Cancer* **71**:1039, 1995.

286. Noel AC, Polette M, Lewalle JM, et al: Coordinate enhancement of gelatinase A mRNA and activity levels in human fibroblasts in response to breast-adenocarcinoma cells. *Intl J Cancer* **56**:331, 1994.

287. Aaltonen M, Lipponen P, Kosma VM, et al: Prognostic value of cathepsin-D expression in female breast. *Anticancer Res* **15**:1033, 1995.

288. Gion M, Mione R, Dittadi R, et al: Relationship between cathepsin D and other pathologic and biochemical parameters in 1752 patients with primary breast cancer. *Eur J Cancer* **31A**:671, 1995.

289. Steeg PS, Bevilacqua G, Kopper L, Thorgeirsson UP, Talmadge JE, Liotta LA, Sobel M: Evidence for a novel gene associated with a low tumor metastatic potential. *J Natl Cancer Inst* **80**:200, 1988.

290. Rosengard AM, Krutzsch HC, Shearn A, Biggs JR, Barker E, Marguilies IMK, King C, Liotta LA, Steeg PS: Reduced nm23/awd protein in tumour metastasis and aberrant Drosophila development. *Nature* **342**:177, 1989.

291. Bevilacqua G, Sobel M, Liotta LA, Steeg PS: Association of low nm23 levels in human proiimary infiltrating ductal breast carcinomas with lymph node involvement and other histopathologic indicators of high metastatic potential. *Cancer Res* **49**:5158, 1989.

292. Leone A, Flatow U, VanHoutte K, Steeg PS: Transfection of human nm23-H1 into the human MDA-MB-435 breast carcinoma cell lines: Effect on tumor metastatic potential, colonization, and enzymatic activity. *Oncogene* **8**:2325, 1993.

293. Steeg PS, de la Rosa A, Flatow U, MacDonald NJ, Benedict M, Leone A: Nm23 and breast cancer metastasis. *Breast Cancer Res Treat* **25**:175, 1993.

294. Howlett AR, Peterson OW, Steeg PS, Bissell MJ: A novel function for the nm23-H1 gene: Overexpression in human breast carcinoma cells to the formation of basement membrane and growth arrest. *J Natl Cancer Inst* **86**:1838, 1994.

295. Postel EH, Berberich SJ, Flint SJ, Ferrone CA: Human c-myc transcription factor identification as nm23-H2 nucleosidase diphosphate kinase, a candidate suppressor of tumor metastasis. *Science* **261**:478, 1993.

296. Chang CL, Zhu X, Thoraval DH, Ungar D, Rawwas J, Hora N, Strahler JR, Hanash S, Radany E: nm23-H1 mutation in neuroblastoma. *Nature* **370**:335, 1994.

297. Hoskins KF, Stopfer JE, Calzone KA, Merajver SD, Rebbeck TR, Garber JE, Weber BL: Assessment and counseling for familial breast cancer risk: A guide for clinicians. *JAMA* **273**:577, 1995.

CHAPTER 31

Colorectal Tumors

Kenneth W. Kinzler ■ Bert Vogelstein

1. Colorectal tumors progress through a series of clinical and histopathologic stages, ranging from single crypt lesions (aberrant crypt foci) to small benign tumors (adenomatous polyps) to malignant cancers (carcinomas). This progression results from a series of genetic changes that involve the activation of oncogenes and the inactivation of tumor-suppressor genes.

2. Several inherited predispositions to colorectal cancer have been described, of which the two best characterized are hereditary nonpolyposis colorectal cancer (HNPCC) (Chap. 17) and familial adenomatous polyposis (FAP). Patients with FAP develop hundreds of benign colorectal tumors, some of which progress to carcinomas. FAP is associated with germ-line mutations of the *APC* gene which generally result in truncation of the encoded protein.

3. The majority of colorectal cancer cases do not have a well-recognized inherited component and therefore are classified as sporadic in nature. These tumors result from a series of somatic genetic mutations. To date, four genetic events which commonly occur in colorectal cancers have been described at the molecular level; these events include activation of *ras* oncogenes and inactivation of tumor-suppressor genes on chromosomes 5q, 17p, and 18q.

4. Activating mutations of one of the *ras* oncogenes occur in about 50 percent of colorectal cancers and in a similar percentage of adenomas larger than 1 cm in diameter. The majority of these mutations affect the c-Ki-*ras* gene, with the rest affecting the N-*ras* gene. The ras proteins are homologous to G proteins and are believed to play a role in signal transduction.

5. The tumor-suppressor gene on chromosome 17p has been identified as the p53 gene. This gene is inactivated in at least 85 percent of colorectal cancers but rarely in benign tumors. Inactivation of p53 is most often due to a missense mutation combined with a loss of the other allele. Biochemical studies of the p53 protein suggest that it functions by binding DNA in a sequence-specific manner and activating the transcription of adjacent genes. Mutant p53 is defective in these activities.

6. Three candidate tumor-suppressor genes, DCC, DPC4, and JV18-1/MADR2, have been isolated from chromosome 18q. At least one copy of these genes is lost in 70 percent of colorectal cancers and over 40 percent of large adenomas with foci of carcinomatous transformation. Somatic alterations, including homozygous deletions, point mutations, and insertions, have been detected in all three candidate genes. Additional studies will be necessary to determine the role of these genes in colorectal tumorigenesis.

7. The tumor-suppressor gene on chromosome 5q has been identified as the *APC* gene. In addition to causing FAP through germ-line transmission, mutations of the *APC* gene occur somatically in over 80 percent of sporadic colorectal tumors, benign or malignant. Almost all these mutations, like the inherited mutations that cause FAP, are predicted to result in truncation of the APC protein. Mutation of the *APC* gene is the earliest genetic event identified in colorectal tumorigenesis, with mutations being identified in lesions as small as a few crypts.

8. The analysis of mutations in colorectal tumors at various stages of their development allows definition of a model for colorectal tumor development. Mutations in the *APC* gene appear to initiate this process, resulting in a small tumor that represents the clonal growth of a single cell. One of the cells in this small tumor may acquire an additional mutation (often in the K-*ras* gene), allowing it to overgrow surrounding cells and resulting in a larger tumor. Subsequent waves of clonal expansion are driven by sequential mutations in the 18q suppressor and p53 genes. Along with this expansion come further cellular disorganization and eventually the ability to invade and metastasize. Understanding this accumulation of genetic events is the first step toward unraveling the complex process of colorectal tumorigenesis.

CLINICAL FEATURES

Incidence and Scope

Colorectal cancer is the second leading cause of cancer deaths in the United States. In 1995, there were about 160,000 new cases of colorectal cancers and 60,000 deaths from this disease.[1] The cases are roughly equally distributed between the sexes. The average age of incidence for colon cancer in the United States is 67 years,[2] and over 90 percent of colon cancer deaths occur in individuals over age 55.[3] Approximately 5 percent of the population develops colorectal cancer, and this figure is expected to rise as life expectancy increases.[3] Furthermore, when nonmalignant colorectal tumors are considered, up to half the population is affected.[4-6]

HISTOPATHOLOGY

A single layer of epithelial cells lines the invaginations (crypts) of the colon and rectum (Fig. 31-1). As is true throughout the digestive tract, these crypts substantially increase the surface area occupied by the epithelium. Four to six stem cells at the base of each crypt give rise to the three major epithelial cell types: absorptive cells, mucus-secreting goblet cells, and neuroepithelial cells. These cells multiply in the lower third of the crypt and differentiate in the upper two-thirds. The journey from the base of the crypt to its apex, where the epithelial cells are extruded, takes 3 to 6 days.[7,8]

Normally, the birthrate of the colonic epithelial cells precisely equals the rate of loss from the crypt apex to the lumen of the bowel. If the birth:loss ratio increases, a tumor results (a tumor is defined as any abnormal accumulation of cells). A tumor of the colon often is first observed clinically as a polyp, a mass of cells protruding from the bowel wall (Fig. 31-2). There are predominantly two types of polyps which can be distinguished only histologically.[9] The nondysplastic or hyperplastic type consists of large numbers of cells which have normal morphology (Fig. 31-3*B*). The cells are lined up in a single row along the basement membrane, and these polyps apparently do not have a tendency to become neoplastic. The other polyp type (adenomatous) is dysplastic, as evidenced by an abnormal intracellular and intercellular organization (Fig. 31-3*C*). Several layers of epithelial cells lie on the basement membrane, the nuclei of the epithelial cells are larger than normal, and their position within the cell is often farther from the basement membrane. Crypts crowd together in a kaleidoscopic pattern. As adenomas grow in size, they become more dysplastic. They also are more likely to contain "villous" components, that is, fingerlike projections of dysplastic crypts which can be distinguished from the smooth contour of the less advanced "tubular" adenomas. As adenomas progress, they are more likely to become malignant, with the ability to invade surrounding tissues and travel to distant organs through direct spread or transport by blood vessels or lymphatics

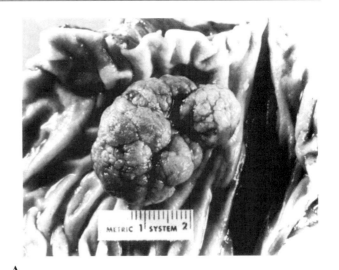

A

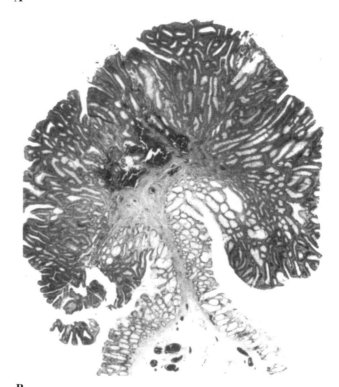

B

FIG. 31-2 Morphology of a colonic polyp showing its pedunculated nature. *A.* A macroscopic view of a large tubular adenoma. *B.* A cross section of a tubular adenoma with a clearly visible stalk. (*From Kent and Mitros with permission.*[9])

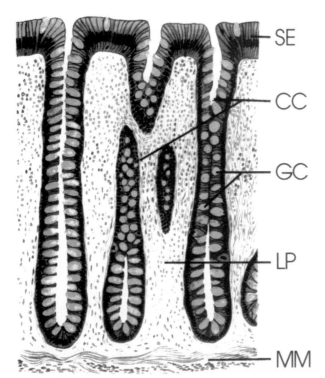

FIG. 31-1 Histology of the normal colon. Examples of surface epithelium (SE), colonic crypts (CC), goblet cells (GC), lamina propria (LP), and muscularis mucosa (MM) are marked. (*From Clara, Herschel, and Gerner with permission.*[271])

(metastasis). Malignant tumors are not necessarily larger or more dysplastic than benign tumors; their sole determining feature is invasiveness. Adenocarcinomas are the most common malignant tumor of the colon, although other cancers (e.g., lymphomas and sarcomas) arising from nonepithelial cell occasionally occur.[10] As was noted above, polyps are the earliest clinical manifestation of colorectal neoplasia, but methylene blue staining or microscopic examination of the colonic mucosa also can detect lesions that affect one or a small number of crypts (Fig. 31-4). These lesions are termed aberrant crypt foci (ACF) and like their larger counterparts can be dysplastic (microadenomas) or nondysplastic.

Colorectal neoplasia is not a rare condition. About 5 percent of individuals less than 50 years old have adenomatous polyps, as do about half of those over 70 years old.[4–6] These figures are even higher when ACF are considered. Adenomas less than 10

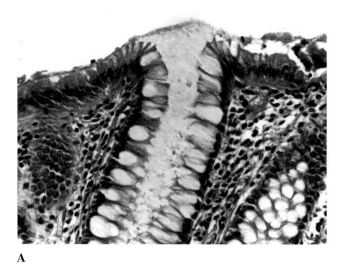

A

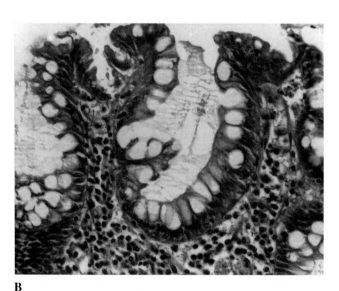

B

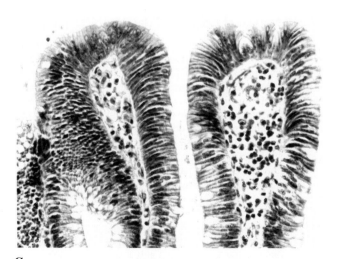

C

FIG. 31-3 Histopathology of colonic polyps. Panels (top, middle, bottom) show high-power views of hematoxylin-eosin-stained sections of normal colonic mucosa, a hyperplastic polyp (nondysplastic), and an adenomatous polyp (dysplastic), respectively. Note the increased disruption of normal architecture in the adenomatous polyp compared to the hyperplastic polyp. (*From Dr. Stanley R. Hamilton, Johns Hopkins University School of Medicine, Baltimore.*)

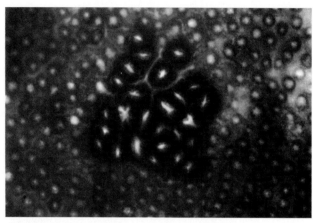

FIG. 31-4 Morphology of an ACF. Macroscopic view of an ACF after staining with methylene blue. (*From Dr. Stanley R. Hamilton, Johns Hopkins University School of Medicine, Baltimore.*)

mm in diameter have a very low probability of developing a focus of malignancy, while tumors larger than 10 mm have a 15 percent chance of becoming malignant over a 10-year period.[11] Benign tumors are easily removed by colonoscopy or surgery. Malignant tumors usually are excisable by surgery, but if they have already metastasized, additional therapy is necessary. The most common site of metastasis is the mesenteric lymph nodes.[2] These lymph nodes usually are excised at the time of the initial surgery for the cancer. If distant metastasis has occurred (to the peritoneal surface or liver), surgery will not be curative. Patients with metastatis disease usually are treated with radiation and/or chemotherapeutic agents (adjuvant therapy). Although such treatments can induce remissions that last many months, they are often not curative, as evidenced by the fact that about 40 percent of patients with colorectal cancer die from the disease within 5 years of the diagnosis.[1]

Inherited Predispositions

Familial colorectal cancers can broadly be divided into two groups: those characterized by the presence of multiple benign colorectal polyps (polyposis) and those characterized by the absence of polyposis. Several types of polyposis syndromes have been described, including familial adenomatous polyposis coli (FAP), Peutz-Jegher's syndrome, familial juvenile polyposis, Cronkhite-Canada syndrome, and hyperplastic polyposis. In this chapter the discussion of the polyposis syndromes is limited to FAP and its variants because its pathogenesis has been proved to be relevant to sporadic colorectal tumorigenesis.

FAP is an autosomal dominant inherited disease in which affected individuals develop hundreds to thousands of adenomatous polyps during the second and third decades of life (Fig. 31-5). These polyps resemble the sporadic adenomatous polyps that develop in the general population. Although an individual FAP polyp is no more likely to progress to cancer than is a sporadic polyp, their large numbers essentially guarantee that some will progress to cancer. Indeed, the median age for colorectal cancer in FAP patients is about 40.[12] Thus, prophylactic colectomies are routinely performed on FAP patients to reduce their risk of cancer. Although about 1 in 5000 to 10,000 individuals are affected with FAP in the United States,[13] less than 1 percent of all colon cancer cases occur in FAP patients, in part because of prophylactic colectomies. Patients with FAP are also at increased risk for cancers of thyroid, small intestine, stomach, and brain.[12,14] Variants of FAP have been described which include all the colonic manifestations of FAP plus varied extracolonic manifestations.[15,16] The most common variant

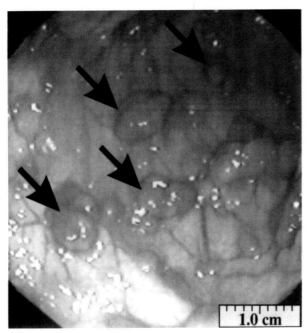

FIG 31-5 Polyposis in a patient with FAP. Colonoscopic view of polyps in a patient with FAP. (*From Kinzler and Vogelstein with permission.*[272])

is Gardner syndrome (GS), which is characterized by soft-tissue tumors, osteomas, dental abnormalities, and congenital hypertrophy of the retinal pigment epithelium (CHRPE).[15] Other attenuated variants of FAP are characterized by a reduced number of intestinal polyps (10 to 100).[17,18] Finally, the majority but not all cases of Turcot syndrome, which is characterized by the presence of central nervous system tumors in combination with a familial predisposition to colorectal cancer, are variants of FAP.[14] As detailed in the section on the *APC* tumor-suppressor gene below, FAP and its variants can now be traced to germ-line mutations of the *APC* gene. Studies of *APC*'s function suggest that the primary defect in FAP syndromes in tumor initiation.

It has been estimated that hereditary nonpolyposis colorectal cancer (HNPCC) accounts for about 2 to 4 percent of colorectal cancers in the western world.[19] Like FAP patients, HNPCC patients develop colorectal cancer at a median age of around 40 (Chap. 13).[20] However, unlike FAP, these patients lack a marked increase in the number of precursor adenomas. Thus, until recently HNPCC kindreds had to be defined operationally by the identification of at least three first-degree relatives in at least two different generations coupled with early-onset colorectal cancer (less than 50 years of age). The recent identification of the underlying genetic defect allows a genetic definition.[21] It is now known that the majority of HNPCC patients inherit defects in DNA mismatch repair genes. Tumors arising in these patients are DNA mismatch repair–deficient and as a result are genetically unstable and rapidly progress to cancer. Thus, in contrast to FAP, the defect in HNPCC primarily affects tumor progression. In addition to colorectal cancer, HNPCC patients are at increased risk for other cancers, including those of the uterus, ovary, and brain.[21] Indeed, the majority of cases of Turcot syndrome not linked to FAP represent HNPCC patients.[14]

Other Genetic Factors

The vast majority of colorectal cancers do not have an easily recognized inherited component and therefore are considered sporadic. Only about 3 to 5 percent of all colorectal cancers occur in individuals with well-characterized inherited predispositions such

as those described above. However, several studies suggest a broader role for inheritance.[22–24] For example, the relatives of patients with "sporadic" colon cancers also have an increased risk for colon cancer, and detailed studies of this phenomenon have suggested a dominant inheritance of susceptibility to adenomatous polyps and associated cancers.[23,24] Furthermore, it has been estimated that such inherited susceptibility could account for 15 to 90 percent of the total colorectal cancer patients in the population at large. Although these studies await identification of the specific genetic factors, it is reasonable to assume that hereditary factors, combined with environmental factors (see below), determine the aggregate risk for colorectal cancer. Whether the hereditary factors turn out to represent a few major genes or a synergistic combination of multiple genes remains to be determined.

Environmental Factors

While inherited genetic factors can clearly play an important role in the development of colon cancers, they are by no means the sole determinant.[25] This point is well illustrated by classic studies of Japanese immigrants to the United States. Historically, the incidence of colon cancer has been low in Japan, whereas the incidence of gastric cancer has been high. Japanese populations that moved to the United States show a progressive increase in colorectal cancer.[26] Today, this change in cancer incidence is being repeated on a larger scale in Japan, where the incidence of gastric cancer is declining while that of colon cancer is increasing.[27] This is believed to be due to the westernization of the Japanese diet. Epidemiologic studies indicate that diets high in animal fat and red meat[28–30] or low in fiber[31,32] are associated with an increased risk for colorectal cancer. The components of animal fat, red meat, and fiber, which are responsible for the effects on risk, and the mechanisms underlying such effects have not been elucidated. Presumably, they affect the incidence of mutations or the ability of mutated cells to expand clonally.

MOLECULAR GENETICS OF COLORECTAL CANCER

Clonal Nature of Colorectal Cancers

The clonal nature of tumors is a critical feature of the somatic mutation–clonal evolution model of carcinogenesis.[33] In this model, a single cell acquires a mutation that provides a selective growth advantage which allows it to outnumber neighboring cells (Fig. 31-6). From within this clonal population, a single cell may acquire a second mutation, providing an additional growth advantage which allows further clonal expansion. Repeated cycles of mutation followed by clonal expansion eventually lead to a fully developed malignant tumor.

The clonal nature of human colorectal tumors was first examined by using techniques based on X-chromosome inactivation in females. Only a single X chromosome is active in any somatic cell of a female. This inactivation occurs early during embryogenesis and is random with regard to which copy of the X-chromosome (maternal or paternal) is inactivated in a given cell. The pattern of X inactivation is transmitted in a highly stable manner to progeny cells. The inactivation is accompanied by changes in the methylation of cytosine residues on the inactivated X chromosome. Thus, methylation-sensitive restriction enzymes in combination with restriction-fragment-length polymorphism can be used to distinguish which copy of X chromosome is inactivated.[34] When this type of analysis is performed on small portions of normal colonic mucosa, the inactivation of X is equally distributed between the maternal

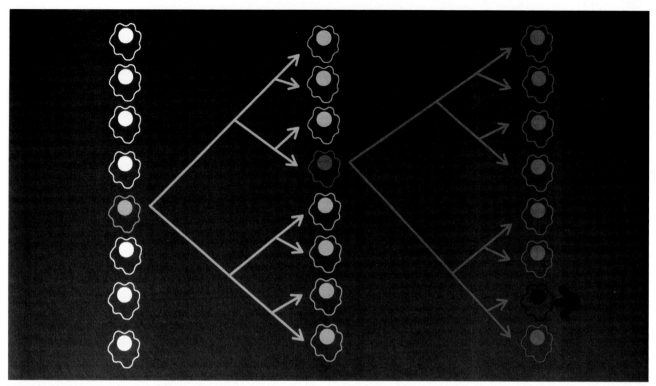

FIG 31-6 Clonal evolution of tumor cells. A normal cell acquires a mutation that gives it a slight growth advantage. With time, this clone expands and one of the progeny cells acquires another mutation that provides an additional growth advantage. After several rounds of mutation followed by expansion, a malignant tumor results. The expansion

phase is important because it provides additional targets for subsequent mutation. Without this expansion, mutations would occur so infrequently that multiple genetic changes would be unlikely to occur and tumors would be very rare.

and paternal copies. In contrast, when benign or malignant colorectal tumors were analyzed, they were each found to display a monoclonal pattern of X inactivation.[35,36] The monoclonal nature of these tumors was further demonstrated by using autosomal polymorphic markers which demonstrated clonal chromosomal losses.[36] These observations were consistent with cytogenetic studies which had demonstrated clonal chromosomal abnormalities in many carcinomas[37–39] and some adenomas.[40–42] Subsequently, the identification of somatic point mutations provided conclusive proof of the monoclonal nature of human colorectal tumors.

The *ras* Oncogenes

The first major breakthrough in the molecular genetics of colorectal tumors was the identification of *ras* gene mutations.[43–45] The first *ras* genes were identified as the transforming components of the Kirsten and Harvey rat sarcoma virus genomes (Chap. 10). Three cellular *ras* genes, K-*ras*, H-*ras*, and N-*ras* were later identified and shown to transform cells in tissue culture when mutated.[46,47] Specific point mutations of K-*ras* or N-*ras* are found in approximately 50 percent of colorectal adenomas larger that 1 cm and 50 percent of carcinomas; *ras* mutations are rarely seen in adenomas less than 1 cm in size (Fig. 31-7).[45] The lack of mutations in smaller adenomas suggests that *ras* mutations are acquired during adenoma progression. Direct evidence for this premise comes from microdissection studies demonstrating subpopulations of adenoma cells which have acquired *ras* mutations.[48] *ras* mutations are not limited to dysplastic colorectal lesions; 100 percent of nondysplastic ACF and 25 percent of hyperplastic polyps have *ras* mutations.[49,50] However, these nondysplastic lesions appear to be largely self-limiting in a clinical context. Most of the mutations identified (85 percent) are in codons 12 and 13 of K-*ras*, with the rest affecting codon 61 of K-*ras* or N-*ras*. These studies clearly indicate that *ras* oncogene mutations play

a role during the development of a significant proportion of colorectal tumors. However, they also suggest that many tumors can develop in the absence of *ras* mutations or fail to progress in their presence. However, the importance of *ras* in colorectal tumorigenesis has been emphasized by the finding that colorectal tumor cells in which the mutated *ras* gene has been removed by homologous recombination lost their tumorigenicity.[51]

The *ras* oncogenes encode 21-kD monomeric proteins with homology to G proteins.[52] Like G proteins *ras* can bind GTP and catalyze its hydrolysis to GDP. *ras* is active only when bound to GTP,

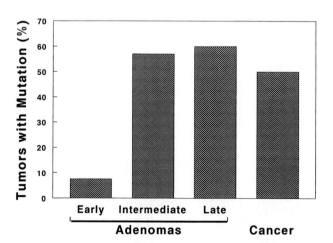

FIG. 31-7 Frequency of *ras* mutations in colorectal tumors. Early adenomas were defined as less than 1 cm, intermediate adenomas were larger than 1 cm but without foci of carcinomatous transformation, and late adenomas were larger than 1 cm and contained at least one focus of carcinomatous transformation; the cancers were adenocarcinomas of the colon. Tumors were assessed for *ras* mutations, as described in Ref. 45.

with the hydrolysis to GDP leading to inactivation. The ratio of GTP-*ras* to GDP-*ras* is higher in cells containing mutant *ras* genes than it is in cells with only wild-type *ras* gene products. The altered ratio is due to decreased hydrolysis of GTP to GDP. However, the intrinsic GTPase activities of wild-type and mutant *ras* usually do not account for this difference. The interaction of *ras* with a cellular GTPase-activating protein (GAP) is apparently responsible for the difference. The GTPase activity of wild-type *ras* is stimulated by GAP, while mutant *ras* does not respond to GAP.[53] Recently, the gene responsible for neurofibromatosis type 1 (NF1) was found to have GAP activity (see Chap. 22).[54–57] This is interesting in light of the fact that many colon cancers do not contain *ras* gene mutations. Accordingly, a mutation of NF1 has been reported to occur in a colon tumor which did not have a *ras* mutation.[58]

Tumor-Suppressor Genes in Colorectal Cancers

The first molecular evidence for the role of tumor-suppressor genes in colorectal tumorigenesis came from the study of allelic losses.[36,45, 59–63] Tumor-suppressor genes can be inactivated in a variety of ways, including point mutations, rearrangements, and deletions. Many of these deletions include entire chromosomal arms or even whole chromosomes. These large deletions can be detected by using polymorphic markers which distinguish the two alleles present in the germ line. Comparison of the alleles in the tumor tissue with those in normal tissue allows the identification of deletions as loss of heterozygosity (LOH). When colorectal cancers were examined by using at least one polymorphic marker for each nonacrocentric autosomal arm, certain arms were found to be frequently lost (Fig. 31-8).[63] Most frequently implicated were chro-

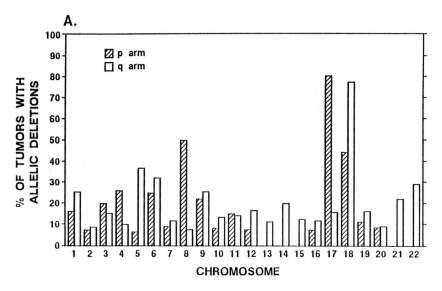

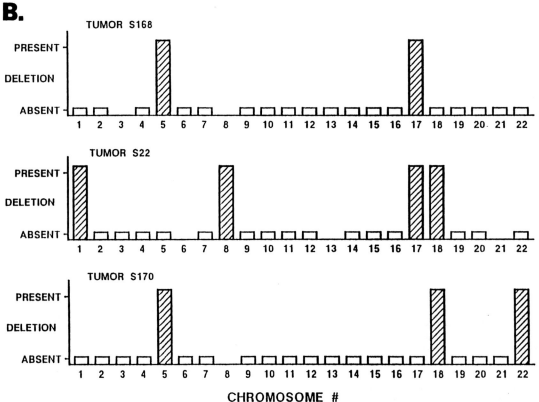

FIG. 31-8 Chromosomal losses in colorectal cancers. *A.* Frequency of allelic deletions for individual chromosome arms in colorectal carcinomas. Allelic losses were scored in 56 colorectal carcinomas by using polymorphic marker for all nonacrocentric autosomal arms.[63] Values for loss are expressed as the percentage of informative cases showing allelic loss. (*From Fearon and Vogelstein with permission.*[248]) *B.* Allelic losses in three individual tumors (S168, S22, and S170). Long bars indicate a deletion, short bars indicate no deletion, and the lack of an informative marker is indicated by the absence of a bar. Note that although there is a significant trend for loss of chromosomes 5, 8, 17, and 18, the exact pattern in individual tumors varies.

mosomes 5q, 8p, 17p, and 18q, which were found to be lost in 36 percent, 50 percent, 73 percent, and 75 percent of the cases, respectively. This frequent loss of specific chromosomes has been taken to represent one step in the inactivation of a tumor-suppressor gene residing on the lost chromosome. The LOH analysis were generally consistent with karyotypic studies which had shown frequent losses of the same chromosomes.[37–39] To date, presumptive tumor-suppressor genes on chromosomes 5q, 17p, and 18q have been identified. Chromosome losses, analyzed by LOH or karyotype, obviously underestimate the prevalence of suppressor gene alterations in colorectal tumors because small deletions, rearrangements, or point mutations are not apparent in such analysis.

Chromosome 17p: The p53 Gene

The first tumor-suppressor gene implicated in the development of colorectal tumors was the p53 gene on chromosome 17p. The existence of a tumor-suppressor gene on 17p came from the aforementioned allelic loss[36,45,60,62,63] and cytogenetic studies.[38,39] Loss of 17p sequences was detected in 75 percent of colorectal cancers, while 17p sequences were rarely lost in colorectal adenomas, suggesting that inactivation of the 17p tumor-suppressor gene was late event (Fig. 31-9).[45]

The p53 gene was originally identified in 1979 by virtue of its expression in cells infected with tumor viruses.[64–66] During the first 10 years of its study, the cellular p53 gene was considered a proto-oncogene, in part because of its increased expression in tumors and also because p53 was apparently able to transform rat embryo fibroblasts in collaboration with *ras* oncogenes.[67–69] However, subsequent studies indicated that the wild-type p53 gene is a tumor-suppressor gene, not a proto-oncogene. The studies in colorectal tumors were critical in this regard.[70] As was mentioned above, chromosome 17p losses were noted frequently in colorectal tumors. To further localize the position of the putative tumor-suppressor gene on this chromosome, a large panel of polymorphic markers was used to analyze numerous colorectal cancer cases. The common region of deletion (i.e., the chromosomal region consistently lost in tumors containing any loss of chromosome 17p) was mapped to a region centered at 17p13.1. Using Knudson's hypothesis, it was hypothesized that the loss of 17p13 removed one copy of a putative suppressor gene from the cell, while the remaining copy was mutant. Because p53 was known to reside at 17p13 and had previously been implicated in neoplasia (although as an oncogene), it was tested to see if it fit Knudson's hypothesis. The remaining p53 gene from a colorectal tumor which had lost one

p53 allele was sequenced. It was found to harbor a missense mutation at codon 143, changing alanine to valine. The mutation was somatic; that is, it was not present in the normal colon of the same patient. Further analysis identified somatic mutations in the remaining p53 gene in 24 of 28 colorectal tumors which had undergone allelic loss of 17p.[71] The majority of these mutations were missense and were clustered in four regions which are conserved among mammals, amphibians, birds, and fish (Figs. 31-10 and 11).

The frequent allelic loss of 17p, coupled with mutation of the remaining copy of p53, strongly suggested that p53 was a tumor-suppressor gene. Several other observations reinforced this idea. Most important, it was found that the wild-type p53 gene but not the mutant p53 gene could inhibit the growth of transformed cells in culture. This was demonstrated first for rodent cell fibroblasts[72,73] and later for human cancers of the colon[74] and other tissues.[75–77] Conversely, it was found that mutant but not wild-type p53 genes could transform rat embryo fibroblasts in cooperation with *ras* oncogenes (the presumable normal p53 genes used for the initial studies on transformation by p53 turned out to contain a mutation).[78,103] In Friend virus-induced erythroleukemias, the p53 gene was found to be inactivated by proviral integration.[79–81] The p53 protein appears to be inactivated by viruses in some human cancers as well. In cervical cancers, the human papillomavirus (HPV) E6 protein binds to the p53 gene product[82] and inhibits its functional properties.[83] Finally, studies of other human tumor types, including lung, breast, brain, bladder, and liver, show that p53 is frequently mutated, just as it is in the colon.[84] In fact, the mutations observed in some of these tumors have provided some clues to the mutagenic event.[85] For example, a specific mutation of codon 249 in liver tumors suggests a role for aflatoxins,[86–88] pyrimidine dimer mutations in skin tumors are consistent with a role for ultraviolet light,[89] and the pattern of mutations in lung cancers suggests mutagens in tobacco smoke as the culprits.[90] It has been estimated that over half the total malignancies in the world involve inactivation of p53. How does p53 exert its tumor-suppressor effect? The biochemical properties of the p53 protein provide some answers to this question. The p53 gene encodes a 393-amino acid phosphoprotein (Fig. 31-11). Biophysical studies of the p53 protein indicate that it exists as a tetramer.[91,92] The region responsible for this tetramerization has been mapped to the carboxy terminus[93] between amino acids 344 and 393, and this tetramerization appears to be critical for defining the biochemical properties of p53.[94] The most compelling property is the ability of wild-type p53 to bind DNA in a sequence-specific manner.[95] Analysis of numerous human and artificially constructed sequences which bind p53 in vitro allowed the definition of a consensus binding site composed to two copies of the 10-bp motif 5′-PuPuPuC(A/T)(A/T)GPyPyPy-3′.[96–98] One copy of this binding site is insufficient for binding, but binding is preserved even when the two copies are separated by as much as 13 bp. The complete p53 binding site is thus composed of four copies of the 5′-bp half site 5′-PuPuPuC(A/T(A/T)-3′ arranged in opposing directions. The ability of p53 to form tetramers could account for the four-fold symmetry of the binding site.

The fact that tumor-derived mutant p53 proteins almost uniformly have altered ability to bind DNA in a sequence-specific manner accentuates the importance of this activity.[95–97, 99,100] The recent determination of the three-dimensional structure of the p53 DNA-binding complex provides a conceptual basis for the effects of these mutations.[101] Indeed, the Arg 248 and Arg 273 residues, which are the most frequently targeted residues for somatic mutations, were observed to directly contact the bound DNA (Fig. 31-12).

What does this DNA binding accomplish in the cell? The amino terminus of p53 (codons 20 through 42) has an acidic domain that is similar to those in other transcription factors (Fig. 31-

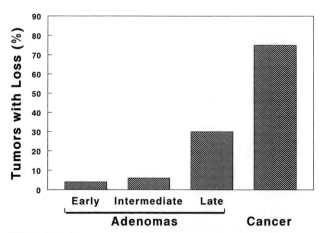

FIG. 31-9 Frequency of 17p losses in colorectal tumors. Tumor classes are defined as in Fig. 31-7. Values for chromosome 17p losses are expressed as the percentage of informative cases showing allelic loss.

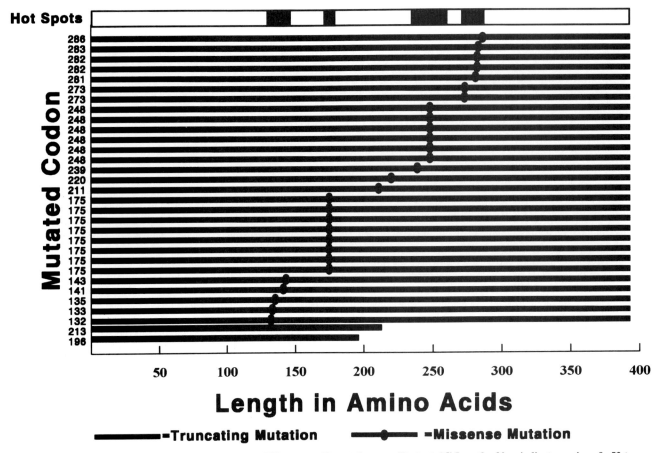

FIG. 31-10 Mutation of p53 in colorectal tumors. Thirty-one p53 mutations are illustrated.[71] Length of bar indicates region of p53 translated until terminated normally or by a somatic nonsense mutation. Cross-bars indicate the locations of somatic missense mutations.

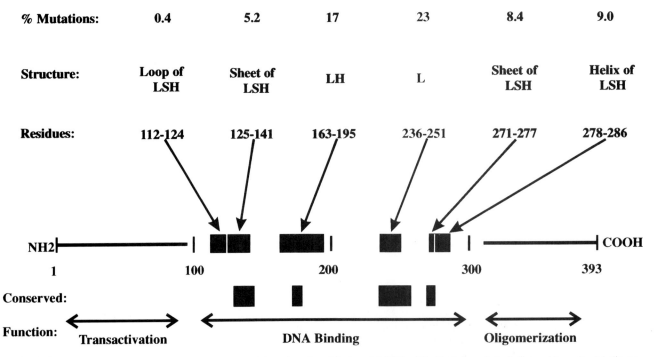

FIG. 31-11 Mutations as they relate to structural domains of p53. Mutations within the indicated region are taken from compiled data (*Greenblatt et al.*[273]). Structural domains were determined by x-ray crystallography of the region indicated in yellow.[101] L (green), LH (blue), and LSH (red) indicate loop, loop-helix, and loop-sheet-helix, respectively. Function domains and conserved domains are indicated at the bottom. (*Modified from Vogelstein and Kinzler with permission.*[274])

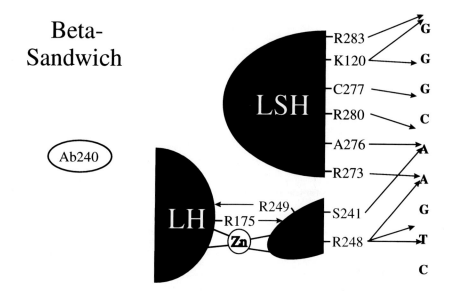

FIG. 31-12 Key structural elements of p53 DNA binding bases on the crystal structure in Cho et al.[101] Structures are shown as they appear in Fig. 31-11. Residues are indicated in single-letter code, and DNA contacts are indicated by arrows. For simplicity, only one strand is shown with arrows pointing to bases indicating a base contact and arrows pointing between bases indicating contacts to sugar or phosphate groups. (*From Vogelstein and Kinzler with permission.*[274])

11).[102–105] When this domain is fused to a DNA-binding protein, it conveys the ability to activate transcription.[102–104] Additional evidence for the role of p53 as a transcription regulatory factor has come from studies of artificial genes containing a p53 binding site upstream of a reporter gene.[97,106] Expression of wild-type p53 in the presence of these reporter constructs results in strong transcriptional activation of the reporter molecule. The activation of transcription is proportional to the strength of p53 binding, and no transactivation is seen with constructs containing mutated binding sites which no longer bind p53. Additionally, p53 can mediate the transactivation of genes containing p53 binding sites in yeast.[106,107] As expected from the lack of specific DNA binding, mutant p53 proteins are devoid of transactivation activity. Moreover, mutant p53 was able to suppress transactivation by wild-type p53 in a dominant negative manner.[106] This suppression was found to be due to the ability of mutant p53 to inhibit wild-type p53 binding to DNA, probably through the formation of inactive hetero-oligomers between wild-type and mutant p53.

Taken together, these properties allow the advancement of a model showing how p53 might function (Fig. 31-13).[108] Wild-type p53 binds to specific sequences within the human genome and activates the transcription of adjacent growth inhibitory genes. If a tumor acquires an inactivating missense mutation in one copy of the p53 gene, the activity of wild-type p53 is greatly reduced (in part because of the dominant negative activity of mutant p53). The resulting decrease in the expression of growth inhibitory genes leads to a selective growth advantage. Eventually, the residual wild-type activity is completely eliminated by loss of the normal copy of p53 gene, resulting in an additional growth advantage and further clonal expansion. This type of scenario is common in tumors of the colon, brain, lung, breast, skin, and bladder. Occasionally p53 is inactivated by nonsense or splice site mutations that lead to truncated proteins or by deletions of one or both copies of the p53 gene. In cervical cancers, it appears that p53 often is inactivated by association with the HPV-produced E6 protein.[82,83] Similarly, p53 appears to be inactivated in some tumors by association with the product of the *MDM2* gene.[109] The MDM2 protein can bind to p53 and conceal its activation domain from the transcriptional machinery.[110] The *MDM2* gene was originally identified by virtue of its amplification in transformed mouse cells[111] and often is amplified in human sarcomas, particularly those in the malignant fibrous histiocytoma subclass.[109]

Direct evidence for this model has come from the identification of genes transcriptionally regulated by p53. To date, at least 10 genes have been identified that are regulated by p53, including the apoptosis-inducing gene *BAX*[112,113] and the growth-arresting gene p21WAF1/CIP1.[114] The best understood of the downstream pathways is that containing p21WAF1/CIP1.[114–117] p53 directly induces the expression of p21WAF1/CIP1 via binding to three consensus binding sites within 2.3 kb of the transcription start site.[114,118] p21WAF1/CIP1 in turn inhibits growth by inducing G1 cell cycle arrest.[114,115] This arrest is due to the ability of p21WAF1/CIP1 to bind to and inhibit the cyclin-dependent kinases.[116,119] Consistent with this, disruption of the p21WAF1/CIP1 genes by homologous recombination eliminates the ability of p53 to induce a G1 arrest in colorectal cancer cells.[120,121]

Although p53 function is beginning to be understood at the cellular and biochemical levels, its role at the organismal levels remains elusive. Mice with both copies of p53 inactivated by homologous recombination are viable and develop normally, although with a predisposition to lymphomas and, to a lesser extent, other tumors.[122–124] Furthermore, individuals with Li-Fraumeni syndrome inherit a mutated p53 gene and are normal except for an increased risk of leukemia, breast carcinoma, soft-tissue sarcoma, brain tumor, and osteosarcoma.[125,126] These results suggest that p53 function is not essential in normal cells. However, evidence suggests that p53 may have an important function in stressed cells. Normal cells arrest in the cell cycle in response to x-ray- or drug-induced DNA damage, whereas cells with mutant p53 are only partially blocked and continue to divide.[127–129] This has prompted the suggestion that p53 in part determines the fate of damaged cells by regulating passage through the cell cycle.[130]

A role for p53 in tumors that is consistent with all the data noted above is as follows. Usually p53 is expressed at negligible levels in normally growing cells, where it is not needed. However, at some point during the evolution of the tumor, p53 expression is induced, perhaps by some form of stress. The stress factors have not been identified but could be related to the cell crowding, hypoxia, acidity, or inflammation that often accompanies tumorigenesis in vivo p53 expression will then result in the transcriptional activation of a variety of genes (e.g., p21WAF1/CIP1) which limit growth. At this time, and not before, a cell acquiring a somatic mutation of p53 will have a selective growth advantage (Fig. 31-14). Indeed, recent studies have identified hypoxia as a potential physiologic inducer of p53. Hypoxia such as that found in tumors can induce p53 expression and p53-dependent apoptosis.[131,132] Moreover, cells lacking p53 were shown to have a selective advantage in such an environment.[132]

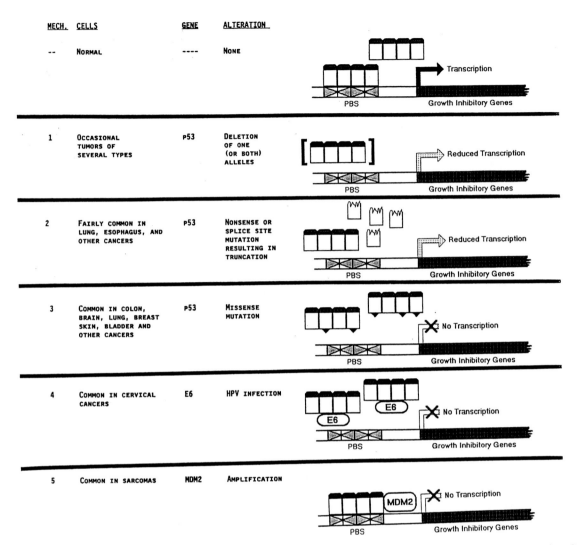

FIG. 31-13 p53 inactivation mechanisms. p53 is postulated to bind as a tetramer to p53 binding sites (PBS) and activate the expression of adjacent genes which inhibit growth and/or invasion. A deletion of one or both p53 alleles reduces the expression of tetramers, resulting in decreased expression of these genes (mechanism 1). Mutations which truncate the protein do not allow oligomerization, resulting in a similar reduction of p53 tetramers (mechanism 2). Missense mutations that have dominant negative effects in an even greater reduction of functionally active tetramers (mechanism 3). The expression of E6 (mechanism 4) and the increased expression of *MDM2* (mechanism 5) result in functional inactivation of p53. *MDM2*–p53 complexes probably bind to PBS, but *MDM2* inhibits transcriptional activation. E6 may promote degradation of p53 through ubiquitin-mediated proteolysis. (*Modified from Vogelstein and Kinzler with permission.*[108])

While a great deal has been learned about the function of p53, several fundamental questions remain unanswered. For example, it is not understood why patients with Li-Fraumeni syndrome do not have a higher incidence of colon cancer, and the intracellular mediators which determine the expression levels of p53 in normal and tumor cells have not been fully elucidated. Finally, while some insights into the ability of p53 to induce growth arrest have been achieved, its ability to induce apoptosis is still mysterious.

Chromosome 18q: The DCC, DPC4, and JV18-1/MADR2 Genes

As with p53, the first evidence for a tumor-suppressor gene on chromosome 18q came from the study of chromosomal loss in colorectal cancers.[36,45,62,63] One copy of chromosome 18q is lost in 73 percent of sporadic colorectal cancers and 47 percent of large adenomas with foci of carcinomatous growth, but the loss occurs infrequently in less advanced adenomas (Fig. 31-15).[45] Several candidate tumor-suppressor genes have been identified in this re-

gion, but efforts to pinpoint positively the culprit gene or genes have been hampered by the inability to identify a candidate gene displaying intragenic mutations in the majority of cases.

The primary structure of *DCC* provides important clues to how *DCC* may function. If initiation occurs at the first methionine of the open reading frame, it will encode a 1447-amino acid protein. DCC protein has several structural features indicating that it is a membrane protein (Fig. 31-16).[133,134] The amino terminal end has a 25-amino acid hydrophobic leader sequence, and an apparent membrane-spanning region divides the protein into a 1100-amino acid extracellular domain and a 324-amino acid intracytoplasmic domain. The intracytoplasmic domain shows no obvious homologies to previously sequenced proteins. The extracellular domain shows extensive homology to the cell adhesion molecule N-CAM and to other related cell-surface glycoproteins. Specifically, the extracellular domain contains four immunoglobulin-like C2 domains and six fibronectin type III repeats. Some of the suspected properties of *DCC* derived from the primary sequence have been confirmed by direct analysis of the DCC protein. Cell-surface labeling studies confirm a cell surface localization for the DCC protein. Immunocytochemical analysis of cells expressing high levels of DCC

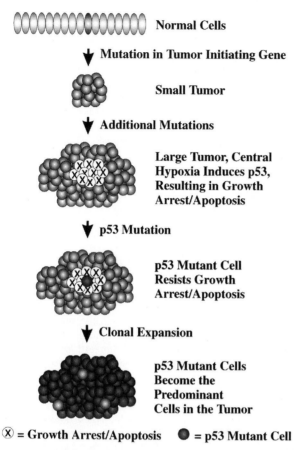

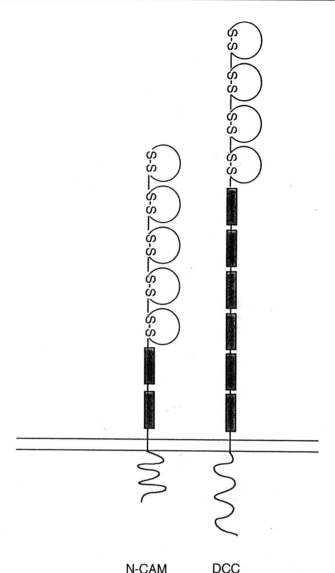

N-CAM   DCC

FIG. 31-14 Function of p53 in tumor development. Model showing why p53 mutations occur late in tumorigenesis and lead to selective survival in the adverse environment of a tumor. In this example, hypoxia is the selecting factor, although other adverse conditions may operate in tumors. (*From Kinzler and Vogelstein.*[275])

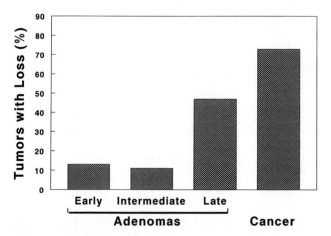

FIG. 31-15 Frequency of 18q losses in colorectal tumors. Tumor classes are defined as in Fig. 31-7. Values for chromosome 18q losses are expressed as the percentage of informative cases showing allelic loss.

FIG. 31-16 *DCC* domain map. *DCC* contains four immunoglobulin-like C2 loops followed by six fibronectin type III repeats. N-CAM contains five immunoglobulin-line C2 loops followed by two fibronectin type III repeats. (*From Hedrick et al.*[136])

revealed membrane staining concentrated at points of cell–cell contact.[134] Immunohistochemical studies of human tissues indicate that DCC protein is expressed in differentiating cells, particularly in the intestinal epithelium and brain.[136]

The precise role of *DCC* in colorectal cancer has been difficult to define, in part because of its large size and lack of expression in colorectal cancers. While the *DCC* transcript is expressed in many tissues, including the colonic mucosa, most colorectal cancers fail to express an intact *DCC* transcript, consistent with its potential role as a tumor suppressor.[133,137] Unfortunately, this lack of expression complicates mutational analysis in that the mutations leading to such loss of expression need not be limited to the coding portions of *DCC*. Despite this, a small number of somatic mutations of *DCC*, including small insertions and point mutations, have been identified in human tumors.[133,135] Southern blot analysis of *DCC* has revealed two intronic point mutations by chance, and detailed analysis of 7 of *DCC*'s 29 coding exons in 30 colorectal cancers identified one somatic missense mutation.[133,135] In addition, three homozygous mutations affecting *DCC* have been described in colorectal cancer cells.[133,137] Homozygous deletions of *DCC* also were observed in 2 of 91 human germ-cell cancers screened by Southern blot analysis.[138] Moreover, the lack of expression of *DCC* in a subset of tumors with mismatch repair deficiency may be due to an unusually large expansion of a repeat in a *DCC* intron.[133,135] To date, no germ-line mutations of *DCC* have been found. Studies employing chromosome transfer demonstrated the ability of chromosome 18q to eliminate or reduce the growth of human colon cancer cells in nude mice.[139,140] The reduction in growth is accompanied by expression of the *DCC* product. More direct evidence for the tumor-suppressive ability of *DCC* comes from antisense studies. When *DCC* expression in rat cells is inhibited by *DCC* antisense sequences, the cells become anchorage-independent in vitro and form tumors in nude mice.[141,142] Conversely, when *DCC* expression vectors are used to express *DCC* in human keratinocytes lacking *DCC* expression, tumorigenicity in nude mice is suppressed.[143] All these observations are consistent with the idea that DCC is a tumor-suppressor gene that is a target of 18q losses. However, the data do not rule out the possibility that other genes on chromosome 18q can function as tumor suppressors alone or in combination with *DCC*.

A second tumor-suppressor gene was identified on chromosome 18q21 during the investigation of chromosome 18q losses in pancreatic cancers.[144] Chromosome 18q losses occur in nearly 90 percent of pancreatic cancers.[145] Detailed analysis of pancreatic tumors losses identified a marker which revealed homozygous deletions that did not overlap with *DCC*. Characterization of this minimally deleted region identified a single expressed gene termed deleted in pancreatic cancer 4 (*DPC4*).[144] Further analysis of *DPC4* revealed that it was homozygously deleted in 25 of 84 pancreatic carcinomas (30 percent). Sequencing analysis of *DPC4* in 27 pancreatic cancers without homozygous mutations identified six intragenic mutations, including one splice site, one missense mutation, and four truncating mutations. Together, these findings suggest a critical role for *DPC4* inactivation in pancreatic cancers. *DPC4* encodes a 552-residue protein with significant homology to the Drosophila mothers against Dpp (Mad) protein as well as *Caenorhabditis elegans* Mad homologues (Fig. 31-17). These proteins have been implicated in the signaling pathway of the transforming growth factor-β (TGF-β) superfamily of signaling polypeptides.[146–148] This is of particular interest in light of the fact that TGF-β suppresses the growth of most normal cells and that many cancer cells are resistant to the growth-suppressing affects of TGF-β.[149,150] Indeed, mutations of the TGF-β receptor have been identified in a subset of human colorectal cancers.[151,152] To date, six human Mad homologues have been identified.[144,148,153,154] One of these, JV18-1/MADR2, was mapped to chromosome 18q21, providing a third candidate tumor-suppressor gene in this region.[153,154]

Mutational analysis of *DPC4* in 18 human colorectal cancers with 18q losses identified one homozygous deletion, one nonsense mutation, and three somatic missense mutations.[137] Analysis of JV18-1/MADR2 in the same 18 tumors identified one homozygous deletion which did not affect *DPC4* or *DCC* and a 42-bp deletion.[153] Intact *DPC4* and JV18-1/MADR2 transcripts were detected in the remaining tumors. In a separate study, analysis of JV18-1/MADR2 in 66 colorectal cancers identified four missense mutations.[154] Three of these mutations were shown to be functionally defective as assessed by their abnormal TGF-β induced phosphorylation and Xenopus mesoderm induction.[154] However, the promising mutational data and intriguing functional links reviewed above are somewhat mitigated by the fact that the majority of colorectal cancers, including those with losses of chromosome 18q21, appear to express wild-type DPC4 and JV18 transcripts. These data also indicate that additional studies will be necessary before the role of 18q losses in colorectal cancer will be as well understood as are those of 17p and 5q.

Chromosome 5q: The *APC* Gene

Two lines of evidence suggested that a putative tumor-suppressor gene on chromosome 5q was of particular interest. One came from the study of allelic losses in sporadic colorectal tumors. Chromosome 5q losses were reported to occur in 20 to 50 percent of colorectal cancers, depending on the region of chromosome 5q assessed.[45,59,62,63,155–158] Even more important, the loss of chromosome 5 sequences occurred as frequently in small benign colorectal tumors as in larger malignant tumors (Fig. 31-18).[45] These observations suggested that inactivation of a tumor-suppressor gene on chromosome 5q occurs frequently and early during tumor formation.

The second line of evidence came from the study of FAP, an inherited predisposition to colorectal cancer. The seminal clue to the location of the gene causing FAP came from a patient with polyposis and a constitutional interstitial deletion of 5q that was visible on cytogenetic analysis.[159] This observation suggested that a suppressor gene on chromosome 5q was responsible for the patient's

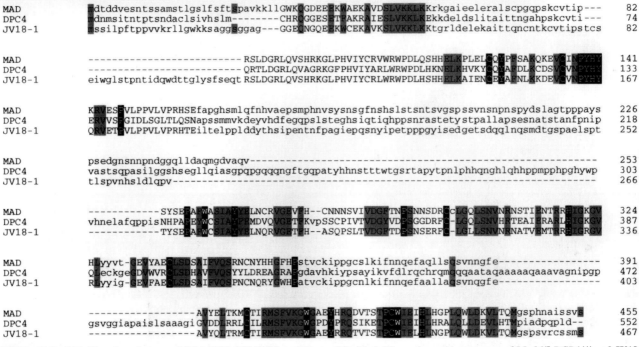

FIG. 31-17 Homology between *DPC4*, JV18-1/MADR2, and Drosophila Mad. The amino acid sequences of Mad,[147] DCP4,[144] and JV18-1/MADR2153 were aligned and shaded by the means of their pairwise scores using the MACAW multiple alignment software.[276]

5q Losses in Colorectal Tumors

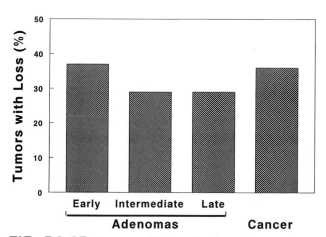

FIG. 31-18 Frequency of 5q losses in colorectal tumors. Tumor classes are defined as in Fig. 31-7. Values for chromosome 5q losses are expressed as the percentage of informative cases showing allelic loss.

condition. This suggestion was confirmed and extended by linkage analysis, which established linkage of FAP to chromosome 5q21 markers in all the kindreds analyzed.[160-162] These two lines of evidence converged with the identification of a small region of chromosome 5q21 which was altered in the germ line of FAP patients and in sporadic colorectal cancers. Four genes were mapped to this region [*MCC*, TB2 (DP1), SRP19, and *APC*].[163,164] One of these genes (*APC*, for adenomatous polyposis coli) was found to be mutated in the germ line of FAP patients[165,166] and in sporadic colorectal tumors.[165] The *APC* gene contains an open reading frame of

8538 bp which would encode a 2843-amino acid protein if translation was initiated at the first methionine. This coding sequence is distributed over 15 exons and is remarkable in that the last exon contains a 6579-bp uninterrupted open reading frame. Several alternatively spliced forms of *APC* are known to exist, including minor variants which affect the coding region.[164,166-168]

The *APC* gene has been examined in over 500 FAP kindreds.[169] The most successful of these analysis identified intragenic mutations in roughly 80 percent of the kindreds examined.[170] The majority of the remaining kindreds also have mutations of the *APC* gene which result in the deletion of large portions of the gene or block its expression.[171] These mutations are difficult to detect because they can be "masked" by the normal allele.[172] The nature of the intragenic mutations identified is quite striking, with over 95 percent predicted to result in truncation of the APC protein (based on 176 mutations compiled in Nagase and Nakamura[169]). The truncating mutations largely result from nonsense point mutations (33 percent) or small insertions (6 percent) and deletions (55 percent) that lead to frameshifts.[169] The majority of mutations occur in the first half of the last exon (Fig. 31-19). A few missense changes were identified, but it is not known whether these changes are functional or merely represent rare variants, and at least one has been shown not to segregate with the disease.[173]

The manifestations of FAP can very considerably and in some cases are due to the specific underlying mutation (Fig. 31-20). For example, CHRPE is associated with truncating mutations between codons 463 and 1387.[174-176] Truncating mutations between codons 1403 and 1578 are associated with increased extracolonic manifestations such as desmoid tumors and mandibular lesions, but patients with such mutations do not exhibit CHRPE.[176-178] Similarly, colonic manifestations have been shown to vary with the position of the mutation. Truncating mutations amino terminal to codon 157 are associated with an attenuated form of FAP in which patients de-

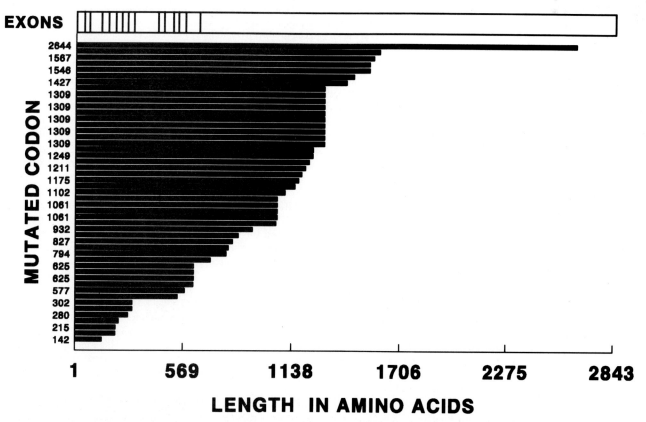

FIG. 31-19 Mutation of the *APC* gene in the germ line of FAP illustrated.[277] Four missense changes are not shown because it is not known whether they represent rare variants or true (functional) muta-tions. Lengths of bars indicate the region of *APC* that is translated until terminated by either a nonsense or a frameshift mutation.

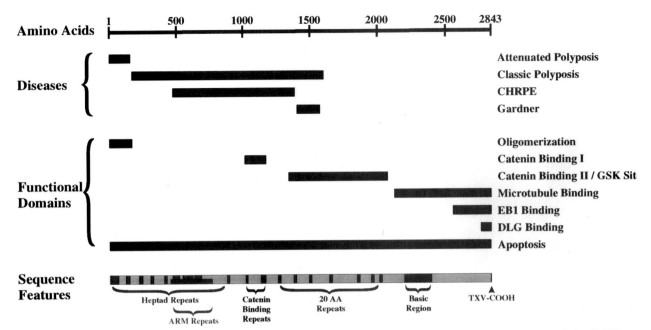

FIG. 31-20 Functional and disease-related domains of *APC*. Disease map: The location of truncating *APC* mutations has been shown to correlate with the extent of colonic and extracolonic manifestations. Truncating mutations before codon 157 are associated with a reduced number of colorectal polyps,[18] whereas the majority of mutations are associated with more pronounced polyposis and occur between codons 169 and 1600.[169] Mutations in codons 463 to 1387 are associated with CHRPE.[174–176] Mutations in codons 1403 to 1578 have been associated with an increased incidence or extracolonic manifestations.[176–178] Functional domains and sequence features: Amino terminal residues 1 to 171 are sufficient for oligomerization.[195,196] This oligomerization is thought to be mediated by the heptad repeats indicated in pink on the sequence features map.[163,166,195] *APC* binds to β-catenin through two motifs, the first including three 15-amino acid repeats indicated in black on the sequence features map and located between residues 1020 and 1169.[199,200] A second region containing "20 amino acid repeats" (indicated in red on the sequence feature map and within residues 1324 to 2075166) binds to β-catenin and also acts as a substrate for GSK phosphorylation.[201,278] Phosphorylation is thought to occur at SXXXS sites within the 20 amino acid repeats.[201] When transiently overexpressed, full-length *APC* decorates the microtubule cytoskeleton. The carboxy terminus of *APC* is required for this association, and residues 2130 to 2843 are sufficient.[184,279] Two proteins have been shown to associate with the carboxy terminus of *APC*. Residues 2560 to 2843 are sufficient to bind EB1, a highly conserved 30-kD protein of unknown function.[197] Residues 2771 to 2843 are sufficient to bind DLG, a human homologue of the Drosophila disks large tumor suppressor gene[198]; the three carboxy terminal residues of *APC* (TXV, indicated in green on the sequence features map) probably mediate this binding. Expression of full-length *APC* in colorectal cancer cell lines results in apoptosis, but the regions required for this activity have not been precisely defined.[193] Residues 453 to 767 contain seven copies of a repeat consensus found in the Drosophila segment polarity gene product Armadillo.[280] and residues 2200 to 2400 correspond to a basic region.[166] (*Modified from Kinzler and Vogelstein with permission.*[272])

velop a relatively small number of polyps (0 to 100).[18] Some studies have suggested that mutations between codons 1250 and 1464 are associated with an increased number of colorectal tumors.[179,180] In contrast, patients with identical mutations can develop dissimilar clinical features. For example, some patients with identical truncating mutations develop features of GS (mandibular osteomas and desmoid tumors) while others do not.[165,181] Similarly, only a small number of patients within a kindred develop brain tumors, hepatoblastomas, or thyroid cancers even though a clear predisposition to these tumors is associated with germ-line *APC* mutations.[12,14]

The role of *APC* in colorectal tumorigenesis is not limited to FAP; *APC* also plays a critical role in the development of sporadic colorectal tumors.[182–184] It has been estimated that at least 80 percent of colorectal tumors have a somatic mutation of the *APC* gene.[182–184] The nature and distribution of somatic mutations identified in sporadic tumors resemble those observed in FAP patients (Fig. 31-21). Over 95 percent of these mutations are predicted to result in truncations of the APC protein as a result of splice site mutations (7 percent), nonsense mutations (40 percent), or insertions (12 percent) or deletions (41 percent) that lead to frameshifts (based on 75 mutations).[182,183] Two observations suggest that mutation of *APC* is an early and perhaps initiating event in sporadic colorectal tumorigenesis. First, the frequency of *APC* mutations is just as high in small benign tumors as in cancers.[50,182,183] This is in marked contrast to mutations of other genes (such as those in *ras* or p53), which appear only as tumors progress. Second,

mutations of *APC* have been found in the earliest sporadic lesions analyzed, including those as small as a few crypts (ACF).[50,185]

Additional evidence of the important role of *APC* in tumorigenesis comes from the study of mice with germ-line inactivation of the murine homologue of *APC* (*mAPC*). Three such mouse lineages have been reported, and all three have an increased risk for intestinal tumors.[186–188] The first and best described of such lines is the multiple intestinal neoplasia (Min) strain in mice.[167] The Min mouse lineage was established from a C57BL/6J male mouse which was treated with ethylnitrosourea and bred for inherited traits. Min mice exhibit an autosomal dominantly inherited predisposition to multiple intestinal neoplasia and on a susceptible background develop an average of 30 to 50 intestinal tumors by age 90 days.[189,190] This phenotype was traced to a single nonsense mutation resulting in the truncation of mAPC protein at codon 850.[186] The other two mouse lineages were derived by the use of homologous recombination to specifically inactivate *mAPC*[187,188] These mutations are highly analogous to mutations in the germ line of FAP patients, making these mice excellent models of FAP at the phenotypic and genotypic levels. Furthermore, because these mouse models share at least one important genetic defect with sporadic human colorectal tumors, they may prove to be a good model for colorectal tumorigenesis in general.

Do both copies of the *APC* gene need to be inactivated for it to exert its effect on tumor development, as Knudson's tumor-

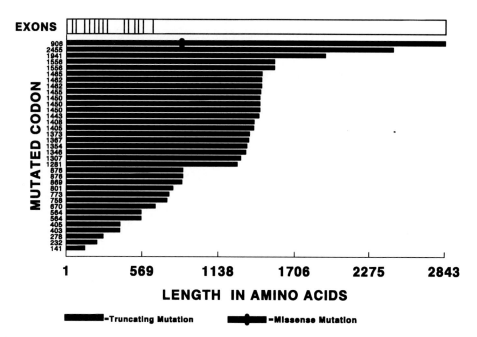

FIG. 31-21 Somatic *APC* mutations in sporadic colorectal tumors. Thirty-five *APC* mutations from 16 adenomas and 26 carcinomas are illustrated.[183] Lengths of bars indicate the region of *APC* translated until terminated by either a nonsense or a frameshift mutation. Crossbar indicates the location of the single somatic missense mutation identified.

suppressor gene model would suggest? Studies of *APC* mutations in primary sporadic colorectal tumors suggest that at least a third of both benign and malignant tumors lack a normally functioning *APC* gene.[182,183] Studies of primary tumors from FAP patients identified a second inactivating mutation in about 80 percent of the tumors. Both studies undoubtedly represent underestimates of the true extent of inactivation of both alleles that were caused by difficulties in analyzing primary human tumors. However, studies of APC protein in colorectal cancer cell lines indicate that about 80 percent (26 of 32) of colon tumor cell lines were totally devoid of full-length APC protein.[184] Similarly, inactivation of both alleles of the *mAPC* gene occurs almost without exception in Min tumors and can be detected in lesions so small that they can be observed only at the microscopic level.[191,192] Together these data suggest that both copies of *APC* must be inactivated during tumorigenesis.

What is *APC*'s normal function that is so critical to the prevention of intestinal tumor development, and how is this function mediated? Expression of wild-type *APC* in colorectal epithelial cells with *APC* mutations results in apoptosis, suggesting that *APC* may control the cell death process.[193] Immunohistochemical analysis indicates that APC protein is apparently located at the basolateral membrane in colorectal epithelial cells, with expression increasing as cells migrate to the top of the crypt.[184,194] As loss of cells from the top of crypts is an important homeostatic process in the colon, it is easy to imagine how disruption of such a "death signal" could clearly lead to neoplasia. The primary structure of *APC* provides few clues to how it might mediate such functions (Fig. 31-20). Residues 453 to 767 contain seven copies of a repeat consensus found in the Drosophila segment polarity gene armadillo. The amino terminal third of *APC* contains several heptad repeats of the type that mediate oligomerization by a coiled structure.[195,196] These regions may mediate homo-oligomerization between mutant and wild-type proteins and could theoretically cause a dominant negative effect, though no such effect has been demonstrated biologically. In addition, seven 20-amino acid repeats have been identified between residues 1324 and 2075.[166]

Although the sequence features described above have provided some insights into the function of *APC*, the identification of proteins which interact with *APC* has yielded even more tantalizing clues. Two proteins which bind to the C terminus of *APC* have been identified. The first was EB1, a highly conserved 30-kD protein of unknown function.[197] The second was the human homologue of the Drosophila tumor-suppressor gene disks large (DLG), which binds the carboxy terminal 72 residues of *APC*.[198] As virtually all *APC* mutations result in the loss of the carboxy terminus of APC protein (Figs. 31-19 and 31-21), these data suggest that DLG and/or EB1 may be essential for *APC*'s growth-controlling function. However, the most penetrating insights into *APC* function have come from studies of the interaction between β-catenin and *APC*.[199,200] The central third of *APC* contains two classes of β-catenin binding repeats, one of which is modulated by phosphorylation (Fig. 31-20).[201] Although many mutant APC proteins retain some β-catenin binding, virtually all these mutant proteins lack at least one type of β-catenin binding repeat.

The β-catenin association links *APC* to two apparently diverse cellular processes. The first process is related to cellular adhesion. The catenins were originally identified as cytoplasmic proteins which bind to cadherins, a family of calcium-dependent homophilic cell-adhesion molecules. Several studies have indicated that β-catenin is necessary for cadherin-mediated cell adhesion.[202] Given that binding of β-catenin to cadherins and binding to *APC* are mutually exclusive, it is possible that *APC* could modulate such adhesion as part of its tumor-suppressing function. *APC* could additionally act as a downstream communicator of adhesion status, linking cadherin–catenin complexes to other cellular components.

The second process involving *APC* has been elucidated by studies of the Wingless (Wg) and Wnt signaling pathways in Drosophila, Zenopus, and the mouse. β-catenin and Armadillo (the Drosophila homologue of β-catenin) have been firmly implicated as signal transducers in these pathways.[203–205] This link was strengthened by the observation that the *APC*–β-catenin complex is physically associated with a second member of this pathway, the ZW3/GSK3β protein kinase.[201] Moreover, this kinase was found to promote β-catenin binding to *APC*, presumably by phosphorylation of *APC* class II binding sites (Fig. 31-20).[201] Epistasis evaluations in Drosophila suggest that Wg signaling inhibits ZW3 function and that active ZW3 can inhibit β-catenin signaling. Finally, studies in Xenopus and the mouse suggest that Wnt signaling ultimately results in the formation of a heteromeric complex containing β-catenin and members of the Tcf/Lef family of HMG box transcription factors.[206,207] Taken together, these studies suggest that *APC* could work in concert with ZW3/GSK3β to inhibit β-catenin-induced transcriptional activity. The relevance of this pathway to neoplasia is strengthened by the ability of truncated β-catenin to transform cells in culture[208] and the involvement of Wnt signaling in breast tumorigenesis in mice.[209] Given the size of *APC*, the biologic manifestations of *APC* inactivation, and the number of proteins already known to associate with *APC*, it is probable that *APC* functions to integrate signals from a variety of sources, potentially transmitting them to the nucleus through β-catenin–Tcf complexes. This conjecture has recently been confirmed by the finding that APC can inhibit β-catenin/Tcf regulated transcription.[209b,209c] The role of this particular APC function in tumor suppression was further accentuated by the identification of activating β-catenin mutations in colorectal cancers[209c] and in melanomas[209d] lacking *APC* mutations.

Other Genetic Changes

MCC   During the search for the gene responsible for FAP, a second gene from chromosome 5q21 was identified which was somatically mutated in sporadic colorectal cancers.[210] The *MCC* (mutated in colorectal cancer) gene is less than 250 kb from the *APC* gene[163,164,211] and was chosen for further study because Southern blot analysis revealed a colon carcinoma with a somatic rearrangement. The *MCC* gene transcript contains a 2511-bp open reading frame which is distributed over 17 exons. Detailed analysis of all 17 coding exons identified specific point mutations in 6 of the 90 colorectal carcinomas examined. All six mutations were predicted to alter the MCC protein by amino acid substitution or altered splicing. As was previously noted, this type of study underestimates the actual mutation rates because of the technical inability to identify all mutations. However, it is unlikely that mutations of *MCC* play a major role in the development of colorectal cancer.[210,212] Comparison of *MCC* to *APC* reveals some interesting similarities in addition to their proximity in the genome. The *MCC* gene would encode an 829-amino acid protein if translation initiation occurred at the first methionine of the open reading frame. Similar to *APC*, the MCC protein sequence displayed weak global homology to myosin and other intermediate-filament protein because of the presence of heptad repeats. In addition, *MCC*, like *APC*, contained a short homology to the region of m3 MAChR that regulates G-protein coupling. Although the significance of *MCC* mutations in colorectal tumors is not clear, these similarities raise the possibility that *MCC* and *APC* function along the same pathway.

Gene Amplification   The specific amplification of a small region of the genome (gene amplification) frequently activates oncogenes in some tumor types. One indication of gene amplification is the cytogenetic observation of double minute chromosomes. These chromosomes are known to harbor amplified sequences. Although double minute chromosome have been reported in a significant proportion of primary colorectal cancers,[213] amplification of specific genes has rarely been described in colon cancers. Isolated cases of c-*myb*,[214] c-*myc*,[215–218] NEU,[217,219,220] and cyclin[221] gene amplification have been reported. It is notable that the few colorectal cancers with demonstrable gene amplification are indistinguishable from other colorectal cancers in terms of histology and behavior. It is likely that amplification of these genes, as well as additional (unidentified) oncogenes, contributes to tumor progression, especially at late stages. It must be remembered that tumors, even malignant ones, are not static entities and eventually evolve

subpopulations that have varying propensities to metastasize, varying resistances to drugs and radiation, and varying biologic and biochemical properties. Although tumors are often said to be genetically unstable, it is more correct to state that they are genetically heterogeneous. Whether this heterogeneity results from an increased mutation rate or enhanced ability of tumor cells with genetic alterations to survive remains to be determined. Regardless, the continuing evolution of tumors, fueled by genetic changes, represents one of the greatest challenges to cancer therapists.

Modifying Loci   The existence of common loci that modify the risk for colorectal cancer has long been suspected, but these loci have been difficult to pinpoint in humans. However, the Min mouse model provides a clear-cut example of a modifying locus. Depending on the inbred mouse strain harboring this mutation, the number of polyps varies significantly.[190] Linkage analysis has demonstrated that a single locus [MOM1 (for modifier of Min)] on mouse chromosome 4 accounts for much of this difference between strains.[222] Recently the MOM-1 gene was identified as that encoding secreted phospholipase A2 (sPLA2).[223] Unfortunately, studies of sPLA2 in humans suggest that it is not a major modifier of colorectal cancer risk.[224]

Gene Expression   One of the most difficult issues in cancer research involves the evaluation of gene expression. Although the expression of numerous genes is different in tumor cells compared to normal cells, the significance of these differences is uncertain. For example, the expression of various oncogenes, particularly c-*myc*,[218,225] a variety of mucins,[226] growth factors and their receptors,[219,227,228] carcinoembryonic antigens,[229] cell-surface glycoproteins,[230,231] and enzymes involved in DNA replication and cell division,[232] increased in neoplastic colon cells. Whether these increases in expression drive the process of tumorigenesis or are simply a result of the abnormal growth of microenvironment of cancer is impossible to determine at present. Some of the abnormally expressed gene products are likely to play an important role in mediating the biologic effects of the mutant genes discussed in this chapter. Others are likely to be insignificant with regard to pathogenesis. The advent of several new technologies for the analysis of gene expression may lead to advances in this important area.[233–236] Indeed, using just one of these new approaches,[235] it was possible to analyze over 600,000 transcripts from human cancer and control cells.[237]

Methylation   The only known covalent modification of DNA in normal mammalian cells occurs at the fifth position of cytosine at 5'-CG-3' dinucleotides. In most somatic cells, 80 percent of these dinucleotides are methylated, and such methylation has been implicated in the control of gene expression and chromosome condensation.[238] In cancer cells, a generalized hypomethylation of the genome occurs relatively early during colorectal tumorigenesis and can be observed even in small adenomas.[239,240] Hypermethylation of a specific 5'-CG-3' rich site also occurs.[241] The causes as well as the effects of these methylation differences are not understood. Hypomethylation probably is not due to the underexpression of methylase activity, because such activity is not decreased in tumors.[242] Changes in the methylation of genes, unlike the mutations of genes noted above, are not clonal changes in that any specific 5'-CG3' dinucleotide is methylated differently in only a fraction of the tumor cell population. Nevertheless, these changes could have significant effects on tumor cell biology. For example, decreased methylation could in part allow the expression of genes which should normally be silent, such as those required for cellular invasion (proteinases) or growth at metastatic sites (cell-surface receptors for growth factors or extracellular matrixes). Conversely, increased methylation could lead to the silencing of genes important for growth suppression. Indeed, methylation changes have been implicated in the silencing of the p16 tumor-suppressor gene.[243,244] Alternatively, it has been experimentally demonstrated that reduced methylation of DNA can lead to aberrant chromosome condensation and adherence of the decondensed regions to one another.[245] This in turn could result in abnormal chromosome segregation, particularly chromosome loss, which, as noted above, is one of the most common mechanisms for inactivating tumor-suppressor genes. The evidence implicating methylation in colorectal tumorigenesis is not limited to the methylation changes observed in tumors but also includes direct experimental evidence. Treatment of cells with the demethylating agent 5-aza-cytidine has been shown to be oncogenic in vitro and in vivo.[246] Moreover, mice with a genetic deficiency of methyltransferase are resistant to intestinal tumors resulting from *mAPC* mutations, and this resistance is potentiated by 5-aza-cytidine.[247] While the evidence implicating methylation changes in tumorigenesis is clear, additional studies will be necessary to clarify the significance of those changes.

A Genetic Model for Colorectal Tumorigenesis

In molecular terms, the process of colorectal tumor evolution represents the acquisition of sequential mutations (Fig. 31-22).[248,249] Mutations in *APC* seem to be required to initiate the adenomatous process, resulting in the clonal growth of a single cell. It appears that both alleles of *APC* need to be inactivated for a small neoplasm to form, but it is not known whether mutation of another gene is also required. A small polyp that results from these initial mutations may remain dormant for decades. Eventually, however, one of the cells of this small tumor acquires an additional mutation (often in the K-*ras* gene), allowing it to overgrow its sister cells and resulting in a larger tumor. Subsequent waves of clonal expansion are driven by further mutations in other genes [particularly the 18q tumor suppressor(s) and p53], and along with this expansion comes further dysplasia. When a cell has acquired enough mutations (generally affecting at least four genes), it acquires the ability to invade and metastasize and is observed clinically as a malignancy.

There are several points worth noting about the model described above. First, not every tumor needs to acquire each of the mutations indicated. For example, only half of all colorectal cancers have *ras* mutations. It is likely that other, unidentified mutated genes can substitute for *ras* mutations. Second, there are likely to be other genetic events required for cancer development. Even so, this model predicts that at least seven genetic events (i.e., one oncogene mutation and six mutations to inactivate three tumor-suppressor genes) are typically required for a cancer to develop. Third, the order of mutations can have a significant impact on the tumorigenic process. For example, as was noted above, nondysplastic ACFs with *ras* gene mutations are amazingly common.[49,50] However, these cells, unlike their dysplastic *APC* mutant counterparts, appear to have little or no potential to form clinically impor-

tant tumors. Similarly, patients with germ-line mutations of p53 do not develop polyposis[250] despite the fact that p53 mutation mutations occur in over 80 percent of colorectal cancers.[71] Therefore, although it is clear that p53 can play a role in colorectal tumorigenesis, it is equally clear that it cannot initiate the process in a fashion similar to that of *APC*. Thus, it appears that it is not simply the accumulation of mutations but also their order that determines the propensity for neoplasia and that only a subset of the genes which can affect cell growth can actually initiate the neoplastic process.

It is notable that the genes identified in colorectal tumors affect almost all the cellular compartments (i.e., *ras* at the inner surface of the cell membrane, *APC* in the cytoplasm, and p53 in the nucleus). This suggests that human cells have evolved several levels of cellular protection against neoplasia and that many of these protective mechanisms must be disassembled before cancer can fully develop. Even at the malignant stage, however, the tumor continues to evolve, developing subclones with varying degrees of aneuploidy, drug or radiation resistance, and metastatic capability. This whole process, from the appearance of a tiny adenomatous tumor to invasion by a carcinoma, takes 20 to 40 years, perhaps reflecting the time required to mutate sequentially the relevant genes.

PROSPECTUS

Despite the advances made in understanding the genetics of colorectal tumorigenesis, many questions remain unanswered. First, chromosomes besides 5q, 17p, and 18q are lost in subsets of colorectal cancers. The identification of the culprit genes on these chromosomes has not been accomplished. It is unclear whether these other genes are simply responsible for the evolution of tumor heterogeneity at late stages of the process or play a more fundamental role in tumorigenesis. Second, about one-half of all colorectal tumors develop without a *ras* mutation, and at least some tumors apparently do not have abnormalities of p53 or *APC*. The mechanism that allows such alterations to be bypassed could prove to be very important. Perhaps such tumors develop mutations of other genes on the same pathway which have the same physiologic effects. Third, the biochemical and physiologic functions of oncogenes and tumor-suppressor genes have not been fully worked out in cells in vitro, much less in the complex environment that exists in tissues in vivo. Fourth, inherited genetic factors affecting colon cancer risk in the general population have not been defined.

Diagnosis

One of the first benefits derived from the study of colorectal cancer genetics was improved diagnosis. Already, knowledge of the genetic bases for FAP and HNPCC is allowing presymptomatic diagnosis in affected families. The demonstration that an individual member of such a family has not inherited the disease can have a significant impact, reducing the discomfort and expense of re-

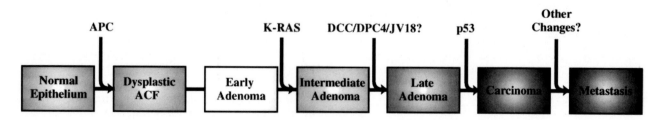

FIG. 31-22 A genetic model for colorectal tumorigenesis. (*Modified from Fearon and Vogelstein.*[248])

peated medial examinations as well as the anxiety associated with disease expectation. Genetic diagnosis could also be performed in utero, although substantial ethical questions are inherent in such diagnoses when the relevant disease is not necessarily lethal and mortality, if it occurs at all, is delayed until adulthood. Presymptomatic testing also will have significant clinical implications with the advent of pharmacologic intervention for the possible prevention of polyposis in FAP patients (see below).

Specific gene mutations also may be used as the basis of a very specific test for presymptomatic diagnosis for colorectal tumors in the general population. Tumor cells shed into the stool can be identified by the presence of their mutant *ras* genes in DNA isolated from stool samples.[251–255] This type of analysis was successful in eight of nine patients whose tumors contained *ras* gene mutations.[251] Mutant genes were detected in stool from patients with benign as well as malignant tumors and could be observed in relatively small tumors as well as large ones. The application of this strategy to other mutations known to occur in colorectal tumors could significantly improve the generality of this test. Numerous additional studies will of course be required to determine whether such assays will lead to improved detection of colorectal neoplasia in a cost-effective manner.

The analysis of genetic changes in colorectal cancers has also been shown to have prognostic value.[256] While *ras* oncogene mutations and chromosome 5q losses do not show any prognostic utility, chromosome 17p and 18q losses each provide independent prognostic information. Chromosome 17p and 18q losses are associated with distant metastasis and a poorer prognosis. This analysis represents the first step in the application of molecular genetics to the management of colorectal cancer patients. In the future, one can imagine that the choice of a chemotherapeutic regimen will depend on the specific genetic changes present in the patient's tumor.

PREVENTION AND TREATMENT

One of the most important purposes of studying colorectal tumorigenesis lies in the hope that this will lead to better treatment and/or prevention of the disease. The notion that more effective drugs to treat colorectal tumors can be developed is furthered by the apparent success of some conventional drug treatments. Several studies/ have indicated that the nonsteroidal anti inflammatory drug (NSAID) sulindac can cause tumor regression in FAP patients.[257–264] The hope that such treatment may prove useful for the general public comes from epidemiology studies of colon cancer and aspirin users.[265–267] Some of these studies have found that the use of aspirin, another NSAID, is associated with a reduced risk of death from colon cancer. Evaluation of these and other drugs may be greatly facilitated by the testing of Min mice. Indeed, several studies have already demonstrated the ability of NSAIDs to reduce the incidence of intestinal tumors in Min mice.[268–270] These mice provide a reasonably accurate model for FAP at the genotypic and phenotypic levels. Furthermore, because *APC* mutations appear to initiate sporadic colorectal tumorigenesis, Min mice may also prove to be a good model for colorectal cancer in general. Ultimately, it is hoped that the study of cancer genes and their biological consequences will lead to the knowledge-based development of much more specific and effective chemopreventive and chemotherapeutic agents.

REFERENCES

1. Parker S, Tong T, Bolden S, Wingo P: Cancer statistics, 1996. *CA Cancer J Clin* **46**:5, 1996.

2. Beart RW: Colorectal cancer, in Holleb AI, Fink DJ, Murphy GP (eds): *American Cancer Society Textbook of Clinical Oncology*. Atlanta, American Cancer Society, 1991, pp 213–218.

3. Cohen AM, Shank B, Friedman MA: Colorectal cancer, in De Vita, Hellman S, Rosenberg S (eds): *Cancer: Principles and Practice of Oncology*. Philadelphia, Lippincott, 1989, p 895.

4. Ransohoff D, Lang C: Screening for colorectal cancer. *N Engl J Med* **325**:37, 1991.

5. Jass JR, Stewart SM: Evolution of hereditary non-polyposis colorectal cancer. *Gut* **33**:783, 1992.

6. Lieberman D: Cost-effectiveness of colon cancer screening. *Am J Gastroenterol* **86**:1789, 1991.

7. Lipkin M, Bell B, Shelrock P: Cell proliferation kinetics in the gastrointestinal tract of man. *J Clin Invest* **42**:767, 1963.

8. Shorter RG, Moertel CG, Titus JL: Cell kinetics in the jejunum and rectum of man. *Am J Dig Dis* **9**:760, 1964.

9. Kent TH, Mitros FA: Polyps of the colon and small bowel, polyp syndromes, and the polyp-carcinoma sequence, in Norris HT (eds): *Pathology of the Colon, Small Intestine, and Anus*. New York, Churchill Livingstone, 1983, vol 2, p 167.

10. Cooper HS: Carcinoma of the colon and rectum, in Norris HT (eds): *Pathology of the Colon, Small Intestine and Anus*. New York, Churchill Livingstone, 1983, vol 2, p 201.

11. Stryker SJ, Wolff BG, Culp CE, Libbe SD, Ilstrup DM, MacCarty RL: Natural history of untreated colonic polyps. *Gastroenterology* **93**:1009, 1987.

12. Giardiello FM: Gastrointestinal polyposis syndromes and hereditary nonpolyposis colorectal cancer, in Rustgi AK (eds): *Gastrointestinal Cancers: Biology, Diagnosis, and Therapy*. Philadelphia, Lippincott-Raven, 1995, pp 367–377.

13. Bussey HJ, Veale AM, Morson DC: Genetics of gastrointestinal polyposis. *Gastroenterology* **74**:1325, 1978.

14. Hamilton SR, Liu B, Parsons RE, et al: The molecular basis of Turcot's syndrome. *N Engl J Med* **332**:839, 1995.

15. Gardner E, Richards R: Multiple cutaneous and subcutaneous lesions occurring simultaneously with hereditary polyposis and osteomatosis. *Am J Hum Genet* **5**:139, 1953.

16. Bulow S: Extracolonic manifestations of familial adenomatous polyposis, in Herrera L (eds): *Familial Adenomatous Polyposis*. New York, Liss, 1990, p 109.

17. Spiro L, Otterud B, Stauffer D, et al: Linkage of a variant or attenuated form of adenomatous polyposis coli to the adenomatous polyposis coli (APC) locus. *Am J Hum Genet* **51**:92, 1992.

18. Spiro L, Olschwang S, Groden J, et al: Alleles of the APC gene: An attenuated form of familial polyposis. *Cell* **75**:951, 1993.

19. Ponz de Leon M, Sassatelli R, Benatti P, Roncucci L: Identification of hereditary nonpolyposis colorectal cancer in the general population: The 6-year experience of a population-based registry. *Cancer* **71**:3493, 1993.

20. Lynch HT, Smyrk T, Jass JR: Hereditary nonpolyposis colorectal cancer and colonic adenomas: aggressive adenomas? *Semin Surg Oncol* **11**:406, 1995.

21. Lynch HT, Smyrk T, Lynch JF: Overview of natural history, pathology, molecular genetics and management of HNPCC (Lynch syndrome). *Int J Cancer* **69**:38, 1996.

22. Burt RW, Bishop DT, Cannon LA, Dowdle MA, Lee RG, Skolnick MH: Dominant inheritance of adenomatous colonic polyps and colorectal cancer. *N Engl J Med* **312**:1540, 1985.

23. Cannon-Albright LA, Skolnick MH, Bishop DT, Lee RG, Burt RW: Common inheritance of susceptibility to colonic adenomatous polyps and associated colorectal cancers. *N Engl J Med* **319**:533, 1988.

24. Houlston RS, Collins A, Slack J, Morton NE: Dominant genes for colorectal cancer are not rare. *Ann Hum Genet* **56**:99, 1992.

25. Willett W: The search for the causes of breast and colon cancer. *Nature* **338**:389, 1989.

26. Haenszel W, Kurihara M: Studies of Japanese migrants: I. Mortality from cancer and other diseases among Japanese in the United States. *JNCI* **40**:43, 1968.

27. Lee JA: Recent trends of large bowel cancer in Japan compared to United States and England and Wales. *Int J Epidemiol* **5**:187, 1976.

28. Armstrong B, Doll R: Environmental factors and cancer incidence and mortality in different countries, with special reference to dietary practices. *Int J Cancer* **15**:617, 1975.

29. Pickle LW, Greene MH, Ziegler RG, et al: Colorectal cancer in rural Nebraska. *Cancer Res* **44**:363, 1984.

30. Willett WC, Stampfer MJ, Colditz GA, Rosner BA, Speizer FE: Relation of meat, fat and fiber intake to the risk of colon cancer in a prospective study among women. *N Engl J Med* **323**:1664, 1990.

31. Burkitt DP: Epidemiology of cancer of the colon and rectum. *Cancer* **28**:3, 1971.

32. Bingham S, Williams DR, Cole TJ, James WP: Dietary fibre and regional large-bowel cancer mortality in Britain. *Br J Cancer* **40**:456, 1979.

33. Nowell PC: The colonal evolution of tumor cell populations. *Science* **194**:23, 1976.

34. Vogelstein B, Fearon ER, Hamilton SR, Feinberg AP: Use of restriction fragment length polymorphisms to determine the clonal origin of human tumors. *Science* **227**:642, 1985.

35. Vogelstein B, Fearon ER, Hamilton SR, et al: Clonal analysis using recombinant DNA probes from the X-chromosome. *Cancer Res* **47**:4806, 1987.

36. Fearon ER, Hamilton SR, Vogelstein B: Clonal analysis of human colorectal tumors. *Science* **238**:193, 1987.

37. Martin P, Levin B, Golomb HM, Riddell RH: Chromosome analysis of primary large bowel tumors: A new method for improving the yield of analyzable metaphases. *Cancer* **44**:1656, 1979.

38. Reichmann A, Martin P, Levin B: Chromosomal banding patterns in human large bowel cancer. *Int J Cancer* **28**:431, 1981.

39. Muleris M, Salmon RJ, Zafrani B, Girodet J, Dutrillaux B: Consistent deficiencies of chromosome 18 and of the short arm of chromosome 17 in eleven cases of human large bowel cancer: A possible recessive determinism. *Ann Genet* **28**:206, 1985.

40. Mark J, Mitelman F, Dencker H, Norryd C, Tranberg KG: The specificity of the chromosomal abnormalities in human colonic polyps: A cytogenetic study of multiple polyps in a case of Gardner's syndrome. *Acta Pathol Microbiol Scand [A]* **81**:85, 1973.

41. Mitelman F, Mark J, Nilsson PG, Dencker H, Norryd C, Tranberg KG: Chromosome banding pattern in human colonic polyps. *Hereditas* **78**:63, 1974.

42. Reichmann A, Martin P, Levin B: Chromosomal banding patterns in human large bowel adenomas. *Hum Genet* **70**:28, 1985.

43. Bos JL, Fearon ER, Hamilton SR, et al: Prevalence of ras gene mutations in human colorectal cancers. *Nature* **327**:293, 1987.

44. Forrester K, Almoguera C, Han K, Grizzle WE, Perucho M: Detection of high incidence of K-ras oncogenes during human colon tumorigenesis. *Nature* **327**:298, 1987.

45. Vogelstein B, Fearon ER, Hamilton SR, et al: Genetic alterations during colorectal-tumor development. *N Engl J Med* **319**:525, 1988.

46. Bishop JM: Molecular themes in oncogenesis. *Cell* **64**:235, 1991.

47. Weinberg RA: Oncogenes and tumor suppressor genes. *CA Cancer J Clin* **44**:160, 1994.

48. Shibata D, Schaeffer J, Li ZH, Capella G, Perucho M: Genetic heterogeneity of the c-K-ras locus in colorectal adenomas but not in adenocarcinomas. *JNCI* **85**:1058, 1993.

49. Pretlow TP, Brasitus TA, Fulton NC, Cheyer C, Kaplan EL: K-ras mutations in putative preneoplastic lesions in human colon. *JNCI* **85**:2004, 1993.

50. Jen J, Powell SM, Papadopoulos N, et al: Molecular determinants of dysplasia in colorectal lesions. *Cancer Res* **54**:5523, 1994.

51. Shirasawa S, Furuse M, Yokoyama N, Sasazuki T: Altered growth of human colon cancer cell lines disrupted at activated Ki-ras. *Science* **260**:85, 1993.

52. Bourne HR, Sanders DA, McCormick F: The GTPase superfamily: Conversed structure and molecular mechanism. *Nature* **349**:117, 1991.

53. Haubruck H, McCormick F: Ras p21: Effects and regulation. *Biochem Biophys Acta* **1072**:215, 1991.

54. Xu GF, Lin B, Tanaka K, et al: The catalytic domain of the neurofibromatosis type 1 gene product stimulates ras GTPase and complements ira mutants of S. cervisiae. *Cell* **63**:835, 1990.

55. Martin GA, Viskochil D, Bollag G, et al: The GAP-related domain of the neurofibromatosis type 1 gene product interacts with ras p21. *Cell* **63**:843, 1990.

56. Ballester R, Marchuk D, Boguski M, et al: The NF1 locus encodes a protein functionally related to mammalian GAP and yeast IRA proteins. *Cell* **63**:851, 1990.

57. Bollag G, McCormick F: Differential regulation of rasGAP and neurofibromatosis gene product activities. *Nature* **351**:576, 1991.

58. Li Y, Bollag G, Clark R, et al: Somatic mutations in the neurofibromatosis 1 gene in human tumors. *Cell* **69**:275, 1992.

59. Solomon E, Voss R, Hall V, et al: Chromosome 5 allele loss in human colorectal carcinomas. *Nature* **328**:616, 1987.

60. Monpezat JP, Delattre O, Bernard A, et al: Loss of alleles on chromosome 18 and on the short arm of chromosome 17 in polyploid colorectal carcinoma. *Int J Cancer* **41**:404, 1988.

61. Okamoto M, Sasaki M, Sugio K, et al: Loss of constitutional heterozygosity in colon carcinoma from patients with familial polyposis coli. *Nature* **331**:273, 1988.

62. Law DJ, Olschwang S, Monpezat JP, et al: Concerted nonsyntenic allelic loss in human colorectal carcinoma. *Science* **241**:961, 1988.

63. Vogelstein B, Fearon ER, Kern SE, et al: Allelotype of colorectal carcinomas. *Science* **244**:207, 1989.

64. DeLeo AB, Jay G, Appella E, Dubois GC, Law LW, Old LJ: Detection of a transformation-related antigen in chemically induced sarcomas and other transformed cells of the mouse. *Proc Natl Acad Sci USA* **76**:2420, 1979.

65. Linzer DI, Levine AJ: Characterization of a 54K dalton cellular SV40 tumor antigen present in SV40-transformed cells and uninfected embryonal carcinoma cells. *Cell* **17**:43, 1979.

66. Lane DP, Crawford LV: T antigen is bound to a host protein in SV40-transformed cells. *Nature* **278**:261, 1979.

67. Eliyahu D, Raz A, Gruss P, Givol D, Oren M: Participation of p53 cellular tumor antigen in transformation of normal embryonic cells. *Nature* **312**:646, 1984.

68. Parada LF, Land H, Weinberg RA, Wolf D, Rotter V: Cooperation between gene encoding p53 tumor antigen and ras in cellular transformation. *Nature* **312**:649, 1984.

69. Jenkins JR, Rudge K, Currie GA: Cellular immortalization by a cDNA clone encoding the transformation-associated phosphoprotein p53. *Nature* **312**:651, 1984.

70. Baker SJ, Fearon ER, Nigro JM, et al: Chromosome 17 deletions and p53 gene mutations in colorectal carcinomas. *Science* **244**:217, 1989.

71. Baker SJ, Preisinger AC, Jessup JM, et al: p53 gene mutations occur in combination with 17p allelic deletions as late events in colorectal tumorigenesis. *Cancer Res* **50**:7717, 1990.

72. Finlay CA, Hinds PW, Levine AJ: The p53 proto-oncogene can act as a suppressor of transformation. *Cell* **57**:1083, 1989.

73. Eliyahu D, Michalovitz D, Eliyahu S, Pinhasi-Kimhi O, Oren M: Wild-type p53 can inhibit oncogene-mediated focus formation. *Proc Natl Acad Sci USA* **86**:8763, 1989.

74. Baker SJ, Markowitz S, Fearon ER, Willson JK, Vogelstein B: Suppression of human colorectal carcinoma cell growth by wild-type p53. *Science* **249**:912, 1990.

75. Diller L, Kassel J, Nelson CE, et al: p53 functions as a cell cycle control protein in osteosarcomas. *Mol Cell Biol* **10**:5772, 1990.

76. Mercer WE, Shields MT, Amin M, et al: Negative growth regulation in a glioblastoma tumor cell line that conditionally expresses human wild-type p53. *Proc Natl Acad Sci USA* **87**:6166, 1990.

77. Chen PL, Chen YM, Bookstein R, Lee WH: Genetic mechanisms of tumor suppression by the human p53 gene. *Science* **250**:1576, 1990.

78. Hinds PW, Finlay CA, Quartin RS, et al: Mutant p53 DNA clones from human colon carcinomas cooperate with ras in transforming primary rat cells: A comparison of the "hot spot" mutant phenotypes. *Cell Growth Diff* **1**:571, 1990.

79. Mowat M, Cheng A, Kimura N, Bernstein A, Benchimol S: Rearrangements of the cellular p53 gene in erythroleukaemic cells transformed by Friend virus. *Nature* **314**:633, 1985.

80. Hicks GG, Mowat M: Integration of Friend murine leukemia virus into both alleles of the p53 oncogene in an erythroleukemic cell line. *J Virol* **62**:4752, 1988.

81. Ben David Y, Prideaux VR, Chow V, Benchimol S, Bernstein A: Inactivation of the p53 oncogene by internal deletion or retroviral integration in erythroleukemic cell lines induced by Friend leukemia virus. *Oncogene* **3**:179, 1988.

82. Werness BA, Levine AJ, Howley PM: Association of human papillomavirus types 16 and 18 E6 proteins with p53. *Science* **248**:76, 1990.

83. Scheffner M, Werness BA, Huibregtse JM, Levine AJ, Howley PM: The E6 oncoprotein encoded by human papillomavirus types 16 and 18 promotes the degradation of p53. *Cell* **63**:1129, 1990.

84. Hollstein M, Shomer B, Greenblatt M, et al: Somatic point mutations in the p53 gene of human tumors and cell lines: Updated compilation. *Nucleic Acids Res* **24**:141, 1996.

85. Vogelstein B, Kinzler KW: Carcinogens leave fingerprints. *Nature* **355**:209, 1992.

86. Hsu IC, Metcalf RA, Sun T, Welsh JA, Wang NJ, Harris CC: Mutational hotspot in the p53 gene in human hepatocellular carcinomas. *Nature* **350**:427, 1991.

87. Bressac B, Kew M, Wands J, Ozturk M: Selective G to T mutations of p53 gene in hepatocellular carcinoma from southern Africa. *Nature* **350**:429, 1991.

88. Ozturk M: p53 mutation in hepatocellular carcinoma after aflatoxin exposure. *Lancet* **338**:1356, 1991.

89. Brash DE, Rudolph JA, Simon JA, et al: A role for sunlight in skin cancer: UV-induced p53 mutations in squamous cell carcinoma. *Proc Natl Acad Sci USA* **88**:10124, 1991.

90. Hollstein M, Sidransky D, Vogelstein B, Harris CC: p53 mutations in human cancers. *Science* **253**:49, 1991.

91. Stenger JE, Mayr GA, Mann K, Tegtmeyer P: Formation of stable p53 homotetramers and multiples of tetramers. *Mol Carcinog* **5**:102, 1992.

92. Jeffrey PD, Gorina S, Pavletich NP: Crystal structure of the tetramerization domain of the p53 tumor suppressor at 1.7 angstroms. *Science* **267**:1498, 1995.

93. Milner J, Medcalf EA: Cotranslation of activated mutant p53 with wild type drives the wild-type p53 protein into the mutant conformation. *Cell* **65**:765, 1991.

94. Hupp TR, Meek DW, Midgley CA, Lane DP: Regulation of the specific DNA binding function of p53. *Cell* **71**:875, 1992.

95. Kern SE, Kinzler KW, Bruskin A, et al: Identification of p53 as a sequence-specific DNA-binding protein. *Science* **252**:1708, 1991.

96. El-Deiry WS, Kern SE, Pietenpol JA, Kinzler KW, Vogelstein B: Definition of a consensus binding site for p53. *Nat Genet* **1**:45, 1992.

97. Funk WD, Pak DT, Karas RH, Wright WE, Shay JW: A transcriptionally active DNA-binding site for human p53 protein complexes. *Mol Cell Biol* **12**:2866, 1992.

98. Tokino T, Thiagalingam S, El-Deiry WS, Waldman T, Kinzler KW, Vogelstein B: p53 tagged sites from human genomic DNA. *Hum Mol Genet* **3**:1537, 1994.

99. Bargonetti J, Friedman PN, Kern SE, Vogelstein B, Prives C: Wild-type but not mutant p53 immunopurified proteins bind to sequences adjacent to the SV40 origin of replication. *Cell* **65**:1083, 1991.

100. Kern SE, Kinzler KW, Baker SJ, et al: Mutant p53 proteins bind DNA abnormally in vitro. *Oncogene* **6**:131, 1991.

101. Cho Y, Gorina S, Jeffrey PD, Pavletich NP: Crystal structure of a p53 tumor suppressor-DNA complex: Understanding tumorigenic mutations. *Science* **265**:346, 1994.

102. Fields S, Jang SK: Presence of a potent transcription activating sequence in the p53 protein. *Science* **249**:1046, 1990.

103. Raycroft L, Wu HY, Lozano G: Transcriptional activation by wild-type but not transforming mutants of the p53 anti-oncogene. *Science* **249**:1049, 1990.

104. O'Rourke RW, Miller CW, Kato GJ, et al: A potential transcriptional activation element in the p53 protein. *Oncogene* **5**:1829, 1990.

105. Unger T, Nau MM, Segal S, Minna JD: p53: A transdominant regulator of transcription whose function is ablated by mutations occurring in human cancer. *EMBO J* **11**:1383, 1992.

106. Kern SE, Pietenpol JA, Thiagalingam S, Seymour A, Kinzler KW, Vogelstein B: Oncogenic forms of p53 inhibit p53-regulated gene expression. *Science* **256**:827, 1992.

107. Scharer E, Iggo R: Mammalian p53 can function as a transcription factor in yeast. *Nucleic Acids Res* **20**:1539, 1992.

108. Vogelstein B, Kinzler KW: p53 function and dysfunction. *Cell* **70**:523, 1992.

109. Oliner JD, Kinzler KW, Meltzer PS, George DL, Vogelstein B: Amplification of a gene encoding a p53-associated protein in human sarcomas. *Nature* **358**:80, 1992.

110. Oliner JD, Pietenpol JA, Thiagalingam S, Gyuris J, Kinzler KW, Vogelstein B: Oncoprotein MDM2 conceals the activation domain of tumor suppressor p53. *Nature* **362**:857, 1993.

111. Fakharzadeh SS, Trusko SP, George DL: Tumorigenic potential associated with enhanced expression of a gene that is amplified in a mouse tumor cell line. *EMBO J* **10**:1565, 1991.

112. Miyashita T, Krajewski S, Krajewska M, et al: Tumor suppressor p53 is a regulator of bcl-2 and bax gene expression in vitro and in vivo. *Oncogene* **9**:1799, 1994.

113. Miyashita T, Reed JC: Tumor suppressor p53 is a direct transcriptional activator of the human bax gene. *Cell* **80**:293, 1995.

114. El-Deiry WS, Tokino T, Velculescu VE, et al: WAF1, a potential mediator of p53 tumor suppression. *Cell* **75**:817, 1993.

115. Harper JW, Adami GR, Wei N, Keyomarsi K, Elledge SJ: The p21 Cdk-interacting protein Cip1 is a potent inhibitor of G1 cyclin-dependent kinases. *Cell* **75**:805, 1993.

116. Xiong Y, Hannon GJ, Zhang H, Casso D, Kobayashi R, Beach D: p21 is a universal inhibitor of cyclin kinases. *Nature* **366**:701, 1993.

117. Noda A, Ning Y, Venable SF, Pereira-Smith OM, Smith JR: Cloning of senescent cell-derived inhibitors of DNA synthesis using an expression screen. *Exp Cell Res* **211**:90, 1994.

118. El-Deiry WS, Tokino T, Waldman T, et al: Topological control of p21 (Waf1/Cip1) expression in normal and neoplastic tissues. *Cancer Res* **55**:2910, 1995.

119. Elledge SJ, Harper JW: Cdk inhibitors: On the threshold of checkpoints and development. *Curr Opin Cell Biol* **6**:847, 1994.

120. Waldman T, Kinzler KW, Vogelstein B: p21 is necessary for the p53-mediated G1 arrest in human cancer cells. *Cancer Res* **55**:5187, 1995.

121. Waldman T, Lengauer C, Kinzler KW, Vogelstein B: Uncoupling of S phase and mitosis induced by anticancer agents in cells lacking p21. *Nature* **381**:713, 1996.

122. Lowe SW, SChmitt EM, Smith SW, Osborne BA, Jacks T: p53 is required for radiation-induced apoptosis in mouse thymocytes. *Nature* **362**:847, 1993.

123. Clarke AR, Purdie CA, Harrison DJ, et al: Thymocyte apoptosis induced by p53-dependent and independent pathways. *Nature* **362**:849, 1993.

124. Donehower LA, Harvey M, Slagle BL, et al: Mice deficient for p53 are developmentally normal but susceptible to spontaneous tumors. *Nature* **356**:215, 1992.

125. Malkin D, Li FP, Strong LC, et al: Germ line p53 mutations in a familial syndrome of breast cancer, sarcomas, and other neoplasms. *Science* **250**:1233, 1990.

126. Srivastava S, Zou ZQ, Pirollo K, Blattner W, Chang EH: Germ-line transmission of a mutated p53 gene in a cancer-prone family with Li-Fraumeni syndrome. *Nature* **348**:747, 1990.

127. Kastan MB, Onyekwere O, Sidransky D, Vogelstein B, Craig RW: Participation of p53 protein in the cellular response to DNA damage. *Cancer Res* **51**:6304, 1991.

128. Kuerbitz SJ, Plunkett BS, Walsh WV, Kastan MB: Wild-type p53 is a cell cycle checkpoint determinant following irradiation. *Proc Natl Acad Sci USA* **89**:7491, 1992.

129. Kastan MB, Zhan Q, El-Deiry WS, et al: A mammalian cell cycle checkpoint pathway utilizing p53 and GADD45 is defective in ataxia-telangiectasia. *Cell* **71**:587, 1992.

130. Lane DP: Cancer: p53, guardian of the genome. *Nature* **358**:15, 1992.

131. Graeber TG, Peterson JF, Tsai M, Monica K, Fornace AJ Jr, Giaccia AJ: Hypoxia induces accumulation of p53 protein, but activation of a G1-phase checkpoint by low-oxygen conditions is independent of p53 status. *Mol Cell Biol* **14**:6264, 1994.

132. Graeber TG, Osmanian C, Jacks T, et al: Hypoxia-mediated selection of cells with diminished apoptotic potential in solid tumors. *Nature* **379**:88, 1996.

133. Fearon ER, Cho KR, Nigro JM, et al: Identification of a chromosome 18q gene that is altered in colorectal cancers. *Science* **247**:49, 1990.

134. Hedrick L, Cho KR, Fearon ER, Wu TC, Kinzler KW, Vogelstein B: The DCC gene product in cellular differentiation and colorectal tumorigenesis. *Genes Dev* **8**:1174, 1994.

135. Cho KR, Oliner JD, Simons JW, et al: The DCC gene: Structural analysis and mutations in colorectal carcinomas. *Genomics* **19**:525, 1994.

136. Hedrick L, Cho KR, Boyd J, Risinger J, Vogelstein B: DCC: A tumor suppressor gene expressed on the cell surface. *Cold Spring Harb Symp Quant Biol* **57**:345, 1992.

137. Thiagalingam S, Lengauer C, Leach FS, et al: Evaluation of chromosome 18q in colorectal cancers. *Nat Genet* **13**:343, 1996.

138. Murty VV, Li RG, Houldsworth J, et al: Frequent allelic deletions and loss of expression characterize the DCC gene in male germ cell tumors. *Oncogene* **9**:3227, 1994.

139. Tanaka K, Oshimura M, Kikuchi R, Seki M, Hayashi T, Miyaki M: Suppression of tumorigenicity in human colon carcinoma cells by introduction of normal chromosome 5 or 18, *Nature* **349**:340, 1991.

140. Goyette MC, Cho K, Fasching CL, et al: Progression of colorectal cancer is associated with multiple tumor suppressor gene defects but inhibition of tumorigenicity is accomplished by correction of any single defect via chromosome transfer. *Mol Cell Biol* **12**:1387, 1992.

141. Narayanan R, Lawlor KG, Schaapveld RQ, et al: Antisense RNA to the putative tumor-suppressor gene DCC transforms Rat-1 fibroblasts. *Oncogene* **7**:553, 1992.

142. Lawlor KG, Telang NT, Osborne MP, et al: Antisense RNA to the putative tumor suppressor gene "deleted in colorectal cancer" transforms fibroblasts. *Ann NY Acad Sci* **660**:283, 1992.

143. Klingelhutz AJ, Hedrick L, Cho KR, McDougall JK: The DCC gene suppresses the malignant phenotype of transformed human epithelial cells. *Oncogene* **10**:1581, 1995.

144. Hahn SA, Schutte M, Hoque ATMS, et al: Dpc4, a candidate tumor suppressor gene at human chromosome 18q21.1. *Science* **271**:350, 1996.

145. Hahn SA, Seymour AB, Hoque AT, et al: Allelotype of pancreatic adenocarcinoma using xenograft enrichment. *Cancer Res* **55**:4670, 1995.

146. Hursh DA, Padgett RW, Gelbart WM: Cross regulation of decapentaplegic and Ultrabithorax transcription in the embryonic visceral mesoderm of Drosophila. *Development* **117**:1211, 1993.

147. Sekelsky JJ, Newfeld SJ, Raftery LA, Chartoff EH, Gelbart WM: Genetic characterization and cloning of mothers against dpp, a gene required for decapentaplegic function in Drosophila melanogaster. *Genetics* **139**:1347, 1995.

148. Savage C, Das P, Finelli AL, et al: Caenohabditis elegans genes Sma2, Sma-3, and Sma-4 define a conserved family of transforming growth factor beta pathway components. *Proc Natl Acad Sci USA* **93**:790, 1996.

149. Fynan TM, Reiss M: Resistance to inhibition of cell growth by transforming growth factor-beta and its role in oncogenesis. *Crit Rev Oncog* **4**:493, 1993.

150. Brattain MG, Howell G, Sun LZ, Willson JK: Growth factor balance and tumor progression. *Curr Opin Oncol* **6**:77, 1994.

151. Markowitz S, Wang J, Myeroff L, et al: Inactivation of the type II TGF-beta receptor in colon cancer cells with microsatellite instability. *Science* **268**:1336, 1995.

152. Parsons R, Myeroff LL, Liu B, et al: Microsatellite instability and mutations of the transforming growth factor beta type II receptor gene in colorectal cancer. *Cancer Res* **55**:5548, 1995.

153. Riggins GJ, Thiagalingam S, Rozenblum E, et al: Mad-related genes in the human. *Nat Genet* **13**:347, 1996.

154. Eppert K, Scherer SW, Ozcelik H, et al: MADR2 maps to 18q21 and encodes a TGF-beta-regulated MAD-related protein that is mutated in colorectal carcinoma. *Cell* **86**:543, 1996.

155. Ashton-Rickardt PG, Dunlop MG, Nakamura Y, et al: High frequency of APC loss in sporadic colorectal carcinoma due to breaks clustered in 5q21-22. *Oncogene* **4**:1169, 1989.

156. Delattre O, Olschwang S, Law DJ, et al: Multiple genetic alterations in distal and proximal colorectal cancer. *Lancet* **2**:353, 1989.

157. Sasaki M, Okamoto M, Sato C, et al: Loss of constitutional heterozygosity in colorectal tumors from patients with familial polyoposis coli and those with nonpolyposis colorectal carcinoma. *Cancer Res* **49**:4402, 1989.

158. Ashton-Rickardt PG, Wyllie AH, Bird CC, et al: MCC, a candidate familial polyposis gene in 5q.21, shows frequent allele loss in colorectal and lung cancer. *Oncogene* **6**:1881, 1991.

159. Herrera L, Kakati S, Gibas L, Pietrzak E, Sandberg A: Gardner syndrome in a man with an interstitial deletion of 5q. *Am J Med Genet* **25**:473, 1986.

160. Leppert M, Dobbs M, Scambler P, et al: The gene for familial polyposis coli maps to the long arm of chromosome 5. *Science* **238**:1411, 1987.

161. Bodmer W, Bailey C, Bodmer J, et al: Localization of the gene for familial adenomatous polyposis on chromosome 5. *Nature* **328**:614, 1987.

162. Nakamura Y, Lathrop M, Leppert M, et al: Localization of the genetic defect in familial adenomatous polyposis within a small region of chromosome 5. *Am J Hum Genet* **43**:638, 1988.

163. Kinzler KW, Nilbert MC, Su LK, et al: Identification of FAP locus genes from chromosome 5q21. *Science* **253**:661, 1991.

164. Joslyn G, Carlson M, Thliveris A, et al: Identification of deletion mutations and three new genes at the familial polyposis locus. *Cell* **66**:601, 1991.

165. Nishisho I, Nakamura Y, Miyoshi Y, et al: Mutations of chromosome 5q21 genes in FAP and colorectal cancer patients. *Science* **253**:665, 1991.

166. Groden J, Thliveris A, Samowitz W, et al: Identification and characterization of the familial adenomatous polyposis coli gene. *Cell* **66**:589, 1991.

167. Horii A, Nakatsuru S, Ichii S, Nagase H, Nakamura Y: Multiple forms of the APC gene transcripts and their tissue-specific expression. *Hum Mol Genet* **2**:283, 1993.

168. Thliveris A, Samowitz W, Matsunami N, Groden J, White R: Demonstration of promoter activity and alternative splicing in the region 5′ to exon 1 of the APC gene. *Cancer Res* **54**:2991, 1994.

169. Nagase H, Hakamura Y: Mutations of the APC (adenomatour polyposis coli) gene. *Hum Mutat* **2**:425, 1993.

170. Powell SM, Petersen GM, Krush AJ, et al: Molecular diagnosis of familial adenomatous polyposis. *N Engl J Med* **329**:1982, 1993.

171. Laken S, Vogelstein B, Kinzler KW. Unpublished observation, 1996.

172. Papadopoulos N, Leach FS, Kinzler KW, Vogelstein B: Monoallelic mutation analysis (MAMA) for identifying germ line mutations. *Nat Genet* **11**:99, 1995.

173. Groden J, Gelbart L, Thliveris A, et al: Mutational analysis of patients with adenomatous polyposis: Identical inactivating mutations in unrelated individuals. *Am J Hum Genet* **52**:263, 1993.

174. Olschwang S, Tiret A, Laurent-Piug P, Muleris M, Parc R, Thomas G: Restriction of ocular fundus lesions to a specific subgroup of APC mutations in adenomatous polyposis coli patients. *Cell* **75**:959, 1993.

175. Wallis YL, Macdonald F, Hulten M, et al: Genotype-phenotype correlation between position of constitutional APC gene mutation and CHRPE expression in familial adenomatous polyposis. *Hum Genet* **94**:543, 1994.

176. Caspari R, Olschwang S, Friedl W, et al: Familial adenomatous polyposis: Desmoid tumours and lack of ophthalmic lesions (CHRPE) associated with APC mutations beyond codon 1444. *Hum Mol Genet* **4**:337, 1995.

177. Davies D, Armstrong J, Thakker N, et al: Severe Gardner syndrome in families with mutations restricted to a specific region of the APC gene. *Am J Hum Genet* **57**:1151, 1995.

178. Dobbie Z, Spycher M, Mary J-L, et al: Correlation between the development of extracolonic manifestations in FAP patients and mutations beyond codon 1403 of the APC gene. *J Med Genet* **33**:274, 1996.

179. Gayther S, Wells D, SenGupta S, et al: Regionally clustered APC mutations are associated with a severe phenotype and occur at a high frequency in new mutation cases of adenomatous polyposis coli. *Hum Mol Genet* **3**:53–56, 1994.

180. Nagase H, Miyoshi Y, Horii A, et al: Correlation between the location of germ-line mutations in the APC gene and the number of colorectal polyps in familial adenomatous polyposis patients. *Cancer Res* **52**:4055, 1992.

181. Giardiello FM, Krush AJ, Petersen GM, et al: Phenotypic variability of familial adenomatous polyposis in 11 unrelated families with identical APC gene mutation. *Gastroenterology* **106**:1542, 1994.

182. Miyoshi Y, Nagase H, Ando H, et al: Somatic mutations of the APC gene in colorectal tumors: Mutation cluster region in the APC gene. *Hum Mol Genet* **1**:229, 1992.

183. Powell SM, Zilz N, Beazer-Barclay Y, et al: APC mutations occur early during colorectal tumorigenesis. *Nature* **359**:235, 1992.

184. Smith KJ, Johnson KA, Bryan TM, et al: The APC gene product in normal and tumor cells. *Proc Natl Acad Sci USA* **90**:2846, 1993.

185. Smith AJ, Stern HS, Penner M, et al: Somatic APC and K-ras codon 12 mutations in aberrant crypt foci from human colons. *Cancer Res* **54**:5527, 1994.

186. Su LK, Kinzler KW, Vogelstein B, et al: Multiple intestinal neoplasia caused by a mutation in the murine homolog of the APC gene. *Science* **256**:668, 1992.

187. Fodde R, Edelmann W, Yang K, et al: A targeted chain-termination mutation in the mouse APC gene results in multiple intestinal tumors. *Proc Natl Acad Sci USA* **91**:8969, 1994.

188. Oshima M, Oshima H, Kitagawa K, Kobayashi M, Itakura C, Taketo M: Loss of APC heterozygosity and abnormal tissue building in nascent intestinal polyps in mice carrying a truncated APC gene. *Proc Natl Acad Sci USA* **92**:4482, 1995.

189. Moser AR, Pitot HC, Dove WF: A dominant mutation that predisposes to multiple intestinal neoplasia in the mouse. *Science* **247**:322, 1990.

190. Moser AR, Dove WF, Roth KA, Gordon JIL The Min (multiple intestinal neoplasia) mutation: Its effect on gut epithelial cell differentiation and interaction with a modifier system. *J Cell Biol* **116**:1517, 1992.

191. Luongo C, Moser AR, Gledhill S, Dove WF: Loss of APC+ in intestinal adenomas from Min mice. *Cancer Res* **54**:5947, 1994.

192. Levy DB, Smith KJ, Beazer-Barclay Y, Hamilton SR, Vogelstein B, Kinzler KW: Inactivation of both SPC alleles in human and mouse tumors. *Cancer Res* **54**:5953, 1994.

193. Morin PJ, Vogelstein B, Kinzler KW: Apoptosis and APC in colorectal tumorigenesis. *Proc Natl Acad Sci USA* **93**:7950, 1996.

194. Miyashiro I, Senda T, Matsumine A, et al: Subcellular localization of the APC protein: Immunoelectron microscopic study of the association of the APC protein with catenin. *Oncogene* **11**:89, 1995.

195. Joslyn G, Richardson DS, White R, Alber T: Dimer formation by an N-terminal coil coiled in the APC protein. *Proc Natl Acad Sci USA* **90**:11109–11113, 1993.

196. Su LK, Johnson KA, Smith KJ, Hill DE, Vogelstein B, Kinzler KW: Association between wild-type and mutant APC gene products. *Cancer Res* **53**:2728, 1993.

197. Su LK, Burrell M, Hill DE, et al: APC binds to the novel protein EB1. *Cancer Res* **55**:2972, 1995.

198. Matsumine A, Ogai A, Senda T, et al: Binding of APC to the human homolog of the drosphila discs large tumor suppressor protein. *Science* **272**:1020–1023, 1996.

199. Rubinfeld B, Souza B, Albert I, et al: Association of the APC gene product with beta-catenin. *Science* **262**:1731, 1993.

200. Su LK, Vogelstein B, Kinzler KW: Association of the APC tumor suppressor protein with catenins. *Science* **262**:1734, 1993.

201. Rubinfeld B, Albert I, Porfiri E, Fiol C, Munemitsu S, Polakis P: Binding of GSK3-beta to the APC-beta-catenin complex and regulation of complex assembly. *Science* **272**:1023, 1996.

202. Kemler R: From cadherins to catenins: Cytoplasmic protein interactions and regulation of cell adhesion. *Trends Genet* **9**:317, 1993.

203. Perrimon N: The genetic basis of patterned baldness in Drosophila. *Cell* **76**:781, 1994.

204. Gumbiner BM: Signal transduc tion of beta-catenin. *Curr Opin Cell Biol* **7**:634, 1995.

205. Peifer M: Regulating cell proliferation: As easy as APC. *Science* **272**:974, 1996.

206. Behrens J, von Kries JP, Kuhl M, et al: Functional interaction of beta-catenin with the transcription factor LEF-1. *Nature* **382**:638, 1996.

207. Molenaar M, van de Wetering M, Oosterwegel M, et al: XTcf-3 transcription factor mediates beta-catenin-induced axis formation in xenopus embryos. *Cell* **86**:391, 1996.

208. Whitehead I, Kirk H, Kay R: Expression cloning of oncogenes by retroviral transfer of cDNA libraries. *Mol Cell Biol* **15**:704, 1995.

209. Nusse R, Varmus HE: Wnt genes. *Cell* **69**:1073, 1992.

209b. Korinek V, Barker N, Morin PJ, van Wichen D, de Weger R, Kinzler KW, Vogelstein B, Clevers H: Constitutive transcriptional activation by a beta-catenin-Tcf complex in APC-/-colon carcinoma. *Science* **275**:1784, 1997.

209c. Morin PJ, Sparks AB, Korinek V, Barker N, Clevers H, Vogelstein B, Kinzler KW: Activation of beta-catenin-Tcf signaling in colon cancer by mutations in beta-catenin or APC. *Science* **275**:787, 1997.

209d. Rubinfeld B, Robbins P, El-Gamil M, Albert I, Porfiri E, Polakis P: Stabilization of beta-catenin by genetic defects in melanoma cell lines. *Science* **275**:1790, 1997.

210. Kinzler KW, Nilbert MC, Vogelstein B, et al: Identification of a gene located at chromosome 5q21 that is mutated in colorectal cancers. *Science* **251**:1366, 1991.

211. Hampton GM, Ward JR, Cottrell S, et al: Yeast artificial chromosomes for the molecular analysis of the familial polyposis APC gene region. *Proc Natl Acad Sci USA* **89**:8249, 1992.

212. Curtis LJ, Bubb VJ, Gledhill S, Morris RG, Bird CC, Wyllie AH: Loss of heterozygosity of MCC is not associated with mutation of the retained allele in sporadic colorectal cancer. *Hum Mol Genet* **3**:443, 1994.

213. Barker PE: Double minutes in human tumor cells. *Cancer Genet Cytogenet* **5**:81, 1982.

214. Alitalo K, Winqvist R, Lin CC, de la Chapelle A, Schwab M, Bishop JM: Aberrant expression of an amplified c-myb oncogene in two cell lines from a colon carcinoma. *Proc Natl Acad Sci USA* **81**:4534, 1984.

215. Alitalo K, Schwab M, Lin CC, Varmus HE, Bishop JM: Homogeneously staining chromosomal regions contain amplified copies of an abundantly expressed cellular oncogene (c-myc) in malignant neuroendocrine cells from a human colon carcinoma. *Proc Natl Acad Sci USA* **80**:1707, 1983.

216. Alexander RJ, Buxbaum JN, Raicht RF: Oncogene alterations in primary human colon tumors. *Gastroenterology* **91**:1503, 1986.

217. Meltzer SJ, Ahnen DJ, Battifora H, Yokota J, Cline MJ: Protooncogene abnormalities in colon cancers and adenomatous polyps. *Gastroenterology* **92**:1174, 1987.

218. Finley GG, Schulz NT, Hill SA, Geiser JR, Pipas JM, Meisler AI: Expression of the myc gene family in different stages of human colorectal cancer. *Oncogene* **4**:963, 1989.

219. Tal M, Wetzler M, Josefberg Z, et al: Sporadic amplification of the HER2/neu protooncogene in adenocarcinomas of various tissues. *Cancer Res* **48**:1517, 1988.

220. D'Emilia J, Bulovas K, Wolf B, Steele G Jr, Summerhayes IC: Expression of the c-erbB-2 gene product (p185) at different stages of neoplastic progression in the colon. *Oncogene* **4**:1233, 1989.

221. Leach FS, Elledge SJ, Sherr CJ, et al: Amplification of cyclin genes in colorectal carcinomas. *Cancer Res* **53**:1986, 1993.

222. Dietrich WF, Lander ES, Smith JS, et al: Genetic identification of Mom-1, a major modifier locus affecting Min-induced intestinal neoplasia in the mouse. *Cell* **75**:631, 1993.

223. MacPhee M, Chepenik K, Liddell R, Nelson K, Siracusa L, Buchberg A: The secretory phospholipase A2 gene is a candidate for the Mom1 locus, a major modifier of ApcMin-induced intestinal neoplasia. *Cell* **81**:957, 1995.

224. Riggins GJ, Markowitz S, Wilson JK, Vogelstein B, Kinzler KW: Absence of secretory phospholipase a(2) gene alterations in human colorectal cancer. *Cancer Res* **55**:5184, 1995.

225. Melhem MF, Meisler AI, Finley GG, et al: Distribution of cells expressing myc proteins in human colorectal epithelium, polyps, and malignant tumors. *Cancer Res* **52**:5853, 1992.

226. Ogata S, Uehara H, Chen A, Itzkowitz SH: Mucin gene expression in colonic tissues and cell lines. *Cancer Res* **52**:5971, 1992.

227. Ciardiello F, Kim N, Saeki T, et al: Differential expression of epidermal growth factor-related proteins in human colorectal tumors. *Proc Natl Acad Sci USA* **88**:7792, 1991.

228. Koenders PG, Peters WH, Wobbes T, Beex LV, Nagengast FM, Benraad TJ: Epidermal growth factor receptor levels are lower in carcinomatous than in normal colorectal tissue. *Br J Cancer* **65**:189, 1992.

229. Gold P, Freedman SO: Demonstration of tumor-specific antigens in human colonic carcinomata by immunological tolerance and absorption techniques. *J Exp Med* **121**:439, 1965.

230. Ransom JH, Pelle B, Hanna MG Jr: Expression of class II major histocompatibility complex molecules correlates with human colon tumor vaccine efficacy. *Cancer Res* **52**:3460, 1992.

231. Tsioulias G, Godwin TA, Goldstein MF, et al: Loss of colonic HLA antigens in familial adenomatous polyposis. *Cancer Res* **52**:3449, 1992.

232. Calabretta B, Kaczmarek L, Ming PM, Au F, Ming SC: Expression of c-myc and other cell cycle-dependent genes in human colon neoplasiaa. *Cancer Res* **45**:6000, 1985.

233. Adams MD, Kerlavage AR, Fleischmann RD, et al: Initial assessment of human gene diversity and expression patterns based upon 83 million nucleotides of cDNA sequence. *Nature* **377**:3, 1995.

234. Liang P, Pardee AB: Differential display of eukaryotic messenger RNA by means of the polymerase chain reaction. *Science* **257**:967, 1992.

235. Velculescu VE, Zhang L, Vogelstein B, Kinzler KWL: Serial analysis of gene expression. *Science* **270**:484, 1995.

236. Schena M, Shalon D, Davis RW, Brown PO: Quantitative monitoring of gene expression patterns with a complementary DNA microarray. *Science* **270**:467, 1995.

237. Zhang L, Zhou W, Vogelstein B, Kinzler KW: Unpublished result, 1996.

238. Bird A: The essentials of DNA methylation. *Cell* **70**:5–8, 1992.

239. Goelz SE, Vogelstein B, Hamilton SR, Feinberg AP: Hypomethylation of DNA from benign and malignant human colon neoplasms. *Science* **228**:187, 1985.

240. Feinberg AP, Gehrke CW, Kuo KC, Ehrlich M: Reduced genomic 5-methylcytosine content in human colonic neoplasia. *Cancer Res* **48**:1159, 1988.

241. Silverman AL, Park JG, Hamilton SR, Gazdar AF, Luk GD, Baylin SB: Abnormal methylation of the calcitonin gene in human colonic neoplasms. *Cancer Res* **49**:3468, 1989.

242. El-Deiry WS, Nelkin BD, Celano P, et al: High expression of the DNA methyltransferase gene characterizes human neoplastic cells and progression stages of colon cancer. *Proc Natl Acad Sci USA* **88**:3470, 1991.

243. Baylin SB, Makos M, Wu JJ, et al: Abnormal patterns of DNA methylation in human neoplasia: Potential consequences for tumor progression. *Cancer Cells* **3**:383, 1991.

244. Herman JG, Merlo A, Mao L, et al: Inactivation of the CDKN2/p16/MTS1 gene is frequently associated with aberrant DNA methylation in all common human cancers. *Cancer Res* **55**:4525, 1995.

245. Schmid M, Haaf T, Grunert D: 5-Azacytidine-induced undercondensations in human chromosomes. *Hum Genet* **67**:257, 1984.

246. Landolph JR, Jones PA: Mutagenicity of 5-azacytidine and related nucleosides in C3H/10T 1/2 clone 8 and V79 cells. *Cancer Res* **42**:817, 1982.

247. Laird P, Jackson-Grusby L, Fazeli A, et al: Suppression of intestinal neoplasia by DNA hypomethylation. *Cell* **81**:197, 1995.

248. Feron ER, Vogelstein B: A genetic model for colorectal tumorigenesis. *Cell* **61**:759, 1990.

249. Vogelstein B, Kinzler KW: The multistep nature of cancer. *Trends Genet* **9**:138, 1993.

250. Garber JE, Goldstein AM, Kantor AF, Dreyfus MG, Fraumeni JF Jr, Li FP: Follow-up study of twenty-four families with Li-Fraumeni syndrome. *Cancer Res* **51**:6094, 1991.

251. Sidransky D, Tokino T, Hamilton SR, et al: Identification of *ras* oncogene mutations in the stool of patients with curable colorectal tumors. *Science* **256**:102, 1992.

252. Smith-Raven J, England J, Talbot IC, Bodmer W: Detection of c-Ki-*ras* mutations in faecal samples from sporadic colorectal cancer patients. *Gut* **36**:81, 1995.

253. Hasegawa Y, Takeda S, Ichii S, et al: Detection of K-*ras* mutations in DNAs isolated from feces of patients with colorectal tumors by mutant-allele-specific amplification (MASA). *Oncogene* **10**:1441, 1995.

254. Villa E, Dugani A, Rebecchi AM, et al: Identification of subjects at risk for colorectal carcinoma through a test based on K-*ras* determination in the stool. *Gastroenterology* **110**:1346, 1996.

255. Nollau P, Moser C, Weinland G, Wagener C: Detection of K-*ras* mutations in stools of patients with colorectal cancer by mutant-enriched PCR. *Int J Cancer* **66**:332, 1996.

256. Jen J, Kim H, Piantadosi S, et al: Allelic loss of chromosome 18q and prognosis in colorectal cancer. *N Engl J Med* **331**:213, 1994.

257. Waddell WR. Ganser GF, Cerise EJ, Loughry RW: Sulindac for polyposis of the colon. *Am J Surg* **157**:175, 1989.

258. Rigau J, Pique JM, Rubio E, Planas R, Tarrech JM, Bordas JM: Effects of long-term sulindac therapy on colonic polyposis. *Ann Intern Med* **115**:952, 1991.

259. Labayle D, Fischer D, Vielh P, et al: Sulindac causes regression of rectal polyps in familial adenomatous polyposis. *Gastroenterology* **101**:635, 1991.

260. Giardiello FM, Hamilton SR, Krush AJ, et al: Treatment of colonic and rectal adenomas with sulindac in familial adenomatous polyposis. *N Engl J Med* **328**:1313, 1993.

261. Nugent K, Farmer K, Spigelman A, Williams C, Phillips R: Randomized controlled trial of the effect of sulindac on duodenal and rectal polyposis and cell proliferation in patients with familial adenomatous polyposis. *Br J Surg* **80**:1618, 1993.

262. Winde G, Gumbinger HG, Osswald H, Kemper F, Bunte H: The NSAID sulindac reverses rectal adenomas in colectomized patients with familial adenomatous polyposis: Clinical results of a dose-finding study on rectal sulindac administration. *Int J Colorectal Dis* **8**:13, 193.

263. Debinski H, Trojan J, Nugent K, Spigelmann A, Phillips R: Effect of sulindac on small polyps in familial adenomatous polyposis. *Lancet* **345**:855, 1995.

264. Winde G, Schmid K, Schlegel W, Fischer R, Osswald H, Bunte H: Complete reversion and prevention of rectal adenomas in colectomized patients with familial adenomatous polyposis by rectal low-dose sulindac maintenance treatment: Advantages of a low-dose nonsteroidal anti-inflammatory drug regimen in reversing adenomas exceeding 33 months. *Dis Colon Rectum* **38**:813, 1995.

265. Kune GA, Kune S, Watson LF: Colorectal cancer risk, chronic illnesses, operations, and medications: Case control results from the Melbourne Colorectal Cancer Study. *Cancer Res* **48**:4399, 1988.

266. Rosenberg L, Palmer JR, Zauber AG, Warshauer ME, Stolley PD, Shapiro S: A hypothesis: Nonsteroidal anti-inflammatory drugs reduce the incidence of large-bowel cancer. *J Natl Cancer Inst* **83**:355, 1991.

267. Thun MJ, Namboodiri MM, Heath CW Jr: Aspirin use and reduced risk of fatal colon cancer. *N Engl J Med* **325**:1593, 1991.

268. Beazer-Barclay Y, Levy DB, Moser AM, et al: Sulindac suppresses tumorigenesis in the Min mouse. *Carcinogenesis* **17**:1757, 1996.

269. Jacoby RF, Marshall DJ, Newton MA, et al: Chemoprevention of spontaneous intestinal adenomas in the APC-Min mouse by the nonsteroidal anti-inflammatory drug piroxicam. *Cancer Res* **56**:710, 1996.

270. Boolbol SK, Dannenberg AJ, Chadurn A, et al: Cyclooxygenase-2 overexpression and tumor formation are blocked by sulindac in a murine model of familial adenomatous polyposis. *Cancer Res* **56**:2556, 1996.

271. Clara M, Herschel K, Ferner H: *Atlas of Normal Microscopic Anatomy of Man.* München, Urban & Schwarzenberg, 1974.

272. Kinzler KW, Vogelstein B: Lessons from hereditary colon cancer, 1966. *Cancer Cell* **87**:159, 1996.

273. Greenblatt MS, Bennett WP, Hollstein M, Harris CC: Mutations in thje p53 tumor suppressor gene: Clues to cancer etiology and molecular pathogenesis. *Cancer Res* **54**:4855, 1994.

274. Vogelstein B, Kinzler K: Tumour-suppressor genes: X-rays strike p53 again. *Nature* **370**:174, 1994.

275. Kinzler KW, Vogelstein B: Life (and death) in a malignant tumour. *Nature* **379**:19, 1996.

276. Altschul SF, Gish W, Miller W, Myers EW, Lipman DJ: Basic local alignment search tool. *J Mol Biol* **215**:403, 1990.

277. Miyoshi Y, Ando H, Nagase H, et al: Germ-line mutations of the APC gene in 53 familial adenomatous polyposis patients. *Proc Natl Acad Sci USA* **89**:4452, 1992.

278. Munemitsu S, Albert I, Souza B, Rubinfeld B, Polakis P: Regulation of intracellular beta-catenin levels by the adenomatour polyposis coli (APC) tumor-suppressor protein. *Proc Natl Acad Sci USA* **92**:3046, 1995.

279. Munemitsu S, Souza B, Muller O, Albert I, Rubinfeld B, Polakis P: The APC gene product associates with microtubules in vivo and promotes their assembly in vitro. *Cancer Res* **54**:3676, 1994.

280. Peifer M, Berg S, Reynolds AB: A repeating amino acid motif shared by proteins with diverse cellular roles. *Cell* **76**:789, 1994.

MANAGING FAMILIAL CANCER SYNDROMES

CHAPTER 32

Genetic Testing for Familial Cancer

Gloria M. Petersen ▪ Ann-Marie Codori

1. **Recent cancer gene discoveries are leading to important changes in the clinical practice of cancer risk assessment. Genetic tests, in conjunction with family history information, will be used to clarify the diagnosis of inherited cancer syndromes in patients with tumors, and provide information about cancer susceptibility to asymptomatic persons in high-risk families.**

2. **Cancer gene testing can include a variety of modalities, including linkage, direct detection when the mutation is known, and sequencing of relevant genes when the mutation is not known. In addition, tests for microsatellite instability in colon tumors may provide indirect evidence supporting a diagnosis of hereditary nonpolyposis colorectal cancer.**

3. **Commercial availability of germline cancer gene tests (i.e., *BRCA1, BRCA2, APC, hMSH2, hMLH1, p16, NF2*) has outpaced the awareness among health professionals of the need for careful implementation of testing algorithms and patient education.**

4. **For persons who are at risk for cancer, testing algorithms and gene test interpretations will depend on whether the specific germline cancer gene mutation is known for the family. Careful evaluation of the pedigree for characteristic aggregation of tumor types among affected individuals, and availability of affected persons for testing are important issues in implementing genetic testing.**

5. **There are numerous psychosocial and ethical issues in cancer gene testing. The impact of gene tests and risk perception on cancer screening/prevention behavior, and psychological distress are being actively investigated; preliminary results suggest that most persons are willing to be tested, and that there is no significant short-term (1–3 month) psychological distress following disclosure of results. Other issues include those related to gene test performance, genetic discrimination, informed consent, genetic testing of children, and privacy of genetic status information.**

6. **Genetic counseling is an essential component of cancer genetic risk assessment services. The genetic counseling process includes patient education (specific cancer-related issues, prevention/intervention options), discussion of the gene test itself, exploration of patient risk perception and sources of anxiety related to cancer risk, and consequences of various gene test outcomes.**

The phenomenal increase in discoveries related to the genetic and molecular basis of cancer, especially hereditary forms, has spawned efforts to apply them clinically, primarily in the form of gene tests. There is no doubt that information derived from genetic testing will lead in many instances to an improvement in cancer risk assessment and clinical management of cancer patients and their families. In conjunction with family history information, gene tests likely will be used to clarify the diagnosis of inherited cancer syndromes in patients with tumors, and provide information about cancer susceptibility to asymptomatic persons in high-risk families. Table 32-1 summarizes some hereditary cancer syndromes, detailed elsewhere in this volume, for which genetic testing potentially can improve cancer risk management of patients and their families.

Genetic testing for cancer holds the promise of reducing cancer mortality through timely screening and early intervention in those with predisposing mutations. The anticipated health benefits of testing rest on the assumption that persons at increased risk for cancer will be given options for preventive screening regimens or other interventions (such as prophylactic surgery or chemoprevention).

Thus, it is thus becoming apparent that gene tests will change the way in which cancer risk assessment will be performed.[1–5] Indeed, certain gene tests (*APC, RET, RB1, VHL*) now may be considered part of the standard management of the respective hereditary cancer syndrome families, whereas the medical benefit of other gene tests (*hMSH2, hMLH1, hPMS1, hPMS2, BRCA1, BRCA2,* and *p53*) is presumed but not established.[6] The gene test outcome for an individual patient or family member can lead to more informed and directed recommendations for preventive interventions. As a general example, Figure 32-1 illustrates the way in which colon cancer risk assessment is conventionally performed. That is, the health professional often evaluates a family history of a person at-risk for colon cancer seeking consultation for the risk, or less often, a patient with colon cancer. Risk assessment is based almost exclusively on evaluation of the family history, after which cancer screening recommendations can be made, tailored according to whether an inherited syndrome can be diagnosed. Figure 32-2 illustrates a potential scenario in which colon cancer gene tests will alter this process. By offering gene tests in conjunction with family history evaluation, the two sources of information not only will help make a firmer diagnosis, but clinical management of colon cancer patients may be influenced by this diagnosis. Likewise, more refined follow-up recommendations may be given to at-risk persons, whether they test positive or negative for a colon cancer gene.

Table 32-1 Hereditary Syndromes with Increased Cancer Risk and Identified Susceptibility Gene and/or Chromosomal Localization

Syndrome	Predominant tumor types	Chromosome	Gene	Reference
Ataxia telangiectasia	Breast cancer, chromosome breakage/rearrangement syndrome	11q22.3	*ATM*	78
Familial adenomatous polyposis	Multiple colorectal adenomas	5q21	*APC*	79–80
Familial melanoma	Melanoma, glioblastoma, lung	9p21	*CDKN (p16)*	81
Gorlin syndrome	Nevoid basal cell carcinoma of the skin	9q	*NBCCS*	82–84
Hereditary breast-ovarian cancer syndrome	Breast, ovarian, prostate carcinoma increased risk of other tumors	17q21 13q12-q13	*BRCA1* *BRCA2*	12–13
Hereditary nonpolyposis colorectal cancer	Colon, endometrial, ovarian, stomach, small bowel, ureter carcinomas	2p16 3p21 2q31-q33 7q11.2	*hMSH2* *hMLH1* *hPMS1* *hPMS2*	34–36
Hereditary prostate cancer	Prostate carcinoma	1q24-25	*HPC1*	85
Li-Fraumeni syndrome	Leukemia, soft-tissue sarcoma, osteosarcoma, brain tumor, breast and adrenal cortical carcinomas	17p13	*TP53*	86
Multiple endocrine neoplasia type 1	Parathyroid, endocrine pancreas and pituitary tumors	11q	*MEN-1*	87
Multiple endocrine neoplasia type 2a	Medullary thyroid carcinoma, pheochromocytoma	10q11.2	*RET*	88
Multiple endocrine neoplasia	Familial medullary thyroid carcinoma	10q11.2	*RET*	89–90
Neurofibromatosis type 1 type 2b	Multiple peripheral neurofibromas, optic glioma, neurofibrosarcoma	17q11.2	*NF1*	91–95
Neurofibromatosis type 2	Central schwannomas and meningiomas, acoustic neuromas	22q11.2	*NF2*	96
Retinoblastoma	Retinoblastomas, osteosarcomas	13q14	*RB*	97–98
von Hippel-Lindau syndrome	Renal cell carcinoma, pheochromocytoma, hemangioblastoma	3p25-p26	*VHL*	99

However, it is important to note that genetic testing for cancer risk also carries psychosocial implications that should be communicated through careful genetic counseling to persons considering cancer gene tests, both patients and family members. On the one hand, genetic counseling will entail directive counseling toward cancer prevention where indicated, but on the other, it will entail communication about complex issues related to heredity, genetic test performance, probabilities, and uncertainty of outcome.

A variety of issues have converged on cancer gene testing, including those related to clinical applications (gene test algorithms, follow-up management), genetic counseling (informed consent, psychological impact, family relationships), social, legal, and ethical implications (privacy of gene test results, genetic discrimination). In this nascent period of gene testing for cancer risk, few of these issues are fully resolved, and many continue to arise. This chapter outlines the current status of these issues.

INDICATIONS FOR CANCER GENE TESTS

At this time, cancer gene tests have two primary clinical applications. When affected individuals are tested, gene tests may be used to molecularly diagnose an inherited cancer syndrome. When asymptomatic persons are tested, gene tests may be used to identify whether or not they are at increased risk if they should carry a known predisposing mutation. The appropriate use of gene tests, particularly in determining who should be tested, is relatively straightforward in clearcut hereditary cancer syndrome families. However, this distinction rapidly is becoming blurred, as further characterization of cancer gene loci may indicate that gene tests may be used in familial cancers (those that may be owing to mutations associated with lower penetrance, and the pedigrees do not fit known criteria for hereditary syndromes), or in screening specific populations where cancer susceptibility genes occur in high frequency.

Colon Cancer Risk Assessment: Conventional

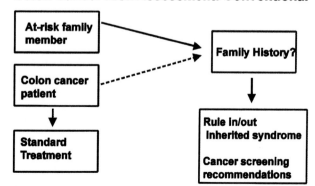

FIG. 32-1 Current view of colon cancer risk assessment.

Colon Cancer Risk Assessment: Future

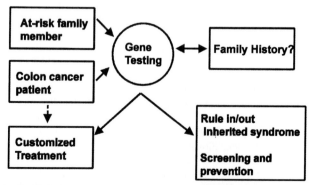

FIG. 32-2 Future view of colon cancer risk assessment.

Testing Affected Individuals to Clarify the Diagnosis

A patient with cancer might be offered gene testing to rule in or out a suspected inherited syndrome. In this case, there may be indications from family history or from clustering of specific tumors in family members suggestive of a hereditary syndrome (e.g., leukemia, soft-tissue sarcoma, brain tumors, and breast cancer in Li-Fraumeni syndrome).[7] Table 32-1 lists some of the tumor types that are associated with known cancer syndromes. Gene tests also may be offered to patients with apparently sporadic cancer if the cancer occurs at an unusually young age or if the patient has other stigmata suggestive of a hereditary syndrome. For example, familial adenomatous polyposis (FAP) might be suspected in a patient who has multiple colonic adenomas, congenital hypertrophy of the retinal pigment epithelium, and desmoid tumor, but no family history of colon polyps or cancer.[8] APC gene testing is an indicated diagnostic test, as this patient could have a de novo mutation in the APC gene.[9] If the APC gene test is positive, this patient can be presumed to have FAP, and his or her children are at 50 percent risk for inheriting the mutation.

Because genetic heterogeneity is seen in some hereditary cancer phenotypes, gene tests may be used help to identify the specific locus that is involved. For example, Turcot syndrome, a rare colon polyposis/cancer syndrome associated with central nervous system malignancies, has been shown to be genetically heterogeneous, with at least three loci (APC, hMLH1, or hPMS2) that independently produce a similar clinical picture.[10] Patients from suspected hereditary breast cancer families may need to be tested for at least two genes, *BRCA1* and *BRCA2,* because both genes may produce similar family histories.[11-13]

Testing At-risk Individuals for Inherited Susceptibility to Cancer

Asymptomatic at-risk persons from known hereditary cancer syndrome families may benefit from gene testing. In particular, when a mutation in a cancer gene is known to be segregating in the family, at-risk persons who test negative for the mutation may be relieved of years of surveillance, whereas persons who test positive for the mutation may approach the screening regimen with greater willingness to adhere to the recommendations.[9,14,15]

When a mutation is not known to segregate in a cancer family, or if the diagnosis of a cancer syndrome is less clearcut, gene tests of at-risk persons in these families is more problematic. Often, there may not be a living family member with cancer who can be gene tested to identify the mutation. In such instances a negative gene test result in an at-risk person is not a "true" negative result that places him or her at the general population risk for that cancer. Rather, this person has an "inconclusive" or "uninformative" negative test result that does not rule out other cancer gene loci, or even other mutations in the tested locus that the gene test was not able to detect. A person receiving an inconclusive test result should continue to maintain a cancer surveillance regimen as though no gene test was ever done.

It has been found that certain types of mutations in cancer genes occur with higher frequency in certain populations; these may lead to genetic screening tests targeted to specific populations. For example, two mutations in *BRCA1,* 185delAG and 5382insC, and a mutation in *BRCA2,* 6174delT, occur with high enough frequency in the Ashkenazi Jewish population that genetic screening for these mutations directed to Ashkenazi Jewish persons may be possible.[16-17] Indeed, a gene test for 185delAG has already been developed by at least one commercial enterprise, with marketing specifically directed to this population.[18]

CANCER GENE TESTS

One of the most consistent patterns to emerge from genetic studies of inherited cancer syndromes is that there are many causal mutations in associated loci, and many families have unique mutations. Thus, testing laboratories will have to develop a variety of different strategies for detecting mutations in patients or diagnosing at-risk individuals in cancer families. These tests range from linkage analysis to single-stranded conformational polymorphism analysis, to protein truncation tests, to direct DNA sequencing and allele specific oligonucleotide assays.[19-26] The relative merits and drawbacks of mutation detection approaches have been reviewed elsewhere, and different laboratories vary in their strategies for gene testing.[27-30]

Because of the relatively high sophistication of current mutation analysis technology, it is not necessarily a simple process for the clinician to understand and interpret the potential implications of gene test results. The Task Force on Genetic Testing of the NIH-DOE Working Group of the Ethical, Legal, and Social Implications of Human Genome Research has set forth general principles on gene testing relative to gene test validation and testing laboratory quality control.[31] This group argues that gene tests are different from other clinical tests because of the complexities in assessment and interpretation, and require more intake information. In addition, health care providers must describe to patients the features of the genetic test, including potential consequences prior to testing. When a clear-cut test result is obtained either because a disease-predisposing mutation is detected (positive gene test), or a mutation is not detected in an at-risk person from a family where a known mutation is segregating (true negative gene test), the subsequent counseling and management options are more apparent. Inconclusive or uninformative negative gene tests will occur when no mutation is detected in a cancer family, but because of the limitations of the testing method, a mutation in the tested locus (or elsewhere) cannot be ruled out. At-risk members in these families should not reduce their vigilance in cancer screening.

Tissue Sources for Clinical Gene Testing

The most common tissue source for gene testing is leukocyte DNA; a simple blood sample often is all that is required to perform a gene test. DNA obtained from paraffin-embedded tissue blocks obtained at surgery is also an option, if an affected relative is deceased or obtaining a blood sample is not feasible.

Specific tumor DNA studies also may yield information to aid in the diagnosis of inherited susceptibility to cancer. In the case of hereditary nonpolyposis colorectal cancer (HNPCC), a special tumor analysis to identify microsatellite instability or replication error (RER) can be performed.[32-33] In this analysis, DNA from both normal tissue and tumor tissue are analyzed using highly polymorphic microsatellite DNA markers and their banding patterns compared. Allele alterations (band shifts) seen between tumor and normal DNA suggest that the patient may have an impaired ability to repair DNA (mismatch repair), which is an indirect assessment of forms of HNPCC that are owing to mutations in mismatch repair genes (hMSH2, hMLH1, hPMS1, and hPMS2).[33-36] Because RER analysis is less time-consuming and expensive than gene tests based on mutation analysis, it offers a possible first screening test for HNPCC.[33]

Commercial Availability of Testing

With the discovery of specific genes responsible for inherited cancer syndromes, commercial laboratories have been quick to invest in the development of marketable gene tests. Among the cancers that may affect a larger segment of the population, gene tests now are commercially available for hereditary breast and ovarian cancer (*BRCA1, BRCA2*), hereditary nonpolyposis colorectal cancer (*hMSH2, hMLH1*), familial adenomatous polyposis (*APC*), hereditary melanoma (*p16*), and neurofibromatosis type 2 (*NF2*).[6,18,37]

The widening commercial availability of germline cancer gene tests has outpaced the awareness among health professionals of the need for careful implementation of testing algorithms and patient education of the issues.[37] There have been calls for caution in moving genetic tests out of the research labs and into the commercial labs until their impact and the effectiveness of cancer prevention strategies can be studied.[6,38–43] Specifically, some professional organizations recommend that genetic testing and counseling for cancer risk may be safely integrated into clinical practice only after there have been studies of gene frequencies and associated cancer risks, test sensitivity and specificity, the efficacy of interventions to decrease cancer morbidity and mortality, counseling methods, and genetic discrimination among those found to be at high risk.[41–43] Efforts to investigate all of these issues are ongoing.

CANCER RISK ASSESSMENT AND GENE TESTING ALGORITHM

With due consideration given to the issues surrounding cancer gene testing, a basic algorithm for integrating gene tests in cancer risk assessment is shown in Figure 32-3. In this algorithm, eligible

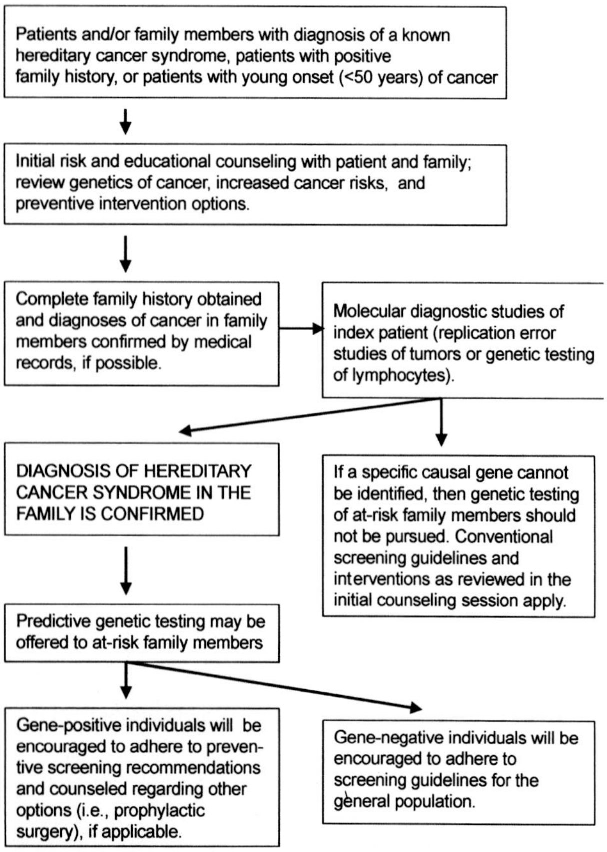

FIG. 32-3 Basic algorithm for cancer risk assessment that employs gene testing.

persons might include patients and family members with a diagnosis of a known hereditary cancer syndrome, patients with a positive family history, or patients with young onset of cancer (generally under age 50). Such patients should receive an initial face-to-face counseling session about cancer risk, with an educational component that includes a review of genetics of the specific cancers relevant to the patient, factors influencing increased cancer risk, and preventive intervention options, all adjusted to the patients' level of understanding. If not already done, a detailed family history should be elicited, and follow-up confirmation of cancer diagnoses in family members obtained, if possible.

The novel aspect of cancer risk assessment is genetic testing. The gene test may consist of mutation analysis or of tumor analysis for RER (in the case of colorectal cancer). Following the initial counseling, a careful explanation of the risks and benefits of the gene test should be given to the patient, and ample opportunity given to check understanding and to answer questions or concerns. Genetic testing may not necessarily be the best option for some patients or families, and gene testing should be entered into voluntarily, after careful deliberation of the implications.

If a specific causal gene mutation cannot be identified, then genetic testing of at-risk family members should not be pursued. Conventional screening guidelines and interventions as reviewed in the initial counseling session apply. If a specific causal gene mutation is identified, then the diagnosis of the corresponding hereditary cancer syndrome can be confirmed. In this instance, genetic counseling and predictive gene testing may be offered to at-risk family members who may wish to have this test done.

If an at-risk person tests positive for the gene, then he or she will be encouraged to adhere to preventive screening recommendations specific to the hereditary syndrome, and counseled regarding other options, such as prophylactic surger or chemoprevention, if applicable. In the case of FAP, hereditary breast and ovarian cancer and hereditary nonpolyposis colon cancer, recommendations have been developed, mostly based on expert opinion.[9,44–47]

If an at-risk person from a family where the mutation in the cancer gene is known to segregate tests negative for the mutation, then he or she will be encouraged to adhere to cancer screening guidelines for the general population.

PSYCHOSOCIAL AND ETHICAL ISSUES IN CANCER GENE TESTING

Widespread cancer genetic screening of the general population is not likely in the near future. Rather, genetic testing is being targeted to selected cancer patients and cancer families. From surveys of such persons, it appears that there is great interest in being gene tested for cancer risk.[48–51] Cancer risk perception is increased among those with a positive family history, and these individuals may be more likely to choose this option for learning more about their cancer risk. Generally, those with a family history of a given disorder are more likely to engage in disease prevention behaviors for that disorder.[52–54] Adherence with screening recommendations after genetic testing is likely to be associated with pre-genetic-testing screening behavior, and with previous symptoms suggestive of cancer.[52–56]

Psychological Consequences of Positive Gene Tests

A favorable balance of health benefits versus costs depends on determining whether the medical benefits will outweigh any psychological "side effects." For at-risk persons, cancer gene testing is not without potential "side effects," as it may pose adverse risks to psychological well-being and to the very cancer prevention practices it is meant to promote. These risks derive from several factors, including the predictable stress reaction that can follow the delivery of unfavorable medical information.

Surveys of persons at risk for cancer have shown that they expect significant distress in the face of a positive cancer gene-test. Eighty percent of 121 female first-degree relatives of ovarian cancer patients reported that they would become depressed if they tested positive for a breast cancer mutation; 77 percent reported that they would become anxious.[50] Similarly, 60 percent of male and female first-degree relatives of colon cancer patients reportedly expected to become depressed, and 52 percent anxious upon receiving a positive gene test.[57] It is possible that distress caused by a positive gene test may interfere with subsequent preventive health behavior. This has been shown in other situations: In women notified of an abnormal mammogram, those who experienced high levels of psychological distress after notification were less likely to perform subsequent breast self-exam than those with moderate levels of distress, persons psychologically-distressed after having been notified of their risk for hypertension adhered less to their medication regimens, and distressed persons delay seeking medical attention for possible cancer symptoms.[58–60]

There is concern that persons distressed by their cancer risk will make irrevocable decisions to have unproven prophylactic surgeries.[61] This prediction has some support from a study of first-degree relatives of breast cancer patients. Those who subsequently chose prophylactic mastectomy were more anxious and had higher levels of cancer-worry than women who later chose continued screening or a chemoprevention trial.[62] The finding suggests that women undertake prophylactic surgery to more fully eliminate their cancer risk. However, prophylactic mastectomy does not eliminate breast cancer risk, and some of the women studied may never develop cancer.[45–46] Moreover, basing decisions on probabilistic genetic information means that short-term relief from cancer-worry could be followed by regret if later, more definitive, information reveals that the surgery was unnecessary.

A positive genetic test can have favorable psychological consequences, including removal of uncertainty, and being better able to prepare for future events, as has been seen in Huntington disease and FAP.[2,63,64] Surveys of persons at risk for cancer suggest that they anticipate benefits from "bad news." For example, 68 percent of first-degree relatives of ovarian cancer patients reported that they would feel more "in control" of their lives even if they tested positive.[50] Two studies that measured psychological parameters at baseline and 1 to 3 months following gene testing have found no adverse reactions in persons who received positive test results: Lerman et al. studied 279 male and female members of *BRCA1*-linked hereditary breast-ovarian cancer families, and found no short-term increased depression or functional impairment in those who tested gene positive.[15] In a study of 42 children at risk for FAP and their parents, Codori et al. also did not observe any significant increase in distress or behaviorial problems in the gene-positive children.[65]

Psychological Consequences of Negative Gene Tests

Those who receive negative gene tests often experience relief at removal of uncertainty and doubt.[2,15,65] These persons are likely to be spared anxiety-provoking, costly and sometimes invasive screening procedures, and relief at knowing that their children's and their own personal risk for cancer is no greater than in the general population.[2,66]

It is possible that some proportion of those who learn that they do not carry the cancer gene mutation in their family may be at risk for psychological distress. In Huntington disease, "survivor guilt" was reported in 25 percent of people who tested negative and individual cases of depression and marital disruption have been reported.[67–68] Twenty-five percent of persons at risk for colon cancer predict feeling guilty and 50 percent expect continued worrying about cancer even after learning that they are noncarriers.[57] Similar rates were reported by women at risk for breast and ovarian cancer.[50]

Risk of Genetic Discrimination

Persons at risk for cancer face other risks in the form of genetic discrimination. Insurance companies may use genetic information, much as they use any other medical information, to underwrite an insurance policy. In these cases, insurance companies may deny insurance to those they consider to be at too great a risk for an illness, or to those with pre-existing conditions.[69,70] Such denials are likely to become more commonplace as new predictive tests are developed.[71,72] Billings et al. and Lapham et al. have identified cases where insurance or employment discrimination have occurred.[70,71] They found discrimination against the "asymptomatic ill"—those with a genetic predisposition who remain healthy—who usually lost their insurance after undertaking preventive care. Overall, the problems encountered included difficulty obtaining coverage, finding or retaining employment, and being given permission for adoptions. Insurance problems often arose when people tried to alter existing policies because of relocations or job changes. Information provided by physicians often had little or no influence on the adverse outcomes. Many people dealt with this by giving incomplete or dishonest information.[70,71]

With respect to discrimination in the work-place, there may be risk of loss of employability if gene status or genetic risk of cancer is known or required by employers.[73] Although the United States Equal Employment Opportunity Commission stated in its 1995 compliance manual that healthy people carrying abnormal genes will be protected against employment discrimination by the Americans with Disabilities Act, protection from loss of insurance awaits additional legislation.

Genetic Testing of Children

There has been debate on the appropriateness of genetic testing of minors, particularly for cancers that have onset later in adulthood or for which there is no intervention to change the outcome. The medical and legal ramifications need to be explored, and the interests of the children and their parents weighed.[40,74] Some issues to consider include assessment of the significance of the potential benefits and harms of the gene test, determination of the decision-making capacity of the child, and advocacy on behalf of the child.[74] Certainly, the medical benefit to the child should be the primary justification for gene testing children.

Certain hereditary cancer syndromes (multiple endocrine neoplasia type 2, FAP, and retinoblastoma) have onset of tumors in childhood, and warrant genetic testing of children, because interventions are feasible.[2,4,40,75] Genetic testing of children requires special counseling adjusted to their age level, and taking into consideration their awareness of cancer risk and perceptions of family attitudes toward cancer.[2] Although screening and prophylactic surgery for gene-positive persons currently are available modalities, there is potential for chemoprevention or other interventions where initiation in childhood is most effective.[76] This would re-open the issue of performing gene tests in childhood for cancer syndromes that have onset in adulthood.[1]

Privacy of Genetic Information

Genetic information should be considered confidential, and it is incumbent on health professionals and laboratories to exercise all means to prevent unauthorized disclosure of gene test results to third parties. In practice, it is recommended that results should be released only to those individuals to whom the patient has consented or subsequently requested in writing, and care should be taken to minimize the likelihood that results will become available to unauthorized persons or organizations.[31] Garber and Patenaude point out that physicians may breach confidentiality unintentionally, however, by placing information in medical charts that may be reviewed by insurers or other third parties.[77] The dilemma is that by omitting this information, the patient's future medical care is compromised, while including the information would compromise the ability of the patient or family members to obtain health, life, or disability insurance (and therefore coverage for preventive screening tests or procedures).

Another crucial issue is the revelation of gene test results to family members. As shown in Figure 32-3, the optimal algorithm for gene testing at-risk persons is to first test a family member who is affected with cancer: This patient must be willing to have the resulting genetic information shared with relatives. It is an important principle of gene testing that health care providers have an obligation to the person being tested not to inform other family members without the permission of the person tested.[31,40] There are also circumstances in which certain individuals may not want their test results known, yet by virtue of the pedigree structure, this information will become known (i.e., an identical twin of a gene-positive patient), or family members may refuse to have their gene test result shared. The resolution of these issues may not always be easy, but will call for careful planning and thorough genetic counseling with the family members involved, well before gene test results are made available.

In summary, the available data suggest that requests for predictive testing for cancer risk will be numerous, but the data also suggest that psychological risks from genetic testing for cancer risk include emotional distress from positive and negative test results, unintended and inappropriate decreases in cancer screening behavior, irrevocable decisions made in a state of anxiety, false reassurances about cancer risk, distressing and unwanted genetic knowledge, and insurance and employment discrimination. These are not reasons for banning genetic testing for cancer risk, but do warrant carefully planned implementation of testing protocols. These factors, in large measure, call for sensitive, thorough preparation and follow-up, including education and psychological evaluation and support.

GENETIC COUNSELING IN CANCER GENE TESTING

Genetic counseling must accompany genetic testing, because of the implications for family members and for reproductive decision-making. Although a conventional non-genetic diagnostic test pertains, primarily, to the health of the person who has been tested, a genetic test often has implications for the health of other relatives, such as offspring, parents, and siblings. For example, a person who learns that he has a gene for an autosomal dominant form of cancer immediately puts all of his offspring at 50 percent risk of

having inherited the mutation and puts his grandchildren at 25 percent risk. When an affected person tests positive, without prior evidence that the cancer was hereditary, the entire family may suddenly be suspected to be at increased risk for cancer. An identical twin cannot be tested without automatically informing the other, whether or not she or he wants the information. Similarly, a person at 25 percent risk for cancer (i.e., affected grandparent, healthy at-risk parent) who tests positive for the mutation automatically gives a genetic diagnosis to the unaffected parent. Thus, genetic information may have serious implications for many persons who were not even tested.

Pretest Counseling

Genetic counseling accompanying gene tests for inherited cancer risk should include:

1. Educating the family about the clinical and management aspects of hereditary cancer, the risks of cancer within the syndrome, the consequences of receiving gene-positive or gene-negative test results, including the recommended screening guidelines for each possible test outcome.

2. Exploration of the issues related to the family history and experiences with cancer. These experience can be multigenerational, and include personal involvement with relatives who have died from cancer and/or who had oncologic or surgical interventions. Family relationships can be profoundly marked by issues such as guilt and blame, and personal and familial identity may be strongly linked with cancer status. Other issues include the denial of disease risk or stigmatization of cancer within the family, and the acceptability, convenience, or affordability of screening regimens. Thus, genetic testing is imbued with meaning for certain patients much beyond its ostensible function as a simple determiner of genetic status. The at-risk patient may have pre-formed, well-entrenched conceptions of what having cancer entails, and family relationships and identity may be strongly linked with disease or gene status. Understanding of the patient's perspective is crucial so that it can be taken into account in assisting her or him to adjust to genetic test results.

3. Exploration of the perception of risk and its meaning, and anticipated meaning of any test results. With parents of at-risk minor children, time also should be devoted to discussing how and when the test results and risk will be communicated to children. In certain countries, employability or loss of insurability (life or health) is a risk, although the magnitude of this risk is unknown at present.

Informed Consent for Gene Testing

The decision to move forward with the gene test should be freely made by the at-risk person after carefully considering the consequences of genetic testing. It is strongly recommended that a consent form that outlines the meaning of test results and the consequences of the gene test be utilized.[6,31,40] If patients are to make fully informed decisions about gene testing, the informed-consent process must include discussions of several complex issues, listed in the following. This is a time-consuming process, and can require at least 1 hour of counseling time. The genetic counseling process that should accompany gene testing should incorporate the basic elements of informed consent, including:[6]

1. information on the specific test being performed

2. implications of a positive and negative result

3. possibility that the test will not be informative

4. options for risk estimation without genetic testing

5. risk of passing a mutation to children

6. technical accuracy of the test

7. fees involved in testing and counseling

8. risks of psychological distress

9. risks of insurance or employer discrimination

10. confidentiality issues

11. options and limitations of medical surveillance and screening following testing

Disclosure and Postdisclosure Counseling

Disclosure of gene test results, which can occur 2 weeks to 2 months later, depending on the laboratory, provides another opportunity to meet again with the at-risk family member and explore the meaning of the test and to discuss in a more subtstantial way the likely follow-up regimen, and cancer risks to future offspring.

For persons who test positive for the tested cancer gene, we recommend a third, follow-up session (either by telephone or in person), in which the patient is allowed a second opportunity, removed from the initial emotional reaction to the test result, to ask questions about clinical management and so the clinician can determine if referral to a mental health professional for additional support is indicated.

SUMMARY

In summary, new research developments in the molecular genetics of cancer have led to the feasibility of cancer genetic testing for many patients and family members. Gene test results have clinical implications for cancer risk management: Conventional preventive recommendations can be modified in light of gene test results such that those at higher risk for cancer (e.g., gene-positive) will be identified for increased cancer surveillance, whereas those at lower risk (true gene-negative) may potentially be reassured. There is the very real potential for misinterpretation of inconclusive gene test results. The new genetic technology also has psychological and social consequences for patients and families. Genetic counseling is an important added component in cancer risk assessment and management, particularly in helping those at risk to understand the implications of gene test results in the context of their experience with cancer and surveillance.

REFERENCES

1. Knudson AG: Hereditary cancers: From discovery to intervention. *J Natl Inst Canc Monogr* **17**:5, 1995.

2. Petersen GM, Boyd PA: Gene tests and counseling for colorectal cancer risk: Lessons from familial polyposis. *J Natl Inst Canc Monogr* **17**:67, 1995.

3. Li FP, Garber JE, Friend SH, Strong LC, Patenaude AF, Juengst ET, et al: Recommendations on predictive testing for germ line p53 mutations among cancer-prone individuals. *J Natl Canc Inst* **84**:1156, 1992.

4. Neumann HPH, Eng C, Mulligan LM, Glavac D, Zäuner I, Ponder BAJ, et al: Consequences of direct genetic testing for germline muta-

tions in the clinical management of families with multiple endocrine neoplasia, type II. *JAMA* **274**:1149, 1995.

5. Hodgson SV, Maher ER: *A Practical Guide to Human Cancer Genetics.* Cambridge, Cambridge University Press, 1993.

6. American Society of Clinical Oncology: Statement of the American Society of Clinical Oncology:Genetic testing for cancer susceptibility. *J Clin Oncol* **14**:1730, 1996.

7. Li FP, Fraumeni JF Jr., Mulvihill JJ, Blattner WA, Dreyfus MG, Tucker MA, et al: A cancer family syndrome in twenty-four kindreds. *Cancer Res* **48**:5358, 1988.

8. Herrera L (ed): *Familial Adenomatous Polyposis.* New York, Liss, 1990.

9. Petersen GM, Brensinger J: Gene tests and genetic counseling in familial adenomatous polyposis. *Oncology* **10**:89, 1996.

10. Hamilton SR, Liu B, Parsons RE, Papadopoulos N, Jen J, Powell SM, et al: The molecular basis of Turcot's syndrome. *N Engl J Med* **332**:839, 1995.

11. Ford D, Easton DF. The genetics of breast and ovarian cancer. *Br J Cancer* **72**:805, 1995.

12. Futreal PA, Liu Q, Shattuck-Eidens D, Cochran C, Harshman K, Tavtigian S, Bennett LM, et al.: BRCA1 mutations in primary breast and ovarian carcinomas. *Science* **266**:120, 1994.

13. Tavtigian SV, Simard J, Rommens J, Couch F, Shattuck-Eidens D, Neuhausen S, et al: The complete BRCA2 gene and mutations in chromosome 13q-linked kindreds. *Nat Genet* **12**:333, 1996.

14. Smith KR, Croyle RT: Attitudes toward genetic testing for colon cancer risk. *Am J Publ Health* **85**:1435, 1995.

15. Lerman C, Narod S, Schulman K, Hughes C, Gomez-Caminero A, Bonney G, et al: BRCA1 testing in families with hereditary breast-ovarian cancer: A prospective study of patient decision making and outcomes. *JAMA* **275**:1885, 1996.

16. Struewing JP, Beliovich D, Peretz T, Avishai N, Kaback MM, Collins FS, et al: The carrier frequency of the BRCA1 185delAG mutation is approximately 1 percent in Ashkenazi Jewish individuals. *Nat Genet* **11**:198, 1995.

17. Neuhausen S, Gilewski T, Norton L, Tran T, McGuire P, Swensen J, et al: Recurrent BRCA2 6174delT mutations in Ashkenazi Jewish women affected by breast cancer. *Nat Genet* **13**:126, 1996.

18. Hubbard R, Lewontin RC: Pitfalls of genetic testing. *N Engl J Med* **334**:1192, 1996.

19. Petersen GM, Slack J, Nakamura Y: Screening guidelines and premorbid diagnosis of familial adenomatous polyposis using linkage. *Gastroenterology* **100**:1658, 1991.

20. Maher ER, Bentley E, Payne SJ, Latif F, Richards FM, Chiano M, et al: Presymptomatic diagnosis of von Hippel-Lindau disease with flanking DNA markers. *J Med Genet* **29**:902, 1992.

21. Shimotake T, Iwai N, Yanagihara J, Tokiwa K, Tanaka N, Yamamoto M, et al: Prediction of affected MEN2A gene carriers by DNA linkage analysis for early total thyroidectomy: A progress in clinical screening program for children with hereditary cancer syndrome. *J Pediatr Surg* **27**:444, 1992.

22. Gayther SA, Sud R, Wells D, Tsioupra K, Delhanty JD: Rapid detection of rare variants and common polymorphisms in the APC gene by PCR-SSCP for presymptomatic diagnosis and showing allele loss. *J Med Genet* **32**:568, 1995.

23. Powell SM, Petersen GM, Krush AJ, Booker S, Jen J, Giardiello FM, et al: Molecular diagnosis of familial adenomatous polyposis. *N Engl J Med* **329**:1982, 1993.

24. Luce MC, Binnie CG, Cayouette MC, Kam-Morgan LN: Identification of DNA mismatch repair gene mutations in hereditary nonpolyposis colon cancer patients. *Int J Cancer* **20**:50, 1996.

25. Luce MC, Marra G, Chauhan DP, Laghi L, Carethers JM, Cherian SP, et al: In vitro transcription/translation assay for the screening of hMLH1 and hMSH2 mutations in familial colon cancer. *Gastroenterology* **109**:1368, 1995.

26. Heim RA, Kam-Morgan LN, Binnie CG, Corns DD, Cayouette MC, Farber RA, et al: Distribution of 13 truncating mutations in the neurofibromatosis 1 gene. *Hum Mol Genet* **4**:975, 1995.

27. Forrest S, Cotton R, Landegren U, Southern E: How to find all those mutations. *Nat Genet* **10**:375, 1996.

28. Cotton R: Current methods of mutation detection. *Mutat Res* **285**:125, 1993.

29. Dianzani I, Camaschella C, Ponzone A, Cotton RGH: Dilemmas and progress in mutation detection. *Trends Genet* **9**:403, 1993.

30. Cotton RGH: Detection of unknown mutations in DNA: A catch-22. *Am J Hum Genet* **59**:289, 1996.

31. Interim principles of the Task Force on Genetic Testing of the NIH-DOE Working Group on Ethical, Legal, and Social Implications of Human Genome Research. http://infonet.welch.jhu.edu/policy/genetics/.

32. Aaltonen LA, Peltomäki P, Leach FS, Sistonen P, Pylkkänen L, Mecklin J-P, et al: Clues to the pathogenesis of familial colorectal cancer. *Science* 260:812, 1993.

33. Liu B, Parsons R, Papadopoulos N, Nicolaides NC, Lynch HT, Watson P, et al: Analysis of mismatch repair genes in hereditary non-polyposis colorectal cancer patients. *Nat Med* 2:169, 1996.

34. Leach FS, Nicolaides N, Papadopoulos N, Liu B, Jen J, Parsons R, et al: Mutations of a MutS homolog in hereditary non-polyposis colorectal cancer. *Cell* 75:1215, 1993.

35. Papadopoulos N, Nicolaides NC, Wei Y-F, Ruben SM, Carter KC, Rosen CA, et al: Mutation of a mutL homolog in hereditary colon cancer. *Science* 263:1625, 1994.

36. Nicolaides NC, Papadopoulos N, Liu B, Wei Y-F, Carter KC, Ruben SM, et al: Mutations of two PMS homologues in hereditary nonpolyposis colon cancer. *Nature* 371:75, 1994.

37. Giardiello FM, Brensinger JD, Petersen GM, Luce MC, Hylind LM, Bacon JA, et al: The use and interpretation of commercial *APC* gene testing for familial adenomatous polyposis. *N Engl J Med* 336:823, 1997.

38. Nelson NJ: Caution guides genetic testing for hereditary cancer genes. *J Natl Canc Inst* 88:70, 1996.

39. Holtzman NA: *Proceed with Caution.* Baltimore, Johns Hopkins University Press, 1989.

40. Andrews LB, Fullarton JE, Holtzman NA (eds): *Assessing Genetic Risks: Implications for Health and Social Policy.* Washington, DC: National Academic Press, 1994.

41. National Advisory Council for Human Genome Research: Statement on use of DNA testing for presymptomatic detection of cancer risk. *JAMA* 271:785, 1994.

42. Statement of the American Society of Human Genetics on Genetic testing for breast and ovarian cancer predisposition. *Am J Hum Genet* 55:i, 1994.

43. National Action Plan on Breast Cancer: Position paper: Hereditary susceptibility testing for breast cancer. *J Clin Oncol* 14:1738, 1996.

44. Lynch HT, Smyrk T: Hereditary nonpolyposis colorectal cancer (Lynch syndrome). An updated review. *Cancer* 78:1149, 1996.

45. King M-C, Rowell S, Love SM: Inherited breast and ovarian cancer. What are the risks? What are the choices? *JAMA* 269:1975, 1993.

46. Burke W, Daly M, Garber J, Botkin J, Kahn MJE, Lynch P, et al: Recommendations for follow-up care of individuals with an inherited predisposition to cancer. II. *BRCA1* and *BRCA2*. *JAMA* 277:997, 1997.

47. Burke W, Petersen G, Lynch P, Botkin J, Daly M, Garber J, et al: Recommendations for follow-up care of individuals with an inherited predisposition to cancer. I. Hereditary nonpolyposis colon cancer. *JAMA* 277:915, 1997.

48. Croyle RT, Lerman C: Interest in genetic testing for colon cancer susceptibility: Cognitive and emotional correlates. *Prev Med* 22:284, 1993.

49. Grana G, Daly M, Lerman C, et al: Attitudes toward genetic testing in a cancer risk counseling program. *Proc Annu Meet Am Soc Clin Oncol* 13:A392, 1994.

50. Lerman C, Daly M, Masney A, Balshem A: Attitudes about genetic testing for breast-ovarian cancer susceptibility. *J Clin Oncol* 12:843, 1994.

51. Lerman C, Seay J, Balshem A, Audrain J: Interest of genetic testing among first-degree relatives of breast cancer patients. *Am J Med Genet* 57:385, 1995.

52. Rodriguez C, Plasencia A, Schroeder DG: Predictive factors of enrollment and adherence in a breast cancer screening program in Barcelona. *Soc Sci Med* 40:1155, 1995.

53. Kelly RB, Shank JC: Adherence to screening flexible sigmoidoscopy in asymptomatic patients. *Med Care* 30:1029, 1992.

54. Kendall C, Hailey BJ: The relative effectiveness of three reminder letters on making and keeping mammogram appointments. *Behav Med* 19:29, 1993.

55. Kash KM, Holland JC, Halper MS, Miller DG: Psychological distress and surveillance behaviors of women with a family history of breast cancer. *J Natl Cancer Inst* 84:24, 1992.

56. Champion VL: Compliance with guidelines for mammography screening. *Cancer Detect Prev* 16:253, 1992.

57. Lerman C, Marshall J, Audrain J, Gomez-Caminero A: Genetic testing for colon cancer susceptibility: Anticipated reactions of patients and challenges to providers. *Int J Cancer* 69:58, 1996.

58. Lerman C, Trock B, Rimer BK, Jepson C, Brody D, Boyce A: Psychological side effects of breast cancer screening. *Health Psychol* 10:259, 1991.

59. Macdonald LA, Sackett DL, Haynes RB, Taylor DW: Labelling in hypertension: A review of the behavioural and psychological consequences. *J Chron Dis* 37:933, 1984.

60. Greenwald HP, Becker SW, Nevitt MC: Delay and noncompliance in cancer detection: A behavioral perspective for health planners. *Milbank Mem Fund Quart* 56:212, 1978.

61. Biesecker BB, Boehnke M, Calzone K, Markel DS, Garber JE, Collins FS, et al: Genetic counseling for families with inherited susceptibility to breast and ovarian cancer. *JAMA* 269:1970, 1993.

62. Stefanek ME, Helzlsouer KJ, Wilcox PM, Houn F: Predictors of and satisfaction with bilateral prophylactic mastectomy. *Prev Med* 24:412, 1995.

63. Codori AM, Brandt J: Psychological costs and benefits of predictive testing for Huntington's disease. *Am J Med Genet* 54:174, 1994.

64. Wiggins S, Whyte P, Huggins M, Adam S, Theilmann J, Bloch M, et al: The psychological consequences of predictive testing for Huntington's disease. *N Engl J Med* 327:1401, 1992.

65. Codori A-M, Petersen GM, Corazzini K, Bacon J, Loth DM, Boyd PA, et al: Genetic testing for cancer in children: Short-term psychological impact. *Arch Pediatr Adolesc Med* 150:1131, 1996.

66. Lerman C, Rimer BK: Psychosocial impact of cancer screening. *Oncology* 7:67–75, 1993.

67. Codori AM, Brandt J: Psychological costs and benefits of predictive testing for Huntington's disease. *Am J Med Genet* 54:174, 1994.

68. Huggins M, Bloch M, Wiggins S, Adam S, Suchowersky O, Trew M, et al: Predictive testing for Huntington disease in Canada: Adverse effects and unexpected results in those receiving a decreased risk. *Am J Med Genet* 42:508, 1992.

69. ASHG Background Statement: Genetic testing and insurance. *Am J Hum Genet* 56:327, 1995.

70. Lapham EV, Kozma C, Weiss JO: Genetic discrimination: Perspectives of consumers. *Science* 274:621, 1996.

71. Billings PR, Kohn MA, deCuevas M, Beckwith J, Alper JS, Natowicz MR: Discrimination as a consequence of genetic testing. *Am J Hum Genet* 50:476, 1992.

72. Natowicz MR, Alper JK, Alper JS: Genetic discrimination and the law. *Am J Hum Genet* 50:465–475, 1992

73. Billings PR, Beckwith J: Genetic testing in the workplace: A view from the USA. *Trends Genet* 8:198, 1992.

74. The American Society of Human Genetics Board of Directors and the American College of Medical Genetics Board of Directors: ASHG/ACMG Report. Points to consider: Ethical, legal, and psychosocial implications of genetic testing in children and adolescents. *Am J Hum Genet* 57:1233, 1995.

75. Gallie BL, Dunn JM, Chan HSL, Hamel PA, Phillips RA: The genetics of retinoblastoma: relevance to the patient. *Pediatr Clin North Am* 38:299, 1991.

76. Giardiello FM, Hamilton SR, Krush AJ, Piantadosi S, Hylind LM, Celano P, et al: Treatment of colonic and rectal adenomas with Sulindac in familial adenomatous polyposis. *N Engl J Med* 328:1313, 1993.

77. Garber JE, Patenaude AF: Ethical, social and counseling issues in hereditary cancer susceptibility. *Cancer Surv* 25:381, 1995.

78. Savitsky K, Bar-Shira A, Gilad S, Rotman G, Ziv Y, Vanagaite L, et al: A single ataxia telangiectasia gene with a product similar to PI-3 kinase. *Science* 268:1749, 1995.

79. Kinzler KW, Nilbert MC, Su L-K, Vogelstein B, Bryan TM, Levy DB, et al: Identification of FAP locus genes from chromosome 5q21. *Science* 253:661, 1991.

80. Groden J, Thliveris A, Samowitz W, Carlson M, Gelbert L, Albertsen H, et al: Identification and characterization of the familial adenomatous polyposis coli gene. *Cell* 66:589, 1991.

81. Kamb A, Shattuck-Eidens D, Eeles R, Liu Q, Gruis NA, Ding W, et al: Analysis of the p16 gene (CDKN2) as a candidate for the chromosome 9p melanoma susceptibility locus. *Nat Genet* 8:23, 1994.

82. Farndon PA, Del Mastro RG, Evans DGR, Kilpatrick MW: Location of the gene for Gorlin syndrome. *Lancet* 339:581, 1992.

83. Reis A, Kuster W, Linss G, Gebel E, Fuhrmann W, Groth W, et al: Localization of the gene for the nevoid basal cell carcinoma syndrome. *Lancet* 339:617, 1992.

84. Gailani MR, Bale SJ, Leffell DJ, DiGiovanna JJ, Peck GL, Poliak S, et al: Developmental defects in Gorlin syndrome related to a putative tumor suppressor gene on chromosome 9. *Cell* 69:111, 1992.

85. Smith JR, Freije D, Carpten JD, Grönberg H, Xu J, Isaacs SD, et al: Major susceptibility locus for prostate cancer on chromosome 1 suggested by a genome-wide search. *Science* **274**:1301, 1996.
86. Malkin D, Li FP, Strong LC, Fraumeni JF Jr., Nelson CE, Kim DH, et al: Germ line p53 mutations in a familial syndrome of breast cancer, sarcomas, and other neoplasms. *Science* **250**:1233, 1990.
87. Larsson C, Skogseid B, Oberg K, Nakamura Y, Nordenskjold M: Multiple endocrine neoplasia type 1 gene maps to chromosome 11 and is lost in insulinoma. *Nature* **332**:85, 1988.
88. Mulligan LM, Kwok JBJ, Healey CS, Elsdon MJ, Eng C, Gardner E, et al: germ-line mutations of the RET proto-oncogene in multiple endocrine neoplasia type 2A. *Nature* **363**:458, 1993.
89. Hofstra RM, Landsvater RM, Ceccherini I, Stulp RP, Stelwagen T, Luo Y, et al: A mutation in the RET proto-oncogene associated with multiple endocrine neoplasia type 2B and sporadic medullary thyroid carcinoma. *Nature* **367**:375, 1994.
90. Carlson KM, Dou S, Chi D, Scavarda N, Toshima K, Jackson CE, et al: Single missense mutation in the tyrosine kinase catalytic domain of the RET protooncogene is associated with multiple endocrine neoplasia type 2B. *Proc Natl Acad Sci USA* **91**:1579, 1994.
91. Rouleau GA, Wertelecki W, Haines JL, Hobbs WJ, Trofatter JA, Seizinger BR, et al: Genetic linkage of bilateral acoustic neurofibromatosis to a DNA marker on chromosome 22. *Nature* **329**:246, 1987.
92. Barker D, Wright E, Nguyen K, Cannon L, Fain P, Goldgar D, et al: Gene for von Recklinghausen neurofibromatosis is in the pericentromeric region of chromosome 17. *Science* **236**:1100, 1987.
93. Seizinger BR, Rouleau GA, Ozelius LJ, Lane AH, Faryniarz AG, Chao MV, et al: Genetic linkage of von Recklinghausen neurofibromatosis to the nerve growth factor receptor gene. *Cell* **49**:589, 1987.
94. Wallace MR, Marchuk DA, Andersen LB, Letcher R, Odeh HM, Saulino AM, et al: Type 1 neurofibromatosis gene: Identification of a large transcript disrupted in three NF1 patients. *Science* **249**:181, 1990.
95. Cawthon RM, Weiss R, Xu GF, Viskochil D, Culver M, Stevens J, et al: A major segment of the neurofibromatosis type 1 gene: cDNA sequence, genomic structure, and point mutations. *Cell* **62**:193, 1990.
96. Trofatter JA, MacCollin MM, Rutter JL, Murrell JR, Duyao MP, et al: A novel moesin-, ezrin-, radixin-like gene is a candidate for the neurofibromatosis 2 tumor suppressor. *Cell* **75**:826, 1993.
97. Cavenee WK, Hansen MF, Nordenskjold M, Kock E, Maumenee I, Squire JA, et al: Genetic origin of mutations predisposing to retinoblastoma. *Science* **228**:501, 1985.
98. Lee W-H, Bookstein R, Hong F, Young L-J, Shew J-Y, Lee EYP: Human retinoblastoma susceptibility gene: cloning, identification, and sequence. *Science* **235**:1394, 1987.
99. Latif F, Tory K, Gnarra J, Yao M, Duh F-M, Orcutt ML, et al: Identification of the von Hippel-Lindau disease tumor suppressor gene. *Science* **260**:1317, 1993.

Part 4

CANCER BY SITE

CHAPTER 33

Pancreatic Cancer

Ralph H. Hruban ▪ Charles J. Yeo ▪ Scott E. Kern

1. **Pancreatic ductal adenocarcinoma is the fifth leading cause of cancer death in the United States. It is estimated that approximately 26,300 Americans will be diagnosed with pancreas cancer in 1996. It is a nearly uniformly fatal disease, and the mortality rate closely follows that of the incidence. Pancreatic cancer presents clinically with pain, with symptoms related to obstruction of the biliary or pancreatic ducts, or with protean symptoms related to the distant effects of the carcinoma.**

2. **Although most carcinomas of the pancreas appear to be sporadic, a number of anecdotal case reports and case-control studies suggest that as many as 10% of all cases of pancreatic carcinoma are hereditary. The gene or genes responsible for the familial aggregation of pancreatic cancer largely are unknown, but germ line mutations in the BRCA2 gene and, less commonly, in the p16 gene, have been shown to predispose to pancreatic cancer, but with incomplete penetrance.**

3. **The profile of genetic mutations in pancreatic cancer is distinct from other neoplasms. The K-*ras* oncogene is commonly activated by somatic mutations in pancreatic cancer, whereas three tumor suppressor genes are commonly inactivated. Ninety percent or more of pancreatic cancers harbor activating point mutations in codon 12 of K-*ras*. The p16 tumor suppressor gene is inactivated in 80% of pancreatic cancers, p53 in 50–75%, and DPC4 in 50%. Occasional somatic mutations of the RB1 gene have also been reported.**

4. **Inactivation of the DPC4 gene may be rather specific for pancreatic neoplasia. DPC4 is inactivated in as few as 15% of colorectal cancers and in less than 10% of other major cancer types. DPC4 belongs to a class of proteins that mediate signals of the TGF-β superfamily.**

5. **Pancreatic cancer is likely to harbor changes in additional, yet uncharacterized genes. Chromosome arms with unexplained losses of heterozygosity at frequencies of greater than 40% in pancreatic cancer include 1p, 6p, 8p, 12q, 13q, 21q, and 22q.**

6. **A large number of pancreatic cancers have been karyotyped. Double minute chromosomes, possibly representing gene amplification, were identified in 8% of pancreatic cancers in one study.**

7. **The diagnosis of pancreatic cancer is suspected based on clinical findings, and often can be confirmed with radiologic and endoscopic techniques. Effective screening tests are not available yet.**

Adenocarcinoma of the pancreas is one of the most aggressive of human malignancies. It typically presents late in the course of the disease with nonspecific symptoms. As a result, patients with pancreatic cancer have an extremely poor prognosis, with an overall 5-year survival rate of less than 5%.[1] However, those patients with early, surgically resectable carcinomas have a substantially improved prognosis. Clearly, early detection of the carcinoma, before it has spread beyond the pancreas, is the key to the successful treatment of patients with pancreatic carcinoma. A better understanding of the molecular genetic alterations in pancreatic cancer may lead to the development of new tests to detect this cancer earlier.

Until recently, our understanding of the genetics of pancreatic cancer was very incomplete. In large part, this was owing to difficulties presented by the carcinomas themselves. Pancreatic cancers induce a prominent non-neoplastic reaction by the host tissues. As a result, the neoplastic cells constitute only a small minority of the cells in the tumor. This problem of low neoplastic cellularity has hampered the molecular analyses of pancreatic cancer. Recent efforts, however, have overcome this obstacle largely by selectively enriching for neoplastic cells by propagating the cancers in tissue culture or in immunodeficient mice. Once a mutation is identified in these enriched populations, it can be confirmed by a sensitive assay of the original primary tumor. Indeed, these techniques are a major advance in our ability to analyze pancreatic cancers, and pancreatic cancer now boasts an extensive molecular description. Whereas much of what is known about pancreatic cancer has been learned by the study of sporadic pancreas cancers, some genes that have been identified in sporadic carcinomas also have been found to play a role in the development of inherited forms of the cancer.

In this chapter we will focus primarily on the recent advances in our understanding of the genetic alterations in human ductal adenocarcinoma of the pancreas, as this tumor type accounts for the majority of pancreatic neoplasms.

CLINICAL ASPECTS OF ADENOCARCINOMA OF THE PANCREAS

Incidence

Adenocarcinoma of the pancreas is the fifth leading cause of cancer death in the United States.[1] This year 26,300 new cases of pancreas cancer will be diagnosed in the United States and nearly the same number will die from it.[1] These patients will mostly be elderly. The incidence of pancreatic cancer increases steadily with age and approximately 80% of the cancers occur in the seventh and eight decades of life.[2] Pancreatic cancer is extremely uncommon before the age of 40, although cases have been reported in children.[3] Pancreatic cancer appears to occur slightly more commonly in men than in women, and, in the United States, in African-Americans more frequently than in whites.[2] The incidence of pancreatic cancer is higher among Jews than among non-Jews and it is higher in Western industrialized countries than it is in the the third world.[4,5] Among white males, the incidence and mortality rates from pancreatic cancer have been decreasing slowly since the 1970s, but, during this same period of time, the mortality rates among African-American women have increased slightly.[1]

A variety of environmental factors have been studied as possible etiologic agents in the development of pancreatic cancer, and cigarette smoking has the highest association with pancreatic cancer.[6-9] For example, smoking during college has been associated with a 2.6-fold risk of developing pancreatic cancer.[10] In addition, the risk of developing pancreatic cancer increases in relation to the duration of smoking and the number of cigarettes smoked.[2,11]

Diets high in meat and fat and low in fiber may also predispose to the development of pancreas cancer, but the role of alcohol consumption is less clear.[2,11-15] Based on an early well-publicized study coffee was once thought to be a possible risk factor for the development of pancreatic cancer, however, this study had serious methodological flaws and coffee is now not felt to be a risk factor.[13,14] Thus, age and cigarette smoking remain the greatest risk factors for developing pancreatic cancer.

Familial Patterns of Pancreatic Cancer

Almost all cancers show a tendency to aggregate in families, but the fraction of cancer that is hereditary varies substantially among different cancer types.[16] There have been a number of case reports in the literature which suggest that there is a familial form of pancreatic cancer.[17-32] For example, Lynch et al. described 47 individuals with pancreatic cancer in 18 families in which multiple family members had pancreatic cancer.[18] The age of onset (median 70 years), histologic types and survival times of these 47 patients were comparable to published data on unselected patients with pancreas cancer, and there appeared to be an autosomal dominant mode of transmission in several of the families.[18,32] Based on these family studies, it has been suggested that as many as 10% of the cases of pancreatic cancer are hereditary.[22] Similarly, Ghadirian et al. interviewed 179 patients with pancreas cancer and 179 controls matched for gender and age, and they reported that 7.8% of the patients with pancreatic cancer had a family history of pancreatic cancer, compared to only 0.6% of control patients without pancreatic cancer ($p < 0.01$).[33] Fernandez et al, also studied the relationship of family history and the development of pancreatic cancer.[34] They conducted a case control study in northern Italy of 362 patients with histologically confirmed pancreatic cancer and 1408 controls admitted to the hospital for acute, non-neoplastic, nondigestive tract disorders.[34] Significantly more of the patients with pancreatic cancer had a family history of pancreatic cancer than did the controls ($RR = 3.0$). From their data they estimated that 3% of newly diagnosed pancreatic cancers were familial.[34]

Thus anecdotal reports and several case-control studies suggest that between 3–10% of pancreatic cancers are caused by inherited factors.

Diagnosing Pancreatic Cancer

Although the pancreas is located deep in the retroperitoneal space it can be visualized with sophisticated imaging tech-

niques.[35] These techniques include real-time ultrasonography, dynamic contrast-enhanced computed tomography, magnetic resonance imaging, angiography, endoscopic retrograde cholangiopancreatography, and endoscopic ultrasonography. Despite the introduction of these new techniques the death rate for pancreatic carcinoma has not changed significantly. This is not surprising because the biggest determinant of patient outcome is stage at presentation, and these tools do not currently influence the timing of patient presentation.[35] The survival rate for pancreatic cancer will not improve significantly until new tests are developed to screen for the disease before the patients become symptomatic.

Although all of the imaging techniques may reveal a suspicious mass in the pancreas, the gold standard for diagnosing pancreatic cancer remains histopathology. Tissue for microscopic examination can be obtained either by fine needle aspiration, tissue needle core biopsy or by excisional biopsy at the time of laparotomy.[35,36] Again, as was true for imaging, the need for biopsy is likely to be apparent only after the disease has advanced.[1]

Pathology of Pancreatic Cancer

The most common type of exocrine pancreatic cancer is the duct cell adenocarcinoma.[37] The majority of these cancers are localized to the head of the pancreas (60%) and the remainder arise in the body (13%) or tail (5%) or infiltrate diffusely throughout the gland (21%).[38] By light microscopy, adenocarcinomas of the pancreas are composed of neoplastic glands infiltrating a dense non-neoplastic stroma (Figs. 33-1 A, and B). Numerous inflammatory cells, including lymphocytes, also are frequently admixed with the tumor cells. This non-neoplastic host response is characteristic of pancreatic cancers and it must be considered when conducting molecular analyses of allelic loss, since DNA isolated from most pancreatic cancers contains predominantly normal DNA. Perineural (Fig. 33-2) and vascular invasion frequently are seen in pancreatic cancers, as is infiltration of adjacent structures and metastases to regional lymph nodes (Fig 33-3).

Infiltrating adenocarcinoma of the pancreas frequently is associated with dramatic histologic changes in the pancreatic ducts and ductules. The normal pancreatic ducts and ductules are linked by a single layer of cuboidal epithelial cells, but in most pancreata with cancer this epithelium is regionally replaced by a proliferative epithelium with varying degrees of cytologic atypia.[37] There is no uniform nomenclature for these duct lesions, but the term flat hyperplasia refers to a uniform increase in the mucin content of the epithelial cells. The term papillary hyperplasia without atypia refers to the presence of papillae lined by columnar cells. The term atypical papillary hyperplasia designates papillary lesions with nuclear enlargement, and increased nuclear to cytoplasmic ratio, loss of cellular polarity, and nuclear pleomorphism.[39,40] The histology of selected examples is illustrated in Figs. 33-4A–F.

These various duct lesions are more common in pancreata with cancer than they are in pancreata without cancer.[39-42] For example, Cubilla and Fitzgerald compared the duct changes in 227 pancreata with pancreatic cancer with the duct changes in 100 age- and sex-matched controls without pancreatic cancer.[39] They found that papillary lesions were three times more common in the pancreata obtained from patients with pancreatic cancer than they were in pancreata obtained from patients without pancreatic cancer and that atypical papillary lesions were seen only in pancreata with pancreas cancer.[39] These finidngs have been confirmed by Kozuka et al. and Pour et al.[41,42] More recently Furukawa et al., using three-dimensional mapping techniques, have demonstrated a stepwise progression from mild dysplasia to severe dysplasia in pancreatic duct lesions. These results suggest that, just as there is a progression

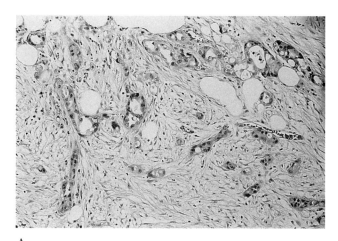

A

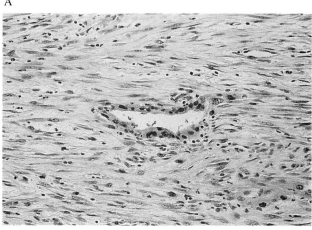

B

FIG. 33-1 Infiltrating adenocarcinoma of th pancreas. Note the haphazard arrangement of markedly atypical glands *(A)* and the intense non-neoplastic infammatory and fibroblastic response elicited by teh carcinoma *(B)*. (*A,B* both hematoxylin and eosin).

from adenoma to infiltrating adenocarcinoma in colonic neoplasia, so too is there a progression in the pancreas from flat mucinous lesions (Fig. 33-4A), to papillary lesions without atypia (Figs. 33-4A–C), to papillary lesions with atypia (Fig. 33-4D), to infiltrating adenocarcinoma (Figs. 33-1 and 33-2).[37] Furthermore, these results suggest that these lesions are not in acutality hyperplasias, but instead represent part of the neoplastic process.

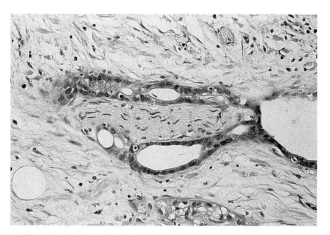

FIG. 33-2 Infiltrating adenocarcinoma of the pancreas growing along a nerve. Pain is a common symptom of pancreatic cancer (hematoxylin and eosin).

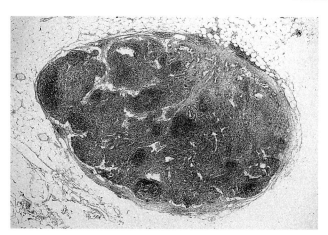

FIG. 33-3 Metastatic adenocarcinoma of the pancreas in a lymph node. The carcinoma has metastasized to the upper right hand corner of this node (hematolylin and eosin).

GENETIC LOCI

Genetic Loci Involved in Hereditary Pancreatic Cancer

It has proven difficult to perform classical linkage studies in families with pancreatic cancer due to the small size of most kindreds and the short life expectancy of patients with carcinoma of the pancreas. Nonetheless, analyses of families in which there is an aggregation of pancreatic cancer may provide clues as to which genes are involved in hereditary pancreatic cancer.

Families with an aggregation of pancreatic cancer can be divided into three general groups: (1) those associated with known syndromes; (2) those in which there is an aggregation of pancreatic cancers, but not part of a known syndrome; and (3) those in which there is an association of pancreatic with nonpancreatic cancers.

Syndromes Associated with Pancreatic Cancer. Several well-characterized genetic syndromes have been shown to predispose affected family members to the development of pancreatic cancer.[31] These include hereditary pancreatitis, ataxia telangiectasia, hereditary nonpolyposis colorectal carcinoma (HNPCC; Lynch Syndrome), a subset of the familial atypical mole-multiple melanoma (FAMMM) syndrome and the Peutz-Jeghers Syndrome.[31,32]

Hereditary pancreatitis is an autosomal dominant disorder with incomplete penetrance characterized by recurrent episodes of severe pancreatitis in blood-related family members over two generations.[43–46] There is often an early age of onset of the pancreatitis and the patients frequently develop chronic pancreatitis. Men are affected at the same rate as women.[32] Familial pancreatitis has recently been attributed to a gene at 7q35 by D. Whitcomb et al.[46] They constructed a 500-member pedigree from a US kindred centered in eastern Kentucky and Western Virginia, and, using microsatellite markers and linkage analysis, they were able to establish cosegregation between the familial pancreatitis phenotype and the 7q35 locus.[46] The mechanism by which the genetic alteration in hereditary pancreatitis predisposes carriers to pancreatic cancer is not clear, however, some have suggested that the increased risk of pancreatic cancer observed in patients with chronic pancreatitis is secondary to chronic injury and regeneration from the pancreatitis itself.[31,47,48]

Patients with ataxia telangiectasia may also be at increased risk for developing pancreatic cancer.[31,32] Ataxia-telangiectasia is characterized by progressive cerebellar-ataxia with degeneration of Purkinje cells, telangiectasias (primarily conjuctival), thymic hypoplasia with cellular and humoral immunodeficiencies, and ocu-

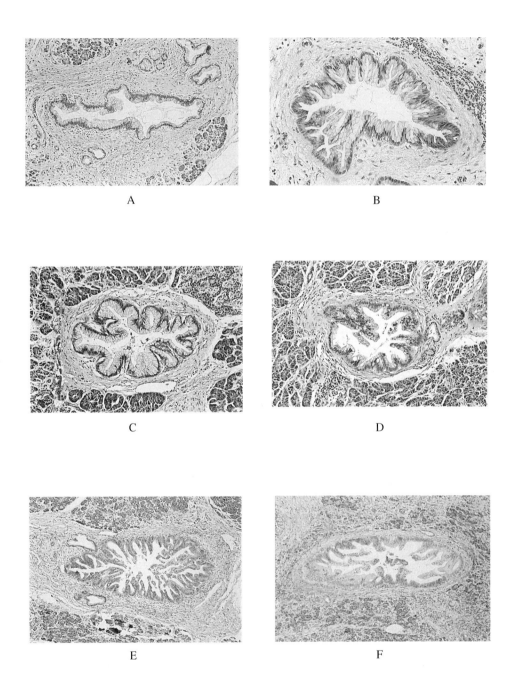

A

B

C

D

E

F

FIG. 33-4 Duct lesions, also called hyperplasias, from pancreata with cancer. Note the progression from (top row, A–C) flat lesions (A), to papillary lesions without atypia (B and C), to (bottom row, D–F) papillary lesion with atypia (D), to papillary lesions with marked atypia (E and F, carcinoma *in situ*) (all hematoxylin and eosin).

lomotor apraxia. Ataxia telangiectasia is inherited in an autosomal recessive pattern and the gene responsible for this syndrome has recently been cloned. The ATM gene resides on chromosome 11q22–23 and it encodes for a protein that is similar to several yeast and mammalian phosphatidylinositol 3' kinases involved in mitogenic signal transduction, meiotic recombination, and cell-cycle control.[49] Patients with ataxia-telangiectasia are at increased risk for developing a number of neoplasms, including ovarian cancer, biliary cancer, gastric cancer, leukemia, lymphoma, and possibly pancreatic cancer.[31,32,49]

HNPCC is another syndrome that predisposes affected individuals to pancreatic cancers.[17,32] This syndrome is characterized by the autosomal dominant transmission of a predisposition to colonic cancer in association with other cancers, including breast, endometrial, ovarian, and pancreatic cancer.[50–53] Recently HNPCC has been shown to be associated with replication errors or microsatellite instability caused by mutations in the human mismatch repair system.[54–56] Of note, replication errors, such as those found in HNPCC, are rare in sporadic pancreatic cancers (<1 in 100 cancers).[57,58]

The Peutz-Jeghers syndrome is an autosomal dominant hereditary disease characterized by hamartomatous polyps of the gastrointestinal tract and by mucocutaneous melanin deposits.[59] Forty-eight percent of thirty-one patients with Peutz-Jeghers syndrome followed by Giardiello et al. developed cancer and four of these cancers were pancreatic cancer.[60] This represents a 100-fold excess of pancreatic cancer compared to that expected.

Finally, a subset of patients with the FAMMM syndrome appear to be at increased risk for developing pancreatic cancer.[19,31,32] The FAMMM syndrome is inherited in an autosomal dominant fashion and it is characterized by multiple nevi, multiple atypical nevi, and multiple cutaneous malignant melanomas.[19,61–62] Germline mutations in p16 have been shown to segregate with the increased risks of pancreatic cancer in some kindreds with the FAMMM syndrome.[61–62] Of interest, although the risk of pancreatic cancer is increased in these kindreds, it is not a highly penetrate trait. In these families there may be a tendency for mutations at the C-terminal end of the p16 gene to be associated with a high penetrance for pancreatic cancer.[63]

Families with an Aggregation of Pancreatic Cancer. Although a number of syndromes have been associated with an increased risk of pancreatic cancer, the majority of pancreatic cancers cannot be explained in this way. In many families pancreatic cancer occurs independent of a known syndrome. Henry Lynch at Creighton University has pioneered this idea and has reported over 30 extended families with multiple cases of pancreatic carcinoma.[17–23,32] He identified a suspected autosomal dominant mode of transmission in some of his pedigrees and estimated that between 5–10% of all pancreatic cancers have a hereditary origin.[22,32] Lynch notes, however, that the clustering of a cancer in a family does not necessarily mean that the cancer is hereditary. Environmental exposures need to be excluded. For example, it is possible that several members of a family developed cancer because they each had smoked cigarettes.[31] Nonetheless, these families provide a unique opportunity to study efficiently the clinical patterns and the genetics of pancreatic cancer.

In addition to the published experience at Creighton University, another well-studied collection of familial pancreatic cancer is the National Familial Pancreas Tumor Registry (NFPTR) at Johns Hopkins. The registry is currently collecting families in which more than one family member is affected with pancreatic cancer (see footnote).* Fifty-six families with two or more first-degree relatives having cancer of the pancreas have enrolled in this registry. The average age at diagnosis for patients with pancreatic cancer in these families (65.5 years) does not appear to differ from the age of onset of apparently sporadic cases of pancreatic carcinoma. Thirty of the pedigrees involved two family members: 16 parent-child pairs and 14 sibling-sibling pairs. Twenty-six of the 56 pedigrees had three to five affected family members.

Members of the registries, as well as those of registries created for other cancer types, are an important resource that can be used to determine the contribution of environmental risk factors, the patterns of inheritance of pancreatic cancer, and the types and prevalence of other tumor types (such as melanoma, breast cancer, and ovarian cancer) in familial pancreatic cancer. The results of these analyses should provide a basis for counseling families with a familial aggregation of pancreatic cancer.

Families in which There Is an Association of Pancreatic with Nonpancreatic Cancers. Several other cancers, including those of the breast and ovary, have been associated with pancreatic cancer in some families.[32] Tulinius et al. analyzed the cancer risk for family members of 947 randomly selected female breast cancer patients in the Icelandic Cancer Registry.[64] They found more cases of pancreas cancer than expected in male first-degree relatives of the breast cancer patients (relative risk 1.66).[64] Kerber and Slattery, in a case-control study of the Utah Population Database, found that a family history of pancreatic cancer is significantly associated with an increased risk of ovarian cancer.[65] From this Kerber and Slattery estimate that a family history of pancreatic cancer accounted for 4.8% of the cases of ovarian cancer.[65] Similarly, genetically defined subsets of families with familial melanoma and with familial breast cancer have been found to have an increased incidence of pancreatic cancer.[61,62,66–69]

Currently, a minority of the cases in which there is an aggregation of pancreatic cancer can be accounted for by known syndromes or by an association of nonpancreatic with pancreatic cancers. Each form of familial pancreatic cancer has, however, provided insights and fresh opportunities to study the genetics of pancreatic cancer. In turn, the results of these analyses will provide insight into the etiology of apparently sporadic pancreatic cancers.

Genetic Loci Involved in Sporadic Pancreatic Cancer

Three general approaches have been taken in the search for the genetic loci involved in the development of pancreatic cancer. The identity of specific chromosomes lost or gained by the pancreatic cancer can be determined by the karyotypes of metaphase spreads obtained from fresh cancers. These cytogenetic studies provide structural information about the mechanisms responsible for the loss or gain of genetic material, but the resolution of this technique is limited. More detailed information can be obtained by looking for loss of heterozygosity (LOH) using a panel of molecular probes specific for each chromosome arm. Such allelotypes were used in the identification of the novel DPC4 tumor suppressor gene in a panel of pancreatic cancers and in defining the roles of the p16 and p53 genes. Finally, the relatively new technique of representational difference analysis (RDA) has been applied to pancreatic cancer. RDA is a method for isolating DNA fragments that are present in only one of two nearly identical complex genomes. It utilizes subtraction hybridization methods and has been shown to enrich for difference products over 1,000,000-fold. RDA is a particularly attractive technique for isolating new tumor suppressor genes, because it can strongly favor the enrichment of ho-

*The National Familial Pancreas Tumor Registry, The Johns Hopkins Hosptial, Department of Pathology, Meyer 7-181, 600 N. Wolfe Street, Baltimore, MD 21287. (410) 955-9132; (410) 955-0115 (fax); e-mail: rhruban@welchlink.welch.jhu.edu.

mozygously deleted regions. Homozygous deletions are smaller than most heterozygous losses and so this technique promises to focus attention on smaller regions of the genome to serve as candidate loci for new tumor suppressor genes.

Karyotype of Sporadic Pancreatic Cancer. A number of recurrent chromosome abnormalities have been identified in sporadic pancreatic cancers, providing clues to the specific genes involved in the pathogenesis of pancreatic cancer. Griffin et al. have karyotyped 62 primary pancreatic cancers resected at The Johns Hopkins Hospital and found clonally abnormal karyotypes in 44 of the cancers.[70–71] The karyotypes were generally complex and included both numerical and structural changes. Losses were more frequent than gains and included a high prevalence of losses of chromosomes 18, 13, 12, 17, and 6. The losses of chromosome 6q were confirmed by flourescent *in situ* hybridization using a biotin-labeled microdissection probe from 6q24-ter. The most frequent whole chromosome gains were of chromosomes 20 and 7. Recurrent structural abnormalities most frequently involved 1p, 3p, 11p, 17p, 1q, 6q and 19q.[70,71] In addition, double-minute chromatin bodies suggestive of gene amplification were identified in six of the cancers. These karyotype studies, when combined with smaller reports by Johansson et al., suggest that chromosomes 1p, 3p, 6q, and 11p may harbor as yet unidentified tumor suppressor genes.[70–72]

Allelotype of Sporadic Pancreatic Cancer. Hahn et al. and Seymour et al. have allelotyped two series of pancreatic cancers.[57,73] High frequencies (>60%) of allelic loss were found at 1p, 9p, 17p, and 18q, whereas moderate frequencies (40–60%) of allelic loss were seen at 3p, 6p, 8p, 10q, 12q, 13p, 18p, 21q, and 22q.[57,73] These patterns of allelic loss suggest regions of the genome as candidate tumor suppressor loci. For example, the p53 gene is located on 17p, and 17p was lost in 100% of the cancers allelotyped by Hahn et al.[57] Similarly, the DPC4 gene on 18q and the p16 gene on 9p each suffered loss of heterozygosity in nearly 90% of the tumors.[57] In these studies, chromosome 1p had the highest frequency of allelic loss (67%) not accounted for by a known tumor suppressor gene.

Allelotype and karyotype studies produce different kinds of information, and a comparison of these results provides new insight into the structural basis of the molecular genetic alterations. Brat et al. recently compared the chromosomal abnormalities of primary pancreatic adenocarcinomas, as determined by classical cytogenetics, with the molecular changes, as determined by the studies of LOH, in the same cancers.[74] In the 14 cancers with abnormal karyotypes, 65% (123 of 188) of the chromosomal arms with molecular LOH were associated with karyotypic structural abnormalities. Karyotypic changes accounting for these losses included 83 whole chromosomal losses, 18 partial deletions, nine isochromosomes, eight additions, and five translocations. The greatest degree of correlation between the cytogenetic and molecular studies were found at sites of known tumor suppressor genes such as p53, DPC4, p16, and BRCA2. These results generally validate both techniques, and indicate that, in pancreatic cancer, structural abnormalities can account for two-thirds of the LOH. Of note, there were 13 chromosomes that had extensive regions of LOH, yet appeared normal on karyotypic analysis. This finding suggests that chromosome loss with reduplication of the remaining chromosome occurs in pancreatic cancer.[74]

RDA Applied to Sporadic Pancreas Cancer. As discussed previously, RDA is a powerful new technique which can be used to isolate small regions of homozygous deletion in a cancer. Schutte et al. applied RDA to a sporadic pancreatic cancer and identified a homozygous deletion which mapped to a 180-kb region on chromosome 13q.[75] This deletion mapped to the area of the BRCA2 locus. Indeed, the map of this deletion provided the first published partial sequences of the BRCA2 gene, including exon 2 and intron 24.[75] The mapping of this deletion was a critical advance in the discovery of the BRCA2 gene by Stratton et al. and its characterization by Myriad Genetics, and it provided the first clue that the BRCA2 was a tumor suppressor gene as opposed to a proto-oncogene, and that BRCA2 served such a role in the pancreas.[76,77]

SPECIFIC GENES

Specific Genes Involved in Hereditary Pancreatic Cancer

The short life expectancy of patients with pancreatic carcinoma has made it difficult to perform classical linkage studies on families with pancreatic cancer. Simply put, it is extremely unusual to find more than one patient alive with disease at a time in any family. Because of these difficulties, most studies of familial pancreatic cancer have relied on the candidate gene approach. In this approach, a tumor suppressor gene which is known to be inactivated in sporadic pancreatic cancers is selected as the candidate gene, and then germline tissues from affected individuals from families with familial pancreatic cancer can be tested for mutations in this candidate gene. This approach is possible because, at the molecular level, familial and sporadic forms of cancer often involve the same genes.[78] For example, familial adenomatous polyposis (FAP) has been shown to be caused by inherited mutations in the APC gene and inactivation of APC is a common and early event in sporadic adenocarcinomas of the colon.[79,80] Similarly, missense germline mutations in the RET proto-oncogene are responsible for the multiple endocrine neoplasia-2 (MEN2) syndrome and these same mutations have been identified in sporadic medullary carcinomas.[81,82]

The candidate gene approach has been applied to familial pancreatic cancer and in a few of the families the pancreatic cancers appear to be caused by germ line mutations in the p16 or BRCA2 genes.[83,84] In contrast, a number of families have been examined for germ line mutations in DPC4, but, to date, none have been found.[63]

Germ Line p16 Mutations in Pancreatic Cancer Families. The multiple tumor suppressor 1 (MTS1/p16/CDKN2) gene is inactivated in almost 80% of sporadic adenocarcinomas of the pancreas.[58] In forty-one percent of these cnacers these inactivations are owing to homozygous deletions of the gene and in 38% to sequence changes. p16 therefore would appear to be a good candidate to examine in patients with familial pancreatic cancers. Moskaluk et al. analyzed 21 kindreds with familial pancreatic carcinoma for germ line mutations in p16 and in the related CDK4 gene.[83] Kindreds with the FAMMM syndrome were excluded. Germline CDK4 mutations were not seen and germ line p16 mutation were identified in only one family. The mutation was found in two individuals affected with pancreas cancer in this family, and the alteration destroyed the donor splice site of intron 2, causing premature termination after the addition of two new codons at the 3 end of exon 2.[83] Of interest, one of the two carriers in this kindred also had a melanoma. All other patients in this series were found to be wild-type for both p16 and for CDK4.[83] Thus, germ line p16 mutations could account for the pancreatic cancers in only one (<5%) of the 21 kindreds studied with familial pancreatic cancer, and they were seen in a patient who also had melanoma. As discussed previously, germline mutations in p16 have also been shown to segregate with an increased risk of pancreatic cancer in some kindreds with familial melanoma.[61,62]

Germ Line BRCA2 Mutations in Pancreatic Cancer Families.
The BRCA2 gene is another logical choice for the candidate gene
approach. BRCA2 may play a role in the development of sporadic
pancreatic cancer. Twenty-five to thirty-five percent of sporadic
cancers show LOH at the BRCA2 locus on 13q and karyotypic
losses of chromosome 13 are common in pancreatic cancer.[57,70–73]
Furthermore, a critical advance in the discovery of BRCA2 was
the identification of a homozygous deletion of the BRCA2 locus
in a pancreatic cancer.[75,76] Finally, as noted previously, there have
been some reports suggesting that the risk of pancreatic cancer is
increased in families of breast cancer patients and in carriers of
BRCA2 mutations.[64,66–69] Goggins et al. therefore screened a panel
of 41 adenocarcinomas of the pancreas for BRCA2 mutations.[84]
Four of the 41 cancers had both a loss of one allele of BRCA2 and
a mutation in the second allele. Three of these four mutations were
germ line. The three germ line mutations identified included two
germline 6174 delT at codon 1982 and a germ line 2481 insT mutation.[84] Because of these findings, the utility of a cross-sectional
population screen was evaluated. Normal tissues from 245 consecutive surgical patients with adenocarcinoma of the pancreas
were screened near the 6174 nucleotide. Sequence analysis of this
limited region of the BRCA2 gene revealed two additional germ
line mutations, a 6174delT mutation and a second nearby 6158
insT mutation. Thus, a total of 5 germ line mutations were identified. Remarkably, only one of the 5 patients with germ line mutations had a relative with breast cancer, and one had a relative with
prostate cancer. None had a family history of pancreatic cancer.[84]

Germ line muations in BRCA2 represent the most common inherited predisposition to pancreatic carcinoma identified to date,
and the results of screening for BRCA2 mutations suggest that the
classic definition of a familial case of pancreatic cancer is too
stringent. Clearly, some cases of pancreatic cancer which appear
sporadic, are, in fact, caused by inherited mutations in BRCA2.

**Absence of Germ Line DPC4, K-*ras* and p53 Mutations in
Pancreatic Cancer Families.** The recently discovered DPC4
gene was an attractive candidate gene to study in families with
pancreatic cancer.[85] DPC4 was identified in a locus of consensus
homozygous deletions in sporadic pancreatic carcinomas and is
biallelically inactivated in almost 50% of pancreatic carcinomas.[85]
Moskaluk et al. sequenced the complete DPC4 coding sequence of
25 individuals from 11 separate kindred with a familial aggregation of pancreatic carcinoma, but no mutations were found.[63] Similarly, the K-*ras* oncogene frequently is activated and the p53 tumor suppressor frequently is inactivated in pancreatic carcinomas,
but, to date, germ line mutations have not been identified in either
of these two genes in patients with familial or sporadic cancer.[85,86]

In summary, the gene or genes responsible for the majority of
cases of familial pancreatic cancer have not yet been identified. A
small minority of these cases may be owing to germ line mutations in p16, particularly in cases in which there is a family history
of melanoma. Germ line mutations in BRCA2 also predispose to
the development of pancreatic cancer, and, owing to their low
penetrance, these mutations may also be responsible for some
cases of pancreatic cancer that appear to be sporadic.

Specific Genes Involved in Sporadic Pancreatic Cancer

The development of an adenocarcinoma of the pancreas is complex and involves the accumulation of mutations in the K-*ras*
oncogene and in numerous tumor suppressor genes. K-*ras* appears
to be activated in the vast majority of pancreatic cancers, whereas
the tumor suppressor genes p53, p16, DPC4, and BRCA2 frequently are inactivated.[86] These mutations disregulate the cell cy-

cle and lead to inappropriate cell proliferation. Of interest, a high
concordance of DPC4 and p16 inactivation ($p = 0.007$) has been
reported in pancreatic cancer, suggesting that inactivation of the
p16/RB pathway increases the selective pressure for subsequent
mutations of DPC4 in this tumor type.[87] This section will begin
with a discussion of K-*ras*, the most frequently altered gene in
pancreatic cancer, and it will then be followed by a discussion of
the three tumor suppressor genes that are mostly frequently inactivated in pancreatic cancer; p53, p16, and DPC4.

Activation of K-*ras*. Oncogenes encode for proteins that, when
overexpressed or activated by a mutation, possess transforming
properties. In normal cells, K-*ras* is a proto-oncogene that encodes for a G protein involved in signal transduction.[88] Point mutations in codons 12, 13, or 61 of K-*ras* activate the gene product.
These mutations impair the intrinsic GTPase activity of this protein and cause it to be constitutively active in signal transduction.[88] K-*ras* is the most frequently mutated gene in pancreatic
cancer, with reported mutation rates ranging 71–100%.[86,89–102] This
is the highest reported prevalence of K-*ras* mutations in any tumor
type. The vast majority of these mutations occur in codon 12 of
K-*ras*.[86] These mutations appear to be early events in the development of pancreatic neoplasia. This has been demonstrated by studies of the noninvasive intraductal lesions that are found in the pancreata with and without cancer. In humans and in the Syrian
golden hamster animal model of pancreatic neoplasia, these duct
lesions have been shown to harbor activating point mutations in
K-*ras*.[103–107] For example, several investigators have microdissected the pancreatic duct lesions from pancreata obtained from
patients without cancer, and they have shown that these noninvasive duct lesions can harbor activating clonal mutations in
K-*ras*.[105–107] Thus, activation of the K-*ras* oncogene appears to be
a fairly early event in the development of adenocarcinoma of the
pancreas. Furthermore, as will be discussed later, the high prevalence of K-*ras* mutations in invasive cancers, their presence early
in the neoplastic process, and the limitation of these mutations
largely to a pair of codons, all make K-*ras* a promising marker for
a molecular-based test to detect early pancreatic carcinomas.

Tumor Suppressor Genes. Tumor suppressor genes differ from
oncogenes in that tumor suppressor genes normally function to restrict cell proliferation. Their loss, by deletion or mutation, may
lead to disregulated cell growth.

p53 Inactivation. The p53 tumor suppressor gene is inactivated
in slightly more than half of all pancreatic carcinomas.[87,95,108–114]
This usually occurs by loss of one allele and mutation of the other.
Evidence for the loss of one allele comes from allelotyping and
karyotyping studies that have identified 17p as a site of frequent
loss in pancreatic cancers.[57,70,71,73] When sequenced, the second allele of p53 is mutated in about 50–75% of the cancers.[87,99,111] The
majority of mutations reported have been transitions (pyrimidine
to pyrimidine or purine to purine) in the conserved regions of the
gene. Redston et al. and Rozenblum et al. also noted a high prevalence of small intragenic mutations in the p53 gene in pancreatic
cancers.[87,111] p53 is a nuclear binding protein that acts as a G1/S
checkpoint, and it also plays a role in the induction of apoptosis.[115]
Inactivation of p53 in pancreatic cancers therefore results in the
loss of two important controls of the cell life cycle, the initiation
of replication and the induction of cell death.

p16 Inactivation. p16 is a recently identified tumor suppressor
gene that is inactivated in a variety of tumors.[116] p16 resides on
chromosome 9p and, as noted earlier, 9p was found to be a frequent site of allelic loss in the pancreatic cancer allelotypes.[57,73]
Recently, Caldas et al. demonstrated sequence changes in p16 in

38% of tumors.[58] Furthermore, Caldas et al. demonstrated homozygous deletions of p16 in nearly 40% of the tumors. Therefore, p16 would appear to be inactivated in as many as 80% of pancreatic cancers. p16 inhibits the promotion of the cell cycle by binding to the cyclin–CDK4 complex, preventing CDK4 from phosphorylating the RB protein. Hypophosphorylated RB protein binds and may sequester transcription factors that otherwise promote the G1/S transition, whereas hyperphosphorylation of RB releases these factors.[117] Therefore, the inactivation of p16 in pancreatic cancer disregulates another important cell cycle checkpoint.

DPC4. One of the most frequently lost chromosome arms in both the allelotypes and karyotypes of pancreatic cancer is 18q.[57,70,71,73] Based on this observation, Hahn et al. performed detailed genome scanning of 18q on a panel of pancreatic carcinomas.[85] These analyses not only confirmed the high frequency of LOH on 18q, but they also revealed a consensus locus of homozygous deletions. These homozygous deletions did not include the DCC locus. Further positional cloning of the locus lead to the discovery of the DPC4 gene. This tumor suppressor gene is biallelically inactivated in almost 50% of pancreatic carcinomas. In thirty percent, this inactivation is by homozygous deletion, and in 20%, by loss of one allele and mutation of the other.[85] Remarkably, although DPC4 appears to be a common target of inactivation in pancreatic cancer, it is only infrequently inactivated in other neoplasms.[118] The specificity of DPC4 inactivation for pancreatic cancer suggests that DPC4 might be useful in determining if a particular metastatic carcinoma in a patient arose in the pancreas.

The precise function of DPC4 is not known, but DPC4 has homology to the *mad* family of proteins. These proteins play a role in signal transduction from TGF-β superfamily cell surface receptors. Indeed, DPC4 may be one of the terminal steps in TGF-β signaling pathways, as DPC4 has been shown to be active in transcriptional assays.[119] TGF-β downregulates the growth of epithelial cells. It is reasonable to expect that inactivation of a similar pathway, owing to inactivation of DPC4, would promote cell growth.

Mutations in Multiple Genes in Pancreatic Cancer. Rozenblum et al. have recently determined the status of K-ras, p53, p16, DPC4 and BRCA2 in a series of 42 pancreatic carcinomas.[87] This extensive molecular analysis of a series of cancers provides a unique opportunity to determine if there are any relationships among the mutations in these various genes. All 42 carcinomas harbored a mutation in codon 12 of K-*ras* and inactivation of all three tumor suppressor genes occurred in 37% of the cancers.[87] A high concordance was found between DPC4 and p16 inactivation ($p = 0.007$) suggesting that inactivation of the p16/RB pathway increased the selective pressure for subsequent mutations of DPC4. Of note, one tumor had a germline mutation in BRCA2 and eight additional selected genetic events, highlighting the complexity of the molecular genetic events responsible for the development of pancreatic cancer. Furthermore, small homozygous deletions appear to be a common mechanism for inactivating tumor suppressor genes in pancreatic cancer. One or more homozygous deletions have been found in 64% of pancreatic cancers.[58,85,118,120]

Other Tumor Suppressor Genes. A number of other tumor suppressor genes appear to be inactivated in only a small minority of pancreatic carcinomas. For example, although one report suggested that APC might be inactivated in pancreatic cancers, more recent studies, which examined large numbers of pancreatic cancers, demonstrated that inactivation of APC is rare to absent in pancreatic cancers.[73,121,122,123] APC is almost universally mutated in colorectal neoplasia and the absence of APC inactivation in pancreatic cancer demonstrates further that the mutation spectrum of pancreatic carcinoma is distinct from that seen in other gastrointestinal neoplasms.

There have been conflicting reports on the expression levels of the DCC gene product in pancreatic carcinomas, but no genetic alterations, including homozygous deletions, have been reported for DCC in pancreatic cancer.[57,85,124]

Mutations of RB are reported in pancreatic cancer, but at a very low rate. Huang et al. found that immunohistological staining for RB expression was lost in three of 30 pancreatic cancers. In one of these three cases a truncating mutation found and in a second a missense mutation was verified by DNA sequencing.[73,124–126]

IMPLICATIONS FOR DIAGNOSIS

There are no molecular tests currently being used to screen for pancreatic carcinomas, but the recent advances in our understanding of how molecular biology can be used to screen for cancer, and in the molecular genetics of this tumor, provide several avenues for developing such a test.[127] Probably the best example is the K-*ras* oncogene. K-*ras* is a particulary attractive target for a molecular screening test for pancreatic cancer for three reasons. First, the vast majority of pancreatic carcinomas harbor mutations in K-*ras*, suggesting that K-*ras* will be a sensitive genetic marker.[86,89–102] Second, mutations in this oncogene essentially are limited to two codons, and so a limited number of probes can be employed to detect these mutations, greatly simplifying the analyses.[86] Finally, as discussed earlier, these mutations appear to be early events in the development of pancreatic neoplasia, suggesting that K-*ras* could be used to detect early and therefore curable cancers.[103–108] Indeed, K-*ras* mutations have been used to identify cells shed from pancreatic cancers in pancreatic juice samples, in cytologic preparations, and in stool and blood specimens.[107,128–130] For example, Caldas et al. screened stool specimens obtained from patients with chronic pancreatitis, cholangiocarcinoma, and pancreatic cancer.[107] They found K-*ras* mutations in stool specimens from nine patients. Six of these nine patiens had pancreatic cancer, and in five of the six cases the mutation found in the patients invasive pancreatic cancer was the same as the one identified in the stool. In the remaining four patients, mutations identified in the stool were identical to those present in intraductal lesions (duct hyperplasias) present in the patient's resected pancreatic specimens. [107] This study established that screening for K-*ras* can be used to detect rare cells shed from pancreatic cancers and from pancreatic duct lesions in the stool. However, in this study, K-*ras* mutations were identified the stool of a patient with duct lesions, but no infiltrating cancer. Clearly, we need to advance our understanding of the molecular genetics of pancreatic cancer, so that new tests can be developed that are both sensitive and specific for early stages of this disease.

ACKNOWLEDGMENT

The authors would like to thank Michele Heffler for her assistance, energy, and enthusiasm in preparing this manuscript. For the latest on pancreatic cancer, visit our Web site (http://www.path.jhu.edu/pancreas).

REFERENCES

1. Cancer Facts and Figures: 1996. The American Cancer Society.
2. Gold EB: Epidemiology of and risk factors for pancreatic cancer. *Surg Clin No Am* **75**:819, 1995.
3. Taxy JB: Adenocarcinoma of the pancreas in childhood. *Cancer* **37**:1508, 1976.
4. Newill VA: Distribution of cancer mortality among ethnic subgroups of the white population in New York City, 1953–1958. *J Natl Cancer Inst* **26**:405, 1961.
5. Seidman H: Cancer death rates by site and sex for religions and socioeconomic groups in New York City. *Environ Res* **3**:235, 1970.
6. Durbec JP, Chevillotte C, Bidart JM, Berthezene P, Sarles H: Diet, alcohol, tobacco, and risk of cancer of the pancreas: A case-control study. *Br J Cancer* **43**:463, 1983.
7. Ghadirian P, Simard, A, Baillargeon J: Tobacco, Alcohol, and coffee and cancer of the pancreas. *Cancer* **67**:2664, 1991.
8. Doll R, Peto R: Mortality in relation to smoking: Twenty years observation on male British doctors. *Br Med J* **2**:1525, 1976.
9. Kahn HA: The Dorn study of smoking and mortality among US Veterans: Report on eight and one-half years of observation. *Natl Cancer Inst Monogr* **19**:1, 1966.
10. Whittemore AS, Paffenbarger RS Jr, Anderson D, Lee JE: Early precursors of pancreatic cancer in college men. *J Chron Dis* **36**:251, 1983.
11. Howe, GR, Ghadirian P, Bueno de Mesquita HB, Zatonski WA, Baghurst PA, Miller AB, Simard A, Baillargeon J, de Waard F, Przewozniak K, McMichael AJ, Jain M, Hsieh CC, Maisonneuve P, Boyle P, Walker AM: Collaborative case-control study of nutrient intake and pancreatic cancer within the search program. *Int J Cancer* **51**:365, 1992.
12. Hirayama T: Epidemiology of pancreatic cancer in Japan. *Jpn J Clin Oncol* **19**:208, 1989.
13. Gold EB, Gordis L, Diener M, Seltser R, Boitnott JK, Bynum TE, Hutcheon DF: Diet and other risk factors for cancer of the pancreas. *Cancer* **55**:460, 1985.
14. LaVecchia C, Liati P, Decarlie A: Coffee consumption and risk of pancreatic cancer. *Int J Cancer* **40**:309, 1987.
15. Velema JP, Walker AM, Gold EB: Alcohol and pancreatic cancer: Insufficient epidemiologic evidence for a causal relationship. *Epidemiol Rev* **8**:28, 1986.
16. Li FP: Molecular epidemiology studies of cancer in families. *Br J Cancer* **68**:217, 1993.
17. Lynch HT, Voorhees GJ, Lanspa SJ, McGreevy PS, Lynch JF: Pancreatic carcinoma and hereditary nonpolyposis colorectal cancer: A family study. *Br J Cancer* **52**:271, 1985.
18. Lynch HT, Fitzsimmons ML, Smyrk TC, Lanspa SJ, Watson P, McClellan J, Lynch JF: Familial pancreatic cancer: Clinicopathologic study of 18 nuclear familes. *Am J Gastroent* **85**:54, 1990.
19. Lynch HT, Fusaro RM: Pancreatic cancer and the familial atypical multiple mole melanoma (FAMMM) syndrome. *Pancreas* **6**:127, 1991.
20. Lynch HT, Fusaro L, Lynch JF: Familial pancreatic cancer: A family study. *Pancreas* **7**:511, 1992.
21. Lynch HT, Smyrk TC, Watson P, Lanspa SJ, Lynch JF, Lynch PM, Cavalieri RJ, Boland CR: Genetics, natural history, tumor spectrum, and pathology of hereditary nonpolyposis colorectal cancer: An updated review. *Gastroenterology* **104**:1535, 1993.
22. Lynch HT: Genetics and pancreatic cancer. *Arch Surg* **129**:266, 1994
23. Lynch HT, Fusaro L, Smyrk TC, Watson P, Lanspa S, Lynch JF: Medical genetic study of eight pancreatic cancer-prone families. *Cancer Invest* **13**:141, 1995.
24. Bergman W, Watson P, de Jong J, Lynch HT, Fusaro RM: Systemic cancer and the FAMMM syndrome. *Br J Cancer* **61**:932, 1990.
25. Dat NM, Sontag SJ: Pancreatic carcinoma in brothers [Letter]. *Ann Intern Med* **97**:282, 1987.
26. Ehrenthal D, Haeger L, Griffin T, Compton C: Familial pancreatic adenocarcinoma in three generations. *Cancer* **59**:1661, 1987.
27. Grajower MM: Familial pancreatic cancer [Letter]. *Ann Intern Med* **98**:111, 1983.
28. Kakhouda N, Mouiel J: Pancreatic cancer in mother and daughter [Letter]. *Lancet* **2**:747, 1986.
29. MacDermott RP, Kramer P: Adenocarcinoma of the pancreas in four siblings. *Gastroenterology* **63**:137, 1973.
30. Reimer RR, Fraumeni Jr, JF, Ozols RF, Bender R: Pancreatic cancer in father and son [Letter]. *Lancet* **1**:911, 1977.
31. Lumadue JA, Griffin CA, Osman M, Hruban RH: Familial pancreatic cancer and the genetics of pancreatic cancer. *Surg Clin N Am* **75**:845, 1995.
32. Lynch HT, Smyrk T, Kern SE, Hruban RH, Lightdale CJ, Lemon SJ, Lynch JE, Fusaro LR, Fusaro RM, Ghadirian P: Familial pancreatic cancer: A review. *Semin Oncol* **23**:251, 1996.
33. Ghadirian P, Boyle P, Simard A, Baillargeon J, Maisonneuve P, Perret C: Reported family aggregation of pancreatic cancer within a population-based case-control study in the francophone community in Montreal, Canada. *Int J Pancreatol* **10**:183, 1991.
34. Fernandez E, La Vecchia C, D Avanzo B, Negri E, Franceschi S: Family history and the risk of liver, gallbladder, and pancreatic cancer. *Cancer Epidemiol Biomarkers Prev* **3**:209, 1994.
35. Moossa AR, Gamagami RA: Diagnosis and staging of pancreatic neoplams. *Surg Clin N Am* **75**:871, 1995.
36. Christoffersen P, Poll P: Peri-operative pancreas aspiration biopsies. *Acta Pathol Microbiol Scand* (Suppl) **22**:28, 1970.
37. DiGiuseppe JA, Yeo CJ, Hruban RH: Molecular biology and the diagnosis and treatment of adenocarcinoma of the pancreas. *Advan Anat Pathol* **3**:139, 1996.
38. Cubilla AL, Fitzgerald PJ: Tumors of the exocrine pancreas. 2nd series, fascicle 19. Washington, DC: *Armed Forces Institute of Pathology,* 1984.
39. Cubilla A, Fitzgerald PJ: Morphological lesions associated with human primary invasive nonendocrine pancreas cancer. *Cancer Res* **36**:2690, 1976.
40. Furukawa T, Chiba R, Kobari M, Matsuno S, Nagura H, Takahashi T: Varying grades of epithelial atypia in the pancreatic ducts of humans. *Arch Pathol Lab Med* **118**:227, 1994.
41. Kozuka S, Sassa R, Taki T, Masamoto K, Nagasawa S, Saga S, Hasegawa K, Takeuchi M: Relation of pancreatic duct hyperplasia to carcinoma. *Cancer* **43**:1418, 1979.
42. Pour PM, Sayed S, Sayed G: Hyperplastic, preneoplastic and neoplastic lesions found in 83 human pancreases. *Am J Clin Pathol* **77**:137, 1982.
43. Madrazo-de la Garza J, Hill ID, Lebenthal E: Hereditary pancreatitis, in Go VLW, DiMango EP, Gardner JD, Lebenth E, Reber A, Scheele A (eds): *The Pancreas: Biology, Pathobiology, and Disease,* 2nd ed. New York, Raven Press, 1993, p.1095.
44. Davidson P, Costanza D, Swieconek JA, Harris JB: Hereditary pancreatitis: A kindred without gross aminoaciduria. *Ann Int Med* **68**:88, 1968.
45. Comfort MW, Steinberg AG: Pedigree of a family with hereditary chronic relapsing pancreatitis. *Gastroenterology* **21**:54, 1952.
46. Whitcomb DC, Preston RA, Aston CE, Sossenheimer MJ, Barua PS, Zhang Y, Wong-Chong A, White GJ, Wood PG, Gates LK Jr, Ulrich C, Martin SP, Post JC, Ehrlich GD: A gene for hereditary pancreatitis maps to chromosome 7q35. *Gastroenterology* **110**:1975, 1996.
47. Ekbom A, McLaughlin JK, Karlsson B, Nyren O, Gridley G, Adami HO, Fraumeni JF Jr: Pancreatitis and pancreatic cancer: A population-based study. *J Natl Cancer Inst* **86**:625, 1994.
48. Lowenfels AB, Maisonneuve P, Cavallini G, Ammann RW, Lankisch PG, Andersen JR, Dimango EP, Andren-Sandberg A, Domellof L: Pancreatitis and the risk of pancreatic cancer. *N Engl J Med* **328**:1433, 1993.
49. Savitsky K, Bar-Shira A, Gilad S, Rotman G, Ziv Y, Vanagaite L, Tagle DA, Smith S, Uziel T, Sfez S, Ashkenasi M, Pecker I, Frydman M, Harnik R, Patanjali SR, Simmons A, Clines GA, Sartiel A, Gatti RA, Chessa L, Sanal O, Lavin MF, Jaspers NGJ, Taylor AMR, Arlett CF, Miki T, Weissman SM, Lovett M, Collins FS, Shiloh Y: A single ataxia telangiectasia gene with a product similar to PI-3 kinase. *Science* **268**:1749, 1995.
50. Lynch HT, Smyrk TC, Watson P, Lanspa SJ, Lynch JF, Lynch PM, Cavalieri RJ, Boland CR: Genetics, natural history, tumor spectrum and pathology of hereditary nonpolyposis colorectal cancer: An updated review. *Gastroenterology* **104**:1535, 1993.
51. Lynch HT, Krush AJ: Heredity and adenocarcinoma of the colon. *Gastroenterology* **53**:517, 1967.
52. Lynch HT, Krush AJ, Guirgis H: Genetic factors in families with combined gastrointestinal and breast cancer. *Am J Gastroenterol* **59**:31, 1973.
53. Lynch HT, Schuelke GS, Kimberling WJ, Albano WA, Lynch JF, Biscone KA, Lipkin ML, Deschner EE, Mikol YP, Sandberg AA, Elston RC, Bailey-Wilson JE, Danes BS: Hereditary non-polyposis colorectal cancer (Lynch syndromes I and II). II. Biomarker studies. *Cancer* **56**:934, 1985.

54. Aaltonen LA, Peltomaki P, Mecklin JP, Jarvinen H, Jass JR, Green JS, Lynch HT, Watson P, Tallqvist G, Juhola M, Sistonen P, Hamilton SR, Kinzler KW, Vogelstein B, de la Chapelle A: Replication errors in benign and malignant tumors from hereditary nonpolyposis colorectal cancer patients. *Cancer Res* **54**:1645, 1994.

55. Thibodeau SN, Bren G, Schaid D: Microsatellite instability in cancer of the proximal colon. *Science* **260**:816, 1993.

56. Ionov Y, Peinado MA, Malkhosyan S, Shibata D, and Perucho M: Ubiquitous somatic mutations in simple repeated sequences reveal a new mechanism for colonic carcinogenesis. *Nature* (Lond). **363**:558, 1993.

57. Hahn SA, Seymour AB, Hoque ATMS, Schutte M, da Costa LT, Redston MS, Caldas C, Weinstein CL, Fischer AY, Yeo CJ, Hruban RH, Kern SE: Allelotype of pancreatic adenocarcinoma using xenograft enrichment. *Cancer Res* **55**:4670, 1995.

58. Caldas C, Hahn SA, da Costa LT, Redston MS, Schutte M, Seymour AB, Wienstein CL, Hruban RH, Yeo CJ, Kern SE: Frequent somatic mutations and homozygous deletions of the p16 (MTS1) gene in pancreatic adenocarcinoma. *Nat Genet* **8**:27, 1994.

59. Bowlby LS: Pancreatic adenocarcinoma in an adolescent male with Peutz-Jeghers syndrome. *Hum Pathol* **17**:97, 1986.

60. Giardiello FM, Welsh SB, Hamilton SR, Offerhaus GJA, Gittelsohn AM, Booker SV, Krush AJ, Yardley JH, Luk GD: Increased risk of cancer in the Peutz-Jeghers syndrome. *N Engl J Med* **316**:1511, 1987.

61. Whelan AJ, Bartsch D, Goodfellow PJ: Brief report: a familial syndrome of pancreatic cancer and melanoma with a mutation in the CDKN2 tumor-suppressor gene. *N Engl J Med* **333**:975, 1995.

62. Goldstein AM, Fraser MC, Struewing JP, Hussassian CJ, Ranade K, Zametkin DP, Fontaine LS, Organic SM, Dracopoli NC, Clark WHC Jr, Tucker MA: Increased risk of pancreatic cancer in melanoma-prone kindred with p16[INK4] mutation. *N Engl J Med* **333**:970, 1995.

63. Moskaluk CA, Hruban RH, Schutte M, Lietman A, Smyrk T, Fusaro L, Fusaro R, Lynch J, Yeo CJ, Jackson CE, Lynch HT, Kern SE: Polymerase chain reaction and cycle sequencing of DPC4 in the analysis of familial pancreatic carcinoma. *Diag Mol Pathol,* 1996, *in press.*

64. Tulinius H, Olafsdottir GH, Sigvaldason H, Tryggvadottir L, Bjarnadottir K: Neoplastic diseases in families of breast cancer patients. *J Med Genet* **31**:621, 1994.

65. Kerber RA, Slattery ML: The impact of family history on ovarian cancer risk. *Arch Int Med* **155**:905, 1995.

66. Thorlacius S, Olafsdottir G, Tryggvadottir L, Neuhausen S, Jonasson JG, Tavtigian SV, Tulinius H, Ogmundsdottir HM, Eyfjord JE: A single BRAC2 mutation in male and female breast carcinoma families from Iceland with varied cancer phenotypes. *Nat Genet* **13**:117, 1996.

67. Phelan CJ, Lancaster JM, Tonin P, Gumbs C, Cochran C, Carter R, Chadirian P, Perret C, Moslehi R, Dion F, Faucher MC, Dole K, Kaimi S, Foulkes W, Lounis H, Warner E, Ggoss P, Anderson D, Larsson C, Naarod SA, Futreal PA: Mutation analysis of the BRCA2 gene in 49 site-specific breast cancer families. *Nat Genet* **13**:120, 1996.

68. Couch FJ, Farid LM, DeShano ML, Tavtigian SV, Calzone K, Campeau L, Peng Y, Bogden B, Chen Q, Neuhausen S, Shattuck-Eidens D, Goodwin AK, Daly M, Radford DM, Sedacek S, Rommens J, Simard J, Garber J, Merajver S, Weber B: BRAC2 germline mutations in male breast cancer cases and breast cancer families. *Nat Genet* **13**:123, 1996.

69. Berman DB, Costalas J, Schultz DC, Grana G, Daly M, Godwin AK: A common mutation in BRAC2 that predisposes to a variety of cancers is found in both Jewish Ashkenazi and non-Jewish individuals. *Cancer Res* **56**:3409, 1996.

70. Griffin CA, Hruban RH, Long PP, Morsberger LA, Douna-Issa F, Yeo CJ: Chromosome abnormalities in pancreatic adenocarcinoma. *Genes Chrom Cancer* **9**:93, 1994.

71. Griffin CA, Hruban RH, Morsberger LA, Ellingham T, Long PP, Jaffee EM, Hauda KM, Bohlander SK, Yeo CJ: Consistent chromosome abnormalities in adenocarcinoma of the pancreas. *Cancer Res* **55**:2394, 1995.

72. Johansson B, Bardi G, Heim S, Mandahl N, Mertens F, Bak-Jensen E, Andren-Sandberg A, Mitelman F: Nonrandom chromosomal rearrangements in pancreatic carcinomas. *Cancer* **69**:1674, 1992.

73. Seymour AB, Hruban RH, Redston M, Caldas C, Powell SM, Kinzler KW, Yee CJ, Kern SE: Allotype of pancreatic adenocarcinoma. *Cancer Res* **54**:2761, 1994.

74. Brat DJ, Hahn SA, Griffin CA, Kern SE, Hruban RH: A comparison of karotypic abnormalities and allelic loss in surgically resected human pancreatic human pancreatic adenocarcinoma. *Mod Pathol* **9**:134A, 1996.

75. Schutte M, daCosta LT, Hahn SA, Moskaluk C, Hoque ATMS, Rozenblum E, Weinstein CL, Bittner M, Meltzer PS, Trent JM, Yeo CJ, Hruban RH, Kern SE: Identification by representational difference analysis of a homozygous deletion in pancreatic carcinoma that lies within the BRCA2 region. *Proc Natl Acad Sci USA* **92**:5950, 1995.

76. Wooster R, Bibnell G, Lancaster J, Swift S, Seal S, Mangion J, Collins N, Gregory S, Gumbs C, Micklem G, Barfoot R, Hamoudi R, Patel S, Rice C, Biggs P, Hashim Y, Smith A, Connor F, Arason A, Gudmundsson J, Ficenec D, Kelsell D, Ford D, Tonin P, Bishop DT, Spurr NK, Ponder BAJ, Eeles R, Peto J, Devilee P, Cornelisse C, Lynch H, Narod S, Lenoir G, Egilsson V, Bardkardottir RB, Easton DF, Bentley DR, Futreal PA, Ashworth A, Stratton MR: Identification of the breast cancer susceptibility gene BRCA2. *Nature* **378**:789, 1995.

77. Tavtigian SV, Simard J, Rommens, J, Couch F, Shattuck-Eidens D, Neuhausen S, Merajver S, Thorlacius S, Offit K, Stoppa-Lyonnet D, Belanger C, Bell R, Berry S, Bogden R, Chen Q, Davis T, Dumont M, Frye C, Hattier T, Jammulapati S, Janecki T, Jiang P, Kehrer R, Leblanc FJ, Mitchell JT, McArthur-Morrison J, Nguyen K, Peng Y, Samson C, Schroeder M, Snyder SC, Steele L, Stringfellow M, Stroup C, Swedlund B, Swensen J, Teng D, Thomas A, Tran T, Tran T, Tranchant M, Weaver-Feldhaus J, Wong AKC, Shizuya H, Eyfjord JE, Cannon-Albright L, Labrie F, Skolnick MH, Weber B, Kamb A, Goldgar DE: The complete BRCA2 gene and mutations in chromosome 13q linked kindreds. *Nat Genet* **12**:333, 1996.

78. Knudson AG: Mutation and cancer, statistical study of retinoblastoma. *Proc Natl Acad Sci Usa* **68**:820, 1971.

79. Powell SM, Petersen GM, Krush AJ, Booker S, Yen J, Giardiello FM, Hamilton SR, Vogelstein B, Kinzler KW: Molecular diagnosis of familial adenomatous polyposis. *N Engl J Med* **329**:1982, 1993.

80. Powell SM, Zilz N, Beazer-Barclay Y, Bryan TM, Hamilton SR, Thibodeau SN, Vogelstein B, Kinzler KW: APC mutations occur early during colorectal tumorigenesis. *Nature* **359**:235, 1992.

81. Mulligan LM, Kwok JBJ, Healey CS, Elsdon MJ, Eng C, Gardner E. Love DR, Mole SE, Moore JK, Papi L, Ponder MA, Telenius H, Tunnacliffe A, Ponder BAJ: Germline mutations of the RET proto-oncogene in multiple endocrine neoplasia type 2A. *Nature* **363**:458, 1993.

82. Blaugrund JE, Johns Jr MM, Eby YJ, Ball DW, Baylin SB, Hruban RH, Sidransky D: *RET* proto-oncogene mutations in inherited and sporadic medullary thyroid cancer. *Hum Mol Gen* **3**:1895, 1994.

83. Moskaluk CA, Hruban RH, Lietman A, Jackson C, Yeo CJ, Lynch HT, Kern SE: Low prevalence of p16[INK4a] and CDK4 mutations in familial pancreatic carcinoma. *Hum Mutat,* 1996, *in press.*

84. Goggins M, Schutte M, Lu J, Moskaluk CA, Weinstein CL, Petersen GM, Yeo CJ, Jackson CE, Lynch HT, Hruban RH, Kern SE: Germline BRCA2 gene mutations in patients with apparently sporadic pancreatic carcinomas. 1996, submitted.

85. Hahn SA, Schutte M, Hoque ATMS, Moskaluk CA da Costa LT, Rozenblum E, Weinstein CL, Fischer A, Yeo CJ, Hruban RH, Kern SE: DPC4, a candidate tumor-suppressor gene at 18q21.1. *Science* **271**:350, 1996.

86. Hruban RH, van Mansfeld AD, Offerhaus GJ, van Weering DH, Allison DC, Goodman SN, Kensler TW, Bose KK, Cameron JL, Bos JL: K-*ras* oncogene activation in adenocarcinoma of the human pancreas. A study of 82 carcinomas using a combination of mutant-enriched polymerase chain reaction analysis and allele-specific oligonucleotide hybridization. *Am J Pathol* **143**:545, 1993.

87. Rozenblum E, Schutte M, Goggins M, Hahn SA, Lu J, Panzer S, Zahurak M, Goodman SN, Yeo CJ, Hruban RH, Kern SE: Co-existent inactivations infer distinct tumor-suppressive pathways in pancreatic cancer. 1996, submitted.

88. Barbacid M: *Ras* genes. *Ann Rev Biochem* **56**:779, 1987.

89. Perucho M: Most human carcinomas of the exocrine pancreas contain mutant c-K-*ras* genes. *Cell* **53**:549, 1988.

90. Smit VTHBM, Book AJM, Smits AMM, Fleuren GJ, Cornelisse SJ, Bos JL: K-*ras* codon 12 mutations occur very frequently in pancreatic adenocarcinomas. *Nucl Acids Res* **16**:7773, 1988.

91. Mariyama M, Kishi K, Nakamura K, Obata H, Nishimura S: Frequency and types of point mutations at the 12th codon of the c-Ki-*ras* gene found in pancreatic cancers from Japanese patients. *Jpn J Cancer Res* **80**:622, 1989.

92. Grunewald K, Lyons J, Frohlich A, Feichtinger H, Weger RA, Schwab G, Janssen JW, Bartram CR: High frequency of Ki-*ras* codon 12 mutations in pancreatic adenocarcinomas. *Int J Cancer* **43**:1037, 1989.

93. Nagata Y, Abe M, Motoshima K, Nakayama E, Shiku H: Frequent glycine to aspartic acid mutations at codon 12 of c-Ki-*ras* gene in human pancreatic cancer in Japanese. *Jpn J Cancer Res* **81**:135, 1990.

94. Tada M, Yokosuka O, Omata M, Ohto M, Isono K: Analysis of *ras* gene mutations in biliary and pancreatic tumors by polymerase chain reaction and direct sequencing. *Cancer* **66**:930, 1990.

95. Berrozpe G, Schaeffer J, Peinado MA, Real FX, Perucho M: Comparative analysis of mutations in the p53 and K-*ras* genes in pancreatic cancer. *Int J Cancer* **58**:185, 1994.

96. Motojima K, Urano T, Nagata Y, Shiku H, Tsunoda T, Kanematsu T: Mutations in the Kirsten-*ras* oncogene are common but lack correlation with prognosis and tumor stage in human pancreatic carcinoma. *Am J Gastroenterol* **86**:1784, 1991.

97. Motojima K, Urano T, Nagata Y, Shiku H, Tsurifune T, Kanematsu T: Deletion of point mutation in the Kirsten-*ras* oncogene provides evidence for the multicentricity of pancreatic carcinoma. *Ann Surg* **217**:138, 1993.

98. Pallegata NS, Losekoot M, Fodde R, Pugliese V, Saccomanno S, Renault B, Bernini LF, Ranzani GN: Detection of K-*ras* mutations by denaturing gradient gel electrophoresis (DGGE): A study on pancreatic cancer. *Anticancer Res* **12**:1731, 1992.

99. Pellegata NS, Sessa F, Renault B, Bonato M, Leone BE, Solcia E, Ranzani GN: K-*ras* and p53 mutations in pancreatic cancer: Ductal and non-ductal tumor progress through different genetic lesions. *Cancer REs* **54**:1556, 1994.

100. Suzuki H, Yoshida S, Ichikawa Y, Yokota H, Mutoh H, Koyama A, Fukazawa M, Todoroki T, Fukao K, Uchida K, Miwa M: Ki-*ras* mutations in pancreatic secretions and aspirates from two patients without pancreatic cancer. *J Natl Cancer Inst* **86**:1547, 1994.

101. Tabata T, Fujimori T, Maeda S, Yamamoto M, Saitoh Y: The role of Ras mutation in pancreatic cancer, precancerous lesions, and chronic pancreatitis. *Int J Pancreatol* **14**:237, 1993.

102. Yashiro T, Fulton N, Hara H, Yasuda K, Montag A, Yashiro N, Straus F, Ito K, Aiyoshi Y, Kaplan EL: Comparison of mutations of *ras* oncogene in human pancreatic exocrine and endocrine tumors. *Surgery* **114**:758, 1993.

103. Cerny IWL, Mangold KA, Scarpelli DG: K-*ras* mutations in an early event in pancreatic duct carcinogenesis in the Syrian golden hamster. *Cancer Res* **52**:4507, 1992.

104. Tada M, Omata M, Ohto M: *Ras* gene mutations in intraductal papillary neoplasms of the pancreas. *Cancer* **67**:634, 1991.

105. DiGiuseppe JA, Hruban RH, Offerhaus GJA, Clement MJ, van den Berg FM, Cameron JL: Detection of K-*ras* mutations in mucinous pancreatic duct hyperplasia from a patient with a family history of pancreatic carcinoma. *Am J Pathol* **144**:889, 1994.

106. Yanagisawa A, Ohtake K, Ohashi E, Hori M, Kitagawa T, Sugano H, Kato Y: Frequent c-Ki-*ras* oncogene activations in mucous cell hyperplasias of pancreas suffering from chronic inflammation. *Cancer Res* **53**:953, 1993.

107. Caldas C, Hahn SA, Hruban RH, Redston MS, Yeo CJ, Kern SE: Detection of K-*ras* mutations in the stool of patients with pancreatic adenocarcinoma and pancreatic ductal hyperplasia. *Cancer Res* **54**:3568, 1994.

108. DiGiuseppe JA, Hruban RH, Goodman SN, Polak M, van den Berg FM, Allison DC, Cameron JL, Offerhaus GJA: Overexpression of p53 protein in adenocarcinoma of the pancreas. *Am J Clin Pathol* **101**:684, 1994.

109. Casey G, Yamanaka Y, Freiss H, Kobrin MS, Lopez ME, Buchler M, Berger HG, Korc M: p53 mutations are common in pancreatic cancer and are absent in chronic pancreatitis. *Cancer Lett* **69**:151, 1993.

110. Nakamori S, Yashima K, Murakami Y, Ishikawa O, Ohigashi H, Imaoka S, Yaegashi S, Kinoshi Y, Sekiya T: Association of p53 gene mutations with short survival in pancreatic adenocarcinoma. *Jpn J Cancer Res* **86**:174, 1995.

111. Redston MS, Caldas C, Seymour AB, Hruban RH, da Costa L, Yeo CJ, Kern SE: p53 mutations in pancreatic carcinoma and evidence of common involvement of homocopolymer tracts in DNA microdeletions. *Cancer Res* **54**:3025, 1994.

112. Scarpa A, Capelli P, Mukai K, Zamboni G, Oda T, Iacono C, Hirohashi S: Pancreatic adenocarcinomas frequently show p53 gene mutations. *Am J Pathol* **142**:1534, 1993.

113. Suwa H, Yoshimura T, Yamaguchi N, Kanehira K, Manabe T, Imamura M, Hiai H, Fukumoto M: K-*ras* and p53 alterations in genomic DNA and transcripts of human pancreatic adenocarcinoma cell lines. *Jpn J Cancer Res* **85**:1005, 1994.

114. Weyrer K, Feichtinger H, Haun M, Weiss G, Ofner D, Wegner AR, Umlauft F, Grunewald K: p53, Ki-*ras*, and DNA ploidy in human pancreatic ductal adenocarcinomas. *Lab Invest* **74**:279, 1996.

115. Yonish-Rouach E, Resnitzky D, Lotem J, Sachs L, Kimchi A, Oren M: Wild-type p53 induces apoptosis of myeloid leukemic cells that is inhibited by interleukin-6. *Nature* **352**:345, 1991.

116. Kamb A, Gruis NA, Weaver-Feldhaus J, Liu Q, Harshman K, Tavtigian SV, Stockert E, Day RS III, Johnson BE, Skolnick MH: A cell cycle regulator potentially involved in genesis of many tumor types. *Science* **264**:436, 1994.

117. Whyte P: The retinoblastoma protein and its relatives. *Semin Cancer Biol* **6**:83, 1995.

118. Schutte M, Hruban RH, Hedrick L, Cho KR, Nadasdy GM, Weinstein CL, Bova GS, Isaacs WB, Cairns P, Nawroz H, Sidransky D, Casero RA Jr., Meltzer PS, Hahn SA, Kern SE: DPC4 gene in various tumor types. *Cancer Res* **56**:2527, 1996.

119. Liu F, Hata A, Baker JC, Doody J, Carcamo J, Harland RM, Massague J: A human *Mad* protein acting as a BMP-regulated transcriptional activator. *Nature* **381**:620, 1996.

120. Hahn SA, Hoque ATMS, Moskaluk CA, Da Costa LT, Schutte M, Rozenblum E, Seymour AB, Weinstein CL, Yeo CJ, Hruban RH, Kern SE: Homozygous deletion map at 18q21.1 in pancreatic cancer. *Cancer Res* **56**:490, 1996.

121. Horii A, Nakatsuru S, Miyoshi Y, Ichii S, Nagase H, Ando H, Yanagisawa A, Tsuchiya E, Kato Y, Nakamura Y: Frequent somatic mutations of the APC gene in human pancreatic cancer. *Cancer Res* **52**:6696, 1992.

122. Yashima K, Nakamori S, Murakami Y, Yamaguchi A, Hayashi K, Ishikawa O, Konishi Y, Sekiya T: Mutations of the adenomatous polyposis coli gene in the mutation cluster region: Comparison of human pancreatic and colorectal cancers. *Int J Cancer* **59**:43, 1994.

123. McKie AB, Filipe MI, Lemoine NR: Abnormalities affecting the APC and MCC tumor suppressor gene loci on chromosome 5q occur frequently in gastric cancer but not in pancreatic cancer. *Int J Cancer* **55**:598, 1994.

124. Barton CM, McKie AB, Hogg A, Bia B, Elia G, Phillips SM, Ding SF, Lemoine NR: Abnormalities of the RB1 and DCC tumor suppressor genes: Uncommon in human pancreatic adenocarcinoma. *Mol Carcinog* **13**:61, 1995.

125. Ruggeri B, Zhang SY, Caamano J, Di Rado M, Flynn SD, Klein-Szanto AJ: Human pancreatic carcinomas and cell lines reveal frequent and multiple alterations in the p53 and Rb-1 tumor-suppressor genes. *Oncogene* **7**:1503, 1992.

126. Huang L, Lang D, Geradts J, Obara T, Klein-Szanto AJ, Lynch HT, Ruggeri BA: Molecular and immunochemical analyses of RB1 and cyclin D1 in human ductal pancreatic carcinomas and cell lines. *Mol Carcinog* **15**:85, 1996.

127. Hruban RH, van der Riet P, Erozan YS, Sidransky D: Molecular biology and the early detection of carcinoma of the bladder. The case of Hubert H Humphrey. *N Engl J Med* **330**:1276, 1994.

128. Slebos RJC, Sturm PDJ, Noorduyn LA, Polak MM, Musler A, Caspers E, Ramsoekh TB, Huibregtse K, Hruban RH, Offerhaus GJA: K-*ras* oncogene mutations in cytologic brush specimens from tumors in the head region of the human pancreas. 1996, submitted.

129. Tada M, Omata M, Kawai S, Saisho H, Ohto M, Saiki RK, Sninsky JJ: Detection of ras gene mutations in pancreatic juice and peripheral blood of patients with pancreatic adenocarcinoma. *Cancer Res* **53**:2472, 1993.

130. Apple SK, Hecht JR, Novak JM, Nieberg RK, Rosenthal DL, Grody WW: Polymerase chain reaction-based K-*ras* mutation detection of pancreatic adenocarcinoma in routine cytology smears. *Am J Clin Pathol* **105**:321, 1996.

131. Wilentz RE, Chung CH, Polak MM, Offerhaus GJA, Hruban RH, Slebos RJC: Detection of K-*ras* mutations in duodenal fluid derived DNA from patients with pancreatic cancer. *Mod Pathol* **9**:139A, 1996.

CHAPTER 34

Ovarian Cancer

Louis Dubeau

1. Ovarian carcinomas are the fifth leading cause of death from cancer among women. These tumors are morphologically similar to those arising from Müllerian-derived gynecological organs in spite of the fact that the ovary itself is not embryologically derived from Müllerian ducts.

2. Ovarian carcinomas are thought to arise from the mesothelial layer lining the ovarian surface. This theory does not account for the Müllerian-like appearance of these tumors and remains unproven.

3. The development of a suitable animal model for ovarian carcinomas is complicated by the low frequencies of these tumors in lower mammals. The observation that such tumors are associated with frequent ovulation in birds supports theories linking incessant ovulation to risk of ovarian cancer in humans.

4. In vitro cultures of cells regarded as possible candidates for the origin of ovarian tumors are available, providing experimental systems to clarify the association between these different cell types and ovarian tumorigenesis.

5. Ovarian epithelial tumors are a good model to study tumor development because they are subdivided into benign, low malignant potential, and different grades of malignant subgroups which can each be regarded as representing a specific stage of tumorigenesis.

6. Although most ovarian carcinomas occur sporadically, a significant proportion arise in individuals with familial predisposition to this disease. The best characterized genetic determinants of such predisposition are inherited mutations in either the BRCA-1 gene (familial breast/ovarian cancer syndrome) or in genes coding for mismatch repair enzymes (Lynch II syndrome).

7. Molecular genetic changes distinguishing ovarian cystadenomas, LMP tumors, and different grades of carcinomas from each other have been described. A gene which possibly escapes X-chromosome inactivation may control the development of tumors of low malignant potential. Abnormalities in the same gene may be associated with increased biological aggressiveness in carcinomas.

8. Molecular genetic studies suggest that benign and malignant ovarian epithelial tumors are usually not part of a disease continuum. Benign tumors that progress to malignancy are probably those that are predisposed to such progression from their onset because of the presence of molecular genetic abnormalities associated with malignancy.

9. A genetic model for ovarian epithelial tumor development can be formulated based on known molecular genetic differences between benign, low malignant potential, and malignant tumors.

Ovarian carcinomas are an important cause of death from cancer among women. Their heterogeneity as well as uncertainties about their cell of origin impede progress in understanding their molecular genetic mechanisms. However, they are an attractive model to study tumor development because they can be subdivided into phenotypically stable and well-defined benign, low malignant potential, and malignant subgroups. This chapter reviews current data about molecular genetic changes associated with sporadic (nonfamilial) ovarian epithelial tumors and formulates a genetic model for ovarian tumorigenesis based on this knowledge.

CLINICOPATHOLOGICAL FEATURES

Ovarian carcinoma is the fifth leading cause of death from cancer among women in the United States. These tumors are a heterogeneous group which includes several histopathological subtypes such as serous, mucinous, endometrioid, clear cell, as well as other less common forms.[1] One of the most intriguing features of these different subtypes is their striking resemblance to carcinomas arising from other organs of the female genital tract. For example, serous ovarian carcinomas are morphologically similar to epithelial tumors arising in the fallopian tubes. Mucinous carcinomas resemble those arising in endocervix. Endometrioid ovarian carcinomas are similar to carcinomas of the endometrium. Clear cell tumors are likewise similar to a variant of endometrial carcinomas. These morphological similarities are difficult to reconcile with the fact that there are no fallopian, endocervical, or endometrial-like epithelia present in normal ovaries. In addition, whereas the above organs are derived embryologically from the Müllerian ducts, the ovary is thought to have a different embryological origin. The histogenesis of ovarian epithelial tumors is therefore still unclear, greatly complicating the development of suitable experimental models (see below).

Current Theories about the Cell of Origin of Ovarian Epithelial Tumors

Ovarian epithelial tumors are derived from the mesothelial layer lining the ovarian surface (surface epithelium) according to the currently favored theory.[1] This cell layer may invaginate to create small cysts which eventually lose their connection to the ovarian surface and may give rise to ovarian tumors. The fact that ovarian epithelial tumors resemble tumors of Müllerian origin (see above) is often explained by the suggestion that the ovarian surface epithelium is not the direct precursor of ovarian epithelial neoplasms but instead must first undergo metaplasia to become Müllerian-like. If this hypothesis is correct, knowledge of the factors responsible for such metaplastic changes could lead to effective approaches for the prevention of ovarian cancer. Indeed, if metaplasia of the ovarian surface epithelium is a necessary step preceding tumor development, controlling this step would put us one step ahead of the cancer. However, the above theory is largely based on morphological observations and remains unproven. A possible role of the tubular structure near the ovarian hilum known as rete ovarii as well as other hypotheses merit further consideration.

Animal Models

Development of a suitable animal model for spontaneous ovarian carcinoma is complicated by the fact that these tumors are rare in most animals including lower mammals. Knowledge of the reasons for the relatively low incidence of spontaneous ovarian epithelial tumors in lower mammals compared to humans could provide important clues about the origin and risk factors of the human tumors. The fact that tumors resembling human ovarian carcinomas are frequently present in the domestic hen[2] may therefore prove particularly relevant. The high frequency of ovarian tumors in those animals has been linked to the activity of incessant egg production.[2] Wild hens or other wild birds, in whom continuous egg production is not artificially induced, do not develop ovarian tumors. These observations are interesting in light of the extensive epidemiological data suggesting an association between incessant ovulation and risk of ovarian cancer in humans.[3] Such studies indicate that interruption of chronic menstrual cycling by either pregnancy or anovulatory drugs has an important protective effect against this disease.[3] The recent findings that the BRCA1 gene, which is important for familial predisposition to breast and ovarian cancer, is strongly expressed in cells responding to pituitary gonadotropin hormones[4] and that ovaries from patients with familial predisposition to the above cancers show various changes related to ovulatory activity[5] provide additional support for a link between ovulatory activity and ovarian cancer development. These observations raise the possibility that ovarian carcinomas result from an artifact of civilization, that of incessant ovulation, as chronic menstrual cycling was unlikely in early humans due to more frequent pregnancies and longer lactation periods.

In Vitro Models

Several authors succeeded in culturing mesothelial cells lining the surface of ovaries of either adult humans or experimental animals and were able to keep the cells in culture over several passages.[6–8] Cultures of epithelial cells derived from rete ovarii were also reported.[9] Godwin et al.[10] reported a high transformation rate in cultured ovarian surface epithelial cells, suggesting that they may indeed be prone to malignant development. Support for the

hypothesis (see above) that cells lining the ovarian surface may be prone to undergo metaplastic changes was provided by the demonstration that steroid hormone responsiveness, a characteristic of Müllerian-derived epithelia, was induced by v-*ras* transformation in cultured ovarian surface epithelial cells.[11]

Ovarian Epithelial Tumors as a Model for Tumor Development

In addition to being an important clinical entity, ovarian epithelial tumors are attractive for studying tumor development because they can be subdivided into well-defined and phenotypically stable categories that may be regarded as representing varying degrees of neoplastic transformation. (Fig. 34-1). Cystadenomas are made up of the same cell type as carcinomas but are readily distinguished from the latter based on their total absence of invasive or metastatic abilities. Ovarian tumors of low malignant potential (LMP) are histologically more complex than cystadenomas and show some histopathological features normally associated with carcinomas, but have absent (or greatly reduced) invasive and metastatic abilities.[1,12] The further subdivision of ovarian carcinomas into low and high histological grades in Fig. 34-1 reduces their phenotypic complexities and facilitates studies of their molecular determinants. Low-grade carcinomas form organized structures such as glandular acini while high-grade lesions form solid, poorly organized cell masses according to the criteria used in Fig. 34-1. These criteria are a measure of cellular differentiation and are related to tumor biological aggressiveness. They were adopted in the author's laboratory because of their simplicity, which should facilitate their reproducibility.

Familial Predisposition to Ovarian Carcinoma

Although this review focuses primarily on sporadic ovarian epithelial tumors, it is estimated that up to 10 percent of ovarian carcinomas occur in individuals with familial predisposition to this disease. Most familial ovarian cancers appear to fall into one of two major syndromes. The first one is the familial breast and ovarian cancer syndrome associated with inherited mutations in the BRCA1 gene. The second is Lynch II syndrome characterized by predisposition to cancers of the colon, endometrium, and ovary, which is associated with inherited abnormalities in genes coding for mismatch repair enzymes. Both syndromes are described more fully in other chapters of *MMBID* and will not be discussed further here.

Molecular Changes Distinguishing Different Subtypes of Ovarian Epithelial Tumors

A number of abnormalities involving cellular protooncogenes, including HER-2/*neu*,[13] AKT2,[14] c-*fms*,[15] Bcl-2,[16] FGF-3,[17] and *met*[18] were described in ovarian carcinomas. Abnormalities involving tumor suppressor genes such as p53,[19–22] SPARC,[23] and nm23[24] were also reported. Data on frequencies of losses of heterozygosity on various chromosomes are extensive, including several complete allelotypes.[25–27] In addition, comprehensive cytogenetic analyses of ovarian tumors have been reported.[28–31] Specific molecular abnormalities were shown to be associated with disease prognosis,[16,17,32,33] and specific genes, such as HER-2/*neu*[4–36] and p53,[37] have been evaluated as potential targets for gene therapy. A comprehensive review of this data is beyond the scope of this article, which focuses on molecular genetic studies presented in the context of the ovarian epithelial tumor model as described above (Fig. 34-1). The intent is to obtain insights into the molecular genetic changes controlling the different tumor subtypes shown in Fig. 34-1, in order to develop a molecular genetic model for ovarian tumorigenesis similar to what was first achieved with colorectal cancer.[38]

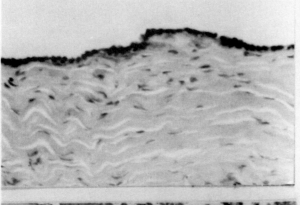

Cystadenoma:
   Incessant but
   Ordered Cell
   Proliferation

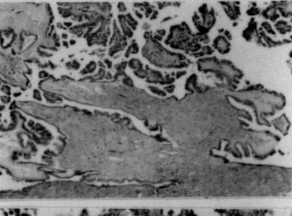

Low Malignant Potential:
   Disorganized Cell
   Proliferation
   Resulting in Complex
   Histologic
   Architectures

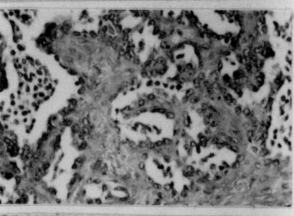

Low Grade Carcinoma:
   Invasive and Metastatic.
   Incessant but Ordered
   Cell Proliferation
   Allowing Maintenance of
   Glandular or other
   Specialized Structures

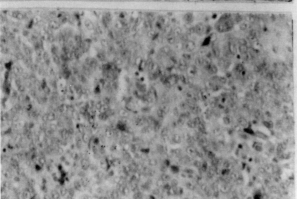

High Grade Carcinoma:
   Invasive and Metastatic.
   Disorganized Cell
   Proliferation Resulting in
   Solid and Amorphous
   Tumor Blocks

FIG. 34-1 Components of the ovarian epithelial tumor model.

The complexity of molecular genetic changes present in ovarian carcinomas clearly increases with increasing tumor histological grades.[27,29,39,40] This observation is in agreement with classical tumor progression theories.[41] Grades of ovarian carcinomas, however, are not only a function of the mere number of molecular genetic abnormalities present in a given tumor genome as specific molecular abnormalities appear strongly associated with high histological grades.[27,29,39,40,42,43] Thus, whereas losses of heterozygosity affecting certain chromosomes such as 6q, 17p, and 17q appear frequent in ovarian tumors of all histological grades,[27] losses in chromosome 13 are frequent only in those of high histological grades.[42,43] It may be that the gene(s) targeted by losses of heterozygosity in chromosome 13 control(s) a different cellular pathway associated perhaps not with cell cycle regulation, but with differentiation or other determinants of tumor grade. Proof of this hypothesis awaits identification and characterization of the gene(s) targeted by the above losses of heterozygosity.

Recent data[27,29] also provide insights into the molecular genetic differences distinguishing ovarian carcinomas from the noninvasive and nonmetastatic ovarian epithelial tumors (Fig. 34-1). Examination of the distribution and frequencies of losses of heterozygosity in these various tumor subtypes showed that such losses, which are frequent in ovarian carcinomas, are rare in the biologically less aggressive ovarian epithelial tumors (with the exception of losses affecting the X chromosome in LMP tumors, discussed below).[27] Thus, the underlying defects responsible for loss of heterozygosity usually result in malignancy, implying that tumor suppressor gene inactivation, which is an important consequence of such losses, is not a feature of cystadenoma or LMP tumor development.[27] Other published molecular genetic differences between the different subtypes of ovarian tumors mentioned in Fig. 34-1 include the presence of p53 mutations,[21,44] which is strongly associated with malignant tumors, and changes in DNA methylation,[45] which are associated with both LMP tumors and carcinomas but not with cystadenomas.

The only exception to the rarity of losses of heterozygosity in LMP tumors are losses affecting the X chromosome, which are present in about 50 percent of the cases.[27] The target(s) of the allelic losses involving this chromosome in LMP tumors is/are still not known. However, the fact that the reduced allele invariably affects the inactive copy of this chromosome suggest that the targeted gene(s) escape(s) X inactivation. This suggestion is attractive because individuals born with a single X chromosome (Turner syndrome)[46] show abnormal ovarian development (gonadal dysgenesis). Thus, the presence of the inactive X chromosome is necessary for normal ovarian development, and it is conceivable that abnormalities in the same gene during adult life may lead to tumorigenesis. The X chromosome is also thought to be important for the establishment of in vitro immortality[47,48] and has recently been implicated in the development of prostate cancer.[49]

Are Ovarian Cystadenomas, LMP Tumors, and Carcinomas Part of a Disease Continuum?

The question of whether ovarian cystadenomas, LMP tumors, and carcinomas represent distinct disease processes or are part of a disease continuum is not only important for our understanding of ovarian tumor development, but is also relevant for the clinical management of cystadenomas and LMP tumors. Arguments in favor of a continuum come from morphological observations that areas histologically indistinguishable from typical ovarian cystadenomas are sometimes found contiguous to carcinomas.[50] The most straightforward interpretation for these lesions, which are sometimes called cystadenocarcinomas, is that the histologically

malignant areas arose from the preexisting morphologically benign areas. This interpretation implies that any molecular genetic change associated with carcinomas but normally not present in solitary cystadenomas should be confined to the histologically malignant portions of cystadenocarcinomas. However, losses of heterozygosity and p53 mutations, which are both frequent in carcinomas and absent or at least very rare in solitary cystadenomas, are usually concordant in all portions of ovarian cystadenocarcinomas including the morphologically benign areas.[21,51] More recently concordance for aneuploidy was likewise shown in different regions of cystadenocarcinomas using interphase cytogenetic approaches.[52] It seems clear based on these observations that histologically benign portions of cystadenocarcinomas are genetically different from typical (solitary) cystadenomas.[21,51] This conclusion supports the idea that cystadenomas do not generally progress to malignancy unless they carry a genetic predisposition to such progression such as a mutation in the p53 gene.[21]

A GENETIC MODEL FOR NONFAMILIAL OVARIAN EPITHELIAL TUMOR DEVELOPMENT

The genetic model shown in Fig. 34-2 is a working hypothesis based on information reviewed in the last section. Little is known about the genetic determinants of ovarian cystadenomas. These tumors appear to share few features with their malignant counterparts and may arise from a different mechanism. In contrast, some molecular changes, such as global changes in DNA methylation, appear to be shared both by LMP tumors and carcinomas.[45] These observations emphasize the merit of subdividing the biologically less aggressive ovarian tumors into cystadenomas and LMP tumors, in spite of the apparent clinically benign nature of the latter.[53] LMP tumors also show frequent losses of heterozygosity, targeting a specific region of the inactive copy of the X chromosome. These changes, by themselves, are not sufficient to induce invasive and metastatic behavior because they occur in LMP tumors. However, if losses affecting the X chromosome occur in tumors where the malignant phenotype is already present, these may result in increased biological aggressiveness. This last conclusion accounts for the observation that losses affecting the X chromosome, although rare in low-grade carcinomas, are frequent in high-grade tumors.[27] Mutations in p53 as well as multiple losses of heterozygosity, the latter presumably resulting from cell cycle errors which may be facilitated by the former, lead to the development of carcinomas. Specific losses of heterozygosity (such as in chromosome 13 or Xq) may be associated with specific features of the malignant phenotype such as cellular differentiation and lead to higher tumor histological grades. In contrast, losses in chromosomes 6q or 17 may be more directly associated with malignant transformation per se and are compatible with all histological grades.

The nature of the specific genes targeted by the allelic deletions mentioned in the above model as well as the exact consequences of other molecular genetic changes such as in DNA methylation are still largely unknown. These questions are the focus of current research efforts in various laboratories and significant progress is likely to be made in the foreseeable future. These advances will not only result in a more comprehensive understanding of the mechanisms of ovarian epithelial tumors at the molecular level, but should also provide a basis for novel screening, diagnostic, and therapeutic approaches likely to improve the clinical management of these important tumors of women.

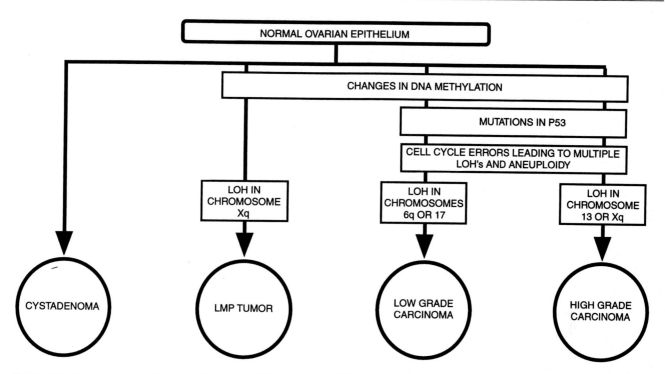

FIG. 34-2 A genetic model for sporadic (nonfamilial) ovarian epithelial tumor development. LOH = loss of heterozygosity.

REFERENCES

1. Scully RE: Ovarian tumors. *Am J Pathol* **87**:686, 1977.
2. Fredrickson TN: Ovarian tumors of the hen. *Environ Health Perspect* **73**:35, 1987.
3. Whittemore AS, Harris R, Intyre J, Collaborative Cancer Group: Characteristics relating to ovarian cancer risk: Collaborative analysis of 12 US case-control studies. *Am J Epidemiol* **136**:1184, 1992.
4. Wan M, Sangiorgi F, Felix JC, Dubeau L: Association of BRCA1 with gonadotropin-responsive cells. *Lancet* **348**:192, 1996.
5. Salazar H, Godwin AK, Daly MB, Laub PB, Hogan WM, Rosenblum N, Boente MP, Lynch HT, Hamilton TC: Microscopic benign and invasive neoplasms and a cancer-prone phenotype in prophylactic oophorectomies. *J Natl Cancer Inst (in press)*.
6. Nicosia SV, Johnson JH, Streibel EJ: Growth characteristics of rabbit ovarian mesothelial (surface epithelial) cells. *Int J Gynecol Pathol* **4**:58, 1985.
7. Siemens CH, Auersperg N: Serial propagation of human ovarian surface epithelium in tissue culture. *J Cell Physiol* **134**:347, 1988.
8. Tsao SW, Mok SC, Fey EG, Fletcher JA, Wan TS, Chew EC, Muto MG, Knapp RC, Berkowitz RS: Characterization of human ovarian surface epithelial cells immortalized by human papilloma viral oncogenes (HPV-E6E7 ORFs). *Exp Cell Res* **218**:499, 1995.
9. Dubeau L, Velicescu M, Sherrod AE, Schreiber G, Holt G: Culture of human fetal ovarian epithelium in a chemically-defined, serum-free medium: a model for ovarian carcinogenesis. *Anticancer Res* **10**:1233, 1990.
10. Godwin AK, Testa JR, Handel LM, Liu Z, Vanderveer LA, Tracey PA, Hamilton TC: Spontaneous transformation of rat ovarian surface epithelial cells: association with cytogenetic changes and implications of repeated ovulation in the etiology of ovarian cancer. *J Natl Cancer Inst* **84**:592, 1992.
11. Pan J, Roskelley CD, Luu The V, Rojiani M, Auersperg N: Reversal of divergent differentiation by ras oncogene-mediated transformation. *Cancer Res* **52**:4269, 1992.
12. Bell DA: Ovarian surface epithelial-stromal tumors. *Hum Pathol* **22**:750, 1991.
13. Press MF, Jones LA, Godolphin W, Edwards CL, Slamon DJ: HER-2/neu oncogene amplification and expression in breast and ovarian cancers. *Prog Clin Biol Res* **354A**:209, 1990.
14. Bellacosa A, DeFeo D, Godwin AK, Bell DW, Cheng JQ, Altomare DA, Wan M, Dubeau L, Scambia G, Masciullo V, Ferrandina G, Panici PB, Mancuso S, Neri G, Testa JR: Molecular alterations of the AKT2 oncogene in ovarian and breast carcinomas. *Int J Cancer* **64**:280, 1995.
15. Chambers SK, Wang Y, Gertz RE, Kacinski BM: Macrophage colony-stimulating factor mediates invasion of ovarian cancer cells through urokinase. *Cancer Res* **55**:1578, 1995.
16. Herod JJ, Eliopoulos AG, Warwick J, Niedobitek G, Young LS, Kerr DG: The prognostic significance of Bcl-2 and p53 expression in ovarian carcinomas. *Cancer Res* **56**:2178, 1996.
17. Rosen A, Sevelda P, Klein M, Dobianer K, Hruza C, Czerwenka K, Hanak H. Vavra N, Salzer H, Leodolter S, Medl M, Spona J: First experience with FGF-3 (INT-2) amplification in women with epithelial ovarian cancer. *Br J Cancer* **67**:1122, 1993.
18. Di-Renzo MF, Olivero M, Katsaros D, Crepaldi T, Gaglia P, Zola P, Sismondi P, Comoglio PM: Overexpression of the Met/HGF receptor in ovarian cancer. *Int J Cancer* **58**:658, 1994.
19. Teneriello MG, Ebina M, Linnoila RI, Henry M, Nash JD, Park RC, Birrer MJ: p53 and K-ras gene mutations in epithelial ovarian neoplasms. *Cancer Res* **53**:3103, 1993.
20. Mazars R, Pujol P, Maudelonde T, Jeanteur P, Theillet C: p53 mutations in ovarian cancer: a late event? *Oncogene* **6**:1685, 1991.
21. Zheng J, Benedict WF, Xu H-J, Hu S-X, Kim TM, Velicescu M, Wan M, Cofer KF, Dubeau L: Genetic disparity between morphologically benign cysts contiguous to ovarian carcinomas and solitary cystadenomas. *J Natl Cancer Inst* **87**:1146, 1995.
22. Kohler MF, Marks JR, Wiseman RW, Jacobs IJ, Davidoff AM, Clarke-Pearson DL, Soper JT, Bast RC, Berchuck A: Spectrum of mutation and frequency of allelic deletion of the p53 gene in ovarian cancer. *J Natl Cancer Inst* **85**:1513, 1993.
23. Mok SC, Chan WY, Wong KK, Muto MG, Berkowitz RS: SPARC, an extracellular matrix protein with tumor-suppressing activity in human ovarian epithelial cells. *Oncogene* **12**:1895, 1996.
24. Mandai M, Konishi I, Koshiyama M, Mori T, Arao S, Tashiro H, Okamura H, Nomura H, Hiai H, Fukumoto M: Expression of metastasis-related nm23-H1 and nm23-H2 genes in ovarian carcinomas: correlation with clinicopathology, EGFR, c-erbB-2, and c-erbB-3 genes, and sex steroid receptor expression. *Cancer Res* **54**:1825, 1994.
25. Sato T, Saito H, Morita R, Koi S, Lee JH, Nakamura Y: Allelotype of human ovarian cancer. *Cancer Res* **51**:5118, 1991.
26. Cliby W, Ritland S, Hartmann L, Dodson M, Halling KC, Keeney G, Podratz KC, Jenkins RB: Human epithelial ovarian cancer allelotype. *Cancer Res* **53**:2393, 1993.
27. Cheng PC, Gosewehr JA, Kim TM, Velicescu M, Wan M, Zheng J, Felix JC, Cofer KF, Luo P, Biela BH, Godorov G, Dubeau L: Potential

role of the inactivated X chromosome in ovarian epithelial tumor development. *J Natl Cancer Inst* **88**:510, 1996.

28. Pejovic T: Genetic changes in ovarian cancer. *Ann Med* **27**:73, 1995.

29. Iwabuchi H, Sakamoto M, Sakunaga H, Ma YY, Carcangiu ML, Pinkel D, Yang Feng TL, Gray JW: Genetic analysis of benign, low-grade, and high-grade ovarian tumors. *Cancer Res* **55**:6172, 1995.

30. Thompson FH, Emerson J, Alberts D, Liu Y, Guan XY, Burgess A, Fox S, Taetle R, Weinstein R, Makar R, Powell D, Trent J: Clonal chromsome abnormalities in 54 cases of ovarian carcinoma. *Cancer Genet Cytogenet* **73**:33, 1994.

31. Persons DL, Hartmann LC, Herath JF, Borell TJ, Cliby WA, Keeney GL, Jenkins RB: Interphase molecular cytogenetic analysis of epithelial ovarian carcinomas. *Am J Pathol* **142**:733, 1993.

32. Henriksen R, Wilander E, Oberg K: Expression and prognostic significance of Bcl-2 in ovarian tumors. *Br J Cancer* **72**:1324, 1995.

33. Berchuck A, Kamel A, Whitaker R, Kerns B, Olt G, Kinney R, Soper JT, Dodge R, Clarke Pearson DL, Marks P, McKenzie S, Yin S, Bast RC: Overexpression of HER-2/neu is associated with poor survival in advanced epithelial ovarian cancer. *Cancer Res* **50**:4087, 1990.

34. Yu D, Matin A, Xia W, Sorgi F, Huang L, Hung MC: Liposome-mediated in vivo E1 A gene transfer suppressed dissemination of ovarian cancer cells that overexpress HER-2/neu. *Oncogene* **11**:1383, 1995.

35. Hung MC, Matin A, Zhang Y, Xing X, Sorgi F, Huang L, Yu D: Her-2/neu-targeting gene therapy—a review. *Gene* **159**:65, 1995.

36. Pietras RJ, Fendly BM, Chazin VR, Pegram MD, Howell SB, Slamon DJ: Antibody to HER-2/neu receptor blocks DNA repair after cisplatin in human breast and ovarian cancer cells. *Oncogene* **9**:1829, 1994.

37. Mujoo K, Maneval DC, Anderson SC, Gutterman JU: Adenoviral-mediated p53 tumor suppressor gene therapy of human ovarian carcinoma. *Oncogene* **12**:1617, 1996.

38. Fearon ER, Vogelstein B: A genetic model for colorectal tumorigenesis. *Cell* **61**:759, 1990.

39. Zheng JP, Robinson WR, Ehlen T, Yu MC, Dubeau L: Distinction of low grade from high grade human ovarian carcinomas on the basis of losses of heterozygosity on chromosomes 3, 6, and 11 and HER-2/neu gene amplification. *Cancer Res* **51**:4045, 1991.

40. Dodson MK, Hartmann LC, Cliby WA, DeLacey KA, Keeney GL, Ritland SR, Su JQ, Podratz KC, Jenkins RB: Comparison of loss of heterozygosity patterns in invasive low-grade and high-grade epithelial ovarian carcinomas. *Cancer Res* **53**:4456, 1993.

41. Nowell PC: The clonal evoulation of tumor cell populations. *Science* **194**:23, 1976.

42. Kim TM, Benedict WF, Xu H-J, Shu S-X, Gosewehr J, Velicescu M, Yin E, Zheng J, D'Ablaing G, Dubeau L: Loss of heterozygosity on chromosome 13 is common only in the biologically more aggressive subtypes of ovarian epithelial tumors and is associated with normal retinoblastoma gene expression. *Cancer Res* **54**:605, 1994.

43. Dodson MK, Cliby WA, Xu H-J, DeLacey KA, Hu S-X, Keeney GL, Li J, Podratz KC, Jenkins RB, Benedict WF: Evidence of functional RB protein in epithelial ovarian carcinomas despite loss of heterozygosity at the RB locus. *Cancer Res* **54**:610, 1994.

44. Wertheim I, Muto MG, Welch WR, Bell DA, Berkowitz RS, Mok SC: P53 gene mutation in human borderline epithelial ovarian tumors. *J Natl Cancer Inst* **86**:1549, 1994.

45. Cheng PC, Schmutte C, Cofer KF, Felix JC, Yu MC, Dubeau L: Alterations in DNA methylation are early, but not initial events in ovarian tumorigenesis. *Br J Cancer* (*in press*).

46. Turner HH: A syndrome of infantilism, congenital webbed neck, and cubitus valgus. *Endocrinol* **23**:566, 1938.

47. Klein CB, Conway K, Wang XW, Bhamra RK, Lin XH, Cohen MD, Annab L, Barrett JC, Costa M: Senescence of nickel-transformed cells by an X chromosome: possible epigenetic control. *Science* **251**:796, 1991.

48. Wang XW, Lin X, Klein CB, Bhamra RK, Lee YW, Costa M: A conserved region in human and Chinese hamster X chromosomes can induce cellular senescence of nickel-transformed Chinese hamster cell lines. *Carcinogenesis* **13**:555, 1992.

49. Monroe KA, Yu MC, Kolonel LN, Coetzee GA, Wilkens LR, Ross RK, Henderson BE: Evidence of an X-linked or recessive genetic component to prostate cancer risk. *Nature Med* **1**:827, 1995.

50. Puls LE, Powell DE, DePriest PD, Gallion HH, Hunter JE, Kryscio RJ, van Nagell JR: Transition from benign to malignant epithelium in mucinous and serous ovarian cystadenocarcinoma. *Gynecol Oncol* **47**:53, 1992.

51. Zheng J, Wan M, Zweizig S, Velicescu M, Yu MC, Dubeau L: Histologically benign or low-grade malignant tumors adjacent to high-grade ovarian carcinomas contain molecular characteristics of high-grade carcinomas. *Cancer Res* **53**:4138, 1993.

52. Wolf NG, Abdul-Karim FW, Schork NJ, Schwartz S: Origins of heterogeneous ovarian carcinomas. A molecular cytogenetic analysis of histologically benign, low malignant potential, and fully malignant components. *Am J Pathol* **149**:511, 1996.

53. Kurman RJ, Trimble CL: The behavior of serous tumors of low malignant potential: are they ever malignant? *Int J Gynecol Pathol* **12**:120, 1993.

CHAPTER 35

Endometrial Cancer

Lora Hedrick

1. Endometrial carcinoma is the most common malignancy of the female genital tract in the United States. In 1996 it is estimated that there will be 34,000 newly diagnosed cases of endometrial carcinoma and 6000 deaths will occur as a result of this cancer.

2. Endometrial carcinoma is the most common noncolorectal carcinoma in women belonging to hereditary nonpolyposis colorectal carcinoma (HNPCC) families. Therefore, mutations in the DNA mismatch repair genes (*hMSH2, hMLH1, hPMS1*, and *hPMS2*) that cause HNPCC are also thought to cause endometrial carcinoma in this setting.

3. Endometrial carcinoma encompasses two broad categories of malignant epithelial tumors that arise from endometrial epithelium. They can be distinguished by epidemiological and clinical features. More recently it has been recognized that there are distinct histological features of endometrial carcinomas that correlate, for the most part, with the two categories. The histological types are called endometrioid carcinoma and uterine serous carcinoma. Recent molecular studies have suggested that there may be differences in the molecular profiles of the two categories of endometrial carcinoma. Furthermore, it has been suggested that these molecular differences may contribute to the differences in the clinical behavior of the tumor types.

4. Approximately 20 percent of sporadic endometrial carcinomas demonstrate microsatellite instability, yet only a fraction of these tumors have been shown to have mutations in one of the four known DNA mismatch repair genes that cause HNPCC. Microsatellite instability has not been identified in uterine serous carcinomas and may represent a molecular phenotype confined to endometrioid carcinomas.

5. The three most common molecular abnormalities identified, to date, in endometrial carcinomas are microsatellite instability, K-*ras* mutations, and p53 gene mutations. K-*ras* mutations are thought to occur in approximately 10 to 30 percent of endometrial carcinomas and may represent a relatively early alteration in the development of endometrioid carcinoma as mutations are present in atypical hyperplastic lesions, the precursors of endometrioid carcinoma.

6. p53 mutations are found in 10 to 30 percent of endometrial carcinomas. Recent data suggest that the majority occur in uterine serous carcinoma and in high-grade and high-stage endometrioid carcinomas. p53 mutations are very common in endometrial intraepithelial carcinoma, the precursor of uterine serous carcinoma, and may, therefore, occur early in the pathogenesis of this aggressive type of endometrial carcinoma. Statistical analyses of p53 overexpression by immunohistochemistry have found that it is an independent indicator of poor prognosis.

7. The molecular genetics of endometrial carcinoma are just beginning to be elucidated. To date, only p53 overexpression offers promise as a useful molecular diagnostic tool.

CLINICAL ASPECTS

Incidence

Endometrial cancer is the fifth leading cause of cancer in women worldwide, with approximately 150,000 cases diagnosed each year. In the United States, it is the most common malignancy of the female genital tract, with 34,000 newly diagnosed cases and roughly 6000 deaths estimated in 1996.[1] It should be noted that the term endometrial cancer encompasses both malignant epithelial tumors (carcinomas) and malignant mesenchymal tumors (sarcomas). Since more than 95 percent of endometrial cancers are carcinomas, the terms endometrial cancer and endometrial carcinoma are often used synonymously in the literature.

Most cases of endometrial carcinoma are thought to be sporadic; however some clearly have a hereditary basis. Mothers and sisters of women with endometrial carcinoma have 2.7 times the risk of developing endometrial carcinoma when compared to controls.[2] The vast majority of endometrial carcinomas recognized as inherited occur in affected women belonging to hereditary nonpolyposis colorectal cancer (HNPCC) families. HNPCC is an autosomal dominantly inherited disease, and members of HNPCC families have an increased risk of developing a number of different types of cancer, especially colorectal cancer.[3] Notably, endometrial carcinoma is the most common extracolonic cancer in HNPCC families.[4] Women who are gene carriers of HNPCC have a tenfold increased risk, compared to the general population, of developing endometrial carcinoma; however, the percentage of endometrial cancers due to HNPCC is not well defined.[5] A small amount of literature has suggested the possibility of a site-specific form of inherited endometrial carcinoma, but there are insufficient data at the present time to conclusively prove its existence as a clinical genetic entity.[6]

Clinical Behavior and Histology

The endometrium forms the lining of the uterine cavity and is a complex tissue composed of both glandular epithelial and stromal components. Endometrial carcinoma arises from the epithelial component, with most tumors displaying glandular differentiation. It most commonly arises in perimenopausal and postmenopausal women. In most cases women with endometrial carcinoma seek medical attention for abnormal vaginal bleeding, and endometrial tissue is obtained by biopsy or curettage for a definitive microscopic diagnosis.

Although endometrial carcinoma is classically thought of as a single disease, there is substantial evidence to support that it consists of two broad categories of malignant epithelial tumors. The initial data suggesting the existence of two distinct types of endometrial carcinoma came from epidemiological and clinical studies.[7] More recently it has become apparent that these clinically defined categories of tumors correlate, for the most part, with specific light microscopic features.

Briefly, the initial clinical studies recognized that one group of women with endometrial carcinoma often have a history of exposure to estrogen, are slightly younger (mean age of 59) than the overall mean for the disease, and have tumors that usually behave in a relatively indolent manner. This group has been designated Type I endometrial carcinoma and is often referred to as "estrogen-related."[8] Histologically, the majority of Type I tumors tend to have architectural features that resemble the appearance of normal endometrial glands, and are called endometrioid carcinomas to denote this resemblance. They are generally low-grade (i.e., well-differentiated), low-stage (confined to the uterus), and have a good prognosis. Both epidemiological and light microscopic studies have suggested that this type of carcinoma develops from normal epithelium, under the influence of estrogen stimulation, through a continuum of histopathologically recognizable lesions called hyperplasias (Fig. 35-1). Hyperplasia is defined as a proliferation of endometrial glands, of abnormal shapes and sizes, that leads to an imbalance in the normal glandular/stromal ratio of the endometrium. This proliferative process can, over time, undergo an increase in architectural complexity and cytological atypia until it is difficult to distinguish from carcinoma, with the notable exception that there is a lack of detectable stromal invasion.[9] Hyperplasia, at any stage, can cause abnormal vaginal bleeding. As a result, many cases come to clinical attention and are treated prior to the development of frankly invasive carcinoma.

Type II carcinoma, in contrast to Type I, is unrelated to estrogenic stimulation (non-estrogen-related), occurs in older women (mean age of 68), and demonstrates aggressive behavior. Virtually all Type II carcinomas are composed of cuboidal cells showing marked cytological atypia and nuclear pleomorphism that grow in either a glandular or papillary architecture.[10] These features are strikingly similar to those of the more common serous carcinoma of the ovary, giving rise to the name uterine serous carcinoma to distinguish them from primary serous ovarian tumors. By definition serous carcinomas of the endometrium are all high-grade, frequently have extrauterine spread by the time of diagnosis, and carry a poor prognosis, behaving much like ovarian serous carcinomas.[11] Serous tumors of the endometrium generally arise in the setting of an atrophic, not a hyperplastic, endometrium. Recently, a putative precursor of uterine serous carcinoma has been described and termed endometrial intraepithelial carcinoma (Fig. 35-1).[12] It is characterized by a replacement of the preexisting endometrial epithelium with markedly atypical cells that are virtually indistinguishable from the cells found in invasive uterine serous carcinoma. Endometrial intraepithelial carcinoma, even in the absence of definitive invasion in the uterus, can be associated with intrabdominal carcinoma illustrating the aggressive nature of this neoplastic endometrial process.

It is important to recognize that the histology of endometrial carcinoma is more complicated than presented above. For example, there are several other minor histological variants of endometrial carcinoma (e.g., mucinous, villoglandular, and clear cell). The appropriate category in which these histological variants belong is not well established. These histological variants are rare and poorly understood and will not be considered further in this chapter.

The fact that the two major types of endometrial carcinoma are distinct has been further supported by recent molecular studies, as will be discussed in detail below. Until recently, many of the molecular genetic studies of endometrial carcinoma have failed to adequately recognize and separately study the two major types of tumors, creating a body of literature that is often difficult to interpret, as will become evident later in this chapter.

HEREDITARY ENDOMETRIAL CARCINOMA

The only well-established form of inherited endometrial carcinoma is associated with HNPCC. Over the past several years the genes responsible for the majority of families that meet the clinical criteria for HNPCC have been identified and cloned. Furthermore, the HNPCC families in which linkage studies have been informative demonstrate linkage to loci that have subsequently been found to harbor one of the known genes. For these reasons, the discussion of the genetic loci and the specific genes involved in inherited endometrial carcinoma will be combined.

HNPCC has been covered in great detail in the chapter on hereditary colorectal cancer (see Colorectal Cancer, Chap. 31). Therefore, it will be presented only briefly here, with an emphasis on endometrial carcinoma. HNPCC is the most common hereditary family cancer syndrome and is transmitted as an autosomal dominant trait. It is clinically defined by the following criteria: (1) at least three relatives with colorectal cancer with one a first-degree relative of the other two, (2) the presence of tumors in at least two successive generations, and (3) one family member affected by colorectal cancer before the age of 50.[13] Of note is the fact that endometrial carcinoma is not a required criterion for the clinical definition of HNPCC. However, the International Collaborative Group on HNPCC has recognized that if these criteria are strictly followed, families with a high incidence of endometrial carcinoma, as well as colorectal carcinoma, would be excluded. Although the actual percentage of all endometrial carcinoma due to HNPCC is not known, it has been shown that the cumulative incidence of endometrial carcinoma in women belonging to HNPCC kindreds is 20 percent by age 70, in contrast to 3 percent in the general population.[5]

Genetic Loci and Specific Genes

As previously stated, endometrial carcinoma is the most common extracolonic tumor that occurs in HNPCC families. Linkage analysis of several large HNPCC kindreds identified susceptibility loci on the short arms of chromosomes 2 and 3.[14,15] Informative linkage studies have determined linkage to either of these two chromosomal arms in the majority of HNPCC families. However, in a small number of families linkage to either of these regions is lacking.

Over the past several years four genes have been identified that cause HNPCC in most of the kindreds meeting the clinical criteria

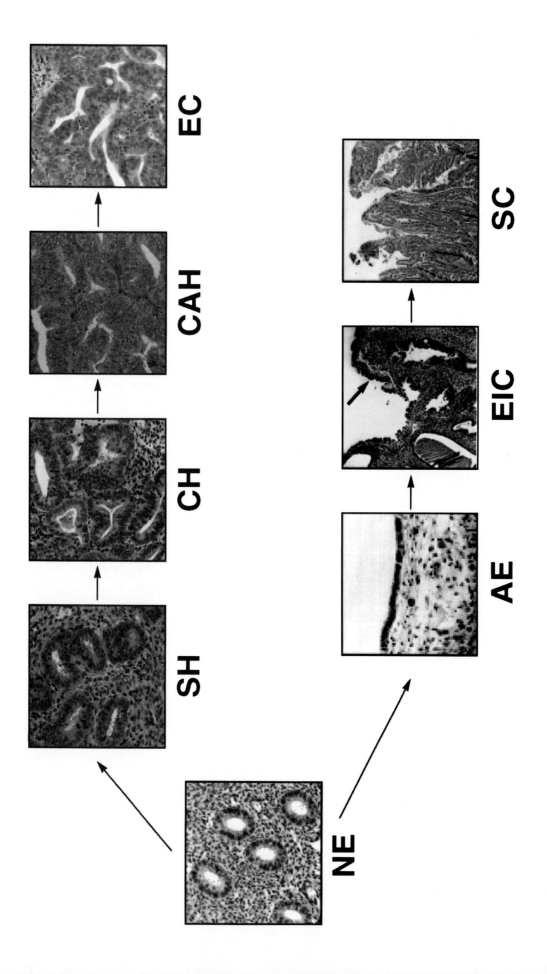

FIG. 35.1 Progression model of the two types of endometrial carcinoma. The development of endometrioid carcinoma (EC) from normal epithelium (NE) arises over time through a series of hyperplastic lesions that increase in both architectural complexity and cytologi- cal atypia from simple hyperplasia (SH) to complex hyperplasia (CH) and finally complex atypical hyperplasia (CAH). Uterine serous carci- noma (SC) develops in the setting of atrophic endometrium (AE) from a precursor lesion called endometrial intraepithelial carcinoma (EIC).

of this inherited family cancer syndrome. The cloning of these genes resulted from the propitious coincidence of several different lines of scientific investigation, including studies aimed at identifying genes that play a role in human tumors and others aimed at understanding fundamental molecular processes in microbial organisms.

Investigators were analyzing microsatellites (small repetitive sequences) in DNA isolated from tumors arising in HNPCC family members and found alterations in the length of microsatellite DNA sequences when compared to germ line DNA from the same patients.[16] Other investigators reported a similar molecular phenotype in approximately 20 percent of sporadic colorectal tumors.[17,18] This molecular phenotype was referred to as microsatellite instability or replication errors. Microsatellite instability and its role, if any, in the neoplastic process was unclear. Shortly after the discovery of microsatellite instability in both sporadic and HNPCC-associated colorectal carcinomas a study was published demonstrating that mutations in DNA mismatch repair genes led to a 100- to 700-fold increase in the instability of simple dinucleotide repeat sequences in the simple eukaryote *S. cerevisiae*.[19] This observation, along with previous work in both *E. coli* and *S. cerevisiae*, provided a crucial connection between microsatellite instability and mutations in DNA mismatch repair genes. This connection led to the ultimate identification of human DNA mismatch repair genes and opened a new avenue of cancer research.

In a very short time four human homologues of microbial DNA mismatch repair genes were cloned. At a somewhat later date a fifth gene involved in DNA mismatch repair, *GTPB*, was cloned, but it will not be discussed here as it is not presently known to be involved in endometrial carcinoma.[20,21] The four human DNA mismatch repair genes known to cause HNPCC were named *hMSH2, hMLH1, hPMS1,* and *hPMS2*, in keeping with their microbial homologues, and are located on chromosomes 2p, 3p, 2q, and 7q, respectively.[22–26] The physical maps of *hMSH2* and *hMLH1* have shown that their locations correlate with chromosomal loci determined to have genetic linkage to HNPCC. The linkage and physical mapping data provided additional information suggesting that DNA mismatch repair genes play a role in the pathogenesis of neoplasms arising in HNPCC kindreds. Subsequent studies documented germ line mutations in one of these four human mismatch repair genes in affected members of most HNPCC kindreds, with the *hMSH2* and *hMLH1* genes accounting for the vast majority. At present, there is not a reported difference in the frequency of endometrial carcinoma among the HNPCC kindreds that carry mutations in the different genes.

The contribution of how microsatellite instability and defects in the DNA mismatch repair system contributed to tumorigenesis remained unproved. In microorganisms the DNA mismatch repair system was known to detect and repair mispaired bases introduced during replication of the cellular genome. Furthermore, microbial organisms lacking a functional DNA mismatch repair system have a marked increase in the rate at which mutations accumulate. In mammalian cells the DNA mismatch repair system has been much less well characterized, but it is thought to have a similar function to its microbial counterpart. Microsatellite DNA sequences, both in humans and microorganisms, are prone to undergo alterations in their length (explaining their highly polymorphic nature) during DNA replication. Therefore, it follows that microsatellite DNA sequences might demonstrate numerous alterations in the absence of an intact DNA mismatch repair system. This suggests that microsatellite instability may simply serve as a marker of an increased rate of mutation cuased by an underlying defect in the DNA mismatch repair system. This lead directly to the notion that lack of a functional mismatch repair

system would result in an increased rate of mutations in oncogenes and tumor suppressor genes, thus predisposing cells to the accumulation of mutations now thought to be a cornerstone of the neoplastic process. In support of this idea, studies have demonstrated an increase in the rate of point mutations in an expressed gene (HPRT) in a mismatch repair-deficient mammalian cell line. The identification of mutations in DNA mismatch repair genes in human tumors created a new class of cancer causing genes called mutator genes.

The high frequency of endometrial carcinoma in HNPCC families indicates that the genes responsible for HNPCC are involved in the pathogenesis of endometrial carcinoma in this setting. A review of the literature does not provide a straightforward analysis of mutations in women with endometrial carcinoma belonging to HNPCC families. Clearly, further studies of HNPCC-associated endometrial carcinomas are needed.

Sporadic Endometrial Carcinoma

As alluded to earlier, the identification and characterization of the genetic loci and specific genes involved in endometrial tumorigenesis have been hampered by the inadequate recognition of the distinct types of endometrial carcinomas. Much of the problem is related to the fact that the classification scheme, described earlier, was initially described in 1983 and has only recently gained widespread acceptance. In addition, uterine serous (Type II) carcinomas are relatively rare, comprising approximately 10 percent of all sporadic endometrial carcinomas. Consequently, and understandably, many of the studies have not clearly stated the type (or types) of endometrial carcinomas that were included. Additionally, many studies that have classified the tumors lack significant numbers to allow the results of the different tumor types to be assessed independently. An attempt has been made in this chapter, when possible, to discuss the molecular genetics of sporadic endometrial carcinoma in the context of the two tumor types.

Genetic Loci

Over the past several years a number of loss of heterozygosity (LOH) studies have attempted to locate regions of the genome that may harbor tumor suppressor genes that play a role in endometrial tumorigenesis. In combining the results of the major studies LOH has been detected on the following chromosomes: 1, 3, 6, 8p, 9p, 9q, 10q, 11, 13, 14q, 15, 16q, 17p, 18p, 18q, 20, 21, and 22q.[28–32] A review of the literature reveals substantial variation in the regions that have been found to undergo LOH in endometrial carcinoma, and there are only several regions from this long list that have shown significant LOH in more than one study. These include loci on chromosomes 3p, 10q, 17p, and 18q. The 3p LOH is striking, as several candidate tumor suppressor genes and the *hMLH1* gene map to this chromosome. The target(s) of 3p LOH have not yet been determined in endometrial carcinoma. Two separate groups of investigators have reported between 35 to 40 percent LOH of a region of 10q, and one group has suggested that there may be two discrete regions of 10q that undergo LOH.[29,31] A range of 9 to 35 percent of endometrial carcinomas have been reported to show 17p LOH. A recent study of uterine serous carcinoma detected LOH of 17p, specifically 17p13.1, in 100 percent of informative cases.[33] Since most of the LOH studies did not specify the tumor type, it will be of interest in the future to determine the percentage of each type that have 17pLOH. LOH of chromosome 18q has been found in three studies, all of which included tumors from Japanese women, with the highest reported frequency of 33 percent.[28,30,32] Other studies have failed to detect 18q LOH, including two studies confined to the analysis of tumors from American women, as well as one exclusively of Japanese women. Although 14q LOH has been identified in only one study, the association of 14q LOH with a poor prognosis led the authors to suggest that 14q LOH may indicate aggressive tumor behavior.[30] Interestingly, the authors note that several of the tumors with 14q LOH were uterine serous carcinomas. Further studies are necessary to confirm the possible association of 14q LOH and aggressive behavior of endometrial carcinoma.

As one can easily imagine the variability among the LOH studies has hindered the identification of novel regions of the genome that may be important in the development of endometrial carcinoma. The reason(s) for the variability between studies are uncertain, but there are many possible explanations. For example, the polymorphic markers used in the various studies are not identical, and if relatively small deletions are responsible for LOH in endometrial carcinoma the critical regions may only be detected with very specific markers. Furthermore, many of the studies have failed to carefully report the histological types of the tumors analyzed. If the histological types, which reflect the distinct categories of endometrial carcinoma, have different underlying molecular genetic alterations the results of such studies may depend heavily on the types of tumors studied. This point is of further interest, as many studies have included tumors from Japanese and American patients and there is some evidence suggesting differences in the molecular basis of endometrial carcinomas in the two populations.

Specific Genes

The discussion of the specific genes has been divided into three sections according to the general classification of genes currently recognized as cancer-causing genes: (1) mutator genes, (2) oncogenes, and (3) tumor suppressor genes.

Mutator Genes. Due to the association of endometrial carcinoma and HNPCC, presumably sporadic cases of endometrial carcinoma were analyzed for instability of microsatellite DNA sequences. In several studies microsatellite instability was detected in approximately 20 percent of endometrial tumors.[34-36] Given the association of microsatellite instability and mutations in human DNA mismatch repair genes it seemed likely that mutations in these genes may be involved in the development of sporadic endometrial carcinomas that displayed microsatellite instability. A mutational analysis of four of the known DNA mismatch repair genes (*hMSH2, hMLH1, hPMS1,* and *hPMS2*) found that only a small number of sporadic endometrial carcinomas with microsatellite instability had mutations in one of these four genes.[37] In addition, mutations of *hMSH2* and *hMLH1* have been found in two endometrial carcinoma cell lines (HEC59 and AN$_{3CA}$) that demonstrate microsatellite instability.[38] These findings are similar to those seen in cases of microsatellite instability–positive sporadic colorectal cancers. It appears that mutations in the known mismatch repair genes are not the only genes that can cause microsatellite instability in sporadic colorectal and endometrial cancer. Clearly, there are additional genetic alterations that can give rise to the identical molecular phenotype. These target genes are actively being sought and it will be of interest to determine whether they, too, play a role in both sporadic colorectal and endometrial tumorigenesis.

Finally, it should be noted that a recent study found that 34 cases of uterine serous carcinoma failed to demonstrate microsatel-

lite instability.[39] The observed difference in the frequency between endometrial and uterine serous carcinoma is statistically significant and provides support for differences in the molecular pathogenesis of the two most common types of endometrial carcinoma.

Oncogenes. A number of oncogenes have been studied over the years, yet there are very few that have been found to be altered in a substantial number of endometrial carcinomas. The proto-oncogene recognized as mutated most commonly in endometrial carcinoma is K-*ras*. It has been shown, in a number of independent studies, to be mutated in 10–30 percent of endometrial carcinomas.[40-45] K-*ras* is a member of the ras gene family that consists of three closely related genes (H-*ras*, K-*ras*, and N-*ras*). The H-*ras* gene was discovered due to its ability to transform an immortalized rodent cell line, and its identification led to the cloning of the two other family members. Each of the *ras* genes encodes a 21-kD guanine nucleotide-binding protein (p21) that transduce signals from activated transmembrane receptors to protein kinases that regulate cell growth and differentiation. The oncogenic mutations occur most commonly at codons 12, 13, and 61 and result in a gain-of-function. The mutant *ras* proteins have a decreased ability to interact with the GTPase-activating protein called *ras*-GAP, reducing their ability to interact with GTPase-activating protein called *ras*-GAP, reducing their ability to hydrolyze guanosine triphosphate (GTP) to guanosine diphosphate (GDP). Hence, the mutant *ras* protein remains in the GTP-bound or activated state. In endometrial carcinoma most mutations are found in codon 12. A recent study of American patients, that separated the two types of endometrial carcinoma, found that 11.6 percent of endometrioid carcinomas contained codon 12 mutations, whereas uterine serous carcinomas were all negative for codon 12 mutations.[46] The numbers were not statistically significant; however, it suggests that K-*ras* mutations may be differentially mutated in the different types of endometrial carcinoma. K-*ras* mutations have also been found in complex atypical hyperplasia (the precursor of endometrioid carcinoma) leading investigators to suggest that K-*ras* mutations may be a relatively early event in endometrial tumorigenesis.[43-45] Investigators have analyzed the association of K-*ras* mutations with prognosis, but the results have been conflicting.

There are a small number of studies showing alterations in the expression and/or amplification of the *HER-2/neu* gene in endometrial carcinoma. *HER-2/neu* is a member of the epidermal growth factor receptor gene family. It encodes a transmembrane tyrosine kinase receptor and it has been found to be overexpressed in a subset of breast and ovarian cancers. The data on this gene in endometrial carcinoma are limited, but several studies have shown that it is overexpressed in 11 to 59 percent and amplified in 14 to 21 percent of tumors.[47,48] One study revealed that overexpression and amplification of *HER-2/neu* were associated with a poor prognosis and multivariate analysis indicated that overexpression was an independent prognostic factor.[49,50] Independent studies have suggested that overexpression may be more common in uterine serous carcinomas.[51]

Recently, there have been several studies looking at expression of the *bcl-2* gene in endometrial carcinomas and hyperplasias. The *bcl-2* gene product prevents cells from undergoing apoptosis and has been found to be overexpressed in a number of different types of human tumors. The results of the studies in endometrial carcinoma are contradictory, with some demonstrating increased expression in endometrial carcinomas and others finding it decreased.[52,53] However, the results of several studies have found expression in normal proliferative endometrium and an absence of expression in normal secretory endometrium. These results suggest that *bcl-2* may play a role in the normal endometrial cycle. Hence, further studies on endometrial carcinoma seem needed to determine if *bcl-2* has a role in endometrial tumorigenesis.

Tumor Suppressor Genes. As is true in many tumors, the p53 gene has been the most extensively studied gene in endometrial carcinoma. p53 is the prototype tumor suppressor gene and it is the most frequently mutated gene in human cancers. It encodes a nuclear phosphoprotein with an apparent molecular weight of 53 kD. For obvious reasons this gene has been under intensive investigation for many years. Recent studies have begun to elucidate the mechanisms by which p53 controls cell growth (reviewed in ref. 54). Briefly, it has been found that p53 expression increases, posttranscriptionally, in response to DNA damage, resulting in a G1/S cell cycle arrest. It is thought that this arrest gives cells the opportunity to repair the damaged DNA such that mutations are not fixed in the genomic template and, in turn, passed to daughter cells after cell division is complete. It has also been found that elevations in p53 gene expression can lead to apoptosis. It is not yet clear how p53 imparts the appropriate signal for these two different cellular responses to DNA damage. However, recent data suggest that transcriptional activation of p21[WAF1] by p53 is important in the G1/S arrest but is not essential for apoptosis. Evidently, given its ubiquitous involvement in human tumorigenesis, mutations that inactivate the p53 gene provide a significant growth-promoting affect on many cell types.

Evaluation of p53 in endometrial carcinoma has largely been by immunohistochemistry, and overexpression of the protein has been reported in anywhere from 11 to 45 percent of endometrial carcinomas.[55–57] Evaluation of the data is troublesome due to lack of description of the staining patterns (intensity and percent of cells staining) and the types of tumors analyzed. The staining pattern may be of utmost importance, as it is thought that detection of p53 by immunohistochemistry reflects the presence of mutations in the gene. Many studies have shown that there is considerable variability in staining and that only intense, diffuse staining may accurately predict the presence of mutations. One large study demonstrated that positive staining was more common in high-grade (41.7 percent) than in low-grade (12 percent) tumors and another study revealed it more frequently in high-stage (41 percent) than in low-stage (9 percent) tumors.[56,58] Furthermore, when the tumor types have been separated a higher frequency of staining is noted in uterine serous carcinomas (66 to 86 percent) as compared to the endometrioid type (Fig. 35-2).[33,59] Several studies have shown that overexpression of p53 by immunohistochemistry is an independent prognostic variable, predicting a poor prognosis.[57,60]

Analyses have also shown a wide range (9.5 to 23 percent) in the frequency of p53 mutations in endometrial carcinoma.[59,61] Again, these differences may be due to the types, grades, and stages of tumors analyzed. Many of the mutational studies have consistently shown that mutations are more common in high-grade tumors, and a recent study analyzing only uterine serous carcinomas detected mutations in 90 percent of tumors.[33] The strong association of p53 mutations and uterine serous carcinoma may offer an explanation for the prognostic significance of p53 overexpression and its association with a poor outcome.

Many of the p53 studies have focused on the clinical utility of the results. Recent studies suggest that they may also provide meaningful information about the molecular pathogenesis of endometrial carcinoma. As mentioned earlier, a putative precursor of uterine serous carcinoma has been described and p53 immunohistochemical studies revealed positivity in a very high percentage of endometrial intraepithelial carcinoma (Fig. 35-2).[62] This finding is in contrast to the very infrequent staining of atypical hyperplasia, the precursor of endometrioid carcinoma. Mutational analyses

have shown that mutations in exons 5-8 of the p53 gene are present in a majority of endometrial intraepithelial carcinomas (78 percent), suggesting, along with the high frequency of p53 mutations in uterine serous carcinoma, that p53 mutations occur early in the pathogenesis of this tumor type.[33] It is reasonable to speculate that early mutation of the p53 gene may be an important determinant of the aggressive biological behavior of uterine serous carcinoma resulting in the poor outcome of patients with this tumor type.

The only other tumor suppressor gene that has received significant attention in endometrial carcinoma is the putative tumor suppressor gene, *DCC*. This gene is located on the long arm of chromosome 18 and encodes a transmembrane protein with homology to cell adhesion molecules of the Ig supergene family. Since this region of 18q has been shown, in some studies, to undergo LOH in 26 to 33 percent of endometrial carcinomas, *DCC* is an obvious candidate for the target of such losses. Studies have shown that a majority of endometrial carcinomas, like several other tumors including colorectal cancer, lose expression of the *DCC* mRNA.[63,64] It should be noted that one study using *DCC*-specific probes did not find significant LOH in 30 endometrial carcinomas.[65] Recently, several other tumor suppressor genes on 18q have been identified.[66,67] Future studies are needed to determine the target of the 18q LOH seen in some cases of endometrial carcinoma.

Finally, a recent study has shown that mutations in *PTEN*, a recently identified tumor suppressor gene located on chromosome 10q23.3, are common in endometrial carcinoma.[68] Although the number of endometrial carcinomas analyzed to date is small it appears that approximately 40% of endometrioid carcinomas contain *PTEN* mutations and that the incidence of *PTEN* mutations may be higher in microsatellite instability positive tumors than in those that lack microsatellite instability. The predicted amino acid sequence of *PTEN* reveals significant homology to both tensin, a protein located in focal cell adhesions, and tyrosine phosphatases.[69] This has led to the speculation that *PTEN* may play a role in the transduction of signals from the cell surface. Clearly, the role of *PTEN* in the development of endometrial carcinoma will be actively pursued in the near future.

IMPLICATIONS FOR DIAGNOSIS

As endometrial carcinoma remains poorly understood at the molecular level, there are very few molecular markers that are currently helpful in its diagnosis. The only gene, at present, with potential usefulness as a diagnostic tool is p53. It is very possible that p53 immunohistochemistry may aid in the recognition of uterine serous carcinoma and its precursor lesion endometrial intraepithelial carcinoma. The ability to consistently recognize this tumor, particularly in its early stages, may lead to better treatment approaches for this very aggressive tumor type. However, future studies are needed to better define the quality and quantity of p53 immunostaining that accurately identify this type of tumor in the endometrium. In addition, p53 staining may help to identify the more aggressive subset of endometrioid tumors that should perhaps be treated more rigorously than those that lack positive staining.

SUMMARY

The role of steroid hormones and their receptors in the development of endometrial carcinoma has been excluded from this chap-

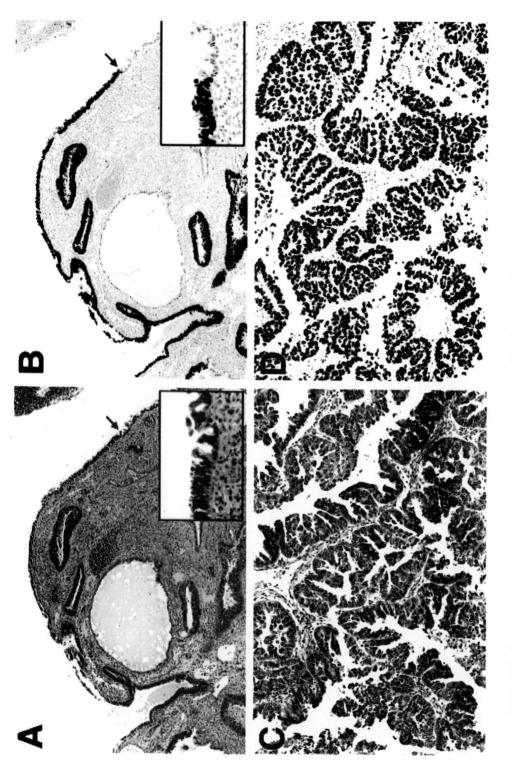

FIG. 35-2 Immunohistochemistry of p53 in uterine serous carcinoma and its precursor endometrial intraepithelial carcinoma. Endometrial intraepithelial carcinoma (EIC) arises abruptly from atrophic endometrium (A) and shows intense positive staining (B). A typical uterine serous carcinoma (C) also shows intense, diffuse staining for p53 protein (D).

627

ter. This has not been an oversight, but little is known at the genetic level about how they contribute to the neoplastic phenotype in the endometrium. It is an area that deserves attention in the future. Finally, there is much to be learned about the molecular basis of endometrial carcinoma. Hopefully, future investigations will more vigilantly include a record of the distinct histologic types of endometrial carcinoma and their specific molecular genetic alterations so that we can come to understand the distinct genetic differences, and similarities, of the two major types of endometrial carcinoma. If the molecular underpinnings of these two types of carcinoma can be determined, perhaps new tools can be developed for more effective diagnosis and treatment of this common malignancy of women.

REFERENCES

1. Parker SL, Tong T, Bolden S, Wingo PA: Cancer Statistics. *Cancer J Clin* **46**:5, 1996.
2. Schildkraut JM, Risch N, Thompson WD: Evaluating genetic association among ovarian, breast, and endometrial cancer: Evidence for a breast/ovarian cancer relationship. *Am J Hum Genet* **45**:521–529, 1989.
3. Watson P, Lynch HT: The tumor spectrum in HNPCC. *Anticancer Res* **14**:1635, 1994.
4. Watson P, Lynch HT: Extracolonic cancer in hereditary nonpolyposis colorectal cancer. *Cancer* **71**:679–685, 1993.
5. Watson P, Vasen HFA, Mecklin JP, Jarvinen H, Lynch HT: The risk of endometrial cancer in hereditary nonpolyposis colorectal cancer. *Am J Med* **96**:516, 1994.
6. Sandles LG, Shulman LP, Elias S, Photopulos GJ, Smiley LM, Posten WM, Simpson JL: Endometrial adenocarcinoma: Genetic analysis suggesting heritable site-specific uterine cancer. *Gynecol Oncol* **47**:167, 1992.
7. Bokhman JV: Two pathogenetic types of endometrial carcinoma. *Gynecol Oncol* **15**:10, 1983.
8. Kurman RJ: *Blaustein's Pathology of the Female Genital Tract.* New York: Springer-Verlag, 1994.
9. Kurman RJ, Kaminski PF, Norris HJ: The behavior of endometrial hyperplasia: A long-term study of "untreated" hyperplasia in 170 patients. *Cancer* **56**:403, 1985.
10. Sherman ME, Bitterman P, Rosenheim NB, Delgado G, Kurman RJ: Uterine serous carcinoma. A morphologically diverse neoplasm with unifying clinicopathologic features. *Am J Surg Pathol* **16**:600, 1992.
11. Hendrickson M, Ross J, Eifel P, Martinez A, Kempson R: Uterine papillary serous carcinoma a highly malignant form of endometrial adenocarcinoma. *Am J Surg Pathol* **6**:93, 1982.
12. Ambros RA, Sherman ME, Zahn CM, Bitterman P, Kurman RJ: Endometrial intraepithelial carcinoma: A distinctive lesion specifically associated with tumors displaying serous differentiation. *Hum Pathol* **26**:1260, 1995.
13. Vasen HFA, Mecklin JP, Meera Khan P, Lynch HT: Hereditary nonpolyposis colorectal cancer. *Lancet* **338**:877, 1991.
14. Lindblom A, Tannergard P, Werelius B, Nordenskjold M: Genetic mapping of a second locus predisposing to hereditary non-polyposis colon cancer. *Nat Genet* **5**:279, 1993.
15. Peltomäki P, Aaltonen LA, Sistonen P, Pylkkänen L, Mecklin J-P, Jarvinen H, Green JS, JR, J, Weber JL, Leach FS, Petersen GM, Hamilton SR, de la Chapelle A, Vogelstein B: Genetic mapping of a locus predisposing to human colorectal cancer. *Science* **260**:810, 1993.
16. Aaltonen LA, Peltomäki P, Leach FS, Sistonen P, Pylkkänen L, Mecklin JP, Jarvinen H, Powell SM, Jen J, Hamilton SR, Petersen GM, Kinzler KW, Vogelstein B, de la Chapelle A: Clues to the pathogenesis of familial colorectal cancer. *Science* **260**:812, 1993.
17. Thibodeau SN, Bren G, Schaid D: Microsatellite instability in cancer of the proximal colon [see comments]. *Science* **260**:816, 1993.
18. Ionov Y, Peinado MA, Malkhosyan S, Shibata D, Perucho M: Ubiquitous somatic mutations in simple repeated sequences reveal a new mechanism for colonic carcinogenesis. *Nature* **363**:558, 1993.
19. Strand M, Prolla TA, Liskay RM, Petes TD: Destabilization of tracts of simple repetitive DNA in yeast by mutations affecting DNA mismatch repair. *Nature* **365**:274, 1993.
20. Palombo F, Gallinari P, Iaccarino I, Lettieri T, Hughes M, D'Arrigo A, Truong O, Hsuan JJ, Jiricny J: GTBP, a 160-kilodalton protein essential for mismatch-binding activity in human cells. *Science* **268**:1912, 1995.
21. Papadopoulos N, Nicolaides NC, Liu B, Parsons R, Lengauer C, Palombo F, D'Arrigo A, Markowitz S, Willson JK, Kinzler KW, et al.: Mutations of GTBP in genetically unstable cells [see comments]. *Science* **268**:1915, 1995.
22. Papadopoulos N, Nicolaides NC, Wei YF, Ruben SM, Carter KC, Rosen CA, Haseltine WA, Fleischmann RD, Fraser CM, Adams MD, et al.: Mutation of a mutL homolog in hereditary colon cancer [see comments]. *Science* **263**:1625, 1994.
23. Nicolaides NC, Papadopoulos N, Liu B, Wei YF, Carter KC, Ruben SM, Rosen CA, Haseltine WA, Fleischmann RD, Fraser CM, et al.: Mutations of two PMS homologues in hereditary nonpolyposis colon cancer. *Nature* **371**:75, 1994.
24. Broner CE, Baker SM, Morrison PT, Warren G, Smith LG, Lescoe MK, Kane M, Earabino C, Lipford J, Lindblom A, et al.: Mutation in the DNA mismatch repair gene homologue hMLH1 is associated with hereditary non-polyposis colon cancer. *Nature* **368**:258, 1994.
25. Fishel R, Lescoe MK, Rao MR, Copeland NG, Jenkins NA, Garber J, Kane M, Kolodner R: The human mutator gene homolog MSH2 its association with hereditary nonpolyposis colon cancer. *Cell* **75**:1027, 1993.
26. Leach FS, Nicolaides NC, Papadopoulos N, Liu B, Jen J, Parsons R, Peltomaki P, Sistonen P, Aaltonen LA, Nystrom LM, et al: Mutations of a mutS homolog in hereditary nonpolyposis colorectal cancer. *Cell* **75**:1215, 1993.
27. Eshleman JR, Markowitz SD, Donover S, Lang EZ, Lutterbaugh JD, Li G, Longley M, Modrich P, Veigl ML, Sedwick WD: Diverse hypermutability of multiple expressed sequence motifs present in a cancer with microsatellite instability. *Oncogene* **12**:1425, 1996.
28. Imamura T, Arima T, Kato H, Miyamoto S, Sasazuki T, Wake N: Chromosomal deletions and K-ras gene mutations in human endometrial carcinomas. *Int J Cancer* **51**:47, 1992.
29. Jones MH, Koi S, Fujimoto I, Hasumi K, Kato K, Nakamura Y: Allelotype of uterine cancer by analysis of RFLP and microsatellite polymorphisms: Frequent loss of heterozygosity on chromosome arms 3p, 9q, 10q, 17p. *Genes Chrom Cancer* **9**:119, 1994.
30. Fujino T, Risinger JI, Collins NK, Liu F-S, Nishii H, Takahashi H, Westphal E-M, Barrett JC, Sasaki H, Kohler MF, Berchuck A, Boyd J: Allelotype of endometrial carcinoma. *Cancer Res* **54**:4294, 1994.
31. Peiffer SL, Herzog TJ, Tribune DJ, Mutch DG, Gersell DJ, Goodfellow PJ: Allelic loss of sequences from the long arm of chromosome 10 and replication errors in endometrial cancers. *Cancer Res* **55**:1922, 1995.
32. Okamoto A, Sameshima Y, Yamada Y, Teshima S-I, Terashima Y, Terada M, Yokota J: Allelic loss on chromosome 17p and p53 mutations in human endometrial carcinoma of the uterus. *Cancer Res* **51**:5632, 1991.
33. Tashiro H, Isacson C, Levine R, Kurman RJ, Cho KR, Hedrick L: p53 gene mutations are common in uterine serous carcinoma and occur early in their pathogenesis. *Am J Path* **150**:177, 1997.
34. Burks RT, Kessis TD, Cho KR, Hedrick L: Microsatellite instability in endometrial carcinoma. *Oncogene* **9**:1163, 1994.
35. Duggan BD, Felix JC, Muderspach LI, Tourgeman D, Zheng J, Shibata D: Microsatellite instability in sporadic endometrial carcinoma. *J Natl Cancer Inst* **86**:1216, 1994.
36. Risinger JI, Berchuck A, Kohler MF, Watson P, Lynch HT, Boyd J: Genetic instability of microsatellites in endometrial carcinoma. *Cancer Res* **53**:5100, 1993.
37. Katabuchi H, van Rees B, Lambers AR, Ronnett BM, Blazes MS, Leach FS, Cho KR, Hedrick L: Mutations in DNA mismatch repair genes are not responsible for microsatellite instability in most sporadic endometrial carcinomas. *Cancer Res* **55**:5556, 1995.
38. Boyer JC, Umar A, Risinger JI, Lipford JR, Kane M, Yin S, Barrett JC, Kolodner RD, Kunkel TA: Microsatellite instability, mismatch repair deficiency, and genetic defects in human cancer cell lines. *Cancer Res* **55**:6063, 1995.
39. Tashiro H, Lax SF, Gaudin PB, Isacson C, Cho KR, Hedrick L: Microsatellite instability is uncommon in uterine serous carcinoma. *Am J Pathol* **150**:75, 1997.

40. Mizuuchi H, Nasim S, Kudo R, Silverberg SG, Greenhouse S, Garrett CT: Clinical implications of k-ras mutations in malignant epithelial tumors of the endometrium. *Cancer Res* **52**:2777, 1992.

41. Ignar-Trowbridge D, Risinger JI, Dent GA, Kohler M, Berchuck A, McLachlan JA, Boyd J: Mutations of the Ki-ras oncogene in endometrial carcinoma. *Am J Obstet Gynecol* **167**:227, 1992.

42. Fujimoto I, Shimizu Y, Hirai Y, Chen J-I, Teshima H, Hasumi K, Masubuchi K, Takahashi M: Studies on ras oncogene activation in endometrial carcinoma. *Gynecol Oncol* **48**:196, 1993.

43. Duggan BD, Felix JC, Muderspach LI, Tsao J-L, Shibata DK: Early mutational activation of the c-Ki-ras oncogene in endometrial carcinoma. *Cancer Res* **54**:1604, 1994.

44. Enomoto T, Fujita M, Inoue M, Rice JM, Nakajima R, Tanizawa O, Nomura T: Alterations of the p53 tumor suppressor gene and its association with activation of the c-K-ras-2 protooncogene in premalignant and malignant lesions of the human uterine endometrium. *Cancer Res* **53**:1883, 1993.

45. Sasaki H, Nishii, Takahashi H, Tada A, Furusato M, Terashima Y, Siegal GP, Parker SL, Kohler MF, Berchuck A, Boyd J: Mutations of the ki-ras protooncogene in human endometrial hyperplasia and carcinoma. *Cancer Res* **53**:1906, 1993.

46. Caduff RF, Johnston CM, Frank TS: Mutations of the Ki-ras oncogene in carcinoma of the endometrium. *Am J Pathol* **146**:182, 1995.

47. Esteller M, Garcia A, Martinez i Palones JM, Cabero A, Reventos J: Detection of c-erbB-2/neu and fibroblast growth factor-3/INT-2 but not epidermal growth factor receptor gene amplification in endometrial cancer by differential polymerase chain reaction. *Cancer* **75**:2139, 1995.

48. Czerwenka K, Lu Y, Heuss F: Amplification and expression of the c-erbB-2 oncogene in normal, hyperplastic, and malignant endometria. *Int J Gynecol Pathol* **14**:98, 1995.

49. Pisani AL, Barbuto DA, Chen D, Ramos L, Lagasse LD, Karlan BY: Her-2/neu, p53, and DNA analyses as prognosticators for survival in endometrial carcinoma. *Obstet Gynecol* **85**:729, 1995.

50. Saffari Jones LA, El-Naggar A, Felix JC, George J, Press MF: Amplification and overexpression of HER2/neu (c-erbB2) in endometrial cancers: Correlation with overall survival. *Cancer Res* **55**:5693, 1995.

51. Khalifa MA, Mannel RS, Haraway SD, Walker J, Min K-W: Expression of EGFR, HER-2/neu, p53, and PCNA in endometrioid, serous papillary, and clear cell endometrial adenocarcinomas. *Gynecol Oncol* **53**:84, 1994.

52. Yamauchi N, Sakamoto A, Uozaki H, Iihara K, Machinami R: Immunohistochemical analysis of endometrial adenocarcinoma for bcl-2 and p53 in relation to expression of sex steroid receptor and proliferative activity. *Int J Gynecol Pathol* **15**:202, 1996.

53. Henderson GS, Brown KA, Perkins SL, Abbott TM, Clayton F: bcl-2 Is down-regulated in atypical endometrial hyperplasia and adenocarcinoma. *Mod Pathol* **9**:430, 1996.

54. Kastan MB, Canman CE, Leonard CJ: P53, cell cycle control and apoptosis: Implications for cancer. *Cancer Metastasis Rev* **14**:3, 1995.

55. Inoue M, Okayama A, Fujita M, Enomoto T, Sakata M, Tanizawa O, Ueshima H: Clinicopathological characteristics of p53 overexpression in endometrial cancers. *Int J Cancer* **58**:14, 1994.

56. Kohler MF, Berchuck A, Davidoff AM, Humphrey PA, Dodge RK, Iglehart JD, Soper JT, Clarke-Pearson DL, Bast RC, Marks JR: Overexpression and mutation of p53 in endometrial carcinoma. *Cancer Res* **52**:1622, 1992.

57. Ito K, Watanabe K, Nasim S, Sasano H, Sato S, Yajima A, Silverberg SG, Garrett CT: Prognostic significance of p53 overexpression in endometrial cancer. *Cancer Res* **54**:4667, 1994.

58. Jiko K, Sasano H, Ito K, Ozawa N, Sato S, Yajima A: Immunohistochemical and in situ hybridization analysis of p53 in human endometrial carcin of the uterus. *Anticancer Res* **13**:305, 1993.

59. Kihana T, Hamada K, Inoue Y, Yano N, Iketani H, Murao S-I, Ukita M, Matsuura S: Mutation and allelic loss of the p53 gene in endometrial carcinoma. *Cancer* **76**:72, 1995.

60. Geisler JP, Wiemann MC, Zhou Z, Miller GA, Geisler HE: p53 as a prognostic indicator in endometrial cancer. *Gynecol Oncol* **61**:245, 1996.

61. Honda T, Kato H, Imamura T, Gima T, Nishida J, Sasaki M, Hosi K, Sato A, Wake N: Involvement of p53 gene mutations in human endometrial carcinomas. *Int J Cancer* **53**:963, 1993.

62. Sherman ME, Bur ME, Kurman RJ: p53 in endometrial cancer and its putative precursors: Evidence for diverse pathways of tumorigenesis. *Hum Pathol* **26**:1268, 1995.

63. Enomoto T, Fujita M, Cheng C, Nakashima R, Ozaki M, Inoue M, Nomura T: Loss of expression and loss of heterozygosity n the DCC gene in neoplasms of the human female reproductive tract. *Br J Cancer* **71**:462, 1995.

64. Gima T, Kato H, Honda T, Imamura T, Sasazuki T, Wake N: DCC gene alteration in human endometrial carcinomas. *Int J Cancer* **57**:480, 1994.

65. Ronnett BM, Burks RT, Cho KR, Hedrick L: DCC genetic alterations and expression in endometrial carcinoma. *Mod Pathol* **10**:38, 1997.

66. Eppert K, Scherer SW, Ozcelik H, Pirone R, Hoodless P, Kim H, Tsui L, Bapat B, Gallinger S, Andrulis IL, Thomsen GH, Wrana JL, Attisano L: MADR2 maps to 18q21 and encodes a TGFB-regulated MAD-related protein that is functionally mutated in colorectal carcinoma. *Cell* **86**:543, 1996.

67. Hahn SA, Schutte M, Shamsul Hoque ATM, Moskaluk CA, da Costa LT, Rozenblum E, Weinstein CL, Fischer A, Yeo CJ, Hruban RH, Kern SE: DPC4, a candidate tumor suppressor gene at human chromosome 18q21.1. *Science* **271**:350, 1996.

68. Tashiro H, Blazes MS, Wu R, Cho KR, Bose S, Wang SI, Li J, Parsons R, Hedrick Ellenson L: Mutations in *PTEN* are frequent in endometrial carcinoma, but rare in other common gynecological malignancies. *Cancer Res* (in press).

69. Li J, Yen C, Liaw D, Podsypanina K, Bose S, Wang SI, Puc J, Miliaresis C, Rodgers L, McCombie R, Bigner SH, Giovanella BC, Ittmann M, Tycko B, Hibshoosh H, Wigler MH, and Parsons R: *PTEN*, a putative protein tyrosine phosphatase gene mutated in human brain, breast, and prostate cancer. *Science* **275**:1943, 1997.

CHAPTER 36

Cervical Cancer

Kathleen R. Cho

1. Based on available worldwide statistics, cervical cancer is the second most common cause of cancer-related mortality in women. Cervical cancers are curable when detected early, and the implementation of effective screening programs has reduced the incidence of and mortality from cervical cancer in industrialized countries substantially.

2. Neoplastic processes undoubtedly are complex, and cervical tumorigenesis is no exception. Like other adult solid tumors, cervical cancer appears to develop and progress largely as a consequence of activating mutations of oncogenes coupled with inactivation of tumor suppressor genes. Alterations of such genes have profound effects on the exquisite control of cell growth and differentiation present in normal cells. Based on currently available information, it appears that inherited factors do not play a major role in cervical tumorigenesis.

3. Cervical cancer is different from most other common malignancies in that it is strongly associated with an infectious agent (human papillomavirus, HPV). This strong association has been used to great advantage in the research laboratory because the HPVs provide tools with which to examine the molecular mechanisms by which the tumors arise.

4. Most studies have focused on the E6 and E7 transforming proteins of the oncogenic HPV types. E6 and E7 interfere with function of the cellular tumor suppressor proteins p53 and pRB via protein-protein interactions. By interfering with cell cycle control and DNA repair mechanisms, oncogenic HPVs appear to contribute indirectly to cervical tumorigenesis, by promoting genetic instability and the accumulation of mutations in HPV-infected cells.

5. Relatively few specific genes have been identified that are often altered in cervical carcinomas, although frequent amplification of c-*myc* and *HER 2-neu* has been reported. However, other cytogenetic and molecular genetic studies suggest that genes on chromosomes 1, 3, 5, 11, and others, are likely to play important roles in cervical tumorigenesis. Intensive efforts are currently underway to identify specific genes targeted by alterations of these chromosomes.

6. Animal models of papillomavirus-associated tumorigenesis have been developed, including several species-specific systems. More recently, production of transgenic animals expressing HPV transforming proteins have provided new insights into the mechanisms by which HPVs contribute to cervical cancer.

7. Cervical cancers are particularly attractive targets for preventive and antitumor vaccines because they virtually always contain tumor-specific antigens (HPV proteins).

CLINICAL ASPECTS

Incidence

Of cancers affecting women worldwide, cervical cancer is second only to breast cancer in both incidence and mortality.[1] Nearly 500,000 women are diagnosed with cervical cancer each year, and many die of the disease. The majority of cervical cancer patients are socioeconomically disadvantaged and thus without access to routine gynecological care and screening for precancerous lesions. As a result, cervical cancer is particularly prevalent in many developing nations.

Notably, carcinomas of the cervix usually are curable if detected early. In the United States, the incidence and death rate from cervical cancer have decreased markedly over the last few decades, largely because of early detection and effective treatment of noninvasive precursor lesions and minimally invasive carcinomas. In the United States during 1996, 15,700 new cervical cancer cases and 4900 cervical cancer deaths are anticipated.[2] Estimates of the prevalence of precursor lesions, collectively referred to as *squamous intraepithelial lesions* (SILs), range from 0.5 to 6.5% of the American female population and include at least 50,000 new cases of carcinoma *in situ* each year.

Histopathology

The cervix includes both vaginal (ectocervical) and internal (endocervical) portions. The ectocervix is covered by stratified squamous epithelium, whereas the endocervix is lined by mucin-producing columnar epithelium that invaginates into the underlying stroma to form gland-like structures. Most cervical cancers are of squamous-type differentiation and arise within a specific region of the cervix referred to as the transformation zone. The transformation zone is an area in which, via a process called squamous metaplasia, the columnar epithelium located at the junction between the ectocervix and endocervix is replaced by squamous epithelium. Less commonly, cervical carcinomas arise from the endocervical columnar/glandular epithelium (adenocarcinomas).

During the development of squamous carcinomas, metaplastic squamous cells within the transformation zone undergo distinctive morphological changes reflecting a progression from normal epithelium to carcinoma (Fig. 31-1). Lesions confined to the epithelium can be categorized as low grade or high grade squamous intraepithelial lesions (LSILs and HSILs) depending on their specific morphological features. Histopathologically, the intraepithelial lesions are characterized by changes reflecting abnormal cellular proliferation and differentiation. LSILs (previously called mild or low grade dysplasias) show mild expansion of the proliferative zone in the basal and parabasal portions of the epithelium. Cells toward the surface are arranged haphazardly, and often contain enlarged, pleomorphic, and hyperchromatic nuclei surrounded by clear halos. Collectively these changes are referred to as koilocytotic atypia. The HSILs show even greater expansion of the proliferative zone, with mitotic figures often identified in the mid- and upper portions of the epithelium. Koilocytotic atypia usually is less prominent than in LSILs, but the cells are more crowded and disorganized, have higher nuclear to cytoplasmic ratios, and show loss of polarity. The HSIL category includes lesions previously characterized as moderate and high grade dysplasias as well as *in situ* carcinomas. Although HSILs may not always arise from pre-existing LSILs, virtually all invasive squamous carcinomas arise from untreated HSILs.[3]

Biological Behavior

If left untreated, SILs can either regress spontaneously, persist, or progress to a more advanced lesion. Based on several previous studies, it appears that the likelihood a LSIL will regress is about 60%, whereas the likelihood of progression to invasive carcinoma is only 1%.[4] In contrast, the highest grade of intraepithelial lesions regress only 33% of the time, and progression to invasive carcinoma occurs in greater than 12% of cases. Clearly, high grade lesions are much more likely to progress to frank malignancy than those of low grade, but not all HSILs will progress to carcinoma, even if left untreated. Presently, lesions that will progress cannot be distinguished from those that will regress based on morphological features alone.

Women with preinvasive and even early invasive cervical lesions usually are asymptomatic. Hence, without a strategy for early detection, those who develop cervical cancer would be more likely to be diagnosed with late stage and often incurable disease. Fortunately, exfoliated cervical cells can be collected easily and microscopically examined following staining with the method originally described by Papanicolaou. Detection of abnormal cells on these "pap smears" is followed by diagnostic biopsy. Although some clinicians elect to closely follow patients with LSILs, some low grade and virtually all high grade lesions are treated by excisional biopsy or other ablative modalities such as laser, cryotherapy, or electrocautery.

Even invasive cancers, when detected early, usually are cured by surgery alone. The 5-year survival of patients with tumors showing <3 mm stromal invasion and maximum width <7 mm (FIGO Stage IA1) is nearly 100%.[5] Unfortunately, a substantial fraction of women in the United States fail to obtain even routine gynecological care. As a consequence, nearly 50% of U.S. women with cervical cancer are diagnosed when the disease is Stage II or higher.[6] Women with clinically visible cancers almost always report abnormal vaginal bleeding. Patients with high stage disease usually are treated with surgery or radiation.

Cervical Cancer as an Infectious Disease

Essentially all human tumors are thought to arise because of mutations in oncogenes, tumor suppressor genes, and genes encoding proteins involved in DNA damage recognition and repair. These mutations may be acquired somatically or inherited in the germ line. Based on the information available to date, it appears that inherited factors do not play a major role in cervical tumorigenesis, although some investigators have noted an association between the incidence of cervical cancer and particular MHC (major histocompatibility complex) alleles (HLA-DQ3 and to a lesser extent, HLA-DR6).[7,8] However, cervical cancer is particularly notable because it is one of few common human cancers that is strongly associated with an infectious agent. The past few years have seen a remarkable convergence of several lines of investigation convincingly implicating involvement of certain types of HPVs in the development of cervical carcinoma. More recent molecular studies have also provided insight into probable mechanisms by which oncogenic HPVs contribute to cervical neoplasia.

Although cervical cancer may, in some respects, be thought of as an infectious disease, it is important to recognize that of the millions of women infected by human papillomaviruses, only a small subset actually develop cervical cancer. This observation suggests that in the majority of patients, host immune surveillance may play an important role in limiting the growth and promoting regression of HPV-induced lesions. Humoral immunity does not appear to be a critical factor in controlling viral infection, particularly once the virus has entered the cell. Rather, HPV infection is more likely limited in most patients by the cell-mediated immune response.[9]

The Role of Human Papillomavirus Infection in Cervical Tumorigenesis

Over 90% of invasive cervical carcinomas have been shown to contain DNA sequences from particular HPV types.[10] Papillomaviruses are small DNA viruses composed of an approximately 8 kb double stranded circular genome enclosed by a 55-nm viral capsid. Over 100 different HPV types have been characterized on the basis of differences in DNA sequence, and a single host may be infected by multiple different HPVs. Based on extensive examination of the association of different HPV types with exophytic condylomas (genital warts), SILs, and cervical cancers, genital HPVs can be broadly classified into two groups: those associated with benign lesions (primarily HPVs 6 and 11) and those associated with invasive carcinomas (primarily HPVs 16 and 18). This classification into low-risk (non-cancer-associated) and high-risk (cancer-associated) types is reflected by in vitro evidence that cloned DNA of high-risk, but not low-risk HPVs will efficiently immortalize primary human keratinocytes.[11-13] Moreover, only the E6 and E7 open reading frames of the high-risk HPV genome are required for this immortalization function.[14]

Nearly all invasive cervical cancers contain high-risk HPV sequences, providing compelling evidence for HPV infection as a causative factor. However, several lines of evidence suggest that HPV infection alone is insufficient to generate the fully malignant phenotype. First, while the HPV E6 and E7 genes from high-risk viruses can cooperate to efficiently immortalize primary cells in culture, a fully transformed phenotype is only seen after many in vitro cell doublings. Second, although infection with high-risk HPV types is very common, only a small percentage of infected women develop invasive cervical cancer. Third, those who develop cancer generally do so long after initial infection with HPV (many years in most cases). These observations suggest that in addition to infection with a high-risk HPV type, other events are required for the development of cervical cancer. Presumably, these events include alterations of oncogenes and tumor suppressor genes in cervical cells harboring the HPV genome.

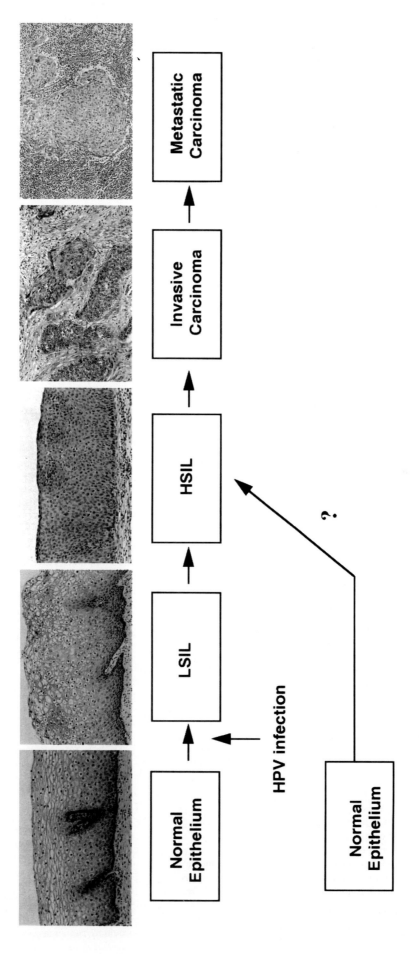

FIG. 36-1 Cervical tumorigenesis is associated with distinctive morphological changes that reflect a progression from normal epithelium to carcinoma. HPV infection is an early, if not initiating, event in this process. Although all high-grade squamous intraepithelial lesions (HSILs) may not arise from low-grade lesions (LSILs), invasive carcinomas are almost always found in association with their HSIL precursors.

Functional Consequences of HPV Oncoprotein Expression

Given that infection with high-risk HPVs contributes to the pathogenesis of cervical cancer, studies over the past decade have sought to investigate the molecular mechanisms underlying HPV-associated tumor development. The HPV E6 and E7 oncoproteins have been shown to interact directly with tumor suppressor gene products. Specifically, the E6 oncoprotein of the high risk HPV types 16 and 18 binds the tumor suppressor protein p53 with much higher affinity than E6 of the low risk types 6 and 11, and this binding appears to promote the ubiquitin mediated degradation of p53.[15,16] Similarly, the HPV16 E7 protein has been shown to bind the retinoblastoma tumor suppressor protein p105-RB (and other members of the RB family) with much greater affinity than its low-risk counterpart, presumably inactivating pRB's tumor suppressor function.[17–19] Since high-risk HPV infection provides a means with which to inactivate these tumor suppressors through protein-protein interactions, it is not surprising that most HPV-positive cervical carcinomas and carcinoma-derived cell lines lack p53 and pRB mutations.[20,21] However, a few HPV-positive tumors have been shown to contain p53 gene mutations, suggesting that in at least some cases, the gene mutation confers an additional growth advantage to the HPV-infected cell.[22–24] Other studies support the notion that p53 gene mutation may play a role in the progression of at least some cervical tumors since p53 point mutations have been identified more frequently in metastases arising from HPV positive cervical carcinomas than in primary tumors.[25]

The functional consequences of p53 and pRB inactivation by HPV oncoproteins have been addressed by several studies. Cells damaged by irradiation or DNA strand-breaking drugs arrest in the G1-S portion of the cell cycle, presumably allowing the cells to repair DNA damage and avoid the accumulation of genetic lesions.[26–28] This cell cycle arrest is temporally associated with accumulation of wild-type p53 protein, and is not seen in cells lacking p53 or in those expressing mutant p53 genes. When the HPV16 E6 protein is expressed in cells exhibiting a normal DNA damage response, baseline p53 protein levels are reduced dramatically and the cell cycle arrest following DNA damage is abolished.[29,30] Hence, high-risk HPVs may indirectly contribute to cervical tumorigenesis, by promoting genomic instability and the accumulation of mutations in HPV-infected cells. HPV16 E7 also has been shown to effectively abrogate the p53-dependent growth arrest in response to DNA damage.[31–33] Several studies suggest that this may be explained by a role for pRB downstream of p53 in the growth arrest pathway (Fig. 36-2). Abrogation of this important cellular response by the HPV transforming proteins suggests a plausible mechanism for the accelerated accumulation of genetic alterations necessary for cervical tumor progression that occurs in the setting of high-risk HPV infection.

There are several types of genetic alterations that might arise as a consequence of p53 and pRB inactivation and the resultant abrogation of the growth arrest in response to DNA damage. When high-risk (HPV16) E6 is introduced into human fibroblasts, the cells show a marked increase in their ability to amplify drug resistance genes in response to drug treatment.[34] In contrast, low-risk (HPV6) E6 has no effect. The idea that high-risk HPV infection might enhance gene amplification is particularly interesting, because frequent amplification of c-*myc*, *HER2-neu*, and as yet unidentified gene(s) on the long arm of chromosome 3 (3q) has been reported in cervical cancers.[35–38] At least one study suggests that c-*myc* amplification may be a useful marker of poor prognosis, since patients whose tumors had c-*myc* amplification suffered early relapse more frequently than those whose tumors lacked the alteration.[36] The gains of chromosome 3q sequences also are particularly interesting because they appear to occur at the transition from

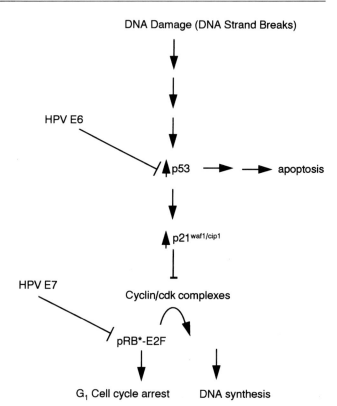

FIG. 36-2 A proposed representation of the DNA damage-induced cell cycle checkpoint pathway in mammalian cells. DNA damage results in accumulation of the p53 protein. Accumulation of wtp53 increases levels of p21$^{waf1/cip1}$, which in turn inhibits activation of cyclin-cdk complexes, preventing phosphorylation of pRB (and perhaps pRB-related proteins p107 and p130). E2F transcription factors therefore remain associated with hypophosphorylated pRB and are unable to activate transcription of genes required for progression from G$_1$ into S phase. Consequently, cells arrest in G1. High-risk HPVs can disrupt the pathway at two separate points: through interaction of E6 with p53, and, further downstream, through interactions of E7 with pRB. Apoptotic cell death is another response to DNA damage that may also be influenced by HPV oncoprotein expression. (Modified with permission from Slebos et al., *Proc Natl Acad Sci USA* 91:5320–5324, 1994.)

severe dysplasia (HSIL) to invasive squamous carcinoma. Specifically, overrepresentation of chromosome 3q sequences was observed in 90% of carcinomas but in less than 10% of HSILs, suggesting that the 3q gains may confer the potential for stromal invasion to affected cells.

Another genetic alteration that occurs frequently at the transition from HSIL to invasive carcinoma is integration of the viral genome into the host DNA. In condylomas and most SILs, the HPV genome is maintained as an episome (a free circular molecule replicating independently of the cellular genome). Regardless of HPV type, the production of progeny virions in these lesions is tightly linked to squamous epithelial differentiation.[39] In contrast, the majority of invasive carcinomas contain high-risk HPV DNA integrated into human chromosomal DNA as one or multiple tandem copies.[40,41] During the process of integration, substantial portions of the HPV genome may be deleted, but the E6 and E7 open reading frames virtually always are retained. Although several studies have failed to find a common site in the host genome where the virus integrates, viral integration almost invariably disrupts elements of the HPV genome (i.e., E1 and/or E2) that regulate expression of the E6 and E7 transforming genes.[42] Not surprisingly, integration of HPV16 DNA into the genome of cervical epithelial cells recently was found to correlate with a selective growth advantage in vitro, providing further support for the notion that viral integration is an important step for in vivo tumor progression.[43] High-risk HPVs may themselves contribute to integration of HPV DNA into the host genome. Indeed, recent studies have shown that the frequency of foreign DNA integration is enhanced in cells expressing high-risk but now low-risk HPV E6 and E7.[44]

In other studies, inactivation of p53 by the HPV16 E6 protein was found to increase the rate of spontaneous mutagenesis (particularly point mutations and small insertions or deletions) in human cells.[45] Interestingly, HPV16 E7 expression had no effect on the rate of mutagenesis, suggesting that the type of genetic alteration detected by this assay is enhanced by p53 but not by pRB inactivation. A plausible explanation for this finding may be provided by the observation that p53's role in suppressing tumorigenesis is not likely to be restricted to its participation in the DNA damage response pathway. p53 is thought to play a more direct role in DNA repair also, because it has been found to be associated with other proteins involved in DNA repair such as the DNA helicases ERCC3/XPB and RPA.[45]

Clearly, we are beginning to develop an understanding of the molecular mechanisms underlying the difference in oncogenic potential between the high- and low-risk HPVs. The E6 and E7 proteins encoded by the low-risk HPVs appear to have substantially less impact on p53 and pRB function than their high-risk counterparts. However, it remains possible, if not likely, that the oncogenic potential of the various HPV types is owing to additional factors beyond their abilities to directly interfere with p53 and pRB function. For example, expression of HPV16 E7 leads to increased cellular levels of cyclin A, cyclin B, and p34cdc2, as well as cyclin E.[46,47] These findings suggest that the HPV oncoproteins affect other portions of the cell cycle besides the G_1S checkpoint. Moreover, the role of other HPV proteins in cellular transformation is being actively investigated. E5 has been shown to act as a mitogen, presumably through growth factor receptor signal transduction pathways. HPV16 E5 also has been shown to be capable of inducing anchorage independent growth of immortalized fibroblasts in an EGF (epidermal growth factor)-dependent fashion.[49]

Other Genetic Loci Implicated in Cervical Tumorigenesis

Both cytogenetic and molecular genetic analyses have been used in an attempt to identify additional loci frequently altered during cervical tumorigenesis. In general, cytogenetic studies have failed to identify consistent specific chromosomal rearrangements or other karyotypic abnormalities in cervical cancer cells. Structural and numerical abnormalities of chromosome 1 have been reported most frequently.[50,51]

Other investigators have performed allelotype analyses of cervical carcinomas in an attempt to localize tumor supressor loci. In one study of 35 uterine cancers (including both endometrial and cervical carcinomas), high frequencies of allelic loss (i.e., >35%) were found at loci on chromosomes 3p, 9q, 10q, and 17p.[52] In another study of 53 primary cervical carcinomas, >25% of informative tumors had allelic losses involving chromosomes 1q, 3p, 3q, 4p, 5p, 5q, 6p, 10q, 11p, 18p, and Xq.[53] Frequent deletions on 3p and 11p have been confirmed by other studies.[54-56] Deletion mapping of chromosome 3p has localized common regions of deletion to 3p13-14.3 and 3p13-p21.1.[54,55] The 3p losses are particularly interesting, in part because deletions of this region are common not only in cervical carcinomas, but also in several other tumor types including clear cell renal carcinomas, lung carcinomas, and nasopharyngeal carcinomas. Recently, a candidate tumor suppressor gene *FHIT* at 3p14.2 was cloned.[59] Aberrant *FHIT* transcripts have been identified in several different tumor types, including

esophageal, stomach, breast, and colon carcinomas.[57,58] The gene spans a fragile site called *FRA3B,* that was independently found to contain a spontaneous HPV16 integration site.[59] Collectively, these data suggest that genetic alterations in this region (including *FHIT* mutation, chromosome deletions, chromosome translocations, and HPV integration) play an important role in cervical tumorigenesis.

Functional studies have provided yet additional evidence suggesting involvement of tumor suppressor genes in the development and progression of cervical cancer. For example, transfer of chromosome 11 into HeLa cells (derived from an HPV18 positive cervical carcinoma) and SiHa cells (derived from an HPV16 positive cervical carcinoma) resulted in complete suppression of tumorigenicity.[60,61] Similarly, expression of the *DCC* gene in keratinocytes transformed by HPV18 and nitrosomethylurea resulted in suppression of tumorigenicity, and tumorigenic reversion was associated with loss or rearrangement of transfected *DCC* sequences.[62]

Animal Models

A better understanding of the role of HPV infection in the pathogenesis of cervical cancer undoubtedly will enhance our ability to effectively manage patients with this disease. Although in vitro systems are very powerful, they are often limited in their ability to provide insights into the processes driving neoplastic progression. Thus, a long-standing goal of HPV and cervical cancer researchers has been to develop effective animal models of HPV-induced tumors. Such models, in addition to leading to improved preventive, diagnostic, and therapeutic strategies may also facilitate the identification of genetic and environmental cofactors that may profoundly influence both tumor development and progression.

The strong association of HPV infection with cervical tumorigenesis led to great optimism that useful animal models of cervical cancer could be developed easily. In general, animal models of viral diseases require a source of infectious virus and a susceptible host. Unfortunately, both have been problematic with respect to HPVs. These viruses are notoriously difficult to culture, largely because HPV virions are only produced in highly differentiated keratinocytes. Successful culture of HPV was not achieved until 1992.[63] To further complicate matters, infection with the various types of papillomaviruses is species-specific, and human papillomaviruses do not infect nonhuman species. Thus, several models of papillomavirus-associated oncogenesis have been developed in species-specific systems, including those in rabbits, rodents, cattle, dogs, and nonhuman primates.[64,65] The rabbit model has been particularly useful since it mimics human disease quite closely.

Fortunately, many researchers have successfully circumvented the species specificity of papillomaviruses by expressing viral genes in transgenic animals. Several groups have produced transgenic mice expressing high-risk HPV transforming genes.[64,65] Increased propensity to develop tumors has been observed in all transgenic lineages, with the specific location and type of tumor determined largely by the nature of the promoter used to express the transgenes. Transgenic mice expressing the E6 and E7 oncogenes of HPV16 under control of the β-actin promoter or α-A-crystallin promoter develop neuroepithelial carcinomas and lens tumors, respectively.[66,67] In one study, mice expressing the same genes under the control of the mouse mammary tumor virus promoter develop large testicular seminomas, whereas another group reported the development of salivary gland carcinomas, lymphomas, and cutaneous histiocytomas.[68,69] In the latter study, 77% of the female transgenic mice also developed dysplastic and/or hyperplastic changes in the cervix and vagina, although no anogenital tumors were observed. Probably the most illustrative transgenic model system is that recently described by Arbeit, Howley, and Hanahan.[70] These investigators generated transgenic mice expressing the early region of the HPV16 genome under the control of the human keratin-14 promoter. The mice developed squamous carcinomas exclusively in the vagina and cervix when treated chronically with 17β estradiol. Although the mechanisms for the synergism between chronic estrogen exposure and expression of HPV oncoproteins in squamous carcinogenesis remain to be determined, this animal model system is likely to prove invaluable in future studies.

IMPLICATIONS FOR DIAGNOSIS AND TREATMENT

Human papillomavirus proteins provide tumor-specific antigens in the great majority of cervical carcinomas, and hence, it should be feasible to develop prophylactic or antitumor vaccines to effectively prevent or treat cervical cancer. The development of such vaccines has been hindered, at least in part, by the difficulty in propagating HPVs in culture and by only relatively recent availability of good animal model systems. Nonetheless, substantial progress has been made in the last few years. Noncapsid papillomavirus antigens (those consistently present in cervical cancer cells) are preferentially routed for MHC Class I presentation, which typically is deficient in cervical cancer cells.[9] Thus, a reasonable approach for an anti-tumor vaccine is one that attempts to route such antigens into the MHC Class II processing and presentation pathway via the endosomal and lysosomal cellular compartments. In a recent study, Wu and colleagues fused a target tumor antigen (HPV16 E7) to a sequence of the lysosomal protein LAMP-1 in order to direct the antigen into the endosomal and lysosomal compartments and enhance MHC Class II presentation of E7 peptides.[72] Expression of the fusion protein in appropriate recipient cells resulted in enhanced presentation to CD4+ cells in vitro. Moreover, in vivo immunization experiments using recombinant vaccinia viruses in mice demonstrated that immunization with the chimeric protein resulted in increased E7-specific lymphoproliferative activity, antibody titers, and cytotoxic T lymphocyte activity compared to immunization with wild-type E7. In more recent studies, these investigators were able to use the same recombinant viral vaccines to cure mice with small established tumors.[73] Clinical trials of this type of vaccine in cervical cancer patients are likely to follow in the near future.

Certainly, another major goal of cervical cancer researchers in the future will be to identify specific genes involved in the progression of premalignant lesions. The identification of such genes is critical for developing potential screening protocols to augment those currently based on cytopathological screening of Papanicolau smears alone. The knowledge gained may also prove useful for designing novel and more sensible therapeutic strategies as well as more reliable methods that can be used to predict which intraepithelial lesions may be more likely to progress to invasive disease.

REFERENCES

1. Beral V, Hermon C, Muñoz N, Devesa SS: Cervical cancer. *Cancer Surv* **19–20**:265–285, 1994.
2. Parker SL, Tong T, Bolden S, Wingo PA: Cancer Statistics, 1996. *Ca Cancer J Clin* **46**:5–27, 1996.
3. Kiviat N, Critchlow CW, Kurman RJ: Reassessment of the morphological continuum of cervical intraepithelial lesions: does it reflect differ-

ent stages in the progression to cervical carcinoma? In: Muñoz N, Bosch FX, Shah KV, Meheus A: *The Epidemiology of Cervical Cancer and Human Papillomavirus,* Lyon: International Agency for Research on Cancer, 59–66, 1992.
4. Östör AG: Natural history of cervical intraepithelial neoplasia—a critical review. *Int J Gynecol Pathol* **12**:186–192, 1993.
5. Benedet JL, Anderson GH: Stage IA carcinoma of the cervix revisited. *Obstet Gynecol* **87**:1052–1059, 1996.
6. Jessup J, McGinnis LS, Winchester DP, Eyre H, Fremgen A, Murphy GP, Menck HR: Clinial highlights from the National Cancer Data Base: 1996. *Ca Cancer J Clin* **46**:185–192, 1996.
7. Wank R, Thomssen C: High risk of squamous cell carcinoma of the cervix for women with HLA-DQw3. *Nature* **352**:723–725, 1991.
8. Helland A, Borresen AL, Kaern J, Ronningen KS, Thorsby E: HLA antigens and cervical carcinoma. *Nature* **356**:23, 1992.
9. Altmann A, Jochmus I, Rösl F: Intra- and extracellular control mechanisms of human papillomavirus infection. *Intervirology* 180–188, 1994.
10. Bosch FX, Manos MM, Muñoz N, Sherman M, Jansen AM, Peto J, Schiffman MH, Moreno V, Kurman R, Shah KV: Prevalence of human papillomavirus in cervical cancer: a worldwide perspective. International biological study on cervical cancer (IBSCC) Study Group. *J Natl Cancer Inst* **87**:796–802, 1995.
11. Pirisi L, Yasumoto S, Feller M, Doniger J, DiPaolo J: Transformation of human fibroblasts and keratinocytes with human papillomavirus type 16 DNA. *J Virol* **61**:1061–1066, 1987.
12. Pecoraro G, Morgan D, Defendi V: Differential effects of human papillomavirus type 6, 16, and 18 DNAs on immortalization and transformation of human cervical epithelial cells. *Proc Natl Acad Sci USA* **86**:563–567, 1989.
13. Woodworth CD, Doniger J, DiPaolo A: Immortalization of human foreskin keratinocytes by various human papillomavirus DNAs corresponds to their association with cervical carcinoma. *J Virol* **63**:159–564, 1989.
14. Hawley-Nelson P, Vousden KH, Hubbert NL, Lowy DR, Schiller JT: HPV16 E6 and E7 proteins cooperate to immortalize human foreskin keratinocytes. *EMBO J* **8**:3905–3910, 1989.
15. Werness BA, Levine AJ, Howley PM: Association of human papillomavirus types 16 and 18 E6 proteins with p53. *Science* **248**:76–79, 1990.
16. Scheffner M, Werness BA, Huibregste JM, Levine AJ, Howley PM: The E6 oncoprotein encoded by human papillomavirus types 16 and 18 promotes the degradation of p53. *Cell* **63**:1129–1136, 1990.
17. Dyson N, Howley P, Munger K, Harlow E: The human papillomavirus-16 E7 oncoprotein is able to bind to the retinoblastoma gene product. *Science* **243**:934–937, 1989.
18. Dyson N, Guida P, Mnger K, Harlow E: Homologous sequences in adenovirus E1A and human papillomavirus E7 proteins mediate interaction with the same set of cellular proteins. *J Virol* **66**:6893–6902, 1992.
19. Davies R, Hicks R, Crook T, Morris J, Vousden K: Human papillomavirus type 16 E7 associates with a histone H1 kinase and with p107 through sequences necessary for transformation. *J Virol* **67**:2521–2528, 1993.
20. Scheffner M, Mgner K, Byrne JC, Howley PM: The state of the p53 and retinoblastoma genes in human cervical carcinoma cell lines. *Proc Natl Acad Sci USA* **88**:5523–5527, 1991.
21. Crook T, Wrede D, Vousden KH: p53 point mutation in HPV negative human cervical carcinoma cell lines. *Oncogene* **6**:873–875, 1991.
22. Helland A, Holm R, Kristensen G, Kern J, Karlsen F, Trope C, Nesland JM, Borresen AL: Genetic alterations of the tp53 gene, p53 protein expression and HPV infection in primary cervical carcinomas. *J Pathol* **171**:105–114, 1993.
23. Fujita M, Inoue M, Tanizawa O, Iwamoto S, Enomoto T: Alterations of the p53 gene in human primary cervical carcinoma with and without human papillomavirus infection. *Cancer Res* **52**:5323–5328, 1992.
24. Kessis T, Slebos R, Han S, Shah K, Bosch FX, Muñoz N, Hedrick L, Cho K: p53 gene mutations and mdm2 amplification are uncommon in primary carcinomas of the uterine cervix. *Am J Pathol* **143**:1398–1405, 1993.
25. Crook T, Vousden KH: Properties of p53 mutations detected in primary and secondary cervical cancers suggest mechanisms of metastasis and involvement of environmental carcinogens. *EMBO J* **11**:3935–3940, 1992.
26. Kastan MB, Onyekwere O, Sidransky D, Vogelstein B, Craig RW: Participation of p53 protein in the cellular response to DNA damage. *Cancer Res* **51**:6304–6311, 1991.

27. Keurbitz SJ, Plunkett BS, Walsh WV, Kastan MB: Wild-type p53 is a cell cycle checkpoint determinant following irradiation. *Proc Natl Acad Sci USA* **89**:7491–7495, 1992.

28. Kastan M, Zhan Q, Eli-Deiry WS, Carrier F, Jacks T, Walsh W, Plunkett B, Vogelstein B, Fornace A: A mammalian cell cycle checkpoint pathway utilizing p53 and GADD45 is defective in ataxia-telangiectasia. *Cell* **71**:587–598, 1992.

29. Kessis TD, Slebos RJ, Nelson WG, Kastan MB, Plunkett BS, Han SM, Lorincz AT, Hedrick L, Cho KR: Human papillomavirus 16 E6 expression disrupts the p53-mediated cellular response to DNA damage. *Proc Natl Acad Sci USA* **90**:3988–3992, 1993.

30. Foster SA, Demers GW, Etscheid BG, Galloway DA: The ability of human papillomavirus E6 proteins to target p53 for degradation in vivo correlates with their ability to abrogate actinomycin D-induced growth arrest. *J Virol* **68**:5698–5705, 1994.

31. Hickman ES, Picksley SM, Vousden KH: Cells expressing HPV16 E7 continue cell cycle progression following DNA damage induced by p53 activation. *Oncogene* **9**:2177–2818, 1994.

32. Demers GW, Foster SA, Halbert CL, Galloway DA: Growth arrest by induction of p53 in DNA damaged keratinocytes is bypassed by human papillomavirus 16 E7. *Proc Natl Acad Sci USA* **91**:4382–4386, 1994.

33. Slebos RJ, Lee MH, Plunkett BS, Kessis TD, Williams BO, Jacks T, Hedrick L, Kastan MB, Cho KR: p53-dependent G1 arrest involves pRB-related proteins and is disrupted by the human papillomavirus 16 E7 oncoprotein. *Proc Natl Acad Sci USA* **91**:5320–5324, 1994.

34. White AE, Livanos EM, Tlsty TD: Differential disruption of genomic integrity and cell cycle regulation in normal human fibroblasts by the HPV oncoproteins. *Gene Dev* **8**:666–677, 1994.

35. Baker VV, Hatch KD, Shingleton HM: Amplification of the c-myc proto-oncogene in cervical carcinoma. *J Surg Oncol* **39**:225–228, 1988.

36. Ocadiz R, Sauceda R, Cruz M, Graef AM, Gariglio P: High correlation between molecular alterations of the c-myc oncogene and carcinoma of the uterine cervix. *Cancer Res* **47**:4173–4177, 1987.

37. Mitra AB, Murty VV, Pratap M, Sodhani P, Chaganti RS: ERBB2 (HER2/neu) oncogene is frequently amplified in squamous cell carcinoma of the uterine cervix. *Cancer Res* **54**:637–639, 1994.

38. Heselmeyer K, Schrock E, Dumanoir S, Blegen H, Shah K, Steinbeck R, Auer G, Ried T: Gain of chromosome 3q defines the transition from severe dysplasia to invasive carcinoma of the uterine cervix. *Proc Natl Acad Sci USA* **93**:479–484, 1996.

39. Chow LT, Broker TR: Papillomavirus DNA replication. *Intervirology* **37**:150–158, 1994.

40. Drst M, Kleinheinz A, Hotz M, Gissman L: The physical state of human papillomavirus type 16 DNA in benign and maligant genital tumors. *J Gen Virol* **66**:1515–1522, 1985.

41. Cullen AP, Reid R, Champion M, Lirincz AT: Analysis of the physical state of different human papillomavirus DNAs in intraepithelial and invasive cervical neoplasms. *J Virol* **65**:606–612, 1991.

42. Choo KB, Pan CC, Han SH: Integration of human papillomavirus type 16 into cellular DNA of cervical carcinoma: preferential deletion of the E2 gene and invariable retention of the long control region and the E6/E7 open reading frames. *Virology* **161**:259–261, 1987.

43. Jeon S, Allen-Hoffmann BL, Lambert PF: Integration of human papillomavirus type 16 into the human genome correlates with a selective growth advantage of cells. *J Virol* **69**:2989–2997, 1995.

44. Kessis TD, Connolly DC, Hedrick L, Cho KR: Expression of HPV16 E6 or E7 increases integration of foreign DNA. *Oncogene* **13**:427–431, 1996.

45. Havre PA, Yuan JL, Hedrick L, Cho KR, Glazer PM: P53 inactivation by HPV16 E6 results in increased mutagenesis in human cells. *Cancer Res* **55**:4420–4424, 1995.

46. Steinmann KE, Pei XF, Stoppler H, Schlegel R: Elevated expression and activity of mitotic regulatory proteins in human papillomavirus-immortalized keratinocytes. *Oncogene* **9**:387–394, 1994.

47. Zerfass K, Schulze A, Spitkovsky D, Friedman V, Henglein B, Jansen-Durr P: Sequential activation of cyclin E and cyclin A gene expression by human papillomavirus type 16 E7 through sequences necessary for transformation. *J Virol* **69**:6389–6399, 1995.

48. Stöppler H, Stöppler C, Schlegel R: Transforming proteins of the papillomaviruses. *Intervirology* **37**:168–179, 1994.

49. Straight SW, Hinkle PM, Jewers RJ, McCance DJ: The E5 oncoprotein of human papillomavirus type 16 transforms fibroblasts and effects the downregulation of the epidermal growth factor receptor in keratinocytes. *J Virol* **67**:4521–4532, 1993.

50. Atkin NB, Baker MC: Chromosome 1 in 26 carcinomas of the cervix uteri: structural and numerical changes. *Cancer* **44**:604–613, 1979.

51. Sreekantaiah C, De Braekeleer M, Haas O: Cytogenetic findings in cervical carcinoma. A statistical approach. *Cancer Genet Cytogenet* **53**:75–81, 1991.

52. Jones MH, Koi S, Fujimoto I, Hasumi K, Kato K, Nakamura Y: Allelotype of uterine cancer by analysis of RFLP and microsatellite polymorphisms—frequent loss of heterozygosity on chromosome arms 3p, 9q, 10q, and 17p. *Genes Chrom Cancer* **9**:119–123, 1994.

53. Mitra AB, Murty VVVS, Li RG, Pratap M, Luthra UK, Chaganti RSK: Allelotype analysis of cervical carcinoma. *Cancer Res* **54**:4481–5487, 1994.

54. Jones MH, Nakamura Y: Deletion mapping of chromosome 3p in female genital tract malignancies using microsatellite polymorphisms. *Oncogene* **7**:1631–1634, 1992.

55. Kohno T, Takayama H, Hamaguchi M, Takano H, Yamaguchi N, Tsuda H, Hirohashi S, Vissing H, Shimizu M, Oshimura M, Yokota J: Deletion mapping of chromosome-3p in human uterine cervical cancer. *Oncogene* **8**:1825–1832, 1993.

56. Srivatsan ES, Misra BC, Venugopalan M, Wilczynski SP: Loss of heterozygosity for alleles on chromosome 11 in cervical carcinoma. *Am J Hum Genet* **49**:868–877, 1991.

57. Ohta M, Inoue H, Cotticelli MG, Kastury K, Baffa R, Palazzo J, Siprashvili Z, Mori M, Mccue P, Druck T, Croce CM, Huebner K: The FHIT gene, spanning the chromosome 3p14.2 fragile site and renal carcinoma-associated t(3-8) breakpoint, is abnormal in digestive tract cancers. *Cell* **84**:587–597, 1996.

58. Negrini M, Monaco C, Vorechovsky I, Ohta M, Druck T, Baffa R, Huebner K, Croce CM: The FHIT gene at 3p14.2 is abnormal in breast carcinomas. *Cancer Res* **56**:3173–3179, 1996.

59. Wilke CM, Hall BK, Hoge A, Paradee W, Smith DI, Glover TW: FRA3B extends over a broad region and contains a spontaneous HPV16 integration site—direct evidence for the coincidence of viral integration sites and fragile sites. *Hum Mol Genet* **5**:187–195, 1996.

60. Oshimura M, Kugoh H, Koi M, Shimizu M, Yamada H, Satoh H, Barrett JC: Transfer of a normal human chromosome 11 suppresses tumorigenicity of some but not all tumor cell lines. *J Cell Biochem* **42**:135–142, 1990.

61. Saxon PJ, Srivatsan ES, Stanbridge EJ: Introduction of human chromosome 11 via microcell transfer controls tumorigenic expression of HeLa cells. *EMBO J* **5**:3461–3466, 1986.

62. Klingelhutz AJ, Hedrick L, Cho KR, McDougall JK: The DCC gene suppresses the malignant phenotype of transformed human epithelial cells. *Oncogene* **10**:1581–1586, 1995.

63. Meyers C, Frattini M, Hudson J, Laimins L: Biosynthesis of human papillomavirus from a continuous cell line upon epithelial differentiation. *Science* **257**:971–973, 1992.

64. Brandsma JL: Animal models of human-papillomavirus-associated oncogenesis. *Intervirology* **37**:189–200, 1994.

65. Griep AE, Lambert PF: Role of papillomavirus oncogenes in human cervical cancer—transgenic animal studies. *Proc Soc Exp Biol Med* **206**:24–34, 1994.

66. Arbeit JM, Mnger K, Howley PM, Hanahan D: Neuroepithelial carcinomas in mice transgenic with human papillomavirus type 16 E6/E7 ORFs. *Am J Pathol* **142**:1187–1197, 1993.

67. Griep AK, Herber R, Jeon S, Lohse JK, Dubielzig RR, Lambert PF: Tumorigenicity by human papillomavirus type 16 E6 and E7 in transgenic mice correlates with alterations in epithelial cell growth and differentiation. *J Virol* **67**:1373–1384, 1993.

68. Kondoh G, Murata Y, Aozasa K, Yutsudo M, Hakura A: Very high incidence of germ cell tumorigenesis (seminomagenesis) in human papillomavirus type 16 transgenic mice. *J Virol* **65**:3335–3339, 1991.

69. Sasagawa T, Kondoh G, Inoue M, Yutsudo M, Hakura A: Cervical/vaginal dysplasia of transgenic mice harbouring human papillomavirus type 16 E6-E7 genes. *J Gen Virol* **75**:3057–3065, 1994.

70. Arbeit JM, Howley PM, Hanahan D: Chronic estrogen-induced cervical and vaginal squamous cercinogenesis in human papillomavirus type 16 transgenic mice. *Proc Natl Acad Sci USA* **93**:2930–2935, 1996.

71. Galloway DA: Human papillomavirus vaccines: a warty problem. *Infect Agents Dis* **3**:187–193, 1994.

72. Wu TC, Guarnieri FG, Staveleyocarroll KF, Viscidi RP, Levitsky HI, Hedrick L, Cho KR, August JT, Pardoll DM, Engineering an intracellular pathway for major histocompatibility complex class II presentation of antigens. *Proc Natl Acad Sci USA* **92**:11671–11675, 1995.

73. Lin KY, Guarnieri FG, Staveleyocarroll KF, Levitsky HI, August JT, Pardoll DM, Wu TC: Treatment of established tumors with a novel vaccine that enhances major histocompatibility class II presentation of tumor antigen. *Cancer Res* **56**:21–26, 1996.

CHAPTER 37

Bladder Cancer

Paul Cairns ▪ David Sidransky

1. **Bladder cancer is the fifth most common cancer among Americans. Almost all bladder cancer in the United States is composed of transitional cell carcinoma. Familial cases are rare and usually part of the Lynch syndrome. Smoking is perhaps the greatest risk factor for sporadic disease.**

2. **Cytogenetic studies have identified a number of chromosomal changes in bladder cancer. Low grade, noninvasive tumors are usually diploid, whereas high grade invasive tumors often contain gross aneuploidy. Monosomy of chromosome 9 is the most common abnormality seen in this disease.**

3. **Few proto-oncogene mutations or amplifications have been frequently described in bladder cancer. However, chromosomal deletions are very common on chromosomes 9p, 17p, and 13q. Candidate genes inactivated at these loci include *p16*, *p53*, and *Rb*, respectively. Moreover, *p53* and *Rb* mutations usually are seen in flat (carcinoma *in situ*) or invasive lesions and are correlated with a poor prognosis.**

4. **Many bladder cancers appear as multifocal disease at presentation. Molecular studies have shown that multiple tumors in the same patient arise from the uncontrolled spread of a single progenitor cell. These tumors then proceed through variable genetic events during progression. A preliminary molecular progression model for bladder cancer suggests that chromosome 9p is an early loss event in most tumors. Conversely, loss of chromosome 17p and 14q are more often associated with flat lesions and invasive tumors.**

5. **Genetic alterations can be detected in the urine sediment of patients with bladder cancer. Microsatellite analysis allows detection of LOH or genomic instability in primary tumor and urine DNA. Pilot studies suggest that most bladder tumors can be detected by DNA analysis. Moreover, these approaches are amenable to automated techniques suitable for the clinical setting.**

BLADDER CANCER

Clinical Aspects

Bladder cancer is the fifth most common cancer among Americans.[1] There are over 50,000 new cases diagnosed yearly, with a male to female ratio of almost 3:1. There is no pathognomonic sign or symptom for bladder cancer, but most patients present with microscopic hematuria. Occasionally gross hematuria and pain also can lead to the diagnosis. This year alone over 11,000 patients will die from advanced and/or metastatic disease.[1]

There are few reports of familial bladder cancer.[2] Clinical cases of bladder cancer owing to hereditary predisposition probably represent 1% or less of all tumors. The estimated relative risk of developing the disease, even with an affected family member under the age of 45, is only 1.45 per person.[3] The greatest risk for inherited urothelial cancer probably occurs as part of the Lynch syndrome (Hereditary Nonpolyposis Colorectal Cancer; HNPCC).[4] In this syndrome, there is a high risk of bladder cancer, but it is often overshadowed by the high risk of other neoplasms, including colon cancer and uterine cancer.

Almost all bladder cancers in the United States are composed of transitional cell carcinoma (TCC). Bladder irritation or infections such as Schistosomiasis, can predispose to specific types of bladder cancer. In areas such as Egypt where these infection rates are high, squamous carcinoma is very common.[5] Exposure to certain chemical compounds including analgesics may also predispose to an increased risk of urothelial cancer.[6,7]

In the United States, cigarette smoking is perhaps the single greatest risk factor for bladder cancer. Compared with nonsmokers, smokers have been estimated to have a twofold increased risk of developing the disease. It is also clear that this risk may be dose related, and in a similar fashion to lung cancer, patients who stop smoking develop an intermediate risk that begins to subside with increasing age.[8-10]

Pathology

The vast majority of bladder cancer originates in the urothelium, the characteristic transitional cell urothelial lining in the urinary tract.[11] Moreover, many tumors are already multifocal at presentation. A major and overwhelming distinction between superficial and invasive disease involves penetration into the lamina propria. The prognosis for invasive disease is much worse and depends on grade and stage. Although 85–95% of bladder cancers are transitional cell carcinomas, mixed tumors occasionally with squamous cell or adenocarcinoma elements are also found. Despite its low frequency in the United States, squamous cell carcinoma, for the reasons mentioned earlier, may be the most common malignancy in Egypt. Adenocarcinoma, thought to arise from the trigone of the bladder, occurs in less than 2% of all bladder cancer. A particular subset of adenocarcinomas may also arise from the urachus remnant located over the dome of the bladder.

There are two separate and clearly defined entities of superficial bladder cancer presentation.[12,13] The treatment for these two distinct clinical entities of bladder cancer is quite unique since the outcome and prognosis of each is quite different.

Primary flat lesions with carcinoma *in situ* are notorious for their high likelihood of recurrence and progression.[14,15] A large retrospective study demonstrated that 40% of the patients with carcinoma *in situ* developed invasive disease within 5 years.[13] Papillary tumors have a strong propensity to recur and over 70% of patients have a second primary lesion, usually within 2 years.[16,17] However, these lesions have no more than a 20% lifetime risk of progression to invasive tumors. Molecular studies have already shed some light as to the different genetic changes that may determine the morphologic appearance and progression of these two very different clinical and pathological presentations of superficial bladder cancer.[18–20]

Chromosomal Abnormalities

Neoplastic cells of the transitional cell epithelium contain many structural and numerical chromosomal changes that appear with some consistency.[21,22] These chromosomal changes in tumor cells include the under-representation or abnormally high numbers of chromosomes (aneuploidy) and the presence of easily identifiable, structurally abnormal chromosomes that are stably inherited from one cell to another (markers). In general, it has been found that low grade, noninvasive tumors are associated with a normal (diploid) number of 46 chromosomes or with numerical deviations of only a few chromosomes. High grade invasive tumors on the other hand are usually associated with gross aneuploidy and often contain marker chromosomes. The presence of marker chromosomes in low grade noninvasive tumors has been associated with a strong tendency for recurrence and progression.[22]

Cytogenetic reports on bladder cancer have demonstrated the consistent gain or loss of specific chromosomes or chromosomal regions in most tumors.[22] Cytogenetic studies have identified loss of chromosome 9 as a very frequent change in bladder tumors.[23–25] These studies often described monosomy of chromosome 9 as the most common karyotypic change.[23] Loss of chromosome 10 or deletions of only a portion of 10q have also been described as the only karyotypic abnormality.[24,25] Another specific chromosomal abnormality in bladder cancer was first reported as an isochromosome of chromosome 5p. This appears cytogenetically as a symmetrical duplication of the short arm of chromosome 5, specific for a subset of bladder cancers. Deletions and translocations of chromosome 5 are also frequently reported.[24,26]

In addition to traditional cytogenetics, novel methods now allow easier identification of genomic amplifications. A method called comparative genomic hybridization (CGH) allows fluorescent identification of amplified genomic regions in human cancers.[27,28] Recent CGH analysis of bladder cancer identified several areas of amplification and confirmed other areas of deletions.[29] Amplifications not previously seen by cytogenetics or molecular studies were identified on chromosomes 3p, 10p, 12q, 17q, 18p, and 22q. Thus, in many ways, CGH has become complementary to traditional cytogenic and molecular studies.

Genetic Loci

As mentioned previously, there have been very few reported cases of inherited bladder cancer. Families have been described without any evidence of cytogenetic abnormalities.[2] Recently, a family was identified with a translocation of 20q and 5p.[30] In addition to bladder cancer, this family also demonstrated metastatic mela-

noma. In this family, however, a putative oncogene or tumor suppressor gene has not been identified.

Sporadic Loci

Proto-oncogenes. Despite the initial discovery of a *ras* mutation in a bladder carcinoma cell line, very few *ras* gene mutations have been detected in primary transitional cell carcinoma of the bladder.[31] It now appears that less than 10% of primary bladder tumors contain *ras* gene mutations.[32,33] Some investigators have observed increased expression of *ras* protein, but this result remains unproven because of questions about the specificity of the antibodies used.[34]

Growth factors are a class of protein that bind to specific cell surface receptors, inducing a variety of responses including mitoses in susceptible target cells. Several laboratories have independently studied the expression of urothelial epidermal growth factor receptors using either immunohistochemistry to detect message with antibodies to various portions of EGFR or autoradiography with isotope labeled ligand.[18] Most groups have found a higher density of receptors on malignant cells compared to normal epithelium.[18,35] Moreover, epidermal growth factors are excreted in high concentrations in human urine, allowing incubation continually with normal premalignant and malignant urothelial cells. EGF receptors are normally found only on the basal cell layer of the bladder epithelium. They can also be richly expressed on the superficial layers of malignant tissue. This malignant distribution of receptors presumably allows greater access of malignant transitional cells to urinary EGF, and has led investigators to suspect that EGF plays a role in the development and growth of bladder cancer.[18] Others have reported that the EGFR gene is expressed mostly in high grace invasive tumors, and increased staining has been correlated with increased stage and death from disease in patients with Ta or T1 lesions.[36,37] However, other investigators have found no gross abnormalities at the DNA level, thus overexpression may be owing to an increase in mRNA transcription alone.[38] The c-*erb*B1 proto-oncogene that maps to chromosome 7 encodes the EGFR gene. Interestingly, trisomy of chromosome 7 is a frequent genetic observation in bladder tumors and could lead to an increase in EGFR expression in tumor cells.[21,22]

Although many proto-oncogenes have been identified in human tumors very few have been found to be consistently altered in bladder cancer. Increased levels of expression of growth factors such as c-*erb*B have been described as well as alterations for c-*myc* and c-*src*.[39–43] However, gross alterations or amplifications of genes have rarely been described in these primary tumors. In contrast, chromosomal loss and inactivation of tumor suppressor genes have been found to play a significant role in progression of bladder tumors.

Chromosomal Deletions and Tumor Suppressor Genes. Southern analysis with RFLP markers followed by the recent availability of highly polymorphic small repeat sequences known as microsatellites has allowed genome-wide assessment of chromosomal loss in bladder cancer.[44–48] The most common loss is the genetic event identified as loss of chromosome 9.[49] Deletion of chromosome 9 appears to be just as common in superficial tumors and invasive tumors. Inactivation of a putative tumor suppressor gene on chromosome 9 is therefore a key candidate for the initiating event in bladder carcinoma. Careful mapping of chromosome 9 with microsatellite markers has revealed that there are at least two distinct regions of loss: one on chromosome 9p21 and the second on chromosome 9q.[50–52] Southern blot analysis, multiplex comparative PCR, and FISH analysis have revealed the presence of small homozygous deletions of 9p21 in primary bladder tumors.[53,54] These deletions have also been seen in cell lines and have been implicated in the genesis of a variety of tumor types.[55,56]

Another common area of allelic loss is on chromosome 17p. Losses of 17p have correlated with mutations of *p53* and occur predominantly in invasive bladder tumors.[57,58] However, a subset of superficial tumors, especially flat lesions, have been found to contain a higher rate of 17p loss.[19,59]

Southern analysis of primary bladder tumors with polymorphic markers has revealed frequent loss of chromosome 13q at the *Rb* locus.[45] Loss of 13q has also been associated with tumors of high stage, and immunohistochemical studies have recently confirmed that *Rb* is the major target of 13q deletions in bladder tumors (see the following).[60]

A variety of other areas of allelic loss have been identified in bladder cancer. Chromosome 11p loss was originally described by Southern blot analysis and has been confirmed by microsatellite analysis.[44,47,48] Although both Wilms tumor loci are candidate targets for the deletion of 11p observed in bladder cancer, bladder tumors are not seen in the spectrum of urogenital abnormalities or as second primary malignancies in Wilms tumors.[61]

Losses of 3p, 4, 5q, 8, 14q and 18q have also been reported.[19,47,48,62] Two distinct regions of loss have been identified on chromosome 4, one on 4p and one on 4q.[63,64] There has also been a report of two distinct regions of loss on chromosome 14, one on proximal and one on distal 14q. These losses of chromosome 14q correlated closely with increasing grade and stage.[65]

The Clonal Origin of Bladder Cancer

Many bladder tumors present as multi focal disease at diagnosis. The concept of field cancerization was originally described by Slaughter to explain the occurrence of multiple skip lesions and second primary tumors in patients with aerodigestive tract tumors.[66] This hypothesis was also extended to bladder tumorigenesis to describe the possible presence of a field defect secondary to continued exposure of exogenous and endogenous compounds excreted in urine.[11]

We have examined the hypothesis of field cancerization in bladder cancer using molecular genetic techniques.[67] We tested tumors from four female patients with a method that analyses *x* chromosome inactivation, which can determine whether tumors were derived from the same precursor cell. This technique was complimented by analysis of allelic loss on various chromosomes as described previously. In each patient examined, all tumors had the same *x* chromosome inactivation, whereas normal bladder retained the same polyclonal *x* chromosome inactivation pattern as expected. Moreover, each of the evaluable tumors from a given patient had lost the same chromosome 9 allele, commonly found early in progression. Later events in progression, such as 17p and 18q, loss were not shared by different tumors from the same patient, implying that multiple tumors in the same patient arose from the uncontrolled early spread of a single transformed cell. These tumors then proceeded through independent and variable genetic events during progression. If a field defect existed, one would expect multiple independent transforming events in each tumor, implying a multiclonal origin for these lesions.

Sine this study, other investigators have confirmed the hypothesis that most multiple tumors in the bladder arise from a single progenitor cell. In another study, multiple tumors from 28 out of 30 patients were found to contain the same *x* chromosome inactivation pattern implying evolution from the same progenitor cell.[68] This understanding about bladder cancer genesis has implications for our understanding of tumor progression and may be useful for cancer diagnosis (see the following). It has also al-

lowed the designation of a preliminary progression model for bladder cancer.

Molecular Progression Model. As mentioned previously, careful characterization of genetic alterations within histopathological lesions at various stages of progression allows the delineation of a molecular progression model. We have previously defined a simple progression model for bladder cancer.[18] In this model, critical allelic losses have been placed in various steps of progression, but oncogenes are not demonstrated because they are involved, so far, in only a minority of primary bladder tumors at the genetic level. Critical steps in this model include initiation of bladder cancer owing to the inactivation of a putative tumor suppressor gene on chromosome 9, loss of *p53* function from the preinvasive to invasive state, and a variety of other genetic alterations associated with invasion and metastasis.

One interesting aspect of this progression model is the distinct differences between the progression of flat and papillary superficial lesions. Both of these lesions share a high frequency of chromosome 9 loss that remains almost unchanged during the progression to invasive tumors. However, loss of chromosome 17p is far more frequent in flat lesions and has been associated with inactivation of the *p53* gene.[19,59,69] This is intriguing because inactivation of *p53* may lead to accumulation of further genetic changes and the propensity of these lesions to acquire a more invasive phenotype. Another distinct change is loss of chromosome 14q. 14q deletion is almost exclusively seen in flat lesions or invasive tumors and virtually absent in papillary lesions.[69] Interestingly, the frequency of 14q loss is even higher in flat lesions than in invasive tumors suggesting that not all invasive tumors arise from flat lesions. 14q loss thus may lead to the initiation of flat lesions, from which only a fraction may continue to progress to invasive tumors. In this way, invasive tumors may be the final progression pathway for some papillary lesions and many flat lesions. Further characterization of the critical gene on chromosome 14q may lead to a better understanding of the events that lead to the development of flat lesions and their propensity for invasion.[65]

Specific Genes

Germ Line Mutations. Although there is no common or defined syndrome for familial bladder cancer, familial uroepithelial tumors have been reported. Often these cases appear as a manifestation of the cancer family syndrome, known as Lynch syndrome (HNPCC).[4] Of the many neoplasms that occur in these families, transitional cell carcinoma is the fourth most common, affecting individuals who manifest TCC alone, TCC and colon cancer, or TCC and other carcinomas.[70,71] Interestingly, in Lynch syndrome, TCC is predominant in the upper tract in contrast to sporadic TCC.

Mutations of mismatch repair genes, including MSH, MUT, PMS, and PMS have been found to be responsible for the majority of cases.[72-75] These genes are involved in DNA mismatch repair and belong to a highly conserved group of repair proteins. As in other sporadic tumors from this syndrome, bladder tumors display characteristic genetic instability manifested by shifts or changes in the repeat size of microsatellite markers.[76] These shifts are actually expansions and contractions of small DNA repeat elements. Approximately 2% of all sporadic bladder tumors display characteristic microsatellite instability associated with HNPCC and mismatch repair.[76]

Somatic Mutation. A candidate gene on chromosome 9p21, *p16* (*CDKN2/MTS-1*), is the most common inactivated gene in bladder cancer.[56,77] This gene has been found to be mutated in familial melanoma and pancreatic cancer.[78,79] Although a few point mutations are observed in bladder cancer cell lines, the vast majority of primary tumors with loss of heterozygosity of 9p21 do not contain obvious mutations of *p16*.[80,81] This finding pointed to alternative mechanisms for gene inactivation or potentially that a second tumor suppressor gene resided nearby. Recently, we have shown that homozygous deletions of chromosome 9p21 stretching into the *p16* locus are quite common in primary bladder tumors.[54] Much of the controversy surrounding this locus stems from difficulty in identifying homozygous deletions in primary tumors because of contaminating non-neoplastic cells. However, using the strategy of fine microsatellite mapping, homozygous deletions can be identified by the apparent retention of one or two closely spaced markers among a large region demonstrating loss of heterozygosity.[54] These results were confirmed in a number of cases by Southern blot and FISH analysis demonstrating the specificity of the technique. It is now clear that at least 50% of all bladder tumors contain a homozygous deletion that includes *p16*. Moreover, we have demonstrated other alternative mechanisms of inactivation including methylation of the *p16* promoter leading to transcriptional block and inactivation of *p16*.[82] Although methylation is common in many other tumor types, inactivation of *p16* by methylation is still uncommon in bladder cancer. Further analysis of a putative second tumor suppressor locus on chromosome 9 is hampered in bladder cancer by the wide occurrence of monosomy, perhaps indicating inactivation of a gene on chromosome 9q. Although the *patched* gene, inactivated in Gorlin's syndrome and sporadic basal cell carcinoma, has been found on chromosome 9q, any role in bladder cancer has not been defined.[83–85] Mutations of *p53* are ubiquitous in human cancer and bladder cancer is no exception.[86] Losses of 17p have correlated well with sequence analysis of *p53* mutations and occur predominantly in invasive bladder tumors.[57] However, a subset of superficial tumors, especially flat lesions, have been found to contain these mutations. Importantly, a large study based on immunohistochemical analysis of *p53* demonstrated a significant decrease in overall survival for *p53* positive patients versus those with tumors that were *p53* negative.[87] It was implied that mutation of *p53* was an independently poor prognostic factor regardless of stage or therapy.

Inactivation of *p53* is critical in many tumor types.[86] It has been postulated that *p53* is a critical regulator of response to DNA damage.[88] The appropriate presence of wild-type *p53* leads to growth arrest in the presence of damage and perhaps to apoptosis with excessive damage. Cells that lack *p53* protein are unable to undergo a normal G_1S arrest and perhaps propagate further accumulated genetic damage.

A number of lines of evidence also point to a role for the *Rb* gene in bladder carcinogenesis. Immunohistochemical studies have confirmed that *Rb* is the target of 13q deletions in most bladder cancers.[60] A substantially worse prognosis for those tumors with negative standing has also been reported.[89,90] Moreover, reintroduction of the *Rb* gene leads to slowing of cell growth and tumorigenicity in bladder carcinoma cells.[91] The regulatory function of the *Rb* protein appears to be controlled by phosphorylation during the G_1S phase of the cell cycle.[92] *p16*, one of a number of CDK inhibitors, is also critical for this pathway. In many ways, inactivation of both *p16* and *Rb* may be redundant and in fact, tumors have demonstrated inactivation of one or the other of these genes but generally not both.[88] Analysis of *Rb* and *p16* status directly in bladder cancer have not been done on the same tumors. It is tempting to speculate however, that the Cyclin D1/*p16*/*Rb* pathway is vital in bladder cancer as in many other tumor types.

In Vitro Systems

In vitro models have been essential for much of the molecular work done on bladder cancers. Transformation of bladder epithelial cell lines that harbor allelic losses similar to those seen in primary human tumors have helped in the cloning of critical tumor suppressor genes.[93,94] Transfection of human cell lines followed by reintroduction into animal bladders or renal capsules also have been important models.[95] Transfection of indolent transitional cell carcinoma with protooncogenes will not only increase expression of epidermal growth factor receptors but also can increase proliferate responses to EGF as well.[96] Moreover, transfection of tumor suppressor genes leads to diminished growth in these models. Furthermore, these models may be useful to test therapeutic efficacy before clinical trials.[97]

Implications for Diagnosis

Microsatellite DNA markers are not only used for mapping primary tumors but also can be used for tumor detection. Microsatellite markers allow detection of loss of heterozygosity or genomic instability in primary tumors.[98] In a blinded study, urine samples from 25 patients with suspicious bladder lesions were analyzed by microsatellite analysis and compared to normal DNA from the same patients. Microsatellite changes matching those in the tumor were detected in the urine sediment in 19 of the 20 patients (95%) who were diagnosed with bladder cancer. Urine cytology detected cancer cells in only 50% of these same samples.

The most common microsatellite abnormality detected in urine was loss of heterozygosity at critical chromosomal loci.[98] As mentioned earlier in the molecular progression model, early changes including loss of chromosome 9p and 14q were instrumental in the diagnosis of these patients. Moreover, although widespread microsatellite instability is only associated with HNPCC, occasional microsatellite alterations are not uncommon. These microsatellite expansions or deletions are rare in small repeats but are more common in larger repeats, including tri- and tetranucleotides repeat sequences.[99] It appears that certain repeats are more susceptible to alterations and can be found with a relatively high frequency in many sporadic tumors including bladder cancers. At least 15% of the patients in this study were diagnosed by microsatellite alterations that would not have been diagnosed by loss of heterozygosity.[98]

In the study, tumors of all grades and stages were detected, including the difficult to diagnose low grade papillary tumors.[98] In many cases that were considered atypical but not diagnostic for cancer by cytology, the correct diagnosis was established by molecular analysis. Importantly, control patients without cancer did not demonstrate any of the abnormalities. Followup studies have continued to suggest that the molecular analysis of urine will be an important and accurate addition for the detection of tumor recurrences. Moreover, the ability to automate this technique with fluorescent labeling and microcapillary electrophoresis may make this a rapidly useful clinical test.[100] The final implementation awaits the completion of large prospective clinical trials to assess overall efficacy.

SUMMARY

The recent explosion in our understanding of the genetic events that underlie the progression of human cancer have allowed us to consider novel approaches for diagnosis and treatment. For bladder cancer, a preliminary progression model already suggests specific genetic differences between papillary and flat lesions that may be critical for the treatment of these patients. These models have also led to the development of molecular markers that promise exquisite specificity and sensitivity for the early detection of cancer and for diagnosis of recurrent cases. The fact that most recurrent disease is owing to the expansion of a single progenitor cell may allow us to develop rational therapeutic targets. Critical changes like *p53* that may lead to a poor outcome, might also yield novel, specific therapeutic strategies. It is certain that the future promises to bring exciting new discoveries that will bring molecular biology closer to the forefront of clinical medicine.

REFERENCES

1. Parker SL, Tong T, Bolden S, Wingo PA: Cancer statistics 1996. *CA Cancer J Clin* **5**:27, 1996.
2. Schulte PA: The role of genetic factors in bladder cancer *Cancer Detect Prev* **11**(3–6):379–388, 1988.
3. Kantor AF, Hartge P, Hoover RN, et al: Familial and environmental interaction in bladder cancer. *Int J Cancer* **35**:703–706, 1985.
4. Lynch HT: Genetics, natural history, tumor spectrum, and pathology of hereditary nonpolyposis colorectal cancer: An updated review. *Gastroenterology* **104**(5):1535–1549, 1993.
5. Tawfik HN: Carcinoma of the urinary bladder associated with schistosomaisis in Egypt: The possible causal relationship. *International Symposium of the Princes Takamatsu Cancer Research Fund* **18**:197–199, 1987.
6. McCredie M, Stewart JH, Ford JM, et al: Phenacetin analgesics and and cancer of the bladder or renal pelvis in women. *Br J Urol* **55**:220–224, 1983.
7. Piper JM, Tonocia J, Matanoski GM: Heavy phenacetin use and bladder cancer in women aged 20 to 49 years. *N Engl J Med* **313**:292–295, 1985.
8. Silverman DT, Hartge P, Morrison AS, et al: Epidemiology of bladder cancer. *Hematol Oncol Clin North Am* **6**:1–30, 1992.
9. Augustine A, Hebert JR, Kabat GC, et al: Bladder cancer in relation to cigarette smoking. *Cancer Res* **48**:4405–4408, 1988.
10. Burch JD, Rohan TE, Howe GR, et al: Risk of bladder cancer by source and type of tobacco exposure: A case study. *Int J Cancer* **44**:622–628, 1989.
11. Fair WR, Fuks ZY, Scher HI: Cancer of the bladder, in Devita VT, Hellman S, Rosenberg SA (eds.): *Cancer: Principles and Practices of Oncology*. 1052–1072. Philadelphia, J.B. Lippincott, 1993.
12. Friedell GH, Soloway MS, Hilgar AG, et al: Summary of workship on carcinoma in situ of the bladder. *J Urol* **136**:1047–1048.
13. Tannenbaum M, Romas NA, Droller MJ: The pathobiology of early urothelial cancer, in Skinner DG, Leiskovsky G. (eds.): *Genitourinary Cancer*. Philadelphia, W.B. Saunders, 1988.
14. Althausen AF, Prout GR, Jr, Daly JJ: Noninvasive papillary carcinoma of the bladder associated with carcinoma in situ. *J Urol* **116**:575–579, 1976.
15. Farrow GM, Utz DC, Rife CC, et al: Clinical observation of sixty cases of in situ carcinoma of the urinary bladder. *Cancer Res* **37**:2794–2798, 1977.
16. Heney NM, Ahmed S, Flanagan MJ: Superficial bladder cancer: Progression and recurrence. *J Urol* **130**:1083–1086, 1983.
17. Fitzpatrick JM, West AB, Butler MR: Superficial bladder tumors (Stage pTa, Grade 1 and 2): The importance of recurrence pattern following initial resection *J Urol* **135**:920–922, 1986.
18. Sidransky D, Messing E: Molecular genetics and biochemical mechanisms in bladder cancer: Oncogenes, tumor suppressor genes, and growth factors. *Urol Clin North Am* **19**(4):629–639, 1992.
19. Dalbagni S, Presti JC, Reuter VE, Fair WR, and Cordon-Cardo, C: Genetic alterations in bladder cancer. *Lancet* **342**:469, 1993.
20. Spruck CH, Ohneseit PF, Gonzalez M, et al: Two molecular pathways to transition cell carcinoma of the bladder. *Cancer Res* **54**:784–788, 1994.
21. Sandberg AA: *The Chromosomes in Human Cancer and Leukemia*, 2nd ed. Elsevier Science Publishing Co., New York, 1990.

22. Sandberg AA: Chromosome changes in bladder cancer: Clinical and other correlations. *Cancer Genet Cytogenet* **19**(1–2), 163–175, 1986.
23. Smeets W, Pauwels R, Laarakkers L, Debruyne F, & Geraedts J: Chromosomal analysis of bladder cancer. III. Nonrandom alterations. *Cancer Genet Cytogenet* **29**(1), 29, 1987.
24. Berger CS, Sandberg AA, Todd IAD, Pennington RD, Haddad FS, Hecht BK, Hecht F: Chromosomes in kidney, ureter, and bladder cancer. *Cancer Genet Cytogenet* **23**:1, 1986.
25. Gibas Z, Prout GJ, Connolly JG, Prontes JE, & Sandberg AA: Nonrandom chromosomal changes in transitional cell carcinoma of the bladder. *Cancer Res* **44**(3):1257, 1984.
26. Gibas Z, Prout GR, Pontes JE, Connolly JG, & Sandberg AA: A possible specific chromosome change in transitional cell carcinoma of the bladder. *Cancer Genet Cytogenet* **19**(3), 229, 1986.
27. Kallioniemi A, Kallioniemi OP, Sudar D, Rutovitz D, Gray JW, Waldman F, Pinkel D: Comparative genomic hybridization for molecular cytogenetic analysis of solid tumors. *Science* **258**(5083):818, 1992.
28. du Manoir S, Speicher MR, Joos S, Schrock E, Popp S, Dohner H, Kovacs G, Robert M, Lichter P, Cremer T: Detection of complete and partial chromosome gains and losses by comparative genomic in situ hybridization. *Human Genetics* **90**(6):590, 1993.
29. Voorter C, Joos S, Vallinga M, Bringuier P, Poddighe P, Schalken J, du Manior S, Ramaekers F, Lichter P, Hopman A: Detection of chromosomal imbalances in transitional cell carcinoma of the bladder by comparative genomic hybridization. *Am J Pathol* **146**(6):1341, 1995.
30. Schoenberg M, Kiemeney L, Walsh PC, Griffin CA, Sidransky D: Germline translocation t(5)(p15) and familial transitional cell carcinoma. *J Urol* **155**(3):1035, 1996.
31. Reddy EP, Reynolds RK, Santos E, & Barbacid M: A point mutation is responsible for the acquisition of transforming properties by the T24 human bladder carcinoma oncogene. *Nature* **300**(5888):149, 1982.
32. Knowles MA, Williamson M: Mutation of H*ras* is infrequent in bladder cancer: Confirmation by single conformation polymorphism analysis, designed restriction fragment length polymorphisms, and direct sequencing. *Cancer Res* **53**:133, 1993.
33. Fujita J, Srivastava SK, Kraus MH, Rhim JS, Tronick SR, & Aaronson SA: Frequency of molecular alterations affecting *ras* protooncogenes in human urinary tract tumors. *PNAS USA* **82**(11):3849, 1985.
34. Viola MV, Fromowitz F, Oravez S, Deb S, and Schlom J: *ras* oncogene p21 expression is increased in premalignant lesions and high gradebladder carcinoma. *J Exp Med* **161**:1213, 1985.
35. Messing EM and Reznikoff CA: Normal and malignant urothelium: In effects of epidermal growth factor. *Cancer Res* **47**:2230, 1987.
36. Neal DE, Marsh C, Bennett MK, Abel PD, Hall RR, Sainsbury JR, & Harris, AL: Epidermal receptors in human bladder cancer: Comparison of invasive and superficial tumours. *Lancet* **1**(8425):366, 1985.
37. Neal DE, Sharples L, Smith K, Fennelly J, Hall RR and Harris AL: The epidermal growth factor receptor and the prognosis of bladder cancer. *Cancer* **65**:1619, 1990.
38. Berger MS, Greenfield C, Gullick WJ, Haley J, Downward J, Neal DE, Harris AL and Waterfieldm MD: Evaluation of epidermal growth factor receptors in bladder tumours. *Br J Cancer* **56**:533, 1987.
39. Coombs LM, Pigott DA, Sweeney E, Proctor AJ, Eydmann ME, Parkinson C, & Knowles MA: Amplification and over of c-erbB2 in transitional cell carcinoma of the urinary bladder. *Cancer* **63**(4):601, 1991.
40. Wright C, Mellon K, Neal DE, Johnston P, Corbett IP and Horne CH: Expression of c-erbB2 protein product in bladder cancer. *Br J Cancer* **62**:764, 1990.
41. Masters JR, Vesey SG, Munn CF, Evan GI, & Watson, JV: c-myc oncoprotein levels in bladder cancer. *Urol Res* **16**(5):341, 1988.
42. Del-Senno L, Maestri I, Piva R, Hanau S, Reggiani A, Romano A and Russo, G: Differential hypomethylation of the c-myc proto in bladder cancers at different stages and grades. *J Urol* **142**:146, 1989.
43. Fanning P, Bulovas K, Saini KS: Elevated expression of pp60[c-src] in low grade bladder carcinomas. *Cancer Res* **52**:1457, 1992.
44. Fearon ER, Feinberg AP, Hamilton SH, & Vogelstein B: Loss of genes on the short arm of chromosome 11 in bladder cancer. *Nature* **318**(6044):377, 1985.
45. Cairns P, Proctor AJ and Knowles MA: Loss of heterozygosity at the Rb locus is frequent and correlates with muscle invasion in bladder carcinoma. *Oncogene* **6**:2305, 1991.

46. Tsai YC, Nichols PW, Hiti AL, Williams Z, Skinner DG & Jones PA: Allelic losses of chromosomes 9, 11, and 17 in human bladder cancer. *Cancer Res* **50**:44, 1990.

47. Presti JC, Reuter VW, Galan T, Fair WR and Cordon C: Molecular genetic alterations in superficial and locally advanced human bladder cancer. *Cancer Res* **51**:5405, 1991.

48. Knowles MA, Elder PA, Williamson M, Cairns JP, Shaw ME, and Law MG: Allelotype of human bladder cancer. *Cancer Research* **54**:531, 1994.

49. Cairns P, Shaw ME, Knowles MA: Initiation of bladder cancer may involve deletion of a tumor suppressor gene on chromosome 9. *Oncogene* **8**:1083, 1993.

50. Ruppert JM, Tokino K and Sidransky D: Evidence for two bladder cancer suppressor loci on human chromosome 9. *Cancer Res* **53**:5093–5094, 1993. *Cancer Res* **54**(6):1422, 1994.

51. Cairns P, Shaw ME and Knowles MA: Preliminary mapping of the deleted region of chromosome 9 in bladder cancer. *Cancer Res* **53**:1230, 1993.

52. Linnenbach AJ, Pressler LB, Seng BA, Kimmel BS, Tomaszewski JE, and Malkowicz SB: Characterization of chromosome 9 deletions in transitional cell carcinoma by microsatellite assay. *Hum Mol Genet* **2**(9):1407, 1993.

53. Cairns P, Tokino K, Eby Y, Sidransky D: Homozygous deletions of 9p21 in primary human bladder tumors detected by comparative multiplex PCR. *Cancer Res* **54**(6):1422, 1994.

54. Cairns P, Polascik TJ, Eby Y, Tokino K, Califano J, Merlo A, Mao L, Herath J, Jenkins R, Westra W, Rutter JL, Buckler A, Gabrielson E, Tockman M, Cho KR, Hedrick L, Bova GS, Issacs W, Schwab D, Sidransky D: Frequency of homozygous deletion at p16/CDKN2 in primary human tumors. *Nat Genet* **11**(2):210, 1995.

55. Olopade OI, Buchhagen DL, Malik K, Sherman J, Nobori T, Bader S, Nau MM, Gazdar AF, Minna JD and Diaz MO: Homozygous loss of the interferon genes defines the critical region on 9p that is deleted in lung cancers. *Cancer Res* **53**:2410, 1993.

56. Kamb A, Gruis NA, Weaver-Feldhaus J, Liu Q, Harshman K, Tavtigian SV, Stockert E, Day RS, Johnson BE and Skolnick MH: A cell cycle regulator potentially involved in genesis of many tumor types. *Science* **264**:436, 1994.

57. Sidransky D, von Eschenbach A, Tsai YC, Jones P, Summerhayes I, Marshall F, Paul M, Green P, Hamilton SR, Frost P and Vogelstein B: Identification of p53 gene mutations in bladder cancers and urine samples. *Science* **252**:706–709, 1991.

58. Habuchi T, Ogawa O, Kaheki Y, Sugiyama T, and Yoshida O: Allelic loss of chromosome 17p in urothelial cancer: Strong association with invasive phenotype. *J Urol* **148**:1595, 1992.

59. Fujimoto K, Yamada Y, Okajima E: Frequent association of p53 mutation in invasive bladder cancer. *Cancer Res* **52**:1393, 1992.

60. Xu HJ, Cairns P, Hu SX, Knowles MA, Benedict WF: Loss of Rb protein expression in primary bladder cancer correlates with loss of heterozygosity at the Rb locus and tumor progression. *Int J Cancer* **53**(5):781, 1993.

61. Hawkins MM, Draper GJ, & Smith RA: Cancer among 1,348 offspring of survivors of childhood cancer. *Int J Cancer* **43**(6):975, 1989.

62. Wu S, Storer BE, Bookland EA, Klingelhutz AJ, Gilchrsit KW, Meisner LF, Oyasu R, and Reznikoff CA: Nonrandom chromosome losses in stepwise neoplastic transformation in vitro of human uroepithelial cells. *Cancer Res* **51**:3323, 1991.

63. Elder PA, Bell SM, Knowles MA: Deletion of two regions on chromosome 4 in bladder carcinoma: Definition of a critical 750KB region at 4p16.3. *Oncogene* **9**(12):3433, 1994.

64. Polascik TJ, Cairns P, Chang WY, Schoenberg MP, Sidransky D: Distinct regions of allelic loss on human chromosome 4 in primary bladder carcinoma. *Cancer Res* **55**(22):5396, 1995.

65. Chang WY, Cairns P, Schoenberg MP, Polasick TJ, Sidransky D: Novel suppressor loci on chromosome 14q in primary bladder cancer. *Cancer Res* **55**(15):3246, 1995.

66. Slaughter DL, Southwick HW, and Smejkal W: Field cancerization in oral stratified squamous epithelium: Clinical implications of multicentric origin. *Cancer* **6**:963, 1953.

67. Sidransky D, Frost P, Von Eschenbach A, Oyasu R, Preisinger AC and Vogelstein B: Clonal origin of bladder cancer. *N Engl J Med* **326**:737, 1992.

68. Hiyao N, Tsai YC, Lerner SP, Olumi AF, Spruck CH, 3rd, Gonzalez M, Nichols PW, Skinner DG, Jones PA: Role_ocRole of chromosome 9 in human bladder cancer. *Cancer Res* **53**(17):4066, 1993.

69. Rosin MP, Cairns P, Epstein JI, Schoenberg MP, Sidransky D: An allelotype of carcinoma in situ of the human bladder. *Cancer Res* **55**:5213, 1995.

70. Vasen HF, Offerhaus GJ, den Hartog Jager FC, Menko FH, Nagengast FM, Griffioen G, van Role_oc Hogezand RB, Heintz AP: The tumour spectrum in hereditary non-polyposis colorectal cancer: A study of 24 kindreds in the netherlands. *Int J Cancer* **46**(1):31, 1990.

71. Lynch HT, Ens JA, Lynch JF: The Lynch Syndrome II and urological malignancies. *J Urol* **143**:24, 1990.

72. Cleaver JE: It was a very good year for DNA repair. *Cell* **76**:1, 1994.

73. Bronner CE, Baker SM, Morrison PT, Warren G, Smith LG, Lescoe MK, Kane M, Earabino C, Lipford J, Lindblom A, Tannergard P, Bollag RJ, Godwin AR, Ward DC, Nordenskjold M, Fishel R, Kolodner R, Liskay RM: Mutation in the DNA mismatch repair gene homologue hMLH1 is associated with hereditary non-polyposis colon cancer. *Nature* **368**:258, 1994.

74. Nicolaides NC, Popadopoulos N, Liu B, Wel Y, Carter KC, Ruben SM, Rosen CA, Haseltine WA, Fleischmann RD, Fraser CM, Adams MD, Venter JC, Dunlop MG, Hamilton SR, Petersen GM, de la Chapelle A, Vogelstein B, Kinzler K: Mutations of two PMS homologues in hereditary nonpolyposis colon cancer. *Nature* **371**:75, 1994.

75. Liu B, Parsons R, Papadopoulos N, Nicolaides NC, Lynch HT, Watson P, Jass JR, Dunlop M, Wyllie A, Peltomaki P, de la Chapelle A, Hamilton SR, Vogelstein B, Kinzler KW: Analysis of mismatch repair genes in hereditary non-polyposis colorectal cancer patients. *Nat Med* **2**(2):169, 1996.

76. Gonzalez M, Ruppert JM, Tokino K, Tsai YC, Spruck CH, III, Miyao N, Nichols PW, Hermann GG, Horn T, Steven K, Summerhayes IC, Sidransky D, Jones PW: Microsatellite instability in bladder cancer. *Cancer Research* **53**:5620, 1993.

77. Serrano M, Hannon GJ, Beach D: A new regulatory motif in cell control causing specific inhibition of Cyclin D^{CDK4}. *Nature* **366**:704, 1993.

78. Hussussian CJ, Struewing JP, Goldstein AM, Higgins PAT, Ally DS, Sheahan MD, Clark Jr., WH, Tucker MA, and Dracopoli NC: Germline p16 mutations in familial melanoma. *Nat Genet* **8**:15, 1994.

79. Caldas C, Hahn SA, da Costa LT, Redston MS, Schutte M, Seymour AB, Weinstein, CL, Hruban RH, Yeo CJ, and Kern SE: Frequent somatic mutations and homozygous deletions of the p16 (MTS1) gene in pancreatic adenocarcinoma. *Nat Genet* **8**:27, 1994.

80. Cairns P, Mao L, Merlo A, Lee D, Schwab D, Eby Y, Tokino K, van der Reit P, Blaugrund J, and Sidransky D: Rates of p16 (MTS1) mutations in primary tumors with 9p loss. *Science* **256**:415, 1994.

81. Spruck CH, Gonzalez-Zuleta M, Shibata A, Simoneau AR, Lin M-F, Gonzales F, Tsai Y and Jones PA: p16 gene in uncultured tumors. *Nature* **370**:183, 1994.

82. Merlo A, Herman JG, Mao L, Lee DJ, Schwab D, Burger PC, Baylin SB, Sidransky D: 5′ CpG island methylation is associated with transcriptional silencing of the tumour suppressor p16/CDKN2/MTS1 in human cancers. *Nat Med* **7**(1):686, 1995.

83. Johnson RL, Rothman AL, Xie J, Goodrich LV, Bare JW, Bonifas JM, Quinn AG, Myers RM, Cox DR, Epstein EH, Scott MP: Human homolog of patched, a candidate gene for the basal cell nevus syndrome. *Science* **272**:1668, 1996.

84. Hahn H, Wicking C, Zaphiropoulos PG, Gailani MR, Shanley S, Chidambaram A, Vorechovsky I, Holmberg E, Unden AB, Gillies S, Negus K, Smyth I, Pressman C, Leffell DJ, Gerrard B, Goldstein AM, Den M, Toftgard R, Chenevix G, Wainwright B, Bale AE: Mutations of the human homolog of drosphila patched in the nevoid basel cell carcinoma syndrome. *Cell* **85**:841, 1996.

85. Gailani MR, StÂhleckdahl M, Leffell DJ, Glynn M, Zaphiropoulos PG, Pressman C, UndEn AB, Dean M, Brash DE, Bale AE, ToftgÂrd R: The role of the human homologue of drosphila patched in sporadic basal cell carcinomas. *Nature Genetics, in press,* 1996.

86. Hollstein M, Sidransky D, Vogelstein B, Harris C: p53 mutations in human cancer. *Science* **253**:49, 1991.

87. Esrig D, Elmajian D, Groshen S, Freeman JA, Stein JP, Chen S, Nichols PW, Skinner DG, Jones PA, Cote RJ: Accumulation of nuclear p53 and tumor progression in bladder cancer. *N Engl J Med* **331**(19):1259, 1994.

88. Hartwell LH, Kastan MB: *Science* **266**(5192):1821, 1994.

89. Cordon C, Wartinger D, Petrylak D, et al: Altered expression of retinoblastoma gene product: Prognostic indicator in bladder cancer. *J Nat Cancer Inst* **84**:1251, 1992.

90. Logothetis CJ, Xu HJ, Ro JY, et al: Altered expression of retinoblastoma protein and known prognostic variables in locally advanced bladder cancer. *J Nat Cancer Inst* **84**:1256, 1992.
91. Takahashi R, Hashimoto T, Hu HJ, et al: The retinoblastoma gene functions as a growth and tumor suppressor in human bladder carcinoma cells. *Proc Natl Acad Sci (USA)* **88**:5257, 1991.
92. Mihara K, Cao XR, Yen A, et al: Cell cycle regulation of phosphorylation of human Rb gene product. *Science* **246**:1300, 1989.
93. Reznikoff CA, Kao C, Messing EM, Newton M, Swaminathan S: A molecular genetic model of human bladder carcinogenesis. *Sem Cancer Biol* **4**(3):143, 1993.
94. Kao C, Wu SQ, Bhatthacharya M, Meisner LF, Reznikoff CA: Losses of 3p, 11p, and 13q in EJ/*ras* simian virus 40 human uroepithelial cells. *Genes, Chromosomes Cancer* **4**(2):158, 1992.
95. Theodorescu D, Cornil I, Fernandez BJ, Kerbel RS: Overexpression of normal and mutated forms of HRAS induces orthotopic bladder invasion in a human transitional cell carcinoma. *Proc Natl Acad Sci USA* **87**(22):9047, 1990.
96. Theodorescu D, Cornil I, Sheehan C, Man MS, Kerbel RS: Ha-ras induction of the invasive phenotype results in up of epidermal growth factor receptors and altered responsiveness to epidermal growth factor in human papillary transitional cell carcinoma cells. *Cancer Res* **51**(16):4486, 1991.
97. Theodorescu D, Connors KM, Groce A, Hoffman RM, Kerbel RS: Lack of influence of c-*ras* expression on the drug sensitivity of human bladder cancer histocultured in three. *Anticancer Res* **13**(4):941, 1993.
98. Mao L, Schoenberg MP, Scicchitano M, Erozan YS, Merlo A, Schwab D, Sidransky D: Molecular detection of primary bladder cancer by microsatellite analysis. *Science* **271**:659, 1996.
99. Mao L, Tockman MS, Erozan YS, Askin F, Sidransky D: Microsatellite alterations as clonal markers in the detection of human cancer. *Proc Natl Acad Sci (USA)* **91**:9871, 1994.
100. Wang Y, Ju J, Carpenter BA, Atherton JM, Sensabaugh GF, Mathies RA: Rapid sizing of short tandem repeat alleles using capillary array electrophoresis and energy fluorescent primers. *Anal Chem* **67**(1):1197, 1995.

CHAPTER 38

Stomach Cancer

Steven M. Powell

1. Adenocarcinoma comprises the vast majority of malignant tumors arising from the stomach. Gastric adenocarcinoma is a significant worldwide health burden, second only to lung tumors as a leading cause of cancer deaths. Significant geographic and temporal variances is observed in this cancer's incidence, predominantly of the intestinal type. Epidemiologic studies indicate a strong environmental component in the acquisition of this cancer. Developing countries which are noted to have a high prevalence of *Helicobacter pylori* infection early in life are distinctly prone to having high rates of gastric adenocarcinomas. Most gastric cancers are identified in advanced stages that present in the later decades of adult life and result in a lethal outcome shortly thereafter.

2. Gastric cancers exhibit heterogeneity in clinical, biologic, and genetic aspects. Multiple pathological classifications of gastric adenocarcinomas exist including those with morphologic and histologic criteria. The TNM staging system is generally used as the basis for prognostication in this cancer with depth of infiltration being an important parameter in this matter. Most cases of stomach cancer are sporadic in nature, with rare reports of an apparent inherited gastric cancer predisposition trait, usually in conjunction with the hereditary nonpolyposis colon cancer disease entity.

3. Cytogenetic studies have been unsuccessful in identifying an obvious significant chromosomal aberration in gastric cancers. Loss of heterozygosity studies have identified several loci with significant allelic loss, thus indicating the possibility of harboring a tumor suppressor gene important in gastric tumorigenesis. The exact target(s) of loss in most of these chromosomal regions of significant loss including 5q and 18q remains to be clarified. Additionally, evidence of Epstein-Barr virus infection can be found in a minority of gastric cancer cases.

4. Multiple somatic alterations have been described in gastric carcinomas at the molecular level. The significance of these changes in gastric tumorigenesis remains to be established in most instances. The p53 gene is consistently altered in a majority of gastric cancer cases. Microsatellite instability and associated alteration of the transforming growth factor β II receptor gene are found in a subset of gastric carcinomas. Cell adhesion abnormalities such as E-cadherin or associated molecule alterations may play an important role in diffuse type gastric cancer development. A detailed, clear working model of gastric tumorigenesis has yet to be formulated. Thus, improved diagnostic, prognostic, therapeu-tic, and preventive strategies are eagerly awaited for gastric carcinomas. Critical molecular alterations which are prevalent in these cancers once fully characterized may ultimately provide new avenues to combat this lethal disease.[1]

CLINICAL ASPECTS

Gastric adenocarcinoma is the predominant cancer of the stomach, accounting for over 95 percent of cases. Lymphomas, leiomyosarcomas, and carcinoid lesions represent only a minority of stomach tumors. Once the leading cause of cancer deaths in the United States, the incidence of gastric cancer in developed countries has declined dramatically. Adenocarcinomas of the gastroesophageal junction which commonly arise from Barrett's esophagus, on the other hand, appear to be on the rise most recently in several populations for unclear reasons.[2,3] Adenocarcinoma of the stomach remains a leading cause of cancer death worldwide and continues to be responsible for the majority of cancer deaths in developing countries.[4,5]

Most cases of gastric cancer appear to occur sporadically without an obvious inherited component. The only well-characterized inherited predisposition syndrome potentially involving gastric cancer development is hereditary nonpolyposis colon cancer (HNPCC), which includes potential tumor development in a variety of tissue types.[6] Germ line genetic abnormalities of mismatch repair genes underlying this disease entity have recently been unveiled, as discussed in Chap. 17. The isolation of these genes should allow better definition of the fraction of gastric cancers which result from this inherited cancer predisposition trait. Interestingly, fewer gastric cancers have been noted to be associated with HNPCC, correlating with the recent general decline in incidence of gastric cancer in developed countries. Rare kindreds exhibiting site-specific gastric cancer predilection have been reported, occasionally associated with other inherited abnormalities.[7-9] Case-control studies suggest a small but consistent increased risk of gastric cancer in first-degree relatives of patients with gastric adenocarcinoma with some familial clustering also exhibited.[10-12] Notably, Napoleon Bonaparte's family was afflicted with this cancer.

Epidemiology

Significant geographic variability in incidence both internationally and intranationally is observed. In the early 1990s incidence rates varied from 60.1 per 100,000 in Costa Rica to 7.3 per 100,000 in the United States.[13] Epidemiologic studies which include migration and temporal analyses indicate that environmental factors, especially in the first decades of life, are important in the etiology of gastric cancers.[14,15] Notably, a consistent predominance of gastric cancers in males (approximately 2:1 ratio) is seen across worldwide populations.

Helicobacter pylori infection has recently been implicated as an etiologic factor in gastric cancer development, both adenocarcinoma and primary Non-Hodgkin lymphoma.[16–18] Evidence continues to accumulate that this infection, especially when contracted early in life as commonly occurs in developing countries, leads to chronic gastric inflammation with subsequent fivefold to sixfold risk of gastric cancer development.[19] This risk of cancer development in infected persons is dependent on as yet unidentified cofactors and its pathophysiologic mechanism remains to be elucidated. Similarly, chronic gastritis and resultant atrophy from pernicious anemia appear to be associated with an increased risk, albeit small, of gastric cancer development.[20]

Evidence of Epstein-Barr virus (EBV) infection has been demonstrated in a small proportion (approximately 10 percent) of gastric carcinomas by *in situ* hybridization with specific RNA probes.[21–24] The monoclonal nature of EBV genomes in virtually all neoplastic cells of these tumors along with signficiant prior antibody levels suggests infection by this virus may not be so latent. The classic proteins associated with cell transformation of EBV infection, LMP1 and EBNA2, do not appear to be expressed in these gastric cancers; however, EBNA1 was shown to be expressed in most virus-associated tumor cells.[24,25] A significant lymphoid infiltration and tendency toward prolonged survival has been observed in gastric cancers harboring detectable EBV. Further studies are needed to determine the role of this infection in human gastric tumorgenesis.

Dietary irritants (i.e., salts or preservatives) and potential carcinogens (i.e., nitrates) have been suggested as etiologic factors of gastric cancer,[26] yet no specific agent has been definitively indicted. Additionally, several protective factors such as fruits, vegetables, ascorbic acid, alpha-tocopherol, onions, and gastric acidity have been indicated; yet the specific agents responsible for mechanism of action remains elusive. Molecular studies may help clarify these issues.

Pathology

Gastric adenocarcinomas display several distinct morphologic, histologic, and biologic characteristics. Thus, multiple tumor classification systems have been created to characterize these lesions pathologically in attempts to confer their natural history. Lauren described histopathologic subtypes of gastric adenocarcinomas as intestinal type (expansive or gland-forming) or diffuse type (infiltrative or scattered neoplastic cells), and this classification is widely applied.[27] Evidence continues to accumulate suggesting that these two subtypes of gastric cancer arise in different settings and have distinctive biologic behavior.[28] Intestinal-type gastric adenocarcinomas tend to predominante in high-risk geographic regions, arise in association with precursor lesions (i.e., chronic atrophic gastritis or intestinal metaplasia), and occur more distally and later in life (usually after the sixth decade of life); whereas the diffuse type of gastric cancers appear to have a relatively constant incidence, arise without identifiable precursor lesions, and present earlier in life and more diffusely in the stomach. Additionally, intestinal-type gastric cancers tend to spread hematogenously to the liver, while diffuse-type gastric cancers tend to spread more contiguously into the peritoneum. Moreover, although some mol-

ecular alterations are shared, distinct genetic abnormalities appear to occur with specific biological phenotypes (see below).

Additional histologic classifications for gastric carcinoma have been developed (i.e., World Health Organization[29] and Ming[30]), which involve tissue architecture and differentiation criteria. The traditional classification of Borman is based on morphologic criteria.[31] Goeski has even developed criteria which examine mucin content and degree of cellular atypia as potentially distinctive prognostic features of gastric tumors.[32,33]

The TMN staging classification[34] is primarily used in staging cancers at diagnosis, to assess resectability and prognoses. The primary tumor's depth is one of the most important parameters in this determination. The concept of early gastric adenocarcinomas[35] (tumors confined to the mucosa or submucosa) originated in Japan,[35] and patients are observed to have much better 5-year survival rates (over 90 percent) versus more advanced lesions (less than 20 percent for stage III or IV). Unfortunately most cases of gastric cancer are diagnosed in more advanced stages for which effective systemic therapy is limited and surgery reserved for palliation. Mass screening programs in high-risk regions such as Japan have helped in diagnosing some of these cancers at earlier stages, but significant improvements in diagnosis, prognostication, and therapy are eagerly awaited to make a substantial impact on this cancer's mortality.

ALTERED GENETIC LOCI

Other than those cases associated with HNPCC and mismatch repair gene alterations, no germ line genetic abnormality has been convincingly linked to an inherited predisposition toward the development of gastric carcinoma. Large kindreds with an obvious highly penetrant inherited predisposition for the development of this cancer, having the potential power to link disease markers, are rare. Of note, the blood group A phenotype was reported to be associated with gastric cancers[36,37] and the blood group O phenotype with gastric ulcers.[38] Interestingly, *Helicobacter pylori* was shown to adhere to the Lewis[b39] blood group antigen[39] and may be an important host factor which facilitates this chronic infection and subsequent risk of gastric cancer development. Further studies are awaited to clarify this or any other host factor with genetic determinants that might predispose toward the development of gastric cancer.

Most molecular analyses of this cancer have involved studies of sporadic tumors for critical, acquired alterations. Cytogenetic studies of gastric adenocarcinomas are few in number and have failed to identify any consistent or noteworthy chromosomal abnormalities. A variable number of numerical or structural aberrations have been reported in gastric cancer cells including those involving chromosome 3 (rearrangements), 6 (deletion distal to 6q21), 8 (trisomy), 11 (11p13-p15 aberrations), 13 (monosomy and translocations).[40–43] Alone, these findings are not compelling for a specific role in gastric tumorigenesis and may represent only nonspecific changes accompanying transformation.

Loss of heterozygosity analyses have identified several arms and regions of chromosomes which may contain tumor suppressor genes important in gastric tumorigenesis. Genetic loci observed to be significantly lost in gastric tumors include those located on the following chromosomal arms: 17p (over 60 percent at p53's locus),[43] 18q (over 60 percent at DCC's locus),[44] and 5q (30 to 40 percent at or near APC's locus).[45–47] Less frequent but significant allelic losses have been reported on 1p, 1q, 7q, and 13q chromosomal arms.[48] Known, as well as candidate, tumor suppressor genes have been isolated in some of these frequently lost regions, as described below, but the actual targets of genetic loss that provide gastric neoplastic cells with additional survival or growth advantages for clonal expansion remain to be clarified for many of these loci.

SPECIFIC MOLECULAR ALTERATIONS

The p53 gene has consistently been demonstrated to be significantly altered in gastric adenocarcinomas. Allelic loss occurs in over 60 percent of cases and mutations are identified in approximately 30 to 50 percent of cases depending on the mutational screening method employed (i.e., single-stranded conformational polymorphism (SSCP) assay or degenerative gradient gel electrophoresis assay) and sample sizes.[49] Some mutations of p53 have even been identified in early dysplastic and apparent intestinal metaplasia gastric lesions. In general, however, alterations of this gene occur more frequently in the advanced stages of dysplasia in both histopathologic subtypes. The spectrum of mutations in this gene within gastric tumors appears similar to that which occurs in other cancers with a predominance of base transitions, especially at CpG dinucleotides. Inactivation of this important cell cycle regulator appears to confer a growth advantage and allow clonal expansion of transformed cells. Many studies have used immunohistochemical analysis of tumors in an effort to detect excessive expression of p53 as an indirect means to identify mutations of this gene; but this assay does not appear to have consistent prognostic value in patients with gastric cancers.[50,51]

Microsatellite instability has been found in a significant portion of sporadic gastric carcinomas.[52–54] Variability in classification of instability or histopathologic subtype and number of loci examined in studies account for some variation of this phenotype's frequency, with a trend toward more frequent occurrence in intestinal-type cancers at more advanced stages observed, although noted in early lesions as well (i.e., adenomas). The degree of genome-wide instability also varies, with more severe instability (e.g., ≥2 abnormal loci) associated with subcardial intestinal or atypical types. A negative association with p53 alterations has also been suggested indicating different paths of alterations accumulating in individual gastric tumors. Studies have indicated less frequent lymph node or vessel invasion, prominant lymphoid infiltration, and better prognosis in those gastric cancers which displayed significant microsatellite instability;[52,55,56] however it remains to be proven if this phenotype is a prognostic marker for improved survival as suggested in colon cancers. The alterations responsible for producing this phenotype in a subset of sporadic gastric cancers remain to be elucidated.

At least one important target of the instability in those cancers displaying abnormal sized microsatellites appears to be the transforming growth factor beta (TGF-β) type II receptor. A study of gastric cancers displaying the microsatellite instability phenotype revealed that a majority (5 of 7) contained mutated TGF-β type II receptors at a polyadenine tract within its gene.[57] Moreover, altered TGF-β type II receptor genes could be found in gastric cancers not displaying microsatellite instability. Several gastric cancer cell lines resistant to the growth inhibitory and apoptotic effects of TGF-β were shown to have altered TGF-β type II genes (deletions and amplifications) and transcripts (truncated or absent).[58] Thus, TGF-β type II receptor mutation appears to be a critical event in the development of at least a subset of gastric cancers, allowing escape from the growth control of TGF-β.

Reduced E-cadherin expression determined by immunohistochemical analysis was noted often (92 percent of 60 cases) in gastric carcinomas and observed to be significantly associated with

diffuse-type cancers and more undifferentiated neoplastic cells (i.e., signet ring cells).[59] Genetic abnormalities of the E-cadherin gene (located on chromosome 16q22.1) and transcripts have also been demonstrated in diffuse gastric cancers.[60] Half of 26 diffuse gastric carcinomas had abnormal E-cadherin transcripts detected by reverse transcription-PCR (RT-PCR) analysis which were not seen in noncancerous tissue from the same patients. Moreover, a study of 10 gastric cancer cell lines displaying loose intracellular adhesion found absent E-cadherin transcripts in four lines, and insertions or deletions in two other lines.[61] Splice site alterations producing exon deletion and skipping, large deletions including allelic loss, and point mutations of the E-cadherin gene were all demonstrated in these diffuse-type cancers, some even exhibiting alterations in both alleles. In comparison of RT-PCR products from normal tissue and tumor tissue from patients, allelic expression imbalance of E-cadherin has also been shown in a porportion (42 percent of 35 informative cases) of gastric carcinomas.[62] E-cadherin is a transmembrane, calcium ion-dependent adhesion molecule (important in epithelial cell homotypic interactions) which, when decreased in expression, is associated with invasive properties.[63] Additionally, alpha-catenin, which binds to the intracellular domain of E-cadherin and links it to actin-based cytoskeletal elements, was noted to have reduced immunohistochemical expression in 70 percent of 60 gastric carcinomas and correlated with infiltrated growth and poor differentiation.[64]

Loss of heterozygosity studies suggest that chromosome 5q harbors at least one tumor suppressor gene important in the development of gastric cancers.[45–47,65,66] The exact target(s), however, of this loss in gastric tumors is not fully clarified. Several somatic APC mutations, mostly missense in nature and of relatively low frequency, have been reported in Japanese patients gastric adenocarcinomas and adenomas using ribonuclease protection or SSCP assays for partial screening.[67] On the other hand, several other reports including Japanese patients have not identified significant APC mutations in gastric carcinomas on similar partial screening analysis of the commonly mutated region and include direct nucleotide sequencing and the sensitive in vitro synthesis protein assays.[66,68,69] Interestingly, an increased risk of gastric cancer associated with familial adenomatous polyposis (patients with germ line APC mutations) has been reported in high-risk regions such as Asia,[70,71] whereas no increased risk was exhibited in other populations.[72,73] Significant allelic loss (30 percent) at APC's loci suggests the existence of a tumor suppressor gene important in gastric tumorigenesis nearby. Indeed, alternative loci have been mapped to commonly deleted regions in gastric cancers (the interferon regulatory factor-1 loci and D5S428)[65] and esophageal cancers (5q31.1).[74] Thus, future studies should help define the important gene(s) on chromosome 5q, which is critically involved in gastric tumorigenesis.

The targets of loss on other chromosomes implicated to harbor important tumor suppressor gene(s) in gastric cancer also remain to be defined. Significant allelic loss (60 percent) has been noted at DCC's loci on 18q in gastric cancers,[44] but there have been no reports of gene mutations or mutational analyses in this region. The recently isolated DPC4 gene as well as several madd human homologues are good candidate tumor suppressor genes in this region which may play an important role in gastric tumorigenesis.[75,76] Similarly, a 13 cM region between D1S201 and D1S197 on chromosome 1p commonly lost in gastric cancers has been delineated, but the critical target remains to be identified.[77] Moreover, a locus on 7q (D7S95) has been associated with peritoneal metastasis when lost.[78] Furthermore, evidence of tumor suppressor loci on chromosome 3p has accumulated from a variety of studies including allelic loss in primary gastric tumors (46 percent) and homozygous deletion in a gastric cancer cell line (KATO III).[79] The candidate tumor suppressor gene FHIT recently isolated from 3p14.2

was reported to have abnormal transcripts of deleted exons in 5 of 9 gastric cancers in addition to transcript abnormalities noted in esophagus and colon cancers as well.[80] However, abnormalities of the *FHIT* gene were not confirmed in a subsequent study of 29 colorectal cancer cases.[81]

Fusion transcripts of a rearrangement involving the translocation promoter region locus on chromosome 1 of the 5′ region of the c-*met* gene on chromosome 7 have been identified by RT-PCR analysis in several gastric cancer cell lines, a portion of gastric cancers, and even preoplastic lesions such as gastritis.[82] This rearrangement was first described in an osteosarcoma cell line transformed by exposure to *N*-methyl-*N*-nitro-*N*-nitrosoguanidine which also induces gastric tumors in rodents. The c-*met* gene encodes a tyrosine kinase receptor for the hepatocyte growth factor. Amplification of the c-*met* gene was reported for the hepatocyte growth factor. Amplification of the c-*met* gene was reported to be associated with scirrhous type gastric cancers.[83] Northern blot analyses of gastric cancer cell lines and resected primary carcinomas compared to paired nonneoplastic tissue showed overexpression of a 7.0-kb transcript of the c-*met* in 48 percent of 31 cancers, predominantly of the well-differentiated type.[84] Moreover, a 6.0-kb c-*met* transcript appeared to be preferentially expressed in scirrhous gastric tumor cells and correlated with latter stages of tumor development. Tumor and stromal cell interactions have been implicated with this growth factor and receptor signal system as well as involvement of multiple others including epidermal growth factor (EGF) (expressed in approximately a quarter of gastric cancers) and its receptor, TGF-α, interleukin-1-α, criptor, amphiregulin, platelet-derived growth factor, K-*sam*, and others.[85,86] Specific alterations and the true prevalence of significant changes in these genes or gene products in gastric tumors remains to be characterized.

Telomerase activity has been detected by a PCR-based assay frequently in the late stages of gastric tumors (85 percent of 66 cases) and is associated with a poor prognosis.[87] The expression of telomerase, a ribonucleoprotein DNA polymerase, and stabilization of telomeres have been noted to be concomitant with immortalization in tumor cells.[88] Another potential marker of poor prognosis is overexpression of c-*erb*B-2, a transmembrane tyrosine kinase receptor protooncogene. Several reports have shown amplification or increased expression of *erb*B-2 immunohistochemically in gastric tumors to be associated with a worse prognosis.[89] Furthermore, enhanced expression of *erb*B-2 has recently been demonstrated to occur more frequently in gastric cancers displaying microsatellite instability.[90] The specific genetic or epigenetic alteration(s) underlying this immunohistochemical finding remains uncharacterized.

A number of other alterations have been reported in gastric carcinomas which remain to be defined as well as the role they play in gastric tumorigenesis. Several splice variants of a transmembrane glycoprotein, CD44, seem to be preferentially expressed in gastric tumors cells.[91] Membrane-type matrix metalloproteinase was preferentially expressed in some gastric cancer cells with colocalization and activation of the zymogen, proMMP-2.[92] Both loss and overexpression of Bc1-2 and nm23 have been reported in several gastric cancers, making their role unclear. Amplification of cyclin E and increased plasminogin activation have been reported as well in several gastric tumors.[93] A somatic mitochondrial deletion of 50 bp was even demonstrated in four gastric adenocarcinomas.[94]

Activation of the oncogene *ras* appears to be rare in gastric tumorigenesis.[69,95,96] Although allelic loss was noted in 18 percent of gastric tumors at the locus for p16 on chromosome 9p, no inactivating somatic mutations were detected in over 70 cases screened by PCR-SSCP analysis.[97] No methylation abnormalities or genetic alterations of other cycle regulators such as p21 or p27 have as yet been reported.

IMPLICATIONS

Identification of important genetic alterations in gastric tumorigenesis has important practical as well as biologic implications. As evident from molecular genetic characterization of colorectal tumor development, genetic markers with potential clinical utility in diagnosis, prognosis, and therapeutic guidance can be discovered. A clear molecular working model of gastric tumorigenesis has yet to be delineated, but as genetic alterations are better characterized in these cancers, critical changes may emerge to provide new opportunities of earlier diagnosis, improved prognostication, and more rational design of therapeutic agents and preventive strategies. As most gastric cancers are diagnosed in late stages of development with concomitant poor prognosis and little chance of cure, genetic changes occurring early and frequently might enable identification of truly premalignant gastric lesions which would be beneficial to remove or warrant intervention in some manner. Directed screening efforts for this cancer is a pressing issue and molecular markers may help address this matter.

Characterization of somatic changes in these gastric tumors might also expose specific environmental factors (e.g., fingerprints[98]) and strongly indict agents for further mechanistic studies. Additionally, identification of a genetic predisposition marker for the development of gastric cancer might facilitate more effective preventive and screening programs. Identifying critical molecular alterations and defining the role played in gastric tumorigenesis may also provide unique opportunities for improved chemopreventive or chemotherapeutic agents to be developed and given at more opportune times.

Finally, as gastric cancer appears to be a rather heterogeneous disease biologically and genetically, characterization of the various pathways and events along the way should afford multiple opportunities to design more specific and therefore more effective therapies in the treatment of this tumor. For example, antibodies to the oncogene *erb*B2 and EGF receptor have shown promise in inhibiting growth of gastric cancer cell lines and xenografts.[86,99] Moreover, current systemic therapies are generally ineffective in controlling gastric cancer growth. Opportunities to explore whether a genetic marker's status such as p53 in these tumors will guide more effective therapy are welcomed. Improved prognostic markers are also eagerly awaited to help guide more aggressive surgical or systemic therapies (i.e., chemotherapy and/or radiotherapy) and may ultimately be derived from molecular alterations indicated above or from as yet unidentified critical change in gastric cancer cells.

ACKNOWLEDGMENTS

The author is grateful to Elaine Lowe for assistance in the preparation of this chapter. This work was supported in part by NIH grant 1R29CA67900-01 and a Foundation AGA Research Scholarship award.

REFERENCES

1. Correa P, Chen V: Gastric cancer. *Cancer Surv* 1994, p. 55.
2. Blot WJ, Devesa SS, Kneller RW: Rising incidence of adenocarcinoma of the esophagus and gastric cardia. *JAMA* **265**:1287, 1991.
3. Locke RG, Talley NJ, Carpenter HA, Harmsen WS, Zinsmeister AR, Melton LJ: Changes in the site- and histology-specific incidence of gastric cancer during a 50-year period. *Gastroenterol* **109**:1750, 1995.

4. Parkin DM, Pisani P, Ferlay J: Estimates of the worldwide incidence of eighteen major cancers in 1985. *Int J Cancer* **54**:594, 1993.
5. Boffetta P, Parkin DM: Cancer in Developing Countries. *CA* **44**:81, 1994.
6. Lynch HT, Smyrk TC, Watson P, Lanspa SJ, Lynch JF, Lynch PM, Cavalieri RJ, Boland CR: Genetics, natural history, tumor spectrum, and pathology of hereditary nonpolyposis colorectal cancer. *Gastroenterology* **104**:1535, 1993.
7. Maimon SN, Zinninger MM: An analysis of 5 stomach cancer families in the state of Utah. *Cancer* **14**:1005, 1953.
8. Woolf CM, Isaacson EA: An analysis of 5 stomach cancer families in the state of Utah. *Cancer* **1961**:1005, 1961.
9. Triantafillidis JK, Kosmidis P, Kottardis S: Genetic studies of gastric cancer in humans: An appraisal. *Cancer* **11**:957, 1958.
10. La Vecchia C, Negri E, Franceschi S, Gentile A: Family history and the risk of stomach and colorectal cancer. *Cancer* **70**:50, 1992.
11. Zangheiri G, Di Gregorio C, Sacchetti C, et al: Familial occurrence of gastric cancer in the 2-year experience of a population-based registry. *Cancer* **66**:2047, 1990.
12. Graham S, Lilienfeld AM: Genetic studies of gastric cancer in humans: An appraisal. *Cancer* **11**:957, 1958.
13. Parker SL, Tong T, Bolden S, Wingo PA: Cancer statistics. *CA* **46**(1):5, 1996.
14. Haenszel W, Kurihara M, Segi M, Lee RK: Stomach cancer among Japanese in Hawaii. *J Natl Cancer Inst* **49**:969, 1972.
15. Correa P, Haenszel W: Epidemiology of gastric cancer, in Correa P, Haenszel W (eds): *Epidemiology of Cancer of the Digestive Tract*. The Hague, The Netherlands: Martinus Hijhoff, 1972, p. 58.
16. Parsonnet J, Hansen S, Rodriguez L, Gelb AB, Warnke RA, Jellum E, Orentreich N, Vogelman JH, Friedman GD: Helicobacter pylori infection and gastric lymphoma. *N Engl J Med* **330**:1267, 1994.
17. Parsonnet J, Friedman GD, Vandersteen DP, Chang Y, Vogelman JH, Orenreich N, Sibley RK: Helicobacter pylori infection and the risk of gastric carcinoma. *N Engl J Med* **325**:1127, 1991.
18. Nomura A, Stemmerman GN, P-HC, Kato I, Perez-Perez GI, Blaser MJ: Helicobacter pylori infection and gastric carcinoma among Japanese Americans in Hawaii. *N Engl J Med* **325**:1132, 1991.
19. Blaser MJ, Chyou PH, Nomura A: Age at establishment of helicobacter pylori infection and gastric carcinoma, gastric ulcer, and duodenal ulcer risk. *Cancer Res* **55**:562, 1995.
20. Elsborg L, Mosbech J: Pernicious anaemia as a risk factor in gastric cancer. *Acta Med Scand* **206**:315, 1979.
21. Rowlands DC, Ito M, Mangham DC, Reynolds G, Herlost H, Fielding JWL, Newbold KM, Jones EL, Young LS, Niedobitek G: Epstein-Barr virus and carcinomas: Rare association of the virus with gastric adenocarcinomas. *Br J Cancer* **68**:1014, 1993.
22. Shibata D, Weiss LM: Epstein-Barr virus-associated gastric adenocarcinoma. *Am J Pathol* **140**:769, 1992.
23. Imai S, Koizumi S, Sugiura M, Toyunaga M, Uemura Y, Yanamoto N, Tanaka S, Sato E, Osato T: Gastric carcinoma: Monoclonal epithelial malignant cells expressing Epstein-Barr virus latent infection protein. *Proc Natl Acad Sci* **91**:9131, 1994.
24. Gulley ML, Pulitzer DR, Eagan PA, Schneider BG: Epstein-barr virus infection is an early event in gastric carcinogenesis and is independent of bcl-2 expression and p53 accumulation. *Human Pathol* **27**(1):19, 1996.
25. Murray PG, Nieddobitek G, Kremmer E, Grasser F, Reynolds GM, Cruchley A, Williams DM, Muller-Lantzsh N, Young LS: In situ detection of the epstein-barr virus-encoded nuclear antigen 1 in oral hairy leukoplakia and virus-associated carcinomas. *J Pathol* **178**:44, 1996.
26. Fuchs, CS and Mayer RJ: Gastric Carcinoma. *N Engl J Med* **333**(1):32, 1995.
27. Lauren P: The two histological main types of gastric carcinoma: Diffuse and so-called intestinal-type carcinoma. *Acta Pathol Microbiol Scand* **64**:31, 1965.
28. Correa P, Shiao YH: Phenotypic and genotypic events in gastric carcinogenesis. *Cancer Res* **54**:1941, 1994.
29. Oota K, Sobin LH: Histological typing gastric and esophageal carcinogenesis, in International histological classification of tumors. Geneva: World Health Organization, 1977.
30. Ming S-C: Gastric carcinoma: A pathobiological classification. *Cancer* **39**:2475, 1977.
31. Borrmann R, Gushwulste de Magens and Duodenums, in Henke F, Lubarsh O (eds): *Handbuch der Speziellen Pathologischen Anatomie und Histologie*. Springer: Berlin, 1926, p. 865.
32. Dixon MF, Martin JG, Sue-Ling HM, Wyatt JI, Quirke P, Johnston D: Goseki grading in gastric cancer: Comparison with existing systems of grading and its reproducibility. *Histopathology* **25**:309, 1994.
33. Goseki N, Takizawa T, Koike M: Differences in the mode of extension of gastric cancer classified by histological type: New histological classification of gastric carcinoma. *Gut* **33**:606, 1992.
34. Kennedy BJ: The unified international gastric cancer staging classification. *Gastroenterology* **22**:1, 1987.
35. Hirota T, Ming SC, Itabashi M: Pathology of early gastric cancer. *Gastric Cancer* **66**, 1993.
36. Aird I, Bentall H: A relationship between cancer of stomach and ABO groups. *Br J Med* **1**:799, 1953.
37. Haenszel W, Kurihara M, Locke F, Shimuzu K, Segi M: Stomach Cancer in Japan. *J Natl Cancer Inst* **56**:265, 1976.
38. Clarke CA, Cowan WK, Edwards JW, Howel-Evans AW, McConnell RB, Woodrow JC, Sheppard PM: The relation of ABO bloodgroups to duodenal and gastric ulceration. *Br Med J* **4940**:643, 1955.
39. Boren T, Per F, Roth KA, Larson G, Normark S: Attachment of Helicobacter pylori to human gastric epithelium mediated by blood group antigens. *Science* **262**:1892, 1993.
40. Seruca R, Castedo S, Correia C, Gomes P, Carneiro F, et al: Cytogenetic findings in eleven gastric carcinomas. *Cancer Genet Cytogenet* **68**:42, 1993.
41. Rodriguez E, Ladanyi M, Altorki N, Albino AP, Kelsen DP, et al: *11p13-15* is a specific region of chromosomal rearrangement in gastric esophageal adenocarcinomas. *Cancer Res* **50**:6410, 1990.
42. Ochi H, Douglass H, Sandberg AA: Cytogenetic studies in primary gastric cancer. *Cancer Genet Cytogenet* **22**:295, 1986.
43. Panani AD, Ferti A, Malliaros S, Raptis S: Cytogenetic study of 11 gastric adenocarcinomas. *Cancer Genet Cytogenet* **81**:169, 1995.
44. Uchino S, Hitoshi T, Masayuki N, Jun Y, Terada M, Saito T, Kobayashi M, Sugimura T, Hirohashi S: Frequent loss of heterozygosity at the *DCC* locus in gastric cancer. *Cancer Res* **52**:3099, 1992.
45. Sano T, Tsujino T, Yoshida K, Nakyama H, Haruma K, Ito H, Nakamura Y, Kajiyama G, Tahara E: Frequent loss of heterozygosity on chromosomes 1q, 5q and 17q human gastric carcinomas. *Cancer Res* **51**:2926, 1991.
46. McKie AB, Filipe I, Lemoine NR: Abnormalities affecting the APC and MCC tumour suppressor gene loci on chromosome 5q occur frequently in gastric cancer but not in pancreatic cancer. *Int J Cancer* **55**:598, 1993.
47. Rhyu MG, Park WS, Jung YJ, Choi SW, Meltzer SJ: Allelic deletions of MCC.APC and p53 are frequent late events in human gastric carcinogenesis. *Gastroenterology* **106**:1584, 1994.
48. Sipponen P, Kekki M, Haapakoski J, Ihamaki T, Siurala M: Gastric cancer risk in chronic atrophic gastritis: Statistical calculations of cross-sectional data. *Int J Cancer* **35**:173, 1985.
49. Hollstein MC, Sidransky D, Vogelstein B, Harris CC: p53 mutations in human cancers. *Science* **253**:49, 1991.
50. Gabber HE, Muller W, Schneiders A, Meier S, Hommel G: The relationship of p53 expression to the prognosis of 418 patients with gastric carcinoma. *Cancer* **76**(5):720.
51. Hurlimann J, Saraga EP: Expression of p53 protein in gastric carcinomas. *Am J Surg Pathol* **18**(12):1247, 1994.
52. Seruca R, Santos NR, David L, Constancia M, Barroca H, Carneiro F, Seixas M, Peltomaki P, Lothe R, Sobrinho-Simoes M: Sporadic gastric carcinomas with microsatellite instability display a particular clinicopathological profile. *Ubt H Cancer* **64**:32, 1995.
53. Strickler JG, Zheng J, Shu Q, Burgart LJ, Alberts SR, Shibata D: p53 mutations and microsatellite instability in sporadic gastric cancer: When guardians fail. *Cancer Res* **54**:4750, 1994.
54. Chong J-M, Fukayama M, Hayashi Y, Takizawa T, Koike M, Konishi M, Kikuchi-Yanoshita R, Miyaki M: Microsatellite instability in the progression of gastric carcinoma. *Cancer Res* **54**:4595, 1994.
55. Nakashima H, Hiroshi I, Mori M, Ueo H, Ikeda M, Akiyoshi T: Microsatellite instability in Japanese gastric cancer. *Cancer (Suppl)* **75**(6):1503, 1995.
56. Dos Santos NR, Seruca R, Constancia M, Seixas M, Sobrinho-Simoes M: Microsatellite instability at multiple loci in gastric carcinoma: Clinicopathologic implications and prognosis. *Gastroenterology* **110**:38, 1996.
57. Myeroff LL, Ramon P, Kim S-J, Hedrick L, Cho KR, Orth K, Mathis M, Kinzler K, Lutterbaugh J, Park K, Bang Y-J, Lee HY, Park J-G, Lynch H, Roberts AB, Vogelstein B, Markowitz SD: A transforming growth factor B receptor type II gene mutation common in colon and gastric but rare in endometrial cancers. *Cancer Res* **55**:5545, 1995.
58. Park K, Kim S-J, Bang Y-J, Park J-G, Kim NK, Roberts AB, Sporn MB: Genetic changes in the transforming growth fact Beta (TGF-b) type II receptor gene in human gastric cancer cells: correlation with

sensitivity to growth inhibition by TGF-B. *Proc Natl Acad Sci* **91**:8772, 1994.

59. Mayer B, Johnson JP, Leitl F, Jauch KW, Heiss MM, Schildberg FW, Birchmeier W, Funke I: E-cadherin expression in primary and metastatic gastric cancer: Down regulation correlates with cellular dedifferentiation and glandular disintegration. *Cancer Res* **53**:1690, 1993.

60. Becker KF, Atkinson MJ, Reich U, Becker I, Nekarda H, Siewart JR, Hofler H: E-cadherin gene mutations provide clues to diffuse type gastric carcinomas. *Cancer Res* **54**:3845, 1994.

61. Oda T, Kanai Y, Oyama T, Yoshiura K, Shimoyama Y, Birchmeier W, Sugimura T: E-cadherin gene mutations in human gastric carcinoma cell lines. *Proc Natl Acad Sci* **91**:1858, 1994.

62. Becker KF, Hofler H: Frequent somatyic allelic inactivation of the E-cadherin gene in gastric carcinomas. *J Natl Cancer Inst* **87**(14):1082, 1995.

63. Birchmeier W, Behrens J: Cadherin expression in carcinomas: Role in the formation of cell junctions and the prevention of invasiveness. *Biochem Biophys Acta* **1198**:11, 1994.

64. Matsui S, Shiozaki H, Masatoshi I, Shigeyuke T, Doki Y, Kadowaki T, Iwazawa T, Shimaya K, Nagafuchi A, Tsukita S, Mori T: Immunohistochemical evaluation of alpha-catenin expression in human gastric cancer. *Virchows Arch* **424**:375.

65. Tamura G, Ogaswara S, Nishizuka S, Sakata K, Maesawa C, Suzuki Y, Tershima M, Saito K, Satodate R: Two distinct regions of deletion on the long arm of chromosome 5 in differentiated adenocarcinomas of the stomach. *Cancer Res* **56**:612, 1996.

66. Powell SM, Cummings OW, Mullen JA, Asghar A, Fuga G, Piva P, Minacci C, Megha T, Piero T, Jackson CE: Characterization of the *APC* gene in sporadic gastric adenocarcinomas. *Oncogene* **12**:1953, 1996.

67. Nagase H, Nakamura Y: Mutation of the APC (Adenomatous Polyposis Coli) gene. *Hum Mutat* **2**:425, 1993.

68. Ogaswara S, Maesawa C, Tamura G, Satodate R: Lack of mutations of the adenomatous polyposis coli gene in oesophageal and gastric carcinomas. *Virchows Arch* **424**(6):607, 1994.

69. Maesawa C, Tamura G, Suzuki Y, Ogaswara S, Sakata K, Kashiwaba M, Satodate R: The sequential accumulation of genetic alterations characteristic of the colorectal adenoma-carcinoma sequence does not occur between gastric adenoma and adenocarcinoma. *J Pathol* **176**:249, 1995.

70. Utsunomiya J: The concept of hereditary colorectal cancer and the implications of its study, in Utsunomiya J, Lynch HT (eds): *Hereditary Colorectal Cancer*. Tokyo: Springer-Verlag, 1990, p. 3.

71. Park JG, Park KJ, Ahn YO, Song IS, Choi KW, Moon HY, Choo SY, Kim JP: Risk of gastric cancer among Korean familial adenomatous polyposis patients. *Dis Colon Rectum* **53**:996, 1992.

72. Offerhaus GJA, Giardello FM, Krush AJ, Booker SV, Tersmette AC, Kelley NC, Hamilton SR: The risk of upper gastrointestinal cancer in familial adenomatous polyposis. *Gastroenterology* **102**:1980, 1992.

73. Burt RW: Polyposis syndromes, in Yamada T, Alpers TH (eds): *Textbook of Gastroenterology*. New York, J.B. Lippincott Company, 1991.

74. Ogaswara S, Tamura G, Maesawa C, Suzuki Y, Iishida K, Satoh N, Uesugi N, Saito K, Satodate R: Common deleted region of the long arm of chromosome 5 in esophageal carcinoma. *Gastroenterology* **110**:52, 1996.

75. Riggins GJ, Thiagalingam S, Rozenblum E, Weinstein CL, Kern SE, Hamilton SR, Willson JKV, Markowitz SD, Kinzler KW, Vogelstein B: *Mad*-related genes in the human. *Nat Genet* **13**:347, 1996.

76. Hahn SA, Schutte M, Shamsul Hoque ATM, Moskaluk CA, da Costa LT, Rozenblum E, Weinstein CL, Fischer A, Yeo CJ, Hruben RH, Kern SE: *DPC4*, a candidate tumor suppressor gene at human chromosome 18q21.1. *Science* **271**:350, 1996.

77. Ezaki T, Yanagisawa A, Ohta K, Aiso S, Watanabe M, Hibi T, Kato Y, Nakajima T, Ariyama T, Inzawa J, Nakamura Y, Horii A: Deletion mapping chromosome 1p in well-differentiated gastric cancer. *Br J Cancer* **73**:424, 1996.

78. Kuniyasu H, Yasui W, Yokosaki H: Frequent loss of heterozygosity of the long arm of chromosome 7 is often associated with progression of human gastric carcinoma. *Cancer* **59**:597, 1994.

79. Kastury K, Baffa R, Druck T, Cotticelli MG, Inoue H, Massimo N, Rugge M, Huang D, Croce CM, Palazzo J, Huebner K: Potential gastrointestinal tumor suppressor locus at the 3p14.2FRA3b site identified by homozygous deletions in tumor cell lines. *Cancer Res* **56**:978, 1996.

80. Ohta M, Hiroshi I, Citticelli MG, Kastury K: The *FHIT* gene, spanning the chromosome 3p14.2 fragile site and renal carcinoma-associated t(3;8) breakpoint, is abnormal in digestive tract cancers. *Cell* **84**:587, 1996.

81. Thiagalingam S, Lisitsyn NA, Hamaguchi M, Wigler MH, Willson JKV, Markowitz SD, Leach FS, Kinzler KW, Vogelstein B: Evaluation of *FHIT* gene in colorectal cancers. *Cancer Res* **56**:2936, 1996.

82. Soman NR, Correa P, Ruiz BA, Wogan GN; The *TPR-MET* oncogenic rearrangement is present and expressed in human gastric carcinoma and precursor lesions. *Proc Natl Acad Sci* **88**:4892, 1991.

83. Kuniyasu H, Yasui W, Kitadai Y, Yokosaki H, Ito H, Tahara E: Frequent amplification of the *c-met* gene in scirrhous type stomach cancer. *Biochem Biophys Res Commun* **189**:227, 1992.

84. Kuniyasu H, Yasui W, Kitadai Y, Tahar E: Aberrant expression of c-met mRNA in human gastric carcinomas. *Int J Cancer* **55**:72, 1993.

85. Tahara E, Semba S, Tahara H: Molecular biological observations in gastric cancer. *Semin Oncol* **23**(3):307, 1996.

86. Tokunaga A, Onda M, Okuda T, Teramoto T, Fijita I, Mizutani T, Kiyama T, Yoshiyuki T, Nishi K, Matsukura N: Clinical significance of epidermal growth factor (EGF), EGF Receptor, and c-erbB-2 in human gastric cancer. *Cancer* **75**:1418, 1995.

87. Hiyama E, Yokoyama T, Tatsumato N, Hiyama K, Imamura Y, Murakami Y, et al: Telomerase activity in gastric cancer. *Cancer Res* **55**:3258, 1995.

88. Kim JW, Piatyszek MA, Prowse MA, Harley KR, West CB, Peter LC, Ho GMC, Woodring EN, Weinrich SL, Shay JW: Specific association of human telomerase activity with immortal cells and cancer. *Science* **266**:2011, 1994.

89. Mizutani T, Onda M, Tokunaga A, Yamanaka N, Sugisaka Y: Relationship of c-erb B-2 protein expression and gene amplification to invasion and metastasis in human gastric cancer. *Cancer* **72**:2083, 1993.

90. Lin J-T, Wu MS, Shun C-T, Lee W-J, Wang T-H: Occurrence of microsatellite instability in gastric carcinoma is associated with enhanced expression of erbB-2 oncoprotein. *Cancer Res* **55**:1428, 1995.

91. Dammrich J, Vollmers HP, Heider K-H, Muller-Hermelink H-K: Importance of different CD44v6 expression in human gastric intestinal and diffuse type cancers for metastatic lymphogenic spreading. *J Mol Med* **73**:395, 1995.

92. Nomura H, Hiroshi S, Motoharu S, Masyoshi M, Yasunori O: Expression of membrane-type matrix metalloproteinase in human gastric carcinomas. *Cancer Res* **55**:3263, 1995.

93. Tahara E: Molecular mechanism of stomach carcinogenesis. *J Cancer Res Clin Oncol* **119**:265, 1993.

94. Burgart LJ, Zheng J, Shu Q, Strickler JG, Shibata D: A somatic mitochondrial mutation in gastric cancer. *Am J Pathol* **147**(4):1105, 1995.

95. Kihana T, Tsuda H, Teruyuki H, Shimosato Y, Hiromi S, Terada M, Hirohashi S: Point mutation of c-Ki-*ras* oncogene in gastric adenoma and adenocarcinoma with tubular differentiation. *Jpn J Cancer Res* **82**:308, 1991.

96. Koshiba M, Ogawa O, Habuchi T, Hamazaki S, Thoshihide S, et al: Infrequent *ras* mutation in human stomach cancers. *Jpn J Cancer Res* **84**:163, 1993.

97. Igaki H, Sasaki H, Tachimori Y, Watanabe H, Kimura T, Harada Y, Sugimura T, Tarada M: Mutation frequency of the *p16*/CDKN2gene in primary cancers in the upper digestive tract. *Cancer Res* **55**:3421, 1995.

98. Vogelstein B, Kinzler KW: Carcinogens leave finger prints. *Nature* **355**:209, 1992.

99. Kasprzyk PG, Song SU, Di Fiore PP, King CR: Therapy of an animal model of human gastric cancer using a combination of Anti-*erb*B-2 monoclonal antibodies. *Cancer Res* **52**:2771, 1992.

CHAPTER 39

Prostate Cancer

William B. Isaacs ▪ G. Steven Bova

1. **Prostate cancer is the most common cancer diagnosed in men in the U.S. The incidence of this disease shows strong age, race, and geographical dependence, being diagnosed in older men, with African Americans being at high risk and Asians being at low risk.**

2. **Although no hereditary prostate cancer loci have been identified, familial clustering data and segregation analysis suggest the existence of autosomal dominant high-risk alleles for prostate cancer.**

3. **Deletion of sequences from the short arm of chromosome 8 is a very frequent chromosomal alteration in prostate cancer, occurring at high frequency even in precursor lesions. Gain of sequences on chromosome 8q and loss of sequences on 13q are only slightly less common than 8p LOH. Gain and deletion of chromosome 7 sequences, along with deletions of chromosomes 5q, 6q, 10q, and 16q also are frequent events in the prostate cancer cell genome. The genes driving the apparent selection of these abnormalities largely are unknown.**

4. **Methylation of a CpG island in the promoter of the *GSTP1* gene is the most common genomic alteration yet identified in prostate cancer, occurring in virtually every case.**

5. **Although mutations of *p53, Rb, ras, CDKN2,* and other tumor suppressor genes and oncogenes have been detected in prostate cancer, no single gene has been identified as being mutated in the majority of prostate cancers.**

6. **The androgen receptor gene, when either mutated or amplified, may play a critical role in prostate tumorigenesis, both at the early stages and during progression to androgen-independent disease. Polymorphic variants of the androgen receptor that differ in their biologic activity may confer increased risk for prostate cancer, or for more aggressive forms of this disease.**

7. **Prostate cancers vary tremendously in their biologic aggressiveness. The ability of various genetic alterations to serve as much-needed molecular diagnostic and prognostic indicators is being evaluated.**

CLINICAL ASPECTS

Incidence

In 1990, prostate cancer became the most common form of cancer (other than skin cancer) diagnosed in the U.S. male. In 1996, there were over 300,000 new prostate cancer cases diagnosed, accounting for over 35% of all cancers affecting men, and over 40,000 deaths will result from this disease.[1] The number of prostate cancers diagnosed in the United States has been increasing since 1972, and in particularly dramatic fashion since 1988. This increase is owing primarily to changes in methods used to detect the disease (e.g., the use of serum prostate specific antigen [PSA]) as well as interest in detecting this disease (increased awareness and screening), coupled with what appears to be an actual but slight increase in the true incidence rate.[2]

The incidence of prostate cancer shows strong age, race, and geographical dependence. It is a disease of older men, with an incidence rate for men over 65 being 20-fold greater than that for men 50–54 years of age. Less than 1% of cases are diagnosed under the age of 40, reaching a peak frequency of approximately one in seven in the eighth and ninth decades of life.[3] This disease is uncommon in Asian populations, high in Scandinavian countries, and the highest incidence (and mortality) rates known are in African American males; the latter being twofold higher than for American white males.[4]

The *initiation* of prostate cancer, that is, the formation of a histologically identifiable lesion, is a very frequent event, occurring in nearly one-third of men over age 45.[5] Fortunately, the majority of such lesions do not progress to clinically detectable tumors. Interestingly, the rate of histological cancer incidence is roughly the same worldwide, suggesting an important role for environmental factors as potential promoting agents to explain the observed regional differences in incidence of clinically detectable disease.[6–8] In contrast, studies of familial aggregation of this disease have suggested that 5–10% of prostate cancers may be directly attributable to the inheritance of prostate cancer susceptibility alleles (see the following), which can act as genetic factors driving this progression potentially independent of environmental exposure. Thus, as with numerous other cancers, there is evidence for both genetic and environmental factors in the etiology of prostate cancer, with the majority of disease most likely being a result of the interaction the two.[9]

Prostate cancer develops in two different regions of the gland, with most lesions (75–80%) found in the periphery, where the majority of glands show multiple lesions, and the remainder in a periurethral region, termed the transition zone.[10] Curiously, it is the latter region of the prostate in which the virtually ubiquitous process of benign prostatic hyperplasia (BPH) occurs.[11] Based primarily on this regional difference in benign and malignant growth incidence, and the fact that stromal cell proliferation typically is a major component of BPH, these benign lesions are not thought to be the precursor lesions of invasive adenocarcinoma in the prostate. Instead, prostatic intraepithelial neoplasia or PIN is the term given to characteristic foci of dysplastic ductal and acinar cells thought to be the precursor lesions of this disease.[12]

Diagnostic Criteria

As the prostate is not visible or readily available to self-examination, the development of symptoms, either owing to local disease resulting primarily in voiding dysfunction, or disseminated disease, commonly resulting in bone pain, has historically been the initial sign of malignancy, with many men being diagnosed with advanced disease. This situation has changed dramatically with the use of PSA as a screening tool which, when combined with digital rectal exam and transrectal ultrasound, results in a much greater ability to detect prostate cancer while still confined to the gland. The use of these latter methods is primarily responsible for the approximately threefold increase in incidence rates observed since 1988.[2]

PSA is a serine protease with a chymotrpysin-like substrate specificity that is normally secreted by the prostate in large amounts into the seminal plasma.[13] Normally its level in the bloodstream of men is below 4 ng/mL, although this varies with age.[14] With prostate pathology these levels can increase, in particularly dramatic fashion in the case of carcinoma. A current focus of intense research effort is on the ability to accurately interpret slightly elevated PSA levels that can be indicative of either benign or malignant disease.[15] Serum PSA detection after prostatectomy or other treatment for prostate cancer is a very reliable indication of disease progression.[16]

Prostate cancer is graded based on tissue architectural patterns according to the system proposed by DF Gleason.[17] Because of the common morphological heterogeneity, two different grades are given for the first and second most prevalent patterns, and the sum of these two grades is the Gleason score. Staging is done using a TNM (tumor, node, metastasis) classification.[18]

Unique Features of Prostate Carcinoma

Several features tend to distinguish adenocarcinoma of the prostate from other common cancers. This list is not exhaustive but serves to highlight important questions in prostate cancer biology for which there is little understanding at the molecular level.

1. *Extreme age dependency of incidence.* Although the most common malignancy in men, this disease does not appear (at least in a clinically detectable form) at significant rates until the sixth decade of life (incidence of 1 in 2,000,000 below the age of 40).[3]

2. *Slow growth rate.* Doubling times measured in years are not uncommon.

3. *Sensitivity to androgens.* Most prostate cancers respond to androgen ablation therapy, although virtually all become insensitive to this treatment.

4. *Multifocality.* The prostate of a man diagnosed with prostate cancer contains an average of five apparently independent lesions.[19] These lesions are genetically heterogeneous, both inter- and intratumorally.[20–22] This multifocality is independent of family history of prostate cancer.[19]

5. *Lack of ability to establish cell lines from clinical specimens of prostate cancer.* After hundreds of attempts by numerous investigators only a handful of cell lines exist.

GENETIC LOCI

Hereditary Versus Sporadic Disease

Although no prostate cancer susceptibility genes have been cloned, there is substantial evidence that a hereditary form of this disease exists. Numerous studies indicate that family history of prostate cancer perhaps is the strongest risk factor identified for this disease, and segregation analysis of familial aggregation patterns suggests that these observations are most consistent with the existence of one or more hereditary prostate cancer genes that act in an autosomal dominant fashion to confer greatly increased risk of disease.[23–27] It is estimated that approximately 9% of all prostate cancer is attributable to such gene(s), although in the case of early onset disease (i.e., diagnosis before 55), a much greater proportion (40%) may be owing to an inherited susceptibility.[27,28] More precise information on inherited prostate cancer will have to await the cloning of the responsible genes.

Chromosomal Alterations in Sporadic Disease

Initial LOH studies indicated that chromosomes 8p, 10q, and 16q may harbor prostate tumor suppressor genes. These studies have been confirmed and extended to include chromosomes 7q and 13q as regions of frequent allelic loss.[29]

Chromosome 8. Of the regions analyzed, the short arm of chromosome 8 has received the most attention, as it appears to be the most frequent site of LOH in prostate cancers, occurring in the majority of cases examined. Two or possibly three distinct regions of LOH occur on this chromosomal arm with region 8p21-12 being deleted in the majority of prostate cancer precursor lesions (PIN), and more distally, 8p22 is deleted in most adenocarcinomas.[30–35] In this latter region, a homozygous deletion of approximately 1 mb has been observed.[36]

The first reports of chromosome 8p abnormalities in prostate cancer were cytogenetic studies that suggested that loss of chromosome 8p material was correlated with loss of androgen responsiveness.[37] The finding of chromosome 8p LOH was first described by Bergerheim et al. in a study of primary and metastatic deposits of prostate cancer.[38] Since then, subregional deletion analysis of chromosome 8p in prostate cancer has been performed using a variety of molecular methods, including Southern analysis, microsatellite analysis, fluorescence *in situ* hybridization (FISH), and comparative genomic hybridization (CGH), all of which have confirmed a high frequency of loss in this region, especially but not exclusively within chromosome band 8p22.[21,30–33,38–45] The rate of 8p22 loss reported in these regions varies 32–65% in primary tumors, and 65–100% in DNA derived from metastases.

Separate discrete regions of loss in more proximal regions including 8p21 and 8p12 have been described.[32,33,35] Frequent loss (63%) of portions of 8p21-p12 have been identified in PIN lesions, suggesting that a gene in this area frequently may become inactivated at a relatively early stage in prostate tumorigenesis.[34] Evidence of heterogeneity of 8p LOH among different PIN lesions within the same gland was observed.[34] A combined CGH, Southern, and microsatellite study has shown loss of chromosome 8p22-p12 in 80% of prostate cancer lymph node metastases, and microcell transfer of human chromosome 8 into a rat prostate cancer cell line has been reported to suppress metastatic ability.[46,47] An association of chromosome 8p loss and higher stage has been reported.[33]

Recently, a candidate tumor suppressor gene, termed N33, located in a homozygously deleted region of chromosome 8p22, has been identified that is expressed in many normal tissues, but not in some cancers, most notably those of the colon.[48] The contribution of this gene to prostatic carcinogenesis awaits further clarification.

The frequent loss of sequences on chromosome 8p provides a marker to determine the similarity or difference between primary prostate cancers and their metastases. This approach has been used to determine the concordance rates for 8p loss in a series of PIN, primary, and metastatic lesions obtained from the same patient.[21] Cases were observed in which there was a complete concordance in that all samples of cancer had retained or lost the same 8p marker, but there were also cases in which the PIN sample would show loss, but not the primary tumor or the lymph node tumor samples. In addition, there were cases that showed differences among the multiple primary lesions within the prostate. These data and similar findings demonstrate the complex genetic relationship that exists between primary and metastatic lesions and suggest that the primary prostate cancer that gives rise to a given metastatic deposit is not predicted easily on the basis of morphological characteristics.[20]

Concomitant with deletion of sequences from the short arm, chromosome 8 frequently is affected by gain of sequences on the long arm. First observed by Southern analysis, a CGH study of lymph node metastases indicated that 85% of such tumors showed evidence of 8q gain, making this the most common numerical alteration observed in this study.[30,46] Van den Berg et al. reported that gain of 8q sequences in prostate cancer was highly correlated with disease progression, and similarly, in the CGH study of Visakorpi et al., gain of 8q sequences was seen in 89% of tumor recurrences after hormonal therapy, whereas only 6% of primary tumors showed this alteration.[44,49] An obvious candidate gene which may be the target of these amplification events in prostate cancer is the oncogene, c-*myc*, located at 8q24, although most of the amplification events on 8q are large, suggesting that many genes are affected. At present the overall contribution of the c-*myc* gene to progression of prostate cancer is undefined.

Chromosome 7. Similar to chromosome 8, chromosome 7 also frequently undergoes both gain and loss events in prostate cancer. Trisomy 7 is common in both PIN, and cancer lesions, and gain of chromosome 7 has been observed in 30–56% of cases in CGH studies.[20,44,45,50,54] The association of chromosome 7 aneusomy with advanced stage, and poor prognosis indicates that gain of chromosome 7 material may play an important role in progression of some prostate cancers.[53–55] Likewise, loss of discrete portions of chromosome 7q in prostate cancer, with the most frequent region of deletion appearing at 7q31.1, suggests that this region also may harbor a gene important in tumor progression, as tumors deleting this region usually are high grade and stage.[56–59]

Chromosome 10. Cytogenetic analyses of prostate cancer have not revealed consistent chromosomal deletions, which might provide information regarding the location of tumor suppressor genes.[52,60–62] However, an early study employing direct preparations of prostate cancer cells, showed that four of four patients with late-stage prostate carcinomas exhibited chromosome 10q deletions, and three of four exhibited chromosome 7q deletions.[63] Since that time, alterations of the long arm of chromosome 10, although by no means ubiquitous, have been the most consistently observed karyotypic abnormalities in prostate cancer. Initial studies examining chromosome 10 by RFLP analysis found losses solely on 10q, or both arms of chromosome 10.[38,64] A number of reports since then, using both RFLP and microsatellite analysis, have found loss of chromosome 10 in 29–48% of informative cases, with a complex pattern of loss being observed, including monosomy and loss of 10p alone, loss of portions of 10p and 10q, and loss of sequences on 10q alone.[65–68] The most common region of

deletion on the short and long arms has been mapped to 10p11.2 and 10q23.1, respectively.

Chromosome 16q. Carter et al. observed LOH of markers on chromosome 16q in approximately 30% of clinically localized tumors, whereas Bergerheim et al. found a higher rate (56%) in a series of metastatic and localized tumors.[38,64] Deletion mapping data presented in this latter study suggested that the critical region was located between D16S4 and 16qter. Employing a series of cosmid contigs in a FISH analysis, Cher et al. suggested that the common region of loss was more distally located between 16q23.1 and 16qter.[69]

Chromosome 17. Studies of loss of chromosome 17 sequences have focused primarily on two regions, one in the vicinity of the *p53* gene at 17p13.1, and the other in the area of the *BRCA1* gene on the proximal long arm. Allelic loss the *p53* gene and distal markers generally is low in low stage primary prostate cancer (<20%), a finding consistent with the low frequency of *p53* gene mutations found in these tumors (see the following). A study by Brooks et al. demonstrates that here is a higher rate of 17p loss in higher grade and stage prostate cancers, but that this loss is not correlated with an increasing frequency of *p53* mutations, suggesting the presence of perhaps another tumor suppressor gene that may contribute to the LOH events on this chromosomal arm.[70]

Brothman et al. and Williams et al. recently used a variety of approaches to implicate a region on the proximal long arm of chromosome 17 in the vicinity of the BRCA1 gene at 17q21 as harboring a gene important in prostate carcinogenesis.[71,72] By using a series of P1 clones in a FISH analysis, these workers were able to demonstrate that the common region of loss did not include BRCA1, but was more distal, implicating a different gene in this region. These results are critical, as it has been suggested repeatedly that the BRCA1 gene may play an important role in prostate carcinogenesis.

Chromosome 18. Initial studies implicating chromosome 18 as harboring prostate tumor suppressor gene found LOH of markers in the vicinity of the DCC gene at band 21.2 on the long arm of this chromosome at rates of 20–40%. A more recent study found that one-third of clinically localized prostate cancers show loss of markers on 18q and suggests that the common region of deletion lies between the centromere and D18S19, located at 18q22.1, although a subsequent study narrowed this region, excluding DCC.[39] A recent examination of the DPC4 gene at 18q21.1 in prostate cancer revealed an absence of inactivating mutations of this pancreatic tumor suppressor gene.

CGH Studies in Prostate Cancer

Visakorpi et al. utilized CGH to survey the genome of a series of both untreated, localized prostate cancers as well as tumors from patients failing hormonal therapy.[44] This study found chromosome 8p to be the most frequently deleted, followed by 13q, 6q, 16q, 18q, and 9p. In a series of nine advanced prostate cancers, there was a significant increase in deletions of chromosome 5q and gains of chromosomes 7p, 8q, and X, when compared to untreated primary tumor samples. Similarly, Cher et al. used CGH combined with Southern and microsatellite analysis to study a series of over 31 advanced prostate cancers (primarily lymph node deposits of prostate cancer).[46] As expected, a high frequency of chromosome 8p loss was seen (71%). This study also revealed that portions of chromosome 13 were just as commonly deleted (65%) followed by chromosomes 17p (52%), 10q22.1-qter (42%), 2cen-q31 (42%),

16q (42%), 5cen-q23.3 (39%), and 6q14-q23.2 (39%). Increases in copy number of sequences on chromosome 8q were observed in 81% of the cases, with gains of chromosomes 1q, 2p, 3p and q, 7p and q, and 11p observed in over 40% of the samples. Thus, these studies confirm previous studies of the allelic loss in prostate cancer, and at the same time, greatly expands the chromosomal regions implicated as harboring prostate cancer genes.

SPECIFIC GENES

Sporadic Disease

A number of genes have been found to be mutated in prostate cancer including *p53, Rb, ras, CDKN2*, androgen receptor (*AR*), *MXI1*, and *POLB*, although the latter two, located on chromosomes 10q25 and 8p11.2, respectively, remain to be confirmed; *ras* mutations are uncommon (<5% of cases) as are point mutations of *Rb*, although loss of one copy of *Rb* readily occurs.[73–76] To date the most consistently observed site of point mutations is the *p53* gene, and these mutations are common only in advanced disease. Microsatellite instability is uncommon but detectable in prostate cancer, and the hPMS2 gene has been shown to be mutated in a prostate cancer cell line which exhibits this phenotype.[77,78]

p53. *p53* Mutations are uncommon in localized disease but become quite frequent in deposits of metastatic prostate cancer, particularly those to bone.[79–85] Observed heterogeneity of *p53* mutations within different tumors in the same gland, and within different regions of the same gland appears to be a unique feature of prostate cancer.[22] Furthermore, LOH and point mutation of *p53* do not appear to be tightly coupled in this disease.[70]

Rb. The importance of *Rb* gene inactivation in prostate cancer was initially suggested by the studies of Bookstein et al., who demonstrated the presence of inactivating mutations in the *Rb* gene in clinical specimens of prostate cancer, as well as the ability of reintroduction of a cloned copy of *Rb* to suppress the tumorigenicity of DU145 prostate cancer cells, which had been shown to produce a non-functional truncated *Rb* protein.[86,87] Combined CGH and LOH studies reveal that one copy of *Rb* is lost in advanced prostate cancer at rates approaching 80%, although limited sequencing studies suggest that point mutations are present in <20% of clinical samples.[46,76] Immunohistochemical studies of *Rb* expression demonstrate lack of expression in 10–22% of tumors, with a questionable correlation between tumor LOH of *Rb* and lack of expression.[88,89] These data, together with LOH events on 13q that do not include *Rb*, suggest the presence of an additional or alternative prostate tumor suppressor gene near the *Rb* locus.[89]

CDKN2. Much attention has been focused upon the *p16/CDKN2* gene, a negative regulator of cell cycle progression located at chromosome 9p21, since the finding of frequent homozygous deletions in a wide variety of cancer cell lines.[90] A relatively high frequency of homozygous (~20%) and hemizygous losses of *CDKN2* have been observed in clinical specimens of prostate cancer.[91,92] In the latter case, loss events in the vicinity of the *CDKN2* gene are more common in metastatic deposits of prostate cancer (43 vs. 20% in primary tumors), and in a small but detectable fraction of tumors (~15%) the *CDKN2* gene shows evidence of inactivation by pro-

moter methylation. Whether all of the allelic loss events at 9p21 in prostate cancer are associated with *CDKN2* inactivation, or whether they reflect inactivation of a neighboring gene, for example, *p15*, has not been determined.

Androgen Receptor. The role of androgen in normal prostate physiology is unquestioned, as these hormones are strictly required for normal development and maintenance of prostate growth and function. However, the role of androgens and androgen receptors (AR) in prostate cancer is much less clear, and recent studies have generated a great deal of renewed interest in this pathway and its role in the critical progression of prostate cancer to androgen independence.[93] An initial hypothesis that loss of *AR* gene expression may be important in androgen independent disease was not supported by several studies that showed continued or even elevated *AR* gene expression in androgen independent tumors.[94,95] Newmark et al. were the first to report a mutated androgen receptor in a clinical specimen of prostate cancer, found curiously in a localized cancer prior to any hormonal therapy.[96] This and other findings of mutations prior to hormonal therapy would suggest that mutant *AR* might provide a growth advantage even in the presence of normal androgen levels.[97] Kelly and Scher. described a number of patients that underwent a paradoxical response to withdrawal of the antiandrogen, flutamide, in that a number of clinical parameters (e.g., PSA levels, bone pain) improved on cessation of drug treatment.[98] One explanation proposed for this response is that such patients harbor *AR* gene mutations similar to that found in the prostate cancer cell line LNCaP (Thr to Ala change at codon 868), which alters the ligand specificity of the receptor such that both estrogens and antiandrogens, as well as androgens, can now act as agonists.[99,100] The frequency of such mutations in prostate cancer patients is unknown but a study by Taplin et al. found five of ten samples of hormone refractory prostate cancer metastatic to bone had mutations of the *AR* and at least two of these mutations resulted in a shift in hormone specificity of the *AR*.[101] Finally, Visakorpi et al. demonstrated that up to 30% of prostate cancer specimens from men failing hormonal therapy are characterized by increases in copy number of X chromosomal region (q11-q13) containing the androgen receptor.[102] These results suggest that instead of being insensitive to androgen, such tumors may become supersensitive to androgen, by an as yet undetermined mechanism, or perhaps sensitive to a different nonandrogen steroid hormone. Thus, whereas the precise role of androgen and the androgen receptor in this disease is not known, these studies imply a potential role of this pathway at a critical step in prostate cancer progression.

Bcl-2: An Inhibitor of Apoptosis. The *bcl-2* gene, located on chromosome 18q21, is unique among oncogenes in that its expression does not enhance the rate of cell proliferation, but instead decreases the rate of cell death.[103,104] The role of *bcl-2* in the development and progression of carcinoma of the prostate has been examined by McDonnell et al.[105] Using immunohistochemical techniques, *bcl-2* usually was not expressed in androgen-dependent prostatic cancer cells, whereas it was expressed in androgen-independent prostatic cancer cells.[105] This observation has been confirmed by Colombel et al.[106] These findings suggest that enhanced expression of bcl-2 protein in carcinomas of the prostate is associated with the transition to androgen independence, although Furuya et al. demonstrated that there are *bcl-2*-independent pathways to this state as well.[107]

E-Cadherin and KAI-1. Genes whose downregulation has been implicated in prostate cancer progression include the cell adhesion molecule genes, E-cadherin and KAI-1, located at chromosomes 16q22.1 (a frequent site of LOH) and 11p11.2, respectively.[108] E-cadherin protein is frequently reduced or absent in high-grade prostate cancers, and this finding has prognostic significance.[109–111] KAI-1 was identified by its ability to suppress metastasis in experimental animal studies.[112,113] Although the predominant mechanism for downregulation of these genes has not been determined, in the case of E-cadherin, gene inactivation via promoter methylation has been commonly found in prostate cancer cell lines, and at a low but detectable rate in clinical specimens of prostate cancer.

GSTπ. Similarly, the gene for the phase II detoxification enzyme, glutathione S-transferase π, has also been found to be extensively methylated in the promoter region, in a completely cancer-specific fashion, with concomitant absence of expression.[114] In fact, this methylation event, being found in over 90% of all prostate cancers, is the most common genomic alteration yet observed in prostate cancer. The mechanism by which this region becomes specifically methylated in prostate cancer, and the basis for its apparent selection in the carcinogenic pathway is unclear at present. As this enzyme is a key part of an important cellular pathway to prevent damage from a wide range of carcinogens, the inactivation of this activity may result in increased susceptibility of prostate tissue to both tumor initiation and progression resulting from an increased rate of accumulated DNA damage.

Hereditary Cases

To date, no germ line mutations have been identified that confer increased risk for prostate cancer, although multiple efforts are underway to identify such changes in prostate cancer families. One gene, however, the androgen receptor gene, has been implicated as a potentially important gene in modifying prostate cancer risk owing to polymorphisms within the gene which result in variable androgen receptor activity. Specifically, there are two polymorphic triplet repeats in exon 1 that code for polyglutamine and polyglycine repeats of varying lengths between 11-31 and 10-22 residues, respectively.[115–118] Although variations in the polyglycine repeat length are of unknown biological consequence, it has been demonstrated that the polyglutamine repeat length is inversely related to the ability of the androgen receptor to stimulate androgen-specific transcriptional activity.[119–121] This is of particular interest since the population with the shortest average glutamine repeat length observed is the African American population, which has the highest incidence and mortality rates reported for prostate cancer, whereas the Asian population, which has low risk for prostate cancer, tends to have longer repeat lengths.[115,116] Hakimi et al. have suggested that *AR* genes with shorter repeat lengths may increase the risk of developing more aggressive prostate cancer, by virtue of conferring greater sensitivity to androgenic stimulation.[93] Further study will be necessary to determine the overall role of androgen receptor polymorphisms in determining or modifying prostate cancer risk.

IMPLICATIONS FOR DIAGNOSIS

Whereas localized prostate cancer is readily curable by prostatectomy, presently there is no effective curative therapy for disseminated disease.[1] Thus, early detection is a critical aspect in prostate cancer treatment, although it is confounded by the presence of neoplastic lesions of limited clinical relevance in most aging men. Thus, once detected, the ability to accurately determine the biological aggressiveness of a given prostate cancer is a prime research goal. As mentioned earlier, certain molecular alterations, such as gain and loss of sequences on chromosomes 7 and 8, have been

shown to have prognostic significance, and loss of expression of the cell adhesion molecules, E-cadherin, and possibly KAI1, is strongly associated with more aggressive disease. In terms of diagnosis, PCR-based detection of methylation of the *GSTP1* promoter offers great potential as a highly sensitive and specific prostate cancer detection tool.

New therapeutic approaches based on genetic alterations in prostate cancer cells have been limited, primarily because of lack of progress in the identification of genes that are mutated at high frequency in this disease. However, *p53* gene replacement and PSA (and other prostate-specific) promoter-based targeting of toxic gene expression to the prostate are examples of novel strategies that are under development.

REFERENCES

1. Wingo PA, Tong T, Bolden BA: *Cancer Statistics* **43**:8, 1995.
2. Brawley OW, Kramer BS: Epidemiology of prostate cancer, in Vogelsang NJ, Scardino PT, Shipley WU, Coffey DS, (eds): *Comprehensive Textbook of Genitourinary Oncology*. Baltimore, Williams & Wilkins, 1996, pp. 565–572.
3. National Cancer Institute: SEER Program, 1996.
4. Boring CC, Squires TS, Tong T: Cancer statistics, 1992 [published erratum appears in CA Cancer J Clin Mar–Apr: 42(2):127–128, 1992.] *CA Cancer J Clin* **42**:19, 1992.
5. Dhom G: Epidemiologic aspects of latent and clinically manifest carcinoma of the prostate. *J Cancer Res Clin Oncol* **106**:210, 1983.
6. Breslow N, Chan CW, Dhom G, Drury RA, Franks LM, Gellei B, Lee YS, Lundberg S, Sparke B, Sternby NH, Tulinius H: Latent carcinoma of prostate of autopsy in seven areas. *Int J Cancer* **20**:680, 1977.
7. Yatani R, Chigusa I, Akazaki K, Stemmermann GN, Welsh RA, Correa P: Geographic pathology of latent prostatic carcinoma. *Int J Cancer* **29**:611, 1982.
8. Carter BS, Carter HB, Isaacs JT: Epidemiologic evidence regarding predisposing factors to prostate cancer. [Review]. *Prostate* **16**:187, 1990.
9. Taylor JA: Epidemiologic evidence of genetic susceptibility to cancer. [Review]. *Birth Defects* **26**:113, 1990.
10. McNeal JE, Redwine EA, Freiha FS, Stamey TA: Zonal distribution of prostatic adenocarcinoma. Correlation with histologic pattern and direction of spread. *Am J Surg Pathol* **12**:897, 1988.
11. McNeal JE: Origin and evolution of benign prostatic enlargement. *Invest Urol* **15**:340, 1978.
12. Bostwidk DG: Prostatic intraepithelial neoplasia (PIN). *Urology* **34**:16, 1989.
13. Lilja H, Abrahamsson PA: Three predominant proteins secreted by the human prostate gland. *Prostate* **12**:29, 1988.
14. Dalkin BL, Ahmann FR, Kopp JB: Prostate specific antigen levels in men older than 50 years without clinical evidence of prostatic carcinoma. *J Urol* **150**:1837, 1993.
15. Oesterling JE: Prostate specific antigen: a critical assessment of the most useful tumor marker for adenocarcinoma of the prostate. [Review]. *J Urol* **145**:907, 1991.
16. Oesterling JE, Chan DW, Epstein JI, Kimball AW, Jr., Bruzek DJ, Rock RC, Brendler CB, Walsh PC: Prostate specific antigen in the preoperative and postoperative evaluation of localized prostatic cancer treated with radical prostatectomy. *J Urol* **139**:766, 1988.
17. Gleason DF: Histologic grading of prostate cancer. A perspective. [Review]. *Hum Pathol* **23**:273, 1992.
18. Montie JE: 1992 staging system for prostate cancer. [Review]. *Semin Urol* **11**:10, 1993.
19. Bastacky SI, Wojno KJ, Walsh PC, Carmichael MJ, Epstein JI: Pathological features of hereditary prostate cancer. *J Urol* **153**:987, 1995.
20. Qian JQ, Bostwick DG, Takahashi S, Borell TJ, Herath JF, Lieber MM, Jenkins RB; Chromosomal anomalies in prostatic intraepithelial neoplasia and carcinoma detected by fluorescence in situ hybridization. *Cancer Res* **55**:5408, 1995.
21. Sakr WA, Macoska JA, Benson P, Grignon DJ, Wolman SR, Pontes JE, Crissman JD: Allelic loss in locally metastatic, multisampled prostate cancer. *Cancer Res* **54**:3273, 1994.

22. Mirchandani D, Zheng J, Miller GJ, Ghosh AK, Shibata DK, Cote RJ, Roy-Burman P: Heterogeneity in intratumor distribution of p53 mutations in human prostate cancer. *Am J Pathol* **147**:92, 1995.

23. Cannon L, Bishop DT, Skolnick M, Hunt S, Lyon JL, Smart CR: Genetic epidemiology of prostate cancer in the Utah Mormon genealogy. *Cancer Surveys* **1**:47, 1982.

24. Meikle AW, Smith JA, West DW: Familial factors affecting prostatic cancer risk and plasma sex-steroid levels. *Prostate* **6**:121, 1985.

25. Spitz MR, Currier RD, Fueger JJ, Babaian RJ, Newell GR: Familial patterns of prostate cancer: A case-control analysis. *J Urol* **146**:1305, 1991.

26. Steinberg GD, Carter BS, Beaty TH, Childs B, Walsh PC: Family history and the risk of prostate cancer. *Prostate* **17**:337, 1990.

27. Carter BS, Beaty TH, Steinberg GD, Child B, Walsh PC: Mendelian inheritance of familial prostate cancer. *Proc Natl Acad Sci USA* **89**:3367, 1992.

28. Carter BS, Bova GS, Beaty TH, Steinberg GD, Childs B, Isaacs WB, Walsh PC: Hereditary prostate cancer: epidemiologic and clinical features. [Review]. *J Urol* **150**(3):797, 1993.

29. Isaacs WB: Molecular genetics of prostate cancer, in Ponder BA, Cavenee WK, Solomon E, (eds): *Genetics and Cancer: A Second Look,* Plainview, New York: Cold Spring Harbor Laboratory Press, 1995, pp. 357–380.

30. Bova GS, Carter BS, Bussemakers MJ, Emi M, Fujiwara Y, Kyprianou N, Jacobs SC, Robinson JC, Epstein JI, Walsh PC, et al: Homozygous deletion and frequent allelic loss of chromosome 8p22 loci in human prostate cancer. *Cancer Res* **53**:3869, 1993.

31. MacGrogan D, Levy A, Bostwick D, Wagner M, Wells D, Bookstein R: Loss of chromosome arm 8p loci in prostate cancer: mapping by quantitative allelic imbalance. *Genes Chromosom Cancer* **10**:151, 1994.

32. Trapman J, Sleddens HF, van der Weiden MM, Dinjens WN, Konig JJ, Schroder FH, Faber PW, Bosman FT: Loss of heterozygosity of chromosome 8 microsatellite loci implicates a candidate tumor suppressor gene between the loci D8S87 and D8S133 in human prostate cancer. *Cancer Res* **54**:6061, 1994.

33. Suzuki H, Emi M, Komiya A, Fujiwara Y, Yatani R, Nakamura Y, Shimazaki J: Localization of a tumor suppressor gene associated with progression of human prostate cancer within a 1.2 Mb region of 8p22-p21.3. *Genes Chrom Cancer* **13**:168, 1995.

34. Emmert-Buck MR, Vocke CD, Pozzatti RO, Duray PH, Jennings SB, Florence CD, Zhuang Z, Bostwick DG, Liotta LA, Linehan WM: Allelic loss on chromosome 8p12-21 in microdissected prostatic intraepithelial neoplasia. *Cancer Res* **55**:2959, 1995.

35. Macoska JA, Trybus TM, Benson PD, Sakr WA, Grignon DJ, Wojno KD, Pietruk T, Powell IJ: Evidence for three tumor suppressor gene loci on chromosome 8p in human prostate cancer. *Cancer Res* **55**:5390, 1995.

36. Bova GS, MacGrogan D, Levy A, Pin SS, Bookstein R, Isaacs WB: Physical mapping of chromosome 8p22 markers and their homozygous deletion in a metastatic prostate cancer. *Genomics* **35**:46, 1996.

37. Konig JJ, Kamst E, Hagemeijer A, Romijn JC, Horoszewicz J, Schroder FH: Cytogenetic characterization of several androgen responsive and unresponsive sublines of the human prostatic carcinoma cell line LNCaP. *Urol Res* **17**:79, 1989.

38. Bergerheim US, Kunimi K, Collins VP, Ekman P: Deletion mapping of chromosomes 8, 10, and 16 in human prostatic carcinoma. *Genes Chromosom Cancer* **3**:215, 1991.

39. Latil A, Baron JC, Cussenot O, Fournier G, Soussi T, Boccon-Gibod L, Le Duc A, Rouesse J, Lidereau R: Genetic alterations in localized prostate cancer: identification of a common region of deletion on chromosome arm 18q. *Genes Chromosom Cancer* **11**:119, 1994.

40. Macoska JA, Trybus TM, Sakr WA, Wolf MC, Benson PD, Powell IJ, Pontes JE: Fluorescence in situ hybridization analysis of 8p allelic loss and chromosome 8 instability in human prostate cancer. *Cancer Res* **54**:3824, 1994.

41. Cher ML, MacGrogan D, Bookstein R, Brown JA, Jenkins RB, Jensen RH: Comparative genomic hybridization, allelic imbalance, and fluorescence in situ hybridization on chromosome 8 in prostate cancer. *Genes Chrom Cancer* **11**:153, 1994.

42. Matsuyama H, Pan Y, Skoog L, Tribukait B, Naito K, Ekman P, Lichter P, Bergerheim US: Deletion mapping of chromosome 8p in prostate cancer by fluorescence in situ hybridization. *Oncogene* **9**:3071, 1994.

43. Massenkeil G, Oberhuber H, Hailemariam S, Sulser T, Diener PA, Bannwart F, Schafer R, Schwarte-Waldhoff I: P53 mutations and loss

of heterozygosity on chromosomes 8p, 16q, 17p, and 18q are confined to advanced prostate cancer. *Anticancer Res* **14**:2785, 1994.

44. Visakorpi T, Kallioniemi A, Syvanen AC, Hyytinen ER, Karhu R, Tammela T, Isola JJ, Kallioniemi OP: Genetic changes in primary and recurrent prostate cancer by comparative genomic hybridization. *Cancer Res* **55**:342, 1995.

45. Joos S, Bergerheim USR, Pan Y, Matsuyama H, Bentz M, Dumanoir S, Lichter P: Mapping of chromosomal gains and losses in prostate cancer by comparative genomic hybridization. *Genes Chrom Cancer* **14**:267, 1995.

46. Cher ML, Bova GS, Moore DH, Small EJ, Carroll PR, Pin SS, Epstein JI, Isaacs WB, Jensen RH: Genetic alterations in untreated prostate cancer metastases and androgen independent prostate cancer detected by comparative genomic hybridization and allelotyping. *Cancer Res* **56**:3091, 1996.

47. Ichikawa T, Nihei N, Suzuki H, Oshimura M, Emi M, Nakamura Y, Hayata I, Isaacs JT, Shimazaki J: Suppression of metastasis of rat prostatic cancer by introducing human chromosome 8. *Cancer Res* **54**:2299, 1994.

48. MacGrogan D, Levy A, Bova GS, Isaacs WB, Bookstein R: Structure and methylation-associated silencing of a gene within a homozygously deleted region of human chromosome band 8p22. In: *35 Ed.* **55**, 1996.

49. Van Den Berg C, Guan XY, Von Hoff D, Jenkins R, Bittner M, Griffin C, Kallioniemi O, Visakorpi T, McGill J, Herath J, Epstein J, Sarosdy M, Meltzer P, Trent J: DNA sequence amplification in human prostate cancer identified by chromosome microdissection: Potential prognostic implications. *Clin Cancer Res* **1**:11, 1995.

50. Macoska JA, Micale MA, Sakr WA, Benson PD, Wolman SR: Extensive genetic alterations in prostate cancer revealed by dual PCR and FISH analysis. *Genes Chromosom Cancer* **8**:88, 1993.

51. Micale MA, Sanford JS, Powell IJ, Sakr WA, Wolman SR: Defining the extent and nature of cytogenetic events in prostatic adenocarcinoma: paraffin FISH vs. metaphase analysis. *Cancer Genet Cytogenet* **69**(1):7, 1993.

52. Arps S, Rodewald A, Schmalenberger B, Carl P, Bressel M, Kastendieck H: Cytogenetic survey of 32 cancers of the prostate. *Cancer Genet Cytogenet* **66**(2):93, 1993.

53. Bandyk MG, Zhao L, Troncoso P, Pisters LL, Palmer JL, van Eschenbach AC, Chung LWK, Liang JC, Chung LW: Trisomy 7: A potential cytogenetic marker of human prostate cancer progression. *Genes Chromosom Cancer* **9**:19, 1994.

54. Alcaraz A, Takahashi S, Brown JA, Herath JF, Bergstralh, EJ, Larson-Keller JJ, Lieber MM, Jenkins RB: Aneuploidy and aneusomy of chromosome 7 detected by fluorescence in situ hybridization are markers of poor prognosis in prostate cancer. *Cancer Res* **54**:3998, 1994.

55. Zitzelsberger H, Szucs S, Weier HU, Lehmann L, Braselmann H, Enders S, Schilling A, Breul J, Hofler H, Bauchinger M: Numerical abnormalities of chromosome 7 in human prostate cancer detected by fluorescence in situ hybridization (FISH) on paraffin-embedded tissue sections with centromere-specific DNA probes. *J Pathol* **172**:325, 1994.

56. Zenklusen JC, Thompson JC, Troncoso P, Kagan J, Conti CJ: Loss of heterozygosity in human primary prostate carcinomas: A possible tumor suppressor gene at 7q31.1. *Cancer Res* **54**(24):6370, 1994.

57. Takahashi S, Shan AL, Ritland SR, Delacey KA, Bostwick DG, Lieber MM, Thibodeau SN, Jenkins RB: Frequent loss of heterozygosity at 7q31.1 in primary prostate cancer is associated with tumor aggressiveness and progression. *Cancer Res* **55**(18):4114, 1995.

58. Watson DL, Mashal R, Krithivas K, Corless C, Kantoff P, Richie JP, Sklar J: Loss of heterozygosity at chromosomal locus 7q21-q31 in metastatic prostate cancer. *153 Ed.* 271A, 1995.

59. Takahashi S, Qian J, Brown JA, Alcaraz A, Bostwick DG, Lieber MM, Jenkins RB: Potential markers of prostate cancer aggressiveness detected by fluorescence in situ hybridization in needle biopsies. *Cancer Res* **54**:3574, 1994.

60. Brothman AR, Peehl DM, Patel AM, McNeal JE: Frequency and pattern of karyotypic abnormalities in human prostate cancer. *Cancer Res* **50**:3795, 1990.

61. Lundgren R, Mandahl N, Heim S, Limon J, Henrikson H, Mitelman F: Cytogenetic analysis of 57 primary prostatic adenocarcinomas. *Genes Chromosom Cancer* **4**:16, 1992.

62. Micale MA, Mohamed A, Sakr W, Powell IJ, Wolman SR: Cytogenetics of primary prostatic adenocarcinoma. Clonality and chromosome instability. *Cancer Genet Cytogenet* **61**:165, 1992.

63. Atkin NB, Baker MC; Chromosome study of five cancers of the prostate. *Hum Genet* **70**:359, 1985.

64. Carter BS, Ewing CM, Ward WS, Treiger BF, Aalders TW, Schalken JA, Epstein JI, Isaacs WB: Allelic loss of chromosomes 16q and 10q in human prostate cancer. *Proc Natl Acad Sci USA* **87**:8751, 1990.

65. Ittmann M: Allelic loss on chromosome 10 in prostate adenocarcinoma. *Cancer Res* **56**:2143, 1996.

66. Gray IC, Phillips SMA, Lee SJ, Neoptolemos JP, Weissenbach J, Spurr NK: Loss of the chromosomal region 10q23-25 in prostate cancer. *Cancer REs* **55**:4800, 1995.

67. Eagle LR, Yin X, Brothman AR, Williams BJ, Atkin NB, Prochownik EV: Mutation of the MXI1 gene in prostate cancer. *Nat Genet* **9**:249, 1995.

68. Trybus TM, Burgess AC, Wojno KJ, Glover TW, Macoska JA; Distinct areas of allelic loss on chromosomal regions 10p and 10q in human prostate cancer. *Cancer Res* **56**:2263, 1996.

69. Cher ML, Ito T, Weidner N, Carroll PR, Jensen RH: Mapping of regions of physical deletion on chromosome 16q in prostate cancer cells by fluorescence *in situ* hybridization (FISH). *J Urol* **153**(1):249, 1995.

70. Brooks JD, Bova GS, Ewing CM, Epstein JI, Carter BS, Piantadosi S, Robinson JC, Isaacs WB: An uncertain role for p53 alterations in human prostate cancers. *Cancer Res* **56**:3814, 1996.

71. Brothman AR, Steele MR, Williams BJ, Jones E, Odelberg S, Albertsen HM, Jorde LB, Rohr LR, Stephenson RA; Loss of chromosome 17 loci in prostate cancer detected by polymerase chain reaction quantitation of alleli markers. *Genes Chrom Cancer* **13**:278, 1995.

72. Williams BJ, Jones E, Zhu XL, Steele MR, Stephenson RA, Rohr LR, Brothman AR: Prostatic neoplasm, genes, tumor, in situ hubridization, chromosome deletion. Evidence for a tumor suppressor gene distal to brca1 in prostate cancer. *J Urol* **155**:720, 1996.

73. Carter BS, Epstein JI, Isaacs WB: *ras* gene mutations in human prostate cancer. *Cancer Res* **50**:6830, 1990.

74. Gumerlock PH, Poonamallee UR, Meyers FJ, de Vere White RW: Activated ras alleles in human carcinoma of the prostate are rare. *Cancer Res* **51**:1632, 1991.

75. Moul JW, Friedrichs PA, Lance RS, Theune SM, Chang EH: Infrequent RAS oncogene mutations in human prostate cancer. *Prostate* **20**:327, 1992.

76. Kubota Y, Fujinami K, Uemura H, Dobashi Y, Miyamoto H, Iwasaki Y, Kitamura H, Shiuin T: Retinoblastoma gene mutations in primary human prostate cancer. *Prostate* **27**:314, 1995.

77. Bussemakers MJG, Bova GS, Schoenberg MP, Hakimi JM, Barrack ER, Isaacs WB: Microsatellite instability in human prostate cancer. *J Urol* **151**:469A, 1995.

78. Boyer JC, Umar A, Risinger JI, Lipford JR, Kane M, Yin S, Barrett JC, Kolodner RD, Kunkel TA: Microsatellite instability, mismatch repair deficiency, and genetic defects in human cancer cell lines. *Cancer Res* **55**:6063, 1995.

79. Visakorpi T, Kallioniemi OP, Heikkinen A, Koivula T, Isola J: Small subgroup of aggressive, highly proliferative prostatic carcinomas defined by p53 accumulation. *J Natl Cancer Inst* **84**:883, 1992.

80. Bookstein R, MacGrogan D, Hilsenbeck SG, Sharkey F, Allred DC: p53 is mutated in a subset of advanced-stage prostate cancers. *Cancer Res* **53**:3369, 1993.

81. Navone NM, Troncoso P, Pisters LL, Goodrow TL, Palmer JL, Nichols WW, von Eschenbach AC, Conti CJ: p53 protein accumulation and gene mutation in the progression of human prostate carcinoma. *J Natl Cancer Inst* **85**:1657, 1993.

82. Aprikian AG, Sarkis AS, Fair WR, Zhang ZF, Fuks Z, Cordon-Cardo C: Immunohistochemical determination of p53 protein nuclear accumulation in prostatic adenocarcinoma. *J Urol* **151**:1276, 1994.

83. Dinjens WN, van der Weiden MM, Schroeder FH, Bosman FT, Trapman J: Frequency and characterization of p53 mutations in primary and metastatic human prostate cancer. *Int J Cancer* **56**:630, 1994.

84. Voeller HJ, Sugars LY, Pretlow T, Gelmann EP: p53 oncogene mutations in human prostate cancer specimens. *J Urol* **151**:492, 1994.

85. Chi SG, de Vere White RW, Meyers FJ, Siders DB, Lee F, Gumerlock PH: p53 in prostate cancer: frequent expressed transition mutations. *J Natl Cancer Inst* **86**:926, 1994.

86. Bookstein R, Shew JY, Chen PL, Scully P, Lee WH: Suppression of tumorigenicity of human prostate carcinoma cells by replacing a mutated RB gene. *Science* **247**:712, 1990.

87. Bookstein R, Rio P, Madreperla SA, Hong F, Allred C, Grizzle WE, Lee WH: Promoter deletion and loss of retinoblastoma gene expression in human prostate carcinoma. *Proc Natl Acad Sci USA* **87**:7762, 1990.

88. Ittmann MM, Wieczorek R: Alterations of the retinoblastoma gene in clinically localized, stage B prostate adenocarcinomas. *Hum Pathol* **27**:28, 1996.

89. Cooney KA, Wetzel JC, Merajver SD, Macoska JA, Singleton TP, Wojno KJ: Distinct regions of loss of 13q in prostate cancer. *Cancer Res* **56**:1142, 1996.

90. Kamb A, Gruis NA, Weaver-Feldhaus J, Liu Q, Harshman K, Tavtigian SV, Stockert E, Day RS, Johnson BE, Skolnick MH: A cell cycle regulator potentially involved in genesis of many tumor types [see comments]. *Science* **264**:436, 1994.

91. Cairns P, Polascik TJ, Eby Y, Tokino K, Califano J, Merlo A, Mao L, Herath J, Jenkins R, Westra W, Bova GS, et al: Frequency of homozygous deletion at p16/CDKN2 in primary human tumours. *Nat Genet* **11**:210, 1995.

92. Jarrard D, Bova GS, Ewing CM, Pin SS, Nguyen SH, Baylin SB, Cairns P, Sidransky D, Herman JG, Isaacs WB: Deletional, mutational, and methylation analyses of CDKN2 (p16/MTS1) in primary and metastatic prostate cancer. *Genes Chrom Cancer* 1996, *in press*.

93. Hakimi JM, Rondinelli RH, Schoenberg MP, Barrack ER: Androgen-receptor gene structure and function in prostate cancer. *World J Urol* 1996, *in press*.

94. Hobisch A, Culig Z, Radmayr C, Bartsch G, Klocker H, Hittmair A: Distant metastases from prostatic carcinoma express androgen receptor protein. *Cancer Res* **55**:3068, 1995.

95. Ruizeveld de Winter JA, Janssen PJ, Sleddens HM, Verleun-Mooijman MC, Trapman J, Brinkmann AO, Santerse AB, Schroder FH, van der Kwast TH: Androgen receptor status in localized and locally progressive hormone refractory human prostate cancer. *Am J Pathol* **144**:735, 1994.

96. Newmark JR, Hardy DO, Tonb DC, Carter BS, Epstein JI, Isaacs WB, Brown TR, Barrack ER: Androgen receptor gene mutations in human prostate cancer. *Proc Natl Acad Sci USA* **89**:6319, 1992.

97. Tilley WD, Buchanan G, Hickey TE, Bentel JM: Mutations in the androgen receptor gene are associated with progression of human prostate cancer to androgen independence. *Clin Cancer Res* **2**:277, 1996.

98. Kelly WK, Scher HI: Prostate specific antigen decline after antiandrogen withdrawal; the flutamide withdrawal syndrome. *J Urology* **149**:607–609, 1993.

99. Harris SE, Rong Z, Harris MA, Lubahn DD: Androgen receptor in human prostate adenocarcinoma LNCaP/ADEP cells contains a mutation which alters the specificity of the steroid-dependent transcriptional activation region. *Endocrinology* **126**:93, 1990.

100. Veldscholte J, Berrevoets CA, Ris-Stalpers C, Kuiper GG, Jenster G, Trapman J, Brinkmann AO, Mulder E: The androgen receptor in LNCaP cells contains a mutation in the ligand binding domain which affects steroid binding characteristics and response to antiandrogens. [Review]. *J Steroid Biochem Mol Biol* **41**:665, 1992.

101. Taplin ME, Bubley GJ, Shuster TD, Frantz ME, Spooner AE, Ogata GK, Keer HN, Balk SP: Mutation of the androgen-receptor gene in metastatic androgen-independent prostate cancer [see comments]. *N Engl J Med* **332**:1393, 1995.

102. Visakorpi T, Hyytinen E, Koivisto P, Tanner M, Keinanen R, Palmberg C, Palotie A, Tammela T, Isola J, Kallioniemi OP: In vivo amplification of the androgen receptor gene and progression of human prostate cancer. *Nat Genet* **9**(4):401, 1995.

103. Reed JC, Cuddy M, Slabiak T, Croce CM, Nowell PC: Oncogenic potential of bcl-2 demonstrated by gene transfer. *Nature* **336**:259, 1988.

104. Hockenbery DM: The bcl-2 oncogene and apoptosis. [Review]. *Semin Immunol* **4**:413–420, 1992.

105. McDonnell TJ, Troncoso P, Brisbay SM, Logothetis C, Chung LW, Hsieh JT, Tu SM, Campbell ML: Expression of the protooncogene bcl-2 in the prostate and its association with emergence of androgen-independent prostate cancer. *Cancer Res* **52**:6940, 1992.

106. Colombel M, Symmans F, Gil S, OToole KM, Chopin D, Benson M, Olsson CA, Korsmeyer S, Buttyan R: Detection of the apoptosis-suppressing oncoprotein bcl-2 in hormone-refractory human prostate cancers. *Am J Pathol* **143**:390, 1993.

107. Furuya Y, Krajewski S, Epstein JI, Reed JC, Isaacs JT: Expression of bcl2 in the progression of human and rodent prostatic cancers. *Clin Cancer Res* **2**:398, 1996.

108. Dong J-T, Suzuki H, Pin SS, Bova GS, Schalken JA, Isaacs WB, Barrett JC, Isaacs JT: Down-regulation of the KAI1 metastasis suppressor gene during the progression of human prostatic cancer infrequently involves gene mutation and allele loss. *Cancer Res* (*in press*), 1996.

109. Umbas R, Isaacs WB, Bringuier PP, Schaafsma HE, Karthaus HF, Oosterhof GO, Debruyne FM, Schalken JA: Decreased E-cadherin expression is associated with poor prognosis in patients with prostate cancer. *Cancer Res* **54**:3929, 1994.

110. Umbas R, Schalken JA, Aalders TW, Carter BS, Karthaus HF, Schaafsma HE, Debruyne FM, Isaacs WB: Expression of the cellular adhesion molecule E-cadherin is reduced or absent in high-grade prostate cancer. *Cancer Res* **52**:5104, 1992.

111. Morton RA, Ewing CM, Nagafuchi A, Tsukita S, Isaacs WB: Reduction of E-cadherin levels and deletion of the alpha-catenin gene in human prostate cancer cells. *Cancer Res* **53**:3585, 1993.

112. Ichikawa T, Ichikawa Y, Dong J, Hawkins AL, Griffin CA, Isaacs WB, Oshimura M, Barrett JC, Isaacs JT: Localization of metastasis suppressor gene(s) for prostatic cancer to the short arm of human chromosome 11. *Cancer Res* **52**:3486, 1992.

113. Dong J-T, Lamb PW, Rinker-Schaeffer CW, Vukanovic J, Isaacs JT, Barrett JC: KAI-1, A Metastasis Suppressor Gene for Prostate Cancer on Human Chromosome 11p11.2. *Science* **268**:884, 1995.

114. Lee WH, Morton RA, Epstein JI, Brooks JD, Campbell PA, Bova GS, Hsieh WS, Isaacs WB, Nelson WG: Cytidine methylation of regulatory sequences near the pi-class glutathine S-transferase gene accompanies human prostatic carcinogenesis. *Proc Natl Acad Sci USA* **91**(24):11733, 1994.

115. Edwards A, Hammond HA, Jin L, Caskey CT, Chakraborty R: Genetic variation at five trimeric and tetrameric tandem repeat loci in four human population groups. *Genomics* **12**:241, 1992.

116. Irvine RA, Yu MC, Ross RK, Coetzee GA: The CAG and GGC microsatellites of the androgen receptor gene are in linkage disequilibrium in men with prostate cancer. *Cancer Res* **55**:1937, 1995.

117. Macke JP, Hu N, Hu S, Bailey M, King VL, Brown T, Hamer D, Nathans J: Sequence variation in the androgen receptor gene is not a common determinant of male sexual orientation. *Am J Hum Genet* **53**:844, 1993.

118. Sleddens HF, Oostra BA, Brinkmann AO, Trapman J: Trinucleotide (GGN) repeat polymorphism in the human androgen receptor (AR) gene. *Hum Mol Genet* **2**:493, 1993.

119. Chamberlain NL, Driver Ed, Misefeld RL: The length and location of CAG trinucleotide repeats in the androgen receptor N-terminal domain affect transactivation function. *Nucleic Acids Res* **22**:3181, 1994.

120. Kazemi-Esfarjani P, Trifiro MA, Pinsky L: Evidence for a repressive function of the long polyglutamine tract in the human androgen receptor: possible pathogenetic relevance for the (CAG)n-expanded neuronopathies. *Hum Mol Genet* **4**:523, 1995.

121. Sobue G, Doyu M, Morishima T, Mukai E, Yasuda T, Kachi T, Mitsuma T: Aberrant androgen action and increased size of tandem CAG repeat in androgen receptor gene in X-linked recessive bulbospinal neuronopathy. *J Neurol Sci* **121**:167, 1994.

CHAPTER 40

Brain Tumors

Sandra H. Bigner ∎ Roger E. McLendon ∎ Naji Al-dosari ∎ Ahmed Rasheed

1. Glioblastoma multiforme, the most common malignant primary brain tumor of adults, is characterized by gains of chromosome 7 and losses of chromosome 10, which are seen in up to 80 to 90 percent of cases. More than half of these tumors also contain abnormalities of genes involved in cell cycle control. Specifically, about one-third of cases contain homozygous deletions of the CDKN2A gene, while some tumors with intact CDKN2A have loss of expression of the retinoblastoma gene or have amplification of the CDK4 gene. In addition, approximately one-third of cases contain amplification, often with rearrangement of the epidermal growth factor receptor (EGFR) gene.

2. Lower-grade astrocytomas, particularly anaplastic astrocytomas, as well as low-grade tumors which progress to glioblastomas, contain mutations of the TP53 gene in up to 50 percent of cases in some series. Oligodendrogliomas are frequently characterized by losses of 1p and 19q. The target genes for loss of these regions remain unknown. A subset of ependymomas has loss of 22q. Mutation of the neurofibromatosis Type 2 (NF2) gene has been described in a single case of an ependymoma. Therefore, whether or not this gene is the target of the 22q loss in these tumors remains speculative.

3. The most consistent finding in medulloblastomas, the most common primary malignant brain tumor of children, is loss of 17p. Mapping of the deleted region to distal 17p, and a low incidence of TP53 gene mutations, suggest that the TP53 is not the target of 17p loss in these tumors.

4. The incidence of gene amplification has variously been reported from less than 5 percent to 22 percent in medulloblastomas. The amplified gene is usually c-myc, with a few examples of N-myc gene amplification. Approximately 60 percent of meningiomas and schwannomas have loss of 22q, which is usually associated with NF2 gene mutations (Table 40-1).

Table 40-1 Chromosomal and Genetic Alterations Characteristic of Specific Types of Brain Tumors

Tumor Type	Chromosomal or LOH Abnormality	Genetic Alteration
Glioblastoma	+7	Unknown
	−9p	CDKN2A, CDKN2B
	−10	Unknown
	−17p	p53 gene mutation
	Dmins	EGFR gene amplification and rearrangement
Oligodendroglioma	−1p, −19q	Unknown
Ependymoma	−22	?NF2 gene mutation
Medulloblastoma	−17p	Unknown
	Dmins	c-myc, N-myc gene amplification
Meningioma	−22	NF2 gene mutation
Schwannoma	−22	NF2 gene mutation

is approximately 7.0 per 100,000,[1] which means that nearly 20,000 Americans will have an astrocytoma diagnosed each year. The World Health Organization (WHO) classification[2] recognizes four grades of astrocytoma (Fig. 40-1). Grade I astrocytomas are slow-growing, noninfiltrative neoplasms, occurring mainly in children and young adults, and include juvenile pilocytic astrocytomas and gangliogliomas. Grade II astrocytomas are mainly well-differentiated fibrillary astrocytomas, while the grade III astrocytoma, the anaplastic astrocytoma, is a more aggressive neoplasm.[3] The most malignant form of astrocytoma, the grade IV tumor, is the glioblastoma multiforme, which is the most common primary malignant brain tumor of adults. Although these tumors most commonly occur in the cerebral hemispheres of older individuals, they can be seen throughout the brain and spinal cord of patients of all ages.

ASTROCYTOMAS

The astrocyte, one form of glial cell which comprises much of the background substance of the brain and spinal cord, is believed to give rise to a large category of primary brain tumors, the astrocytomas. These neoplasms can occur in all areas of the brain and spinal cord in children and adults. The incidence of astrocytomas

Chromosomal Abnormalities in Astrocytomas

The most consistent chromosomal changes in glioblastomas are gains of chromosome 7, seen in about 80 percent of tumors with abnormal stemlines; losses of chromosome 10, seen in 60 percent of tumors; losses of 9p, seen in about a third of cases; and the presence of double minute chromosomes (Dmins), reported in up to 50 percent of cases[4–9] (Figs. 40-2 and 40-3). Loss of heterozygosity

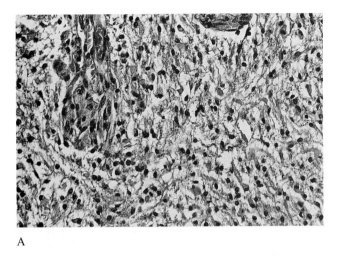

A

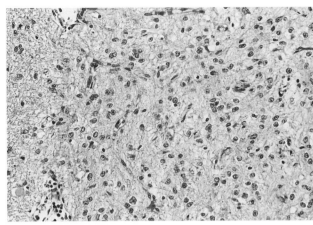

B

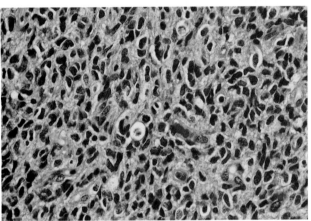

C

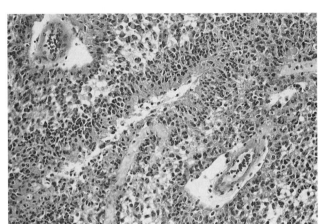

D

FIG. 40-1 Histology of astrocytomas. *A*. WHO grade I astrocytomas are largely represented by pilocytic astrocytomas which are moderately cellular neoplasms formed of bipolar astrocytes that occasionally produce Rosenthal fibers. *B*. WHO grade II astrocytomas, also known as well-differentiated fibrillary astrocytomas, are composed of unipolar and stellate astrocytes with simplified processes that exhibit mild nuclear pleomorphism and a proliferation index of 1 percent or less. *C*. Grade III astrocytomas, or anaplastic astrocytomas, are highly cellular neoplasms composed largely of unipolar astrocytes exhibiting nuclear pleomorphism and a brisk proliferation index but lacking in tumor necrosis and vascular proliferation. *D*. Grade IV astrocytomas, or glioblastomas, form the most malignant end of the spectrum and are characterized by astrocytic neoplasms exhibiting nuclear pleomorphism, brisk proliferation index, vascular proliferation, and/or necrosis with pseudopalisading.

(LOH) analyses have confirmed losses of all or part of chromosome 10 in more than 90 percent of cases (Fig. 40-4) in some series, and have narrowed the smallest region of overlapping deletion to 10q25.[10,11] Most series have also identified a second region on 10p and a third site on proximal 10q has also been targeted by some observers.[12–14] Candidate genes in the 10q25 region include the *MXI1* and *PAX-2*.[15,16] Whether or not these genes are involved in glioblastomas remains to be determined.

Genetic Alterations in Astrocytomas

LOH analyses of astrocytomas revealed that approximately one-third of these tumors have loss of all or part of 17p.[17–28] Unlike the chromosomal deviations described above, which are seen mainly in glioblastomas, LOH for 17p occurs in astrocytomas of all grades. Point mutations of the p53 gene can be demonstrated in the majority of astrocytomas with 17p loss. The mutations are clustered in the same hot spots as are seen in colon, breast, and lung carcinomas. The incidence of TP53 mutations confirmed by sequence data is about 25 percent (73 of 295) in glioblastomas, 34 percent (49 of 144) in anaplastic astrocytomas and 30 percent (33 of 111) in astrocytomas.[21–23;28–36] Most of the TP53 studies have

concentrated on the conserved exons,[5–8] but studies which included the entire coding sequence (exons 2-11) have uncovered only a handful of mutations outside of exons 5-8.[21,23,29,30,33] Similar to colon cancer, codons 175, 248, and 273 are frequently mutated in brain tumors; however the codon which is most frequently mutated in brain is codon 273, whereas in colon it is codon 175.[37] TP53 mutations are associated with age of the patient. These alterations are rare among paediatric patients,[26,28,33,35,38,39] but occur in nearly 50 percent of tumors in the young adult, with a much lower incidence (<20 percent) in the patient over 50 years of age. Most of the TP53 mutations identified in astrocytomas are G:C→A:T transitions located at CpG sites and resemble the pattern of mutations found in colon cancer, sarcomas, and lymphomas.

The cytogenetic observation of 9p loss in gliomas prompted evaluation of the A and B interferon genes which are located at 9p22. Hemizygous or homozygous deletion of interferon genes was reported in glioma cell lines and in biopsies of high grade astrocytomas,[40,41] but it was not clear in these early studies whether the interferon genes were the target of 9p deletions in gliomas or were simply located near the region of the target gene. In 1994, the *CDKN2A* and *CDKN2B* genes which are located at 9p21 were found to be homozygously deleted in various types of tumors.[42] In combined data collected on tumor biopsies

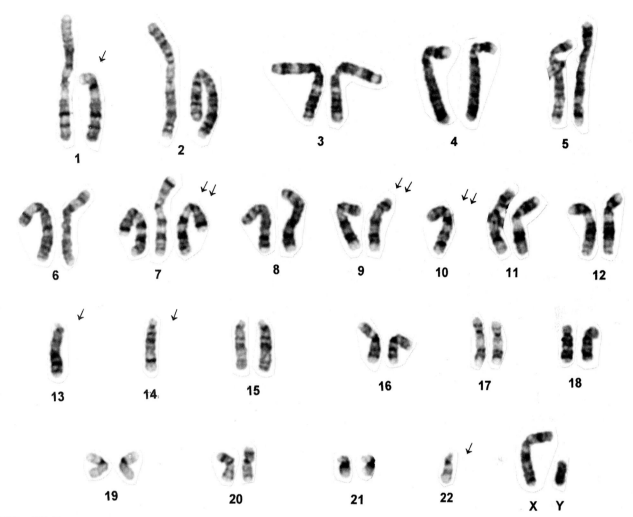

FIG. 40-2 Karyotype of glioblastoma. This giemsa-trypsin banded karyotype of glioblasoma xenograft D-643 MG shows gain of chromosome 7, a deletion of 9p, and loss of a chromosome 10 (double arrows). Additional, nonspecific changes are marked with single arrows.

in several laboratories the overall incidence of homozygeous deletions is 33 percent (98 of 300) in glioblastomas; 24 percent in anaplastic astrocytomas (19 of 79); and for hemizygous deletion or LOH for 9p loci is 24 percent of glioblastomas and 18 percent of anaplastic astrocytomas. The incidence of homozy-

gous deletions of both *CDKN2A* and *CDKN2B* is higher in xenografts, approaching 80 percent in some studies.[43] Among the 23 low-grade astrocytoma biopsies analyzed none exhibited homozygous deletion, although 5 showed LOH. Altogether there have been only three cases of mutations, all in glioblas-

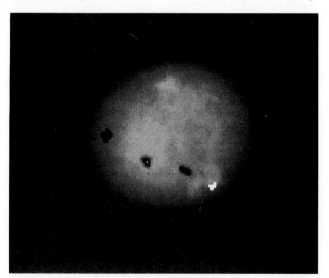

FIG. 40-3 FISH of glioblastoma. This interphase nucleus from a glioblastoma contains three chromosome 7 centromere signals (dark) and one centromere 10 signal (light).

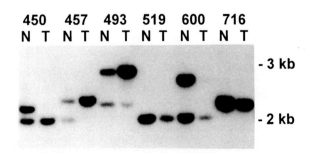

FIG. 40-4 LOH of glioblastoma chromosome 10. A Southern blot of Taq I digested DNA (5 mg) from blood (N) and glioblastoma tumor (T) was hybridized to the 10q marker D10S25. This marker showed LOH in tumors 450, 457, 493, and 600, and was uninformative in tumors 519 and 716. The size of the alleles ranged from 1.9 to 3 kb.

tomas.[44–53] The high frequency of homozygous deletions on chromosome 9 and the inclusion of *CDKN2A* and *CDKN2B* gene sequences in the deleted region in most cases has led most observers to believe that *CDKN2A* and *CDKN2B* are the target suppressor genes for 9p loss in gliomas. Unlike the p53 gene, which usually undergoes point mutation, the most common mechanism for *CDKN2A* gene inactivation in gliomas is homozygous deletions. However, alternative mechanisms such as transcriptional silencing by hypermethylation of CpG islands may be responsible for reduced expression in some gliomas with intact *CDKN2A/CDKN2B* genes.[54]

The majority of glioblastomas which possess Dmins contain amplification of the *EGFR* gene.[55] The *EGFR* gene has been shown to be amplified in one-third to one-half of glioblastomas, but only in isolated cases of anaplastic astrocytomas and rarely in other lower-grade tumors. In many glioblastomas, the amplified *EGFR* gene is also rearranged[56,57] (Fig. 40-5). The most common class of mutants bear deletion of exons 2–7 of the gene, resulting in an in-frame deletion of 801 base pairs of coding sequence and generation of a glycine residue at the fusion point. This variant receptor, designated EGFRvIII, has been reported in 17 to 62 percent of glioblastomas.[58–63] The tumor cell membrane fractions, containing the mutant 140-kDa receptor, show a significant elevation in tyrosine kinase activity without its ligand.[64] The mutant is still capable of binding with its ligand, but at a significantly reduced affinity.[65]

Relationship Between Cell Cycle Regulators in Astrocytomas

In addition to deletions of the *CDKN2A* and *CDKN2B* genes as discussed above, alterations of other genes involved in cell cycle regulation have been described in subsets of astrocytomas. LOH for 13q or loss of expression of the retinoblastoma (Rb) gene

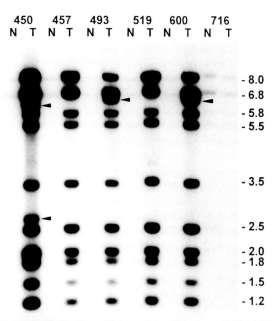

FIG. 40-5 Southern blot gene amplification, glioblastoma. A Southern blot of EcoRI digested DNA (5 mg) from blood (N) and glioblastoma tumor (T) was hybridized with *EGFR* gene probe pE7. The hybridizing fragments, in samples with normal copy number of the gene (all blood and tumor 716), appear as faint bands, and their sizes (in kb) are indicated on the right. In tumors 457 and 519 the gene was amplified, and in 450, 493, and 600 the gene was amplified and rearranged. Arrows indicate variant bands resulting from gene rearrangement.

product has been described in 20 to 40 percent of glioblastomas,[12,13,20,53,66–69] and amplification of the *CDK4* gene has been described in up to 15 percent of glioblastomas.[47,70] Furthermore, He et al.[69] and Ueki et al.[53] have shown that most glioblastomas contain only one of these three alterations: (1) *CDKN2A/CDKN2B* deletion, (2) LOH for 13q or loss of RB expression, or (3) *CDK4* gene amplification or increased expression.

Genetic Alterations in the Progression of Gliomas

It has long been recognized that there are two patterns for the development of glioblastomas. The majority of these tumors occur in patients over 50 years of age, in individuals with no previous indication of a brain tumor. A second group of cases involves younger people whose glioblastomas evolve out of lower-grade astrocytomas. Recent studies have provided molecular markers which in many cases distinguish between these two clinical patterns. The de novo pathway, occurring in older patients, includes tumors over 50 percent of which contain *EGFR* gene amplification and the majority of which lack TP53 gene mutations.[25–27,71] Glioblastomas evolving through progression, in contrast, seldom have *EGFR* gene amplification and more than 50 percent contain *TP53* gene mutations.[24,70,72–74] Other molecular markers, including LOH for chromosome 10, *CDKN2A* and *CDKN2B* deletions, Rb and *CDK4* abnormalities, and amplification of other oncogenes, do not appear to differ in tumors arising through these two pathways.

OLIGODENDROGLIOMAS

Oligodendrogliomas are a type of glioma which occur mainly in the cerebral hemispheres of adults and which are derived from the oligodendrocyte. Lesions with benign cytologic features are considered grade II according to the WHO classification (Fig. 40-6), while tumors with anaplastic characteristics (abundant mitotic activity), necrosis without pseudopalisading and glomeruloid vascular proliferation are considered grade III tumors (anaplastic oligodendrogliomas). According to data collected by the Surveillance, Epidemiology, and End Results (SEER) project, the age-adjusted incidence of oligodendroglioma is 0.33 per 100,000.[1]

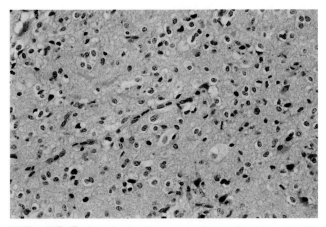

FIG. 40-6 Oligodendrogliomas are characterized by cells with round to oval nuclei surrounded by perinuclear cytoplasmic halos and usually associated with a fine arcuating network of tubular vessels.

Chromosomal Abnormalities in Oligodendrogliomas

Although most cytogenetic analyses of oligodendrogliomas have failed to demonstrate consistent findings, LOH studies have shown that loss of 1p and 19q occur in a substantial proportion of these tumors. Bello et al.[75] reported LOH for loci on 1p in up to 100 percent (6 of 6) oligodendrogliomas and in most (5 of 6) anaplastic oligodendrogliomas. Among other types of glioma only 2 of 11 glioblastomas exhibited 1p LOH, suggesting that 1p LOH is characteristic of tumors of oligodendroglial origin. A high incidence of 1p loss in tumors of oligodendroglial origin has been confirmed by Reifenberger et al.[76] using LOH techniques. Using in situ hybridization, Hashimoto et al.[77] found deletion of a 1p locus in 9 of 9 oligodendrogliomas.

Analysis with restriction fragment length polymorphism and microsatellite markers showed loss of markers on chromosome 19 in about 63 percent (17 of 27) of grade II oligodendrogliomas, 75 percent (18 of 24) of grade III or anaplastic oligodendrogliomas, and in 48 percent (21 of 43) of mixed oligoastrocytomas.[76,78,79] This abnormality has also been reported in about 16 percent (4 of 25) of astrocytomas, 38 percent (13 of 34) of anaplastic astrocytomas, and 28 percent (37 of 130) of glioblastomas tested.[78,79] Loss of loci on 19q was more frequent among oligodendroglial tumors, whereas astrocytic tumors mostly lost 19p alleles.[79] The 19q minimal deletion region has been mapped to a 425-kb region on 19q13.3.[80,81]

EPENDYMOMAS

Ependymomas are a category of glioma which can occur at many locations within the brain and spinal cord of adults and children. Favored sites include the posterior fossa in children and the cauda equina in patients of all ages. Most lesions are classified histologically as grade II (Fig. 40-7), while tumors with anaplastic features (anaplastic ependymomas, grade III) are sometimes seen. SEER data indicate an age-adjusted incidence of 0.18 per 100,000.[1]

Chromosomal Abnormalities in Ependymomas

The most common cytogenetic abnormality in ependymomas is loss or structural alteration of chromosome 22, seen as an isolated finding in some cases and as part of a more complex picture in others.

This alteration characterizes approximately 10 to 20 percent of cases with abnormal stemlines in most cytogenetic studies, and a similar incidence of chromosome 22 loss has been described in LOH studies.[82–93] Some observers, however, have noted this abnormality in a high proportion of cases by karyotype[86,87,91] or by LOH analysis[94,95] Since the *NF2* gene is located on 22q, it has been considered as a possible target for loss of this chromosomal region in ependymomas. However, since only one somatic mutation of this gene has been reported among 25 ependymomas which were studied, the role of *NF2* mutations in ependymomas remains speculative.[90,96]

MEDULLOBLASTOMAS

Medulloblastomas, the most common malignant primary brain tumor of childhood, are small cell neoplasms which arise in the cerebellum. Due to the primitive morphology of the cells, their lack of differentiation, and their resemblance to some poorly differentiated supratentorial neoplasms, these tumors have been called primitive neuroectodermal tumors (PNETs) by some observers. They are characterized by sheets of small cells with scant cytoplasm and a high mitotic rate (Fig. 40-8). In the United Kingdom, the incidence of medulloblastoma has been estimated at 0.5 per 100,000 children less than 15 years old, 97 with an overall age-adjusted incidence reported by the Central Brain Tumor Registry of the United States (CBTRUS) of 0.2 per 100,000.[98]

Chromosomal Abnormalities in Medulloblastomas

The most common specific chromosomal abnormality in medulloblastomas is loss of 17p, through formation of isochromosome 17q [i(17q)] or by unbalanced translocations[84,85,92,99–104] (Fig. 40-9). By karyotype as well as LOH studies, the indicence of this feature is approximately 30 to 40 percent.[94,105–110] Despite the location of the *TP53* gene on 17p, *TP53* gene mutations are uncommon in these tumors, seen in abut 5 percent of cases.[107,109,111–116] This observation, along with mapping of the deleted region to 17p13.1-13.3, which is distal to the p53 gene, suggests that another, as yet undescribed, gene is likely to be the target of 1p loss in these tumors.

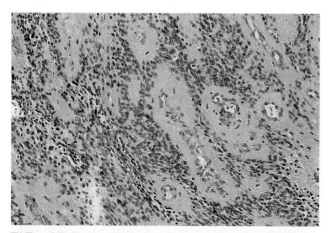

FIG. 40-7 Ependymomas often form perivascular pseudorosettes in which the tumor cells project slender fibrillar processes toward vessels while the nuclei appear excluded to a certain distance.

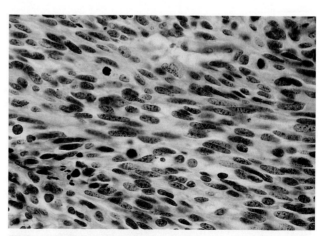

FIG. 40-8 Medulloblastomas are embryonal neoplasms that are markedly cellular with tumor cells generally exhibiting minimal amounts of cytoplasm. Although the classic growth pattern is that of dirffuse sheets of tumor cells, up to a third of cases will show a nodular growth pattern, of uncertain significance.

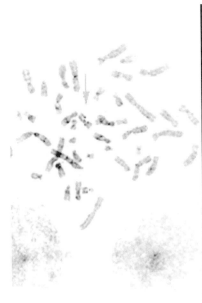

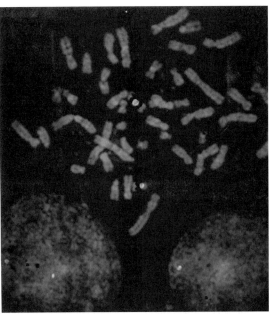

FIG. 40-9 Medulloblastoma with i(17q). The dark label, which corresponds to a 17q probe, stains the normal q arm of one chromosome 17 and both q arms of the i(17q). The light label marks the 17 centromere in both the normal chromosome 17 and i(17q).

Genetic Alterations in Medulloblastomas

Dmins are seen in about 5 percent of medulloblastoma biopsies, but can be identified in almost all permanent cultured cell lines and xenografts derived from these.[99,117] In most samples with Dmins, amplification of the c-*myc*, or less often the N-*myc*, gene can be demonstrated[109,117–123] (Fig. 40-10). The true incidence of myc gene amplification is difficult to determine in these tumors because the observed incidence differs according to the method of analysis. However, a recent analysis by comparative genomic hybridization suggests that it may be as high as 18 percent.[124]

MENINGIOMAS AND SCHWANNOMAS

Meningiomas are slow-growing neoplasms derived from the meningothelial cell which forms the arachnoid membrane. These tumors are composed of swirling sheets of cells with oval nuclei, often forming whorls and psammoma bodies (Fig. 40-11). They are generally considered to be benign, because they can often be completely excised surgically, but occasional cases recur and can show aggressive clinical characteristics. SEER data indicate an age-adjusted incidence of 0.13 per 100, 000 although data reported by CBTRUS support a much higher incidence of 2.5 per 100,000.[97,98]

Schwannomas are benign neoplasms, derived from the schwann cell which forms myelin in the peripheral nervous system. They are found attached to cranial or peripheral nerves, with favored sites being the acoustic and other sensory nerves. CBTRUS data report an overall incidence of nerve sheath tumors of 0.7 per 100,000.[98] Histologically they form masses of spindle-shaped cells and are usually benign (Fig. 40-12). Both schwannomas, particularly bilateral lesions involving the acoustic nerves,

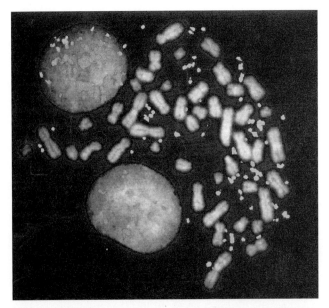

FIG. 40-10 Medulloblastoma with c-*myc* gene amplification. The c-*myc* probe, labeled darkly, is duplicated numerous times, as seen in the interphase nuclei and in the Dmins of a chromosomal spread.

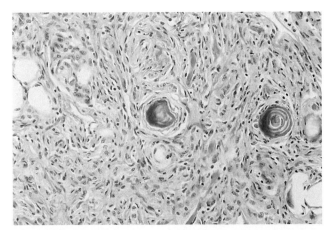

FIG. 40-11 Meningiomas are dural based neoplasms that grow as noninfiltrating masses, pushing brain away. These spindle cell tumors are often arranged in whorls and cords separated by collagen and are occasionally associated with eosinophilic psammoma bodies.

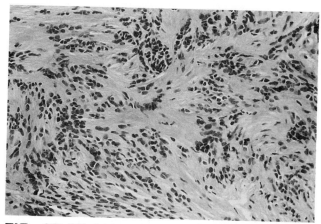

FIG. 40-12 Schwannomas also grow as solid, noninfiltrating tumors but are found along peripheral, and some cranial, nerves. The histologic hallmark of the schwannoma is the Verocay body, an aneuclear zone formed by palisading tumor cell nuclei.

and meningiomas are components of central von Recklinghausen neurofibromatosis or NF2.

Genetic Alterations in Meningiomas and Schwannomas

One of the first chromosomal abnormalities described in a solid human tumor was monosomy for a G group chromosome.[125] With the implementation of banding techniques, the missing chromosome was identified in the early 1970s as a number 22.[126,127] Loss or deletion of chromosome 22 is the most consistent karyotypic abnormality seen in this tumor type, occurring in about 60 percent of cases[128] (Fig. 40-13). LOH studies confirmed loss of 22q in 40 to 60 percent of both meningiomas and schwannomas.[129–135] This observation, taken together with the occurrence of these tumors in NF2 and linkage studies which localized the *NF2* locus to 22q, raised the possibility that the *NF2* gene was the target of chromosome 22 loss in these two tumor types. Isolation of the *NF2* gene

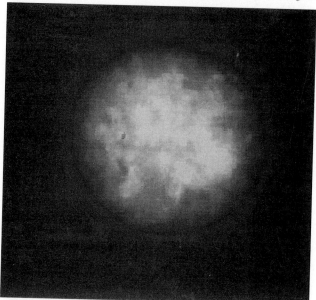

FIG. 40-13 FISH using a chromosome 22 probe in a meningioma. This interphase nucleus from a meningioma contains only one chromosome 22 signal.

and sequencing of this gene in these tumors confirmed that 40 to 60 percent of sporadic meningiomas and schwannomas contain *NF2* gene mutations.[136–142]

REFERENCES

1. Velema JP, Percy CL: Age curves of central nervous system tumor incidence in adults: Variation of shape by histologic type. *JNCI* **79**:623, 1987.
2. Kleihues P, Burger PC, Scheithauer BW: *Histological Typing of Tumours of the Central Nervous System.* 2nd ed. New York: Springer-Verlag, 1993.
3. Burger PC, Scheithauer BW, Vogel FS: *Surgical Pathology of the Nervous System and Its Coverings.* New York: Churchill Livingstone, 1991
4. Rey JA, Bellow J, deCampos JM, Kusak EM, Ramos C, Benitez, J: Chromosomal patterns in human malignant astrocytomas. *Cancer Genet Cytogenet* **29**:201, 1987.
5. Bigner SH, Mark J, Burger P, Mahaley MS Jr, Bullard DE, Muhlbaier LH, Bigner DD: Specific chromosomal abnormalities in malignant human gliomas. *Cancer Res* **48**:405, 1988.
6. Jenkins RJ, Kimmel DW, Moertel CA, Schultz CG, Schiethauer BW, Kelly PJ, Dewald GW: A cytogenetic study of 53 human gliomas. *Cancer Genet Cytogenet* **39**:253, 1989.
7. Thiel G, Losanowa T, Kintzel D, Nisch G, Martin H, Vorpahl K, Witkowski R: Karyotypes in 90 human gliomas. *Cancer Genet Cytogenet* **58**:109, 1992.
8. Hecht BK, Turc-Carel C, Chatel M, Grellier P, Gioanni J, Attias R, Gaudray P, Hecht F: Cytogenetics of malignant gliomas: 1. The autosomes with reference to rearrangements. *Cancer Genet Cytogenet* **84**:1, 1995.
9. Debiec-Rychter M, Alwasiak J, Liberski PP, Nedoszytko B, Babinska M, Mrózek, K, Imielinski B, Borowska-Lehman J, Limon J: Accumulation of chromosomal changes in human glioma progression. *Cancer Genet Cytogenet* **85**:61, 1995.
10. Fults, D, Pedone C: Deletion mapping of the long arm of chromosome 10 in glioblastoma multiforme. *Genes Chrom Cancer* **7**:173, 1993.
11. Rasheed BK, McLendon RE, Friedman HS, Friedman AH, Fuchs HE, Bigner DD, Bigner SH: Chromosome 10 deletion mapping in human gliomas: A common deletion region in 10q25. *Oncogene* **10**:2243, 1995.
12. Ransom DT, Ritland SR, Moertel CA, Dahl RJ, O'Fallon JR, Scheithauer BW, Kimmel DW, Kelly PJ, Olopade OI, Diaz MO, Jenkins RB: Correlation of cytogenetic analysis and loss of heterozygosity studies in human diffuse astrocytomas and mixed oligo-astrocytomas. *Genes Chrom Cancer* **5**:357, 1992.
13. Karlbom AE, James CD, Boethius J, Cavenee WK, Collins VP, Nordenskjold M, Larsson C: Loss of heterozygosity in malignant gliomas involves at least three distinct regions on chromosome 10. *Hum Genet* **92**:169, 1993.
14. Kimmelman AC, Ross DA, Liang BC: Loss of heterozygosity of chromosome 10p in human gliomas. *Genomics* **34**:250, 1996.
15. Eagle LR, Yin X, Brothman AR, Williams BJ, Atkin NB, Prochownik EV: Mutation of the MXI1 gene in prostate cancer. *Nat Genet* **9**:249, 1995.
16. Stapleton P, Weith A, Urbanek P, Kozmik Z, Busslinger, M: Chromosomal localization of seven PAX genes and cloning of a novel family member, PAX-9. *Nat Genet* **3**:292, 1993.
17. El-Azouzi M, Chung RY, Farmer GE, Martuza RL, Black PM, Rouleau GA, Hettlilch C, Hedley-Whyte ET, Zervas NT, Panagopoulos K, Nakamura Y, Gusella JF, Seizinger BR: Loss of distinct regions on the short arm of chromosome 17 associated with tumorigenesis of human astrocytomas. *Proc Natl Acad Sci USA* **86**:7186, 1989.
18. Fults D, Tippets RH, Thomas RJ, Nakamura Y, White R: Loss of heterozygosity for loci on chromosome 17p in human malignant astrocytoma. *Cancer Res* **49**:6572, 1989.
19. James CD, Carlbom E, Nordenskjold M, Collins VP, Cavenee WK: Mitotic recombination of chromosome 17 in astrocytomas. *Proc Natl Acad Sci USA* **86**:2858, 1989.

20. Venter DJ, Bevan KL, Ludwig RL, Riley TEW, Jat PS, Thomas DGT, Noble MD: Retinoblastoma gene deletions in human glioblastomas. *Oncogene* **6**:445, 1991.

21. Fults D, Brockmeyer D, Tullous MW, Pedone CA, Cawthon RM: P53 mutation and loss of heterozygosity on chromosomes 17 and 10 during human astrocytoma progression. *Cancer Res* **52**:674, 1992.

22. von Deimling A, Eibl RH, Ohgaki H, Louis DN, von Ammon K, Petersen I, Kleihues P, Chung RY, Wiestler OD, Seizinger BR: p53 mutations are associated with 17p allelic loss in grade II and grade III astrocytoma. *Cancer Res* **52**:2987, 1992.

23. Frankel RH, Bayona W, Koslow M, Newcomb EW: p53 Mutations in human malignant gliomas: Comparison of loss of heterozygosity with mutation frequency. *Cancer Res* **52**:1427, 1992.

24. Lang FF, Miller DC, Koslow M, Newcomb EW: Pathways leading to glioblastoma multifome: A molecular analysis of genetic alterations in 65 astrocytic tumors. *J Neurosurg* **81**:427, 1994.

25. Leenstra S, Bijlsma EK, Oosting J, Westerveld A, Bosch D, Huslebos TJM: Allele loss on chromosomes 10 and 17p and epidermal growth factor receptor amplification in human malignant astrocytoma related to prognosis. *Br J Cancer* **70**:684, 1994.

26. Rasheed, BK, McLendon RE, Herndon JE, Friedman HS Friedman AH, Bigner DD, Bigner SH: Alterations of the TP53 gene in human gliomas. *Cancer Res* **54**:1324, 1994.

27. Tenan M. Colombo BM, Pollo B, Cajola L, Broggi G, Finocchiaro G: P53 mutations and microsatellite analysis of loss of heterozygosity in malignant gliomas. *Cancer Genet Cytogenet* **74**:139, 1994.

28. Hermanson M, Funa K, Koopmann J, Maintz D, Waha A, Westermark B, Heldin CH, Wiestler OD, Louis DN, von Deimling A, Nister M: Association of loss of heterozygosity on chromosome 17p with high platelet-derived growth factor alpha receptor expression in human malignant gliomas. *Cancer Res* **56**: 164, 1996.

29. Chung R, Whaley J, Kley N, Anderson K, Louis D, Menon A, Hettlich C, Freiman R, Hedley-Whyte ET, Martuza R, Jenkins R, Yandell D, Seizinger BR: TP53 gene mutations and 17p deletions in human astrocytoma. *Genes Chrom Cancer* **3**:323, 1991.

30. Mashiyama S, Murakami Y, Yoshimoto T, Sekiya T, Hayashi F: Detection of p53 gene mutations in human brain tumors by single-strand conformation polymorphism analysis of polymerase chain reaction products. *Oncogene* **6**:1313, 1991.

31. Louis, DN: The p53 gene and protein in human brain tumors. *J Neuropathol Exp Neurol* **53**:11, 1994.

32. Kraus JA, Bolln C, Wolf HK, Neumann J, Kindermann D, Fimmers R, Forster F, Baumann A, Schlegel U: TP53 alterations and clinical outcome in low grade astrocytomas. *Genes Chrom Cancer* **10**:143, 1994.

33. Lang FF, Miller DC, Pisharody S, Koslow M, Newcomb E: High frequency of p53 protein accumulation without p53 gene mutation in human juvenile pilocytic, low grade and anaplastic astrocytomas. *Oncogene* **9**:949, 1994.

34. Alderson LM, Castleberg RL, Harsh GR, Louis DN, Henson JW: Human gliomas with wild-type p53 express bcl-2. *Cancer Res* **55**:999, 1995.

35. Chen P, Iavarone A, Fick J, Edwards M, Prados M, Israel MA: Constitutional p53 mutations associated with brain tumors in young adults. *Cancer Genet Cytogenet* **82**:106, 1995.

36. Kyritsis AP, Xu R, Bondy ML, Levin V, Bruner JM: Correlation of p53 immunoreactivity and sequencing in patients with glioma. *Mol Carcinog* **15**:1, 1996.

37. Bogler O, Huang H-J S, Kleihues P, Cavenee WK: The p53 gene and its role in human brain tumors. *Glia* **15**:308, 1995.

38. Litofsky NS, Hinton D, Raffel C: The lack of a role for p53 in astrocytomas in pediatric patients. *Neurosurgery* **34**:967, 1994.

39. Willert JR, Daneshvar L, Sheffield VC, Cogen PH: Deletion of chromosome arm 17p DNA sequences in pediatric high-grade and juvenile pilocytic astrocytomas. *Genes Chrom Cancer* **12**:165, 1995.

40. Miyakoshi J, Dobler KD, Allalunis-Turner J, McKean JD, Petruk K, Allen PBR, Aronyk KN, Weir B, Huyser-Wierenga D, Fulton D, Urtsun RC, Day RS III: Absence of IFNA and IFNB genes from human malignant glioma cell lines and lack of correlation with cellular sensitivity to interferons. *Cancer Res* **50**:278, 1990.

41. Olopade OI, Jenkins RB, Ransom DT, Malik K, Pomykala H, Nobori T, Cowan JM, Rowley JD, Diaz MO: Molecular analysis of deletions of the short arm of chromosome 9 in human gliomas. *Cancer Res* **52**:2523, 1992.

42. Kamb A, Grui, NA, Weaver-Feldhaus J, Liu Q, Harshman K, Tavtigian SV, Stockert E, Day RS, Johnson BE, Skolnick MH: A cell cycle regulator potentially involved in genes of many tumor types. *Science* **264**:436, 1994.

43. Jen J, Harper JW, Bigner SH, Bigner DD, Papadopoulos N, Markowitz S, Wilson JKV, Kinzler KW, Vogelstein B: Deletion of p16 and p15 genes in brain tumors. *Cancer Res* **54**:6353, 1994.

44. Ueki K, Rubio MP, Ramesh V, Correa KM, Rutter JL, von Deimling A, Buckler AJ, Gusella JF, Louis DN: MTS1/CDKN2 gene mutations are rare in primary human astrocytomas with allelic loss of chromosome 9p. *Hum Mol Genet* **3**:1841, 1994.

45. Giani C, Finocchiaro G: Mutation rate ofthe CDKN2 gene in malignant gliomas. *Cancer Res* **54**:6338, 1994.

46. He J, Allen JR, Collins VP, Allalunis-Turner MJ, Godbout R, Day RS, James CD: CDK4 amplifications is an alternative mechanism to p16 gene homozygous deletion in glioma cell lines.*Cancer Res* **54**:5804, 1994.

47. Schmidt EE, Ichimura K, Reifenberger G, Collins VP: CDKN2 (p16/MTS1) gene deletion or CDK4 amplification occurs in the majority of glioblastomas. *Cancer Res* **54**:6321, 1994.

48. Moulton T, Samara G, Chung WY, Yuan L, Desai R, Sist, Bruce J, Tyco B: MTS1/p16/CDKN2 lesions in primary glioblastoma multiforme. *Am J Pathol* **145**:613, 1995.

49. Nishikawa R, Furnari FB, Lin H, Arap W, Berger MS, Cavenee WK, Su Huang HJ: Loss of P16INK4 expression is frequent in high grade gliomas. *Cancer Res* **55**:1941, 1995.

50. Walker DG, Duan W, Popovic EA, Kaye AH, Tomlinson FH, Lavin, M: Homozygous deletions of the multiple tumor suppressor gene 1 in the progression of human astrocytomas. *Cancer Res* **55**:20, 1995.

51. Sonoda Y, Yoshimoto T, Sekiya T: Homozygous deletion of the MTS1/p16 and MTS2/p15 genes and amplification of the CDK4 gene in glioma. *Oncogene* **11**:2145, 1995.

52. Li YJ, Hoang-Xuan K, Delattre JY, Poisson M, Thomas G, Hamelin R: Frequent loss of heterozygosity on chromosome 9, and low incidence of mutations of cyclin-dependent kinase inhibitors p15 (MTS2) and p16 (MTS1) genes in gliomas. *Oncogene* **11**:597, 1995.

53. Ueki K, Ono Y, Henson JW, Efird JT, von Deimling A, Louis DN: CDKN2/p16 or RB alterations occur in the majority of glioblastomas and are inversely correlated. *Cancer Res* **56**:150, 1996.

54. Herman JG, Merlo A, Mao L, Lapidus RG, Issa JPJ, Davidson NE, Sidransky D, Baylin SB: Inactivation of the CDKN2/p16/MTS1 gene is frequently associated with aberrant DNA methylation in all common human cancers. *Cancer Res* **55**:4525, 1995.

55. Bigner SH, Wong AJ, Mark J, Muhlbaier LH, Kinzler KW, Vogelstein B, Bigner DD: Relationship between gene amplification and chromosomal deviations in malignant human gliomas. *Cancer Genet Cytogenet* **29**:165, 1987.

56. Wong AJ, Bigner SH, Bigner DD, Kinzler KW, Hamilton SR, Vogelstein B: Increased expression of the epidermal growth factor receptor gene in malignant gliomas is invariably associated with gene amplification. *Pro Natl Acad Sci USA* **84**:6899, 1993.

57. Bigner SH, Humphrey PA, Wong AJ, Vogelstein B, Mark J, Friedman HS, Bigner DD: Characterization of the epidermal growth factor receptor in human glioma cell lines and xenografts. *Cancer Res* **50**:8017, 1990.

58. Humphrey PA, Wong AJ, Vogelstein B, Zalutsky MR, Fuller GN, Archer GE, Friedman HS, Kwatra MM, Bigner SH, Bigner DD: Antisynthetic peptide antibody reacting at the fusion junction of deletion-mutant epidermal growth factor receptors in human glioblastoma. *Pro Natl Acad Sci USA* **87**:4207, 1990.

59. Sugawa N, Ekstrand A, James CD, Collins VP: Identical splicing of aberrant epidermal growth factor receptor transcripts from amplified rearranged genes in human glioblastomas. *Pro Natl Acad Sci USA* **8**:8602, 1990.

60. Ekstrand AJ, James CD, Cavenee WK, Seliger B, Pettersson RF, Collins VP: Genes for epidermal growth factor receptor, transforming growth factor alpha, and epidermal growth factor and their expression in human gliomas in vivo. *Cancer Res* **51**:2164, 1991.

61. Ekstrand AJ, Sugawa N, James CD, Collins VP: Amplified and rearranged epidermal growth factor receptor genes in human glioblastomas reveal deletions of sequences encoding portions of the N- and/or C-terminal tails. *Pro Natl Acad Sci USA* **89**:4309, 1992.

62. Moscatello DK, Holgado-Madruga M, Godwin AK, Ramirez G, Gunn G, Zoltick PW, Biegel J, Hayes RL, Wong AJ: Frequent expression of a mutant epidermal growth factor receptor in multiple human tumors. *Cancer Res* **55**:5536, 1995.

63. Wikstrand CJ, Hale LP, Batra SK, Hill ML, Humphrey PA, Kurpad SN, McLendon RE, Moscatello D, Pegram CN, Reist CJ, Traweek T, Wong AJ, Zalutsky MR, Bigner DD: Monoclonal antibodies against EGFRvIII are tumor specific and react with breast and lung carcinomas and malignant gliomas. *Cancer Res* **55**:3140, 1995.

64. Yamazaki H, Fukui Y, Ueyama Y, Tamaoki N, Kawamoto T, Taniguchi S, Shibuya M: Amplification of the structurally and functionally altered epidermal growth factor receptor gene (c-erbB) in human brain tumors. *Mol Cell Biol* **8**:1816, 1988.

65. Batra SK, Castelino-Prabhu S, Wikstrand CJ, Zhu X, Humphrey PA, Friedman HS, Bigner DD: Epidermal growth factor ligand-independent, unregulated, cell-transforming potential of a naturally occurring human mutant EGFRvIII gene. *Cell Growth Differ* **6**:1251, 1995.

66. James CD, He J, Carlbom E, Dumanski JP, Hansen M, Nordenskjöld M, Collins VP, Cavenee WK: Clonal genomic alterations in glioma malignancy stages. *Cancer Res* **48**:5546, 1988.

67. Fults D, Pedone CA, Thomas GA, White R: Allelotype of human malignant astrocytoma. *Cancer Res* **50**:5784, 1990.

68. Henson JW, Schnitker BL, Correa KM, von Deimling A, Fassbender F, Xu HJ, Benedict WF, Yandell DW, Louis DN: The retinoblastoma gene is involved in malignant progression of astrocytomas. *Ann Neurol* **3**:714, 1994.

69. He J, Olson JJ, James CD: Lack of p16INK4 or retinoblastoma protein (pRb), or amplification-associated overexpression of cdk4 is observed in distinct subsets of malignant glial tumors and cell lines. *Cancer Res* **55**:4833, 1995.

70. Reifenberger G, Reifenberger J, Ichimura K, Meltzer PS, Collins VP: Amplification of multiple genes from chromosomal region 12q13-14 in human malignant gliomas: Preliminary mapping of the amplicons shows preferential involvement of CDK4, SAS, and MDM2. *Cancer Res* **54**:4299, 1994.

71. von Deimling A, von Ammon K, Schoenfeld D, Wiestler OD, Seizinger BR, Louis DN: Subsets of glioblastoma multiforme defined by molecular genetic analysis. *Brain Pathol* **3**:19, 1993.

72. Ohgaki H, Schauble B, zur Hausen A, von Ammon K, Kleihues P: Genetic alterations associated with the evolution and progression of astrocytic brain tumors. *Virchows Arch* **427**:113, 1995.

73. Watanabe K, Tachibana O, Sato K, Yonekawa Y, Kleihues P, Ohgaki H: Overexpression of the EGF receptor and p53 mutations are mutually exclusive in the evolution of primary and secondary glioblastomas. *Brain Pathol* **6**:217, 1996.

74. Louis DN: Clinicopatho-genetic subsets of glioblastoma multiform: From both sides now. *Brain Pathol* **6**:217, 1996.

75. Bello MJ, Vaquero J, de Campos JM, Kusak ME, Sarasa JL, Szez-Castresana J, Pestana A, Rey JA: Molecular analysis of chromosome 1 abnormalities in human gliomas reveals frequent loss of 1p in oligodendroglial tumors. *Int J Cancer* **57**:172, 1994.

76. Reifenberger J, Reifenberger G, Liu L, James CD, Wechsler W, Collins VP: Molecular genetic analysis of oligodendroglial tumors shows preferential allelic deletions on 19q and 1p. *Am J Pathol* **145**:1175, 1994.

77. Hashimoto N, Ichikawa D, Arakawa Y, Date K, Ueda S, Nakagawa Y, Horil A, Nakamura Y, Abe T, Inazawa J: Frequent deletions of material from chromosome arm 1p in oligodendroglial tumors revealed by double-target fluorescence in situ hybridization and microsatellite analysis. *Genes Chrom Cancer* **14**:295, 1995.

78. von Deimling A, Nagel J, Bender B, Lenartz D, Schramm J, Louis DN, Wiestler OD: Deletion mapping of chromosome 19 in human gliomas. *Int J Cancer* **57**:676, 1994.

79. Ritland SR, Ganju V, Jenkins RB: Region-specific loss of heterozygosity on chromosome 19 is related to the morphologic type of human glioma. *Genes Chrom Cancer* **12**:277, 1995.

80. Rubio MP, Correa KM, Ueki K, Mohrenweiser HW, Gusella JF, von Deimling A, Louis DN: The putative glioma tumor suppressor gene on chromosome 19q maps between APOC2 and HRC. *Cancer Res* **54**:4760, 1994.

81. Yong WH, Chou D, Ueki K, Harsh, GR IV, von Deimling A, Gusella JF, Mohrenweiser HW, Louis DN: Chromosome 19q deletions in human gliomas overlap telomeric to D19S219 and may target a 425 kb region centromeric to D19S112. *Neuropathol Exp Neurol* **54**:622, 1995.

82. Brown NP, Pearson ADJ, Davison EV, Gardner-Medwin D, Crawford P, Perry R: Multiple chromosome rearrangements in a childhood ependymoma. *Cancer Genet Cytogenet* **36**:25, 1988.

83. Stratton MR, Darling J, Lantos PL, Cooper CS, Reeves BR: Cytogenetic abnormalities in human ependymomas. *Int J Cancer* **44**:579, 1989.

84. Chadduck WM, Boop FA, Sawyer JR: Cytogenetic studies of pediatric brain and spinal cord tumors. *Pediatr Neurosurg* **17**:57, 1991-1992.

85. Vagner-Capodano AM, Gentet JC, Gambarelli D, Pellissier JF, Gouzien M, Lena G, Genitori L, Choux M, Raybaud C: Cytogenetic studies in 45 pediatric brain tumors. *Pediatr Hematol Oncol* **9**:223, 1992.

86. Weremowicz S, Kupsky WJ, Morton CC, Fletcher JA: Cytogenetic evidence for a chromosome 22 tumor suppressor gene in ependymoma. *Cancer Genet Cytogenet* **61**:193, 1992.

87. Rogatto SR, Casartelli C, Rainho CA, Barbieri-Neto J: Chromosomes in the genes and progression of ependymomas. *Cancer Genet Cytogenet* **69**:146, 1993.

88. Neumann E, Kalousek DK, Norman MG, Stienbok P, Cochrane DD, Goddarad K: Cytogenetic analysis of 109 pediatric central nervous system tumors. *Cancer Genet Cytogenet* **71**:40, 1993.

89. Sawyer JR, Sammartino G, Husain M, Boop FA, Chadduck WM: Chromosome aberrations in four ependymomas. *Cancer Genet Cytogenet* **74**:132, 1994.

90. Bijlsma EK, Voesten AMJ, Bijleveld EH, Troost D, Westerveld A, Mérel P, Thomas G, Huslebos TJM: Molecular analysis of genetic changes in ependymomas. *Genes Chrom Cancer* **13**:272, 1995.

91. Wernicke C, Thiel G, Lozanova T, Vogel S, Kintzel D, Jänisch W, Lehmann K, Witkowski R: Involvement of chromosome 22 in ependymomas. *Cancer Genet Cytogenet* **79**:173, 1995.

92. Agamanolis DP, Malone JM: Chromosomal abnormalities in 47 pediatric brain tumors. *Cancer Genet Cytogenet* **81**:125, 1995.

93. Blaeker H, Rasheed BKA, McLendon RE, Friedman H, Batra SK, Fuchs HE, Bigner SH: Microsatellilte analysis of childhood brain tumors. *Genes Chrom Cancer* **15**:54, 1996.

94. James CD, Carlbom E, Mikkelsen T, Ridderheim PA, Cavenee WK, Collins VP: Loss of genetic information in central nervous system tumors common to children and young adults. *Genes Chrom Cancer* **2**:94, 1990.

95. Ransom DT, Ritland SR, Kimmel DW, Moertel CA, Dahl RJ, Scheithauer BW, Kelly PJ, Jenkins RB: Cytogenetic and loss of heterozygosity studies in ependymomas, pilocytic astrocytomas, and oligodendrogliomas. *Genes Chrom Cancer* **5**:348, 1992.

96. Rubio M, Correa KM, Ramesh V, MacCollin MM, Jacoby B, von Deimling A, Gusella JF, Louis DN: Analysis of the neurofibromatosis 2 gene in human ependymomas and astrocytomas. *Cancer Res* **54**:45, 1994.

97. Stevens MCG, Cameron AH, Muir KR, Parkes SE, Reid H, Whitwell H: Descriptive epidemiology of primary central nervous system tumours in children: A population-based study. *Clin Oncol* **3**:323, 1991.

98. *Central Brain Tumor Registry of the United States. Annual Report.* Chicago, 1995.

99. Bigner SH, Mark J, Friedman HS, Biegel JA, Bigner DD: Structural chromosomal abnormalities in human medulloblastomas. *Cancer Genet Cytogenet* **30**:91, 1988.

100. Griffin CA, Hawkins AL, Packer RJ, Rorke LB, Emanuel BS: Chromosome abnormalities in pediatric brain tumors. *Cancer Res* **48**:175, 1988.

101. Biegel JA, Rorke LB, Packer RJ, Sutton LN, Schut L, Bonner L, Emanuel S: Isochromosome 17q in primitive neuroectodermal tumors of the central nervous system. *Genes Chrom Cancer* **1**:139, 1989.

102. Krames PS, Tra TN, Cui MY, Raffel C, Gilles FH, Barranager JA, Ying KL: Cytogenetic analysis of 39 pediatric central nervous system tumors. *Cancer Genet Cytogenet* **59**:12, 1992.

103. Neumann E, Kalousek DK, Norman MG, Stienbok P, Cochrane DD, Goddard K: Cytogenetic analysis of 109 pediatric central nervous system tumors. *Cancer Genet Cytogenet* **71**:40, 1993.

104. Fuji Y, Hongo T, Hayashi Y: Chromosome analysis of brain tumors in childhood. *Genes Chrom Cancer* **11**:205, 1994.

105. Thomas GA, Raffel C: Loss of heterozygosity on 6q, 16q and 17p in human central nervous system primitive neuroectodermal tumors. *Cancer Res* **51**:639, 1991.

106. Cogen P, Daneshvar L, Metzger AK, Edwards MSB: Deletion mapping of the medulloblastoma locus on chromosome 17p. *Genomics* **8**:279, 1990.

107. Biegel JA, Burk CD, Barr FG, Emanuel BS: Evidence for a 17p tumor related locus distinct from p53 in pediatric primitive neuroectodermal tumors. *Cancer Res* **52**:3391, 1992.

108. Albrecht S, von Deimling A, Pietsch T, Giangaspero F, Brandnert S, Kleiheust P, Wiestler OD: Microsatellite analysis of loss of heterozy-

gosity on chromosomes 9q, 11p, and 17p in medulloblastoma. *Neuropathol Appl Neurobiol* **20**:74, 1994.

109. Batra SK, McLendon RE, Koo JS, Castelino-Prabhu S, Fuchs E, Krischer JP, Friedman HS, Bigner DD, Bigner SH: Prognostic implications of chromosome 17q deletions in human medulloblastomas. *J Neuro Oncology* **24**:39, 1995.

110. Scheurlen WG, Senf L: Analysis of the GAP-related domain of the neurofibromatosis type 1 (NF1) gene in childhood brain tumors. *Int J Cancer* **64**:234, 1995.

111. Ohgaki H, Eibl RH, Wiestler OD, Yasargil MG, Newcomb EW, Kleihues P: P53 mutations in nonastrocytic human brain tumors. *Cancer Res* **51**:6202, 1991.

112. Saylors R, Sidransky D, Friedman HS, Bigner SH, Bigner DD, Vogelstein B, Brodeur GM: Infrequent p53 gene mutations in medulloblastomas. *Cancer Res* **51**:4721, 1989.

113. Cogen PH, Daneshvar L, Metzgar AK, Geoffrey D, Edwards MSB, Sheffield VC: Involvement of multiple chromosome 17p loci in medulloblastoma tumorigenesis. *Am J Hum Genet* **50**:584,1992.

114. Badiali M, Iolascon A, Loda M, Scheithauer B, Basso G, Trentini G, Giangaspero F: p53 gene mutations in medulloblastoma, immunohistochemistry, gel shift analysis and sequencing. *Diagn Mol Pathol* **2**:23, 1993.

115. Raffel C, Thomas GA, Tishler DM, Lassof S, Allen JC: Absence of p53 mutations in childhood central nervous system primitive neuroectodermal tumors. *Neurosurgery* **33**:301, 1993.

116. Adesina AM, Nalbantoglu J, Cavenee, WK: p53 Gene mutation and mdm2 gene amplification are uncommon in medulloblastoma. *Cancer Res* **54**:5649. 1994.

117. Bigner SH, Friedman HS, Vogelstein B, Oakes WJ, Bigner DD: Amplification of the c-myc gene in human medulloblastoma cell lines and xenografts. *Cancer Res* **50**:2347, 1990.

118. Raffel C, Gilles FE, Weinberg KI: Reduction to homozygosity and gene amplification in central nervous system primitive neuroectodermal tumors of childhood. *Cancer Res* **50**:587, 1990.

119. Badiali M, Pession A, Basso G, Andreini L, Rigobello L, Galassi E, Giangaspero F: N-myc and c-myc oncogenes amplification in medulloblastomas. Evidence of particularly aggressive behavior of a tumor with c-myc amplification. *Tumori* **77**:118, 1991.

120. Friedman HS, Burger PC, Bigner SH, Trojanowski JQ, Brodeur GM, He X, Wikstrand CJ, Kurtzberg J, Berens ME, Halperin EC, Bigner DD: Phenotypic and genotypic analysis of a human medulloblastoma cell line and transplantable xenograft (D341 Med) demonstratig amplification of c-myc. *Am J Pathol* **130**:472, 1988.

121. Wasson JC, Saylors RL, Zelter P, Friedman HS, Bigner SH, Burger PC, Bigner DD, Look AT, Douglass EC, Brodeur GM: Oncogene amplification in pediatric brain tumors. *Cancer Res* **50**:2987, 1990.

122. Batra SK, Rasheed A, Bigner SH, Bigner DD: Oncogenes and antioncogenes in human central nervous system tumors. *Lab Invest* **71**:621, 1994.

123. Pietsch T, Scharman T, Fonatsch CF, Schmidt D, Ockler R, Freihoff D, Albrecht S, Wiestler OW, Zeltzer P, Riehm H: Characterization of five new cell lines derived from human primitive neuroectodermal tumors of the central nervous system. *Cancer Res* **54**:3278, 1994.

124. Schröck E, Blume C, Meffeert M-C, du Manoir S, Bersch W, Kiessling M, Lozanowa T, Thiel G, Witkowski R, Cremer T: Recurrent gain of chromosome arm 7q in low grade astrocytic tumors studied by comparative genomic hybridization. *Genes Chrom Cancer* **15**:199, 1996.

125. Zang KD, Singer H: Chromosomal constitution of meningiomas. *Nature* **216**:84, 1967.

126. Mark J, Levan G, Mitelman F: Identification by fluorescence of the G chromosome lost in human meningiomas. *Hereditas* **71**:163, 1972.

127. Zankl H, Zang KD: Cytological and cytogenetical studies on brain tumors. IV. Identification of the missing G chromosome in human meningiomas as No. 22 by fluorescence technique. *Hum Genet* **14**:167, 1972.

128. Zang KD: Cytological and cytogenetical studies on human meningioma. *Cancer Genet Cytogenet* **53**:271, 1991.

129. Seizinger BR, De la Monte S, Atkins L, Gusella JF, Martuza RL: Molecular genetic approach to human meningioma: Loss of genes on chromosome 22. *Pro Natl Acad Sci USA* **84**:5419, 1987.

130. Dumanski JP, Carlbom E, Collins VP, Nordenskjöld M: Deletion mapping of a locus on human chromosome 22 involved in the oncogenesis of meningioma. *Pro Natl Acad Sci USA* **84**:9275, 1987.

131. Seizinger BR, Rouleau G, Ozelius LJ, Lane AH, St. George-Hyslop P, Huson S, Gusella JF, Martuza RL: Common pathogenetic mechanism for three tumor types in bilateral acoustic neurofibromatosis. *Science* **236**:317, 1987.

132. Rouleau GA, Wertlecki W, Haines JL, Hobbs WJ, Trofatter JA, Seizinger BR, Martuza RL, Superneau DW, Conneally PM, Gusella JF: Genetic linkage of bilateral acoustic neurofibromatosis to a DNA marker on chromosome 22. *Nature* **329**:246, 1987.

133. Wertelecki W, Rouleau GA, Superneau DW, Forehand LW, Williams JP, Haines JL, Gusella JF: Neurofibromatosis 2: Clinical and DNA linkage studies of a large kindred. *N Engl J Med* **319**:278, 1988.

134. Dumanski JP, Rouleau GA, Nordenskjöld M, Collin VP: Molecular genetic analysis of chromosome 22 in 81 cases of meningioma. *Cancer Res* **50**:5863, 1990.

135. Cogen PH, Daneshvar L, Bowcock AM, Metzger AK, Cavalli-Sforza LL: Loss of heterozygosity for chromosome 22 DNA sequences in human meningioma. *Cancer Genet Cytogenet* **53**:271, 1991.

136. Rouleua GA, Merel P, Lutchman M, Sanson M, Zucman J, Marineau C, Hoang-Xuan K, Demczuk S, Desmaze C, Plougastel B, Pulst SM, Lenoir G, Bijlsma E, Fashold R, Dumanski J, deJong P, Parry D, Eldridge R, Aurias A, Delattre O, Thomas G: Alteration in a new gene encoding a putataive membrane-organizing protein causes neurofibromatosis type 2. *Nature* **363**:515, 1993.

137. Deprez RHL, Bianchi AB, Groen NA, Seizinger BR, Hagemeijer A, vanDrunen E, Bootsma D, Koper JW, Avezaat CJJ, Kley N, Zwarthoff EC: Frequent NF2 gene transcript mutations in sporadic meningiomas and vestibular schwannomas. *Am J Hum Genet* **54**:1022, 1994.

138. Ruttledge MH, Xie Y-G, Han F-Y, Peyrard M, Collins V, Nordenskjöld M, Dumanski JP: Deletions on chromosome 22 in sporadic meningioma. *Genes Chrom Cancer* **10**:122, 1994.

139. Ruttledge MH, Sarrazin J, Rangaratnam S, Phelan CM, Twist E, Merel P, Delattre O, Thomas G, Nordenskjöld M, Collins VP, Dumanski JP, Rouleau GA: Evidence of the complete inactivation of the NF2 gene in the majority of sporadic meningiomas. *Nat Genet* **6**:180, 1994.

140. Jacoby LB, MacCollin M, Louis DN, Mohney T, Rubio M-P, Pulaski K, Trofatter JA, Kley N, Seizinger B, Ramesh V, Gusella JF: Exon scanning for mutations of the NF2 gene in schwannomas. *Hum Mol Genet* **3**:413, 1994.

141. Irving RM, Moffat DA, Hardy DG, Barton DE, Xuereb JH, Raher ER: Somatic NF2 gene mutations in familial and non-familial vestibular schwannoma. *Hum Mol Genet* **3**:347, 1994.

142. Bijlsma EK, Mérel P, Bosch DA, Westerveld A, Delattre O, Thomas G, Hulsebos TJM: Analysis of mutations in the SCH gene in schwannomas. *Genes Chrom Cancer* **11**:7, 1994.

CHAPTER 41

Lung Cancer

Mack Mabry ■ Barry D. Nelkin ■ Stephen B. Baylin

1. Lung cancer is the leading cause of cancer related death for both men and women in the United States and the solid tumor with the most defined relationship to a known environmental cause, cigarette smoking. The clinical and biologic aspects of this disease are complex in that 4 major histologic cancer types, all related to smoking, can arise from the bronchial epithelium, including large cell undifferentiated-, squamous cell-, adeno- and small cell lung carcinomas. The first three types, collectively known as non-small cell lung cancer (NSCLC) metastasize later than the small cell tumors (SCLC) and can be cured by early surgery. SCLC is one of the most highly metastatic tumors in man and has less than a 5% five year survival rate.

2. Hereditary aspects of lung cancer are probably less well understood than for any of the other common forms of solid tumors. There are no well-defined syndromes for inherited lung cancer. However, a growing body of evidence suggests that a complex Mendelian dominant inheritance pattern for genetic predisposition may play a significant role in determining which smokers eventually will get lung tumors. Animal models for carcinogen induced lung cancers, particularly in mice, suggest a major locus for genetic predisposition to lung adenocarcinoma and may prove useful for defining a gene(s) important to the human disease. The specific gene(s) involved have not been defined nor have the genetic loci involved been delineated.

3. In part, because of the poorly defined hereditary aspects of lung cancer, little is known about the precise gene alterations that underlly the earliest steps for lung carcinogenesis. However, multiple genetic alterations, in candidate gene regions (LOH at chromosomes 3p, 9p, 13q, 17p) or in specific candidate genes (p16, p53, K-*ras* genes), have been elucidated for established lung cancers. The most frequent of these changes, and those that occur earliest in disease progression, provide clues for genes involved in both the initial steps and hereditary aspects of lung neoplasia.

4. Further definition of the genes mediating the evolution of lung cancers is essential to establish critically needed markers to facilitate risk assessment for, and design of novel tests for early diagnosis of, these neoplasms.

CLINICAL AND BIOLOGICAL ASPECTS

In 1996, 177,000 people in the United States were diagnosed with lung cancer and over 158,000 deaths resulted. Thus, lung cancer is the leading cause of cancer related death in this country.[1] Ironically, considering the tremendous impact of this disease, lung cancer is arguably the most preventable solid tumor, since 90% of all patients with these malignancies develop their disease because of exposure to tobacco products, and in virtually all instances through cigarette smoking.[2,3]

One of the difficulties in defining genetic predisposition for lung cancer, for making the diagnosis of this disease, and for treatment, is that four major histologies of lung tumors evolve from the bronchial epithelium of smokers and the precise cellular relationships between these tumor types still are not elucidated. From a clinical perspective, lung cancer can be divided into two treatment groups of four histological types.[4] Squamous cell-, adeno-, and large cell carcinomas are collectively referred to as non-small cell lung cancers (NSCLC) and comprise approximately 75% of all lung tumors. These are different in their treatment approaches and responses from a fourth type, small cell lung cancer (SCLC), which constitutes the remaining 25% of lung neoplasms. Each of these major forms of lung cancer is intimately related to cigarette smoking. Of great interest for consideration of genetic predisposition to lung cancer, and for studies of the genetic changes in these diseases, is that only 10% of all smokers at risk develop lung carcinoma.[3] This is despite the fact that virtually all of these individuals have a degree of preneoplastic histologic changes in their bronchial epithelium.[5] Also, the average age for diagnosis of lung cancer is approximimately 60 years. All of these data suggest that the evolution of lung cancer occurs over a protracted period of time and involves multiple genetic changes.

For all of the lung cancer types, current therapeutic approaches are less than optimal as reflected in the high death rate from these malignancies. The initial diagnosis for each tumor type almost always stems from clinical evaluation of a chronic cough, weight loss, dyspnea, hemoptysis, hoarseness, or chest pain in patients with a long history of smoking.[6] For the NSCLC group, successful therapies center on early surgery since metastases occur later than for SCLC. For patients with the most limited stage of NSCLC at the time of initial diagnosis and surgery, 5-year cure rates are approximately 50%.[7,8] For patients with nonresectable initial NSCLC, and with recurrent disease, chemotherapy and irradiation are employed, but long term response rates are only 35% with a median survival time of only 25 weeks.[9,10]

The clinical course for SCLC is very different than that for NSCLC, as is the mode of, and response pattern to, treatment. This cancer is one of the most metastatic of all solid tumors and is extremely lethal.[11] Tumor spread occurs so early in the course of the disease that surgery is seldom used as a primary approach even for patients with no objective signs of metastasis at the time of initial diagnosis.[12,13] Treatment approaches rely, primarily, on combination chemotherapy with thoracic irradiation added in patients with nonmetastatic disease.[14,15] Ironically, this highly lethal cancer has among the highest initial sensitivity among solid tumors to these approaches.[16] However, recurrent and resistant disease virtually always ensues and the 5-year survival rate is only 5%, with an average survival time of 13 months, even for extensively treated patients presenting with detectable disease limited to the chest.[16]

The division of NSCLC and SCLC into two separate categories is useful for consideration of clinical behavior but is simplistic from a biological standpoint and for considerations of inherited predisposition for these neoplasms. The heterogeneous histologic types of lung cancers may reflect different cells of origin for each tumor type within the bronchial epithelium.[17] For example, as discussed in a section that follows on animal models of lung carcinogenesis, the parent cell for bronchoalveolar carcinomas, a subtype of adenocarcinomas, appears to be the type II pneumocyte within the bronchial eptithelium. The cellular origins of SCLC are less certain, although they have been of particular interest since this tumor is characterized by having a neuroendocrine phenotype that most closely resembles that of a sparse population of normal neuroendocrine cells found throughout the bronchial epithelium.[18] The complex biology underlying lung cancer evolution is illustrated by the fact that it is not uncommon for individual lung cancers to manifest biochemical features of both SCLC and NSCLC, such as sharing of neuroendocrine features.[19,20] This fact suggests that lung cancers are capable of a transdifferentiation that reflects a common differentiation lineage in which they may arise.[20] This biology, as well as the discussed clinical aspects, must be taken into account in all studies to define the gene defects responsible for evolution of sporadic and inherited forms of these diseases. As will be discussed later, there are some patterns of genetic loci abnormalities, and of altered function of tumor suppressor genes and oncogenes, that suggest segregation of specific genetic changes to NSCLC and SCLC.

GENETIC LOCI

Hereditary Cases—Linkage Analyses

The contribution of hereditary factors to the development of lung cancer is probably less well understood than for any of the common forms of solid tumors in humans. Unlike for breast, colon, renal, and other cancers, no distinct familial forms of the common types of lung cancer have been defined. Therefore, specific genetic loci responsible for predisposition to lung tumor development have not been elucidated. However, a building body of evidence indicates that there may be an exceedingly important role for genetic predisposition in determining risk of lung cancer development among smokers. This section briefly reviews the progress in this area and the prospects for defining the specific genetic loci responsible.

Proof that the familial occurrence of lung cancer has a genetic basis is complicated by the central role of cigarette smoking in causing these neoplasms. Smoking rates increased dramatically after World War I in American men and this trend was followed by a later increase in the incidence of women who smoke.[21] Since there is a lag period of at least 20 years from the initiation of smoking

until the development of lung cancer, smoking habits must be taken into account in analyzing multiple family generations.[22] This is especially important for the occurrence of lung cancer in women, since their incidence of smoking has increased dramatically over the past 40 years.[23,24] Finally, there is evidence that the likelihood of an individual choosing to smoke can be highly influenced on a familial basis and this must be taken into account in all studies of familial lung cancer.[25]

Despite the discussed problems, a growing number of studies over the past 30 years, using increasingly sophisticated statistical methods to factor in influence of smoking and other environmental factors, have demonstrated a twofold or more risk of lung cancer in relatives of patients with this disease.[25] However, the firm link to actual Mendelian inheritance of lung cancer itself still was difficult to establish. The most significant step in documenting this probability has come from the detailed investigations of Sellers and colleagues of a large number of families in southern Louisiana. Using sophisticated epidemiology approaches which factor in pre- and post–World War I smoking histories of families, and effects of age, sex, and environment, these authors found validation for a Mendelian, codominant inheritance pattern for lung cancer among smokers.[25–27] In fact, their data predict, in the population studied, that all smokers eventually develop lung cancer because they inherit a gene(s) that may have a high incidence in the general population.[25–27] As the authors are careful to point out, these results must be verified through studies of other families in other regions. However, the implications are enormous for considering approaches to control of lung cancer and for identifying specific genetic loci involved in predisposition to these neoplasms.

The cited evidence for the role of true inheritance in development of lung cancer must be translated into formal searches for the involved genetic loci. The job will not be an easy one for multiple reasons. First, as discussed, the inheritance patterns for lung cancer even within a given family appear complex and multiple loci may be involved. Second, although an earlier age of onset may be a result of inheriting lung cancer risk genes, particularly in women, disease onset still occurs primarily in older individuals.[25–27] These factors make standard linkage analysis of large kindreds with multiple generations very difficult. Early age onset lung cancer certainly occurs.[28–30] However, it remains to be determined whether patients with this phenotype develop their disease via the same mechanisms as do patients with typical late age onset lung cancer, and whether familial patterns for this phenotype can be delineated to facilitate the search for lung cancer predisposition genes.

In addition, the complex array of lung cancer histologies dictates the need to decipher whether hereditary factors contribute to occurrence of each major subtype. Recent studies indicate that adenocarcinoma of the lung may be the histologic type most linked to definite familial occurrence.[31,32] Interestingly, this is also the type that has been most associated with the few instances of early age onset.[28–30,33,34]

Therefore, for all the reasons articulated, definition of the actual genetic loci involved for inherited forms of lung cancer will require acquisition of large numbers of families to facilitate nonclassical linkage analyses, such as segregation analyses and sib-pair linkage approaches. Consortium arrangements to conduct such studies are now being established and will hopefully yield, at least chromosome assignment, for lung cancer predisposition genes within the next several years.

Genetic Loci For Sporadic Forms Of Lung Cancer

Cytogenetic Changes. The karyotypes of both SCLC and NSCLC exhibit extensive abnormalities. Whang-Peng et al. showed the first consistent cytogenetic abnormality in lung cancer, deletions on the short arm of chromosome 3, in virtually all SCLC cell lines examined.[35] As discussed in the following section, this observation has been confirmed and extended at the molecular level, using polymorphic probes. Testa et al. have shown that in NSCLC primary tumors, an average of 31 clonal karyotypic abnormalities were evident.[36] Among the most common abnormalities were loss of chromosomes 9 and 13 (65 and 71%, respectively).

Loss of Heterozygosity (LOH). As suggested by the extensive cytogenetic abnormalities, LOH is common in lung cancers, as in other solid tumors, and has been extensively studied. Although some LOH loci occur in all lung cancer types, several have distinct incidence differences between subtypes.

LOH areas commonly found in lung cancer are listed in Table 36-1 and those most extensively studied are discussed below. For SCLC, there is a very high incidence (90–100% of specimens) of LOH on chromosome 3p in the previously discussed area of frequent cytogenetic loss.[37,38] This last change also often occurs, but is less frequent (50–80%), in NSCLC. The individual regions of chromosome 3p that are lost differ somewhat among the histologic lung cancer subtypes. Chromosome areas within 3p21 are lost in NSCLC, whereas more distal regions, at 3p25-p26, and more proximal regions at 3p12-p14, are more often lost in SCLC.[37,38] Studies of SCLC cell lines also have demonstrated areas of homozygous deletion within 3p21 and 3p12-14.[39,40] Importantly, this region is the site for the most common fragile site in the genome, Fra3B. Delineation of these distinct and frequent chromosome 3 LOH areas in lung tumors has prompted intense efforts to identify associated tumor suppressor genes. As discussed in a section that follows, the search has been difficult and few, if any, real candidate genes have been delineated, to date.

LOH for chromosome region 17p also is extremely frequent in all types of lung cancer and especially in DNA from SCLC (90%).[41] The tumor suppressor gene, p53, is located at region 17p13.1 and as discussed in a later section, is clearly a gene involved in the pathogenesis of established lung cancer.

13q also has a high frequency (75%) of LOH in SCLC but low frequency (15%) in NSCLC.[41] As noted in a later section in the text, and in Table 41-1, this locus includes the site of the retinoblastoma susceptibility gene (Rb), which is almost always aberrantly expressed or mutated in SCLC.

As previously discussed, 9p is an area of frequent cytogenetic abnormality in NSCLC but not in SCLC. This site is the locus of two separate cyclin dependent kinase inhibitors (CDKIs), p15 and p16. These genes are described in more detail in a section that follows. Also there is some evidence that a third tumor suppressor gene may be located at 9p22-23 and a number of laboratories are attempting to identify genes in this region.[42]

LOH for chromosome 5q is observed in approximately half of the SCLC cases studied and is most commonly localized to 5q13-21.[43] The region of loss has been intriguing because the tumor suppressor gene APC, which plays a major role in colon cancer, is located within this region. However, analyses of lung cancers for inactivating mutations of APC using an RNAse protection screen have not identified any lesions despite the frequent LOH for this locus.[44]

Listed in Table 41-1 are additional, less well-characterized LOH loci that occur with significant frequency (30–50%) in lung cancer. These lesions presumably include loci for tumor suppressor genes that may be of biological importance, but more work is required to validate this assumption and to document the importance of these changes within the full spectrum of genetic alterations in lung tumors.

Timing of LOH during Lung Cancer Progression. Several studies have attempted to examine the stages in NSCLC tumor progression at which various genetic lesions accrue. Two groups have shown that 3p loss occurs early in NSCLC and is detectable in hyperplastic, precancerous bronchial lesions.[45,46] Similarly, 9p and 17p loss could be detected in preoplastic hyperplasia.[47] In one study, K-*ras* mutations were found to occur later in NSCLC development than the above LOH changes, and were not detectable until the later carcinoma *in situ* stage; another study suggested that the *ras* mutations may occur earlier.[48,49] Allelic loss on chromosomes 2q, 18q, and 22q were relatively uncommon (20–33%) in primary NSCLC, but often (63–83%) were found in brain metastases.[50] These results suggest that these latter genetic lesions provide growth advantages to NSCLC cells late in tumor development. The timing of genetic events in lung carcinogenesis needs much further study and will help to define genes for tumor initiation and clues to those involved in genetic predisposition.

Microsatellite Instability. In hereditary nonpolyposis colon cancer, defects in the mismatch repair pathway, which lead to instability changes in microsatellite repeat sequences, recently have been delineated (Chapter 17). Instability in microsatellite markers have also been studied by several groups in lung cancers with diverse

Table 41-1 Commonly Altered Chromosomal Loci in Lung Cancer

Locus	Histological Subtype	Gene	Frequency
A. Loci with defined tumor suppressor gene			
9p21-p22	SCLC, NSCLC	p15, p16	60–70%
13q14	SCLC > NSCLC	Rb	75–80%*
17p13.1	SCLC > NSCLC	p53	50**–95%*
B. Loci without defined tumor suppressor gene			
3p12-p14	SCLC > NSCLC		80**–100%*,***
3p21	NSCLC > SCLC		" "
3p25	SCLC > NSCLC		" "
5q21	SCLC, NSCLC		50%
11q12-q24	NSCLC		65%**
22q	SCLC, NSCLC		55%
C. Other loci commonly (30–50%) altered in lung cancer			
1p, 1q, 2q, 3q, 6q, 7q, 8p, 9p, 9q, 11p, 12p, 17q, 18q, 19p, 21q			

* SCLC
** NSCLC
***Combined frequency for LOH on 3p

and occasionally conflicting results. Initial reports indicated that microsatellite markers were more likely to be altered in SCLC compared to NSCLC.[51-53] However, other investigators have found no significant differences. Most recently, it has been reported that microsatellite instability is not observed in SCLC but frequently observed in NSCLC and that the replication error phenotype was more likely in NSCLC metastases and in clinically advanced lung cancers.[52] Whether these conflicting results are dependent on the microsatellite markers selected for analyses, differences in the selection of cases for study, or technical factors in the assays remains to be determined.

SPECIFIC GENES

Genes Involved in Hereditary Lung Cancer

As mentioned previously, there are no distinct genetic syndromes for lung cancer to help identify gene mutations that specify absolute genetic predisposition to these malignancies. However, there are a few clues to genes for which inherited mutations or patterns of inherited polymorphisms could play a role.

Germline Mutations in Genes Involved in Sporadic Lung Cancer. As noted in a section that follows, mutations in the Ha-*ras* gene occur with frequency in sporadic forms of non-small cell lung cancers. A rare polymorphism in this gene, which involves differences in numbers of a tandemly arranged reiterated sequence, has been reported to occur with increased frequency in patients with lung cancer.[54] However, subsequent studies have provided conflicting results for the actual linkage of this *ras* polymorphism to lung cancer.[55] The majority of the most recent studies have failed to reveal a predictive relationship and more work will be required to resolve this issue.

Genetic Syndromes for Other Types of Cancer and the Occurrence of Lung Cancer

There are at least three genetic syndromes that predominantly predispose to other forms of cancer, in which lung cancer also may occur. Since these syndromes are so rare, it is not yet clear whether a specific histologic type of lung cancer is favored; moreover, the few reported cases have not yet reached the statistical significance to prove that there is increased incidence of lung cancer associated with these genetic disorders.

Lung cancer may occur with increased frequency in the Li-Fraumeni syndrome (LFS), caused by a germ line mutation in the p53 tumor suppressor gene on chromosome 17p.[56] A substantial fraction of the lung cancers in LFS appear in nonsmokers and young (<45 years) patients, suggesting a biological effect of LFS on lung cancer development. Similarly, transgenic mice expressing a mutant p53 gene, or lacking p53 genes, can develop lung adenocarcinomas.[57,58]

Patients harboring an inactivating mutation in the Rb tumor suppressor gene on chromosome 13q commonly develop retinoblastoma and osteosarcoma.[59] Primary relatives of bilateral retinoblastoma patients, many of whom are carriers of the mutation, have been reported to develop a variety of secondary cancers, including lung cancer.[60,61] In these studies, several of the lung cancers developed in relatively young (<55 years) patients.

Bloom syndrome is an exceedingly rare recessive genetic disorder (165 patients reported) that is associated with defects in DNA repair (Chapter 15). Leukemias and other cancers are quite common in this syndrome. One case of squamous cell carcinoma

of the lung has been reported in a 38-year-old Bloom syndrome patient.[62]

Genetic Differences in Capacity to Metabolize Tobacco Carcinogens

Since cigarette smoking is so intimately involved in the development of lung cancer, it has been logical to search for specific lung cancer predisposition genes by investigating genetic differences between individuals in their capacity to metabolize the major carcinogens present in tobacco and in cigarette smoke. Clues to a role for such differences in determining lung cancer risk have emerged. Several enzymes associated with the cytochrome P450 system (CYP) are responsible for metabolizing tobacco carcinogens to forms that can be excreted readily from the body.[63] In so doing, however, functional groups can be altered on the parent molecules that result in enhancement of carcinogenicity through increased propensity to form bulky DNA adducts. Certain polymorphisms in the discussed enzymes are being associated with differing degrees of metabolic capacity between individuals and increased risk of developing lung cancer. For example, the ability to induce activity of the enzyme CYP2D6 by the antihypertensive drug, debrisoquine, has been associated with lung cancer risk.[63] The major tobacco carcinogen 4-(methylnitrosoamino)-1-(3-pyridyl)-1-butanone (NNK) is a substrate for CYP2D6.[64] High ability for induction of this enzyme now has been correlated with increased incidence of lung cancer (odds ratio of about 7.5 in one study) in several studies.[65,66] Poor ability to induce CYP2D6 is associated with mutations and polymorphisms in the gene.[67] Controversy exists about how tightly the debrisoquine polymorphisms actually relate to lung cancer risk and how useful this marker will be for determining predisposition among smokers.[63,66,68] Work is ongoing to match allelotypes for these gene changes, using sensitive PCR based assays, with lung cancer incidence in larger populations, and continued study should resolve these issues over the next several years.

Another cytochrome system enzyme, CYP1A1 (aromatic hydrocarbon hydroxylase-AHH), also demonstrates genetically determined differences between individuals for basal activity, and inducibility by tobacco smoke.[63] This enzyme metabolically activates polyaromatic hydrocarbons (PAHs) and levels have been reported to be higher in patients with lung cancer than in control individuals without cancer.[69] Differences in activity of and association of polymorphisms for other CYP enzymes to lung cancer risk alone have been reported.[63] However, for all of these enzymes, subsequent studies have yielded conflicting results with regard to tightness of linkage to predisposition and occurrence of lung cancer and future investigations will be required to resolve these issues.[63]

In addition to the described enzymes that may form carcinogenic metabolites from tobacco related compounds, other enzymes can influence lung cancer risk by catalyzing detoxication reactions that enhance elimination of the described toxic products. Low or absent activity of one such enzyme, the M1 isoform of glutathione-S-transferase (GSTM1), which arises through autosomal recessive inheritance for homozygous deletion of the gene, has been linked to high lung cancer risk.[70] Again, this relationship has been challenged by some studies.[71] However, a recent report of PCR-detected deletion of the GSTM1 gene showed an odds ratio of approximately 1.5 for linkage of the null phenotype with SCLC and adenocarcinoma of the lung.[70] Future studies will, again, be necessary to establish the precise relationships between GSTM1 status and lung cancer risk.

In summary, there is a growing body of data for linking genetic differences in capacity to metabolize tobacco carcinogens with risk for developing lung cancer. The odds ratios being reported indicate that no one of the factors being studied has an overwhelming role in predisposition for an individual smoker to be at the highest risk for lung cancer susceptibility. However, a profile of each of the genetic differences in a given smoker might well define a truly significant indicator of risk status. It is clear, from the studies to date, that existing PCR assays for detecting genetic status of each important metabolizing enzyme require much additional refinement. As these improve, monitoring of inherited capacity for carcinogen metabolism may provide a significant way to assess predisposition to lung cancer in large populations.

Genes Involved in Sporadic Lung Cancer

Despite the large body of data for altered genetic loci in sporadic lung cancer, discussed earlier, few specific genes in these regions have been shown to have an role in lung tumorigenesis. However, as outlined below, alterations in both dominantly acting oncogenes and tumor suppressor genes do occur in established lung tumors and provide clues to the progression steps for these cancers.

Oncogenes Involved in Sporadic Lung Cancer

Ras Family Genes. As for other solid tumors discussed in this book, mutations in ras family genes (see Chapter 10) occur frequently in lung cancer. In NSCLC tumors, ras mutations, primarily of K-ras, are observed at frequencies that may approach 50% of cases as detected by sensitive PCR-based methods.[72] H-ras mutations are observed in NSCLC at a very low frequency and mutations in N-ras are rare.[73–75] K-ras mutations are common in adenocarcinomas, less common in squamous cell lung cancers, extremely rare in bronchoalveolar carcinomas and have not been described in SCLC.[76–81] In NSCLC, the presence of ras mutations has been reported to be a negative prognostic factor, especially in patients with adenocarcinomas.[72,79,82]

myc Family Genes. Members of the myc family of oncogenes, c-myc, N-myc, and L-myc (see Chapter 10), represent another dominant oncogene family that can be activated in lung cancer, usually by gene amplification. C-myc amplification in SCLC appears to be a negative prognostic factor; c-myc amplification is three times more common in cancers obtained from treated patients than in tumor specimens from untreated patients.[83–85] Amplification of c-myc also correlated with a twofold reduction in median patient survival.[85] A number of investigators have suggested that this poor prognosis occurs because increased c-myc protein modifies intrinsic drug resistance to certain treatment modalities.[86,87] Amplification or overexpression of L-myc and N-myc are also found in SCLC and SCLC cell lines but the prognostic implications of this overexpression are not certain.[88–90]

Tumor Suppressor Genes Involved in Sporadic Lung Cancer

As discussed in a previous section, there are many common sites of LOH, suggestive of alterations in tumor suppressor loci in the major forms of lung cancer. However, the specific genes that may have altered function in these chromosome regions have, in the main, not been characterized. Several well-described tumor suppressor genes are altered in established lung cancers and almost certainly play a role in the evolution of these tumors, especially for progression stages of these cancers. These genes, summarized in Table 41-1, are as follows.

p53 Gene. Perhaps, the best defined tumor suppressor gene change in lung cancer is mutation of the p53 gene. This loss of gene function appears to be the major correlate to the previously discussed very frequent LOH that occurs for chromosome region 17p13.1 in all lung cancer types.[41] p53 mutations are obviously one of the most common genetic changes in all types of human cancer and these have been found in 50% of NSCLC and 90% of SCLC tumors.[91,92] The most frequently observed mutations in these tumors are G-T transversions and these may reflect bulky DNA adducts resulting from carcinogens found in cigarette smoke.[91] Recently, it has been reported that the tobacco carcinogen, benzo[a]pyrenediolepoxide (BPDE), binds directly to the hot spots for the mutations in the p53 gene found in lung carcinomas.[92a] Some studies suggest that lung cancers with p53 mutations have a worse clinical prognosis, but this relationship remains to be clarified.[93,94]

p16 Gene. Alterations in the cyclin dependent kinase inhibitor encoding gene, p16, occur frequently in lung cancers, as they do in most common forms of human cancer.[95–98] This gene is a strong tumor suppressor candidate to account for the previously discussed frequent LOH, and homozygous deletions, which occur at chromosome region 9p21 in lung and other tumor types. As in many tumor types, point mutations in the p16 gene are rare and the homozygous deletions are most common in cell culture lines.[98–100] However, this latter change now has been documented in primary lung cancers, as well.[99–101] In both cultures and primary tumors, loss of p16 gene function also occurs frequently via transcriptional silencing associated with abnormal DNA methylation of the transcription start site region.[102] The methylation change occurs in the absence of p16 gene coding region mutations.[102,103] Both the homozygous deletions of p16, and the methylation changes, occur almost always in NSCLC, rather than in SCLC tumors.[102] This is thought to reflect the fact that the p16 gene functions in the cyclin D-Rb gene pathway for control of cell proliferation. Tumor cells appear to require inactivation of only one gene in this pathway.[104–106] Since Rb gene mutations are very frequent, as noted below, in SCLC, but are much less frequent in NSCLC, inactivation of the cyclin D-Rb pathway by loss of p16 function may be advantageous primarily for NSCLC cells.[104–106]

The precise role for p16 gene changes in the progression of NSCLC tumors has not been delineated yet. However, this loss of gene function may play a very early role since, as discussed earlier, LOH and homozygous deletions of chromosome 9p21 have been found in early lung cancer lesions. Further investigations of the role of the p16 gene in lung carcinogenesis are critical and could be important for understanding of genetic susceptibility for lung cancer.

Rb Gene. The tumor suppressor gene, Rb, which plays a critical role in the cyclin D pathway for cell cycle control, and is located in chromosome region 13q14, is altered in nearly all SCLC tumors, and in 30–40% of NSCLC.[107–109] In NSCLC, aberrant Rb was more common in tumors of higher clinical stage.[109]

FHIT-1 Gene. The intense search for altered genes on chromosome 3p that, as discussed in an earlier section, undergoes frequent LOH changes in both NSCLC and SCLC tumors, has resulted, to date, in a strong proposal for only one candidate gene. Altered transcription splice products for the FHIT-1 gene, located in a frequent region of homozygous deletion at 3p14, and in the fragile site region FRA3B, which is disrupted in some familial renal tumors, recently have been described as a frequent characteristic of lung cancers.[110] However, it remains to be determined whether mutations in tumor DNA actually underlie the majority of these different transcripts and future studies are required to document the importance of FHIT-1 in pulmonary carcinogenesis.

Animal Models for Defining Genetic Aspects of Lung Cancer

Animal models can prove invaluable for clarifying genetic determinants of human cancers especially for tumors such as lung cancer where little is known about the initial molecular steps underlying tumorigenesis. Multiple animal types, including dogs, mice, and rats, are susceptible to development of either spontaneous lung cancers or lung neoplasms induced by exposure to carcinogens. The carcinogen models may be particularly valuable for determining genetic changes that contribute to predisposition to lung neoplasia and have been especially well studied in the mouse.[111] The most important features of the murine lung cancer models with regard to potential contribution to our understanding of human lung neoplasia will be discussed briefly below.

Controlled exposure of mice to tobacco-related carcinogens, such as NNK, and to various forms of irradiation, consistently induce lung tumors. In the main, the lesions have a histology similar to human lung adenocarcinoma and appear to constitute an excellent model for this common form of tumor.[111–113] A particularly important feature of the tumor is that the lesions have been hypothesized to arise in a defined parent cell, the type II pneumocyte.[111,112] This postulation has been further strengthened by the finding that a distinct change, increase in DNA-methyltransferase activity, occurs only in this cell type in the lung immediately after exposure of mice to NNK.[113] Also, following carcinogen exposure, the murine tumors evolve over a distinct course of progression from hyperplasia, to benign appearing adenomas, to frank carcinoma.[111–113] This cellular origin, and the ability to examine defined stages of tumor progression, offer an excellent opportunity to outline molecular steps responsible for multiple stages of lung tumor progression.

Importantly, susceptibility of mice to the described tumor induction is very strain-dependent and this genetically determined response relates specifically to lung cancer.[111] This situation provides an opportunity to outline molecular events for predisposition to multiple stages of lung cancer evolution that may have great ramifications for defining genetic steps for human lung cancer. Several approaches to detecting genes responsible for strain susceptibility have already been utilized. For example, standard linkage analyses have been applied to study generations of mice bred from an initial cross between the A/J mouse, which is very sensitive to tumor induction with NNK exposure, with a resistant strain, the C3H mouse. A major susceptibility locus on distal chromosome 6, termed Pas1, has been identified and confirmed in subsequent studies including crosses between the sensitive strain, and noninbred mice that are resistant to tumor induction.[111,114]

The gene(s) responsible for the contribution of the described Pas1 locus has not yet been identified but obviously will be of great interest for human lung cancer as well. One interesting candidate, the Kras2 gene, is near the locus and has been studied in detail. As noted in a previous section, this gene is mutated in a significant percentage of human lung adenocarcinomas and is mutated in an even higher proportion (70 to over 90%) of spontaneous and carcinogen induced murine lung adenocarcinomas as well.[111,112] Furthermore, the alterations in the murine tumors occur very early in the hyperplasia and adenoma stages.[111,112] Intriguingly, in tumors induced in susceptible offspring from crosses between carcinogen sensitive with resistant mice, the Kras2 gene mutations are always in the allele inherited from the sensitive strain.[111] However, the Kras2 gene does not appear to fall within the tightest area of chromosome linkage on chromosome 6, and the presence of mutations in this gene is as high in tumors from the more resistant strains of mice as in those from sensitive strains.[111] Thus, it is felt, at this time, that, either the Kras2 gene mutations are an important step for early progression of the murine tumors but not for the initial

steps influenced by inherited susceptibility, or, the gene mutations are influenced in some way by a control locus that is contained within the nearby area of tight linkage on chromosome 6.[111]

Studies of LOH frequency throughout the genome also have been employed to search for tumor suppressor genes responsible for initiation of murine lung tumors. The only consistent region for this change has been on chromosome 4, interestingly in an area syntenic to that near the p16 gene on human chromosome 9p.[111] Interestingly, the frequency for p16 gene alterations in the rat lung tumors is extremely high and consists of homozygous deletions and aberrant promoter region hypermethylation. The lack of linkage for the chromosome 4 region to the strain differences in tumor susceptibility suggests that the p16 gene, or other genes in the LOH area, may, as for Kras2 mutations, play more of a role in progression than in tumor initiation. Direct studies of alterations in murine homologues of key tumor suppressor genes for human neoplasia also have been utilized to search for molecular clues to strain differences in lung tumor susceptibility. No significant incidence for Rb or p53 gene mutations have been found in the murine tumors.[111]

In summary, animal models for lung carcinoma, especially those defined in mice, offer an important opportunity to help define genes which may be central to the development of, and genetic predisposition to, particularly, human lung adenocarcinoma. The difficulty in acquiring large numbers of families with inherited human lung cancer that are suitable for standard linkage analyses, emphasizes the importance of using animal models as adjuncts to the study of genetic predisposition to lung cancer in humans. The defined progression stages for the murine carcinogenesis-induced tumors, and the differences in strain susceptibility, all contribute to the inherent value of utilizing these models to define genes for which human homologues can readily be identified. It will not be surprising if some of the genes discovered will have key roles for lung cancer evolution in both the murine and human settings.

IMPLICATIONS OF GENETIC CHANGES FOR THE DIAGNOSIS AND TREATMENT OF LUNG CANCER

The tremendous impact that lung cancer has on society, and the distinct relationship to a known environmental cause for these tumors, make this malignancy a prime target for defining genetic markers of risk and for use in early diagnosis. Hopefully, the evidence for an important role for genetic predisposition in determining which smokers develop lung cancer will be followed in the coming years by elucidation of the molecular events involved. In turn, these genetic changes may serve as the best markers for defining risk and marking the earliest stages of lung cancer.

As the best markers emerge, they can be incorporated into diagnostic strategies that are already providing proof of principle for use of genetic changes to provide for early diagnosis of lung cancer. Detection of p53 and ras gene mutations in sputum DNA months to years before clinical signs of tumor have been reported.[115] These are retrospective studies in which the precise mutations that appeared in the eventual tumors were known and prospective investigations will be needed to validate such approaches. However, the ability to use tissue samples obtained by such noninvasive procedures is most encouraging. In fact, other body fluids, including blood and urine, have now been used to detect genetic changes, such as microsatellite instability, which are present in the established lung tumors of the patients studies.[116] Hopefully, germline DNA changes that reflect increased risk for development of lung cancer also will come to play a role in population screening since the rate of cigarette smoking remains high and is increasing, especially among young people and women, in many regions of the world.

Some of the genetic changes that already have been defined as frequent events in established lung cancers are being investigated as potential therapeutic targets for lung cancer. Recently, in an initial gene therapy study of patients with lung cancer, regression of tumors injected with a retrovirus for expression of the wild-type p53 gene has been reported.[117] Inhibitors of *ras* gene function hold promise for treatment of the many patients with lung cancers that harbor mutations in this family of genes.[118,119] Surely, as other gene alterations important for the various stages of lung cancer progression are discovered, these will present more potential molecular targets for new and novel therapeutic strategies for the current most lethal form of human neoplasia.

REFERENCES

1. Parker SL, Tong T, Bolden S, Wingo PA: Cancer statistics, 1996. *CA Cancer J Clin* **46**:5, 1996.
2. Ferguson MK, Skosey C, Hoffman PL, Golomb HM: Sex differences in presentation and survival in patients with lung cancer. *J Clin Oncol* **8**:1402, 1990.
3. Mattson ME, Pollack ES, Cullen JW: What are the odds that smoking will kill you. *Am J Public Health* **77**:425, 1987.
4. Pass HI, Mitchell JB, Johnson DH, Turrisi AT: *Lung Cancer: Principles and Practice.* Philadelphia, Lippincott, 1996.
5. Fontana RS, Sanderson DR, Taylor WF: Early lung cancer detection: results of the initial (prevalence) radiologic and cytologic screening in the Mayo clinic study. *Am Rev Respir Dis* **130**:561, 1984.
6. Midthun DE, Jett JR: Clinical Presentation of Lung Cancer, in Pass HI, Mitchell JB, Johnson DH, and Turrisi AT (eds): *Lung Cancer: Principles and Practice.* Philadelphia, Lippincott, 1996, p. 421.
7. Williams DE, Pairolero PC, Davis C, Bernatz PE, Payne WS, Taylor WF, Uhenhopp MA, Fontana RS: Survival of patients surgically treated for stage I lung cancer. *J Thoracic Cardiovasc Surg* **82**:70, 1981.
8. Shimizu N, Ando A, Teramoto S, Moritani Y, Nishii K: Outcome of patients with lung cancer detected via mass screening as compared to those presenting with symptoms. *J Surg Oncol* **50**:7, 1992.
9. Einhorn LH, Loehrer PJ, Williams SD, Meyers S, Gabrys T, Nattan SR, Woodburn R, Drasga R, Songer J, Fisher W: Random prospective study of vindesine versus vindesine plus high cisplatin versus vindesine plus cisplatin plus mitomycin C in advanced non lung cancer. *J Clin Oncol* **4**:1037, 1986.
10. Bonomi P: Non cell lung cancer chemotherapy, in Pass HI, Mitchell JB, Johnson DH, and Turrisi AT (eds): *Lung Cancer: Principles and Practice.* Philadelphia, Lippincott, 1996, p. 811.
11. Johnson DH, Greco FA: Small cell carcinoma of the lung. *Crit Rev Oncol Hematol* **4**:303, 1986.
12. Miller AB, Fox W, Tall R: Five year follow-up of the Medical Research Council comparative trial of surgery and radiotherapy for the primary treatment of small-celled or oat-celled carcinoma of the bronchus. *Lancet* **2**:501, 1969.
13. Johnson DH: Chemotherapy of small cell lung cancer, in Pass HI, Mitchell JB, Johnson DH, and Turrisi AT (eds): *Lung Cancer: Principles and Practice.* Philadelphia, Lippincott, 1996, p. 825.
14. Ihde DC: Chemotherapy of lung cancer. *N Engl J Med* **327**:1434, 1992.
15. Murray N, Coy P, Pater J, Hodson I, Arnold Z, Zee BC, Payne D, Kostashuk EC, Evans WK, Dixon P: Importance of timing for thoracic irradiation in the combined modality treatment of limited stage small cell lung cancer. *J Clin Oncol* **11**:336, 1993.
16. Arrigada R, Le Chevalier T, Pignon JP, Riviere A, Monnet I, Chomy P, Tuchais C, Tarayre M, Ruffie P: Initial chemotherapeutic doses and survival in patients with limited small cell lung cancer. *N Engl J Med* **329**:1848, 1993.
17. Gazdar AF, Carney DN, Guccion JG, Baylin SB: Small cell carcinoma of the lung: Cellular origin and relationship to other pulmonary

18. Linnoila RI: in Kaliner MA, Barnes PJ, Kunkel GHH, Baraniuk JN (eds): *Neuropeptides in Respiratory Medicine.* New York, Marcel Dekker, 1994, p. 197.
19. Linnoila RI, Mulshine JL, Steinberg SM, Funa K, Matthews MJ, Cotelingam JD, Gazdar AF: Neuroendocrine differentiation in endocrine and non lung carcinomas. *Am J Clin Pathol* **90**:641, 1988.
20. Mabry M, Nelkin BD, Falco JP, Barr LF, Baylin SB: Transitions between lung cancer phenotypes: implications for tumor progression. *Cancer Cell* **3**:53, 1991.
21. Giovino GA, Schooley MW, Zhu BP, Chrismon JH, Tomar SL, Peddicord JP, Merritt RK, Husten CG, Eriksen MP: Surveillance for selected tobacco behaviors: United States, 1900–1994. *MMWR CDC Surveill Summ* **43**:1, 1994.
22. Schottenfeld D: Epidemiology of lung cancer, in Pass HJ, Mitchell JB, Johnson DH, Turrisi AT (eds): *Lung Cancer: Principles and Practice.* Philadelphia, Lippincott, 1996, p. 305.
23. Ernster VL: The epidemiology of lung cancer in women. *Ann Epidemiol* **4**:102, 1994.
24. Harris RE, Zang EA, Anderson JI, Wynder EL: Race and sex differences in lung cancer risk associated with cigarette smoking. *Int J Epidemiol* **22**:592, 1993.
25. Sellers TA: Familial predisposition to lung cancer, in Roth JA, Cox JP, Hong WK (eds); *Lung Cancer.* Boston, Blackwell, 1993, p. 20.
26. Sellers TA, Bailey JE, Elston RC, Wilson AF, Elston GZ, Ooi WL, Rothschild H: Evidence for mendelian inheritance in the pathogenesis of lung cancer. *J Natl Cancer Inst* **82**:1272, 1990.
27. Sellers TA, Potter JD, Bailey JE, Rich SS, Rothschild H, Elston RC: Lung cancer detection and prevention for an interaction between smoking and predisposition. *Cancer Res* **52**:2694s, 1992.
28. Makimoto T, Tsuchiya S, Nakano H, Watanabe S, Takei Y, Nomoto T, Ishihara S, Saitoh R: Primary lung cancer in young patients. *Nippon Kyobu Shikkan Gakkai Zasshi* **33**:241, 1995.
29. Rocha MP, Fraire AE, Guntupalli KK, Greenberg SD: Lung cancer in the young. *Cancer Detect Prev* **18**:349, 1994.
30. Bourke W, Milstein D, Giura R, Donghi M, Luisetti M, Rubin AH, Smith LJ: Lung cancer in young adults. *Chest* **102**:1723, 1992.
31. Tsuji H, Hara S, Tagawa Y, Kawahara K, Ayabe H, Tomita M: Bilateral bronchiolalveolar carcinoma, showing familial aggregation of lung cancer. *Nippon Kyobu Geka Gakkai Zasshi* **42**:1061, 1994.
32. Ogawa H: Interaction between family history and smoking in lung cancer. *Gan No Rinsho* **33**:575, 1987.
33. Capewell S, Wathen CG, Sankaran R, Sudlow MF: Lung cancer in young patients. *Respir Med* **86**:499, 1992.
34. Larrieu AJ, Jamieson WR, Nelems JM, Fowler R, Yamamoto B, Leriche J, Murray N: Carcinoma of the lung in patients under 40 years of age. *Am J Surg* **149**:602, 1985.
35. Whang-Peng J, Knutsen T, Gazdar A, Steinberg SM, Oie H, Linnoila I, Mulshine J, Nau M, Minna JD: Nonrandom structural and numerical chromosome changes in non-small-cell lung cancer. *Genes Chromosomes Cancer* **3**:168, 1991.
36. Testa JR, Siegfried JM, Liu Z, Hunt JD, Feder MM, Litwin S, Zhou J, Taguchi T, Keller SM: Cytogenetic analysis of 63 non cell lung carcinomas: Recurrent chromosome alterations amid frequent and widespread genomic upheaval. *Genes Chromosomes Cancer* **11**:178, 1994.
37. Hibi K, Takahashi T, Yamakawa K, Ueda R, Sekido Y, Ariyoshi Y, Suyama M, Takagi H, Nakamura Y: Three distinct regions involved in 3p deletion in human lung cancer. *Oncogene* **7**:445, 1992.
38. Brauch H, Tory K, Kotler F, Gazdar AF, Pettengill OS, Johnson B, Graziano S, Winton T, Buys CH, Sorenson GD: Molecular mapping of deletion sites in the short arm of chromosome 3 in human lung cancer. *Genes Chromosomes Cancer* **1**:240, 1990.
39. Rabbitts P, Bergh J, Douglas J, Collins F, Waters J: A submicroscopic homozygous deletion at the D3S3 locus in a cell line isolated from a small cell lung carcinoma. *Genes Chrom Cancer* **2**:231, 1990.
40. Daly MC, Xiang RH, Buchhagen D, Hensel CH, Garcia DK, Killary AM, Minna JD, Naylor SL; A homozygous deletion on chromosome 3 in a small cell lung cancer cell line correlates with a region of tumor suppressor activity. *Oncogene* **8**:1721, 1993.
41. Yokota J, Wada M, Shimosato Y, Terada M, Sugimura T: Loss of heterozygosity of chromosome 3,13 and 17 in small cell carcinoma and on chromosome 3 in adenocarcinoma of the lung. *Proc Natl Acad Sci USA* **84**:9252, 1987.

42. Neville EM, Stewart M, Myskow M, Donnelly RJ, Field JK: Loss of heterozygosity at 9p23 defines a novel locus in non-small cell lung cancer. *Oncogene* **11**:581, 1995.

43. Hosoe S, Ueno K, Shigedo Y, Tachibana I, Osaki T, Kumagai T, Tanio Y, Kawase I, Nakamura Y, Kishimoto T: A frequent deletion of chromosome 5q21 in advanced small cell and non-small cell carcinoma of the lung. *Cancer Res* **54**:1787, 1994.

44. Horii A, Nakatsuru S, Miyoshi Y, Ichii S, Nagase H, Ando H, Yanagisawa A, Tsuchiya E, Kato Y, Nakamura Y: Frequent somatic mutations of APC gene in human pancreatic cancer. *Cancer Res* **52**:6696, 1992.

45. Sundaresan V, Ganly P, Haselton P, Rudd R, Sinha G, Bleehen NM, Rabbitts P: p53 and chromosome 3 abnormalities, characteristic of malignant lung tumours, are detectable in preinvasive lesions of the bronchus. *Oncogene* **7**:1989, 1992.

46. Hung J, Kishimoto Y, Sugio K, Virmani A, McIntire DD, Minna JD, Gazdar AF: Allele-specific chromosome 3p deletions occur at an early stage in the pathogenesis of lung carcinoma. *JAMA* **273**:558, 1995.

47. Kishimoto Y, Sugio K, Hung JY, Virmani AK, McIntire DD, Minna JD, Gazdar AF: Allele loss in chromosome 9p loci in preneoplastic lesions accompanying non-small-cell lung cancers. *J Natl Cancer Inst* **87**:1224, 1995.

48. Sugio K, Kishimoto Y, Virmani AK, Hung JY, Gazdar AF: K-ras mutations are a relatively late event in the pathogenesis of lung carcinomas. *Cancer Res* **54**:5811, 1994.

49. Westra WH, Slebos RJ, Offerhaus GJ, Goodman SN, Evers SG, Kensler TW, Askin FB, Rodenhuis S, Hruban RH: K-ras oncogene activation in lung adenocarcinomas from former smokers. Evidence that K-ras mutations are an early and irreversible event in the development of adenocarcinoma of the lung. *Cancer* **72**:432, 1993.

50. Shiseki M, Kohno T, Nishikawa R, Sameshima Y, Mizoguchi H, Yokota J: Frequent allelic losses on chromosome 2q, 18q, and 22q in advanced non-small cell lung carcinoma. *Cancer Res* **54**:5643, 1994.

51. Merlo A, Mabry M, Gabrielson E, Vollmer R, Baylin SB, Sidransky D: Frequent microsatellite instability in primary small cell lung cancer. *Cancer Res* **54**:2098, 1994.

52. Adachi J, Shiseki M, Okazaki T, Ishimaru G, Noguchi M, Hirohashi S, Yokota J: Microsatellite instability in primary and metastatic lung carcinomas. *Genes, Chrom Cancer* **14**:301, 1995.

53. Shridhar V, Siegfried J, Hunt J, del Mar Alonso M, Smith DI: Genetic instability of microsatellite sequences in many non-small cell lung carcinomas. *Cancer Res* **54**:2084, 1994.

54. Sugimura H, Caporaso NE, Modali RV, Hoover RN, Resau JH, Trump BF, Longeran JA, Krontiris TG, Mann DL, Weston A: Association of rare alleles of the Harvey ras protooncogene with lung cancer. *Cancer Res* **50**:1857, 1990.

55. Vineis P, Caporaso N: The analysis of restriction fragment length polymorphism in human cancer: a review from an epidemiologic perspective. *Int J Cancer* **47**:26, 1991.

56. Li FP, Fraumeni JF, Mulvihill JJ, Blattner WA, Dreyfus MG, Tucker MA, Miller RW: A cancer family syndrome in twenty kindreds. *Cancer Res* **48**:5358, 1988.

57. Lavigueur A, Bernstein A: p53 transgenic mice: Accelerated erythroleukemia induction by Friend virus. *Oncogene* **6**:2197, 1991.

58. Donehower LA, Harvey M, Slagle BL, McArthur MJ, Montgomery CA, Butel JS, Bradley A: Mice deficient for p53 are developmentally normal but susceptible to spontaneous tumours. *Nature* **356**:215, 1992.

59. Goodrich DW, Lee W: The molecular genetics of retinoblastoma. *Cancer Surv* **9**:529, 1990.

60. Strong LC, Herson J, Haas C, Elder K, Chakraborty R, Weiss KM, Majumder P: Cancer mortality in relatives of retinoblastoma patients. *J Natl Cancer Inst* **73**:303, 1984.

61. Sanders BM, Jay M, Draper GJ, Roberts EM: Non-ocular cancer in relatives of retinoblastoma patients. *Br J Cancer* **60**:358, 1989.

62. German J: Bloom syndrome: a mendelian prototype of somatic mutational disease. *Medicine* **72**:393, 1993.

63. Shields PG, Harris CC: Genetic predisposition to cancer, in Roth JA, Cox JD, and Hong WK (eds): *Lung Cancer.* Boston, Blackwell, 1993, p. 3.

64. Crespi CL, Penman BW, Gelboin HV, Gonzalez FJ: A tobacco smoke nitrosamine, 4(methylnitrosamino)(3) is activated by multiple cytochrome P450s including the polymorphic human cytchrome P450 2D6. *Carcinogenesis* **12**:1197, 1991.

65. Caporaso NE, Shields PG, Landi MT, Shaw GL, Tucker MA, Hoover R, Sugimura H, Weston A, Harris CC: The debrisoquine metabolic phenotype and DNA assays: Implications of misclassification for the association of lung cancer and the debrisoquine metabolic phenotype. *Environ Health Perspect* **98**:101, 1992.

66. Caporaso NE, Hayes RB, Dosemeci M, Hoover R, Ayesh R, Hetzel M, Idle J: Lung cancer risk, occupational exposure, and the debrisoquine metabolic phenotype. *Cancer Res* **49**:3675, 1989.

67. Gough AC, Miles JS, Spurr NK, Moss JE, Gaedigk A, Eichelbaum M, Wolf CR: Identification of the primary gene defect at the cytochrome P450 CYP2D locus. *Nature* **347**:773, 1990.

68. Shaw GL, Falk RT, Deslauriers J, Frame JN, Nesbitt JC, Pass HI, Issaq HJ, Hoover RN, Tucker MA: Debrisoquine metabolism and lung cancer risk. *Cancer Epidemiol Biomarkers Prev* **4**:41, 1995.

69. Rudiger HW, Nowak D, Hartmann K, Cerutti PA: Enhanced formation of benzo(a) pyrene: DNA adducts in monocytes of patients with a presumed predisposition to lung cancer. *Cancer Res* **45**:5890, 1985.

70. To J, Gene M, Gomez J, Galan C, Firvida J, Fuentes M, Rodamilans M, Huguet E, Estape J, Corbella J: Glutathione M1 and codon 72 p53 polymorphisms in a northwestern Mediterranean population and their relation to lung cancer susceptibility. *Cancer Epidemiol, Biomarkers Prev* **5**:337, 1996.

71. London SJ, Daly AK, Cooper J, Navidi WC, Carpenter CL, Idle JR: Polymorphism of glutathine S M1 and lung cancer risk among African-Americans and Caucasians in Los Angeles County, California. *J Natl Cancer Inst* **87**:1246, 1995.

72. Clements NC, Nelson MA, Wymer JA, Savage C, Aquirre M, Garewal H: Analysis of K-ras gene mutations in malignant and nonmalignant endobronchial tissue obtained by fiberoptic bronchoscopy. *Am J Respir Crit Care Med* **152**:1374, 1995.

73. Rodenhuis S, Slebos R, Boot AJ, Evers SG, Mooi WJ, Wagenaar SS, van Bodegom PC, Bos JL: Incidence and possible clinical significance of K-ras oncogene activation in adenocarcinoma of the human lung. *Cancer Res* **48**:5738, 1988.

74. Mills NE, Fishman CL, Scholes J, Anderson SE, Rom WN, Jacobson DR: Detection of K-ras oncogene mutations in bronchoalveolar lavage fluid for lung cancer diagnosis. *J Natl Cancer Inst* **87**:1056, 1995.

75. Suzuki Y, Orita M, Shiraishi M, Hayashi K, Sekiya T: Detection of ras gene mutations in human lung cancers by single strand conformation polymorphism analysis of polymerase chain reaction products. *Oncogene* **5**:1037, 1990.

76. Slebos RJC, Evers SG, Wagenaar SS, Rodenhuis S: Cellular protooncogenes are infrequently amplified in untreated non-small cell lung cancer (NSCLC). *Br J Cancer* **59**:76, 1988.

77. Reynolds S, Anna CK, Brown KC, Wiest JS, Beattie EJ, Pero RW, Iglehart JD, Anderson MW: Activated oncogenes in human lung tumors from smokers. *Proc Natl Acad Sci USA* **88**:1085, 1991.

78. Li S, Rosell R, Urban A, Font A, Ariza A, Armengol P, Abad A, Navas JJ, Monzo M: K-ras gene point mutation: a stable tumor marker in non-small cell lung carcinoma. *Lung Cancer* **11**:19, 1994.

79. Rosell R, Li S, Skacel Z, Mate JL, Maestre J, Canela M, Tolosa E, Armengol P, Barnadas A, Ariza A: Prognostic impact of mutated K-ras gene in surgically resected non cell lung cancer patients. *Oncogene* **8**:2407, 1993.

80. Ohshima S, Shimizu Y, Takahama M: Detection of c-Ki-ras gene mutation in paraffin sections of adenocarcinoma and atypical bronchioloalveolar cell hyperplasia of human lung. *Virchows Arch* **424**:129, 1994.

81. Wagner SN, Muller R, Boehm J, Putz B, Wunsch PH, Hofler H: Neuroendocrine neoplasms of the lung are not associated with point mutations at codon 12 of the Ki-ras gene. *Virchows Arch B Cell Pathol Incl Mol Pathol* **63**:325, 1993.

82. Rodenhuis S, Slebos RJ: Clinical significance of ras oncogene activation in human lung cancer. *Cancer Res* **52**:2665s, 1992.

83. Little CD, Nau MM, Carney DN, Gazdar AF, Minna JD: Amplification and expression of the c-myc oncogene in human lung cancer cell lines. *Nature* **306**:194, 1983.

84. Brennan J, O'Connor T, Makuch RW, Simmons AM, Russell E, Linnoila RI, Phelps RM, Gazdar AF, Ihde DC, Johnson BE: Myc family DNA amplification in 107 tumors and tumor cell lines from patients with small cell lung cancer treated with different combination chemotherapy regimens. *Cancer Res* **51**:1708, 1991.

85. Johnson BE, Ihde DC, Makuch RW, Gazdar AF, Carney DN, Oie H, Russell E, Nau MM, Minna JD: c-myc family oncogene amplification in tumor cell lines established from small cell lung cancer patients and its relationship to clinical status and course. *J Clin Invest* **79**:1629, 1987.

86. Sklar MD, Prochownik EV: Modulation of cis resistance in Friend erythroleukemia cells by c-myc. *Cancer Res* **51**:2118, 1991.

87. Niimi S, Nakagawa K, Yokota J, Tsunokawa Y, Nishio K, Terashima Y, Shibuya M, Terada M, Saijo N: Resistance to anticancer drugs in NIH3T3 cells transfected with c-myc and/or c-H-ras genes. *Br J Cancer* **63**:237, 1991.

88. Nau MM, Brooks BJ, Battey J, Sausville E, Gazdar AF, Kirsch IR, McBride OW, Bertness V, Hollis GF, Minna JD: L-myc, a new myc gene amplified and expressed in human small cell lung cancer. *Nature* **318**:69, 1985.

89. Nau MM, Brooks BJ, Carney DN, Gazdar AF, Battey JF, Sausville EA, Minna JD: Human small lung cancers show amplification and expression of the N-myc gene. *Proc Natl Acad Sci USA* **83**:1092, 1986.

90. Johnson BE: The role of MYC, JUN, and FOS oncogenes in human lung cancer, in Pass HI, Mitchell JB, Johnson DH, Turisi AT (eds): *Lung Cancer: Principles and Practice.* Philadelphia, Lippincott, 1996, p 83.

91. Chiba I, Takashi T, Nau MM, D Amico D, Curiel DT, Misudomi T, Buchhagen DL, Carbone D, Piantadosi S, Koga H: Mutations in the p53 gene are frequent in primary, resected non-small cell lung cancer. *Oncogene* **5**:1603, 1990.

92. D Amico D, Carbone D, Mitsudomi T, Nau M, Fedorko J, Russell E, Johnson B, Buchhagen D, Bodner S, and Phelps R: High frequency of somatically acquired p53 mutations in small cell lung cancer cell lines and tumors. *Oncogene* **7**:339, 1992.

92a.Denissenko MF, Pao A, Tang M, and Pfeifer GP: Preferential formation of benzo[a]pyrene adducts at lung cancer mutational hot spots in p53. *Science* **274**:430, 1996.

93. Quinlan DC, Davidson AG, Summers CL, Warden HE, Doshi HM: Accumulation of p53 protein correlates with a poor prognosis in human lung cancer. *Cancer Res* **52**:4828, 1992.

94. McLaren R, Kuzu I, Dunnill M, Harris A, Lane D, Gatter K: The relationship of p53 immunostaining to survival in carcinoma of the lung. *Br J Cancer* **66**:735, 1992.

95. Serrano M, Hannon GJ, Beach D: A new regulatory motif in cell control causing specific inhibition of cyclin D/CDK4. *Nature* **366**:704, 1993.

96. Sherr CJ: G1 phase progression: cycling on cue. *Cell* **79**:551, 1994.

97. Larsen C: p16^INK4a: a gene with a dual capacity to encode unrelated proteins that inhibit cell cycle progression. *Oncogene* **12**:2041, 1996.

98. Kamb A, Gruis NA, Weaver J, Liu Q, Harshman K, Tavtigian SV, Stockert E, Day RS, Johnson BE, Skolnick MH: A cell cycle regulator potentially involved in genesis of many tumor types. *Science* **264**:436, 1994.

99. Cairns P, Mao L, Merlo A, Lee DJ, Schwab D, Eby Y, Tokino K, van der Riet P, Blaugrund JE, Sidransky D: Rates of p16 (MTS1) mutations in primary tumors with 9p loss. *Science* **265**:415, 1994.

100. Okamoto A, Hussain SP, Hagiwara K, Spillare EA, Rusin MR, Demetrick DJ, Serrano M, Hannon GJ, Shiseki M, Zariwala M, Xiong Y, Beach DH, Yokota J, Harris CC: Mutations in the p16^INK4/MTS1/CDKN2, p15^INK4B/MTS2, and p18 genes in primary and metastatic lung cancer. *Cancer Res* **55**:1448, 1995.

101. Packenham JP, Taylor JA, White CM, Anna CH, Barrett JC, Devereux TR: Homozygous deletions at chromosome 9p21 and mutation analysis of p16 and p15 in microdissected primary non cell lung cancers. *Clin Cancer Res* **1**:687, 1995.

102. Merlo A, Herman JG, Mao L, Lee DJ, Gabrielson E, Burger PC, Baylin SB, Sidransky D: 5′ CpG island methylation is associated with transcriptional silencing of the tumour suppressor p16/CDKN2/MTS1 in human cancers. *Nat Med* **1**:686, 1995.

103. Herman JG, Merlo A, Mao L, Lapidus RG, Issa J, Davidson NE, Sidransky D, Baylin SB: Inactivation of the CDKN2/p16/MTS1 gene is frequently associated with aberrant DNA methylation in all common human cancers. *Cancer Res* **55**:4525, 1995.

104. Shapiro GI, Edwards CD, Kobzik L, Godleski J, Richards W, Sugarbaker DJ, Rollins BJ: Reciprocal Rb inactivation and p16^INK4 expression in primary lung cancers and cell lines. *Cancer Res* **55**:505, 1995.

105. Otterson GA, Khleif SN, Chen W, Coxon AB, Kaye FJ: CDKN2 gene silencing in lung cancer by DNA hypermethylation and kinetics of p16INK4 protein induction by 5-aza 2′deoxycytidine. *Oncogene* **11**:1211, 1996.

106. Otterson GA, Kratzke RA, Coxon A, Kim YW, Kaye FJ: Absence of p16INK4 protein is restricted to the subset of lung cancer lines that retains wildtype RB. *Oncogene* **9**:3375, 1994.

107. Sherr CJ: Mammalian G1 cyclins. *Cell* **73**:1059, 1993.

108. Hensel CH, Hsieh CL, Gazdar AF, Johnson BE, Sakaguchi AY, Naylor SL, Lee WH, Lee EY: Altered structure and expression of the retinoblastoma susceptibility gene in small cell lung cancer. *Cancer Res* **50**:3067, 1990.

109. Xu HJ, Hu SX, Cagle PT, Moore GE, Benedict WF: Absence of retinoblastoma protein expression in primary non-small cell lung carcinomas. *Cancer Res* **51**:2735, 1991.

110. Sozzi G, Veronese ML, Negrini M, Baffa R, Cotticelli MG, Inoue H, Tornielli S, Pilotti S, De Gregorio L, Pastorino U, Pierotti MA, Ohta M, Huebner K, Croce CM: The FHIT gene at 3p14.2 is abnormal in lung cancer. *Cell* **85**:17, 1996.

111. Dragani TA, Manenti G, Pierotti MA: Genetics of murine lung tumors. *Adv Cancer Res* **67**:83, 1995.

112. Belinsky SA, Devereux TR, Maronpot RR, Stoner GD, Anderson MW: Relationship between the formation of promutagenic adducts and the activation of K-ras protooncogene in lung tumors from A/J mice treated with nitrosamines. *Cancer Res* **49**:5305, 1989.

113. Belinsky SA, Nikula KJ, Baylin SB, Issa J: Increased cytosine DNA activity is target-cell-specific and an early event in lung cancer. *Proc Natl Acad Sci USA* **93**:4045, 1996.

114. Gariboldi M, Manenti G, Canzian F, Falvella FS, Radice MT, Pierotti MA, Della Porta G, Binelli G, Dragani TA: A major susceptibility locus to murine lung carcinogenesis maps on chromosome 6. *Nat Genet* **3**:132, 1993.

115. Mao L, Hruban RH, Boyle JO, Tockman M, Sidransky D: Detection of oncogene mutations in sputum precedes diagnosis of lung cancer. *Cancer Res* **54**:1634, 1994.

116. qi Chen X, Stroun M, Magnenat J, Nicod LP, Kurt A, Lyautey J, Lederrey C, Anker P: Microsatellite alterations in plasma DNA of small cell lung cancer patients. *Nat Med* **2**:1033, 1996.

117. Roth JA, Nguyen D, Lawrence DD, Kemp BL, Carrasco CH, Ferson DZ, Hong WK, Komaki R, Lee JJ, Nesbitt JC, Pisters KMW, Putnam JB, Schea R, Shin DM, Walsh GL, Dolormente MM, Han C, Martin FD, Yen N, Xu K: Retrovirus wild p53 gene transfer to tumors of patients with lung cancer. *Nat Med* **2**:985, 1996.

118. Sun J, Qian Y, Hamilton AD, Sebti SM: Ras CAAX peptidomimetic FTI276 selectivity blocks tumor growth in nude mice of a human lung carcinoma with K-ras mutation and p53 deletion. *Cancer Res* **55**:4243, 1995.

119. James GL, Goldstein JL, Brown MR, Rawson TE, Somers TC, McDowell RS, Crowley CW, Lucas BK, Levinson AD, Marsters JC: Benzodiazepine peptidomimetics: potent inhibitors of ras farnesylation in animal cells. *Science* **260**:1937, 1993.

CHAPTER 42

Hepatocellular Carcinoma

Lynne W. Elmore ▪ Curtis C. Harris

1. Hepatocellular carcinoma (HCC) is an aggressive malignancy with a poor prognosis. The multifactorial and multistage pathogenesis of HCC has fascinated a wide spectrum of cancer researchers for decades. While a number of etiologic factors have been identified, the elucidation of their mechanistic roles in hepatocarcinogenesis has recently begun. Clearly, in sub-Saharan Africa and Eastern Asia viral and chemical carcinogenic components are involved, with the subsequent inactivation of the p53 tumor suppressor gene playing a central role. A better understanding of the molecular pathogenesis of HCC will provide clues for more effective preventative and therapeutic strategies.

2. HCC is the predominant cause of cancer mortality in Southern China and sub-Saharan Africa. Infection with hepatitis B virus (HBV) and food contamination with aflatoxin B1 (AFB1) are major and possible synergistic risk factors. A number of conditions associated with chronic hepatic inflammation and cirrhosis have also been identified as important etiologic factors worldwide.

3. HBV sequences randomly integrate into host chromosomal DNA resulting in frequent rearrangements. HBV-induced chromosomal aberrations may in part explain the loss of heterozygosity reported on many chromosomes in HCCs. Allelic loss of the short arm of chromosome 17, which includes the p53 tumor suppressor gene, has commonly been found in human HCCs.

4. In specific geographic regions of Asia, Africa, and North America with high HCC risk, e.g., Qidong, China, southern Africa, and Mexico, a G to T transversion at the third position of codon 249 of p53 has provided a molecular link between dietary AFB1 exposure and liver cancer development. Data from laboratory studies indicate that this region of the p53 area is highly sensitive to AFB1-induced DNA damage and that the resulting mutated protein provides a selective growth advantage in liver cells. Inactivation of p53 gene function may also result from its association with the HBV X protein (HBx). p53 and HBx physically associate, resulting in the inability of p53 to bind specific DNA sequences, transcriptionally transactivate p53-effector genes, associate with critical DNA repair proteins, and induce apoptosis. Abnormalities of the retinoblastoma tumor suppressor gene, typically in advanced lesions and associated with loss of p53, have also been reported in HCCs.

5. While mutation and amplification of protooncogenes, e.g., the ras family, are rarely detected in human HCCs, their overexpression is a common finding. c-myc and c-fos overexpression may result in part from HBV-encoded transcriptional transactivators which are often expressed and functionally active in HCCs.

6. Insulin-like growth factor II (IGF-II) and insulin receptor substrate 1 (IRS-I) are frequently expressed at high levels in HCCs. The insulin growth factor signal transduction pathways may contribute to hepatocarcinogenesis by providing a strong proliferative response as well as by preventing transforming growth factor-$\beta1$ (TGF-$\beta1$)-induced apoptosis. Overexpression of transforming growth factor-α also is observed in many HCCs, particularly in those tumors associated with HBV infection.

7. A better understanding of the complex pathobiological process of hepatocarcinogenesis has resulted in more effective preventative measures, including the implementation of HBV vaccination programs. The possibility of p53 as a target for HCC therapy is discussed. Hepatocellular carcinoma (HCC) is one of the most common malignancies worldwide affecting 250,000 to 1,000,000 individuals annually (reviewed in refs. 1 and 2). HCC causes at least 200,000 deaths per year, and in some regions such as Qidong, China, this disease causes 10 percent of all deaths. Both epidemiologists and laboratory researchers have greatly contributed to the understanding of the multifactorial etiology and multistage pathogenesis of HCC[3,4] (Fig. 42-1).

EPIDEMIOLOGY AND ETIOLOGY

The geographic distribution of HCC is highly variable, with Eastern Asia and sub-Saharan Africa being the most prevalent regions (reviewed in refs. 2 and 5). Substantial epidemiologic evidence indicates that hepatitis B virus (HBV) is a major risk factor for the development of HCC (reviewed in ref. 6). HBV carriers with chronic active hepatitis have up to a 200-fold greater risk of developing HCC than age-matched noninfected controls.[7-12] Moreover, an estimated 80 percent of HCCs worldwide are in HBV-infected individuals. Aflatoxin B1 (AFB1) also is considered to be a significant etiologic agent in certain geographic areas (e.g., Asia, southern Africa, and Mexico) where food contaminated by this mycotoxin is consumed.[13-15] In the high-HCC incidence geographic area of China, exposure to dietary AFB1 and chronic HBV infection are synergistic risk factors.[15-17] Other etiologic factors for hepatocar-

MODEL: VIRAL-CHEMICAL INTERACTIONS IN HUMAN LIVER CARCINOGENESIS

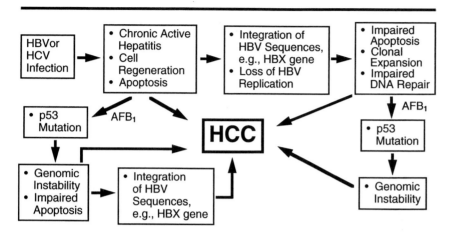

FIG. 42-1 Model of multistage hepatocellular carcinogenesis.

cinogenesis include conditions associated with chronic necroinflammatory liver disease and cirrhosis such as hepatitis C infection (HCV), chronic alcohol-induced liver disease, hemochromatosis, primary biliary cirrhosis, and alpha-1 antitrypsin deficiency.[2,6,18,19] Data from recent case series and case control studies indicate that synergistic interactions may also exist between HBV and HCV in the development of HCC.[20]

CHROMOSOMAL AND GENETIC ABNORMALITIES

Little is known regarding the specific alterations responsible for the development or progression of human HCC. Loss of heterozygosity (LOH) has been associated with inactivation of tumor suppressor genes.[21–27] In human HCCs, LOH has been reported on several chromosome arms including 1p,[28,29] 4q,[29] 5q,[30] 6q,[31] 8p,[32] 8q,[29] 10q,[33] 11p,[34] 13q,[35] 16q,[29,35] and 17p,[29,35,36] with some occurring irrespective of the presence of HBV infection.[33,37] It is noteworthy that four cases have been reported in which HBV-associated rearrangements have affected chromosome 17.[26,27,38,39] In two of these[26,27] the rearrangement mapped in the vicinity of the tumor suppressor gene p53 which is located on chromosome 17p13.1.[40] As described below ("Tumor Suppressor Genes"), p53 is the most common LOH site described in human HCCs,[41–43] and data are accumulating to strongly suggest that inactivation of this gene/protein may significantly contribute to the molecular pathogenesis of human HCC. DeSouza et al.[31] have recently reported a frequent LOH on 6q at the mannose-6-phosphate/insulin-like growth factor II receptor locus in human hepatocellular carcinomas and adenomas. Since this receptor is necessary for both the activation of a growth inhibitor [transforming growth factor β1 (TGF-β1)][44] and the degradation of a potent mitogen [insulin growth factor II (IGF-II)],[45] its loss could facilitate liver cell growth.

Most HCCs in HBV carriers contain HBV DNA sequences integrated into the host chromosomal DNA.[6,46] Unlike woodchuck hepatitis virus DNA, which frequently integrates into the c-*myc* or N-*myc* protooncogenes, resulting in either their rearrangement or overexpression,[47,48] the sites of HBV integration in human HCC are highly variable and random.[49,50] Findings of amplification or a single base mutation of some oncogenes have been reported in human HCCs associated with HBV integration, but their incidence is very rare.[51,52] Instead, the sites of cellular DNA at which HBV inte-

grates frequently undergo rearrangements,[53,54] resulting in translocations,[26,38] inverted duplications,[55] deletions,[34,38,56] and possibly recombinatorial events.[2,57] These HBV-induced chromosomal alterations may result in the loss of relevant cellular genes such as tumor suppressor genes important in cell cycle control and differentiation.

Tumor Suppressor Genes

The p53 tumor suppressor protein is involved in multiple cellular processes including cell cycle control, senescence, DNA repair, genomic stability, and apoptosis (reviewed in refs. 58 and 59). p53 is functionally inactivated by structural mutations, viral proteins, and endogenous cellular mechanisms in the majority of human cancers.[58,60–62] Certain domains of the p53 gene have been highly conserved, reflecting the functional importance and selection of this protein.[63] The majority of base substitutions fall within the highly conserved central portion of the gene[64,65] which mediates sequence-specific DNA binding and transcriptional activation[66] (Fig. 42-2). An extensive analysis of p53 gene mutations indicates that the sites and features of DNA base changes differ among the various human tumor types.[61,64] In the case of HCC, a unique mutational spectrum has provided a strong molecular link between carcinogen exposure and cancer development. When primary HCCs in Qidong, China, were examined we found that 8 of 16 had point mutations at the third position of codon 249, resulting in a G:C to T:A transversion.[67] This finding has been confirmed by others[68,69] and extended to HCCs from southern Africa and North America.[41,70,71] A dose-dependent relationship between dietary AFB1 and codon 249ser p53 mutations is observed in these geographic areas (Fig. 42-3). HCCs from geographic areas of low AFB1 exposure have a different mutational spectrum,[41,72,73] further establishing a positive association between high dietary AFB1 exposure and 249ser mutations. An analysis of p53 mutations in several human HCC and hepatoblastoma cell lines indicates that this mutational hotspot is specific for liver tumors of hepatocellular origin and does not require the genomic integration of HBV.[74]

Using a highly sensitive genotypic mutation assay, Aguilar et al.[75] have demonstrated the relative abundance of the p53 249ser mutant liver cells of nonmalignant specimens from Qidong when compared to specimens from Thailand and the United States. The biological basis for this frequently observed, early mutational event may be due to the high mutability of the third base at codon 249, as suggested by in vitro studies using human liver cells[76,77]

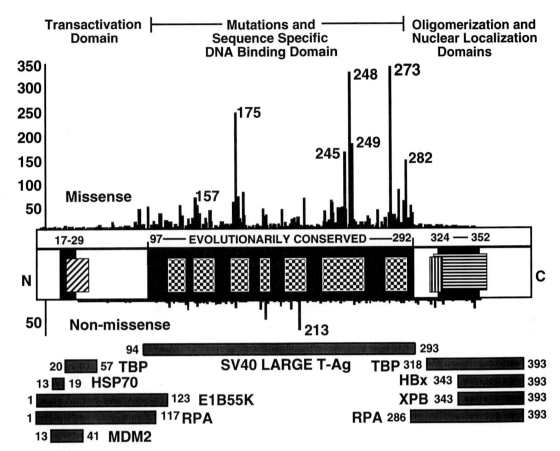

FIG. 42-2 Schematic representation of p53 molecule. The p53 protein consists of 393 amino acids with functional domains, evolutionarily conserved domains and regions designated as mutational hotspots. Functional domains include the transactivation region (amino acids 20–42; diagonal striped block), sequence-specific DNA-binding region (amino acids 100–293), nuclear localization sequence (amino acids 316–325; vertical striped block), and oligomerization region (amino acids 319–360; horizontal striped block). Cellular or oncoviral proteins bind to specific areas of the p53 protein. Evolutionarily conserved domains (amino acids 17–29, 97–292, and 324–352;black areas) were determined using the MACAW program. Seven mutational hotspot regions within the large conserved domain are identified: amino acids 130–142, 151–164, 171–181, 193–200, 213–223, 234–258, and 270–286 checkered blocks). Functional domains and protein binding sites (gray bars underneath) were compiled from references. Vertical lines above the schematic, missense mutations; lines below schematic, nonmissense mutations.

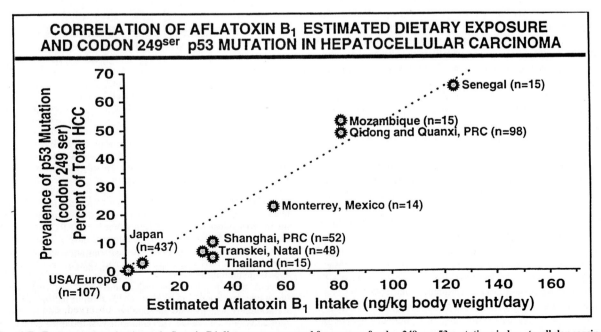

FIG. 42-3 Correlation of estimated aflatoxin B1 dietary exposure and frequency of codon 249ser p53 mutations in hepatocellular carcinoma.

(Mace K, Aguilar F, Harris CC, Pfeifer GP, unpublished results). An alternate, but not mutually exclusive, explanation is that this mutation provides liver cells with a selective growth advantage. Supporting this hypothesis are the following observations: (1) p53-null human liver cancer cells exhibit an enhanced growth rate following transfection with the p53 249ser mutant;[78] (2) introduction of a murine p53 mutation corresponding to human codon 249 into a murine hepatocyte cell line resulted in a selective growth advantage;[79] (3) the 249ser mutant inhibits wild-type p53-mediated apoptosis, resulting in increased cell survival;[80] and (4) the 249ser mutant is more effective than other p53 mutants in inhibiting wild-type p53 transactivation activity in human liver cells[81] (Fig. 42-4). One model concerning the generation of liver cancers with 249ser mutation is that AFB1 is metabolically activated to form the promutagenic N7dG adduct.[82,83] Enhanced cell proliferation due to chronic active hepatitis then allows both fixation of the G:C to T:A transversion in codon 249 of the p53 gene and selective clonal expansion of cells containing this mutated gene.

In some cases of HCC, mutation of p53 can be a late event in tumor progression.[84,94,95] Tanaka et al.[96] have reported that p53 mutations are closely related to the progression of HCC and that in some cases, malignant cells which acquire the p53 mutations might develop into dedifferentiated subpopulations within a single HCC. Further suggesting an involvement of mutant p53 in the progression of liver cancer is the observation that some nodules consist of both p53 LOH and non-LOH, with the former being associated with cells of more severe cellular atypia.[94] It is noteworthy that abnormalities of the retinoblastoma tumor suppressor gene (Rb) have also been reported in advanced HCCs.[37,97,98] In one study, LOH at the Rb gene was detected in 6 of 7 (86 percent) HCCs with a p53 mutation compared to none of 17 HCCs lacking mutation of p53.[97] A possible additive effect of p53 and Rb mutations during the progression of hepatocarcinogenesis is further supported by the finding that in this study all tumors with both abnormalities were poorly or moderately differentiated.

Oncogenes

Although activated protooncogenes are found in many spontaneous and experimentally induced HCCs in animal models,[99] no single oncogene has been shown to be preferentially activated in human HCCs.[100–102] By DNA transfection assay in NIH-3T3 cells, activated N-*ras* has been isolated from human HCC tissue, however, the gene was mutated in only a small fraction of the tumor cells.[103] Overexpression of N-*ras*, usually in the absence of a mutation, is often observed in human HCCs,[100,102] while mutations or overexpression of H- and K-*ras* are rare.[104] New oncogenes have been cloned from human HCC tissue,[5,105,106] but their role in hepatocarcinogenesis is unclear.

Mutations and amplification of c-*myc* are rarely detected in human HCCs, but overexpression of this protooncogene is a common finding.[98,102,107] Small studies have also demonstrated frequent overexpression of c-*fos* with an absence of mutations.[98,107,108] The HBV genome contains four open reading frames, two of which are potential transcriptional transactivators (reviewed in ref. 109). It is well established that HBx is a potent co-transactivator of many viral[110,111] and cellular[110,112–114] promoters including c-*myc*.[115,116] and c-*fos*.[116] The preS2/S region of the HBV genome following 3'-truncation[117] also is able to co-transactivate these two protooncogenes.[118] In most cases of HCC, either or both transactivators are expressed and functionally active,[49,118–122] while the other HBV gene products are infrequently detected.[46,120] These data indicate that the transcriptional co-transactivation function of HBx and/or preS2/S may significantly contribute to the development of HCC. However, considering the multiple functions of

HBx, its role in hepatocarcinogenesis may not be limited to its ability to either inactivate p53 functions or transactivate cellular genes. In this regard, HBx can deregulate cell cycle checkpoints,[123] activate the ras-raf-mitogen-activated protein (MAP) kinase[124,125] and protein kinase C signaling cascades,[126,127] stimulate DNA synthesis[123] and cell cycle progression,[128] bind to the DNA repair gene UV-DDB,[129] complex with cellular transcription factors,[89,130] inhibit hepatic serine proteases,[131–133] neoplastically transform rodent cells in vitro,[134,135] and, as a transgene, induce HCCs in mice.[136]

Growth Factors

The insulin growth factors, which include insulin and insulin-like growth factors I and II (IGF-I and II, respectively), are potent hepatocellular mitogens.[137] IGF-II is overexpressed[45,137–140] and exhibits an allelic-expression imbalance[141] in many human HCCs. Insulin receptor substrate 1 (IRS-1), a main substrate for insulin and insulin-like growth factors I and II, also is highly expressed in many human HCC tumor tissues and cell lines.[141] Moreover, IRS-1 exhibits transforming potential in NIH-3T3 cells, which is dependent in part on the presence of IGF-1.[142] These data suggest that the insulin growth factor signal transduction pathway may provide a critical proliferative stimulus during hepatocarcinogenesis. A recent study[143] reports that overexpression of at least one component of this pathway (i.e., IRS-1) may also contribute to liver cancer development by preventing TGF-β1-induced apoptosis.[144,145]

Transforming growth factor-α (TGF-α), another potent hepatocellular mitogen, is present at elevated levels in human HCCs, with its detection being closely linked to HBV infection.[140,146] Specifically, TGF-α was detected more frequently in patients whose adjacent nontumorous liver had detectable HBV surface

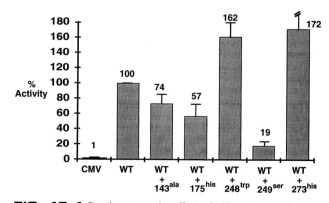

FIG. 42-4 Dominant negative effects of p53 mutants on the transcription of wild-type p53 in a p53-null human liver cancer cell line (Hep-3B). While the p53 249ser mutant in HCCs correlates with high risk exposure to AFB1, the absence of mutations in exons 5–8 of the p53 gene in 50 to 80 percent of HCCs[66,67,70,84] suggests that p53 inactivation may be achieved by another mechanism. The finding that p53 protein and HBx interact,[85–87] prompted us to evaluate the functional consequences of this association. HBx strongly inhibits p53 sequence-specific binding,[86] which is in contrast to the enhanced DNA binding specificity of the transcription factors CREB and AFT-2 when complexed to HBx, a non-DNA binding cotransactivator.[88,89] HBx also blocks p53-mediated transcriptional transactivation in vivo, as well as the in vitro association of p53 with either XPB (ERCC3),[86] or XPD,[90] transcriptional factors involved in nucleotide excision repair.[91,92] Moreover, HBx efficiently abrogates p53-mediated apoptosis[80] (Fig. 42-5). The binding of HBx to the extreme carboxyl-terminal domain of p53 appears to inhibit the association of p53 with two putative downstream effectors of p53-mediated apoptosis, namely XPB and XPD.[93] Based on the above data we speculate that inactivation of p53-mediated transcriptional transactivation and apoptosis by HBx could lead to a disruption of normal cellular surveillance mechanisms for repairing and removing damaged cells, thus contributing to genomic instability.

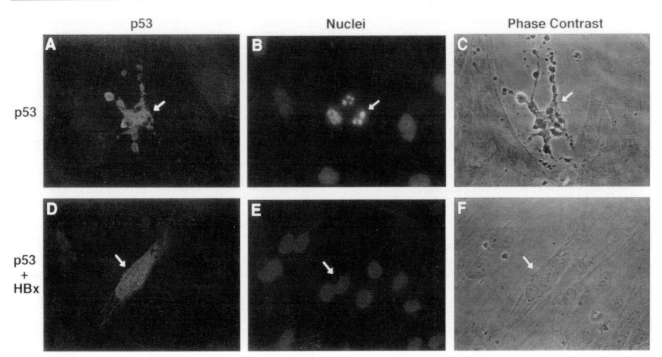

FIG. 42-5 Inhibition of p53-mediated apoptosis by the hepatitis B viral X gene. Induction of apoptosis in normal primary human fibroblasts was achieved by microinjection of a wild-type p53 expression vector. Cells were injected with the wild-type expression vector alone (A–C) or coinjected with wild-type p53 and the HBx gene (D–F). Cells were processed and analyzed as described in ref. 80.

antigen and/or HBV core antigen (91 percent) than in those whose liver lacked these viral protein products (61 percent).[146] It remains unclear, however, whether increased expression of this growth factor is mechanistically related to hepatocarcinogenesis or whether it results from liver regeneration in response to chronic HBV infection. The latter possibility is supported by the finding that elevated TGF-α expression is typically observed in the liver of patients with chronic hepatitis and without HCC.[140]

IMPLICATIONS FOR TREATMENT AND PREVENTION

HCC is regarded as an aggressive tumor with a poor prognosis.[1,147] Of the more than 250,000 cases diagnosed worldwide annually, less than 3 percent will survive 5 or more years. For some patients, surgical resection or orthotopic liver transplantation offers disease-free survival; however, most must rely on other modes of treatment which are currently only palliative.[1]

Our better understanding of the complex pathobiological processes during hepatocarcinogenesis has already resulted in more effective preventive measures. Vaccines for HBV are well developed, and vaccination programs are currently being implemented in many areas of Africa and Asia. Knowing that AFB1 is a significant risk factor in the development of HCC, limiting the exposure to this mycotoxin by improving the storage of food grains, would be another feasible strategy to decrease the incidence of HCC.

The frequent inactivation of p53 in HCCs makes this gene an attractive target for cancer therapy (reviewed in ref. 58). The development of drugs which would inhibit wild-type p53-HBx interactions may provide a means to rescue p53 tumor suppressor function. In those cases where p53 is mutated, agents which mimic wild-type p53 may be effective. Another possibility is p53 gene therapy. Laboratory studies have demonstrated the efficacy of p53 gene therapy in human cancer cells in vitro[148,149] and as a xeno-

graph in athymic nude mice.[150–152] Based on this success, a phase I protocol for non-small cell lung cancer in humans has been approved (Office of Recombinant DNA Activities, National Institutes of Health, Bethesda, Maryland, December, 1995). While the success of this approach is still speculative, it is encouraging that a p53 cDNA expression vector under the control of an α-fetoprotein promoter was successfully transferred into Hep-3B liver cells using a replication-defective retroviral vector, resulting in decreased cell growth and increased sensitivity to chemotherapeutic-induced apoptosis in vitro.[153] Vogelstein and coworkers[154] have recently devised a novel strategy of gene therapy which may also be a future option for HCCs containing mutant p53. This approach relies on the ability of mutant p53 in tumor cells to selectively bind to exogenously introduced gene products resulting in the transcriptional activation of a toxic gene. As we continue to better understand the molecular pathogenesis of human HCC, clues for additional, rational intervention and therapeutic strategies will likely follow.

ACKNOWLEDGMENTS

The editorial and graphic assistance of Dorothea Dudek and Amy Hancock is greatly appreciated.

REFERENCES

1. Haydon GH, Hayes PC: Hepatocellular carcinoma. *Br J Hosp Med* **53**:74, 1995.
2. Sherman M: Hepatocellular carcinoma. *Gastroenterologist* **3**:55, 1995.
3. Harris CC: Solving the viral puzzle of human liver carcinogenesis. *Cancer Epidemiol Biomarkers Prev* **3**:1, 1994.
4. Harris CC: The 1995 Walter Hubert Lecture/Molecular epidemiology of human cancer: insights from the mutational analysis of the p53 tumor suppressor gene. *Br J Cancer* **73**:261, 1996.

5. Okuda K: Hepatocellular carcinoma: recent progress. *Hepatology* **15**:948, 1992.

6. Robinson WS: Molecular events in the pathogenesis of hepadnavirus hepatocellular carcinoma. *Annu Rev Med* **45**:297, 1994.

7. Beasley RP, Hwang LY, Lin CC, Chien CS: Hepatocellular carcinoma and hepatitis B virus. A prospective study of 22707 men in Taiwan. *Lancet* **2**:1129, 1981.

8. Yeh FS, Yu MC, Mo CC, Luo S, Tong MJ, Henderson BE: Hepatitis B virus, aflatoxins, and hepatocellular carcinoma in southern Guangxi, China. *Cancer Res* **49**:2506, 1989.

9. Beasley RP: Hepatitis B virus. The major etiology of hepatocellular carcinoma. *Cancer* **61**:1942, 1988.

10. McMahon BJ, Lanier AP, Wainwright RB, Kilkenny SJ: Hepatocellular carcinoma in Alaska Eskimos: epidemiology, clinical features, and early detection. *Prog Liver Dis* **9**:643, 1990.

11. Iijma T, Saitoh N, Nobutomo K, Nambu M, Sakuma K: A prospective cohort study of hepatitis B surface antigen carriers in a working population. *Gann* **75**:571, 1984.

12. Obata H, Hayashi N, Motoike Y, Hisamitsu T, Okuda H, Kobayashi S, Nishioka K: A prospective study on the development of hepatocellular carcinoma from liver cirrhosis with persistent hepatitis B virus infection. *Int J Cancer* **25**:741, 1980.

13. Wogan GN: Aflatoxins as risk factors for hepatocellular carcinoma in humans. *Cancer Res* **52**:2114s, 1992.

14. Harris CC: Hepatocellular carcinogenesis: recent advances and speculations. *Cancer Cells* **2**:146, 1990.

15. Ross RK, Yuan JM, Yu MC, Wogan GN, Qian GS, Tu JT, Groopman JD, Gao YT, Henderson BE: Urinary aflatoxin biomarkers and risk of hepatocellular carcinoma. *Lancet* **339**:943, 1992.

16. Qian GS, Ross RK, Yu MC, Yuan JM, Gao YT, Henderson BE, Wogan GN, Groopman JD: A follow-up study of urinary markers of aflatoxin exposure and liver cancer risk in Shanghai, People's Republic of China. *Cancer Epidemiol Biomarkers Prev* **3**:3, 1994.

17. Hsia CC, Kleiner DE, Jr, Axiotis CA, Di Bisceglie A, Nomura AM, Stemmermann GN, Tabor E: Mutations of p53 gene in hepatocellular carcinoma: role of hepatitis B virus and aflatoxin contamination in the diet. *J Natl Cancer Inst* **84**:1638, 1992.

18. Tsukuma H, Hiyama T, Tanaka S, Nakao M, Yabuuchi T, Kitamura T, Nakanishi K, Fujimoto I, Inoue A, Yamazaki H, Kawashima T: Risk factors for hepatocellular carcinoma among patients with chronic liver disease. *N Engl J Med* **328**:1797, 1993.

19. Robinson WS: The role of hepatitis B virus in development of primary hepatocellular carcinoma: Part II. *J Gastroenterol Hepatol* **8**:95, 1993.

20. Yu MW, Chen CJ: Hepatitis B and C viruses in the development of hepatocellular carcinoma. *Crit Rev Oncol Hematol* **17**:71, 1994.

21. Shiraishi M, Morinaga S, Noguchi M, Shimosato Y, Sekiya T: Loss of genes on the short arm of chromosome 11 in human lung carcinomas. *Jpn J Cancer Res* **78**:1302, 1987.

22. Kovacs G, Erlandsson R, Boldog F, Ingvarsson S, Muller R, Klein G, Sumegi J: Consistent chromosome 3p deletion and loss of heterozygosity in renal cell carcinoma. *Proc Natl Acad Sci USA* **85**:1571, 1988.

23. Bodmer WF, Bailey CJ, Bodmer J, Bussey HJ, Ellis A, Gorman P, Lucibello FC, Murday VA, Rider SH, Scambler P, et al: Localization of the gene for familial adenomatous polyposis on chromosome 5. *Nature* **328**:614, 1987.

24. Solomon E, Voss R, Hall V, Bodmer WF, Jass JR, Jeffreys AJ, Lucibello FC, Patel I, Rider SH: Chromosome 5 allele loss in human colorectal carcinomas. *Nature* **328**:616, 1987.

25. Johnson BE, Sakaguchi AY, Gazdar AF, Minna JD, Burch D, Marshall A, Naylor SL: Restriction fragment length polymorphism studies show consistent loss of chromosome 3p alleles in small cell lung cancer patients' tumors. *J Clin Invest* **82**:502, 1988.

26. Meyer M, Wiedorn KH, Hofschneider PH, Koshy R, Caselmann WH: A chromosome 17:7 translocation is associated with a hepatitis B virus DNA integration in human hepatocellular carcinoma DNA. *Hepatology* **15**:665, 1992.

27. Zhou YZ, Slagle BL, Donehower LA, vanTuinen P, Ledbetter DH, Butel JS: Structural analysis of a hepatitis B virus genome integrated into chromosome 17p of a human hepatocellular carcinoma. *J Virol* **62**:4224, 1988.

28. Zhang W, Hirohashi S, Tsuda H, Shimosato Y, Yokota J, Terada M, Sugimura T: Frequent loss of heterozygosity on chromosomes 16 and 4 in human hepatocellular carcinoma. *Jpn J Cancer Res* **81**:108, 1990.

29. Kuroki T, Fujiwara Y, Tsuchiya E, Nakamori S, Imaoka S, Kanematsu T, Nakamura Y: Accumulation of genetic changes during de-

30. Ding SF, Habib NA, Dooley J, Wood C, Bowles L, Delhanty JD: Loss of constitutional heterozygosity on chromosome 5q in hepatocellular carcinoma without cirrhosis. *Br J Cancer* **64**:1083, 1991.

31. De Souza AT, Hankins GR, Washington MK, Fine RL, Orton TC, Jirtle RL: Frequent loss of heterozygosity on 6q at the mannose 6-phosphate/insulin-like growth factor II receptor locus in human hepatocellular tumors. *Oncogene* **10**:1725, 1995.

32. Emi M, Fujiwara Y, Nakajima T, Tsuchiya E, Tsuda H, Hirohashi S, Maeda Y, Tsuruta K, Miyaki M, Nakamura Y: Frequent loss of heterozygosity for loci on chromosome 8p in hepatocellular carcinoma, colorectal cancer, and lung cancer. *Cancer Res* **52**:5368, 1992.

33. Fujimori M, Tokino T, Hino O, Kitagawa T, Imamura T, Okamoto E, Mitsunobu M, Ishikawa T, Nakagama H, Harada H: Allelotype study of primary hepatocellular carcinoma. *Cancer Res* **51**:89, 1991.

34. Rogler CE, Sherman M, Su CY, Shafritz DA, Summers J, Shows TB, Henderson A, Kew M: Deletion in chromosome 11p associated with a hepatitis B integration site in hepatocellular carcinoma. *Science* **230**:319, 1985.

35. Nishida N, Fukuda Y, Kokuryu H, Sadamoto T, Isowa G, Honda K, Yamaoka Y, Ikenaga M, Imura H, Ishizaki K: Accumulation of allelic loss on arms of chromosomes 13q, 16q and 17p in the advanced stages of human hepatocellular carcinoma. *Int J Cancer* **51**:862, 1992.

36. Nishida N, Fukuda Y, Kokuryu H, Toguchida J, Yandell DW, Ikenaga M, Imura H, Ishizaki K: Role and mutational heterogeneity of the p53 gene in hepatocellular carcinoma. *Cancer Res* **53**:368, 1993.

37. Fujimoto Y, Hampton LL, Wirth PJ, Wang NJ, Xie JP, Thorgeirsson SS: Alterations of tumor suppressor genes and allelic losses in human hepatocellular carcinomas in China. *Cancer Res* **54**:281, 1994.

38. Hino O, Shows TB, Rogler CE: Hepatitis B virus integration site in hepatocellular carcinoma at chromosome 17;18 translocation. *Proc Natl Acad Sci USA* **83**:8338, 1986.

39. Tokino T, Fukushige S, Nakamura T, Nagaya T, Murotsu T, Shiga K, Aoki N, Matsubara K: Chromosomal translocation and inverted duplication associated with integrated hepatitis B virus in hepatocellular carcinomas. *J Virol* **61**:3848, 1987.

40. McBride OW, Merry D, Givol D: The gene for human p53 cellular tumor antigen is located on chromosome 17 short arm 17p13). *Proc Natl Acad Sci USA* **83**:130, 1986.

41. Ozturk M: p53 mutation in hepatocellular carcinoma after aflatoxin exposure. *Lancet* **338**:1356, 1991.

42. Oda T, Tsuda H, Scarpa A, Sakamoto M, Hirohashi S: Mutation pattern of the p53 gene as a diagnostic marker for multiple hepatocellular carcinoma. *Cancer Res* **52**:3674, 1992.

43. Bressac B, Galvin KM, Liang TJ, Isselbacher KJ, Wands JR, Ozturk M: Abnormal structure and expression of p53 gene in human hepatocellular carcinoma. *Proc Natl Acad Sci USA* **87**:1973, 1990.

44. Takiya S, Tagaya T, Takahashi K, Kawashima H, Kamiya M, Fukuzawa Y, Kobayashi S, Fukatsu A, Katoh K, Kakumu S: Role of transforming growth factor beta 1 on hepatic regeneration and apoptosis in liver diseases. *J Clin Pathol* **48**:1093, 1995.

45. Seo JH, Park BC: Expression of insulin-like growth factor II in chronic hepatitis B, liver cirrhosis, and hepatocellular carcinoma. *Gan To Kagaku Ryoho* 22 Suppl **3**:292, 1995.

46. Diamantis ID, McGandy CE, Chen TJ, Liaw YF, Gudat F, Bianchi L: Hepatitis B X expression in hepatocellular carcinoma. *J Hepatol* **15**:400, 1992.

47. Fourel G, Trepo C, Bougueleret L, Henglein B, Ponzetto A, Tiollais P, Buendia MA: Frequent activation of N-myc genes by hepadnavirus insertion in woodchuck liver tumours. *Nature* **347**:294, 1990.

48. Hsu T, Moroy T, Etiemble J, Louise A, Trepo C, Tiollais P, Buendia MA: Activation of c-*myc* by woodchuck hepatitis virus insertion in hepatocellular carcinoma. *Cell* **55**:627, 1988.

49. Matsubara K, Tokino T: Integration of hepatitis B virus DNA and its implications to hepatocarcinogenesis. *Mol Biol Med* **7**:243, 1990.

50. Rogler CE, Chisari FV: Cellular and molecular mechanisms of hepatocarcinogenesis. *Semin Liver Dis* **12**:265, 1992.

51. de The H, Marchio A, Tiollais P, Dejean A: A novel steroid thyroid hormone receptor gene inappropriately expressed in human hepatocellular carcinoma. *Nature* **330**:667, 1987.

52. Wang J, Chenivesse X, Henglein B, Brechot C: Hepatitis B virus integration in a cyclin A gene in a hepatocellular carcinoma. *Nature* **343**:555, 1990.

53. Ogata N, Tokino T, Kamimura T, Asakura H: A comparison of the molecular structure of integrated hepatitis B virus genomes in hepato-

cellular carcinoma cells and hepatocytes derived from the same patient. *Hepatology* **11**:1017, 1990.

54. Hino O, Kajino K: Hepatitis virus hepatocarcinogenesis. *Intervirology* **37**:133, 1994.
55. Hino O, Nomura K, Ohtake K, Kawaguchi T, Sugano H, Kitagawa T: Instability of integrated hepatitis B virus DNA with inverted repeat structure in a transgenic mouse. *Cancer Genet Cytogenet* **37**:273, 1989.
56. Nakamura T, Tokino T, Nagaya T, Matsubara K: Microdeletion associated with the integration process of hepatitis B virus DNA. *Nucleic Acids Res* **16**:4865, 1988.
57. Hino O, Tabata S, Hotta Y: Evidence for increased in vitro recombination with insertion of human hepatitis B virus DNA. *Proc Natl Acad Sci USA* **88**:9248, 1991.
58. Harris CC: Structure and function of the p53 tumor suppressor gene: clues for rational cancer therapeutic strategies. *J Natl Cancer Inst* **88**:1442, 1996.
59. Ko LJ, Prives C: p53: puzzle and paradigm. *Genes Devel* **10**:1054, 1996.
60. Levine AJ, Momand J, Finlay CA: The p53 tumour suppressor gene. *Nature* **351**:453, 1991.
61. Hollstein M, Sidransky D, Vogelstein B, Harris CC: p53 mutations in human cancers. *Science* **253**:49, 1991.
62. Greenblatt MS, Bennett WP, Hollstein M, Harris CC: Mutations in the p53 tumor suppressor gene: clues to cancer etiology and molecular pathogenesis. *Cancer Res* **54**:4855, 1994.
63. Soussi T, Caron de Fromentel C, May P: Structural aspects of the p53 protein in relation to gene evolution. *Oncogene* **5**:945, 1990.
64. Hollstein M, Rice K, Greenblatt MS, Soussi T, Fuchs R, Sorlie T, Hovig E, Smith B, Montesano R, Harris CC: Database of p53 gene somatic mutations in human tumors and cell lines. *Nucleic Acids Res* **22**:3547, 1994.
65. Hollstein M, Shomer B, Greenblatt M, Soussi T, Hovig E, Montesano R, Harris CC: Somatic point mutations in the p53 gene of human tumors and cell lines: updated compilation. *Nucleic Acids Res* **24**:141, 1996.
66. Murakami Y, Hayashi K, Sekiya T: Detection of aberrations of the p53 alleles and the gene transcript in human tumor cell lines by single conformation polymorphism analysis. *Cancer Res* **51**:3356, 1991.
67. Hsu IC, Metcalf RA, Sun T, Welsh JA, Wang NJ, Harris CC: Mutational hotspot in the p53 gene in human hepatocellular carcinomas. *Nature* **350**:427, 1991.
68. Scorsone KA, Zhou YZ, Butel JS, Slagle BL: p53 mutations cluster at codon 249 in hepatitis B virus-positive hepatocellular carcinomas from China. *Cancer Res* **52**:1635, 1992.
69. Li D, Cao Y, He L, Wang NJ, Gu J: Aberrations of p53 gene in human hepatocellular carcinoma from China. *Carcinogenesis* **14**:169, 1993.
70. Bressac B, Kew M, Wands J, Ozturk M: Selective G to T mutations of p53 gene in hepatocellular carcinoma from southern Africa. *Nature* **350**:429, 1991.
71. Soini Y, Chia SC, Bennett WP, Groopman JD, Wang JS, DeBenedetti VM, Cawley H, Welsh JA, Hansen C, Bergasa NV, Jones EA, DiBisceglie AM, Trivers GE, Sandoval CA, Calderon IE, Munoz Espinosa LE, Harris CC: An aflatoxin-associated mutational hotspot at codon 249 in the p53 tumor suppressor gene occurs in hepatocellular carcinomas from Mexico. *Carcinogenesis* **17**:1007, 1996.
72. Oda T, Tsuda H, Scarpa A, Sakamoto M, Hirohashi S: p53 gene mutation spectrum in hepatocellular carcinoma. *Cancer Res* **52**:635, 1992.
73. Kress S, Jahn UR, Buchmann A, Bannasch P, Schwarz M: p53 Mutations in human hepatocellular carcinomas from Germany. *Cancer Res* **52**:3220, 1992.
74. Hsu IC, Tokiwa T, Bennett W, Metcalf RA, Welsh JA, Sun T, Harris CC: p53 gene mutation and integrated hepatitis B viral DNA sequences in human liver cancer cell lines. *Carcinogenesis* **14**:987, 1993.
75. Aguilar F, Harris CC, Sun T, Hollstein M, Cerutti P: Geographic variation of p53 mutational profile in nonmalignant human liver. *Science* **264**:1317, 1994.
76. Aguilar F, Hussain SP, Cerutti P: Aflatoxin B1 induces the transversion of G →T in codon 249 of the p53 tumor suppressor gene in human hepatocytes. *Proc Natl Acad Sci USA* **90**:8586, 1993.
77. Cerutti P, Hussain P, Pourzand C, Aguilar F: Mutagenesis of the H-ras protooncogene and the p53 tumor suppressor gene. *Cancer Res* **54**:1934s, 1994.
78. Ponchel F, Puisieux A, Tabone E, Michot JP, Froschl G, Morel AP, Frebourg T, Fontaniere B, Oberhammer F, Ozturk M: Hepatocarcinoma mutant p53 induces mitotic activity but has no effect on trans-

forming growth factor beta 1-mediated apoptosis. *Cancer Res* **54**:2064, 1994.
79. Dumenco L, Oguey D, Wu J, Messier N, Fausto N: Introduction of a murine p53 mutation corresponding to human codon 249 into a murine hepatocyte cell line results in growth advantage, but not in transformation. *Hepatology* **22**:1279, 1995.
80. Wang XW, Gibson MK, Vermeulen W, Yeh H, Forrester K, Sturzbecher HW, Hoeijmakers JHJ, Harris CC: Abrogation of p53-induced apoptosis by the hepatitis B virus X gene. *Cancer Res* **55**:6012, 1995.
81. Forrester K, Lupold SE, Ott VL, Chay CH, Band V, Wang XW, Harris CC: Effects of p53 mutants on wild-type p53-mediated transactivation are cell type dependent. *Oncogene* **10**:2103, 1995.
82. Guengerich FP, Johnson WW, Ueng Y-F, Yamazaki H, Shimada T: Involvement of cytochrome P450, glutathione S-transferase, and epoxide hydrolase in the metabolism of aflatoxin B1 and relevance to risk of human liver cancer. *Environ Health Perspect* **104**:557, 1996.
83. Buss P, Caviezel M, Lutz WK: Linear dose-response relationship for DNA adducts in rat liver from chronic exposure to aflatoxin B1. *Carcinogenesis* **11**:2133, 1990.
84. Hosono S, Chou MJ, Lee CS, Shih C: Infrequent mutation of p53 gene in hepatitis B virus positive primary hepatocellular carcinomas. *Oncogene* **8**:491, 1993.
85. Feitelson MA, Zhu M, Duan LX, London WT: Hepatitis B x antigen and p53 are associated in vitro and in liver tissues from patients with primary hepatocellular carcinoma. *Oncogene* **8**:1109, 1993.
86. Wang XW, Forrester K, Yeh H, Feitelson MA, Gu JR, Harris CC: Hepatitis B virus X protein inhibits p53 sequence-specific DNA binding, transcriptional activity, and association with transcription factor ERCC3. *Proc Natl Acad Sci USA* **91**:2230, 1994.
87. Ueda H, Ullrich SJ, Gangemi JD, Kappel CA, Ngo L, Feitelson MA, Jay G: Functional inactivation but not structural mutation of p53 causes liver cancer. *Nat Genet* **9**:41, 1995.
88. Maguire HF, Hoeffler JP, Siddiqui A: HBV X protein alters the DNA binding specificity of CREB and ATF-2 by protein-protein interactions. *Science* **252**:842, 1991.
89. Williams JS, Andrisani OM: The hepatitis B virus X protein targets the basic region zipper domain of CREB. *Proc Natl Acad Sci USA* **92**:3819, 1995.
90. Jia L, Wang XW, Sun Z, Harris CC: Interactive effects of p53 tumor suppressor gene and hepatitis B virus in hepatocellular carcinogenesis. *Cancer Surveys,* 1997. (*in press*)
91. Schaeffer L, Roy R, Humbert S, Moncollin V, Vermeulen W, Hoeijmakers JH, Cambon P, Egly JM: DNA repair helicase: a component of BTF2 (TFIIH) basic transcription factor. *Science* **260**:58, 1993.
92. Weeda G, van Ham RC, Vermeulen W, Bootsma D, Van der Eb AJ, Hoeijmakers JH: A presumed DNA helicase encoded by ERCC is involved in the human repair disorders xeroderma pigmentosum and Cockayne's syndrome. *Cell* **62**:777, 1990.
93. Wang XW, Yeh H, Schaeffer L, Roy R, Moncollin V, Egly JM, Wang Z, Friedberg EC, Evans MK, Taffe BG, Bohr VA, Hoeijmakers JH, Forrester K, Harris CC: p53 modulation of TFIIH-associated nucleotide excision repair activity. *Nature Genet* **10**:188, 1995.
94. Teramoto T, Satonaka K, Kitazawa S, Fujimori T, Hayashi K, Maeda S: p53 gene abnormalities are closely related to hepatoviral infections and occur at a late stage of hepatocarcinogenesis. *Cancer Res* **54**:231, 1994.
95. Jaskiewicz K, Banach L, Izycka E: Hepatocellular carcinoma in young patients: histology, cellular differentiation, HBV infection and oncoprotein p53. *Anticancer Res* **15**:2723, 1995.
96. Tanaka S, Toh Y, Adachi E, Matsumata T, Mori R, Sugimachi K: Tumor progression in hepatocellular carcinoma may be mediated by p53 mutation. *Cancer Res* **53**:2884, 1993.
97. Murakami Y, Hayashi K, Hirohashi S, Sekiya T: Aberrations of the tumor suppressor p53 and retinoblastoma genes in human hepatocellular carcinomas. *Cancer Res* **51**:5520, 1991.
98. Tabor E: Tumor suppressor genes, growth factor genes, and oncogenes in hepatitis B virus-associated hepatocellular carcinoma. *J Med Virol* **42**:357, 1994.
99. Pascale RM, Simile MM, Feo F: Genomic abnormalities in hepatocarcinogenesis. Implications for a chemopreventive strategy. *Anticancer Res* **13**:1341, 1993.
100. Gu JR: Molecular aspects of human hepatic carcinogenesis. *Carcinogenesis* **9**:697, 1988.
101. Zhang XK, Huang DP, Chiu DK, Chiu JF: The expression of oncogenes in human developing liver and hepatomas. *Biochem Biophys Res Commun* **142**:932, 1987.

102. Gu JR, Hu LF, Cheng YC, Wan DF: Oncogenes in human primary hepatic cancer. *J Cell Physiol* Suppl **4**:13, 1986.

103. Takada S, Koike K: Activated N gene was found in human hepatoma tissue but only in a small fraction of the tumor cells. *Oncogene* **4**:189, 1989.

104. Ogata N, Kamimura T, Asakura H: Point mutation, allelic loss and increased methylation of c gene in human hepatocellular carcinoma. *Hepatology* **13**:31, 1991.

105. Yang SS, Modali R, Parks JB, Taub JV: Transforming DNA sequences of human hepatocellular carcinomas, their distribution and relationship with hepatitis B virus sequence in human hepatomas. *Leukemia* **2**:102S, 1988.

106. Yuasa Y, Sudo K: Transforming genes in human hepatomas detected by a tumorigenicity assay. *Jpn J Cancer Res* **78**:1036, 1987.

107. Arbuthnot P, Kew M, Fitschen W: c-fos and c-myc oncoprotein expression in human hepatocellular carcinomas. *Anticancer Res* **11**:921, 1991.

108. Farshid M, Tabor E: Expression of oncogenes and tumor suppressor genes in human hepatocellular carcinoma and hepatoblastoma cell lines. *J Med Virol* **38**:235, 1992.

109. Feitelson MA: Biology of hepatitis B virus variants. *Lab Invest* **71**:324, 1994.

110. Twu JS, Schloemer RH: Transcriptional trans-activating function of hepatitis B virus. *J Virol* **61**:3448, 1987.

111. Spandau DF, Lee CH: Trans-activation of viral enhancers by the hepatitis B virus X protein. *J Virol* **62**:427, 1988.

112. Twu JS, Lai MY, Chen DS, Robinson WS: Activation of protooncogene c-jun by the X protein of hepatitis B virus. *Virology* **192**:346, 1993.

113. Aufiero B, Schneider RJ: The hepatitis B virus X-gene product transactivates both RNA polymerase II and III promoters. *EMBO J* **9**:497, 1990.

114. Natoli G, Avantaggiati ML, Chirillo P, Costanzo A, Artini M, Balsano C, Levrero M: Induction of the DNA-binding activity of c-jun/c-fos heterodimers by the hepatitis B virus transactivator pX. *Mol Cell Biol* **14**:989, 1994.

115. Balsano C, Avantaggiati ML, Natoli G, De Marzio E, Will H, Perricaudet M, Levrero M: Full-length and truncated versions of the hepatitis B virus (HBV) X protein (pX) transactivate the cmyc protooncogene at the transcriptional level. *Biochem Biophys Res Commun* **176**:985, 1991.

116. Levrero M, Balsano C, Avantaggiati ML, Natoli G, De Marzio E, Will H: Hepatitis B virus and hepatocellular carcinoma: a possible role for the viral transactivators. *Ital J Gastroenterol* **23**:576, 1991.

117. Caselmann WH, Meyer M, Kekulî AS, Lauer U, Hofschneider PH, Koshy R: A trans-activator function is generated by integration of hepatitis B virus preS/S sequences in human hepatocellular carcinoma DNA. *Proc Natl Acad Sci* **87**:2970, 1990.

118. Kekulî AS, Lauer U, Meyer M, Caselmann WH, Hofschneider PH, Koshy R: The preS2/S region of integrated hepatitis B virus DNA encodes a transcriptional transactivator. *Nature* **343**:457, 1990.

119. Unsal H, Yakicier C, Marcais C, Kew M, Volkmann M, Zentgraf H, Isselbacher KJ, Ozturk M: Genetic heterogeneity of hepatocellular carcinoma. *Proc Natl Acad Sci USA* **91**:822, 1994.

120. Paterlini P, Poussin K, Kew M, Franco D, Brechot C: Selective accumulation of the X transcript of hepatitis B virus in patients negative for hepatitis B surface antigen with hepatocellular carcinoma. *Hepatology* **21**:313, 1995.

121. Caselmann WH: Transactivation of cellular gene expression by hepatitis B viral proteins: a possible molecular mechanism of hepatocarcinogenesis. *J Hepatol* **22**:34, 1995.

122. Wei Y, Etiemble J, Fourel G, Vitvitski-Trepo L, Buendia MA: Hepadna virus integration generates virus-cell cotranscripts carrying 3' truncated X genes in human and woodchuck liver tumors. *J Med Virol* **45**:82, 1995.

123. Benn J, Schneider RJ: Hepatitis B virus HBx protein deregulates cell cycle checkpoint controls. *Proc Natl Acad Sci USA* **92**:1121, 1995.

124. Benn J, Schneider RJ: Hepatitis B virus HBx protein activates Ras-GTP complex formation and establishes a Ras, Raf, MAP kinase signaling cascade. *Proc Natl Acad Sci USA* **91**:1035, 1994.

125. Doria M, Klein N, Lucito R, Schneider RJ: The hepatitis B virus HBx protein is a dual specificity cytoplasmic activator of Ras and nuclear activator of transcription factors. *EMBO J* **14**:4747, 1995.

126. Kekulî AS, Lauer U, Weiss L, Luber B, Hofschneider PH: Hepatitis B virus transactivator HBx uses a tumor promoter signalling pathway. *Nature* **361**:742, 1993.

127. Luber B, Lauer U, Weiss L, Hohne M, Hofschneider PH, Kekulî AS: The hepatitis B virus transactivator HBx causes elevation of diacylglycerol and activation of protein kinase C. *Res Virol* **144**:311, 1993.

128. Koike K, Moriya K, Yotsuyanagi H, Iino S, Kurokawa K: Induction of cell cycle progression by hepatitis B virus HBx gene expression in quiescent mouse fibroblasts. *J Clin Invest* **94**:44, 1994.

129. Lee TH, Elledge SJ, Butel JS: Hepatitis B virus X protein interacts with a probable cellular DNA repair protein. *J Virol* **69**:1107, 1995.

130. Lucito R, Schneider RJ: Hepatitis B virus X protein activates transcription factor NF-kappa B without a requirement for protein kinase C. *J Virol* **66**:983, 1992.

131. Fischer M, Runkel L, Schaller H: HBx protein of hepatitis B virus interacts with the C-terminal portion of a novel human proteasome alpha-subunit. *Virus Genes* **10**:99, 1995.

132. Takada S, Kido H, Fukutomi A, Mori T, Koike K: Interaction of hepatitis B virus X protein with a serine protease, tryptase TL2 as an inhibitor. *Oncogene* **9**:341, 1994.

133. Takada S, Tsuchida N, Kobayashi M, Koike K: Disruption of the function of tumor-suppressor gene p53 by the hepatitis B virus X protein and hepatocarcinogenesis. *J Cancer Res Clin Oncol* **121**:593, 1995.

134. Höhne M, Schaefer S, Seifer M, Feitelson MA, Paul D, Gerlich WH: Malignant transformation of immortalized transgenic hepatocytes after transfection with hepatitis B virus DNA. *EMBO J* **9**:1137, 1990.

135. Shirakata Y, Kawada M, Fujiki Y, Sano H, Oda M, Yaginuma K, Kobayashi M, Koike K: The X gene of hepatitis B virus induced growth stimulation and tumorigenic transformation of mouse NIH3T3 cells. *Jpn J Cancer Res* **80**:617, 1989.

136. Kim CM, Koike K, Saito I, Miyamura T, Jay G: HBx gene of hepatitis B virus induces liver cancer in transgenic mice. *Nature* **351**:317, 1991.

137. Macaulay VM: Insulin-like growth factors and cancer. *Br J Cancer* **65**:311, 1992.

138. Su Q, Liu YF, Zhang JF, Zhang SX, Li DF, Yang JJ: Expression of insulin-like growth factor II in hepatitis B, cirrhosis and hepatocellular carcinoma: its relationship with hepatitis B virus antigen expression. *Hepatology* **20**:788, 1994.

139. Cariani E, Lasserre C, Seurin D, Hamelin B, Kemeny F, Franco D, Czech MP, Ullrich A, Brechot C: Differential expression of insulin-like growth factor II mRNA in human primary liver cancers, benign liver tumors, and liver cirrhosis. *Cancer Res* **48**:6844, 1988.

140. Park BC, Huh MH, Seo JH: Differential expression of transforming growth factor alpha and insulin-like growth factor II in chronic active hepatitis B, cirrhosis and hepatocellular carcinoma. *J Hepatol* **22**:286, 1995.

141. Takeda S, Kondo M, Kumada T, Koshikawa T, Ueda R, Nishio M, Osada H, Suzuki H, Nagatake M, Washimi O, Takagi K, Takahashi T, Nakao A: Allelic-expression imbalance of the insulin-like growth factor 2 gene in hepatocellular carcinoma and underlying disease. *Oncogene* **12**:1589, 1996.

142. Ito T, Sasaki Y, Wands JR: Overexpression of human insulin receptor substrate 1 induces cellular transformation with activation of mitogen protein kinases. *Mol Cell Biol* **16**:943, 1996.

143. Tanaka S, Wands JR: Insulin receptor substrate 1 overexpression in human hepatocellular carcinoma cells prevents transforming growth factor beta 1 apoptosis. *Cancer Res* **56**:3391, 1996.

144. Oberhammer FA, Pavelka M, Sharma S, Tiefenbacher R, Purchio AF, Bursch W, Schulte R: Induction of apoptosis in cultured hepatocytes and in regressing liver by transforming growth factor beta 1. *Proc Natl Acad Sci USA* **89**:5408, 1992.

145. Chuang LY, Hung WC, Chang CC, Tsai JH: Characterization of apoptosis induced by transforming growth factor beta 1 in human hepatoma cells. *Anticancer Res* **14**:147, 1994.

146. Hsia CC, Axiotis CA, Di Bisceglie AM, Tabor E: Transforming growth factor-alpha in human hepatocellular carcinoma and coexpression with hepatitis B surface antigen in adjacent liver. *Cancer* **70**:1049, 1992.

147. Di Bisceglie AM, Rustgi VK, Hoofnagle JH, Dusheiko GM, Lotze MT: NIH conference: Hepatocellular carcinoma. *Ann Intern Med* **108**:390, 1988.

148. Harris CC: p53 Tumor suppressor gene: from the basic research laboratory to the clinic: An abridged historical perspective. *Carcinogenesis*, 1996. (*in press*)

149. Lee JM, Bernstein A: Apoptosis, cancer and the p53 tumor suppressor gene. *Cancer Metastasis Rev* **14**:149, 1995.

150. Mullen CA, Blaese RM: Gene therapy of cancer. *Cancer Chemother Biol Response Modif* **15**:176, 1994.

151. Clayman GL, el-Naggar AK, Roth JA, Zhang WW, Goepfert H, Taylor DL, Liu TJ: In vivo molecular therapy with p53 adenovirus for microscopic residual head and neck squamous carcinoma. *Cancer Res* **55**:1, 1995.

152. Liu TJ, el-Naggar AK, McDonnell TJ, Steck KD, Wang M, Taylor DL, Clayman GL: Apoptosis induction mediated by wild-type p53 adenoviral gene transfer in squamous cell carcinoma of the head and neck. *Cancer Res* **55**:3117, 1995.

153. Xu GW, Sun ZT, Forrester K, Wang XW, Coursen J, Harris CC: Tissue growth suppression and chemosensitivity promotion in human hepatocellular carcinoma cells by retroviral-mediated transfer of the wild-type p53 gene. *Hepatology,* 1996. (*in press*)

154. da Costa LT, Jen J, He TC, Chan TA, Kinzler KW, Vogelstein B: Converting cancer genes into killer genes. *Proc Natl Acad Sci USA* **93**:4192, 1996.

CHAPTER 43

Clinical and Biological Aspects of Neuroblastoma

Garrett M. Brodeur

- Neuroblastoma, a tumor of the postganglionic sympathetic nervous system, is the most common extracranial solid tumor of childhood.

- No environmental exposures or agents have been associated with an increased risk of neuroblastoma. However, a subset has a genetic predisposition that follows an autosomal dominant pattern of inheritance.

- Primary tumors generally arise in the adrenal medulla (50%) or elsewhere in the abdomen or pelvis (30%). Only 20 percent arise in the chest.

- Metastases usually are found in the regional lymph nodes, bone, bone marrow, skin, or liver. Paraneoplastic syndromes characteristic of neuroblastomas are seen in a small percentage of patients.

- Neuroblastomas are diagnosed by tissue biopsy or characterization of cells in the bone marrow. Catecholamine metabolites are elevated in the urine in over 90 percent of cases.

- There is an international neuroblastoma staging system for categorizing the extent of the primary tumor and the presence or absence of metastases.

- A number of prognostic variables have been identified that allow better prediction of clinical behavior: *MYCN* amplification, allelic loss of 1p36, expression of *TRK-A*, tumor cell ploidy, and tumor pathology.

- Histologically neuroblastic tumors can be immature (neuroblastomas), partially mature (ganglioneuroblastomas), or completely mature (ganglioneuromas). However, other features (such as the presence or absence of schwannian stroma, mitoses, or karyorrhectic cells) may have more prognostic importance.

- Localized, resectable tumors can be cured by surgery alone. Unresectable tumors or metastatic disease in infants require mild to moderately intensive chemotherapy. Metastatic disease in older patients, and regional tumors with unfavorable biological features in any age, require intensive chemotherapy, frequently with bone marrow rescue.

- Screening of infants for neuroblastoma by measuring urinary catecholamine metabolites has resulted in a doubling of the apparent incidence rate in infants with no decrease in advanced disease in older children.

- Future therapeutic approaches may be aimed at the induction of differentiation or programmed cell death through neurotrophin receptor pathways. Alternate approaches may focus on the *MYCN* gene or the 1p36 suppressor gene.

Neuroblastoma is the most common solid tumor of childhood. This tumor has the propensity to regress spontaneously in some infants or to differentiate into a benign ganglioneuroma in some older patients. Unfortunately, neuroblastoma is metastatic at the time of diagnosis in the majority of patients, and it usually leads to rapid tumor progression and a fatal outcome. Recent advances in understanding the biology of neuroblastoma have provided considerable insight into the genetic and biochemical mechanisms underlying these seemingly disparate behaviors. High expression of the nerve growth factor receptor (called *TRK-A*) is found in the majority of infants, and this may mediate either apoptosis or differentiation in these tumors. On the other hand, amplification of the *MYCN* oncogene is found in a substantial number of patients with advanced stages of disease and a poor prognosis. Finally, two neuroblastoma patients have been reported with constitutional rearrangements of 1p36, a site that is frequently deleted in the tumors of advanced stage patients. This suggests that a constitutional predisposition gene may reside at this locus. These and other biological observations have given us tremendous insight into mechanisms of malignant transformation and progression, as well as spontaneous differentiation and regression. The challenge of the next decade will be to translate this information into more effective and less toxic therapy for these patients.

Few tumors have engendered as much fascination and frustration for clinical and laboratory investigators as neuroblastoma. This tumor of the post-ganglionic sympathetic nervous system is the most common solid tumor in childhood. However, despite dramatic improvements in the cure rate for other common pediatric neoplasms, such as acute lymphoblastic leukemia or Wilms tumor, there has been relatively little improvement in the overall survival rate of patients with neuroblastoma. Surprisingly, some infants with metastatic disease can experience complete regression of their disease without therapy, and some older patients have complete maturation of their tumor into a benign ganglioneuroma. Unfortunately, the majority of patients have metastatic tumor that grows relentlessly despite even the most intensive multimodality therapy.

Recently there has been considerable progress in elucidating the genetic basis for these diverse clinical behaviors. This progress has come from the analysis of tumors at the cytogenetic and molecular level. Specific genetic changes have been identified that allow tumors to be classified into subsets with distinct biological features and clinical behavior (see the following). Indeed, certain genetic abnormalities are very powerful predictors of response to therapy and outcome, and as such they have become essential components of tumor characterization at diagnosis. Thus, neuroblastoma serves as a model solid tumor in which the cytogenetic and molecular analysis of the tumor cells has become a conventional determinant of optimal patient management.

In this chapter, the epidemiological, genetic, and pathologic features of neuroblastomas will be reviewed. In addition, the essential clinical features of tumor presentation and management will be discussed, including several paraneoplastic syndromes that are associated with neuroblastomas. The cytogenetic and molecular genetic features of the tumor cells and their implications will be reviewed. Finally, the current results of mass screening for neuroblastoma, and the implications for understanding the genetic heterogeneity of this disease, will be presented.

EPIDEMIOLOGY

Incidence

Neuroblastomas account for 8 to 10 percent of all childhood cancers. The prevalence is about one case per 8,000 live births, and there are about 550 new cases of neuroblastoma per year in the United States.[6] This corresponds to an incidence of 10.5 per million per year in white children and 8.8 per million per year in Black children less than 15 years of age.[6,7] Evidence indicates that this incidence is fairly uniform throughout the world, at least for industrialized nations. The tumor is slightly more common in boys than in girls, with a male:female sex ratio of 1.2:1 in most large studies.

The median age at diagnosis of 1,001 consecutive children with neuroblastoma seen at Pediatric Oncology Group (POG) institutions from 1981 to 1989 is 22 months.[8] Thus, 37 percent of patients are less than 1 year of age, 81 percent are less than 4 years, and 97 percent are diagnosed by 10 years of age (Figure 43-1). Some studies have shown a bimodal age distribution, with an initial peak before 1 year and a second peak between 2 and 4 years of age.[7] This observation suggests that there may be at least two subpopulations of neuroblastoma, one of which may represent a genetically predisposed subset, as seen in retinoblastoma. Alternatively, there may be two genetically distinct types of neuroblastoma with different ages of onset. However, a bimodal age distribution is not always seen.

Embryology

In 1963, Beckwith and Perrin reported that microscopic neuroblastic nodules, resembling neuroblastoma in situ, were found frequently in infants less than 3 months of age who died of other causes.[9] This finding was interpreted initially to indicate that neuroblastomas develop up to 40 times more often than they are detected clinically, but that the tumor regresses spontaneously in the vast majority of cases. However, others have demonstrated that

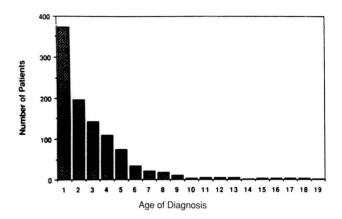

FIG. 43-1 Age at diagnosis in 1,001 consecutive patients diagnosed with neuroblastoma in the Pediatric Oncology Group (POG) between 1981 and 1989. (From Brodeur GM: Neuroblastoma and other peripheral neuroectodermal tumors, in Fernbach DJ, Vietti TJ (eds): *Clinical Pediatric Oncology*. St. Louis, Mosby Year Book, 1991, p. 337, with permission.)

these neuroblastic nodules occurred uniformly in all fetuses studied, peaked between 17 and 20 weeks of gestation, and gradually regressed by the time of birth or shortly after.[10,11] Thus, the microscopic neuroblastic nodules seen in the earlier study were more likely remnants of fetal adrenal development. Nevertheless, these neuroblastic cell rests may be the cells from which neuroblastomas develop, at least in the adrenal medulla. Although some controversy still exists concerning the phenomenon of in situ neuroblastoma, the latter interpretation is generally accepted.

Microscopic neuroblastic nodules as described above would never be detected clinically, nor would they be detected by screening infants for neuroblastoma by measuring urinary catecholamine metabolites. However, the concept of "in situ" neuroblastoma has been used to support the argument that many neuroblastomas arise and regress spontaneously. Indeed, there are a number of well-documented cases in infants with neuroblastoma that have had complete regression of tumor.[12–14] The actual frequency of neuroblastomas that are detected clinically and subsequently regress without treatment probably is much lower than was suggested by this earlier report, and more likely represents 2 to 5 percent of all neuroblastoma patients.[9,15–17] However, the frequency of development and regression of true neuroblastomas that never cause symptoms is probably much higher, based on estimates from the mass screening studies, and is perhaps a number equal to those detected clinically.[18,19]

Environmental Studies

The etiology of neuroblastoma is unknown in most cases, but, based on current information, it appears unlikely that environmental exposures play a major role. There have been a few reports of neuroblastoma associated with the fetal hydantoin, phenobarbitol or alcohol syndromes,[20–22] suggesting that prenatal exposure to these substances may increase the risk of neuroblastoma. However, this association has not been confirmed with certainty. There have been two studies that have reported a weak association between neuroblastoma and paternal occupational exposure to electromagnetic fields, but this was not confirmed in another study.[23–25] The latter group previously had shown an association between maternal use of hair coloring products, but this also has not been confirmed.[26] Moreover, no prenatal or postnatal exposure to drugs, chemicals, or radiation has been either strongly or consistently associated with an increased incidence of neuroblastoma.

CONSTITUTIONAL GENETICS

Genetic Predisposition

A subset of patients with neuroblastoma exhibits a predisposition to develop this disease, and this predisposition follows an autosomal dominant pattern of inheritance. Knudson and Strong have estimated that as many as 22 percent of all neuroblastomas could be the result of a germinal mutation.[27] Regression analysis of these data from neuroblastoma fits the two-mutation hypothesis proposed by Knudson for the origin of childhood cancer.[28] According to this hypothesis, the nonhereditary form of neuroblastoma would result from two postzygotic (somatic) mutations in a single cell, causing malignant transformation of the cell that then develops into a single tumor. Hereditary tumors would arise in individuals in whom the first mutation is acquired as a prezygotic (germinal) event, so it is present in all cells. Only one additional mutation in any cell of the target tissue would be needed to induce malignant transformation, so these individuals have a higher incidence of neuroblastoma with a peak incidence at an earlier age. In addition, they may develop tumors at multiple primary sites, either simultaneously or sequentially. If such persons survive, one-half of their offspring should be carriers of the germinal mutation, with an estimated 63 percent chance of developing neuroblastoma.[27,29]

There have been a number of reports of familial neuroblastoma, as well as bilateral or multifocal disease, consistent with hereditary predisposition, and these were viewed recently by Kushner and colleagues.[30] The median age at diagnosis of patients with familial neuroblastoma is 9 months, which contrasts with a median age of 22 months for neuroblastoma in the general population. At least 20 percent of patients with familial neuroblastoma have bilateral adrenal or multifocal primary tumors. The concordance for neuroblastoma in monozygotic siblings during infancy suggests that hereditary factors may be predominant, whereas the discordance in older twins suggests that random mutations or other factors may play a role.[31] There has been a recent report examining the genetic linkage of neuroblastoma predisposition to two candidate loci in several families segregating the disease, but linkage has not yet been found.[32]

Constitutional Chromosome Abnormalities

A constitutional predisposition syndrome or associated congenital anomalies have not yet been identified in human neuroblastoma.[33,34] Several cases of constitutional chromosome abnormalities detected by banding have been reported in individuals with neuroblastoma, but no consistent pattern has emerged as yet (Table 43-1).[35–48] There have been two reports of constitutional abnormalities involving the short arm of chromosome 1, which frequently is deleted or rearranged in neuroblastoma cells. Laureys and colleagues described a patient with neuroblastoma who had a constitutional translocation between chromosomes 1 and 17, with the breakpoint on chromosome 1 in the region frequently deleted in neuroblastoma cells.[44] A second interesting case was reported by Biegel and colleagues.[47] This patient had a constitutional deletion of 1p36 and neuroblastoma, confirmed by both cytogenetic and molecular analysis. Together, these cases suggest that constitutional deletions or rearrangements involving a gene on 1p36 may be important in malignant transformation or predisposition to neuroblastoma. However, a recent report that familial neuroblastoma is not linked to 1p36 suggests that the predisposition locus lies elsewhere.[32]

Two series reporting the routine constitutional karyotype analysis of a series patients with neuroblastoma have identified several cases with balanced translocations (Table 43-1).[38,46] However, no consistent breakpoint has been identified, so routine karyotypic analysis is unlikely to be rewarding. Individuals with neuroblastoma who also have mental retardation, dysmorphic features, or other evidence of gross genetic abnormalities should be examined cytogenetically, because this may help identify the neuroblastoma predisposition locus (or loci).[47]

Other Genetic Syndromes

Neuroblastoma has been associated with neurofibromatosis and aganglionosis of the colon, suggesting that it might be part of a spectrum of syndromes involving maldevelopment of the neural crest.[27,29,49–53] However, a recent analysis of the simultaneous occurrence of neuroblastoma and neurofibromatosis in the same patient suggests that the reported coincidence probably can be accounted for by chance alone.[53] A variety of other congenital anomalies and genetic syndromes have been reported in associa-

Table 43-1 Constitutional Chromosome Abnormalities in Patients with Neuroblastoma

Chromosome Abnormality	Comments	Ref.
del(21)(p11); inv(11)(q21q23)	One from each parent	35–37
t(4;7)(p?;q?)	Balanced; normal phenotype	38
t(11;16)(q?;q?)	Balanced; normal phenotype	38
Partial trisomy 2p and monosomy 16p	Congenital anomalies	39
Partial trisomy 3q and monosomy 8p	Congenital anomalies	39
Partial trisomy 15q and monosomy 13q	Congenital anomalies	40
Trisomy 18	Congenital anomalies	41
fra(1)(p13.1)	Hereditary fragile site	42
t(1;?)(p36;?)	Mosaic?	43
t(1;17)(p36;q12-21)	Balanced	44
t(1;13)(q22;q12)	Balanced	45
t(8;11)(q22.1;q21)	Balanced	46
t(2;11)(p23;q22)	Balanced	46
t(2;6)(q32.2;q25.3)	Balanced	46
del(1)(p36.2-p36.3)	Dysmorphic, retarded	47
t(1;10)(p22;q21)	Balanced	48

tion with neuroblastoma, but no specific abnormality has been identified with increased frequency.[54–56]

TUMOR CYTOGENETICS AND MOLECULAR GENETICS

Considerable progress has been made in the past 10 to 15 years in understanding human neuroblastoma at a cellular and molecular level.[57–60] These studies have contributed to better methods of tumor diagnosis and subclassification, and they provide information that is useful in predicting clinical behavior and following disease activity. In addition to providing insights into mechanisms of malignant transformation and progression, these studies promise to generate novel approaches to treatment that may be more effective and less toxic than current therapeutic modalities.

Tumor Karyotype

Neuroblastomas are characterized cytogenetically by deletion of the short arm of chromosome 1 (1p), double-minute chromatin bodies (dmins), and homogeneously staining regions (HSRs) (Figure 43-2).[33,61–65] The former cytogenetic abnormality may represent deletion of a tumor suppressor gene, whereas the latter two abnormalities are cytogenetic manifestations of gene amplification.[66] To date, the only other specific karyotypic abnormality that has been detected is trisomy for the long arm of chromosome 17 (17q).[62,65] Although the majority of tumors that have been karyotyped are in the diploid range, a substantial number of tumors from patients with lower stages of disease are hyperdiploid or near triploid. The modal karyotype number has been shown to have prognostic value.[67–69] However, karyotypic analysis of tumor cells is a somewhat tedious process that is generally successful in less than 25 percent of the cases attempted.

DNA Index

Flow cytometric analysis of DNA content is a simple and semiautomated way of measuring total cell DNA, which correlates well with modal chromosome number. Recent studies by Look and colleagues, and others have demonstrated that determination of the DNA index (DI) of neuroblastomas from infants provides important information that can be predictive of response to particular chemotherapeutic regimens as well as outcome.[70–76] Interestingly, tumors with a "hyperdiploid" DNA content (DI > 1) are more likely to have lower stages of disease and to respond to cyclophosphamide and doxorubicin, whereas those with a "diploid" DNA content (DI = 1) more likely have advanced stages of disease and do not respond to this combination.[70,71] Although this analysis cannot detect specific chromosome rearrangements, such as deletions, translocations, or even gene amplification, it is a relatively simple test that correlates with biologic behavior, at least in subsets of patients. Unfortunately, the DNA index loses its prognostic significance for patients over 2 years of age.[71] This is probably because hyperdiploid tumors from infants generally have whole chromosome gains without structural rearrangements, whereas in older patients there are usually a number of structural rearrangements as well.

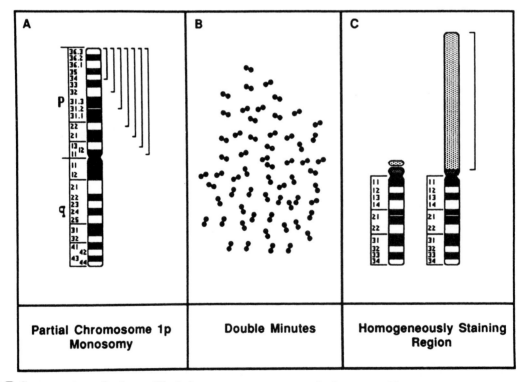

FIG. 43-2 Common cytogenetic abnormalities in human neuroblastomas. Shown are diagrammatic representations of the three most common cytogenetic abnormalities seen in human neuroblastomas. (A) Deletions of the short arm of chromosome 1. The brackets indicate that the region deleted in different tumors is variable in terms of its proximal breakpoint, but the distal short arm appears to be deleted in all cases, resulting in partial 1p monosomy. (B) Extrachromosomal double-minute chromatin bodies (dmins). Dmins are seen at about 30 percent of primary neuroblastomas and are a cytogenetic manifestation of gene amplification. (C) Homogeneously staining region (HSR). A representative HSR on the short arm of chromosome 13 is shown in this example. HSRs are a cytogenetic manifestation of gene amplification in which the amplified sequences are chromosomally integrated. (From Brodeur GM: Neuroblastoma: Clinical applications of molecular parameters. *Brain Pathol* 1:47, 1990, with permission.)

MYCN AMPLIFICATION

Extrachromosomal dmins and chromosomally integrated HSRs are cytogenetic manifestations of gene amplification, but the gene or genetic region amplified was not known initially. The region amplified is known now to be derived from the distal short arm of chromosome 2, and it contains the proto-oncogene *MYCN*. Brodeur and colleagues have demonstrated that *MYCN* amplification (Figures 43-3 and 43-4) occurs in about 25 percent of primary neuroblastomas from untreated patients, and amplification is associated predominantly with advanced stages of disease (Table 43-2).[33,77,78] Seeger and colleagues have shown that *MYCN* amplification was associated with rapid tumor progression and a poor prognosis.[79–82] Amplification is found in 5 to 10 percent of patients with low stages of disease and stage IV-S but 30 to 40 percent of advanced disease patients.[33,34,78] *MYCN* amplification is almost always present at the time of diagnosis, if it is going to occur, so it appears to be an intrinsic biologic property of a subset of very aggressive tumors that are destined to have a poor outcome.[83]

Oncogene Expression

The expression of *MYCN* and other oncogenes also may have clinical utility for diagnosis and prognosis. There is a correlation between *MYCN* copy number and expression, and tumors with amplification generally express *MYCN* at much higher levels than are seen in tumors without amplification. There is heterogeneity in the level of expression among the tumors that have a single copy of *MYCN*, but higher-expressing, single-copy tumors do not appear to be a particularly aggressive subset.[80,84–86] Expression of other oncogenes, such as *HRAS*, correlate generally with lower stages of disease and differentiated tumors, but *RAS* family genes rarely are activated by base-pair mutations of critical codons in neuroblastomas.[87–91] The pattern of oncogene expression may be used to distinguish neuroblastomas from other histologically similar tumors, such as neuroepithelioma.[92] However, the ultimate clinical

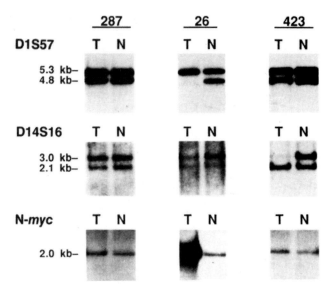

FIG. 43-4 Patterns of genetic change in neuroblastomas. The first row shows assessment of LOH for the short arm of chromosome 1 (1p34) using the hypervariable probe D1S57 and the enzyme *Taq*I. The second row shows assessment of LOH for the long arm of chromosome 14 (14p32) using the probe D14S16 and the enzyme *Taq*I. The third row shows assessment of *MYCN* amplification using the pNB-1probe and *Eco*RI digestion of the DNAs. The first column (patient no. 287) shows no LOH for 1 p or 14q, and normal *MYCN* copy number. The second column (patient no. 26) shows LOH for 1p and *MYCN* amplification, without allelic loss for 14q. The third column (patient no. 423) shows LOH for 14q, without LOH for 1p or *MYCN* amplification, which was the second most common pattern of genetic change. (T = tumor DNA; N = normal DNA from the same patient). (From Fong CT, White PS, Peterson K, Sapienza C, Cavenee WK, Kern S, Vogelstein B, Cantor AB, Look AT, Brodeur GM: Loss of heterozygosity for chromosome 1 or 14 defines subsets of advanced neuroblastomas. *Cancer Res* 52:1780, 1992, with permission.)

utility of the analysis of oncogene expression in neuroblastomas remains to be determined.

Chromosome Deletion or Allelic Loss

1p deletions are found in 70 to 80 percent of the near-diploid tumors that have been karyotyped (Figure 43-2).[33,63–65,67–69,93,94] Although near-diploid karyotypes with 1p deletions are associated commonly with advanced stages of disease, tumors from patients with lower stages are more likely to be hyperdiploid or triploid, with very few structural rearrangements. The deletions of chromosome 1 are somewhat variable in their proximal breakpoints, but the region of consistent deletion has been mapped to subbands of 1p36 using restriction fragment length polymorphisms that revealed loss of heterozygosity (LOH) for the deleted allele (Figure 43-4).[95,96] This 1p36 region may contain a suppressor gene that is important in malignant transformation or progression (Figure 43-5).[97]

There is evidence that allelic loss occurs with increased frequency on the long arm of chromosome 14 in neuroblastomas, suggesting that there may be another suppressor gene involved in the pathogenesis of neuroblastomas.[98] This finding has been confirmed by several other studies, which suggest that LOH of 1p, 14q, and possibly other loci occur with increased frequency in patients with neuroblastoma.[98–101] Studies have shown a strong correlation between LOH for 1p and *MYCN* amplification, suggesting that these two genetic events may be related, but 14q LOH does not occur with *MYCN* amplification, unless there is 1p LOH as well (Figure 43-6).[95,99]

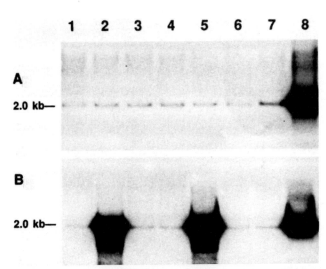

FIG. 43-3 Southern blots showing *MYCN* amplification. In both rows, lane 1 represents DNA from a normal lymphoblastoid cell line as a single-copy control, and lane 8 represents DNA from the NGP cell line, with 150 copies of *MYCN* per haploid genome. (Row A) Lanes 2–7 represent 6 neuroblastomas with a single copy of *MYCN* per haploid genome. (Row B) Lanes 2 and 5 show examples of tumors with *MYCN* amplification, whereas the other tumors have the normal single-copy signal. (From Brodeur GM: Neuroblastoma: Clinical application of molecular parameters. *Brain Pathol* 1990, with permission.)

Table 43-2 Correlation between *MYCN* Amplification and Stage in Three Thousand Neuroblastomas

Stage at Diagnosis	*MYCN* Amplification, %	3-year Survival, %
Benign ganglioneuromas	0/64 (0)	100
Low stages (1, 2)	31/772 (4)	90
Stage 4-S	15/190 (8)	80
Advanced stages (3, 4)	612/1,974 (31)	30
TOTAL	658/3,000 (22)	50

SOURCE: Brodeur GM, Azar C, Brother M, Hiemstra J, Kaufman B, Marshall H, Moley J, Nakagawara A, Saylors R, Scavarda N, Schneider S, Wasson J, White P, Seeger R, Look T, Castleberry R: Neuroblastoma: Effect of genetic factors on prognosis and treatment. *Cancer* **70**:1685, 1992.
Brodeur GM, Nakagawara A: Molecular basis of clinical heterogeneity in neuroblastoma. *Am J Pediat Hematol/Oncol* **14**:111, 1992.
Brodur GM, Castleberry RP: Neuroblastoma, in Pizzo PA, Poplack DG (eds): *Principles and Practice of Pediatric Oncology.* Philadelphia, JB Lippincott, 1993, p. 739.
Brodeur GM: Molecular pathology of human neuroblastomas. *Sem Diag Pathol* **11**:118, 1994.
Brodeur GM: Molecular basis for heterogeneity in human neuroblastomas. *Eur J Cancer* **31A**:505, 1995.

PATHOLOGY AND NEURONAL DIFFERENTIATION

Pathology

Neuroblastomas arise from primitive, pluripotential sympathetic nerve cells (sympathogonia), which are derived from the neural crest. These cells differentiate into the different normal tissues of the sympathetic nervous system, such as the spinal sympathetic ganglia, the supporting Schwannian cells, and adrenal chromaffin cells. The three classic histopathologic patterns of neuroblastoma, ganglioneuroblastoma, and ganglioneuroma reflect a spectrum of morphologic and biochemical differentiation. The typical neuroblastoma is composed of small but uniformly sized cells containing dense, hyperchromatic nuclei and scant cytoplasm. The presence of neuritic processes, or neuropil, is a pathognomonic feature of all but the most primitive neuroblastoma. The fully differentiated, and benign, counterpart of neuroblastoma is the ganglioneuroma. It is composed of mature ganglion cells, surrounded by a matrix of Schwannian cells and neuropil. Ganglioneuroblastomas are a heterogeneous group of tumors with histopathologic features spanning the extremes of maturation represented by neuroblastoma and ganglioneuroma. Histopathologic characteristics range from a predominance of neuroblastic elements with rare maturing cells, to those neoplasms comprised almost exclusively of ganglioneuroma containing occasional rests of neuroblasts. Ganglioneuroblastomas may be either focal or diffuse, depending on the pattern seen, but diffuse ganglioneuroblastoma is associated with less aggressive behavior.[102]

Immunohistochemistry and electron microscopy are helpful adjuncts to light microscopy in confirming a diagnosis of neuroblas-

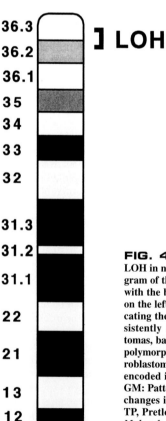

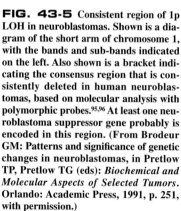

FIG. 43-5 Consistent region of 1p LOH in neuroblastomas. Shown is a diagram of the short arm of chromosome 1, with the bands and sub-bands indicated on the left. Also shown is a bracket indicating the consensus region that is consistently deleted in human neuroblastomas, based on molecular analysis with polymorphic probes.[95,96] At least one neuroblastoma suppressor gene probably is encoded in this region. (From Brodeur GM: Patterns and significance of genetic changes in neuroblastomas, in Pretlow TP, Pretlow TG (eds): *Biochemical and Molecular Aspects of Selected Tumors.* Orlando: Academic Press, 1991, p. 251, with permission.)

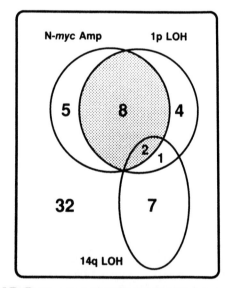

FIG. 43-6 Venn diagram of the relationship between different types of genetic change in neuroblastomas. Fifteen patients had *MYCN* amplification, 15 patients had 1p LOH, and ten of these patients had both genetic abnormalities (shaded area). Ten patients had 14q LOH, which generally occurred independent of the other two genetic changes (seven of 10 cases). From Fong CT, White PS, Peterson K, Sapienza C, Cavenee WK, Kern S, Vogelstein B, Cantor AB, Look AT, Brodeur GM: Loss of heterozygosity for chromosome 1 or 14 defines subsets of advanced neuroblastomas. *Cancer Res* **52**:1780, 1992, with permission.)

toma.[103] Neuroblastoma will stain with monoclonal antibodies recognizing neurofilaments, synaptophysin, and neuron-specific enolase.[104,105] Electron microscopy typically demonstrates dense core, membrane-bound neurosecretory granules as well as neurofilaments and parallel arrays of microtubules within the neuropil.[106] Several pathologic classification systems of neuroblastoma have been proposed that have some value in predicting the behavior of the tumor. Some utilize features of neuronal differentiation, whereas others consider the amount of Schwannian stroma, mitotic figures, karyorrhexis, or tumor calcification.[102,107–111] However, at the current time the "Shimada classification" and its variants appear to be the most popular.[102,111]

Neuronal Differentiation

Neuroblastoma cells are derived from sympathetic neuroblasts, and they frequently exhibit features of neuronal differentiation. Indeed, neuroblastomas may show spontaneous or induced differentiation to ganglioneuroblastoma or ganglioneuroma, so the malignant transformation of these cells may result in part from a failure to respond fully to the normal signals to undergo this maturation process. The factors responsible for regulating normal differentiation are not understood well at present, but they probably involve one or several neurotrophin receptor pathways that signal the cell to differentiate, such as nerve growth factor and its receptor.

Chromogranin A and neuropeptide Y are two markers of neuronal differentiation. Chromogranin A is an acidic protein that was identified first from the chromaffin cells of the adrenal medulla, and it is a component of neurosecretory granules of neuroendocrine cells, tissues, and tumors.[112,113] It is released from storage vesicles along with catecholamines, and its expression is regulated developmentally.[113,114] It is present in the serum of patients with neuroblastoma, so it may serve as a sensitive and specific serum marker for disease activity and response to treatment.[115] Neuropeptide Y is another neurosecretory protein whose expression is regulated developmentally and is restricted to the nervous system.[116,117] These and other developmentally regulated, neural-specific proteins may be useful in characterizing neuroblastomas in terms of their state of differentiation.[114,118]

Expression of the Neurotrophin Receptors: *TRK-A*, *TRK-B*, and *TRK-C*

Neuroblastoma is derived from the sympathoadrenal lineage of the neural crest. Neurotrophic factors and their receptors have been implicated in the pathogenesis of neuroblastoma, but their role has been obscure. Recently, three tyrosine kinase receptors for a homologous family of neurotrophin factors have been cloned. The main ligand for the TRK-A, TRK-B and TRK-C receptors is nerve growth factor (NGF), brain-derived neurotrophic factor (BDNF), and neurotrophin-3 (NT-3), respectively, and neurotrophin-4/5 (NT-4) appears to function through TRK-B.[119–128] Another transmembrane receptor binds all the neurotrophins with low affinity (LNTR), but its role in mediating responses to the presence or absence of these homologous ligands is controversial.[119,129–132]

To evaluate the clinical significance of *TRK-A* expression in neuroblastomas, we studied the relationship between patient survival and their mRNA expression in frozen tissue samples. We studied tumors from 77 children with neuroblastomas and five children with ganglioneuromas that had been diagnosed in Japan and the United States from 1982 to 1991.[133] *TRK-A* expression was detected in 70 of the 77 neuroblastomas (91%), and a high level of expression ($\geq$100 density units) was observed in 63 (82%). All 46 tumors in stages I, II, and IVS (according to the Evans staging system) that had no *MYCN* amplification showed a high level of *TRK-A* expression. However, 10 of 11 tumors with *MYCN* amplification had an extremely low level of *TRK-A* expression. One tumor that had *MYCN* amplification but showed a high level of *TRK-A* expression was obtained from an infant patient in stage IVS, and the tumor was regressing at the time of surgery. The expression of *TRK-A* correlated strongly with survival: The 5-year cumulative-survival rate of the group with a high level of *TRK-A* expression was 86 percent, whereas that of the group with a low level of *TRK-A* expression was 14 percent ($p < 0.001$).

The combination of *TRK-A* expression and *MYCN* amplification had a strong influence on overall survival. The group with high levels of *TRK-A* expression and no *MYCN* amplification showed a cumulative 5-year survival of 87 percent ($n = 62$). Four patients whose tumors had a normal *MYCN* copy number had a low level of expression of *TRK-A*, and their survival was significantly worse than that of the group with a high level of *TRK-A* expression ($p = 0.03$). Ten of the 11 patients with *MYCN* amplification had low or undetectable levels of *TRK-A* expression, and all eleven died within 2 years. Similar results have been obtained independently by others, providing further support for the strong correlation between high *TRK-A* expression and a favorable outcome.[134–137]

The NGF/*TRK-A* pathway may be playing an important role in the biological behavior of some neuroblastomas, namely, their propensity to regress or differentiate in selected patients. The association of *TRK* expression with tumors that have a favorable outcome suggests that it may play some role in the behavior of the tumors. Indeed, the expression of *TRK-A* is required for biological responsiveness to NGF. In the presence of ligand, neuronal differentiation is induced and survival is promoted.[138] However, neurotrophic factor deprivation may lead to programmed cell death (apoptosis) at this stage.[139,140] Thus, the in vivo differentiation or regression that is seen either spontaneously or in response to treatment may be mediated by the NGF/TRK-A pathway.[133]

Recently we have examined the expression and function of *TRK-B* and *TRK-C* in neuroblastomas. Both of these neurotrophin receptors can be expressed in a truncated form (lacking the tyrosine kinase) and a full-length form. Interestingly, expression of full-length *TRK-B* was strongly associated with *MYCN*-amplified tumors.[141] Since these tumors also express the TRK-B ligand (BDNF), this may represent an autocrine or paracrine loop providing some survival or growth advantage.[142–144] Maturing tumors were more likely to express the truncated *TRK-B*, whereas the most immature, nonamplified tumors expressed neither.[141] In contrast, the expression of *TRK-C* was found predominantly in lower stage tumors, and, like *TRK-A*, was not expressed in *MYCN* amplified tumors.[145] This suggests that favorable tumors are characterized by the expression of *TRK-A*, with or without *TRK-C*, but unfavorable tumors express full-length TRK-B plus its ligand BDNF.

CLINICAL MANIFESTATIONS AND PATTERN OF SPREAD

Primary Tumors

About half of all neuroblastomas originate in the adrenal medulla; 30 percent occur in nonadrenal abdominal sites in the paravertebral ganglia, pelvic ganglia, or the organ of Zuckerkandl; and 20 percent occur in the paravertebral ganglia of the thorax.[3,8] Most primary tumors cause symptoms of abdominal mass or pain. However, because of the midline location of many tumors, they may invade the spinal canal through neural foramina and cause compression of the spinal cord. In the thoracic or upper lumbar region this usually leads to paraplegia, where lower lumbar invasion leads to a cauda equina syndrome with loss of bowel or bladder function. Midline tumors can displace or compress other structures, such as the trachea or esophagus, and lead to obstructive symptoms. Finally, involvement of the superior cervical ganglion can produce Horner syndrome, which consists of unilateral ptosis, myosis, and anhydrosis.

Metastatic Disease

Most neuroblastomas are metastatic at the same time of diagnosis. Frequent sites of metastasis are: regional or distant lymph nodes, cortical bone, bone marrow, liver, and skin. In infants (≤1 year old), a characteristic pattern of small primary tumors with dissemination limited to liver and skin (with or without minimal marrow involvement) is associated with a favorable outcome. This special pattern is referred to as stage IVS or 4S.[146–149] However, in older patients (>1 year old), the dissemination most frequently involves bone marrow and bone, particularly the bones of the skull and orbits. Rarely, disease may spread to lung and brain parenchyma, usually as a manifestation of relapsing or end-stage disease. The outlook for these older patients is very poor, even with intensive multimodality therapy. However, there has been recent progress in elucidating the genetic and biochemical basis of these very different patterns of behavior.

Paraneoplastic Syndromes

Several paraneoplastic syndromes have been associated with neuroblastoma, although each is seen in only 1 to 5 percent of patients. Intractable secretory diarrhea and abdominal distention, sometimes associated with hypokalemia and dehydration (Kerner-Morrison syndrome), is a manifestation of tumor secretion of vasoactive intestinal peptide (VIP).[150,151] VIP is a 28 amino acid polypeptide hormone that is related in structure to glucagon, secretin, and several other polypeptide hormones.[152] It is encoded by the third exon of a large, 6-exon gene that also encodes a closely related polypeptide hormone PHM-27 in exon 4.[153] However, these two proteins are expressed differentially in some cells.[154] The biological functions of VIP are relaxation of smooth muscle, stimulation of intestinal water and electrolyte secretion, and the stimulation of release of other polypeptide hormones.[152] The VIP syndrome usually is associated with ganglioneuroblastoma or ganglioneuroma, and these symptoms usually resolve after eradication of the tumor.[150,151]

Opsomyoclonus, sometimes called myoclonic encephalopathy, is a syndrome that consists of myoclonic jerking and random eye movement, sometimes associated with cerebellar ataxia. This syndrome has been observed in up to 4 percent of patients.[155,156] Other neuromuscular disorders have been seen in association with neuroblastoma as well, but they are less common.[157] These symptoms may diminish or even disappear with eradication of the tumor, and these usually have a favorable outcome from the oncologic perspective.[156] However, it is becoming increasingly apparent that many patients have residual neurologic abnormalities.[158,159] The symptoms may vary in severity, especially worsening in association with intercurrent illnesses. Recent evidence suggests that the

opsoclonus syndrome may be caused by antineuronal autoantibodies.[160–162]

The third paraneoplastic syndrome is due to increased secretion of catecholamines, but this appears to occur in less than 1 percent of patients. The syndrome consists of episodes of tachycardia, palpitations, profuse sweating, and flushing, which are produced by secretion of norepinephrine.[163] Indeed, symptoms attributed to excess catecholamine secretion reportedly were seen in a mother who had a fetus with a neuroblastoma.[164] This syndrome is more common in patients with pheochromocytomas, because these tumors secrete epinephrine, which is a more potent inducer of these symptoms than norepinephrine.

METHODS OF DIAGNOSIS

Diagnostic Criteria

To confirm a diagnosis of neuroblastoma, usually some histologic evidence is required that demonstrates neural origin or differentiation by light microscopy, electron microscopy, or immunohistology. Alternatively, since the bone marrow is involved frequently, some patients are considered to have neuroblastoma based on the presence of "compatible" tumor cells involving the bone marrow, accompanied by increased urinary catecholamine metabolites. Differences in diagnostic criteria used by different groups or countries have led to some difficulties in comparing studies. However, proposals have been made to develop international criteria to confirm a diagnosis of neuroblastoma.[148,149]

Catecholamine Metabolism

When sensitive techniques are used, usually 90 to 95 percent of tumors produce sufficient catecholamines to result in increased urinary metabolites. This provides a great diagnostic advantage in confirming the diagnosis of neuroblastoma, as well as in following disease activity in those patients whose tumors are secreters.[165–168] A diagrammatic representation of catecholamine synthesis and metabolism is depicted in Figure 43-7. Although the major pathways and products of catecholamine catabolism are shown, the actual pathways of intracellular and extracellular catecholamine breakdown are more complex.

The precursor amino acids for catecholamine synthesis are phenylalanine and tyrosine. Phenylalanine is converted by phenylalanine hydroxylase to tyrosine (Figure 43-7). Tyrosine is then converted by tyrosine hydroxylase to 3,4-dihydroxyphenylalanine (DOPA), which is a catecholamine precursor. DOPA is converted by DOPA decarboxylase to the first catecholamine in the pathway, dopamine. Dopamine is converted by dopamine-β-hydroxylase to norepinephrine, which is then converted by phenylethanolamine-N-methyltransferase to epinephrine. Neuroblastoma cells lack this last enzyme, which is present in adrenal chromaffin cells and pheochromocytomas. The two enzymes primarily responsible for the catabolism of catecholamines are catechol-O-methyl transferase and monamine oxidase. DOPA and dopamine are converted primarily to homovanillic acid (HVA), whereas norepinephrine and epinephrine are converted primarily to vanillylmandelic acid (VMA). Most laboratories involved in neuroblastoma diagnosis measure both urinary VMA and HVA.

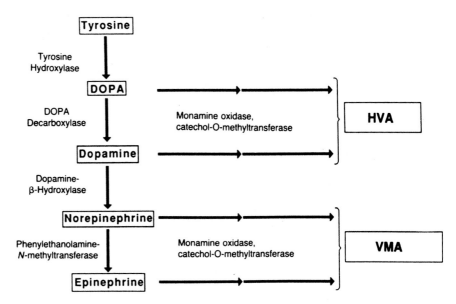

FIG. 43-7 Pathway of catecholamine metabolism. Shown is a simplified diagram of catecholamine synthesis and metabolism. HVA and VMA are the urinary catecholamine metabolites usually measured. (From Brodeur GM: Neuroblastoma and other peripheral neuroectodermal tumors, in Fernbach DJ, Vietti TJ (eds): *Clinical Pediatric Oncology*. St. Louis, Mosby Year Book, 1991, p. 337, with permission.)

Differential Diagnosis

Because of the many potential clinical presentations, neuroblastoma may be confused with a variety of other neoplasms as well as non-neoplastic conditions. This is a problem particularly in the 5 to 10 percent of tumors that to do not produce catecholamines as well as the 1 percent or so who do not have an obvious primary tumor.[169–172] Patients with the VIP syndrome can be confused with infectious or inflammatory bowel disease, and those with the opsoclonus-myoclonus and ataxia syndromes can resemble primary neurologic disease.[150,151,156,157,173,174] Histologically, neuroblastoma tissue from primary or metastatic sites may be quite undifferentiated, and may be confused with other embryonal pediatric cancers, such as rhabdomyosarcoma, Ewing sarcoma, neuroepithelioma, lymphoma, or leukemia (especially megakaryoblastic leukemia). Fortunately, a battery of monoclonal antibodies are being developed that should allow these various disease entities to be made with greater objectivity and confidence.[106,175–178]

CLINICAL EVALUATION AND STAGING

Diagnostic Testing

A standard set of recommended tests to define the clinical stage or extent of disease has been established.[148,149] Certainly, the more tests that are done, the greater the likelihood of finding disseminated disease. This applies particularly to the number of bone marrow aspirates and biopsies that are done, and the manner in which marrow disease is detected.[179–181] For this purpose, a standard set of immunologic reagents to detect occult neuroblastoma are being developed.[149] This immunocytological approach may obviate the need for multiple aspirates and biopsies in the future. Uniformity with respect to minimum testing should improve the comparability of studies, but the tests recommended should be available in most medical centers.

The conventional diagnostic imaging modalities include plain radiographs, bone scintigraphy, ultrasound, computerized tomography (CT scan), and magnetic resonance imaging (MRI scan).[182–189] In addition, the potential specificity and sensitivity of meta-iodobenzylguanidine (MIBG) scintigraphy for evaluation of

bone and soft tissue involvement by neuroblastoma is attractive.[190,191] This compound is taken up by catecholaminergic cells, which includes most neuroblastomas. Radiolabeled MIBG scintigraphy thus becomes potentially a very specific and sensitive method of assessment of the primary tumor and focal metastatic disease. Unfortunately, MIBG scintigraphy is not readily available throughout the industrialized countries of the world at the current time.

Staging

The distribution of patients by stage or extent of disease differs depending on the age at diagnosis. For instance, in a consecutive series of 1001 patients enrolled on POG protocols from 1981 to 1989 and staged by the POG staging system, only about 40 percent of patients less than 1 year of age had unresectable or metastatic disease, whereas almost 80 percent of older patients had advanced stages of disease.[3,8,192] These findings explain in part the generally better outcome of infants with neuroblastoma compared to their older counterparts, but biological differences of the tumors in the two age groups appear to be very important also.

Until recently there were several different staging systems used for neuroblastoma throughout the world.[146,192–196] In general, the various staging systems give comparable results in distinguishing low-stage, good-prognosis patients from high-stage, poor-prognosis patients. However, some of the differences between the staging systems are substantial, particularly as applied to patients with intermediate stages. Therefore, a group of individuals met in 1986 and again in 1991 to formulate an International Neuroblastoma Staging System that would lead to uniformity in staging of patients with neuroblastoma for clinical trials and biological studies around the world.

International Neuroblastoma Staging System

The International Neuroblastoma Staging System (INSS) is based on clinical, radiographic, and surgical evaluation of children with neuroblastoma.[148] This staging system (Table 43-3) utilizes the most important components of previous systems. In order to distinguish the INSS from previous systems, Arabic numbers are used rather than Roman numerals or letters of the alphabet. Recently, modifications have been proposed in this system to clarify defini-

Table 43-3 International Neuroblastoma Staging System

Stage 1	Localized tumor with complete gross excision, with or without microscopic residual disease; representative ipsilateral lymph nodes negative for tumor microscopically. (Nodes attached to and removed with the primary tumor may be positive.)
Stage 2A	Localized tumor with incomplete gross excision; representative ipsilateral nonadherent lymph nodes negative for tumor microscopically.
Stage 2B	Localized tumor with or without complete gross excision, with ipsilateral nonadherent lymph nodes positive for tumor. Enlarged contralateral lymph nodes must be negative microscopically.
Stage 3	Unresectable unilateral tumor infiltrating across the midline,* with or without regional lymph node involvement; *or* localized unilateral tumor with contralateral regional lymph node involvement; *or* midline tumor with bilateral extension by infiltration (unresectable) or by lymph node involvement.
Stage 4	Any primary tumor with dissemination to distant lymph nodes, bone, bone marrow, liver, skin, and/or other organs (except as defined for Stage 4S).
Stage 4S	Localized primary tumor (as defined for Stage 1, 2A or 2B), with dissemination limited to skin, liver, and/or bone marrow† (limited to infants <1 year of age).

Multifocal primary tumors (e.g., bilateral adrenal primary tumors) should be staged according to the greatest extent of disease, as defined above, and followed by a subscript "M" (e.g., 3_M).

*The midline is defined as the vertebral column. Tumors originating on one side and "crossing the midline" must infiltrate to or beyond the opposite side of the vertebral column.

†Marrow involvement in Stage 4S should be minimal, that is, less than 10 percent of total nucleated cells identified as malignant on bone marrow biopsy or on marrow aspirate. More extensive marrow involvement would be considered to be Stage 4. The MIBG scan (if done) should be negative in the marrow.

SOURCE: Brodeur GM, Seeger RC, Barrett A, Berthold F, Castleberry RP, D'Angio G, De Bernardi B, Evans AE, Favrot M, Freeman AI, Haase G, Hartmann O, Hayes FA, Helson L, Kemshead J, Lampert F, Ninane J, Ohkawa H, Philip T, Pinkerton CR, Pritchard J, Sawada T, Siegel S, Smith EI, Tsuchida Y, Voute PA: International criteria for diagnosis, staging and response to treatment in patients with neuroblastoma. *J Clin Oncol* **6**:1874, 1988.

tions of stages, as well as criteria for diagnosis and response to treatment.[148,149] In addition, suggestions were made to develop biologic risk groups that incorporate clinical and laboratory variables in determining prognosis.[149]

PROGNOSTIC CONSIDERATIONS: CLINICAL VARIABLES

The most important clinical variables are the stage of disease, the age of the patient at diagnosis, and the site of the primary tumor.[73,108,197–206] The overall prognosis of patients with stage 1, 2, and 4S is between 75 and 90 percent, whereas those with stages 3 and 4 have a 2-year disease-free survival range of 10 to 30 percent. The outcome of infants less than 1 year of age is substantially better than older patients with the same stage of disease, particularly those with more advanced stages of disease. Patients with primary tumors in the adrenal gland appear to do worse than patients with tumors originating at other sites, particularly the thorax, but this does not appear to add substantially to the prognosis once the variables of age and stage are considered.

PROGNOSTIC CONSIDERATIONS: BIOLOGICAL VARIABLES

A variety of biological variables (pathology, serum markers, genetic features) have been studied that appear to have predictive value as independent prognostic markers in patients with neuroblastoma. The serum markers include ferritin, neuron-specific enolase (NSE), a cell membrane ganglioside (G_{D2}), and lactate dehydrogenase (LDH). The genetic features of the tumor that have been proposed as prognostic markers include tumor cell DNA index, *MYCN* oncogene copy number, and deletion or LOH involving 1p.

Additional markers have been proposed, such as expression of the H-*ras* oncogene, the multidrug resistance gene, or the multidrug resistance related protein, but the value of these markers is still unclear.[87,88,207–212] Moreover, no study to date has examined all variables in a large set of patients, so it is somewhat difficult to say which single variable or combination of variables are the most powerful predictors of outcome, in addition to the more conventional clinical features of patient age and stage.

Tumor Pathology

Differentiated histology, such as ganglioneuroblastoma, generally is associated with localized tumors, but this type of histologic classification does not have prognostic value that adds substantially to age and stage.[107–110] More detailed analysis of histology, such as the classifications by Shimada or Joshi, take into consideration the amount of Schwannian stroma, mitotic figures, karyorrhexis, and calcification.[102,111] These classifications appear to be more powerful predictors of outcome. Soon there will be an international neuroblastoma pathology classification (INPC) that will supersede the mentioned systems and become the international standard for histopathologic classification, particularly as a prognostic variable.[149]

Serum Markers

Serum Ferritin. Analysis of serum from patients with neuroblastoma has determined that ferritin levels are increased in some patients with actively growing tumors.[213–217] Ferritin levels are rarely elevated in patients with low stages of disease, whereas up to half of patients with advanced stages have significant elevations and a much worse outcome.[213–217] In vitro evidence suggests that this ferritin may be produced by the tumor cells. Increased ferritin levels may be simply a marker of rapid tumor growth or large tumor burden. On the other hand, ferritin or iron may be particularly important for growth of neuroblastoma cells. In this regard, it is interesting that some therapeutic approaches are targeting the increased levels of ferritin and iron in patients with advanced disease.

Serum NSE. NSE is a cytoplasmic protein with enolase activity that is associated with neural cells. Analysis of serum NSE from patients with neuroblastoma has indicated that survival is substantially worse in advanced patients with high serum NSE levels.[218–221] Although marked increases in serum NSE were associated with neuroblastomas, mild to moderate elevations were seen with other pediatric tumors, also. Thus, NSE is not as specific as was once thought, but it may have prognostic value, and perhaps it may be useful to follow disease activity and response to treatment in individual patients.

Ganglioside G$_{D2}$. Several independently derived monoclonal antibodies against neuroblastoma cells recognize gangliosides, which are sialic acid-containing glycosphingolipids. The most characteristic ganglioside on human neuroblastoma cell membranes is called G$_{D2}$. Not only is the presence of this ganglioside useful for identifying neuroblastoma cells, but also increased levels have been found in the plasma of patients with neuroblastoma. Measurement of circulating G$_{D2}$ may serve as another useful marker of disease activity or response to treatment.[222–225] Indeed, gangliosides shed by tumor cells may play a role in accelerating tumor progression, and antibodies against G$_{D2}$ may be useful for therapy of neuroblastoma as well.[226,227]

LDH. Although it is not specific to neuroblastoma, serum LDH level has been proposed as a prognostic marker for neuroblastoma. Increased LDH levels may be a reflection of rapid cellular turnover or of large tumor burden. Increased levels are more common in patients with extensive or progressive disease, and levels of greater than 1,500 u/mL have been associated with a poor prognosis in infants with neuroblastoma.[228–230]

Genetic Markers

Tumor Cell DNA Index. Tumor cells with an increased DNA content (or "hyperdiploid" karyotype) have been associated with a favorable outcome in infants with neuroblastoma.[67–76,93,231–233] In addition, hyperdiploid tumors are more likely to have lower stages of disease and to respond to cyclophosphamide and doxorubicin, whereas those with a "diploid" DNA content more likely have advanced stages of disease and do not respond to this combination. However, this variable appears to be useful primarily for patients less than 1 year of age with advanced stages of disease.[71]

MYCN Amplification. The presence of *MYCN* amplification in tumor cells is found predominantly in patients with advanced stages of disease.[77] However, *MYCN* amplification is associated with rapid tumor progression and a poor prognosis, regardless of the age of the patient or the stage of the disease.[33,71,76,77,79–82,84–86,234] Although not all patients with a poor outcome have *MYCN* amplification, virtually all patients with amplification treated with conventional therapy have rapid progression and die (Figures 43-8 and 43-9).[3,8]

Allelic Loss for 1p or 14q. Finally, although these studies are still preliminary, there appears to be a strong correlation between 1p deletion and poor survival.[33,67,94,95,99] Because there is an association between *MYCN* amplification and 1p deletion, it remains controversial as to whether this finding has independent prognostic significance.[235–239] However, 14q LOH does not appear to have

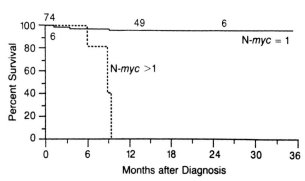

FIG. 43-8 *MYCN* amplification and survival in infants. Survival according to *MYCN* copy number in 133 infants with POG stages B, C, D, and DS neuroblastoma. (From Brodeur GM, Castleberry RP: Neuroblastoma, in Pizzo PA, Poplack DG (eds): *Principles and Practice of Pediatric Oncology.* Philadelphia, JB Lippincott, 1993, p. 739, with permission.)

prognostic significance, other than its association with advanced stages of disease in some studies.[98–101]

TRK Gene Expression. Recent studies suggest that high levels of expression of the *TRK-A* gene are associated with a favorable outcome in neuroblastoma patients.[98,133,135–137] Although prospective studies need to be done to confirm these observations, current evidence suggests that high *TRK-A* gene expression may be a very powerful prognostic marker, and it may predict the propensity of selected tumors to undergo either programmed cell death, leading to regression, or neuronal differentiation, leading to a benign ganglioneuroma. Similar results have been obtained by analysis of *TRK-C*, which is also associated with biologically favorable outcome.[145] However, the *TRK-C* expressing tumors appear to be a subset of the *TRK-A* positive tumors, so *TRK-C* expression does not have independent prognostic significance.[145] In contrast, *TRK-B* expression is associated with advanced stage tumors with *MYCN* amplification.[141] Tumors expressing TRK-B, along with its ligand BDNF, may have an autocrine pathway survival pathway that provides them with a survival advantage.[141–144]

Genetic and Clinical Subsets of Neuroblastomas

In summary, there is increasing evidence for at least three genetic subsets of neuroblastomas that are highly predictive of clinical behavior. One classification that has been proposed recently takes into account abnormalities of 1p, *MYCN* copy number, and assessment of DNA content, and three distinct genetic subsets of neuro-

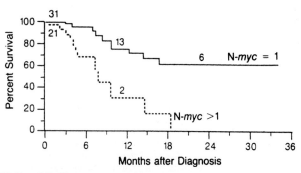

FIG. 43-9 *MYCN* amplification and survival in children with advanced neuroblastoma. Survival according to *MYCN* copy number in 106 children over 1 year of age with unresectable or metastatic neuroblastoma (POG stages C and D). (From Brodeur GM, Castleberry RP: Neuroblastoma, in Pizzo PA, Poplack DG (eds): *Principles and Practice of Pediatric Oncology.* Philadelphia, JB Lippincott, 1993, p. 739, with permission.)

blastomas can be identified (Table 43-4).[1,2,4,5] The first is characterized by a hyperdiploid or near-triploid modal karyotype, with few if any cytogenetic rearrangements. They lack specific genetic changes like *MYCN* amplification or 1p LOH, and they have high *TRK-A* expression. These patients are generally less than 1 year of age with localized disease and a very good prognosis (≥95% survival). The second has a near-diploid karyotype, with no consistent abnormality identified to date, and they lack *MYCN* amplification, although they may have 1p or 14q LOH. *TRK-A* expression generally is low or absent. They generally are older patients with more advanced stages of disease that progress slowly and are often fatal (25–50% survival). The third group has amplification of *MYCN*, usually with 1p36 LOH, and their DI is usually diploid. *TRK-A* expression is low or absent, but *TRK-B* plus *BDNF* expression may be present. These patients generally are older with advanced stages of disease, which is rapidly progressive and almost always fatal (≤5% survival). This general subclassification has been validated by two recent studies.[71,240] Thus, genetic analysis of neuroblastoma cells provides prognostic information that can direct more appropriate choice of treatment. It is unknown if a tumor from one type ever converts to a less favorable type, but current evidence suggests that they are genetically distinct.[71,83]

THERAPEUTIC APPROACHES

The treatment modalities traditionally employed in the management of neuroblastoma are surgery, chemotherapy, and radiotherapy. The role of each is determined by the natural history of individual cases considering stage, age, and biological features. With few exceptions (e.g., completely resected primary tumors and infants with stable 4S disease), chemotherapy remains the backbone of the multimodality treatment plan. In this section, stage is defined by the INSS criteria (Table 43-3).[148,149]

Surgery

Surgery plays a pivotal role in the management of neuroblastoma. Depending on the timing, operative procedures can have diagnostic as well as therapeutic functions.[241] The goals of primary surgical procedures, performed prior to any other therapy, are to establish the diagnosis, provide tissue for biological studies, stage the tumor surgically, and excise the tumor, if feasible. In delayed primary or second-look surgery, the surgeon will determine response to therapy and remove residual disease when possible.

Chemotherapy

Chemotherapy is the predominant modality of management in neuroblastoma. Single agent, phase II trials conducted in patients with recurrent or advanced neuroblastoma have identified a number of effective drugs.[3] Cyclophosphamide, cisplatin, doxorubicin (Adriamycin), and the epipodophyllotoxins (teniposide, VM-26; and etoposide, VP-16) yield complete and partial response rates of 25 to 50 percent and have become the cornerstone of multiagent regimens. Drug combinations have been developed that take advantage of drug synergism, mechanisms of cytotoxicity, and differences in side effects. The drug pairs cyclophosphamide + doxorubicin and cisplatin + teniposide, used separately and in combination, take advantage of combining non-cell cycle specific agents (cyclophosphamide, cisplatin), followed by cell cycle dependent drugs (doxorubicin, teniposide).[242,243] Treatment of children with advanced stage neuroblastoma using these combinations resulted in improved response rates with minimal increase in toxicity.[244–246] Newer generations of the discussed agents, such as ifosphamide and carboplatin, have been incorporated in the multiagent regimens, but it is not clear that they have altered the long-term survival of advanced stage patients significantly.[247]

Table 43-4 Biological/Clinical Types of Neuroblastoma

Feature	Type 1	Type 2	Type 3
MYCN	Normal	Normal	Amplified
DNA Ploidy	Hyperdiploid	Near diploid	Near diploid
	Near triploid	Near tetraploid	Near tetraploid
1p LOH	<5%	25–50%	80–90%
14q LOH	<5%	25–50%	<5%
TRK-A exp.	High	Low or absent	Low or absent
TRK-B exp.	Truncated	Low or absent	High (full length)
TRK-C exp.	High	Low or absent	Low or absent
Age	Usually <1 year	Usually >1 year	Usually 1–5 year
Stage	Usually 1,2,4S	Usually 3,4	Usually 3,4
3-year Survival	95%	25–50%	<5%

SOURCE: Brodeur GM, Azar C, Brother M, Hiemstra J, Kaufman B, Marshall H, Moley J, Nakagawara A, Saylors R, Scavarda N, Schneider S, Wasson J, White P, Seeger R, Look T, Castleberry R: Neuroblastoma: Effect of genetic factors on prognosis and treatment. *Cancer* **70**:1685, 1992.
Brodeur GM, Nakagawara A: Molecular basis of clinical heterogeneity in neuroblastoma. *Am J Pediat Hematol/Oncol* **14**:111, 1992.
Brodeur GM, Castleberry RP: Neuroblastoma, in Pizzo PA, Poplack DG (eds): *Principles and Practice of Pediatric Oncology*. Philadelphia, JB Lippincott, 1993, p. 739.
Brodeur GM: Molecular pathology of human neuroblastomas. *Sem Diag Pathol* **11**:118, 1994.
Brodeur GM: Molecular basis for heterogeneity in human neuroblastomas. *Eur J Cancer* **31A**:505, 1995.

Radiation Therapy

Neuroblastoma is considered a radiosensitive tumor, and radiation therapy is very effective in achieving local control or palliation. However, long-term control of neuroblastoma is seldom achieved with radiation therapy alone because of the propensity of this tumor to widespread metastases.[248,249] Historically, radiation has been used in the multimodality management of residual neuroblastoma, bulky unresectable tumors, and palliation. More recently, the role of radiotherapy in neuroblastoma continues to be refined with the improvement in multiagent chemotherapy and the increasing trend toward developing risk-related treatment groups based on age, stage, and biological features.

Bone Marrow Transplantation

Attempts have been made to improve on the modest gains of intensive, combined-modality therapy to increase intensity of therapy. Dose-limiting marrow toxicity can be ameliorated to some extent by the use of colony stimulating factors for the granulocyte or granulocyte-macrophage lineages, which increase the rate of marrow recovery. However, more intensive therapy can be administered if accompanied by bone marrow transplantation (BMT). Although allogeneic BMT is practiced by some centers, the most popular approach is autologous BMT, frequently with a purged marrow.[250–261] Marrow purging usually is accomplished by covalently attaching a cocktail of antineuroblastoma antibodies to magnetic beads and mixing beads with the marrow, followed by passing the marrow over powerful magnets.[251,260,261] A variation on this approach that is undergoing clinical trials currently is the use of peripheral blood stem cells (with or without CD34 positive selection) as the source of cells for marrow rescue. Although these approaches may increase the median survival of older patients with advanced stages of neuroblastoma, it is not clear that the long-term, disease-free survival has been affected appreciably.

Biologically Based Risk Groups

In future studies, the development of risk groups for neuroblastoma must take into account various biological features (histopathology, serum markers, tumor ploidy, and *MYCN* copy number) in addition to stage and age. Preliminary data, adjusted for age and stage, indicate that analysis of DNA content in infants and *MYCN* copy number in all patients, allow more precise determination of risk.[70,71,78,262] Tumor histopathology also appears to be an important independent prognostic marker, at least for certain subsets of patients. Judging the prognostic impact of these biological variables relative to other, more simply evaluated features (serum ferritin and LDH) must await prospective therapeutic and biological studies. Based on current trends, Table 43-5 details a proposed prognostic stratification model for determining therapy that is under evaluation that utilized *MYCN* copy number and DNA ploidy. It is likely that tumor histopathology as determined by the Shimada or INPC classification also will be incorporated into biologic risk assessment.[102]

Future Treatment Strategies

The use of dose intensified chemotherapy combinations, with or without autologous bone marrow transplantation, has produced better immediate disease control in neuroblastoma. Unfortunately, this has not translated into durable remissions in children with high-risk tumors. Future treatment strategies will address: 1) the identification of new drugs and drug combinations; 2) the use of biological agents targeted at killing neuroblastoma cells, such as radiolabeled MIBG or antineuroblastoma antibodies;[263–268] 3) agents that might induce differentiation, like retinoic acid or NGF;[269–272] 4) the cytotoxic and maturational effects of iron chelation[273,274] or other novel approaches.

Table 43-5 Proposed Prognostic Strata for Neuroblastoma Therapy Based on Clinical and Biological Tumor Features

	Clinical and Biologic Features			
	Patient INSS		*MYNCDNA*	
Risk Category	Age (year)	Stage	Copy	Index
Low	≤1	1,2A,2B,3,4,4S	1	>1
	≤1	1,2A	1	1
	>1	1,2A	1	NA*
Intermediate	≤1	2B,3,4,4S	1	1
	>1	2B,3	1	NA
High	≤1	2B,3,4,4S	>1	NA
	>1	4	1	NA
	>1	2B,3,4	>1	NA
Unclear	≤1	1,2A	>1 and/or	1
	>1	1,2A	>1	NA

*NA = not applicable

SOURCE: Brodeur GM, Castleberry RP: Neuroblastoma, in Pizzo PA, Poplack DG (eds): *Principles and Practice of Pediatric Oncology*. Philadelphia, JB Lippincott, 1993, p. 739.

COMPLICATIONS OF NEUROBLASTOMA AND ITS TREATMENT

A variety of complications of neuroblastoma and its treatment may occur that are not particularly unique to this tumor. These include bone marrow replacement, with symptoms of bone marrow failure such as anemia, bleeding leading to anemia or hypotension, or leukopenia leading to increased risk of infection. In addition, increased catecholamine secretion leading to hypertension, and coagulopathies leading to bleeding or thrombosis have been reported.[275-277] Hypercalcemia has been reported also, but is uncommon.[278] Neurologic complications are fairly common and can take on several forms. These are discussed in more detail, along with second malignant neoplasms in patients with neuroblastoma.

Neurological Complications

Because of its origin next to the spinal column, neuroblastomas have a tendency to invade through neural foramina into the spinal canal and cause spinal cord compression. This situation can be a medical emergency, and there is controversy as to the optimum approach to managing spinal cord compression. Many of these patients are quite young, and so extensive laminectomies or radiation to the spine can result in long-term morbidity later in life. Hayes and colleagues have reported their experience with 18 such patients who were managed primarily by chemotherapy, and their results appear to be excellent.[279,280] Thus, chemotherapy appears to be a safe and effective initial modality to manage spinal canal invasion or cord compression, and it has less long-term morbidity in infants or small children than surgery or radiation therapy. Newer approaches, such as laminotomy with replacement or very targeted, low-dose radiation, remain effective options.

In addition to cord compression, neuroblastoma can disseminate to the central nervous system. This occurs most commonly by inward compression on the brain from cranial metastases, but it can occur also as meningeal involvement.[281-283] Unfortunately, the development of meningeal dissemination is a very ominous sign.

Telander and colleagues reported the clinical outcome of 10 children with neuroblastoma and acute cerebellar encephalopathy, a characteristic but uncommon paraneoplastic syndrome associated with neuroblastoma.[158] All had localized tumors, mostly ganglioneuroblastomas, and all were surviving free of tumor at the time of the report. Although most had improvement of their neurologic deficits with ACTH or steroid therapy, as well as tumor removal, seven of the 10 had some persistent neurologic sequellae. Three recent reports provide further support to the notion that substantial neurologic abnormalities may persist after the tumor is removed.[159,162,284] Thus, a better understanding of the pathogenesis (presumably immunologic) of these neurologic problems may be necessary before they can be avoided or ameliorated.

Second Malignant Neoplasms

Other malignant diseases have been observed in individuals with neuroblastoma, such as pheochromocytoma, brain tumors, acute leukemia, and renal cell carcinoma.[285-289] However, none of these second cancers have occurred with sufficient frequency to indicate a specific relationship between neuroblastoma and any other neoplasm.[290] Furthermore, it is not clear if second malignant neoplasms are more common in survivors who had hereditary predisposition to develop neuroblastoma. Analysis of this question will require more precise methods to detect predisposed individuals, as well as improved patient survival.

NEUROBLASTOMA SCREENING STUDIES

Another proposed approach to improve the long-term outcome of patients with neuroblastoma is to identify patients with this disease earlier in the course of their disease. This assumes that patients with more advanced stages of disease and a higher risk of treatment failure "progress" from more localized disease over time. Since neuroblastomas frequently produce increased levels of catecholamines whose metabolites are detectable in the urine, mass urinary screening of infants for neuroblastoma has been proposed. Indeed, such a screening program has been underway in Japan for almost 20 years.[172,291-293] This was initially a program localized to certain prefectures, but it has been expanded to a nationwide program because of the apparent success of the effort. An effort is underway in North America, particularly the Canadian province of Quebec, to answer questions concerning the feasibility and utility of screening for neuroblastoma.[19,170,171,294]

Recent studies of the clinical and cytogenetic features of tumors identified as a result of mass screening of infants for neuroblastomas in Japan suggest that the majority of patients identified have lower stages of disease, and virtually all of the tumors are in the hyperdiploid or near-triploid range.[231,232] Previous studies have demonstrated that such findings generally are associated with a very favorable outcome.[67-75,93] Therefore, the results of the screening study have suggested at least two possibilities; either all neuroblastomas begin as tumors with a more favorable genotype and phenotype, and some evolve into more aggressive tumors with adverse genetic features, or there are at least two or three different subsets of neuroblastoma, and the more favorable group presents earlier and therefore is the predominant group detected by screening. The accumulating body of genetic information, as discussed in (Table 43-4), is more consistent with the latter explanation.[18,33,34,68,71,78,94,95,233,240,295]

In addition to the genetic data, the accumulating evidence suggests that the prevalence of neuroblastoma in screened populations is increased by 50 to 100 percent over that seen in unscreened populations, and the prevalence of neuroblastoma in patients over 1 year of age has not changed appreciably.[18,233,295] Taken together with the biologic information, this suggests that screening is detecting tumors in a substantial number of patients who likely would never develop symptomatic disease because their tumors would have regressed or matured without therapy. Many of the tumors detected by screening at 6 months of age have favorable biologic features and could be cured easily with relatively mild therapy. A few patients with unfavorable biologic features have presented clinically during the first 6 to 12 months of age in the screened population, and they have had an unfavorable outcome. It remains to be determined if screening will permit early detection of tumors with intermediate or unfavorable biological features and thereby improve their prognosis.

FUTURE CONSIDERATIONS

In addition to the improvements and prospects for future therapy discussed herein, there are a variety of areas in which improvement in the management of patients with neuroblastoma may come. These include: 1) the identification of individuals with a genetic predisposition to develop this disease; 2) general population screening approaches for early detection and treatment; 3) additional markers besides urinary catecholamine metabolites to follow tumor response to treatment; and 4) better biologic and immunologic characterization of tumors for classification and prognostication.

As improvements occur in the long-term outcome of patients with neuroblastoma, it will become increasingly important to identify individuals who are predisposed to develop this tumor. Not only will this be useful for the siblings of neuroblastoma patients, but also it will provide useful information for genetic counseling of patients and their offspring. No predisposition locus has been identified as yet, although several loci have been excluded recently, including 1p36.[32] Thus, it appears the familial neuroblastoma predisposition gene resides elsewhere, although there is the formal possibility that more than one predisposition locus exists. In any case, it may take a genome-wide search with a large battery of polymorphic markers to identify the familial neuroblastoma predisposition gene.

The urinary VMA screening programs initiated in Japan, and underway in North America and Europe, initially were very promising, leading to cautious optimism. However, there are certain epidemiological and statistical problems with many of the studies underway that will have to be addressed. Furthermore, preliminary characterization of the tumors identified by screening indicate that the majority of these tumors have favorable biologic features, more like those seen in infants with lower stages of disease. Indeed, the screening may just be increasing the prevalence of neuroblastoma by detection of tumors that might regress spontaneously. Finally, it is not clear if genetically unfavorable, aggressive tumors are detected by screening, it will ultimately improve their outcome.

Following the levels of catecholamine metabolites in the urine of patients with neuroblastoma does not appear to be as sensitive as α-fetoprotein or β-human chorionic gonadotropin for following germ cell tumors. Additional markers have been proposed, including serum ferritin, NSE, G_{D2}, chromogranin A, and others, but none have yet emerged as superior. As more is understood about the biology of neuroblastomas, additional candidates might emerge that could be used to follow response to treatment and to predict early relapse. Such markers might obviate the need for multiple-diagnostic imaging studies and marrow sampling in patients in remission.

The development of serum markers, such as ferritin, and genetic features such as DNA index, *MYCN* amplification, 1 p LOH, and *TRK-A* expression, have provided powerful prognostic variables. It remains to be determined which of these is the most powerful when subjected to multivariate analysis, and whether these or other variables will supplant more conventional clinical features such as age, stage, and primary site of tumor. It is possible that these biological features will become more important than clinical distinctions, such as lymph node involvement, crossing the midline or microscopic bone marrow involvement. The mandate for the future is to translate promising biological studies into clinical applications, and to continue to look for new insights into mechanisms of neuroblastoma transformation and progression that can be used to clinical advantage.

ACKNOWLEDGMENTS

Some of this material has been published previously.[1–5]

REFERENCES

1. Brodeur GM, Azar C, Brother M, Hiemstra J, Kaufman B, Marshall H, Moley J, Nakagawara A, Saylors R, Scavarda N, Schneider S, Wasson J, White P, Seeger R, Look T, Castleberry R: Neuroblastoma: Effect of genetic factors on prognosis and treatment. *Cancer* **70**:1685, 1992.
2. Brodeur GM, Nakagawara A: Molecular basis of clinical heterogeneity in neuroblastoma. *Am J Pediat Hematol/Oncol* **14**:111, 1992.
3. Brodeur GM, Castleberry RP: Neuroblastoma, in Pizzo PA, Poplack DG (eds): *Principles and Practice of Pediatric Oncology*. Philadelphia, JB Lippincott, 1993, p. 739.
4. Brodeur GM: Molecular pathology of human neuroblastomas. *Sem Diag Pathol* **11**:118, 1994.
5. Brodeur GM: Molecular basis for heterogeneity in human neuroblastomas. *Eur J Cancer* **31A**:505, 1995.
6. Young JLJ, Ries LB, Silverberg E, Horm JW, Miller RW: Cancer incidence, survival and mortality for children younger than 15 years. *Cancer* **58**:598, 1986.
7. Voute PA: Neuroblastoma, in Sutow WW, Fernbach DJ, Vietti TJ (eds): *Clinical Pediatric Oncology*. St. Louis, CV Mosby, 1984, p. 559.
8. Brodeur GM: Neuroblastoma and other peripheral neuroectodermal tumors, in Fernbach DJ, Vietti TJ (eds): *Clinical Pediatric Oncology*. St. Louis, Mosby Year Book, 1991, p. 337.
9. Beckwith J, Perrin E: In situ neuroblastomas: A contribution to the natural history of neural crest tumors. *Am J Pathol* **43**:1089, 1963.
10. Turkel SB, Itabashi HH: The natural history of neuroblastic cells in the fetal adrenal gland. *Am J Pathol* **76**:225, 1975.
11. Ikeda Y, Lister J, Bouton JM, Buyukpamukcu M: Congenital neuroblastoma, neuroblastoma in situ, and the normal fetal development of the adrenal. *J Pediat Surg* **16**:636, 1981.
12. Schwartz AD, Dadash-Zadeh M, Lee H, Swaney JJ: Spontaneous regression of disseminated neuroblastoma. *J Pediatr* **85**:760, 1974.
13. Altman AC, Gross S: Progression from stage IVS to stage IV neuroblastoma with eventual spontaneous resolution. *Am J Pediatr Hematol Oncol* **3**:441, 1981.
14. Haas D, Ablin AR, Miller C, Zoger S, Matthay KK: Complete pathologic maturation and regression of the stage IVS neuroblastoma without treatment. *Cancer* **62**:818, 1988.
15. Evans AE, Baum E, Chard R: Do infants with stage IV-S neuroblastoma need treatment? *Arch Dis Child* **56**:271, 1981.
16. McWilliams NB: Stage IV-S neuroblastoma: treatment controversy revisited. *Med Pediat Oncol* **14**:41, 1986.
17. Carlsen NLT: How frequent is spontaneous remission of neuroblastomas? Implications for screening. *Br J Cancer* **61**:441, 1990.
18. Bessho F, Hashizume K, Nakajo T, Kamoshita S: Mass screening in Japan increased the detection of infants with neuroblastoma without a decrease in older children. *J Pediatr* **119**:237, 1991.
19. Woods WG, Tuchman M, Bernstein ML, Leclerc J-M, Brisson L, Look T, Brodeur GM, Shimada H, Hann HL, Robison LL, Shuster JJ, Lemieux B: Screening for neuroblastoma in North America. 2-year results from the Quebec project. *Am J Pediat Hematol/Oncol* **14**:312, 1992.
20. Allen RW, Ogden B, Bentley FL, Jung AL: Fetal hydantoin syndrome, neuroblastoma, and hemorrhagic disease in a neonate. *JAMA* **244**:1464, 1980.
21. Kinney H, Faix R, Brazy J: The fetal alcohol syndrome and neuroblastoma. *Pediatrics* **66**:130, 1980.
22. Seeler RA, Israel JN, Royal JE, Kaye CI, Rao S, Abulaban M: Ganglioneuroblastoma and fetal hydantoin-alcohol syndromes. *Pediatrics* **63**:524, 1979.
23. Spitz MR, Johnson CC: Neuroblastoma and paternal occupation. A case-control analysis. *Am J Epidemiol* **121**:924, 1985.
24. Wilkins JRI, Hundley VD: Paternal occupational expsoure to electromagnetic fields and neuroblastoma in offspring. *Am J Epidemiol* **131**:995, 1990.
25. Bunin GR, Ward E, Kramer S, Rhee CA, Meadows AT: Neuroblastoma and parental occupation. *Am J Epidemiol* **131**:776, 1990.
26. Kramer S, Ward E, Meadows AT, Malone KE: Medical and drug risk factors associated with neuroblastoma: A case-control study. *J Nat Cancer Insti* **78**:797, 1987.
27. Knudson AGJ, Strong LC: Mutation and cancer: Neuroblastoma and pheochromocytoma. *Am J Hum Genet* **24**:514, 1972.
28. Knudson AG: Mutation and cancer: Statistical study of retinoblastoma. *Proc Nat Acad Sci USA* **68**:8820, 1971.
29. Knudson AGJ, Meadows AT: Developmental genetics of neuroblastoma. *J Nat Cancer Inst* **57**:675, 1976.
30. Kushner BH, Gilbert F, Helson L: Familial neuroblastoma: Case reports, literature review, and etiologic considerations. *Cancer* **57**:1887, 1986.
31. Kushner BH, Helson L: Monozygotic siblings discordant for neuroblastoma: Etiologic implications. *J Pediatr* **107**:405, 1985.

32. Maris JM, Kyemba SM, Rebbeck TR, White PS, Sulman EP, Jensen SJ, Allen C, Biegel JA, Yanofsky RA, Feldman GL, Brodeur GM: Familial predisposition to neuroblastoma does not map to chromosome band 1p36. *Cancer Res* **56**:3421, 1996.

33. Brodeur GM, Fong CT: Molecular biology and genetics of human neuroblastoma. *Cancer Genet Cytogenet* **41**:153, 1989.

34. Brodeur GM: Molecular biology and genetics of human neuroblastoma, in Pochedly C (eds): *Neuroblastoma: Tumor Biology and Therapy.* Boca Raton, FL: CRC Press, 1990, p. 31.

35. Pegelow CH, Ebbin AJ, Powars D, Towner JW: Familial neuroblastoma. *J Pediatr* **87**:763, 1975.

36. Hecht F, Kaiser-McCaw B: Chromosomes in familial neuroblastoma [letter]. *J Pediatr* **98**:334, 1981.

37. Hecht F, Hecht BK, Northrup JC, Trachtenberg N, Wood ST, Cohen JT: Genetics of familial neuroblastoma: Long-range studies. *Cancer Genet Cytogenet* **7**:227, 1982.

38. Moorhead PS, Evans AE: Chromosomal findings in patients with neuroblastoma. *Prog Cancer Res Ther* **12**:109, 1980.

39. Nagano H, Kano Y, Kobuchi S, Kajitani T: A case of partial 2p trisomy with neuroblastoma. *Jpn J Hum Genet* **25**:39, 1980.

40. Sanger WG, Howe J, Fordyce R, Purtilo DT: Inherited partial trisomy #15 complicated by neuroblastoma. *Cancer Genet Cytogenet* **11**:153, 1984.

41. Robinson MG, McCorquodale MM: Trisomy 18 and neurogenic neoplasia. *J Pediatr* **99**:428, 1981.

42. Rudolph B, Harbott J, Lampert F: Fragile sites and neuroblastoma: Fragile site at 1p13.1 and other points on lymphocyte chromosomes from patients and family members. *Cancer Genet Cytogenet* **31**:83, 1988.

43. Lampert F, Rudolph B, Christiansen H, Franke F: Identical chromosome 1p breakpoint abnormality in both the tumor and the constitutional karyotype of a patient with neuroblastoma. *Cancer Genet Cytogenet* **34**:235, 1988.

44. Laureys G, Speleman F, Opdenakker G, Leroy J: Constitutional translocation t(1;17)(p36;q12-21) in a patient with neuroblastoma. *Genes Chrom Cancer* **2**:252, 1990.

45. Michalski AJ, Cotter FE, Cowell JK: Isolation of chromosome-specific DNA sequences from an Alu polymerase chain reaction library to define the breakpoint in a patient with a constitutional translocation t(1;13)(q22;q12) and ganglioneuroblastoma. *Oncogene* **7**:1595, 1992.

46. Bown NP, Pearson ADJ, Reid MM: High incidence of constitutional balanced translocations in neuroblastoma. *Cancer Genet Cytogenet* **69**:166, 1993.

47. Biegel JA, White PS, Marshall HN, Fujimori M, Zackai EH, Scher CD, Brodeur GM, Emanuel BS: Constitutional 1p36 deletion in a child with neuroblastoma. *Am J Hum Genet* **52**:176, 1993.

48. Mead RS, Cowell JK: Molecular characterization of a (1;10)(p22;q21) constitutional translocation from a patient with neuroblastoma. *Cancer Genet Cytogenet* **81**:151, 1995.

49. Knudson AGJ, Amromin GD: Neuroblastoma and ganglioneuroma in a child with multiple neurofibromatosis. Implications for the mutational origin of neuroblastoma. *Cancer* **19**:1032, 1966.

50. Bolande R, Towler WF: A possible relationship of neuroblastoma to von Recklinghausen's disease. *Cancer* **26**:162, 1970.

51. Bolande RP: The neurocristopathies: A unifying concept of disease arising in neural crest maldevelopment. *Hum Pathol* **5**:409, 1974.

52. Witzleben CL, Landy RA: Disseminated neuroblastoma in a child with von Recklinghausen's disease. *Cancer* **34**:786, 1974.

53. Kushner BH, Hajdu SI, Helson L: Synchronous neuroblastoma and von Recklinghausen's disease: A review of the literature. *J Clin Oncol* **3**:117, 1985.

54. Miller RW, Fraumeni JFJ: Neuroblastoma: Epidemiologic approach to its origin. *Am J Dis Child* **115**:253, 1968.

55. Sy WM, Edmonson JH: The developmental defects associated with neuroblastoma—Etiologic implications. *Cancer* **22**:234, 1968.

56. Nakissa N, Constine LS, Rubin P, Strohl R: Birth defects in three common pediatric malignancies: Wilms' tumor, neuroblastoma and Ewing's sarcoma. *Oncology* **42**:358, 1985.

57. Evans AE, D'Angio GJ, Knudson AGJ, Seeger RC: *Advances in Neuroblastoma Research*, 2nd ed. New York: Alan R. Liss, 1988.

58. Evans AE, D'Angio GJ, Knudson AGJ, Seeger RC: *Advances in Neuroblastoma Research*, 3rd ed. New York: Wiley-Liss, 1991.

59. Evans AE, Brodeur GM, D'Angio GJ, Nakagawara A: *Advances in Neuroblastoma Research*, 4th ed. New York, Wiley-Liss, 1994.

60. Schwab M, Tonini GP, Benard J: *Human Neuroblastoma. Recent Advances in Clinical and Genetic Analysis.* Chur. Switzerland, Harwood Academic Publishers, 1993.

61. Balaban-Malenbaum G, Gilbert F: Relationship between homogeneously staining regions and double minute chromosomes in human neuroblastoma cell lines. *Progr Cancer Res Ther* **12**:97, 1980.

62. Biedler JL, Ross RA, Shanske S, Spengler BA: Human neuroblastoma cytogenetics: Search for significance of homogeneously staining regions and double minute chromosomes. *Prog Cancer Res Ther* **12**:81, 1980.

63. Brodeur GM, Sekhon GS, Goldstein MN: Chromosomal aberrations in human neuroblastomas. *Cancer* **40**:2256, 1977.

64. Brodeur GM, Green AA, Hayes FA, Williams KJ, Williams DL, Tsiatis AA: Cytogenetic features of human neuroblastomas and cell lines. *Cancer Res* **41**:4678, 1981.

65. Gilbert F, Feder M, Balaban G, Brangman D, Lurie DK, Podolsky R, Rinaldt V, Vinikoor N, Weisband J: Human neuroblastomas and abnormalities of chromosome 1 and 17. *Cancer Res* **44**:5444, 1984.

66. Brodeur GM, Seeger RC: Gene amplification in human neuroblastomas: Basic mechanisms and clinical implications. *Cancer Genet Cytogenet* **101**, 1986.

67. Christiansen H, Lampert F: Tumour karyotype discriminates between good and bad prognostic outcome in neuroblastoma. *Br J Cancer* **57**:121, 1988.

68. Hayashi Y, Hanada R, Yamamoto K, Bessho F: Chromosome findings and prognosis in neuroblastoma. *Cancer Genet Cytogenet* **29**:175, 1986.

69. Kaneko Y, Kanda N, Maseki N, Sakurai M, Tsuchida Y, Takeda T, Okabe I, Sakurai M: Different karyotypic patterns in early and advanced stage neuroblastomas. *Cancer Res* **47**:311, 1987.

70. Look AT, Hayes FA, Nitschke R, McWilliams NB, Green AA: Cellular DNA content as a predictor of response to chemotherapy in infants with unresectable neuroblastoma. *N Eng J Med* **311**:231, 1984.

71. Look AT, Hayes FA, Shuster JJ, Douglass EC, Castleberry RP, Brodeur GM: Clinical relevance of tumor cell ploidy and N-myc gene amplification in childhood neuroblastoma. A Pediatric Oncology Group Study. *J Clin Oncol* **9**:581, 1991.

72. Gansler T, Chatten J, Varello M, Bunin GR, Atkinson B: Flow cytometric DNA analysis of neuroblastoma. Correlation with histology and clinical outcome. *Cancer* **58**:2453, 1986.

73. Oppedal BR, Storm-Mathisen I, Lie SO, Brandtzaeg P: Prognostic factors in neuroblastoma. Clinical, histopathologic immunohistochemical features and DNA ploidy in relation to prognosis. *Cancer* **72**:772, 1988.

74. Taylor SR, Blatt J, Constantino JP, Roederer M, Murphy RF: Flow cytometric DNA analysis of neuroblastoma and ganglioneuroma. A 10-year retrospective study. *Cancer* **62**:749, 1988.

75. Taylor SR, Locker J: A comparative analysis of nuclear DNA content and N-myc gene amplification in neuroblastoma. *Cancer* **65**:1360, 1990.

76. Cohn SL, Rademaker AW, Salwen HR, Franklin WA, Gonzales-Crussi F, Rosen ST, Bauer KD: Analysis of DNA ploidy and proliferative activity in relation to histology and N-myc amplification in neuroblastoma. *Am J Pathol* **136**:1043, 1990.

77. Brodeur GM, Seeger RC, Schwab M, Varmus HE, Bishop JM: Amplification of N-myc in untreated human neuroblastomas correlates with advanced disease stage. *Science* **224**:1121, 1984.

78. Brodeur GM: Neuroblastoma: Clinical applications of molecular parameters. *Brain Pathol* **1**:47, 1990.

79. Seeger RC, Brodeur GM, Sather H, Dalton A, Siegel SE, Wong KY, Hammond D: Association of multiple copies of the N-myc oncogene with rapid progression of neuroblastomas. *N Engl Med* **313**:1111, 1985.

80. Seeger RC, Wada R, Brodeur GM, Moss TJ, Bjork RL, Sousa L, Slamon DJ: Expression of N-myc by neuroblastomas with one or multiple copies of the oncogene. *Prog Clin Biol Res* **271**:41, 1988.

81. Brodeur GM, Seeger RC, Sather H, Dalton A, Siegel SE, Wong KY, Hammond D: Clinical implications of oncogene activation in human neuroblastomas. *Cancer* **58**:541, 1986.

82. Brodeur GM, Fong CT, Morita M, Griffith RC, Hayes FA, Seeger RC: Molecular analysis and clinical significance of N-myc amplification and chromosome 1 abnormalities in human neuroblastomas. *Prog Clin Biol Res* **271**:3, 1988.

83. Brodeur GM, Hayes FA, Green AA, Casper JT, Wasson J, Wallach S, Seeger RC: Consistent N-myc copy number in simultaneous or consecutive neuroblastoma samples from sixty individual patients. *Cancer Res* **47**:4248, 1987.

84. Bartram CR, Berthold F: Amplification and expression of the N-myc gene in neuroblastoma. *Eur J Pediatr* **146**:162, 1987.

85. Nisen PD, Waber PG, Rich MA, Pierce S, Garvin JRJ, Gilbert F, Lanzkowsky P: N-myc oncogene RNA expression in neuroblastoma. *J Nat Cancer Inst* **80**:1633, 1988.

86. Slavc I, Ellenbogen R, Jung W-H, Vawter GF, Kretschmar C, Grier H, Korf BR: myc gene amplification and expression in primary human neuroblastoma. *Cancer Res* **50**:1459, 1990.

87. Tanaka T, Slamon DJ, Shimoda H, Waki K, Kawaguchi Y, Tanaka Y, Ida N: Expression of Ha-ras oncogene products in human neuroblastomas and the significant correlation with a patient's prognosis. *Cancer Res* **48**:1030, 1988.

88. Tanaka T, Slamon DJ, Shimada H, Shimoda H, Fujisawa T, Ida N, Seeger RC: A significant association of Ha-ras p21 in neuroblastoma cells with patient prognosis. *Cancer* **68**:1296, 1991.

89. Ballas K, Lyons J, Jannsen JWG, Bartram CR: Incidence of ras gene mutations in neuroblastoma. *Eur J Pediatr* **147**:313, 1988.

90. Ireland CM: Activated N-ras oncogenes in human neuroblastoma. *Cancer Res* **49**:5530, 1989.

91. Moley JF, Brother MB, Wells SA, Spengler BA, Biedler JL, Brodeur GM: Low frequency of *ras* gene mutations in neuroblastomas, pheochromocytomas and medullay thryroid cancers. *Cancer Res* **51**:1596, 1991.

92. Thiele CJ, McKeon C, Triche TJ, Ross RA, Reynolds CP, Israel MA: Differential protoocogene expression characterizes histopathologically indistinguishable tumors of the peripheral nervous system. *J Clin Invest* **80**:804, 1987.

93. Franke F, Rudolph B, Christiansen H, Harbott J, Lampert F: Tumour karyotype may be important in the prognosis of human neuroblastoma. *J Cancer Res Clin Oncol* **111**:266, 1986.

94. Hayashi Y, Kanda N, Inaba T, Hanada R, Nagahara N, Muchi H, Yamamoto K: Cytogenetic findings and prognosis in neuroblastoma with emphasis on marker chromosome 1. *Cancer* **63**:126, 1989.

95. Fong CT, Dracopoli NC, White PS, Merrill PT, Griffith RC, Housman DE, Brodeur GM: Loss of heterozygosity for the short arm of chromosome 1 in human neuroblastomas: Correlation with N-myc amplification. *Proc Nat Acad Sci USA* **86**:3753, 1989.

96. Weith A, Martinsson T, Cziepluch C, Bruderlein S, Amler LC, Berthold F: Neuroblastoma consensus deletion maps to 1p36.1-2. *Genes, Chromosomes and Cancer* **1**:159, 1989.

97. Brodeur GM: Patterns and significance of genetic changes in neuroblastomas, in Pretlow TP, Pretlow TG (eds): *Biochemical and Molecular Aspects of Selected Tumors.* Orlando: Academic Press, 1991, p. 251.

98. Suzuki T, Yokota J, Mugishima H, Okabe I, Ookuni M, Sugimura T, Terada M: Frequent loss of heterozygosity on chromosome 14q in neuroblastoma. *Cancer Res* **49**:1095, 1989.

99. Fong CT, White PS, Peterson K, Sapienza C, Cavenee WK, Kern S, Vogelstein B, Cantor AB, Look AT, Brodeur GM: Loss of heterozygosity for chromosome 1 or 14 defines subsets of advanced neuroblastomas. *Cancer Res* **52**:1780, 1992.

100. Takayama H, Suzuki T, Mugishima H, Fujisawa T, Ookuni M,Schwab M, Gehring M, Nakamura Y, Sugimura T, Terada M, Yokota J: Deletion mapping of chromsomes 14q and 1p in human neuroblastoma. *Oncogene* **7**:1185, 1992.

101. Srivatsan ES, Ying KL, Seeger RC: Deletion of chromosome 11 and 14q sequences in neuroblastoma. *Genes, Chrom Cancer* **7**:32, 1993.

102. Shimada H, Chatten J, Newton WA, Jr., Sachs N, Hamoudi AB, Chiba T, Marsden HB, Misugi K: Histopathologic prognostic factors in neuroblastic tumors: Definition of subtypes of ganglioneuroblastoma and an age-linked classification of neuroblastomas. *J Nat Cancer Inst* **73**:405, 1984.

103. Shimada H: Transmission and scanning electron microscopic studies on the tumors of neuroblastoma group. *Acta Pathol Jpn* **32**:415, 1982.

104. Dehner LP: Pathologic anatomy of classic neuroblastoma: Including prognostic features and differential diagnosis, in Pochedly C (eds): *Neuroblastoma: Tumor Biology and Therapy.* Boca Raton, FL: CRC Press, 1990, p. 111.

105. Delellis RA: The adrenal glands, in Sternbert SS (eds): *Diagnostic Surgical Pathology.* New York, Raven, 1989, p. 445.

106. Triche TJ, Askin FB, Kissane JM: Neuroblastoma, Ewing's sarcoma, and the differential diagnosis of small-, round-, blue-cell tumors, in Finegold M (eds): *Pathology of Neoplasia in Children and Adolescents.* Philadelphia: WB Saunders, 1986, p. 145.

107. Hughes M, Marsden HB, Palmer MK: Histologic patterns of neuroblastoma related to prognosis and clinical staging. *Cancer* **34**:1706, 1974.

108. Hassenbusch S, Kaizer H, White JJ: Prognostic factors in neuroblastic tumors. *J Pediatr Surg* **11**:287, 1976.

109. Thomas PRM, Lee JY, Fineberg BB, Razek AA, Perez CA, Land VJ, Vietti TJ: An analysis of neuroblastoma at a single institution. *Cancer* **53**:2079, 1984.

110. Standstedt B, Jereb B, Eklund G: Prognostic factors in neuroblastomas [Abstract]. *Acta Pathol Microbiol Immunol Scand* **91**:365, 1983.

111. Joshi V, Cantor A, Altshuler G, Larkin E, Neill J, Shuster J, Holbrook T, Hayes A, Castleberry R: Prognostic significance of histopathologic features of neuroblastoma: A grading system based on the review of 211 cases from the Pediatric Oncology Group [Abstract]. *Proc Am Soc Clin Oncol* **10**:311, 1991.

112. O'Connor DT, Deftos LJ: Secretion of chromogranin A by peptide-producing endocrine neoplasms. *N Eng J Med* **314**:1145, 1986.

113. Helman LJ, Gazdar AF, Park J-G, Cohen PS, Cotelingam JD, Israel MA: Chromogranin A expression in normal and malignant human tissues. *J Clin Invest* **82**:686, 1988.

114. Cooper MJ, Hutchins GM, Cohen PS, Helman LJ, Mennie RJ, Israel MA: Human neuroblastoma tumor cell lines correspond to the arrested differentiation of chromaffin adrenal medullary neuroblasts. *Cell Growth Diff* **1**:149, 1990.

115. Hsiao RJ, Seeger RC, Yu AL, O'Connor DT: Chromogranin A in children with neuroblastoma. *J Clin Invest* **85**:1555, 1990.

116. O'Hare MMT, Schwartz TW: Expression and precursor processing of neuropeptide Y in human pheochromocytoma and neuroblastoma tumors. *Cancer Res* **49**:7010, 1989.

117. Cohen PS, Cooper MJ, Helman LJ, Thiele CJ, Seeger RC, Israel MA: Neuropeptide Y expression in the developing adrenal gland and in childhood neuroblastoma tumors. *Cancer Res* **50**:6055, 1990.

118. Tsokos M, Scarpa S, Ross RA, Triche TJ: Differentiation of human neuroblastoma recapitulates neural crest development. *Am J Pathol* **128**:484, 1987.

119. Hempstead BL, Martin-Zanca D, Kaplan DR, Parada LF, Chao MV: High-affinity NGF binding requires coexpression of the trk proto-oncogene and the low-affinity NGF receptor. *Nature* **350**:678, 1991.

120. Kaplan DR, Hempstead BL, Martin-Zanca D, Chao MV, Parada LF: The trk proto-oncogene product: A signal transducing receptor for nerve growth factor. *Science* **252**:554, 1991.

121. Kaplan DR, Martin-Zanca D, Parada LF: Tyrosine phosphorylation and tyrosine kinase activity of the trk proto-oncogene product induced by NGF. *Nature* **350**:158, 1991.

122. Klein R, Jing S, Nanduri V, O'Rourke E, Barbacid M: The trk proto-oncogene encodes a receptor for nerve growth factor. *Cell* **65**:189, 1991.

123. Klein R, Nanduri V, Jing S, Lamballe F, Tapley P, Bryant S, Cordon-Cardo C, Jones KR, Reichardt LF, Barbacid M: The trkB tyrosine protein kinase is a receptor for brain-derived neurotrophic factor and neurotrophin-3. *Cell* **66**:395, 1991.

124. Lamballe F, Klein R, Barbacid M: trkC, a new member of the trk family of tyrosine protein kinases, is a receptor for neurotrophin-3. *Cell* **66**:967, 1991.

125. Squinto SP, Stitt TN, Aldrich TH, Davis S, Bianco SM, Radziejewski C, Glass DJ, Masiakowski P, Furth ME, Valenzuela DM, DiStefano PS, Yancopoulos GC: trkB encodes a functional receptor for brain-derived neurotrophic factor and neurotrophin-3 but not nerve growth factor. *Cell* **65**:885, 1991.

126. Ip NY, Ibanex CF, Nye SH, McClain J, Jones PF, Gies DR, Belluscio L, Le Beau MM, Espinosa III R, Squinto SP, Persson H, Yancopoulos GD: Mammalian neurotrophin-4: Structure, chromosomal localization, tissue distribution, and receptor specificity. *Proc Nat Acad Sci USA* **89**:3060, 1992.

127. Berkemeier LR, Winslow JW, Kaplan DR, Nikolics K, Goeddel DV, Rosenthal A: Neurotrophin-5: A novel neurotrophic factor that activates trk and trkB. *Neuron* **7**:857, 1991.

128. Soppet D, Escandon E, Maragos J, Middlemas DS, Reid SW, Blair J, Burton LE, Stanton BR, Kaplan DR, Hunter T, Nikolics K, Parada LF: The neurotrophic factors brain-derived neurotrophic factor and neurotrophin-3 are ligands for the trkB tyrosine kinase receptor. *Cell* **65**:895, 1991.

129. Green SH, Greene LA: A single Mr ≈ 103,000 ^{125}I-β-nerve growth factor-affinity-labeled species represents both the low and high affinity forms of the nerve growth factor receptor. *J Biol Chem* **261**:15316, 1986.

130. Chao MV, Bothwell MA, Ross AH, Koprowski H, Lanahan AA, Buch CR, Sehgal A: Gene transfer and molecular cloning of the human NGF receptor. *Science* **232**:518, 1986.

131. Radeke MJ, Misko TP, Hsu C, Herzenberg LA, Shooter EM: Gene transfer and molecular cloning of the rat nerve growth factor receptor. *Nature* **325**:593, 1987.

132. Hempstead BL, Patil N, Olson K. Chao MV: Molecular analysis of the nerve growth factor receptor. *Cold Spring Harbor Symp Quant* **53**:477, 1988.

133. Nakagawara A, Arima-Nakagawara M, Scavarda NJ, Azar CG, Cantor AB, Brodeur GM: Association between high levels of expression of the TRK gene and favorable outcome in human neuroblastoma. *N Engl J Med* **328**:847, 1993.

134. Suzuki T, Bogenmann E, Shimada H, Stram D, Seeger RC: Lack of high-affinity nerve growth factor receptors in aggressive neuroblastomas. *J Nat Cancer Inst* **85**:377, 1993.

135. Kogner P, Barbany G, Dominici C, Castello MA, Raschella G, Persson H: Coexpression of messenger RNA for TRK protooncogene and low affinity nerve growth factor receptor in neuroblastoma with favorable prognosis. *Cancer Res* **53**:2044, 1993.

136. Borrello MG, Bongarzone I, Pierotti MA, Luksch R, Gasparini M, Collini P, Pilotti S, Rizzetti MG, Mondellini P, DeBernardi B, DiMartino D, Garaventa A, Brisgotti M, Tonini GP: TRK and RET protooncogene expression in human neuroblastoma specimens: high-frequency of trk expression in non-advanced stages. *Int J Cancer* **54**:540, 1993.

137. Tanaka T, Hiyama E, Sugimoto T, Sawada T, Tanabe M, Ida N: trkA gene expression in neuroblastoma. *Cancer* **76**:1086, 1995.

138. Levi-Montalcini R: The nerve growth factor 35 years later. *Science* **237**:1154, 1987.

139. Martin DP, Schmidt RE, DiStefano PS, Lowry OH, Carter JG, Johnson EMJ: Inhibitors of protein synthesis and RNA synthesis prevent neuronal death caused by nerve growth factor deprivation. *J Cell Biol* **106**:829, 1988.

140. Koike T, Tanaka S: Evidence that nerve growth factor dependence of sympathetic neurons for survival in vitro may be determined by levels of cytoplasmic free Ca^{2+}. *Proc Nat Acad Sci USA* **88**:3892, 1991.

141. Nakagawara A, Azar CG, Scavarda NJ, Brodeur GM: Expression and function of TRK-B and BDNF in human neuroblastomas. *Mol Cell Biol* **14**:759, 1994.

142. Kaplan DR, Matsumoto K, Lucarelli E, Thiele CJ: Induction of TrkB by retinoic acid mediates biologic responsiveness to BDNF and differentiation of human neuroblastoma cells. *Neuron* **11**:321, 1993.

143. Acheson A, Conover JC, Fandi JP, DeChiara TM, Russell M, Thadani A, Squinto SP, Yancopoulos GD, Lindsay RM: A BDNF autocrine loop in adult sensory neurons prevents cell death. *Nature* **374**:450, 1995.

144. Matsumoto K, Wada RK, Yamashiro JM, Kaplan DR, Thiele CJ: Expression of brain-derived neurotrophic factor and p145TrkB affects survival, differentiation, and invasiveness of human neuroblastoma cells. *Cancer Res* **55**:1798, 1995.

145. Yamashiro DJ, Nakagawara A, Ikegaki N, Liu X-G, Brodeur GM: Expression of TrkC in favorable human neuroblastomas. *Oncogene* **12**:37, 1996.

146. Evans AE, D'Angio GJ, Randolph JA: A proposed staging for children with neuroblastoma. Children's Cancer Study Group A. *Cancer* **27**:374, 1971.

147. D'Angio GJ, Evans AE, Koop CE: Special pattern of widespread neuroblastoma with a favorable prognosis. *Lancet* **1**:1046, 1971.

148. Brodeur GM, Seeger RC, Voute PA, et al: International criteria for diagnosis, staging and response to treatment in patients with neuroblastoma. *J Clin Oncol* **6**:1874, 1988.

149. Brodeur GM, Pritchard J, Berthold F, Carlsen NLT, Castel V, Castleberry RP, De Bernardi B, Evans AE, Favrot M, Hedborg F, Kaneko M, Kemshead J, Lampert F, Lee REJ, Look AT, Pearson ADJ, Philip T, Roald B, Sawada T, Seeger RC, Tsuchida Y, Voute PA: Revisions of the international criteria for neuroblastoma diagnosis, staging and response to treatment. *J Clin Oncol* **11**:1466, 1993.

150. Kaplan S, Holbrook C, McDaniel H, Buntain W, Crist W: Vasoactive intestinal peptide secreting tumors of childhood. *Am J Dis Child* **134**:21, 1980.

151. El Shafie M, Samuel D, Lippel CH, Robinson MG, Cullen BJ: Intractable diarrhea in children with VIP-secreting ganglioneuroblastomas. *J Pediatr Surg* **18**:34, 1983.

152. Said SI: Vasoactive intestinal peptide (VIP): Current status. *Peptides* **5**:143, 1984.

153. Bodmer M, Fridkin M, Gozes I: Coding sequences for vasoactive intestinal peptide and PHM-27 peptide are located on two adjacent exons in the human genome. *Proc Nat Acad Sci USA* **82**:3548, 1985.

154. Beinfeld MC, Brick PL, Howlett AC, Holt IL, Pruss RM, Moskal JR, Eiden LE: The regulation of vasoactive intestinal peptide synthesis in neuroblastoma and chromaffin cells. *Ann NY Acad Sci* **527**:68, 1988.

155. Roberts KB, Freeman JM: Cerebellar ataxis and "occult neuroblastoma" without opsoclonus. *Pediatrics* **56**:464, 1975.

156. Altman AJ, Baehner RL: Favorable prognosis for suvival in children with coincident opsomyoclonus and neuroblastoma. *Cancer* **37**:846, 1976.

157. Robinson MJ, Howard RN: Neuroblastoma, presenting as myasthenia gravis in a child aged 3 years. *Pediatrics* **43**:111, 1969.

158. Telander RL, Smithson WA, Groover RV: Clinical outcome in children with acute cerebellar encephalopathy and neuroblastoma. *J Pediatr Surg* **24**:11, 1989.

159. Koh PS, Raffensperger JG, Berry S, Larsen MB, Johnstone HS, Chou P, Luck SR, Hammer M, Cohn SL: Long-term outcome in children with opsoclonus-myoclonus and ataxia and coincident neuroblastoma. *J Pediatr* **125**:712, 1994.

160. Noetzel MJ, Cawley LP, James VL, Minard BJ, Agrawal HC: Antineurofilament protein antibodies in opsoclonus-myoclonus. *J Neuroimmunol* **15**:137, 1987.

161. Budde-Steffen C, Anderson NE, Rosenblum MK, Graus F, Ford D, Synek BJ, Wray SH, Posner JB: An antineuronal autoantibody in paraneoplastic opsoclonus. *Ann Neurol* **23**:528, 1988.

162. Pranzatelli MR: The neurobiology of the opsoclonus-myoclonus syndrome. *Clin Neuropharmacol* **3**:186, 1992.

163. Kedar A, Glassman M, Voorhess ML, Fisher J, Allen J, Jenis E, Freeman AI: Severe hypertension in a child with ganglioneuroblastoma. *Cancer* **47**:2077, 1981.

164. Mason GA, Hart-Mercer J, Miller EJ, Strang LB, Wynne NA: Adrenaline-secreting neuroblastoma in an infant. *Lancet* **2**:322, 1957.

165. Graham-Pole J, Salmi T, Anton AH, Abramowsky C, Gross S: Tumor and urine catecholamines (CATS) in neurogenic tumors. Correlations with other prognostic factors and survival. *Cancer* **51**:834, 1983.

166. Itoh T, Ohmori K: Biosynthesis and storage of catecholamines in pheochromocytoma and neuroblastoma cells. *J Lab Clin Med* **81**:887, 1973.

167. LaBrosse EH, Com-Nougue C, Zucker JM, Comoy E, Bohuon C, Lemerle J, Schweisguth O: Urinary excretion of 3-methoxy-4-hydroxymandelic acid and 3-methoxy-4-hydroxyphenylacetic acid by 288 patients with neuroblastoma and related neural crest tumors. *Cancer Res* **40**:1995, 1980.

168. Laug WE, Siegel SE, Shaw KNF, Landing B, Baptista J, Gutenstein M: Initial urinary catecholamine metabolite concentrations and prognosis in neuroblastoma. *Pediatrics* **62**:77, 1978.

169. Prasad KN, Mandal B, Kumar S: Demonstration of cholinergic cells in human neuroblastoma and ganglioneuroma. *J Pediatr* **82**:677, 1973.

170. Tuchman M, Fisher EJ, Heisel MA, Woods WG: Feasibility study for neonatal neuroblastoma screening in the United States. *Med Pediatr Oncol* **17**:258, 1989.

171. Tuchman M, Lemieux B, Auray-Blais C, Robinson LL, Giguere R, McCann MT, Woods WG: Screening for neuroblastoma at 3 weeks of age: Methods and preliminary results from the Quebec neuroblastoma screening project. *Pediatrics* **86**:765, 1990.

172. Sawada T, Hirayama M, Nakata T, Takeda T, Takasugi N, Mori T, Maeda K, Koide R, Hanawa Y, Tsunoda A, Shimizu K, Nagahara N, Yamamoto K: Mass screening for neuroblastoma in infants in Japan. *Lancet* **2**:271, 1984.

173. Kinast M, Levin HS, Rothner AD, Erenberg G, Wacksman J, Judge J: Cerebellar ataxia, opsoclonus, and occult neural crest tumor. Abdominal computerized tomography in diagnosis. *Am J Dis Child* **134**:1057, 1980.

174. Nickerson BG, Hutter JJ: Opsoclonus and neuroblastoma. Response to ACTH. *Clin Pediatr* **18**:446. 1979.

175. Kemshead JT, Goldman A, Fritschy J, Malpas JS, Pritchard J: Use of panels of monoclonal antibodies in the differential diagnosis of neuroblastoma and lymphoblastic disorders. *Lancet* **1**:12, 1983.

176. Sugimoto T, Sawada T, Arakawa S, Matsumura T, Dakamoto I. Takeuchi Y, Reynolds CP, Kemshead JT, Helson L: Possible differential diagnosis of neuroblastoma from rhabdomyosarcoma and Ewing's sarcoma by using a panel of monoclonal antibodies. *Jpn J Cancer Res* **76**:301, 1985.

177. Donner K, Triche TJ, Israel MA, Seeger RC, Reynolds CP: A panel of monoclonal antibodies which discriminate neuroblastoma from Ewing's sarcoma, rhabdomyosarcoma, neuroepithelioma, and hematopoietic malignancies. *Prog Clin Biol* **175**:367, 1985.

178. Moss TJ, Seeger RC, Kindler-Rohrborn A, Marangos PJ, Rajewsky MF, Reynolds CP: Immunohistologic detection and phenotyping of neuroblastoma cells in bone marrow using cytoplasmic neuron spe-

cific enolase and cell surface antigens. *Prog Clin Biol Res* **175**:367, 1985.

179. Bostrom B, Nesbit ME, Brunning RD: The value of bone marrow trephine biopsy in the diagnosis of metastatic neuroblastoma. *Am J Pediatr Hematol Oncol* **7**:303, 1985.

180. Franklin IM, Pritchard J: Detection of bone marrow invasion by neuroblastoma is improved by sampling at two sites with both aspirates and trephine biopsies. *J Clin Pathol* **36**:1215, 1983.

181. Moss TJ, Reynolds CP, Sather HN, Romansky SG, Hammond GD, Seeger RC: Prognostic value of immunocytologic detection of bone marrow metastases in neuroblastoma. *N Engl J Med* **324**:219, 1991.

182. Daubenton JD, Fisher RM, Karabus CD, Mann MD: The relationship between prognosis and scintigraphic evidence of bone metastases in neuroblastoma. *Cancer* **59**:1586, 1987.

183. Heisel MA, Miller JH, Reid BS, Siegel SE: Radionuclide bone scan in neuroblastoma. *Pediatrics* **71**:206, 1983.

184. Podrasky AE, Stark DD, Hattner RS, Gooding CA, Moss AA: Radionuclide bone screening in neuroblastoma: Skeletal metastases and primary tumor localization of 99mTc-MDP. *Am J Roentgenol* **141**:469, 1983.

185. White SJ, Stuck KJ, Blane CE, Silver TM: Sonography of neuroblastoma. *Am J Roentgenol* **141**:465, 1983.

186. Couanet D, Hartmann O, Pickarski JD, Vanel D. Masselot J: The use of computed tomography in the staging of neuroblastomas in childhood. *Arch Francaises Pediatrie* **38**:315, 1981.

187. Golding SJ, McElwain TJ, Husband JE: The role of computed tomography in the management of children with advanced neuroblastoma. *Br J Radiol* **57**:661, 1984.

188. Fletcher BD, Kopiwoda SY, Strandjord SE, Nelson AD, Pickering SP: Abdominal neuroblastoma: magnetic resonance imaging and tissue characterization. *Radiology* **155**:699, 1985.

189. Smith FW, Cherryman GR, Redpath TW, Crosher G: The nuclear magnetic resonance appearances of neuroblastoma. *Pediatr Radiol* **15**:329, 1985.

190. Geatti O, Shapiro B, Sisson JC, Hutchinson RJ, Mallette S, Eyre P, Beierwaltes WH: Iodine-131 metaiodobenzylguanidine (131-I-MIBG) scintigraphy for the location of neuroblastoma: Preliminary experience in ten cases. *J Nucl Med* **26**:736, 1985.

191. Voute PA, Hoefnagel CA, Marcuse HR, de Kraker J: Detection of neuroblastoma with 131I-meta-iodobenzylguanidine. *Prog Clin Biol Res* **175**:389, 1985.

192. Nitschke R, Smith EI, Shochat S, Altshuler G, Travers H, Shuster JJ, Hayes FA, Patterson R, McWilliams N: Localized neuroblastoma treated by surgery—A Pediatric Oncology Group Study. *J Clin Oncol* **6**:1271, 1988.

193. Hayes FA, Green AA, Hustu HO, Kumar M: Surgicopathologic staging of neuroblastoma: Prognostic significance of regional lymph node metastases. *J Pediatr* **102**:59, 1983.

194. De Bernardi B, Rogers D, Carli M, Madon E, de Laurentis T, Bagnulo S, di Tullio MT, Paolucci G, Pastore G: Localized neuroblastoma. Surgical and pathological staging. *Cancer* **60**:1066, 1987.

195. Sawaguchi S, Suganuma Y, Watanabe I, et al: Studies of the biological and clinical characteristics of neuroblastoma. III. Evaluation of the survival rate in relation to 17 factors. *Nippon Shoni Geka Gakkai Zasshi* **16**:51, 1980.

196. Nakagawara A, Morita K, Okabe I, Uchino J, Ohi R, Iwafuchi M, Matsuyama S, Nagashima K, Takahashi H, Nakajo T, Hirai Y, Tshchida Y, Saeki M, Yokoyama J, Nishi T, Okamoto E, Suita S: Proposal and assessment of Japanese Tumor Node Metastasis postsurgical histopathological staging system for neuroblastoma based on an analysis of 495 cases. *Jpn J Clin Oncol* **21**:1, 1990.

197. Altman AJ, Schwartz AD: Tumors of the sympathetic nervous system, in *Malignant Disease of Infancy, Childhood and Adolescence.* Philadelphia: WB Saunders, 1983, p. 368.

198. Carlsen NLT, Christensen IJ, Schroeder H, Bro PV, Erichsen G, Hambort-Pedersen B, Jensen KB, Nielsen OH: Prognostic factors in neuroblastomas treated in Denmark from 1943 to 1980. A statistical estimate of prognosis based on 253 cases. *Cancer* **58**:2726, 1986.

199. Coldman AJ, Fryer CJH, Elwood M, Sonley MJ: Neuroblastoma: Influence of age at diagnosis, stage, tumor size, and sex on prognosis. *Cancer* **46**:1896, 1980.

200. Evans AE, D'Angio GJ, Propert K. Anderson J, Hann H-WL: Prognostic factors in neuroblastoma. *Cancer* **59**:1853, 1987.

201. Filler RM, Traggis DG, Jaffe N, Vawter GF: Favorable outlook for children with mediastinal neuroblastoma. *J Pediatr Surg* **7**:136, 1972.

202. Grosfeld JL, Schartzlein M, Ballantine TVN, Weetman RM, Baehner RL: Metastatic neuroblastoma: Factors influencing survival. *J Pediatr Surg* **13**:59, 1978.

203. Grosfeld JL: Neuroblastoma in infancy and childhood, in Hays DM (ed): *Pediatric Surgical Oncology.* New York: Grune & Stratton, 1986, p. 63.

204. Jaffe N: Neuroblastoma: Review of the literature and an examination of factors contributing to its enigmatic character. *Cancer Treat Rev* **3**:61, 1976.

205. Jereb B, Bretsky SS, Vogel R, Helson L: Age and prognosis in neuroblastoma. Review of 112 patients younger than 2 years. *Am J Pediatr Hematol/Oncol* **6**:233, 1984.

206. Kinnier-Wilson LM, Draper GJ: Neuroblastoma, its natural history and prognosis: A study of 487 cases. *Br Med J* **3**:301, 1974.

207. Bourhis J, Benard J, Hartmann O, Boccon-Gibod L, Lemerle J, Riou G: Correlation of MDR1 gene expression with chemotherapy in neuroblastoma. *J Natl Cancer Inst* **81**:1401, 1989.

208. Goldstein LJ, Fojo AT, Ueda K, Crist W, Green A, Brodeur G, Pastan I, Gottesman MM: Expression of the multidrug resistance, *MDR1,* gene in neuroblastomas. *J Clin Oncol* **8**:128, 1990.

209. Nakagawara A, Kadomatsu K, Sato S-I, Kohno K, Takano H, Akazawa K, Nose Y, Kuwano M: Inverse correlation between expression of multidrug resistance gene and N-myc oncogene in human neuroblastomas. *Cancer Res* **50**:3043, 1990.

210. Corrias MV, Cornaglia-Ferraris P, Di Martino D, Stenger AM, Lanino E, Boni L, Tonini GP: Expression of multidrug resistance gene, MDR1, and N-myc oncogene in an Italian population of human neuroblastoma patients. *Anticancer Res* **10**:897, 1990.

211. Chan HSL, Haddad G, Thorner PS, DeBoer G, Lin YP, Ondrusek N, Yeger H, Ling V: P-glycoprotein expression as a predictor of the outcome of therapy for neuroblastoma. *N Engl J Med* **325**:1608, 1991.

212. Norris MD, Bordow SB, Marshall GM, Haber PS, Haber M: Association between high levels of expression of the multidrug resistance-associated protein (*MRP*) gene and poor outcome in primary human neuroblastoma. *N Engl J Med* **334**:231, 1996.

213. Hann HWL, Evans AE, Cohen IJ, Leitmeyer JE: Biologic differences between neuroblastoma stage IVS and IV. Measurement of serum ferritin and E-rosette inhibition in 30 children. *N Engl J Med* **305**:1981.

214. Hann HWL, Evans AE, Siegel SE, Wong KY, Sather H, Dalton A, Hammond D, Seeger RC: Prognostic importance of serum ferritin in patients with stages III and IV neuroblastoma. The Children's Cancer Study Group Experience. *Cancer Res* **45**:2843, 1985.

215. Hann HWL, Stahlhut MW, Evans AE: Serum ferritin as a prognostic indicator in neuroblastoma: Biological effects of isoferritins. *Prog Clin Biol Res* **175**:331, 1985.

216. Hann HWL, Stahlhut MW, Evans AE: Basic and acidic isoferritins in the sera of patients with neuroblastoma. *Cancer* **62**:1179, 1988.

217. Silber JH, Evans AE, Fridman M: Models to predict outcome from childhood neuroblastoma: the role of serum ferritin and tumor histology. *Cancer Res* **51**:1426, 1991.

218. Marangos P: Clinical studies with neuron specific enolase. *Prog Clin Biol Res* **175**:285, 1985.

219. Tsuchida Y, Honna T, Iwanaka T, Saeki M, Taguchi N, Kaneko T, Koide R, Tsunematsu Y, Shimizu KI, Makino SI, Hashizume K, Nakajo T: Serial determination of serum neuron-specific enolase in patients with neuroblastoma and other pediatric tumors. *J Pediatr Surg* **22**:419, 1987.

220. Zeltzer PM, Parma AM, Dalton A, Siegel SE, Marangos PJ, Sather H, Hammond D, Seeger RC: Raised neuron-specific enolase in serum of children with metastatic neuroblastoma. *Lancet* **2**:361, 1983.

221. Zeltzer PM, Marangos PJ, Evans AE, Schneider SL: Serum neuron-specific enolase in children with neuroblastoma. Relationship to stage and disease course. *Cancer* **57**:1230, 1986.

222. Ladisch S, Wu Z-L: Circulating gangliosides as tumor markers. *Prog Clin Biol Res* **175**:277, 1985.

223. Ladisch S, Wu ZL: Detection of a tumour-associated ganglioside in plasma of patients with neuroblastoma. *Lancet* **1**:136, 1985.

224. Schengrund CL, Repman MA, Shochat SJ: Ganglioside composition of human neuroblastomas—correlation with prognosis. A Pediatric Oncology Group Study. *Cancer* **56**:2640, 1985.

225. Schulz G, Cheresh DA, Varki NM, Yu A, Staffileno LK, Reisfeld RA: Detection of ganglioside GD2 in tumor tissues and sera of neuroblatoma patients. *Cancer Res* **44**:5914, 1984.

226. Ladisch S, Kitada S, Hays EF: Gangliosides shed by tumor cells enhance tumor formation in mice. *J Clin Invest* **79**:1879, 1987.

227. Valentino L, Moss T, Olson E, Wang H-J, Elshoff R, Ladisch S: Shed tumor gangliosides and progression of human neuroblastoma. *Blood* **75**:1564, 1990.

228. McWilliams NB, Hayes FA, Shuster JJ, Smith EI, Green A, Castleberry R: Prognostic indicators in babies less than 1 with stage D neuroblastoma [Abstract]. *Pediat Res* **23**:344A, 1988.

229. Quinn JJ, Altman AJ, Frantz CN: Serum lactic dehydrogenase, an indicator of tumor activity in neuroblastoma. *J Pediatr* **97**:89, 1980.

230. Woods WG: The use and significance of biologic markers in the evaluation and staging of a child with cancer. *Cancer* **58**:442, 1986.

231. Hayashi Y, Habu Y, Fujii Y, Hanada R, Yamamoto K: Chromsome abnormalities in neuroblastomas found by VMA mass screening. *Cancer Gen Cytogenet* **22**:363, 1986.

232. Hayashi Y, Inabada T, Hanada R, Yamamoto K: Chromsome findings and prognosis in 15 patients with neuroblastoma found by VMA mass screening. *J Pediatr* **112**:67, 1988.

233. Kaneko Y, Kanda N, Maseki N, Nakachi K, Okabe I, Sakuri M: Current urinary mass screening or catecholamine metabolites at 6 months of age may be detecting only a small portion of high-risk neuroblastomas: A chromosome and N-myc amplification study. *J Clin Oncol* **8**:2005, 1990.

234. Grady-Leopardi EF, Schwab M, Ablin AR, Rosenau W: Detection of N-myc oncogene expression in human neuroblastoma by in situ hybridization and blot analysis: Relationship to clinical outcome. *Cancer Res* **46**:3196, 1986.

235. Caron H: Allelic loss of chromosome 1 and additional chromosome 17 material are both unfavourable prognostic markers in neuroblastoma. *Med Pediatr Oncol* **24**:215, 1995.

236. Caron H, van Sluis P, de Kraker J, Bokkerink J, Egeler M, Laureys G, Slater R, Westerveld A, Voute PA, Versteeg R: Allelic loss of chromsome 1p as a predictor of unfavorable outcome in patients with neuroblastoma. *N Engl J Med* **334**:225, 1996.

237. Maris JM, White PS, Beltinger CP, Sulman EP, Castleberry RP, Shuster JJ, Look AT, Brodeur GM: Significance of chromosome 1p loss of heterozygosity in neuroblastoma. *Cancer Res* **55**:4664, 1995.

238. Gehring M, Berthold F, Edler L, Schwab M, Amler LC: The 1p deletion is not a reliable marker for the prognosis of patients with neuroblastoma. *Cancer Res* **55**:5366, 1995.

239. Martinsson T, Shoberg P-M, Hedborg F, Kogner P: Deletion of chromosome 1p loci and microsatellite instability in neuroblastomas analyzed with short-tandem repeat polymorphisms. *Cancer Res* **55**:5681, 1995.

240. Bourhis J, De Vathaire F, Wilson GD, Hartmann O, Terrier-Lascombe MJ, Boccon-Gibod L, McNally NJ, Lemerle J, Riou G, Bernard J: Combined analysis of DNA ploidy index and N-myc genomic content in neuroblastoma. *Cancer Res* **51**:33, 1991.

241. Smith EI, Castleberry RP: Neuroblastoma, in Wells SA, Jr (ed): *Current Problems in Pediatric Surgery*. St. Louis: CV Mosby, 1990, p. 577.

242. Green AA, Hustu HO, Kumar M: Sequential cyclophosphamide and doxorubicin for induction of complete remission in children with disseminated neuroblastoma. *Cancer* **48**:2310, 1981.

243. Hayes FA, Green AA, Casper J, Cornet J, Evans WE: Clinical evaluation of sequentially scheduled cisplatin and VM26 in neuroblastoma; response and toxicity. *Cancer* **48**:1715, 1981.

244. Ninane J, Pritchard J, Malpas JS: Chemotherapy of advanced neuroblastoma; does Adriamycin contribute? *Arch Dis Child* **56**:544, 1981.

245. Bernard JL, Philip T, Zucker JM, Frappaz D, Robert A, Margueritte G, Boilletot A, Philippe N, Lutz P, Roche H, Pinkerton R: Sequential cisplatin/VM26 and vincristine/cyclophosphamide/doxorubicin in metastatic neuroblastoma; an effective alternating non-cross resistant regimen? *J Clin Oncol* **5**:1952, 1987.

246. Berthold F, Brandeis WE, Lambert F: Neuroblastoma; diagnostic advances and therapeutic results in 370 patients. *Monog Pediatr* **18**:206, 1985.

247. Castello MA, Donfrancesco A, Clerico A, Cozza R, Dominici C, De Laurentis C, Properzi E, De Sio L, Schiavetti A, Deb G: High-dose carboplatin with etoposide (JET regimen) in children with advanced neuroblastoma, in Evans AE, D'Angio GJ, Knudson AGJ, Seeger RC (eds): *Advances in Neuroblastoma Research*, 3rd ed. New York, Wiley-Liss, 1991, p. 535.

248. Weichselbaum RR, Epstein J, Little JB: In vitro cellular radiosensitivity of human malignant tumors. *Eur J Cancer* **36**:47, 1976.

249. Halperin E: Neuroblastoma, in Halperin E, Kun L, Constine L, Tarbell N (eds): *Pediatric Radiat Oncol* New York, Raven Press, 1989, p. 134.

250. August CS, Serota FT, Koch PA, Burkey E, Schlesinger H, Elkins WL, Evans AE, D'Angio GJ: Treatment of advanced neuroblastoma with supralethal chemotherapy, radiation and allogeneic or autologous marrow reconstitution. *J Clin Oncol* **2**:609, 1984.

251. Gee AP, Graham Pole J: Use of bone marrow purging and bone marrow transplantation for neuroblastoma, in Pochedly C (eds): *Neuroblastoma: Tumor Biology and Therapy*. Boca Raton, FL: CRC Press, 1990, p. 317.

252. Graham-Pole J, Gee AP, Gross S, Casper J, Graham M, Harvey W, Kapoor N., Koch P, Mendenhall N, Norris D, Pick T, Thomas P: Bone marrow transplantation (BMT) for advanced neuroblastoma (NBL): A multicenter POG study. *Prog Clin Biol Res* **271**:215, 1988.

253. Graham-Pole J, Casper J, Elfenbein G, Gee A, Gross S, Janssen W, Koch P, Marcus R, Pick T, Shuster J, Spruce W, Thomas P, Yeager A: High-dose chemoradiotherapy supported by marrow infusions for advanced neuroblastoma: A Pediatric Oncology Group study. *J Clin Oncol* **9**:152, 1991.

254. Hartmann O, Kalifa C, Benhamou E, Patte C, Flamank F, Jullien C, Beaujean F, Lemerle J: Treatment of advanced neuroblastoma with high-dose melphalan and autologous bone marrow transplantation. *Cancer Chemother Pharmacol* **16**:165, 1986.

255. Hartmann O, Benhamou E, Beaujean F, Kalifa C, Lejars O, Patte C, Behard C, Flamant F, Thyss A, Deville A, Vannier JP, Pautard-Muchemble B, Lemerle J: Repeated high-dose chemotherapy followed by purged autologous bone marrow transplantation as consolidation therapy in metastatic neuroblastoma. *J Clin Oncol* **5**:1205, 1987.

256. Philip T, Bernard JL, Zucker JM, Pinkerton R, Lutz P, Bordigoni P, Plouvier E, Robert A, Carton R, Philippe N, Philip I, Chauvin F, Favrot M: High-dose chemoradiotherapy with bone marrow transplantation as consolidation treatment in neuroblastoma: An unselected group of stage IV patients over 1 year of age. *J Clin Oncol* **5**:266, 1987.

257. Philip T, Zucker JM, Bernard JL, et al: Bone marrow transplantation in an unselected group of 65 patients with stage IV neuroblastoma, in Dickie KA, Spitzer G, Jagannath S (eds): *Autologous Bone Marrow Transplantation III*. Houston: Univ. of Texas, 1987, p. 407.

258. Pinkerton CR, Philip T, Biron P, Frapaz D, Philippe N, Zucker JM, Bernard JL, Philip I, Kemshead J, Favrot M: High-dose melphalan, vincristine and total-body irradiation with autologous bone marrow transplantation in children with relapsed neuroblastoma: A phase II study. *Med Pediatr Oncol* **15**:236, 1987.

259. Pritchard J, McElwain TJ, Graham-Pole J: High dose melphalan with autologous marrow for treatment of advanced neuroblastoma. *Br J Cancer* **45**:86, 1982.

260. Seeger R, Moss TJ, Feig SA, Lenarsky C, Seleh M, Ramsay N, Harris R, Wells J, Sather W, Reynolds CP: Bone marrow transplantation for poor prognosis neuroblastoma. *Prog Clin Biol Res* **271**:203, 1988.

261. Treleaven JG, Gibson FM, Ugelstad J, Rembaum A, Philip T, Caine GD, Kemshead JT: Monoclonal antibodies and magnetic microspheres for the removal of tumor cells from bone marrow. *Lancet* **i**:70, 1984.

262. Bowman LC, Castleberry RP, Alshuler G, Smith EI, Cantor A, Shuster J, Yu A, Look AT, Hayes FA: Therapy based on DNA index (DI) for infants with unresectable and disseminated neuroblastoma (NB): Preliminary results of the Pediatric Oncology Group "Better Risk" study [Abstract]. *Med Pediatr Oncol* **18**:364, 1990.

263. Voute PA, Hoefnagel CA, de Kraker J, Olmost RV, Bakker DJ, van de Kleij AJ: Results of treatment with 131 I-metaiodobenzylguanidine (131 I-MIBG) in patients with neuroblastoma, future prospects of zetotherapy, in Evans AE, D'Angio GJ, Knudson AGJ, Seeger RC (eds): *Advances in Neuroblastoma Research*, 3rd ed. New York, Wiley-Liss, 1991, p. 439.

264. Troncone L, Rufini V, Danza FM: Radioiodinated metaiodobenzylguanidine (I-MIBG) scintigraphy in neuroblastoma: A review of 160 studies. *J Nucl Med All Sci* **34**:279, 1990.

265. Sisson JC, Hutchinson RJ, Shapiro B, Zasadny KR, Normolle D, Wieland DM, Wahl RL, Singer DA, Mallette SA, Mudgett EE: Iodine-125-MIBG to treat neuroblastoma: Preliminary report. *J Nucl Med* **31**:1479, 1990.

266. O'Donoghue JA, Wheldon TE, Babich JW, Moyes JSE, Barrett A, Meller ST: Therapeutic implications of the uptake of radiolabeled mIBG for the treatment of neuroblastoma, in Evans AE, D'Angio GJ, Knudson AGJ, Seeger RC (eds): *Advances in Neuroblastoma Research*, 3rd ed. New York, Wiley-Liss, 1991, p. 455.

267. Cheung N-KV, Burch L, Kushner BH, Munn DH: Monoclonal antibody 3F8 can effect durable remissions in neuroblastoma patients refractory to chemotherapy: a phase II trial, in Evans AE, D'Angio GJ,

Knudson AGJ, Seeger RC (eds): *Advances in Neuroblastoma Research*, 3rd ed. (New York, Wiley-Liss, 1991, p. 395.)

268. Yu AL, Gillies SD, Reisfeld RA: Phase I clinical trial of CH14.18 in patients with refractory neuroblastoma [Abstract]. *Proc Am Soc Clin Oncol* **10**:318, 1991.

269. Seeger RC, Siegel SE, Sidell N: Neuroblastoma: Clinical perspectives, monoclonal antibodies, and retinoic acid. *Ann Int Med* **97**:873, 1982.

270. Sidell N, Sarafian T, Kelly M, Tsuchida T, Haussler M: Retinoic acid-induced differentiation of human neuroblastoma, a cell variant system showing two distinct responses. *Exp Cell Biol* **54**:287, 1986.

271. Thiele CJ, Reynolds CP, Israel M: Deceased expression of N-myc precedes retinoic acid-induced morphological differentiation of human neuroblastoma. *Nature* **313**:404, 1986.

272. Kumar S, Steward JK, Waghe M, Pearson D, Edwards DC, Fenton EL, Griffith AH: The administration of the nerve growth factor to children with widespread neuroblastoma. *J Pediatr Surg* **5**:18, 1970.

273. Iyer J, Korones DN, Ikegaki N, Kennett RH, Frantz CN: Regulation of N-myc gene expression in human neuroblastoma, in Evans AE, D'Angio GJ, Knudson AGJ, Seeger RC (eds): *Advances in Neuroblastoma Research*, 3rd ed. New York, Wiley-Liss, 1991, p. 55.

274. Donfrancesco A, Deb G, Dominici C. Pileggi D, Castello MA, Helson L: Effects of a single course of deferoxamine in neuroblastoma patients. *Cancer Res* **50**:4929, 1990.

275. Scott JP, Morgan E: Coagulapathy of disseminated neuroblastoma. *J Pediatr* **103**:219, 1983.

276. Labotka RJ, Morgan ER: Myelofibrosis in neuroblastoma. *Med Pediatr Oncol* **10**:21, 1982.

277. Quinn JJ, Altman AJ: The multiple hematologic manifestations of neuroblastoma. *Am J Pediatr Hematol/Oncol* **1**:201, 1979.

278. Al-Rashid RA, Cress C: Hypercalcemia associated with neuroblastoma. *Am J Dis Child* **133**:838, 1979.

279. Hayes FA, Green AA, O'Connor DM: Chemotherapeutic management of epidural neuroblastoma. *Med Pediatr Oncol* **17**:6, 1989.

280. Hayes FA, Thompson E, Hvizdala E, O'Connor D, Green AA: Chemotherapy as an alternative to laminectomy and radiation in the management of epidural tumor. *J Pediatr* **104**:221, 1984.

281. de la Monte SM, Moore GW, Hutchins GM: Nonrandom distribution of metastases in neuroblastic tumors. *Cancer* **52**:915, 1983.

282. Feldges AJ, Stanisic M, Morger R, Waidelich E: Neuroblastoma with meningeal involvement causing increased intracranial pressure and coma in two children. *Am J Pediatr Hematol/Oncol* **8**:355, 1986.

283. Rohrlich P, Hartmann O, Couanet D, Caillaud JM, Valleau D, Brugieres L, Kalifa C, Lemerle J: Secondary metastatic neuromeningeal localization of neuroblastoma in children. *Arch Francaises Pediatrie* **46**:5, 1989.

284. Mitchell WG, Snodgrass SR: Opsoclonus-ataxia due to childhood neural crest tumors: A chronic neurologic syndrome. *J Child Neurol* **5**:153, 1990.

285. Fairchild RS, Kyner JL, Hermreck A, Schimke RN: Neuroblastoma, pheochromocytoma and renal cell carcinoma. Occurrence in a single patient. *JAMA* **242**:2210, 1979.

286. Secker-Walker LM, Stewart EL, Todd A: Acute lymphoblastic leukaemia with t(4;11) follows neuroblastoma: A late effect of treatment? *Med Pediatr Oncol* **13**:48, 1985.

287. Shah NR, Miller DR, Steinherz PG, Garbes A, Farber P: Acute monoblastic leukemia as a second malignant neoplasm in metastatic neuroblastoma. *Am J Pediatr Hematol/Oncol* **7**:309, 1983.

288. Weh HJ, Kabisch H, Landbeck G, Hossfeld DK: Translocation (9;11)(p21;q23) in a child with acute monoblastic leukemia following 2 1/2 years after successful chemotherapy for neuroblastoma. *J Clin Oncol* **4**:1518, 1986.

289. Ben-Arush MW, Doron Y, Braun J, Mendelson E, Dar H, Robinson E: Brain tumor as a second malignant neoplasm following neuroblastoma stage IV-S. *Med Pediatr Oncol* **18**:240, 1990.

290. Meadows AT, Baum E, Fossati-Bellani F, Green D, Jenkin RDT, Marsden B, Nesbit M, Newton W, Oberlin O, Sallan SG, Siegel S, Strong LC, Voute PA: Second malignant neoplasms in children: An update from the Late Effects Study Group. *J Clin Oncol* **3**:532, 1985.

291. Nishi M, Miyake H, Takeda T, Shimada M, Takasugi N, Sato Y, Hanai J: Effects of the mass screening of neuroblastoma in Sapporo City. *Cancer* **60**:433, 1987.

292. Sawada T, Kidowaki T, Sakamoto I, Hashida T, Matsumura T, Nakagawara M, Kusunoki T: Neuroblastoma. Mass screening for early detection and its prognosis. *Cancer* **53**:2731, 1984.

293. Takeda T, Hatae Y, Nakadate H, Nishi M, Hanai J, Sato Y, Takasugi N: Japanese experience of screening. *Med Pediatr Oncol* **17**:368, 1989.

294. Woods WG, Tuchman M: Neuroblastoma: The case for screening infants in North America. *Pediatrics* **79**:869, 1987.

295. Nakagawara A, Zaizen Y, Ikeda K, Suita S, Ohgami H, Nagahara N, Sera Y, Akiyama H, Kawakami K, Uchino J-I: Different genomic and metabolic patterns between mass screening-positive and mass screening-negative later-presenting neuroblastomas. *Cancer* **68**:2037, 1991.

INDEX

O

NOTES

NOTES

NOTES

NOTES

NOTES

NOTES

NOTES

NOTES

NOTES

NOTES

NOTES

NOTES

NOTES

NOTES

NOTES

ISBN 0-07-067596-1

90000>